T3-AKE-748

VOLUME ONE

DIAGNOSTIC ULTRASOUND

SECOND EDITION

Edited by

John P. McGahan

Department of Radiology

University of California, Davis Medical Center

Sacramento, California, USA

Barry B. Goldberg

Department of Radiology

Thomas Jefferson University

Philadelphia, Pennsylvania, USA

informa

healthcare

New York London

Informa Healthcare USA, Inc.
52 Vanderbilt Avenue
New York, NY 10017

10 9 8 7 6 5 4 3 2 1

International Standard Book Number-10: 1-4200-6978-0 (Hardcover: Volume 1)
International Standard Book Number-13: 978-1-4200-6978-5 (Hardcover: Volume 1)

International Standard Book Number-10: 1-4200-6979-9 (Hardcover: Volume 2)
International Standard Book Number-13: 978-1-4200-6979-2 (Hard cover: Volume 2)

International Standard Book Number-10: 0-8493-3076-9 (Hardcover: Set)
International Standard Book Number-13: 978-0-8493-3076-6 (Hardcover: Set)

International Standard Book Number-10: 1-4200-6742-7 (Hardcover: Set)
International Standard Book Number-13: 978-1-4200-6742-2 (Hardcover: Set)

Library of Congress Cataloging-in-Publication Data

Diagnostic ultrasound / edited by John P. McGahan, Barry B. Goldberg. – 2nd ed.
p. ; cm.
Includes bibliographical references and index.
ISBN-13: 978-1-4200-6742-2 (set : hardcover : alk. paper)
ISBN-10: 1-4200-6742-7 (set : hardcover : alk. paper)
ISBN-13: 978-1-4200-6978-5 (v. 1 : hardcover : alk. paper)
ISBN-10: 1-4200-6978-0 (v. 1 : hardcover : alk. paper)
ISBN-13: 978-1-4200-6979-2 (v. 2 : hardcover : alk. paper)
ISBN-10: 1-4200-6979-9 (v. 2 : hardcover : alk. paper)
1. Diagnosis, Ultrasonic. 2. Ultrasonics in obstetrics. I. McGahan, John P. II. Goldberg, Barry B., 1937-
[DNLM: 1. Ultrasonography–methods. WN 208 D536 2007]
RC78.7.U4D5145 2007
616.07′543–dc22 2007023721

For Corporate Sales and Reprint Permissions call 212-520-2700 or write to:
Sales Department, 52 Vanderbilt, 16th floor, New York, NY 10017.

Visit the Informa Web site at
www.informa.com

and the Informa Healthcare Web site at
www.informahealthcare.com

Printed in India

Preface

Diagnostic ultrasound is recognized worldwide as the premier cross-sectional imaging modality. Although other imaging modalities have advantages over sonography in certain anatomical regions, none are more readily available or more widely used throughout the world than sonography. Therefore, there is a growing need in every country to learn ultrasound.

Our text is a practical, comprehensive teaching and reference work on ultrasound. Our aim has been for the text to include detailed coverage of all anatomical structures accessible to ultrasound, including obstetrical applications. We have also included thorough coverage of such topics as the physics of ultrasound, artifacts, invasive and intraoperative ultrasound, endoscopic ultrasound, and three-dimensional sonographic imaging. The prior edition folded pediatric chapters into other anatomical areas. This second edition includes dedicated pediatric ultrasound chapters on the head, neck, spine, chest, abdomen, pelvis, and musculoskeletal system. We included these chapters to make this text more comprehensive in all facets of sonography. This approach has been taken to reduce redundancy and foster unified, comprehensive analyses of the organ or system under discussion. Artifacts that occur in all anatomical regions are addressed in a separate chapter, but artifacts or pitfalls that occur in site-specific regions are presented to the reader in those site-specific chapters, so as to avoid errors that we or others already have encountered.

We felt that it was vital that the chapters exploring organs or organ systems assess normal anatomy and pathology by using the logic inherent in most ultrasound examinations. The way in which we approach ultrasound imaging is by deciding if a particular finding truly represents an abnormality. We then determine the best choice or best differential of possibilities of what this abnormality represents. We have organized the chapters on anatomical regions into explorations based on this logic, which is used by most experienced ultrasound practitioners. First, we take the reader through the normal sonographic anatomy of the region. We then examine artifacts and pitfalls that are uniquely site-specific to that region. We elaborate on disease entities occurring within each organ system, but place emphasis on how we encounter ultrasound abnormalities in our daily practice. For instance, if on an ultrasound examination we visualize a solid lesion in a parenchymal organ, it may have pathopneumonic features that are listed within this text. More often, we have a number of possibilities that may be considered in the different diagnosis. Such ultrasound features as solid or cystic, single or multiple lesions, location, and the Doppler features may all be helpful in establishing a most probable diagnosis. We emphasize utilization of numerous tables, flow charts, and figures to help the reader to logically approach a differential diagnosis. If no specific diagnoses can be made by ultrasound, we suggest other imaging modalities that may be useful. We conclude each chapter with presentation of the ultrasound features of pathological entities. We also show how ultrasound may be used to guide biopsy, aspiration, drainage, operative, or percutaneous therapy for a variety of abnormalities.

We have placed heavy emphasis on pedagogy in developing the chapters. You will find frequent use of tables and flow charts to summarize important decision-making processes, key comparisons and relationships, and vital factual data. The tables are highlighted for quick reference, and outlines are placed at the beginning of each chapter for easy access.

We have tried to produce a volume that will serve as an accessible reference tool and teaching aid for any application of ultrasound in widespread practice. We hope that readers find the discussion, tables, differentials, and numerous figures to be a good background and reference for a logical approach to the daily practice of ultrasonography.

John P. McGahan, M.D.
Barry B. Goldberg, M.D.

Acknowledgments

This book is a selection of chapters written by an outstanding group of international experts in the field of diagnostic ultrasound, without whose efforts this book would not have been possible. We offer sincere thanks to each of these individuals for their contributions. Their years of hard work and experience have created both a valued reference text and a logical approach to the understanding of ultrasound.

We thank those individuals at Informa Healthcare USA, Inc., who were instrumental in the development of this textbook, especially Andrea Seils, who had the vision and gave us the encouragement and impetus to move forward on this text. Equally instrumental in the success of this endeavor was Vanessa Sanchez, who helped us with words of encouragement to produce high-quality work and to meet deadlines in spite of our busy work schedules.

In addition, we thank those individuals who are not often recognized but who contribute greatly in the development of any text by both transcribing and editing chapters. These individuals include, among others, Elisa Valenton, Angela Michelier, and Marilyn Lin-Kempeter.

Our many co-workers, including sonologists and sonographers, who provided case material for this text also deserve our sincere gratitude.

Finally, we thank our immediate and extended families for their patience while we were busy and, at times, distracted during the completion of this work.

Contents

PART VII MUSCULOSKELETAL SYSTEM

VOLUME TWO

PART VIII PELVIS/GENITOURINARY TRACT

PART IX OBSTETRICS

Contributors

Andrei V. Alexandrov, M.D. ■ Comprehensive Stroke Center, Neurovascular Ultrasound Laboratory, University of Alabama Hospital, Birmingham, Alabama, U.S.A.

Sandra J. Allison, M.D. ■ Department of Radiology, Georgetown University Hospital, Washington, D.C., U.S.A.

John Amodio, M.D. ■ SUNY Downstate Medical Center, Brooklyn, New York, U.S.A.

Beryl R. Benacerraf, M.D. ■ Department of Radiology and Department of Obstetrics/Gynecology, Harvard Medical School, Boston, Massachusetts, U.S.A.

Carol B. Benson, M.D. ■ Department of Radiology, Harvard Medical School, Brigham and Women's Hospital, Boston, Massachusetts, U.S.A.

Lincoln L. Berland, M.D. ■ Department of Radiology, University of Alabama at Birmingham, Birmingham, Alabama, U.S.A.

Shweta Bhatt, M.D. ■ Department of Radiology, University of Rochester Medical Center, Rochester, New York, U.S.A.

William E. Brant, M.D. ■ Department of Radiology, Division of Thoraco-Abdominal Imaging, University of Virginia Health System, Charlottesville, Virginia, U.S.A.

Robert L. Bree, M.D. ■ Department of Radiology, University of Washington Medical Center, Seattle, Washington, U.S.A.

Étienne Cardinal, M.D. ■ Department of Radiology, Centre Hospitalier de l'Universite de Montreal, Pavillon Saint-Luc, Montreal, Quebec, Canada

Dru E. Carlson, M.D. ■ Department of Obstetrics and Gynecology, UCLA School of Medicine and Department of Reproductive Genetics, Cedars Sinai Medical Center, Los Angeles, California, U.S.A.

Frank A. Chervenak, M.D. ■ Department of Obstetrics and Gynecology, Division of Maternal Fetal Medicine, New York Hospital-Cornell Medical College, New York, U.S.A.

Rethy K. Chhem, M.D., Ph.D. ■ Department of Radiology and Nuclear Medicine, Schulich School of Medicine and Dentistry, University of Western Ontario, London, Ontario, Canada

W. K. Chooi, M.D. ■ Department of Radiology, University of British Columbia and St. Paul's Hospital, Vancouver, British Columbia, Canada

Terry L. Coates, M.D. ■ Department of Radiology, University of California, Davis Medical Center, Sacramento, California, U.S.A.

Dennis L. Cochlin, MB., BCh., FRCR ■ Radiology Department, University Hospital of Wales, Cardiff, U.K.

Peter L. Cooperberg, M.D. ■ Department of Radiology, University of British Columbia, and St. Paul's Hospital, Vancouver, British Columbia, Canada

Sidney M. Dashefsky, M.D. ■ Department of Radiology, University of Manitoba, Section of Diagnostic Ultrasound, Health Sciences Centre, Winnipeg, Manitoba, Canada

Greggory R. DeVore, M.D. ■ Fetal Diagnostic Center of Pasadena, Pasadena, California, U.S.A.

Vasudha Dhar, M.D. ■ Department of Gastroenterology New York-Presbyterian Hospital/Columbia University, New York, New York, U.S.A.

Vikram S. Dogra, M.D. ■ Department of Imaging Sciences, University of Rochester School of Medicine, Rochester, New York, U.S.A.

Peter M. Doubilet, M.D. ■ Department of Radiology, Harvard Medical School, Brigham and Women's Hospital, Boston, Massachusetts, U.S.A.

Harris J. Finberg, M.D. ■ Phoenix Perinatal Associates, Phoenix, Arizona and Department of Radiology, Mayo Medical School, Rochester, Minnesota, U.S.A.

Verlee L. Fines-Dailey, M.D. ■ Department of Obstetrics and Gynecology, Norton Maternal-Fetal Hospital, Louisville, Kentucky, U.S.A.

Flemming Forsberg, Ph.D. ■ Department of Radiology, Thomas Jefferson University, Philadelphia, Pennsylvania, U.S.A.

Wilbert Fortson, M.D. ■ Department of Obstetrics and Gynecology, Maternal-Fetal Medicine, Dekalb Medical Center, Decatur, Georgia, U.S.A.

Mary C. Frates, M.D. ■ Department of Radiology, Harvard Medical School, Brigham and Women's Hospital, Boston, Massachusetts, U.S.A.

Eugenio O. Gerscovich, M.D. ■ Department of Radiology, University of California, Davis Medical Center, Sacramento, California, U.S.A.

Marijo A. Gillen, M.D. ■ Department of Radiology, University of California, Davis Medical Center, Sacramento, California, U.S.A.

Barry B. Goldberg, M.D. ■ Department of Radiology, Thomas Jefferson University, Philadelphia, Pennsylvania, U.S.A.

Ruth B. Goldstein, M.D. ■ Department of Radiology, Obstetrics, Gynecology and Reproductive Science, University of California Medical Center, San Francisco, California, U.S.A.

Lawrence P. Gordon, M.D. ■ Department of Pathology, Crouse Hospital and Department of Pathology, Upstate Medical University, Syracuse, New York, U.S.A.

Lyndon M. Hill, M.D. ■ Department of Obstetrics and Gynecology, University of Pittsburgh School of Medicine and Magee-Women's Hospital of UPMC Health System, Pittsburgh, Pennsylvania, U.S.A.

Javine Horani, M.D. ■ Department of Obstetrics and Gynecology, Colorado Springs Health Partners, Colorado Springs, Colorado, U.S.A.

R. Brooke Jeffrey, M.D. ■ Department of Radiology, Stanford University Medical Center, Stanford, California, U.S.A.

Robert A. Kane, M.D. ■ Department of Radiology, Beth Israel Deaconess Medical Center, Boston, Massachusetts, U.S.A.

Mira L. Katz, Ph.D., M.P.H. ■ Division of Health Behavior and Health Promotion, The Ohio State University, Columbus, Ohio, U.S.A.

Ada Kessler, M.D. ■ Department of Radiology, Souraski-Tel Aviv Medical Center, Sackler School of Medicine, Tel Aviv University, Tel Aviv, Israel

Vijay P. Khatri, M.B.Ch.B.., FACS ■ Division of Surgical Oncology, University of California, Davis Cancer Center, Sacramento, California, U.S.A.

Viviane Khoury, M.D. ■ Department of Radiology, McGill University Health Center, Montreal, Quebec, Canada

Ercan Kocakoc, M.D. ■ Department of Radiology, Faculty of Medicine, Firat University, Elazig, Turkey

Ewa Kuligowska, M.D. ■ Department of Radiology, Boston University School of Medicine, Boston, Massachusetts, U.S.A.

Annabelle Lao, M.D. ■ Departments of Neurology and Psychiatry, University of Santo Tomas Hospital, Manila, Philippines and Department of Neurology, Barrow Neurological Institute, St. Joseph Hospital, Phoenix, Arizona, U.S.A.

Clifford S. Levi, M.D. ■ Department of Radiology, University of Manitoba, Section of Diagnostic Ultrasound, Health Sciences Centre, Winnipeg, Manitoba, Canada

Deborah Levine, M.D. ■ Department of Obstetric and Gynecologic Ultrasound, Beth Israel Deaconess Medical Center, Harvard Medical School, Boston, Massachusetts, U.S.A.

Anna S. Lev-Toaff, M.D. ■ Department of Radiology, Thomas Jefferson University, Philadelphia, Pennsylvania, U.S.A.

Ji-Bin Liu, M.D. ■ Department of Radiology, Thomas Jefferson University, Philadelphia, Pennsylvania, U.S.A.

Mark E. Lockhart, M.D., M.P.H. ■ Department of Radiology, University of Alabama at Birmingham, Birmingham, Alabama, U.S.A.

Edward A. Lyons, M.D. ■ Department of Radiology, Obstetrics and Gynecology, and Anatomy, University of Manitoba, Section of Diagnostic Ultrasound, Health Sciences Centre, Winnipeg, Manitoba, Canada

John P. McGahan, M.D. ■ Department of Radiology, University of California, Davis Medical Center, Sacramento, California, U.S.A.

Daniel A. Merton, B.S., RDMS, FSDMS, FAIUM ■ Department of Radiology, Thomas Jefferson University, Philadelphia, Pennsylvania, U.S.A.

Valdair Muglia, M.D., Ph.D. ■ Department of Radiology, Ribeiro Preto School of Medicine, Sao Paulo, Brazil

Laurence Needleman, M.D. ■ Department of Radiology, Thomas Jefferson University, Philadelphia, Pennsylvania, U.S.A.

Thomas R. Nelson, Ph.D. ■ Department of Radiology, University of California, San Diego, San Diego, California, U.S.A.

Matilde Nino-Murcia, M.D. ■ Department of Radiology, Stanford University School of Medicine, Stanford, California, U.S.A.

Suhas G. Parulekar, M.D. ■ Department of Radiology, The University of Texas, M. D. Anderson Cancer Center, Houston, Texas, U.S.A.

Catherine W. Piccoli, M.D. ■ Diagnostic Radiology, Turnersville and Voorhees, New Jersey; Philadelphia and Scranton, Pennsylvania; and Virginia Beach, Virginia, U.S.A.

Lawrence D. Platt, M.D. ■ Center for Fetal Medicine and Women's Ultrasound, Los Angeles, California, U.S.A.

Joseph F. Polak, M.D., M.P.H. ■ Department of Radiology, Tufts University School of Medicine, and Department of Cardiovascular Imaging, Tufts-New England Medical Center, Boston, Massachusetts, U.S.A.

M. Porto, M.D. ■ Department of Obstetrics and Gynecology, University of California-Irvine, Orange, California, U.S.A.

Myron A. Pozniak, M.D. ■ Department of Radiology, University of Wisconsin Clinical Science Center, Madison, Wisconsin, U.S.A.

Mladen Predanic, M.D. ■ Department of Obstetrics and Gynecology, Jamaica Hospital Medical Center, Jamaica, New York; and Department of Obstetrics and Gynecology of Weill Medical College of Cornell University, New York, New York, U.S.A.

Dolores H. Pretorius, M.D. ■ Department of Radiology, University of California-San Diego, San Diego, California, U.S.A.

John R. Richards, M.D. ■ Department of Emergency Medicine, University of California-Davis, Davis, California, U.S.A.

Ashley J. Robinson, M.D. ■ Department of Radiology, University of California Medical Center, San Francisco, California, U.S.A.

Henrietta Kotlus Rosenberg, M.D. ■ Department of Radiology and Pediatrics, Mt. Sinai School of Medicine, Mt. Sinai Medical Center, New York, New York, U.S.A.

Philip D. Schneider, M.D. ■ Department of Oncology, University of California-Davis, Davis, California, U.S.A.

Vijay K. Sharma, M.D. ■ Division of Neurology, National University Hospital, Singapore

Marilyn J. Siegel, M.D. ■ Mallinckrodt Institute of Radiology, Washington University School of Medicine, St. Louis, Missouri, U.S.A.

Beverly A. Spirt, M.D. ■ Oneida Medical Imaging Center, Oneida, New York; and Department of Radiology, Upstate Medical University, Syracuse, New York, U.S.A.

R. M. Steiger, M.D. ■ Department of Obstetrics and Gynecology, University of California-Irvine, Orange, California, U.S.A.

Rebecca Stein-Wexler, M.D. ■ Department of Radiology, University of California, Davis Medical Center and U.C. Davis Children's Hospital, Sacramento, California, U.S.A.

Peter D. Stevens, M.D. ■ Department of Clinical Medicine, Columbia University, New York, New York, U.S.A.

James F. Stinchon, M.D. ■ Department of Radiology, Boston University Medical Center, Boston, Massachusetts, U.S.A.

Mitchell E. Tublin, M.D. ■ Department of Radiology, University of Pittsburgh School of Medicine, Pittsburgh, Pennsylvania, U.S.A.

Vijay Viswanathan, M.D. ■ Department of Radiology, Harvard Medical School, Brigham and Women's Hospital, Boston, Massachusetts, U.S.A.

Peter N. T. Wells, F.R.S. ■ The Institute of Medical Engineering and Medical Physics, Cardiff University School of Engineering, Cardiff, U.K.

Annina N. Wilkes, M.D. ■ Department of Radiology, Thomas Jefferson University, Philadelphia, Pennsylvania, U.S.A.

Sandra L. Wootton-Gorges, M.D. ■ Department of Radiology, University of California, Davis Medical Center and U.C. Davis Children's Hospital, Sacramento, California, U.S.A.

Physics and Bioeffects

Peter N. T. Wells

1

HISTORY[a]

The fact that ultrasound has biological effects was first noticed three-quarters of a century ago by scientists experimenting with techniques for the underwater detection of obstacles at sea (1). The early sonar (sound navigation and ranging) transmitters produced beams that were intense enough to kill small fish which had the misfortune to swim into them. Later, ultrasound was widely used in physiotherapy and this is an application that has a long-established niche in current clinical practice (2,3). During World War II, the ultrasonic pulse-echo method was developed for the detection of cracks in metal. With the cessation of hostilities, interest soon grew in the possibility that the technique could be used for medical diagnosis (4,5). By the 1960s, two-dimensional imaging had become practicable, albeit with slow, manually operated scanners (6). With the inventions of real-time scanning and gray-scale display (7,8), ultrasonic imaging began to be accepted quite widely; steady improvements, resulting from developments in transducer materials, signal processing, and display, led to a competitive commercial market with the potential to revolutionize radiology. Most recently, color flow imaging, three-dimensional display, and the use of contrast agents, along with the development of specialized scanning systems for intracavitary, intraluminal, and intraoperative examinations, have further strengthened the importance of diagnostic ultrasound in clinical medicine. Indeed, today, ultrasound accounts for one out of every four imaging studies performed worldwide.

Because ultrasound can affect living systems, the possibility that diagnostic ultrasonic techniques might under some circumstances be hazardous has always to be remembered (9). Much research into ultrasonic bioeffects has been carried out (10,11); there is no evidence that any of the methods used in contemporary practice carries any risk.

THE PHYSICS OF ULTRASOUND

Propagation of Ultrasound in Tissues

When ultrasound travels through media such as the soft tissues of the body, it does so at particular speeds and the energy carried by the ultrasonic waves is progressively attenuated. The ultrasound is also reflected and scattered, depending on the properties of the different tissues in the body.

Ultrasonic waves have frequencies above the range of human hearing, beginning at about 20,000 cycles per second (20 kHz). Because ultrasound travels at a particular speed (c) in a given medium, the wavelength (λ) (the distance occupied by a single cycle of the wave) depends on the frequency (f) of the wave, according to the following equation:

$$\lambda = \frac{c}{f} \tag{1}$$

[a]Detailed references are provided for this section and for the section on Bioeffects of Ultrasound. For other sections, please consult the Bibliography.

The wavelength in soft tissues, in which the speed is about 1540 m/sec, is about 1.54 mm at 1 MHz and proportionately shorter at higher frequencies. The wavelength is one of the factors that control the spatial resolution of ultrasonic imaging. In abdominal scanning, for example, a resolution of a millimeter or better is needed, so that frequencies of 1.5 MHz or higher are necessary.

The attenuation of ultrasound increases with frequency. This means that the penetration of ultrasound into the body decreases as the frequency is increased, because sufficient ultrasound has to remain to be detected. In pulse-echo ultrasonic techniques, brief pulses of ultrasound are transmitted into the body and echoes are detected from reflecting and scattering structures. The half-power distance in soft tissues is about 30 mm at a frequency of 1 MHz. In other words, the attenuation for the go-and-return travel distance is about 0.5 dB/(cm MHz): the dB (decibel) unit is explained in the next section. In practice, frequencies of up to about 5 MHz can be used for examinations at depths of up to about 10 cm; the corresponding wavelength is about 0.3 mm. Higher frequencies, with proportionately shorter wavelengths and higher resolutions, can be used in situations where less penetration is acceptable.

The amount of ultrasound that is reflected at the boundary between two media depends on the acoustic properties of the media on each side of the boundary. The relevant property is the "characteristic acoustic impedance," which is equal to the product of the density of the medium and the speed of propagation of ultrasound within it. Although the speeds in different soft tissues are quite similar (ranging from about 1480 m/sec in fat to about 1600 m/sec in muscle) and the densities of the different tissues are also not very different, the characteristic impedance variations are fortunately large enough to give rise to detectable echoes. For normal incidence on a flat interface,

$$R = \left(\frac{Z_2 - Z_1}{Z_2 + Z_1}\right)^2 \tag{2}$$

where R is the ratio of the power of the reflected wave to that of the incident wave and Z_1 and Z_2 are the characteristic impedances of the media on the incident and other sides of the interface, respectively. Of course, even extensive interfaces within the body can only approximate to this ideal condition. Generally, interfaces are curved and the physical sizes of the characteristic impedance discontinuities within homogeneous tissues are often similar to, or smaller than, the wavelength. Ultrasound is scattered, rather than reflected in a mirror-like or "specular" fashion, by such small structures.

Besides the echoes from soft tissues, there are two other extreme conditions that are of practical relevance to ultrasonic imaging. These relate to the situations where soft tissues interface with bone or with gas. Bone has a relatively high characteristic impedance, whereas that of gas is low. In both these conditions, ultrasound is almost totally reflected at the interface; this limits penetration into and beyond bone and gas.

An ultrasonic wave consists of a progression of compressions and rarefactions of the medium through which it travels. In compression, the density of the medium increases—albeit slightly—and vice versa in rarefaction. The wave actually travels slightly faster in the denser region and slightly slower in the less dense regions. Thus, the wave becomes distorted and adopts a saw-tooth shape as a result of this nonlinearity in the medium. This means that some of the energy transmitted into the medium is transferred to frequencies that are harmonics (and, at higher intensities, subharmonics) of the original frequency. The second harmonic is of particular importance in ultrasonic imaging, for reasons that are explained later.

The Decibel Scale

The strength of an ultrasonic wave is described, at fundamental level, in terms of its oscillating pressure, particle displacement amplitude, intensity, or any other measure relevant to the particular phenomenon under consideration. In ultrasonic diagnosis, however, it is often not the actual strength of the wave which is of direct importance, but the amplitude of the signal in relation to some particular reference level such as the amplitude of another signal. Under circumstances such as this, it is more convenient to express signal levels as the logarithms of the ratios of the particular amplitudes or powers to that of the reference. Thus, the ratio of the powers P_1 and P_2 can be expressed in logarithmic units of decibels as follows:

$$[\mathrm{dB}] = 10\log\left(\frac{P_1}{P_2}\right) \tag{3}$$

The use of decibels to express signal levels has two advantages. First, the ratios of powers differing by many orders of magnitude (such as are commonly experienced in ultrasonic diagnosis) correspond to quite small numbers of decibels. Second, adding and subtracting signal levels expressed in decibels correspond to the processes of amplification and attenuation, respectively, thus avoiding the need for calculations involving multiplication and division.

Generation and Detection of Ultrasound

A transducer is a device that converts one form of energy to another. In medical ultrasonics, piezoelectric ceramics or composites of piezoelectric ceramics and plastics are generally used to convert between electrical energy and mechanical vibrations. A piezoelectric transducer can operate both as a transmitter and as a receiver of ultrasonic waves.

The shape of an ultrasonic beam is determined by the size of the aperture, measured in terms of wavelengths, from which it originates. One of the simplest shapes is a disk, which produces a beam that is circular in cross-section. The diametrical distribution of the beam depends on the distance from the transducer which forms the aperture. Figure 1 represents the beam produced by a disk with a diameter equal to $2a$; essentially, the beam is cylindrical in the near field and diverges at a half-angle

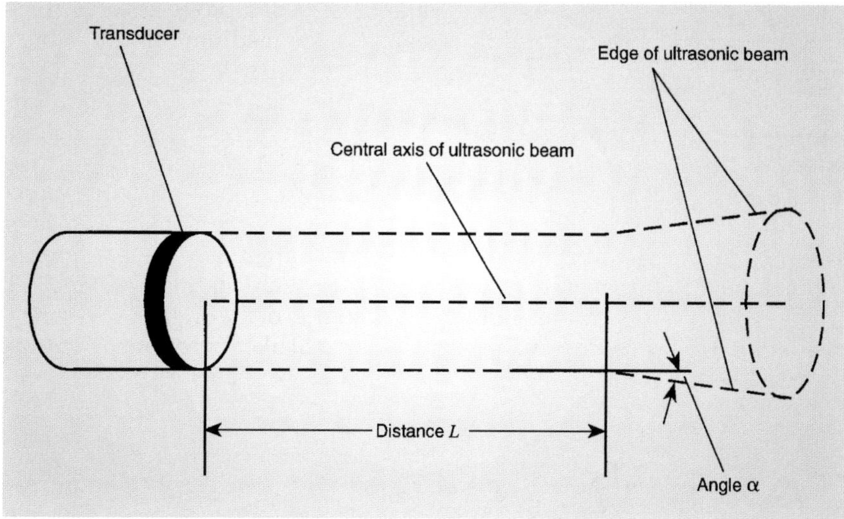

FIGURE 1 ■ Diagram showing the beam produced by a disk transducer. The beam is roughly cylindrical in the near field and diverges in the far field. In the near field, the beam is inhomogeneous; it consists of annuli, the number of which decreases as the distance from the transducer increases until, in the far field, the beam has a smooth profile peaking on the central axis.

equal to α in the far field. The length of the near field is equal to L and the following equations apply:

$$L = \frac{a}{\lambda} \tag{4}$$

$$\alpha = \sin^{-1}\left(0.6\frac{\lambda}{a}\right) \tag{5}$$

In the near field, between the transducer and the distance L, an ultrasonic beam can be focused to reduce its diameter over a distance (the depth-of-focus) which depends on the strength of the focusing. This is illustrated in Figure 2. Focusing can be achieved either with a lens, constructed from material (typically a plastic) in which the speed of sound differs from that in the surrounding media, or by tailoring the time delays of the signal paths associated with the separate elements of a transducer divided into an array. With an array, as with a lens, the position of the focus of the transmitted beam cannot be changed during the process of echo acquisition. On reception, however, an array allows the position of the focus to be swept continuously to coincide with the changing depth from which echoes are originating. This is done by making appropriate changes in the particular delay times associated with each of the individual elements in the array. Although this idea may seem to be simple, the physics and engineering behind the successful realization of practical instruments are challenging, and, currently, the subject of beam forming is one of intense research activity.

PULSE-ECHO TECHNIQUES

General Principles

When a pulse of ultrasound is transmitted along a beam into the body, the ultrasound is scattered and reflected as it encounters changes in characteristic acoustic impedance. This gives rise to echoes which can be detected by the same transducer as that from which the beam originated. Since ultrasound travels at similar speeds in the different soft tissues of the body, the time delays between

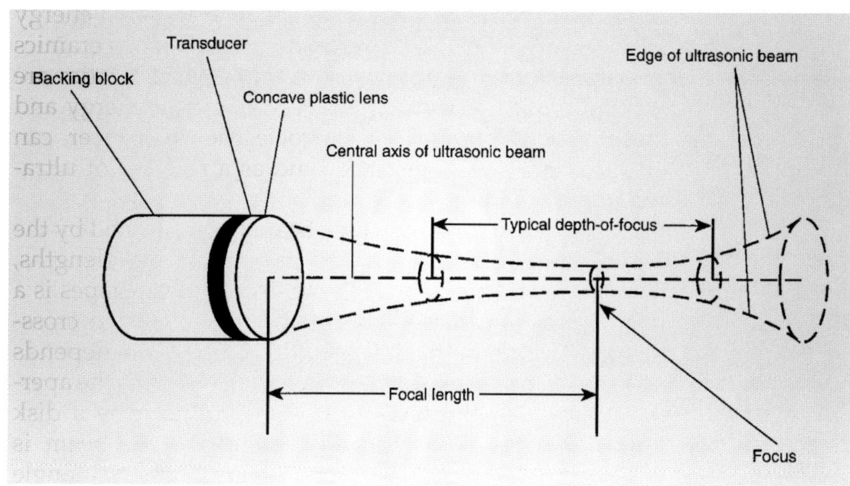

FIGURE 2 ■ Diagram showing the beam produced by a disk transducer, focused in the near field by means of a lens attached to the transducer.

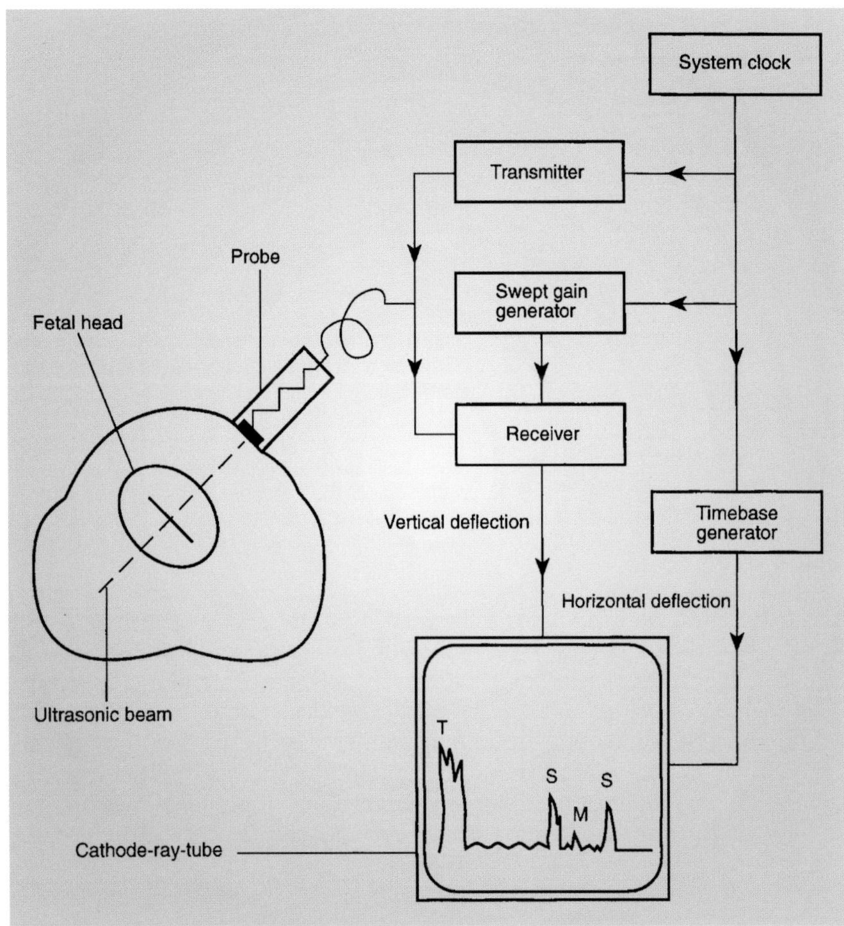

FIGURE 3 ■ Block diagram of an ultrasonic A-scope system. The A-scan is used primarily for pulse-echo measurements of distance and it is shown here being used to measure the diameter of a fetal head. On the display, S are the echoes from the parietal bones of the fetal skull and M is the echo from the midline structures of the fetal brain. T corresponds to the transmission of the ultrasonic pulse into the patient.

the transmission of an ultrasonic pulse and the reception of echoes can be measured and used to calculate the depths along the ultrasonic beam of the echo-producing structures. Moreover, the amplitudes of the individual echoes depend on the nature of the "targets," although they are, of course, also subject to increasing attenuation with increasing penetration.

Since an ultrasonic beam is directional, it can be used to explore the internal structures of the body by observing the echoes received from different directions within the body. The simplest technique for doing this is illustrated in Figure 3. The A-scan produced by this instrument carries information only about the depths of echo-producing structures and the strengths of the echoes, but not about the direction of the beam. As far as the strengths of the echoes are concerned, compensation for increasing attenuation with depth is to a large extent provided by the swept gain control (also known as the time gain control). This increases the gain of the receiver amplifier with time following the transmission of the pulse. The interpretation of the A-scan depends on the knowledge of the position and orientation of the ultrasonic probe on the body and the likely anatomy within the body. It is only in a limited number of clinical situations that interpretation is easy or even possible. The technique is perhaps most useful when accurate measurements of distance are required, as, for example, in the measurement of the fetal biparietal diameter and, even then, it may not be obvious to the operator that the measurement which is being made with modern scanners is directly derived from the original A-scan approach.

Time–Position Recording

When an ultrasonic beam passes through moving structures in the body, the changing axial positions of echo-producing targets can be seen on an A-scan display. The movements can be studied in detail, both qualitatively and quantitatively, by means of an M-mode recording. Figure 4 shows a common arrangement for producing this kind of display. The ultrasonic timebase is connected to the vertical deflection circuit of the display and the output from the receiver controls the brightness, rather than the deflection of the spot on the display. A second timebase generator is connected to the horizontal deflection circuit. This drives the lines of ultrasonically obtained depth information across the display to produce a time–position recording that allows the patterns of movements of structures along the beam to be studied.

Two-Dimensional Scanning

The principles of two-dimensional ultrasonic scanning are illustrated in Figure 5. As in the M-mode technique,

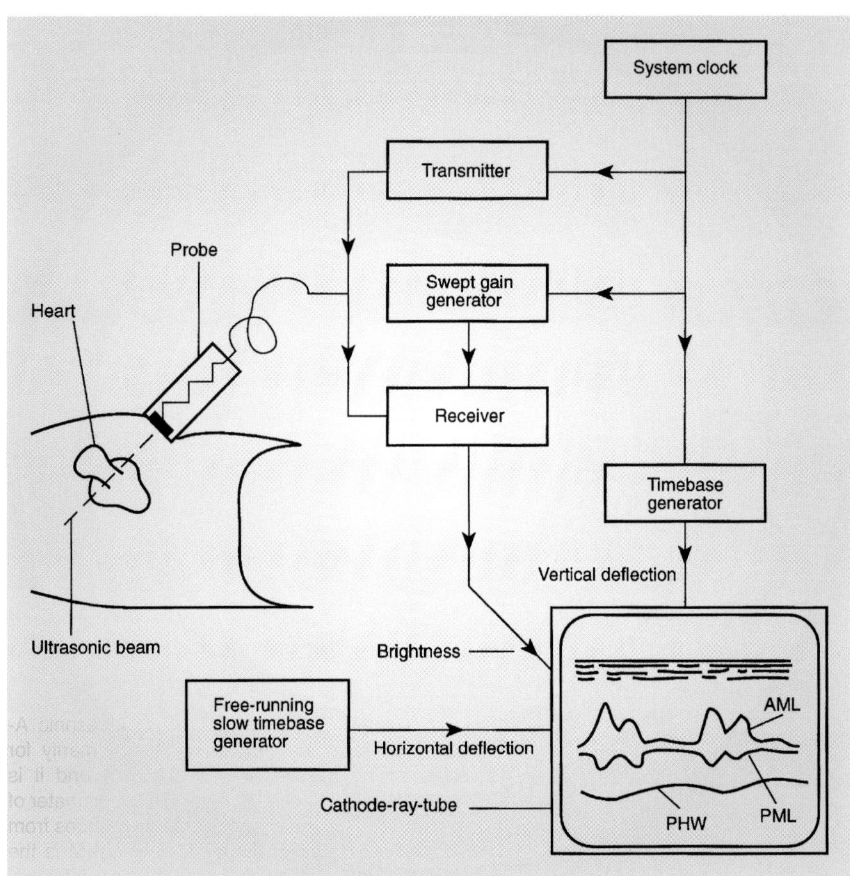

FIGURE 4 ■ Block diagram of an ultrasonic system for M-mode display. The system consists of the essential elements of the A-scope, as illustrated in Figure 3, with the addition of a slow horizontal timebase to allow the motion of echoes, displayed as bright spots instead of deflections, to be observed as corresponding structures move in the body. PHW, posterior heart wall; AML, anterior mitral valve leaflet; PML, posterior mitral valve leaflet.

the brightness of spots on the ultrasonic timebase corresponding to echo-producing targets in the body is controlled by the strength of the ultrasonic echoes. The direction of the timebase on the display, however, is linked to the direction of the ultrasonic beam within a plane of section through the patient. The beam is swept through the plane to produce a cross-sectional image.

In modern ultrasonic imaging, scanning is almost always accomplished in real time. The ultrasonic image can be considered to be made up of discrete lines of information, each line being acquired by a separate pulse of transmitted ultrasound. For a penetration of, for example, 15 cm, the go-and-return travel time for the acquisition of an echo from the maximum depth is 200 μsec. Since there are 5000 intervals of 200 μsec in one second, up to 5000 lines of ultrasonic image information can be acquired per second. In this example, if there are 100 lines of image information per frame, the frame rate is up to 50 per second, which is more than fast enough to be flicker-free to the observer.

Two-dimensional scanning can be accomplished either by mechanical movement of an ultrasonic transducer producing an axially directed beam or by electronic control of an array of transducer elements. Two examples of probes for two-dimensional scanning are shown in Figure 6. Although the mechanical probes are simpler in principle and have a number of advantages, such as low cost and simplicity of the associated electronics, their disadvantages are such that modern ultrasonic scanners almost exclusively employ transducer arrays. As shown in Figure 7, the simplest kind of transducer array produces a scan with a rectangular format. Rather more complicated, because of the additional complexity of the electronics, is the curvilinear array, which produces a sector scan such as that shown in Figure 8. The electronic circuitry to drive a curvilinear array is simpler than that needed for the phased array, which also produces a sector scan but which has a surface shape that is not only flat but smaller than the corresponding curvilinear array.

Second Harmonic Imaging

The discovery that energy is transferred into the second harmonic frequency of the transmitted ultrasound as a result of the nonlinear propagation through tissue led to the development of what is often called "tissue harmonic imaging." In this process, the principles are the same as those for traditional ultrasonic imaging techniques, except that the receiver is tuned to receive echoes at twice the frequency of the transmitted ultrasound. This has several advantages. First, the spatial resolution is better than that which can be obtained for a given depth of penetration using traditional (or "fundamental") imaging. Second, the beam-distorting effects of the body wall are less troublesome for the outward passage of the ultrasonic pulse, since tissue inhomogeneities, especially those due to fat, are less pronounced at lower frequencies. Finally, although the central lobes of the ultrasonic beams are coincident on

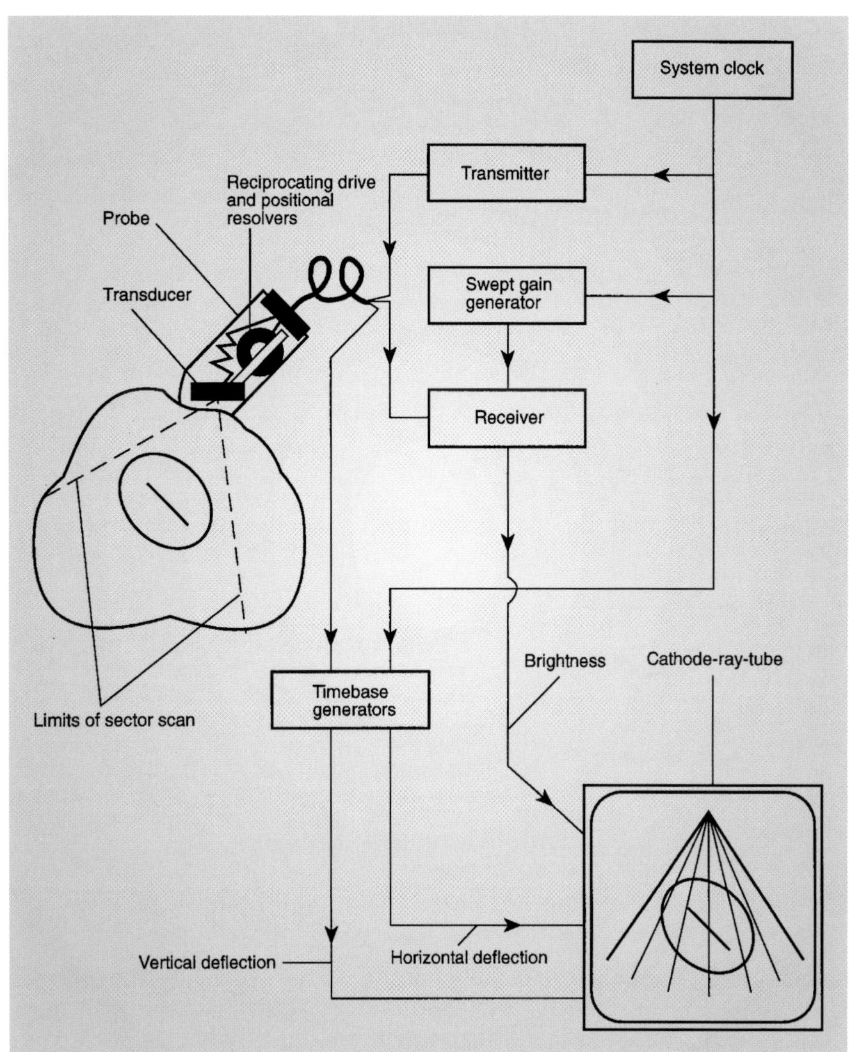

FIGURE 5 ■ Block diagram of an ultrasonic system for two-dimensional real-time scanning. The pulse-echo system is arranged to control the brightness of the display on which the position and direction of the timebase is determined by resolvers mounted in the mechanical scanning head. A single-element disk transducer is arranged to sweep the ultrasonic beam repetitively in a sector within the patient.

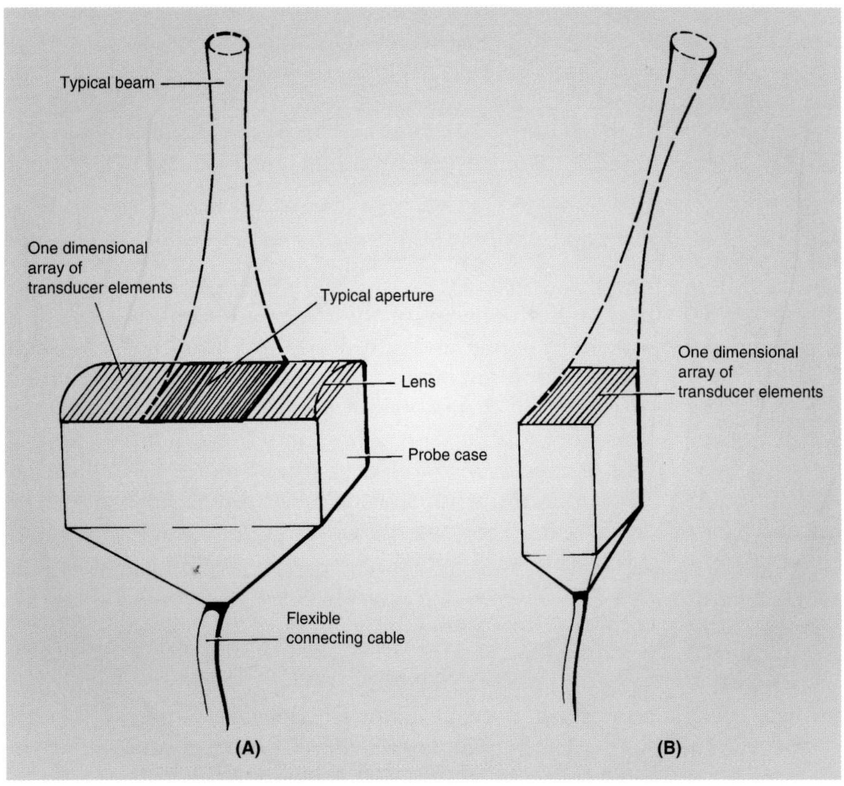

FIGURE 6 A AND B ■ Two types of transducer arrays for two-dimensional scanning by electronic beam control. (**A**) A linear array, producing a scan with a rectangular format. A cylindrical lens provides fixed focusing in elevation and, in azimuth, there is electronically controlled focusing at a fixed distance on transmission and swept dynamically on reception. (**B**) A phased array, producing a scan with a sector format.

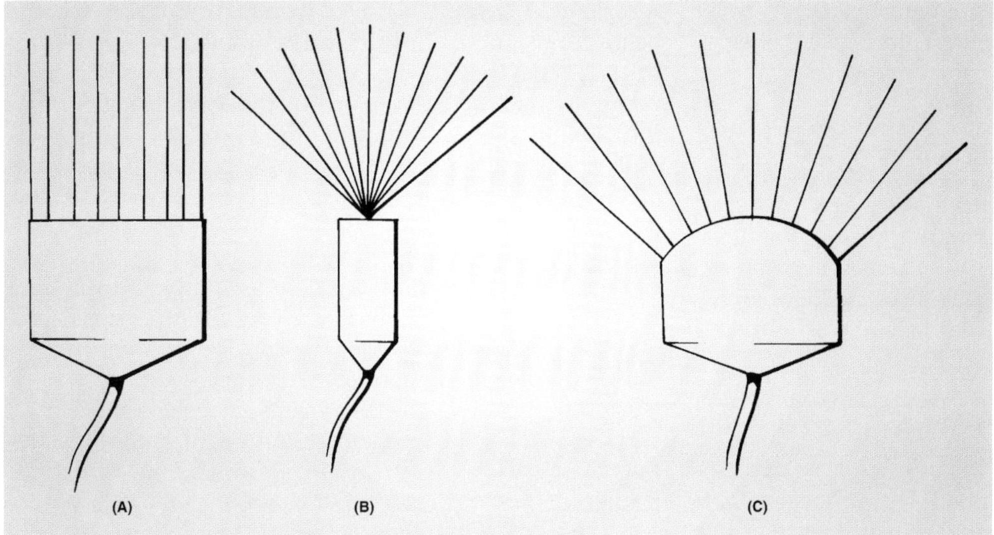

FIGURE 7 A–C ■ Three examples of scan formats produced by electronically controlled transducer arrays. (**A**) Rectangular format, produced by a linear array. (**B**) Sector format, produced by a phased array. (**C**) Truncated sector format, produced by a curvilinear array.

both transmission and reception, the same is not true for the side lobes, because their positions are frequency dependent. It is the side lobes which often cause artifacts which reduce the contrast in the image and thus this problem is diminished by tissue harmonic imaging.

DOPPLER TECHNIQUES

The Doppler Effect

The frequency of ultrasound received after reflection by a stationary target is the same as that of the ultrasonic transmitter. If the target has a component of motion along the axis of the ultrasonic beam (as shown in Fig. 9), however,

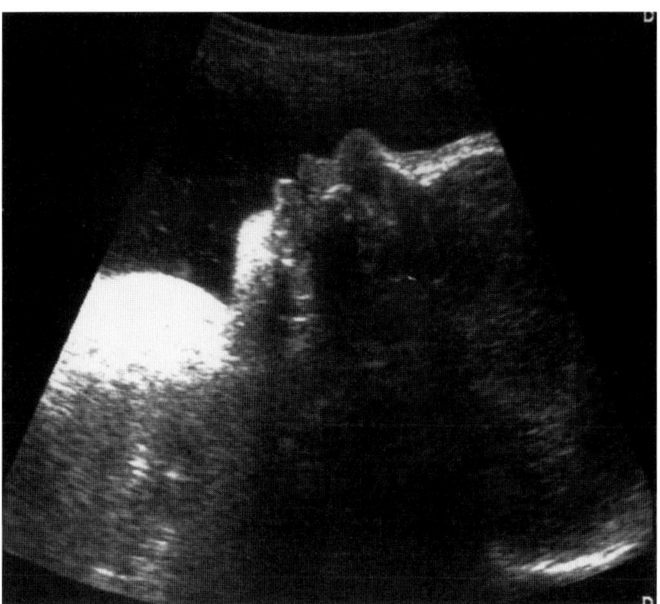

FIGURE 8 ■ Fetal scan, produced by a curvilinear transducer array. Features of the midline section of the fetal face can be clearly seen at 32 weeks, gestation. *Source*: Courtesy of H. S. Andrews.

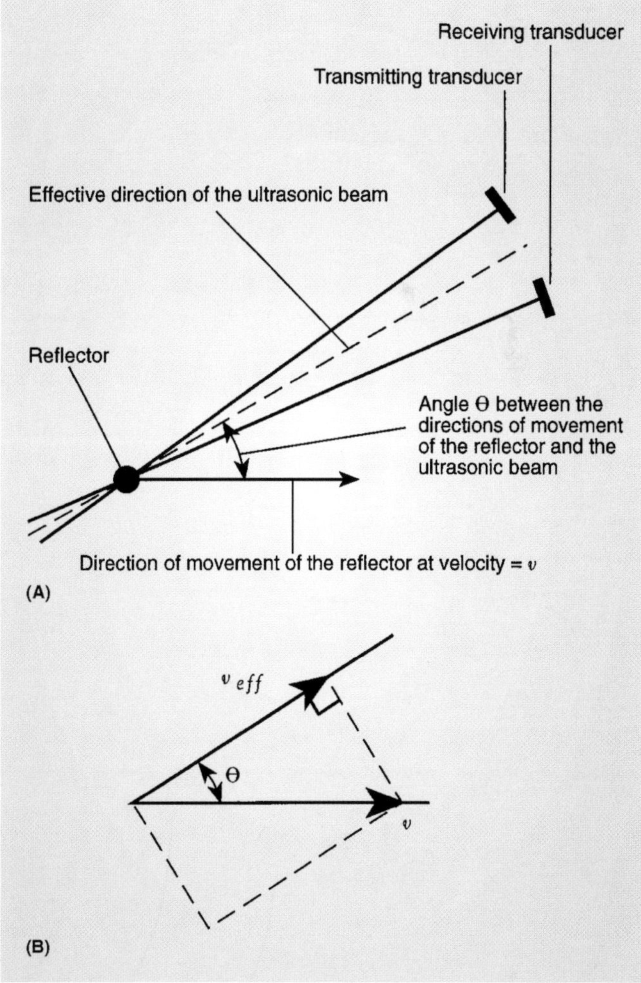

FIGURE 9 A AND B ■ Diagrams illustrating the situation in which an ultrasonic beam is used to acquire Doppler signals from a moving structure or from flowing blood. (**A**) The effective direction of the ultrasonic beam lies between the beams of the transmitting and receiving transducers, at a measurable angle to the direction of motion within the patient. (**B**) Diagram showing the corresponding vector relationships; v_{eff} is the velocity that gives rise to the measured Doppler frequency shift which, after correction by the cosine of the angle θ, allows the motion velocity v to be calculated according to Equation 6.

the received signal is shifted in frequency by the Doppler effect according to the following equation:

$$f_D = 2v(\cos\theta)\frac{f}{c} \qquad (6)$$

where f_D is the difference between the received and the transmitted ultrasonic frequencies, v is the speed of the target, and θ is the angle between the directions of the ultrasonic beam and the movement of the target. Fortunately, for typical ultrasonic frequencies and the speeds at which targets move within the body, the difference frequency usually lies in the audible range.

Continuous Wave Doppler Techniques

Figure 10 is a block diagram of the simplest type of medical ultrasonic Doppler instrument. The probe contains two separate transducers, one for transmission and one for reception. This is necessary because the transmitting transducer is excited to produce continuous waves and the voltage needed to do this is much larger than the voltage produced by the echoes detected by the receiving transducer: the echoes would be masked if the same transducer were to be used for both transmission and reception. Figure 11 is a schlieren photograph of the beams of the transducers in such a probe. The signals from the receiving transducer, however, do include substantial components at the frequency of the transmitter, so that the mixing which occurs in the signal processing circuitry produces an output which, after filtering, consists of the Doppler shift frequencies from moving targets lying in the beam.

The Doppler signals are usually audible and an experienced listener can derive much qualitative information from them. To obtain quantitative information, it is necessary for the signals to be analyzed, usually by a process involving the calculation of the Doppler frequency spectrum, although a simple ratemeter suffices in some clinical situations. There are various methods to obtain the frequency spectra, as illustrated in Figure 12. The fast Fourier transform analyzer is the most common.

The simple Doppler instrument illustrated in Figure 10 provides information only about the amplitude of the echo and the magnitude of the Doppler frequency shift, but not about the direction of movement of the target. Movement toward the transducer results in an upward shift in frequency, and vice versa for movement in the opposite direction. Whether the Doppler-shifted frequency is higher or

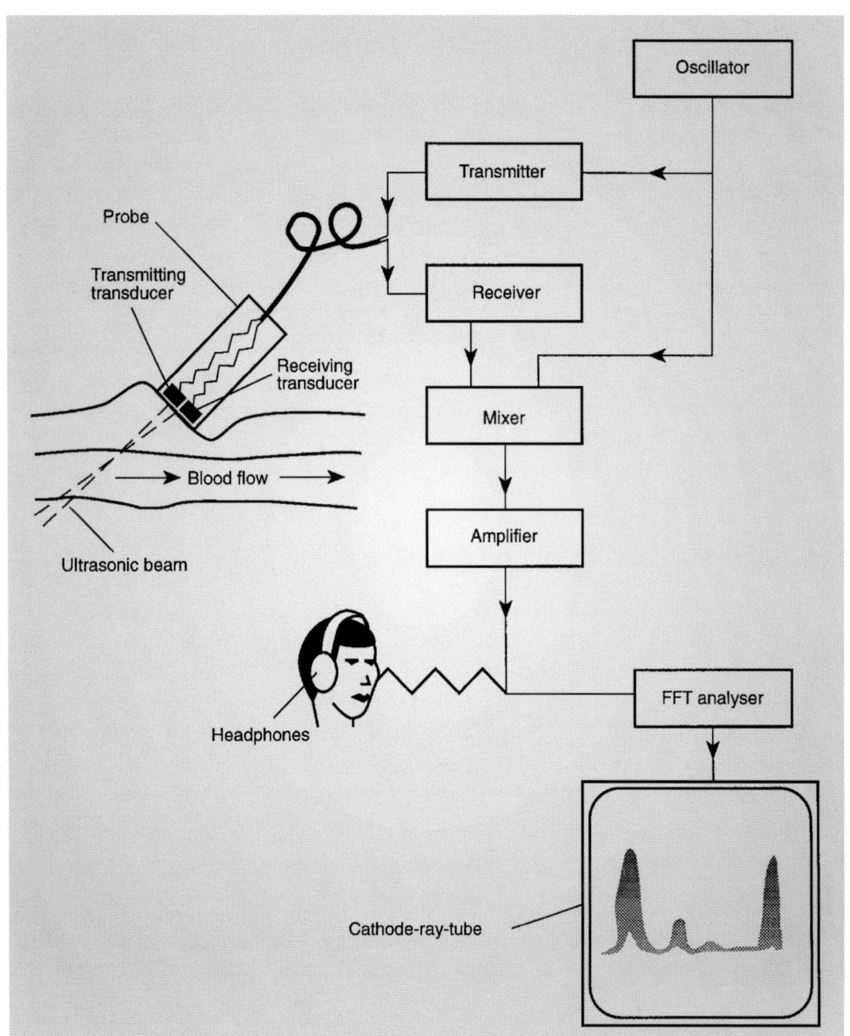

FIGURE 10 ■ Block diagram of an ultrasonic Doppler system using continuous waves, without directional detection. Echoes, including Doppler-shifted signals, are amplified in the receiver and mixed with signals at the transmitted frequency, the result of which can be filtered to provide the audible Doppler shift signal. This signal can be analyzed by the fast Fourier transform (FFT) analyzer and displayed as a frequency spectrum.

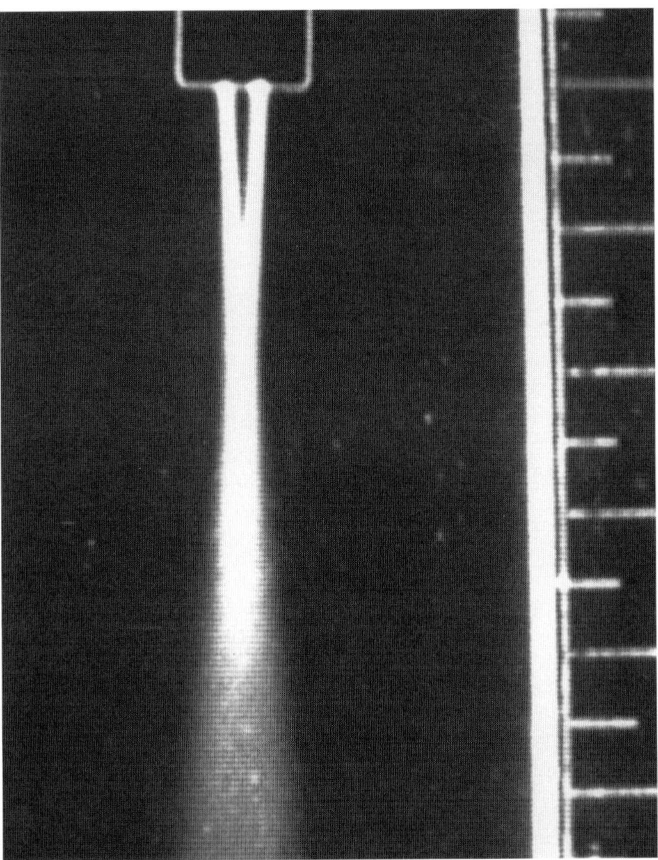

FIGURE 11 ■ The beams of the transducers in a typical probe for continuous wave ultrasonic Doppler blood flow studies, made visible by schlieren photography. The tip of the probe was immersed in a tank of water through which a parallel beam of light traveled, subsequently to be brought to a focus on an occluding spot. When each of the transducers was excited in turn to make the double-exposure photograph, the water through which the beam passed experienced a change in refractive index, so that the beam became visible beyond the occluding spot. The region of crossover of the beams can be seen, and standing waves resulting from reflection at the bottom of the tank can also be seen. *Source*: Courtesy of D. H. Follett.

lower than that of the transmitter can be determined by phase quadrature detection. A phase quadrature detector operates by determining whether the phase of the received signal leads or lags that of the transmitted signal.

Pulsed Doppler Techniques

Apart from the steady reduction in signal strength which occurs with increasing penetration into the body, simple continuous wave Doppler techniques lack depth selectivity. By pulsing the transmitted ultrasound, depth information can be obtained in the same way as with pulse-echo imaging methods. In Figure 13 , an example of a pulsed Doppler instrument is shown. The position of the Doppler sample volume along the ultrasonic beam can be chosen by the operator, as can its length.

There is an upper limit to the unambiguously detectable shift frequency in a pulsed Doppler system. This is because sampling theory requires that the sampling frequency should be more than twice the sampled frequency. This condition is known as the Nyquist criterion. Just as the pulse repetition frequency determines the compromise between depth of penetration, image line density, and image frame rate in pulse-echo imaging, so in pulsed Doppler studies the ultrasonic frequency usually has to be selected to ensure that the maximum Doppler shift frequency falls within the Nyquist limit.

When the anatomical situation is well defined, a pulsed Doppler probe can provide additional information to that obtained with a continuous wave probe. The interpretation of Doppler signals, unguided by imaging, is, however, of limited clinical utility.

DUPLEX SCANNING

General Principles

Although a hand-held Doppler probe without imaging guidance can provide useful information in a few clinical situations, usually it is necessary to have an image in order to provide the confidence of target identification. Duplex scanning makes this possible, as shown in Figure 14. Real-time pulse-echo imaging, performed in the traditional way, allows the locations within which flow or motion are to be measured to be visualized. Thus, the ultrasonic beam can accurately be directed through the region-of-interest. By a process involving time sharing, the Doppler signals from targets moving in the region-of-interest can be acquired and analyzed, as already explained. The process of time sharing can involve either the complete cessation of image acquisition during Doppler studies, or a switching between the two modes of operation that is fast enough for both modes apparently to proceed simultaneously. Simultaneous image and Doppler acquisition is generally only possible, however, with transducer array scanning, because most mechanical scanners cannot be started and stopped fast enough or without the accompaniment of troublesome vibration. Indeed, such are the practical limitations of the technique that, nowadays, it is really mainly of historical interest.

Duplex Instrument Design

The designer of the duplex scanner is faced by the necessity to make numerous compromises. The ultrasonic frequencies can be taken as the starting point for the design. For imaging, the highest frequency which provides adequate penetration is usually considered to be the optimum. The same frequency is unlikely to be best for pulsed Doppler operation, however, because the Doppler shift frequency associated with the fastest-moving targets would probably exceed the Nyquist limit. This, together with the attenuation of Doppler-shifted signals in the intervening tissue, means that a lower frequency is usually needed for satisfactory Doppler operation. With mechanical duplex scanners, different transducers can often be used for imaging and for Doppler signal acquisition. The same transducer array, however, has to serve for both purposes when electronic scanning is employed and differences between the frequencies for imaging and Doppler studies have to be accommodated within the

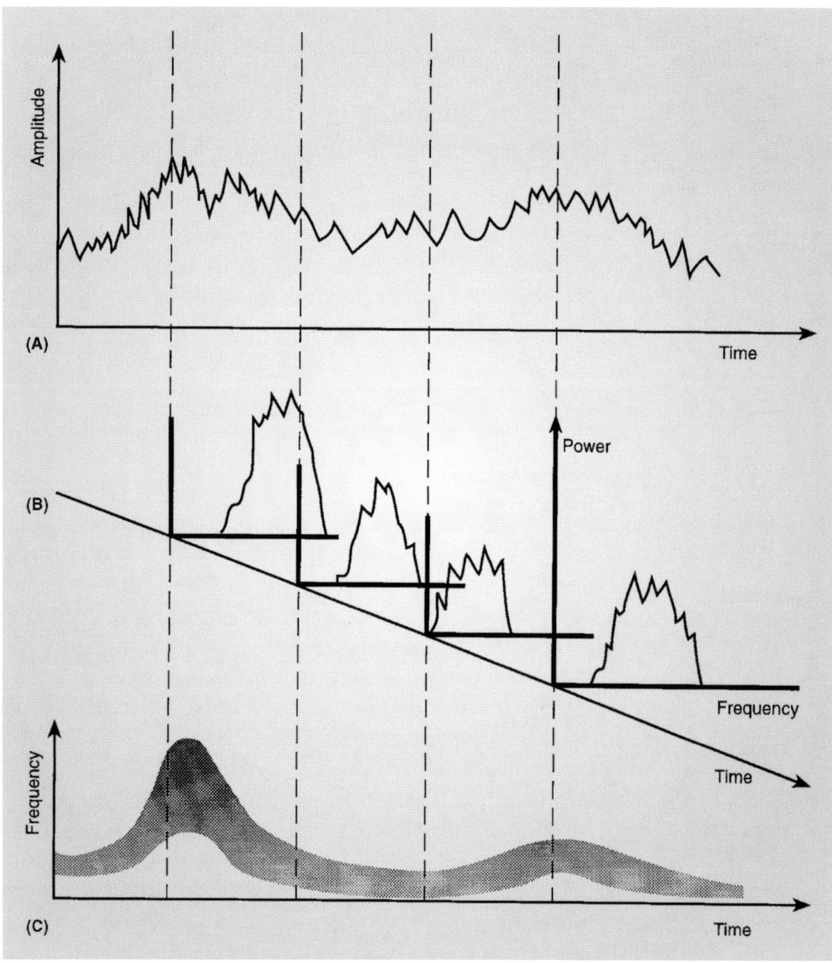

FIGURE 12 A–C ■ The Doppler signal and its frequency spectrum. (**A**) The raw signal, in which variations in both amplitude and frequency can be seen, although they are hard to interpret. (**B**) The distribution of signal power with frequency at several brief periods separated in time. (**C**) The traditional frequency spectrum, in which frequency is shown vertically, time is shown horizontally, and the intensity of the recording corresponds to the instantaneous signal power.

bandwidth of the transducer. Nowadays, this is becoming less of a problem as transducer bandwidths continue to be increased: indeed, bandwidths of 4 to 12 MHz are now not uncommon.

In a typical duplex scan, the position of the ultrasonic beam for Doppler signal acquisition is highlighted against the background of the real-time gray-scale image. On this line, the sample volume position and length are also indicated. This allows the observer appropriately to place the Doppler sample volume. In the example shown in Figure 14, there is a cursor which the operator can orientate so that it lies parallel to the presumed direction of flow within the sample volume. In this way, the relative directions of the ultrasonic beam and the flow can be taken into account by the system software in calculating the speed of the target from Equation 6. For convenience, the Doppler frequency spectrum corresponding to the target motion in the region-of-interest is often displayed on the same screen as the real-time duplex scan. In addition, the system software is able to calculate indices derived from the Doppler signal. In this way, the operator can interpret the results of the examination whilst it is being carried out. It should be noted that these indices are generally the ratios of Doppler frequencies (for example, the frequencies corresponding to systolic and diastolic blood flow velocities) and, since these measurements are made with the ultrasonic beam in a fixed position, there is no need to make any correction for the actual angle between the beam and the flow direction.

COLOR FLOW IMAGING

General Principles

Although technically challenging to achieve, the idea of producing an image in which two-dimensional blood flow information is superimposed on cross-sectional anatomical details in real time is a simple concept. It can be considered to be an extension of duplex scanning, with the Doppler sample volume somehow placed simultaneously at every point in the image with the corresponding flow measurements coded in a way that can easily be perceived by the observer. Color provides a convenient method of coding.

Figure 15 shows how color flow imaging can be realized in practice. The anatomical information is provided by a traditional real-time pulse-echo gray-scale scanner. In principle, there are two methods by which the color flow information can be obtained. Currently, the most commonly used method is what is usually described as a Doppler technique which uses phase domain processing.

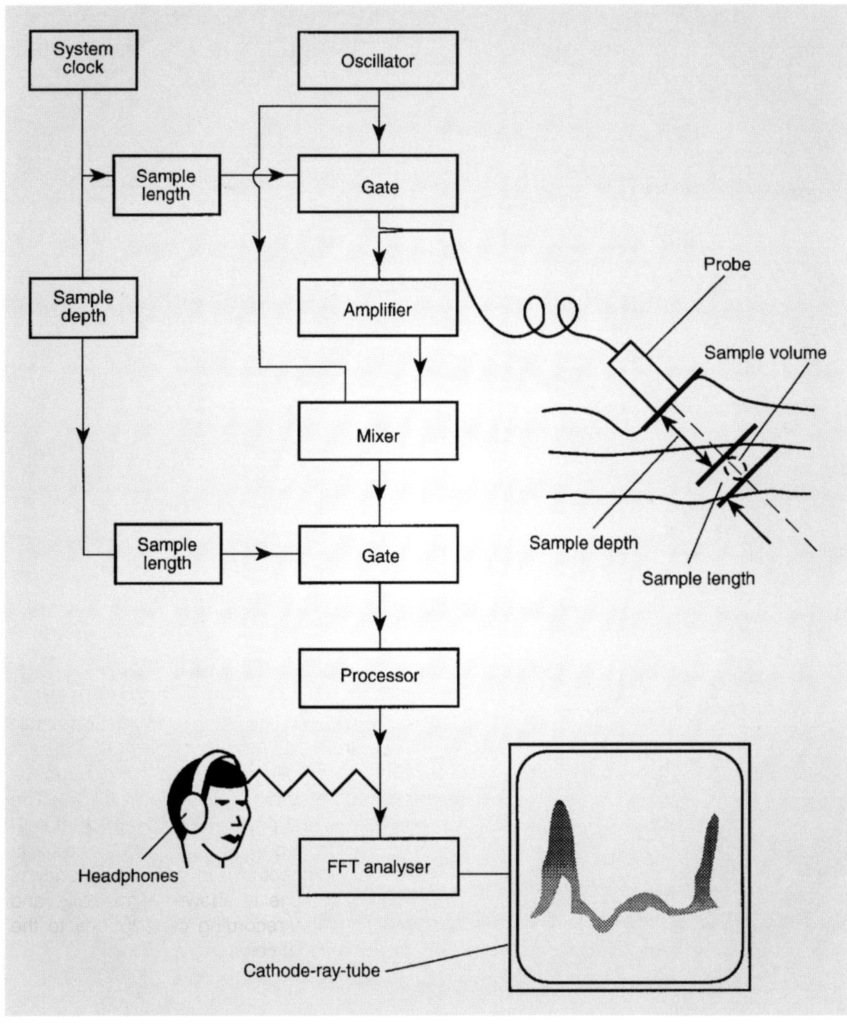

FIGURE 13 ■ Block diagram of ultrasonic pulsed Doppler system. The system clock controls the pulse repetition rate. The clock triggers both the sample length and sample depth time interval generators. The first sample length generator opens the first gate for a brief period, allowing signals from the oscillator to be transmitted as an ultrasonic pulse into the patient. Echoes are received by the probe from this pulse and fed to the amplifier. In the mixer, the amplified signals and the transmitted frequency combine to produce a Doppler-shifted wavetrain. The segment of this wavetrain corresponding to the sample volume within the patient is selected by the second sample length generator which is triggered at the appropriate instant by the sample depth generator. The output from the second gate consists of the sampled Doppler signal, which is processed into an audible form or subjected to Fourier transform (FFT) analysis and displayed as a frequency spectrum.

Similar flow information can also be obtained, however, by time domain processing. These two techniques are described in more detail in the following paragraphs.

Phase Domain Processing

Phase domain processing for color flow imaging can be considered to be a pulsed Doppler technique. As a result of flow, the echoes from successive ultrasonic pulses arrive at the receiving transducer shifted in phase by an amount which depends on the flow velocity. The phase shift is measured by a process of "autocorrelation detection," in which an electronically generated delay, exactly equal to the interval between consecutively transmitted pulses, is applied so that the echo wavetrains from consecutively transmitted pulses can be multiplied together in a coherent fashion. If the two consecutive wavetrains are identical, as they are if they originate from stationary structures, their product remains constant. If, however, the phases of parts of the wavetrains change as a result of flow, the magnitude of the corresponding product changes and this is, in fact, equivalent to the Doppler shift signal. Autocorrelation detection is a process which can be achieved at high speed, making real-time operation possible. There are limits, however, to the maximum speed of imaging and these are discussed later.

Time Domain Processing

In the M-mode method, velocity can be measured by observing the distance which a target moves in the known time interval between the transmissions of consecutive ultrasonic pulses. This forms the basis of time domain processing for color flow imaging. Consecutive echo wavetrains are compared by "cross-correlation detection."

Comparison of Phase and Time Domain Processing

The fundamental difference between phase and time domain processing is that the former is a narrow frequency band technique, whereas the latter is wide band. The implications of this fundamental difference on the image frame rate, sensitivity, and spatial resolution are important in clinical practice.

For a given number of lines in each image frame, the maximum image frame rate is controlled by the time which is necessary for the ultrasonic beam to remain stationary at each point in the scan plane in order to acquire sufficient information to allow the lowest blood flow velocity of interest to be estimated. Here, phase domain processing is at a disadvantage in comparison with time domain processing, because it requires the lowest Doppler

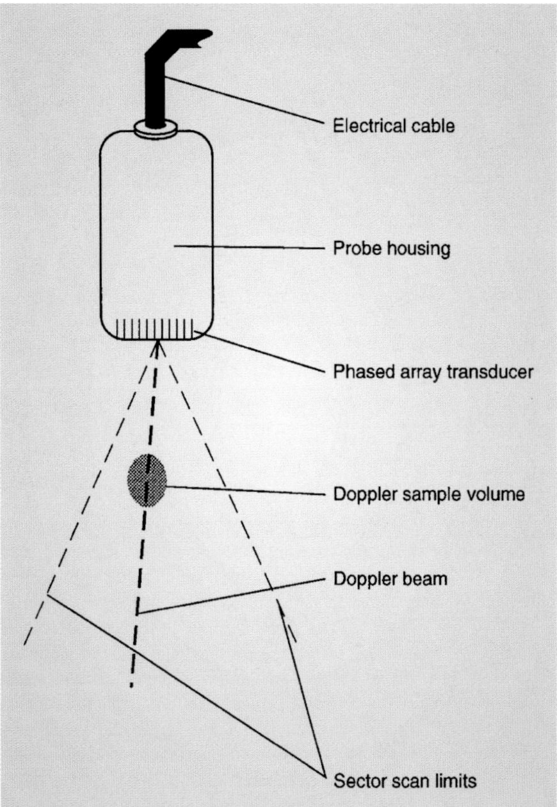

FIGURE 14 ■ Diagram showing the principle of the ultrasonic duplex scanner using a phased array transducer. The probe produces a sector scan within which a particular beam direction can be selected and used for the acquisition of signals from the sample volume of a pulsed Doppler system.

frequency shift to be estimated, whereas time domain processing only requires the target to move a measurable distance. The sensitivity of the phase domain system is inherently better than that of time domain processing because, being a narrow band technique, the noise performance of the receiver is better. For the same reason, the phase domain technique is associated with a longer-duration ultrasonic pulse and so it has a poorer axial resolution than that with time domain processing. Moreover, as in all other pulsed Doppler methods, phase domain processing is subject to the aliasing ambiguity if the pulse repetition frequency is less than twice the highest Doppler shift frequency. The lateral resolution depends on the width of the ultrasonic beam, which is, in principle, not dependent on whether phase or time domain processing is used.

Consideration is seldom given to the potentially different bioeffects of phase and time domain processing in color flow imaging. For similar performance, the pulse transmitted for phase domain processing is both of longer duration and lower intensity than that with time domain processing. Consequently, different emphasis has to be given to the various factors, discussed later, which affect the safety of ultrasonic diagnosis.

Color Coding Schemes

There are two color coding schemes which are in general use in color flow imaging. One option is to color-code the image according to the velocity of blood flow. Increasing velocity toward the probe is usually coded on a red-orange-yellow scale, whereas increasing reverse flow

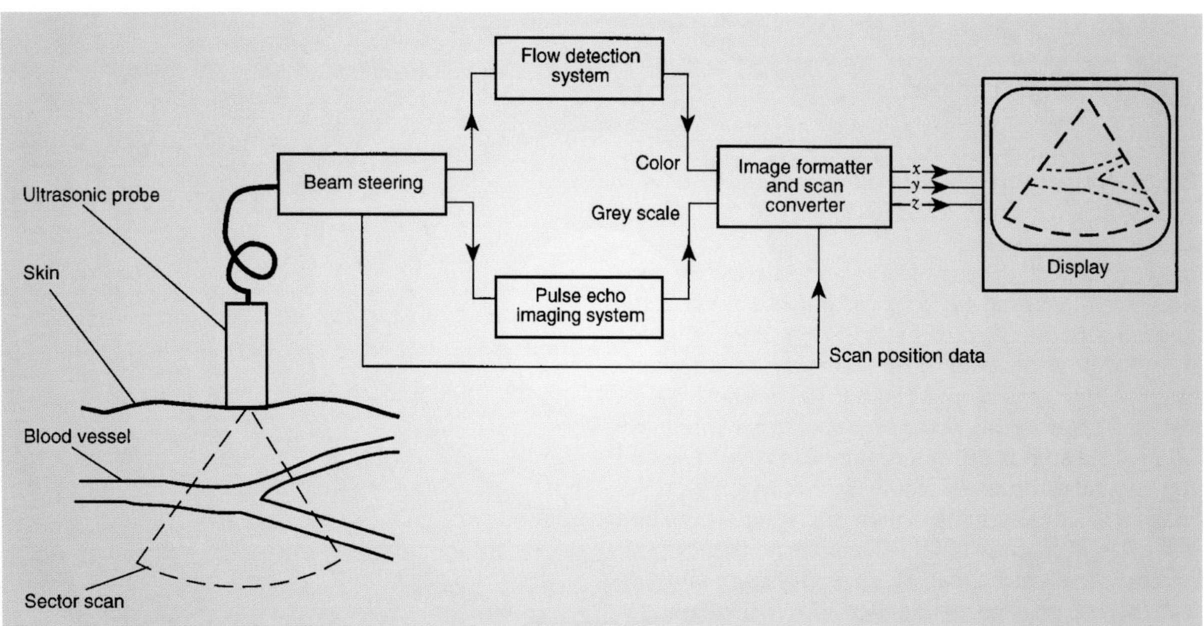

FIGURE 15 ■ Block diagram of an ultrasonic color flow imaging system. In this example, an ultrasonic probe containing a phased array transducer produces a sector scan. Echoes from within the scan plane are processed by a traditional imaging system to produce a gray-scale display in real time. The flow detection system, which can use either phase or time domain processing, produces a two-dimensional color-coded scan which is superimposed on the gray-scale display, also in real time although not so rapidly as is possible with gray-scale imaging alone.

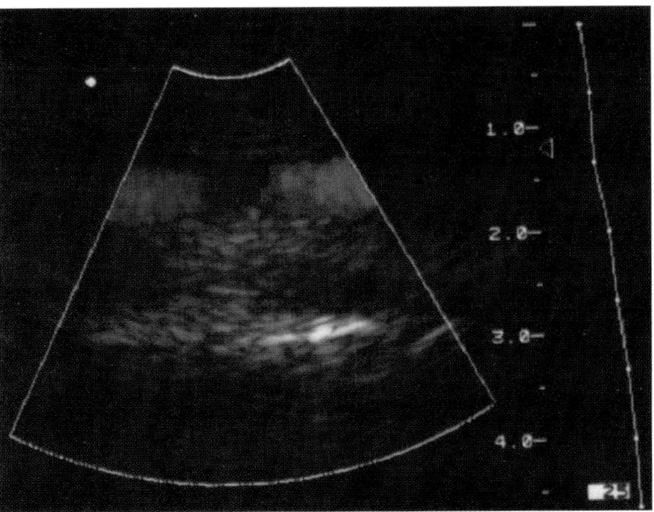

FIGURE 16 ■ Color velocity image of flow in a large superficial vein. In the vein, the flow is unidirectional during the time of signal acquisition. The image sector, however, is orientated so that the relative direction of the ultrasonic beam and that of the flow actually reverse across the scan plane. This results in the display of both approaching and receding flow, with the absence of flow display when the ultrasonic beam is approximately normal to the flow direction.

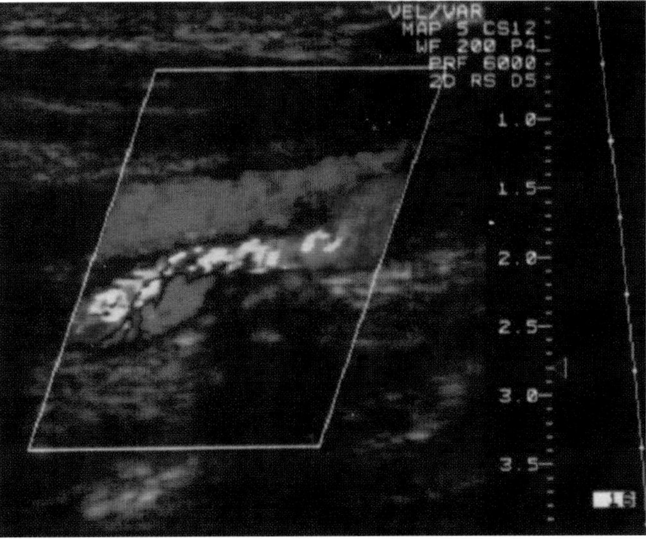

FIGURE 17 ■ Color velocity image of flow in the jugular vein and in the region of the carotid artery bifurcation in a patient with an atherosclerotic plaque in the carotid. The flows in the two vessels are predominantly in opposite directions, although there is some reversal of flow in the carotid. There is also flow disturbance around the plaque, as is evident from the increase in the displayed variance of the velocity signal.

velocity is coded in increasingly lighter blue. Figure 16 shows why, in interpreting color flow velocity images, whether obtained by phase or time domain processing, it is essential to take account of the relative directions of the ultrasonic beam and the flow.

In the second of the main color coding schemes, the power (or amplitude) of the flow signal is used to control the brightness of a monochromatic hue (or wavelength). The hue can be chosen according to the individual preference of the user. It is also worth noting that most modern color flow imaging systems partially suppress the real-time two-dimensional pulse-echo image information in the color-coded region of the display. Consequently, the use of color is not really necessary, since the blurry nature of the flow information is sufficiently characteristic for it to be distinguished from a traditional B-scan when both are displayed in gray scale.

In a color-coded velocity image, green, which contrasts well with both red-yellow and blue, is sometimes used to highlight lines of equal velocity, or to mark regions where there are abnormally high values of velocity variance. The velocity variance is a statistical measure of the spread of velocities in the corresponding sample volume in the image and so it is related to the degree of flow disturbance or actual turbulence. This is illustrated in Figure 17. An artifact in color flow imaging is due to the fact that, if the pulse repetition rate is less than twice the highest Doppler shift frequency, so that the Nyquist limit is exceeded, the color scale reverses and the interpretation of the image becomes problematic.

Color-coded power images represent merely the presence and the amount of flowing blood. They are unaffected by the direction of flow, the vector relationship between the directions of the ultrasonic beam and the flow, flow disturbance or turbulence, or the existence of aliasing when the Nyquist limit is exceeded. Superficially, at least, they resemble X-ray contrast or magnetic resonance angiograms and they provide a crude qualitative representation of blood perfusion.

SPECIALIZED AND EMERGING PROCEDURES

Endoluminal and Intravascular Scanners

Although it is true that a large majority of ultrasonic investigations are carried out transcutaneously, there are a growing number of applications in which the probe is introduced either into a body cavity, by puncture into a blood vessel, or intraoperatively. The main advantage of these approaches is that the distance between the probe and the tissue under investigation is reduced, so that a higher frequency can be used. Moreover, the distortion due to overlying tissues is also reduced. This makes it easier for high quality images, with high resolution, to be produced.

Figure 18 gives some examples of probes for intracavitary and intraluminal scanning. The intracavitary probes (Fig. 18A–C) are for the esophagus, rectum, and vagina, respectively. Figure 18D is an endoluminal probe, primarily for intravascular studies. For intraoperative imaging, small high-resolution arrays are generally used: they may be sterilized (for example, by gas) or fitted into a sterile sheath.

Three-Dimensional Scanners

Currently, two-dimensional scanning is the mainstay of ultrasonic imaging. There are two important reasons for this: imaging specialists are familiar with cross-sectional anatomy and the process can generally be performed in

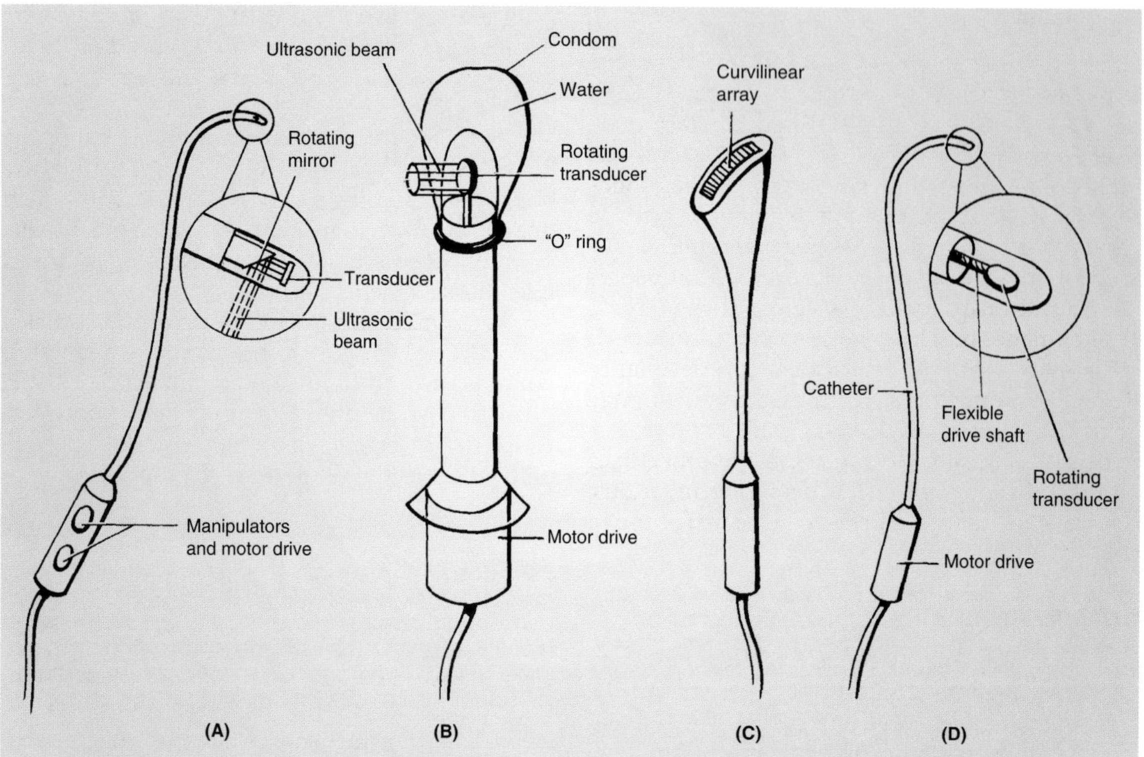

FIGURE 18 A–D ■ Some examples of probes for intracavitary and intraluminal scanning. (**A**) Ultrasonic endoscope for intraesophageal scanning, by means of a rotating mirror directing the beam from a disk transducer into a radial scan plane. (**B**) Endorectal probe, using a mechanically rotating disk transducer. (**C**) Endovaginal probe, using a curvilinear array. (**D**) Intravascular probe, with a small rotating transducer mounted within the probe at its tip to produce a radial scan.

real time. Imaging specialists do not often confine themselves to single two-dimensional image planes, however, but they change the scan plane whilst interactively observing the display. Thus, they build up, in their mind's eye, a three-dimensional image of the scanned anatomy.

As illustrated in Figure 19, a three-dimensional image data set can be acquired in the form of contiguous two-dimensional scans. There are numerous other scanning schemes which are also practicable in addition to the one shown. For example, probes with two-dimensional arrays of transducers are beginning to become available and these make it possible to acquire three-dimensional image volumes without any mechanical motion, because the ultrasonic beam can be steered in any direction. Whatever scheme is adopted, the total scanning time is necessarily at least as long as the product of the two-dimensional frame time multiplied by the number of frames in the image data set. Consequently, the process is relatively slow. Moreover, the display of the information in the image data set poses several problems. Because of their speckly nature, ultrasonic images are not easily segmented into, for example, organs and structures with well-defined boundaries. Volume rendering with rotation of the image to provide depth cues is quite a satisfactory option. Alternatively, the operator may select for display any two-dimensional plane within the data set, thus exploring the three-dimensional volume by interacting with the computer rather than with the patient.

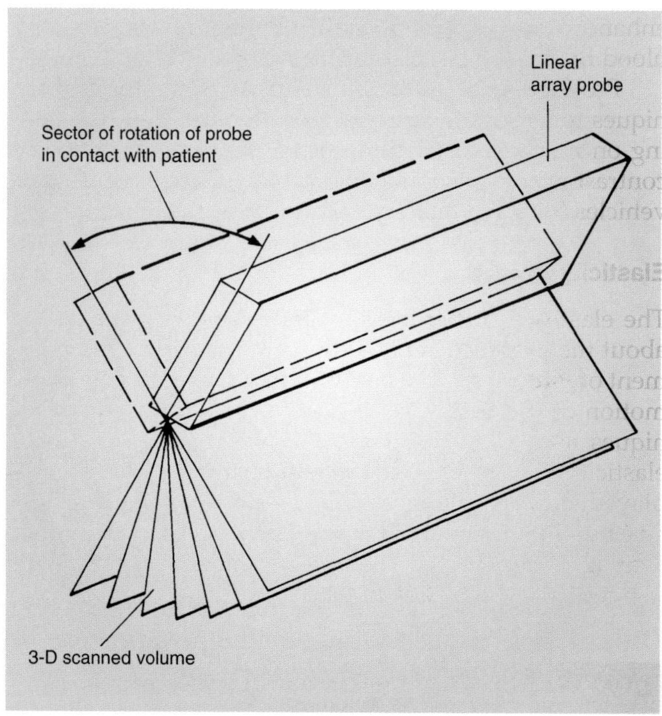

FIGURE 19 ■ Diagram showing a typical method for the acquisition of a three-dimensional scan. In this example, a linear array is rotated about its long axis in contact with the patient to produce a set of contiguous two-dimensional rectangular scans that are stored in an image processing computer for subsequent display.

Image Management

In the past, ultrasonic scanning was largely an interactive process; the operator tried to reach a diagnostic conclusion during the scanning procedure and photographic hard copies were made mainly for record purposes. Nowadays, however, most ultrasonic scanners have solid-state image stores that enable the information to be reviewed at leisure; some have sufficient memory capacity to allow sequences of images to be studied retrospectively. Ultrasonically acquired images are managed, often in parallel with images obtained by other techniques such as computed tomography (CT) and magnetic resonance imaging (MRI), on networks with associated storage devices and distributed displays. This has greatly increased both the efficiency of imaging specialists and the accessibility of the images and their interpretations. Moreover, ultrasound is now a prime candidate for use in telemedicine.

Contrast Agents

Specialized contrast agents, particularly those based on microbubbles, are beginning significantly to expand the clinical applications of diagnostic ultrasound. The bubbles are small enough to cross over capillary beds and they can exist for times long enough to allow venous injection to produce contrast effects in the systemic circulation. Another promising development depends on the phenomenon in which bubbles scatter ultrasound not only at the same frequency as that of the transmitted pulses but also at twice this frequency. This is the basis of "harmonic imaging" with contrast agents, which is associated with greatly enhanced sensitivity to small volumes of low velocity blood flow.

Progress is being made in the development of techniques to target contrast agents to specific sites, depending on metabolic and pathological processes. Ultrasonic contrast agents are also beginning to show promise as a vehicles for drug delivery and gene transfection.

Elasticity Imaging

The elasticity, or hardness, of tissues often gives a clue about the presence of pathology. By applying a displacement or vibration to tissue structures, the relative internal motion of the tissues can be tracked by ultrasonic techniques and, from these data, information about tissue elasticity can be derived. This information can be displayed, for example, as a map of elasticity superimposed on a two-dimensional ultrasonic scan of the corresponding anatomical structures. The first commercial system with this capability is now available.

QUALITY CONTROL IN ULTRASONIC IMAGING

Modern ultrasonic scanners are advanced devices with great reliability and excellent stability. It is necessary, however, to carry out initial acceptance tests when a new machine comes into service and then to institute a regular program of quality control. The latter is important, because operators become accustomed to their scanners and often fail to notice if the performance is gradually deteriorating.

There are several aspects of performance that should be monitored. The sensitivity and spatial registration can be checked by using a variety of phantoms which provide images in which there are not only objects at known positions but also scatterers of various strengths chosen to give measurements of contrast.

For quality control of Doppler, flow measurement, and color imaging systems, there are several phantoms with targets and fluids which move at known velocities. There is also a family of acoustically coupled devices which inject signals into the transducer that simulate defined conditions experienced in scanning.

ARTIFACTS IN ULTRASONIC IMAGING

It is important that both operators and those concerned with ultrasonic image interpretation should be aware of the numerous artifacts that can occur. Many of these artifacts are due to the physics of the image-forming process; others arise because of limitations in scanner performance.

In pulse-echo imaging, there are several common artifacts. Shadowing or enhancement of echoes from beyond a structure is due to its attenuation being higher or lower than that of its surroundings. Reverberation, with which banding appears in the image, arises from multiple echoes associated with strong reflectors oriented normal to the beam. Duplications of image features are caused by strong reflectors lying obliquely to the direction of the beam, whereas side lobes of the beam lead to misregistration.

Pulsed Doppler systems are prone to the same artifacts as pulse-echo systems, although the problems may not be so immediately obvious. In addition, aliasing of Doppler signals occurs when the pulse repetition rate is less than twice the Doppler shift frequency. Motion and flow detection by time domain processing suffer from mainly different artifacts, due to, for example, targets passing through the beam so fast that they cannot be tracked as echoes from consecutive pulses.

The time required for the acquisition of a frame of color-flow image information has already been discussed. An artifact caused by this is illustrated in Figure 20A, in which it appears that blood flow in a short segment of artery is in both directions at the same time. Figure 20B shows the spectrum of the Doppler frequency shift observed over several cardiac cycles at a particular anatomical site within the artery. Forward flow occurs in systole, but this reverses in diastole. The explanation of the appearance in Figure 20A is that the time required to acquire the image was such that, on the left, systolic flow was occurring, whereas, on the right, time had moved on so that, when it was imaged here, the flow had become diastolic.

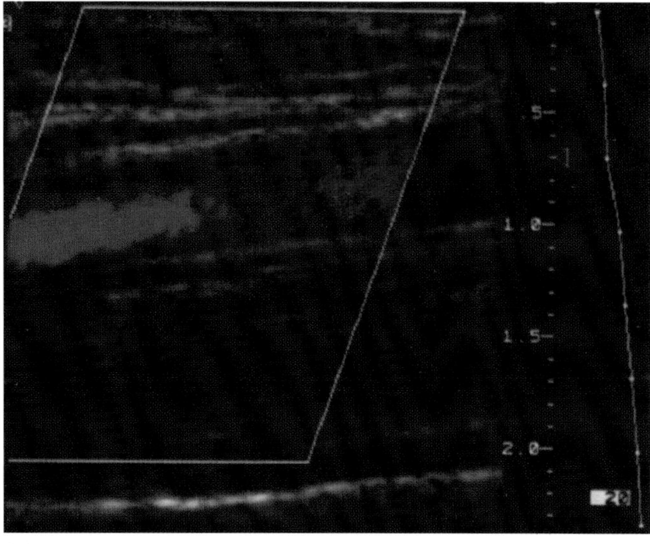

(A)

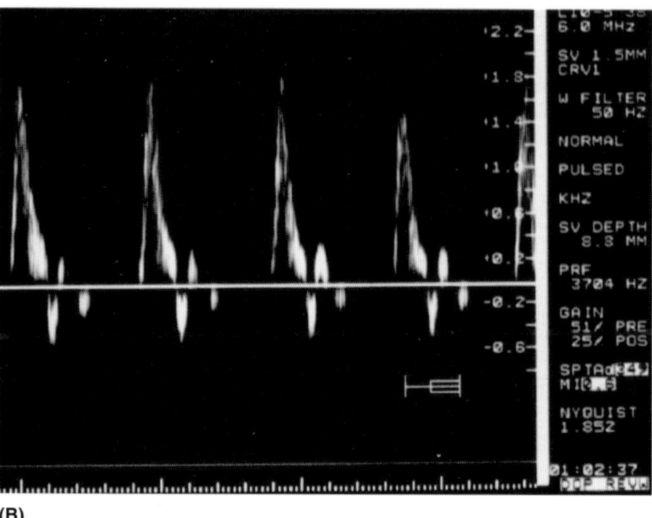

(B)

FIGURE 20 A AND B ■ A common artifact in color flow imaging. (**A**) Color-coded velocity image showing flow in a superficial artery, observed by a linear array probe steered to produce a trapezoidal scan format. The apparent coexistence of flow in opposite directions is an artifact that arises because a significant time is required to acquire the color flow image information. (**B**) The Doppler frequency spectrum, acquired from a fixed anatomical site within the same artery but with the scanner operating in duplex mode, shows that flow reversal occurs during diastole. The explanation of the artifact is that the color flow image acquisition time extends throughout systole and well into diastole.

BIOEFFECTS OF ULTRASOUND

Mechanisms of Bioeffects

Ultrasonic waves carry energy into the patient. Even in diagnostic applications, most of this energy is converted into heat as it is absorbed in the tissues. In fact, the amount of energy that is actually reflected to provide the diagnostic information is only a tiny fraction of the energy transmitted into the patient.

The quantity of energy and the rate of its delivery in ultrasonic diagnosis are determined primarily by the necessity to produce a satisfactory image or other kinds of useful information. Although the quantity of energy is small, it is appropriate to review the mechanisms by which ultrasound may have effects on biological systems, as a preliminary to considering the safety of diagnostic levels of exposure.

The heat produced in tissue by ultrasonic irradiation is fundamentally dependent on two factors: the power density and the cooling conditions. For a given rate of attenuation, it is possible to calculate the rate of heat deposition for given exposure conditions of frequency and intensity. The cooling conditions, however, are less predictable: they depend, for example, on thermal conduction and blood perfusion. It is important to note that the possibility of biological effects and, by implication, the risk of damage increase nonlinearly with increasing temperature (12). Moreover, as the temperature increases, the time for harmful effects to occur is shorter.

There is also evidence that ultrasound can produce bioeffects by direct mechanical action associated with wave motion (13,14). Although much research remains to be done, it seems probable that these effects are unlikely to be significant at diagnostic exposure levels unless gas bubbles are present and, even then, the risks have not been quantified. Most likely, damage would occur as the result of streaming velocity gradients on a minute scale. Such velocity gradients are known to be amplified in the presence of bubbles of appropriate dimensions. It is reassuring to note that bubbles of these dimensions, typically a few micrometers in diameter, do not appear to be commonplace, if they exist at all, in the intact body, except when deliberately introduced for use as contrast or drug delivery agents.

Safety of Diagnostic Ultrasound

Because bioeffects, some of which are harmful, may be caused by ultrasound under certain exposure conditions, it is necessary to consider the hypothetical possibility that ultrasonic diagnosis may not be completely safe (15). It is first worth noting that the last three decades have seen a steady increase in both the time-averaged intensities and the peak pressures used in diagnostic procedures (16). Consequently, both regulatory authorities and prudent physicians do not take the subject lightly.

The World Federation for Ultrasound in Medicine and Biology (17) has published the following statements on thermal effects in clinical applications:

B-Mode Imaging

Known diagnostic ultrasound equipment as used today for simple B-mode imaging operates at acoustic outputs that are not capable of producing harmful temperature rises. Its use in medicine is therefore not contraindicated on thermal grounds. This includes endoscopic, transvaginal, and transcutaneous applications.

Doppler

It has been demonstrated in experiments with unperfused tissue that some Doppler diagnostic equipment has the potential to produce biologically significant temperature rises, specifically at bone/soft tissue interfaces. The effects of elevated temperatures may be minimized by keeping the time for which the beam passes through any one point in tissue as short as possible. Where output power can be controlled, the lowest available power level consistent with obtaining the desired diagnostic information should be used.

Although the data on humans are sparse, it is clear from animal studies that exposures resulting in temperatures less than 38.5 °C can be used without reservation on thermal grounds. This includes obstetric applications.

Transducer Heating

A substantial source of heating may be the transducer itself. Tissue heating from this source is localized to the volume in contact with the transducer.

The situation relating to nonthermal effects and their relevance to exposure conditions in contemporary ultrasonic diagnostic procedures is currently more hotly debated (9). Acoustic cavitation, defined as the formation and/or activity of gas- or vapor-filled cavities (bubbles) in a medium exposed to an ultrasonic field, is the phenomenon of principal concern. Other possible nonthermal mechanisms include radiation pressure, radiation force, acoustic torque, and acoustic streaming.

Pragmatically, users of ultrasound for diagnosis should apply the as low as reasonable achievable (ALARA) principle to the exposures to which they subject their patients. The exposure levels should be at the lowest intensities and for the briefest times consistent with imaging of adequate diagnostic quality. In order to assist in this, a predictor of cavitation known as the "mechanical index" (MI) has been developed (18), given by the expression

$$\mathrm{MI} = \frac{P_r 3Z_{sp}}{\sqrt{f_c}} \tag{7}$$

where $P_r3(Z_{sp})$ is the peak rarefactional pressure (in MPa) derated by 0.3 dB/(cm MHz) to the point on the beam axis (Z_{sp}) where the pulse intensity integral is maximum and f_c is the center frequency (in MHz). Modern scanners display the value of MI on the screen, so that the operator can aim to minimize it.

It is important to realize that the consequences of misdiagnosis are likely to be the greatest hazard of ultrasonic investigation (15). Other risks must not be discounted, but they should always be viewed in the proper perspective.

In summary, the modern approach (19) is to use ultrasonic diagnostic procedures only when justified by reasonable expectation that the information to be obtained will be likely to be of clinical benefit to the patient. Moreover, even when justified in this way, the ultrasonic exposure used should be as low as reasonably practicable to obtain useful information. This is sometimes referred to as the application of the ALARA principle.

REFERENCES

1. Wood RW, Loomis AL. The physical and biological effects of high-frequency sound waves of great intensity. Phil Mag 1927; 7(4):417.
2. Summer W, Patrick MK. Ultrasonic Therapy. Amsterdam: Elsevier, 1964.
3. Warden SJ, McMeeken JM. Ultrasound usage and dosage in sports physiotherapy. Ultrasound Med Biol 2002; 28:1075.
4. Howry DH, Bliss WR. Ultrasonic visualization of soft tissue structures of the body. J Lab Clin Invest 1952; 40:579.
5. Wild JJ, Reid JM. Further pilot echographic studies of the histologic structure of tumors of the living intact human breast. Am J Path 1952; 28:839.
6. Wells PNT. Developments in medical ultrasonics. Wld Med Electron 1966; 4:272.
7. Griffith JM, Henry WL. A sector scanner for real time two-dimensional echocardiography. Circulation 1974; 49:1147.
8. Kossoff G. Display techniques in ultrasound pulse echo investigations: a review. J Clin Ultrasound 1974; 2:61.
9. Whittingham TA. The safety of ultrasound. Imaging 1994; 6:33.
10. Barnett SB, ter Haar GR, Ziskin MC, Nyborg WL, Maeda K, Bang J. Current status of research on biological effects of ultrasound. Ultrasound Med Biol 1994; 20:205.
11. Simpson DG, Ho M-H, Yang Y, Zhou J, Zachary JF, O'Brien WD. Excess risk thresholds in ultrasound safety studies: statistical methods for data on occurrence and size of lesions. Ultrasound Med Biol 2004; 30:1289.
12. Edwards MJ. Hyperthermia as a teratogen: a review of experimental studies and their clinical significance. Teratogen Carcinogen Mutagen 1986; 6:563.
13. Wells PNT, ed. The Safety of Diagnostic Ultrasound. London: Br J Radiology, suppl 20, 1987.
14. Nyborg WL. Biological effects of ultrasound: development of safety guidelines. Part II: General review. Ultrasound Med Biol 2001; 27:301.
15. Wells PNT. The prudent use of diagnostic ultrasound. Br J Radiol 1986; 59:1143.
16. Duck FA, Martin K. Trends in diagnostic ultrasound exposure. Phys Med Biol 1991; 16:1423.
17. World Federation for Ultrasound in Medicine and Biology. Statements on thermal effects and clinical applications. Ultrasound Med Biol 1992; 18:731.
18. American Institute of Ultrasound in Medicine/National Electronics Manufacturers' Association. Standard for the Display of Thermal and Acoustic Output Indices on Diagnostic Ultrasound Equipment. Rockville: American Institute of Ultrasound in Medicine, 1992.
19. Barnett SB, ter Haar GR, Ziskin MC, Rott H-D, Duck FA, Maeda K. International recommendations and guidelines for the safe use of diagnostic ultrasound in medicine. Ultrasound Med Biol 2000; 26:355.

BIBLIOGRAPHY

Burns PN. Contrast agents for Doppler ultrasound. In: Taylor KJW, Burns PN, Wells PNT, eds. Clinical Applications of Doppler Ultrasound. 2nd ed. New York: Raven Press, 1995:367.

Duck FA, Baker AC, Starritt HC. Ultrasound in Medicine. Bristol: Institute of Physics, 1998.

Evans DH, McDicken WN. Doppler Ultrasound: Physics, Instrumentation and Clinical Applications. 2nd ed. Chichester: Wiley, 2000.

Fish P. Physics and Instrumentation of Diagnostic Medical Ultrasound. Chichester: Wiley, 1990.

Hedrick W, Hykes D, Starchman D. Ultrasound Physics and Instrumentation. 4th ed. St Louis: Mosby, 2005.

Hill CR ed. Physical Principles of Medical Ultrasonics. Chichester: Ellis Horwood, 1986.

Hoskins P, Thrush A, Martin K, Whittingham A, eds. Diagnostic Ultrasound. Cambridge: Cambridge University Press, 2002.

Kremkau FW. Doppler Ultrasound. Principles and Instruments. Philadelphia: Saunders, 1990.

McDicken WN. Diagnostic Ultrasonics: Principles and Use of Instruments. 3rd ed. Edinburgh: Churchill Livingstone, 1991.

Wells PNT. Biomedical Ultrasonics. London: Academic Press, 1977.

Wells PNT ed. Advances in Ultrasound Techniques and Instrumentation. New York: Churchill Livingstone, 1993.

Williams AR. Ultrasound: Biological Effects and Potential Hazards. London: Academic Press, 1983.

Ziskin MC, Lewin PA, eds. Ultrasonic Exposimetry. Baco Raton: CRC Press, 1993.

Artifacts

W. K. Chooi, Valdair Muglia, and Peter L. Cooperberg

2

INTRODUCTION

Despite the significant technological advances in diagnostic ultrasound equipment, artifacts still represent a challenge for the radiologist and the sonographer. Artifacts are echoes that appear on the image and do not correspond in location or intensity to actual interfaces in the patient. Some artifacts are undesired and interfere with interpretation. Others help to identify certain structures. It is important to appreciate that artifacts are inherent to the diagnostic method and can occur despite appropriate technique and machine settings. Both education and experience can alert the operator to the possibility of these artifacts and result in their appropriate identification (1–3).

All methods of radiological imaging are associated with artifacts. Nonetheless, artifacts are particularly common and can be particularly troublesome in ultrasonography. In most cases, the artifacts can be recognized for what they are but occasionally an artifact can lead to a missed diagnosis or obscure a real abnormality.

The physical basis of ultrasound is the key to understanding artifacts. Artifacts obey the same physical principles as ultrasonography and are difficult to eliminate completely despite new technological advances. Therefore, it is important to recognize them, appreciate their significance, and thus avoid potentially important diagnostic errors.

BASIC ASSUMPTION

Despite the greatly increased sophistication of state-of-the-art ultrasound equipment, the production of an image still relies on basic principles (Fig. 1) (see Chapter 1 for a more detailed discussion).

1. A pulse of sound travels from the transducer in a straight line to an interface in the body, and the reflected echo returns in the reverse direction back to the transducer.
2. The time taken for this round trip, *time of flight*, is used to calculate the depth of the interface as a simple equation: $D = V \times T$, where V, the speed of sound in biologic tissue, is assumed to be constant, the same in all tissues, and is set at 1540 m/sec.
3. All of the returning echoes are presumed to arise from the center of the sound beam and are, therefore, displayed along the central vector representing the beam.
4. The intensity of the displayed echo relates to the acoustic properties and the size of the interface modified only by the time gain compensation (TGC).

The machine cannot differentiate deviations from these assumptions and displays an echo that may not correspond to the position or intensity of the original interface. For example, if the beam is reflected by an interface to another outside the plane of section, the returning echo will be displayed as if it were indeed directly under the transducer. The distance is determined by the actual time of flight of the sound pulse.

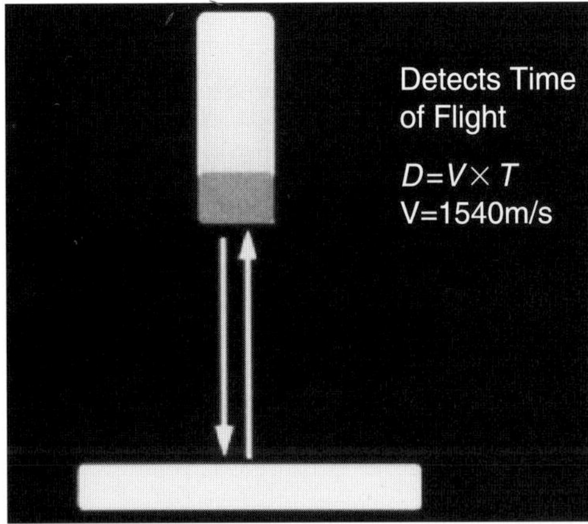

FIGURE 1 ■ Basic principle of linear propagation and reflection of ultrasound. The assumption is that all returning echoes come from interfaces in the direction that the sound beam was pointing and at a distance corresponding to the time of flight between the transducer and the interface.

REVERBERATION ARTIFACTS

In reverberation artifacts, the sound bounces back and forth between two interfaces. This prolongs the time of flight, producing an artifact deep to the interface. In this situation, some of the sound returning to the transducer is reflected back into the patient. That pulse strikes the same interface in the patient and is reflected back to the transducer a second time. The first reverberation artifact is, therefore, twice as far from the skin surface as the original interface was from the transducer (Fig. 2). This phenomenon often occurs when the sound beam is perpendicular to a strong reflector, such as a soft tissue–air interface or the abdominal wall deep to a considerable depth of subcutaneous adipose tissue. Depending on the intensity of the reflection of the interface and the degree of echogenicity of the tissue deep to the interface, a second and even a third reverberation artifact can occur. All of these will be equally spaced reflecting the distance from the transducer to the actual interface.

Generally, the reverberation artifacts caused by the abdominal wall do not cause confusion. If there is a fluid collection deep to the abdominal wall, such as the bladder, there should be no difficulty appreciating the artifactual nature of the echoes. There can be real echoes from sludge in the dependent portion of fluid collections. Echoes in the superficial (nondependent) aspect of the bladder are easily appreciated as artifacts. On the other hand, reverberation artifacts can be superimposed over the superficial portion of the liver. This gives the appearance of increased echogenicity. Although the TGC may be manipulated to balance the echogenicity in the near and the far portions of the liver, the near echo may not represent true interfaces in the liver. When watching during real-time scanning, the true echoes can be seen to move with respiration, whereas the artifactual echoes appear like a haze through which the liver is being viewed. These artifacts, however, can easily obscure superficial metastases and superficial cysts (Fig. 3).

The superimposition of this reverberation artifact on certain structures can cause diagnostic difficulty. For example, a first reverberation artifact could be superimposed over the lateral aspect of the kidney to simulate a subcapsular hematoma (Fig. 4). Once again, watching the kidney move during real-time scanning and moving

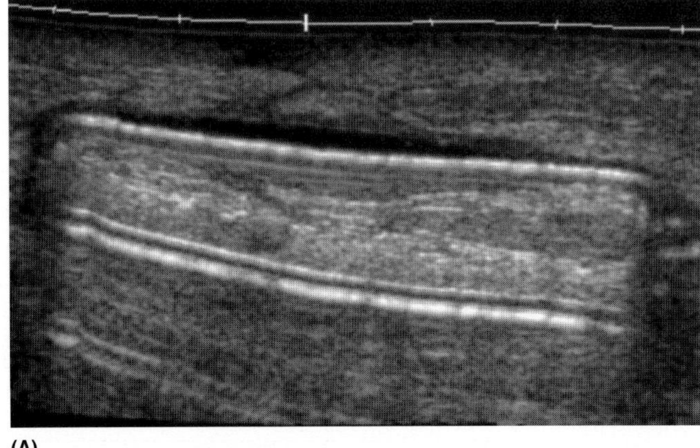

(A)

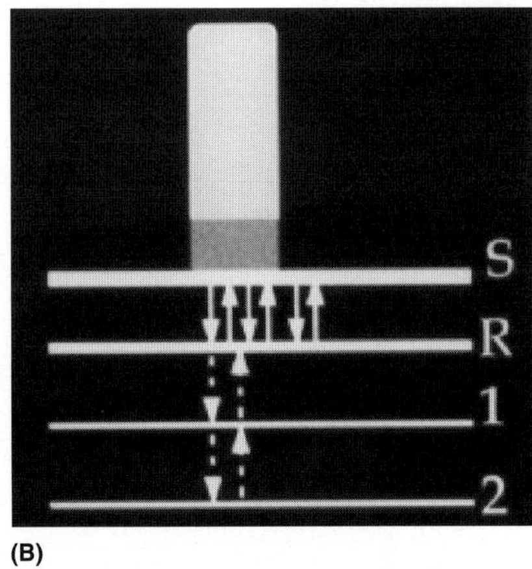

(B)

FIGURE 2 A AND B ■ Reverberation artifact. (A) This patient has a pacemaker in the chest wall. Note the multiple reverberations coming from the metallic interface approximately 13 mm deep to the transducer–skin interface. Multiple reverberation artifacts were caused by the sound bouncing back and forth between the transducer and the real interface. Note that the distance to the interface is greater to the right of the image. This increased distance is magnified with successive reverberation artifacts. (B) Diagram explaining the reverberation artifact. Note that the sound may bounce back and forth between the transducer/scan (S) and the real interface (R). As it returns the second time, the first reverberation artifact (1) is displayed in equal distance deep to the real interface. A second reverberation artifact (2) may occur twice as deep as the original interface.

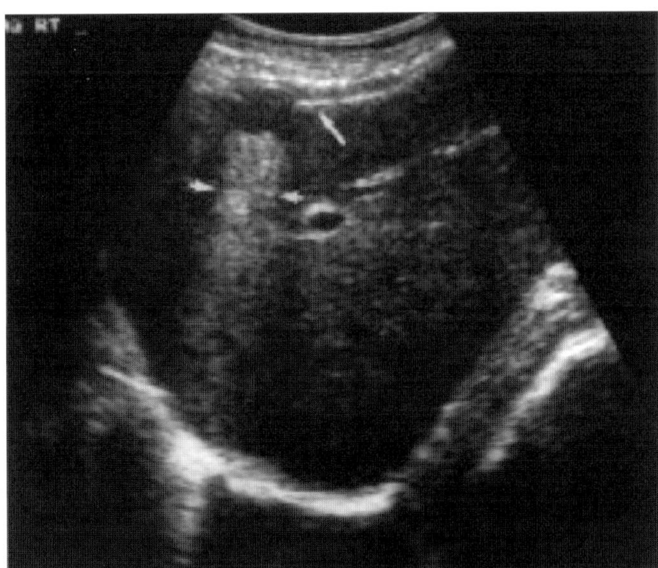

FIGURE 3 ■ Reverberation artifact. The diffuse reverberating artifacts from the abdominal wall almost completely obscure the superficial cyst. The cyst is detected by the enhanced through transmission and the deformity of the liver surface. A metastasis in the location would be missed completely.

the plane of section of the transducer should help clarify the issue. The hard copy image, however, can be confusing.

Ultrasound experts usually have had the experience of being mistaken, or at least perplexed, by an artifactual fluid collection simulating a real pelvic cyst or abscess (Fig. 5). In this case, the combination of two artifacts simulates the fluid collection. The reverberation is generally caused by air within the rectum or other loop of bowel. The air not only reflects the sound back to cause the reverberation artifact, but also causes distal acoustic shadowing, resulting in an echo-free shadow. The reverberation artifact is then superimposed on the echo-free shadow to simulate the deep wall of the fluid collection. In this situation, the first step is to consider the possibility that the fluid collection in the pelvis could be an artifact. Attempting different angulations of the plane of section from different windows on the abdominal wall may be helpful. Partially emptying the bladder can show that the artifactual fluid collection also decreases in size. This is because the difference from the transducer to the air interface deep to the bladder decreases, the distance from the air interface to the artifactual wall also decreases. It is important not to empty the bladder completely lest gas-filled bowel interposes, hiding a real fluid collection. A mirror image artifact (see the section entitled Mirror Image Artifacts) can cause a similar appearance, so that the depth of the deep wall of the cyst may not be the same as the distance from the transducer to the bowel air.

Tissue harmonic imaging (THI), now widely available, is a useful technique for removing reverberation artifacts. Tissue harmonics are sound waves formed within the body by interaction of the fundamental pulse with tissue. The image is then formed by these low

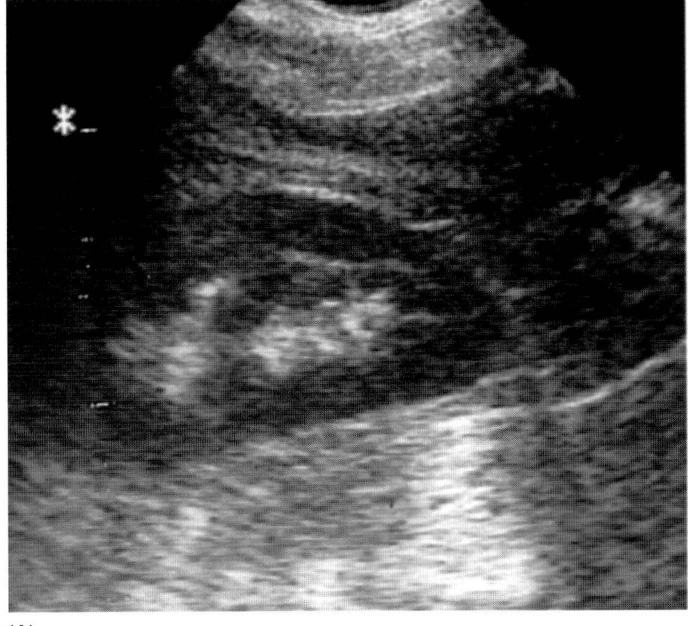

(A)

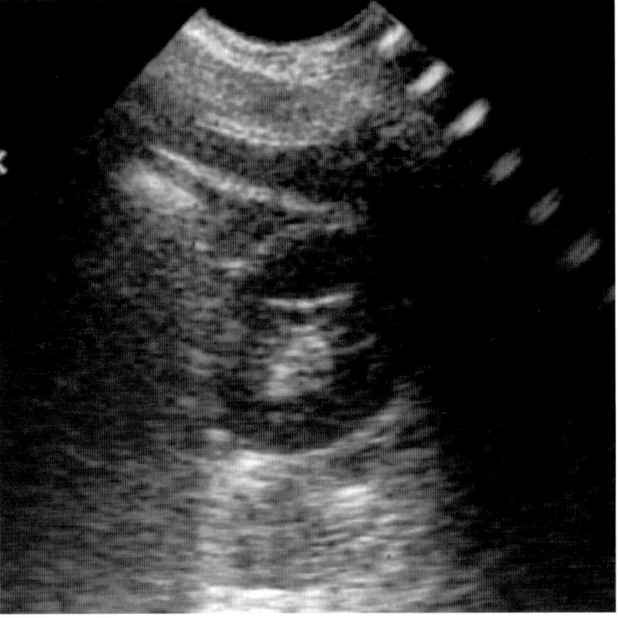

(B)

FIGURE 4 A AND B ■ (A) Longitudinal and (B) transverse images showing reverberation artifact simulating a subcapsular hematoma of the kidney. Note that the slightly curved echo imitating the interface between the subcapsular hematoma and the renal parenchyma is caused by the slightly less curved line halfway back to the transducer representing an interface between that and abdominal wall musculature. Note that the artifact crosses the echo of the renal capsule indicating that it cannot be a true finding and must be an artifact.

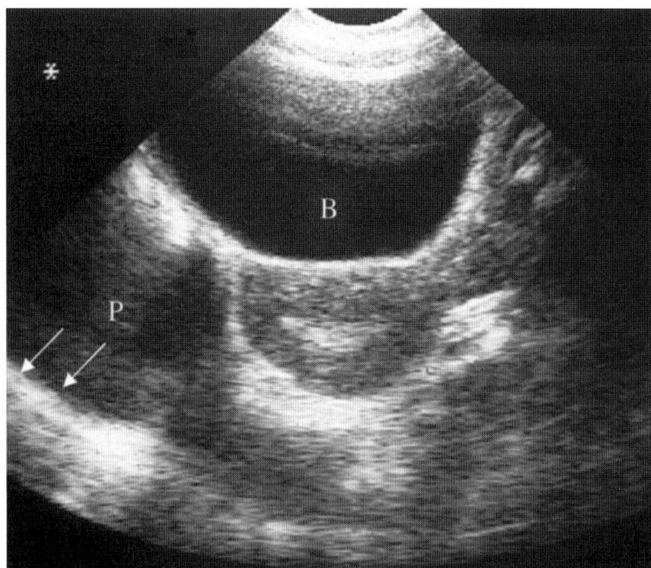

FIGURE 5 ■ Reverberation artifact simulating a pelvic fluid collection. Air in the rectum to the left of the uterus is causing the shadow. Deep to the shadow there is a collection of echoes (*arrows*) that is the first reverberation artifact from the gas/bowel interface. This is a very common artifact. P, pseudofluid; B, bladder.

amplitude, high frequency sound waves while the fundamental frequency is suppressed by various means (e.g., pulse inversion, pulse encoding) (4). Thus, the conditions for reverberations are largely removed and the amplitude of other artifactual sound waves is so low as to be negligible. Tissue harmonics are useful for producing a cleaner image and are particularly effective at clearing cysts (Fig. 6).

MIRROR IMAGE ARTIFACTS

The mirror image artifact is similar to the reverberation artifact. In a reverberation artifact, the sound pulse is reflected back into the body from the transducer–skin interface. In the mirror image artifact, the extra reflection comes from within the body itself. Furthermore, although the extra reflection may be within the line of the sound beam, more commonly, the sound is reflected off at an angle to another interface so that like a real mirror, the artifact shows up as the virtual object. An example of this is the situation where there is a hemangioma in the liver that appears to be a lesion within the lung above the diaphragm (Fig. 7). The sound is reflected off the diaphragm back into the liver. The angle of reflection is equal to the angle of incidence, and the sound pulse then hits the interfaces within the hemangioma to be reflected back to the diaphragm once again with an angle of reflection equal to the angle of incidence and then back to the transducer. The machine "straightens" out the path of the returning echo assuming that the interfaces were coming from the direction the transducer was pointing and at a distance corresponding to the actual time of flight.

As mentioned earlier, the mirror image artifact may also simulate a pelvic fluid collection similar to the reverberation artifact (Fig. 8). The sound may be reflected off the rectal air at an angle so that the deep wall of the artifactual cyst represents the mirror image of the inferior and anterior walls of the bladder. In this case, it is not helpful to measure the distances from the transducer. Especially in the transverse image, only a short segment of the bladder is traversed and yet the "fluid collection" may seem very large (Fig. 8B). That is because the sound is reflected out of the plane of section to hit the inferior wall of the bladder.

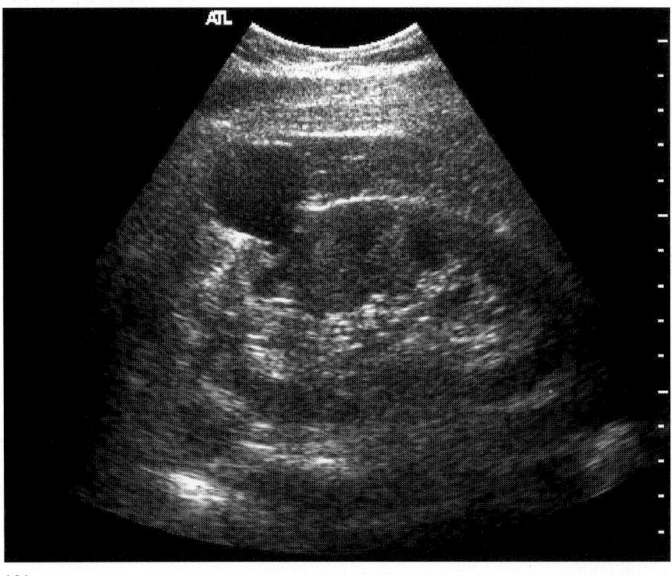

(A)

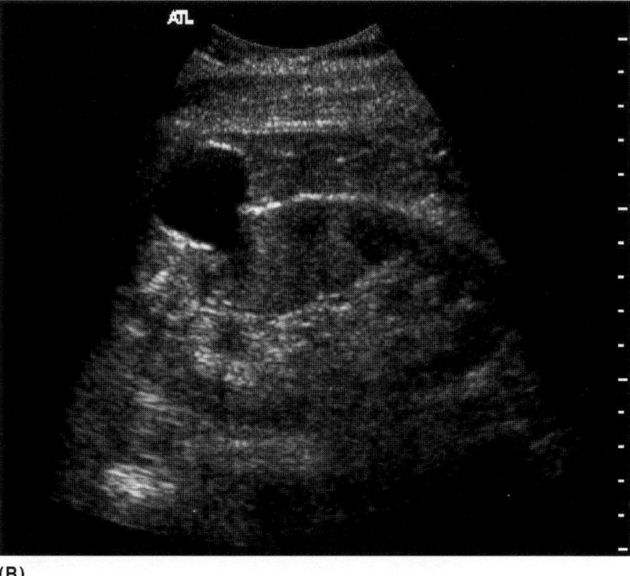

(B)

FIGURE 6 A AND B ■ (**A**) Tissue harmonic imaging. The initial image showed a probable cyst on the right kidney but internal echoes were evident. (**B**) Application of tissue harmonic imaging "cleaned-up" the image, removing the internal echoes and demonstrating a simple renal cyst.

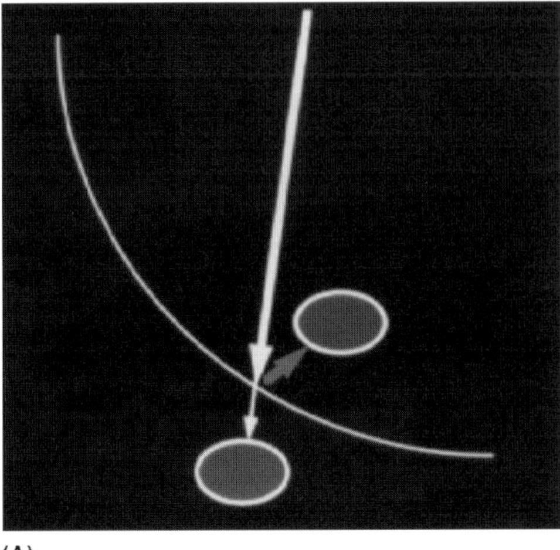

(A)

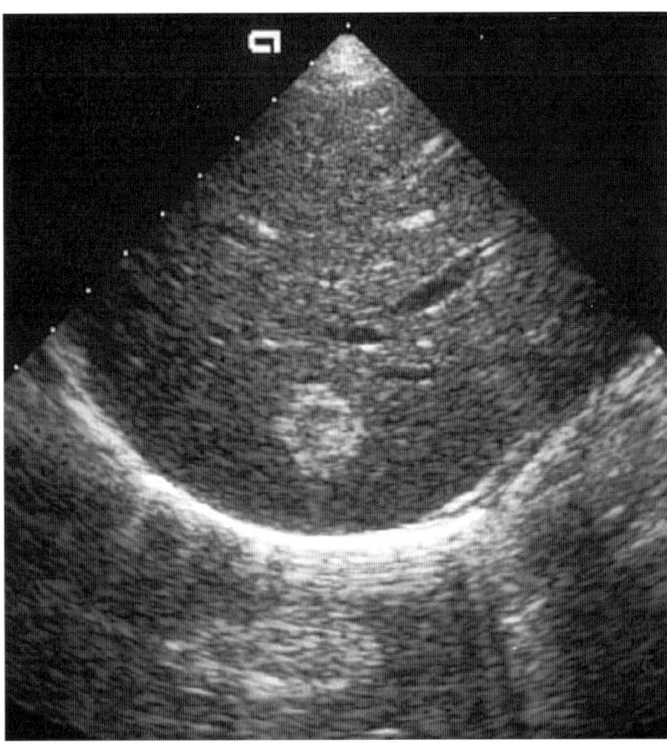

(B)

FIGURE 7 A AND B ■ (**A**) Diagram of a mirror image artifact. Note the main sound beam (*long arrow*) reflecting off the diaphragm (*short arrow*) at an angle of reflection equal to the angle of incidence back to the hemangioma within the liver. The machine does not know that the sound beam was deflected and displays the image of the lesion as though it were in the base of the lung. (**B**) Ultrasound image showing the mirror artifact.

Mirror image artifacts can cause other strange appearances such as invasion of a transitional cell carcinoma through the bladder wall (Fig. 9). A mirror image artifact of a hepatic cyst can simulate an empyema or lung abscess (Fig. 10).

RING-DOWN ARTIFACTS

The ring-down artifact, also known as the comet tail artifact, appears as a line in the direction of the sound beam and deep to a strong reflector (5–7). The cause can be a

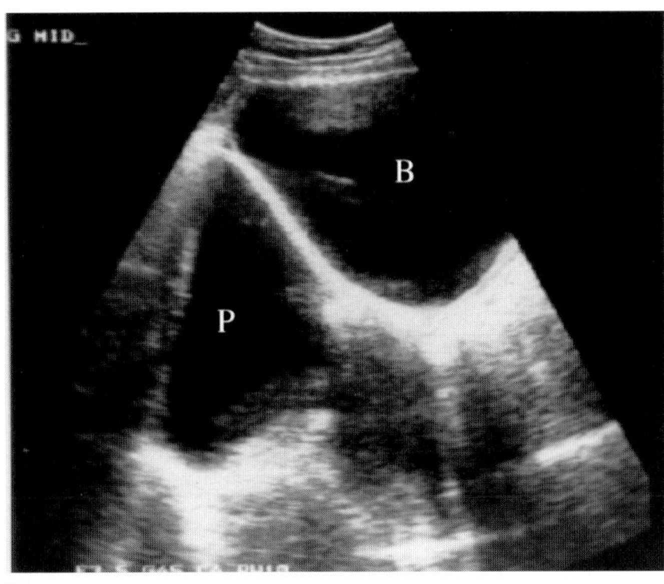

(A)

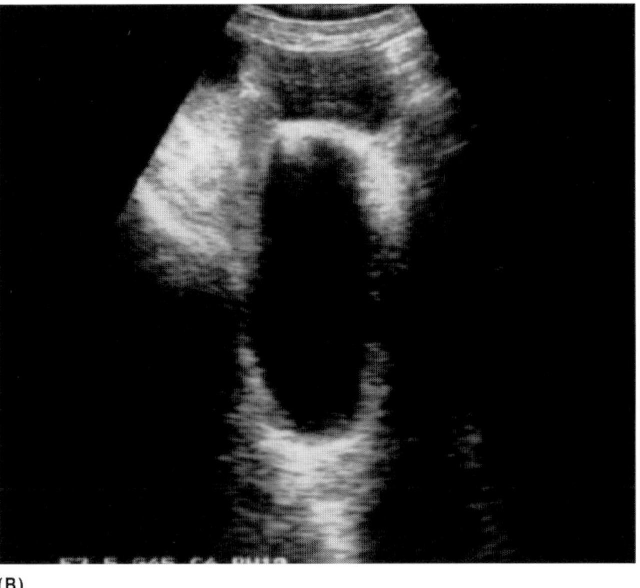

(B)

FIGURE 8 A AND B ■ (**A**) Longitudinal and (**B**) transverse scans showing a mirror image artifact. This appearance of pseudofluid collection is similar to the reverberation artifact shown in Figure 5. In this case, however, the distance between the rectal air interface and the artifact is significantly greater than the distance from the transducer to the interface, especially on the transverse image. In the longitudinal image, the artifactual echo appears as a mirror image of the anterioinferior wall of the bladder. P, pseudofluid collection; B, bladder.

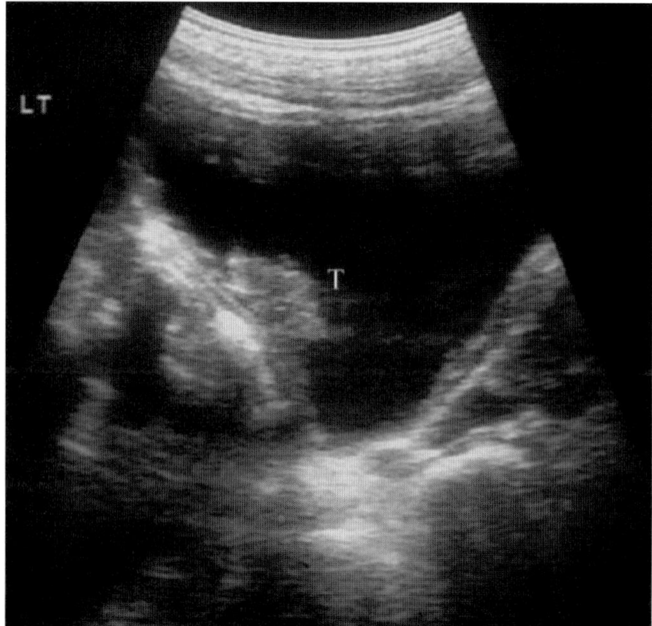

FIGURE 9 ■ Mirror image transitional cell carcinoma of the bladder simulating spread through the bladder wall. The rectal air interface behind the bladder serves as the mirror. This could be misinterpreted as spread of tumor through the bladder wall. T, transitional cell carcinoma.

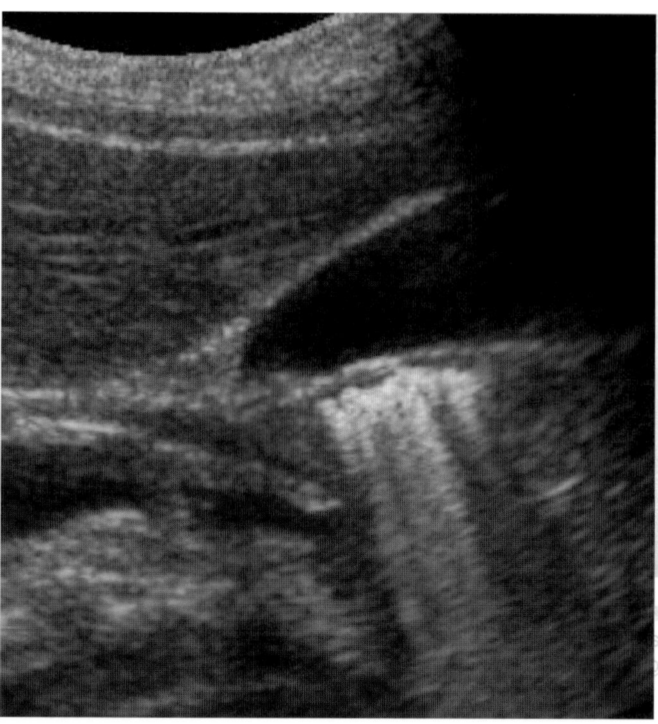

FIGURE 11 ■ Ring-down artifact. Note the closely spaced, short perpendicular artifacts simulating a vertical line along a vector deep to bubbles in the duodenal cap. The explanation for why this occurs in some situations and not others is the "bubble tetrahedron" theory, explained in the text.

piece of metal in the body such as a surgical clip or lead shot. More commonly, the ring-down artifact is seen deep to a collection of gas (Fig. 11). In fact, the artifact is not an echogenic line, but rather a collection of closely spaced perpendicular echoes along one or two vectors in the ultrasound image. Originally, these were thought to be sound entering the metal or gas bubble and reverberating back and forth within the structure, each time sending some of the sound back to the transducer. This explanation would account for a series of closely spaced echoes equal to the depth of the piece of metal or gas bubble. However, a more plausible explanation is equivalent to the ringing of a bell. The sound pulse "insonates" the metal causing it to ring. Interestingly, the artifact does not occur deep to calcification or calculi.

With gas bubbles, there is a slightly different explanation. Not all collections of gas produce ring-down artifacts, but the ring-down artifact can be characteristic of certain configurations of gas bubbles. It has been shown (8) that the "bugle" of fluid trapped between four small bubbles (the bubble tetrahedron) is the source of the artifact. The sound pulse insonates the "bugle" and causes it to vibrate and send a prolonged sound wave back to the transducer. The presence of ring-down artifact in an unusual place may help diagnose pneumobilia or pneumoperitoneum, and its absence when scanning the thorax can be a clue to pneumothorax (Figs. 12 and 13) (9–11).

A variant of this artifact occurs deep to cholesterol crystals, usually in the wall of the gallbladder. This has been referred to as the "V-shaped artifact" (Fig.14) (12). The characteristic appearance of these artifacts is as only two or three "rings" and the more distal ones always smaller than the proximal ones. It is thought that the plate-like cholesterol crystals must be oriented perpendicular to the beam to cause the ringing (13).

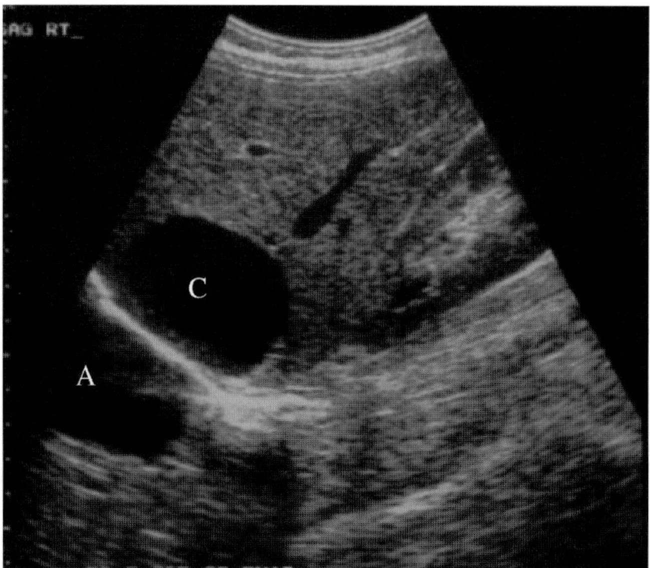

FIGURE 10 ■ Mirror image of the liver cyst. Note that the deep echoes of the artifactual cyst (A) represent the anterior wall of the liver cyst (C). Note also that the echoes deep to the artifactual cysts represent mirror image artifacts of actual liver echoes. If the cysts were not there, the "noises" that are normally seen above the diaphragm are actually mirror image artifacts of normal liver cell interfaces.

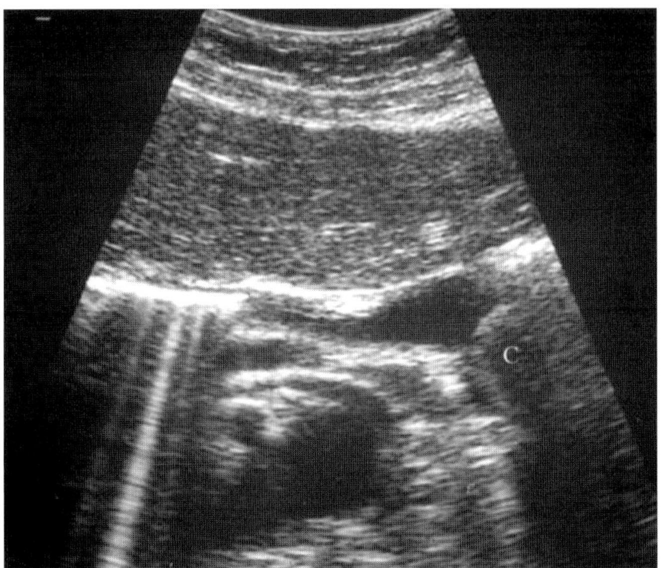

FIGURE 12 ■ Pneumobilia causing ring-down. When echogenic foci are noted in the bile ducts, the presence of ring-down is helpful to distinguish pneumobilia from calculi (C).

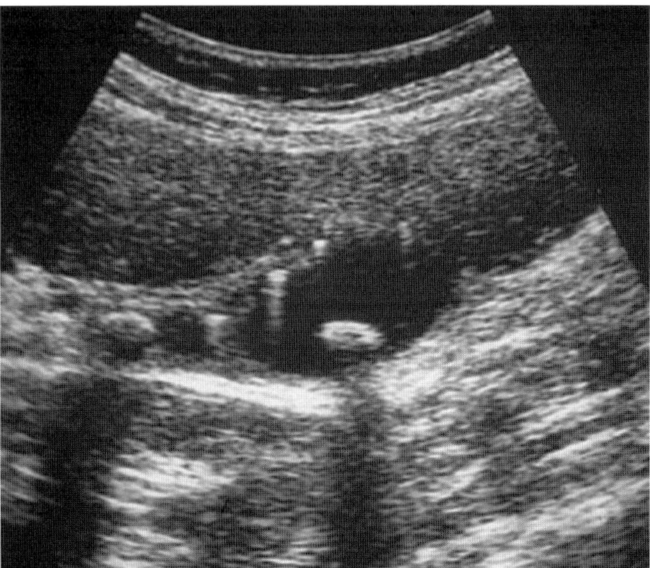

FIGURE 14 ■ A shorter, V-shaped ring-down can occur deep to cholesterol crystals. When this is seen in association with a thickened gallbladder wall, it is indicative of adenomyomatosis. Also note the presence of a gallstone.

REFRACTION ARTIFACTS

Refraction is the bending of the sound beam at an oblique interface between tissues of different acoustic velocity. One type of refractive artifact has the appearance of a refractive shadow caused by defocusing of the sound beam at the edge of a cyst. Another type involves displacement of the distal structure by a more proximal refraction of the beam.

In a duplication artifact, the sound beam is refracted by a more proximal interface. For example, the image of the superior mesenteric artery (SMA) may be duplicated when the transducer is held in transverse plane of section over the midline. When the beam is pointing toward the right, the sound could be refracted back toward the midline by the oblique interface between the posterior aspect of the rectus muscle and the triangular fat pad behind it. This causes the SMA to be shifted toward the right. Also, when the sound beam is directed toward the left, it is also refracted back toward the midline and, therefore, displays another image of the SMA toward the left (Fig. 15). If the transducer is moved to one side or the other, the artifactual duplication can be eliminated. This type of duplication artifact could also occur in the pelvis causing a single early gestational sac to appear as twins. A copper 7 intrauterine device (IUD) in the uterus can also appear duplicated. We, therefore, call this the "copper-14" artifact (Fig. 15D) (14–16).

Refraction can also displace the position of the echo of a deeper interface such as the diaphragm deep to a small cyst in the liver. Since the sound travels more slowly in fluid than in the liver parenchyma, a large cyst can delay the passage of sound causing the diaphragm to appear further away than it is (17). A small cyst, however, can cause a peculiar effect on the echo of the diaphragm. At the superior aspect of the cyst, the sound beam is refracted inferiorly where the diaphragm is actually further way. From the inferior aspect of the cyst, the sound beam is refracted superiorly where the diaphragm is closer. Therefore, the segment of the diaphragm can appear rotated due to refraction (18).

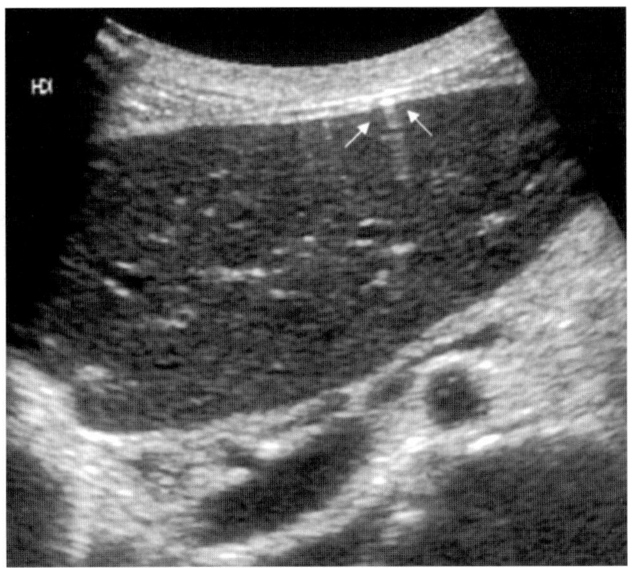

FIGURE 13 ■ Pneumoperitoneum with ring-down superficial to the liver (*arrows*). While sonography is not the ideal modality to diagnose pneumoperitoneum, the presence of this artifact in an unusual place can enable one to make this important diagnosis.

SHADOWING AND ENHANCEMENT

The intensity of an echo is determined not only by the strength of the reflection but also by the acoustic characteristics of the tissue between the transducer and the

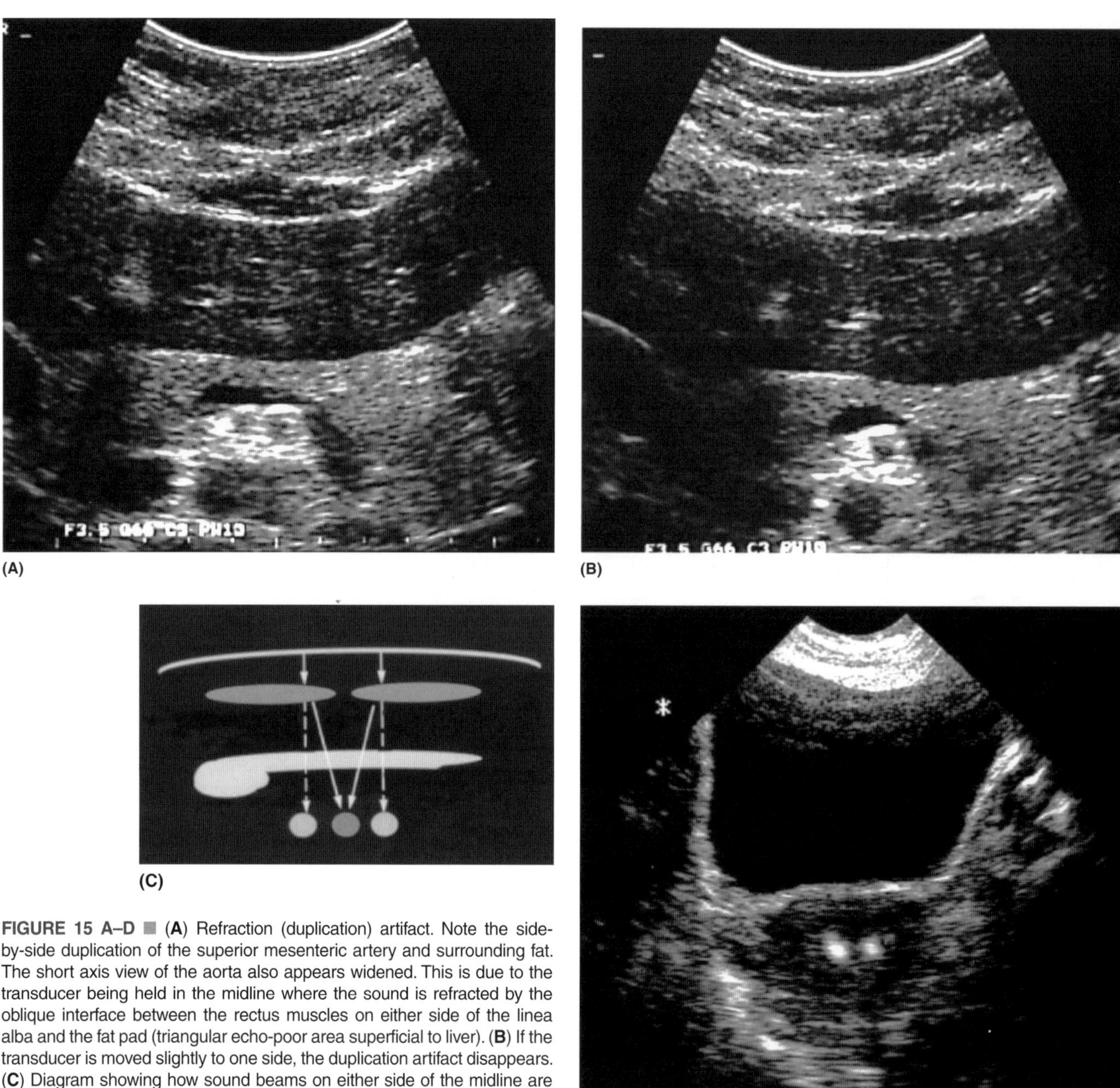

(A) (B) (C) (D)

FIGURE 15 A–D ■ (**A**) Refraction (duplication) artifact. Note the side-by-side duplication of the superior mesenteric artery and surrounding fat. The short axis view of the aorta also appears widened. This is due to the transducer being held in the midline where the sound is refracted by the oblique interface between the rectus muscles on either side of the linea alba and the fat pad (triangular echo-poor area superficial to liver). (**B**) If the transducer is moved slightly to one side, the duplication artifact disappears. (**C**) Diagram showing how sound beams on either side of the midline are refracted back to where the superior mesenteric artery actually is, but artifactually displays them separately. (**D**) The same phenomenon causing side-by-side duplication of a copper 7 IUD—hence the "copper 14 artifact."

interface. The sound travels through the intervening tissue on the way down to the interface and the returning echo must also traverse the same tissue. The intervening tissue may attenuate or appear to enhance the intensity of the returning echo.

Enhancement Through Transmission

An increase in the amplitude of the echoes deep to a structure is called "enhanced through transmission" (19,20). This is a characteristic of cysts but is actually a misnomer. The fluid only attenuates the sound less than the surrounding tissue. The cystic fluid causes almost no attenuation of the sound. Adjacent to the cyst, the liver parenchyma, for example, does cause some attenuation. This is compensated by the TGC, making the liver echoes uniform from superficial to deep. The TGC overcompensates through the cyst causing the deeper echoes to be brighter (Fig. 16). The great value of this artifact is that it greatly increases confidence in the diagnosis of a cyst.

Sometimes a cyst is too small for the enhancement to be explained only by the absence of attenuation. In fact, the small cyst can act as a lens, refocusing the sound beam (Fig. 17). This would correspond to using a magnifying glass to focus the sun's rays to burn a hole in a dead leaf. The refocusing of the sound beam also causes enhanced through transmission.

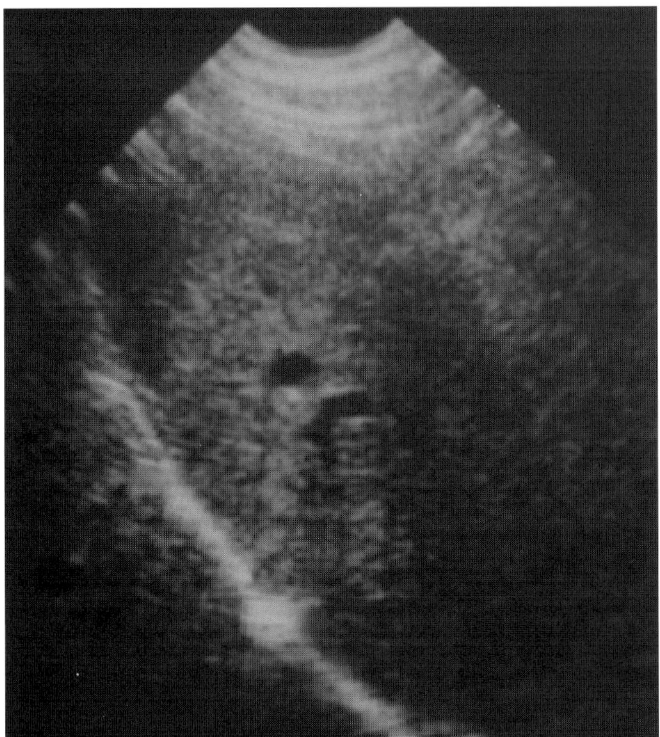

FIGURE 16 ■ Refractive artifact causing displacement. Although it is true that sound goes slower in cysts than in the liver and could account for the diaphragm being displaced deeper than it should be, the explanation in this case is different. The sound beam at the superior edge at the cyst is refracted inferiorly where the diaphragm is further away. The sound beam is refracted by the inferior aspect of the cyst superiorly where the diaphragm is closer. This gives the impression that a segment of the diaphragm has swiveled around so that its superior aspect is deeper and its inferior aspect is closer.

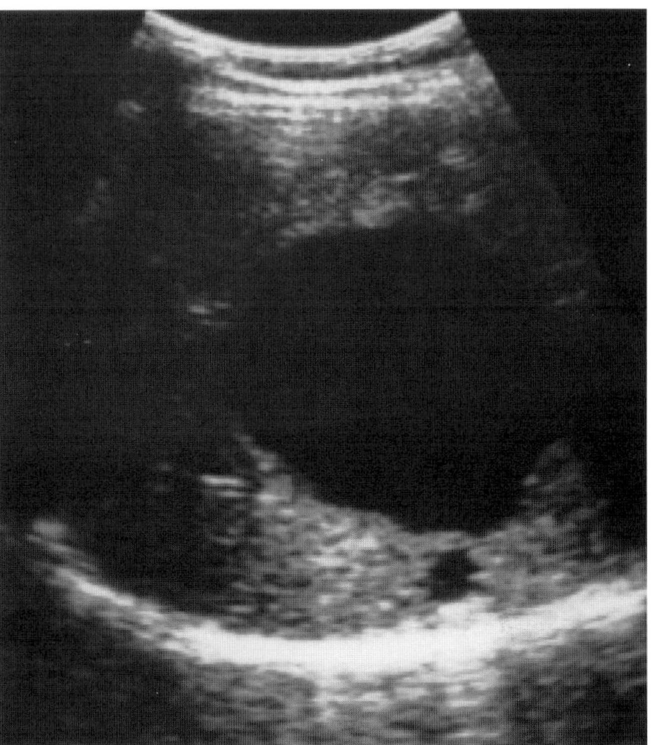

FIGURE 17 ■ Enhancement deep to hepatic cysts (large and small). Note the enhancement deep to the large cyst in the liver. The easy explanation is that the sound is not as attenuated by the fluid in the cyst as it is through the hepatic parenchyma on either side. However, note that there is increased enhancement deep to the smaller cyst than is deep to the large cyst. The explanation for this is refractive refocusing (like a lens) by the small cyst.

Acoustic Shadowing

When there is acoustic shadowing (e.g., deep to a gallstone), the sound pulse does not reach the deeper tissues to produce an echo (21). Complete shadowing does not cause confusion and can be helpful in confirming a gallstone or a renal stone. In fact, one should be wary of making the diagnosis of a calculus without its tell-tale shadow. There are situations in which a shadow may not be complete deep to a calculus. This is due to the difference between the width of the beam and the diameter of the calculus. If the calculus is smaller than the beam, an echo will be received from the calculus, but some of the sound will go around the stone and echoes will return from the deeper structures. There may be no shadow at all. It is important to use the appropriate transducer and to adjust the transmit focus to the depth of the stone to appreciate the shadow. Focusing plays an important role in the production of acoustic shadows (Fig. 18).

In clinical practice, it is important to differentiate shadows due to gas-filled structures from calcified objects. Hard or calcified structures, including bone, reflect about 30% of the sound and absorb the rest; thus the shadows are relatively "clean." Gas collections reflect about 99% of the sound energy, so diffuse reverberations can fill the shadow with noise making it relatively "dirty." For example, it is important to differentiate gas in the biliary tree (pneumobilia) from calculi. In addition to the different characteristics of the shadows, the gas bubbles tend to have caps from short off-axis artifacts, whereas gallstones have curved proximal surfaces.

It is more difficult to appreciate the artifactual nature of relative shadowing. For example, if the sound beam is attenuated but not completely blocked, an area of the liver may look echo poor and simulate a metastasis or focal sparing of fatty infiltration (Fig. 18D) (21).

Acoustic shadowing can also occur deep to oblique interfaces due to refraction (19,22,23). Refraction has already been discussed in terms of deflecting the whole of the sound beam to interfaces deep to the edge of a cyst. However, the edge of a cyst can also refract parts of the sound beam away from the other parts not traversing the edge of the cyst. The effect is defocusing. A defocused beam will have less intense sound, less intense returning echoes, and therefore a relative shadow (Fig. 19).

The refractive shadowing can also cause confusion if it is more diffuse and only relatively attenuating. This can occur frequently through the lower uterine segment due to the oblique interface of the superior aspect of the bladder (Fig. 20). In the liver, the fissure for the ligamentum venosum may contain some fat and the oblique interface can cause relative shadowing of the caudate lobe simulating a metastasis (23). Portions of the pancreas can appear

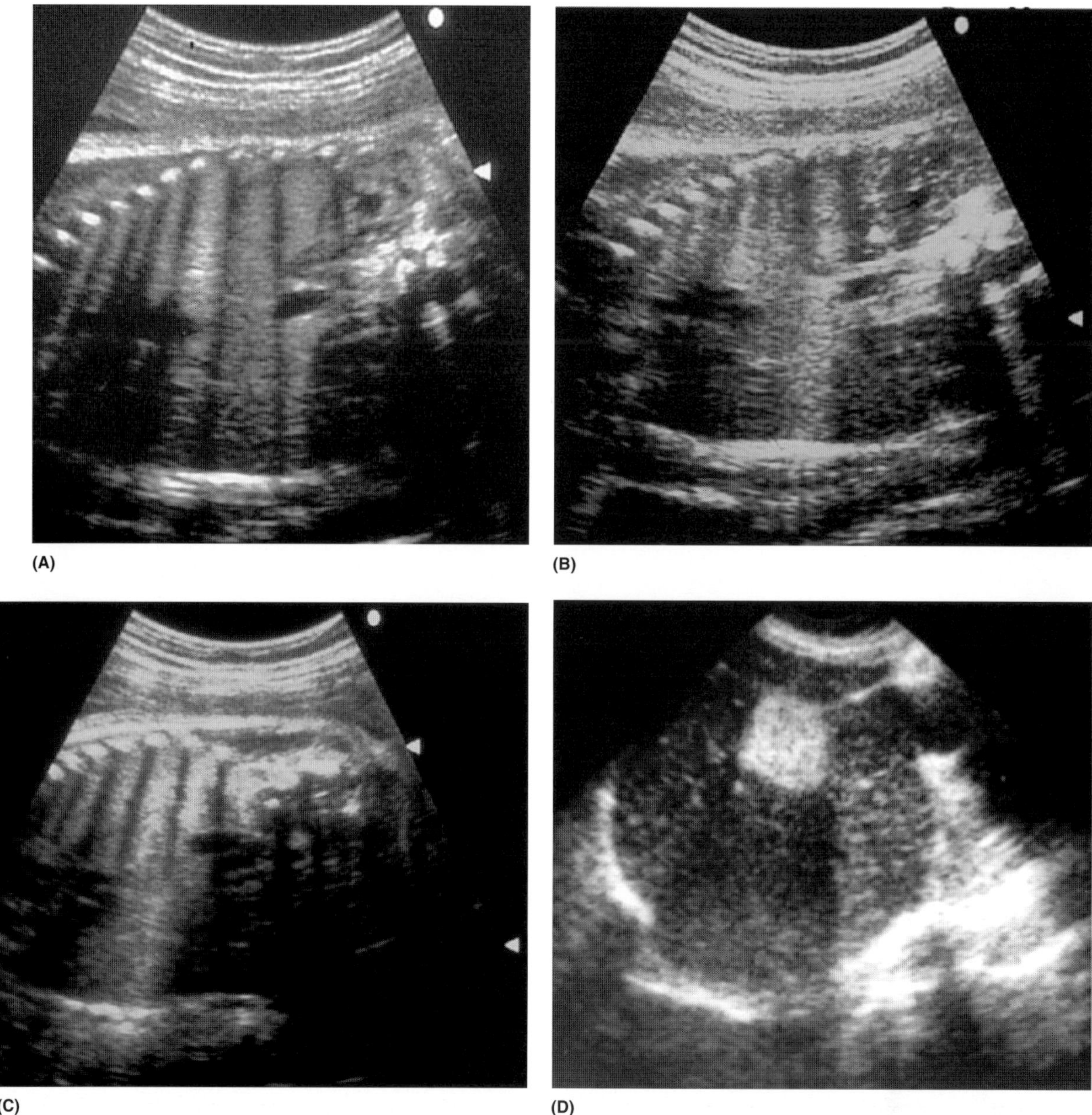

FIGURE 18 A–D ■ (**A**) Acoustic shadowing, the effect of focusing. Note that the transmit focal zone is at the level of the fetal ribs. Thus, the ribs block most of the sound and cause sharp acoustic shadows. (**B**) The transmit focal zone has been shifted deeper. The beam is wider as it traverses the ribs and the shadows are less distinct. (**C**) There are two focal zones. Note the sharp shadows in the upper focal zone and the complete lack of shadows in the lower focal zone with an abrupt change. This is due to separate pulses along the same vector for the first and second focal zones. (**D**) Hepatic lipoma causing relative shadowing by the increased absorption of the sound beam. The hepatic echoes deep to it are echo poor but not because any characteristic of the hepatic interfaces. Note also the posterior displacement of the diaphragm since the sound is slower through the fat than through the adjacent liver (Fig. 16).

echo poor due to interposed fat deep to the left lobe of the liver. A relatively uncommon, but interesting artifact is the "two-tone testis" caused by refraction of the testicular artery (Fig. 21) (24).

Compound real-time imaging is another recent development to improve image quality by suppressing image artifacts. The technique involves acquiring multiple frames from different viewing angles that are then combined to form a real-time compound image on the display (25). Scanning from different angles produces different artifact patterns. Averaging these independent frames diminishes the random artifacts and reinforces true echoes, producing a smoother image. Compound real-time imaging has a significant effect of reducing both acoustic shadowing and enhancement through transmission. This is best demonstrated in the case of a linear probe that is traditionally associated with acoustic shadowing which is perpendicular to the surface of the transducer. With real-time compound imaging the acoustic shadowing is diminished resulting in a "v" configuration.

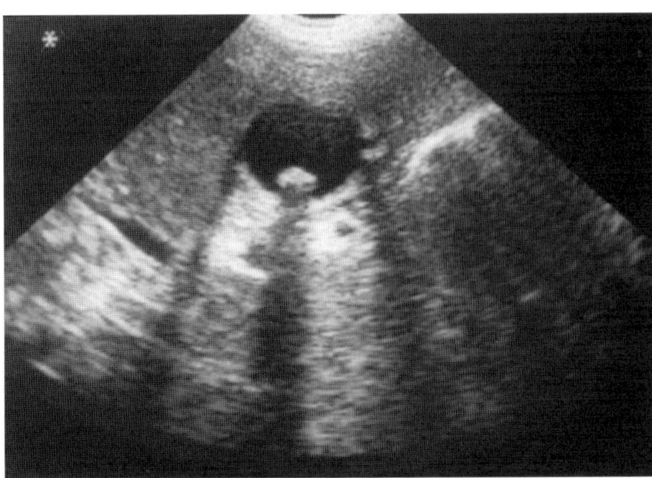

FIGURE 19 ■ Shadowing—reflective and refractive. Note the three shadows in this image. One comes from absorption and reflection of the sound by the gallstone. The other two are caused by the edge of the gallbladder due to a refractive defocusing of the sound beam on either side.

BEAM-WIDTH ARTIFACT

Low-level echoes may appear within cystic structures, mimicking sludge, pus, or debris; in these situations, it is called beam-width or slice thickness artifact (27). Beam-width artifact is a partial volume effect and is analogous to the artifact described for computed tomography (CT). Its occurrence can be diminished by using the correct transmit focal zone making the slice as thin as possible.

Although the sound beam is displayed on the image as a very narrow vector, the beam does have a finite width. It is at least several millimeters wide in the focal zone and even wider in the near and the far zones. The intensity is higher in the center of the beam, decreasing toward the periphery. The periphery of the sound beam can be reflected by adjacent structures. When the center of the beam is aimed beside a strong reflector, an off-axis echo can be displayed along the vector representing the center of the beam (26). Side-lobes of the main beam can cause echoes to appear from structures as much as 45° away from the central vector (Fig. 22). The same artifact can be detected when the plane of section is aimed away from the strong reflector. Then the cause of the artifact is less apparent. Side-lobe artifacts are much more prone to occur with phased array and curved linear array transducers. Fortunately, they are usually easily differentiated from real septations.

Side-lobe and grating-lobe artifacts can be diminished by using the same maneuvers described for beam-width artifacts, since they are also dependent on the incident angle and not on gravity. Furthermore, grating lobes can be avoided, when apodization is used in the transducer. In this process the lateral transducer elements have less energy than central elements. Another process, called spatial filtering, makes the echoes from the peripheral transducer elements less amplified, again making grating lobes less likely to occur. Dynamic focusing of the returning echo likewise tends to enhance echoes along the central axis and diminish the effects of off-axis interfaces.

Aside from the beam-width and side-lobes, a third artifact can induce the presence of low-level echoes in cystic structures. This is the range-ambiguity artifact (28,29).

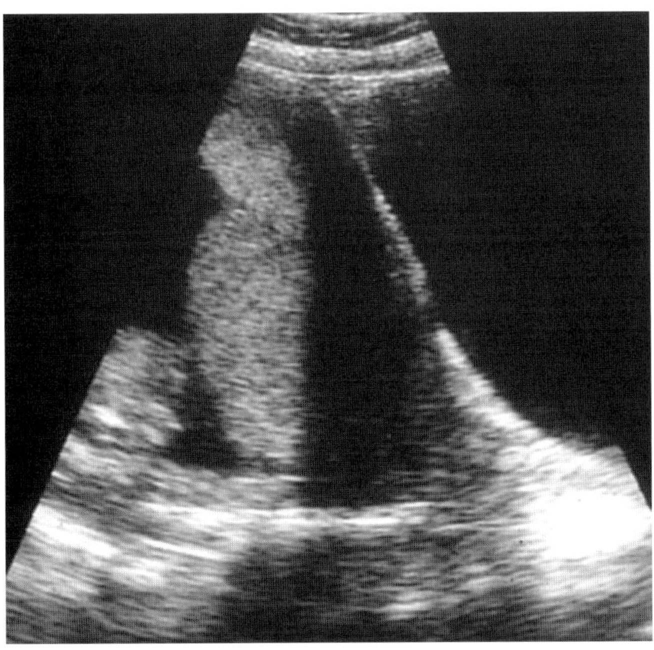

(A)

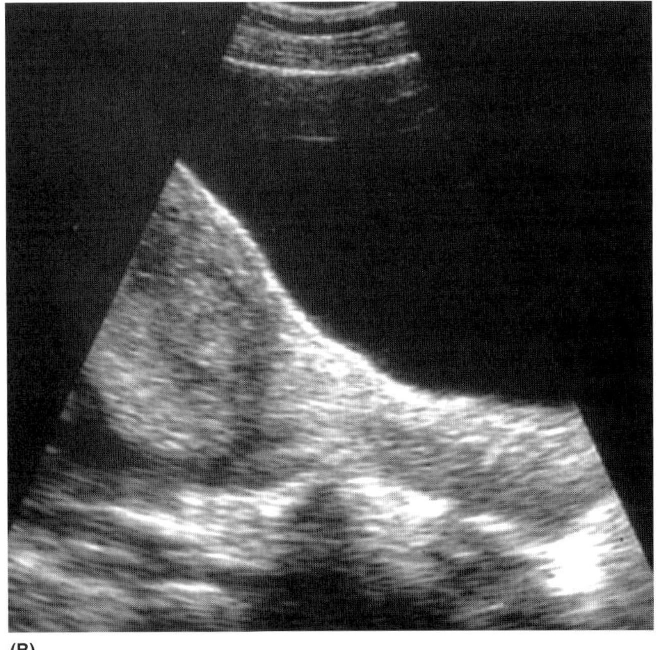

(B)

FIGURE 20 A AND B ■ (**A**) Longitudinal scan through the bladder and lower uterine segment. Note the broad refractive shadow caused by the oblique interface between the bladder and uterus. (**B**) Note when the bladder is full and the interface closer to perpendicular, the shadow is markedly diminished.

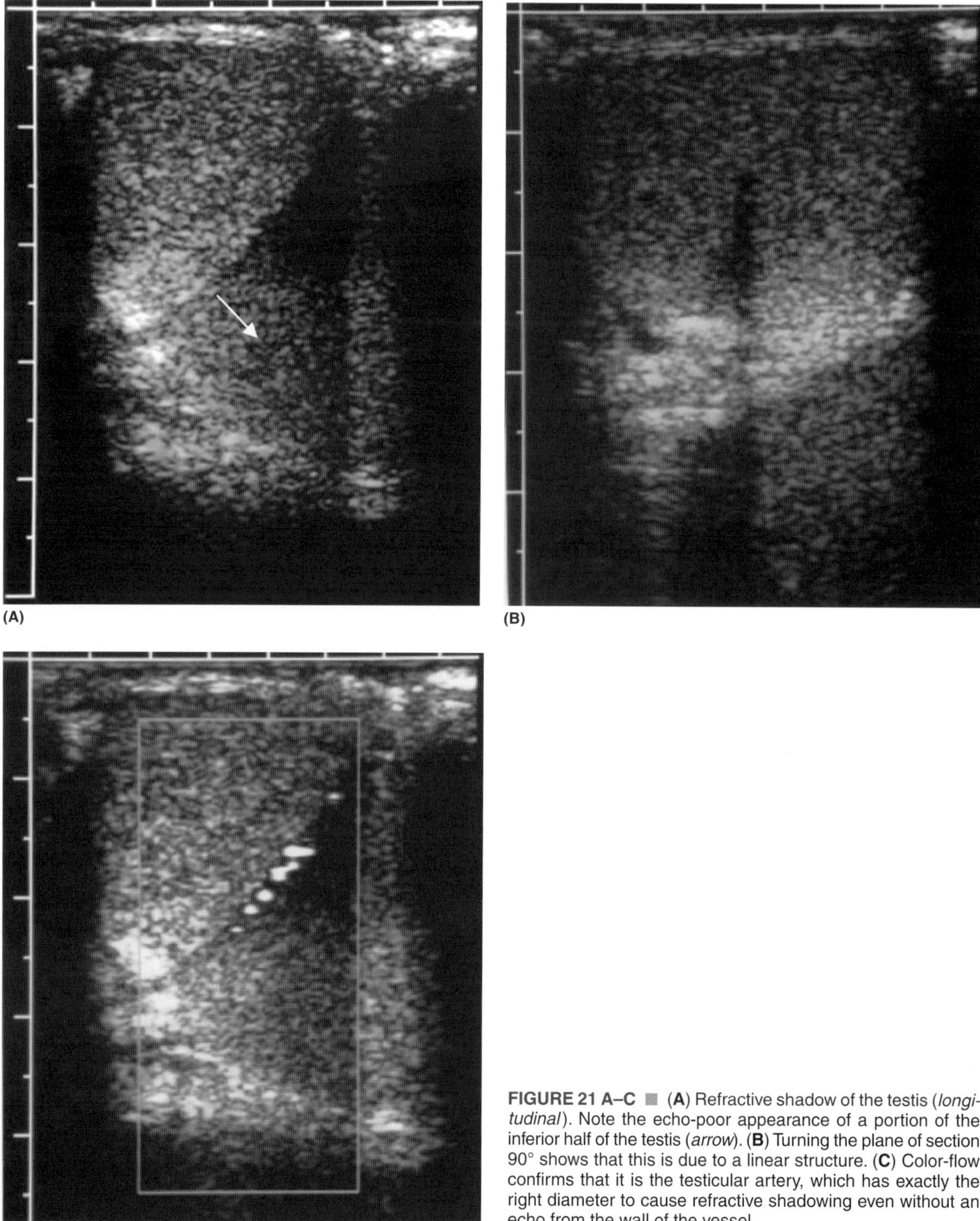

FIGURE 21 A–C ■ (**A**) Refractive shadow of the testis (*longitudinal*). Note the echo-poor appearance of a portion of the inferior half of the testis (*arrow*). (**B**) Turning the plane of section 90° shows that this is due to a linear structure. (**C**) Color-flow confirms that it is the testicular artery, which has exactly the right diameter to cause refractive shadowing even without an echo from the wall of the vessel.

These echoes are related to the use of fast frame rates and high pulse repetition frequency (PRF). If the depth setting is low, as for superficial structures, echoes from deeper interfaces may return to the transducer after the next pulse has been fired. This echo will be interpreted as an interface much closer to the transducer. Usually these are not noted because they are low intensity echoes that are lost in echogenic tissue. However, if there is a large cystic structure, for example, on an endovaginal scan, they can be misinterpreted as representing the far wall of the cyst. For objects situated deep in the body, or even for the dorsal skin, the time of the returning echoes can be very long, and they can reach the transducer just after a second pulse had been emitted. The machine interprets these echoes as originating in superficial structures. They can also be second reverberation echoes. They are only noted if they are superimposed over cystic structures (e.g., gall bladder, bladder, cysts).

(A)

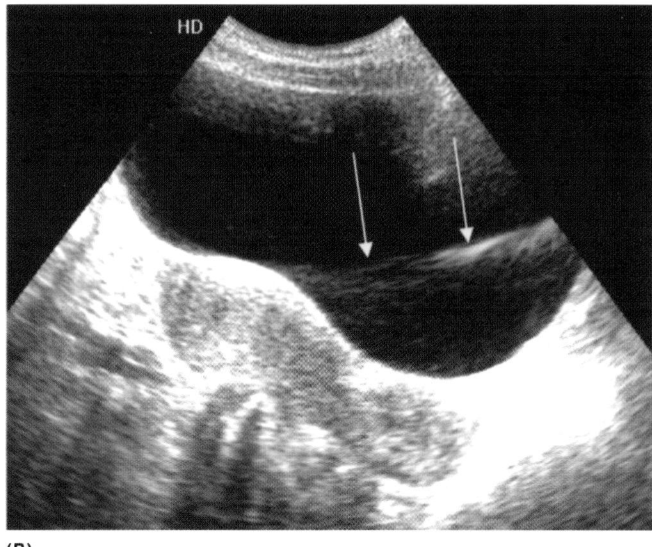

(B)

FIGURE 22 A AND B ■ Side-lobe artifact. (**A**) Note the curvilinear artifact projecting off the "promontory" of the uterus in both directions. Even when the central axis of the beam is pointing inferior or superior to the strong reflector, some of the off-axis or side-lobe sound energy is reflected back from the strong perpendicular interface. Nonetheless, it is still displayed along the central vector. (**B**) Another example of an extensive side-lobe artifact from a phased array transducer.

PROPAGATION SPEED ERRORS

As stated previously, ultrasound machines assume that the sound speed in all organic tissues is constant, about 1504 m/sec, but actually sound velocities in organic tissues are quite variable (27). When an area containing tissues with different velocities is scanned, incorrect depth assignments are seen distally to the tissue with lower velocity. Fat (21) and fluid-filled structures (18) are usually seen as the cause of this artifact. The most striking example is when a liver lesion with a velocity of less than 1540 m/sec is scanned. The echoes that travel through the lesion arrive back at the transducer after a relative delay, and are assigned a deeper position. This can simulate a "break" in the structure located posteriorly to the lesion, such as the diaphragm (Fig. 18D) or the kidney.

PULSED DOPPLER ARTIFACTS

Two main types of artifacts are seen on spectral tracings of pulsed Doppler. Both cause patterns to be seen on the other side of the baseline even though there is no flow in that direction (30).

The most important of these is aliasing. As discussed in the section on color-flow, aliasing always occurs when analog waveforms are digitized to determine their frequencies. The sine waves must be sampled at a frequency (the Nyquist limit) that should be at least twice the highest Doppler frequency. If the PRF is less than twice the Doppler frequency, the highest velocities will be displayed below the baseline. This usually does not cause diagnostic difficulty, since the lowest velocities above the Nyquist limit are furthest from the baseline. Velocities even higher are closer to the baseline. Aliasing is analogous to wagon wheels seeming to rotate backwards in early movies with slow frame rates. For a systolic peak above the Nyquist, the appearance is that of a truncated cone, with the apex below the baseline and pointing up.

Aliasing does not usually cause diagnostic difficulties. In fact the presence of aliasing alerts the sonographer to the likelihood of a poststenotic jet.

The other type of artifact seen on spectral tracings of pulsed Doppler images occurs when the sound beam is perpendicular to the direction of flow. The appearance is a symmetrical tracing on the other side of the baseline. This is because the beam is not narrow enough. The side-lobes will hit the flowing blood both upstream and downstream. Thus, the flow will be detected both toward and away from the transducer. The tracing will show symmetrical waveforms above and below the baseline.

COLOR DOPPLER ARTIFACTS

As much as artifacts can be a problem with gray-scale imaging, they can cause even more trouble with color-flow Doppler imaging. Color Doppler can show the presence of the flow, the direction of flow, and turbulent flow to help identify stenotic lesions (31). Power Doppler is more sensitive at detecting flow, particularly slow flow, but is unable to demonstrate direction or velocity of flow.

The color Doppler artifacts can be grouped into three types: (*i*) color appearing where there is no flow; (*ii*) no color appearing where there is flow; and (*iii*) appearance of the wrong color or shade of color, confusing the direction and velocity of flow (32,33).

No Color Where There Is Flow

Even more than gray-scale imaging, Doppler and color-flow Doppler are greatly dependent on the intensity of the sound energy reaching an interface. Since the Doppler echoes are reflected back from moving blood cells, the interfaces are very small and are all nonspecular reflectors. If the blood vessel is deep, it is very difficult to demonstrate flow. This is particularly true for large vessels like the inferior vena cava and aorta in moderate-sized to large patients. Flow in the kidney can be difficult to identify unless the patient is very thin or the kidney is superficial as with a renal transplant.

Transducer selection and fine control of the settings on the machine are essential to produce adequate color-flow imaging. High-frequency transducers are much better at detecting the low intensity reflections from individual blood cells. However, as there is greater sound attenuation at higher frequency, lower frequency transducers must be used. The transducer frequency necessary to demonstrate color-flow Doppler is generally lower than the frequency needed for gray-scale imaging. For example, the carotid artery can be visualized on gray-scale with a 7.5 MHz transducer, whereas a 5 MHz transducer is needed for color-flow imaging. Similarly, a 3 MHz central frequency transducer may be necessary for color-flow imaging in situations in which 5 MHz is adequate for gray-scale imaging. Some machines may use a lower frequency with the same transducer for the color-flow pulse and a higher frequency for the gray-scale pulses.

It is important to use adequate gain and TGC. Although this is also true for gray-scale, color-flow is much more sensitive. Similarly, as discussed later, excessive gain or power settings will cause color noise artifacts.

Frequency filters and other algorithms are used to decrease color tissue noise. When the filters are set too high, however, slow flowing blood does not show color.

Color–echo priority is a control that some manufacturers set automatically. Other companies allow the operator to set it manually. It is not possible to display a color-flow pixel in the same location as a gray-scale echo. The machine, therefore, has to determine which should receive priority. The color–echo priority can be set so that color is only shown where the lumen is otherwise echo free. Or, the sensitivity for color-flow can be prioritized so that color will show up even where no vessel was visible on gray-scale imaging (Fig. 23). Clearly, if the color–write priority is set too low, some flow may be missed.

The scale control is probably the most important setting to adjust in color-flow imaging. In gray-scale imaging, for each vector on the screen, only one pulse is necessary. However, with color-flow, the data from several pulses are necessary to correctly interpret the frequencies and hence velocities. Three to eight pulses (ensemble length) may be necessary per gray-scale pulse to adequately characterize slow flow. Faster flow can be characterized with fewer additional pulses. Increasing the number of pulses, however, decreases the pulse repetition rate for the gray-scale image and the frame rate as seen on the screen. This will cause a jerky image, and the transducer must be moved very slowly. One can decrease the size of the color box on the image to regain a faster frame rate.

The ability to show slow flow at a lower scale is accompanied by aliasing and inability to determine direction of flow with the higher velocities. For example, if the color scale is set appropriately to demonstrate homogeneous color in the common carotid artery, the slow flow in

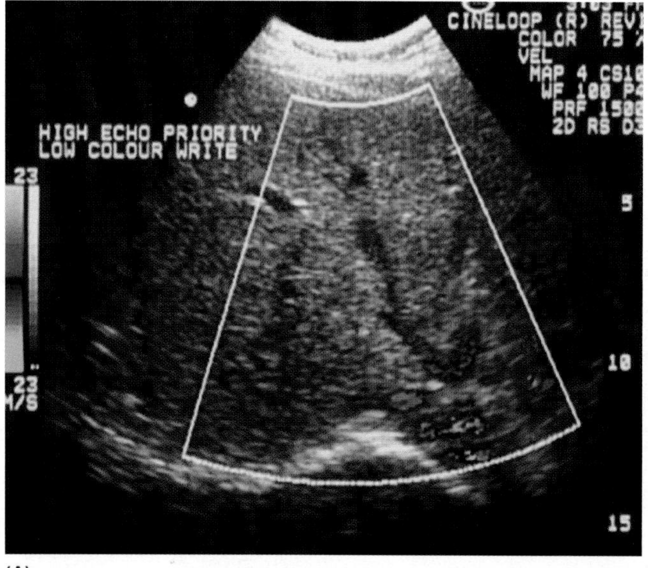

(A)

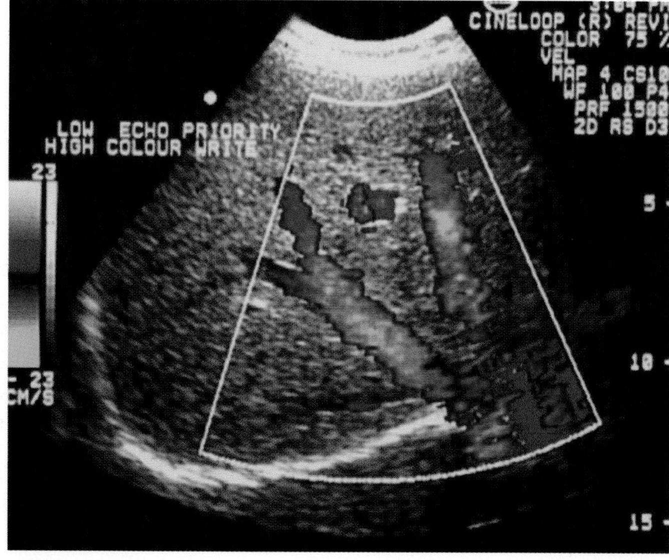

(B)

FIGURE 23 A AND B ■ Color–echo priority. **(A)** The system is set to have a low threshold for inserting an echo rather than color in a relatively echo-poor area. **(B)** Color–echo priority now demonstrates hepatic venous flow. If the color priority is higher, flow will be displayed even where there are stationary echoes. However, the images can become very noisy if there is any motion. If the color priority is decreased, flow only appears in echo-free areas.

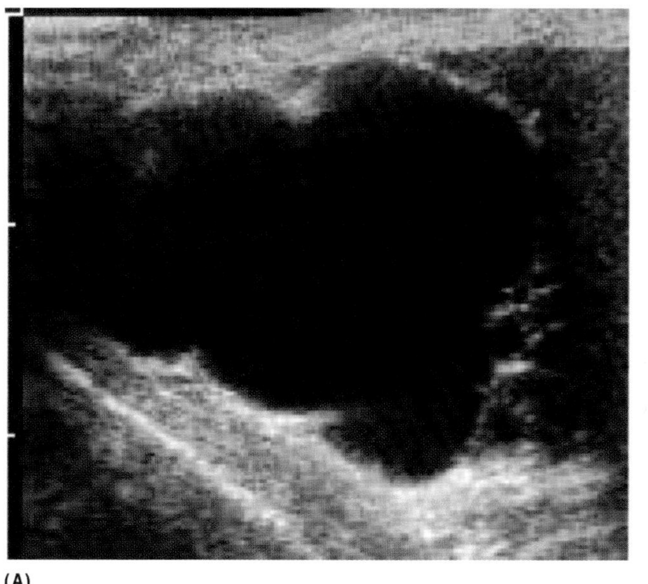
(A)

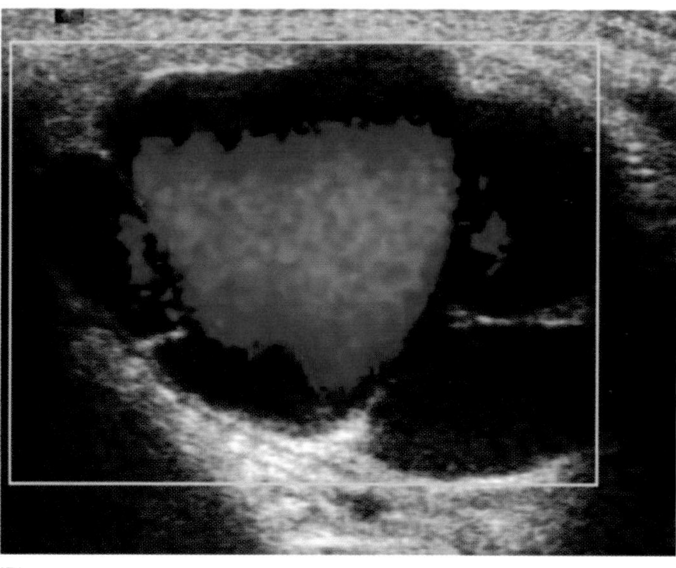
(B)

FIGURE 24 A AND B ■ Epididymal cyst. (**A**) Gray-scale image showing a cystic structure in the head of the epididymis. (**B**) Color-flow Doppler showing artifactual flow due to movement of the transducer.

the periphery of the carotid bulb may not be detected and can simulate thrombus.

Another example that can be frustrating is trying to determine if there is a Budd-Chiari syndrome (hepatic vein thrombosis). If no color is seen in the hepatic veins, it is important to have confidence that color would be detected if flow existed. This is a problem in general with color-flow imaging. The lack of color does not always mean that there is no flow. Lack of color is significant only when slow flow can be demonstrated in adjacent vessels.

Color Where There Is No Flow (Color Noise)

Any moving structure can cause a Doppler shift. The detected Doppler shifts can be displayed on screen as color and therefore may simulate flow. Structures adjacent to the heart, particularly in the left lobe of the liver, can exhibit artifactual color noise (33). Movement of the transducer or even bowel peristalsis can similarly cause color noise (Figs. 24 and 25). Filters and algorithms can decrease the noise since the characteristics of moving blood cells are clearly different from that of interfaces that move back and forth such as in the left lobe of the liver adjacent to the heart. Nonetheless, difficulties can arise.

A special circumstance exists in tissue adjacent to a vessel with extremely high flow. This can occur around an arterial venous fistula (29). This is the color-flow Doppler equivalent to a palpable thrill or an auscultatory "bruit." The tissues actually do vibrate. The fistula will, therefore, appear larger than it is. On the other hand, it is easier to detect the fistula since the surrounding color noise makes it more noticeable.

Although intravenous contrast agents for enhancement of color-flow Doppler imaging has not as yet become common practice in most countries, a similar artifact can occur. The stable microbubbles that make up the contrast agent can cause significant color noise. Burns et al. (34) have shown that this particular type of noise can be eliminated by filtering out the main frequency so that only the harmonics of the main frequency are detected (35).

Movement of the transducer can set up its own Doppler shift. Color noise can appear throughout the image when the transducer is moved. For example, in trying to screen for portal systemic collaterals, movement of the transducer can prevent detection of the abnormal vessels. This can be corrected by moving the transducer slower. That would limit its usefulness in searching for abnormal vessels.

Some of the machine settings are important to prevent color noise. Obviously, the color gain and power must be

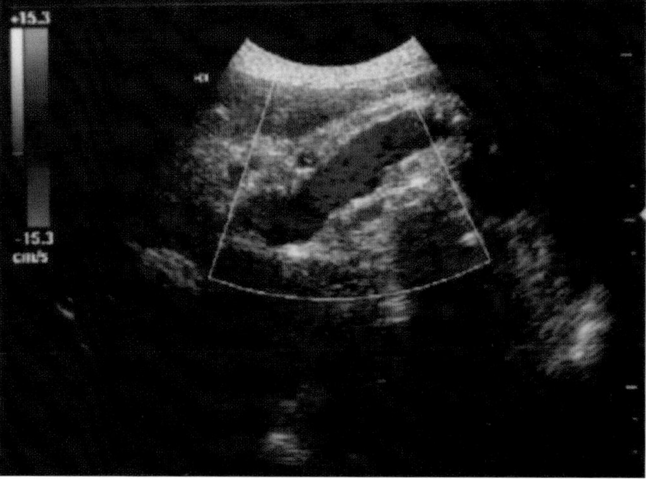

FIGURE 25 ■ Artifactual pseudo-flow in a dilated pancreatic duct. This was due to transmitted pulsations from the adjacent left lobe of the liver and heart. Computed tomography confirmed that it was a dilated pancreatic duct.

set appropriately to minimize artifactual color. Filters and appropriate algorithms can be used to separate true flow from other, more vibratory type of motion.

The color–echo priority setting is important for differentiating true flow from artifactual color. As was mentioned earlier, however, the settings must be carefully adjusted so that real flow is not missed.

To illustrate the problem of color noise, the Budd-Chiari syndrome case can be revisited. All of the settings must be maximized to show the slow flow of the hepatic veins at a considerable distance from the transducer. This area is adjacent to the heart, however, which causes color noise artifacts. Furthermore, the patients with Budd-Chiari syndrome are frequently tachypneic, which adds to the difficulties.

Although color noise interferes with the detection of real flow, it is usually easy to tell that this is an artifact and not real. Because the motion is vibratory and not in one direction, the color shows random pixels of blue and red (color speckle) as opposed to the homogeneous color one expects in a vessel. Interestingly, in the cases illustrated in Figures 24 and 25, the color was homogeneous and not speckled. This facilitated misinterpretation. Pulse Doppler with spectral analysis is usually helpful by demonstrating a vascular flow pattern for vessels which is not the case with color noise.

A mirror image artifact is another condition that can cause color to appear where there is no flow. The principle is exactly the same as with gray-scale imaging. For example, the subclavian artery lies on the apex of the lung. The air in the lung serves as the acoustic mirror. The sound is reflected from the surface of the lung, to the moving blood cells in the subclavian artery and the resulting Doppler shift is reflected back to the surface of the lung and then to the transducer. The extra time taken causes the appearance of a second vessel deep to the real subclavian vessel (Fig. 26) (36,37). Rarely, the direction of flow can appear reversed in the mirror image artifact (38).

Another phenomenon is the color Doppler "twinkling artifact." This is described as a rapidly changing mixture of red and blue color Doppler signal deep to a relatively strong granular reflector such as a urinary calculus (39). The twinkling effect is usually readily recognizable as an artifact and can be helpful in the detection of small renal calculus (Fig. 27).

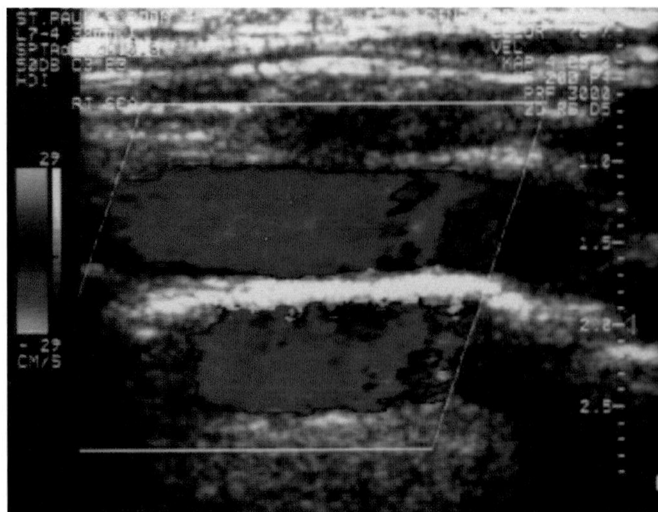

FIGURE 26 ■ Color-flow mirror image artifact. There is flow (away from the transducer) in the right subclavian artery. However, the artery is adjacent to the apex of the right lung. The air/pleura interface serves as the acoustic mirror causing the mirror image of not only the vessel but also the flow within the lumen.

Artifacts that Confuse Velocity or Direction of Flow

Generally, flow in the vessel is homogeneously red toward the transducer and homogeneously blue away from the transducer. During diastole, the slower flow will appear darker, and, during systole, the faster flow should appear brighter.

Several factors interfere with this facile understanding. First, the colors can be reversed with a switch on most machines (Fig. 28), causing the flow toward the transducer to appear blue, and the flow away from the transducer to appear red. Furthermore, turning the transducer around can have the same effect.

Although the angle of flow on pulse Doppler imaging must be adjusted to appreciate the velocity, this is not possible on standard color-flow imaging. Therefore, the color can relate more to the direction of flow than to the velocity. If the vessel curves on the image, where it is pointing more directly in the direction of the sound beam, the velocity will be perceived as faster. Where the direction is more horizontal or perpendicular to the direction of the beam, the color will be darker. Toward the center of the vessel, the flow is faster and, therefore, the color can be brighter. Toward the periphery, the theory of laminar flow dictates that the flow is slower, and therefore, the color is darker.

Also, many assume that the entire image is formed instantaneously, but this is not true. It may take as much as 250 msec to produce the whole image if there is a relatively slow frame rate. Therefore, part of the color-flow image may have been obtained at end diastole and the later part in the beginning of systole. Especially in structures such as the hepatic veins, this can show two directions of flow in the same vessel!

The last and most complicated artifact to understand is that of aliasing. This is related to the flow velocity and the PRF. The Nyquist frequency limit is defined as two times the Doppler frequency. If the PRF is below the Nyquist frequency, aliasing will occur. This will cause the other color to appear where the flow is faster. If the velocity is just above the Nyquist limit, the flow will appear to be slow (dark in the other color). Even faster flow will show up as brighter in the other color (Fig. 28).

Generally, aliasing and bright colors indicate turbulence and flow jets related to arterial stenoses or arterial venous fistulas. It is extremely important, however, to appreciate the direction of flow. The same velocity flow appears much faster and even shows aliasing in the direction of the sound beam (Fig. 29).

(A)

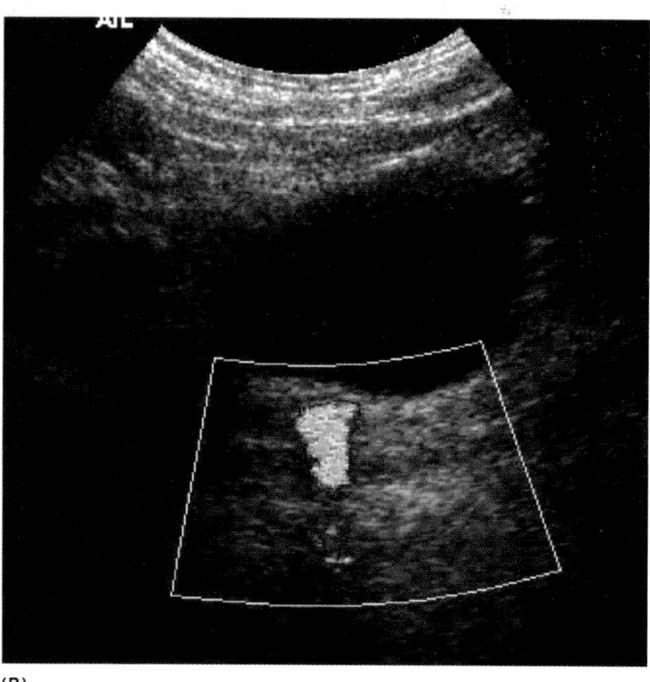

(B)

FIGURE 27 A AND B ■ Twinkle artifact. (**A**) A calculus seen within the vesicoureteric junction. (**B**) A bright mixture of various colors is noted deep to an echogenic focus (calculus). The artifact may be seen adjacent to any focal echogenic lesion.

Power Doppler Imaging

Power Doppler utilizes the same Doppler shift information in a slightly different manner. As opposed to detecting the velocity and direction of flow, power Doppler is much more sensitive in detecting the presence and volume of flow. It is important to appreciate that the brightness of a color in color Doppler is related to only the velocity not the number of blood cells at that velocity. Conversely, in power Doppler, the brightness of the color is related to the number of blood cells moving, but not the velocity.

Power Doppler is even more sensitive to artifactual motion such as movement of the transducer. The frame rate is even lower than with color Doppler. However,

FIGURE 28 ■ Aliasing and effects of eddies. Flow in vessels tends to be laminar, i.e., faster in the center of the vessel than in the periphery. The color scale is set too low and is causing aliasing in the center of the vessel (blue color). At correct color setting, aliasing helps identify high flow due to stenoses.

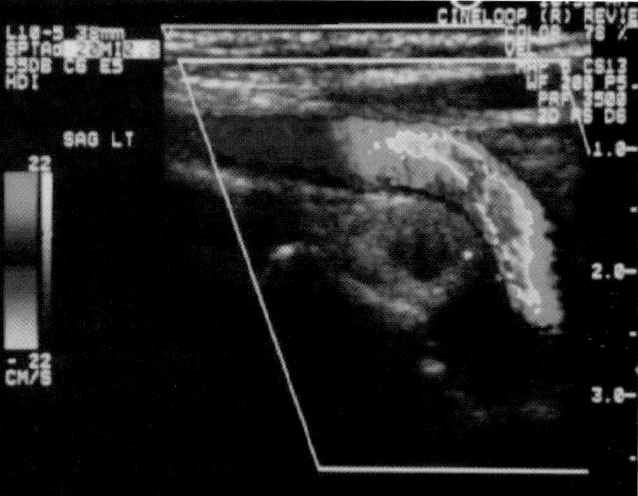

FIGURE 29 ■ Color-flow Doppler image of the left common carotid artery displaying aliasing. The flow is going toward the transducer and, therefore, should be blue. The centre of the lumen where the blood is flowing more directly toward the transducer (i.e., inferiorly) is red and yellow. Around the yellow is cyan. The slower flow is demonstrated by a darker blue color. This is a combination of laminar flow with faster flow toward the center of the vessel and the curvature of the vessel. There is a larger Doppler shift if the direction of flow is closer to parallel to the beam. It is important to realize that aliasing can occur due to the direction of flow in the absence of a stenotic jet.

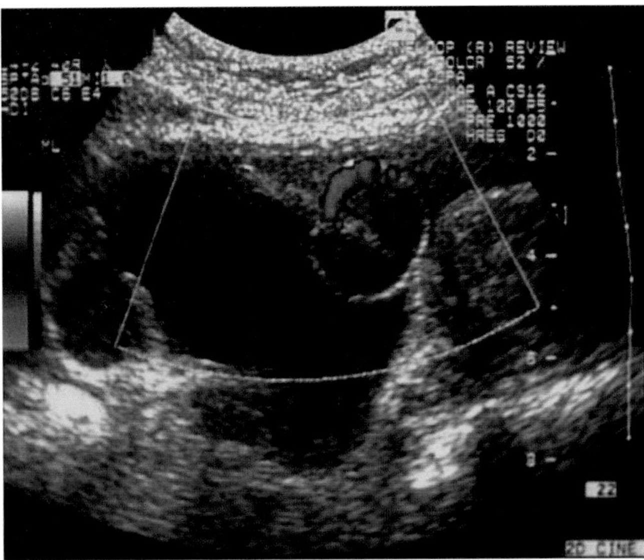

FIGURE 30 ■ Power Doppler is even more sensitive to artifactual motion than conventional color Doppler. In addition, power Doppler "flow" can occur where there are strong spectral reflectors, for example in the yolk sac or, as in this case, a Foley catheter.

slow flow can be detected even in small vessels such as in the periphery of the kidney or lymph nodes. Exquisite images can be made of the neonatal cerebral circulation.

With power Doppler, color can appear where there are strong specular reflectors. This is different from color Doppler ultrasound, in which the color–write priority determines that color will appear in preference where there is no echo. With power Doppler, the opposite is true. It was impressive in the earlier days of power Doppler to think that we could detect flow in the tiny vessels of the yolk sac. This turned out to be an artifact. A similar appearance can be seen in the wall of a Foley catheter! (Fig. 30).

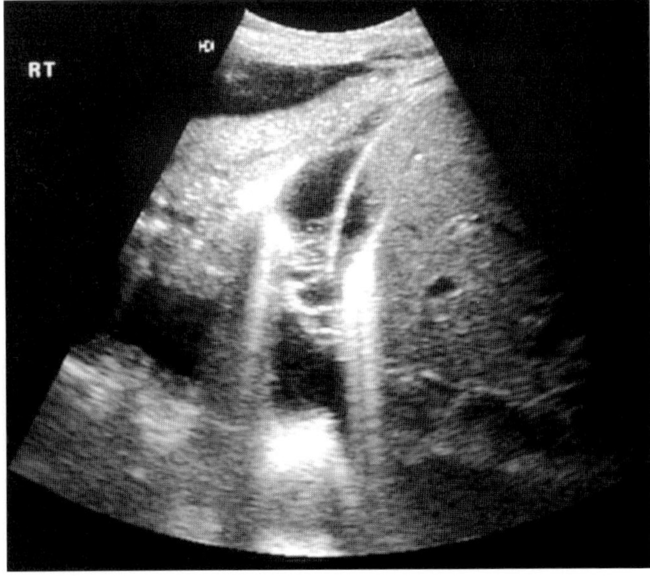

FIGURE 31 ■ Quiz case. Is there a subphrenic abscess?

SUMMARY

Despite the continued improvement and sophistication of ultrasound technology, artifacts have not disappeared. Some of the newer transducer shapes and geometry can cause increased artifact problems. Some artifacts can help in certain circumstances. If an artifact appears in the wrong place at the wrong time, however, misdiagnoses can be made. Appropriate machine settings can eliminate only some artifacts. The best defense against misinterpretation of artifacts is education and experience.

Figure 31 represents a quiz case. Spend a minute looking at the image. It is not a subphrenic abscess. The image shows a loculated, septated right pleural effusion with a partially consolidated right lower lobe. A refractive shadow deep to the right hemidiaphragm can be seen. The mirror image of the air in the lung is superimposed over the refractive shadow simulating a subphrenic abscess with gas. Did you get it right?

REFERENCES

1. Kremkau FW, Taylor KJW. Artifacts in ultrasound imaging. J Ultrasound Med 1986; 5:227.
2. Cooperberg PL. Artifacts in US. Ultrasound Syllabus. Radiological Society of North America, Inc., 1991.
3. Laing FC. Commonly encountered artifacts in clinical ultrasound. Seminars in Ultrasound 1983; 4:27.
4. Desser TS, Jeffrey RB, Lane MJ, Palls PW. Tissue harmonic imaging: utility in abdominal and pelvic sonography. J Clin Ultrasound 1999; 27:135–142.
5. Ziskin MC, Thickman DI, Goldenberg NJ, et al. The comet-tail artifact. J Ultrasound Med 1982; 1:1.
6. Wendell BA, Athey PA. Ultrasonic appearance of metallic foreign bodies in parenchymal organs. J Clin Ultrasound 1981; 9:133.
7. Thickman DI, Ziskin MC, Goldenberg NJ, Linder BE. Clinical manifestations of the comet tail artifact. J Ultrasound Med 1983; 2:225.
8. Avruch L, Cooperberg PL. The ring-down artifact. J Ultrasound Med 1985; 4:21.
9. Lee DH, Kim JH, Ko YT, Yoon Y. Sonographic detection of pneumoperitoneum in patients with acute abdomen. Am J Roentgenol 1990; 154:107–109.
10. Goodman TR, Traill ZC, Philips AJ, Berger J, Gleeson FV. Ultrasound detection of pneumothorax. Clin Rad 1999; 54:736–739.
11. Rowan KR, Kirkpatrick AW, Liu D, Forkheim KE, Mayo JR, Nicolaou S. Traumatic pneumothorax detection with thoracic US: correlation with chest radiography and CT—initial experience. Radiology 2002; 225:210–214.
12. Lafortune M, Gariépy G, Dumont A, Breton G, Lapointe R. The V-shaped artifact of the gallbladder wall. AJR Am J Roentgenol 1986; 147:505.
13. Shapiro RS, Winsberg F. Comet-tail artifact from cholesterol crystals: observations in the postlithotripsy gallbladder and an in vitro model. Radiology 1990; 177:153.
14. Müller N, Cooperberg PL, Rowley VA, Mayo J, Ho B, Li DKB. Ultrasonic refraction by the rectus abdominis muscles: the double image artifact. J Ultrasound Med 1984; 3:515.
15. Sauerbrei EE. The split image artifact in pelvic ultrasonography: the anatomy and physics. J Ultrasound Med 1985; 4:29.
16. Middleton WD, Melson GL. Renal duplication artifact in US imaging. Radiology 1989; 173:427.
17. Mayo J, Cooperberg PL. Displacement of the diaphragmatic echo by hepatic cysts: a new explanation with computer simulation. J Ultrasound Med 1984; 3:337.
18. Pierce G, Golding RH, Cooperberg PL. The effects of tissue velocity changes on acoustical interfaces. J Ultrasound Med 1982; 1:185.

19. Robinson DE, Wilson LS, Kossoff G. Shadowing and enhancement in ultrasonic echograms by reflection and refraction. J Clin Ultrasound 1981; 9:181.
20. Filly RA, Sommer FG, Minton MJ. Characterization of biological fluids by ultrasound and computed tomography. Radiology 1980; 134:167.
21. Richman TS, Taylor KJW, Kremkau FW. Propagation speed artifact in a fatty tumor (myelolipoma): significance for tissue differential diagnosis. J Ultrasound Med 1983; 2:45.
22. Sommer FG, Filly RA, Minton MJ. Acoustic shadowing due to refractive and reflective effects. AJR Am J Roentgenol 1979; 132:973.
23. Mitchell SE, Gross BH, Spitz HB. The hypoechoic caudate lobe: an ultrasonic pseudolesion. Radiology 1982; 144:569.
24. Nicolaou S, Cooperberg PL. The two-tone testis is due to refractive shadowing of the intratesticular artery. J Ultrasound Med 1995; 14:963–965.
25. Entrekin RR, Porter BA, Sillesen HH, Wong AD, Cooperberg PL, Fix C. Real-Time Spatial Compound Imaging: applications to breast, vascular and musculoskeletal ultrasound. Seminars in US CT MRI 2001; 22:50–64.
26. Laing FC, Kurtz AB. The importance of ultrasonic side-lobe artifacts. Radiology 1982; 145:763.
27. Goldstein A, Madrazo BL. Slice-thickness artifacts in gray-scale ultrasound. J Clin Ultrasound 1981; 9:365.
28. Goldstein A. Range ambiguities in real-time ultrasound. J Clin Ultrasound 1981; 9:83.
29. Middleton WD, Erickson S, Melson GL. Perivascular color artifact: pathologic significance and appearance on color Doppler US images. Radiology 1989; 171:647.
30. Pozniak MA, Zagzebski JA, Scanlan KA. Spectral and color Doppler artifacts. RadioGraphics 1992; 12:35.
31. Mitchell DG. Color Doppler imaging: principles, limitations, and artifacts. Radiology 1990; 177:1.
32. Burns PN. Doppler ultrasound: principles and artifacts. In: Ultrasound: Categorical Course Syllabus. ARRS, 1993:281–300.
33. Mitchell DG, Burns P, Needleman L. Color Doppler artifact in anechoic regions. J Ultrasound Med 1990; 9:255.
34. Forsberg F, Liu JB, Burns PN, Merton DA, Goldberg BB. Artifacts in ultrasonic contrast agent studies. Ultrasound Med 1991; 10:691.
35. Burns PN. Harmonic imaging with ultrasound contrast agents. Clin Rad 1996; 51(suppl 1):50.
36. Reading CC, Charboneau JW, Allison JW, Cooperberg PL. Color and spectral Doppler mirror-image artifact of the subclavian artery. Radiology 1990; 174:41.
37. Middleton WD, Melson GL. The carotid ghost: a color Doppler ultrasound duplication artifact. J Ultrasound Med 1990; 9:487.
38. Gooding GA, Saloner D, Eisert W, Nagarkar S. Color Doppler artifact from metallic carotid clamp. J Ultrasound Med 1994; 13:357–365.
39. Rahmouni A, Bargoin R, Herment A, Bargoin N, Vasile N. Color Doppler twinkling artifact in hyperechoic regions. Radiology 1996; 199:269–271.

Contrast-Enhanced Ultrasound Imaging

Ji-Bin Liu, Daniel A. Merton, Flemming Forsberg, and Barry B. Goldberg

3

Contrast enhancement has become a routine part of clinical radiography, computed tomography (CT), and magnetic resonance imaging (MRI), increasing their diagnostic capabilities. During the last two decades, contrast-enhanced ultrasound (CEUS) imaging has been investigated and has gradually emerged in clinical settings. Concurrent with technological improvements in ultrasound (US) scanning equipment, contrast agents have been developed to meet the demands of this rapidly expanding field of imaging.

The rapid development of contrast agents for sonography is precipitated by the performance limits of grayscale imaging and Doppler techniques. As US imaging is used to study smaller and deeper structures in the body, the spatial resolution of grayscale imaging and Doppler sensitivity becomes critical to the degree that it impacts the clinical utility of sonography. Contrast agents promise to improve the sensitivity and the specificity of current sonographic diagnoses and have the potential to expand the already broad range of its applications. This chapter is intended to provide an overview of the principles behind contrast-specific US imaging technology and a review of clinical applications that are currently being used or are under investigation.

BASIC PRINCIPLES OF CONTRAST AGENTS

All current intravascular US contrast agents are based on microbubbles of a specific gas encapsulated in various types of shells. Various biochemical techniques have been adopted to produce stabilized gas-filled microbubbles for use as US contrast agents. Different shell compositions have an important influence upon the performance of the agent. This is evident in both acoustic behavior and in vivo stability. Materials employed in contrast agent design include polymeric, phospholipids, surfactants, and galactose as well as perfluorocarbon emulsions.

US contrast agents should have some characteristics that are independent of a specific application. They should (*i*) be as echogenic as possible, producing a detectable response that allows improved visualization of the blood circulation; (*ii*) be small enough to cross the pulmonary circulation for intravenous (i.v.) injection; (*iii*) be persistent enough to permit sufficient examination times; (*iv*) be nontoxic, biodegradable, and have no side effects; (*v*) be user-friendly for easy dosage, storage, and preparation; and (*vi*) be affordable so as to provide a cost-effective diagnosis.

During the last decade, many new US contrast agents have been developed. These are characterized by both smaller microbubble mean sizes (<10 μm) and prolonged persistence (as much as 10 minutes) within the systemic circulation. Various techniques are used to combine materials that control the microbubble surface (i.e., the encapsulating shell) with gases that inhibit diffusion and dissolution (e.g., heavy gasses such as

TABLE 1 ■ Partial List of Ultrasound Contrast Agents

Name	Shell composition	Gas	Manufacturer
AI-700	Polymer	Perfluorocarbon	Acusphere
biSphere	Gelatin/polymer	Air	Point Biomedical
BR14	Phospholipid	Perfluorobutane	Bracco Diagnostics
BY 963	Lipid	Air	Byk-Gulden
Levovist	Galactose/palmitic acid	Air	Schering
Definity	Lipid	Perfluoropropane	Bristol-Myers Squibb
Imagent	Surfactant	Perfluorocarbon	Imcor Pharmaceuticals
Optison	Albumin	Perfluoropropane	GE Healthcare
Sonazoid	Lipid	Perfluorobutane	GE Healthcare
SonoVue	Surfactant	SF6	Bracco Diagnostics
MRX-408	Lipid/ligand oligopeptide	Perfluoropropane	ImaRx Therapeutics
Quantison	Albumin	Air	Andaris Ltd.
QFX	Albumin	Perfluorocarbon	Guangzhou Nanfang Hospital

perfluorocarbons). At present, several contrast agents have been approved for clinical use whereas others are in various stages of development (Table 1). This table is by no means a complete inventory of all of the products being tested.

Vascular US contrast agents consist of gas-filled microbubbles stabilized by a thin shell (Fig. 1). They are typically less than 8 μm in diameter, which allows them to pass through the pulmonary circulation and the systemic capillary beds (1). When administered intravenously, US contrast agents improve the detection of blood flow and depiction of the vasculature in a variety of structures compared to conventional (i.e., noncontrast) sonography due to the increased signal-to-noise ratio (SNR). These agents significantly enhance the acoustic backscatter from blood in both Doppler and grayscale modes, which results from the large impedance difference between the gas-filled microbubbles and the surrounding blood. In certain contrast-specific imaging modes, the SNR can be further improved by suppression of tissue signals. The improved SNR can also be exploited in nonvascular structures such as the genitourinary tract, gastrointestinal (GI) tract, fallopian tubes, and lymphatic system.

CONTRAST-SPECIFIC IMAGING TECHNOLOGY

Conventional US scanners have technical limitations when used with US contrast agents. These limitations can ultimately reduce the clinical usefulness of contrast enhancement. Thus, US scanners have been and will continue to be modified to optimize their use with a variety of US contrast agents.

When an acoustic wave hits a microbubble, it alternately compresses the microbubble on the positive portion of the pressure wave and the microbubble expands in the negative portion. Therefore, the microbubble becomes symmetrically larger and smaller in response to the

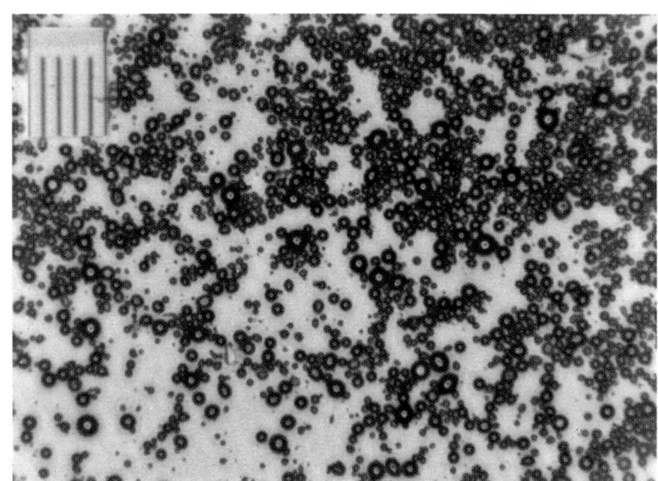

FIGURE 1 ■ Microscopic view of microbubbles with sizes ranging from 2 to 8 μm.

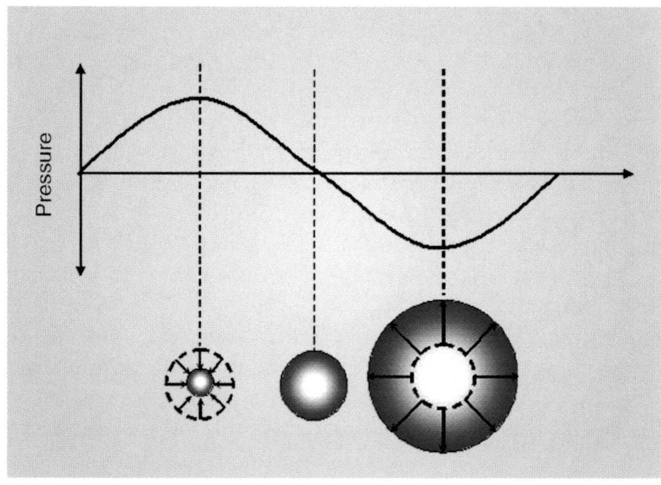

FIGURE 2 ■ An illustration of the microbubble behavior in an acoustic field.

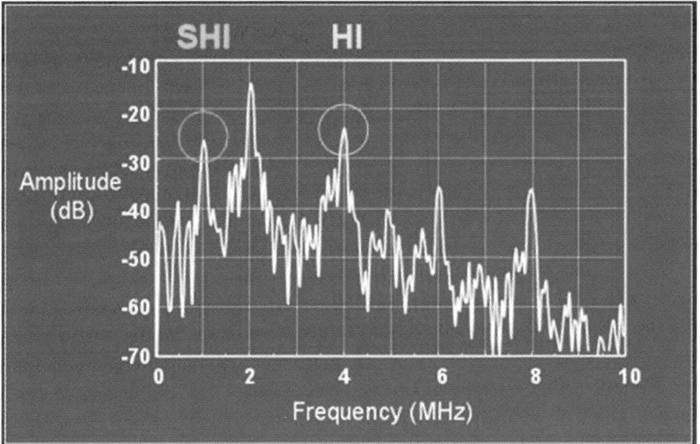

FIGURE 3 ■ Spectrum of a microbubble agent showing the fundamental (f = 2 MHz), second harmonic (HI at 4 MHz), and subharmonic (SHI at 1 MHz) components. HI, harmonic imaging; SHI, subharmonic imaging.

oscillations of the pressure caused by the incident wave (Fig. 2). Furthermore, the vibration of the microbubble in an acoustic field is frequency dependent.

In general, during insonation, US contrast agents produce a linear response at low acoustic pressures (<50 kPa), which means the microbubbles will undergo rhythmic oscillations at a resonant frequency (f_0). A nonlinear contrast agent response occurs at intermediate pressures (from approximately 50–500 kPa depending on the agent). This nonlinear response consists of an asymmetric change in microbubble size due to greater resistance to compression than expansion, which produces harmonic and subharmonic signal components (i.e., frequency components at $2f_0$, $3f_0$, $4f_0$, etc. and at $1/2f_0$, $1/3f_0$, etc.) (Fig. 3) (2). Eventually, at higher acoustic pressures (>500 kPa; although these pressure levels vary significantly from agent to agent), the contrast microbubbles will be disrupted and destroyed.

Initially, the enhancement of Doppler flow signals (either spectral, color Doppler or power Doppler) was used to detect contrast enhancement in the vessels or organs of interest. However, color flow imaging (CFI) artifacts (e.g., color blooming and poor spatial resolution) often result from the addition of contrast agents, so this is not always an ideal method for flow imaging. Recent advances in contrast-specific imaging technologies have been shown to improve the utility of grayscale CEUS.

Harmonic Imaging

Harmonic imaging (HI) is a contrast-specific imaging mode originally developed for CEUS. The phenomenon of harmonic signal generation is not confined to microbubble-based contrast agents but can also be induced in native tissue and this forms the basis of native tissue harmonic imaging (THI). HI uses the same broadband transducers used for conventional imaging, but the US system is configured to preferentially receive echoes at the second harmonic frequency (i.e., twice the transmit frequency). HI provides a way to better differentiate areas with and without contrast microbubbles. Therefore, contrast-enhanced HI has the potential to demonstrate, in real-time, grayscale blood-flow imaging (i.e., perfusion imaging) (Fig. 4). The frequencies and parameters of HI that are used depend on the specific characteristics (e.g., microbubble size and shell composition) of the US contrast agent being utilized. Selection of the appropriate agent and imaging mode optimizes the utility of CEUS (3).

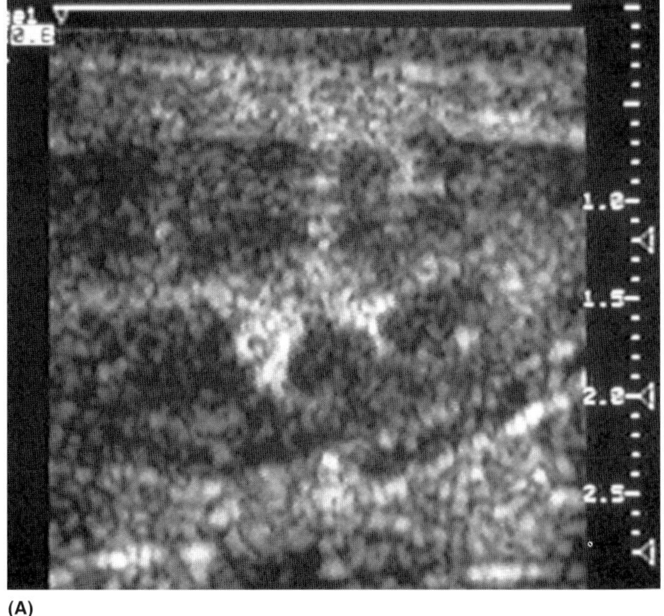

(A)

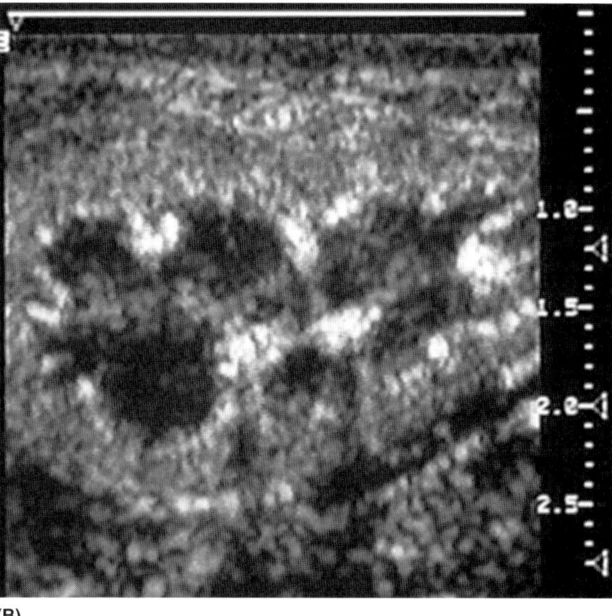

(B)

FIGURE 4 A AND B ■ Compared with fundamental imaging (**A**), second harmonic imaging (**B**) of a kidney after contrast injections shows better enhancement and vascular definition.

Initially HI relied on simple filtering techniques to extract the returning harmonic signals from microbubble signals, but more sophisticated processing schemes have emerged in recent years. In order to better separate grayscale echoes arising from those arising from the contrast agent from tissue, tissue signal suppression has to be carried out. This can be achieved by phase/pulse cancellation, coded pulses, or amplitude modulation. Although there are various commercial methods available with differing levels of sophistication and technology, grayscale phase/pulse inversion HI (PIHI) is the basis of most of the "contrast-specific" modes used for grayscale imaging with US contrast agents (4,5). This technique cancels first harmonic (linearly scattered echoes at the fundamental frequency) signals by transmitting a pulse sequence where each pulse is an inverted copy of the previous pulse, and then summing the echoes from subsequent pulses (resulting in zero under linear scattering conditions). Hence, echoes from stationary tissue will be suppressed whereas nonlinear echoes arising from contrast microbubbles will combine and, thus, be preferentially detected and displayed. The PIHI technique depicts signals from microbubbles with good accuracy and spatial resolution (6–8). Additional details on the equipment and software available for US contrast imaging may be found in the recent European Federation of Societies for Ultrasound in Medicine and Biology (EFSUMB) guideline paper (9).

Intermittent Imaging

In order to optimally enhance detection of tumor neovascularity with contrast agents, a sufficient amount of the microbubbles must enter the tumor microvasculature. Conventional US systems, however, often deliver power levels that are sufficient to destroy contrast microbubbles. If the microbubbles are destroyed before they reach the neovasculature, the desired enhancement of flow in the tumor vessels will not be observed. A potential solution to this problem is the use of intermittent US imaging, which has been shown to increase US contrast enhancement (10–12). The degree of enhancement provided with intermittent imaging is dependent upon flow rate, acoustic power output, and the frequency of insonation (13). With continuous grayscale sonography, contrast microbubbles within the imaging plane may be destroyed during each frame used to form the image. Since a typical grayscale US image is refreshed at approximately 30 frames per second, the available contrast agent for each new image frame is that amount that enters the imaging plane in 1/30th of a second. In this short time, contrast may enter larger vessels but will not generally reach the microcirculation. With intermittent imaging, the US beam is turned off for longer periods between each image frame. More contrast microbubbles enter the imaging field during this interscan delay period resulting in increased echo enhancement. Furthermore, the contrast material will have time to traverse further into the capillary bed to provide enhancement from the neovascular vessels.

Flash echo imaging (FEI) is a particular combination of real-time and intermittent grayscale imaging technology, consisting of low-power real-time monitor pulses transmitted continuously, while microbubble destruction is achieved with intermittent higher power flash pulses (14). These two modes are displayed simultaneously (occasionally in a dual screen format). Each sequence of multiple-frame (1–15 frames) flash pulses can be triggered manually or electronically (e.g., every 1–8 seconds). The principle of microbubble destruction in intermittent mode has been used by investigators to measure mean myocardial microbubble velocity and to assess the microvascular cross-sectional area during constant infusion of contrast (15). The product of these two estimates is the mean myocardial blood flow (i.e., a measure of myocardial perfusion). To date, FEI is the only quantitative method for US perfusion estimation (in mL/min/g) that has been developed.

Continuous Imaging

Although intermittent imaging can obtain high contrast within a single frame, this imaging mode is not real time, which may impair the visualization of some structures and the utility of the modality. In the last few years, a number of other methods have been introduced (some commercially), such as PIHI, superharmonic imaging, power harmonics, coded harmonic angio, and agent detection imaging (ADI) (16–20), which employ low acoustic power settings and contrast-specific signal processing to produce a real-time display. The visualization of the contrast-enhancement pattern of the normal and the abnormal tissues can significantly improve the diagnostic capability of sonography.

Other Imaging Methods

When imaging small vessels or if the concentration of contrast is low, the level of enhancement can be limited. However, collecting images over an extended period of time (e.g., 3–10 seconds) using alternative postprocessing techniques (e.g., maximum intensity projection) can achieve a temporally summed (or compounded) enhanced image. This is the basis of a commercially available technique (21), which has currently been implemented by some manufacturers (Figs. 5 and 6).

Under specific conditions, gas microbubbles generate subharmonics, which occur mainly at half the transmitted frequency. Compared to superharmonic imaging, an advantage of subharmonic imaging is that tissue signal is minimal, resulting in a high agent-to-tissue ratio (i.e., high SNR). Reports have described the feasibility and implementation of subharmonic US imaging (22,23) (Fig. 7). Currently, subharmonic imaging is still in its early development.

CLINICAL APPLICATIONS

US contrast agents can potentially be utilized for assessment of any body region that is evaluated with conventional US. Currently, the primary applications of US contrast agents are in cardiac and hepatic imaging. Other

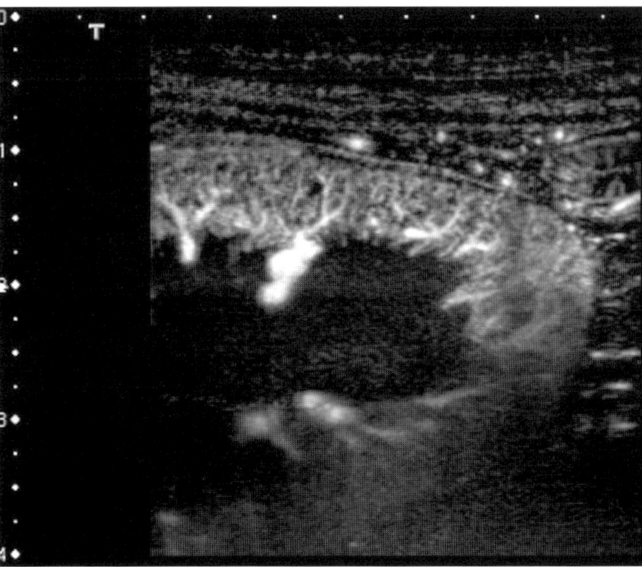

FIGURE 5 ■ Contrast-enhanced imaging using the micro-flow-imaging mode (MFI, Toshiba, Japan) shows a high-resolution depiction of normally perfused kidney parenchyma in an animal model.

applications are being explored, although there are currently fewer reports on their clinical use. The assessment of vascularity by demonstration of microvessels or increased parenchymal signal intensity provides a new parameter for diagnostic evaluation just as i.v. contrast has improved CT and MRI as well as nuclear imaging.

Hepatic Applications

The sonographic detection of hepatic lesions and other hepatic abnormalities can be limited by patient body habitus, examiner expertise, and other factors. Conventional sonography is limited in its ability to detect small (<10 mm), isoechoic, and/or peripherally located lesions, particularly in patients with diffuse liver disease. Additionally, sonography is not as effective as CT or MRI for characterization of hepatic tumors. Numerous reports on the use of CEUS

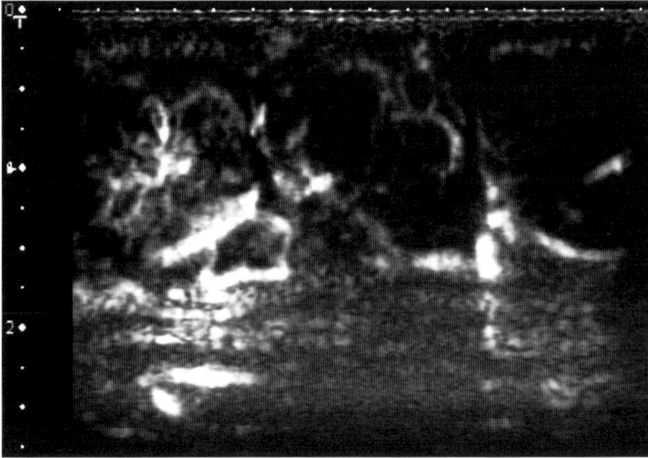

FIGURE 6 ■ Contrast-enhanced imaging using the micro-flow-imaging mode (MFI, Toshiba, Japan) shows a high-resolution depiction of tumor neovascularity in an animal model.

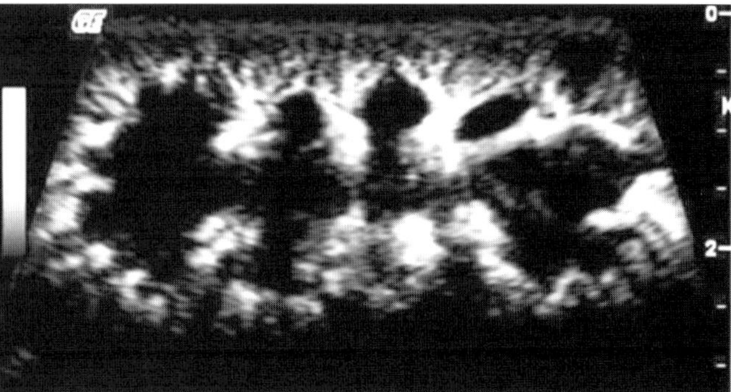

FIGURE 7 ■ Subharmonic image of a canine kidney shows the perfusion pattern of vasculature of the kidney with suppression of background tissue. *Source*: From Ref. 23.

for hepatic applications have described the potential to enhance the detection of lesions as well as to improve the ability to characterize hepatic masses (24–30).

Using CEUS, it is possible to distinguish specific phases of hepatic blood flow (as can be done with contrast CT and MRI). Scanning the liver after i.v. administration of a US contrast agent will demonstrate contrast-enhanced blood flow initially in branches of the hepatic artery (arterial or early vascular phase), which is then followed by the portal venous phase identified as contrast-enhanced flow in the portal veins. The late vascular phase is identified by detection of flow in the hepatic capillaries, which is seen as a parenchymal blush. If a reticuloendothelial system (RES)–specific contrast agent is utilized, it is possible to identify a fourth phase, commonly referred to as the delayed or the parenchymal enhancement phase representing contrast enhancement arising from the stationary microbubbles that have been phagocytosed by the RES (31).

Similar diagnostic criteria currently used for contrast-enhanced CT or MRI, including evaluation of the phase, degree, and pattern of vascularity in and around hepatic tumors can also be applied to CEUS (24,25). In fact, CEUS, because of its ability to image dynamic events in real time, may prove to be better than CT or MRI in the evaluation of hemodynamics that occurs in the various hepatic vascular phases. Numerous published reports suggest that CEUS can improve the detection and the characterization of liver lesions (26–30).

Cavernous hemangiomas are common benign hepatic tumors. The "classic" sonographic appearance of a hemangioma is that of a homogeneously hyperechoic round mass with well-defined margins. However, not all hemangiomas meet those criteria; therefore, they are inaccurately characterized sonographically. Several recent reports have suggested that CEUS can improve the characterization of hemangiomas and reduce the need for other more costly imaging studies as well as biopsies (32,33). Weskott reported using US contrast and interval delay grayscale HI to identify the hemodynamic patterns most consistent with hemangiomas (32). Before and after i.v. administration of Levovist® (Schering AG, Berlin, Germany), 15 atypical hemangiomas were evaluated, with CT or MRI correlation obtained. The authors concluded that most atypical hemangiomas imaged with the interval delay technique show rapid refilling of contrast, suggesting that their blood supply was via arterial supply. Early and late vascular phase imaging improved the ability to characterize hemangiomas. Solbiati et al. (33) used SonoVue to study seven atypical hemangiomas (1.5–6.5 cm in size) with grayscale HI. On baseline (noncontrast) sonography, four lesions appeared hypoechoic or anechoic whereas the other three were isoechoic and "almost undistinguishable." Imaging in the arterial phase detected only peripheral enhancement around all lesions. The portal and the late vascular phases demonstrated progressive centripetal filling lasting from five to seven minutes. The study suggests that multiphase sonography is necessary for accurate diagnosis of atypical hemangiomas.

Several reports have described the contrast-enhanced appearance of hepatocellular carcinoma (HCC) as having intense enhancement in the early arterial phase and relatively rapid wash-out of contrast in the portal phase (29,34,35). With the use of an RES-specific agent, HCC lesions can have a similar appearance to focal nodular hyperplasia (FNH) in the early arterial phase. However, on delayed phase imaging, the HCC tumor will be hypoechoic compared to the surrounding normal liver parenchyma whereas FNH will be isoechoic to the surrounding normal liver tissue. The central feeding artery and spoke-wheel radiating branches that are characteristic of FNH on dynamic computed tomographic angiography (CTA) can also be depicted by CEUS, which can help to differentiate these two types of hepatic tumors (34).

CEUS has been shown to improve the detection and/or delineation of liver metastases (26). However, accurate characterization of metastatic liver tumors with CEUS can be problematic because the degree of vascularity in these lesions is related to the primary cancer (29). Therefore, some metastatic liver lesions will be hypervascular while others are hypovascular. One imaging characteristic of liver metastases that has been identified during delayed phase imaging using an RES-specific contrast agent is an echogenic rim around the tumor. The echogenic rim is thought to reflect the higher concentration of Kupffer cells around metastases and/or a higher degree of contrast that results from compression of the normal liver parenchyma around the metastases (25).

By providing a means to detect and differentiate the various vascular enhancement patterns (e.g., degree, architecture, and phasicity) in and around hepatic lesions, CEUS has the ability to improve characterization of liver lesions including HCC, FNH, and hemangiomas.

Other studies suggest that CEUS is useful for evaluation of liver transplant recipients (36,37). Leutoff et al. reported their findings of 21 patients (31 examinations) who received orthotopic liver transplants (36). After Levovist was administered, significantly better arterial flow signals were detected in the porta hepatis as well as in the right and the left lobes of the liver. The study suggests that the use of contrast-enhanced CFI significantly improves the detection of hepatic arterial flow in transplant recipients. This is a clinically important application of CEUS because of the frequent use of sonography to evaluate organ recipients in the immediate postoperative period. Although X-ray angiography remains the gold-standard imaging examination to assess patency of the transplanted hepatic artery, it is invasive and not without potential complications. A contrast agent used post-operatively could enhance the detection of hepatic artery flow and potentially reduce the number of unnecessary angiograms.

The use of US contrast agents for evaluation of the liver has become widespread and can be considered routine in parts of Europe and Asia (3). Currently available microbubble-based agents are essentially blood pool agents. The type of enhancement demonstrated in the liver is similar to that shown with contrast-enhanced CT and MR imaging. Hence, the interpretation of enhancement patterns depicted with CEUS is similar to that performed with contrast-enhanced CT or MR. In addition, continuous scanning at low acoustic pressures may reveal dynamic contrast enhancement that can be quite helpful for survey scanning to localize lesions as well as for characterization of a variety of focal liver lesions (Fig. 8).

Hepatic pathology can be considered in two main groups: focal lesions and diffuse disease. The characteristic patterns of enhancement in benign and malignant liver lesions have been described (38–40). There is good concordance between the enhancement characteristics of focal liver lesions using CEUS and those that have been described for CT and MR studies (39,40). This is true for benign and malignant hepatic tumors (41). CEUS performs better for characterization of some focal lesions (e.g., HCC) (Fig. 9) and metastatic lesions (Fig. 10) compared to an unenhanced US scan (42). This is especially the case for small (<2 cm) focal liver lesions. Contrast agents have been shown to be useful for improving the detection of HCC (Fig. 11), differentiating HCC from regenerating nodules and for detection of recurrence in treated lesions. Complementary information may be obtained when compared to contrast-enhanced CT scans (43). This improvement shows good interobserver agreement (44). FNH has a central star-like pattern of enhancement that can be observed with continuous CEUS (Fig. 12) (45). Due to the transient nature of enhancement, the star-like pattern may not be seen in all examinations, especially if an intermittent mode is used.

In some cases, there is overlap of the benign and malignant features in focal liver lesions on CEUS but the use of additional parameters may provide advantages over CT and MR. For example, hepatic transit time has been found to be useful in monitoring post-radiofrequency (RF) ablation procedures (46) and contrast-enhanced power Doppler imaging for radiotherapy (47). For diffuse liver disease such as cirrhosis, global parameters such as hepatic transit time show promise in being able to diagnose cirrhosis without biopsy. In an initial study of patients with biopsy-proven cirrhosis, the hyperdynamic circulatory state was demonstrated using contrast-enhanced spectral Doppler of the hepatic veins. Patients with cirrhosis were found to have contrast arrival transit time from antecubital vein into the hepatic veins within

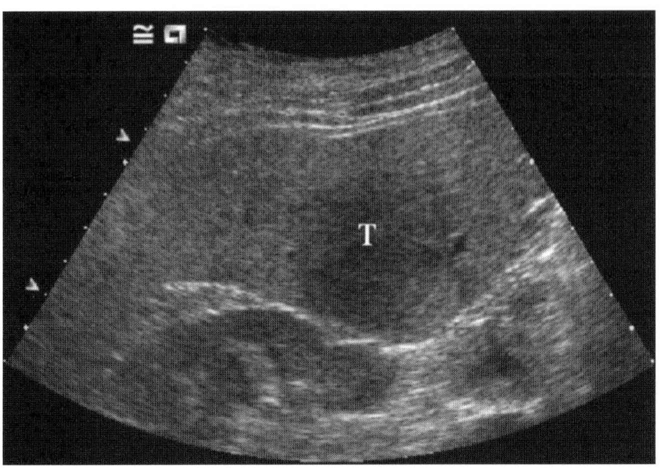

(A)

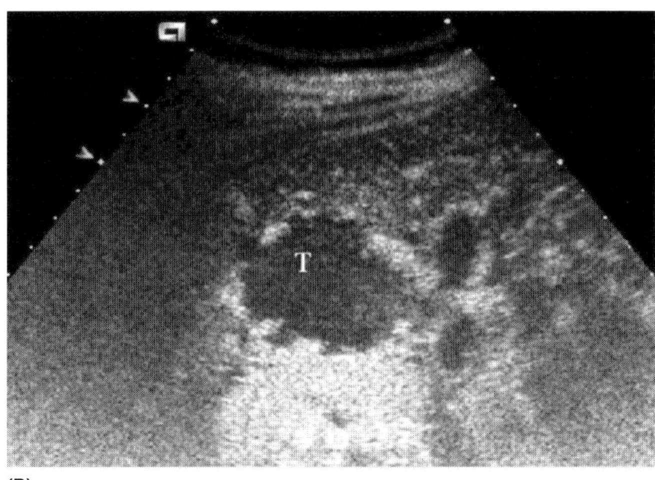

(B)

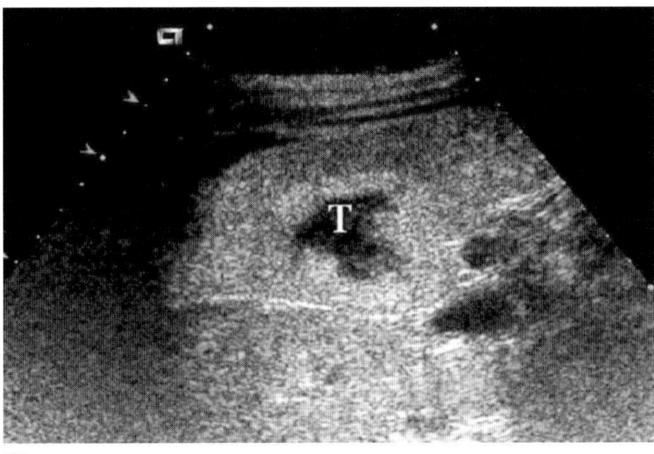

(C)

FIGURE 8 A–C ■ (**A**) Baseline imaging shows a heterogeneous liver mass (T). (**B**) Following a bolus injection of Sonovue (Bracco, Milan, Italy), characteristic peripheral globular enhancement of the tumor (T) is present. (**C**) After several minutes, centripetal filling of the tumor (T) is observed. This enhancement pattern is consistent with a hemangioma. *Source*: Bracco Diagnostics.

24 seconds, while the mean transit times for control subjects and patients with noncirrhotic diffuse liver disease were 49.8 and 35.8 seconds, respectively (48).

A prospective study to assess the diagnostic accuracy of transhepatic circulatory time with an US contrast agent demonstrated that the hepatic artery to hepatic vein and portal vein to hepatic vein interval times were significantly shorter in the cirrhosis group (7.4 ± 1.7 and 1.9 ± 1.5 seconds, respectively) compared with those in the noncirrhosis group (normal: 15.6 ± 2.1 and 11.1 ± 1.7 seconds,

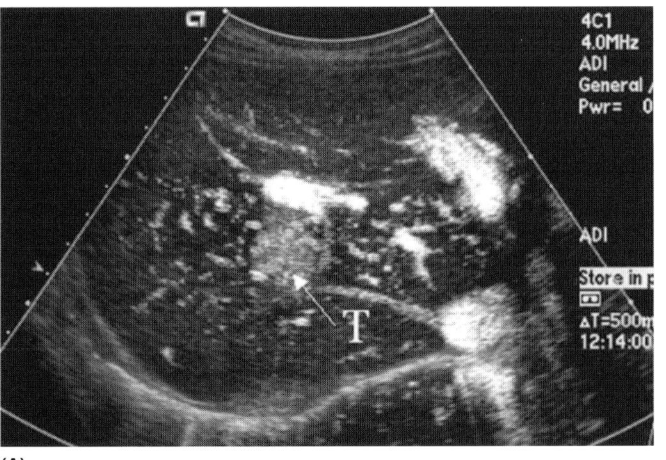

(A)

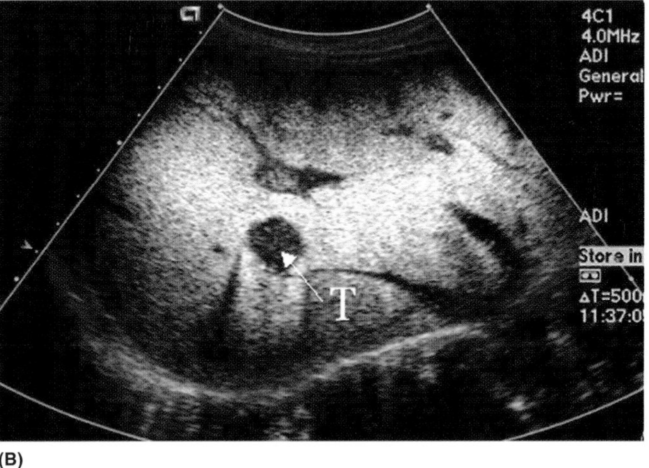

(B)

FIGURE 9 A AND B ■ (**A**) Harmonic imaging of a hepatocellular carcinoma demonstrates tumor enhancement in its arterial phase using agent detection imaging mode. *Source*: ADI, Siemens. (**B**) In its delayed phase, the tumor appears as a hypoechoic lesion within the contrast-enhanced parenchyma. *Source*: Bracco Diagnostics. T, tumor.

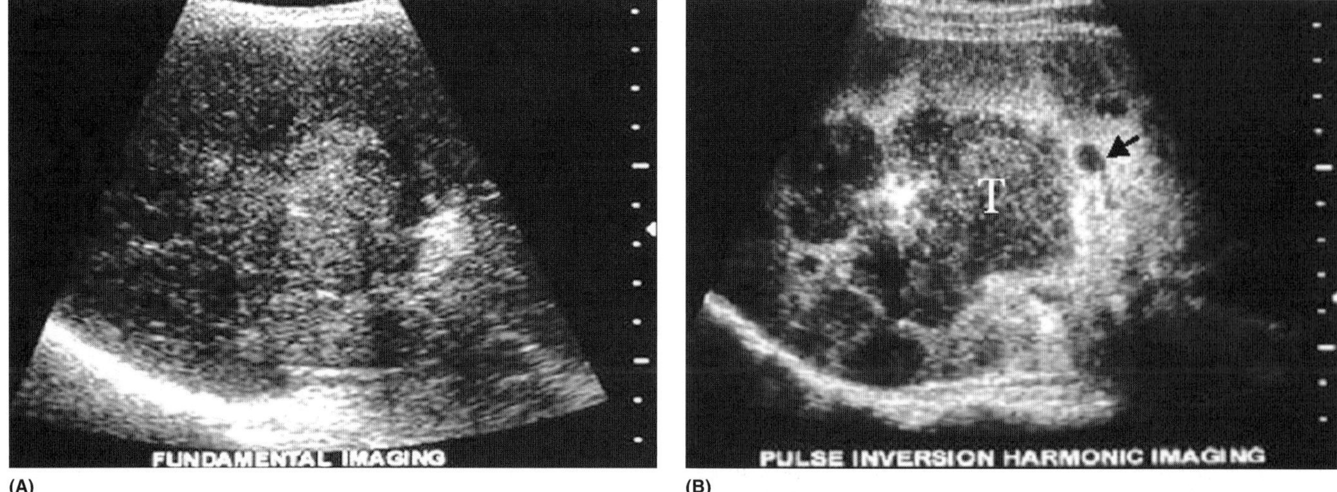

FIGURE 10 A AND B ■ (**A**) Conventional grayscale imaging shows suspicious masses within a heterogenous liver in a patient with colon cancer. (**B**) Contrast-enhanced pulse inversion harmonic imaging improved the delineation of multilobulated tumors within the enhanced liver parenchyma. T, tumor.

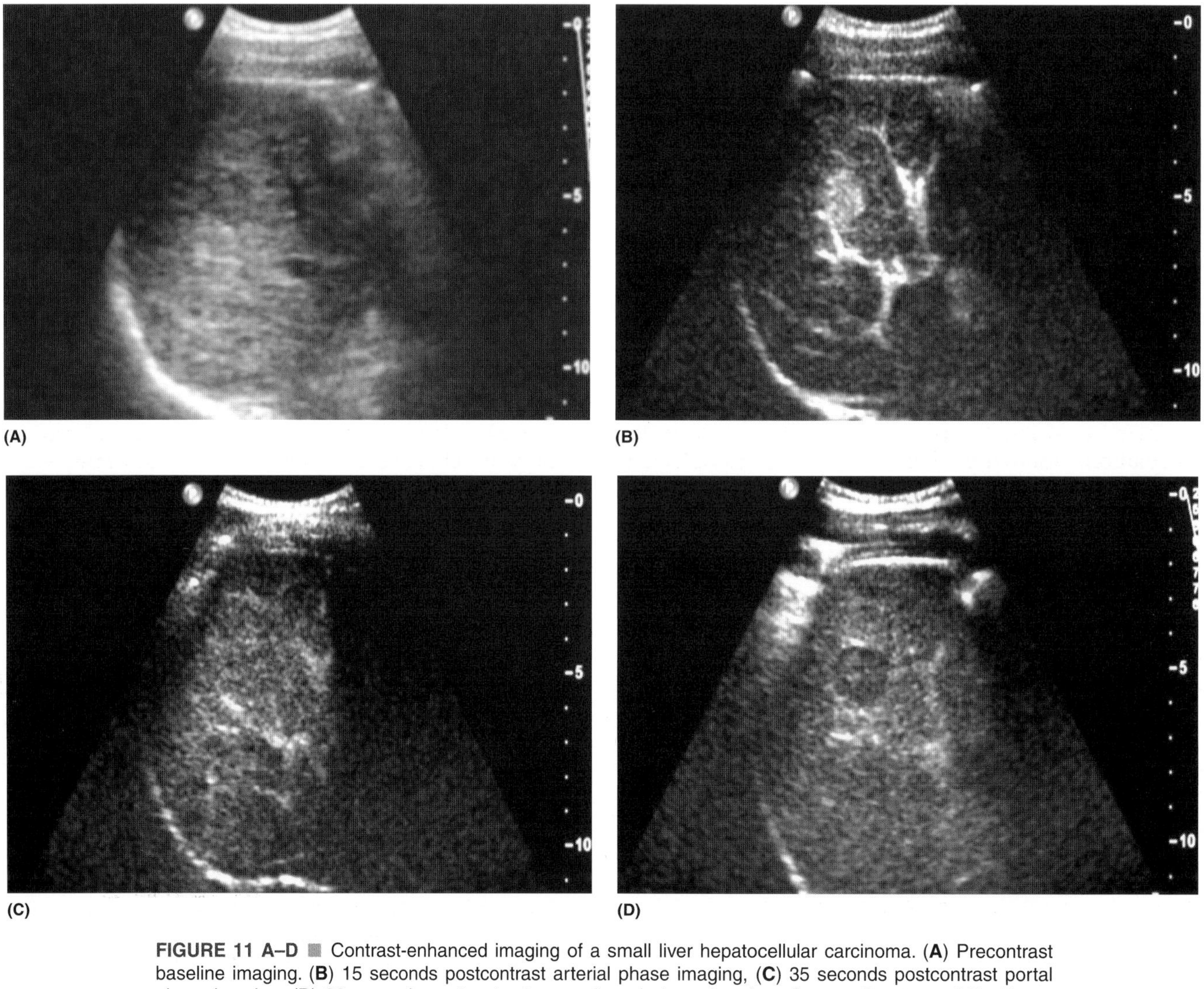

(A) (B)

(C) (D)

FIGURE 11 A–D ■ Contrast-enhanced imaging of a small liver hepatocellular carcinoma. (**A**) Precontrast baseline imaging. (**B**) 15 seconds postcontrast arterial phase imaging, (**C**) 35 seconds postcontrast portal phase imaging, (**D**) 98 seconds postcontrast parenchymal phase imaging. *Source*: Courtesy of Dr. Zheng Rongqin, Guangzhou, China.

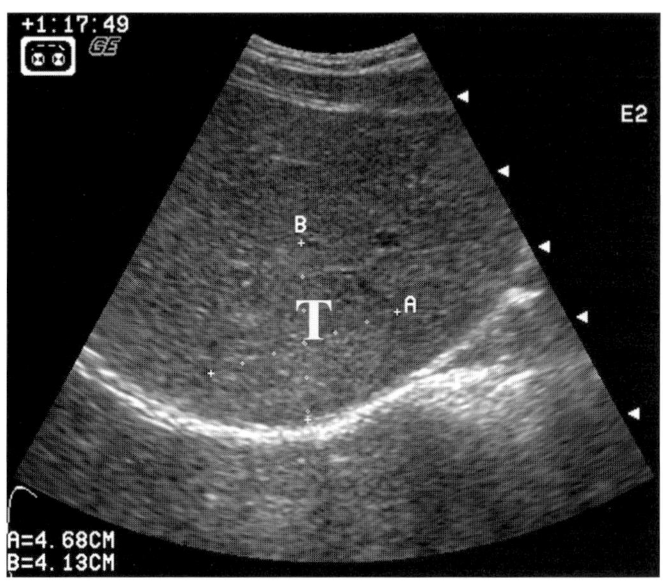

(A)

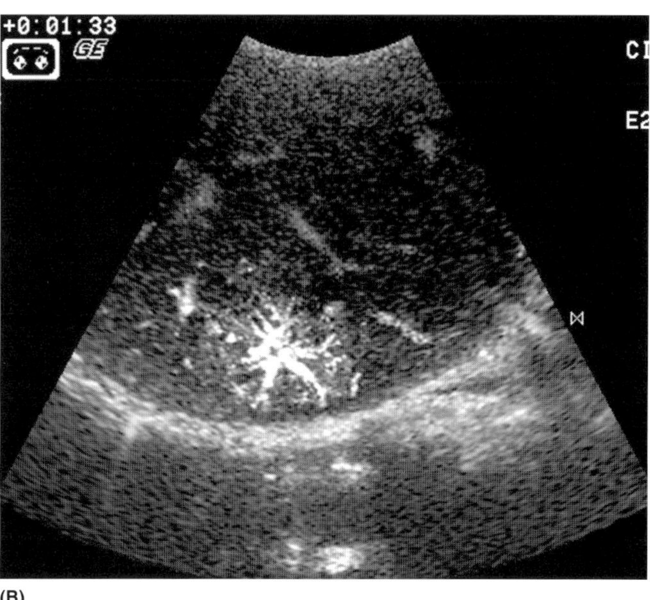

(B)

FIGURE 12 A AND B ■ (**A**) Conventional grayscale imaging shows an isoechoic lesion (T) in the right lobe of liver. (**B**) After a bolus injection of contrast agent, the tumor demonstrates a central star-like pattern of enhancement, consistent with a diagnosis of focal nodular hyperplasia. *Source*: Courtesy of Dr. Ding Hong, Shanghai, China.

$P < 0.001$ and $P < 0.001$ and hepatitis: 12.8 ± 4.1 and 7.8 ± 4.4 seconds, $P < 0.001$ and $P < 0.002$, respectively) (49). Hepatic transit time can also distinguish between cirrhosis and severe hepatitis from mild hepatitis although there is overlap between severe hepatitis and cirrhosis (48,49).

Interventional and Intraoperative Applications

The ablation of lesions with RF is a technique that is increasing in popularity, especially in the treatment of unresectable liver lesions. The ideal method for monitoring ablation during the procedure itself as well as for postablation followup has not been established. Conventional sonography, even when combined with color/power Doppler, does not accurately predict the effectiveness of ablation treatments. In fact, the assessment of vascularization and tissue perfusion is crucial to differentiate necrosis from residual viable tumor. Clinically, CEUS has been used in diagnosis of lesions before ablation as well as for monitoring the outcome of ablation procedures in the liver (Fig. 13) (50).

When sonography is used as the imaging modality for guiding ablations, the addition of a US contrast agent can provide important information including (*i*) pretreatment assessment of lesion vascularity and delineation of lesions poorly visualized with conventional imaging; (*ii*) guidance of the ablation needle into lesions not visualized or well delineated; (*iii*) immediate detection of blood flow in residual viable tumor; and (*iv*) postablation followup to assess treatment effectiveness.

CEUS has the potential to be very useful as it allows real-time assessment of lesion vascularity (51) and is similar to dynamic CT in its sensitivity and specificity (52,53). Grayscale PIHI is superior to contrast-enhanced power Doppler imaging (54) and both are superior to conventional sonography (55) in demonstrating residual tumor after thermal ablation. Similar findings have been described in a preliminary report on ablation of renal lesions (56). The use of CEUS for intraoperative evaluation of focal liver lesions should improve detection of subcentimeter nodules, show nodular vascularity with greater detail and, potentially, improve clinical outcomes (57).

Given the multifocal nature of prostate cancer, treatment of localized prostate cancer requires the destruction of the entire gland. Radiation therapy and radical prostatectomy are effective treatments but are associated with significant morbidity. In order to minimize the complications of therapy for prostate cancer, several alternative treatments for localized prostate cancer have emerged. Based on the biological behavior of prostate cancer, we proposed and performed research to evaluate a new therapeutic strategy for the treatment of prostate cancer: RF ablation of the whole prostate with CEUS guidance to monitor and control ablation in an animal model (58).

Our study demonstrated that CEUS can be used to differentiate thermal lesions from viable tissue during RF ablation of the prostate. We found that PIHI dramatically improved the visualization of the thermal RF lesions. The lesions appeared as hypoechoic avascular areas within the contrast-enhanced hyperechoic prostate parenchyma. Although i.v. infusion of contrast was useful for real-time monitoring of the ablation, bolus injection of contrast provides better definition of the thermal lesion and viable tissue. The thermal lesion volume was proportional to the power and time of ablation. There was no significant difference in the measured thermal

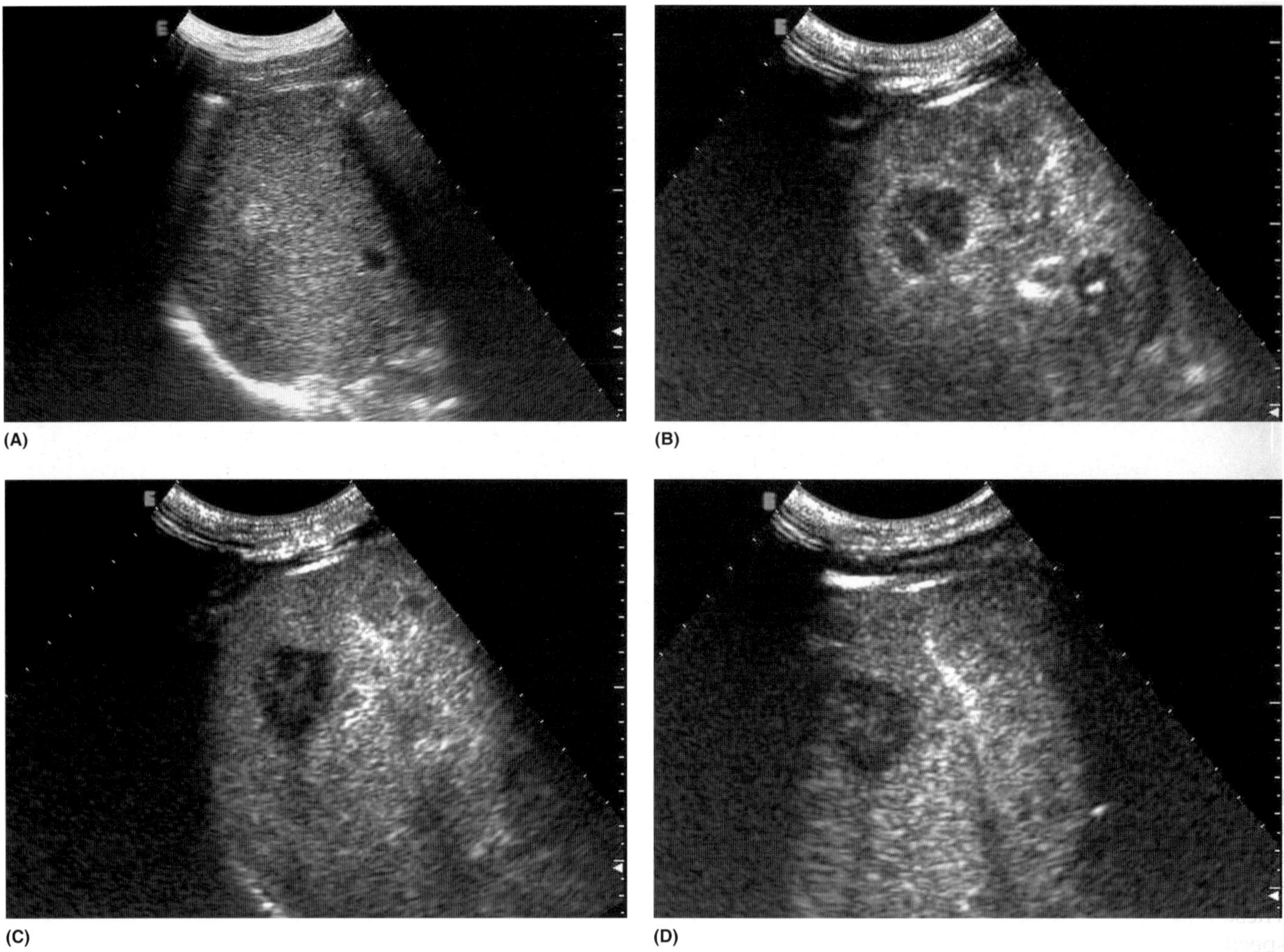

FIGURE 13 A–D ■ Pulse inversion harmonic images of a small liver tumor post-radiofrequency ablation demonstrates the avascular thermal lesion at (**A**) the baseline, (**B**) arterial phase (14 seconds post injection), (**C**) portal phase (47 seconds post injection), and (**D**) parenchymal phase (140 seconds post injection). *Source*: Courtesy of Dr. Zheng Rongqin, Guangzhou, China.

lesion size between US and pathology (US: 1.51 cm^3 ± 0.74 SD; Pathology: 1.46 cm^3 ± 0.74 SD; $p = 0.56$); likewise for the residual viable tissue (US: 0.43 cm^3 ± 0.043 SD; Pathology: 0.41 cm^3 ± 0.291 SD; $p = 0.21$) (Fig. 14). The average volume of prostate ablation achieved was 96.3% (Fig. 15) (58). The initial results showed that CEUS is a useful means to guide and monitor the RF ablation of the entire prostate. RF thermal ablation of the entire prostate guided by contrast US imaging could potentially provide a minimally invasive method for alternative treatment of prostate cancer.

Echocardiographic Applications

The U.S. Food and Drug Administration (FDA) and the European Union have approved several contrast agents for use during echocardiography to provide improved ventricular opacification and endocardial border definition in patients with technically suboptimal echocardiograms (Fig. 16). Contrast echocardiography includes applications for the right ventricle such as demonstration of shunts, abnormalities in the position or presence of the great vessels, and for the left ventricle such as cardiac structure, valvular function, and wall motion. Additional applications include perfusion quantification and reperfusion assessment of the myocardium (59,60).

The administration of contrast agents has been shown to enable more accurate measurement of left ventricular volume, ejection fraction, diagnosis and grading of valvular disease, intracardiac thrombus detection, aortic dissection, detection of complications of myocardial infarction (e.g., ventricular rupture and aneurysm formation), and improved assessment of systolic function compared to conventional echocardiography. In stress echocardiography, contrast agents increase the number of interpretable segments, which allows accurate assessment of left ventricular function (61). At the myocardial level, contrast agents can be used to diagnose infarction and assess tissue viability. Coronary artery stenoses can be localized and their severity quantified using intermittent HI. Coronary perfusion rates may be calculated using microbubble destruction and reperfusion techniques (62).

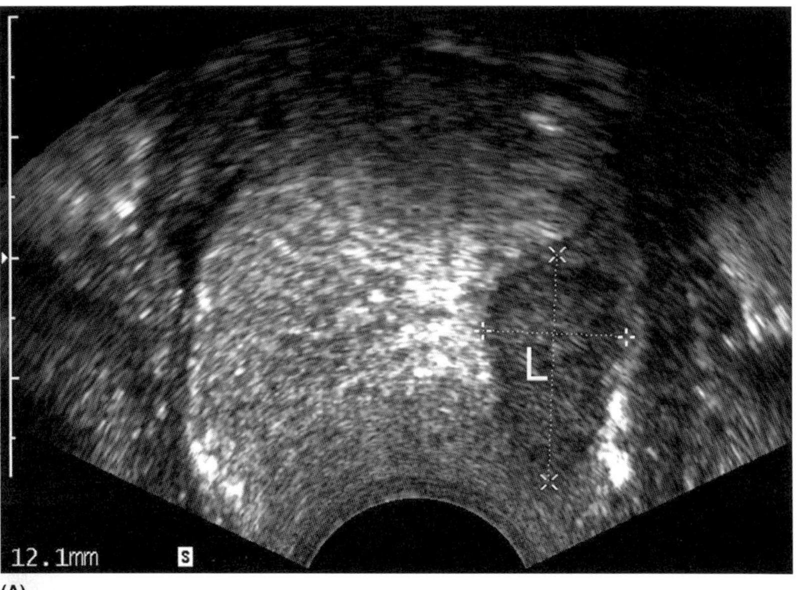

(A)

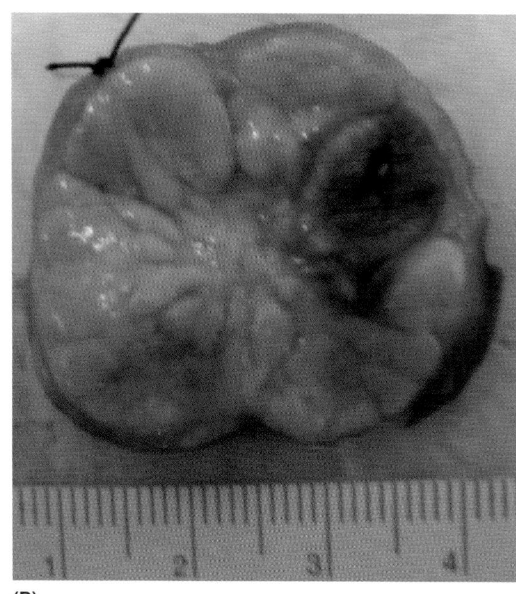

(B)

FIGURE 14 A AND B ■ (**A**) Contrast-enhanced pulse inversion harmonic imaging of a canine prostate after radiofrequency ablation identifies a demarcated thermal lesion within contrast-perfused normal parenchyma. This information is useful for monitoring RF ablation of the entire prostate. (**B**) Pathological specimen showing the coagulated lesion corresponding to the ultrasound findings. L, thermal lesion.

A recent study, led by Firschke in Germany, assessed the degree of infarction and ischemia of heart following a myocardial infarction with real-time myocardial contrast echocardiography (MCE) and compared the results to single photon emission computed tomography (SPECT). These researchers found that the overall sensitivity and specificity of MCE for detecting an abnormal segment on SPECT were 87% and 91%, respectively and intraobserver and interobserver agreement were 94% ($\kappa = 0.84$) and 92% ($\kappa = 0.83$), respectively. This study demonstrated that real-time MCE is a promising technique to determine infarct size after successful mechanical reperfusion of acute myocardial infarction (63).

Cerebrovascular Applications

Significant limitations exist in current transcranial Doppler US examinations; these include low reproducibility, inter-investigator variability, and inadequate access through the skull. Thus, transcranial Doppler examinations can be markedly improved with the addition of US contrast agents (64). US contrast agents provide better delineation

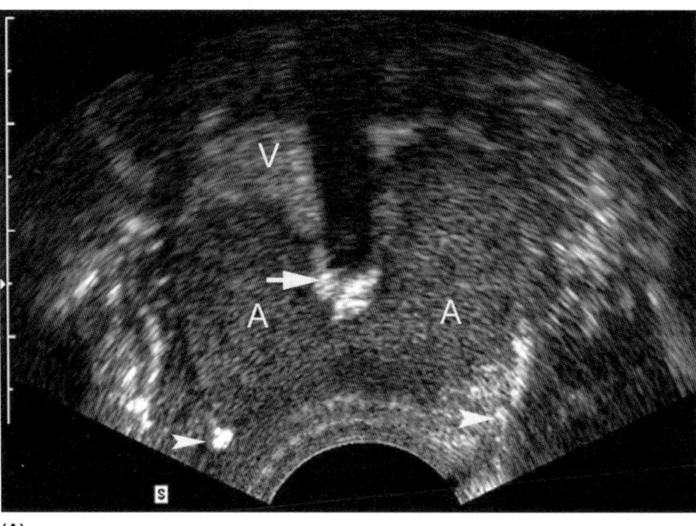

(A)

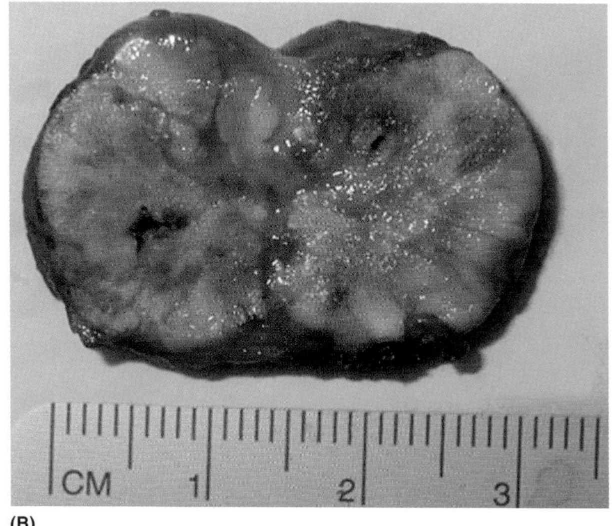

(B)

FIGURE 15 A AND B ■ (**A**) Contrast-enhanced phase/pulse inversion showed a residual viable area and radiofrequency-ablated area of the prostate with normal flow (*arrow*) of the urethral wall and the neovascular bundle areas (*arrowheads*). (**B**) Pathological examination confirmed ultrasound findings. V, viable area; A, RF-ablated area.

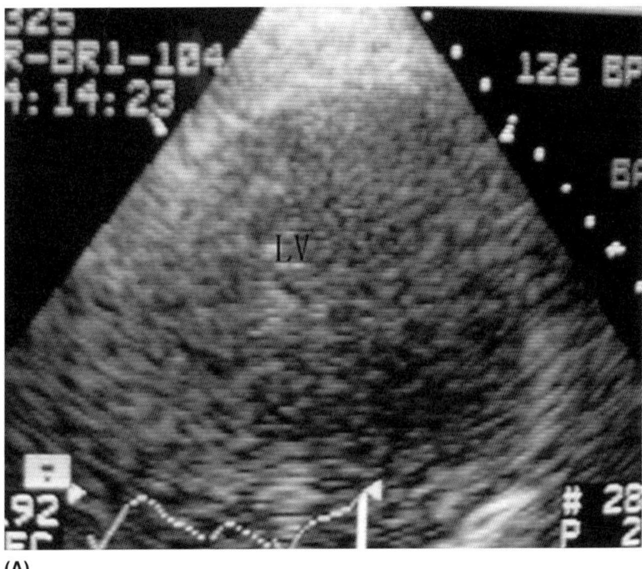

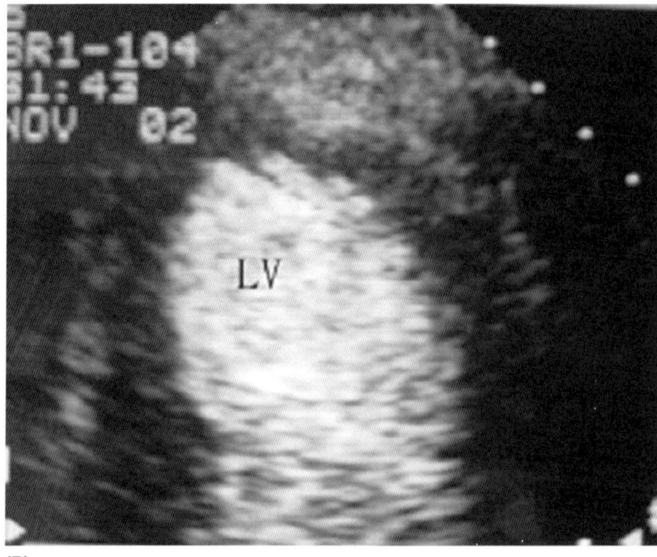

(A) (B)

FIGURE 16 A AND B ■ (**A**) Suboptimal echocardiography of the left ventricle (LV) shows inadequate endocardial border definition. (**B**) After intravenous contrast injection, complete opacification of the LV is obtained and the endocardial borders are clearly seen. *Source*: Courtesy of Dr. Shu Xianhong, Shanghai, China.

of normal blood flow, occlusions, pseudo-occlusions, stenoses, and collaterals in the extracranial and intracranial vascular beds (65). For examination of the extracranial carotid arteries, contrast administration can increase visualization of the residual lumen, increase diagnostic confidence, and decrease the number of indeterminate examinations. However, the applications of contrast agents to the carotid artery are in their infancy. Clinical trials are necessary to determine optimal techniques for contrast-enhanced carotid imaging.

Stroke is one of the leading causes of death and disabilities in Western countries. Although US imaging is a relatively simple, affordable, and widespread bedside imaging technique, evaluation of brain perfusion with conventional US imaging techniques is usually not reliable. However, the introduction of US contrasts agents and development of contrast-specific imaging modalities have helped to improve the diagnostic quality of transcranial US. CEUS techniques are used not only to aid the visualization of large cerebral vessels but also to assess the perfusion of the small vasculature that is not easily imaged by conventional US techniques (66).

Several studies on the visualization of cerebral perfusion in healthy human subjects after contrast injection have been published (67–69). These studies were predominantly conducted using harmonic grayscale imaging and evaluating the bolus kinetics. With bolus injection kinetics, different parameters of the CEUS can be extracted such as the time to peak intensity (TPI) and the peak intensity (PI). These parameters can be displayed as parametric images (70). A number of studies in patients with acute ischemic stroke demonstrated that CEUS showed sufficient insonation conditions for performing a perfusion study using HI modes (71–73). A combination of PI and TPI proved to be most helpful in detecting the area of infarction, with a sensitivity between 75% and 86% as well as a specificity between 96% and 100% (72,73).

Development of specifically targeted contrast agents could be useful for thrombus discrimination and brain tumor detection. Aside from diagnosis, therapeutic applications using contrast microbubbles as a drug carrier are under investigation. The expected outcome of these studies is that association of contrast microbubbles and a therapeutic substance should provide a synergistic thrombolytic effect (74,75). The concomitant monitoring with CEUS and thrombolytic agent therapy may be an efficient means for treating ischemic stoke patients with reduced systemic side effects.

Thyroid and Parathyroid Applications

US contrast agents have been used to obtain time-intensity curves of flow through thyroid nodules. Carcinomas showed a significantly earlier arrival time of the contrast agent than nodular hyperplastic benign nodules and adenomas (8.1 ± 1.41 seconds vs. 19.6 ± 2.2 and 16.1 ± 2.8 seconds; $P < 0.0001$). This technique has the potential to differentiate benign from malignant lesions and characterize hypovascularized malignant nodules, which could not be observed without contrast (76). In parathyroid lesions that do not show flow with conventional sonography, contrast agents can provide useful information by visualizing typical color Doppler signals of the parathyroid lesions. This can help to distinguish parathyroid nodules from thyroid lesions (77).

Gastrointestinal Applications

CEUS has been used to evaluate patients with portal hypertension by enhancing the Doppler signal and permitting better visualization of esophageal varices using transabdominal imaging (78) and perforating veins in recurrent varices (79). This technique has great potential for improving early detection of visceral varices and monitoring therapeutic response.

Bowel pathology may be diagnosed on the basis of altered vascularity. CEUS can be useful to detect bowel ischemia (80) and help differentiate benign from malignant GI stromal tumors (81). Assessment of inflammatory bowel disease can also be improved with the use of contrast agents by demonstrating increased vascularity in affected segments (82). This is of benefit in determining if active disease is present or only fibrosis even when the bowel wall does not show significant thickening (83). The same reasoning applies in the evaluation of pathologic hyperemic bowel (e.g., acute appendicitis) (84).

The common methods for examination of the GI tract are X ray with barium and endoscopy. Their shortcomings include the fact that they often cannot delineate submucosal mural structures of the GI tract. Limitations to the sonographic assessment of the upper GI tract and adjacent organs include patient body habitus and the presence of gas-filled bowel, which can produce shadowing artifacts. Although ingestion of degassed water has been used to improve sonographic assessments of the GI tract and such retroperitoneal structures as the pancreas, water simply displaces gas within the GI tract and can produce inconsistent results. Imaging water-filled bowel usually results in an increase in through transmission, which may cause tissues of otherwise normal echogenicity to appear more echogenic than expected, creating a potential source of diagnostic error. The ideal oral contrast agent should have the ability to improve the assessment of the GI tract and adjacent structures by absorbing and displacing bowel gas that limits visualization of structures such as pancreas, renal arteries, or para-aortic lymphadenopathy. One such agent is SonoRx™ (Bracco Diagnostics, Princeton, New Jersey, U.S.A.), which contains simethicone-coated cellulose. Ingestion of this agent results in a homogeneous transmission of sound through the contrast-filled stomach. SonoRx does not pass through the GI tract as quickly as water, and its acoustic attenuating properties more closely approximate those of soft tissue. Clinical trials have demonstrated that the administration of SonoRx increases diagnostic capabilities and, at times, obviates the need for additional imaging studies (85). Although SonoRx received U.S. FDA approval and was marketed for several years, it is no longer commercially available.

Another oral contrast agent SW-85 (Huqingyutang Pharmaceuticals Co., Hangzhou, China) has similar characteristics as SonoRx. Before an US examination, the patient can easily swallow the agent, filling the stomach. An enema of this agent can also be used for the examination of the lower GI tract. It produces uniform reflections within the bowel and reduces or eliminates artifacts due to bowel gas. In China, this agent has been used clinically for the diagnosis of GI tumors (Fig. 17), gastric and duodenal ulcerations (Fig. 18), and abnormalities involving the pancreas, lymph nodes, and other structures adjacent to the stomach (86).

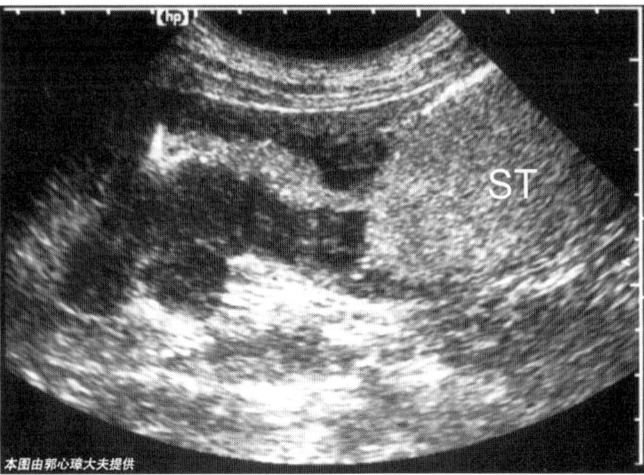

FIGURE 17 ■ Transverse ultrasound imaging of the stomach after ingestion of oral contrast shows irregular thickening of the walls of the pylorus with a narrowed gastric cavity, consistent with gastric cancer in the pyloric region. ST, stomach. *Source*: Courtesy of Dr. Guo Xinzhang, Hangzhou, China.

The use of orally administered US contrast agents for evaluation of bowel has been shown to be of value (87). Oral contrast agents significantly improve the ability to image both normal and abnormal structures in the GI tract and provide an acoustic window for evaluation of adjacent organs such as the pancreas (Fig. 19). Acoustic artifacts associated with bowel gas often prevent complete sonographic evaluation of the pancreas, which has led to CT as being the primary choice for the evaluation of this organ. Evaluation of oral US contrast agents has shown significant improvement in visualization of the stomach, pancreas, and adjacent structures. These oral agents conceivably could be, in the future, administrated prior to using an i.v. contrast agent to improve the ability of US to detect pancreatic tumors.

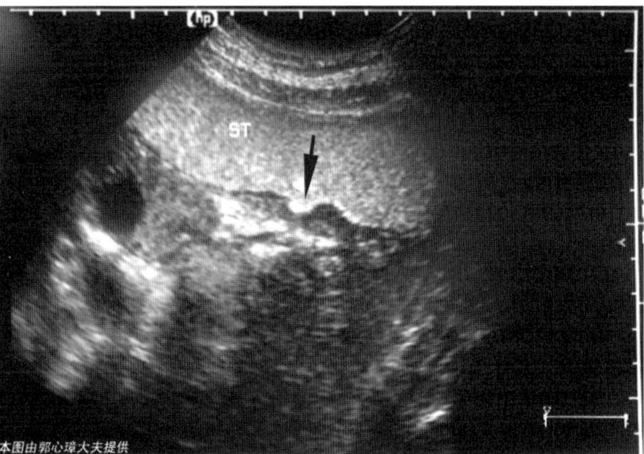

FIGURE 18 ■ Following the ingestion of oral contrast, ultrasound imaging shows a uniform and homogeneous echogenicity within the stomach. Note that a demarcated defect on the posterior wall of the stomach is clearly seen, which corresponds to an ulceration lesion. ST, stomach. *Source*: Courtesy of Dr. Guo Xinzhang, Hangzhou, China.

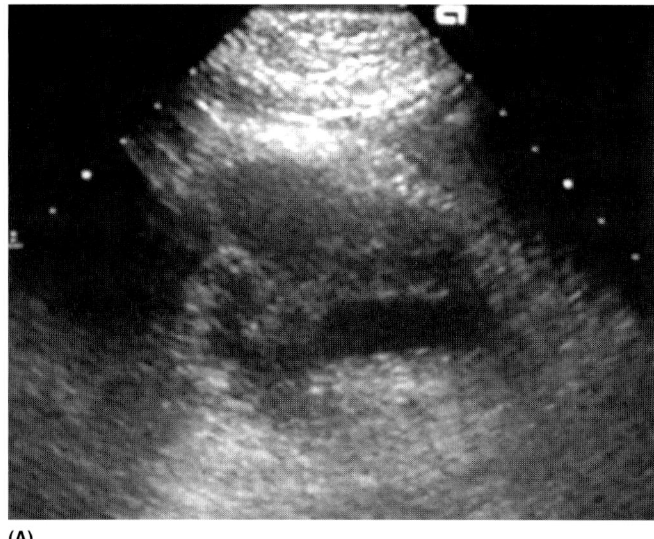

(A)

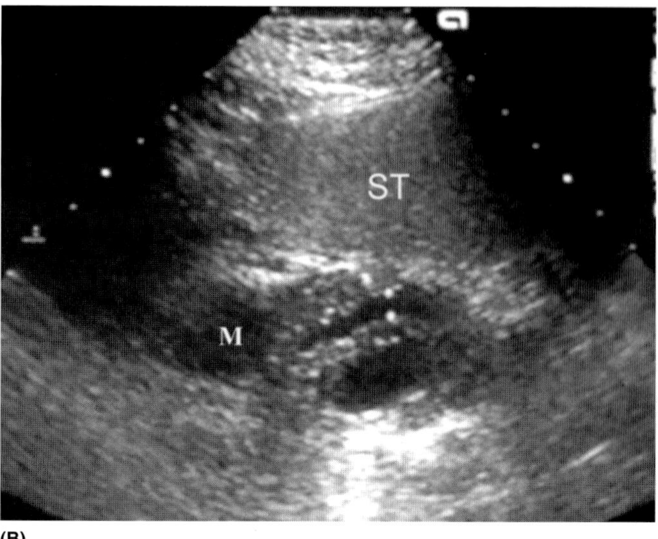

(B)

FIGURE 19 A AND B ■ (**A**) Precontrast transverse imaging of the mid epigastrium reveals partial obscuration of the head of the pancreas. (**B**) Postcontrast imaging shows a hypoechoic mass (M) at the head of the pancreas through a contrast-filled stomach (ST). Dilation of the pancreatic duct is also seen (calibers).

Biliary Applications

A few published reports describe the use of CEUS for the evaluation of abnormalities of the gallbladder and biliary tree (88–90). One report described how the detection and staging of malignant hilar obstructions of the biliary tree was improved by the use of Levovist in the postvascular phase compared to conventional sonography (88). Some studies have described how US contrast agents can improve visualization of blood flow in the gallbladder wall and hyperemia of the liver parenchyma adjacent to gallbladder in cases of acute cholecystitis (89,90).

Genitourinary Applications

CEUS can provide a clear and detailed view of renal vascularity, with early enhancement in the arterial phase followed by an intense, uniform enhancement in the renal cortex (i.e., a form of perfusion imaging). The enhancement then extends to the pyramids until they become isoechoic with the cortex.

The application of CEUS for characterization of renal tumors has great promise. CEUS has the potential to perform dynamic time-intensity curves (91), characterize focal renal lesions (92), and evaluate for the presence of a pseudo capsule in renal-cell carcinoma (93). Other potential renal applications of CEUS include the evaluation of renal perfusion, kidney transplants, and monitoring tumor ablation procedures.

Clinically, the most common diagnostic test for reflux is voiding cystourethrography (VCU). The main disadvantage of this method is the associated radiation exposure. Voiding urosonography (VUS) using a microbubble contrast agent has been introduced as an alternative technique in the diagnosis of vesicoureteral reflux in children (94). This technique uses a microbubble contrast agent administered retrograde into the bladder via an indwelling catheter and continuous sonography of the ureters and kidneys during filling and voiding to detect reflux. Contrast-enhanced VUS has been shown to be an accurate and reliable alternative to VCU and is now routinely used in clinical settings (94,95). Furthermore, the use of contrast-specific imaging technique PIHI can provide stronger and longer signal enhancement than conventional fundamental grayscale imaging, which improves the sensitivity and specificity for detection of vesicoureteral reflux (96–98).

Prostate Applications

The typical grayscale sonographic appearance of prostate cancer is a hypoechoic lesion, but prostate cancer can appear echogenic or isoechoic in up to 50% of cases. Color Doppler imaging (CDI) has been proposed to supplement conventional grayscale imaging in order to increase the overall sensitivity of sonography for the detection of prostate cancer. However, conventional grayscale and color/power Doppler-guided needle biopsy do not substantially improve the detection rate of prostate cancer (99). In order to more accurately detect the presence of prostate cancer, researchers have focused upon the detection of neovascularity in prostate cancer. The vascular supply to malignant prostate tissue differs from the vascularity of normal prostate tissue in density and distribution of microvessels. Studies of the prostate demonstrate a clear association of increased microvessel density with the presence of cancer (100). Quantitative assessment of microvascular density may provide important data to guide therapeutic decisions (101). Unfortunately, the microvessels that proliferate around and within prostate cancers cannot be seen with grayscale sonography and blood flow in the microvessels below the detectable limit of conventional Doppler US modes. One potential solution to this problem may be the use of US contrast agents to detect flow in microvessels associated with cancer. Preliminary studies show that contrast-enhanced grayscale and color flow detection of increased vascularity was associated with the presence of prostate cancer (99,102,103). These preliminary studies suggested that contrast agents might be useful for US evaluation of prostate vascularity to improve the detection of cancer (Fig. 20).

Transrectal US-guided biopsy is the standard method for diagnosing prostate cancer. Improved cancer detection with US contrast agents is related to better detection of tumor vascularity. Both contrast-enhanced color Doppler and harmonic grayscale imaging have been used successfully to improve imaging of prostate cancer and to guide targeted biopsy for definitive diagnosis of prostate cancer (104–107). A study led by Halpern to assess the value of CEUS directed biopsy of the prostate shows that cancer was identified in 30 biopsy sites in 16 of the patients (40%). A suspicious site identified during transrectal CEUS was 3.5 times more likely to have positive biopsy findings than an adjacent site that was not suggestive of malignancy ($p < 0.025$). When a suspicious site was evaluated with an additional biopsy core, the site was five times more likely to have a biopsy with positive findings than a standard sextant site ($p < 0.01$). The study suggests that CEUS improves the sonographic detection of malignant foci in the prostate and the performance of multiple biopsies of suspicious enhancing foci significantly improves the detection of cancer (108).

A recent study evaluated the impact of a combined approach of contrast-enhanced, color Doppler targeted biopsy (CECD) and systematic biopsy (SB) on the prostate cancer detection rate in 380 men with prostate specific antigen (PSA) 4.0 to 10 ng/mL. The cancer detection rate for the CECD, SB, and combined approaches was assessed. Prostate cancer was detected in 143 of 380 patients (37.6%, mean total PSA 6.2 ng/mL). The cancer detection rate of CECD and SB was 27.4% and 27.6%, respectively. The overall cancer detection rate with the two methods combined was 37.6%. For targeted biopsy cores, the detection rate was significantly better than for SB cores (32.6% vs. 17.9%, $p < 0.01$). CECD in a patient with cancer was 3.1-fold more likely to detect cancer than SB. This study suggests that CECD allows for the detection of lesions that cannot be found on grayscale

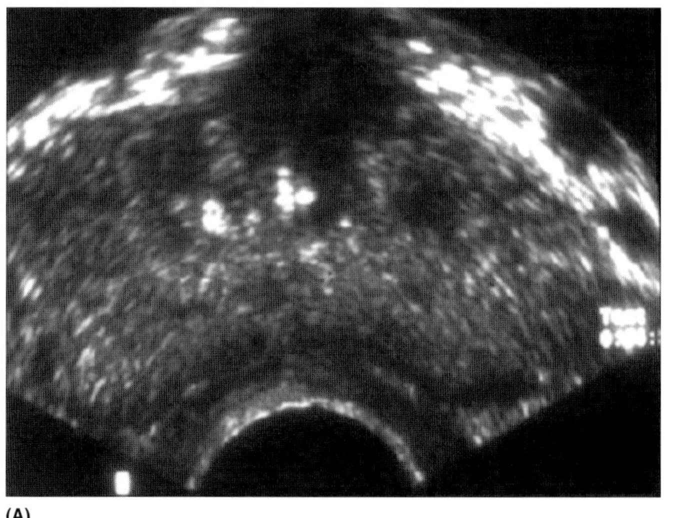

(A)

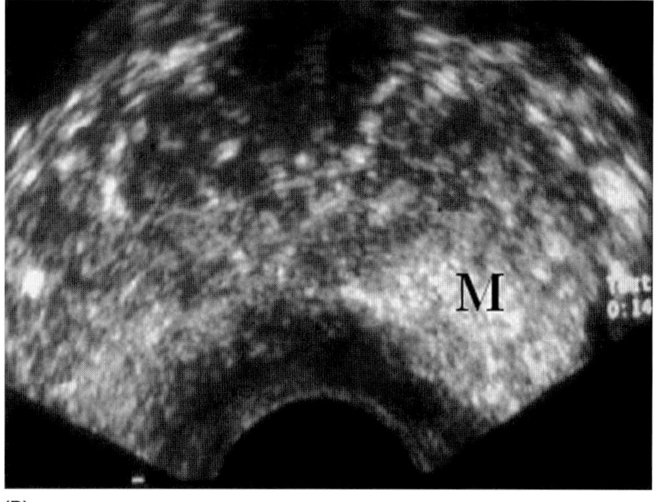

(B)

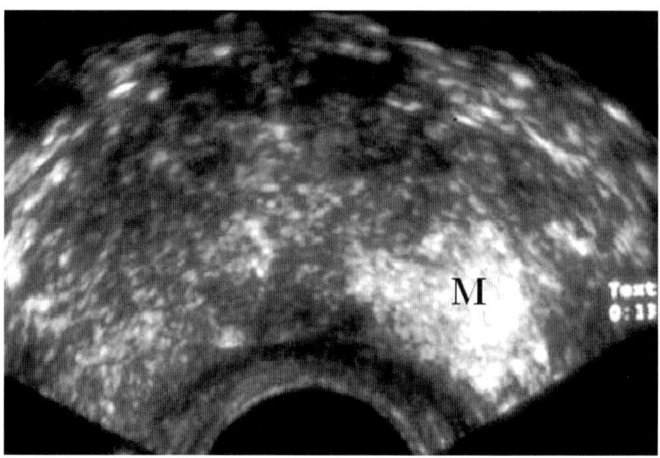

(C)

FIGURE 20 A–C ■ (**A**) Baseline conventional ultrasound imaging of the prostate reveals no evidence of abnormality. (**B**) Contrast-enhanced real-time pulse inversion harmonic imaging shows an enhanced focal area compared with the rest of the gland. (**C**) With intermittent imaging mode, the enhanced area is more dramatically seen. Pathology proved this hypervascular area to be prostate cancer. M, focal area.

US or SB and also allows for assessment of neovascularity associated with prostate cancer (109).

Pancreatic Applications

The diagnosis of pancreatic cancers, particularly their differential diagnosis from chronic pancreatitis, has often been difficult, even when a combination of various imaging modalities such as magnetic resonance cholangiopancreatography, endoscopic retrograde cholangiopancreatography, endosonography, contrast-enhanced CT, and angiography are employed. In a study by Kitano to assess the usefulness of coded PIHI for detection and differential diagnosis of pancreatic tumors, researchers found that CEUS demonstrated tumor vessels in 67% of pancreatic ductal carcinoma (110). In addition, the vascular patterns of tumors obtained with CEUS were closely correlated with those obtained by contrast-enhanced CT. Values for sensitivity in detecting pancreatic tumors 2 cm or less in size were 68% for contrast-enhanced CT and 95% for CEUS (110). Other preliminary reports show that CEUS improves the conspicuity of pancreatic carcinoma compared to conventional sonography (111,112). Quantitative analysis of the amount of contrast enhancement may be useful in separating benign and malignant pancreatic lesions (113). Additional work is needed to validate these preliminary findings.

Vascular Applications

Conventional sonographic detection of blood flow is limited by the depth and size of a vessel, the attenuation properties of intervening tissue, and low velocity flow. Limitations of US equipment sensitivity and the operator dependency of Doppler US can also impact the results of vascular examinations. Microbubble-based contrast agents enhance Doppler flow signals by providing more and better acoustic scatterers. This results in improved detection of blood flow from vessels that, without their use, are often difficult to assess, such as the renal arteries, hepatic arteries, intracranial vessels, and small capillaries within organs (i.e., tissue perfusion). Although US contrast agents can enhance Doppler (color and spectral) signals, it is more likely that grayscale HI will become a more useful alternative since it can provide high-resolution real-time assessment of flow without color Doppler artifacts.

Clinical reports have described how CEUS can improve visualization of the renal arteries and its branches and improve the detection of renal artery stenosis (RAS), reduce examination time, and improve the accuracy of these examinations (114,115). Improved detection of intra- and extrarenal arteries with contrast-enhanced CDI provides a superior roadmap of the vessels themselves and allows for more accurate placement of the spectral Doppler sample volume (Fig. 21). Several clinical contrast studies in the evaluation of RAS have produced encouraging results (99,100). In a multicenter trial, 191 patients referred for renal arteriography were examined with CEUS. The ability to image the renal arteries improved from 75% to 90% after contrast administration ($p < 0.001$). Accuracy in diagnosing RAS above 50% increased from 65% on noncontrast evaluations to 78% with the use of contrast (116,117).

Needleman reported on the use of contrast in a Phase III clinical trial including evaluations of RAS (118). Included in this series were 12 kidneys with dual renal arteries, identified with magnetic resonance angiography (MRA). Only two cases of dual renal arteries were identified with US prior to contrast administration, while nine of these were correctly identified with CEUS. Of the confirmed cases of RAS, three of 12 were only detected with CEUS. Missouris et al. reported their experience with Levovist for evaluation of 21 patients with suspected RAS (113). Sensitivity and specificity for the detection of RAS improved from 85% and 79%, respectively, on precontrast studies to 94% and 88% on Levovist-enhanced examinations.

Levovist was used in the studies of nine patients with suboptimal baseline peripheral arterial color Doppler

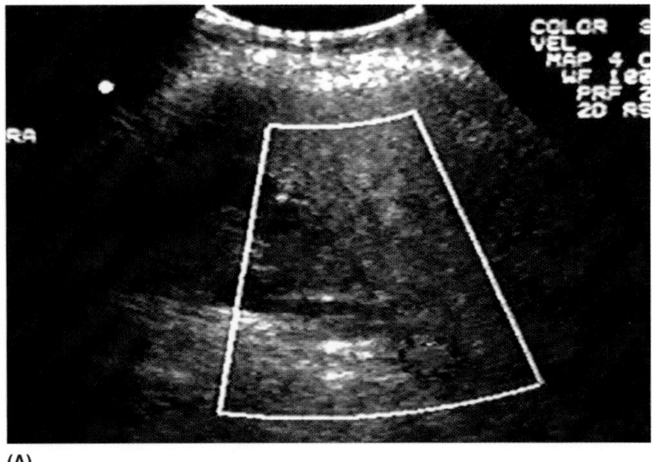

(A)

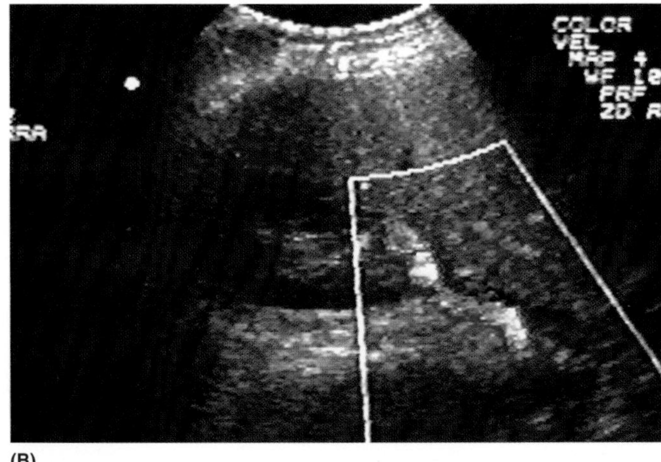

(B)

FIGURE 21 A AND B ■ In a patient with suspected right renal artery stenosis, color Doppler enhancement of the normal renal artery after intravenous injection of a contrast agent is clearly visible. With this information, renal artery stenosis was ruled out. (**A**) preinjection; (**B**) postinjection.

examinations (119). Three of these were examinations of infrainguinal vessels, one studied the digital arteries of the hand, and there was one study of an iliac artery. There were two occlusions and two stenoses. The occlusions showed no flow but collaterals were seen after contrast. In five vessels, no flow was seen at baseline but normal flow was confirmed after contrast administration. Spectral Doppler was entirely adequate in 19% of cases at baseline and significantly improved to 71% after both 200 and 300 mg/mL doses of Levovist.

Schwarz et al. reported the results of a multicenter Phase III trial of Levovist (120). The enrollment criterion was an inadequate baseline arterial Doppler examination. Patients in the peripheral vascular group received one or two doses of 200 mg/mL Levovist. The intensity of the contrast-enhanced pulsed Doppler signal increased compared to baseline. The investigators stated that their diagnostic confidence in the spectral Doppler waveforms increased from 35% pre-contrast to 91% post-contrast.

Hirai et al. (121) reported another multicenter Levovist trial from Japan with 41 patients, 36 with vascular disease and five with tumors of the extremities. The majority (n = 23) were evaluated for lower extremity arterial occlusive disease. A dose of 5 mL Levovist at a concentration of 300 mg/mL produced enhancement in all patients and was considered adequate in 90% of patients. The effect lasted at least two minutes in 85% of cases. The diagnosis was definitely improved in 40 of the 41 patients, all of whom had difficult or inadequate baseline sonography examinations.

Puls et al. (122) evaluated the value of Levovist injection in 31 patients with suspected deep venous thrombosis (DVT) and who had at least one segment that was inadequately evaluated after color Doppler sonography. All patients had a venogram as the gold standard. An inadequately seen segment was described as one where there was an insufficient color Doppler signal without obvious DVT by grayscale or spectral Doppler analysis. Levovist was injected through an arm vein at 300- or 400-mg/mL concentrations. Baseline conventional US was inadequate in 43 of 279 segments. Venous flow enhancement was seen in 40 of the 43 inadequate segments after arterial enhancement. DVT was detected in 27 segments. Accuracy increased from 26 of 43 (60%) precontrast to 37 of 43 (86%) to correctly identifying thrombosed venous segments after contrast administration.

US contrast agents have been used for surveillance of aortic stent grafts. One report described the evaluation of 30 patients who were serially evaluated with CEUS with results compared to either CTA or MRA. All confirmed endoleaks were detected by CEUS (123).

Research is being performed to develop contrast agents that will attach to thrombus and increase their grayscale echogenicity compared to the blood around them (124,125). If these attempts are successful, some of the false-positive conventional sonographic examinations may be avoided. Contrast-enhanced studies using these targeted agents could also be useful for differentiating flow defects that are not related to thrombus (e.g., scars or chronic changes to the vessel wall). Using these agents, the sensitivity of sonography could be improved if the increase in echogenicity can be detected even in technically limited examinations related to difficult-to-image patients or deep vessel location.

Trauma Applications

Traumatic lesions have common enhancement features on cross-sectional imaging, independent of the organ and tissues involved. The arterial tree is invariably involved in all damaged organs and CEUS easily detects parenchymal lesions, such as lacerations and hematomas, providing detailed information (126). Several clinical studies in assessment of liver trauma with CEUS have been reported. Poletti et al. prospectively evaluated CEUS and compared it to conventional US and CT in 210 patients with blunt abdominal trauma. They found that CT findings were positive for 88 solid organ injuries in 71 (34%) of the 210 patients. Conventional US and CEUS had a detection rate for solid organ injury of 57% and 80%, respectively. The improvement in the detection rate between conventional US and CEUS was statistically significant (p = 0.001) (127).

Another study by Catalano et al. showed that contrast enhancement to baseline sonographic survey of abdominal organs improves the effectiveness of sonography in the assessment of liver injuries. CEUS was more sensitive than unenhanced sonography in directly showing hepatic lesions (87% vs. 65%, 100% specificity) and correlated better with CT for injury size and capsule involvement (128).

In the evaluation of trauma to the abdomen, CEUS has the advantage of demonstrating viable tissue and improving contrast resolution to enhance differentiation between traumatic lesions and normal parenchyma. Although superior to conventional sonography, CEUS is not yet a replacement for contrast-enhanced CT (127,128). However, CEUS has several advantages over CT, including the ability to be performed at the bedside within the intensive care unit and to be used for serial evaluations to determine if there is continued active bleeding present. Thus, additional research in this area is warranted.

Lymphatic Applications

The importance of identifying sentinel lymph nodes (SLNs) has long been recognized for the effective treatment of a variety of malignancies including melanoma and breast, colon, and other cancers. The need to localize regional draining lymph nodes (i.e., SLNs) to which tumor cells from a primary tumor potentially can spread has lead to the development and clinical utilization of various techniques and imaging agents including the use of blue dye with surgical dissection and injection of radioactive material and evaluation with a gamma camera (i.e., lymphoscintigraphy). These techniques are used prior to or at the time of surgery, but there are potential limitations and adverse effects with these established approaches.

For instance, the use of blue dye to identify SLNs requires surgical dissection that, in some cases, can be extensive and there is a danger of anaphylactic reactions

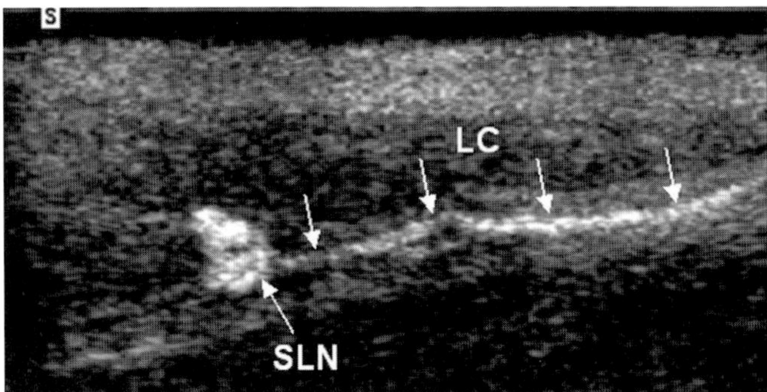

FIGURE 22 ■ Following subcutaneous injection of a contrast agent in an animal model, pulse inversion harmonic imaging identifies a contrast-filled lymphatic channel (LC) (*arrows*) and its sentinel lymph node (SLN). *Source*: From Ref. 134.

to the dye. Lymphoscintigraphy requires the use of radiation; thus, there is exposure to the patient as well as surgeon and support personnel. Furthermore, reports on the use of both of these established methods indicate that there can be leakage of the injected materials beyond the SLNs (i.e., to second echelon nodes), potentially resulting in more time consuming and extensive resection than may be needed (129,130).

The use of US contrast agent to image lymph nodes was proposed and investigated (131). Our group has evaluated the feasibility and usefulness of CEUS with intradermal injections of a tissue-specific microbubble agent for the detection of SLNs in animal models (132,133). The studies were designed to evaluate the potential of CEUS to identify lymphatic channel (LCs) and SLNs using US after subcutaneous or intraparenchymal injection of a US contrast agent in a variety of anatomical locations in animal models. We have termed this technique "lymphosonography."

The tissue-specific US contrast agent Sonazoid (GE Healthcare, Oslo, Norway) was injected intraparenchymally into a variety of organs including the testes, prostate, bowel, and breast as well as subcutaneously into areas around the orbit as well as in the trunk, neck, and extremities. Injections of blue dye at the same sites were used as the gold standard and to guide surgical dissections of the LCs and SLNs with results compared to the lymphosonographic findings.

Using grayscale PIHI at low acoustic power contrast could be detected within the regional draining LCs in some cases just a few seconds after the subcutaneous injections of Sonazoid. The flow of contrast could be seen with real-time PIHI within the LCs, which could then be traced to the SLNs (Fig. 22). Contrast-filled LCs could be followed for distances of up to 38 cm from the injection sites to the regional draining-enhanced SLNs. A variety of lymphatic drainage patterns were identified depending on where the injections were administered (e.g., head, trunk, or limbs). Contrast enhancement of SLNs persisted for up to four hours. The presence of contrast within the LCs and SLNs was confirmed with acoustic emission imaging using higher-power CDI resulting in a typical color pattern only seen within the areas that contained contrast (Fig. 23). When Sonazoid was injected into the testes, prostate, and bowel, the LCs and regional-draining LCs and SLNs of these organs could be detected and followed to their SLNs (Fig. 24). Surgical dissections after blue dye injections confirmed that LCs and SLNs detected with lymphosonography were the regional draining LCs and SLNs.

The presence of metastasis within SLNs is among the strongest known prognostic indicators for the survival and recurrence in patients with breast cancer (135). The ability to detect the draining lymph nodes from tumors (i.e., the SLNs) is an important part of routine clinical

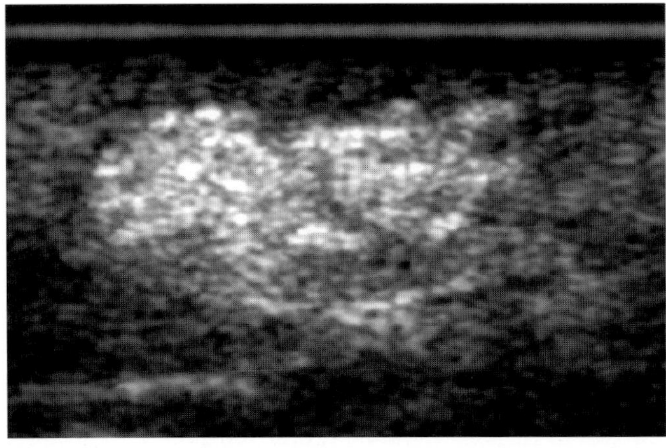

(A)

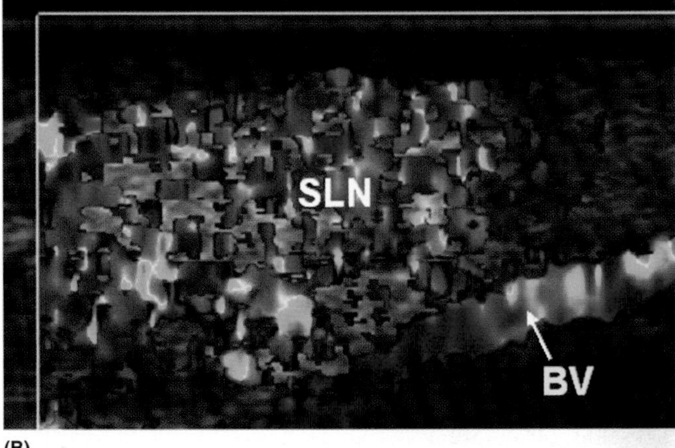

(B)

FIGURE 23 A AND B ■ (A) Grayscale phase/pulse inversion of a normal sentinel lymph node (SLN), demonstrates increased echogenicity of the SLN after subcutaneous injection of a contrast agent. (B) Color Doppler imaging (CDI) with acoustic emission technique showed mosaic color display within the SLN. Acoustic emission imaging provides a means to differentiate structures that contain contrast microbubbles from those that do not. Note how the CDI appearance of the SLN is distinctly different from that of blood flow in an adjacent vessel (BV).

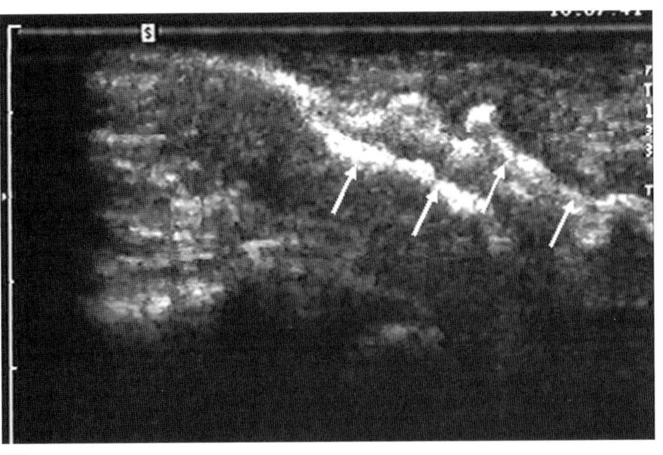

(A)

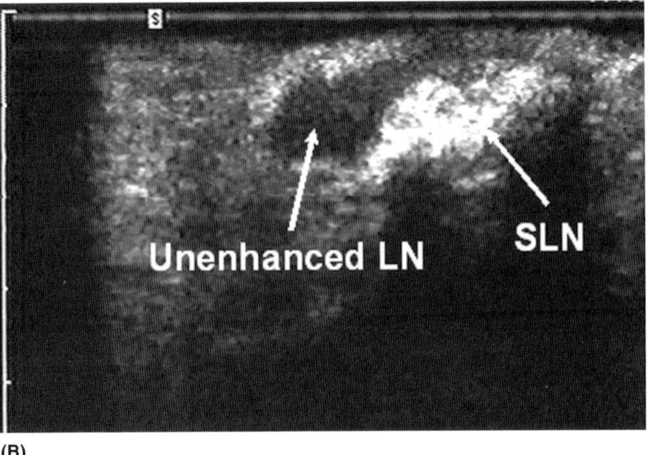

(B)

FIGURE 24 A AND B ■ (**A**) After Sonazoid was injected submucosally into the rectal wall of a canine, multiple relatively lymphatic channel (LCs) (*arrows*) could be identified with transabdominal real-time phase/pulse inversion (PIHI). (**B**) The contrast-filled LCs were followed into the deep pelvis and ultimately drained into a sentinel lymph node (SLN). Note the hypoechoic appearance of an unenhanced lymph node adjacent to the contrast-enhanced SLN. *Source*: From Ref. 134.

management that is considered essential in the care of many patients with malignancies (136,137). With the established methods currently used for clinical practice (e.g., lymphoscintigraphy or injection of blue dye), it is impossible to demonstrate the internal architecture of SLNs (138), which is important for the detection of SLN metastases. We have used a naturally occurring melanoma tumor model (Sinclair swine) to demonstrate that lymphosonography can be used to evaluate SLNs for metastasis (Figs. 25 and 26). In this preliminary study, we found that the accuracy of SLN detection was 90% (28 of 31) for lymphatic US and 81% (25 of 31) for lymphoscintigraphy ($P = 0.29$). Lymphosonography correctly depicted metastases in 19 of 20 SLNs, and five of the eight normal SLNs were correctly characterized, for an accuracy of 86% ($\kappa = 0.62$) (132). These experiments demonstrated lymphosonography could provide a minimally invasive technique that may be used to map lymphatic drainage, localize draining SLNs, and evaluate the SLN for metastases.

FIGURE 25 ■ In a swine melanoma model, contrast-enhanced ultrasound imaging identifies a metastatic sentinel lymph node (*arrows*), which appears as partially enhanced normal lymphatic tissue and hypoechoic tumor deposits. N, lymphatic tissue; T, hypoechoic tumor.

We also performed research to determine the fate of Sonazoid microbubbles after subcutaneous injection and uptake by the lymphatic system in an attempt to explain the mechanism of US contrast retention in, and enhancement of, the SLNs in an animal model (134). With the use of a transmission electron microscope at a magnification range of 3000× to 15,000×, the ultrastructural analysis of the contrast-enhanced SLNs revealed multiple intracytoplasmic spherical vacuoles within histiocytes (i.e., macrophages). The vacuoles ranged in size from 1.07 to 1.99 μm, with variation relating to different planes of section through the spherical structures (Fig. 27). Histiocytes in the control nodes did not contain these vacuoles. Thus, this confirms that the Sonazoid microbubbles are phagocytized and retained within the SLN macrophages in a similar manner as has been shown in the liver RES cells (31,134).

Although it is unlikely that minimal tumor deposits would be detected with lymphosonography, the ability to identify larger tumor deposits could potentially prove useful to indicate the likelihood of the cancer to have spread beyond the SLN. This concept is currently under investigation. Lymphosonography also has the potential to enhance US-guided needle biopsies of SLNs to improve tissue sampling for definitive pathologic assessment.

Gene and Drug Delivery and Targeted Agents

Most of the current contrast agents comprise free-flowing microbubbles (also referred to as intravascular or blood-pool agents). Apart from its diagnostic value, much effort has been made in the development of targeted contrast agents, using ligands (e.g., antibodies or synthetic peptides) to specifically bind and accumulate at a desired site and selectively enhance it by US imaging.

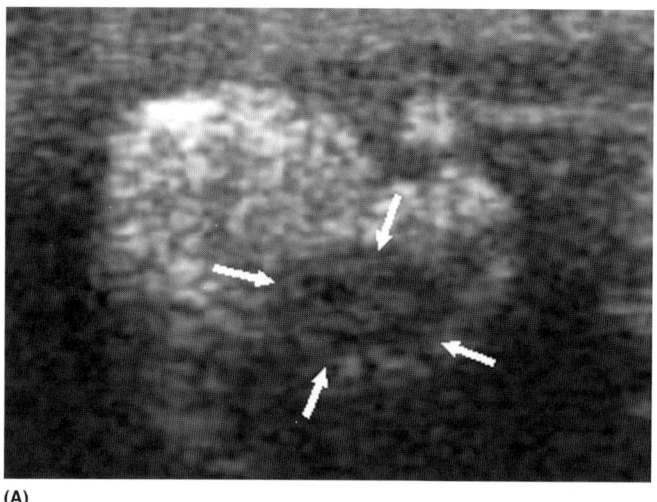

(A)

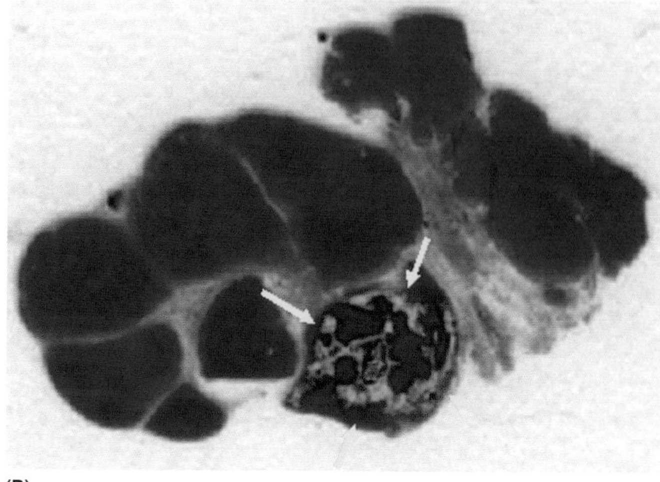

(B)

FIGURE 26 A AND B ■ (**A**) Contrast-enhanced imaging of a small sentinel lymph node (SLN) in a melanoma swine model shows a hypoechogenic metastatic infiltration area (*arrows*) within echogenic normal parenchyma of the lymph node. (**B**) Pathological examination confirmed the ultrasound findings.

Sonographic imaging of specific tissues using targeted microbubbles represents a new approach that departs from the concept that microbubbles passively transit the microcirculation like red blood cells. This involves the design and synthesis of microbubbles that will adhere to the endothelium or other targets under disease-specific conditions (such as inflammation). To the extent that the microbubbles are designed to adhere to molecular epitopes on the surface of the abnormal endothelium, targeted contrast imaging could provide capabilities for in vivo sonographic detection of phenotypic features of endothelium that predate clinical disease and/or are otherwise not detectable using currently available technologies (139–141). Investigators have demonstrated that targeted contrast microbubbles can be phagocytosed intact by activated neutrophils and monocytes and can be detected by US imaging. These findings suggest that contrast-enhanced US may used for molecular imaging as a useful means for the noninvasive assessment of inflammation and for following the response to treatment (142).

FIGURE 27 ■ Electron microscopy of an sentinel lymph node (SLN). Scanning electron microscopy identified multiple spherical empty vacuoles ranging in size from 1.07 to 1.99 μm, which were not present in control SLNs. These vacuoles (V) represent phagocytized intact contrast microbubbles. *Source*: From Ref. 134.

Targeted imaging using US contrast microbubbles has advantages over other molecular imaging methods. Unlike nuclear imaging approaches, blood-pool US contrast microbubbles stay within the vascular space and have a short circulation time. This is useful to the extent that the technique is not susceptible to nonspecific signals resulting from extravasation of the imaging agent or retention in nontarget organs such as the liver. However, these features are intrinsically limited to the interrogation of phenomena occurring on the surface of endothelial cells, thus excluding its application to many important physiologic processes that occur intracellularly and outside the vascular space. Recent reports of acoustically active nanoparticle emulsions (or gas-filled nanobubbles) capable of exiting the vascular space may offer an exciting solution to this challenge (143).

Another possible therapeutic application of US energy and microbubbles is gene delivery. To avoid safety concerns raised with the use of viral vectors, great efforts have been invested in the development of nonviral approaches. One approach for improving efficiency of nonviral delivery of genes is to use US energy. US can enhance gene transfer by increasing cell permeability (144) and sonoporation (145). Several in vivo studies have shown that reporter genes associated with cationic microbubbles can be delivered to the myocardium or to the skeletal muscles after an i.v. injection and an appropriate insonation (141,146). Subsequent protein expression has been observed.

Targeted microbubbles may ultimately have utility beyond their diagnostic attributes. Sonographic destruction

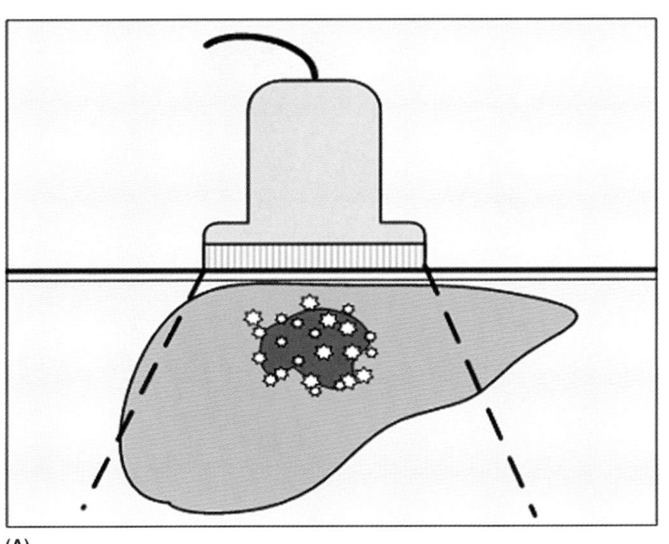

(A)

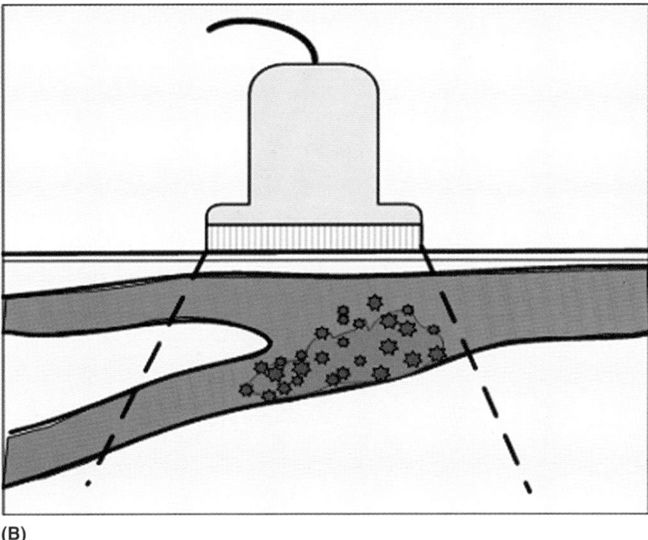

(B)

FIGURE 28 A AND B ■ Diagrams showing a tumor-specific contrast agent (**A**) for liver tumor imaging and therapeutic contrast agent (**B**) for thrombolysis.

of microbubbles appears to enhance delivery of genes, drugs, and lysis of clots (Fig. 28) (147–149). The ability to target therapeutics by designing the delivery agent (microbubbles) to the site of interest may ultimately prove to be another powerful clinical application of this rapidly advancing technology.

SUMMARY

In conclusion, US contrast agents that are nontoxic, administered intravenously, and are stable for recirculation are already being used routinely for a variety of clinical applications. Present and future US contrast agents should provide for increased diagnostic capabilities in a variety of applications. These agents enhance the detection of both normal and abnormal vascularity, delineate areas of ischemia, and improve visualization of many abnormalities, including the detection and characterization of tumors in such organs as the liver. Future developments including the continued modification of US equipment to better exploit the enhancement properties of contrast agents should increase the capability of these agents to improve the sensitivity and specificity of sonography. The field of targeted contrast agents is still in its infancy and, as with the field of molecular imaging in general, much remains to be done to develop this area into a clinical reality.

REFERENCES

1. Harvey CJ, Pilcher JM, Eckersley RJ, et al. Advances in ultrasound. Clin Radiol 2002; 57:157–177.
2. Forsberg F, Shi WT. Physics of contrast microbubbles. In: Goldberg BB, Raichen JS, Forsberg F, eds. Ultrasound Contrast Agents. 2nd ed. London: Martin Dunitz, 2001.
3. Lencioni R, Cioni C, Bartolozzi C. Tissue harmonic and contrast-specific imaging: back to gray scale in ultrasound. Eur Radiol 2002; 12:151–165.
4. Hohmann J, Albrecht T, Oldenburg A, et al. Liver metastases in cancer: detection with contrast-enhanced ultrasonography. Abdom Imaging 2004; 29:669–681.
5. Barr R. Seeking Consensus: contrast ultrasound in radiology. Eur J Radiol 2002; 41:207–216.
6. Simpson DH, Chin CT, Burns PN. Pulse inversion Doppler: a new method for detecting nonlinear echoes from microbubble contrast agents. IEEE Trans Ultrason Ferroelec Freq Contr 1999; 46:372–382.
7. Forsberg F, Liu JB, Chiou HJ, et al. Comparison of fundamental and wideband harmonic contrast imaging of liver tumors. Ultrasonics 2000; 38:110–113.
8. Wilson SR, Burns PN, Muradali D, et al. Harmonic hepatic US with microbubble contrast agent: initial experience showing improved characterization of hemangioma, hepatocellular carcinoma, and metastasis. Radiology 2000; 215:153–161.
9. Albrecht T, Blomley M, Bolondi L, et al. Guidelines for the use of contrast agents in ultrasound. Ultraschall Med 2004; 25:249–256.
10. Porter TR, Xie F. Transient myocardial contrast after initial exposure to diagnostic ultrasound pressures with minute doses of intravenously injected microbubbles. Circulation 1995; 92:2391–2395.
11. Colon PJ, Richards DR, Moreno CA, et al. Benefits of reducing the cardiac cycle-triggering frequency of ultrasound imaging to increase myocardial opacification with FS069 during fundamental and second harmonic imaging. J Am Soc Echocardiogr 1997; 10:602–607.
12. Broillet A, Puginier J, Ventrone R, et al. Assessment of myocardial perfusion by intermittent harmonic power Doppler using SonoVue, a new ultrasound contrast agent. Invest Radiol 1998; 33:209–215.
13. Porter TR, Kricsfeld D, Cheatham S, et al. The effect of ultrasound frame rate on perfluorocarbon-exposed sonicated dextrose albumin microbubble size and concentration when insonifying at different flow rates, transducer frequencies and acoustic outputs. J Am Soc Echocardiogr 1997; 10:593–601.
14. Kamiyama N, Moriyasu F, Mine Y, et al. Analysis of flash echo from contrast agent for designing optimal ultrasound diagnostic systems. Ultrasound Med Biol 1999; 25:411–420.
15. Wei K, Jayaweera AR, Firoozan S, et al. Quantification of myocardial blood flow with ultrasound-induced destruction of microbubbles administered as a constant venous infusion. Circulation 1998; 97:473–483.

16. Bouakaz A, Krenning BJ, Vletter WB, et al. Contrast superharmonic imaging: a feasibility study. Ultrasound Med Biol 2003; 29: 547–553.
17. Kim JH, Eun HW, Lee HK, et al. Renal perfusion abnormality. Coded harmonic angio US with contrast agent. Acta Radiol 2003; 44:166–171.
18. Murthy TH, Locricchio E, Kuersten B, et al. Power Doppler myocardial contrast echocardiography using an improved multiple frame triggered Harmonic Angio technique. Echocardiography 2001; 18:191–196.
19. Kaul S. Instrumentation for contrast echocardiography: technology and techniques. Am J Cardiol 2002; 90(suppl):8J–14J.
20. Van Camp G, Ay T, Pasquet A, et al. Quantification of myocardial blood flow and assessment of its transmural distribution with real-time power modulation myocardial contrast echocardiography. J Am Soc Echocardiogr 2003; 16:263–270.
21. Ro RJ, Forsberg F, Lipcan KJ, et al. Comparing contrast-enhanced US to markers of angiogenesis in a murine glioma model. Proc IEEE US Symp 2005:365–368.
22. Shankar PM, Dala Krishna P, Newhouse VL. Advantages of subharmonic over second harmonic backscatter for contrast-to-tissue echo enhancement. Ultrasound Med Biol 1998; 24:395–399.
23. Forsberg F, Jiu JB, Shi WT, et al. In vivo perfusion estimation using subharmonic contrast microbubble signals. J Ultrasound Med 2006; 25(1):15–21.
24. Isozaki T, Numata K, Kiba T, et al. Differential diagnosis of hepatic tumors by using contrast enhancement patters at US. Radiology 2003; 229(3):798–805.
25. Leen E. Radiological applications of contrast agents in the hepatobiliary system. In Goldberg BB, Raichlen JS, Forsberg F, eds. Ultrasound contrast agents. 2nd ed. London: Martin Dunitz Ltd., 2001:278–288.
26. Blomley MJK, Albrecht T, Cosgrove DO, et al. Improved imaging of liver metastases with stimulated acoustic emission in the late phase of enhancement with the US contrast agent SH U 508A: early experience. Radiology 1999; 210:409–416.
27. Forsberg F, Liu JB, Merton DA, et al. Gray scale second harmonic imaging of acoustic emission signals improves detection of liver tumors in rabbits. J Ultrasound Med 2000; 19:557–563.
28. Koda M, Matsunaga Y, Ueki M, et al. Qualitative assessment of tumor vascularity in hepatocellular carcinoma by contrast-enhanced coded ultrasound: comparison with arterial phase of dynamic CT and conventional color/power Doppler ultrasound. Eur Radiol 2004; 14(6):1100–1108.
29. Wilson SR, Burns PN, Muradali D, et al. Harmonic hepatic US with microbubble contrast agent: initial experience showing improved characterization of hemangioma, hepatocellular carcinoma, and metastasis. Radiology 2000; 215:153–161.
30. Nicolau C, Vilana R, Catala V, et al. Important of evaluating all vascular phases on contrast-enhanced sonography in the differentiation of benign from malignant focal liver lesions. AJR Am J Roentgenol 2006; 186:158–167.
31. Kindberg GM, Tolleshaug H, Roos N, et al. Hepatic clearance of Sonazoid perfluorobutane microbubbles by Kupffer cells does not reduce the ability of liver to phagocytose or degrade albumin microspheres. Cell Tissue Res 2003; 312(1):49–54.
32. Weskott HP. Contrast-enhanced Reperfusion imaging in atypical hepatic hemangiomas. J Ultrasound Med 2001; 20:S9.
33. Solbiati L, Cova L, Ierace T, et al. Diagnosis of atypical hemangioma using contrast-enhanced wideband harmonic sonography (CE-WBHS). J Ultrasound Med 2001; 20:S9.
34. Kim EA, Yoon KH, Lee YH, et al. Focal hepatic lesions: contrast-enhancement patterns at pulse-inversion harmonic US using a microbubble contrast agent. Korean J Radiol 2003; 4:224–233.
35. Solbiati L, Cova L, Ierace T, et al. Characterization of focal lesions in patients with liver cirrhosis using second generation contrast-enhanced (CE) wideband harmonic sonography (WBHS) in different enhancement phases. J Ultrasound Med 2001; 20:S10.
36. Leutoff UC, Scharf J, Richter GM, et al. Use of ultrasound contrast medium Levovist in after-care of liver transplant patients: improved vascular imaging in color Doppler ultrasound. Radiology 1998; 38:399–404.
37. Sidhu PS, Marshall MM, Ryan SM, et al. Clinical use of Levovist, an ultrasound contrast agent, in the imaging of liver transplantation: assessment of the pre- and post-transplant patient. Eur Radiol 2000; 10(7):1114–1126.
38. Bartolotta TV, Midiri M, Quaia E, et al. Benign focal liver lesions: spectrum of findings on SonoVue-enhanced pulse-inversion ultrasonography. Eur Radiol 2005; 15:1643–1649.
39. Passamonti M, Vercelli A, Azzaretti A, et al. Characterization of focal liver lesions with a new ultrasound contrast agent using continuous low acoustic power imaging: comparison with contrast enhanced spiral CT. Radiol Med (Torino) 2005; 9:358–369.
40. Ricci P, Laghi A, Cantisani V, et al. Contrast-enhanced sonography with SonoVue: enhancement patterns of benign focal liver lesions and correlation with dynamic gadobenate dimeglumine-enhanced MRI. AJR Am J Roentgenol 2005; 184:821–827.
41. Luo BM, Wen YL, Yang HY, et al. Differentiation between malignant and benign nodules in the liver: use of contrast C3-MODE technology. World J Gastroenterol 2005; 11:2402–2407.
42. Ignee A, Weiper D, Schuessler G, et al. Sonographic characterisation of hepatocellular carcinoma at time of diagnosis. Z Gastroenterol 2005; 43:289–294.
43. Giorgio A, Ferraioli G, Tarantino L, et al. Contrast-enhanced sonographic appearance of hepatocellular carcinoma in patients with cirrhosis: comparison with contrast-enhanced helical CT appearance. AJR Am J Roentgenol 2004; 183:1319–1326.
44. Kim SH, Lee JM, Lee JY, et al. Value of contrast-enhanced sonography for the characterization of focal hepatic lesions in patients with diffuse liver disease: receiver operating characteristic analysis. AJR Am J Roentgenol 2005; 184:1077–1084.
45. Ding H, Wang WP, Huang BJ, et al. Imaging of focal liver lesions: low-mechanical-index real-time ultrasonography with SonoVue. J Ultrasound Med 2005; 24:285–297.
46. Zhou X, Strobel D, Haensler J, et al. Hepatic transit time: indicator of the therapeutic response to radiofrequency ablation of liver tumours. Br J Radiol 2005; 78:433–436.
47. Niizawa G, Ikegami T, Matsuzaki Y, et al. Monitoring of hepatocellular carcinoma, following proton radiotherapy, with contrast-enhanced color Doppler ultrasonography. J Gastroenterol 2005; 40:283–290.
48. Albrecht T, Blomley MJ, Cosgrove DO, et al. Non-invasive diagnosis of hepatic cirrhosis by transit-time analysis of an ultrasound contrast agent. Lancet 1999; 353:1579–1583.
49. Hirota M, Kaneko T, Sugimoto H, et al. Intrahepatic circulatory time analysis of an ultrasound contrast agent in liver cirrhosis. Liver Int 2005; 25:337–342.
50. Hotta N, Tagaya T, Maeno T, et al. Advanced dynamic flow imaging with contrast-enhanced ultrasonography for the evaluation of tumor vascularity in liver tumors. Clin Imaging 2005; 29:34–41.
51. Solbiati L, Ierace T, Tonolini M, et al. Guidance and monitoring of radiofrequency liver tumor ablation with contrast-enhanced ultrasound. Eur J Radiol 2004; 51(suppl):S19–S23.
52. Vallone P, Gallipoli A, Izzo F, et al. Local ablation procedures in primary liver tumors: levovist US versus spiral CT to evaluate therapeutic results. Anticancer Res 2003; 23(6D):5075–5079.
53. Ding H, Kudo M, Onda H, et al. Evaluation of posttreatment response of hepatocellular carcinoma with contrast-enhanced coded phase-inversion harmonic US: comparison with dynamic CT. Radiology 2001; 221:721–730.
54. Meloni MF, Goldberg SN, Livraghi T, et al. Hepatocellular carcinoma treated with radiofrequency ablation: comparison of pulse inversion contrast-enhanced harmonic sonography, contrast-enhanced power Doppler sonography, and helical CT. AJR Am J Roentgenol 2001; 177:375–380.
55. Minami Y, Kudo M, Kawasaki T, et al. Treatment of hepatocellular carcinoma with percutaneous radiofrequency ablation: usefulness of contrast harmonic sonography for lesions poorly defined with B-mode sonography. AJR Am J Roentgenol 2004; 183:153–156.
56. Johnson DB, Duchene DA, Taylor GD, et al. Contrast-enhanced ultrasound evaluation of radiofrequency ablation of the kidney: reliable imaging of the thermolesion. J Endourol 2005; 19:248–252.
57. Torzilli G, Olivari N, Moroni E, et al. Contrast-enhanced intraoperative ultrasonography in surgery for hepatocellular carcinoma in cirrhosis. Liver Transpl 2004; 10(2 suppl 1):S34–S38.

58. Liu JB, Merton DA, Wansaicheong G, et al. Contrast-Enhanced US for Monitoring Radiofrequency Ablation of Canine Prostates: initial Results. J Urology 2006; 176:1654–1660.
59. Miller AP, Nanda NC. Contrast echocardiography: new agents. Ultrasound Med Biol 2004; 30:425–434.
60. Stewart MJ. Contrast echocardiography. Heart 2003; 89:342–348.
61. Cheng SC, Dy TC, Feinstein SB. Contrast echocardiography: review and future directions. Am J Cardiol 1998; 81(12A):41G–48G.
62. Cwaig J, Xie F, O'Leary E, et al. Detection of angiographically significant coronary artery disease with accelerated intermittent imaging after intravenous administration of ultrasound contrast material. Am Heart J 2000; 139:675–683.
63. Tousek P, Orban M, Martinoff S, et al. Assessment of infarcted myocardium with real time myocardial contrast echocardiography: comparison with technetium-99m sestamibi single photon emission computed tomography. Heart 2005; 91:1568–1572.
64. Della Martina A, Meyer-Wiethe K, Allemann E, et al. Ultrasound contrast agents for brain perfusion imaging and ischemic stroke therapy. J Neuroimaging 2005; 15:217–232.
65. Droste DW, Metz RJ. Clinical utility of echocontrast agents in neurosonology. Neurol Res 2004; 26:754–759.
66. Martina AD, Meyer-Wiethe K, Allemann E, et al. Ultrasound contrast agents for bran perfusion imaging and ischemic stroke therapy. J Neuroimaging 2005; 15:217–232.
67. Meyer K, Seidel G. Transcranial contrast diminution imaging of the human brain: a pilot study in healthy volunteers. Ultrasound Med Biol 2002; 28:1433–1437.
68. Eddying J, Krogias C, Wilkening W, et al. Parameters of cerebral perfusion in phase-inversion harmonic imaging (PIHI) ultrasound examinations. Ultrasound Med Biol 2003; 29:1379–1385.
69. Shiogai T, Takayasu N, Mizuno T, et al, Comparison of transcranial brain tissue perfusion images between ultraharmonic, second harmonic, and power harmonic imaging. Stroke 2004; 35:687–693.
70. Wiesmann M, Meyer K, Albers T, et al. Parametric perfusion imaging with contrast-enhanced ultrasound in acute ischemic stroke. Stroke 2004; 35:508–513.
71. Seidel G, Meyer-Wiethe K, Berdien G, et al. Ultrasound perfusion imaging in acute middle cerebral artery infarction predicts outcome. Stroke 2004; 35:508–513.
72. Seidel G, Albers T, Meyer K, et al. Perfusion harmonic imaging in acute middle cerebral artery infarction. Ultrasound Med Biol 2003; 29:1245–1251.
73. Federlein J, Postert T, Meves SH, et al. Ultrasonic evaluation of pathological brain perfusion in acute stroke using second harmonic imaging. J Neuol Neurosurg Psychiatry 2000; 69:616–622.
74. Viguier A, Rigal M, Petit R, et al. Microbubbles accelerate ultrasound-driven thrombolysis in acute middle cerebral artery stem occlusion. Stroke 2004; 35:297.
75. Garcia MJ. Therapeutic application of ultrasound contrast agents. In: Zamorano JL, Garcia Fernandez MA, eds. Contrast Echocardiography in Clinical Practice. Milan, Italy: Springer-Verlag, 2004:263–286.
76. Spiezia S, Farina R, Cerbone G, et al. Analysis of color Doppler signal intensity variation after levovist injection: a new approach to the diagnosis of thyroid nodules. J Ultrasound Med 2001; 20: 223–231;quiz 233.
77. Mazzeo S, Caramella D, Marcocci C, et al. Contrast-enhanced color Doppler ultrasonography in suspected parathyroid lesions. Acta Radiol 2000; 41:412–416.
78. Tamano M, Yoneda M, Kojima K, et al. Evaluation of esophageal varices using contrast-enhanced coded harmonic ultrasonography. J Gastroenterol Hepatol 2004; 19:572–575.
79. Sato T, Yamazaki K, Toyota J, et al. Perforating veins in recurrent esophageal varices evaluated by endoscopic color Doppler ultrasonography with a galactose-based contrast agent. J Gastroenterol 2004; 39:422–428.
80. Hata J, Kamada T, Haruma K, et al. Evaluation of bowel ischemia with contrast-enhanced US: initial experience. Radiology 2005; 236:712–715.
81. Fukuta N, Kitano M, Maekawa K, et al. Estimation of the malignant potential of gastrointestinal stromal tumors: the value of contrast-enhanced coded phase-inversion harmonics US. J Gastroenterol 2005; 40:247–255.
82. Robotti D, Cammarota T, Debani P, et al. Activity of Crohn disease: value of Color-Power-Doppler and contrast-enhanced ultrasonography. Abdom Imaging 2004; 29:648–652.
83. Rapaccini GL, Pompili M, Orefice R, et al. Contrast-enhanced power Doppler of the intestinal wall in the evaluation of patients with Crohn disease. Scand J Gastroenterol 2004; 39:188–194.
84. Incesu L, Yazicioglu AK, Selcuk MB, et al. Contrast-enhanced power Doppler US in the diagnosis of acute appendicitis. Eur J Radiol 2004; 50:201–209.
85. Lev-Toaff AS, Merton DA, Dumsha J, et al. Evaluation of an oral contrast agent to improve ultrasonic visualization of abdominal anatomy: a phase I trial. J Ultrasound Med 1994; 13:S8.
86. Guo XZ, Zhong SG, Zhang W. A new type of acoustic contrast for visualizing the upper digestive tract walls and pancreas. Program of the 3rd Congress of Asian Federation of Societies for Ultrasound in Medicine and Biology, Seoul, Korea, Aug 30 to Sep 3, 1992:129.
87. Parente F, Greco S, Molteni M, et al. Oral contrast enhanced bowel ultrasonography in the assessment of small intestine Crohn's disease. A prospective comparison with conventional ultrasound, x ray studies, and ileocolonoscopy. Gut 2004; 53:1652–1657.
88. Khalili K, Metser U, Wilson SR. Hilar biliary obstruction: preliminary results with Levovist-enhanced sonography. AJR Am J Roentgenol 2003; 180:687–693.
89. Hirooka Y, Naitoh Y, Goto H, et al. Contrast-enhanced endoscopic ultrasonography in gallbladder diseases. Gastrointest Endosc 1998; 8:406–410.
90. Kim KA, Park CM, Park SW, et al. Contrast-enhanced power Doppler US: is it useful in the differentiation of gallbladder disease? Clin Imaging 2002; 26:319–324.
91. Fischer T, Muhler M, Kroncke TJ, et al. Early postoperative ultrasound of kidney transplants: evaluation of contrast medium dynamics using time-intensity curves. Rofo 2004; 176:472–477.
92. Siracusano S, Quaia E, Bertolotto M, et al. The application of ultrasound contrast agents in the characterization of renal tumors. World J Urol 2004; 22:316–322.
93. Ascenti G, Gaeta M, Magno C, et al. Contrast-enhanced second-harmonic sonography in the detection of pseudocapsule in renal cell carcinoma. AJR Am J Roentgenol 2004; 182:1525–1530.
94. Darge K, Troeger J, Duetting T, et al. Reflex in young patients: comparison of voiding US of the bladder and retrovesical space with echo enhancement versus voiding cystourethrography for diagnosis. Radiology 1999; 210:201–207.
95. Darge K. Diagnosis of vesicoureteral reflex with ultrasonography. Pediatr Nephrol 2002; 17:52–60.
96. Albracht T, Hoffmann CW, Schettler S, et al. B-mode enhancement at phase—inversion US with air-based microbubble contrast agent: initial experience in humans. Radiology 2000; 216:273–278.
97. Kopizko A, Cornely D, Reither K, et al. Low contrast dose voiding urosonography in children with phase inversion imaging. Eur Radiol 2004; 14:2290–2296.
98. Darge K, Moeller RT, Trusen A, et al. Diagnosis of vesicoureteric reflux with low-dose contrast-enhanced harmonic ultrasound imaging. Pediatr Radiol 2005; 35:73–78.
99. Halpern EJ, Frauscher F, Strup SE, et al. Prostate: high Frequency Doppler US Imaging for Cancer Detection. Radiology 2002; 225:71–77.
100. Fregene TA, Khanuja PS, Noto AC, et al. Tumor–associated angiogenesis in prostate cancer. Anticancer Res 1993; 13:2377–2381.
101. Brawer MK. Quantitative microvessel density. A staging and prognostic marker for human prostatic carcinoma. Cancer 1996; 78:345–349.
102. Halpern EJ, Lev Verkh L, Forsberg F, et al. Initial experience with contrast-enhanced sonography of the prostate. AJR Am J Roentgenol 2000; 174:1575–1580.
103. Bogers HA, Sedelaar JPM, Beerlage HP, et al. Contrast-enhanced three-dimensional power Doppler angiography of the human prostate: correlation with biopsy outcome. Urology 1999; 54:97–104.
104. Frauscher F, Klauser A, Halpern EJ, et al. Detection of Prostate Cancer with a Microbubble Ultrasound Contrast Agent. Lancet 2001; 357:1849–1850.

105. Halpern EJ, Rosenberg M, Gomella LG. Prostate cancer: contrast-enhanced US for detection. Radiology 2001; 219:219–225.
106. Halpern EJ, McCue PA, Aksnes AK, et al. Contrast enhanced sonography of the prostate with sonazoid: comparison with whole mount prostatectomy specimens in twelve patients. Radiology 2002; 222:361–366.
107. Frauscher F, Klauser A, Volgger H, et al. Comparison of contrast-enhanced color doppler targeted biopsy to conventional systematic biopsy: impact on prostate cancer detection. J Urol 2002; 167:1648–1652.
108. Halpern EJ, Frauscher F, Rosenberg M, et al. Directed biopsy during contrast enhanced sonography of the prostate. AJR Am J Roentgenol 2002; 178:915–919.
109. Pelzer A, Bektic J, Berger AP, et al. Prostate cancer detection in men with prostate specific antigen 4 to 10ng/ml using a combined approach of contrast enhanced color Doppler targeted and systematic biopsy. J Urol 2005; 173(6):1926–1929.
110. Kitano M, Kudo M, Maekawa K, et al. Dynamic imaging of pancreatic diseases by contrast enhanced coded phase inversion harmonic ultrasonography. Gut 2004; 53:854–859.
111. Rickes S, Unkrodt K, Neye H, et al. Differentiation of pancreatic tumours by conventional ultrasound, unenhanced and echo-enhanced power Doppler sonography. Scand J Gastroenterol 2002; 37:1313–1320.
112. Hohl C, Schmidt T, Haage P, et al. Phase-inversion tissue harmonic imaging compared with conventional B-mode ultrasound in the evaluation of pancreatic lesions. Eur Radiol 2004; 14: 1109–1117.
113. Itoh T, Hirooka Y, Itoh A, et al. Usefulness of contrast-enhanced transabdominal ultrasonography in the diagnosis of intraductal papillary mucinous tumors of the pancreas. Am J Gastroenterol 2005; 100:144–152.
114. Melany ML, Grant EG, Duerinckx AJ, et al. Ability of a phase shift contrast agent to improve imaging of the main renal arteries. Radiology 1997; 205:147–152.
115. Missouris CG, Allen CM, Balen FG, et al. Non-invasive screening for renal artery stenosis with ultrasound contrast enhancement. J Hypertens 1996; 14:519–524.
116. Claudon M, Rohban T. Levovist in the diagnosis of renal artery stenosis: results of a controlled multicenter study. Radiology 1997; 205:242.
117. Drelich-Zbroja A, Jargiello T, Drelich G, et al. Renal artery stenosis: value of contrast-enhanced ultrasonography. Abdom Imaging 2004; 29:518–524.
118. Needleman L. Review of a new ultrasound contrast agent—echoGen emulsion. Appl Rad 1997; 26 (S):8–12.
119. Needleman L, Goldberg BB, Feld RI, et al. Evaluation of arterial diseases in humans using an ultrasound contrast agent. J Ultrasound Med 1994; 13:S48.
120. Schwarz KQ, Becher H, Schimpfky C, et al. Doppler enhancement with SHU 508A in multiple vascular regions. Radiology 1994; 193:195–201.
121. Hirai T, Kichikawa K, Ohishi H, et al. Examination of efficacy of SHU 508A for color Doppler sonography of peripheral vascular disease and soft tissue tumors in the pelvis and extremity. In: Advances in Echo Imaging Using Contrast Enhancement. Nanda NC, Schlief R, Goldberg BB, eds. Dordrecht: Kluwer, 1997: 615–626.
122. Puls R, Hosten N, Bock JS, et al. Signal-enhanced color Doppler sonography of deep venous thrombosis in the lower limbs and pelvis. J Ultrasound Med 1999; 18:185–190.
123. Giannoni MF, Palombo G, Sbarigia E, Speziale F, Zaccaria A, Fiorani P. Contrast-enhanced ultrasound for aortic stent-graft surveillance. J Endovasc Ther 2003; 10(2):208–217.
124. Unger EC, McCreery TP, Sweitzer RH, et al. In vitro studies of a new thrombus-specific ultrasound contrast agent. Am J Cardiol 1998; 81:58G–61G.
125. Lanza GM, Wallace KD, Fischer SE, et al. High-frequency ultrasonic detection of thrombi with a targeted contrast system. Ultrasound Med Biol 1997; 23:863–870.
126. Liu JB, Merton DA, Goldberg BB, et al. Contrast-enhanced 2-D and 3-D sonography for evaluation of intra-abdominal hemorrhage. J Ultrasound Med 2002; 21:161–169.
127. Poletti PA, Platon A, Becker CD, et al. Blunt abdominal trauma: does the use of a second-generation sonographic contrast agent help to detect solid organ injuries? Am J Roentgenol 2004; 183: 1293–1301.
128. Catalano O, Lobianco R, Raso MM, et al. Blunt hepatic trauma, evaluation with contrast-enhanced sonography. J Ultrasound Med 2005; 24:299–310.
129. Bostick PJ, Giuliano AE. Vital dyes in sentinel node localization. Semin Nucl Med 2000; 30:18–24.
130. Goldfarb LR, Alazraki N, Eshima D, et al. Lymphoscintigraphic identification of sentinel lymph nodes: clinical evaluation of 0.22mm filtration of Tc-99m sulfur colloid. Radiology 1998; 208:505–509.
131. Mattrey RF, Kono Y, Baker K, et al. Sentinel lymph node imaging with microbubble ultrasound contrast material. Acad Radiol 2002; 9(suppl 1):S231–S235.
132. Goldberg BB, Merton DA, Liu JB, et al. Sentinel lymph nodes in a swine model with melanoma: contrast-enhanced lymphatic US. Radiology 2004; 230:727–734.
133. Goldberg BB, Merton DA, Liu JB, et al. Contrast-enhanced sonographic imaging of lymphatic channels and sentinel lymph nodes. J Ultrasound Med 2005; 24:953–965.
134. Goldberg BB, Murphy GF, Merton DA, et al. Lymphatic uptake of ultrasound contrast microbubbles. J Ultrasound Med 2004; 23:S31.
135. Zavagno G, De Salvo GL, Bozza F, et al. Number of metastatic sentinel nodes as predictor of axillary involvement in patients with breast cancer. Breast Cancer Res Treat 2004; 86:171–179.
136. Yang JH, Slack NH, Memoto T. Effect of axillary nodal status on the long-term survival following mastectomy for breast carcinoma: nodal metastases may not always suggest systemic disease. J Surg Oncol 1987; 36:243–248.
137. Shivers SC, Wang X, Li W, et al. Molecular staging of malignant melanoma: correlation with clinical outcome. JAMA 1998; 280:1410–1415.
138. Eshima D, Fauconnier T, Eshima I, et al. Radiopharmaceuticals for lymphoscintigraphy: including dosimetry and radiation considerations. Semin Nucl Med 2000; 30:25–32.
139. Price RJ, Kaul S. Contrast ultrasound targeted drug and gene delivery: an update on a new therapeutic modality. J Cardiovasc Pharmacol Ther 2002; 7:171–180.
140. Bekeredjian R, Chen S, Frenkel PA, et al. Ultrasound-targeted microbubble destruction can repeatedly direct highly specific plasmid expression to the heart. Circulation 2003; 108:1022–1026.
141. Shohet RV, Chen S, Zhou YT, et al. Echocardiographic destruction of albumin microbubbles directs gene delivery to the myocardium. Circulation 2000; 101:2554–2556.
142. Lindner JR, Dayton PA, Coggins MP, et al. Noninvasive imaging of inflammation by ultrasound detection of phagocytosed microbubbles Circulation 2000; 102:531–538.
143. Crowder, KC, Hughes MS, Marsh JN, et al. Augmented and selective delivery of liquid perfluorocarbon nanoparticles to melanoma cells with noncavitational ultrasound. Ultrasonics 2003; 1:532–535.
144. Blomley M. Which US microbubble contrast agent is best for gene therapy? Radiology 2003; 229:297–298.
145. Deng CX, Sienling F, Pan H, et al. Ultrasound-induced cell membrane porosity. Ultrasound Med Biol 2004; 30:519–526.
146. Christiansen JP, French BA, Klibanov AL, et al. Targeted tissue transfection with ultrasound destruction of plasmid-bearing cationic microbubbles. Ultrasound Med Biol 2003; 29:1759–1767.
147. Unger EC, Hersh E, Vannan M, et al, Local drug and gene delivery through microbubbles. Prog Cardiovasc Dis 2001; 44:45–54.
148. Tsutsui JM, Xie F, Porter RT. The use of microbubbles to target drug delivery. Cardiovascular Ultrasound 2004; 2:23–29.
149. Xie F, Tsutsui J, Lof J, et al. Effectiveness of lipid microbubbles and ultrasound in declotting thrombosis. Ultrasound Med Biol 2005; 31(7):979–985.

4 Three-Dimensional Ultrasound in Obstetrics

Dolores H. Pretorius, Verlee L. Fines-Dailey, Javine Horani, and Thomas R. Nelson

INTRODUCTION

First introduced in the late 1980s, three-dimensional ultrasound (3DUS) is an evolving technology that has been gaining physicians' acceptance rapidly in the last couple of years. 3DUS allows imaging from volume sonographic data rather than conventional planar data used by two-dimensional ultrasound (2DUS). Each volume can be viewed as three perpendicular slices as well as innumerable arbitrary oblique slices, similar to 2DUS images. However, the volume data can also be displayed as rendered images that combine information from all the slices in the volume to allow curved structures to be visualized more easily. Advantages of 3DUS over 2DUS are summarized in Table 1. As improvements in new technology allowed volume imaging to become a practical clinical tool, clinicians are working to identify the clinical applications in which it will be most useful.

ACQUISITION OF VOLUME DATA

In contrast to 2DUS that uses a single plane of image information acquired with a conventional transducer, a variety of techniques are used to obtain volume data in 3D sonography. Different acquisition techniques include (*i*) volume probe with a mechanical swept transducer, (*ii*) free-hand sweep of a conventional 2D transducer, (*iii*) positional sensors attached to a conventional 2D transducer, and (*iv*) 2D array transducers. The mechanical transducer appears to be the most popular today, since it provides automatic registration of the data, is easy to use, and allows for accurate measurement of structures. Free-hand transducers are less popular because they are less accurate in reconstructing the volumes and therefore in providing measurements needed in clinical medicine. However, free-hand transducers may be generating renewed interest in that they can be used to acquire a volume over a larger area of interest that can then be reviewed easily as a cine loop; multiplanar display of these sweeps is also possible. Position sensors can be very accurate but have other drawbacks, particularly because they can be cumbersome to use. 2D array transducers are currently being developed with echocardiography in mind. However, there is great potential for imaging of the entire fetus. The resolution of planes viewed from the matrix array may be much better than planes reconstructed from volume data sets. However, the resolution of these transducers is currently suboptimal for general imaging although they are being used in echocardiography.

Various terms are used in connection with volume data. 3DUS is a static volume that is acquired in a single sweep of the transducer. Four-dimensional ultrasound (4DUS) is a display of sequential 3D volumes that show movement—the fourth dimension being time. Thick-slice imaging is a display of narrow 3D volumes. Spatial-temporal-image correlation (STIC) imaging displays the heart in a gated method that allows for assessment of a beating heart. True real-time displays of volume

TABLE 1 ■ Advantages of 3DUS compared to 2DUS in Obstetrics

- Standardization of anatomy display
  - Coronal, sagittal, and transverse
  - Face upright
  - Limbs upright
- Simultaneous MPR display of three orthogonal planes
  - Localization of single voxel in three planes
  - Navigation through volume following a structure through planes
- Viewing of arbitrary planes not possible with 2DUS
- Volume-rendering display of surface and skeletal anatomy
- Volume-rendering display of vascular structures
- Improved comprehension of anatomy
- Improved recognition of anomalies by less-experienced physicians
- More accurate identification of the location, extent, and size of anomalies
- Retrospective review or consultation with specialists/clinicians/trainees/family
- Enhanced parental bonding

Abbreviations: 2DUS, two-dimensional ultrasound; 3DUS, three-dimensional ultrasound.

information are acquired using 2D transducer matrix array technology.

THE FIRST TRIMESTER

Sonographic evaluation during the first trimester has become an effective screening method for structural and chromosomal abnormalities (1). 3DUS has been found to be an excellent tool that permits detailed and comprehensive evaluation of the embryo. One of the advantages of 3DUS compared to 2DUS is that the volume data acquired with the transvaginal transducer may be rotated to identify the desired structures irrespective of the plane of acquisition. In the first trimester, fetal head, face, neck, anterior abdominal wall, stomach, and spine can be examined routinely. This is particularly important in cases at risk for chromosomal abnormalities. Hull et al. showed that more anatomic structures were identified with 3DUS than 2DUS (Figs. 1 and 2), and that the length of time needed to obtain the desired structures was significantly less with 3DUS than with the conventional 2DUS (2.7 minutes vs. 14.7 minutes, respectively) (2). Michailidis et al.

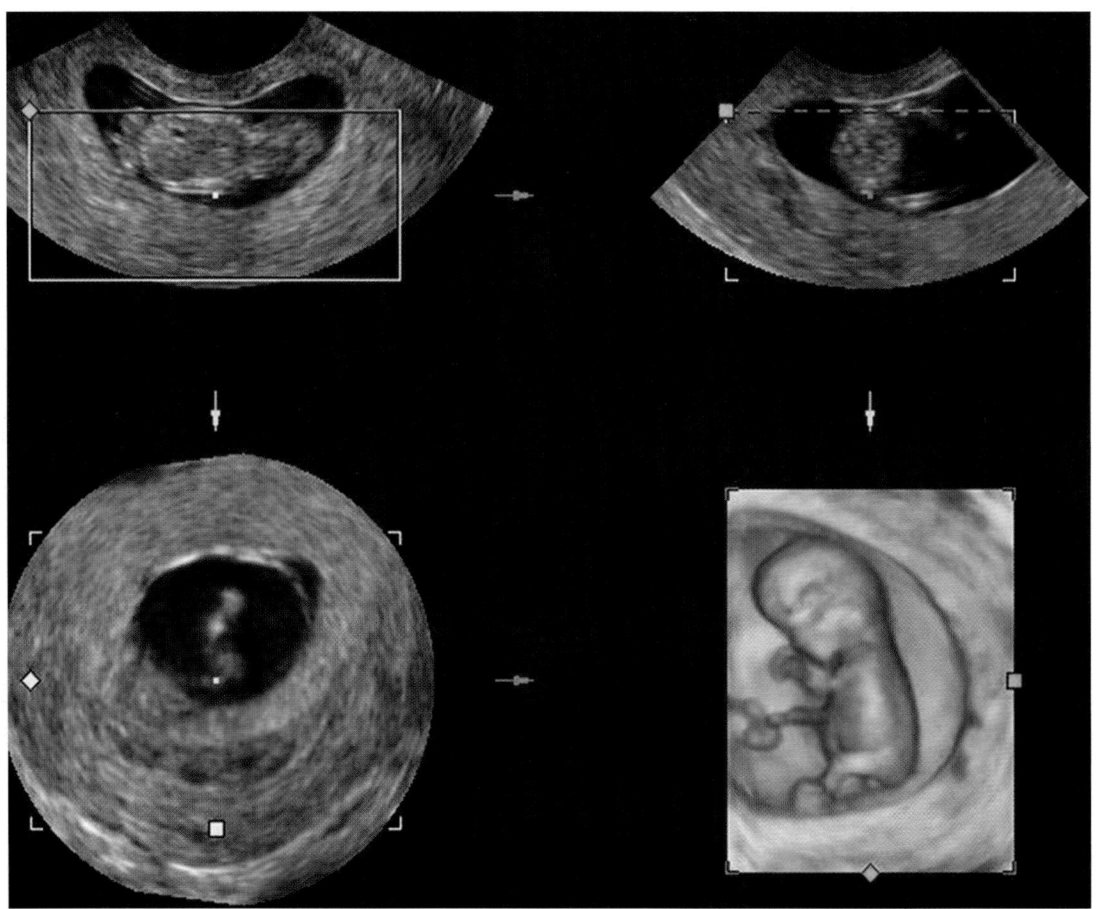

FIGURE 1 ■ Ten-week fetus in multiplanar and rendered view. Upper left image shows fetus in sagittal plane. Upper right image shows fetus embryo in axial transverse plane. Lower left image shows coronal plane of fetal leg. Lower right image shows surface-rendered image of fetus within the uterine cavity. Notice the umbilical cord entering fetus from the left.

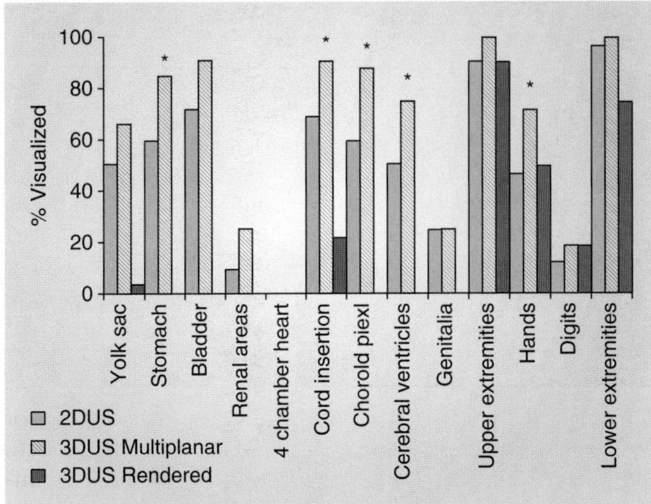

FIGURE 2 ■ Chart showing anatomy identified in first trimester embryos using 2DUS, 3DUS multiplanar display, and rendered displays. 2DUS, two-dimensional ultrasound; 3DUS, three-dimensional ultrasound. *Source*: From Ref. 2.

also demonstrated it was possible to perform a comprehensive anatomical survey of the fetus using 3DUS in the first trimester. They studied 159 women between 12 weeks and 13 weeks 6 days with crown–rump length 56 to 84 mm (3). They found that complete anatomical surveys were possible in 93.7% of cases using 2DUS and in 80.5% of the cases using 3DUS. The scanning time was 12.2 minutes for 2D examination, whereas the mean time for 3D volume acquisition was only 2.9 minutes. The total time for 3DUS, including the time for examining fetal anatomy following the acquisition, was 8.4 minutes. This difference was statistically significant ($p < 0.001$). They concluded that although the anatomical survey was completed in more cases using conventional 2DUS, 3DUS provided maximum information with less scanning time, thus reducing total examination time (3).

3DUS enables all three orthogonal planes to be visualized simultaneously, resulting in easy distinction of fetal skin from the amnion. This makes 3DUS a useful tool for nuchal translucency (NT) measurement in early pregnancy (4,5). Chung et al. showed it was not only effective in obtaining the desired measurement but it was also reproducible with a low intraoperator variability ($p = 0.862$) (4). Clementschitsch et al. performed NT measurements using 2DUS and 3DUS on 229 pregnant women. NT was measured in 96.8% of cases using 2DUS. 3DUS was successful in 98.6% of cases. The correlation between the measurements obtained by the different techniques was very high ($r = 0.97$) (6). However, there is some conflicting information in the literature regarding the effectiveness of 3DUS in obtaining NT measurement. In the study by Michailidis et al., NT was measured in 98.1% of cases using 2DUS, compared to only 91.8% using 3DUS (3). Fetal movement during the examination was responsible for the inability to complete the anatomical survey, including the NT. These limitations could be overcome with newer equipment that allows faster acquisition. Measurement accuracy of the NT may be compromised by 3DUS if the measurement is taken in a plane with suboptimal resolution. It must be remembered that the NT measurement is used along with the biochemistry data to assess risk.

Increased NT measurements suggest aneuploidy or other congenital abnormalities such as congenital heart disease. Figure 3 shows a series of parallel images from a single-volume acquisition of a fetus with an enlarged NT. This type of 3DUS display is very new and is similar to the display used in computed tomography (CT) or magnetic resonance imaging (MRI).

Another benefit of 3DUS is that the surface-rendered images of the embryo are very life-like and very appealing to parents (Fig. 1). In addition, movement of the embryo and the limbs can be seen using the fourth dimension, 4DUS. Although surface display has the most appeal for parents, it is the multiplanar information that generally offers the greatest potential adding diagnostic information.

In the original description of patients with Trisomy 21, Langdon Down reported a flat face accompanied by small noses (7). This finding gave rise to the investigation of the nasal bone length as a marker for Trisomy 21. Multiple studies have been performed and have shown that an absent or short nasal bone (<2.5 percentile) is a sensitive and specific marker for Trisomy 21 (8–11). Rembouskos et al. looked at the benefit of 3DUS in the evaluation of the fetal nasal bone. They examined the fetal nasal bone in 120 stored volumes acquired in transverse, midsagittal, parasagittal, and oblique longitudinal sections of the fetal head. They found that in midsagittal sections, the nasal bone was always visible in a normal fetus when the angle of insonation was within a range of 30° to 60° (Fig. 4). They concluded that in a 3D volume, the extent to which the nasal bone can be demonstrated in a given reconstructed section is entirely dependent on a good initial 2D view (11,12). Therefore, when it is difficult to obtain the nasal bone on 2D imaging, it is reasonable to acquire a volume through the fetal face in a plane close to the sagittal plane of the fetus; if the nasal bone is identified, then it should be measured, but if it is not identified, then the angle of insonation must be scrutinized to determine that it is within 30° to 60°.

Normal brain development of the embryo has been described in detail by O'Rahilly and Muller (13,14). The shape and volume of the embryonic brain cavities can be demonstrated with 3DUS, as shown by Blaas et al. (15). In a series of studies, they demonstrated that 3DUS allows images of the embryonic brain cavities to be reconstructed and that these correlate well with classic human embryology (16,17). This finding is of great clinical importance. The knowledge of the volumes of the various specific structures can aid in the early diagnosis of abnormal fetal development. An example of how this information can lead to early diagnosis of abnormal central nervous system (CNS) development was presented by Blaas et al. in a case of alobar holoprosencephaly in a nine-week gestation (17). An enlarged rhombencephalic cavity was noted

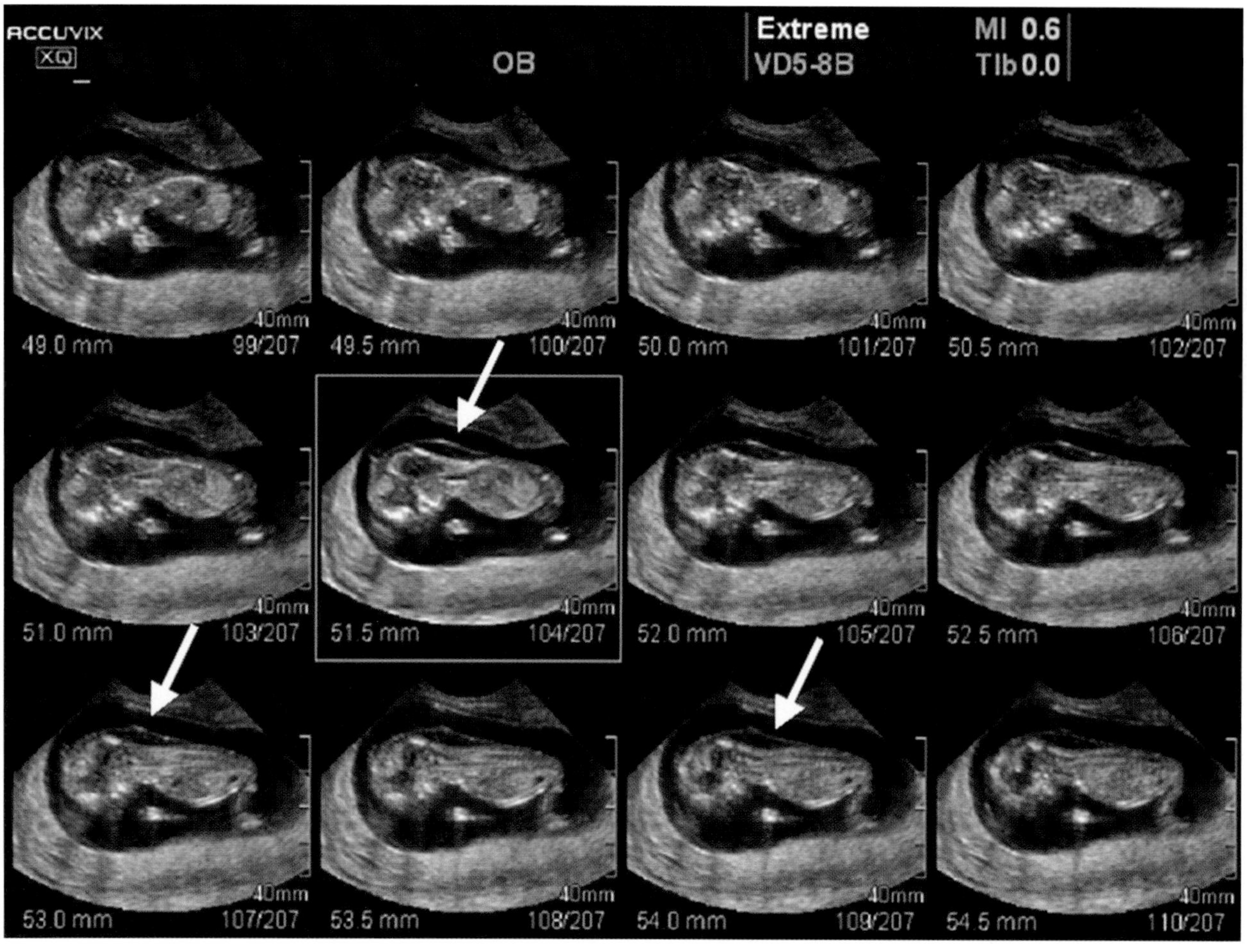

FIGURE 3 ■ Multislice display of a single-volume acquisition showing an abnormal nuchal translucency (*arrows*). The images are displayed at 0.5 mm intervals. *Source*: Courtesy of Medison.

along with a proboscis. The diagnosis was confirmed by postabortem examination. Benoit et al. have also reported on the detection of CNS anomalies such as anencephaly, encephalocele, hydrocephaly, and holoprosencephaly during the first trimester (18).

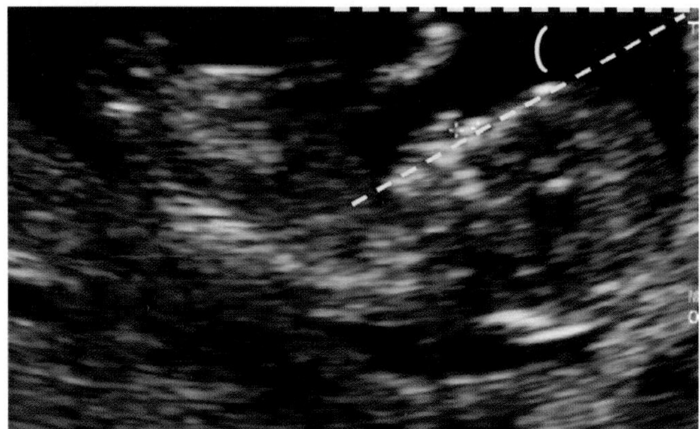

FIGURE 4 ■ Sagittal image through a 12-week fetus showing that the angle of acquisition must be between 30° and 60° as shown in the image.

THE FACE

The human face is so much more than the sum of its parts. It projects our emotions, helps define our personality, and uniquely identifies each and every one of us. One of the most enthralling moments in a mother's life is the first look at her infant's face at the moment of birth. With the introduction of ultrasound, we are now able to offer this experience to parents many months before the birth of their child. Although the primary purpose of the ultrasound examination is to evaluate fetal anatomy and growth, its use has afforded parents a glimpse of their infant prior to birth and a greater understanding of what the future may bring (Fig. 5).

One of the difficulties with 2DUS is that the image is often difficult for the patient to understand without considerable explanation from the examiner. This difficulty is especially problematic if a fetal defect is detected. The introduction of 3D- or 4DUS provides parents a much more easily recognized, life-like image of the way the fetus will look at birth, an example of which is provided in Figure 1. Preliminary data suggests that 3DUS images may increase parental bonding with the infant prior to birth (19,20). 3D images may also provide a

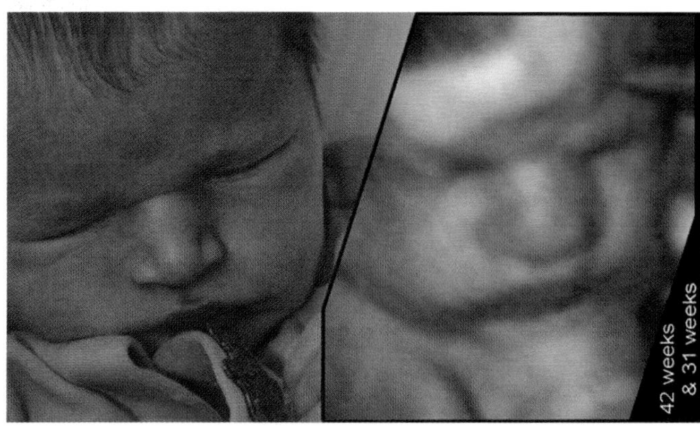

FIGURE 5 ■ Normal face at 31 weeks by 3DUS (*right*) and at birth at 42 weeks (*left*). Notice the similarity in the head position, eyes, and nasal bridge.

greater understanding of birth defects for the family and for consultants.

One of the most valuable functions of ultrasound in the prenatal period is the diagnosis of facial abnormalities. In most centers, routine screening with 2DUS includes evaluation of three traditional planes—sagittal, coronal, and axial. Using this technique to screen for abnormalities leads to a 21% to 30% detection rate that could be increased to 88% with systematic assessment of all three planes added to the standard exam (21). Unfortunately, time limitations do not allow this level of screening on all patients and serial scanning is only added if an anomaly is suspected or if the fetus is at a high risk for a particular anomaly. One of the benefits of 3D-/4DUS is the ability to perform both a screening exam and a full facial analysis in the same exam in less time than it would take to acquire these images in a 2D scan (21).

Diagnosing cleft lip and/or palate is one of the most common uses of 3DUS. We suggest the following sequence of evaluation. First, acquire the volume of the face using the profile-up plane. Second, rotate the volume into a symmetrical orientation of the face by placing the marker dot on the nose and then rotating the orbits to be symmetrical on the axial plane. Third, tip the facial profile posteriorly approximately 45° to obtain the more standard coronal view of the lip seen on 2D images. To view the primary palate on 3DUS, the volume should be acquired in the axial plane to obtain the highest resolution possible and to assess the tooth buds on the axial plane in the multiplanar display. The palate can also be assessed using rendered skeletal images (obtained by increasing the threshold on the surface-rendered images) of the face from a frontal (coronal) view. Examples of multiplanar and rendered 3D images of cleft lip and palate are shown in Figure 6. The right-sided cleft can be appreciated readily on the rendered images by even an inexperienced observer. The cleft palate can be seen on the axial and skeletal view and is shown to involve the primary palate as indicated by the arrow. The green line on the rendered image delineates the reference plane for the axial view on the multiplanar image, thereby decreasing the likelihood of errors in diagnosing a cleft palate or any other defect, for example, misdiagnosing a nasal passage as a cleft. 4D scanning, in which motion is added to the 3D scan, expands the evaluation by allowing the examiner to identify the fetal tongue moving in and out of the cleft. Although the 4D image often offers better surface images, the 3D volume provides greater resolution, which is particularly important when identifying cleft lip and palate.

Currently, only about 21% to 30% of facial clefts are detected antenatally, leaving much room for improvement. As seen in Figure 6, the cosmetic results of corrected cleft lips can be quite impressive. A prenatal consultation with a plastic surgeon using 3D images can help parents plan corrective surgery before the birth of their child. Use of 3DUS has increased detection rates of cleft palate and has provided incomparable information to both practitioners and families, as documented by Johnson et al. (22). In this study, 3DUS was used to rescan 31 fetuses found to have cleft lip and/or palate on 2DUS. Of the 22 (86%) associated cleft palates, 19 were identified by 3DUS in comparison to only 9 (41%) detected by 2DUS ($p < 0.005$). Another important finding of this study was that the images obtained by 3DUS allowed families to have a greater understanding of the extent of the defect. Also, three fetuses were found to have normal lips and palates on 3DUS after diagnosis of cleft lip had been made on 2DUS, leading to obvious relief on the part of the involved families (22). Several other investigators have also found that 3DUS adds significantly to the assessment of cleft lip and palate (23–26).

Visualization of the secondary palate remains problematic using both 2D- and 3DUS. Unfortunately, isolated cleft palate is a difficult diagnosis and is often overlooked due to the lack of a cleft lip that would otherwise clue the operator in to scanning the palate more closely. Although rates of identification of cleft palate associated with cleft lip have increased by the use of 3DUS, the rates of identification of isolated cleft palate have remained the same. One of the reasons for this is the shadowing of surrounding bone and tissue onto the palate as well as shadowing from one side of the palate to the other, making it difficult to separate a true defect from an artifact. One proposed method, by Campbell et al., of identifying defects of the secondary palate more clearly and overcoming the difficulty of shadowing, is referred to as the 3D reverse face view. In order to achieve this view, a frontal view of the face is made and then rotated through 180°. Campbell explains that a true coronal plane must be obtained in which "both eyes are symmetrically placed in the upper part of the image with the nasal cavity in the midline between and just below the eyeballs." The view bar can then be scrolled through the length of the palate, as would be done in the usual rendered view, and used to identify the normal secondary palate, which should be seen as an uninterrupted line between the nasal and the oral cavities (27,28).

Most facial anomalies will be recognized on 2DUS; however, Merz and Welter have shown that occasionally a cleft lip and palate can be detected only on 3DUS (29). 3DUS enhances the exam by allowing the examiner to

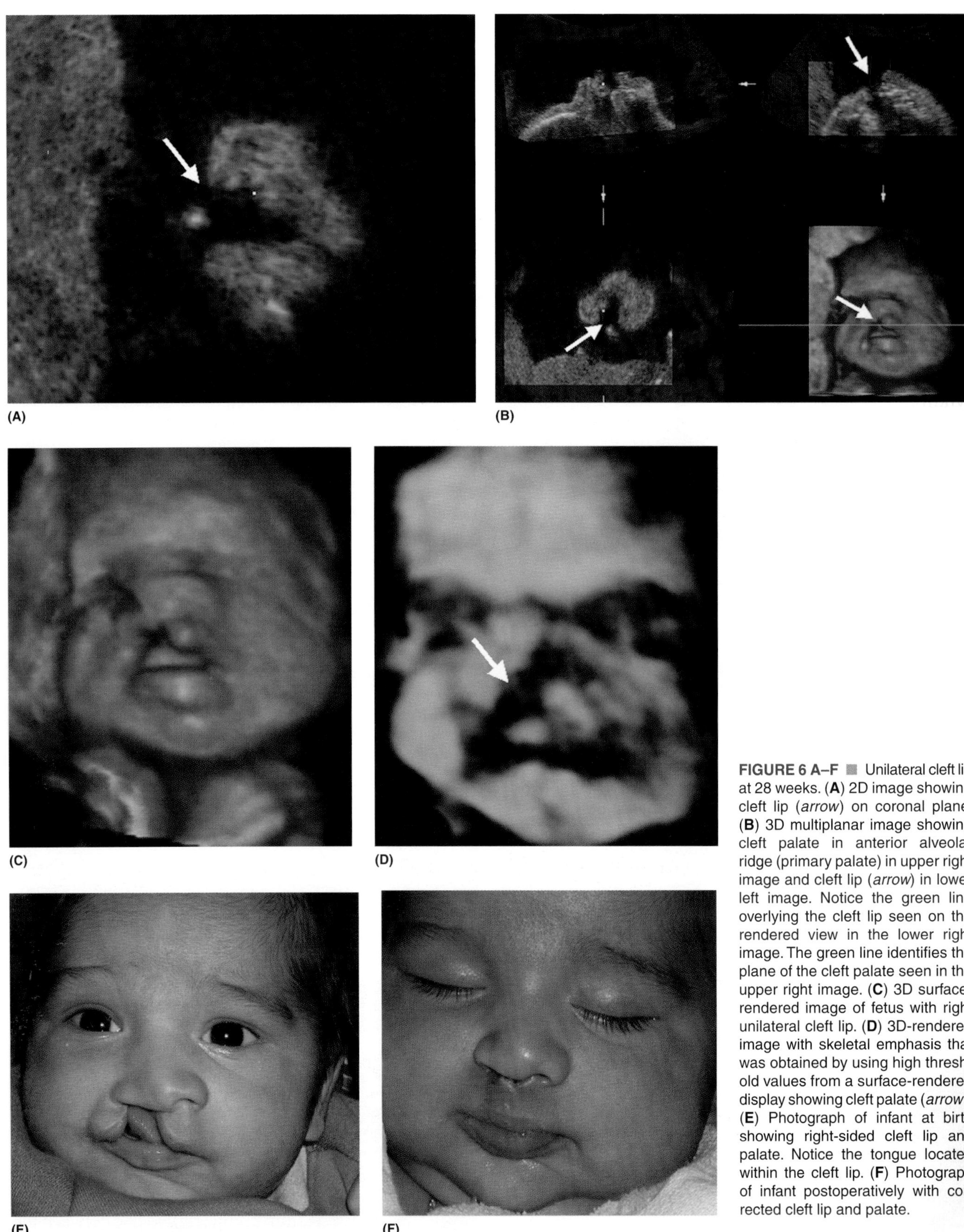

FIGURE 6 A–F ■ Unilateral cleft lip at 28 weeks. (**A**) 2D image showing cleft lip (*arrow*) on coronal plane. (**B**) 3D multiplanar image showing cleft palate in anterior alveolar ridge (primary palate) in upper right image and cleft lip (*arrow*) in lower left image. Notice the green line overlying the cleft lip seen on the rendered view in the lower right image. The green line identifies the plane of the cleft palate seen in the upper right image. (**C**) 3D surface-rendered image of fetus with right unilateral cleft lip. (**D**) 3D-rendered image with skeletal emphasis that was obtained by using high threshold values from a surface-rendered display showing cleft palate (*arrow*). (**E**) Photograph of infant at birth showing right-sided cleft lip and palate. Notice the tongue located within the cleft lip. (**F**) Photograph of infant postoperatively with corrected cleft lip and palate.

scroll through the defect on multiple planes and obtain a more accurate depiction of the anomaly. Also, since the volume can be acquired by a less experienced examiner, consultation in difficult cases is possible without having to rescan the patient or even having the patient present for the evaluation.

3DUS is unquestionably superior in the evaluation of the fetal ear. Abnormalities of the ear are more easily visualized in a 3D image, allowing evaluation of rotation and normal or abnormal lobulation, often not feasible in 2D scanning (30). Since abnormalities of the fetal ear are often involved in syndromes, 3DUS can provide valuable additional diagnostic information.

Another area of increased utility of 3DUS is in the evaluation of fetal tooth germs. Fetal tooth germ abnormalities such as oligodontia or anodontia can be associated with numerous genetic syndromes including Down's syndrome and can be associated with facial clefts. The evaluation of the fetal tooth germs on 3DUS allows for increased visualization of the tooth germs as shown by Ulm et al. in which 45 fetuses were evaluated by both 2D- and 3DUS. 3DUS was successful in clearly visualizing the tooth germs of the maxilla and the mandible in 86% to 94% of cases compared to only 56% to 62% of cases scanned with 2DUS (31).

3DUS is also useful in the diagnosis of other facial anomalies such as micrognathia, retrognathia, orbital hypoplasia, facial masses such as proboscis (Fig. 7), and holoprosencephaly. In micrognathia and retrognathia, early diagnosis can assist in birth planning. The presence of a neonatologist at birth in case of acute respiratory distress syndrome, which often accompanies these anomalies may be critical, as immediate treatment can avert a fatal outcome. In an article by Rotten et al., parameters were defined to assist in the objective diagnosis of micrognathia and retrognathia, since their presence can also be associated with various syndromes such as Pierre Robin Sequence and Treacher Collins Syndrome as well as several chromosomal abnormalities including Trisomy 13 and 18. In most cases, a subjective diagnosis is made based on the sonographic appearance of the fetal chin and jaw on fetal profile. Rotten et al. identified a quantitative method of assessing the profile using a facial angle. Using an inferior facial angle of less than 50° on the sagittal view was positively associated with retrognathia. The use of a ratio of mandible width to maxilla width of less than 0.785 defined micrognathism and remained constant throughout gestation (32). Although these measurements could be acquired on 2DUS, the simplicity of acquiring the correct planes on 3DUS makes the evaluation much more feasible in a relatively short period of time.

In evaluating fetal markers for aneuploidy, the nasal bone has received much attention as a new soft marker in assessing risk for Down's syndrome. 3DUS may provide valuable information as to why false positives and negatives occur in the assessment of absence or hypoplasia of the nasal bone. One of the difficulties with using the nasal bone as a marker is related to the learning curve required

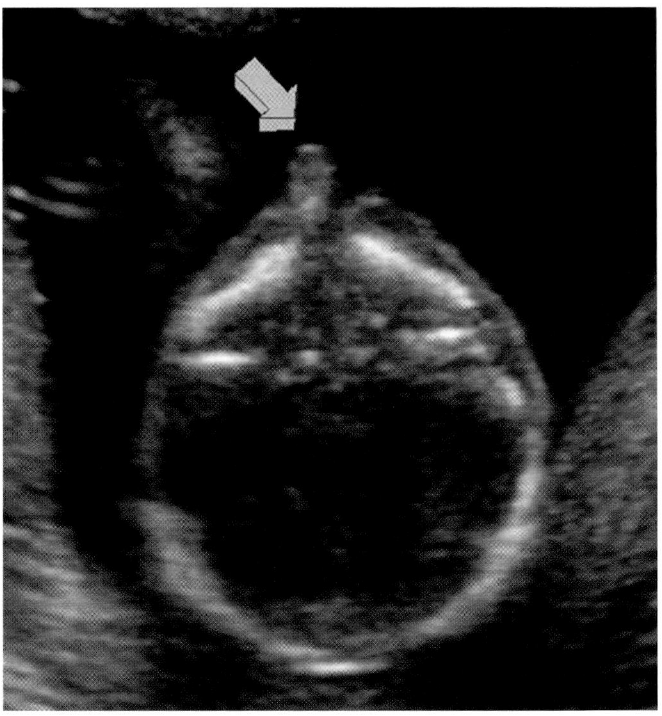

(A)

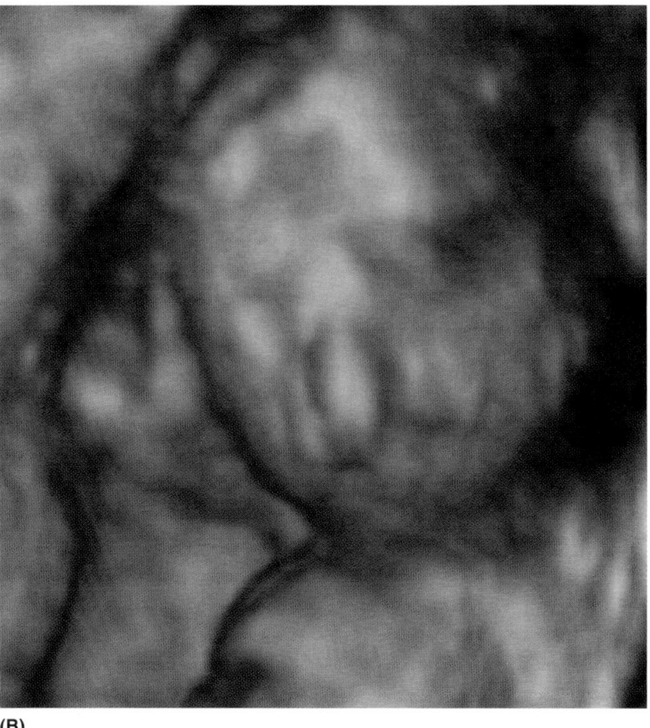

(B)

FIGURE 7 A AND B ■ Abnormal face in fetus with holoprosencephaly and Trisomy 13. (**A**) 2D axial image showing proboscis (*arrow*) in fetus. (**B**) 3D image of fetal face showing proboscis that was clearly visible to the parents. *Source*: Courtesy of Philips Medical Systems.

to accurately capture and assess the image acquired on 2DUS. One confounding factor is the finding of unilateral absence of the nasal bone as described by Benoit and Chaoui (33). Using rendering in the transparent maximal mode to increase visualization of the bony face, the bones of the nose were assessed to diagnose absence or unilateral absence of the nasal bone. In the study by Benoit and Chaoui, nine cases of fetuses with hypoplastic/absent nasal bone analyzed by 2DUS were reviewed by 3DUS. There was a 30% discrepancy between 2D and 3D images, with findings of unilateral absence of the nasal bone, hypoplasia, or normal length of the other nasal bone. This may explain discrepancies in postmortem or neonatal evaluations of fetuses with false-positive and false-negative 2D assessments of the fetal nasal bone. It is possible that the use of 3D rendering will simplify the evaluation of suspected nasal bone hypoplasia and absence, resulting in more accurate prenatal diagnosis and leading to the increased utility of the nasal bone as a marker of aneuploidy (33).

Drawbacks of 3D-/4DUS are similar to those of 2DUS and include difficulty of visualizing the fetus in the setting of oligohydramnios, when the fetus is closely approximated to the uterine wall or placenta or when an extremity is shadowing the face (21). Examiners using 3DUS must be aware of potential artifacts in order to avoid errors in diagnosis. Some of the artifacts specific to 3DUS include overthresholding, leading to an apparent "black eye" or "black nose" (Fig. 8) and inappropriate rendering, leading to loss of normal structures and an erroneous diagnosis of a single nostril or even a cleft lip (34). Artifacts can also occur resulting from motion of the fetus or from structures obscuring the desired view during the acquisition of the volume. Changing the position of the rendering line can assist in eliminating artifacts created by shadowing from bony fetal parts such as the fetal nose, palate, or extremity. Decreasing the threshold can restore an apparent "black eye" to normal.

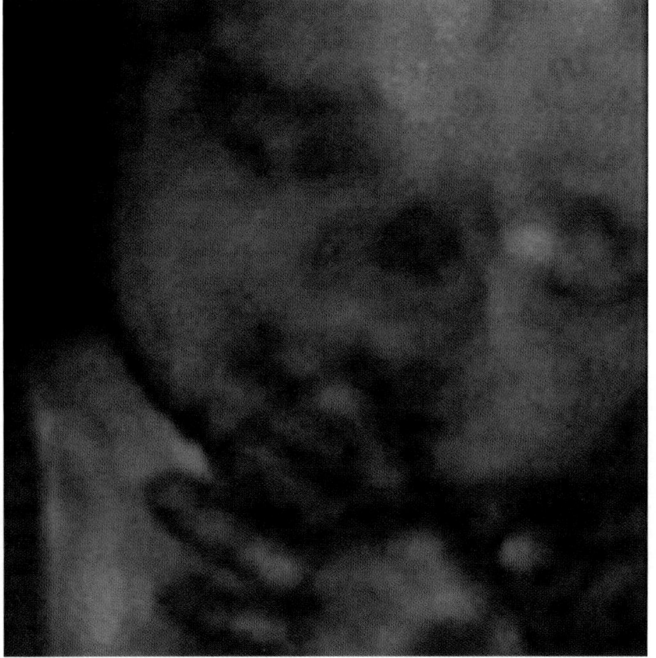

FIGURE 8 ■ Artifact appearing as a "black nose." The rendering algorithm causes the nose not to be seen when in reality it is normal.

The electronic scalpel editing tool may be used to modify images in which a fetal limb, placenta, or portion of the umbilical cord obscures the view. The electronic scalpel function allows the examiner to mask areas of the volume in order to improve images acquired in less than ideal situations. In order to use the electronic scalpel (cut-mode function), the rendered image is rotated into a position where the obscuring structure can easily be viewed, outlined with the cursor, and then cut out (Fig. 9). This process can be repeated until the desired image is achieved and can then be assessed without the obscuring structure. An undo function allows return to the previous position in case of an error. The value of this feature was identified in a study of electronic scalpel use in 80 cases of 3D scans of fetal face abnormalities by Merz et al. In this study, the cutting-mode function was able to achieve superior quality improvement of the rendered image in 72.5% of cases (35). Care must be taken in the use of the electronic scalpel in order to decrease the chance of creating iatrogenic defects. In addition, we have found that it is preferable to tell the patient that we are masking an area of the volume rather than cutting an area of the fetus.

Unfortunately, with all the advances made in prenatal diagnosis, many fetal anomalies are not diagnosed in the prenatal period. One such example is highlighted in a study by Chmait et al. in which associated fetal anomalies were missed when fetuses with cleft lip with or without cleft palate were examined with 2D- and 3DUS. This study found a 35.6% rate of additional structural or syndromic abnormalities. Unfortunately, even with intense screening using both 2D- and 3DUS, 21.6% of the fetuses thought to have isolated cleft lip with or without palate were still found to have additional malformations identified after delivery (26).

THE CNS

CNS abnormalities, including brain and spine anomalies, are among the most common congenital malformations detected using prenatal ultrasound, with an estimated incidence of one per 1000 births (36). They are often associated with poor outcome, and therefore, correct diagnosis is of great importance.

Although 2DUS has proven to be a very sensitive tool in identifying CNS abnormalities, particularly of open neural tube defects, it has some limitations. It depends on the knowledge, skill, and experience of the sonographer (37). Artifacts, such as pseudodysraphism, can be easily created just by subtle angulations of the transducer. Fetal position is critical in the proper visualization of the spine. Furthermore, spine and thorax cannot be imaged in their entirety using one single plane. As part of the routine spine evaluation, one needs to make sure that ossification centers in the vertebral bodies are parallel on longitudinal views and that the posterior elements of the spine are

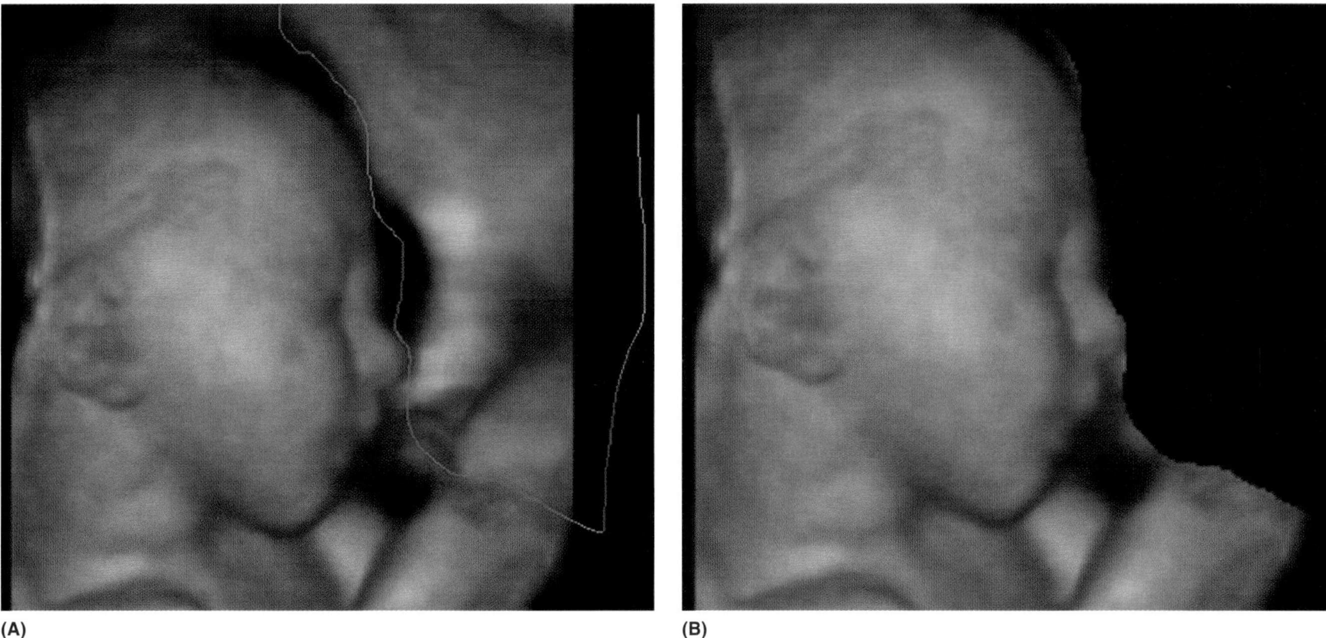

FIGURE 9 A AND B ■ Use of the editing scalpel. (**A**) Profile of face with placenta and arm anterior to face. A red line was drawn by scalpel to outline the region to be removed from the image. (**B**) Image of fetus without placenta and arm seen on (**A**).

paired on transverse views, a process that can be time consuming (38).

Since the introduction of 3DUS, this modality has become a useful tool in the evaluation of the normal and the abnormal brain and spine anatomy. Riccabona et al. evaluated different display modalities and rendering techniques of 3DUS in the evaluation of the fetal spine and the thorax (Fig. 10) (39). With 3DUS, they were able to rotate the obtained volumes into a standard anatomic orientation, scroll through any planes, and evaluate consecutive axial planes using a flight path mode. They also calculated a volume-rendered image. Both the multiplanar display and the rendered image were used together to analyze and interpret the images obtained. Good visualization of continuity and curvature of the spine and ribs was shown. The ribs, clavicles, and cranial sutures were visualized using adequate rotation of the rendered images. Furthermore, they showed that different rendering modalities and postprocessing of 3D volumes of the fetal spine and thorax could be used to evaluate different structures of interest in the same data set. For example, spinal osseous structures were better visualized using maximum intensity weighting, whereas the surface skin continuity was better visualized using surface-weighted rendering. The ability to rotate the volume into anatomic orientation, the use of interactive display of the three orthogonal planes, and the extent of visualized spine in a single data set made abnormalities such as hemivertebra and scoliosis easily recognizable. More so, the ability to visualize the rendered image along with the multiplanar display improved diagnostic confidence and provided better understanding of the anatomy and the spatial relationship. In another study by Johnson et al., the extent of spinal anatomy obtained in a single data set was dependent on gestational age, with the entire spine visualized in younger fetuses (37). In 5 of 16 fetuses with a normal spine, the entire spine was visualized in a single-volume data set, from upper thoracic to lower sacral in 10 and only the lumbosacral area seen in one. Nevertheless, at least five images were needed in 2DUS to visualize the entire spinal anatomy. They also showed, like the previous study, that the adjacent structures such as ribs, clavicles, iliac wings, and scapulae could be visualized without further scanning time. Moreover, their continuity with the spine was also seen.

In a study by Dyson et al., 3DUS provided additional information in 12 of 13 cases of extracerebral CNS anomalies, including open neural tube defects (40). The ability to visualize the rendered image alongside the multiplanar display was most helpful in localizing the lesion. Axial skeletal anomalies, including scoliosis and segmentation defects, were also better visualized using 3DUS rotation of the rendered images. Muller et al. also found the three orthogonal planes to be very helpful in identifying the level of the defect (41). Determining the exact location and extent of a spinal lesion is an important prognostic factor, as it correlates with neurologic and functional deficit (42). This is particularly critical when counseling families (Table 2). 2DUS has been found to estimate the location of the defect within one vertebral body in 79% of the fetuses (43). In the study by Johnson et al., 3DUS was essential in the diagnosis and the location of one of nine cases of open neural tube defects (37). This lesion could not be seen with conventional 2DUS due to fetal position, which was not found to be critical with 3DUS. The volume was obtained by using a transvaginal probe and then rotating the spine into the desired transverse plane. The exact location of the lesion was identified by using the rendered image as a reference: the T12 vertebral body was determined by the adjacent last rib and the S1 vertebral

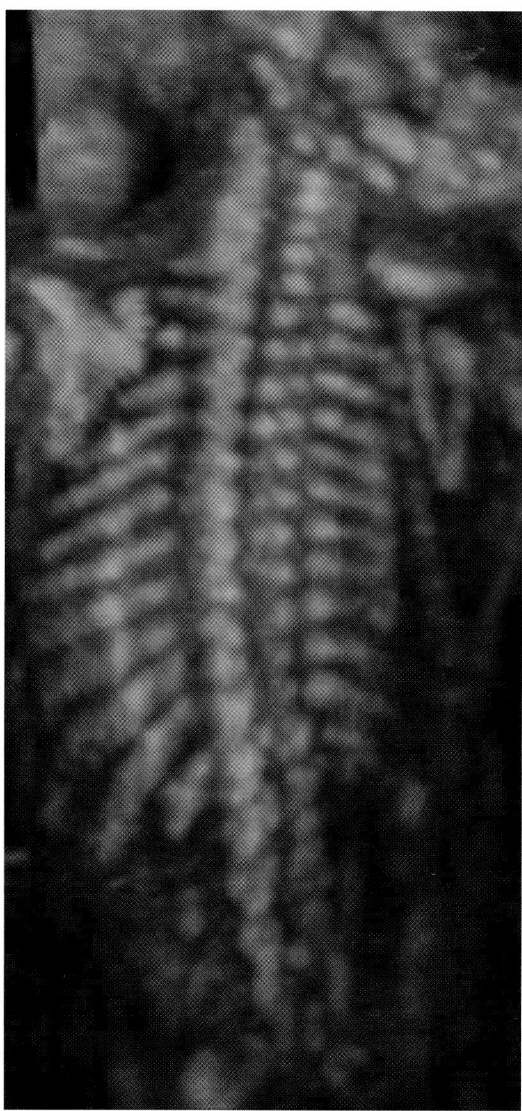

FIGURE 10 ■ Normal spine and thorax. Notice the ribs, spine, and both scapulae.

body determined using the top of the iliac wing. In their study, however, the lesion was localized to two vertebral bodies higher on 3DUS. By contrast, in a study by Lee et al., the spinal level determined by 3D sonography agreed within one vertebral body in eight of nine infants (89%) compared to six of nine (67%) using 2DUS (23). Bony vertebral defects (butterfly vertebrae and left hemivertebra) were clearly shown in two fetuses, and the meningeal sac could be identified using the rendered volume in five of nine fetuses. Although multiplanar views offer more clinically significant information, the simultaneous use of the rendered image ensures that the appropriate area will be visualized. Moreover, the image is easier for parents to visualize and understand during counseling.

Volumes of the fetal brain can also be obtained with the use of 3D sonography. Monteagudo et al., using new views similar to the neonatal transfontanelle approach, showed that 3D sonography was effective for obtaining the fetal neuroscan (44). Using transvaginal ultrasound probes, fetal brain volumes were obtained through either the anterior or the sagittal suture. These were manipulated to obtain the "three-horn" view (3HV) bilaterally. In this view, anterior, posterior, and inferior horns of the lateral ventricle were visualized. 3D sonography allowed visualization of not only the coronal and the sagittal section obtained with 2DUS but also the axial section. The main advantages of using 3DUS versus 2DUS were: (*i*) the ability to navigate within the volume and move through multiple sections in all three planes from a single data set. This contrasts with 2DUS in which a predetermined number of sections need to be obtained creating snapshots, from which the anatomy then needs to be mentally reconstructed; (*ii*) the use of the marker dot that marks the same anatomical spot in all three orthogonal and simultaneously displayed planes. This proved to be valuable when evaluating brain anomalies such as agenesis of the corpus callosum, where following the third ventricle and noticing its upward displacement improved the confidence of

TABLE 2 ■ Neurologic Syndromes with Myelomeningoceles

Lesion level	Spinal-related disability
Above L3	Complete paraplegia and dermatomal para-anesthesia
	Bladder and rectal incontinence
	Nonambulatory
L4 and below	Same as for above L3 except preservation of hip flexors, hip adductors, and knee extensions
	Ambulatory with aids, bracing, and orthopedic surgery
S1 and below	Same as for L4 and below except preservation of feet dorsiflexors and partial preservation of hip extensors and knee flexors
S3 and below	Normal lower extremity motor function
	Saddle anesthesia
	Variable bladder–rectal incontinence

Source: Courtesy of Dr. John Menkes.

the diagnosis; (*iii*) sections obtained are comparable to images obtained from neonatal CT and MRI. This allowed for better understanding of the pathology by the pediatric neurologist and/or the neurosurgeon. The 3HV is used to evaluate the lateral ventricles. The three horns are considered to be abnormal when (*i*) the anterior horn height is more than 8.7 mm at 14 weeks and 6.9 at 40 weeks; (*ii*) the posterior horn height is more than 11 mm at 14 weeks and 14 mm at 40 weeks; (*iii*) the measurement from the posterior tip of the thalamus to the posterior tip of the posterior horn is in excess of 2.6 mm at 14 weeks and 3.4 mm at 40 weeks; and (*iv*) the inferior horn is visible to any degree (45). Timor-Tritsch et al. found that the best predictor of ventriculomegaly was the presence of any dilatation of the inferior horn using the 3HV (45). They also found 3DUS to be paramount in the diagnosis of agenesis of corpus callosum, further confirmed by following the anterior cerebral artery and not being able to follow the entire length of the absent pericallosal artery. 3DUS was also helpful in seeing the normal corpus callosum (Fig. 11). Other major brain anomalies, including anencephaly, holoprosencephaly, Dandy–Walker cyst, and arachnoid cyst have been diagnosed using 3D sonography (45,46).

3D sonography has its limitations when evaluating the fetal CNS. Optimal resolution of the spine is obtained when the volume is acquired in the transverse plane. However, most volumes are acquired in the sagittal plane because more vertebral bodies can be seen in one volume (37). The quality of the volumes acquired will determine the quality of both the planar and the rendered images obtained. One of the major benefits of 3DUS is the fact that fetal position is not as critical since the images obtained can be rotated (39).

THE SKELETON

Visualization of the fetal skeleton with 3DUS has been a valuable addition to the evaluation of the spine, ribs, cranial sutures, and fetal extremities. Multiple anomalies including craniosynostosis, spina bifida, phocomelia, and osteogenesis imperfecta have been diagnosed using 3DUS (47,48). Multiple articles in the literature discuss the many uses of 3DUS in evaluating the fetal skeleton.

Bones can be displayed using any of the following three volume displays: skeletal display, maximal intensity rendering, or increased thresholding on surface rendering. This feature allows the separation of hypoechogenic structures such as viscera from dense, hyperechogenic structures such as the bone. When imaging the bone, 3DUS allows the practitioner to easily view the ribs and spine, particularly on a posterior view, in order to quickly count each rib and vertebra while allowing evaluation of multiple malformations (49). Evaluating the fetal spine is important in determining not only the presence of anomalies such as spina bifida but also the level of the defect. Since the level of the defect correlates directly with the level of impairment expected, this information is vital in counseling parents (Table 2). Lee et al. scanned nine

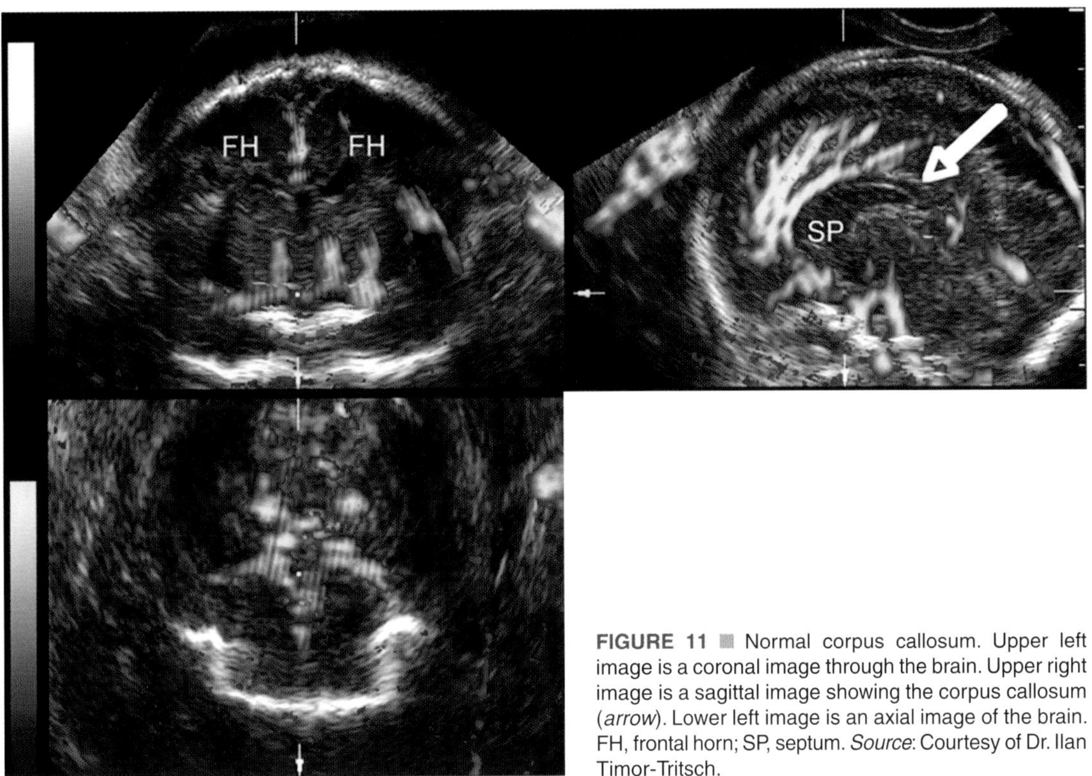

FIGURE 11 ■ Normal corpus callosum. Upper left image is a coronal image through the brain. Upper right image is a sagittal image showing the corpus callosum (*arrow*). Lower left image is an axial image of the brain. FH, frontal horn; SP, septum. *Source*: Courtesy of Dr. Ilan Timor-Tritsch.

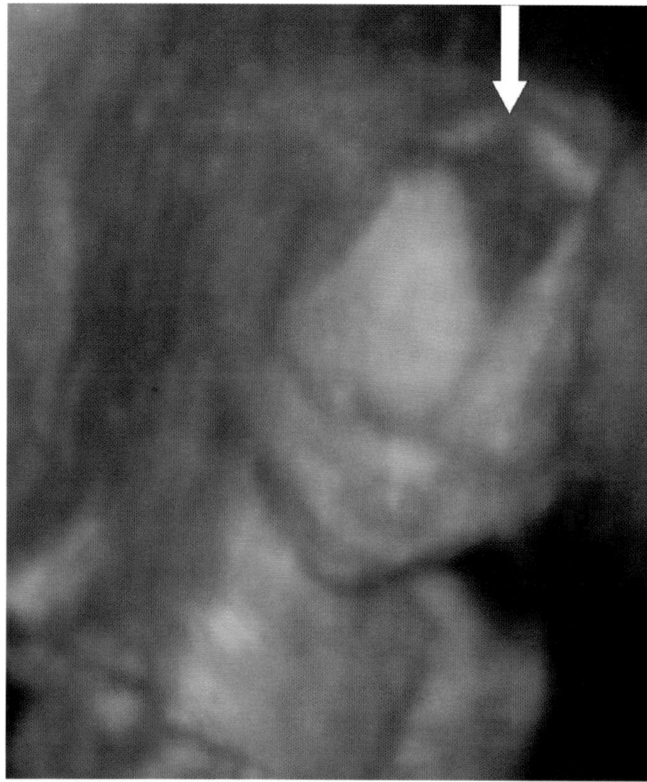

FIGURE 12 ■ Normal anterior fontanelle (*arrow*) at 18 weeks.

fetuses with spinal defects that were confirmed by postnatal MRI and found that 2DUS identified the spinal level within one vertebral segment in six of nine infants compared to 3DUS, which agreed in eight of nine infants. The key to such accuracy lies in the ability to view both the sagittal and the axial images at the same time while using the view bar to evaluate both the presence and the level of the defect (50).

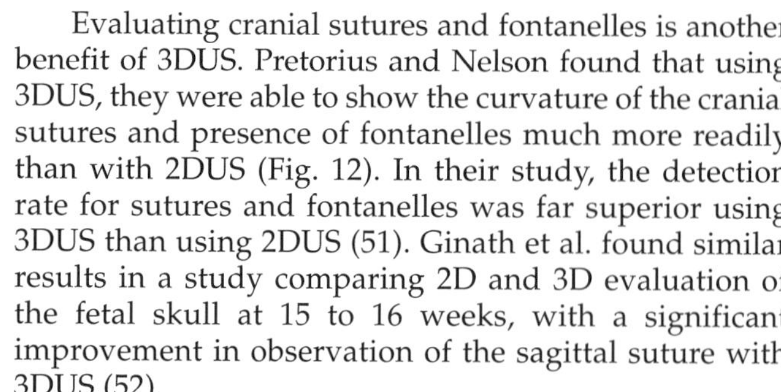

Evaluating cranial sutures and fontanelles is another benefit of 3DUS. Pretorius and Nelson found that using 3DUS, they were able to show the curvature of the cranial sutures and presence of fontanelles much more readily than with 2DUS (Fig. 12). In their study, the detection rate for sutures and fontanelles was far superior using 3DUS than using 2DUS (51). Ginath et al. found similar results in a study comparing 2D and 3D evaluation of the fetal skull at 15 to 16 weeks, with a significant improvement in observation of the sagittal suture with 3DUS (52).

Multiple case reports in the literature have discussed identification of multiple anomalies including a case of a fetus with holoprosencephaly, cyclopia, and a fetal proboscis. The use of 3DUS in this case allowed enhanced visualization of the anomaly in comparison to 2DUS views and allowed determination of the presence of cyclopia not recognized on the initial 2D images (53). An example of both 2DUS and 3DUS images of a fetus with proboscis is shown in Figure 7.

An additional application of skeletal imaging using 3DUS is the evaluation of the fetal limbs as described in a case report of a fetus with phocomelia. In this case, 2DUS was unable to visualize the upper extremities clearly; shortening of the upper limbs was confirmed upon delivery of the infant. Although 2DUS suggested an abnormality, 3DUS allowed enhanced visualization of the extent of the defect and allowed the parents to better understand the anomaly (48). In a study by Garjian et al., 3DUS was valuable in evaluating several skeletal dysplasias. Short ribs, splayed ribs, and absent bones were more easily demonstrated using 3DUS. In two fetuses with facial abnormalities and scapular anomalies, additional information was provided with the use of 3DUS (54). The diagnosis of polydactyly can be made with both multiplanar views and rendered views. 3DUS may also assist in the diagnosis of clubfoot (Fig. 13) and clenched hands (Fig. 14).

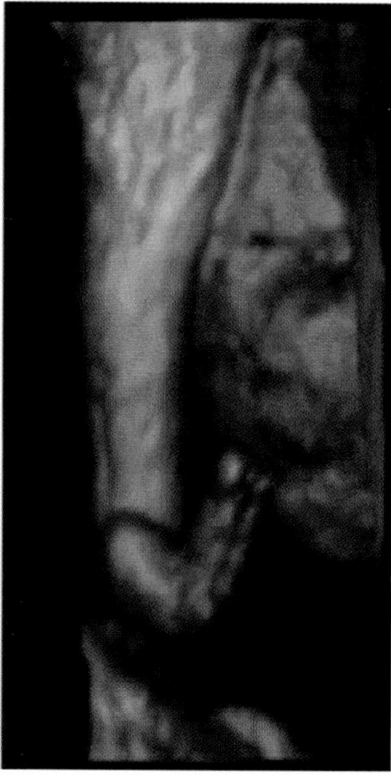

FIGURE 13 ■ Clubfoot. The multiplanar images are seen on the left and the abnormally formed ankle (*arrow*) is shown. The surface-rendered image of the clubfoot is seen on the right.

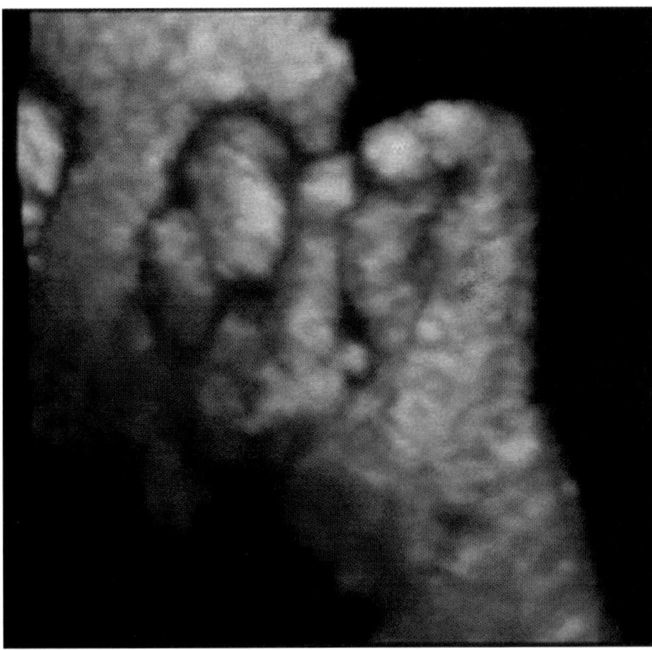

FIGURE 14 ■ Clenched hands of Trisomy 18. *Source*: Courtesy of Dr. Larry Platt.

A unique use of 3DUS is the determination of the fetal iliac angle as a prenatal marker for Down's syndrome. Although difficult to reproduce with 2DUS, an angle of greater than 87° correctly identified 56% of fetuses with Trisomy 21, with excellent reproducibility on 3DUS as described by Lee et al. 3DUS improved the reproducibility by allowing the practitioner to manipulate the volume data into a standardized view in which both ischial tuberosities were visualized and the axial plane adjusted until the longest straightest iliac angles could be visualized (55). This new data may increase the use of the fetal iliac angle as another marker on 3DUS for screening for Trisomy 21.

One of the difficulties with visualizing the fetal skeleton, particularly the extremities, lies in the acquisition of the initial volume. Fetal movements can create artifacts or completely obscure the view being sought. Once an adequate volume is acquired though, the features of 3DUS allow careful sequential evaluation of the skeleton with no further impedance from fetal movement as would continue to be the case in 2D scanning.

THE HEART

Congenital heart defects (CHD) are found in 8 of 1000 live births. Half of those are considered to be major, with long-term impact on morbidity and mortality (56–58). They account for a third of all perinatal mortality from congenital anomalies (59). Most of these occur in "low-risk" pregnancies and therefore the diagnosis relies on an abnormal finding on a routine ultrasound. In an effort to improve prenatal detection of CHD, both the American Institute of Ultrasound in Medicine (AIUM) and the American College of Radiology (ACR) have included the evaluation of the four-chamber view of the heart as part of the standard for an antepartum ultrasound (Standards for the Performance of the Antepartum Obstetrical Ultrasound Examination) (ACR Standard for the Performance of Antepartum Obstetrical Ultrasound). Although the addition of the ventricular outflow tracts (also recently adopted by the AIUM and ACR) has improved prenatal detection of cardiac defects, many defects still go unrecognized.

Studies have demonstrated the value of 3D echocardiography in the diagnosis of CHD in infants, children, and adults (60–63). This led to investigations of this newer technology in the evaluation of the fetal heart and prenatal diagnosis of fetal CHD. The main problem faced was the difficulty in obtaining a fetal electrocardiogram. Results of early work using nongated fetal echocardiography, in which a single static volume is generated from multiple planes obtained from different parts of the cardiac cycle, were mixed. Some authors suggested the technique was promising whereas others believed it to be of little clinical usefulness (64–69). Although Sklansky et al. demonstrated that nongated echocardiography allowed visualization of cardiac structures not visualized with 2DUS, cardiac motion could not be reconstructed (70). Several investigators developed methods for gating the fetal heart. Deng et al. used a simultaneous real-time directed M-mode facility to record the cardiac phases (71). Nelson et al. used Fourier transform analysis of fetal cardiac motion (72). Sklansky et al. compared conventional 2D echocardiography with gated and nongated 3D echocardiography in visualizing cardiac anatomy (67). Nine fetuses were studied, all with normal cardiac anatomy demonstrated on standard 2D echocardiography. Free-hand sweeps were obtained in either transverse or sagittal orientation of the fetal heart. A total of seven transverse and five sagittal sweeps were selected for reconstruction. They showed that, when compared to conventional 2D imaging, both gated and nongated 3D echocardiography exceeded the ability to demonstrate cardiac anatomy. The acquisition time was shorter with 3D echocardiography since a complete volumetric data set could be acquired from a single 13 to 37 second sweep, compared to the multiple views and sweeps required with conventional 2D echocardiography. The major finding of the study was that gated 3D echocardiography allowed better visualization as well as comprehension of fetal cardiac anatomy. By allowing v isualization of cardiac dynamics, gating allowed assessment of cardiac function as well as anatomy. Nevertheless, this technique continued to be limited by fetal movements and breathing.

The use of real-time 3D echocardiography equipment in the evaluation of adult hearts stimulated investigators to work on imaging fetal hearts. This newer technology had the potential to overcome some of the limitations of the earlier methods of fetal 3D echocardiography mentioned. This system uses a 2D matrix-phased array transducer that would acquire a pyramidal volume at 20 volumes/sec. The entire fetal heart was included within this volume data. Any one particular area of interest could

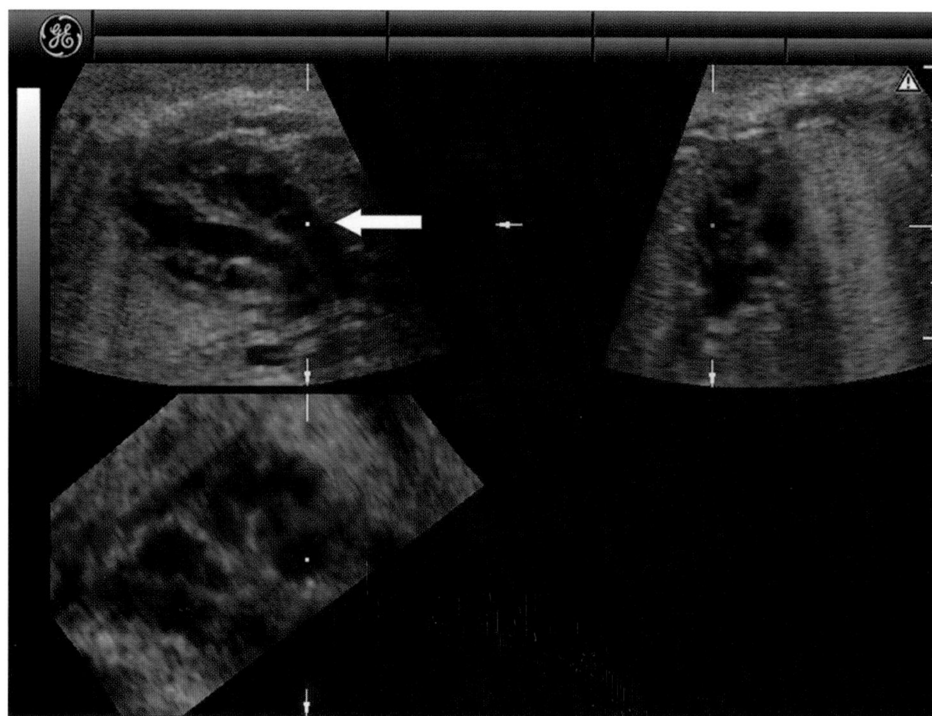

FIGURE 15 ■ Transposition of the great vessels. The marker dot is on the aorta in all three images. Upper left image shows the parallel great vessels with the aorta on top (*arrow*) and the pulmonary artery below, arising from the left ventricle. In the upper right image, the aorta is found anterior to the pulmonary artery. *Source*: Courtesy of Dr. Greggory Devore.

be visualized by moving through the cardiac volumes. Also, motion could be stopped, slowed down, or viewed at actual acquisition speed. Sklansky et al. demonstrated the advantages of this newer technique (73). They showed that the images obtained with real-time 3D echocardiography were good, fast, and easy to interpret. They also showed that gating was no longer needed since the entire fetal heart was contained within the volumetric data. Planes could be selected and oriented in any fashion to visualize the structure of interest. This improved not only the visualization of anatomical relationships but also the understanding of complex CHD. Therefore, real-time 3D echocardiography allowed evaluation of fetal cardiac function as well as anatomy. Another important benefit of this technique was the ability to store the images for later interpretation or send the volumes via Internet to an expert at a distant location for assistance in interpretation.

The concept of a gated fetal heart using heart motion to gate the heart was introduced into clinical practice as spatiotemporal image correlation (STIC). This technology allows for an automatic volume acquisition through the fetal heart that results in a complete fetal cardiac cycle displayed in motion in an endless 3D cine-loop sequence. Several authors have written about the benefits of STIC (74–78). STIC can be used to evaluate the four-chamber view as well as the outflow tracts by sweeping through a single cardiac volume and looking at standardized, reconstructed planes that are reproducible. Abnormal outflow tracts, such as transposition of the great vessels, can be interrogated and identified (Fig. 15). The heart can be evaluated for small defects (such as ventricular septal defects) on images throughout the cardiac cycle as they may be present on only a few of the images. Chaoui et al. and Goncalves et al. showed that color Doppler could be integrated into the volume acquisition to evaluate for congenital heart disease (77,78). Blood pool images of vessels within the cardiac chambers can be displayed using the minimum projection mode or the invert mode (Fig. 16) (79–82).

VOLUME MEASUREMENTS

3DUS has been shown to improve accuracy of length and volume measurements (83,84). A variety of strategies has been used from manual outlining of structures on serial parallel images to semiautomatic and fully automatic

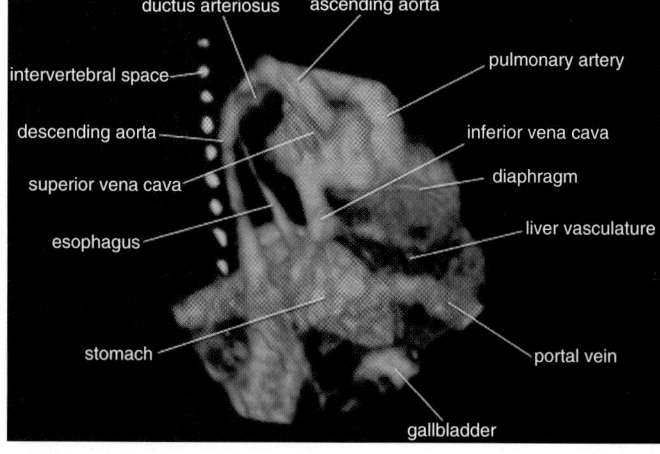

FIGURE 16 ■ Invert mode of the heart and great vessels. *Source*: From Ref. 82.

algorithms that segment organs and structures for analysis. Automated segmentation algorithms are needed in order for such measurements to be clinically useful. Ultrasound poses challenges in developing robust algorithms however, particularly because edges are often obscured by shadows or refractive shadows emanating from curved structures; improvements in image processing should improve capabilities in the future. 3DUS has been used to measure bladder volume, estimate fetal weight and age, fetal lung volume, liver volume, and placental volume (84–89).

CONCLUSION

3DUS has great potential to change the way that ultrasound is practiced. New display techniques including presentation of multiple parallel planar images similar to CT and MRI (Fig. 3) may allow physicians to "see" many more ultrasound images that were previously seen only by the sonographer. In addition, volume data may allow physicians to acquire data more rapidly and review it in a cine-loop mode rather than as individual images (O'Neill MJ, Personal communication, Massachusetts General Hospital).

ACKNOWLEDGMENTS

We thank Vivian Cohen for assistance with manuscript preparation. This study was performed using equipment on loan from General Electric Medical Systems.

REFERENCES

1. Economides D, Braithwaite J. First trimester ultrasonographic diagnosis of fetal structural abnormalities in a low risk population. Br J Obstet Gynaecol 1998; 105(1):53–57.
2. Hull A, James G, Salerno C, et al. Three dimensional ultrasonography and assessment of the first trimester fetus. J Ultrasound Med 2001; 20:287–293.
3. Michailidis G, Papageorgious P, Economides D. Assessment of fetal anatomy in the first trimester using two- and three-dimensional ultrasound. Br J Obstet Gynaecol 2002; 75:215–221.
4. Chung B, Kim H, Lee KL. The application of three-dimensional ultrasound to nuchal translucency measurement in early pregnancy (10–14 weeks): a preliminary study. Ultrasound Obstet Gynecol 2000; 15(2):122–125.
5. Paul C, Krampl E, Skentou C, et al. Measurement of fetal nuchal translucency thickness by three-dimensional ultrasound. Ultrasound Obstet Gynecol 2001; 18(5):481–484.
6. Clementschitsch G, Hasenohrl G, Schaffer H, et al. Comparison between two- and three-dimensional ultrasound measurements of nuchal translucency. Ultrasound Obstet Gynecol 2001; 18(5): 475–480.
7. Down J. Observations on an ethnic classification of idiots. London Hospital Reports 1866; 3:259–262.
8. Cicero S, Curcio P, Papageorghious A, et al. Absence of nasal bone in fetuses with trisomy 21 at 11–14 weeks of gestation: an observational study. Lancet 2001; 358:1665–1667.
9. Cicero S, Sonek J, McKenna D, et al. Nasal bone hypoplasia in trisomy 21 at 15–22 weeks' gestation. Ultrasound Obstet Gynecol 2003; 21:15–18.
10. Sonek J, Nicolaides K. Prenatal ultrasonographic diagnosis of nasal bone abnormalities in three fetuses with Down Syndrome. Am J Obstet Gynecol 2002; 186:139–141.
11. Cicero S, Bindra R, Rembouskos G, et al. Integrated ultrasound and biochemical screening for trisomy 21 using fetal nuchal translucency, absent fetal nasal bone, free B-hCG and PAPP-1 at 11 to 14 weeks. Prenat Diagn 2003; 23:306–310.
12. Rembouskos G, Cicero S, Longo D, et al. Assessment of the fetal nasal bone at 11–14 weeks of gestation by three-dimensional ultrasound. Ultrasound Obstet Gynecol 2004; 23(3):232–236.
13. O'Rahilly R, Muller F. Ventricular system and choroid plexus of the human brain during the embryonic period proper. Z Anat Entwicklungsgesch 1971; 134:1–12.
14. O'Rahilly R, Muller F. Ventricular system and choroid plexuses of the human brain during the embryonic period proper. Am J Anat 1990; 189(4):285–302.
15. Blaas H, Eik-Nes S, Kiserud T, et al. Three-dimensional imaging of the brain cavities in human embryos. Ultrasound Obstet Gynecol 1995; 5(4):228–232.
16. Blaas H, Eik-Nes S, Berg S, et al. In-vivo three-dimensional ultrasound reconstructions of embryos and early fetuses. Lancet 1998; 352(9135):1182–1186.
17. Blaas H, Eik-Nes S, Vainio T, et al. Alobar holoprosencephaly at 9 weeks gestational age visualized by two- and three-dimensional. Ultrasound Obstet Gynecol 2000; 15(1):62–65.
18. Benoit B, Hafner T, Bekavac I, et al. 3-dimensional Sonoembryology. Ultrasound Rev Obstet Gynecol 2001; 1(2):128–37.
19. Ji E, Pretorius D, Newton R, et al. Effects of ultrasound on maternal-fetal bonding: a comparison of 2-dimensional vs. 3-dimensional imaging. J Ultrasound Obstet Gynecol 2005; 25:473–477.
20. Maier B, Steiner H, Wienerroither H, et al. The psychological impact of three-dimensional fetal imaging on the fetomaternal relationship. In: Baba K, Jurkovic D, ed. Three-Dimensional Ultrasound in Obstetrics and Gynecology. New York: Pathenon, 1997:67–74.
21. Rotten D, Levaillant J. Two- and three-dimensional sonographic assessment of the fetal face. 2: systematic analysis of the normal face. Ultrasound Obstet Gynecol 2004; 23:224–231.
22. Johnson D, Pretorius D, Budorick N, et al. Fetal lip and primary palate: three dimensional versus two dimensional US. Radiology 2000; 217:236–239.
23. Lee W, Chaiworapongsa T, Romero R, et al. A diagnostic approach for the evaluation of spina bifida by three-dimensional ultrasonography. J Ultrasound Med 2002; 21:619–626.
24. Rotten D, Levaillant J. Two- and three-dimensional sonographic assessment of the fetal face. 2. Analysis of cleft lip, alveolus and palate. Ultrasound Obstet Gynecol 2004; 24:402–411.
25. Chmait R, Pretorius D, Jones M, et al. Prenatal evaluation of facial clefts with two dimensional and adjunctive three dimensional ultrasonography: a prospective trial. Am J Obstet Gynecol 2002; 187(4):946–949.
26. Chmait R, Pretorius D, Moore T. Prenatal detection of associated anomalies in fetuses diagnosed with cleft lip with or without cleft pallet in utero. Ultrasound Obstet Gynecol 2006; 27:173–176.
27. Campbell S, Lees C. The three-dimensional reverse face (3D RF) view for the diagnosis of cleft palate. Ultrasound Obstet Gynecol 2003; 22(5):552–554.
28. Campbell S, Lees C, Moscoso G, et al. Ultrasound antenatal diagnosis of cleft palate by a new technique: the 3D 'reverse face' view. Ultrasound Obstet Gynecol 2005; 25:12–18.
29. Merz E, Welter C. 2D and 3D ultrasound in the evaluation of normal and abnormal fetal anatomy in the second and third trimesters in level III center. Ultraschall Med 2005; 26:9–16.
30. Shih J, Shyu M, Lee C, et al. Antenatal depiction of the fetal ear with three-dimensional ultrasonography. Obstet Gynecol 1998; 91(4):500–505.
31. Ulm M, Kratochwil A, Ulm B, et al. Three-dimensional ultrasound evaluation of fetal tooth germs. Ultrasound Obstet Gynecol 1998; 12:240–243.
32. Rotten D, Levaillant J, Martinez H, et al. The fetal mandible: a 2D and 3D sonographic approach to the diagnosis of retrognathia and micrognathia. Ultrasound Obstet Gynecol 2002; 19:122–130.

33. Benoit B, Chaoui R. Three-dimensional ultrasound with maximal mode rendering: a novel technique for the diagnosis of bilateral or unilateral absence or hypoplasia of nasal bones in second-trimester screening for Down Syndrome. Ultrasound Obstet Gynecol 2005; 25:19–24.
34. Nelson T, Pretorius D, Hull A, et al. Sources and impact of artifacts on clinical 3DUS imaging. Ultrasound Obstetrics Gynecology 2000; 16(4):374–383.
35. Merz E, Miric-Tesanic D, Welter C. Value of the electronic scalpel (cut mode) in the evaluation of the fetal face. Ultrasound Obstet Gynecol 2000; 16:564–568.
36. Pilu G, Perolo A, Falco P, et al. Ultrasound of the fetal central nervous system. Curr Opin Obstet Gynecol 2000; 12(2):93–103.
37. Johnson DD, Pretorius DH, Riccabona M, et al. Three-dimensional ultrasound of the fetal spine. Obstet Gynecol 1997; 89(3):434–438.
38. Budorick N, Pretorius D, Nelson T. Sonography of the fetal spine: technique, imaging findings, and clinical implications. Am J Roentgenology 1995; 164(2):421–428.
39. Riccabona M, Johnson D, Pretorius DH, et al. Three dimensional ultrasound: display modalities in the fetal spine and thorax. Eur J Radiol 1996; 22(2):141–145.
40. Dyson R, Pretorius D, Budorick N, et al. Three dimensional ultrasound in the evaluation of fetal anomalies. Ultrasound Obstet Gynecol 2000; 16:321–328.
41. Muller F, Weiner C, Yankowitz J. Three dimensional ultrasound in the evaluation of fetal head and spine anomalies. Obstet Gynecol 1996; 88(3):372–378.
42. Menkes J, Sarnat H. Child Neurology. 6th ed. Philadelphia: Lippincott Williams & Wilkins, 2000:316.
43. Kollias SS, Goldstein RB, Cogen H, et al. Prenatally detected myelomeningoceles: sonographic accuracy in estimation of the spinal level. Radiology 1992; 185(1):109–112.
44. Monteagudo A, Timor-Tritsch IE, Mayberry P. Three-dimensional transvaginal neurosonography of the fetal brain: 'navigating' in the volume scan. Ultrasound Obstet Gynecol 2000; 16(4):307–313.
45. Timor-Tritsch IE, Monteagudo A, Mayberry P, Three-dimensional ultrasound evaluation of the fetal brain: the three horn view. Ultrasound Obstet Gynecol 2000; 16(4):302–306.
46. Hata T, Yanagihara T, Matsumoto M, et al. 3 dimensional sonographic features of fetal central nervous system anomaly. Acta Obstet Gynecol Scand 2000; 79:635–639.
47. Benacerraf B, Spiro R, Mitchell G. Using three-dimensional ultrasound to detect craniosynostosis in a fetus with Pfeiffer Syndrome. Ultrasound Obstet Gynecol 2000; 16:391–394.
48. Lee A, Kratochwil A, Deutinger J, et al. Three-dimensional ultrasound in diagnosing phocomelia. Ultrasound Obstet Gynecol 1995; 5:238–240.
49. Benoit B. The value of three-dimensional ultrasonography in the screening of the fetal skeleton. Childs Nerv Syst 2003; 19:403–409.
50. Lee W, McNie B, Chaiworapongsa T, et al. Three-dimensional ultrasonographic presentation of micrognathia. J Ultrasound Med 2002; 21:775–781.
51. Pretorius DH, Nelson TR. Prenatal visualization of cranial sutures and fontanelles with three-dimensional ultrasonography. J Ultrasound Med 1994; 13(11):871–876.
52. Ginath S, Debby A, Malinger G. Demonstration of cranial sutures and fontanelles at 15–16 weeks of gestation: a comparison between two-dimensional and three-dimensional ultrasonography. Prenat Diagn 2004; 24:812–815.
53. Hsu T, Chang S, Ou C, et al. First trimester diagnosis of holoprosencephaly and cyclopia with triploidy by transvaginal three-dimensional ultrasonography. Eur J Obstet Gynecol 2001; 96(2): 235–237.
54. Garjian K, Pretorius D, Budorick N, et al. 3 dimensional ultrasound imaging of fetal skeletal dysplasia: initial experience. Radiology 2000; 214:717–723.
55. Lee W, Blanckaert K, Bronsteen R, et al. Fetal iliac angle measurements by three-dimensional sonography. Ultrasound Obstet Gynecol 2001; 18:150–154.
56. Hoffman J. Incidence of congenital heart disease: I Postnatal Incidence. Pediatr Cardiol 1995; 16(3):103–113.
57. Hoffman J. Incidence of congenital heart disease: II postnatal incidence. Pediatr Cardiol 1995; 16(4):155–165.
58. Hoffman J, Christianson R. Congenital heart disease in a cohort of 19,502 births with long term followup. Am J Cardiol 1978; 42(4):641–647.
59. Centers for Disease Control & Prevention. Infant Mortality–United States. MMWR, Morb Mortal Wkly Rep 1996; 45(10): 211–215.
60. Bates J, Tantengco M, Ryan T, et al. A systematic approach to echocardiographic image acquisition and 3 dimensional reconstruction with subxiphoid rotational scan. J Am Soc Echocard 1996; 9:257–265.
61. Marx G, Fulton D, Pandian N, et al. Delineation of site, relative size and dynamic geometry of atrial septal defects by real time three-dimensional echocardiography. J Am Coll Cardiol 1995; 25(2): 482–490.
62. Salustri A, Spitael S, McGhie J, et al. Transthoracic three-dimensional echocardiography in adult patients with congenital heart disease. J Am Coll Cardiol 1995; 26(3):759–767.
63. Vogel M, Losch S. Dynamic three-dimensional echocardiography with a computed tomography imaging probe: initial clinical experience with transthoracic application in infants and children with congenital heart deficits. Br Heart J 1994; 71(5):462–467.
64. Zosmer N, Jurkovic D, Jauniaux F, et al. Selection and identification of standard cardiac views from three-dimensional volume scans of the fetal thorax. J Ultrasound Med 1996; 15(11):25–32.
65. Meyer-Wittkopf M, Cook A, McLennan A, et al. Evaluation of three-dimensional ultrasonography and magnetic resonance imaging in assessment of congenital heart anomalies in fetal cardiac specimens. Ultrasound Obstet Gynecol 1996; 8:303–308.
66. Chang FM, Hsu KF, Ko HC, et al. Fetal heart volume assessment by three-dimensional ultrasound. Ultrasound Obstet Gynecol 1997; 9(1):42–48.
67. Sklansky MS, Nelson TR, Pretorius DH. Three-dimensional fetal echocardiography: gated versus nongated techniques. J Ultrasound Med 1998; 17(7):451–457.
68. Merz E, Bahlman F, Weber G. Volume scanning in the evaluation of fetal malformations: a new dimension in prenatal diagnosis. Ultrasound Obstet Gynecol 1995; 5:222–227.
69. Leventhal M, Pretorius DH, Sklansky MS, et al. Three-dimensional ultrasonography of normal fetal heart: comparison with two-dimensional imaging. J Ultrasound Med 1998; 17(6):341–348.
70. Sklansky MS, Nelson TR, Pretorius DH. Usefulness of gated three-dimensional fetal echocardiography to reconstruct and display structures not visualized with two-dimensional imaging. Am J Cardiol 1997; 80(5):665–668.
71. Deng J, Gardener J, Rodeck C, et al. Fetal echocardiography in three and four dimensions. Ultrasound Med Biol 1996; 22(8): 979–986.
72. Nelson TR, Pretorius DH, Sklansky M, et al. Three-dimensional echocardiographic evaluation of fetal heart anatomy and function: acquisition, analysis, and display. J Ultrasound Med 1996; 15(1):1–9 quiz 11–2.
73. Sklansky M, Nelson T, Strachan V, et al. Real time three dimensional fetal echocardiography: initial feasibility study. J Ultrasound Med 1999; 18:745–752.
74. Vinals F, Poblete P, Guiliano A. Spatio-temporal image correlation (STIC): a new tool for the prenatal screening of congenital heart defects. Ultrasound Obstet Gynecol 2003; 22(4):388–394.
75. DeVore G, Falkensammer P, Sklansky M, et al. Spatio-temporal image correlation (STIC): new technology for evaluation of the fetal heart. Ultrasound Obstet Gynecol 2003; 22(4):380–387.
76. DeVore G, Polanco B, Sklansky M, et al. The 'spin' technique: a new method for examination of the fetal outflow tracts using three-dimensional ultrasound. Ultrasound Obstet Gynecol 2004; 24(1):72–82.
77. Goncalves L, Romero R, Espinoza J, et al. Four-dimensional ultrasonography of the fetal heart using color Doppler spatio-temporal image correlation. J Ultrasound Med 2004; 23(4): 473–481.
78. Chaoui R, Hoffmann J, Heling K. Three-dimensional (3D) and 4D color Doppler fetal echocardiography using spatio-temporal image correlation (STIC). J Ultrasound Med 2004; 23(6):535–45.

79. Espinoza J, Kalache K, Gonçalves L, et al. Prenatal diagnosis of membranous ventricular septal aneurysms and their association with absence of atrioventricular valve 'offsetting.' Ultrasound Obstet Gynecol 2004; 24(7):787–792.
80. Chaoui R, Kalache K, Heling S. Potential of off-line 4D fetal echocardiography using new acquisition and rendering technique (STIC = Spatio Temporal Image Correlation). Ultrasound Obstetrics Gynecology 2003; 22(S1):661–663.
81. Lee W, Goncalves L, Espinoza J, et al. Inversion mode: a new volume analysis tool for 3-dimensional ultrasonography. J Ultrasound Med 2005; 24(2):201–207.
82. Gonçalves L, Espinoza J, Lee W, et al. Three- and four-dimensional reconstruction of the aortic and ductal arches using inversion mode: a new rendering algorithm for visualization of fluid-filled anatomical structures. Ultrasound Obstet Gynecol 2004; 24(6): 696–698.
83. Riccabona M, Nelson TR, Pretorius DH, et al. Distance and volume measurement using three-dimensional ultrasonography. J Ultrasound Med 1995; 14(12):881–886.
84. Riccabona M, Nelson TR, Pretorius DH, et al. In vivo three-dimensional sonographic measurement of organ volume: validation in the urinary bladder. J Ultrasound Med 1996; 15(9): 627–632.
85. Lee W, Deter R, Ebersole J, et al. Birth weight prediction by three-dimensional ultrasonography: fractional limb volume. J Ultrasound in Medicine 2001; 20(12):1283–1292.
86. Chang CH, Yu C, Ko HC, et al. The efficacy assessment of thigh volume in predicting intrauterine fetal growth restriction by three-dimensional ultrasound. Ultrasound Med Biol 2005; 31(7): 883–887.
87. Sabogal J, Becker E, Bega G, et al. Reproducibility of fetal lung volume measurements with 3-dimensional ultrasonography. J Ultrasound Med 2004; 23(3):347–352.
88. Boito S, Laudy J, Struijk PC, et al. Three-dimensional US assessment of hepatic volume, head circumference, and abdominal circumference in healthy and growth restricted fetuses. Radiology 2002; 223(3): 661–665.
89. Wataganara T, Metzenbauer M, Peter I, et al. Placental volume, as measured by 3-dimensional sonography and levels of maternal plasma cell-free fetal DNA. Am J Obstet Gynecol 2005; 193(2):496–500.

Invasive Ultrasound Principles (Biopsy, Aspiration, and Drainage)

John P. McGahan

5

Although needle puncture and aspiration were described more than 60 years ago, it was not until the early 1970s that Goldberg and Pollack (1) and Holm et al. (2) independently devised transducers that could be used for ultrasound-guided aspiration or biopsy. Since that time, gradual advances have been made in ultrasound instrumentation and refinement of aspiration biopsy and drainage techniques. Most recently, the advances in ultrasound technology, combined with a better understanding of aspiration drainage techniques, have produced unparalleled growth in the field of interventional ultrasound. Therefore, ultrasound has been used not only as a diagnostic tool but also to guide a number of different interventional procedures.

WHY ULTRASOUND?

Some unique features of ultrasound make it an ideal modality to guide a number of different interventional procedures (3–6). These may be arbitrarily separated in terms of importance as primary, secondary, or tertiary (Table 1).

Primary Importance

Probably one of the most important considerations in selecting a guidance method for performance of interventional procedures is the precision for needle placement provided by the guidance system. The inherent precision and safety of the imaging modality outweighs most other considerations. Technologic advances, including specially designed ultrasound needles, allow for precise needle placement into target lesions as small as 1 cm in diameter in critical anatomic areas (Figs. 1 and 2) (6). This precision is necessary to ensure a successful procedure and often makes ultrasound the best choice in guiding a number of interventional techniques.

Secondary Importance

Compact, portable ultrasound units have been developed that can be transported to the intensive care unit or operating room to guide interventional procedures (7,8). Review of more than 100 ultrasound-guided aspiration and drainage procedures performed at our institution revealed that about one-third of these procedures were performed using a portable machine at the patient's bedside. Moving the ultrasound unit to the patient's bedside may avoid the risk and inconvenience of transporting a critically ill patient (Fig. 3).

Color

Color Doppler may be used before needle placement during this procedure or after needle or catheter placement (Table 2).

TABLE 1 ■ Unique Features of Ultrasound in Guiding Interventional Procedures

Primary
- Precision

Secondary
- Portable
- Confirm drainage
- Check for complications
- Color: avoid complications
- Color: confirm catheter position

Tertiary
- Nonionizing radiation
- Inexpensive (widely available)
- Expedient

Reports have demonstrated the utility of ultrasound in avoiding complications of aspiration biopsy (9,10). Color sonography can help to identify vascular structures within the needle path (Fig. 4). Thus, the vascular complications encountered when performing interventional procedures should be decreased using color Doppler ultrasound. Color can be used during the procedure to identify any potential complications (Fig. 5).

Color Doppler can be used to confirm needle or catheter position (Fig. 6). Although needles and guide wires are usually well visualized, with ultrasound, catheters can be more difficult to detect. Observing with color Doppler the rapid injection of small aliquots of normal saline into the catheter after drainage can help to reconfirm catheter position and demonstrate that the catheter has been placed directly into the fluid collection (11). This is especially helpful in situations in which it had been difficult to demonstrate catheter position by real-time ultrasound (Fig. 6).

Tertiary Importance

Another advantage of ultrasound is that it uses nonionizing radiation. This is especially advantageous when dealing with the fetus or in radiation sensitive areas.

Ultrasound is also relatively inexpensive. Ultrasound-guided procedures are usually cost effective compared with interventional procedures performed under computed tomography (CT) guidance or more costly surgical alternatives. Also, because it is inexpensive, ultrasound is often widely available throughout the hospital, allowing procedures to be performed on short notice. Alternatively, it may be difficult to perform an emergent CT-guided aspiration or drainage because of lack of availability of CT as compared with ultrasonography.

Finally, ultrasound is an extremely expedient method of performing needle biopsy or aspiration. In most situations, patient preparation and the ultrasound examination take a much longer time to perform than actual needle placement.

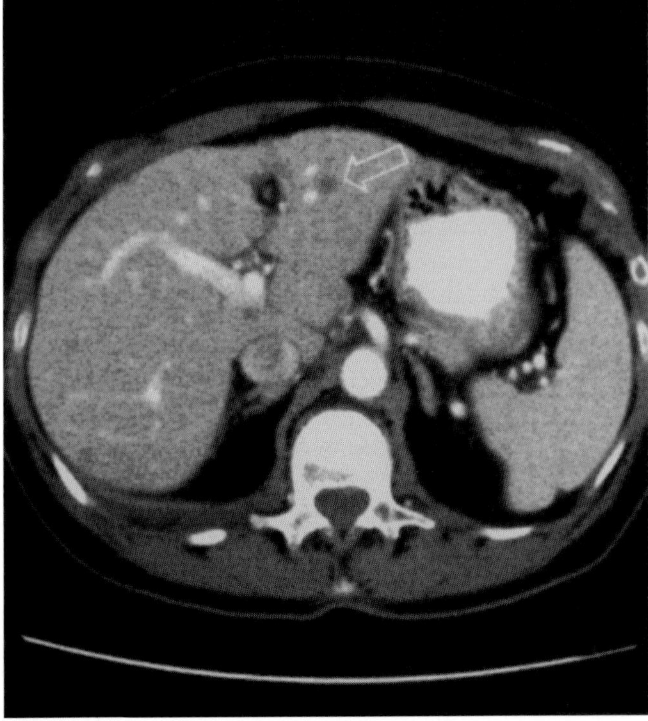
(A)

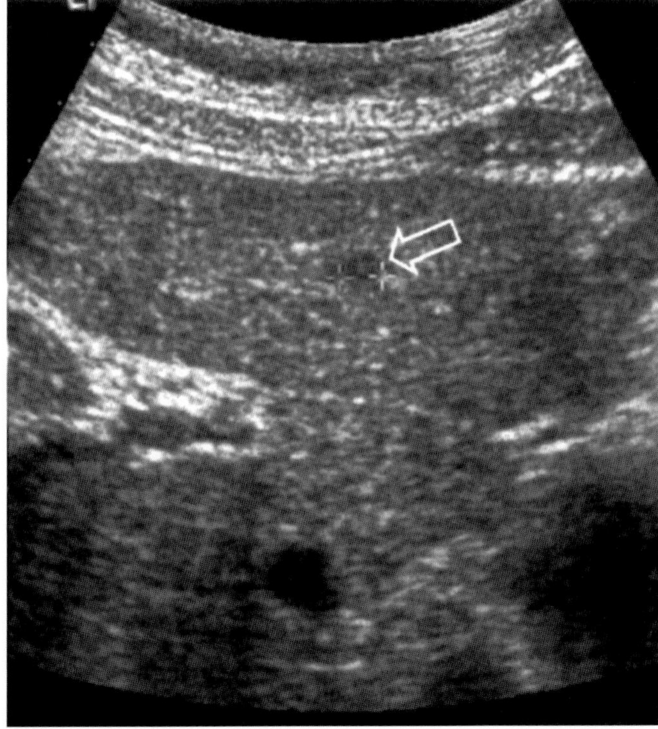
(B)

FIGURE 1 A–E ■ Liver metastasis FNA biopsy. (**A** and **B**) In this patient, there are multiple areas of decreased density seen on CT (*open arrow*) and corresponding hypoechoic regions (*open arrow*) identified on ultrasound. (*Continued*)

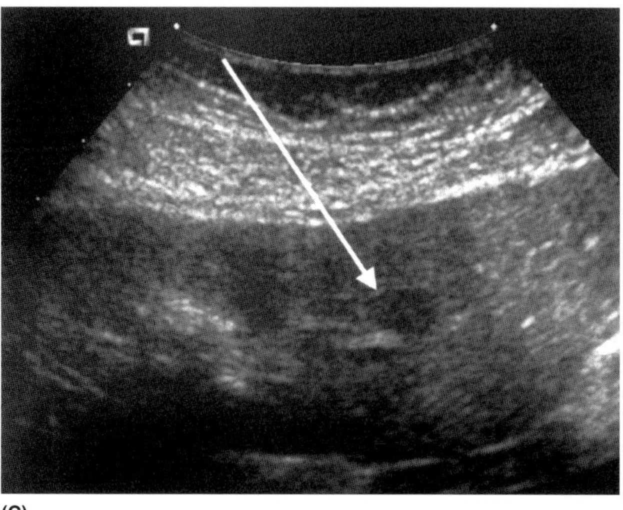

(C)

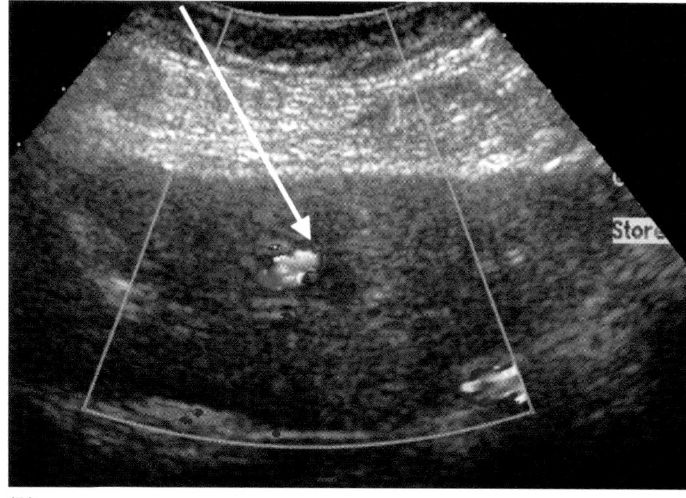

(D)

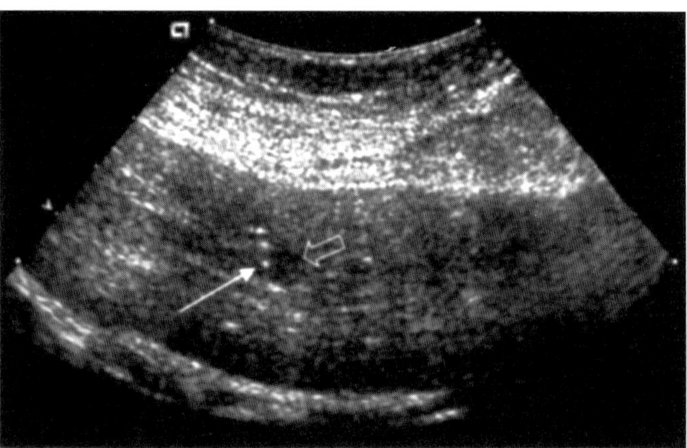

(E)

FIGURE 1 A–E ■ (*Continued*) (**C**) Hypoechoic region identified on ultrasound with possible needle path (*arrow*). (**D**) Using color flow prebiopsy, the possible needle path (*arrow*) showed overlying portal vein branch. (**E**) This portal vein was avoided during fine-needle aspiration. Needle tip (*long arrow*) within the metastatic lesion (*open arrow*). Color flow was helpful in avoiding the portal vein.

PREPROCEDURAL PREPARATION

Patient History and Consent

Proper patient consent must be obtained before aspiration biopsy or drainage. The procedure must be explained in detail, including possible risks, complications, and alternatives to the procedure. This must be documented not only on the consent form but also on the patient's chart. Patients should be questioned about a history of a bleeding disorder, easy bruising, or abnormal bleeding after surgery or during tooth extraction. The patient should be questioned concerning any medication that may prolong bleeding time. The entire procedure should be explained in detail so that the patient understands the length of the procedure as well as possible discomfort that may be encountered during the procedure. Any alternatives to the procedure must be explained. Also, the patient should be questioned concerning pain tolerance and the possible need for anesthesia.

Coagulation Studies

The acceptable range of clotting studies is based on several factors, including the site and nature of the invasive procedure (4). In general, the international ratio (INR) should not be greater than three seconds of the control, and the partial thromboplastin time should be less than 45 seconds. Platelet count should be greater than 75,000/mL for less invasive procedures (e.g., needle aspiration), but it probably should be even higher than this when large-bore drainage catheters are to be placed. A bleeding time is probably the best single test to check for abnormal bleeding. If there is any problem, hematologic consult should always be obtained. Corrective measures for increased INR are administration of vitamin K or fresh-frozen plasma and stoppage of warfarin sodium (Coumadin®) therapy. Platelet transfusions may be used for patients with low platelet counts.

Anesthesia

Simple aspiration procedures, such as thoracentesis or paracentesis, usually require only local anesthesia. Placement of an intravenous catheter before the procedure, however, can be helpful in patients who may require analgesia and monitoring.

Use of anesthesia and premedication is based on the difficulty of the procedure and patient anxiety. Simple

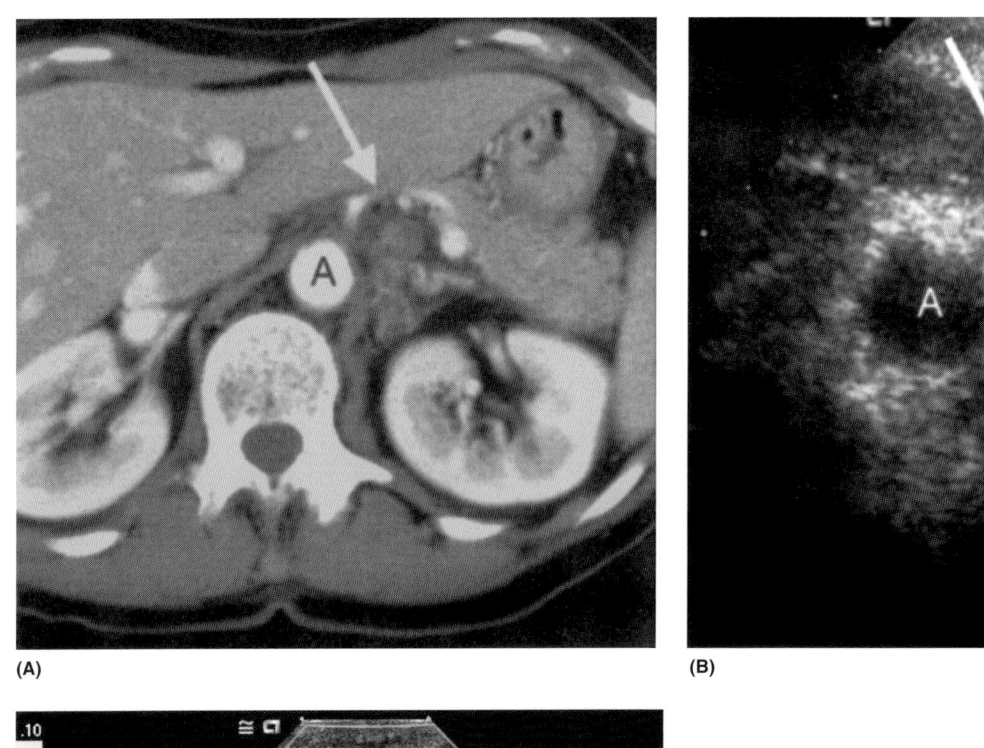

(A)

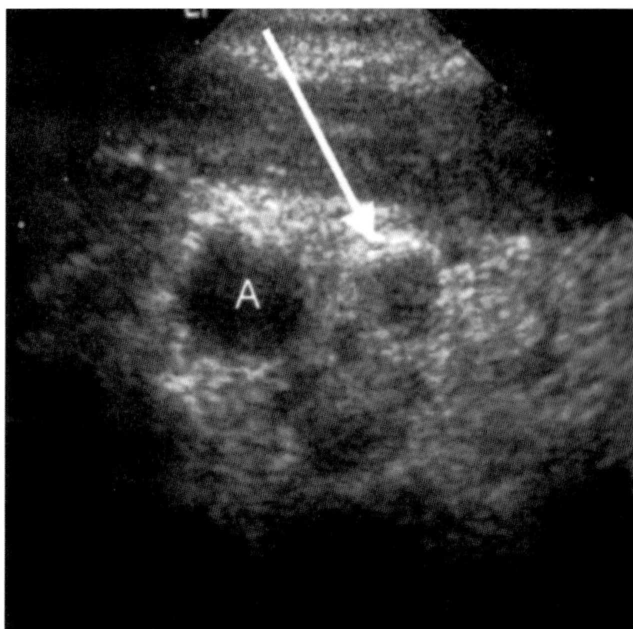

(B)

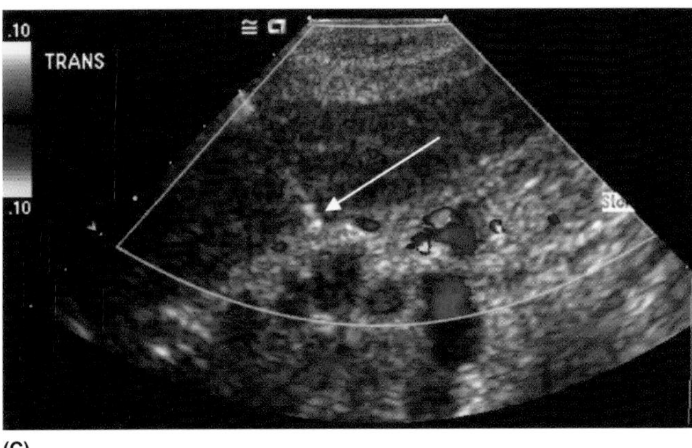

(C)

FIGURE 2 A–C ■ Fine-needle aspiration of gastrohepatic adenopathy. (**A** and **B**) CT scan and corresponding ultrasound demonstrating small node (*arrow*). (**C**) Color flow was utilized to avoid overlying vessels and a needle was placed transhepatic (*arrow*) into this metastatic node. A, aorta.

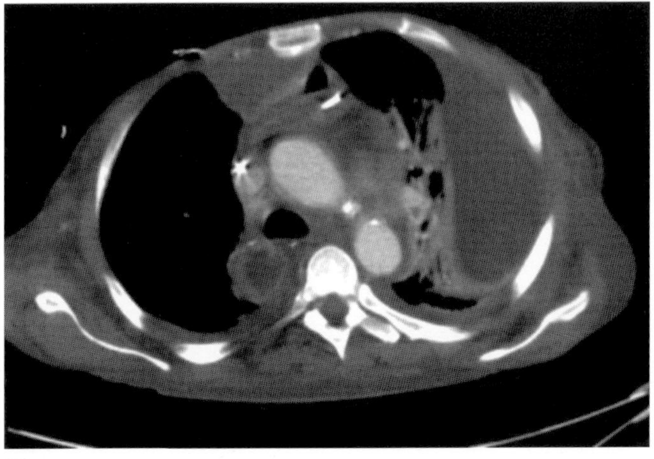

(A)

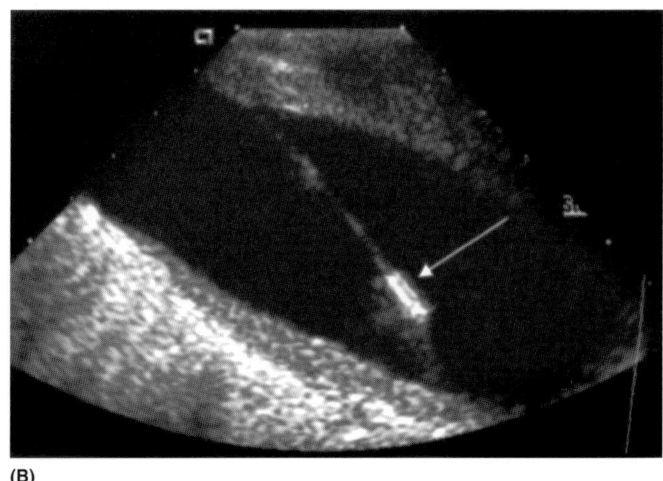

(B)

FIGURE 3 A–E ■ Chest drainage. (**A**) CT scan demonstrating empyema along the left chest wall. (**B**) After initial needle was placed into the fluid collection at the patient's bedside, the guidewire (*arrow*) is pushed through the needle. (*Continued*)

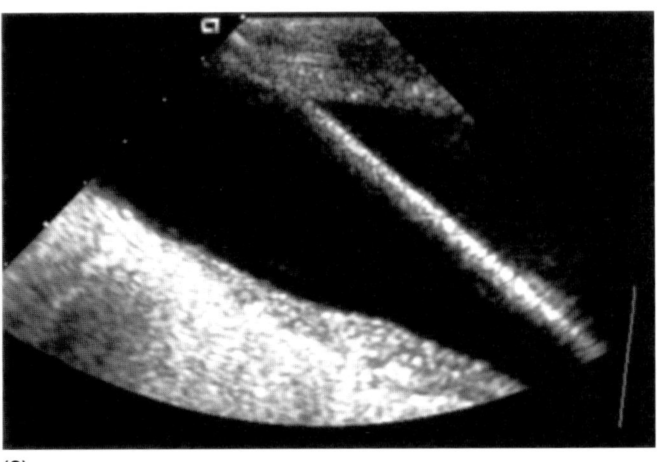

(C)

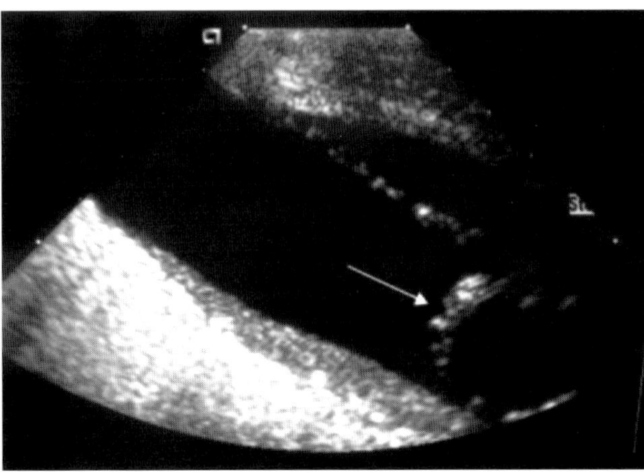

(D)

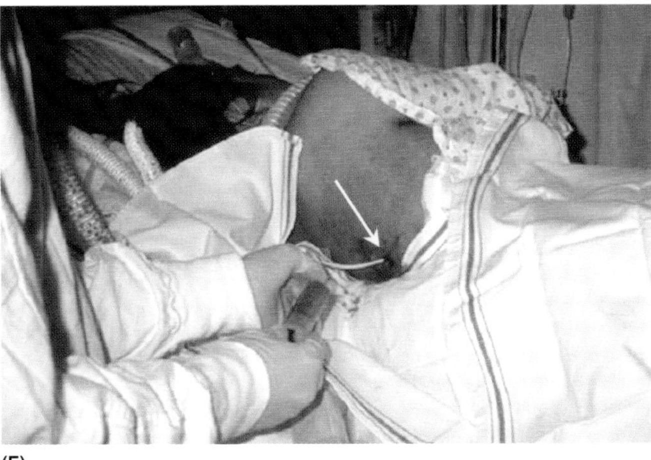

(E)

FIGURE 3 A–E ■ (*Continued*) (**C**) The guidewire is placed in the fluid collection. Using the guidewire exchange technique, the drainage catheter which is looped (*arrow*) is positioned in the fluid collection (**D**). In another patient, bedside empyema drainage catheter (*arrow*) is shown (**E**).

aspiration procedures usually require a single puncture and cause less pain and apprehension than does intramuscular injection. More complicated procedures may require use of either conscious sedation or general anesthesia. Most ultrasound-guided interventional procedures require conscious sedation and thus close patient monitoring and use of intravenous analgesics or tranquilizers.

In general, intravenous medication usually includes a combination of narcotics and tranquilizers. Narcotics that produce analgesia and sedation include fentanyl, morphine sulfate, and meperidine (Demerol). The major side effect of these narcotics is dose-dependent respiratory depression. For this reason, resuscitation equipment, including naloxone hydrochloride (Narcan), must be available.

TABLE 2 ■ Color Doppler for Interventional Procedures

Color Doppler may be used:
Preprocedure
During the procedure
Postprocedure
To avoid vessels, to detect complications, or to check catheter position

Typical tranquilizers administered by the intravenous route include midazolam hydrochloride (Versed) and diazepam (Valium). When using these medications, patients should be continuously monitored for early signs of apnea, which can lead to hypoxia or even cardiac arrest. Flumazenil (Romazicon) can counteract the side effects of diazepam and its derivatives.

GUIDANCE METHODS

The three different methods for guidance of interventional procedures are indirect needle guidance, the freehand technique, and use of a needle guidance system (4,5,12).

Indirect Method

Indirect guidance is used for aspiration or drainage of large fluid collections. It is a blind technique because the needle or catheter is not inserted using real-time guidance. The puncture site is identified, the angle and depth of the puncture are preselected from the ultrasound image, and the site is marked. The biopsy site is then prepared and draped, and the aspiration or drainage is

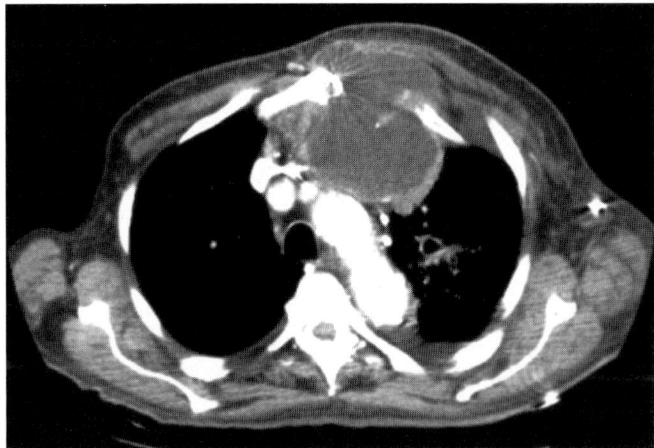
(A)

FIGURE 4 A–C ■ Color flow preprocedure. (**A**) A CT scan demonstrating large fluid collection anterior to the aorta, which eroded the anterior chest wall. (**B** and **C**) Ultrasound image without (**B**) and with (**C**) color flow. Using a color flow, an internal mammary artery graft was visualized (*arrows*) within the fluid collection. Catheter drainage was not performed, after identification of the artery within the fluid.

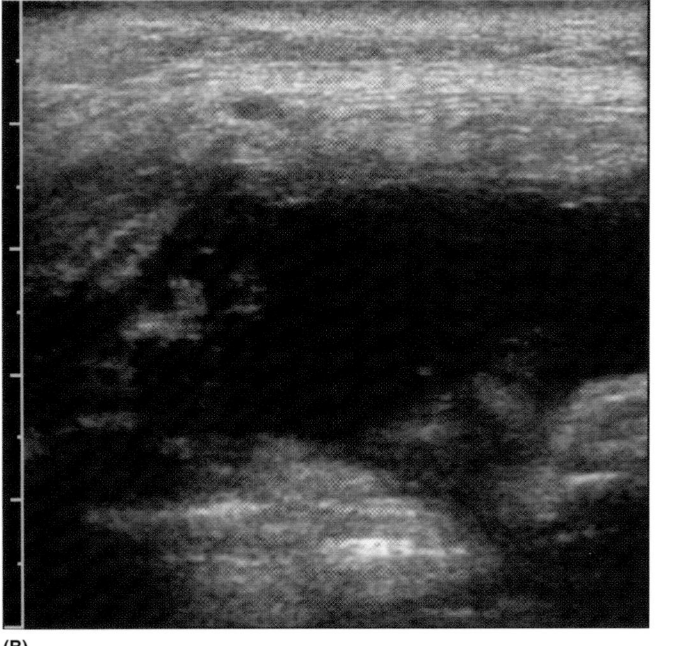
(B)

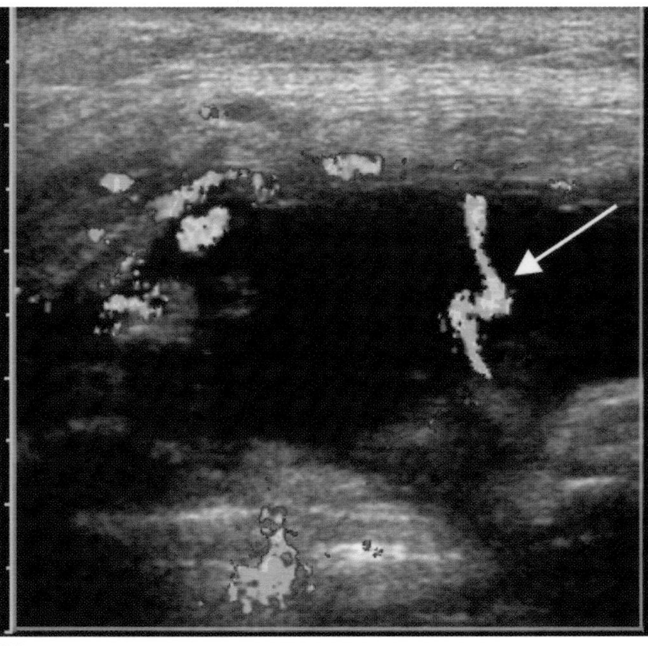
(C)

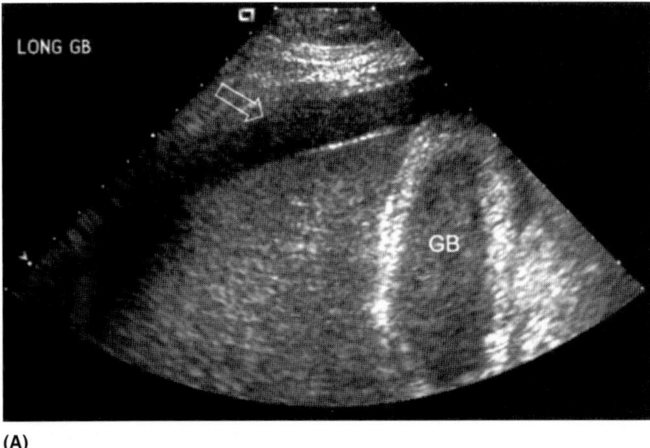

(A)

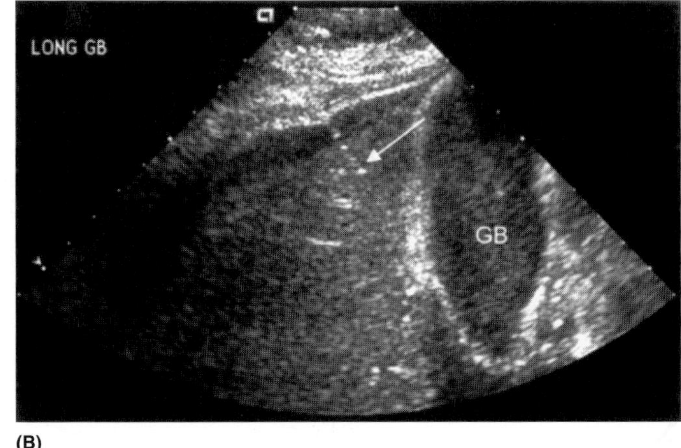

(B)

FIGURE 5 A–D ■ Color flow during the procedure. (**A**) Percutaneous cholecystostomy is to be performed using the transhepatic route with trocar catheter to be placed into the GB through ascites (*open arrow*). (**B**) Trocar catheter tip is visualized within the liver (*arrow*). (*Continued*)

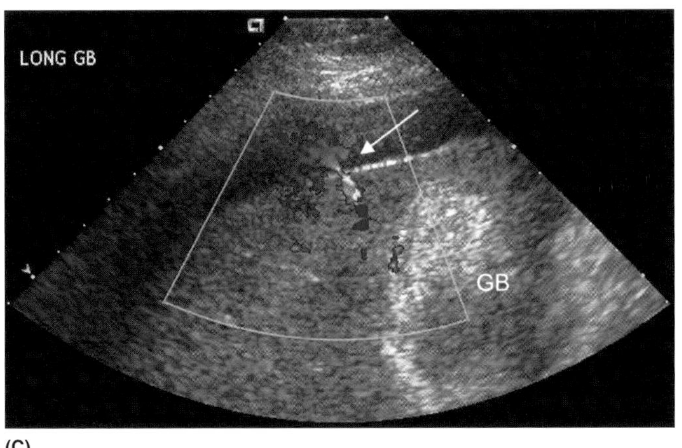

(C)

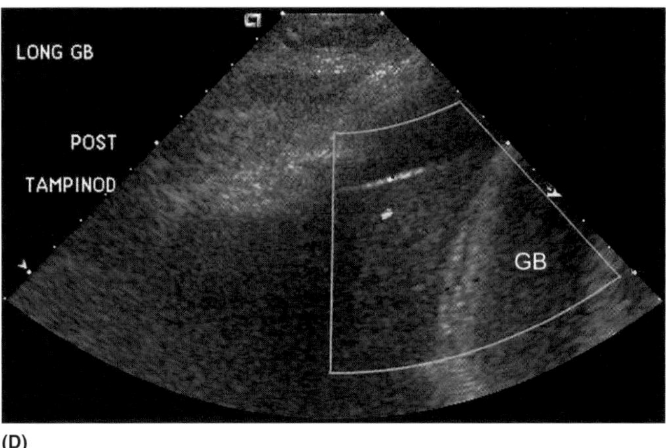

(D)

FIGURE 5 A–D ■ (*Continued*) (**C**) Catheter was removed to be redirected. Real-time image demonstrated no abnormalities. However, color flow demonstrated hemorrhage (*arrow*) into ascitic fluid. (**D**) Ultrasound probe was used to compress site of leakage, and this postcompression image demonstrated the bleeding had stopped. GB, gallbladder.

performed. Alternatively, the ultrasound transducer may be placed in a sterile glove, and a sterile gel or povidone–iodine (Betadine) solution may be used as an acoustic coupling agent after the sterile field is prepared. In this way, the interval between removal of the ultrasound probe and needle placement is decreased. This decreases potential inadvertent patient movement, which could change the needle path.

Freehand Method

The freehand method allows direct needle visualization because the needle is placed with ultrasound guidance. The needle may be either adjacent to or remote from the transducer, parallel or, less frequently, perpendicular to the scan plane (Fig. 7). A sector probe may be used for performance of aspiration or biopsy of deeper lesions, but the linear array transducer is often helpful for needle guidance of superficial lesions. The needle may be placed perpendicular to the ultrasound beam. Placing a sterile glove over the transducer before performing aspiration biopsy protects the ultrasound probe and ensures an entire sterile field if the probe is inadvertently moved into the sterile field. Acoustic gel or povidone–iodine solution may be used as an acoustic coupling agent.

An advantage of the freehand method is that it allows either the needle or the transducer to be independently moved during the procedure. Thus, if the needle is placed too close to the transducer, either the needle site can be reselected or the transducer can be moved. A disadvantage of the freehand technique is that it can be difficult to keep the needle in the same plane as the ultrasound transducer.

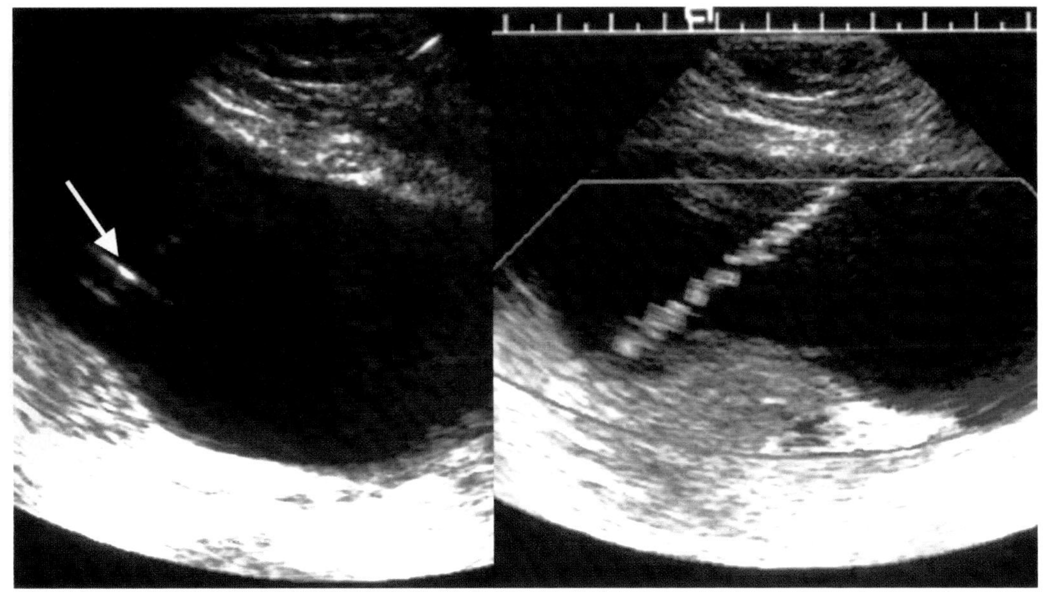

FIGURE 6 ■ Color flow during procedure. Image on the left demonstrates paracentesis needle tip (*arrow*). The rest of the needle was not visualized. On the image to the right using color flow during aspiration, the entire shaft of the paracentesis needle was visualized.

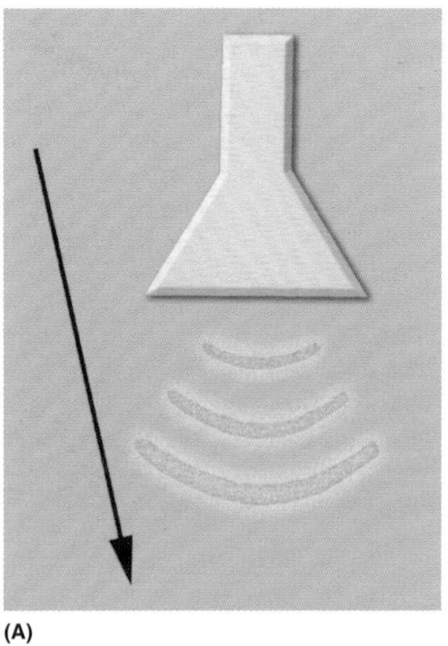
(A)

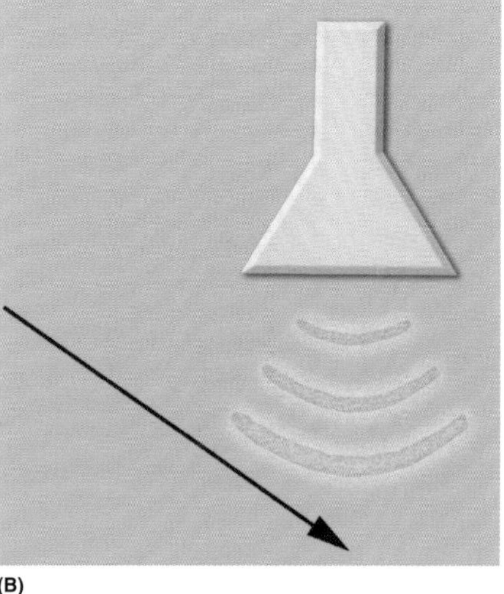
(B)

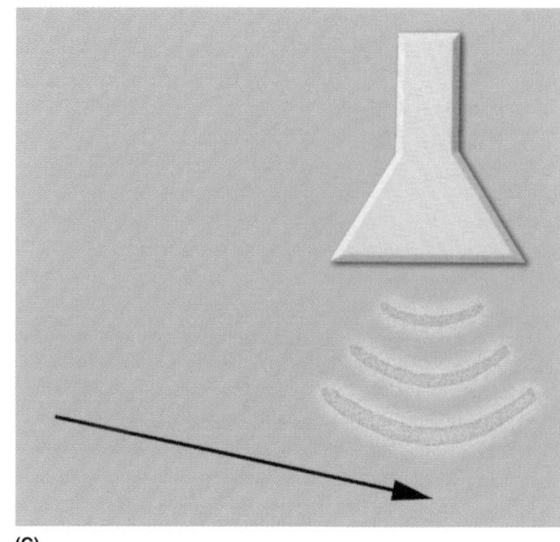
(C)

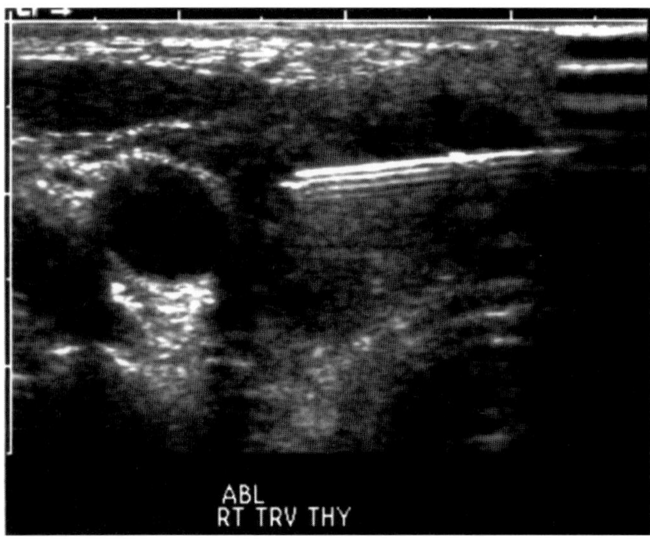

(D)

FIGURE 7 A–D ■ Needle visualization. (**A** and **B**). Needle visualization is improved during the freehand technique if, in fact; the needle can be placed from a position as in (**A**) in which it is parallel to the ultrasound beam, to (**B**) in which it is more angled to the ultrasound beam. (**C**) If it the needle is perpendicular to the ultrasound beam, the entire shaft of the needle may be visualized. (**D**) Needle placement into a thyroid in which the needle is placed perpendicular to the ultrasound beam, in which the entire shaft of the needle is visualized.

The needle or transducer may move, resulting in a needle that is not parallel to the ultrasound plane and thus impossible to visualize (Table 3).

Needle Guidance Systems

Most available needle guidance systems are attached to the transducer. These guidance systems are designed with grooves and slots to allow passage of different needles; some of these are large enough to accompany small catheters. The angle, direction, or depth of the needle can be continuously monitored with real-time guidance. The guidance system holds the needle firmly along a predetermined course, which is displayed as a line or caliper on a video monitor of the ultrasound unit (Fig. 8).

The needle guidance system holds the needle firmly in place, and its position can be monitored as it is placed into a preselected site. Use of a biopsy guide attachment, however, can be cumbersome. The needle must be placed close to the ultrasound transducer and cannot be positioned at a site more remote from the transducer, as with the freehand technique (Table 3).

TABLE 3 ■ Common Guidance Methods

Method	Advantages	Disadvantages
Freehand	Improved needle visualization Needle placed remote from transducers Independent movement of needle and transducer	Difficulty in keeping needle in path of transducer for visualization
Guidance systems	Widely available Preselected path Needle close to predetermined course	Cumbersome Needle close to transducer

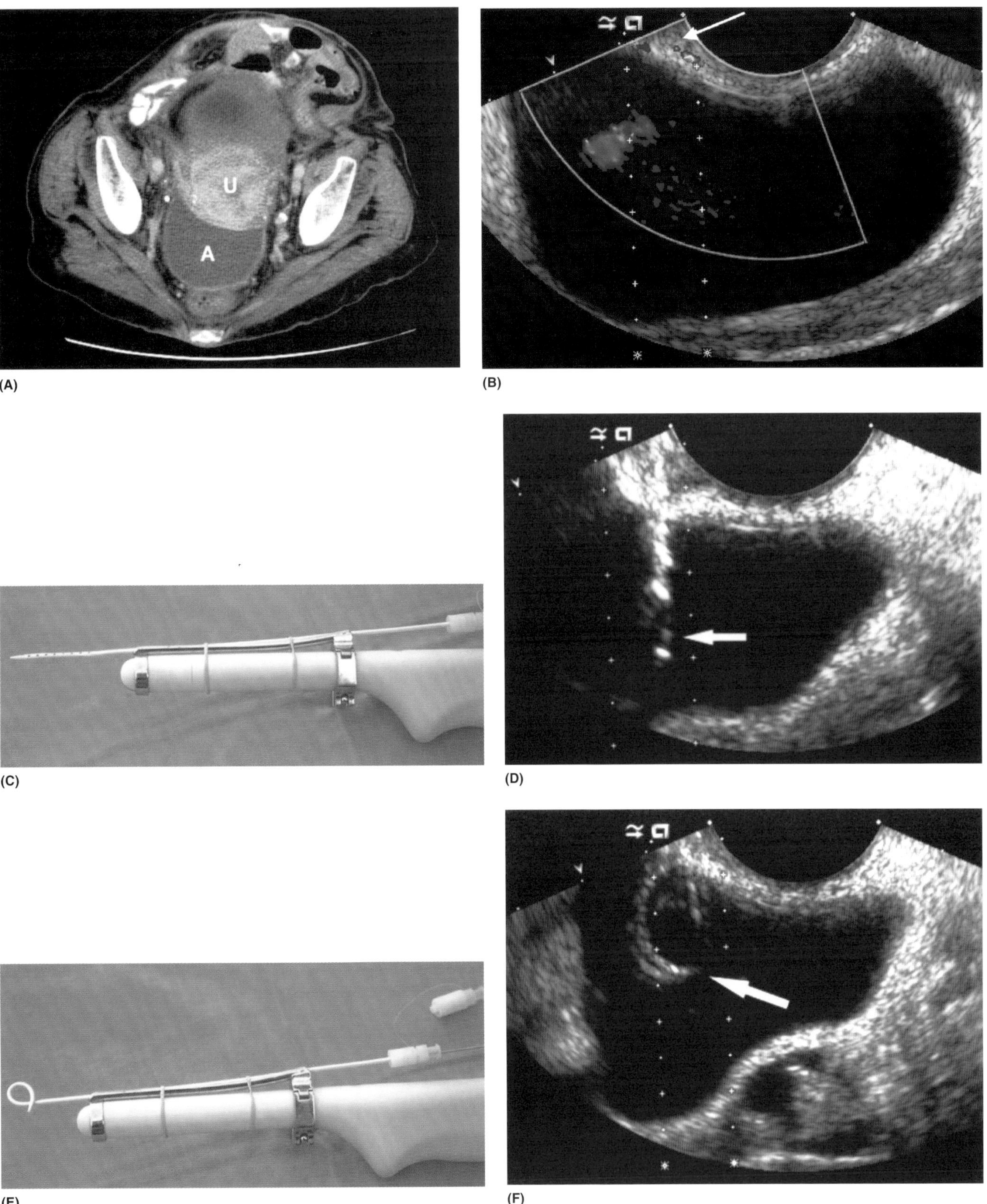

FIGURE 8 A–F ■ Pelvic abscess transvaginal drainage. (**A**) CT scan demonstrating abscesses (A) posterior to the uterus (U). (**B**) Color flow image with biopsy guided attachment, used to identify safe access route (*arrow*) avoiding large vessels. (**C** and **D**)Trocar catheter (*arrow*) is placed using the biopsy guided attachment which is attached with sterile rubber bands. (**E** and **F**) After the trocar is positioned within the fluid collection, the catheter is pushed into the collection to be reformed (*arrow*). Following this, the rubber bands are cut to allow ultrasound probe to be removed and the catheter to be left in the fluid collection.

Alternate Guidance Methods: Ultrasound and Fluoroscopy

Fluoroscopy is often used to guide interventional procedures. In the past, fluoroscopy alone was used to guide procedures such as biliary drainage and nephrostomy. When performing biliary drainage, for example, blind puncture of the liver was performed to attempt puncture of a biliary duct. A combined use of ultrasound and fluoroscopy has several advantages when performing drainage procedures. Ultrasound can be used as the initial method to place the needle into the target area. After this, fluoroscopy can guide catheter placement using the guide wire exchange technique. Thus, the entire procedure can be performed under real-time control, from needle placement with ultrasound to final catheter placement with fluoroscopy.

NEEDLE VISUALIZATION

General Principles

Needle visualization depends on complex interaction between the ultrasound beam and the biopsy needle (13). Visualization is determined by a number of different factors, including the type of tissue or fluid into which the needle is placed. In practice, the echogenicity of the liver may approximate that of most needle shafts, and thus the needle may be difficult to visualize. When the needle is placed in a fluid-filled body cavity, however, it is much more readily apparent.

Visualization is also determined by reflection of the ultrasound beam. Reflection is determined by the acoustic impedance mismatch between the different body tissues, angle of incidence between the needle and ultrasound beam, and size of the needle. Needle visualization is again much more apparent in fluid than in soft tissues or parenchymal organs. If the needle is placed parallel to the ultrasound beam, the major portion of the ultrasound beam is reflected away from the transducer face, making needle visualization more difficult. If the needle is placed perpendicular to the ultrasound beam, much of the beam is reflected back to the transducer face for excellent needle visualization (Fig. 7). Thus, when performing needle placement with a biopsy attachment, the needle is usually more parallel to the ultrasound beam than when using the freehand technique. For instance, in an abdominal biopsy using the freehand technique, the ultrasound transducer can be placed on the anterior abdomen, with the needle placed through the right flank. Thus, the needle intersects the ultrasound beam perpendicularly, allowing for much better acoustic detection than if the needle were placed parallel to the ultrasound beam (Fig. 7) (Table 4).

Large needles are easier to identify with ultrasound than small needles because large needles intersect a greater portion of the width of the ultrasound beam, causing greater reflection. Visualization is also best at the appropriate transducer focal zone. Imaging parameters should be optimized for best needle detection. For example, when using a low-frequency mechanical array transducer, it may be difficult to identify a needle in a superficial soft tissue structures (thyroid). When using a high-frequency linear array ultrasound probe with a good near-field focal zone, however, needle detection is improved. All parameters should be optimized to improve needle detection. This would include optimizing transducer frequency, selecting the proper focal zone, and trying to place the needle perpendicular rather than parallel to the ultrasound beam (Table 4).

TABLE 4 ■ Methods to Improve Needle Detection

- Optimize ultrasound scanning parameters (focal zone, transducer frequency)
- Place needle at angle or perpendicular to scan plane
- Use roughening or abraded needles (commercially available)
- Use "pump" action of inner stylet
- Use color Doppler to identify needle movement
- "Rock" transducer in plane of needle

Needle Shaft and Tip Visualization

The tip of most needles is better visualized in the shaft of the needle. This is probably secondary to the surface of the needle tip causing increased scatter of the ultrasound beam. Reflection is responsible for visualization of most of the shaft of the needle; however, scattering may cause improved detection of the needle tip. Also, a number of needles have been scratched, roughened, abraded, or otherwise altered to increase scattering and thus increase acoustic detection. Grooves may trap gas bubbles within the needle and increase scattering of the beam, thus improving acoustic detection.

Pump Maneuver

Needle detection may also be improved by gently moving the inner stylet up and down. This is the so-called "pump" maneuver, which may improve needle detection (14). The tip of the distal stylet probably scatters the ultrasound beam, leading to increased visualization. Also, a vacuum may be created in the needle, causing air trapping and increased scattering, thereby increasing needle visualization.

Color Doppler

Color Doppler can often detect minute movements of the needle. If the color settings are not appropriate, however, movement of the needle within the tissue can cause color within the entire organ. A commercial ultrasound unit has been developed that can detect minute movements or vibrations of needles but is not utilized (15). Color Doppler is often performed after a needle or catheter is positioned to better identify the needle or catheter position (Fig. 6).

"Rock the Transducer"

If, during needle placement parallel to the plane of the transducer, the shaft of the needle is not seen, the transducer may be "rocked" back and forth to better visualize

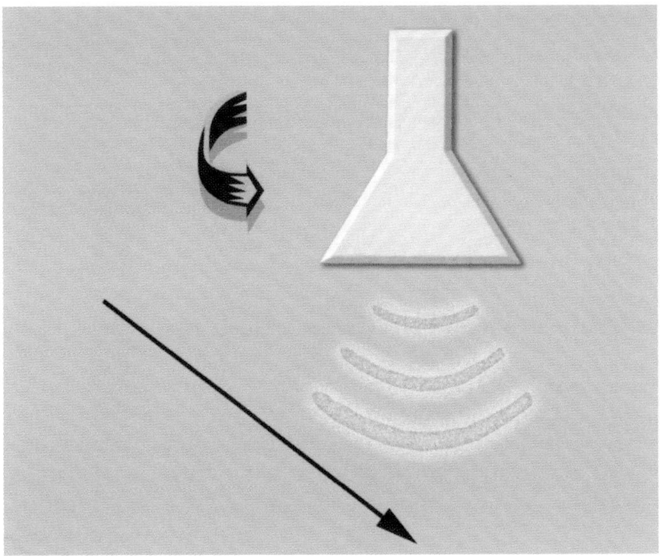

FIGURE 9 ■ "Rocking" maneuver. After the needle is placed, if in fact, the needle cannot be identified, then the transducer may be "rocked" back and forth, as illustrated above, until the needle is identified parallel to the plane of the ultrasound transducer.

the needle. Using this maneuver the transducer is moved over the trajectory of the shaft of the needle until the needle is seen (Fig. 9).

NEEDLE SELECTION

Aspiration

Needle selection depends on the procedure. Specific details for thoracentesis or paracentesis are presented in those sections.

Cytology

A number of different needles are available for percutaneous biopsy for aspiration cytology (16–18). Beveled-edge needles include the Chiba, Menghini, and Turner needles, which have been shown to yield more suitable specimens than nonbeveled-edge needles. The disadvantage of the beveled-edge needle is that it may bend as it courses through tissue, with the bend following the direction of the bevel.

Histology

A number of manufacturers have designed needles to obtain histologic core specimens (19,20). These needles obtain a core of tissue that can be examined for histology, as opposed to the specimens obtained by thin-walled needles, on which only cytologic preparations can be performed. The complication rate associated with taking core specimens is higher, however, because of the larger caliper of these needles. In general, all of these core-specimen needles work in a similar fashion. An automated mechanism rapidly fires the inner stylet with a sample notch, and the outer cannula of the needle slides forward (Fig. 10). As the outer

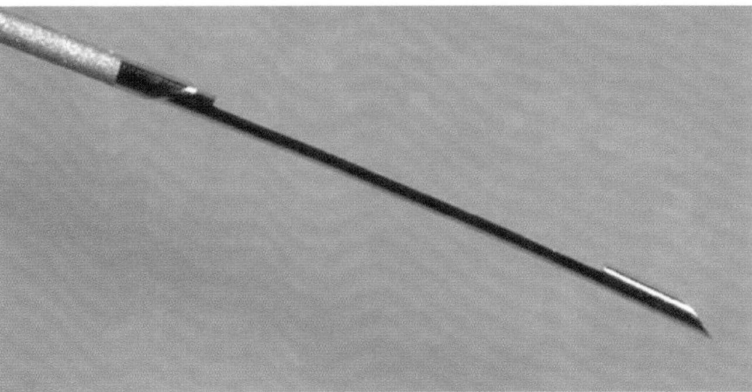

FIGURE 10 ■ Automated biopsy cutting needle. The inner trocar with a sampling notch which is common to all automated tru-cut needles.

cannula moves over the inner stylet, it shears the specimen in the notch of the inner stylet. Thus, a core sample for histology is obtained. These needles use an automated spring-loaded gun that rapidly fires the needle about 2 to 2.5 from its nonfired position into the target area.

TECHNIQUE

Aspiration

The technique for aspiration of fluid depends on the amount of fluid to be aspirated and the consistency of the fluid. Thoracentesis and paracentesis will be discussed later.

Biopsy: Aspiration Cytology

Biopsy may be performed for either cytologic or histologic retrieval. Aspiration cytology was developed by Papanicolaou (21) for examination of the female reproductive tract. This technique involves a staining process and emphasizes the cellular rather than the specific tissue characteristics that are observed on histology. As such, cells from almost any body part demonstrate organ-specific criteria for interpretation of neoplastic and nonneoplastic processes. In this procedure, stained cells are obtained by fine-needle aspiration (FNA) (Figs. 1 and 2).

Cytology is typically performed using either an aspiration or a nonaspiration technique. When performing aspiration cytology, a diagnostic ultrasound examination is performed. The target lesion is visualized, and a path is selected by ultrasound for needle placement. Depending on the size of the lesion and the specific target organ, the indirect, freehand, or biopsy guide method is selected for needle placement. Local anesthesia is placed into the subcutaneous tissue and the organ capsule. Many needles are difficult to insert into the skin and subcutaneous tissue; therefore, the point of a scalpel (no. 11 blade) is used to puncture the skin. The needle is placed under ultrasound guidance. For aspiration cytology, the inner stylet is then removed. This is attached to the syringe, and several milliliters of negative suction are applied with a 10-mL hand-held syringe. Several 1-cm up-and-down movements are made within the lesion. A rotatory motion may be helpful when using thin needles to obtain not only a cytologic specimen but also possible larger fragments for histologic analysis. After several up-and-down movements, suction is released. It is important not to aspirate the specimen into the syringe, which may cause fragmentation of the cells. The needle with the syringe is removed. It is useful to have a cytopathologist or a cytopathology technologist immediately available to place the specimen on a slide for staining. Staining is immediately performed with toluidine blue, and a coverslip is placed on the slide. The slide is then examined immediately by the cytopathologist or the cytopathology technologist. If an adequate specimen is obtained, then the procedure is usually terminated. In most situations, usually one or two additional passes are performed for further analysis in the cytopathology laboratory. Toluidine blue is a temporary stain that also fixes the cell.

After being expressed for smear preparation, some of the material can be placed into a separate container for preparation of a cell block. This usually involves washing the material from the syringe and needle and saving it in either saline or a fixative solution. Later, a cell block is obtained by centrifuge of the solution to obtain the small fragments of compact tissue at the bottom of the container. The cell block is then processed like a biopsy specimen, including fixation, embedding, sectioning, and staining.

Biopsy: Nonaspiration Technique

Cytologic diagnosis has been successfully performed using a nonaspiration technique (16). The accuracy of this technique varies in the literature, but it may be useful to often perform at least one pass using a nonaspiration technique. The technique is similar to the aspiration cytology. The patient is prepared and draped in the usual sterile fashion, and the needle is placed into the targeted lesion. The inner stylet is removed, but no syringe is attached. Several up-and-down motions are performed in the target lesion or until a small amount of fluid returns within the hub of the needle. The needle is then removed and prepared in a similar fashion as with aspiration cytology.

Biopsy: Histology

A number of specially designed needles are available for obtaining core tissue specimens. Most of these are variations of the Tru-Cut needles (19,20,22–25). These automated miniaturized Tru-Cut needles are used for histologic diagnosis. This needle consists of an inner trocar with a sampling notch (Fig. 10). This is common to all needles. The inner trocar is surrounded by an outer cannula. When the spring-loaded biopsy needle is fired, the inner trocar with a sampling notch is thrust forward. This is followed almost simultaneously by a forward thrust of the outer cannula, which shears off tissue for a sample. The needle is easily placed under ultrasound guidance. It can be more difficult to visualize these needles, however, because the inner trocar cannot be removed to perform the pump maneuver, which is easily done with cytologic needles. Also, once the needle is placed in the desired location, allowance must be made for about a 2- to 2.5-cm excursion of the needle as the gun is fired (Fig. 11). I usually use an 18-gauge needle to perform core histologic diagnosis. The specimen is placed in formalin for pathologic review.

These automated biopsy guns have certain advantages and disadvantages. A major advantage over use of cytology is that a histologic specimen is obtained; thus, not only can malignant tissue be distinguished from nonmalignant tissue but also true histologic diagnosis of the target lesion can be obtained. For instance, a histologic assessment is needed to reliably diagnose transplant rejection, but this requires a large-bore (18-gauge cutting vs. 22-gauge cytology) needle, which increases the complication rate. In addition, care must be taken in placing these cutting needles. Performing color Doppler ultrasound before needle placement ensures a safer procedure.

Automated biopsy needles also have advantages over regular Tru-Cut needles. An interesting article on renal transplant biopsy compared using a 14-gauge Tru-Cut needle and palpation for guidance with using an 18-gauge automated needle performed under ultrasound guidance (26). The complication rate was five times greater with the 14-gauge Tru-Cut needle (10%) than with the 18-gauge ultrasound-guided automated needle (2%). Even more impressive was the 99% retrieval rate obtained using the 18-gauge automated needle, compared with a 98% retrieval rate associated with the 14-gauge Tru-Cut. Therefore, the automated needles have demonstrated excellent retrieval and decreased complication rates compared with conventional Tru-Cut needles when under ultrasound guidance.

Biopsy: Coaxial Histology/Cytology

Certain manufacturers have automated Tru-Cut type devices, in which the needle may be separated from the spring-loaded arm of the needle. Thus, once the larger (18-gauge) needle is placed, 22-gauge needles may be placed coaxially for cytology retrieval. After cytology, the 18-gauge needle can be reattached to the firing device for histological retrieval.

Drainage

Percutaneous drainage techniques are usually guided by ultrasound, CT, fluoroscopy, or a combination of these. Whenever possible, drainage procedures at my institution are performed under ultrasound guidance. If a target area can be visualized under ultrasound, usually the drainage procedure is performed under ultrasound control. The advantages of ultrasound are that it can be portable and that the initial needle puncture can be visualized in its entirety. Either ultrasound or fluoroscopy can be used for catheter placement with the guide wire exchange technique. Ultrasound can guide trocar catheter placement for procedures such as percutaneous cholecystostomy and abscess drainage.

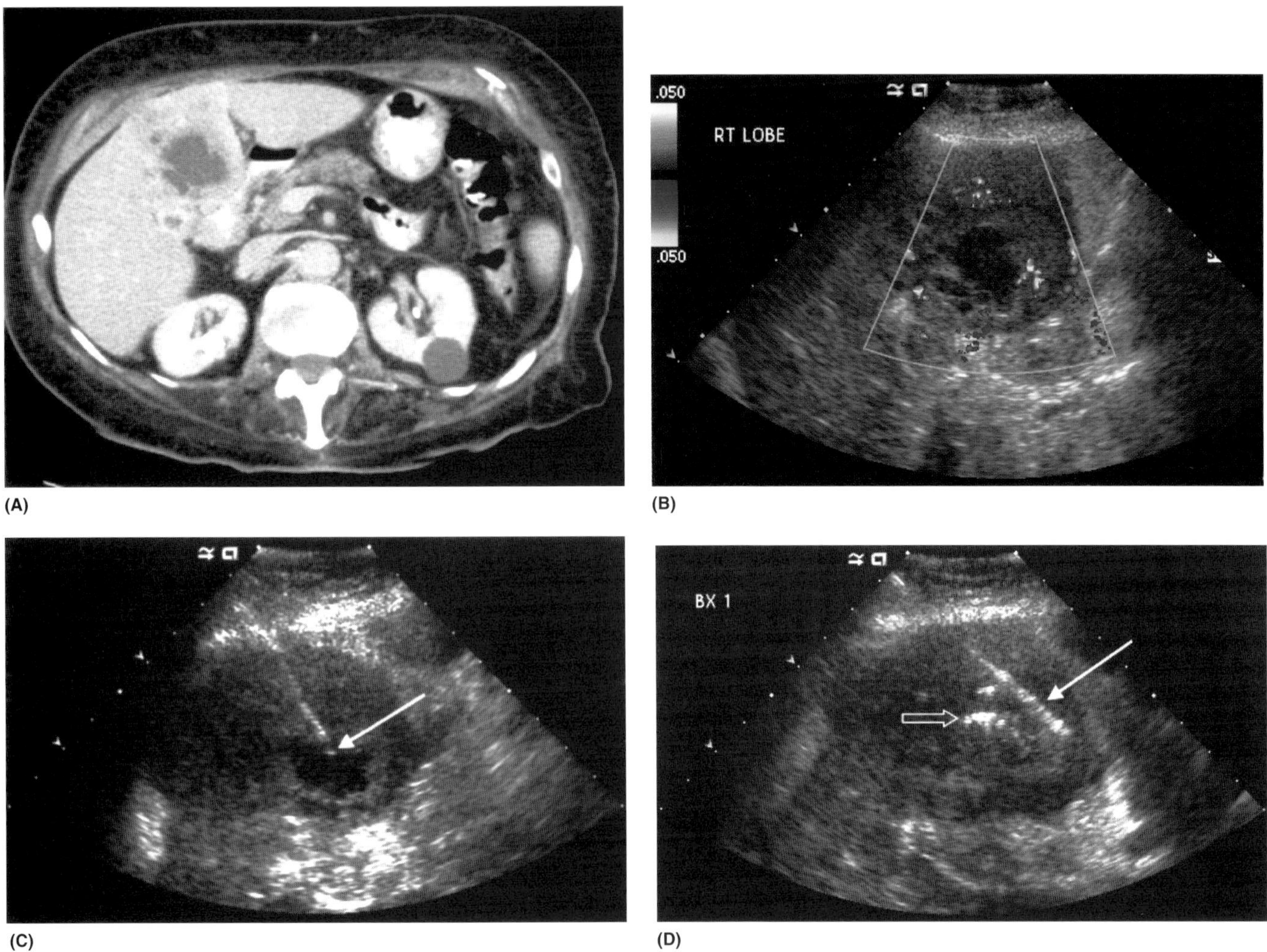

FIGURE 11 A–D ■ Necrotic metastatic sarcoma. (**A**) CT scan demonstrating mass with center of decreased density. (**B**) Color flow was performed, demonstrated solid component of mass to be vascular with surrounding vessels. (**C**) An 18-gauge needle was placed into the central fluid collection, which was aspirated (*arrow*). (**D**) After aspiration, a small collection of air (*open arrow*) was noted within the necrotic cavity. Using an 18-gauge core automated biopsy device (*arrow*), the solid component of the mass was biopsied.

Fluoroscopy is often used to guide drainage procedures (e.g., biliary drainage). The initial needle puncture is often performed blindly, and the catheter placement is performed under fluoroscopy. In other procedures, such as percutaneous nephrostomy, the renal collecting system may be opacified with intravenous contrast and the initial needle puncture guided by fluoroscopy. Ultrasound is increasingly used for initial needle placement in these drainage procedures. There are certain advantages of combined use of ultrasound and fluoroscopy for performance of drainage procedures. Initial needle puncture is performed with ultrasound, and guide wire exchange and catheter manipulation are monitored by fluoroscopy. Therefore, combined use of ultrasound and fluoroscopy allows for complete real-time visualization of needle puncture, guide wire exchange, and final catheter placement. The combined real-time control should ensure a safer procedure. The inherent advantages of ultrasound, including precise needle placement, are combined with the advantages of fluoroscopy to identify guide wires and catheters within a specific body cavity.

Computed Tomography

In many instances, CT is used instead of ultrasound in guidance of interventional procedures. This is especially true in performing aspiration biopsy or drainage procedures in which ultrasound cannot identify the target area. For instance, chest biopsy is usually performed under fluoroscopic or CT control because air within the lungs obscures ultrasound. This is not true for pleural lesions, which are readily identified with ultrasound and thus amenable to ultrasound-guided biopsy. Mid-abdomen abscesses and fluid collections also may be better visualized by CT than ultrasound. CT may better define the extent of intra-abdominal abscess and its relation to overlying bowel, which could be inadvertently transgressed during catheter placement. More simple procedures, such as paracentesis, are performed under ultrasound guidance.

Almost all drainage procedures are performed in a similar fashion, using either trocar catheter placement or the guide wire exchange technique.

Trocar Technique

Small catheters (about 7F) can easily be placed with the trocar method into a target area. For instance, percutaneous cholecystostomy has been performed under complete ultrasound control using the trocar technique. This procedure is performed in a similar fashion to needle biopsy—localizing the target area, preparing and draping the patient, injecting a local anesthetic, and then placing the catheter using the trocar technique into the gallbladder (Fig. 12). Once the trocar is placed within the gallbladder, the catheter is pushed from the stiffening cannula and reformed in the gallbladder for drainage.

Guide Wire Exchange Technique

More commonly, catheters are placed using the guide wire exchange technique. The initial needle puncture is performed under ultrasound control, usually with an 18-gauge needle. Alternatively, smaller (21-gauge) needles can be used with small (0.018-inch) guide wires placed through the needle and progressively dilated for passage of 0.035-inch guide wires. Once the guide wire has been positioned, the tract is progressively dilated, and the catheter is placed under ultrasound or fluoroscopic guidance (Fig. 3).

SPECIFIC ANATOMIC REGIONS: BIOPSY

Neck

FNA cytology of the neck is usually guided by palpation. Ultrasound may be helpful, however, to guide fine-needle placement for biopsy of palpable or nonpalpable neck

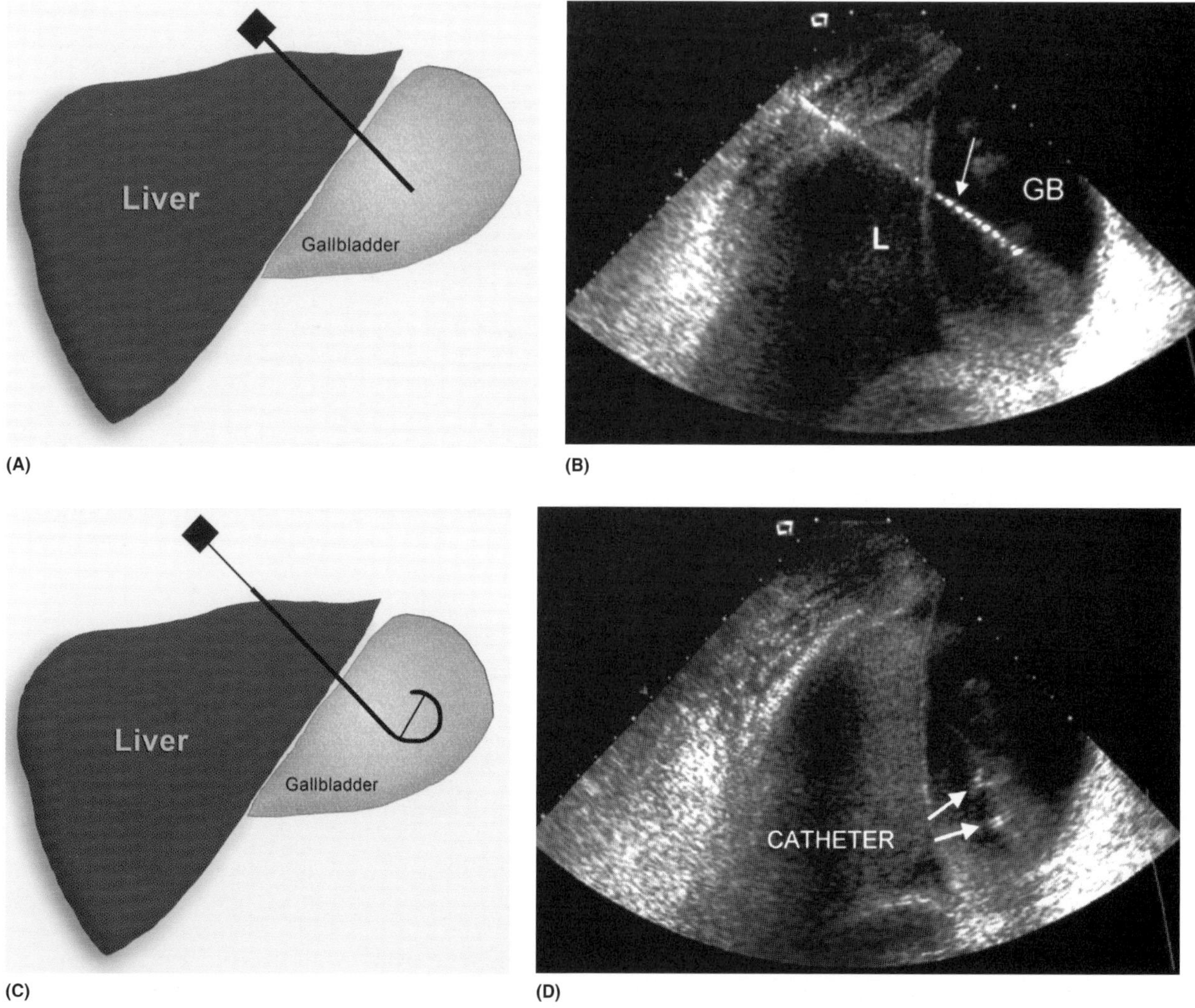

FIGURE 12 A–D ■ Percutaneous cholecystostomy. (**A** and **B**) Line drawing and ultrasound image demonstrating trocar placement of percutaneous cholecystostomy catheter (*arrow*) using the transhepatic route. (**C** and **D**) Once the trocar is positioned within the gallbladder (GB), the catheter is pushed from the stiffening cannula and reformed within the gallbladder (*arrows*). L, liver.

masses (Fig. 7) (27). Ultrasound-guided aspiration cytology may help to exclude nonpalpable thyroid tumors in patients who are at high risk for carcinoma. Patients who are at high risk for developing thyroid carcinoma, such as those that have had head and neck irradiation in childhood, may have a single nodule identified by ultrasound. It may be too small to be palpated, and thus ultrasound is the only method to guide aspiration cytology. Additionally, patients who underwent prior thyroidectomy and who have questionable residual thyroid mass or neck adenopathy may have aspiration cytology performed under ultrasound control.

Parathyroid Localization

Ultrasound helps to localize enlarged parathyroid glands. In most situations, there is clinical or laboratory evidence of parathyroid disease, and aspiration cytology of the parathyroid glands is not always necessary. In some instances, however, aspiration cytology of the parathyroids may be necessary (28), such as in patients who had a prior operation and are considered for reoperation to exclude the presence of parathyroid tissue. In these situations, FNA of the soft tissue mass may demonstrate the presence of a parathyroid tissue. Both parathyroid hormone assay and aspiration cytology have been advocated to determine whether the tissue is parathyroid (28).

Aspiration cytology of thyroid or parathyroid nodules is usually performed in a similar fashion to aspiration cytology of other areas. Some authors, however, advocate using smaller-gauge needles for thyroid aspiration cytology. I usually use the freehand technique with a linear array probe and place sterile coverings over the probe. Others have not advocated use of sterile coverings on the probe. A 23-gauge Menghini-type needle may be used for FNA cytology. Alternatively, a 25-gauge, noncutting beveled-edge needle alone or attached to a 10-mL syringe may be satisfactory. Some have advocated the use of the smaller-gauge needle to prevent trauma to the tissue and thus decrease contamination of the aspirate with blood. Some advocate a nonaspiration technique for thyroid nodules. Needle visualization is improved by inserting the needle perpendicular to the ultrasound plane, if possible (Fig. 7).

Breast

Although FNA cytology has been advocated for suspicious breast masses, there has been a recent trend toward using large gauge automated needles to obtain histologic specimens (29–31).

Chest

Chest lesions amenable to ultrasound-guided biopsy include peripheral lesions that abut the chest wall (32). Rib lesions may be biopsied with ultrasound (Fig. 13). On occasion, it is difficult to scan in the intercostal space and simultaneously place the needle. The linear array transducers give better near-field resolution, but sector scanners allow for intercostal scanning to provide for simultaneous visualization of the target lesion and the needle. FNA cytology has proved safe and effective, whereas core biopsy for histology can also be used but probably has an increased complication rate.

Liver

FNA is a safe and accurate method for cytologic diagnosis of malignancy (17,18). In a large series (17), FNA technique had an accuracy rate of up to 95% in cytologic diagnosis of hepatic malignancy (Fig. 1). With the use of automated Tru-Cut biopsy needles of moderate size (18–20 gauge), the diagnostic yield for malignancy should increase without a significant increase in morbidity (Fig. 11).

Ultrasound may also decrease complication rates and increase diagnostic yield of histologic biopsy procedures on the liver for hepatic architecture. Greiner and Franken (33) compared liver biopsy techniques using blind biopsy and ultrasound-guided biopsy with a 14-gauge cutting needle. Ultrasound knowledge of liver topography reduced the complication rate in this series from 1.4% to 0.2% and reduced the need for analgesia from 4.5% to 1.1% in core liver biopsies. Situations in which bowel may be interposed between liver and the abdominal wall could be disastrous if the blind biopsy is performed using a large bore needle. Use of ultrasound before performance of biopsy may help to prevent this complication.

Pancreas

Percutaneous ultrasound-guided FNA or biopsy for diagnosis of malignancy in the pancreas has been shown to have an accuracy rate slightly less than that for cytologic diagnosis of the liver (17). The use of ultrasound-guided 18-gauge automated biopsy gun has proved highly accurate in the diagnosis of pancreatic malignancy (34). I do not routinely use these larger-bore (18-gauge) needles for pancreatic biopsy because of the possibility of transgressing the colon or inadvertently performing a core biopsy of the highly vascular pancreatic bed. Instead, I usually perform FNA cytology of the pancreas. Ultrasound is also useful in aspirating nodes in, or about the pancreas using the FNA technique (Fig. 2).

Kidney/Adrenal

While CT is often utilized for biopsy of retroperitoneal masses, if they can be identified by sonography, they usually can be biopsied under sonographic guidance. Indeterminate renal lesions are biopsied using a posterior approach with the patient prone. Right adrenal masses may be biopsied using a transhepatic approach under sonographic control (Fig. 14).

Pelvis: Transvaginal Pelvic Mass

Endoluminal transducers that may be placed close to pelvic contents have been developed. Special biopsy guidance systems allow for transvaginal aspiration and biopsy of the pelvis. Most commonly, this is used for transvaginal biopsy of ovarian follicles for oocyte retrieval for in vitro fertilization programs. This technique may also

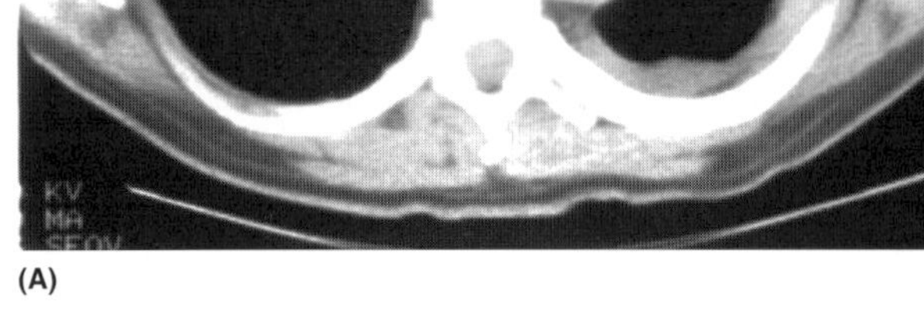

(A)

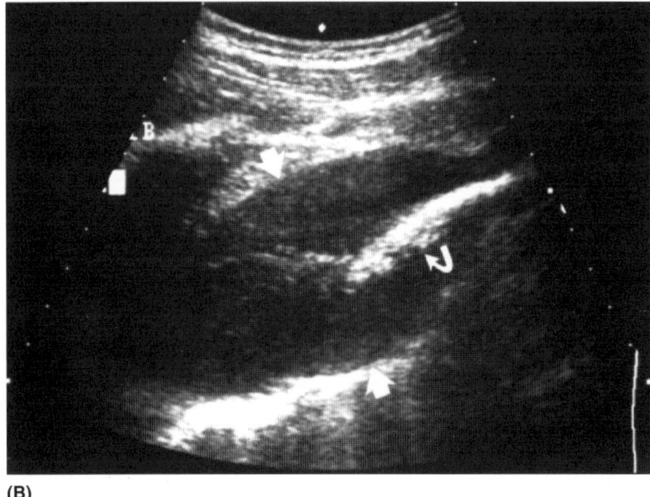

(B)

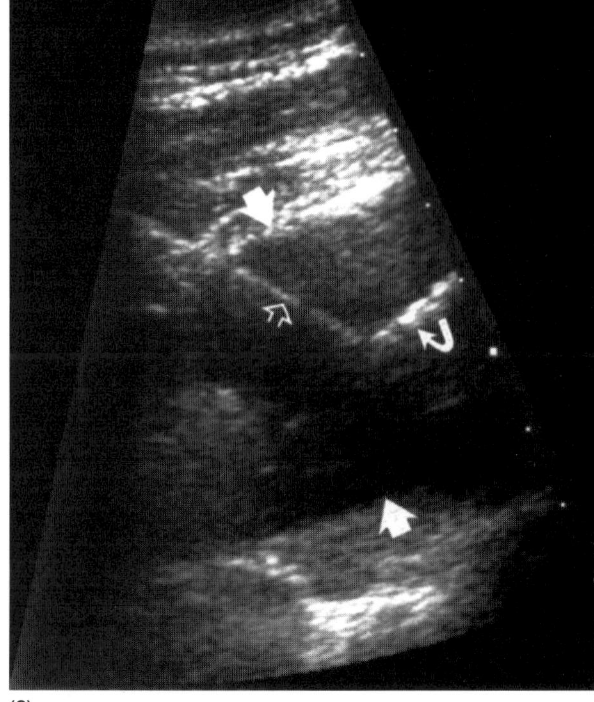

(C)

FIGURE 13 A–C ■ Metastatic tumor to the ribs. (**A**) Soft tissue mass (*arrow*) surrounding destructive lesion of the left rib (*curved arrow*). (**B**) An ultrasound demonstrates soft tissue mass (*arrows*) with destructive rib lesion (*curved arrow*). (**C**) A 22-gauge needle (*open arrow*) placed into the mass, which demonstrated metastatic carcinoma.

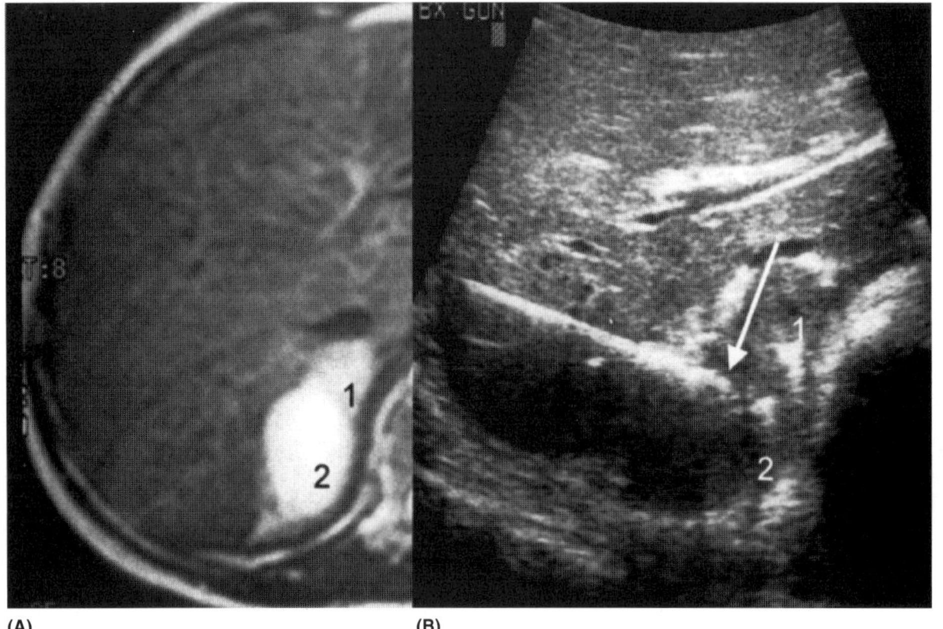

(A) (B)

FIGURE 14 A AND B ■ Adrenal biopsy. Image to the left demonstrates MRI with adrenal mass consisting of two components (1) and (2). In the image to the right, an automated biopsy needle was placed, using the transhepatic route, into the adrenal mass (*arrow*), which demonstrated metastasis into the adrenal.

be used for other applications, such as aspiration or biopsy of pelvic masses (35). Transvaginal ultrasound may also be used for aspiration or drainage of pelvic fluid collections when other routes are inaccessible. Usually, the patient is placed in the Trendelenburg position. The vagina is prepared and draped after a speculum is inserted. The probe is inserted and the biopsy performed, usually without local anesthesia. I usually use FNA for cytologic diagnosis of possible malignancy. Intravenous sedation is used in most instances. Transvaginal ultrasound may also be used for aspiration and drainage of pelvic fluid collection when other routes are inaccessible. Transvaginal aspiration is discussed in more detail later in this chapter.

Transrectal Biopsy: Rectal Mass

The transrectal route may also be used to guide biopsy. Biopsy can be done on rectal masses that can be visualized with the endoluminal probe (35). The method is similar to other endoluminal biopsy procedures. The patient is usually placed on oral antibiotics. If possible, an enema is administered on the morning of the examination. The patient is scanned and the route planned. Either FNA cytology or histology with an automated biopsy type needle can be used.

Transrectal Biopsy: Prostate

The prostate route has become the preferred method over the previously described transperineal route for biopsy of the prostate (23). The retrieval rate is excellent using automated biopsy needles. The patient is placed on oral antibiotics two days before the procedure, and an enema is administered on the morning of the examination. Premedication is optional; local or intravenous anesthesia is not routine. The diagnostic examination is performed and documented. The biopsy is performed with the patient in the decubitus position without local anesthesia. If no specific nodule is identified, a 6- or 10-quadrant biopsy is performed. The needle is advanced to the edge of the prostate, remembering that the automated needle advances 20 to 25 mm when fired. It is important not to move the needle once placed to the prostate edge to prevent tearing of the rectal mucosa. Biopsy too deep or too lateral to the prostate should be avoided so that the periprostatic venous plexus is not inadvertently punctured. The specimens are placed in individual bottles of formalin for pathologic preparation and examination. The prostate is rescanned after biopsy to check for potential complications, and the patient is alerted to the potential risk of hematuria, rectal bleeding, or sepsis. Oral antibiotics are continued for 1.5 to 2 days.

Transplant: Biopsy

Ultrasound can be used to perform core biopsy or histologic diagnosis of possible transplant rejection.

Liver

Liver transplant biopsy is one of the simplest and perhaps one of the safest procedures to perform (36). Needles are placed under ultrasound control transhepatically using an automated biopsy needle. Color Doppler ultrasound is used to identify vessels to avoid transversing hepatic vascularity. Usually, only local anesthesia is needed because the hepatic capsule is denervated with the transplant. This ensures a relatively painless procedure compared with biopsy of the native liver. Usually, two samples are obtained with an 18-gauge automated needle for histologic retrieval (Fig. 15).

Kidney

Renal transplant biopsy is also easily performed under ultrasound guidance. Either the superior or the inferior pole of the kidney is identified for possible biopsy. The site is selected based on overlying bowel and relation to other vital intervening structures. It is important to sample the renal cortex and to not place the needle too deep into the medulla, which may result in cutting a small artery and

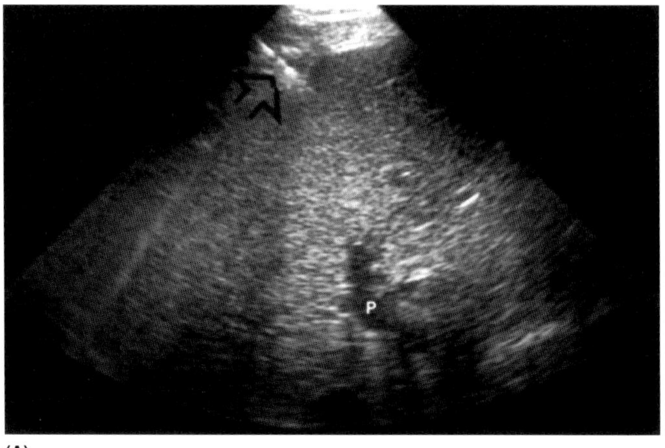

(A)

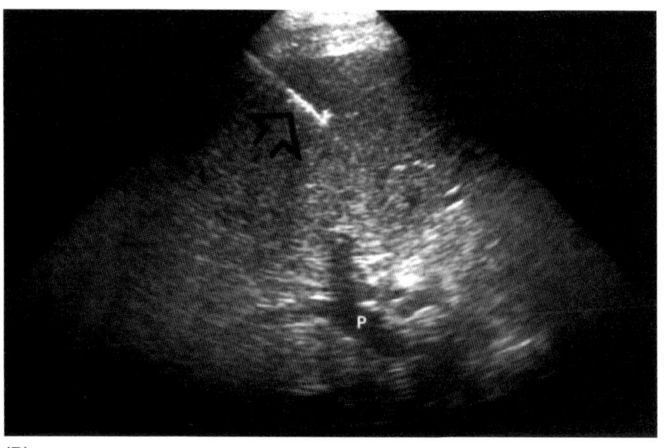

(B)

FIGURE 15 A AND B ■ Histological biopsy of liver transplant. (**A**) An 18-gauge automated biopsy needle is being placed transhepatically into this patient's liver under ultrasound guidance. (**B**) Once the needle is positioned, it is "fired" into the liver (*open arrow*).

vein. This can cause an arterial venous fistula, pseudoaneurysm, or hematoma formation. In one study (26), ultrasound-guided biopsy of renal transplants was easily performed under real-time guidance with a retrieval rate of 99% and a 2% complication rate. This was compared with a blinded technique using a 14-gauge needle, which had a 98% retrieval rate and a 10% complication rate.

Pancreas

Rarely, biopsy of pancreatic transplants is needed. In the situation in which biopsy is to be performed, the exact operation for pancreatic transplant should be known in advance of biopsy. In cases in which the transplanted duodenum and pancreas are sutured into the dome of the bladder, a transcystoscopic technique may be used to biopsy the head of the pancreas. This may be performed under ultrasound guidance. Alternatively, percutaneous biopsy of pancreatic transplants can be done using combined CT and ultrasound guidance (37). CT is used to visualize the region of the pancreas, then color Doppler ultrasound examination is performed to guide needle placement. Color Doppler is extremely helpful in avoiding vital arterial and venous structures that surround the pancreatic transplant. Two samples with an 18-gauge automated needle are usually obtained.

ASPIRATION

Thoracentesis and Paracentesis

A diagnostic thoracentesis can be performed by placing the needle into the collection, removing the inner stylet, attaching a syringe directly to the needle, and aspirating the fluid. In most situations, a 21-gauge thin-walled needle would suffice (Fig. 16). However, diagnostic aspiration of a possible empyema would include use of a larger (18-gauge) needle. Alternatively, attachment of a three-way stop cock with tubing, which then is attached to a drainage bag, provides an effective closed system for therapeutic paracentesis or thoracentesis (Fig. 16). Flexible catheters may also be used, which can be left in place within a fluid collection during aspiration, thus decreasing the possibility or risk of tissue injury. A flexible catheter with side holes as well as an end hole may avoid plugging of the distal catheter tip during therapeutic thoracentesis or paracentesis (Fig. 17). Tubing may be connected via a male-to-male adapter to a needle inserted into a vacuum bottle when performing paracentesis (Fig. 17), the inferior epigastric artery should be avoided (Fig. 18). Therapeutic thoracentesis and paracentesis should be limited to avoid re-expansion of pulmonary edema with thoracentesis or hypotension with larger volume paracentesis.

If aspiration is to be performed before drainage, a 0.035-inch guide wire may be placed through an 18-gauge thin-walled needle into the fluid collection for possible catheter placement using the guide wire exchange technique.

Little difference exists between aspiration of peripancreatic, perihepatic, or pelvic fluid collections and thoracentesis or paracentesis. In all situations, the area is localized, ultrasound guidance is performed, and either diagnostic aspiration or therapeutic aspiration is completed.

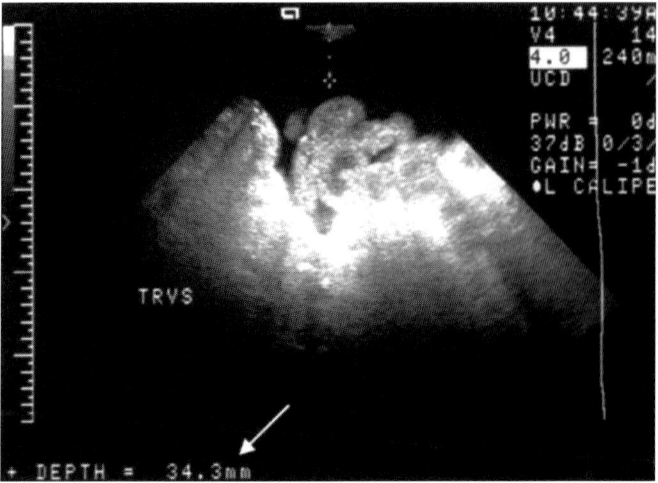

(A)

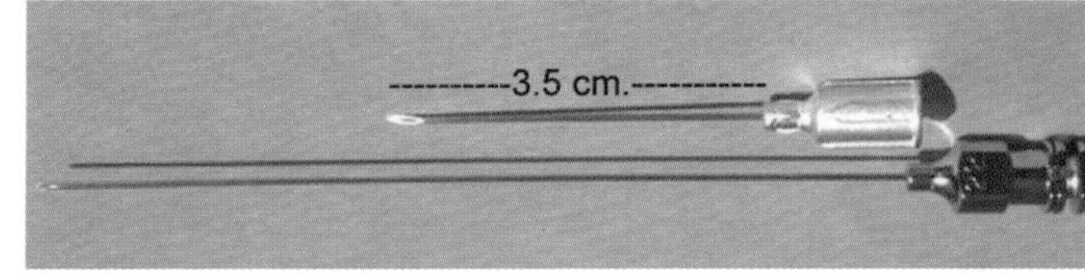

(B)

FIGURE 16 A AND B ■ Diagnostic paracentesis. (**A**) Before performing diagnostic paracentesis, the depth of the fluid is marked. It can be seen in this example, the depth to the center of the fluid is only 3.4 cm. (**B**) A long needle or catheter need not be used for a simple diagnostic paracentesis or thoracentesis, if in fact the depth is less than 3.5 cm. An injection needle, which is approximately 3.5 cm, can be used for aspiration.

Renal Cyst Aspiration

Indications for percutaneous aspiration of a renal cyst include the following:

- Thick or irregular wall
- Wall calcifications
- Internal echoes or presence of septations
- Presence of a solid mass arising from a wall
- Discrepancy in imaging results regarding the cystic or solid nature of a mass (38–42)

Ultrasound-guided percutaneous FNA of the cyst is simple. Using the aseptic technique, a 22-gauge thin-walled needle is passed directly into the cyst under ultrasound guidance. Aspirated cystic fluid should be evaluated by culture and sensitivity, lipids (Sudan stain), lactate dehydrogenase (LDH), protein, and glucose. A small amount of protein (<2.5 g/dL) in association with an LDH level of less than 25.5 μ/L may be obtained from a simple cyst (38). Increased LDH levels are associated with malignancy (41). Cytologic analysis is important for detection of malignancy.

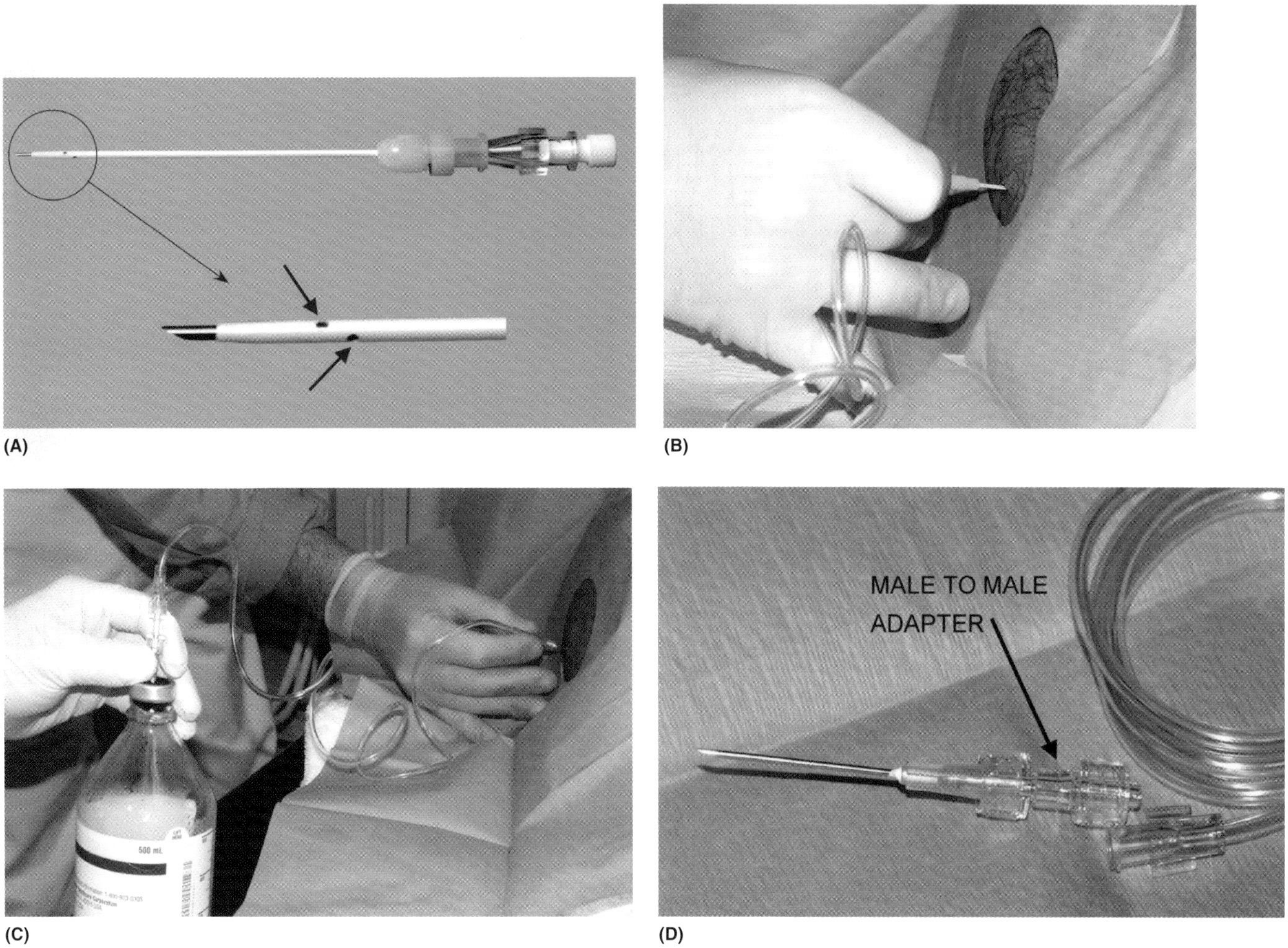

(A) (B)

MALE TO MALE ADAPTER

(C) (D)

FIGURE 17 A–D ■ Therapeutic paracentesis. (**A**) This image demonstrates a Yueh catheter with both an end hole and side holes (*arrow*). (**B**) After puncture, the small catheter is connected to tubing. (**C**) This tubing is connected to a vacuum container. (**D**) A male-to-male adapter is needed for needle placement into a vacuum container.

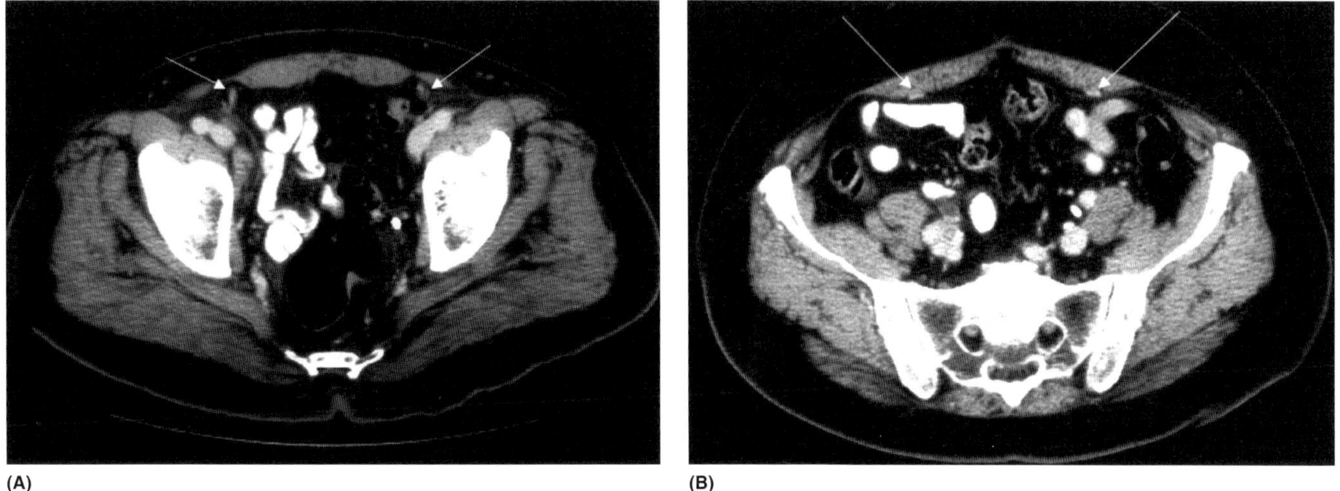

(A) (B)

FIGURE 18 A AND B ■ Paracentesis pitfall—inferior epigastric artery. (**A** and **B**) It must be remembered that inferior epigastric artery (*arrow*) runs posterior to the rectus sheath. These arteries can be seen with color flow sonography and obviously should be avoided when performing diagnostic or therapeutic paracentesis.

Gallbladder Aspiration

Gallbladder aspiration previously was advocated as a method of diagnosis of acute cholecystitis in the hospitalized patient. Using ultrasound guidance, a 22-gauge needle was placed transhepatically into the gallbladder (43,44). A small amount of bile was aspirated, and immediate Gram stain was performed; the remaining bile was sent for culture and sensitivity. The needle was then removed. Subsequently it was shown that a positive gallbladder aspirate was indicative of acute cholecystitis with a specificity of 87%, but there was a low sensitivity (<50%) of gallbladder aspirate in predicting acute cholecystitis in the hospitalized patient (43).

Gallbladder aspiration may be used to classify gallstones as either pigmented or cholesterol stones (45). In two series, fine-needle puncture of the gallbladder with ultrasound guidance was performed in 325 patients without major complications (45,46). These investigators performed biliary analysis and found an elevated cholesterol saturation index in patients with cholesterol gallstones relative to that in patients with pigmented gallstones. These studies reiterate the safety of percutaneous puncture of the gallbladder. However, in most institutions gallbladder aspirate for these purposes is rarely used.

Pancreatic Aspiration

Aspiration of peripancreatic fluid may be performed in a number of situations (47). In most instances, after simple aspiration of a pancreatic pseudocyst, most of the fluid reaccumulates. In patients with necrotizing pancreatitis, however, the timing of the operative intervention may determine the infected versus noninfected nature of the fluid. Therefore, simple aspiration performed under ultrasound or CT guidance can be sent for Gram stain, culture, and sensitivity. In cases of necrotizing pancreatitis, the fluid is usually too viscous to drain completely, and operative intervention is required. Noninfected or infected pseudocysts, however, may be amenable to catheter drainage. This is discussed in more detail in the next section.

DRAINAGE

Percutaneous Cholecystostomy

Cholecystectomy is the accepted method of treatment of both acute and chronic cholecystitis. Although elective cholecystectomy for chronic cholecystitis is associated with low mortality, there are conflicting reports concerning the management of patients with acute cholecystitis, especially with reference to optimal time for intervention. Emergency surgical cholecystostomy has been championed as a life-saving, although temporizing, procedure in the elderly, debilitated, or critically ill patient who presents too great a surgical or anesthetic risk for formal cholecystectomy. Surgical cholecystostomy is a simpler procedure than cholecystectomy, yet it too may be associated with high mortality because of the underlying medical problems in this group of patients (48). A major advantage of ultrasound-guided cholecystostomy is that the procedure can be performed at the patient's bedside. Thus, critically ill patients need not be moved to surgery or the radiology department for cholecystostomy (Fig. 12).

Newer catheters include some type of securing device (49–53). The McGahan drainage catheter set has a distal Cope loop to prevent catheter dislodgement (51). The catheter is easily placed with ultrasound guidance using a transhepatic route by either the trocar method (Fig. 12) or guide wire exchange technique.

Using the trocar method, a small-diameter catheter, adequate in size to decompress the inflamed gallbladder, fits over a stiffening cannula. A sharp inner stylet is placed within the cannula for insertion. The trocar catheter assembly is advanced transhepatically under ultrasonographic control into the gallbladder. The catheter is pushed from the cannula. The distal loop is reformed by tightening the attached string to secure the catheter within the gallbladder lumen (Fig. 12).

With the guide wire exchange technique, the initial puncture needle is placed into the gallbladder. A guide wire is then advanced through the needle and coiled within the gallbladder. The needle is then removed, and the guide wire is used as an anchor for passage of a dilator to widen the catheter tract. The catheter–cannula assembly is placed over the guide wire into the gallbladder. Once the catheter is within the gallbladder, the guide wire and the inner cannula are removed while the catheter is simultaneously advanced. The distal Cope loop of the catheter is reformed to prevent catheter dislodgement.

Both Browning et al. (49) and Boland et al. (54) thought that acute cholecystitis is difficult to diagnose in hospitalized patients and that percutaneous cholecystostomy serves as both a diagnostic and therapeutic maneuver in these patients. It is a safe and effective method to clear the gallbladder as a potential source of sepsis in these patients (54).

Percutaneous cholecystostomy has several other applications, including drainage of the biliary system in patients with failed transhepatic biliary drainage. Percutaneous cholecystostomy may be used as an alternative and is a less invasive procedure than transhepatic cholangiography or drainage in patients in whom transhepatic cholangiography or drainage is difficult or unsuccessful. Creasy et al. (55) performed percutaneous transperitoneal cholecystostomy in 44 patients. Antegrade cholecystography was successful in visualizing the common bile duct in all but two patients in whom there was no cystic duct obstruction. This technique was successful in visualizing common duct calculi in eight of nine patients. These investigators concluded that antegrade cholecystography is an easy and safe method for not only visualizing the gallbladder anatomy but also evaluating the common duct for associated biliary ductal problems or common duct calculi.

Biliary Tract: Percutaneous Transhepatic Drainage

Percutaneous transhepatic cholangiography (PTC) and drainage are traditionally performed using blind cholangiography with fluoroscopy for initial needle placement.

The combined use of ultrasonography for the initial needle puncture and fluoroscopy for final catheter placement using the guide wire exchange technique, however, optimizes the advantages of both guidance systems for performance of PTC, biliary drainage, and other invasive procedures (56). Selected ducts may be punctured under ultrasound guidance either for PTC or as the site of definitive catheter placement. In patients with segmental biliary obstruction, a blind technique allows initial opacification of the biliary system only by chance. Ultrasonography, however, may allow direct puncture of the appropriate biliary duct. Some authors have advocated the use of ultrasound alone for percutaneous transhepatic biliary drainage (57). These authors used complete ultrasound guidance for PTC and drainage in patients with hilar cholangiocarcinoma. Ultrasound was successful for percutaneous puncture and drainage in these patients. There was only one major complication in this group—one patient with ascites and severe cholangitis had bacterial peritonitis (57).

Percutaneous Nephrostomy

Ultrasonography has gained wide acceptance as the imaging modality for initial needle placement for percutaneous nephrostomy (Fig. 19) (39). After the dilated collecting system is accessed, a catheter is placed using the Seldinger technique under fluoroscopic control (58). Saitoh (10) demonstrated that color Doppler flow imaging is useful in supplementing ultrasound guidance in not only renal biopsies but also nephrostomies and renal cyst punctures. Puncture of intrarenal vessels can be avoided by using color Doppler for interventional procedures.

Puncture is similar to other techniques. Initial needle placement is guided either with a freehand technique or with a needle biopsy guide. Small (22-gauge) needles may be used to puncture the renal collecting system, which may then be opacified. A specific calyx then may be identified under fluoroscopy for more precise needle placement. Alternatively, precise needle placement may be performed with the use of an 18-gauge needle placed under ultrasound control into a posterior calyx. Hawkins (Hawkins IF Jr. Personal communication, University of Florida, Gainesville, 1994) has advocated the use of a blunt needle to avoid inadvertent injury to kidney or other organs during placement. Once the needle is in position, the catheter is placed using the guide wire exchange technique.

Pancreatic Drainage

Sonnenberg et al. (59) published their experience with percutaneous drainage of pseudocysts, with excellent results. The overall cure rate by catheter drainage alone was 90.1%; this includes 48 of 51 infected pseudocysts (94%) and 43 of 50 noninfected pseudocysts (86%). In most of these patients, CT rather than ultrasonography was the primary method of guidance, although ultrasonography can be used for guidance of drainage (Figs. 3–12). Although van Sonnenberg most commonly used the transperitoneal or retroperitoneal route for drainage, others have advocated use of transgastric drainage of pseudocysts (60). Kumar et al. (61) published their work with 57 patients, comparing CT with ultrasonography in evaluation and percutaneous intervention in patients with acute pancreatitis. Although CT was considered superior to ultrasound in evaluation of acute pancreatitis, ultrasound provided easy guidance for percutaneous interventional procedures, such as fluid aspiration, in these patients.

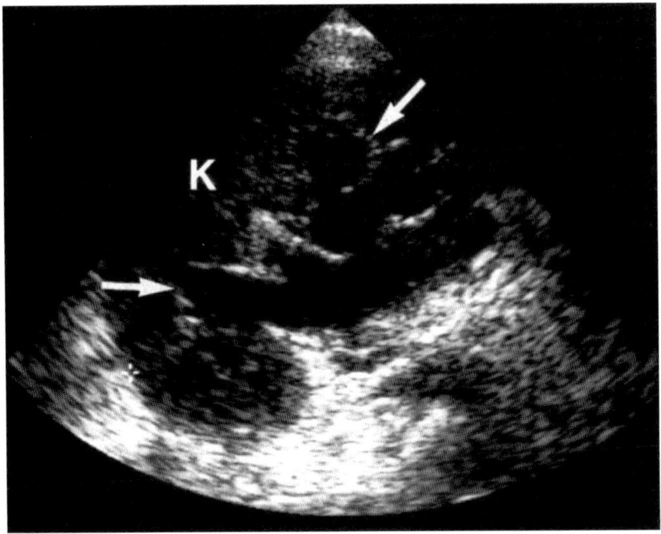

(A)

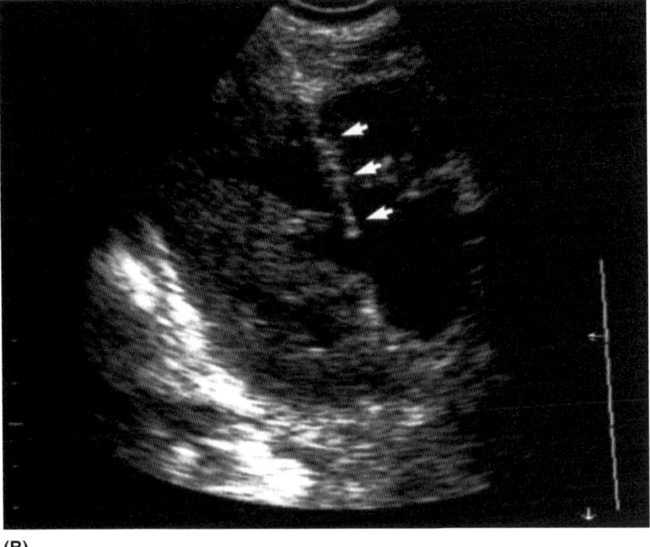

(B)

FIGURE 19 A AND B ■ Percutaneous nephrostomy. (**A**) Images demonstrate dilatation of the renal pelvis collecting system (*arrow*). (**B**) Initial needle (*arrows*) is placed under ultrasound guidance into the dilated renal collecting system. K, kidney.

Abscess Drainage

Percutaneous catheter drainage of abdominal abscesses has been shown to be a safe and effective alternative to operative drainage (62–65). Percutaneous drainage avoids the morbidity associated with operation and the necessity for general anesthesia. Percutaneous abscess drainage has proved an effective alternative to surgical techniques. In general, there are only a few contraindications to percutaneous drainage of abdominal abscesses. These include (*i*) poorly defined abscesses, such as pancreatic phlegmons, that are not amenable to catheter drainage; (*ii*) extensive abdominal abscesses with either multicompartment involvement or in multiple locations within the abdomen; (*iii*) infected necrotic materials, such as pancreatic necrosis, which require surgical débridement; (*iv*) lack of a safe access route, owing to overlying bowel or overlying vascular structures; and (*v*) major bleeding problems, including coagulopathies (63).

When performing catheter drainage, a safe access route must be determined. The cavity is first aspirated, and purulent material is obtained. The catheter is usually inserted using the guide wire exchange technique. Most patients are on broad-spectrum antibiotics for underlying sepsis before drainage. Various catheters may be used for drainage. Nonviscous fluid collections are probably adequately drained with 8- to 10-F catheters. More viscous fluids are best evacuated with a double-lumen sump-type catheter.

After the abscess cavity has been drained, the patient is rescanned with ultrasound or CT to check for adequacy of catheter drainage. The patient is then followed closely for catheter output, decreased pain, normalization of temperature, and laboratory parameters. The patient's antibiotics are adjusted for appropriate culture and sensitivity. A follow-up fluoroscopic abscessogram helps to identify the size and configuration of the abscess cavity and to check for fistulous communications. Most low-output enteric fistulas (outputs <50 mL/day) generally resolve with a combination of percutaneous drainage and antibiotic therapy. Higher-output fistulas (>200 mL/day) may not be cured with catheter drainage alone (62,64,65).

Pelvic Drainage

Several studies have been published advocating use of either ultrasound-guided transrectal or transvaginal route for performance of pelvic drainage (Fig. 8) (66–69).

Classically, CT has been used to guide drainage of pelvic abscesses. More recently, ultrasound guidance has been used not only in the transabdominal route but also in the transrectal or transvaginal route for drainage of pelvic abscesses (68). There has also been a trend toward the use of smaller catheters or even aspiration alone as an effective treatment of pelvic abscesses. Some difficulties have occurred in placement of catheters using the transvaginal route and the guide wire exchange technique. The initial needle puncture is usually simple to perform; however, placement of the dilators and catheters over the guide wire through the tough musculature of the vagina is difficult. Lee et al. (68) have advocated use of a single-step trocar catheter system (Fig. 8). Transrectal aspiration may be performed in a similar fashion. The probe is prepared, and a diagnostic examination is performed. A route for needle or catheter placement is planned. Conscious sedation is necessary for transrectal aspiration, and general anesthesia is often required for transvaginal drainage. A 16- to 18-gauge needle is placed after the area is prepared, and fluid is aspirated and the cavity irrigated.

A modified 6.7-F catheter is used for transvaginal drainage catheter placement using the trocar method (68). The catheter is placed into the groove of a standard endoluminal probe. Instead of replacing the clip of the endoluminal guide, the trocar catheter can be fixed in place with sterile rubber bands. The catheter is placed in a standard fashion using a trocar method and is left in place for two to three days, until the patient defervesces and drainage decreases. This method was curative in 87% of patients.

REFERENCES

1. Goldberg BB, Pollack HM. Ultrasonic aspiration transducer. Radiology 1972; 102:187.
2. Holm HH, Kristensen JK, Rasmussen SN, et al. Ultrasound as a guide in percutaneous puncture technique. Ultrasonics 1972; 10:83.
3. McGahan JP. The history of interventional ultrasound. J Ultrasound Med 2004; 23(6):727–741.
4. McGahan JP. Interventional abdominal ultrasound. In: Mittelstaedt CA, ed. General ultrasound. New York: Churchill Livingstone, 1992:1189.
5. Phal PM, Brooks DM, Wolfe R. Sonographically guided biopsy of focal lesions: a comparison of freehand and probe-guided techniques using a phantom. AJR Am J Roentgenol 2005; 184(5): 1652–1656.
6. Reading CC, Charboneau JW, James EM, et al. Sonographically guided percutaneous biopsy of small (3 cm or less) masses. AJR Am J Roentgenol 1988; 151:189.
7. McGahan JP. Aspiration and drainage procedures in the intensive care unit: percutaneous sonographic guidance. Radiology 1985; 154:531.
8. McGahan JP, Anderson MW, Walter JP. Portable realtime sonographic and needle guidance systems for aspiration and drainage. AJR Am J Roentgenol 1986; 147:1241.
9. McGahan JP, Anderson MW. Pulse Doppler sonography as an aid in ultrasound-guided aspiration biopsy. Gastrointest Radiol 1987; 12:279.
10. Saitoh M. Color Doppler flow imaging in interventional ultrasound of the kidney. Scandinavian J Urol Nephrol 1991; 137(suppl):59.
11. Gerscovich EO, Budenz RW, Lengle SJ. Assessment of catheter placement and patency by color Doppler ultrasonography. J Ultrasound Med 1994; 13:367.
12. McGahan JP, Brant WE. Principles, instrumentation, and guidance systems. In: McGahan JP, ed. Interventional Ultrasound. Baltimore: Williams & Wilkins, 1990:1.
13. McGahan JP. Laboratory assessment of ultrasonic needle and catheter visualization. J Ultrasound Med 1986; 5:373.
14. Bisceglia M, Matalon TA, Silver B. The pump maneuver: an atraumatic adjunct to enhance US needle tip localization. Radiology 1990; 176:867.
15. Jones CD, McGahan JP, Clark KJ. Color Doppler ultrasound detection of a vibrating needle system. J Ultrasound Med 1997; 16:269.
16. Fagelman D, Chess Q. Nonaspiration fine-needle cytology of the liver: a new technique for obtaining diagnostic samples. AJR Am J Roentgenol 1990; 155:1217.
17. Porter B, Karp W, Forsberg L. Percutaneous cytodiagnosis of abdominal masses by ultrasound guided fine-needle aspiration biopsy. Acta Radiol [Diagn] 1981; 22:663.
18. Siu A, Teplitz RL. Fine needle aspiration/cytology for invasive ultrasound techniques. In: McGahan JP, ed. Interventional Ultrasound. Baltimore: Williams & Wilkins, 1990:21.

19. Bernardino ME. Automated biopsy devices: significance and safety. Radiology 1990; 176:615.
20. Parker SH, Hopper KD, Yakes WF, et al. Image-directed percutaneous biopsies with a biopsy gun. Radiology 1989; 171:663.
21. Papanicolaou GN. Epithelial regeneration in uterine glands and on the surface of the uterus. Am J Clin Gynecol 1933; 25:30.
22. Mehrotra P, Hubbard JG, Johnson SJ, Richardson DL, Bliss R, Lennard TW. Ultrasound scan-guided core sampling for diagnosis versus freehand FNAC of the thyroid gland. Surgeon 2005; 3(1):1–5.
23. Ragde H, Aldape HC, Blasko JC. Biopty: an automatic needle biopsy device—its use with an 18-gauge Tru-Cut needle (Biopty-cut) in 174 consecutive prostate core biopsies. Endosonographique 1987; 3:5.
24. Winters SR, Paulson EK. Ultrasound guided biopsy: what's new? Ultrasound Q 2005; 21(1):19–25.
25. Yu SC, Lo DY, Ip CB, Liew CT, Leung TW, Lau WY. Does percutaneous liver biopsy of hepatocellular carcinoma cause hematogenous dissemination? An in vivo study with quantitative assay of circulating tumor DNA using methylation-specific real-time polymerase chain reaction. AJR Am J Roentgenol 2004; 183(2):383–385.
26. Mahoney MC, Racadio JM, Merhar GL, et al. Safety and efficacy of kidney transplant biopsy: tru-cut needle vs sonographically guided Biopty gun. AJR Am J Roentgenol 1993; 160:325.
27. Siewert B, Kruskal JB, Kelly D, Sosna J, Kane RA. Utility and safety of ultrasound-guided fine-needle aspiration of salivary gland masses including a cytologist's review. J Ultrasound Med 2004; 23(6):777–83.
28. Doppman JL, Krudy AG, Marx SJ, et al. Aspiration of enlarged parathyroid glands for parathyroid hormone assay. Radiology 1983; 148:31.
29. Fornage BD. Interventional ultrasound of the breast. In: McGahan JP, ed. Interventional Ultrasound. Baltimore: Williams & Wilkins, 1990:71.
30. Kline TS, Joshi LP, Hunter SN. Fine-needle aspiration of the breast: diagnoses and pitfalls. A review of 3545 cases. Cancer 1979; 44:1458.
31. Palombini L, Fulciniti F, Vetrani A, et al. Fine-needle aspiration biopsies of breast masses: a critical analysis of 1956 cases in 8 years (1976–1984). Cancer 1988; 61:2273.
32. Yang PC, Chang DB, Yu CJ, et al. Ultrasound-guided core biopsy of thoracic tumors. Am Rev Respir Dis 1992; 146:763.
33. Greiner L, Franken FH. Sonographically assisted liver biopsy: replacement for blind needle biopsy? Dtsch Med Wochenschr 1983; 11:108.
34. Elvin A, Andersson T, Scheibenpflug L, et al. Biopsy of the pancreas with a biopsy gun. Radiology 1990; 176:677.
35. Zanetta, Brenna A, Pittelli M, et al. Transvaginal ultrasound-guided fine needle sampling of deep cancer recurrences in the pelvis: usefulness and limitations. Gynecol Oncol 1994; 54:59.
36. Don S, Kopecky KK, Pescoitz MD, et al. Ultrasound-guided pediatric liver transplant biopsy using a spring-propelled cutting needle (biopsy gun). Pediatr Radiol 1994; 24:21.
37. Lee BC, McGahan JP, Perez RV, Boone JM. The role of percutaneous biopsy in detection of pancreatic transplant rejection. Clin Tansplant 2000; 14(5):493–498.
38. Clayman RV, Williams RD, Fraley EE. The pursuit of the renal mass. N Engl J Med 1979; 300:72.
39. Lindsay DJ, Lyons EA, Levi CS. Urinary tract. In: McGahan JP, ed. Interventional Ultrasound. Baltimore: Williams & Wilkins, 1990:199.
40. Nishimura K, Tsujimura A, Matsumiya K, et al. Clinical experience of percutaneous renal cyst puncture in recent six years. Hinyokika Kiyo. Acta Urol Jpn 1993; 39:121.
41. Phillips GN, Kumari-Subaiya S. Renal cyst puncture: LDH as a tumor marker. Annual Meeting of the Radiology Society of North America, Chicago, November, 1986.
42. Zama S. Percutaneous renal cyst puncture and ethanol instillation. Hinyokika Kiyo. Acta Urol Jpn 1994; 40:9.
43. McGahan JP, Lindfors KK. Acute cholecystitis: diagnostic accuracy of percutaneous aspiration of the gallbladder. Radiology 1988; 167:669.
44. McGahan JP, Walter JP. Diagnostic percutaneous aspiration of the gallbladder. Radiology 1985; 155:619.
45. Swobodnik W, Hagert N, Janowitz P, et al. Diagnostic fine-needle puncture of the gallbladder with US guidance. Radiology 1991; 178:755.
46. Tudyka J, Kratzer W, Kunh K, et al. Diagnostic value of fine-needle puncture of the gallbladder: side effects, safety, and prognostic value. Hepatology 1995; 21:1303.
47. Gandini G, Grosso M, Bonardi L, et al. Results of percutaneous treatment of sixty-three pancreatic pseudocysts. Ann Radiol 1988; 31:117.
48. Jurkovich GJ, Dyess DL, Ferrara JJ. Cholecystostomy. Expected outcome in primary and secondary biliary disorders. Am Surg 1988; 54:40.
49. Browning PD, McGahan JP, Gerscovich EO. Percutaneous cholecystostomy for suspected acute cholecystitis in the hospitalized patient. J Vasc Interven Radiol 1993; 4:531.
50. Ito K, Fujita N, Noda Y, Kobayashi G, Kimura K, Sugawara T, Horaguchi J. Percutaneous cholecystostomy versus gallbladder aspiration for acute cholecystitis: a prospective randomized controlled trial. AJR Am J Roentgenol 2004; 183(1):193–196.
51. McGahan JP. A new catheter design for percutaneous cholecystostomy. Radiology 1988; 166:49.
52. McGahan JP, Lindfors KK. Percutaneous cholecystostomy: an alternative to surgical cholecystostomy for acute cholecystitis? Radiology 1989; 173:481.
53. Sosna J, Kruskal JB, Copel L, Goldberg SN, Kane RA. US-guided percutaneous cholecystostomy: features predicting culture-positive bile and clinical outcome. Radiology 2004; 230(3):785–791.
54. Boland GW, Lee MJ, Leung J, et al. Percutaneous cholecystostomy in critically ill patients: early response and final outcome in 82 patients. AJR Am J Roentgenol 1994; 163:339.
55. Creasy TS, Gronvall S, Stage JG. Assessment of the biliary tract by antegrade cholecystography after percutaneous cholecystostomy in patients with acute cholecystitis. Br J Radiol 1993; 66:662.
56. McGahan JP, Raduns K. Biliary drainage using combined ultrasound fluoroscopic guidance. J Interven Radiol 1990; 5:33.
57. Lameris JS, Hesselink EJ, Van Leeuwen PA, et al. Ultrasound-guided percutaneous transhepatic cholangiography and drainage in patients with hilar cholangiocarcinoma. Semin Liver Dis 1990; 10:121.
58. Pedersen H, Juul N. Ultrasound-guided percutaneous nephrostomy in the treatment of advanced gynecologic malignancy. Acta Obstet Gynecol Scan 1988; 67:199.
59. van Sonnenberg E, Wittich GR, Casola G, et al. Percutaneous drainage of infected and noninfected pancreatic pseudocysts: experience in 101 cases. Radiology 1989; 170:757.
60. Ho CS, Taylor B. Percutaneous transgastric drainage for pancreatic pseudocyst. AJR Am J Roentgenol 1984; 143:623.
61. Kumar P, Mukhopadhyay S, Sandhu M, et al. Ultrasonography, computed tomography and percutaneous intervention in acute pancreatitis: a serial study. Australas Radiol 1995; 39:145.
62. Jeffrey RB Jr, Tolentino CS, Federle MP, et al. Percutaneous drainage of perappendiceal abscesses: review of 20 patients. AJR Am J Roentgenol 1987; 149:59.
63. Jeffrey RB Jr. Abdominal abscesses: the role of CT and sonography. In: McGahan JP, ed. Interventional Ultrasound. Baltimore: Williams & Wilkins, 1990:129.
64. Kerlan RJ Jr, Jeffrey RB Jr, Pogany AC, et al. Abdominal abscess with low output fistula: successful percutaneous drainage. Radiology 1985; 155:73.
65. Kerlan RJ Jr, Pogany AC, Jeffrey RB, et al. Radiologic management of abdominal abscesses. AJR Am J Roentgenol 1985; 144:145.
66. Casola G, van Sonnenberg E, D'Agostino HB, et al. Percutaneous drainage of tubo-ovarian abscesses. Radiology 1992; 182:399.
67. Feld R, Eschelman DJ, Sagerman JE, et al. Treatment of pelvic abscesses and other fluid collections: efficacy of transvaginal sonographically guided aspiration and drainage. AJR Am J Roentgenol 1994; 163:1141.
68. Lee BC, McGahan JF, Bijan B. Single-step transvaginal aspiration and drainage for suspected pelvic abscesses refractory to antibiotic therapy. J Ultrasound Med 2002; 21(7):731–738.
69. Kuligowska E, Keller E, Ferrucci JT. Treatment of pelvic abscesses: value of one-step sonographically guided transrectal needle aspiration and lavage. AJR Am J Roentgenol 1995; 164:201.

Invasive Ultrasound Principles (Obstetrics/Gynecology)

Lyndon M. Hill

6

INTRODUCTION

The ability to diagnose fetal disorders has evolved quickly. Amniocentesis made possible the diagnosis of chromosomal abnormalities and an increasing number of inherited metabolic disorders. The development of ultrasonography permitted accurate delineation of normal fetal anatomy and the diagnosis of numerous structural malformations. Sonographically guided procedures soon followed. Transabdominal and transcervical chorionic villus sampling (CVS); percutaneous umbilical blood sampling (PUBS); the aspiration of fetal urine, pleural effusions, and ascites; biopsy of fetal tissues (skin, muscle, and liver); and the guidance of specific fetal surgical procedures (bladder-amniotic shunting) have become more common with improvements in the resolution of sonographic equipment. Initially, prenatal testing meant the diagnosis of potentially fatal conditions that led to either abortion or unremitting progression of a particular malformation or condition. However, as the pathophysiologic features of specific malformations were determined, appropriate fetal treatments were devised. For example, in the early 1960s, Liley (1) first attempted in utero fetal transfusion for severe Rh isoimmunization. Although a review of current in utero therapy is beyond the scope of this chapter, the reader should be cognizant of the shift in emphasis from prenatal diagnosis alone to prenatal diagnosis and therapy.

There have also been significant changes in the utilization of prenatal diagnosis over the past 10 years. Recent advances in prenatal screening include (*i*) the addition of inhibin-A to the second trimester triple screen (i.e., quad screen) (2); (*ii*) the first trimester genetic screening with nuchal translucency and serum screening (3); and (*iii*) the second trimester genetic sonogram with a reported 68.3% (4) to 91% (5) sensitivity in the detection of trisomy 21 with a false positive rate of 14% to 14.7%. At the University of Connecticut Health Center, Benn et al. (6) recorded a 50% decline in genetic amniocenteses and CVS between 1991 and 2002. The number of Down syndrome fetuses detected increased. As a result, the proportion of genetic tests with an abnormal karyotype increased from 1 in 43 to 1 in 14. These changes in prenatal testing require an increase in patient counseling. The changes in relative risk based upon a normal or abnormal screening test (first trimester genetic screen, second trimester quad screen, or second trimester genetic sonogram) must first of all be appreciated by the couple before they can incorporate the information into their decision concerning invasive prenatal testing.

In gynecology, the role of sonography was also initially to diagnose specific disease states. The advantages of sonographically guided follicular aspiration, cyst aspiration, and pelvic abscess drainage soon became apparent. This chapter reviews the current role of sonographically guided procedures in obstetrics and gynecology.

CHORIONIC VILLUS SAMPLING

Transcervical Approach

CVS was first performed by Chinese investigators in 1975. Although this technique was not guided by ultrasound, the authors claimed a high success rate for obtaining villi, with a procedure-related miscarriage rate of 5% (7). In 1982, Kazy et al. (8) emphasized the importance of ultrasound guidance for successful CVS.

Transcervical CVS uses a 27-cm polyethylene catheter with an external diameter of 1.9 mm. The catheter contains a removable stainless steel stylet that is visible sonographically (Fig. 1). The catheter is followed sonographically throughout its course from the cervix to an appropriate position within the placenta (Fig. 2). The tip of the catheter should rest within the chorion frondosum before aspiration and should not abut the myometrium. Sampling near the umbilical cord insertion into the placenta is optimal. When the catheter is placed too close to the chorionic plate, fewer villi are obtained.

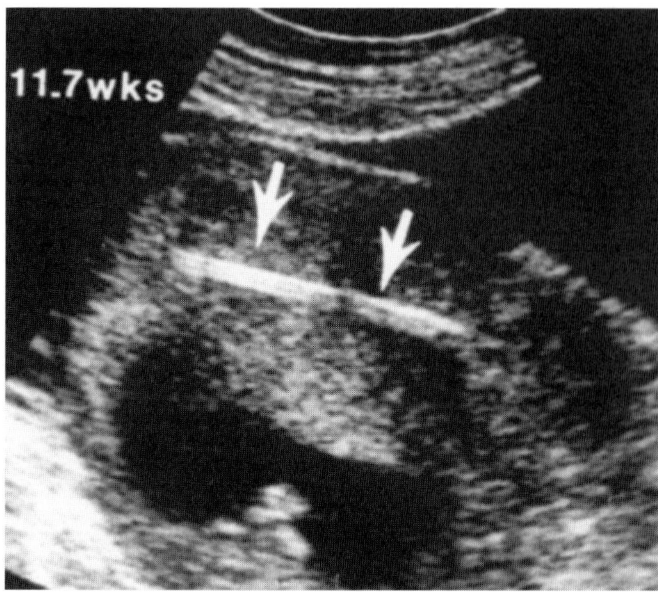

FIGURE 2 ■ Transcervical chorionic villus sampling at 11.7 weeks. The catheter (*arrows*) is appropriately positioned within the anterior placenta.

Transabdominal Approach

Ultrasonically directed transabdominal CVS is performed freehand (Figs. 3–6) or with a biopsy guide. Either filling or serially emptying the maternal bladder may be required before an optimal site for transabdominal CVS is located. The needle is directed into the placenta along its longest axis. Uterine contractions may assist (Fig. 7) or may impede CVS. In the latter instance, waiting 15 to 20 minutes allows for the resolution of a contraction; a site for CVS may then be available. When the placenta is posterior, a transamniotic route with puncture of the membranes should be avoided (11). By almost completely emptying the maternal bladder and by providing counterpressure with the ultrasound transducer, the uterus can be straightened so a posterior placenta can be entered directly from the uterine fundus.

Some authors recommend the use of an 18-gauge spinal needle as a guide through the myometrium (Fig. 8); a 21-gauge needle is then passed coaxially through the 18-gauge needle into the placenta for sampling. In the typical two-person technique, an assistant performs the ultrasound examination. The primary operator inserts the biopsy needle into the placenta, connects a 20-mL syringe to the needle hub, and then aspirates while slowly moving the needle back and forth (Fig. 3) (9). Hill and Laifer (12) modified this technique by attaching a small piece of extension tubing (0.5 mL dead space) to the needle hub. A 12-mL syringe is then connected to the extension tubing (Fig. 9). While the sonologist manipulates the biopsy needle under ultrasound guidance, repeated rapid aspiration of the plunger can then be performed by an assistant.

In experienced hands, transcervical and transabdominal CVS appear to be equally effective and result in comparable fetal loss rates (13). The technique employed,

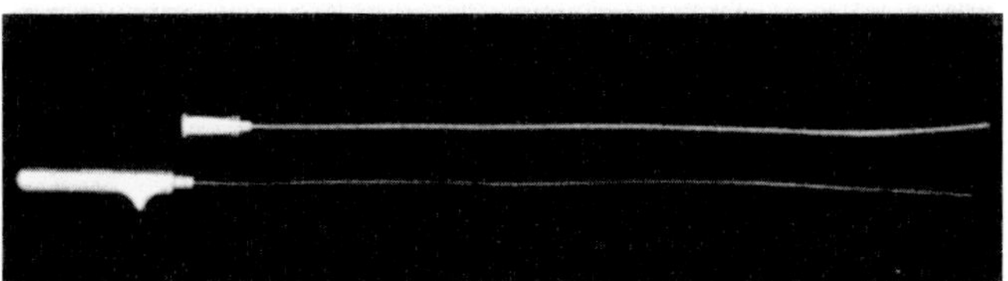

FIGURE 1 ■ A 1.5 mm (16-g) polyethylene chorionic fillus catheter (*top*) with a malleable stainless steel stylet (*bottom*) (Portex, Wilmington, Massachusetts, U.S.A.).

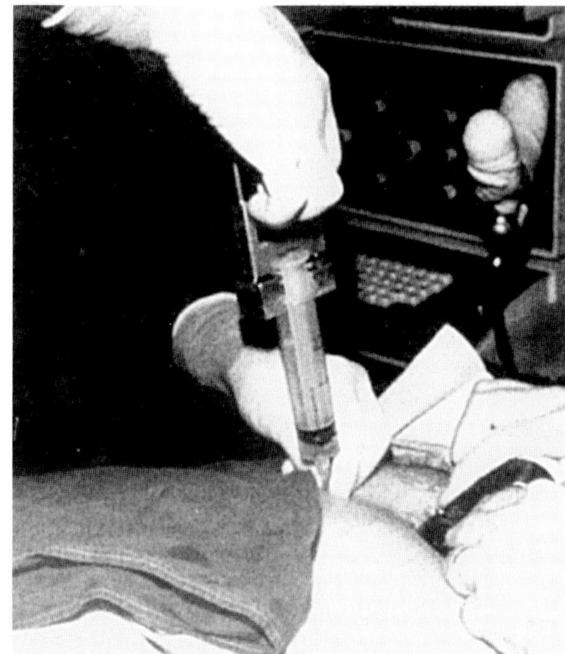

FIGURE 3 ■ Freehand ultrasound-guided chorionic villus sampling method; a 30-mL syringe is set in a syringe holder with ultrasound probe to the side (*arrow*). *Source*: From Ref. 9.

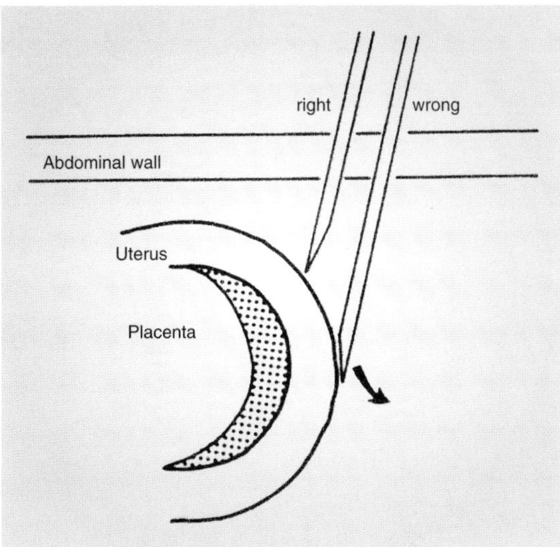

FIGURE 4 ■ Correct position of the guide needle tip: the sharp edge "catches" the uterine surface; the bevel deflects from the uterus in the "wrong" position. *Source*: From Ref. 10.

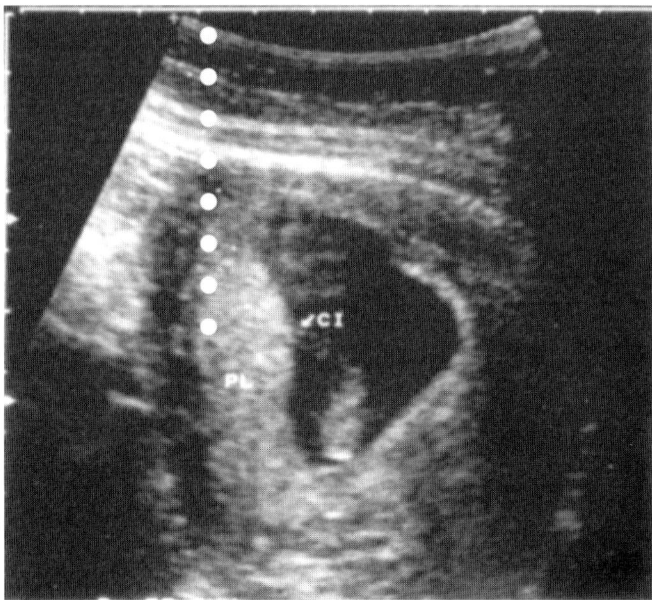

FIGURE 6 ■ Transabdominal scan at 11 weeks' gestation. The markers denote the path for transabdominal chorionic villus sampling. PL, placenta; CI, cord insertion.

therefore, depends on the physician's experience as well as the easiest approach to the placenta at the time of the procedure.

Complications

Any pregnancy loss occurring within 14 days of CVS has generally been considered to be related to the procedure (14). Some losses resulting from infection or rupture of the membranes may not occur until after this arbitrary time limit has passed (15). The procedure-related pregnancy loss rate from CVS of 1% is similar to the loss rate of second trimester genetic amniocentesis (16). Several factors significantly affect the overall miscarriage rate after CVS. Both maternal age and gestational age at the time of the CVS must be considered. For example, the spontaneous miscarriage rate rises from 1.9% at 35 to 36 years of age to 10.9% at age 40 years or older (17). Because most miscarriages occur before 12 weeks' gestation, some authors have suggested delaying CVS until the 12th week of pregnancy.

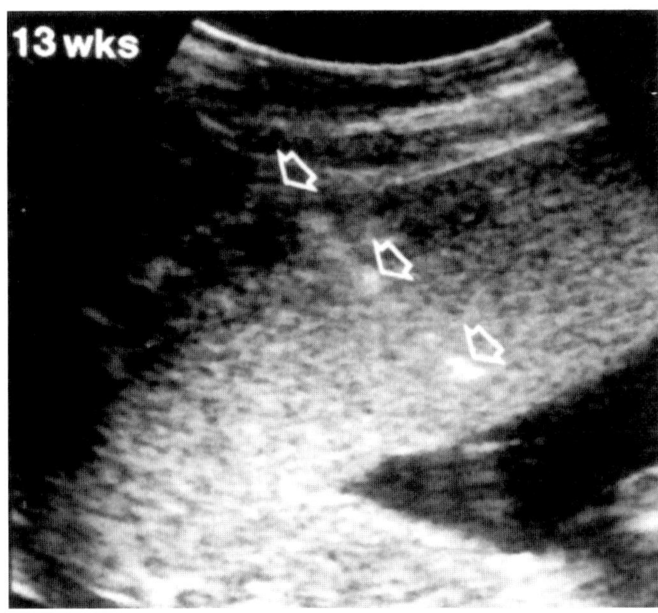

FIGURE 5 ■ Transabdominal chorionic villus sampling at 13 weeks' gestation (*arrows* Identify the needle).

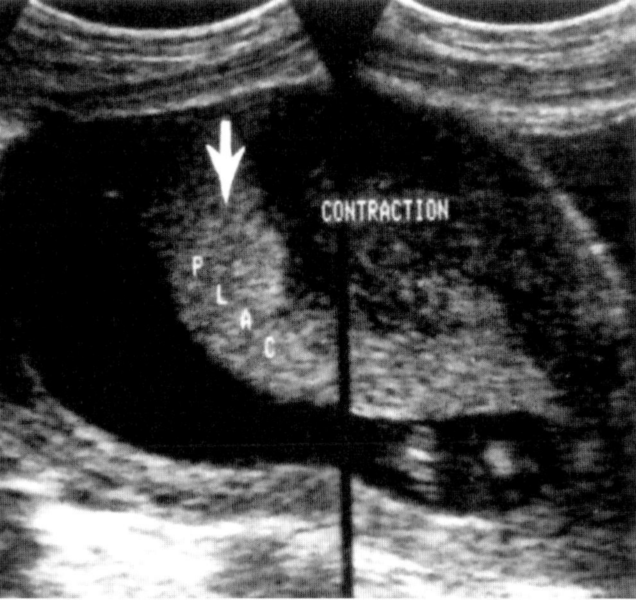

FIGURE 7 ■ A uterine contraction has straightened the placenta, so vertical needle insertion (*arrow*) for chorionic villus sampling is possible. PLAC, placenta.

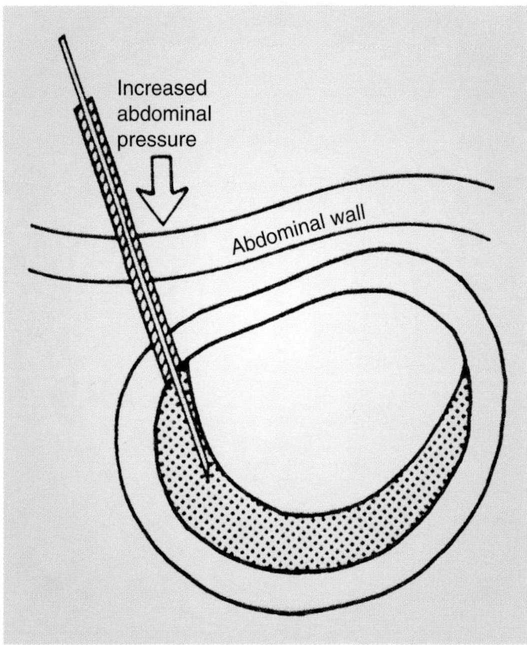

FIGURE 8 ■ Technique of transabdominal chorionic villus sampling for posterior localized placentas in retroflexed uteri. Increased probe and hand pressure on the abdominal wall allows for more direct route for sampling of chorionic villi. *Source*: From Ref. 10.

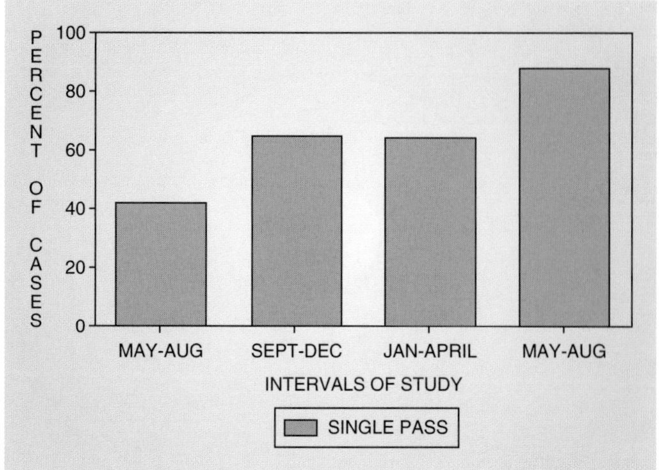

FIGURE 10 ■ Proportion of chorionic villus sampling procedures accomplished in a single aspiration correlated with increasing experience during study intervals ($P < 0.0005$). *Source*: From Ref. 23.

From a practical standpoint, however, most women elect to have CVS between 10 and 11 weeks' gestation.

The sonographic detection of a subchorionic hematoma after CVS or postprocedural vaginal bleeding increases the risk of subsequent miscarriage (18,19).

Rh sensitization, as well as the exacerbation of Rh disease, has been reported with CVS (20). Rh (D) immune globulin is, therefore, given to Rh-negative unsensitized women after CVS. Because of the potential for exacerbation, Rh-sensitized women should consider genetic amniocentesis with avoidance of the placenta rather than CVS for prenatal diagnosis.

Investigators acknowledge a reduction in the pregnancy loss rate after CVS with increasing operator experience. With transcervical CVS, experience with several hundred patients is required before the loss rate stabilizes (18,21,22). Although fetal loss rate is critical in an assessment of a CVS program, other measures of expertise (such as single-pass success rate) (Fig. 10) may be more appropriate indicators of competence (23). The rate of vaginal bleeding is lower with transabdominal than with transcervical CVS (0.2% vs. 2.5%, $p < 0.001$) (24).

A few cases of serious maternal infection have been reported after transcervical CVS. Such an infection is more likely to occur if the same catheter is used for several passes. With better aseptic technique, the risk of maternal infection has been reduced (25,26). Although occurring less frequently, localized peritonitis has been reported after transabdominal CVS (24).

In late 1991, reports from several institutions suggested an increase in the risk of limb reduction defects and in the overall miscarriage rate when CVS was performed before nine weeks' menstrual age (Table 1) (27–29). Trauma to the placental vasculature, and subsequent fetal hypoperfusion, has been suggested as the cause of this specific congenital malformation. Subsequent reports with larger series of patients have not found an increase in distal limb defects after CVS (29). As a result of this controversy, CVS is no longer recommended before 10 weeks' menstrual age (30).

Confined placental mosaicism is an acknowledged disadvantage of CVS. Approximately 1% of CVS samples are mosaic; only 10% to 40% are confirmed in the fetus. The mosaicism rate after second trimester genetic amniocentesis is 0.1% to 0.3%; 70% are confirmed in the fetus (31).

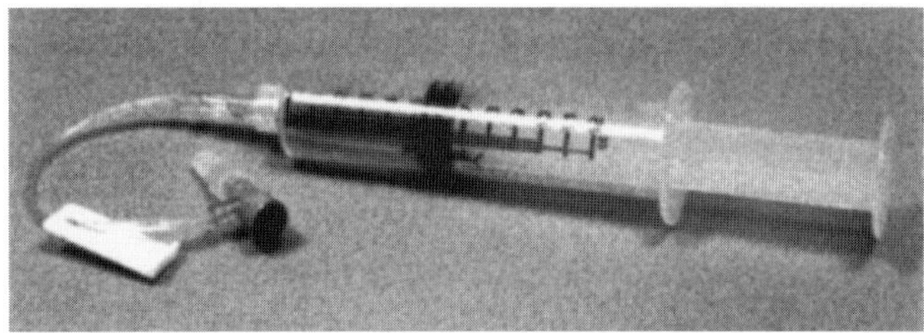

FIGURE 9 ■ A 12-mL syringe filled with 3 mL of media and attached to 0.5 mL of extension tubing. The extension tubing is attached to the chorionic villus sampling needle after it is appropriately positioned within the placenta.

Second and Third Trimester Placental Biopsy

Placental biopsy or late CVS may be performed in the second or third trimester. In cases of oligohydramnios, placental biopsy or PUBS may be the only method available to obtain a fetal karyotype. The risk associated with second or third trimester placental biopsies is no higher than with fetal blood sampling and varies with the reason for sampling (32,33). Patients with and without sonographic

TABLE 1 ■ Gestational Age at CVS and Rates of Fetal Loss, Congenital Malformations, and Limb Defects

	Gestational age at CVS (wk)				
	6–7	8	9–12	>12	Total
Number of cases	256	655	4700	268	5879
Fetal loss					
Number	14	20	108	4	146
Percentage (%)	5.3	3.1	2.3	1.5	2.3
Malformations					
Number	9	12	80	3	104
Percentage (%)	3.5	1.8	1.7	1.1	1.7
Limb defects					
Number	4	1	3	0	8[a]
Percentage (%)	1.58	0.15	0.06	0	0.13

[a]Three of the five limb defects following sampling at 6–8 wk were reported as Möbius-like syndrome cases. Of the five pregnancies, two were terminated after limb defect anomalies were detected at fetal anomaly scanning before voluntary abortion.

Abbreviation: CVS, chorionic virus sampling.

Source: From Ref. 28.

findings suggestive of a fetal karyotypic abnormality have a fetal loss rate of 10% and 2%, respectively (34).

AMNIOCENTESIS

Amniocentesis was suggested more than 100 years ago by Schatz. Not until 1919, however, did Hinkel use this technique to treat a patient with polyhydramnios (35). In 1950, amniotic fluid was first used to assess patients with Rh sensitization (36). Midtrimester amniocentesis (MA) for prenatal diagnosis began in 1967 (37). Since the 1970s, the use of amniocentesis in prenatal diagnosis and for third trimester assessment of fetal lung maturity has increased almost exponentially. Although amniocentesis was performed years before the general availability of ultrasound, the advantages of sonography as a guide for this procedure became readily apparent.

Technique

Initially, ultrasound-directed amniocentesis was performed. In this technique, a site was selected sonographically and the abdomen was marked. After preparation of the patient, the amniocentesis needle was inserted into the predetermined depth and the fluid was removed. Over the past 20 years, continuous ultrasound guidance during amniocentesis has been performed (38). With this approach, the ultrasound transducer is placed in a sterile bag, and the needle is imaged throughout its course from the maternal skin to the amniotic cavity (Fig. 11). When properly performed, this method almost completely eliminates bloody taps and the necessity of performing multiple punctures (39). Ultrasound can also be used to assist the sonologist in moving a fetus out of a pocket of amniotic fluid immediately before amniocentesis (40).

Needle Selection

Needle gauge is a technical aspect of genetic amniocentesis that is not frequently considered. Both the National Institute of Child Health and Development (41) and the Canadian collaborative (42) studies found a higher fetal

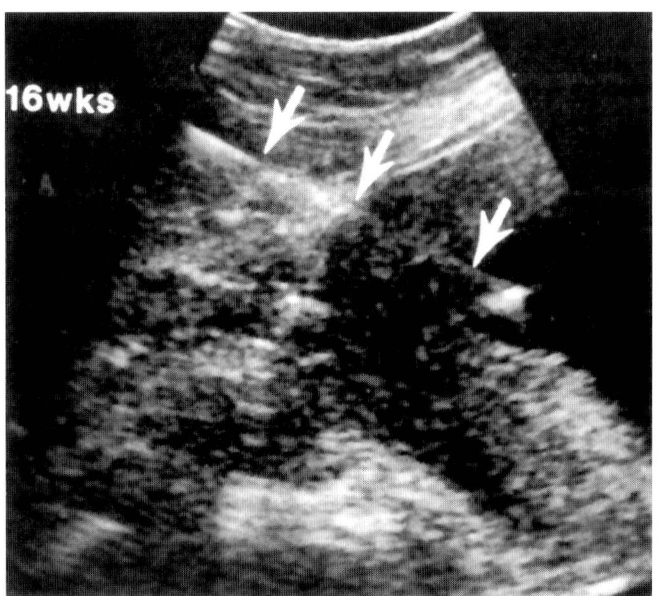

FIGURE 11 ■ Genetic amniocentesis at 16 weeks' gestation. Arrows outline the needle entering the amniotic cavity.

loss rate with needles of 19 gauge or larger. Smaller-bore needles are less painful for the patient and may reduce the frequency of uterine contractions and fluid leakage after the procedure. Active bleeding into the amniotic cavity after transplacental amniocentesis occurs in approximately 8% of patients (Fig. 12A and B) (43–46). The duration of bleeding is an effect of needle gauge (38).

Needles that optimize sonographic visualization have become commercially available. Acoustic visualization is enhanced by roughening the needle. In addition, these needles have side holes to expedite amniotic fluid aspiration when the needle tip may be blocked (Sono-Vu, US, E-Z-EM, Westbury, New York, U.S.A.) (Fig. 13). These apparent advantages are not clinically significant for the obstetrician or perinatologist skilled in continuously guided amniocentesis.

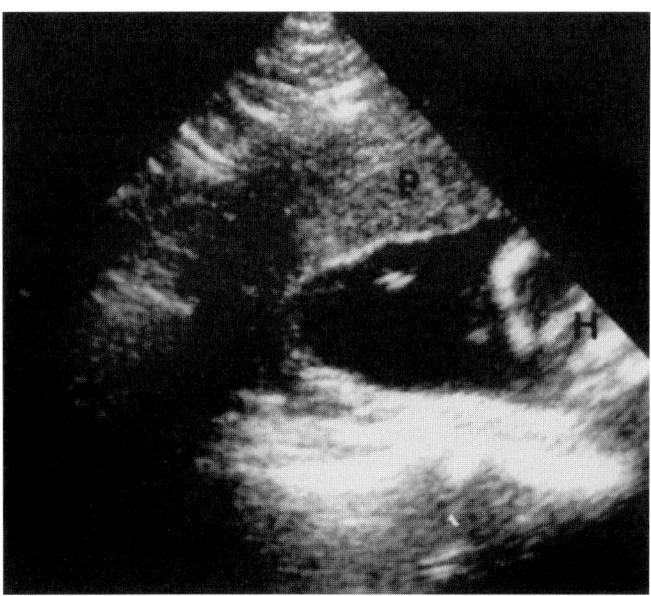

(A)

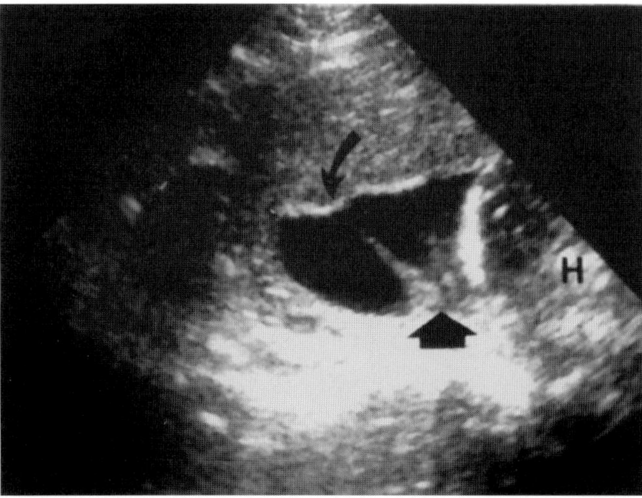

(B)

FIGURE 12 A AND B ■ Intra-amniotic hemorrhage after transplacental amniocentesis. (**A**) Needle traversing the margin of an anterior placenta. Needle (*arrow*) in amniotic cavity. (**B**) After removal of the needle, active intra-amniotic bleeding occurs. Echogenic material originating from the placental puncture site (*curved arrow*) actively streams into the amniotic cavity, hitting the opposite wall (*large arrow*) and dispersing into the amniotic fluid. H, fetal head; P, placenta. *Source*: From Ref. 46.

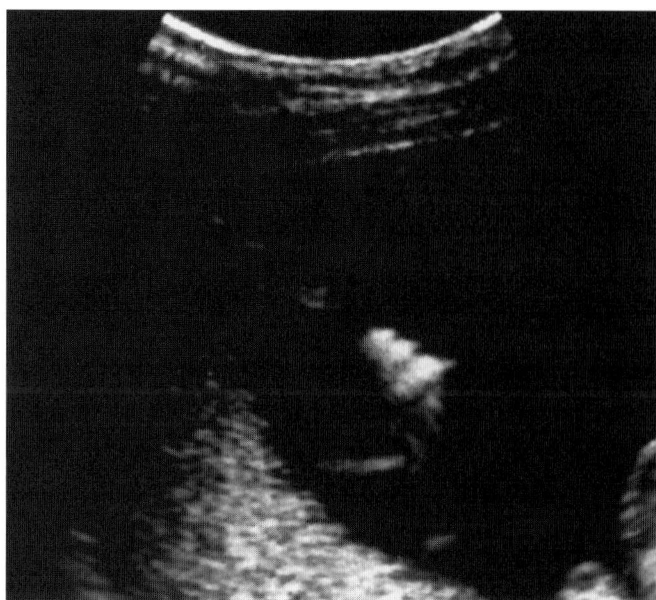

FIGURE 13 ■ Genetic amniocentesis at 17 weeks' gestation using a needle with enhanced acoustic visualization at the tip.

Maternal Complications

Complications associated with amniocentesis include uterine cramping, vaginal spotting, amniotic fluid leakage, and, rarely, intra-amniotic infection (41,42). In cases of vaginal bleeding or amniotic fluid leakage, ultrasound can be used to assess the intrauterine environment. Perinatal outcome is not adversely affected if an amniotic fluid leak stops and the fluid in the amniotic cavity reaccumulates (47).

Fetal Complications

Miscarriage

Controversy exists concerning the procedure-related pregnancy loss rate in transplacental versus nontransplacental genetic amniocentesis. Two earlier reports noted a twofold increase in pregnancy loss when the placenta was traversed (48,49). The first investigation (48) was a collaborative investigation by 10 obstetric departments. The second study by Porreco et al. (49) was published before continual ultrasound guidance during amniocentesis. Two studies by single investigators involving 2136 and 4454 patients, respectively, suggested that transplacental genetic amniocentesis does not result in a higher spontaneous miscarriage rate (50,51). In addition, Giorlandino et al. (51) and Crane and Kopta (43) reported a lower risk of amniotic fluid leakage after transplacental amniocentesis. Fetomaternal hemorrhage appears to be increased with the transplacental approach (52). When transplacental amniocentesis must be performed, surface vessels and intraplacental sonolucent areas that may represent subchorionic lakes or intervillous thrombi should be avoided (53).

A study by Tabor et al. (54) randomized 4606 women into a second trimester amniocentesis group and a control group. The women were between the ages of 25 and 34 and were not at risk of having a child with a chromosomal abnormality. The amniocentesis was performed with a 20-gauge needle under ultrasound guidance. There was a significant increase (2.1% vs. 1.3%; relative risk 1.02–2.52) in spontaneous miscarriage following second trimester genetic amniocentesis.

When attempting to assess the miscarriage rate after amniocentesis, the same confounding variables discussed with CVS must be considered. Advanced maternal age, increasing parity, history of early fetal wastage, and abnormal maternal serum α-fetoprotein concentration have been associated with an increase in the spontaneous miscarriage rate (55,56). Finally, and perhaps most important, is the operator's experience. Leschot et al. (57) have shown a significant difference ($P < 0.001$) in the miscarriage rate between obstetricians who have performed no more than 50 amniocenteses and those who have performed more than 50 procedures (Table 2).

Fetal Trauma

Fetal trauma secondary to amniocentesis was more common before the widespread use of continuous ultrasound guidance. In a prospective study of 460 ultrasonically directed amniocenteses, the needle pierced the fetus in 27 instances (5.9%) (58). Although most fetal punctures are without long-lasting sequelae, some injuries can be devastating. Ocular trauma (59), gangrene of a fetal limb (Fig. 14) (60), ileocutaneous fistula (Fig. 15) (61), porencephalic cyst (62), intestinal atresia (63), and disruption of a patellar tendon (64) have been reported after second trimester amniocentesis. Continuous ultrasound guidance during insertion of the amniocentesis needle minimizes, but cannot completely prevent, the possibility of fetal trauma. The foregoing cases of ocular trauma (59) and intestinal atresia (63) occurred during amniocentesis performed under continuous ultrasound guidance.

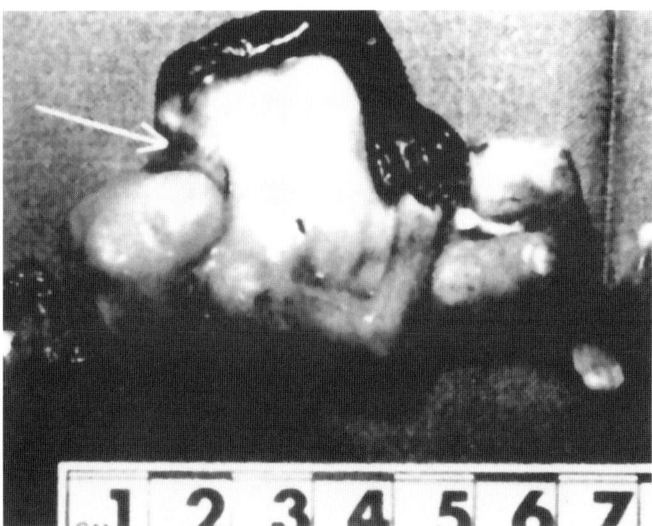

FIGURE 14 ■ Traumatic amniocentesis in an anencephalic fetus with gangrene of left arm. The site of needle puncture in the left supraclavicular region is shown by an arrow. *Source*: From Ref. 60.

EARLY AMNIOCENTESIS

Evans et al. (65) have defined early and very early amniocentesis (EA) as those procedures performed between 12.0 and 13.9 menstrual weeks and before 11.9 menstrual weeks, respectively. The gestational age range for amniocentesis in a given study has a significant effect not only on the ease of the procedure but also on the background miscarriage rate.

Amniotic Fluid Volume

One of the difficulties inherent in EA is the smaller amount of amniotic fluid available for aspiration. In general, the volume of amniotic fluid between the 11th and 15th weeks' menstrual age can be determined by the following equation: volume = 25 (weeks − 10) (66). However, reported amniotic fluid volumes for each week in the first trimester have a wide range (Table 3). The volume of fluid aspirated during EA is generally 1 mL/wk of gestation (68,69). The last two columns in Table 3 indicate the

TABLE 2 ■ Fetal Loss Associated with Amniocentesis in the First Series of 1500 Pregnancies Related to the Experience of the Obstetrician

Total no. of amniocenteses performed by obstetrician	No. of pregnancies	Fetal death or abortion within 3 wk after amniocentesis
10	347	13 (3.7%)[a]
11–50	453	8 (1.8%)
>50	700	2 (0.3%)[a]
Total	1500	23

[a] $P < 0.001$.
Source: From Ref. 57.

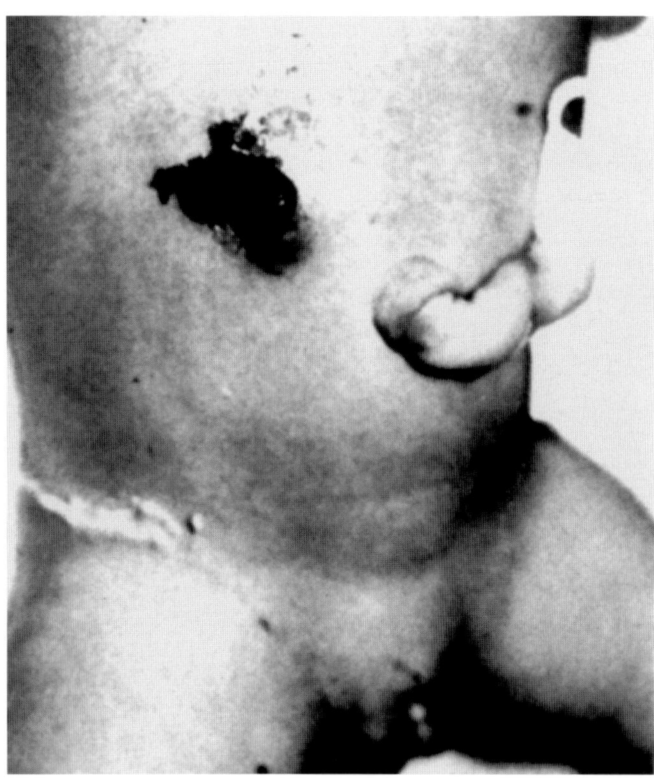

FIGURE 15 ■ Traumatic amniocentesis showing the appearance of the abdomen at birth. An intestinal fistula to the right of the umbilicus is present. *Source*: From Ref. 61.

amount of amniotic fluid removed by the week of gestation as well as the percentage that amount represents of the total volume available. Although the amniotic fluid volume is constantly replaced, the loss of over 18% of the amniotic fluid for even a short period of time has been considered the etiology of the increased incidence of talipes equinovarus with this procedure.

Technique

The technique of continuous ultrasonically guided EA is the same as for traditional amniocentesis. Sundberg et al. (70) addressed the theoretic problem of a reduced amniotic fluid volume before 14 weeks' gestation by using a cell filter through which amniotic fluid is passed before its return to the amniotic cavity. The fetal cells are then flushed from the filter with culture media.

Complications

The likelihood of amniotic fluid leakage is increased if the amnion has not yet attached to the uterine wall, a common finding before 13.9 weeks' menstrual age (71). When the amnion is adherent to the uterine wall, the frequency of fluid leakage after EA is not significantly higher than after conventional amniocentesis (41,71).

The trend appears to be toward an increased pregnancy loss rate when amniocentesis is performed before 12 weeks' gestation (69). Nicolaides et al. (72) compared EA and transabdominal CVS performed between 10 and 13 weeks' menstrual age. Both techniques used continuous ultrasound guidance of a 20-gauge needle. The spontaneous loss rate was significantly higher after EA (5.3%) than after CVS (2.3%).

The Canadian Early and Midtrimester Amniocentesis Trial (CEMAT) randomly allocated pregnant women to EA (11 + 0 – 12 + 6 menstrual weeks) or MA (15 + 0 – 16 + 6 menstrual weeks) (73,74). There was a significant difference between the groups in

1. Total fetal losses (7.6% for EA vs. 5.9% for MA).
2. Prevalence of talipes equinovarus (1.3% in the EA group vs. 0.1% in the MA group).

TABLE 3 ■ Volume of Amniotic Fluid by Week of Gestation

		Amniotic fluid volume				
Week	No.	Mean (mL)	SD	Range (mL)	Amount removed (mL)	Percentage (%)
10	7	29.7	11.2	18–33	10	33
11	9	53.5	16.4	64–76	11	20
12	13	58.0	23.4	35–86	12	20
13	13	71.4	21.3	38–98	13	18
14	14	124.1	42.1	95–218	14	11
15	15	136.8	43.7	64–245	15	11
16	16	191.2	59.7	27–285	20	10
17	20	252.6	98.5	140–573	20	8
18	4	289	150	70–140	20	7
19	14	324.5	65.2	241–470	20	6
20	3	380	39	355–425	20	5

Source: From Ref. 67.

3. Post-procedure amniotic fluid leakage (3.5% for EA vs. 1.7% for MA).
4. Number of repeat amniocenteses (2.2% for EA vs. 0.3% for MA).

The NICHD EATA study (75) compared EA and transabdominal CVS at 13 menstrual weeks. This study also found a significantly increased risk of talipes equinovarus after amniocentesis (0.76%), in contrast to CVS (0.16%). The procedure-related loss rate was slightly higher after earlier amniocentesis.

As a result of these studies, late first trimester amniocentesis has been abandoned in favor of CVS.

AMNIOCENTESIS IN TWIN GESTATIONS

Approximately 1% to 2% of genetic amniocenteses are performed on twin pregnancies (76,77). As with singleton pregnancies, the most frequent indication for genetic amniocentesis is advanced maternal age.

Technique

The technique for tapping twins was described by Elias et al. in 1980 (76). The separate amniotic sacs are distinguished by injecting 1 mL of indigo carmine dye into the sac from which the first sample of amniotic fluid is obtained. A second amniocentesis is then performed; aspiration of clear amniotic fluid indicates that the second sac has been successfully entered. Jeanty et al. (78) proposed an alternative to this technique in which a single needle insertion was used to tap both twin sacs. After tapping the first sac, the stylet is replaced and the needle is advanced under continuous ultrasound guidance through the intra-amniotic membrane into the second sac (Fig. 16). Gilbert et al. (79) cautioned that this technique could theoretically disrupt the dividing membrane and result in a perinatal mortality rate commensurate with true monoamniotic twins. Bahado-Singh et al. (80) have proposed a different technique for genetic amniocentesis in twins. After a needle is inserted in one gestational sac under ultrasound guidance, a second needle is introduced into the second cavity without changing the position of the transducer. This technique permits visualization of the two needles in separate sacs simultaneously. Hence, indigo carmine dye need not be instilled into the first sac. Finally, with the improved resolution of current ultrasound equipment, the course of the dividing membrane can be mapped; two sites for amniocentesis are selected well away from one another. The use of indigo carmine dye is then reserved for only the more difficult cases.

Complications

In 1983, Palle et al. (81) reported that the multiple needle insertions required for successful twin amniocenteses result in a significantly higher miscarriage rate than for singleton pregnancies. The Canadian Collaborative study (42) on singleton amniocenteses found a significantly higher ($P < 0.001$) miscarriage rate when more than two needle insertions were required. Consequently, studies have indicated that twin amniocenteses under continuous sonographic guidance that require two needle insertions are not associated with a higher miscarriage rate (82,83).

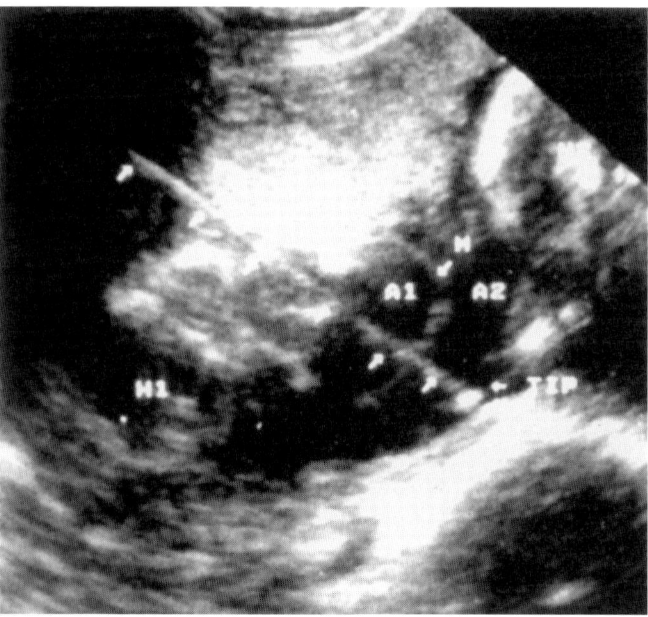

FIGURE 16 ■ Single needle insertion in twin genetic amniocentesis at 16 weeks' gestation. The interamniotic membrane is roughly in a vertical plane and separates the first amniotic cavity on the left from the second amniotic cavity on the right. The two fetal heads are included in the lower left and upper right corner of the scan. The needle (*arrows*) has perforated the membrane, and its tip is in the second amniotic cavity. M, interamniotic membrane; A1, first amniotic cavity; A2, second amniotic cavity; H1 and H2, fetal heads; TIP, needle tip. *Source*: From Ref. 78.

MULTIFETAL PREGNANCY REDUCTION

Perinatal morbidity and mortality, as well as maternal morbidity, increase with fetal number (84). Despite improvements in outcome with modern obstetrical management, the pregnancy risks associated with triplets and higher-order multiple gestations remain significant (85,86). The goal of selective reduction is to improve the perinatal outcome for the remaining fetuses. Although the clinical advantage of multifetal reduction for quadruplets or greater is significant, the procedure is still controversial in twin and triplet pregnancies.

There have not been any randomized controlled trials evaluating the efficacy of multifetal pregnancy reduction (MFPR). Dodd and Crowther (87) performed a meta-analysis of the available nonrandomized studies and concluded that for women with a triplet pregnancy, reduction to twins compared to expectant management results in a reduced rate of pregnancy loss, antenatal complications, and birth before 36 weeks' gestation. However, the authors offered the caveat that these studies may be associated with potential bias and their results should be interpreted with caution.

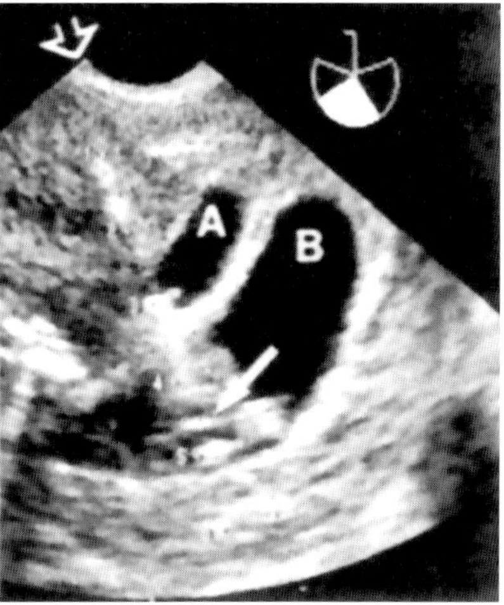

FIGURE 17 ■ Fetal reduction. A four-to-two reduction was performed on this patient. The first fetus to be reduced was fetus A. The tip of the needle is seen within the fetus, at the left side. On the right side, the same needle was advanced into fetus B. The advantage of a single needle insertion is to minimize maternal morbidity. *Source*: From Ref. 91.

The outcomes of higher-order pregnancies reduced to twins are as good as unreduced twins (88). Because the risks associated with a twin pregnancy are more than double that of singletons, it has recently been proposed that one might consider fetal reduction from twins to a singleton (89).

Technique

MFPR is performed by transabdominal fetal intrathoracic injection of potassium chloride (Fig. 17) (90). A freehand technique, a biopsy guide, and an automated spring-loaded puncture device (Fig. 18) (92) have all been used.

Sonographic criteria suggested for fetal selection in MFPR include (*i*) an abnormally small crown–rump length, (*ii*) an anomalous fetus, (*iii*) a thickened nuchal translucency, and (*iv*) monochorionic twins (94,95). An abnormally small crown–rump length has been associated with karyotypic (96) or structural (97) malformations.

Complications

With increasing experience, there has been a significant improvement in outcome from MFPR. Collaborative loss rates of 4.5% for triplets, 7.3% for quadruplets, 11.5% for quintuplets, and 15.4% for sextuplets or higher have been reported (88). The loss rate and the prematurity rate are functions of the starting number of fetuses (90).

There is no difference in loss rate if fetuses near the cervix or near the uterine fundus are targeted for reduction. The miscarriage rate appears to be lower when multifetal reduction is performed before 13 weeks' menstrual age (98,99). The dramatic rise in multiple pregnancies is due to assisted reproductive technologies (ART). MFPR is a therapy aimed at the result of ART, not at the cause. A consensus is finally developing that the number of embryos transferred should be sharply curtailed (100).

FIGURE 18 ■ The automatic puncturing device by Popp fits on the ultrasound probe and automatically advances the needle to a predetermined depth when fired (Labotect, Gottinger, Germany). *Source*: From Ref. 93.

LASER ABLATION OF AN ACARDIAC TWIN

The reversed arterial perfusion sequence (acardiac twin) is a rare complication of monochorionic placentation. The normal twin provides the blood supply to the acardiac twin through an artery-to-artery anastomosis. As the acardiac twin increases in size and requires a larger blood volume, the pump twin becomes anemic and eventually hydropic. Sonographically guided intrafetal radiofrequency (Fig. 19) or laser ablation of a vessel within the acardiac twin has been reported as an effective way to reduce flow to the acardiac twin and improve the survival rate for the normal twin (102).

PERCUTANEOUS UMBILICAL BLOOD SAMPLING

Direct access to the fetal circulation heralded the beginning of a new era of prenatal diagnosis and therapy. Fetal blood was initially obtained by means of fetoscopy (103). In 1983, sonographically guided fetal PUBS

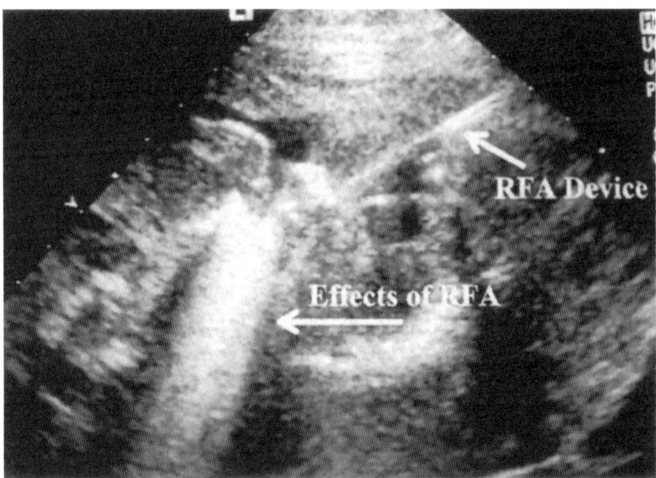

FIGURE 19 ■ Transabdominal intraoperative ultrasound images reveal radiofrequency ablation (RFA) device deployed within the abdomen of the acardiac fetus and the echogenic material that represents the tissue effects of RFA. *Source*: From Ref. 101.

(cordocentesis and funicentesis) was introduced by Daffos et al. (104). This technique is usually performed in the second or third trimester. Cordocentesis has been performed as early as 12 weeks' menstrual age (105). As gestational age advances, the diameter of the umbilical artery and vein increases, making cordocentesis technically easier (Fig. 20) (Table 4) (106). Boulot et al. (107) reported a first-attempt success rate with PUBS of 50%, 75%, 87%, and 92% at up to 20 weeks' gestation, at 20 to 24 weeks' gestation, at 25 to 29 weeks' gestation, and above 30 weeks' gestation, respectively.

Indications

The indications for cordocentesis and their relative frequency as reported to the National Percutaneous Umbilical Blood Sampling Registry in 1988 are outlined in Table 5 (108). At that time, rapid fetal karyotyping and red-cell isoimmunization were the most common indications for PUBS in the United States.

Fetal blood sampling has been used to assess cases of chromosome mosaicism found in amniotic fluid culture. Mosaicism of 30% in amniotic fluid is not confirmed in the fetus (31). Although a detailed fetal anatomic survey is reassuring, structural anomalies may not be present with mosaicism because of the dilutional effect of the normal cell line (109). Fetal blood

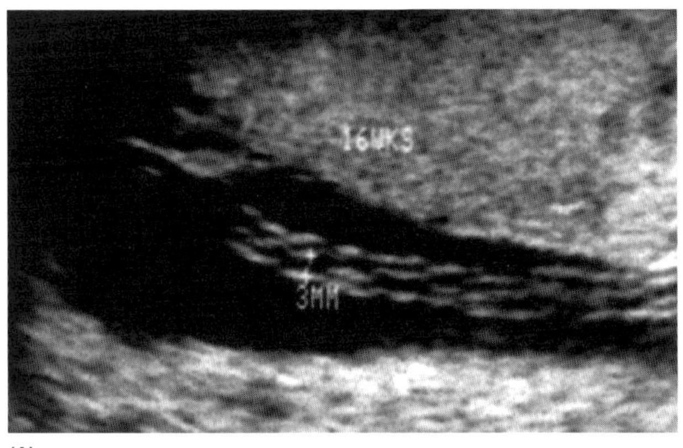

(A)

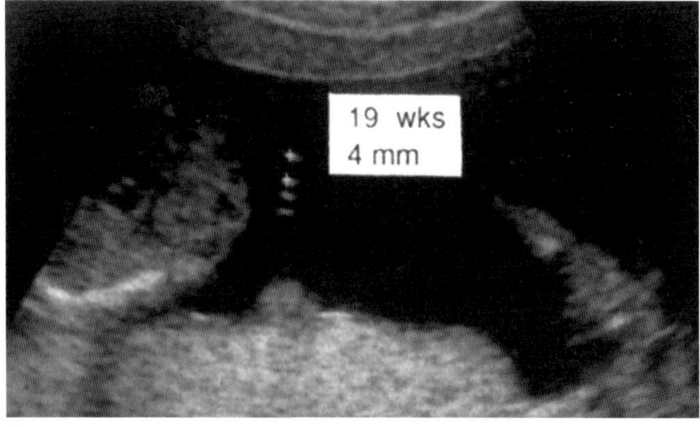

(B)

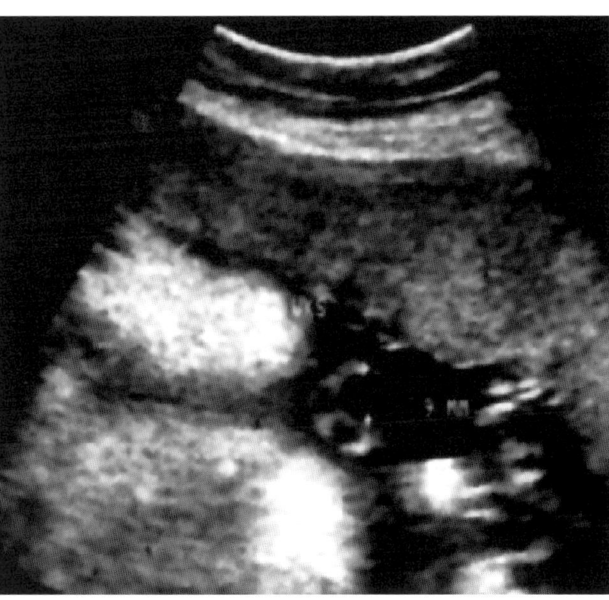

(C)

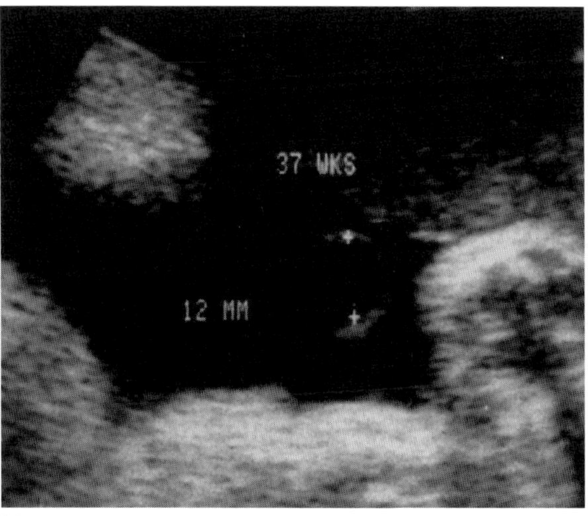

(D)

FIGURE 20 A–D ■ Umbilical vein diameter: (**A**) 3 mm (16 weeks' gestation); (**B**) 4 mm (19 weeks' gestation); (**C**) 9 mm (33 weeks' gestation); and (**D**) 12 mm (37 weeks' gestation).

TABLE 4 ■ Umbilical Vein and Artery Diameters According to Gestational Age

Gestational age (wk)	Umbilical vein diameter (mm)	Umbilical artery diameter (mm)
14–15	2.0	1.2
16–17	2.4	1.1
18–19	3.6	1.9
20–21	4.1	2.0
22–23	4.7	2.4
24–25	5.4	2.6
26–27	6.0	2.8
28–29	6.6	3.1
30–31	7.3	3.4
32–33	7.7	3.6
34–35	7.4	3.3
36–37	7.6	3.7
38–39	8.2	4.2
40–42	7.8	3.9

Source: From Ref. 106.

sampling provides a rapid karyotype of a different fetal tissue. Gosden et al. (110) reported a normal fetal blood karyotype in 15 of 16 cases of mosaic trisomy obtained from amniotic fluid cultures. Although the absence of aneuploid cells in fetal blood does not exclude the possibility of chromosomal mosaicism in other tissues, women in these circumstances generally elect to continue the pregnancy (111).

TABLE 5 ■ Indication for Cordocentesis as Reported at the National Percutaneous Umbilical Blood Sampling Registry (1601 Cases)

Indication	No. of cases	Percentage (%)
Rapid karyotype	620	39
Fetal red-cell isoimmunization	512	32
Idiopathic thrombocytopenia	137	8
Nonimmune hydrops	94	6
Intrauterine fetal infection	44	2.8
Fetal acid–base balance	38	2.3
Coagulation factor deficiency	32	2
Hemoglobinopathies	28	1.8
Immunologic deficiency	26	1.6
Alloimmune thrombocytopenia	23	1.4
Twin–twin transfusion	23	1.4
Fetal drug levels	10	0.6
Diagnosis of fetal thyrotoxicosis	2	0.12
TAR syndrome	2	0.12
Paternity determination	1	0.06
Low platelets (maternal phenytoin)	1	0.06

Abbreviation: TAR, thrombocytopenia–absent radii.
Source: From Ref. 108.

PUBS has also been used to diagnose and manage fetal bleeding disorders. Neonatal alloimmune thrombocytopenia is usually secondary to antibodies directed against the PLA-1 antigen. The maternal level of anti–PLA-1 antibody does not accurately predict the severity of fetal thrombocytopenia. For this indication, platelets should be administered after fetal blood sampling to reduce the likelihood of bleeding from the umbilical cord (112). If a fetus is significantly thrombocytopenic, a subsequent cordocentesis should be performed to assess the effect of treatment with prednisone or high-dose intravenous γ-globulin (113–115).

Medical advances have reduced the frequency with which PUBS is required. Although rapid fetal karyotyping had been a common reason for cordocentesis, amniocentesis results are routinely available in seven days. Fluorescent in situ hybridization (FISH) with chromosome-specific probes (13, 18, 21, x and y) to uncultured amniotic cells can confirm or exclude a specific karyotype abnormality in 48 to 72 hours (116). Because of the limited number of probes available, FISH remains complimentary rather than an alternative to standard karyotyping.

Umbilical blood sampling rapidly became the gold standard for diagnosing fetal anemia. In 2000, Mari et al (117) correlated the peak systolic velocity in the middle cerebral artery (MCA) with fetal hemoglobin values. They reported that the sensitivity of an increased peak systolic velocity in the MCA for predicting moderate-to-severe anemia prior to 35 weeks' gestation was 100% (95% confidence interval 86–100%) with a false positive rate of 12% (118). This method of surveillance is also useful in following fetuses with parvovirus B-19 exposure and suspected anemia (119).

Fetal blood sampling is no longer the primary tool in the evaluation of a fetus at risk for in utero infection. The culture of amniotic fluid is more sensitive for cytomegalovirus than is an assessment of fetal IgM obtained by PUBS (120). In addition, polymerase chain reaction amplification can now identify microorganisms in amniotic fluid (121). Fetal Rh (D type) can also be ascertained by means of polymerase chain reaction amplification of DNA obtained at amniocentesis (122). Finally, most of the hereditary diseases (e.g., hemophilia and metabolic disorders) for which PUBS was performed (123) can now be diagnosed by DNA analysis of a chorionic villus sample (124). Despite these additional advances in antenatal diagnosis, ultrasonically directed PUBS will continue to play a critical role in the diagnosis of fetal conditions as well as in selected treatment regimens. For example, the fetus appears to be "immunoprivileged" up to 18 to 20 weeks' gestation, allowing engraftment of stem cells derived from either adult bone marrow or fetal tissue. In the future, second trimester cordocentesis may be used to administer stem cells for the in utero treatment of specific congenital hematopoietic disorders.

Technique

The preferred site for PUBS is the placental cord insertion, but a free loop of umbilical cord may also be sampled. The location of the placental cord insertion, the position of the fetus relative to the cord insertion, the amniotic fluid volume, the gestational age at the time of sampling, and the maternal habitus are important factors that determine the best site for fetal blood sampling. In severe oligohydramnios, a placental biopsy can be performed for fetal karyotypic information (32). If fetal blood is required for other diagnostic purposes, color Doppler imaging or the instillation of 100 to 300 mL of warmed isotonic saline into the amniotic cavity is frequently helpful in selecting an appropriate sampling site (125). Polyhydramnios with a posterior placenta poses another technical difficulty. In these cases, a longer needle can be used for fetal blood sampling, or an initial therapeutic amniocentesis can be performed to reduce the distance between the maternal abdomen and the placental cord insertion.

Cardiocentesis has been proposed as an alternative method of fetal blood sampling. The fetal loss rate (5.6%) is substantially higher with cardiac puncture than with PUBS (126).

Nicolini et al. (127) recommended the intrahepatic vein as an alternate site for fetal blood sampling or transfusion. In this technique, the needle is advanced through the substance of the liver into the umbilical vein (Fig. 21). The frequency of intraperitoneal bleeding associated with this technique is approximately 2.3%.

The method for PUBS is the same as for amniocentesis. The patient is prepped and draped. The ultrasound transducer is then placed in a sterile bag to image the umbilical cord. The operator holds the transducer in one hand and inserts a 22-gauge needle with the other hand. The entire path of the needle is imaged as it approaches and then enters the umbilical cord (Fig. 22). Alternatively, a sonologist can hold the transducer, or a needle guide can be used. Bovicelli et al. (129) have reported using a 20-gauge needle through a biopsy guide for uterine entry. A 25-gauge needle is then passed through the lumen of the 20-gauge needle for the actual fetal blood sampling. An in vitro model consisting of a fresh placenta

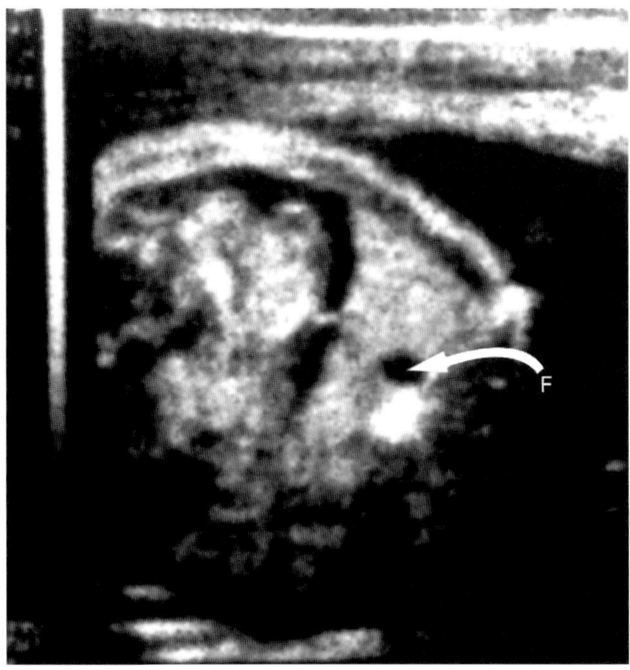

(A)

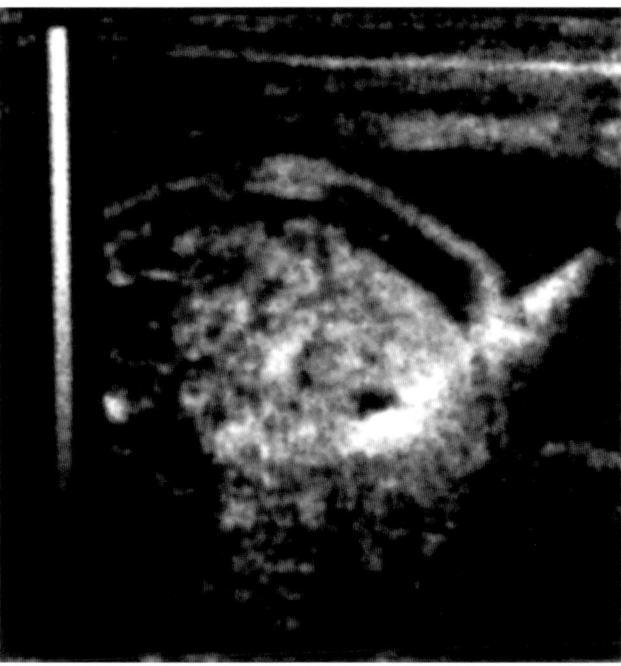

(B)

FIGURE 21 A AND B ■ Ultrasound showing fetal blood sampling at the intrahepatic portion of the umbilical vein. (**A**) The needle tip is identified in the liver parenchyma beyond the umbilical vein. (**B**) The needle was withdrawn and blood aspirated with the needle tip now observed in the umbilical vein. *Source*: From Ref. 128.

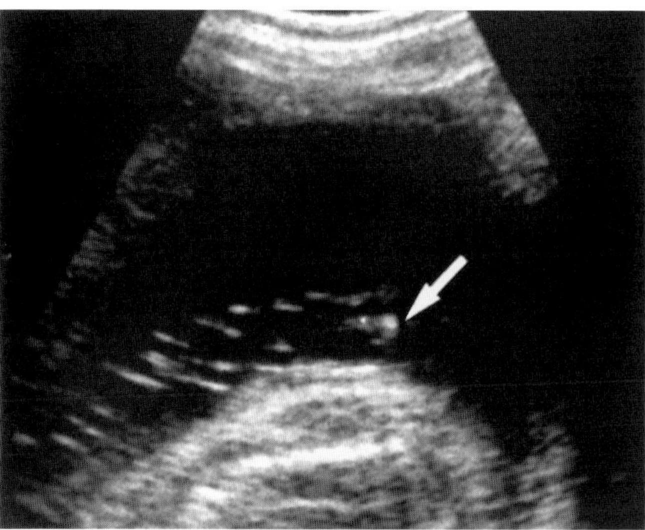

FIGURE 22 ■ Percutaneous umbilical blood sampling in a free loop of umbilical cord at 20 weeks' gestation.

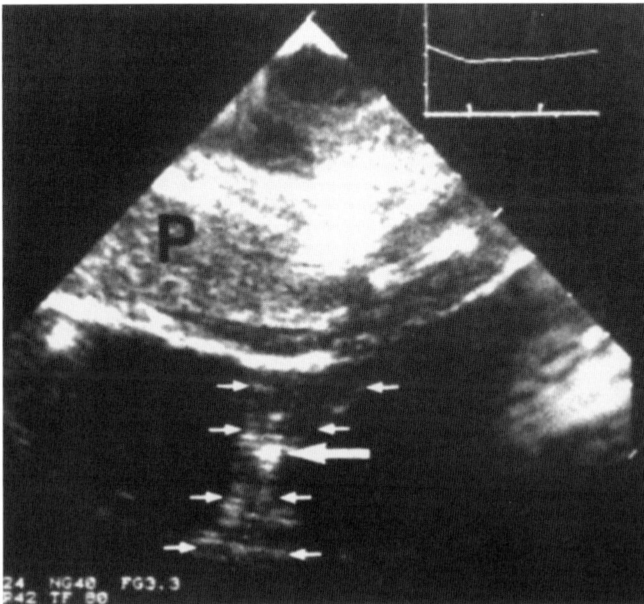

FIGURE 23 ■ Placental model for diagnostic and therapeutic fetal intravascular puncture. *Small arrows*, umbilical cord; *large arrow*, needle. P, placenta. *Source*: From Ref. 130.

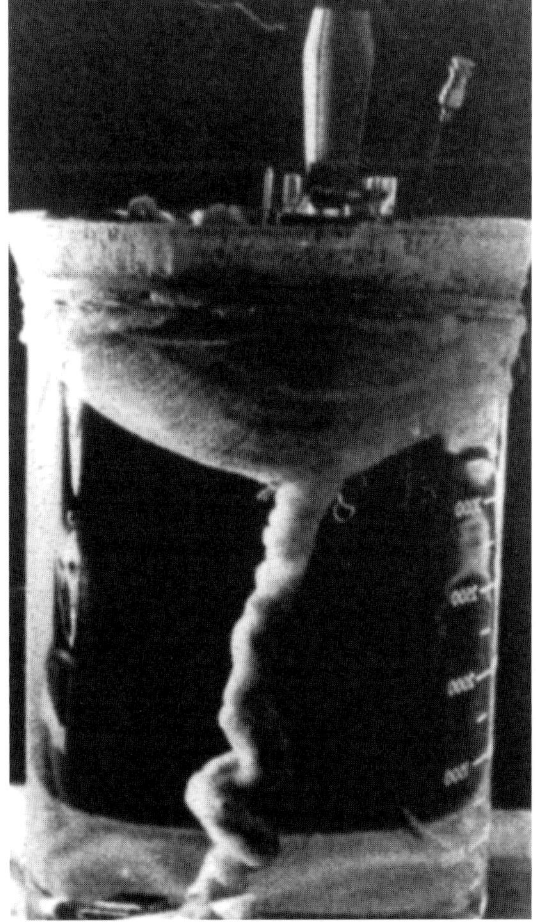

FIGURE 24 ■ Ultrasonographic picture of the placental model in Figure 23. *Source*: From Ref. 130.

in a water bath may be used to train physicians interested in cordocentesis (Figs. 23 and 24) (130). With a posterior placenta, fetal paralysis may be necessary for successful intravascular transfusion. The injection of pancuronium, 0.1 mg/kg (131) or atracurium, 0.4 mg/kg (132) before transfusion results in fetal paralysis for 15 to 130 minutes.

Complications

The complications associated with PUBS include fetal bradycardia (9%), bleeding from the umbilical cord puncture site for longer than two minutes (2%), and intrauterine fetal demise (1.1%) (133). Most instances of bradycardia occur in growth-restricted or malformed fetuses (134). Doppler studies indicate an absence of diastolic flow in the umbilical artery during prolonged fetal bradycardias. When the heart rate returns to normal, diastolic flow is reestablished. These findings suggest that the bradycardia after PUBS is secondary to vascular spasm (134). Fetal blood sampling from the umbilical artery increases the risk of subsequent bradycardia (135).

The elastic consistency of Wharton's jelly (Fig. 25) and the coagulation properties of amniotic fluid help to reduce the frequency of bleeding from the umbilical cord (133,136,137). However, in some cases, hemorrhage into the amniotic cavity may result in significant fetal blood loss. Daffos et al. (133,138) have reported a 2% incidence of cord bleeding lasting longer than two minutes after PUBS with a 20-gauge needle. Bleeding from the umbilical cord occurs more frequently and for a longer period when a 20-gauge, in contrast to a 22-gauge, needle is used for sampling (Table 6). Fetal thrombocytopenia also increases the duration of bleeding from the umbilical cord (112,139). The type of bleeding that occurs after PUBS depends on the vessel punctured. A jet of blood from an

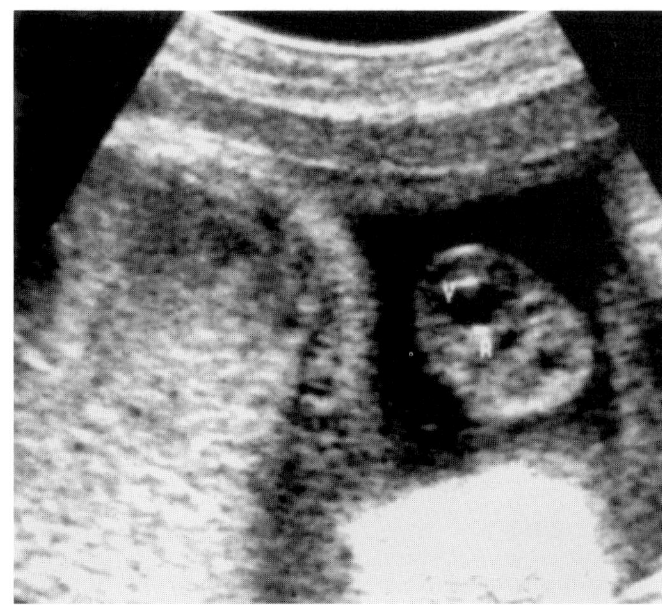

FIGURE 25 ■ Wharton's jelly surrounding the umbilical artery (A) and vein (V) at 31 weeks' gestation.

TABLE 6 ■ Comparison of Bleeding Times with a 22-Gauge Needle vs. a 20-Gauge Needle

Category	No.	Postpuncture bleeding time (sec)	
		Mean	Range
22-gauge needle			
Total cases	85	137	5–720
Venous puncture	72	144	5–450
Arterial puncture	15	95[a]	5–720
Normal platelets	75	123	5–400
Thrombocytopenia	8	375[b]	140–720
20-gauge needle			
Total cases	27	92[c]	5–300
Venous puncture	22	102	20–350
Arterial puncture	5	48[a]	5–350

[a] $P < 0.05$, as compared with venous bleeding time.
[b] $P < 0.05$, as compared with normal platelet count.
[c] $P < 0.05$, as compared with 22-gauge needle puncture.
Source: From Ref. 112.

arterial puncture site ceases abruptly; with umbilical vein puncture, bleeding is slower and is intermittent (112). The volume of blood lost depends on the rate of blood flow through the puncture site and the duration of bleeding. Generally, blood loss is minimal and does not exceed 5% to 10% of fetal blood volume. With prolonged bleeding, fetal exsanguination may occur.

Although the reported incidence of cord hematomas after PUBS is approximately 1%, its occurrence at our institution is no more than 0.5%. This complication primarily occurs when PUBS is attempted in a free loop of umbilical cord (140,141) or after intravascular transfusion (142). Most umbilical cord hematomas are small and do not affect fetal blood flow. Larger hematomas may partially or completely compress the umbilical vessels, resulting in fetal distress or fetal demise.

Infection after PUBS is an uncommon event, occurring once in every 250 procedures (143,144). Placental abruption has occasionally been reported after PUBS.

The rate of complications increases when PUBS takes longer than 10 minutes or when more than three attempts are made (Table 7). The fetal loss rate is also increased (5.2%) when fetal blood sampling is performed before 19 weeks' gestation (105). Healthy fetuses have a significantly lower risk of fetal death (0.58% or 1 of 172) than do fetuses with congenital malformations or those fetuses presumably already compromised (11.24% or 19 of 169) (134,135,140).

TABLE 7 ■ Number of Needle Punctures and Fetal Deaths

No. of punctures	No. of cases	Fetal death		
		Related	Not related	Percentage (%)
1	243	1	8	3.70
2	65	0	4	6.15
3	21	1	2	14.29
>3	13	1	3	33.33

Source: From Ref. 140.

Fetomaternal hemorrhage after PUBS may increase the severity of maternal red-cell alloimmunization. Bowman et al. (145) detected transplacental hemorrhage in 57.5% of nonimmunized women after PUBS. When compared with a control group who underwent neither PUBS nor amniocentesis, fetomaternal hemorrhage of at least 0.5 mL is 185 times and 15 times more likely to occur with PUBS and amniocentesis, respectively.

FETAL SKIN BIOPSY

Fetal skin biopsies for hereditary skin disorders (genodermatoses) can be obtained under continuous ultrasound guidance. Conditions for which skin biopsies have been performed include ichthyosis, Sjogren–Larsson syndrome, and epidermolysis bullosa dystrophica (146). The gluteal region and the back are the preferred sites for biopsy.

There are currently four genes known to be associated with autosomal-recessive congenital ichthyosis. Of individuals with severe (lamellar) ichthyosis, 90% have a mutation in *TGM1*. DNA-based molecular prenatal diagnosis (CVS or amniocentesis) is available for pregnancies with a 25% risk for autosomal-recessive congenital ichthyosis. However, the two disease-causing mutations of *TGM1* must previously have been identified in the proband. Carrier testing for other mutations is not yet available (147–149).

Technique

An adequate fetal tissue sample is often difficult to obtain. The optimum time for biopsy is around 20 weeks' gestation. Since some of the dermatoses have different origins, the selection of a biopsy site may vary with the condition one is trying to diagnose. The use of a needle for skin biopsy does not carry any risk greater than that of amniocentesis. When a trocar and a 2.5-mm forceps are used, sampling success is nearly 100% but at a cost of a miscarriage rate of approximately 5% (150).

Under continuous ultrasound guidance, the biopsy instrument is directed toward an appropriate site. Once a specimen has been obtained, it is immediately viewed under a microscope to determine whether the sample size is sufficient to make a diagnosis.

Complications

Too few fetal skin biopsies have been performed to accurately know the risks. As with other invasive procedures, amniotic fluid leakage, bleeding, infection, and fetal injury should be considered. Shulman and Elias (151) have reported three fetal losses within 20 days of 107 skin biopsies reviewed at the Seventh International Meeting on Prenatal Diagnosis and Fetal Treatment. Unfortunately, this report is currently 20 years old.

FETAL MUSCLE BIOPSY

The dystrophinopathies include a spectrum of muscle diseases that are caused by mutation in the Duchenne muscular dystrophy (*DMD*) gene. DMD is rapidly progressive and results in affected males being wheelchair bound by the age of 12. Cardiomyopathy becomes manifest after age 20. Few affected individuals survive beyond 30 years of age. In Becker muscular dystrophy (BMD), skeletal muscle weakness occurs later; individuals remain ambulatory until their 20s. Cardiomyopathy also occurs. Survival is approximately 10 years longer than with DMD. Both of these conditions have cross-linked recessive inheritance. Sons who inherit the gene mutation are affected, while daughters with the mutation are carriers (152–154).

Fetal muscle biopsy can be performed under direct ultrasound guidance for BMD or DMD. One series of 12 cases had no reported neonatal scars or nerve damage after in utero muscle biopsy. The procedure-related risk of a second-trimester muscle biopsy is estimated to be between 1% and 5% (155). In some cases, prenatal diagnosis by CVS or amniocentesis is possible. If the fetus is 46,xy, DNA can be extracted from fetal cells for analysis. However, the *DMD* mutation must have been identified in a family member or linkage markers established.

Technique

Under continuous ultrasound guidance, a 16-gauge biopsy device is positioned directly over the fetal buttock. A trigger mechanism advances a cutting needle to a predetermined depth to obtain a core of muscle tissue for analysis. If the biopsy gun temporarily opens as it passes through the resistance of the rectus sheath, maternal contamination may occur. An analysis of the sampled tissue (i.e., muscle fiber size) can be used to exclude maternal contamination (156). The puncture success rate is 75% (150).

FETAL LIVER BIOPSY

Prenatal diagnosis of mutations in ornithine transcarbamylase, the most common enzyme defect in the urea cycle, can now be performed by analyzing chorionic villi or amniocytes. Fetal liver biopsy must be used to diagnosis glucose-6-phosphatase deficiency as well as carbamoyl-phosphate synthetase deficiency (151).

Murotsuki et al. (157) used a 20-gauge percutaneous transhepatic cholangiography needle, whereas Rodeck and Nicolaides (146) used a standard 19-gauge needle for liver biopsy. A double cannula system (17-gauge outer, 19-gauge inner) has also been recommended. The larger outer needle is used to stabilize the fetus while the smaller needle is moved back and forth several times in the substance of the liver to obtain a specimen (158). Although no complications have been reported, this method of prenatal diagnosis should be restricted to those hereditary liver diseases with an extremely poor prognosis.

FETOAMNIOTIC SHUNTING

Intrauterine shunting is a rarely performed ultrasound-guided procedure that attempts to prevent compression and subsequent damage to normal tissue by various types of intrafetal cysts or fluid accumulations. Table 8 outlines the number of cases and indications for intrauterine drainage from four European centers. A double-pigtail catheter was used in each case (Figs. 26 and 27). The procedure-related fetal death rate was 8%; occlusion of the catheter or dislodgement occurred in 29% of cases.

Hagay et al. (160) performed a MEDLINE search and found 54 fetuses with a pleural effusion that was managed expectantly and 24 fetuses who had either repeated needle drainage or placement of a shunt (Fig. 28A–C).

TABLE 8 ■ Number of Cases and Indications for Intrauterine Catheter Placement

Indication	No.
Cystic adenomatoid malformation	4
Fetal ascites	8
Hydrothorax	9
Bladder outlet obstruction	13
Total	34

Source: From Ref. 159.

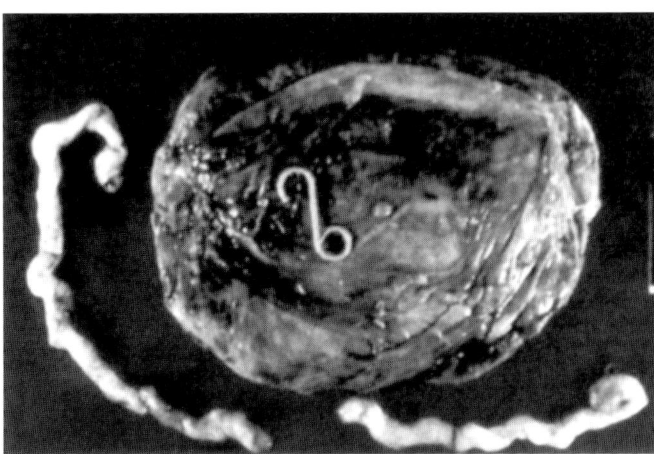

FIGURE 26 ■ Double-pigtailed catheter used for a vesicoamniotic shunt.

The neonatal death rate, excluding terminations, was 37% and 33% for conservative and interventional management, respectively. However, the criteria for intervention and the type of intervention was not consistent between series and case reports.

Spontaneous resolution of a pleural effusion may occur (161).

In the absence of a dramatic improvement in survival with intervention for a fetal pleural effusion, a consensus has evolved that only specific cases should be offered therapy. The four generally accepted criteria for intervention include (*i*) gestational age below 32 weeks with an immature fetal lung profile; (*ii*) hydrops; (*iii*) a risk of pulmonary hypoplasia secondary to compression; and (*iv*) a rapid reaccumulation of a pleural effusion after two needle aspirations (162). Picone et al. (163) evaluated perinatal outcome after thoracoamniotic shunting for fetal pleural effusions with hydrops. Of the 47 pregnancies that continued after shunting, 31 (66%) resulted in children that survived; all 31 survivors had chylothorax. The main morbidities associated with pleuroamniotic shunting were premature rupture of the membranes and preterm delivery. Other reported complications include hypoproteinemia and shunt migration. Pregnancy loss with thoracentesis has been estimated at 0.5% to 1% (164).

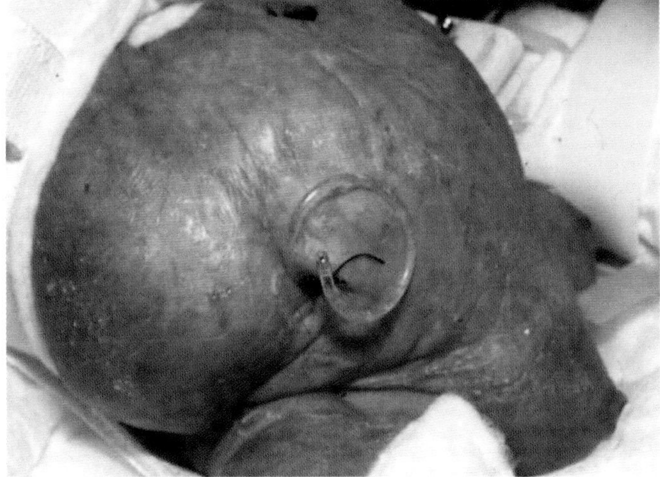

FIGURE 27 ■ Double-pigtailed catheter in the lower abdomen of a neonate with posterior urethral valves.

A failure of the lung to reexpand after removal of pleural fluid is a poor prognostic sign (160).

The catheter should be placed in the lower lateral aspect of the hemithorax in order to permit maximum drainage and reduce the likelihood of tubal occlusion.

Thompson et al (165) evaluated lung function between 3 and 60 months after delivery in 17 infants who had undergone pleuroamniotic shunting between 21 and 35 weeks' menstrual age. Respiratory status did not differ between the study group and a control group who had not undergone shunting.

With respect to macrocystic adenomatoid malformation, an intra-amniotic shunt should only be considered in the presence of developing fetal decompensation (i.e., hydrops) before 32 weeks' menstrual age (162). Antenatal shunting in the second trimester can result in normal neonatal lung growth (166).

With bladder outlet obstruction, shunting should only be considered in an otherwise structurally normal fetus with megacystitis, a subjective decrease in amniotic fluid volume, and normal renal function as assessed by urinary sodium (<100 mEq/L), chloride (<90 mEq/L), and osmolarity (<210 mOsm) (Fig. 29A–C) (159,167). β2 microglobulin is selectively absorbed in the proximal tubule. The presence of large quantities of β2 microglobulin (>4 mg/L) in fetal urine and, therefore, amniotic fluid is indicative of tubular destruction. Hence, an elevated β2 microglobulin would also be a contraindication to shunt placement.

The appearance of the renal parenchyma must also be carefully assessed. The presence of cortical cysts and/or echogenic or thin cortex is a poor prognostic sign that should prevent attempts at vesicoamniotic shunting (168). Unfortunately, ultrasound cannot diagnose all renal dysplasias. Hence, there remains a role for the biochemical evaluation of fetal urine. Fetal karyotyping should be performed before any shunting procedure.

The purpose of vesicoamniotic shunting is to prevent renal dysplasia and pulmonary hypoplasia. McLorie et al. (169) reported the results with eight vesecoamniotic shunts; six fetuses survived (75%). The final diagnosis in the six surviving patients was posterior urethral valves in four, urethral atresia in one, and prune belly with urethral atresia in one. Three of the neonates had normal renal function, one had mild renal impairment, and two had severe renal insufficiency. None of the patients had pulmonary problems. This study illustrates the potential as well as the complications associated with this procedure. Although vesicoamniotic shunting can reverse oligohydramnios in highly selected appropriate candidates, long-term renal function is variable and the mortality rate remains high. In this study, mortality from termination or stillbirth was 3/9 (33%).

Reported complications with vesicoamniotic shunting include chorioamnionitis, shunt migration and/or

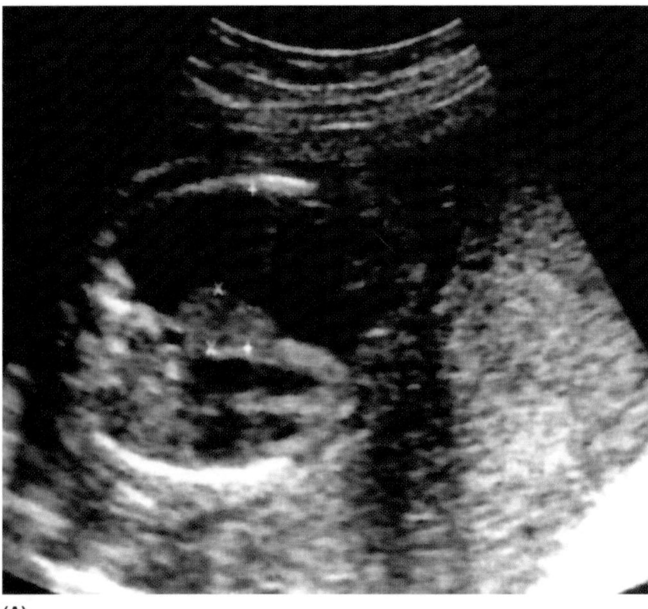

FIGURE 28 A–C ■ Left fetal hydrothorax. (**A**) 24 weeks' gestation. The compressed fetal lung is between the x marks, the heart is deviated into the right thorax. (**B**) Pleuroamniotic shunt (*arrow*) at 25.8 weeks' gestation. (**C**) Pleuroamniotic shunt at 33 weeks' gestation. The hydrothorax is no longer present. Arrows point to the catheter in the chest.

(A)

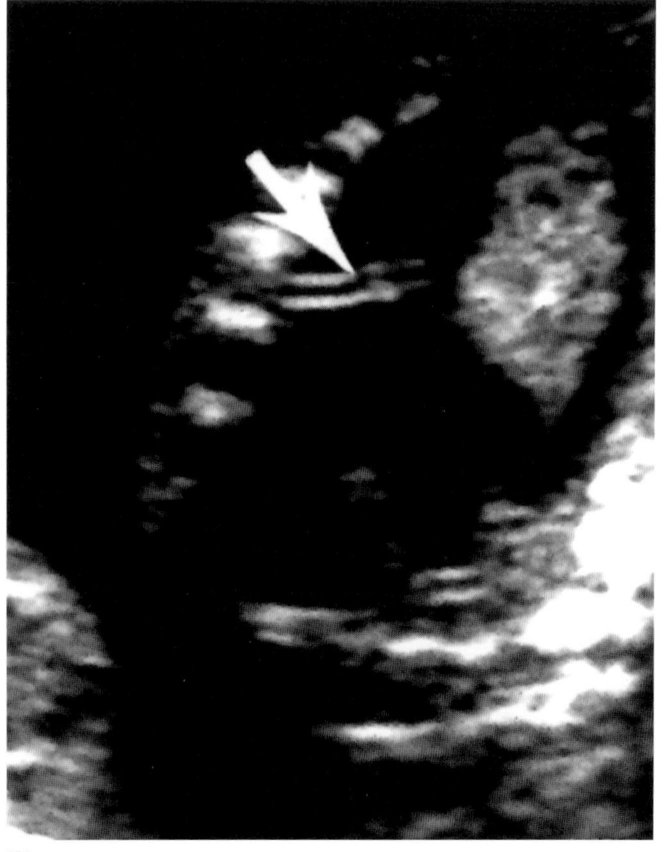

(B)

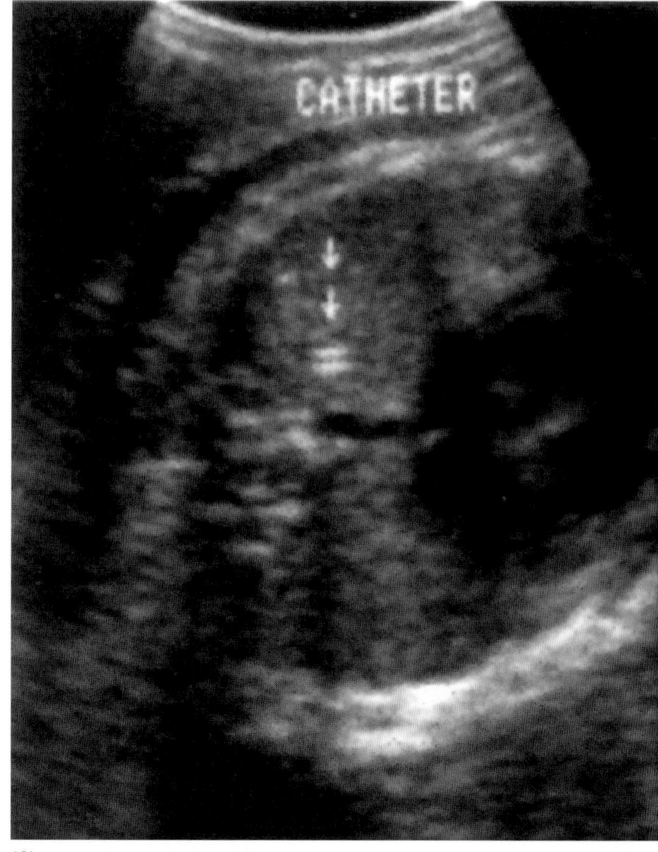

(C)

obstruction, rupture of the membranes, fetal trauma, fetal death, and preterm labor.

Efficacy

There have not been any randomized controlled trials evaluating the efficacy of fetoamniotic shunting. Relatively small study groups have been compared to historical controls that did not undergo treatment. These procedures may be efficacious for a limited number of fetuses. However, strict entry criteria must be followed; otherwise, the maternal and fetal complications will outweigh the benefits of intervention.

Technique

Under ultrasound guidance, a trocar is introduced into the amniotic cavity immediately adjacent to the intrafetal

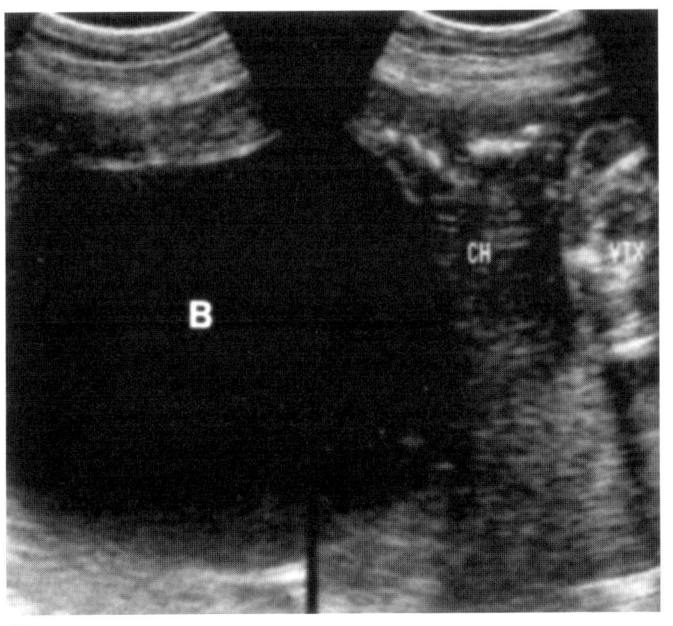

(A)

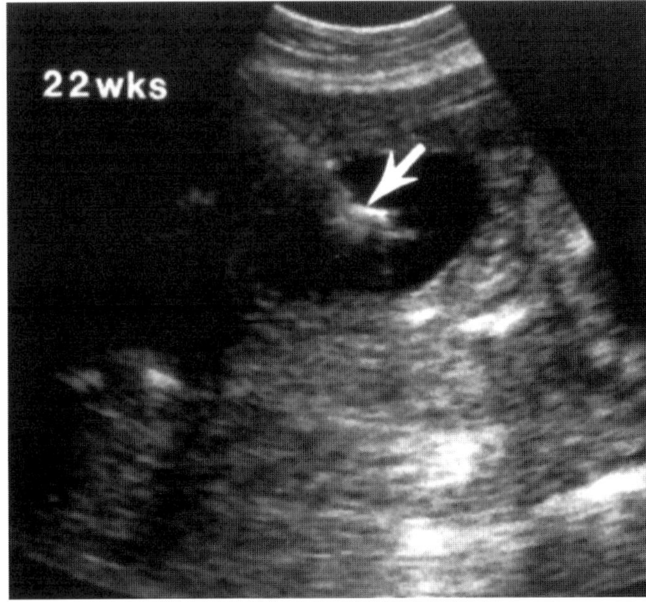

(B)

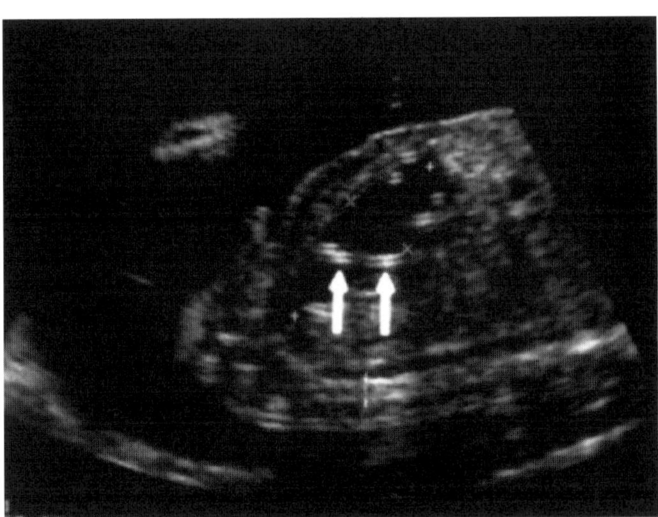

(C)

FIGURE 29 A–C ■ Fetus with posterior urethral valves. (**A**) 21 weeks' gestation, with a massively distended bladder. No amniotic fluid is visible. (**B**) Insertion of a bladder amniotic shunt (*arrow*) at 22 weeks' gestation. (**C**) A bladder amniotic shunt (*arrows*) at 25.4 weeks' gestation. The amniotic fluid volume is normal. B, bladder; CH, chest; VTX, vertex.

cyst or fluid collection that is to be shunted. With a quick thrust, the trocar is inserted into the fluid-filled space. A double-pigtailed catheter is inserted through the trocar and is advanced into the cyst cavity by a plunger of a predetermined length; a second, longer plunger (Fig. 30) is used to position the remaining part of the catheter in the amniotic cavity.

GYNECOLOGY

Oocyte Retrieval

Laparoscopy or laparotomy was initially required for oocyte retrieval (170). Advantages of ultrasound-guided transvaginal oocyte retrieval include avoidance of general anesthesia, lower risk of operative complications, and ability to perform the retrieval in an outpatient setting.

Interactive three-dimensional imaging has recently been employed for follicle retrieval (171). Although this technique permits accurate visualization of the needle tip in three dimensions, it has not yet been shown to significantly improve the success rate of oocyte retrieval.

Technique

The ovary is imaged with transvaginal sonography, and the selected follicle is aligned along the biopsy line of the display screen. A 30-cm, 17- or 18-gauge needle is then quickly advanced through the vaginal wall into the follicle. The follicular contents are then aspirated (Fig. 31). If an oocyte is not obtained, the follicle is flushed with culture media to dislodge the oocyte from the follicle wall. In order to demonstrate competency in transvaginal ultrasound-guided oocyte retrieval (TVUOR), $\geq$ 70% of eggs should be collected per follicle aspiration (172). A failure to collect at least one oocyte from both ovaries has been

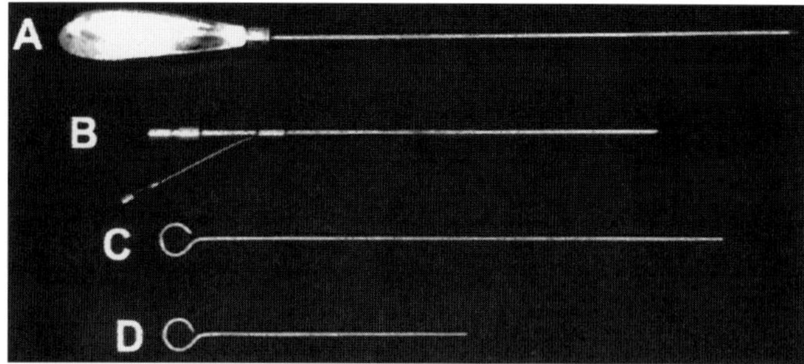

FIGURE 30 A–D ■ Rodeck insertion set for fetal shunting procedures. (**A**) Trocar, which is inserted with a metal guide. (**B**) Metal guide, which is inserted into the fetal cavity with a side port for sampling. (**C**) The longer plunger is used to insert the catheter into the amniotic cavity. (**D**) The shorter plunger is used to advance the catheter into the fetal cystic place.

reported to occur in 0.92% of cycles when human chorionic gonadotropin is given (173).

Complications

Some of the reported complications are outlined in Table 9. The most common complication of TVUOR is hemorrhage and/or hematoma formation. Dessole et al. (174) estimated that the average blood loss associated with this procedure over 24 hours is 230 mL. Minor vaginal hemorrhage occurs in 1.4% to 18.4% of all patients undergoing TVUOR (175). Significant intra-abdominal bleeding rarely occurs (176). Broad ligament hematomas have also been reported (177).

The use of smaller bore needles (18-gauge) and an automatic puncture device may reduce the frequency and severity of hemorrhagic complications. In addition, the aspiration of all of the follicles without removing the needle from the ovary reduces the likelihood of bleeding.

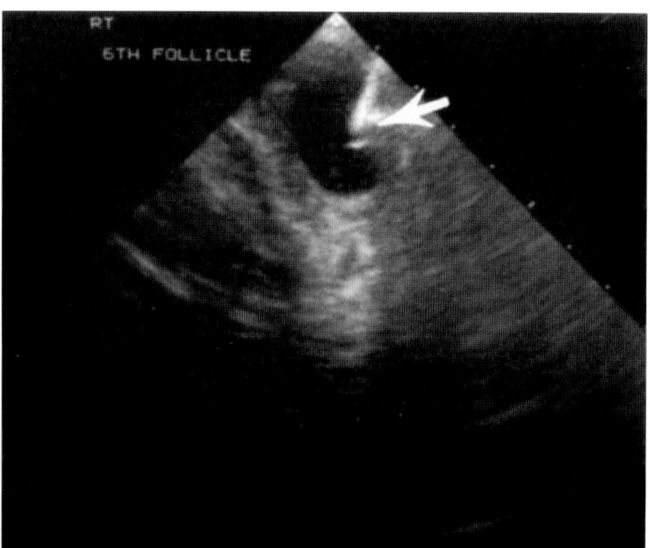

FIGURE 31 ■ Transvaginal oocyte retrieval. The needle (*arrow*) is within the follicle before aspiration.

TABLE 9 ■ Complications of Transvaginal Ultrasound-Guided Oocyte Retrieval

- Hemorrhage
- Trauma
- Infection
- Injury
  - Bowel
  - Ureter
  - Nerves
  - Blood vessels
- Adnexal torsion
- Rupture of ovarian cysts
- Vertebral osteomyelitis

Pelvic infection occurs in 0.6% of oocyte retrievals (176). The risk of infection is increased in patients with a history of prior pelvic inflammatory disease. Some authors advocate routine prophylactic antibiotics (Dicker et al.) (178), while others (Curtis et al.) (179) advocate selective antibiotic for patients at increased risk. In a U.K. survey, just over half of in vitro fertilization units used prophylactic antibiotics during egg retrieval (180).

Uterine Transfer

Intrauterine embryo transfer can be performed under transvaginal sonographic guidance. This technique not only ensures that the tip of the catheter is appropriately positioned but also assists the operator when submucous myomas or uterine anomalies make embryo transfer difficult (Fig. 32) (181). Ultrasound-guided transfer not only significantly increases the embryo implantation rate but also significantly increases the chance of clinical pregnancy (182). Three-dimensional ultrasound has recently been used to locate the optimal transfer area in the uterine cavity (183). A randomized controlled study has not yet been performed to determine if this technique offers any advantage over two-dimensional ultrasound-guided placement. Three-dimensional ultrasound has also been

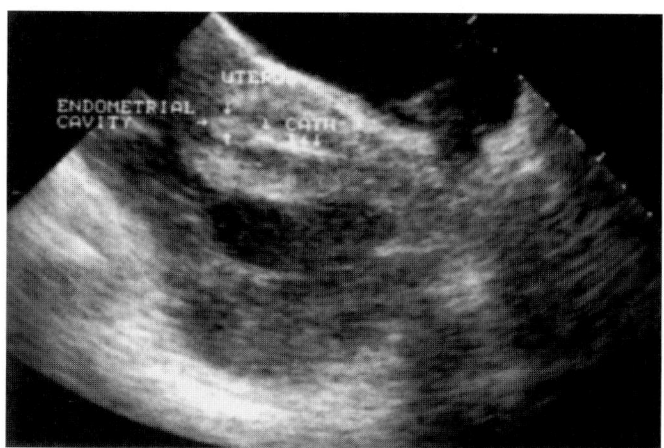

FIGURE 32 ■ Embryo transfer 1.

utilized to determine the location of embryo implantation after transfer. Baba et al. (184) have shown that 48 of 60 (80%) embryos implant in areas to which they are initially transferred; the remaining 20% implant elsewhere in the uterus.

Fallopian Tube Catheterization

Transvaginal fallopian tube catheterization is used for proximal bilateral fallopian tube occlusion. Histologic examination of hysterectomy and salpingectomy specimens has not demonstrated any untoward effects from fallopian tube cannulation (Fig. 33) (185,186).

In preliminary studies, the measurement of tubal perfusion pressures at the time of selective salpingography further improved the evaluation of tubal factors in infertility—patent fallopian tubes with normal compliance result in significantly higher pregnancy rates than patent noncompliant fallopian tubes (188).

Sonohysterography

Tubal occlusion is a frequent cause of infertility. Consequently, hysterosalpingography has been an integral part of any infertility evaluation. Transvaginal sonography has been combined with endometrial fluid instillation to assess tubal patency. When saline solution is used as a contrast agent, usually, only the proximal 2 to 3 cm of the fallopian tubes is visualized. Air has also been successfully employed as a contrast agent. In one study, air sonohysterography and laparoscopy were in agreement with respect to tubal patency 79.4% of the time. With air sonohysterography, shoulder pain is considered a sign of tubal patency; the pain usually subsides within a few hours (189).

Because of flash artifacts, color and power Doppler have not always been shown to be efficacious in detecting tubal patency with either air or saline sonohysterography (Fig. 34A and B).

The availability of sonographic contrast media permits visualization of the entire fallopian tube (190). Duplex and color Doppler imaging have also been used to confirm flow of a contrast agent through the fallopian tube (Fig. 35A and B) (191,192). In some institutions, sonohysterography has replaced hysterosalpingography in the assessment of female infertility (192).

Two-dimensional scanning of the pelvis is limited to the sagittal and the axial planes. With three-dimensional scanning, the coronal plane can be imaged. Although this technique is very effective in the detection of uterine anomalies, it does not offer any advantage over two-dimensional sonohysterography in the assessment of tubal patency (194).

Ovarian Cyst Aspiration

de Crespigny et al. (195) successfully aspirated 100 cysts in 88 women under transvaginal sonographic guidance. In 51 patients, the cyst aspiration was performed because of persistent pain. Of the 16 women with a clear cyst, 15 (94%) reported improvement in their pain; only 7/12 (58%) with blood-stained cyst fluid reported a reduction in pain (195). Over the past several years, the diagnostic accuracy of ultrasound in the differentiation of specific types of ovarian masses has significantly improved. Tailor et al. (196) reported a sensitivity and specificity of 93.3% and 90.4%, respectively, for the prediction of malignancy. As a result, cyst aspiration is no longer considered a diagnostic procedure. Therapeutic cyst aspiration is reserved for a few selective indications.

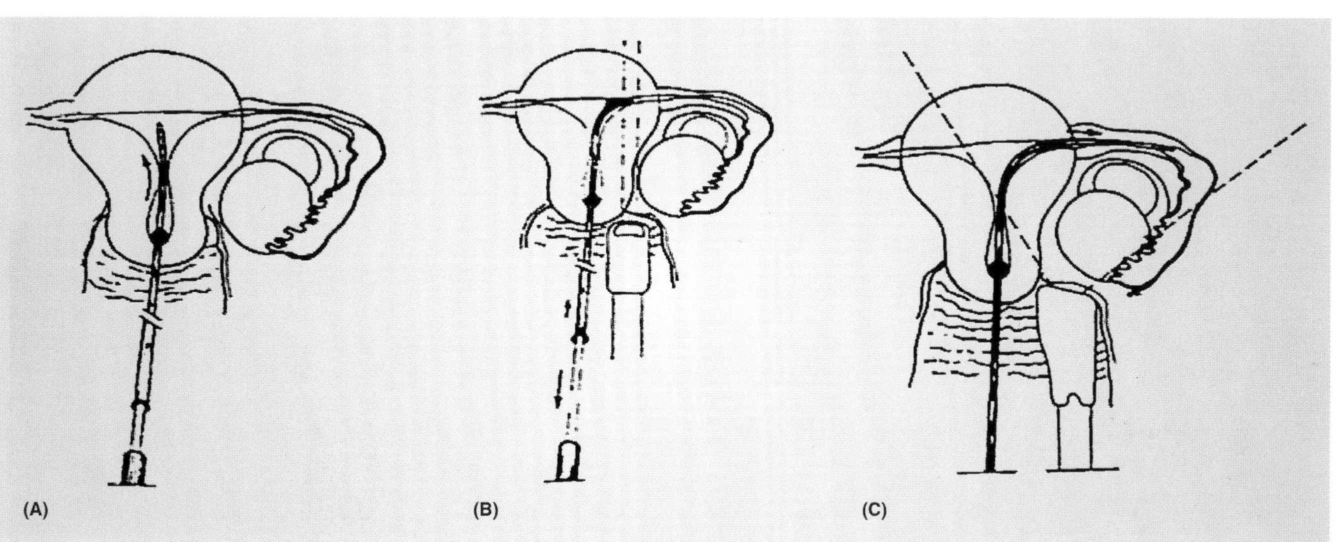

FIGURE 33 A–C ■ System for catheterization of the fallopian tubes under ultrasound guidance. (**A**) A metal obturator is used to guide the cannula through the curve of the cervix into the uterus. (**B**) As the obturator is withdrawn (*large arrow*), the cannula regains its lateral curve and is advanced to the uterotubal junction. (**C**) The catheter is then passed down the cannula and through the isthmus of the fallopian tube (*arrow*). *Source*: From Ref. 187.

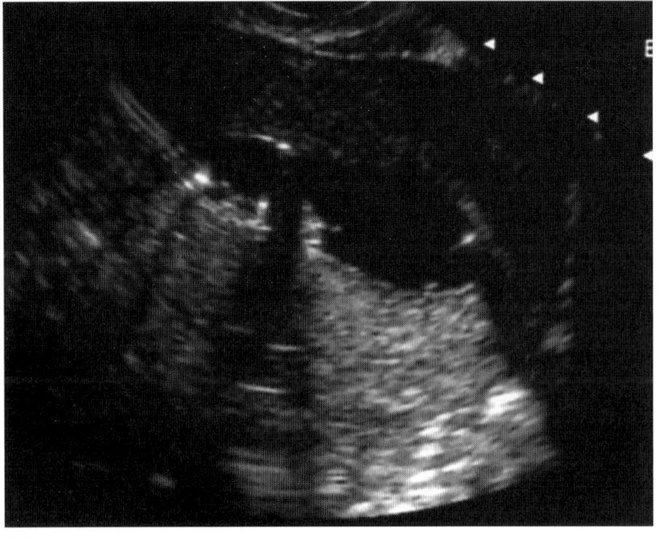

(A)

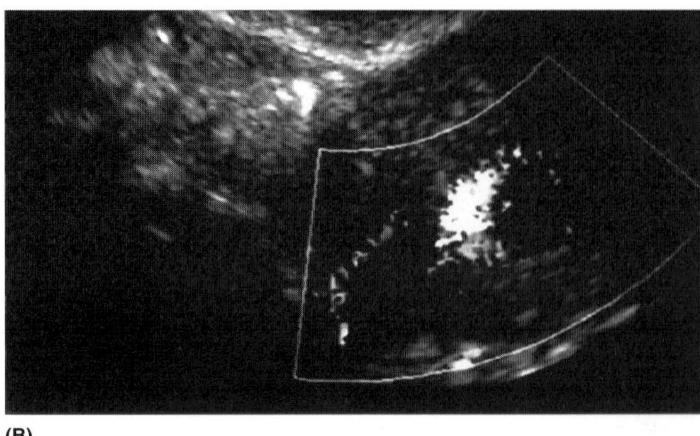

(B)

FIGURE 34 A AND B ■ (A) A balloon-tipped catheter is in the lower uterine segment. The fundus is filled with fluid. (B) A transverse view of the cornua confirms patency of the right fallopian tube with color Doppler.

Technique

The location of the ovarian cyst determines whether transabdominal or transvaginal sonography is indicated to direct the procedure. With either modality, a needle of appropriate length is directed through a needle guide or, in the case of the transabdominal approach, freehand into the cyst. A short piece of extension tubing (0.5-mL dead space) is attached to the needle hub and the fluid is aspirated by an assistant, while the sonologist visualizes the tip of the needle and its location within the cyst.

Complications

The primary concern with needle aspiration of an ovarian cyst is the possible spillage of tumor cells into the peritoneal cavity from an undiagnosed malignant tumor. The combination of transvaginal sonography for morphology assessment and color Doppler waveform analysis has improved the diagnostic abilities of sonography in the detection of malignant ovarian disease (197,198). The likelihood that a clear cyst with a normal Doppler pattern is benign ranges between 90% and 95% (198–200). Hence, even using strict clinical and sonographic guidelines, aspiration of a malignant ovarian tumor is still possible.

An important drawback of cyst aspiration is the recurrence risk between 11% and 67% (201). Dordoni et al. (202) found a trend toward an increase in cyst recurrence with postmenopausal status, incomplete cyst aspiration, and increasing cyst size.

Ovarian cyst cytology has a low sensitivity and negative predictive value for the detection of malignancy (203,204).

Complications associated with ultrasonically guided puncture of gynecologic masses include bleeding, hematoma formation, and infection. Disinfection of the vagina seems to protect against pelvic infections adequately. Hence, antibiotic prophylaxis is not generally used with transvaginal cyst aspiration (205).

Until the controversy over ovarian cyst aspiration as a diagnostic or therapeutic modality is resolved (201,202), restricting cyst aspiration to specific circumstances is appropriate. First and foremost, the cyst should be unilocular. In premenopausal women, ovarian cysts should initially be followed for at least three months before considering aspiration. Over this time interval, 60% of cysts smaller than 8.0 cm in diameter will resolve; even in postmenopausal women, 28.5% of simple cysts will resolve spontaneously (206). A follow-up ultrasound examination in two to three months with color Doppler imaging should be performed. A determination can then be made either to excise or to observe a cyst, depending on its size, the presence or absence of symptoms, the patient's age, her possible risk factors for ovarian carcinoma, and her general medical condition. Cyst aspiration is most applicable to the postmenopausal patient who is a high surgical risk. Finally, postmenopausal patients must be counseled that current sonographic techniques can reduce, but not completely exclude, the possibility of a malignant ovarian tumor.

Drainage of Pelvic Abscesses

Continuous sonographic monitoring permits the precise positioning of a 16- or 18-gauge Chiba needle into a pelvic abscess through the posterior fornix. The needle tip can then be repositioned without repiercing the vaginal vault to aspirate loculated abscess cavities. Occasionally, apparently loculated abscess cavities communicate with each other. Hence, when one loculation is drained, the others collapse as well. The abscess must be within easy reach of the endovaginal probe. Because of patient discomfort, conscious sedation as well as local anesthetic infiltration of the vaginal vault is performed. The vagina is routinely cleansed with povidone–iodine before the procedure. If an abscess is multiloculated or the contents viscous, a catheter is placed into the abscess for irrigation and continuous drainage. In an attempt to avoid dislodgement, a balloon-tipped or pigtail catheter is used (207). Needle drainage is frequently possible with unilocular collections of low viscosity. Transrectal ultrasonographically guided drainage of a pelvic abscess can also be performed (208). When the two approaches are compared, patients seem to tolerate the transrectal approach better (209).

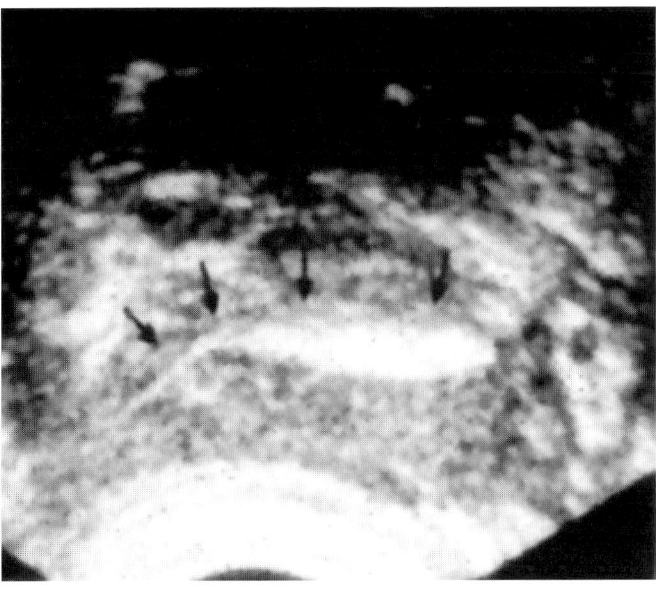

(A)

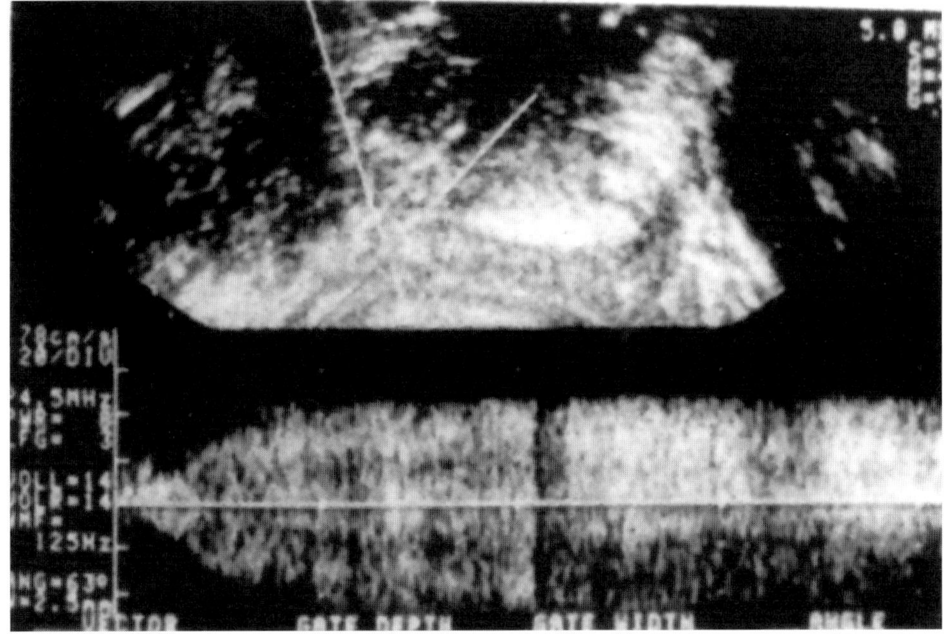

(B)

FIGURE 35 A AND B ■ Demonstration of tubal patency (right tube) by contrast sonography. (**A**) Cross-section of the fundus of the uterus: the cavity, intramural part, and proximal part of the isthmus of the tube are perfused by the contrast agent (*arrows*). (**B**) Confirmation of tubal patency by Doppler signal. The Doppler is positioned over the fallopian tube; with injection. Doppler signals are observed. *Source*: From Ref. 193.

Technique

Feld et al. (210) found transvaginal sonographically guided aspiration of pelvic abscesses to be either curative or temporizing in 78% of cases. Gentle irrigation of an abscess cavity with sterile saline significantly increases the success rate of single-step aspiration drainage. In one study, 51 of 62 (92.3%) abscesses were treated successfully with aspiration and lavage versus 6 of 16 (37.5%) cases treated without irrigation (211). Nelson et al. (212) reported an 83.9% success rate with transvaginal aspiration and saline irrigation of pelvic abscesses. If reaccumulation occurs, a catheter may be placed in the abscess cavity after repeat drainage (210). Overdistension of an abscess cavity with irrigation fluid or vigorous lavage has been associated with an increased risk of bacteremia or sepsis (213).

The patient's discomfort dictates the administration of intravenous sedation immediately before abscess aspiration. Nelson et al. (212) reported that 10% of their patients stopped the procedure before aspiration was completed because of pain. Approximately 10% of patients who initially respond to abscess drainage show signs of unresolved infection within 48 hours and require additional therapy.

Intraoperative Ultrasound Guidance

The intraoperative use of ultrasound has been reported for (*i*) intracavitary cesium implantation (214), (*ii*) difficult postmenopausal dilatation and curettage (215), (*iii*) direction of second trimester abortions (216), and (*iv*) removal of retained products of conception (217). Ultrasound has also been used to direct operative hysteroscopy (218). With this technique, the hysteroscope is directed sonographically to the area of uterine disease. During the hysteroscopic resection of an intracavitary leiomyoma, the depth

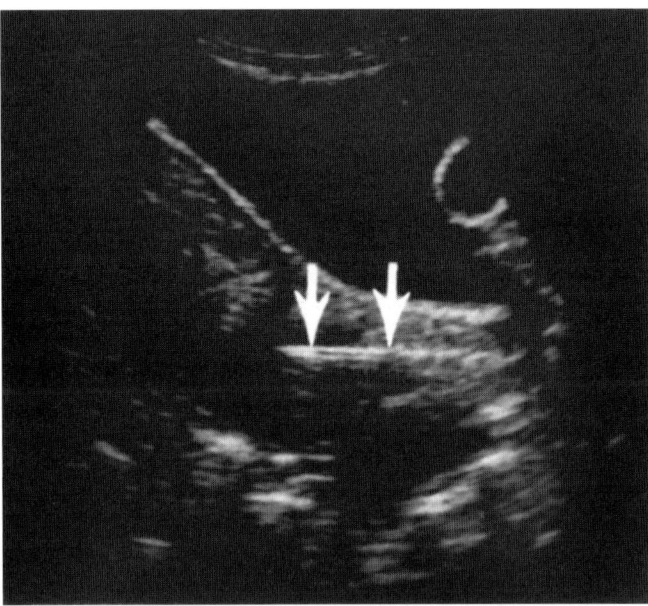

FIGURE 36 ■ Sagittal view of the uterus on transabdominal sonography. A uterine sound (*arrows*) is noted at the level of the lower uterine segment.

of resection can be assessed sonographically. Although all these reports have described the use of transabdominal sonography (Fig. 36), I have found transvaginal sonography particularly helpful for appropriately directing a uterine sound in obese patients or in patients with large leiomyomas that obstruct transabdominal visualization.

This chapter has illustrated the increasing importance of sonographic guidance to obstetrics and gynecology. The rapid development of high-resolution ultrasound equipment permits the recognition of fetal malformations in all three trimesters of pregnancy. Fetal evaluation by means of CVS, amniocentesis, or PUBS is, therefore, an extension of a complete fetal workup. Although fetal therapy is not a new concept, it has only recently been extended beyond transfusion for Rh isoimmunization. Other types of fetal therapy primarily involve techniques to overcome obstruction to fetal fluid dynamics (e.g., posterior urethral valves). A current area of intensive research involves replacing abnormal or missing cell lines by means of in utero stem cell therapy. For these therapeutic techniques to be successful, sonographically guided direct access to the fetal circulation in the early part of the second trimester is required.

In gynecology, transvaginal sonographic guidance was originally used for follicular aspiration and oocyte retrieval. It soon became apparent that this technique could also be used in the treatment of adnexal cysts and pelvic abscesses and in the intraoperative direction of specific uterine procedures. As clinicians become more comfortable with transvaginal sonography and needle aspiration, ultrasound will play a greater role in the treatment of specific gynecologic conditions.

REFERENCES

1. Liley AW. Intrauterine transfusion of the foetus in haemolytic disease. Br Med J 1963; 2(5365):1107–1109.
2. Benn PA, Fang M, Egan JFX, et al. Incorporation of inhibin-A in second-trimester screening for Down syndrome. Obstet Gynecol 2003; 101(3):451–454.
3. Wapner R, Thom E, Simpson JL, et al. First-trimester screening for trisomies 21 and 18. N Engl J Med 2003; 349(15): 1405–1413.
4. Nyberg DA, Luthy DA, Resta RG, et al. Age-adjusted ultrasound risk assessment for fetal Down syndrome during the second trimester: description of the method and analysis of 142 cases. Ultrasound Obstet Gynecol 1998; 12(1):8–14.
5. DeVore GR. Trisomy 21:91% detection rate using second-trimester ultrasound markers. Ultrasound Obstet Gynecol 2000; 16(2): 133–141.
6. Benn PA, Egan JFX, Fang M, et al. Changes in utilization of prenatal diagnosis. Obstet Gynecol 2004; 103(6):1255–1260.
7. Lilford RJ. Chorion villus biopsy. Clin Obstet Gynaecol 1986; 13:611–632.
8. Kazy Z, Rozovsky IS, Bakharev VA. Chorion biopsy in early pregnancy: a method of early prenatal diagnosis for inherited disorders. Prenat Diagn 1982; 2(1):39–45.
9. Brambati B, Lanzani A, Oldrini A. Transabdominal chorionic villus sampling: clinical experience of 1159 cases. Prenat Diagn 1988; 8(8):609–617.
10. Smidt-Jensen S, Hahnemann N. Transabdominal villus sampling for fetal genetic diagnosis. Technical and obstetrical evaluation of 100 cases. Prenat Diagn 1988; 8(1):7–17.
11. Saura R, Longy M, Horovitz J, et al. Risks of transabdominal chorionic villus sampling before the 12th week of amenorrhea. Prenat Diagn 1990; 10(7):461–467.
12. Hill LM, Laifer SA. Transabdominal chorionic villus sampling: a modified freehand ultrasonographically guided technique. Am J Obstet Gynecol 1992; 166(2):512.
13. Jackson LG, Zachary JM, Fowler SE, et al. A randomized comparison of transcervical and transabdominal chorionic-villus sampling. New Engl J Med 1992; 327(9):594–598.
14. Green JE, Dorfman A, Jones SL, et al. Chorionic villus sampling: experience with an initial 940 cases. Obstet Gynecol 1988; 71(2): 208–212.
15. Hogge WA, Schonberg SA, Golbus MS. Chorionic villus sampling: experience of the first 1000 cases. Am J Obstet Gynecol 1986; 154(6):1249–1252.
16. Papp C, Papp Z. Chorionic villus sampling and amniocentesis: what are the risks in current practice? Curr Opin Obstet Gynecol 2003; 15(2):159–165.
17. Cohen-Overbeek TE, Hop WCJ, Den Duden M, et al. Spontaneous abortion rate and advanced maternal age: consequences for prenatal diagnosis. Lancet 1990; 336(88706):27–29.
18. Williams J III, Wang BBT, Rubin CH, et al. Chorionic villus sampling: experience with 3016 cases performed by a single operator. Obstet Gynecol 1992; 80(6):1023–1029.
19. Maxwell DJ, Lilford RJ. An interesting ultrasonic observation following chorionic villus sampling. J Clin Ultrasound 1985; 13(5): 343–344.
20. Jackson LG, Wapner RJ. Risks of chorion villus sampling. Bailliére's Clin Obstet Gynaecol 1987; 1(3):513–531.
21. Wass DM, Brown GA, Warren PS, et al. Completed follow-up of 1000 consecutive transcervical chorionic villus sampling performed by a single operator. Aust NZ J Obstet Gynaecol 1991; 31(3): 240–245.
22. Brambati B, Oldrini A, Ferrazzi E, et al. Chorionic villus sampling: an analysis of the obstetric experience of 1000 cases. Prenat Diagn 1987; 7(3):157–169.
23. Silver RK, MacGregor SN, Sholl JS, et al. An evaluation of the chorionic villus sampling learning curve. Am J Obstet Gynecol 1990; 163(3):917–922.
24. Brambati B, Tului L, Cislaghi C et al. First 10,000 chorionic villus samplings performed on singleton pregnancies by a single operator. Pernat Diagn 1998; 18(3):255–266.
25. Evans MI, Johnson MP, Holzgreve W. Chorionic villus sampling. J Reprod Med 1992; 37(15):389–394.
26. Barela AI, Kleinman GE, Golditch IM, et al. Septic shock with renal failure after chorionic villus sampling. Am J Obstet Gynecol 1986; 154(5):1100–1102.

27. Firth HV, Boyd PA, Chamberlain I, et al. Severe limb abnormalities after chorionic villus sampling at 56–66 days gestation. Lancet 1991; 337(8744):762–763.
28. Kuliev AM, Modell B, Jackson L, et al. Risk evaluation of CVS. Prenat Diagn 1993; 13(3):197–209.
29. Report of National Institute of Child Health and Human Development Workshop on Chorionic Villus Sampling and Limb and Other Defects, 1992. Am J Obstet Gynecol 1993; 169:1–6.
30. Rodeck CH. Prenatal diagnosis: fetal development after chorionic villus sampling. Lancet 1993; 341(8843):468–469.
31. Wilson RD. Amniocentesis and chorionic villus sampling. Curr Opin Obstet Gynecol 2000; 12(2):81–86.
32. Holzgreve W, Miny P, Gerlach B, et al. Benefits of placental biopsies for rapid karyotyping in the second and third trimesters (late chorionic villus sampling) in high-risk pregnancies. Am J Obstet Gynecol 1990; 162(5):1188–1192.
33. Cameron AD, Mathers AM, Wisom S, et al. Second-trimester placental biopsy for rapid fetal karyotyping. Am J Obstet Gynecol 1990; 163(3):931–934.
34. Holzgreve W, Miny P, Schloo R, and participants of the "Late CVS" International Registry. Compilation of data from 24 centres. Prenat Diagn 1990; 10(3):159–167.
35. Scrimgeour JB. Amniocentesis: technique and complications. In: Emery AEH, ed. Antenatal Diagnosis of Genetic Disease. Baltimore: Williams & Wilkins, 1973:11.
36. Bevis DCA. Composition of liquor amnii in haemolytic disease of newborns. Lancet 1950; 2:443.
37. Jacobson CB, Barter RH. Intrauterine diagnosis and management of genetic defects. Am J Obstet Gynecol 1967; 99(6):796–807.
38. Jeanty P, Rodesch F, Romero R, et al. How to improve your amniocentesis technique. Am J Obstet Gynecol 1983; 146(6): 593–596.
39. Romero R, Jeanty P, Reece EA, et al. Sonographically monitored amniocentesis to decrease intraoperative complications. Obstet Gynecol 1985; 65(3):426–430.
40. Hill LM, Breckle R. Real-time ultrasound guidance of fetal manipulation during genetic amniocentesis. J Ultrasound Med 1985; 4(6):267–268.
41. The NICHD National Registry for Amniocentesis Study Group. Midtrimester amniocentesis for prenatal diagnosis: safety and accuracy. JAMA 1976; 236:1471–1476.
42. Simpson NE, Dallaire L, Miller JR, et al. Prenatal diagnosis of genetic disease in Canada: report of a collaborative study. Can Med Assoc J 1976; 115(8):739–748.
43. Crane JP, Kopta MM. Genetic amniocentesis: impact of placental position upon the risk of pregnancy loss. Am J Obstet Gynecol 1984; 150(7):813–816.
44. Perkes EA, Baim RS, Clair MR, et al. Intrauterine bleeding following transplacental amniocentesis. J Ultrasound Med 1983; 2(2):55–57.
45. Lenke RR, Ashwood ER, Cyr DR, et al. Genetic amniocentesis: significance of intra-amniotic bleeding and placental location. Obstet Gynecol 1985; 65(6):798–801.
46. Chinn DH, Towers CV, Beeman RG, et al. Sonographically demonstrated intra-amniotic hemorrhage following transplacental genetic amniocentesis: frequency. J Ultrasound Med 1990; 9(9): 495–501.
47. Gold RB, Goyert GL, Schwartz DB, et al. Conservative management of second-trimester and post-amniocentesis fluid leakage. Obstet Gynecol 1989; 74(5):745–747.
48. Kappel B, Nielsen J, Hansen KB, et al. Spontaneous abortion following mid-trimester amniocentesis: clinical significance of placental perforation and bloodstained amniotic fluid. Br J Obstet Gynaecol 1987; 94(1):50–54.
49. Porreco RP, Young PE, Resnik R, et al. Reproductive outcome following amniocentesis for genetic indications. Am J Obstet Gynecol 1982; 143(6):653–660.
50. Hanson FW, Tennant FR, Zorn EM, et al. Analysis of 2136 genetic amniocenteses: experience of a single physician. Am J Obstet Gynecol 1985; 152(4):436–443.
51. Giorlandino C, Mobili L, Bilacioni E, et al. Transplacental amniocentesis: is it really a higher-risk procedure? Prenat Diagn 1994; 14(9):803–806.
52. Thomsen SG, Isager-Sally L, Lange AP, et al. Elevated maternal serum alpha-fetoprotein caused by midtrimester amniocentesis: a prognostic factor. Obstet Gynecol 1983; 62(3):297–300.
53. Bombard AT, Powers JF, Carter S, et al. Procedure-related fetal losses in transplacental versus nontransplacental genetic amniocentesis. Am J Obstet Gynecol 1995; 172(3):868–872.
54. Tabor A, Philip J, Madsen M et al. Randomized controlled trial of genetic amniocentesis in 4606 low-risk women. Lancet 1986; 1(8493):1287–1293.
55. Harlap S, Shiono PH, Ramcharan S. A life table of spontaneous abortions and effects of age, parity, and other variables. In: Porter IH, Hook EB, eds. Human Embryonic and Fetal Death. New York: Academic Press, 1980:145.
56. Milunsky A, Jick SS, Bruell CL, et al. Predictive values, relative risks and overall benefits of high and low maternal serum alpha-fetoprotein screening in singleton pregnancies: new epidemiologic data. Am J Obstet Gynecol 1989; 161(2):291–297.
57. Leschot NJ, Verjaal M, Treffers PE. Risk of midtrimester amniocentesis: assessment in 3000 pregnancies. Br J Obstet Gynaecol 1985; 92(8):804–807.
58. McArdle CR, Cohen W, Nickerson C, et al. The use of ultrasound in evaluating problems and complications of genetic amniocentesis. J Clin Ultrasound 1983; 11(8):427–429.
59. Admoni M, Ben Ezra D. Ocular trauma following amniocentesis as the cause of leukocoria. J Pediatr Ophthalmol Strabismus 1988; 25:196–197.
60. Lamb MP. Gangrene of a fetal limb due to amniocentesis. Br J Obstet Gynaecol 1975; 82(10):829–830.
61. Rickwood AM. A case of ileal atresia and ileocutaneous fistula caused by amniocentesis. J Pediatr 1977; 91(2):312.
62. Eller KM, Kuller J. Porencephaly secondary to fetal trauma during amniocentesis. Obstet Gynecol 1995; 85(5 Pt 2):865–867.
63. Therkelsen AJ, Rehder H. Intestinal atresia caused by second trimester amniocentesis: case report. Br J Obstet Gynaecol 1981; 88(5):559–562.
64. Epley SL, Hanson JW, Cruikshank DP. Fetal injury with midtrimester diagnostic amniocentesis. Obstet Gynecol 1979; 53(1): 77–80.
65. Evans MI, Johnson MP, Holzgreve W. Early amniocentesis: what exactly does it mean? J Reprod Med 1994; 39(2):77–78.
66. Johnson A, Godmilow L. Genetic amniocentesis at 14 weeks or less. Clin Obstet Gynecol 1988; 31(2):345–352.
67. Elejalde BR et al. Prospective study of amniocentesis performed between weeks 9 and 16 of gestation: its feasibility, risks, complications and use in early genetic prenatal diagnosis. Am J Med Genet 1990; 35:188.
68. Hanson FW, Happ RL, Tennant FR, et al. Ultrasonography-guided early amniocentesis in singleton pregnancies. Am J Obstet Gynecol 1990; 162(6):1376–1381.
69. Penso CA, Frigoletto FD. Early amniocentesis. Semin Perinatol 1990; 14(6):465–470.
70. Sundberg K, Bang J, Brocks V, et al. Early sonographically guided amniocenteses with filtration technique: follow-up on 249 procedures. J Ultrasound Med 1995; 14(8):585–590.
71. Hanson FW, Tennant F, Hune S, et al. Early amniocentesis: outcome, risk and technical problems at 12.8 weeks. Am J Obstet Gynecol 1992; 166(6 Pt 1):1707–1711.
72. Nicolaides K, Brizot Mde L, Patel F, et al. Comparison of chorionic villus sampling and amniocentesis for fetal karyotyping at 10–13 weeks' gestation. Lancet 1994; 344(8920):435–439.
73. The Canadian Early and Mid-Trimester Amniocentesis Trial (CEMAT) Group. Randomized trial to assess safety and fetal outcome of early and midtrimester amniocentesis. Lancet 1998; 351: 242–247.
74. Johnson JM, Wilson RD, Singer J et al. Technical factors in early amniocentesis predict adverse outcome. Results of the Canadian Early (EA) and mid-trimester amniocentesis (MA) trial (CEMAT). Prenat Diagn 1999; 19(8):782–788.
75. Philip J, Silver RK, Wilson RD, et al. First-trimester invasive prenatal diagnosis: results of an international randomized trial. Obstet Gynecol 2004; 103(6):1164–1173.
76. Elias S, Gerbie AB, Simpson JL, et al. Genetic amniocentesis in twins. Am J Obstet Gynecol 1980; 138(2):169–174.

77. Tabsh KM, Crandall B, Lebherz TB, et al. Genetic amniocentesis in twin pregnancy. Obstet Gynecol 1985; 65(6):843–845.
78. Jeanty P, Shah D, Roussis P. Single-needle insertion in twin amniocentesis. J Ultrasound Med 1990; 9(9):511–517.
79. Gilbert WM, Davis SE, Kaplan C, et al. Morbidity associated with prenatal disruption of the dividing membrane in twin gestations. Obstet Gynecol 1991; 78(4):623–630.
80. Bahado-Singh R, Schmitt R, Hobbins JC. New technique for genetic amniocentesis in twins. Obstet Gynecol 1992; 79(2):304–307.
81. Palle C, Andersen JW, Tabor A, et al. Increased risk of abortion after genetic amniocentesis in twin pregnancy. Prenat Diagn 1983; 3(2):83–89.
82. Ghidini A, Lynch L, Hicks C, et al. The risk of second-trimester amniocentesis in twin gestations: a case-control study. Am J Obstet Gynecol 1993; 169(4):1013–1016.
83. Pijpers L, Jahoda MG, Vostas RP, et al. Genetic amniocentesis in twin pregnancies. Br J Obstet Gynaecol 1988; 95(4):323–326.
84. Petrikovsky BM, Vintzileos AM. Management and outcome of multiple pregnancies of higher fetal order: literature review. Obstet Gynecol Surv 1989; 44(8):578–584.
85. Newman RB, Hamer C, Miller MC. Outpatient triplet management: a contemporary review. Am J Obstet Gynecol 1989; 161(3):547–553.
86. Collins MS, Bleyl JA. Seventy-one quadruplet pregnancies: management and outcome. Am J Obstet Gynecol 1990; 162(6):1384–1391.
87. Dodd J, Crowther C. Multifetal pregnancy reduction of triplet and higher order multiple pregnancies to twins. Fertil Steril 2004; 81(5):1420–1422.
88. Evans MI, Berkowitz RL, Wapner RJ, et al. Improvement in outcomes of multifetal pregnancy reduction with increased experience. Am J Obstet Gynecol 2001; 184(2):97–103.
89. Evans MI, Kaufman MI, Urban AJ, et al. Fetal reduction from twins to a singleton: a reasonable consideration? Obstet Gynecol 2004; 104(1):102–109.
90. Evans MI, Krivchenia EL, Gelber SE, et al. Selective reduction. Clin Perinatol 2003; 30(1):103–111.
91. Timor-Tritsch IE, Rottem S. Transvaginal Sonography. 2nd ed, Chapman-Hall Publishers/New York, 1990.
92. Timor-Tritsch IE, Peisner DB, Monteagudo A, et al. Multifetal pregnancy reduction by transvaginal puncture: evaluation of the technique in 134 cases. Am J Obstet Gynecol 1993; 168(3 Pt 1):799–804.
93. Popp LW, Ghirardini G. The role of transvaginal sonography in chorionic villi sampling. J Clin Ultrasound 1990; 18:315.
94. Berkowitz RL, Lynch L, Lapinski R, et al. First trimester transabdominal multifetal pregnancy reduction: a report of two hundred completed cases. Am J Obstet Gynecol 1993; 169(1):17–21.
95. Wapner RJ, Davis GH, Johnson A, et al. Selective reduction of multifetal pregnancies. Lancet 1990; 335(8681):90–93.
96. Drugan A, Johnson MP, Isada NB, et al. The smaller than expected first trimester fetus is at increased risk for chromosome abnormalities. Am J Obstet Gynecol 1992; 167(6):1525–1528.
97. Tchobroutsky C, Breart GL, Rambaud DC, et al. Correlation between fetal defects and early growth delay observed by ultrasound (Letter) Lancet 1985; 1(8430):706–707.
98. Timor-Tritsch IE, Bashiri A, Monteagudo A, et al. Two hundred ninety consecutive cases of multifetal pregnancy reduction: comparison of the transabdominal versus the transvaginal approach. Am J Obstet Gynecol 2004; 191(6):2085–2089.
99. Evans MI, Dommerques M, Wapner RJ, et al. Efficacy of transabdominal multifetal pregnancy reduction: collaborative experience among the world's largest centers. Obstet Gynecol 1993; 82(1):61–66.
100. The Practice Committee of the Society for Assisted Reproductive Technology and the American Society for Reproductive Medicine. Guidelines on the number of embryos transferred. Fertil Steril 2004; 82(3):773–774.
101. Tsao K et al. Selective reduction of acardiac twin by radiofrequency ablation. Am J Obstet Gyn 2002; 187(3):635–640.
102. Tan TYT, Sepulveda W. Acardiac twin: a systematic review of minimally invasive treatment modalities. Ultrasound Obstet Gynecol 2003; 22:409–419.
103. Valenti C. Antenatal detection of hemoglobinopathies: a preliminary report. Am J Obstet Gynecol 1973; 115(6):851–853.
104. Daffos F, Capella-Pavlovsky M, Forestier F. Fetal blood sampling via the umbilical cord using a needle guided by ultrasound: a report of 66 cases. Prenat Diagn 1983; 3(4):271–277.
105. Orlandi F, Damiani G, Jakil C, et al. The risks of early cordocentesis (12–21 weeks): analysis of 500 procedures. Prenat Diagn 1990; 10(7):425–428.
106. Weissman A, Jakobi P, Bronshtein M, et al. Sonographic measurements of the umbilical cord and vessels during normal pregnancies. J Ultrasound Med 1994; 13(1):11–14.
107. Boulot P, Deshamps F, Lefort G, et al. Pure fetal blood samples obtained by cordocentesis: technical aspects of 322 cases. Prenat Diagn 1990; 10(2).93–100.
108. Foley MR, Sonek J, O'Shaughnessy R. Cordocentesis: cracking the diagnostic and therapeutic barrier between fetus and physician. Obstet Gynecol Rep 1989; 1(2):152–166.
109. Sarkar R, Marimuthu KM. Association between the degree of mosaicism and the severity of syndrome in Turner mosaics and Klinefelter mosaics. Clin Genet 1983; 24(6):420–428.
110. Gosden C, Nicolaides KH, Rodeck CH. Fetal blood sampling in investigation of chromosome mosaicism in amniotic fluid culture. Lancet 1988; 1(8685):613–617.
111. Shalev E, Zalel Y, Weiner E, et al. The role of cordocentesis in assessment of mosaicism found in amniotic fluid cell culture. Acta Obstet Gynaecol Scand 1994; 73(2):119–122.
112. Segal M, Manning FA, Harman CR, et al. Bleeding after intravascular transfusion: experimental and clinical observations. Am J Obstet Gynecol 1991; 165(5 Pt 1):1414–1418.
113. Daffos F, Forestier F, Kaplan C, et al. Prenatal diagnosis and management of bleeding disorders with fetal blood sampling. Am J Obstet Gynecol 1988; 158(4):939–946.
114. Wenstrom KD, Weiner CP, Williamson RA. Antenatal treatment of fetal alloimmune thrombocytopenia. Obstet Gynecol 1992; 80(3 Pt 1):433–435.
115. Bussel J, Berkowitz RL, McFarland JG, et al. Antenatal treatment of neonatal alloimmune thrombocytopenia. N Engl J Med 1988; 319(21):1374–1378.
116. Bryndorf T, Christensen B, Philip J, et al. New rapid test for prenatal detection of trisomy 21 (Down's syndrome): preliminary report. Br Med J 1992; 304(6841):1536–1539.
117. Mari G, Deter RL, Carpenter RL, et al. Noninvasive diagnosis by Doppler ultrasonography of fetal anemia due to maternal red-cell alloimmunization. N Engl J Med 2000; 342(1):9–14.
118. Zimmerman R, Carpenter RJ Jr, Durig P et al. Longitudinal measurement of peak systolic velocity in the fetal middle cerebral artery for monitoring pregnancies complicated by red cell alloimmunization: a prospective multicentre trial with intention-to-treat. Br J Obstet Gynaecol 2002; 109(7): 746–752.
119. Delle Chiaie L, Buck G, Grab D, et al. Prediction of fetal anemia with Doppler measurement of the middle cerebral artery peak systolic velocity in pregnancies complicated by maternal blood group alloimmunization or parvovirus B19 infection. Ultrasound Obstet Gynecol 2001; 18(3):232–236.
120. Hogge WA, Buffone GJ, Hogge JS. Prenatal diagnosis of cytomegalovirus (CMV) infection: a preliminary report. Prenat Diagn 1993; 13(2):131–136.
121. Cazenave J, Forestier F, Bessieres MH, et al. Contribution of a new PCR assay to the prenatal diagnosis of congenital toxoplasmosis. Prenat Diagn 1992; 12(2):119–127.
122. Bennett PR, Le Van Kim C, Colin Y, et al. Prenatal determination of fetal RhD type by DNA amplification. N Engl J Med 1993; 329(9):607–610.
123. Forestier F, Daffos F, Solc Y, et al. Prenatal diagnosis of hemophilia by fetal blood sampling under ultrasound guidance. Haemostasis 1986; 16(5):346–351.
124. Old JM, Thein SL, Weatherall DJ, et al. Prenatal diagnosis of the major haemoglobin disorders. Mol Biol Med 1989; 6(1):55–63.
125. Nicolaides KH, Rodeck CH, Gosden CM. Rapid karyotyping in non-lethal fetal malformations. Lancet 1986; 1(8476):283–287.
126. Antsaklis AI, Papantoniou NE, Mesogitis SA, et al. Cardiocentesis: an alternative method of fetal blood sampling for the prenatal diagnosis of hemoglobinopathies. Obstet Gynecol 1992; 72(4):630–633.

127. Nicolini U, Nicolaides P, Fisk NM, et al. Fetal blood sampling from the intrahepatic vein: analysis of safety and clinical experience with 214 procedures. Obstet Gynecol 1990; 76(1):47–53.
128. Romero R, et al. Fetal blood sampling. In: Milunsky A, ed. Genetic Disorders and the Fetus: Diagnosis Prevention and Treatment. The Johns Hopkins University Press, 3rd edt., 1992.
129. Bovicelli L, Orsini LF, Grannum PAT, et al. A new funipuncture technique: two-needle ultrasound and needle biopsy-guided procedure. Obstet Gynecol 1989; 73(3 Pt 1):428–431.
130. Timor-Tritsch IE, Yeh M-N. In vitro training model for diagnostic and therapeutic fetal intravascular needle puncture. Am J Obstet Gynecol 1987; 157(4 Pt 1):858–859.
131. Copel JA, Grannum PA, Harrison D, et al. The use of intravenous pancuronium bromide to produce fetal paralysis during intravascular transfusion. Am J Obstet Gynecol 1988; 158(1):170–171.
132. Bernstein HH, Chitakara U, Plosker H, et al. Use of atracurium besylate to arrest fetal activity during intrauterine intravascular transfusions. Obstet Gynecol 1988; 72(5):813–816.
133. Daffos F, Capello-Pavlovsky M, Forestier F. Fetal blood sampling during pregnancy with use of a needle guided by ultrasound: a study of 606 consecutive cases. Am J Obstet Gynecol 1985; 153(6):655–660.
134. Donner C, Simon P, Karioun A, et al. Experience of a single team of operators in 891 diagnostic funipunctures. Obstet Gynecol 1994; 84(5):827–831.
135. Weiner CP, Wenstrom KD, Sipes SL, et al. Risk factors for cordocentesis and fetal intravascular transfusion. Am J Obstet Gynecol 1991; 165(4 Pt 1):1020–1025.
136. Jauniaux E, Donner C, Simon P, et al. Pathologic aspects of the umbilical cord after percutaneous umbilical cord blood sampling. Obstet Gynecol 1989; 72(2):215–218.
137. Ney JA, Fee SC, Dooley SL, et al. Factors influencing hemostasis after umbilical vein puncture in vitro. Am J Obstet Gynecol 1989; 160(2):424–426.
138. Daffos F, Capello-Pavlovsky M, Forestier F. A new procedure for fetal blood sampling in utero: preliminary results of fifty-three cases. Am J Obstet Gynecol 1983; 146(8):985–987.
139. Ludomirski A, Nemiroff R, Johnson A, et al. Percutaneous umbilical blood sampling: a new technique for prenatal diagnosis. J Reprod Med 1987; 32(4):276–279.
140. Duchatel F, Oury JF, Mennesson B, et al. Complications of diagnostic ultrasound-guided percutaneous umbilical blood sampling: analysis of a series of 341 cases and review of literature. Eur J Obstet Gynecol 1993; 52(2):95–104.
141. Chenard E, Bastide A, Fraser WD. Umbilical cord hematoma following diagnostic funipuncture. Obstet Gynecol 1990; 76(5 Pt 2):994–996.
142. Seeds JW, Chescheir NC, Bowes WA, et al. Fetal death as a complication of intrauterine intravascular transfusion. Obstet Gynecol 1989; 74(3 Pt 2):461–463.
143. Wilkins I, Mezrow G, Lynch L, et al. Amnionitis and life-threatening respiratory distress after percutaneous umbilical blood sampling. Am J Obstet Gynecol 1989; 160(2):427–428.
144. McColgin SW, Hess LW, Martin RW, et al. Group B streptococcal sepsis and death in utero following funipuncture. Obstet Gynecol 1989; 74(3 Pt 2):464–465.
145. Bowman JM, Pollock JM, Peterson LE, et al. Fetomaternal hemorrhage following funipuncture: increase in severity of maternal red-cell alloimmunization. Obstet Gynecol 1994; 84(5): 839–843.
146. Rodeck CH, Nicolaides KH. Ultrasound guided invasive procedures in obstetrics. Clin Obstet Gynaecol 1983; 10(3):515–539.
147. Parmentier L, Blanchet-Bardon C, Nguyen S, et al. Autosomal recessive lamellar ichthyosis: identification of a new mutation in transglutaminose 1 and evidence for genetic heterogeneity. Hum Mol Genet 1995; 4(8):1391–1395.
148. Russell LJ, DeGiovanna JJ, Rogers GR, et al. Mutations in the gene for transglutaminose 1 in autosomal recessive lamellar ichthyosis. Nat Genet 1995; 9:279.
149. Vahlquist A, Ganemo A, Pigg M, et al. The clinical spectrum of congenital ichthyosis in Sweden: a review of 127 cases. Acta Derm Venereol Suppl (Stockh) 2003; 213:34–47.
150. Troyano JM, Clavijo MT, Marco OY, et al. Ultrasound-guided fetal invasive procedures: current status. Ultrasound Rev Obstet Gynecol 2003; 3(3):178–191.
151. Shulman LP, Elias S. Percutaneous umbilical blood sampling, fetal skin sampling and fetal liver biopsy. Sem Perinatol 1990; 14(6):456–464.
152. Bushby KM, Gardner-Medwin D. The clinical, genetic and dystrophin characteristics of Becker muscular dystrophy. I. Natural history. J Neurol 1993; 240(7):98–104.
153. Cox GF, Kunkel LM. Dystrophies and heart disease. Curr Opin Cardiol 1997; 12(3):329–343.
154. Jennekens FG, ten Kate LP, de Visser M, et al. Diagnostic criteria for Duchenne and Becker muscular dystrophy and myotonic dystrophy. Neuromuscul Disord 1991; 1(6):389–391.
155. Evans MI, Hoffman EP, Cadrin C, et al. Fetal muscle biopsy: collaborative experience with varied indications. Obstet Gynecol 1994; 84(6):913–917.
156. Overton TG, Smith RP, Sewry CA, et al. Maternal contamination at fetal muscle biopsy. Fetal Diagn Ther 2000; 15(2):118–121.
157. Murotsuki J, Uehara S, Okamura K, et al. Fetal liver biopsy for prenatal diagnosis of carbamoyl phosphate synthetase deficiency. Am J Perinatol 1994; 11(2):160–162.
158. Fisk NM, Rodeck CH. Fetal liver biopsy. In: Chervenak FA, Isaacson GC, Campbell S, eds. Ultrasound in Obstetrics and Gynecology. Boston: Little, Brown, 1993.
159. Bernaschek G, Deutinger J, Hansmann M, et al. Fetoamniotic shunting: report of the experience of four European centers. Prenat Diagn 1994; 14(9):821–833.
160. Hagay Z, Reece A, Roberts A, et al. Isolated fetal pleural effusion: a prenatal management dilemma. Obstet Gynecol 1993; 81(1):147–152.
161. Rodeck CH, Fisk NM, Fraser DI, et al. Long-term in utero drainage of fetal hydrothorax. N Engl J Med 1988; 319(17):1135–1138.
162. Wilson RD, Baxter JK, Johnson MP, et al. Thoracoamniotic shunts: fetal treatment of pleural effusions and congenital cystic adenomatoid malformations. Fetal Diagn Ther 2004; 19(5): 413–420.
163. Picone O, Benachi A, Mandelbrot L, et al. Thoracoamniotic shunting for fetal pleural effusions with hydrops. Am J Obstet Gynecol 2004; 191(6):2047–2050.
164. Wilson RD, Johnson MP. Prenatal ultrasound guided percutaneous shunts for obstructive uropathy and thoracic disease. Semin Ped Surg 2003; 12(3):182–189.
165. Thompson PJ, Greenough A, Nicolaides KH. Respiratory function in infancy following pleuro-amniotic shunting. Fetal Diagn Ther 1993; 8(2):79–83.
166. Blott M, Nicolaides KH, Greenough A. Postnatal respiratory function after chronic drainage of fetal pulmonary cyst. Am J Obstet Gynecol 1988; 159(4):858–859.
167. Manning FA, Harrison MR, Rodeck CH. Catheter shunts for fetal hydronephrosis and hydrocephalus. N Engl J Med 1986; 315(5):336–340.
168. Mahony BS, Filly RA, Callen PW, et al. Fetal renal dysplasia: sonographic evaluation. Radiology 1984; 152(1):143–146.
169. McLorie G, Walid F, Khoury A, et al. Outcome analysis of vesicoamniotic shunting in a comprehensive population. J Urol 2001; 166(3):1036–1040.
170. Edwards RG, Steptoe PC, Purdy JM. Establishing full-term human pregnancies using cleavage embryos grown in vitro. Br J Obstet Gynaecol 1980; 87(9):737–756.
171. Feichtinger W. Follicle aspiration with interactive three-dimensional digital imaging (Voluson®): a step toward real-time puncturing under three-dimensional ultrasound control. Fertil Steril 1998; 70(2):374–377.
172. Birch H. The extended role of the nurse—opportunity or threat? Human Fertility 2001; 4(3):138–144.
173. Driscoll GL, Tyler JP, Knight DC, et al. Failure to collect oocytes in assisted reproductive technology: a retrospective. Hum Reprod 1998; 13(1):84–87.
174. Dessole S, Rubattu G, Ambrosini G, et al. Blood loss following non-complicated transvaginal oocyte retrieval for IVF. Fertil Steril 2001; 76(1):205–206.

175. Evers JLH, Larsen JF, Gnany GG, et al. Complications and problems in transvaginal sector scan-guided follicle aspiration. Fertil Steril 1988; 49(2):278–282.
176. Bennett SJ, Waterstone JJ, Cheng WC, et al. Complications of transvaginal ultrasound-directed follicle aspiration: a review of 2670 consecutive procedures. J Assisted Reprod Genet 1993; 10(1):72–77.
177. Baber R, Porter R, Picker R, et al. Transvaginal ultrasound-directed oocyte collection for in vitro fertilization: successes and complications. J Ultrasound Med 1988; 7(7):377–379.
178. Dicker D, Ashkenazi J, Feldberg D et al. Severe abdominal complications after transvaginal ultrasonographically guided retrieval of oocyte for IVF and ET. Fertil Steril 1993; 59(6):1313–1315.
179. Curtis P, Amso N, Keith E, et al. Evaluation of the risk of pelvic infection following transvaginal oocyte retrieval. Human Reprod 1991; 6(9):1294–1297.
180. Schenker JG, Ezra Y. Complications of assisted reproductive techniques. Fertil Steril 1994; 61(3):411–422.
181. Hurley VA, Osborn JC, Leoni MA, et al. Ultrasound-guided embryo transfer: a controlled trial. Fertil Steril 1991; 55(3): 559–562.
182. Buckett WM. A meta-analysis of ultrasound-guided versus clinical touch embryo transfer. Fertil Steril 2003; 80(4):1037–1041.
183. Baba K, Ishihara O, Hayashi N, et al. Three-dimensional ultrasound in embryo transfer. Ultrasound Obstet Gynecol 2000; 16(4):372–373.
184. Baba K, Ishihara O, Hayashi N, et al. Where does the embryo implant after transfer in humans? Fertil Steril 2000; 73(1):123–125.
185. Scholtes MCW, Roosenburg BJ, Alberda AT, et al. Transcervical intrafallopian transfer of zygotes. Fertil Steril 1990; 54(2):283–286.
186. Hughes EG, Shekelton P, Leonie M, et al. Ultrasound-guided fallopian tube catheterization per vaginuum: a feasibility study with the use of laparoscopic control. Fertil Steril 1988; 50(6):986–989.
187. Jansen RP, Anderson JC. Catheterisation of the fallopian tubes from the vagina. Lancet 1987; 2(8554):309–310.
188. Papaioannou S, Afnan M, Girling A, et al. The potential values of tubal perfusion pressures measured during selective salpingography in predicting fertility. Human Reprod 2003; 18(2):358–363.
189. Jeanty P, Besnard S, Arnold A, et al. Air-contrast sonohysterography as a first step assessment of tubal patency. J Ultrasound Med 2000; 19(8):519–527.
190. Deichert U, Schlief R, van de Sandt M, et al. Transvaginal hysterosalpingo-contrast-sonography (Hy-Co-Sy) compared with conventional tubal diagnostics. Hum Reprod 1989; 4(4):418–424.
191. Stern J, Peters AJ, Coulam CB. Color Doppler ultrasonography assessment of tubal patency: a comparison study with traditional techniques. Fertil Steril 1992; 58(5):897–900.
192. Volpi E, De Grandis T, Rustichelli S, et al. A new technique to test tubal patency under transvaginal sonographic control. Acta Obstet Gynaecol Scan 1994; 73(10):797–801.
193. Deichert U et al. Transvaginal hysterosalpingo-contrast sonography for the assessment of tubal patency with gray scale imaging and additional use of pulsed wave Doppler. Fertil Steril 1992; 57(1):62–67.
194. Sankpal RS, Confino E, Matzel A et al. Investigation of the uterine cavity and fallopian tubes using three-dimensional saline sonohysterosalpingography. Int J Gynecol Obstet 2001; 73(2):125–129.
195. de Crespigny LC, Robinson HP, Davoren RA, et al. The "simple" ovarian cyst: aspirate or operate? Br J Obstet Gynaecol 1989; 96(9):1035–1039.
196. Tailor A, Jurkovic D, Bourne TH, et al. Sonographic prediction of malignancy in adnexal masses using multivariate logistic regression analysis. Ultrasound Obstet Gynecol 1997; 10(1):41–47.
197. Sassone AM, Timor-Tritsch IE, Artner A, et al. Transvaginal sonographic characterization of ovarian disease: evaluation of a new scoring system to predict ovarian malignancy. Obstet Gynecol 1991; 78(1):70–76.
198. Herrmann UJ Jr, Locher GW, Goldhirsch A. Sonographic patterns of ovarian tumors: prediction of malignancy. Obstet Gynecol 1987; 69(5):777–781.
199. Kurjak A, Schulman H, Sosic A, et al. Transvaginal ultrasound, color flow, and Doppler waveform of the postmenopausal adnexal mass. Obstet Gynecol 1992; 80(6):917–921.
200. Luxman D, Bergman A, Sagi J, et al. The postmenopausal adnexal mass: correlation between ultrasonic and pathologic findings. Obstet Gynecol 1991; 77(5):726–728.
201. Nicklin JL, van Eijkeren M, Athanasatos P, et al. A comparison of ovarian cyst aspirate cytology and histology: the case against aspiration of cystic pelvic masses. Aust NZ J Obstet Gynaecol 1994; 34(5):546–549.
202. Dordoni D, Zaglio S, Zacca S, et al. The role of sonographically guided aspiration in the clinical management of ovarian cysts. J Ultrasound Med 1993; 12(1):27–31.
203. Martinez-Onsurbe P, Villaespesa AR, Anquela JMS, et al. Aspiration cytology of 147 adnexal cysts with histologic correlation. Acta Cytol 2001; 45(5):941–947.
204. Higgins RV, Matkins JF, Marroum M-C. Comparison of fine-needle aspiration cytologic findings of ovarian cysts with ovarian histologic findings. Am J Obstet Gynecol 1999; 180(3 Pt 1): 550–553.
205. Zanetta G, Trio D, Lissoni A, et al. Early and short-term complications after US-guided puncture of gynecologic lesions: evaluation after 1,000 consecutive cases. Radiology 1993; 189(1):161–164.
206. Pinotti JA, deFranzin CMMO, Marussi EF, et al. Evolution of cystic and adnexal tumors identified by echography. Int J Gynaecol Obstet 1988; 26(1):109–114.
207. 199.Varghese JC, O'Neill MJ, Gervais DA, et al. Transvaginal catheter drainage of tuboovarian abscess using the trocar method: technique and literature review. AJR Am J Roentgenol 2001; 177(1):139–144.
208. Nelson AL, Sinow RM, Oliak D. Transrectal ultrasonographically guided drainage of gynecologic pelvic abscesses. Am J Obstet Gynecol 2000; 182(6):1382–1388.
209. Hovsepian DM, Steele JR, Skinner CS, et al. Transrectal versus transvaginal abscess drainage: survey of patient tolerance and effect on activities of daily living. Radiol 1999; 212(1):159–163.
210. Feld R, Eschelman DJ, Sagerman JE, et al. Treatment of pelvic abscesses and other fluid collections: efficacy of transvaginal sonographically guided aspiration and drainage. AJR Am J Roentgenol 1994; 163(5):1141–1145.
211. Scatamacchia SA, Raptopoulos V, Davidson RI. Saline microbubbles monitoring sonography-assisted abscess drainage. Invest Radiol 1987; 22(11):868–870.
212. Nelson AL, Sinow RM, Renslo R, et al. Endovaginal ultrasonographically guided transvaginal drainage for treatment of pelvic abscesses. Am J Obstet Gynecol 1995; 172(6):1926–1932.
213. Jeffrey RB Jr, Wing VW, Laing FC. Real-time sonographic monitoring of percutaneous abscess drainage. AJR Am J Roentgenol 1985; 144(3):469–470.
214. Granai CO, Allee P, Doherty F, et al. Intra-operative real-time ultrasonography during intrauterine tandem placement. Obstet Gynecol 1986; 67(1):112–114.
215. Hunter RE, Reuter K, Kopin E. Use of ultrasonography in the difficult postmenopausal dilation and curettage. Obstet Gynecol 1989; 73(5 Pt 1):813–816.
216. Darney PD, Sweet RL. Routine intraoperative ultrasonography for second trimester abortion reduces incidence of uterine perforation. J Ultrasound Med 1989; 8(2):71–75.
217. Romero R, Copel JA, Jeanty P, et al. Sonographic monitoring to guide the performance of postabortal uterine curettage. Am J Obstet Gynecol 1985; 151(1):51–53.
218. Shalev E, Shimoni YU, Peleg D. Ultrasound controlled operative hysteroscopy. J Am Coll Surg 1994; 179(1):70–71.

Intraoperative Ultrasonography

Robert A. Kane

7

INTRODUCTION

Intraoperative ultrasonography is a dynamic, practical, and clinically effective diagnostic tool that has a direct and immediate impact on patient care and clinical decision making during the time of surgery. This is a highly interactive scan procedure between the sonologist and the surgeon, and there has been a steady increase in demand for intraoperative ultrasonographic scanning because of its clinical efficacy. While more radiologists have become involved with intraoperative ultrasonography, many radiologists are still reluctant to perform these procedures, and, as a result, many intraoperative ultrasound (IOUS) scans are now being performed by the surgeons themselves.

The reluctance of radiologists to perform intraoperative ultrasonography is largely related to concerns about the amount of time away from the department required to perform and interpret these scans. The reimbursement levels for diagnostic IOUS scans are similar to reimbursement for studies performed in the ultrasound suite of the radiology department, but the time requirements for IOUS can be considerably greater. Therefore, strategies for minimizing the total time required for IOUS scanning are important in order to maximize the radiologist's efficiency when performing these scans. We have developed several tactics which, when implemented, can allow the entire scanning procedure to be accomplished in a reasonable time period, typically no more than 30 minutes total time out of the department. Except for emergencies, IOUS scans are scheduled in advance with radiology department, and the relevant prior imaging studies are reviewed in order to understand the clinical concerns and questions to be answered by IOUS. Selecting the appropriate probe or probes and prepositioning the scanner in the operating room (OR) suite when possible can save several minutes of transportation time. Similarly, if the radiologist worked in scrubs, another few minutes can be saved.

The most important time saver is a collegial and mutually respectful interaction between the surgeon and the radiologist so that time is wasted by neither party. In our institution, we have a 10 to 15 minute rule, such that the call from the surgical suite to radiology department for scanning will be initiated 10 to 15 minutes before the surgeon is ready for the intraoperative scans, and the radiologist, technologist, and scanner will be ready to perform the scans within 10 to 15 minutes of receiving the call. In this way, neither the surgeon nor the radiologist is spending an inordinate amount of time waiting for the other, thereby maximizing efficiency.

It is most optimal if the sonologist scrubs in on the case and performs the actual scanning. Typically, a diagnostic scan can be performed and completed in 5 to 10 minutes, and this is facilitated by having reviewed the prior diagnostic imaging studies before performing the scans. An experienced sonologist is much more capable of performing an efficient, complete, and comprehensive study, but another alternative is the surgeon actually performing the scans with the radiologist available in the operating suite to help interpret the study. A third alternative is the surgeon performing and interpreting the scans with the radiologist available for consultation, only if the surgeon is having difficulty in interpreting the scans. Some institutions make this type of consultation available via remote teleradiology or PACS linkage, but, more commonly, the radiologist would come up to the OR to observe and interpret the images being obtained by the surgeon. These latter two alternatives work most effectively when the surgeon is very skilled and experienced but, in most settings, the radiologist's skills and experience in scanning are much greater than the surgeon's and, in particular, their understanding of proper scanning techniques, suppression of imaging artifacts, and appreciation of subtle changes in echo texture, all of which are necessary for optimal detection of disease and interpretation of the findings. Therefore, in most settings, it is appropriate and desirable for the radiologist to scrub in and perform the scans themselves.

The first uses of intraoperative ultrasonography date back to the 1960s when A-mode ultrasound scanning was used to detect renal calculi during nephrolithotomy procedures (1) and gallstones and choledocholithiasis (2,3). Scattered and sporadic reports were found in the literature for the next two decades but it was not until the mid- to late 1980s that IOUS techniques and equipment became an increasingly important imaging tool for the surgeons (4). Miniaturization of equipment, the development of specific IOUS probes, the ability to perform Doppler and color flow imaging, and the development of laparoscopic ultrasound (LUS) probes all have contributed to the rapidly growing demand for IOUS imaging.

GENERAL PRINCIPLES

Equipment

While standard ultrasound probes used for daily scanning in the ultrasound department can also be used for intraoperative ultrasonography, it is preferable to utilize probes specifically designed for intraoperative use. The larger size and configuration of standard ultrasound probes can make it difficult to gain complete access to the target organs, due to the confined spaces available during intraoperative scanning. A variety of probes have been developed for different intraoperative uses (Fig. 1). For intra-abdominal scanning, both end-fire and side-fire probes are necessary. End-fire probes are most optimal for evaluating the gallbladder, extrahepatic bile ducts, pancreas, and other retroperitoneal structures. However, small, flat side-fire probes are required to evaluate the liver and the intrahepatic biliary tract, because of the very confined space available between the liver surface and adjacent rib cage. Broadband or multifrequency probes are optimal since frequencies ranging from 5 to 7.5 MHz are most desirable for intra-abdominal scanning. For renal scanning, typically the window available is quite small and a small end-fire 5 to 7.5 MHz probe is most optimal. For neurosurgical use, both in the head and in the spine, once again end-fire probes are most optimal, with frequencies ranging from 7 to 10 MHz. Very small end-fire probes have been developed for intracranial use to allow successful scanning through entry sites as small as a burr hole. Very small footprint high frequency probes have also been developed for intraoperative vascular ultrasound uses, such as evaluation in patients undergoing carotid endarterectomy.

Finally, a word about LUS probes is necessary. The initial LUS equipment was rigid, using small linear array probes mounted on the end of a long, rigid shaft. This initial design proved unsuitable because of the inability to maintain contact with the target organs. As a result, flexible tipped LUS probes were developed using mechanisms similar to those found on endoscopes. The LUS probe should be of a size that allows passage through the 10 to 11 mm laparoscopic ports. It should have a shaft length of approximately 25 to 30 cm in order to reach all relevant intra-abdominal sites and should have a frequency range from 5 to 7.5 MHz, either via broadband or via multiple frequency transducers. The lower frequencies are required to penetrate large organs, such as the liver, while the higher frequencies are most optimal for imaging superficial structures close to the probe, such as the common bile duct. While both linear array and curvilinear array scanners are available, we prefer a sector format, because it allows for better orientation to the underlying anatomy.

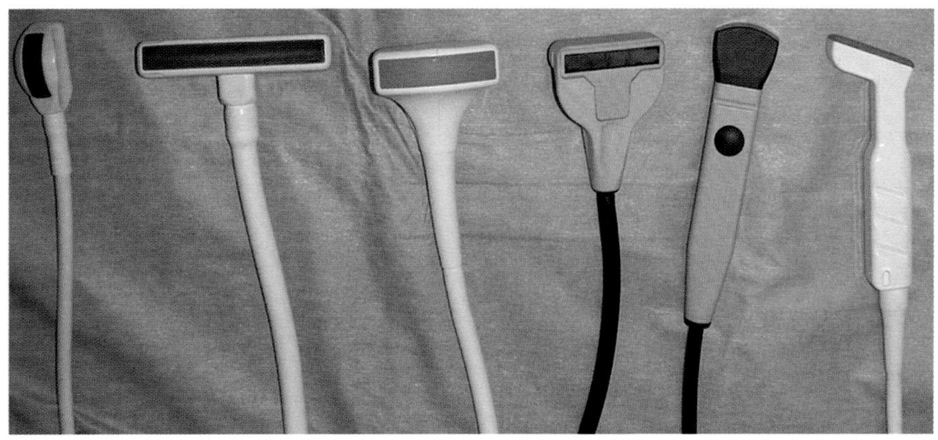

FIGURE 1 ■ Intraoperative ultrasound probes. Both end-fire and side-fire probes are useful, either linear array or curvilinear.

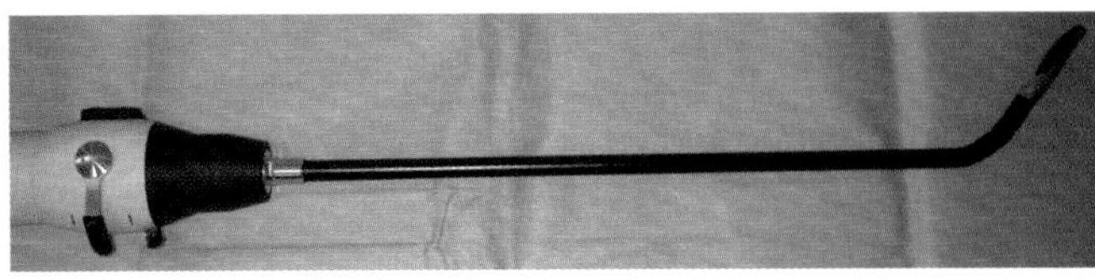

(A)

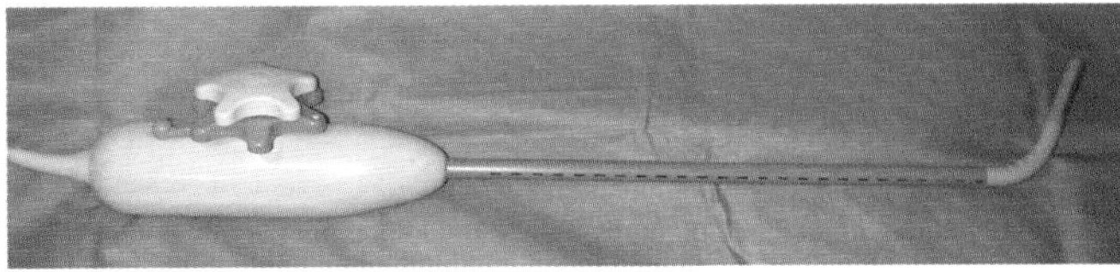

(B)

FIGURE 2 A AND B ■ Laparoscopic ultrasound (LUS) probes. (**A**) Curvilinear LUS probe in flexed position. (**B**) Linear array LUS probe in left deflexion.

This is particularly important with LUS scanning, because the probe is seldom in a precise transverse or sagittal orientation, but is much more often in a variably oblique plane, which can make orientation to the anatomy much more difficult (5).

As mentioned above, the ability to flex and extend the scanning surface is an absolute requirement in order to maintain acoustic contact with the target organ. Many probes also offer a left-to-right deflection, which can also be useful, but is not an absolute necessity (Fig. 2).

Sterilization

It is, of course, an absolute requirement that the equipment used for intraoperative scanning maintain a high level of sterilization at all times. In the most optimal circumstances, the probes themselves are sterilized prior to the examination. In the past, we have successfully used gas sterilization with ethylene oxide for some of our intraoperative probes, but many manufacturers do not support this type of gas sterilization, fearing that the high temperatures during the aeration process might damage the transducer skin. We did not find this to be a problem over many years of use, but there are other problems with ethylene oxide gas sterilization, including a 24-hour turnaround time due to the prolonged aeration cycle (5). We currently use a gas–plasma sterilization technology, the Sterad system, which utilizes low temperature sterilization and is more environmentally acceptable. This still requires a prolonged turnaround time of several hours.

Obviously, rapid sterilization using an autoclave is not feasible for this sensitive electronic equipment. Some institutions will allow prolonged immersion in glutaraldehyde, but this is not deemed sufficiently effective sterilization for internal intraoperative use at our institution. There are also environmental issues with glutaraldehyde fumes and there have been some reported adverse patient reactions to contact with glutaraldehyde, if it has not been sufficiently rinsed off prior to the scans. Sterile probe covers are probably the simplest means of achieving adequate sterilization for intraoperative use. Both the transducer itself and the transducer cord must be covered in sterile sheaths. Optimally, one should use a sheath specifically designed to fit snugly over the probe in use. Some of these have long extensions to cover the transducer cord, but, if not, standard endoscopic sheaths can also be utilized for this purpose in combination with the transducer probe sheath.

Applying the sterile sheath and cord covers takes an additional one to two minutes of OR time in order to maintain meticulous sterile technique while covering the probes with these sheaths. Acoustic coupling must be applied to the transducer prior to insertion into the sheath, using either sterile gel or sterile fluid. The principal problem with the sheaths is the potential for rips or tears in the sheath, which would then compromise the sterile field. This is particularly concerning with use of laparoscopic probes, which must pass through the rather snug skin ports. Therefore, if sterile probe covers are used as the principal means of protection, it is necessary to soak the probes in some sterilizing solution, such as glutaraldehyde or bleach, for 30 minutes prior to the intraoperative scan. The specific solutions must be cleared with the manufacturer of the equipment in order to avoid damage to the ultrasound probes.

Technique

Scanning technique will vary with the choice of transducer and the target organ being studied. Whenever possible, it is important to position the scanner and monitor such that it can be easily viewed while scanning, avoiding the necessity to look over one's shoulder or some other awkward configuration (Fig. 3). With LUS, simple electronic beam splitters are widely available and inexpensive, which can allow a picture-within-picture display of the ultrasound image on the laparoscopic monitors. This is very convenient since visualization of the probe itself is important to help orient the examiner to the ultrasound images, as well as to avoid misplacing the LUS probe into undesirable or vulnerable sites. By a simple switch, the ultrasound image can be made the predominant image on the screen with the laparoscopic image superimposed in one corner, or the positions can be reversed with a small ultrasound image and a larger laparoscopic image (6).

Usually, there is sufficient moisture within the body cavity to provide the necessary acoustic coupling but, if necessary, warmed sterile saline can be applied to the surface of the organ. For neurosurgical applications, usually the surgical entry site is again filled with sterile saline, which provides the necessary acoustic coupling for optimal imaging. When the saline is initially applied, there may be a veritable blizzard of microbubbles, which can interfere with the ultrasound image, but these will rapidly dissipate, usually within 60 seconds, and more optimal imaging will then be obtained. If the sterile water bath contains any debris or hemorrhagic material, fibrin or other reflectors, the site can be aspirated and the debris cleared, and then refilled with more sterile saline. A clear water bath is essential to avoid artifacts

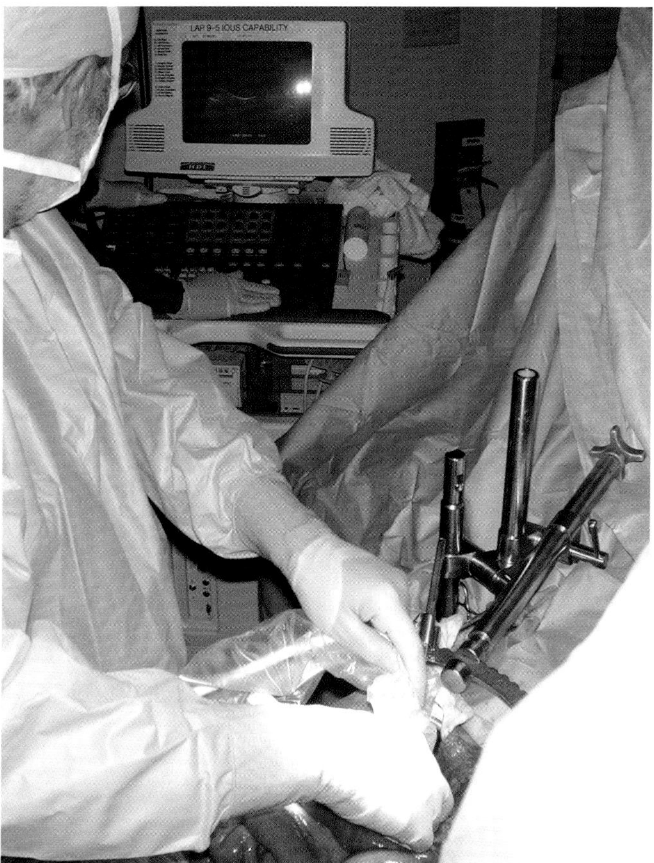

FIGURE 3 ■ IOUS scanning. Note sterile sheath covering transducer cord and nearby positioning of the ultrasound scanner, allowing easy viewing.

from any floating debris, which can interfere with optimal ultrasound imaging.

Since the transducer cord is covered with the sterile sheath, this must be maintained as part of the sterile surgical field and should be clipped onto the surgical drapes with a towel clamp or Kelly clamp, to avoid contamination if the cord falls from the operative field to the side of the surgical table. If this should occur, the cord needs to be redraped and this wastes several minutes of time, which can be avoided by affixing the sterile sheath and cord to the surgical drapes before beginning the scans.

When performing LUS, it is important to select the appropriate laparoscopic port in which to insert the LUS probe. If the port is too close or directly over the target organ, there may be insufficient room to manipulate the probe over the entire organ. Similarly, if the port is too distant from the target, the probe may not be long enough to reach all portions of the organ. Not infrequently, more than one laparoscopic port is required for a complete scan, particularly when imaging the liver (6). A periumbilical port may allow good access to the left lobe and caudate, but may not allow sufficient room to reach the dome of the right lobe, which may require further scanning via a right upper quadrant subcostal port. This same port, however, may render the left lateral segment and caudate lobe inaccessible. Similarly, LUS imaging of the bile duct or pancreas may require the use of more than one port, particularly if the pancreas has a pronounced "S" shape or if both the intrahepatic and the extrahepatic biliary trees must be assessed. The optimal port sites for LUS scanning can be quite variable, and must be individualized from patient to patient.

LIVER

IOUS imaging of the liver is best performed with a 5 MHz sidefire probe, either linear array or curvilinear array. The probe must be sufficiently low profile to fit between the liver surface and the thorax, a surprisingly small and confined space in patients who have not had complete mobilization of the liver. A routine and systematic approach to imaging the liver is essential for optimal lesion detection, when imaging for primary or metastatic liver tumors. Our scanning protocol begins with positioning the probe at the dome of the left lobe of the liver over Segment II along the free edge. We then scan in a cephalad to caudad direction, slowly moving the probe from the dome to the caudal edge of the left lateral segment. The probe is then repositioned once again at the dome of the liver, moving to the patient's right and another sweep is made from the dome to caudal edge of the liver, slightly overlapping the first pass. In this fashion, a series of overlapping scans are obtained from left to right until the entire liver surface is evaluated (Fig. 4). While the lateral segment and caudate lobe may be completely imaged in one or two sweeps, the greater bulk of the left medial segment and right lobe may require two repetitive sweeps, one with the focal zone in the relative near field and a second with a greater depth of field and deeper positioning of the focal zone in order to image the posterior deep aspects of the liver. This is the reason why a 5 MHz frequency probe is optimal, since higher frequencies will lack sufficient power to penetrate through the entire liver.

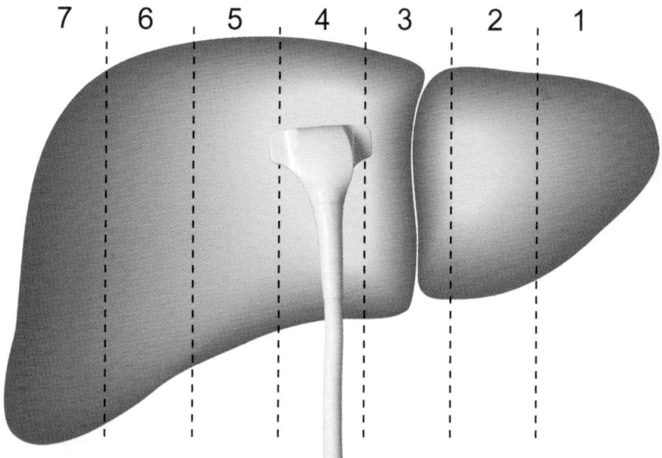

FIGURE 4 ■ Schematic diagram of the systematic approach to liver IOUS scanning with slightly overlapping fields from the extreme left margin of the liver across to the extreme right margin. Typically, five to seven sweeps will encompass the entire liver.

There are several applications for IOUS of the liver: (*i*) the most complete detection and characterization of focal liver lesions; (*ii*) definition of anatomic landmarks which define lobar and segmental liver anatomy, and identification of normal or anomalous liver vasculature; (*iii*) assistance in planning for surgical resection of liver tumors; (*iv*) real-time guidance for interventional procedures, such as biopsies, drainages, and aspirations, and tumor ablation procedures; (*v*) guidance for defining the avascular resection plane during living donor split liver transplant procedures.

IOUS liver imaging is capable of extremely fine spatial resolution, with ability to image cystic structures as small as 1 to 3 mm and solid nodules as small as 5 mm (Fig. 5). Until most recently, IOUS liver imaging consistently would demonstrate 25% to 30% more focal liver lesions than were identified by preoperative imaging with ultrasound, computed tomography (CT), or magnetic resonance imaging (MRI) (7–9). The majority of these additional lesions detected by IOUS are quite small, often 1 cm or less in diameter, and the majority of these small lesions are not detectable by palpation, unless they are immediately subcapsular in position. Since 1990, lesion detection was increased by CT arterial portography (10), but this came at a cost of less specificity, with numerous pseudolesions such as small perfusion defects or tiny cysts, being confused for tumor nodules (11,12).

More recently, preoperative imaging results have improved substantially, with the advent of multidetector CT scans, more powerful and faster MRI scans, and positron emission tomography imaging. There are several recent reports in the literature, which suggest that IOUS imaging may now only detect 5% to 10% more lesions when compared with these state-of-the-art preoperative scanners (13–15). This is concordant with our own experience, but nevertheless, the detection of any additional lesions can be critical in influencing decisions about the resectability of liver tumors, and hence, routine IOUS scanning of the liver is still a recommendation for patients undergoing possible surgical resection of liver cancer.

Many patients will undergo a staging laparoscopy, prior to a planned liver tumor resection. Laparoscopy is capable of detecting certain types of metastatic disease, which are relatively poorly detected even with the best preoperative imaging, particularly identifying peritoneal tumor implants and some instances of lymphadenopathy (16). Very small, flat surface liver metastases can also be visualized and biopsied laparoscopically, but the majority of the liver below the surface cannot be assessed, and, as a result, if staging laparoscopy is to be performed, LUS of the liver can be performed and is capable of similar sensitivity for detection of small liver tumors (Fig. 6) as IOUS (17). However, the technique is more difficult and scanning times are lengthier than IOUS. A typical IOUS liver scan can be performed in 5 to 10 minutes, whereas a complete LUS scan of the liver may take 15 to 20 minutes, since the transducer surface is much smaller with the LUS probes, and, hence, many more overlapping sweeps are required to perform a complete assessment of the liver. Frequently, the LUS probe must often be placed in more than one laparoscopic port in order to gain access to the entire liver surface.

Depiction of the lobar and segmental anatomy of the liver is relatively straightforward, and demonstrating the location of liver tumors relative to these anatomic landmarks helps the surgical decision on the most appropriate type of resection to perform (Fig. 7). While many lesions are amenable to standard segmental or lobar resection, demonstrating the relationship of the tumor to critical vascular structures, such as the hepatic veins, may indicate the need for a more extensive resection in order to obtain clear surgical margins. Alternatively, lesions which straddle both right and left lobes may be better approached with a deep, nonsegmental, wedge-type resection in order to spare as much functioning liver as possible. IOUS imaging is essential for these nonsegmental resections, to depict and define the deep margins

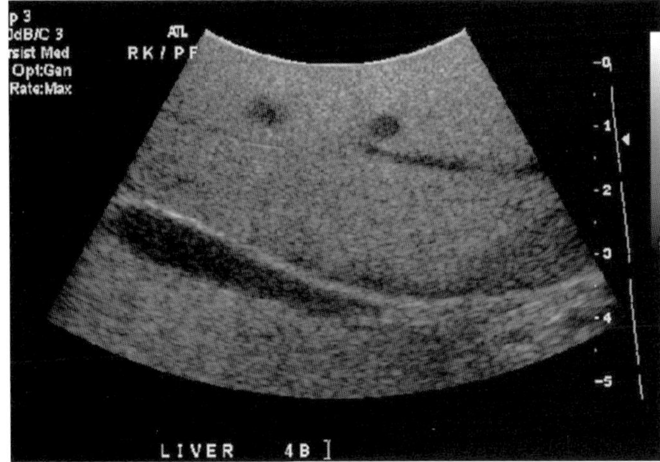

FIGURE 5 ■ IOUS scan showing fatty liver with two 5 mm breast metastases, not seen on preoperative CT scan.

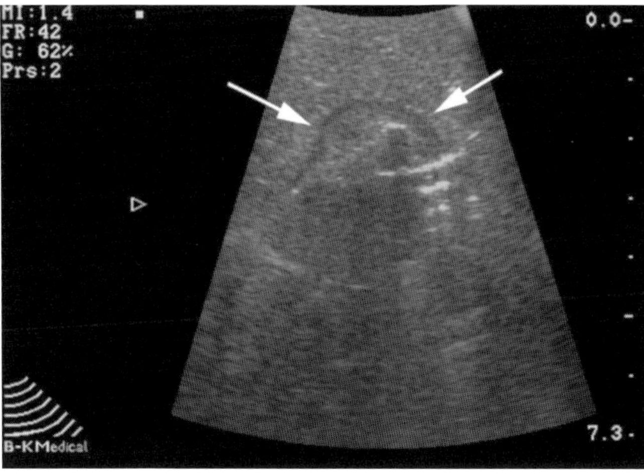

FIGURE 6 ■ Laparoscopic ultrasound image of unsuspected, 1.2 cm, subcapsular metastasis (*arrows*) in a patient with pancreatic carcinoma.

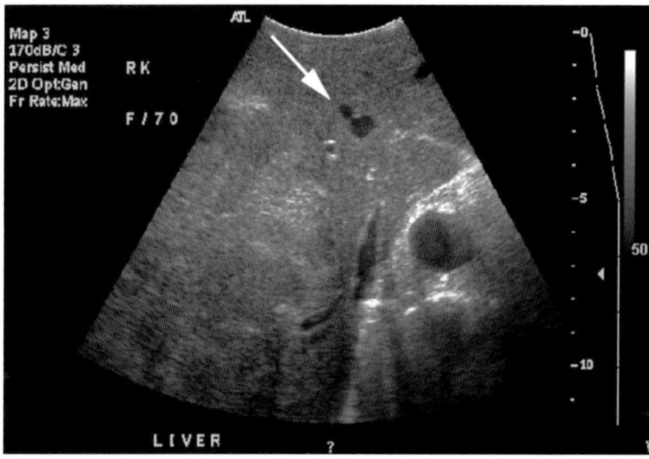

FIGURE 7 ■ Adrenal carcinoma metastasis. A clear, tumor-free margin can be seen between this large, slow-growing mass in Segments VII and VIII and the middle hepatic vein (*arrow*). Therefore, this solitary metastasis could be completely resected by a right hepatic lobectomy.

of the tumor, which are often impalpable. We will often demonstrate the deep margins of the tumor with ultrasound and make appropriate marks on the liver capsule with electrocautery in order to define the optimal margins for deep wedge resection, striving for a 1 cm tumor-free margin in all planes.

Anomalous vasculature is readily identified by intraoperative scanning. Accessory arterial supply is frequently seen with an accessory or replaced right hepatic artery present in up to 25% of individuals, arising from the superior mesenteric artery (SMA) and extending into the liver, deep to the main portal vein. An accessory or replaced left hepatic artery is seen in about 12% of patients, arising from the left gastric artery and entering the liver along the ligamentum venosum (Fig. 8). The hepatic venous confluence has a markedly variable configuration. Most commonly, the left and middle hepatic veins have a common trunk. Also frequently seen is a venous branch draining Segment VIII into the middle hepatic vein. The right hepatic vein may have superior or inferior accessory branches. Identifying the inferior accessory right hepatic vein can be quite important for the surgeon prior to a major hepatic resection, since this vein could be torn inadvertently during complete mobilization of the right lobe of the liver. The portal venous anatomy is somewhat more standard, but, occasionally, the main portal vein immediately trifurcates into left portal, anterior right portal, and posterior right portal branches. This anatomic anomaly is somewhat rare and may be accompanied by anomalous biliary drainage patterns as well. This is an important feature to demonstrate in living related adult liver transplantation procedures, since both vascular and biliary anomalies may lead to difficulties during surgery and postoperative complications, such as ischemia and biliary stenoses.

Evaluation of the portal and hepatic venous vasculature is also extremely important in patients with hepatocellular carcinoma (Fig. 9). These tumors can be quite aggressive and are prone to invade the portal venous system in up to 20% to 30% of patients with large hepatomas (18). These tumors may also invade the hepatic veins and occasionally may invade both systems simultaneously. The hepatic venous invasion may extend all the way into the inferior vena cava and even into the right atrium, and complete depiction of these tumor thrombi is essential. Venous invasion by hepatoma is generally considered a sign of inoperability, although, occasionally, attempts have been made to extract the tumor thrombus from the portal venous system and resect the tumor. Obviously, the venous invasion portends a significantly worse outcome.

With open intraoperative scanning of the liver, real-time guidance can be provided for biopsies, aspirations, and tumor ablation treatments (Fig. 10). With real-time free-hand ultrasound guidance, highly accurate placement of needles, catheters, and probes can be

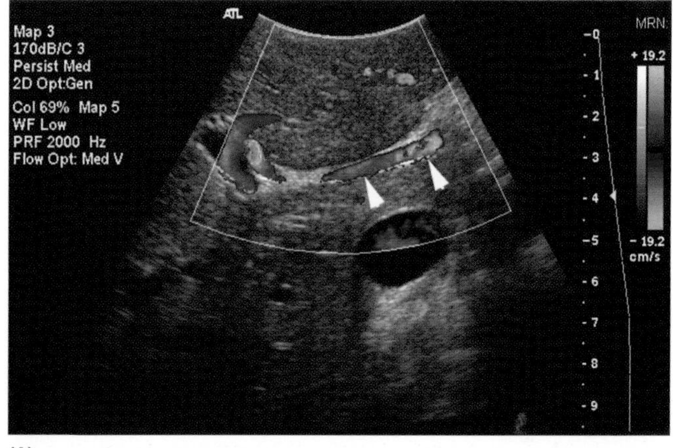

(A)

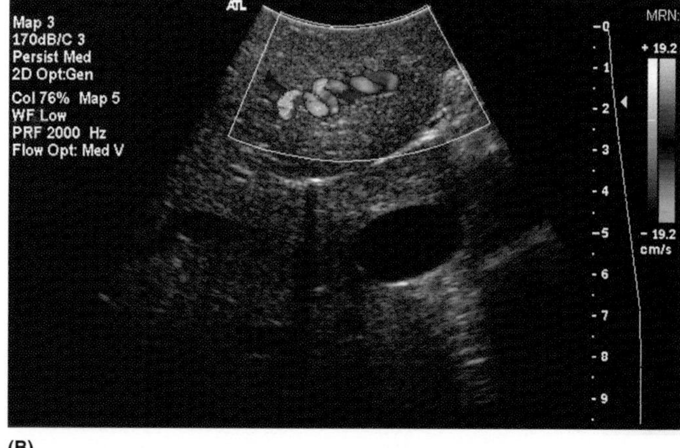

(B)

FIGURE 8 A AND B ■ Accessory left hepatic artery in a patient with focal nodular hyperplasia (FNH). (**A**) Color flow IOUS image shows flow in a replaced left hepatic artery (*arrowheads*), entering the liver via the ligamentum venosum. (**B**) Color flow IOUS image showing tortuous vascular flow in the central FNH scar.

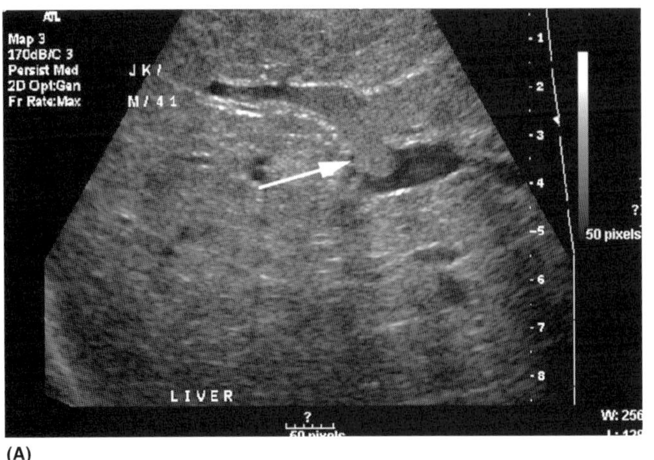

(A)

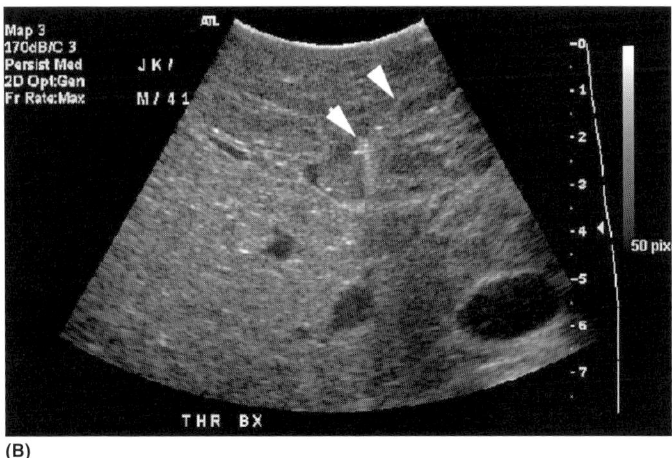

(B)

FIGURE 9 A AND B ■ Hepatocellular carcinoma invading the portal vein. (**A**) Arrow shows tumor thrombus extending into the lumen of the right portal vein. (**B**) IOUS guidance for fine needle aspiration biopsy of the tumor thrombus. Arrowheads indicate the path of the 21-gauge biopsy needle.

expected. The same procedures become more difficult when performed laparoscopically with LUS guidance. Because the biopsy or ablation devices must be placed transabdominally, the distances to the target are significantly greater, and the LUS probes are smaller in size, making the procedures much more difficult. Nevertheless, percutaneous biopsies and positioning of ablation probes can be successfully performed with LUS guidance, with the needle or probe passing through the abdominal wall and entering the liver close to the LUS probe surface, adjusting the angle of entry with real-time guidance (Fig. 11). There is at least one commercially available LUS system with an intrinsic electronic biopsy guidance system for fine needle aspiration procedures, but the system is somewhat cumbersome and arduous to utilize, and we still prefer the free-hand approach when possible.

IOUS imaging during liver transplantation is most important in adult split liver living related transplant procedures. The course of the middle hepatic vein can be readily demonstrated on the surface of the donor's liver, in order to help define the avascular plane for right lobe resection. Frequently, intraoperative scans are also requested after the donor liver is implanted in order to confirm fully patent flow across the anastomosed arteries, portal and hepatic veins, and inferior vena cava. Good color flow and pulsed Doppler capacity is essential for this purpose.

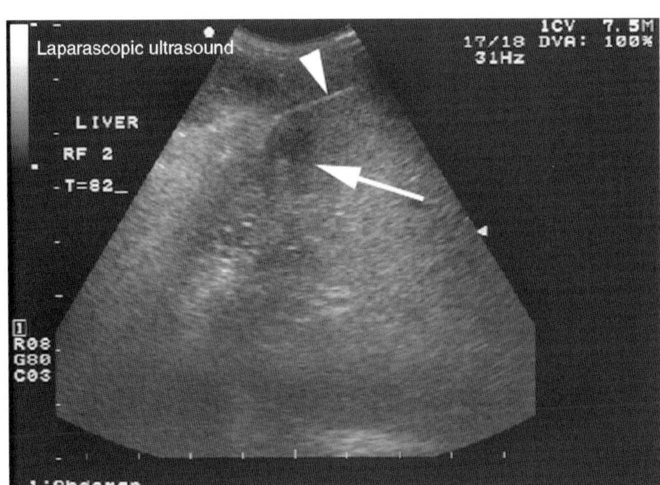

FIGURE 10 ■ Laparoscopic ultrasound guided radiofrequency ablation (RFA) of colorectal metastasis. The RFA probe is indicated by the arrowhead, extending into the mass, as shown by the arrow. The bright signal within the mass is due to cavitation artifact created by tissue heating.

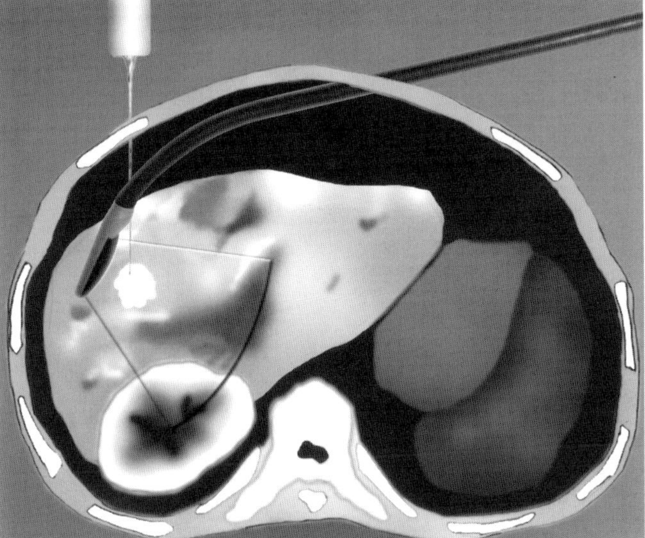

FIGURE 11 ■ Schematic diagram demonstrating transabdominal laparoscopic ultrasound (LUS) guidance technique. The LUS probe is positioned over the target mass in the liver, and the automated biopsy needle is passed through the abdominal wall, adjacent to the imaging array and guided into the mass in real time.

GALLBLADDER/BILIARY

Imaging of the extrahepatic biliary tract (common hepatic and common bile duct) and gallbladder is best achieved using a high frequency end-fire intraoperative probe. Since these structures are fairly superficial, frequencies in the 7 to 10 MHz range are appropriate. However, for complete imaging of the intrahepatic bile ducts, a side-fire liver-type probe with a frequency of 5 MHz is necessary. Because the probe is often in immediate contact with the gallbladder or common duct, near field artifacts may limit the evaluation of the proximal walls of these structures and, if necessary, an acoustic standoff may be achieved either by filling the anatomic site with warm, sterile saline, or by imaging these structures through the liver, when possible.

Imaging of the gallbladder is infrequently required for patients with gallstone disease, since preoperative ultrasound imaging is highly accurate in virtually all patients. The use of IOUS to detect occult gallstones in patients with morbid obesity who are undergoing gastric bypass procedures has been described (19), but even in this group of patients, preoperative ultrasound imaging is usually entirely adequate to detect stones.

The principal use of IOUS of the gallbladder is in evaluation of gallbladder masses, both to characterize unsuspected gallbladder masses and, more importantly, to assess for full extent of disease in patients with gallbladder carcinoma. The extent of invasion into the adjacent liver bed is difficult for the surgeon to detect by inspection and palpation, and can be well portrayed by IOUS (20). An aggressive resection of all contiguous tumors that have invaded into the liver is essential for any hope of long-term survival or surgical cure (21), and IOUS imaging can provide an accurate depiction of the depth of invasion (Fig. 12). In addition, a careful survey should be performed for evidence of distant hepatic metastases or metastases to the lymph nodes in the porta hepatis and peripancreatic regions, since the presence of metastatic disease would preclude a chance for radical curative surgery.

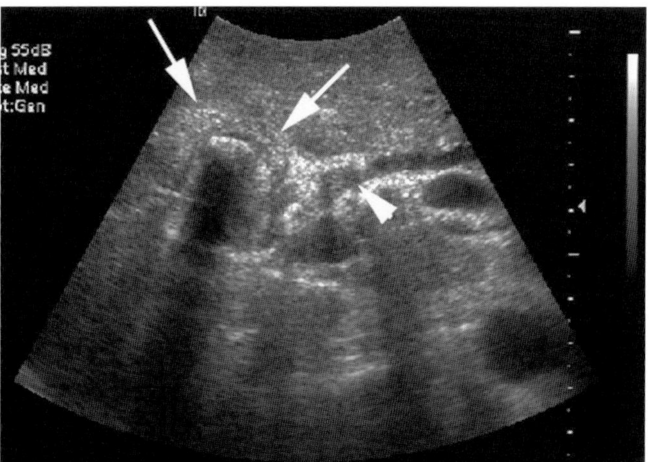

FIGURE 12 ■ Gallbladder carcinoma. IOUS image demonstrates a mass (*arrows*) surrounding a central gallstone. The arrowhead indicates an extension of the tumor to the left hepatic duct, which is partially obstructed and dilated.

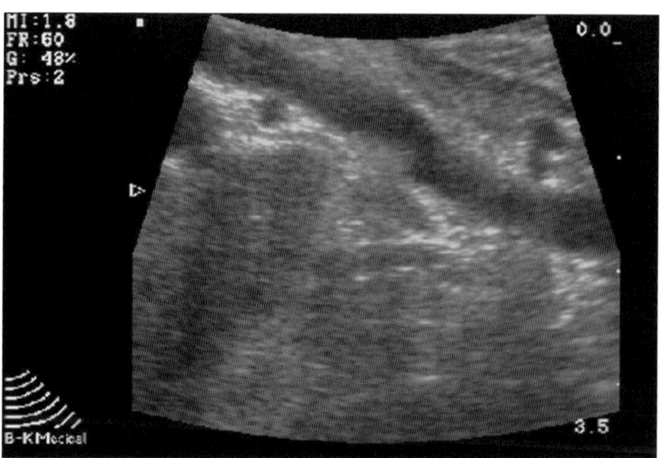

FIGURE 13 ■ Laparoscopic ultrasound image at 7.5 MHz of the common duct in long axis. There is some near-field reverberation artifact, but this is minimized by imaging at the highest possible frequency.

IOUS of the bile ducts has been established as at least as good, if not superior, to intraoperative cholangiography (22), and similar conclusions have been drawn regarding LUS (Fig. 13) for assessment of possible choledocholithiasis (23). In fact, LUS imaging is regarded by many as preferable to laparoscopic cholangiography, which is more technically difficult and time consuming when compared with LUS imaging. In simple choledocholithiasis however, many of these patients have had the diagnosis made preoperatively by ultrasound or MRI, occasionally by CT imaging, and also by endoscopic retrograde cholangiopancreatography. Consequently, the routine use of laparoscopic cholangiography is not advised, since the yield of positive studies has proven to be quite low (24).

There are many other uses for IOUS imaging in the biliary tract, however. In patients with biliary strictures, whether benign or malignant, IOUS or LUS imaging is of great help in determining the extent of the stricture, particularly those which extend into the intrahepatic ductal system, helping to define the optimal surgical approach. With malignant strictures secondary to the so-called Klatzkin-type cholangiocarcinoma, the full extent of the tumor is often difficult to predict with both preoperative and intraoperative imaging due to the extensive sclerotic inflammatory component of these tumors. But, in certain cases, the tumor is well identified with intraoperative imaging (25,26), such that an optimal resection plane and site of hepaticojejunostomy can be facilitated (Fig. 14). Occasionally, when the central tumor is too extensive into both the right and left systems, a peripheral dilated bile duct can be selected for surgical drainage, particularly if there is a large duct draining Segments II and III along the ligamentum teres. Most of these cases, however, will not be amenable to successful surgical drainage and will require percutaneous biliary catheters.

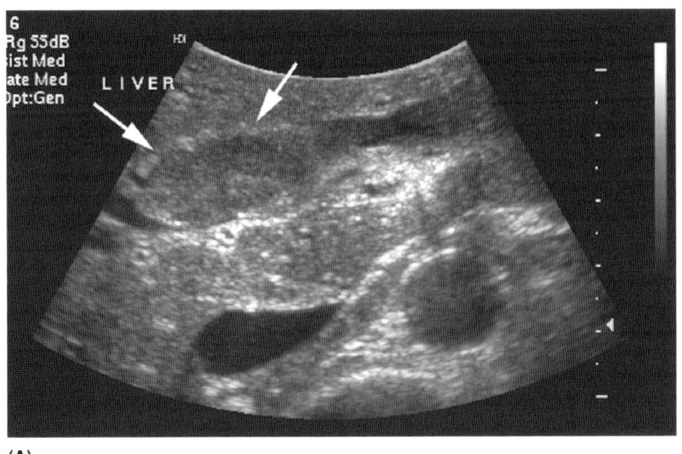

(A)

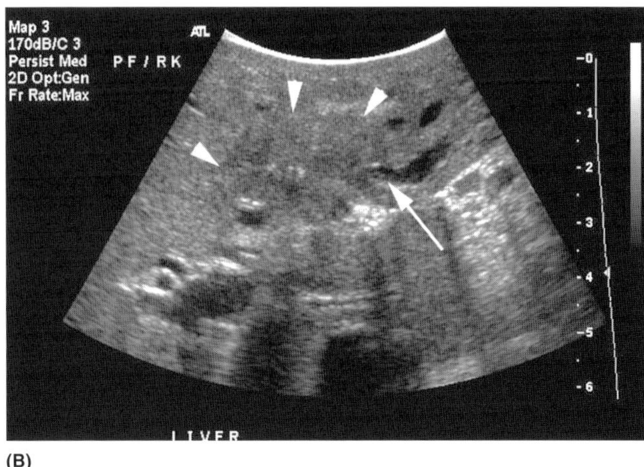

(B)

FIGURE 14 A AND B ■ Cholangiocarcinoma. (A) IOUS demonstrates well-defined cholangiocarcinoma (*arrows*) growing within the lumen of the left hepatic duct. (B) Much more subtle appearance of a Klatztkin tumor (*arrowheads*) obstructing a peripheral left hepatic duct (*arrow*).

IOUS imaging is also useful in other inflammatory and infectious conditions of the biliary tract, including recurrent pyogenic cholangitis and segmental Caroli's disease, both of which may be amenable to a surgical approach of partial hepatectomy and hepaticojejunostomy. Again, the full extent of the disease is essential to depict in order to perform the appropriate surgical procedure or to define those patients in whom a liver resection would not be successful due to residual disease left behind in other portions of the liver. Small intrahepatic biliary stones can be difficult to fully assess with preoperative imaging, but can be readily visualized with IOUS (Fig. 15). Similarly, the surgical approach to choledochal cysts also requires full demonstration of the extent of the disease in order to achieve an adequate resection margin. Since cholangiocarcinoma risk is increased in these conditions, a careful assessment of the entire biliary tract, including the gallbladder, is mandatory to evaluate for any occult sites of tumor.

PANCREAS

For IOUS of the pancreas, an end-fire probe is optimal, either linear or curvilinear array, with frequencies from 5 MHz up to as high as 10 MHz, since the target organ is relatively small. The side-fire probe configuration, favored for liver imaging, is unsuitable for imaging the pancreas because the power cord configuration may prevent adequate contact with the target organ. However, when imaging pancreatic tumors, it is useful to have a side-fire probe available in order to assess for potential liver involvement with metastatic disease. Both IOUS and LUS imaging of the pancreas can be achieved by direct contact

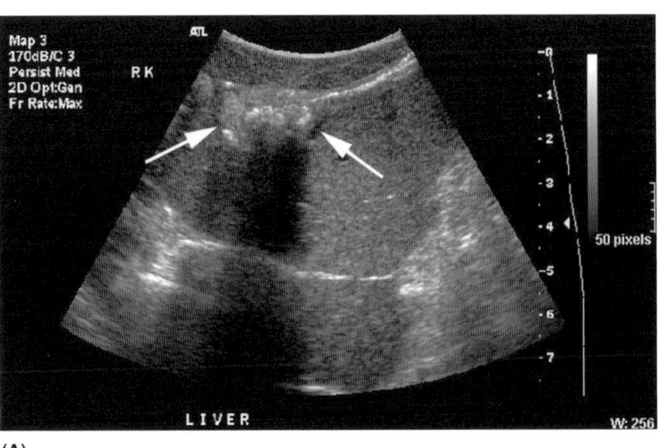

(A)

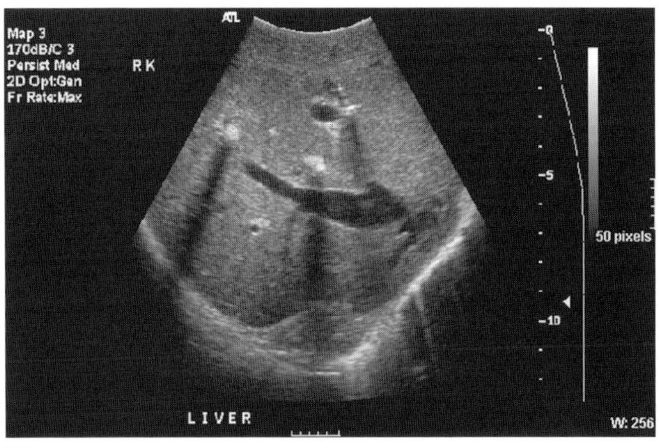

(B)

FIGURE 15 A AND B ■ Recurrent pyogenic cholangitis. (A) IOUS image showing sludge and stones (*arrows*) in a markedly distended left hepatic duct. (B) In the same patient, small right lobe stones are demonstrated by IOUS, which were not visualized on preoperative imaging studies. Note acoustic shadowing behind these 3- to 4-mm stones.

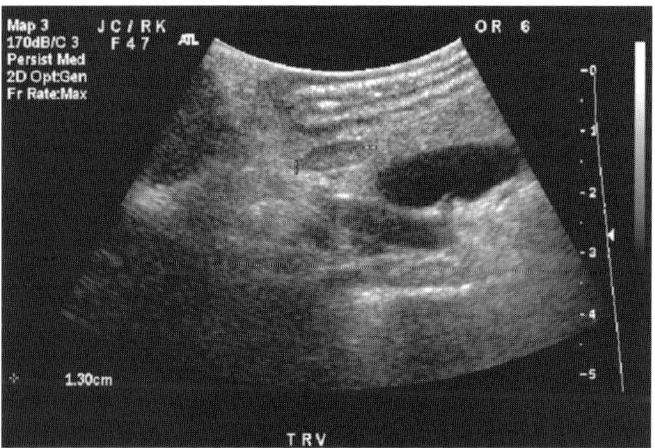

FIGURE 16 ■ Insulinoma. IOUS image of a 5×13mm nonpalpable insulinoma (calipers) in the pancreatic head.

with the overlying peritoneal surface, by scanning through compressed overlying bowel or by filling the deep abdominal cavity with sterile saline for a water standoff. A curvilinear sector array LUS probe is preferable to a straight linear array, since a wider area of anatomy is portrayed in the sector format, which can be helpful in orientation. We prefer to use a left upper quadrant or right upper quadrant port for imaging the pancreas, in order that the probe may be oriented down the long axis of the organ in a relatively transverse orientation.

As with the liver, IOUS imaging of the pancreas has changed substantially in the past 5 to 10 years due to the considerable advances in preoperative multidetector CT and MRI as well as in endoscopic ultrasound and octreotide nuclear medicine scanning. Nevertheless, there remains an important role for IOUS imaging in both benign and malignant tumors of the pancreas.

IOUS imaging is capable of identifying tiny, functioning islet cell tumors as small as 3 to 5mm in diameter, some of which are too small to be palpated by the surgeon. Most islet cell tumors are homogeneous in nature and appear as hypoechoic masses (Fig. 16), standing out against the relatively hyperechoic pancreatic parenchyma (27). Apart from the multiple endocrine neoplasia syndromes, most insulinomas are solitary, benign, and intrapancreatic in location (28). In contrast, gastrinomas are much more frequently malignant, multiple, and are also commonly seen in extrapancreatic locations (29) such as peripancreatic lymph nodes and within the "gastrinoma triangle," which is the area between the common duct, the second and third portions of the duodenum, and the head of the pancreas. Indeed, gastrinomas may be present in the wall of the duodenum in this location. Other types of islet cell tumors, such as glucagonomas and somatostatinomas, are also more often malignant than insulinomas and tend to be more frequently located in the body and tail of the pancreas.

While most islet cell tumors are not locally aggressive, they all possess the potential for metastatic disease, even insulinomas, and therefore the liver should be carefully scanned for occult metastatic disease. Metastasis to local lymph nodes is also occasionally seen in the more aggressive islet cell malignancies. It is rare, however, for islet cell tumors to obliterate or invade surrounding vascular structures. LUS imaging of the pancreas is becoming more important in islet cell tumors of the pancreas (30), since techniques for laparoscopic partial pancreatic resections have been developed, which may allow resection of these small, functional tumors without the necessity for open surgical laparotomy. These tumors can be readily identified and markers can be placed close to the margins of the

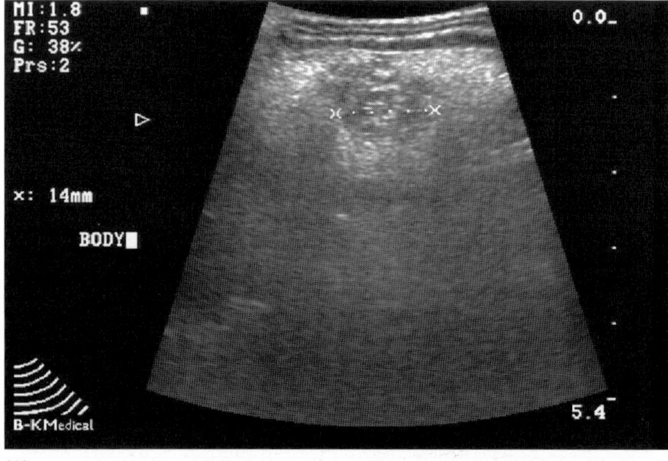

(A)

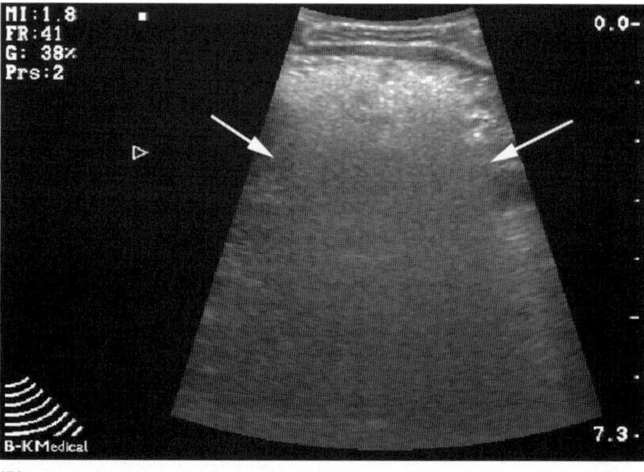

(B)

FIGURE 17 A AND B ■ Pancreatic pseudomass. (**A**) Laparoscopic ultrasound image of a known 1.4cm pancreatic lipoma (*calipers*) seen on preoperative CT and MRI. (**B**) Same patient with ill-defined mass in pancreatic head, suspicious for tumor on preoperative scans. LUS image shows ill-defined mass with acoustic shadowing (*arrows*) consistent with focal fatty infiltration forming a pseudomass in the pancreas. Therefore, no biopsy or further surgery was done and this area has remained stable on follow-up imaging.

tumor for guidance for the surgeon undertaking a laparoscopic resection. Typically, laparoscopic surgical clips are placed on either side of the tumor under direct ultrasound guidance, with confirmation of appropriate clip placement by imaging the acoustic shadow generated from these clips.

Unlike islet cell tumors of the pancreas, ductal adenocarcinoma of the pancreas is typically a highly aggressive tumor, frequently invading the surrounding vasculature, such as the celiac and SMA, the superior mesenteric and portal veins, as well as obstructing the common bile duct or pancreatic duct. The majority of these tumors are inoperable at presentation, and both CT and MRI, and even preoperative ultrasound, are quite accurate in predicting unresectability. In the subset of patients which are judged potentially operable by preoperative imaging, there is a significant role for IOUS (31) or LUS imaging (Fig. 17). Many of these patients will have metastatic disease involving the omentum or mesentery, or even small surface liver metastases (32). These can usually be detected well by laparoscopy and confirmed with laparoscopic biopsies. However, if staging laparoscopy is to be complete, LUS imaging of the liver should also be performed to search for small occult liver metastases which may not have been demonstrated on preoperative studies (33). LUS-guided biopsies of such lesions can be performed to confirm metastatic disease (Fig. 18) and obviate the need for a failed laparotomy in patients with incurable pancreatic carcinoma (34).

In some patients, the preoperative imaging may be equivocal regarding invasion of critical vascular structures, such as the superior mesenteric vein, celiac artery, SMA, or portal vein. LUS or IOUS imaging is often helpful in evaluating these patients, as well. The excellent spatial resolution afforded by high frequency IOUS imaging can accurately depict the extent of tumor and invasion of these critical vascular structures (Fig. 19).

IOUS imaging has a role in cystic pancreatic neoplasms, as well, and is helpful in distinguishing the small, thin-walled cyst cavities of serous microcystic adenomas from the more potentially malignant mucinous cystadenomas (Fig. 20) and cystadenocarcinomas, which typically have thicker, more irregular septa and mural nodularity, which can be very accurately identified by ultrasound (35). Intraductal papillary mucinous tumors of the pancreas can be well assessed by IOUS (36), both by demonstrating echogenic papillary masses growing within the pancreatic ducts (Fig. 21) and by delineating the multiple small side-branch cysts, which help define the extent of the neoplasm, thereby helping in defining the most appropriate plane for surgical resection. Pathologic confirmation of clear surgical margins by frozen section is, of course, essential to confirm completeness of the surgical resection.

In patients with chronic relapsing pancreatitis, IOUS may facilitate surgical drainage of pseudocysts and obstructed pancreatic ducts (37). While most pseudocysts can be drained surgically without any additional imaging, if a Puestow pancreaticojejunostomy-type drainage is required, IOUS imaging can dramatically facilitate this

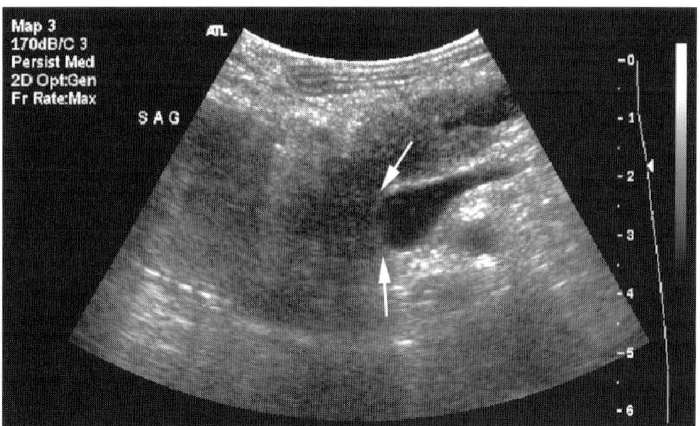

FIGURE 19 ■ Inoperable pancreatic carcinoma. IOUS image shows invasion of the lateral margin of the portal vein (*arrows*), making this an unresectable lesion. SAG, sagittal.

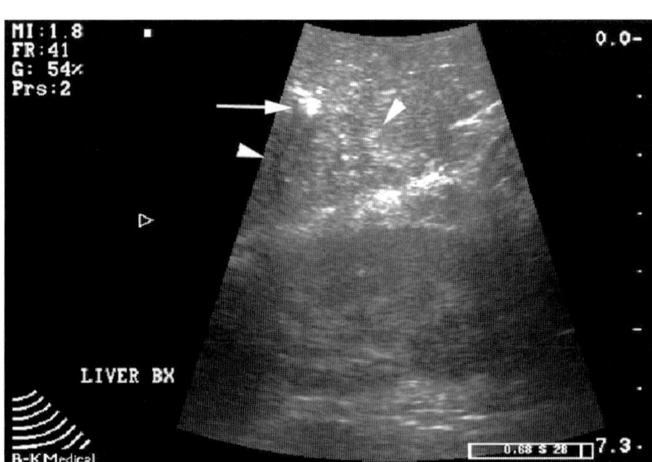

FIGURE 18 ■ Liver metastasis. Laparoscopic ultrasound (LUS) image with arrowheads delineating a subtle metastasis from pancreatic carcinoma. Arrow indicates the advancing LUS-guided biopsy needle, confirming the metastasis and avoiding unnecessary laparotomy.

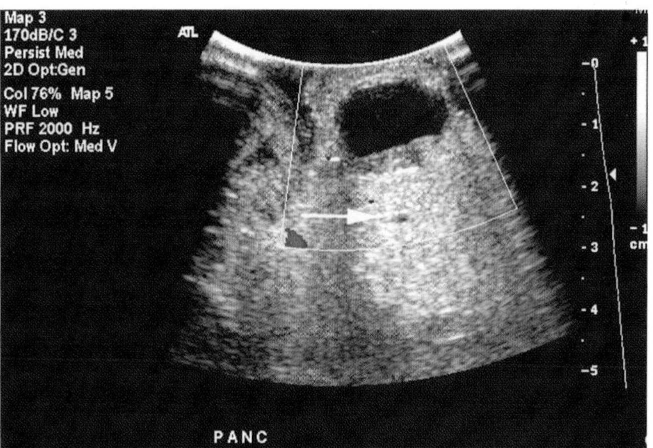

FIGURE 20 ■ Mucinous cystadenoma of the pancreas. IOUS image demonstrates a small, slightly thick-walled, cystic mass. Arrow indicates cross-section of the normal pancreatic duct 8 mm deep to the mass, thereby allowing for a safe, simple wedge resection of the mass, rather than a Whipple procedure. PANC, pancreas.

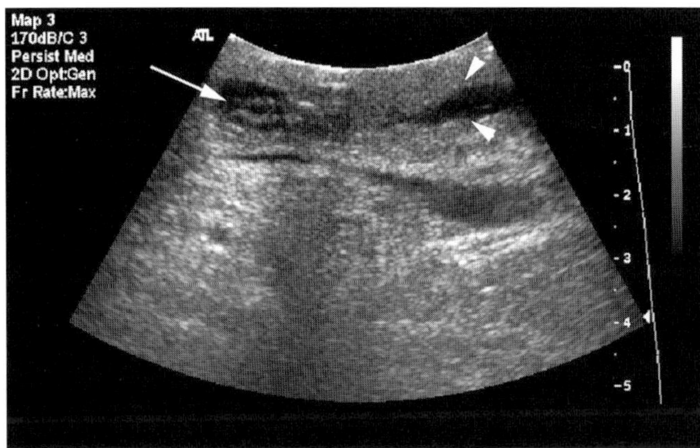

FIGURE 21 ■ Intraductal papillary mucinous tumor. IOUS image demonstrates papillary tumor growing in the pancreatic duct (*arrow*) causing dilatation of the more distal pancreatic duct toward the tail (*arrowheads*).

surgery. The pancreas is frequently rock-hard and both the pancreatic duct and the pancreatic parenchyma are filled with calcifications and stones, such that identification of the position of the pancreatic duct within the fibrotic gland is virtually impossible by palpation. With IOUS imaging, the pancreatic duct is easily identified, even when filled with many stones, and the optimal location for pancreatotomy can be identified. The use of color flow and Doppler imaging is important to ascertain that the incision site selected is in a safe, avascular plane. We will often direct a needle into the pancreatic duct under direct IOUS visualization. This needle can then be used as a visual guide to the surgeon while resecting through the pancreas into the pancreatic duct for Puestow drainage (Fig. 22). IOUS or LUS guidance can also be employed for biopsy of pancreatic masses, to distinguish inflammatory from neoplastic lesions, as well as for drainage of fluid collections or placement of surgical clips for subsequent resection, or as markers for postoperative radiation therapy.

RENAL

The use of IOUS for detection and localization of renal calculi was one of the very first reported uses of this modality. The first report in 1961 by Schlegel described the use of A-mode ultrasonography (1), but more widespread use of IOUS did not occur until B-mode ultrasound scanning was available. In a report by Sigel in 1982, this technique was described as very effective in defining the optimal site for renal cortical incision, reducing total intraoperative time and improving the results of complete stone fragment extraction (38). The widespread use of extracorporal shockwave lithotripsy and percutaneous techniques for stone dissolution and extraction has dramatically reduced the requirement for IOUS in treatment of renal calculi, but surgery is still occasionally required for removal of large staghorn calculi. In this setting, the use of IOUS with color flow and pulsed Doppler is useful in helping to define the optimal avascular plane for making the cortical incision, minimizing damage to the vascular supply, and helping to preserve renal parenchyma from ischemic damage (39,40).

Nephron-sparing partial resection of small renal neoplasms has grown in popularity, particularly as cross-sectional imaging more frequently finds these small, 1 to 3 cm, asymptomatic tumors. Laparoscopic hand-assisted resection of small renal cell carcinomas is a very effective surgical technique, and IOUS imaging is often requested in order to define the deep margins of the tumor and its relationship to surrounding vascular structures and the intrarenal collecting system (Fig. 23). Even for lesions that extend to the cortical surface, the deep margins of the tumor are difficult to assess without IOUS imaging. Adequate surgical margins are required in order to avoid local recurrence, which is estimated to occur in as many as 3% to 13% of patients (41).

For this type of imaging, an end-fire probe of approximately 5 MHz frequency is optimal. Again, a sector format

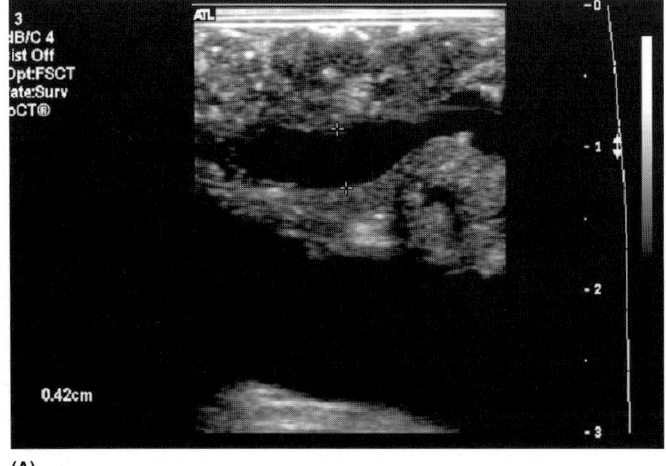

(A)

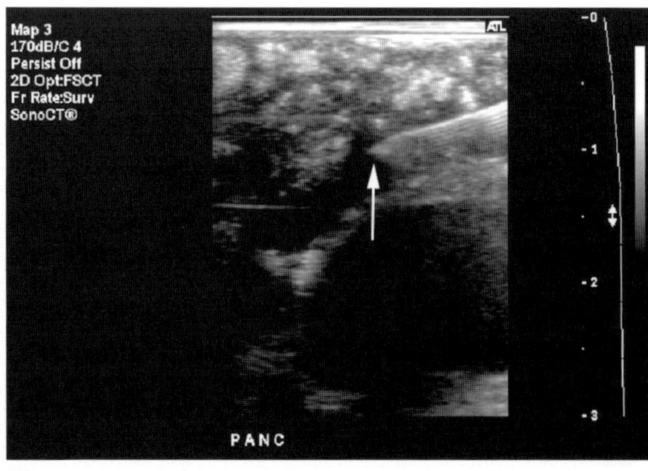

(B)

FIGURE 22 A AND B ■ Chronic pancreatitis. (**A**) IOUS image with calipers demonstrating a dilated pancreatic duct with a stricture in the neck. (**B**) Arrow indicates the tip of a needle guided into the dilated pancreatic duct under real-time IOUS guidance. PANC, pancreas.

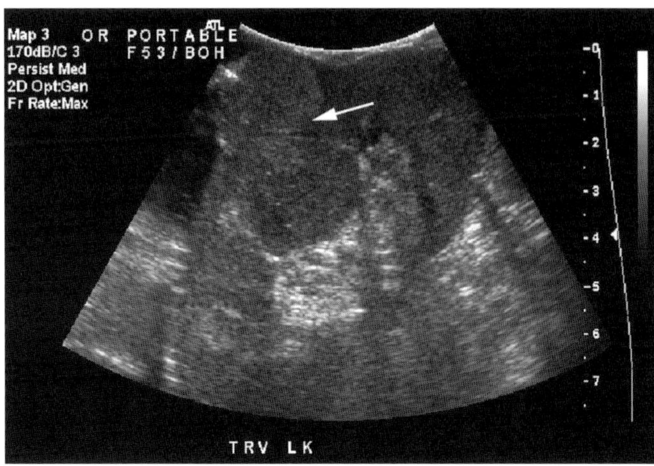

FIGURE 23 ■ Small renal cell carcinoma. IOUS image shows small, slightly hyperechoic renal cell carcinoma, with the deep tumor margin indicated by arrow.

is most desirable in order to obtain proper orientation in a relatively small acoustic field. In larger patients with relatively deep incisions, we have had good success using an end-fire endoluminal probe with appropriate sterile covering, but, in most cases, a standard end-fire intraoperative probe is entirely adequate. The measurement to the deepest portion of the tumor can be determined for the surgeon (42,43) and surgical clips can be placed with ultrasound guidance to mark the edges of the tumor.

With small renal cell carcinomas, the likelihood of venous invasion is minimal, but this occurs frequently in larger tumors. IOUS imaging may be useful in helping to demonstrate tumor invasion into the renal vein and inferior vena cava, and the extent of caval involvement can be well defined (Fig. 24). If the thrombus extends proximally toward the right atrium, a combined retroperitoneal and thoracic surgical approach may be required in order to gain control of the thrombus from above, thereby avoiding the potential for lethal saddle embolus as the thrombus is being extracted.

NEUROSURGERY

Brain

For IOUS brain imaging, end-fire probes in the 5 to 7.5 MHz range are required. Specially designed small footprint probes are available for imaging through very small craniotomy sites or burr holes, but standard endoluminal end-fire probes can also be successfully utilized for imaging and interventional guidance. Initial imaging of the brain is usually performed through the intact dura, which is moistened with sterile saline to provide good acoustic coupling. Sufficient fluid should be placed into the craniotomy site to allow for adequate imaging without requiring pressure on the dura and underlying brain parenchyma.

Many neurosurgeons routinely utilize image guidance systems in the operating suite based on CT or MR scans with stereotactic frame-based systems or virtual reality interactive fusion imaging based on preoperative scans. IOUS can provide the surgeon with an equally effective technique for localizing focal masses in the brain and is much less expensive than the stereotactic or interactive virtual reality systems (44). However, many neurosurgeons are more comfortable with the CT and MR images than with ultrasound, but even using these complex systems, IOUS is occasionally required due to slippage of the stereotactic frame or tissue motion during the surgical procedure (45).

The majority of benign and malignant primary brain tumors, as well as most metastatic brain lesions, are hyperechoic (Fig. 25) in comparison to the surrounding brain tissue (46). The surface of normal brain sulci is moderately echogenic while the deeper tissues are quite hypoechoic and homogeneous. Frequently, a mass is

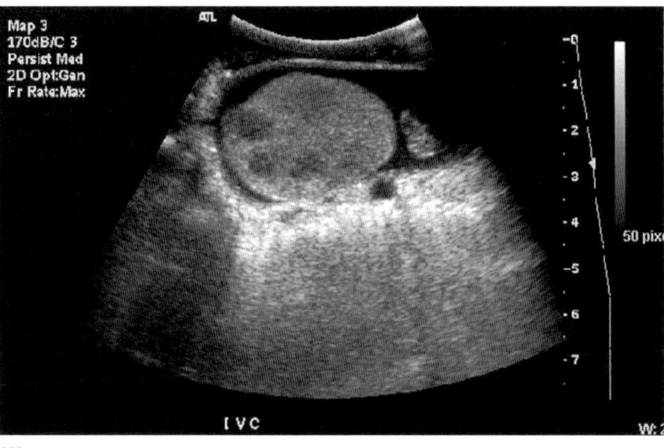

(A)

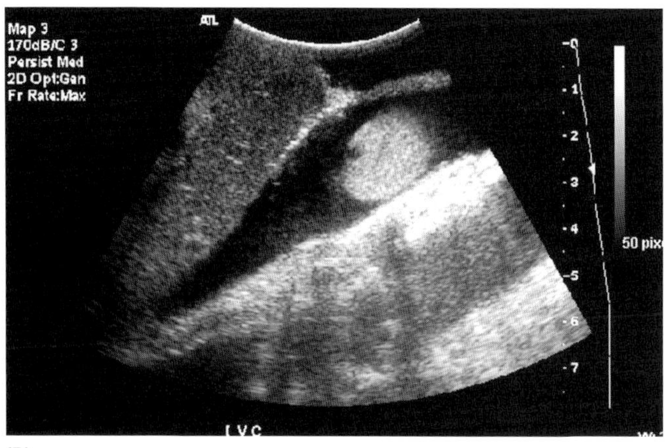

(B)

FIGURE 24 A AND B ■ Tumor thrombus. (A) Large heterogeneous tumor thrombus entering the inferior vena cava (IVC) from the right renal vein. (B) Sagittal view shows thrombus well below the intrahepatic portion of the IVC.

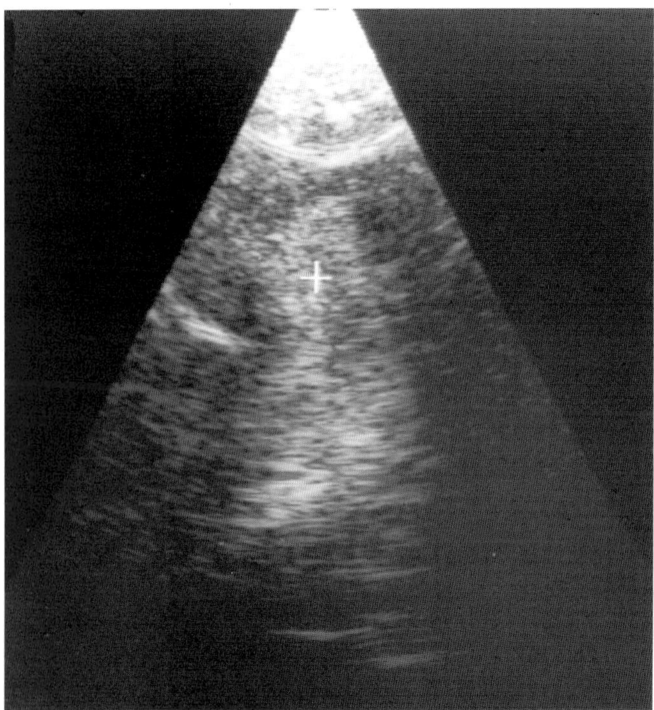

FIGURE 25 ■ Brain metastasis. Hyperechoic lung metastasis is marked by the caliper and readily distinguishable from the surrounding edematous brain parenchyma.

associated with acute edematous swelling of the brain which makes the lesions appear even more echogenic and increases the conspicuity of tumors (47). However, certain patients with longstanding brain tumors may develop a chronic edematous pattern, which may actually increase echogenicity of brain tissue, and this can decrease the conspicuity of focal masses (Fig. 26) (48).

The most highly echogenic brain lesions are usually meningiomas, and especially those with calcifications, which occur frequently. Glioblastomas and other primary

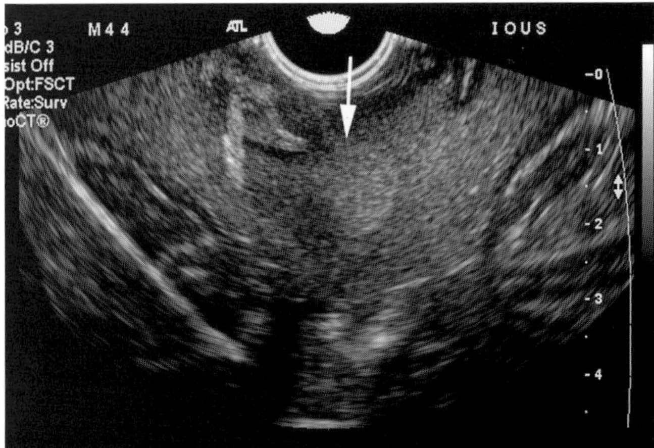

FIGURE 26 ■ Lymphoma. Arrow delineates a hyperechoic B cell lymphoma nodule, which is difficult to identify due to the increased brain echogenicity from chronic edema.

brain tumors, as well as most metastases and even lymphoma tend to be hyperechoic and are usually well circumscribed and sharply marginated. The more aggressive glioblastomas may have less well-defined margins as they infiltrate into surrounding brain parenchyma (49). Hypoechoic areas of fluid accumulation may be seen in brain tumors due to liquefaction necrosis, but cystic spaces are also frequently seen in certain types of cystic astrocytomas. The cyst cavities, septations, and solid components of the cystic tumors may be better depicted by IOUS than by preoperative imaging (Fig. 27). Low grade astrocytomas and some lymphomas and inflammatory/infectious brain lesions are often less echogenic and less well marginated and, hence, may be difficult to precisely identify and delineate with IOUS. Distortion of the sulcal groove pattern or compression of surface brain markings may help identify the tumor, and the use of color flow or power Doppler, demonstrating deformity and displacement of vessels, may also be useful in defining the borders of these subtle lesions (50).

If a complete surgical resection is planned, IOUS is useful in helping to define the most optimal path to expose the lesion with the least amount of damage to surrounding brain tissue and vascular structures. Following resection, the surgical excision site can be evaluated by filling with sterile saline and repeat IOUS imaging to assess for any sites of residual tumor (Fig. 27). If a lesion is unresectable, surgical decompression of cystic or liquefied tumors can be facilitated by IOUS guidance.

Real-time IOUS imaging guidance is extremely accurate and efficient, allowing precise placement of neurosurgical biopsy needles and catheters with real-time guidance (51). This can be done as a free hand technique or with fixed electronic real-time biopsy guides; we frequently use end-fire endoluminal probes with biopsy guides to allow for biopsy of lesions through small craniotomy sites (52) or to direct ventricular shunt catheters (53) or aspiration devices to drain intracranial abscesses and fluid collections (Fig. 28). We routinely use color flow imaging as an adjunct to help define the least vascular path for placing the biopsy needle or catheter in order to minimize damage to major blood vessels in the path between the probe and the target site (Fig. 29).

If biopsies or other interventions are performed, it is useful to reimage the patients after the procedure for several minutes in order to assess for potential acute hemorrhage into the lesion at the site of biopsy or aspiration. Acute bleeding into a tumor or brain parenchyma will typically appear as single or multiple, small, hyperechoic foci, which may enlarge or become confluent over time (54). Occasionally, a fluid/blood level may be seen if there is bleeding into a previous cystic space. Most postprocedure bleeding does not require intervention and will stabilize over time. Therefore, if hemorrhage is identified, the area should be scanned for several minutes to assess for stabilization.

IOUS imaging can be helpful in the surgical approach to AV malformations, many of which are poorly visualized by gray scale imaging. However, the use of color flow and power Doppler imaging may be very helpful in

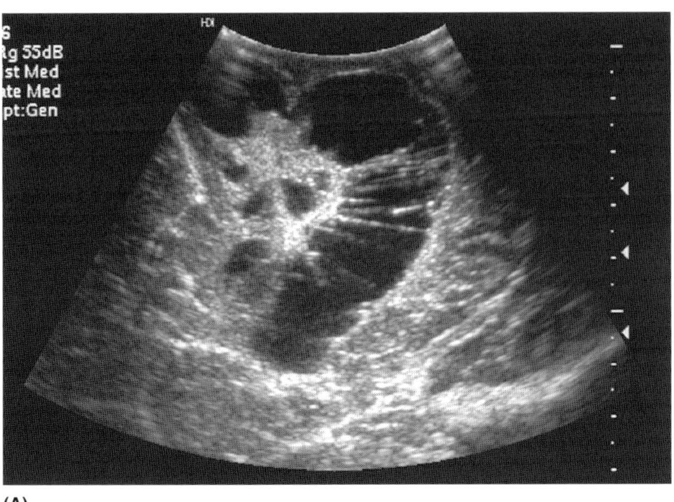

(A)

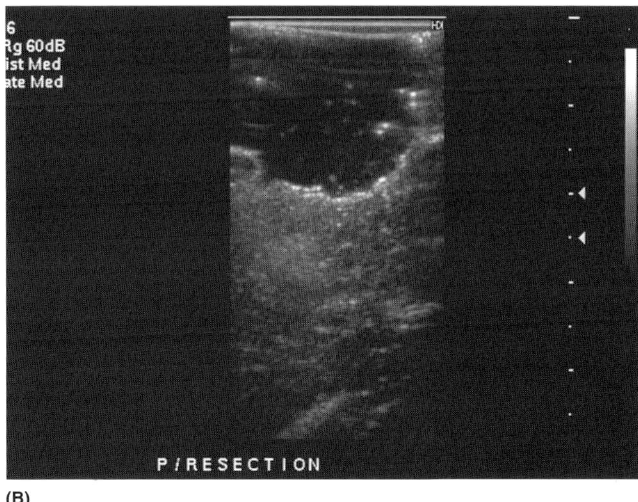

(B)

FIGURE 27 A AND B ■ Cystic glioma. (**A**) The IOUS image elegantly demonstrates the cystic septated and solid portions of this tumor. (**B**) Following resection, the excision site is filled with sterile saline and repeat imaging demonstrates no evidence of residual tumor.

defining the extent of these occult lesions (55). IOUS color flow or power Doppler imaging is also useful in patients who are being treated for intracranial aneurysms, in order to assess the cessation of blood flow after clipping and also to look for any postprocedure hemorrhage.

Spine

As with brain imaging, small footprint end-fire probes are required for IOUS of the spinal cord and surrounding tissues. However, the frequencies can be increased up to 7 to 10 MHz since the depth of tissues being imaged is only a few centimeters. When possible, the laminectomy site is filled with degassed saline to provide an acoustic window for the ultrasound probe, similar to the approach for brain imaging. At times, with cervical spine neurosurgery, the patient is in the upright position, which makes more of a technical challenge to achieve good acoustic coupling. Care should be taken to avoid tearing the sterile probe covers on bony protrusions at the edges of the laminectomy

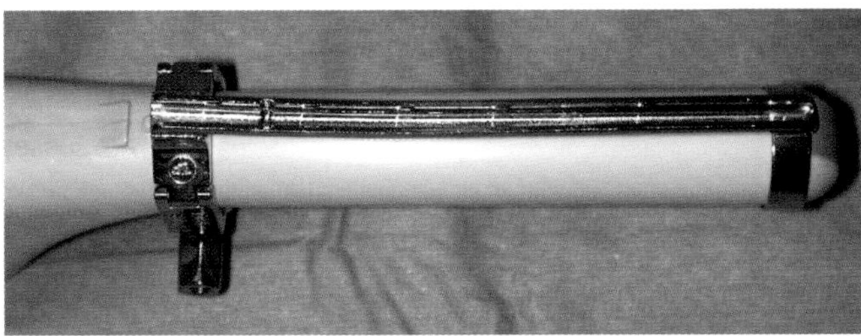

(A)

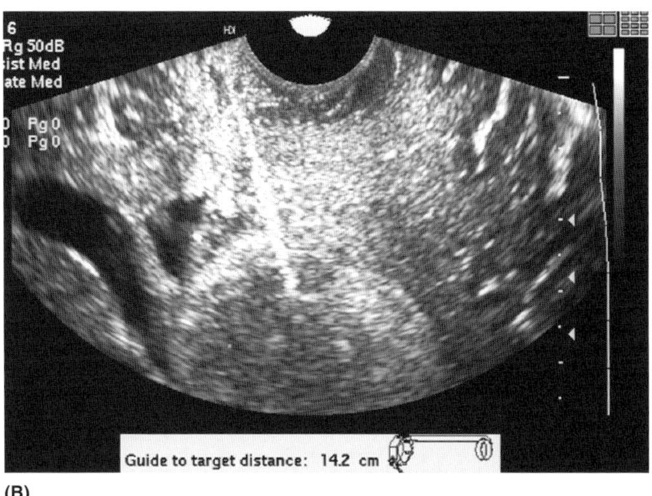

(B)

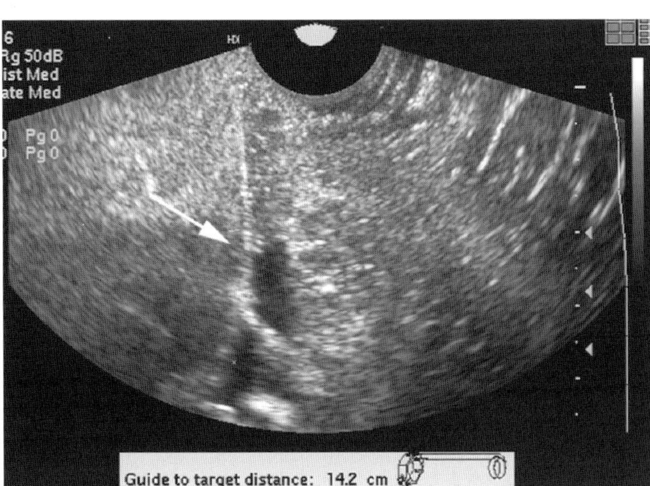

(C)

FIGURE 28 A–C ■ IOUS biopsy. (**A**) Standard endoluminal probe with biopsy guide, which is useful for accurately directing biopsies and drainages through small burr holes. (**B**) The brain biopsy needle course is shown as the echogenic line extending from the brain surface into the target lesion. (**C**) In the same AIDS patient, the needle is then precisely passed into the dilated lateral ventricle (*arrow*) in order to obtain cerebrospinal fluid for culture.

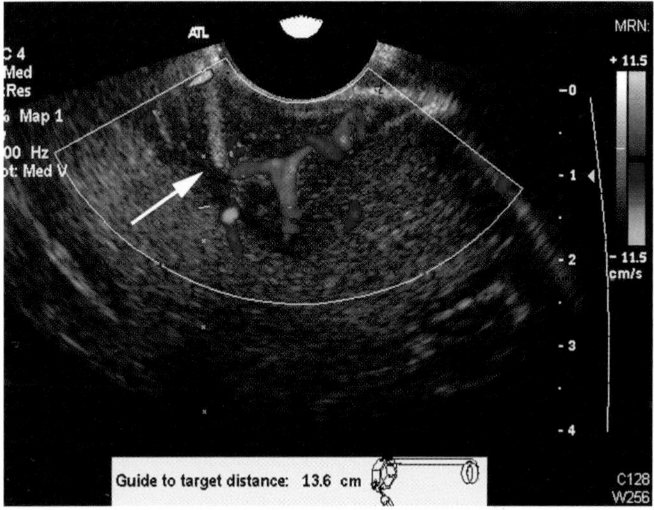

FIGURE 29 ■ Hypervascular glioblastoma. Arrow indicates tip of biopsy needle. The precision of real-time guidance allowed for safe biopsy of the less vascular portions of this lesion.

site, and, again, as in the brain, excess pressure on the dural surface must be avoided since the underlying spinal cord could be injured by excess pressure.

The normal spinal cord is a hypoechoic structure with very little intrinsic architecture defined by IOUS, other than the paired echogenic lines of the central canal, which is readily seen and an important anatomic landmark of normal spinal cord anatomy (56). Other normal anatomic features that may be visualized include the dentate ligaments, which arise from the dorsolateral margins of the cord and are best seen in axial views as thin linear structures. Nerve roots may also be imaged as either single or paired linear structures within the dural sac, and these are especially well seen in the distal regions of the conus medullaris and cauda equina (Fig. 30). The dural sac itself is a brightly echogenic line and can be imaged both posteriorly and anteriorly, as can the cerebrospinal fluid bathing the spinal cord. The arachnoid membrane is closely applied to the cord and is usually not distinctly imaged. The anterior spinal artery may be visualized in gray scale as a pulsating structure and this vessel and other smaller vessels may be imaged using color flow and power Doppler imaging.

The principal use of IOUS imaging in the spine is for localization and definition of the extent of various neoplastic, inflammatory, or infectious masses involving the cord and surrounding spaces and tissue planes (57). Tumors are generally well visualized and can be accurately defined as intramedullary, intradural-extramedullary, and/or extramedullary in location (58,59). The full extent of tumors can be precisely defined (Fig. 31) and those with extramedullary component or extradural component (such as neurofibromas) can be accurately depicted, and this information is extremely helpful for planning surgical resection.

Certain intramedullary tumors of the cord are hyperechoic, including dermoids, ependymomas, and many metastatic lesions. However, more lesions in the cord are relatively isoechoic and, hence, more difficult to precisely define than is seen with intraoperative brain imaging. In particular, spinal cord astrocytomas can be difficult to image since they have poorly defined margins and are similar in echogenicity to the surrounding cord (60). Deformity or obliteration of the central spinal canal may be the only compelling ultrasound feature to indicate the location of some of these subtle astrocytomas. However, similar appearance can also be caused by other conditions, including transverse myelitis and post-traumatic cord injury, which may be indistinguishable from infiltrative astrocytoma (61). The cord swelling and obliteration of the central spinal canal, however, can at least

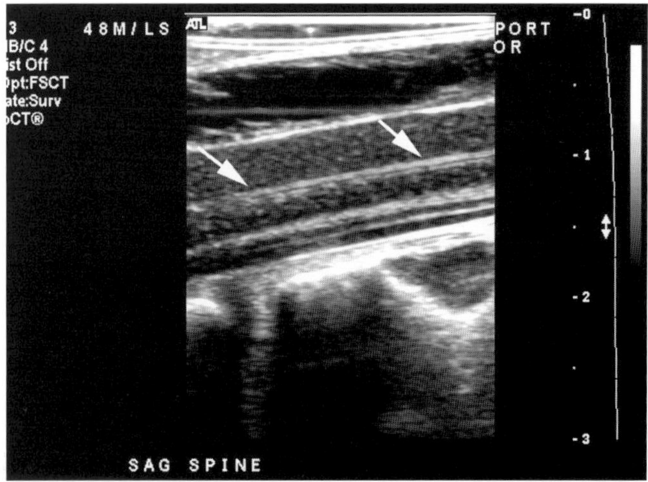

(A)

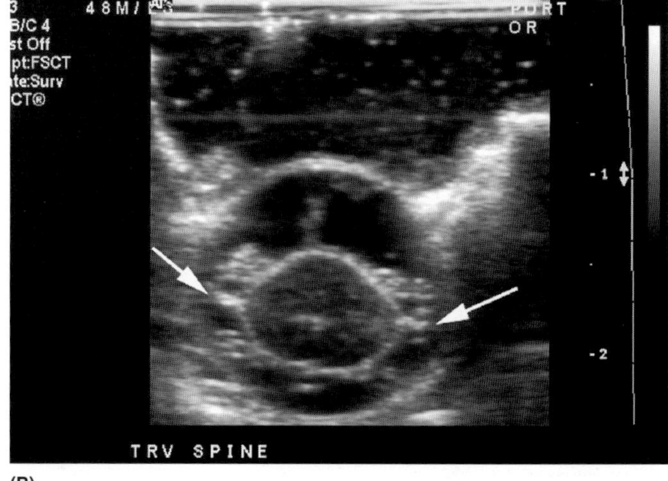

(B)

FIGURE 30 A AND B ■ Normal cervical spinal cord. (A) Sagittal image through the intact dura shows the cord and central spinal canal, as indicated by the arrows. (B) Transverse image at the same level again shows the central canal as an echogenic dot in the middle of the cord. Arrows indicate the dentate ligaments, and several dorsal and ventral nerve roots can be seen within the subarachnoid fluid.

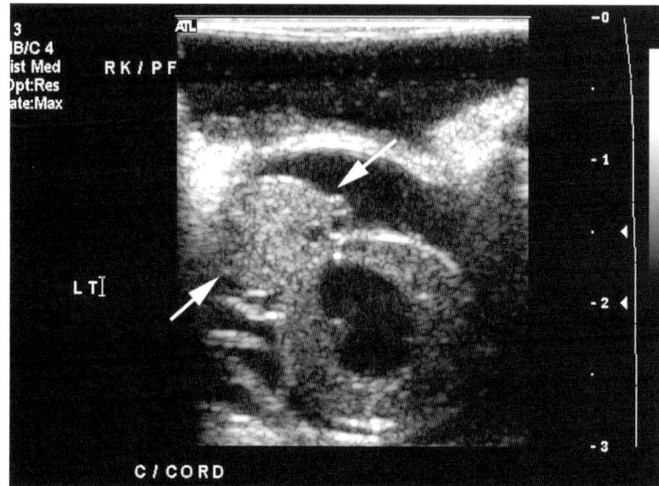

FIGURE 31 ■ Hemangioblastoma. This mass arises from the cervical cord, but also has a large extramedullary intradural extent (*arrows*). Note the distended fluid-filled central spinal canal due to an associated syrinx. LT, left.

define an appropriate site for intraoperative biopsy, which may be the only means to distinguish infiltrative tumor from non-neoplastic inflammatory or post-traumatic myelitis.

Certain intramedullary tumors may show areas of cystic cavity formation, which can be seen with certain astrocytomas, hemangioblastomas, and ependymomas. The cyst cavities are easily imaged with IOUS and usually can be distinguished from a simple syrinx by virtue of thick septations, mural nodules, or solid components of these tumors (62).

Extramedullary tumors can be difficult to assess visually, particularly those that extend anteriorly, but these are usually well imaged by IOUS, including neurofibromas, meningiomas, and lipomas, as well as non–central nervous system tumors from metastatic disease (Fig. 32) or lymphoma, although these tend more often to be extradural, as well. A variety of other extradural masses can be well assessed by IOUS (63), including disc fragments, foreign bodies, abscesses and hematomas, arachnoid cysts, and bony lesions or bone fragments in patients with spine fractures (64). Most of the tumors tend to be moderately echogenic and vascular supply may be recognized with color flow imaging. Foreign bodies, bone fragments, and disc fragments are usually highly echogenic and are frequently associated with acoustic shadows, with the herniated disc fragments being the least echogenic of these conditions. Hematomas have a variable appearance depending on their age and may be difficult to distinguish from epidural abscesses, although the infected collections usually have a more hyperechoic reactive rim. Arachnoid cysts are easily identified as hypoechoic, thin-walled, fluid collections.

As with many other intraoperative sites, IOUS is an excellent method to guide interventional surgical approaches, such as directing biopsies of tumors to the most appropriate site, avoiding areas of cyst formation and liquefaction necrosis, and also avoiding areas of increased vascularity as defined by color flow or power Doppler imaging. Drainage of the cyst cavities of syringomyelia can be easily accomplished with IOUS guidance (Fig. 33) or, alternatively, placement of intracystic shunt catheters can be successfully performed. Drainages of hematoma or abscess cavities can also be facilitated with IOUS and the completeness of the drainage procedure can be accurately assessed. Residual disc fragments or bony fragments may also be easily identified, helping to avoid incomplete surgical extraction.

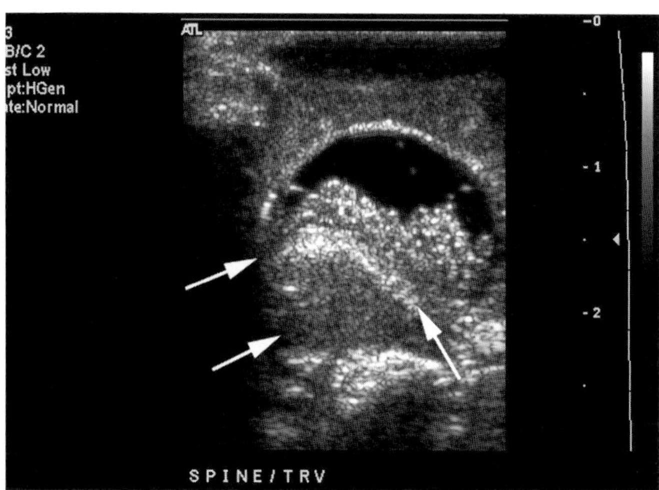

(A)

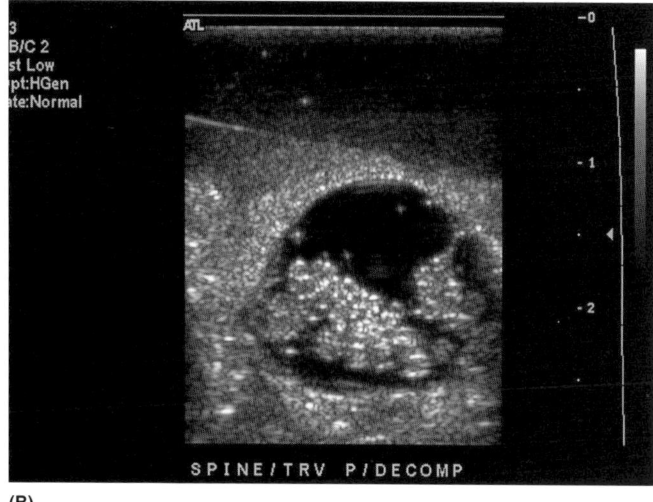

(B)

FIGURE 32 A AND B ■ Metastatic lung cancer. (**A**) Axial IOUS image through the lumbar spinal canal shows a ventral soft tissue mass indenting the spinal canal (*arrows*) secondary to metastatic lung cancer. (**B**) Following surgical resection, the lumbar sac has returned to a normal, rounded configuration with multiple roots of the cauda equina seen within the sac.

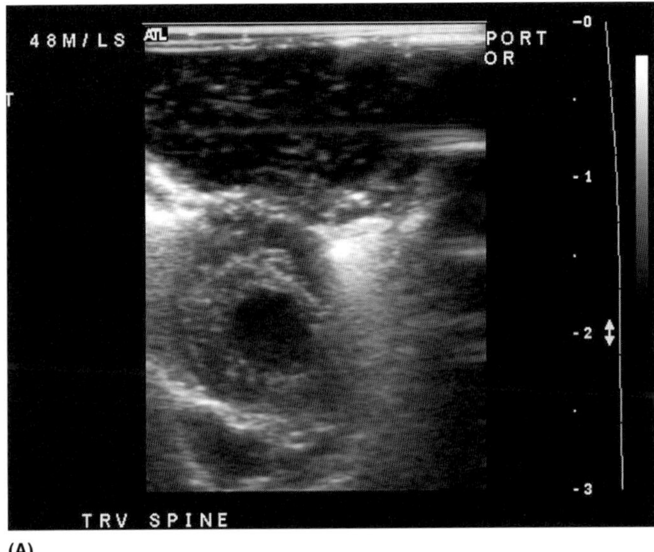

(A)

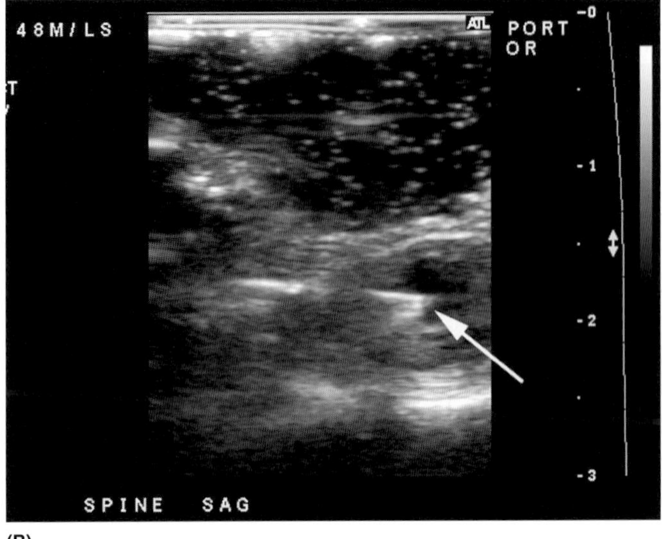

(B)

FIGURE 33 A AND B ■ Syrinx drainage. (**A**) Axial view through the cervical cord shows a central, fluid-filled syrinx cavity. (**B**) Arrow points to the tip of an aspiration needle being positioned in real time within the syrinx cavity.

OTHER APPLICATIONS

There are many other applications for intraoperative ultrasonography, and as familiarity with this technique grows, more and more applications are found. For instance, there are advocates for IOUS localization of nonpalpable breast masses (Fig. 34) which are undergoing surgical excisional biopsy (65). The optimal site for skin incision and the depth from skin to the mass can be readily ascertained for the surgeon. For deeper lesions, real-time placement of localization wires can be performed just prior to the surgical incision.

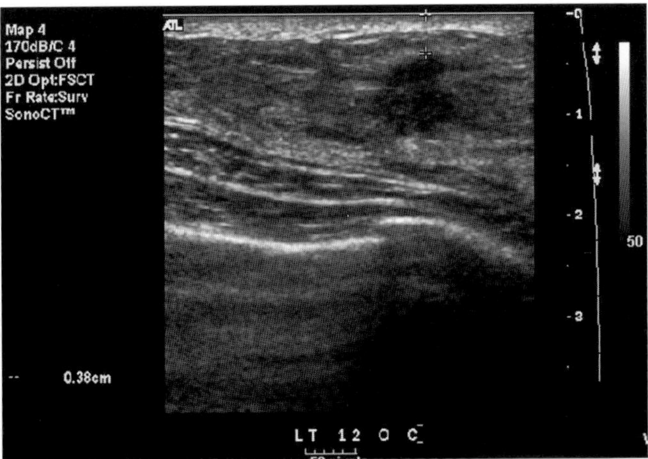

FIGURE 34 ■ Breast carcinoma. Calipers are seen measuring the distance from skin to the anterior margin of a lobulated breast carcinoma. Many surgeons prefer intraoperative ultrasound localization in order to better define the optimal site for skin incision in patients undergoing lumpectomy only.

Similarly, IOUS localization is useful for localization of nonpalpable neck masses, such as recurrent or residual parathyroid adenomas (66), or metastatic lymphadenopathy in patients with papillary carcinoma of the thyroid. Palpation of these masses can be difficult in patients who have had previous neck exploration and/or radiation, and IOUS localization is an excellent method for accurate identification of these lesions and limitation of unnecessary surgical exploration.

While we have discussed renal IOUS scanning in a previous section, there are numerous other uses for IOUS in the genitourinary system. IOUS is often used in the treatment of prostate cancer, either to monitor intraoperative ablation procedures (67), or to guide the placement of radioactive seeds within the prostate for brachytherapy (68,69). During gynecologic surgical procedures, IOUS can play an important role in guiding proper placement of curetting and biopsy instruments into the endocervical or endometrial canal (70), particularly if passage is difficult due to the configuration of the uterus or to the presence of uterine masses, such as fibroids. IOUS monitoring can help avoid perforations of the uterus due to difficult instrumentation. LUS imaging may be useful during endoscopic evaluation of adnexal pathology, such as hydrosalpinx, or for evaluation of the internal architecture and vascularity of adnexal masses.

LUS has also been utilized for staging tumors of the esophagogastric junction and stomach, combined with laparoscopy. Many of these patients had peritoneal metastases or small surface metastases on the liver which were readily seen by laparoscopy (71), but a small percentage had deeper liver metastases only discovered by LUS (72). Confirmation of metastases required biopsy, and, in some cases, this could be accomplished with LUS guidance. In other cases, this was not possible and, for esophagogastric

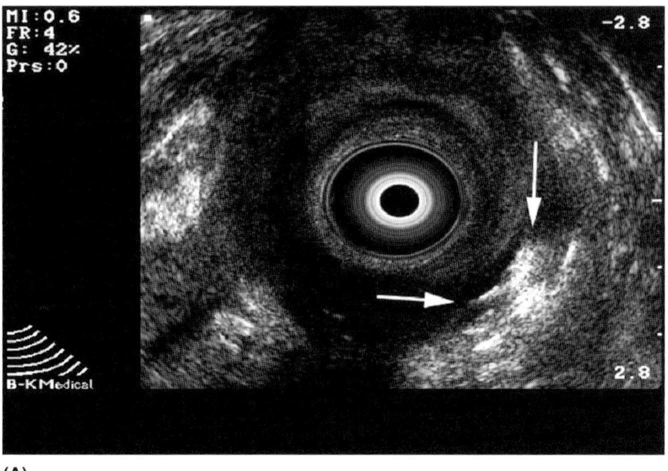

(A)

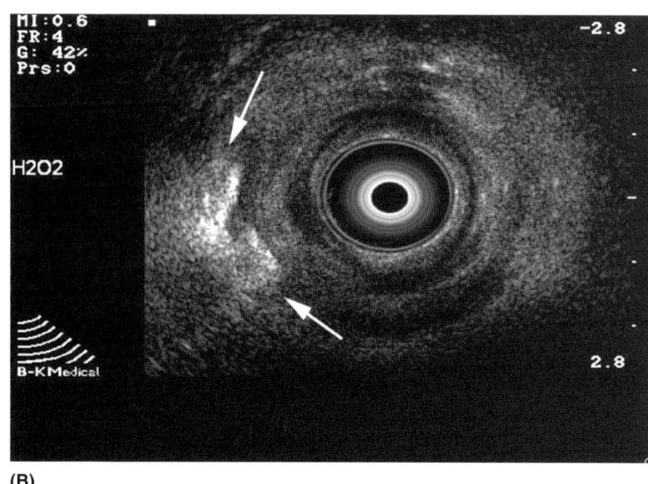

(B)

FIGURE 35 A AND B ■ Horseshoe perianal fistula. (**A**) In a patient with Crohn's disease and multiple failed attempts at fistula drainage and repair, intraoperative transanal ultrasound with H_2O_2 injection demonstrates bubbles within a transsphincteric fistula and abscess in the left posterolateral ischial anal fossa (*arrows*). (**B**) Continued injection demonstrates microbubbles in a right posterolateral transsphincteric abscess (*arrows*), confirming a horseshoe type perianal fistula.

tumors, the overall contribution of LUS in addition to laparoscopy is fairly small (73).

Transanal ultrasound is useful in the intraoperative treatment and drainage of perianal abscesses. Hydrogen peroxide ultrasound fistulography can be performed in the operating suite to delineate the course and complexity of these perianal fistulous tracts (Fig. 35), providing information to help the surgeon select the most appropriate approach to accomplish complete drainage and minimize damage to the perianal sphincter muscles. Transrectal ultrasound for staging of rectal neoplasms is usually accomplished preoperatively but, in the setting of tight anal stenosis, this may be impossible to perform preoperatively, but can be successfully accomplished under anesthesia. Similarly, in patients with tight anal stenosis, ultrasound-guided prostate biopsies may be only achievable in a setting under anesthesia.

Certain institutions highly favor IOUS in assessment vascular surgical procedures (74), such as renal or carotid endarterectomy or bypass grafts. Some studies have demonstrated IOUS findings requiring surgical revision in up to 9% to 11% of reconstructed renal arteries (75). A study from the Mayo Clinic showed minor defects in 30% of IOUS examinations following carotid endarterectomy, and significant abnormalities in 11%, including large intimal flaps or dissections, residual plaque and obstructing thrombus (76). Both gray scale and color flow and Doppler assessments are required for complete evaluation of vascular surgical sites. This use is diminishing somewhat with the proliferation of minimally invasive stent treatment of vascular stenoses.

IOUS imaging has even been proposed as a useful adjunct for patients undergoing chest surgery for resection of pulmonary nodules (77). During video-assisted thoracoscopic surgery, the lung is deflated and the airless lung presents an acoustic signature similar to that of liver. IOUS or LUS has been reported to be successful in localizing pulmonary nodules for wedge resection.

CONCLUSION

Intraoperative and laparoscopic ultrasonography is an exciting and continually developing technique which provides valuable anatomic information to the surgeon, much of which has a critical influence in optimizing surgical decision making (78). This is an efficient and effective technique which helps identify occult lesions, localize known lesions in relation to vascular supply, identify those patients in whom surgical resection would be inappropriate, and guide intraoperative interventional procedures from biopsies and aspirations to intraoperative tumor ablation procedures. The applications continue to grow, particularly with the further development of minimally invasive surgical techniques (79,80). For those interested in ultrasonography and in optimizing patient care, this is a highly satisfying examination which provides invaluable information, and radiologists are encouraged to provide their invaluable assistance in providing and interpreting these scans. Utilizing the strategies presented at the beginning of this chapter, an efficient use of the radiologist's time can be achieved with considerable benefit to patient care.

REFERENCES

1. Schlegel JU, Diggdon P, Cuellar J. The use of ultrasound for localizing renal calculi. J Urol 1961; 86:367–369.
2. Eiseman B, Greenlaw RH, Gallagher JQ. Localization of common duct stones by ultrasound. Arch Surg 1965; 91:195–199.
3. Knight PR, Newell JA. Operative use of ultrasonics in cholelithiasis. Lancet 1963; 1:1023–1025.

4. Kane RA. Intraoperative ultrasonography: history, current state of the art, and future directions. J Ultrasound Med 2004; 23: 1407–1420.
5. Sammons LG, Kane RA. Technical aspect of intraoperative ultrasound. In: Kane RA, ed. Intraoperative, Laparoscopic, and Endoluminal Ultrasound. Philadelphia: Churchill Livingstone/Saunders, 1999:1–11.
6. Kane RA. Laparoscopic ultrasound. In: Kane RA, ed. Intraoperative, Laparoscopic, and Endoluminal Ultrasound, Philadelphia: Churchill Livingstone/Saunders, 1999:90–105.
7. Clarke MP, Kane RA, Steele G Jr, et al. Prospective comparison of preoperative imaging and intraoperative ultrasound in the detection of liver tumors. Surgery 1989; 106:849–855.
8. Gozzetti G, Mazziotti A, Bolondi L, et al. Intraoperative ultrasonography in surgery for liver tumors. Surgery 1989; 99:523–530.
9. Machi J, Isomoto H, Yamashita Y, et al. Intraoperative ultrasonography in screening for liver metastases from colorectal cancer: comparative accuracy with traditional procedures. Surgery 1987; 101:678–684.
10. Soyer P, Levesque M, Elias D, et al. Detection of liver metastases from colorectal cancer: comparison of intraoperative US and CT during arterial portography. Radiology 1992; 183:541–544.
11. Nelson RC, Thompson GH, Chezmar JL, et al. CT during arterial portography; diagnostic pitfalls. RadioGraphics 1992; 12: 705–718.
12. Matsui O, Takahashi S, Kadoya M, et al. Pseudolesion in segment IV of the liver at CT during arterial portography: correlation with aberrant gastric venous drainage. Radiology 1994; 193:31–35.
13. Sahani DV, Kalva SP, Tanabe KK, et al. Intraoperative US in patients undergoing surgery for liver neoplasms: comparison with MR imaging. Radiology 2004; 232:810–814.
14. Rydzewski B, Dehdashti F, Gordon BA, et al. Usefulness of intraoperative sonography for revealing hepatic metastases from colorectal cancer in patients selected for surgery after undergoing FDG PET. AJR Am J Roentgenol 2002; 178:353–358.
15. Milson JW, Jerby BL, Kessler H, et al. Prospective, blinded comparison of laparoscopic ultrasonography vs. contrast-enhanced computerized tomography for liver assessment in patients undergoing colorectal carcinoma surgery. Dis Colon Rectum 2000; 43:41–49.
16. John TG, Greig JD, Crosbie JL, et al. Superior staging of liver tumors with laparoscopy and laparoscopic ultrasound (comments). Ann Surg 1994; 220:709–711.
17. Kane RA, Roizental M, Kruskal JB, et al. Preliminary investigation of liver and biliary imaging with a dedicated laparoscopic US system (abstr.). Radiology 1994; 193(P):287.
18. Kruskal JB, Kane RA. Correlative imaging of malignant liver tumors. Semin Ultrasound CT MR 1992; 13:336–354.
19. Herbst CA, Mittlestaedt CA, Staab EV, et al. Intraoperative ultrasonography evaluation of the gallbladder in morbidly obese patients. Ann Surg 1984; 200:691–692.
20. Azuma T, Yoshikawa T, Araida T, et al. Intraoperative evaluation of the depth of invasion of gallbladder cancer. Am J Surg 1999; 178:381–384.
21. Machi J, Sigel B, Zaren HA, et al. Operative ultrasonography during hepatobiliary and pancreatic surgery. World J Surg 1993; 17:640–645.
22. Sigel B, Machi J, Beitler JG, et al. Comparative accuracy of operative ultrasonography and cholangiography in detecting common duct calculi. Surgery 1983; 94:715–720.
23. Jakimowicz J. Laparoscopic intraoperative ultrasonography, equipment, and technique. Semin Laparosc Surg 1994; 1:52–61.
24. Rothlin MA, Schlumpf R, Largiader F. Laparoscopic sonography. Arch Surg 1994; 129:694–700.
25. Kusano T, Shimabukuro M, Tamai O, et al. The use of intraoperative sonography for detecting tumor extension in bile duct carcinoma. Int Surg 1997; 82:44–48.
26. van Delden OM, de Wit LT, van Dijkum EJMN, et al. Value of laparoscopic ultrasonography in staging of proximal bile duct tumors. J Ultrasound Med 1997; 16:7–12.
27. Zeiger MA, Shawker TH, Norton JA. Use of intraoperative ultrasonography to localize islet cell tumors. World J Surg 1993; 17:448–454.
28. Gorman B, Charboneau JW, James EM, et al. Benign pancreatic insulinoma: preoperative sonographic localization. AJR Am J Roentgenol 1986; 147:929–934.
29. Sugg SL, Norton JA, Fraker DL, et al. A prospective study of intraoperative methods to diagnose and resect duodenal gastrinomas. Ann Surg 1993; 218:138–144.
30. Lo CY, Lo CM, Fan ST. Role of laparoscopic ultrasonography in intraoperative localization of pancreatic insulinoma. Surg Endosc 2000; 14:1131–1135.
31. Alberti A, Dattola P, Littori F, et al. Intraoperative ultrasonography in the staging of pancreatic head neoplasms L'ecografia intraoperatoria nella stadiazione delle neoplasie cefalopancreatiche. Chir Ital 2002; 54:59–64.
32. John TG, Greig JD, Carter DC, et al. Carcinoma of the pancreatic head and periampullary region: tumor staging with laparoscopy and laparoscopic ultrasonography. Ann Surg 1995; 221:156–164.
33. van Delden OM, Smits NJ, Bemelman WA, et al. Comparison of laparoscopic and transabdominal ultrasonography in staging of cancer of the pancreatic head region. J Ultrasound Med 1996; 15:207–212.
34. Hann LE, Conlon KC, Bach AM, et al. Laparoscopic gray-scale spectral Doppler ultrasound: applications in management of pancreatic carcinoma (abstr.). J Ultrasound Med 1996; 15:63.
35. Kubota K, Noie T, Sano K, et al. Impact of intraoperative ultrasonography on surgery for cystic lesions of the pancreas. World J Surg 1997; 21:72–76.
36. Kaneko T, Nakao A, Inoue S, et al. Intraoperative ultrasonography by high-resolution annular array transducer for intraductal papillary mucinous tumors of the pancreas. Surgery 2001; 129:55–65.
37. Printz H, Klotter HJ, Nies C, et al. Intraoperative ultrasonography in surgery for chronic pancreatitis. Int J Pancreatol 1992; 12:233–237.
38. Sigel B, Coelho JCU, Sharifi R, et al. Ultrasonic scanning during operation for renal calculi. J Urol 1982; 127:421–424.
39. Riedmiller H, Thuroff J, Aiken P, et al. Doppler and B-mode ultrasound for avascular nephrotomy. J Urol 1983; 130:224–227.
40. Walther MM, Choyke PL, Hayes W, et al. Evaluation of color Doppler intraoperative ultrasound in parenchymal sparing renal surgery. J Urol 1994; 152:1984–1987.
41. Topley M, Novick AC, Montie JE. Long-term results following partial nephrectomy for localized renal adenocarcinomas. J Urol 1984; 131:1050–1052.
42. Gilbert BR, Russo P, Zirinsky K, et al. Intraoperative sonography: application in renal cell carcinoma. J Urol 1988; 139:582–584.
43. Choyke PL, Pavlovich CP, Daryanani KD, et al. Intraoperative ultrasound during renal parenchymal sparing surgery for hereditary renal cancers: a 10-year experience. J Urol 2001; 165:397–400.
44. Rubin JM, Quint DJ. Intraoperative US versus intraoperative MR imaging for guidance during intracranial neurosurgery. Radiology 2000; 215:917–918.
45. Comeau RM, Fenster A, Peters TM. Intraoperative US in interactive image-guided neurosurgery. RadioGraphics 1998; 18:1019–1027.
46. Knake JE, Chandler WF, McGillicuddy JE, et al. Intraoperative sonography for brain tumor localization and ventricular shunt placement. AJR Am J Roentgenol 1982; 139:733–738.
47. Enzmann DR, Wheat R, Marshall WH, et al. Tumors of the central nervous system studied by computed tomography and ultrasound. Radiology 1985; 154:393–399.
48. Smith SJ, Vogelzang RL, Marzano MI, et al. Brain edema: ultrasound examination. Radiology 1985; 155:379–382.
49. Rubin JM, Dohrmann GJ. Intraoperative neurosurgical ultrasound in the localization and characterization of intracranial masses. Radiology 1983; 148:519–524.
50. Hatfield MK, Rubin JM, Gebarski SS, et al. Intraoperative sonography in low-grade gliomas. J Ultrasound Med 1989; 8:131–134.
51. Tsutsumi Y, Andoh Y, Inoue NI. Ultrasound-guided biopsy for deep-seated brain tumors. J Neurosurgy 1982; 57:164–167.
52. Enzmann DR, Irwin KM, Marshall WH, et al. Intraoperative sonography through a burr hole: guide for brain biopsy. Am J Neuroradiol 1984; 5:243–246.
53. Shkolnik A, McLone DG. Intraoperative real-time ultrasonic guidance of ventricular shunt placement in infants. Radiology 1981; 141:515–517.

54. Shanley DJ, Eline MJ. Intracerebral hematoma localization and removal using intraoperative ultrasound. Milit Med 1992; 157:622–624.
55. Black KL, Rubin JM, Chandler WF, et al. Intraoperative color flow Doppler imaging of AVMs and aneurysm. J Neurosurg 1988; 68:635–639.
56. Quencer RM, Montalvo BM. Normal intraoperative spinal sonography. Am J Neuroradiol 1984; 5:501–505; AJR Am J Roentgenol 1984; 143:1301–1305.
57. Rubin JM, Dohrmann GJ. Intraoperative ultrasonography of the spine. Radiology 1983; 146:173–175.
58. Platt JF, Rubin JM, Chandler WF, et al. Intraoperative spinal sonography in the evaluation of intramedullary tumors. J Ultrasound Med 1988; 7:317–325.
59. Mimatsu K, Kawakami N, Kato F, et al. Intraoperative ultrasonography of extramedullary spinal tumors. Neuroradiology 1992; 34:440–443.
60. Quencer RM, Montalvo BM, Green BA, et al. Intraoperative spinal sonography of soft tissue masses of the spinal cord and spinal canal. AJR Am J Roentgenol 1984; 143:1307–1315.
61. Post MJD, Quencer RM, Montalvo MB, et al. Spinal infection: evaluation with magnetic resonance imaging and intraoperative ultrasound. Radiology 1988; 169:765–771.
62. Hutchins WW, Vogelzang RL, Neiman HL, et al. Differentiation of tumor from syringohydromyelia: intraoperative neurosonography of the spinal cord. Radiology 1984; 151:171–174.
63. Montalvo BM, Quencer RM, Brown MD, et al. Lumbar disk herniation and canal stenosis: value of intraoperative sonography in diagnosis and surgical management. AJR Am J Roentgenol 1990; 154:821–830.
64. Mirvis SE, Geisler FH. Intraoperative sonography of cervical spinal cord injury: results in 30 patients. AJR Am J Roentgenol 1990; 155:603–609.
65. Fornage BD. Intraoperative ultrasound of the breast. In: Kane RA, ed. Intraoperative, Laparoscopic, and Endoluminal Ultrasound, Philadelphia: Churchill Livingstone/Saunders, 1999:142–147.
66. Kern KA, Shawker TH, Doppman JL, et al. The use of high-resolution ultrasound to locate parathyroid tumors during reoperations for primary hyperparathyroidism. World J Surg 1987; 11:579–585.
67. Onik GM, Cohen JK, Reyes GD, et al. Transrectal ultasound-guided percutaneous radical cryosurgical ablation of the prostate. Cancer 1993; 72:1291–1299.
68. Edmundson GK, Yan D, Martinez AA. Intraoperative optimization of needle placement and dwell times for conformal prostate brachytherapy. Int J Radiat Oncol Biol Phys 1995; 33:1257–1263.
69. Wei Z, Wan G, Gardi L, Mills G, et al. Robot-assisted 3D-TRUS guided prostate brachytherapy: system integration and validation. Med Phys 2004; 31:539–548.
70. Letterie GS, Case KJ. Intraoperative ultrasound guidance for hysteroscopic retrieval of intrauterine foreign bodies. Surg Endosc 1993; 7:182–184.
71. Bemelman WA, Van Delden OM, Van Lanschot JJB, et al. Laparoscopy and laparoscopic sonography in staging of carcinoma of the esophagus and gastric cardia. J Am Coll Surg 1995; 181: 421–425.
72. Hünerbein M, Rau B, Schlag PM. Laparoscopy and laparoscopic ultrasound for staging of upper gastrointestinal tumours. Eur J Surg Oncol 1995; 21:50–55.
73. Gouma DJ, De Wit T, Van Dijkum EN, et al. Laparoscopic sonography for staging of gastrointestinal malignancy. Scan J Gastroenterol Suppl 1996; 218:43–49.
74. Dougherty MJ, Hallett JW, Naessens JM, et al. Optimizing technical success of renal revascularization: the impact of intraoperative color flow duplex sonography. J Vasc Surg 1993; 7:849–857.
75. Lantz EJ, Charboneau JW, Hallett JW, et al. Intraoperative color Doppler sonography during renal artery revascularization. AJR Am J Roentgenol 1994; 162:859–863.
76. Hallett JW Jr, Berger MW, Lewis BD. Intraoperative color-flow duplex ultrasonography following carotid endarterectomy. Neurosurg Clin North Am 1996; 7:733.
77. Greenfield AL, Steiner RM, Liu JB, et al. Sonographic guidance for the localization of peripheral pulmonary nodules during thoracoscopy. AJR Am J Roentgenol 1997; 168:1057–1060.
78. Kane RA, Hughes LA, Cua EJ, et al. The impact of intraoperative ultrasonography on surgery for liver neoplasms. J Ultrasound Med 1994; 13:1–6.
79. Boctor EM, Taylor RH, Fichtinger G, et al. Robotically assisted intraoperative ultrasound with application to ablative therapy of liver cancer. In: Robert L. Galloway Jr, ed. Proc. SPIE. Medical Imaging 2003: Visualization, Image-Guided Procedures, and Display. Vol. 5029, 2005:281–291.
80. Ellsmere J, Stoll J, Rattner D, Brooks D, et al. Integrating preoperative CT data with laparoscopic ultrasound images facilitates interpretation. Surg Endosc 2003; 17:S296.

Ultrasound-Guided Percutaneous Tissue Ablation

8

Vijay P. Khatri, John P. McGahan, and Philip D. Schneider

INTRODUCTION

Some patients with hepatic malignancies are not candidates for potentially curative surgery. Investigators have searched for safe, alternative means to treat lesions in situ to control disease and avoid complications associated with surgery. There is early promise that interstitial ablation may provide the means to achieve reasonable local control, with reduced risk compared with standard surgery, and reports of long-term follow-up are awaited.

Ultrasound (US) is the imaging modality of choice to guide needle placement and monitor therapy for percutaneous tissue ablation. US is ideal for several reasons. US is universally available and portable and therefore can be transported to the operating suite for open procedures such as hepatic cryosurgery. It has real-time capabilities that can guide precise needle placement into even small target organs such as enlarged parathyroid glands. Finally, US has been shown to be effective in several instances in monitoring application of therapy such as the freeze with cryotherapy or the diffusion of alcohol with percutaneous ethanol ablation which otherwise may be notably cumbersome with computed tomography (CT) or magnetic resonance guidance.

The limitations of US are subject to operator experience, equipment quality, and patient-related factors such as body habitus, characteristics of the organ being imaged such as inhomogeneity of liver parenchyma due to cirrhosis, steatosis, and postchemotherapy vascular changes. For liver lesions, conventional US has poor resolution for small focal lesions (<1 cm). To overcome the limitations of conventional US and enhance the ability to detect subcentimeter focal lesions, the evolution of contrast-enhanced ultrasound (CEUS) is proving to be a valuable adjunct.

In this chapter, the major percutaneous ablation techniques, concentrating on ethanol ablation, radiofrequency (RF) electrocautery, cryotherapy, laser hyperthermia, and radiotherapy are reviewed. The liver is emphasized as the target organ, although other solid organs may also be considered for treatment with US-guided therapy.

TECHNIQUE FOR PERCUTANEOUS APPROACHES TO ABLATION IN THE LIVER

Materials and Protocol

The steps taken are as follows:

1. Real-time US or CT is used to locate the lesion to be ablated (Fig. 1).
2. Using imaging (US or CT), a Chiba needle is placed in the desired position within or near the tumor. Aspiration biopsy confirms the nature of the lesion.
3. Needle placement is performed into the target lesion under real-time US control. For alcohol ablation techniques, alcohol can be injected at this point, and its tracking through the interstitium is monitored.

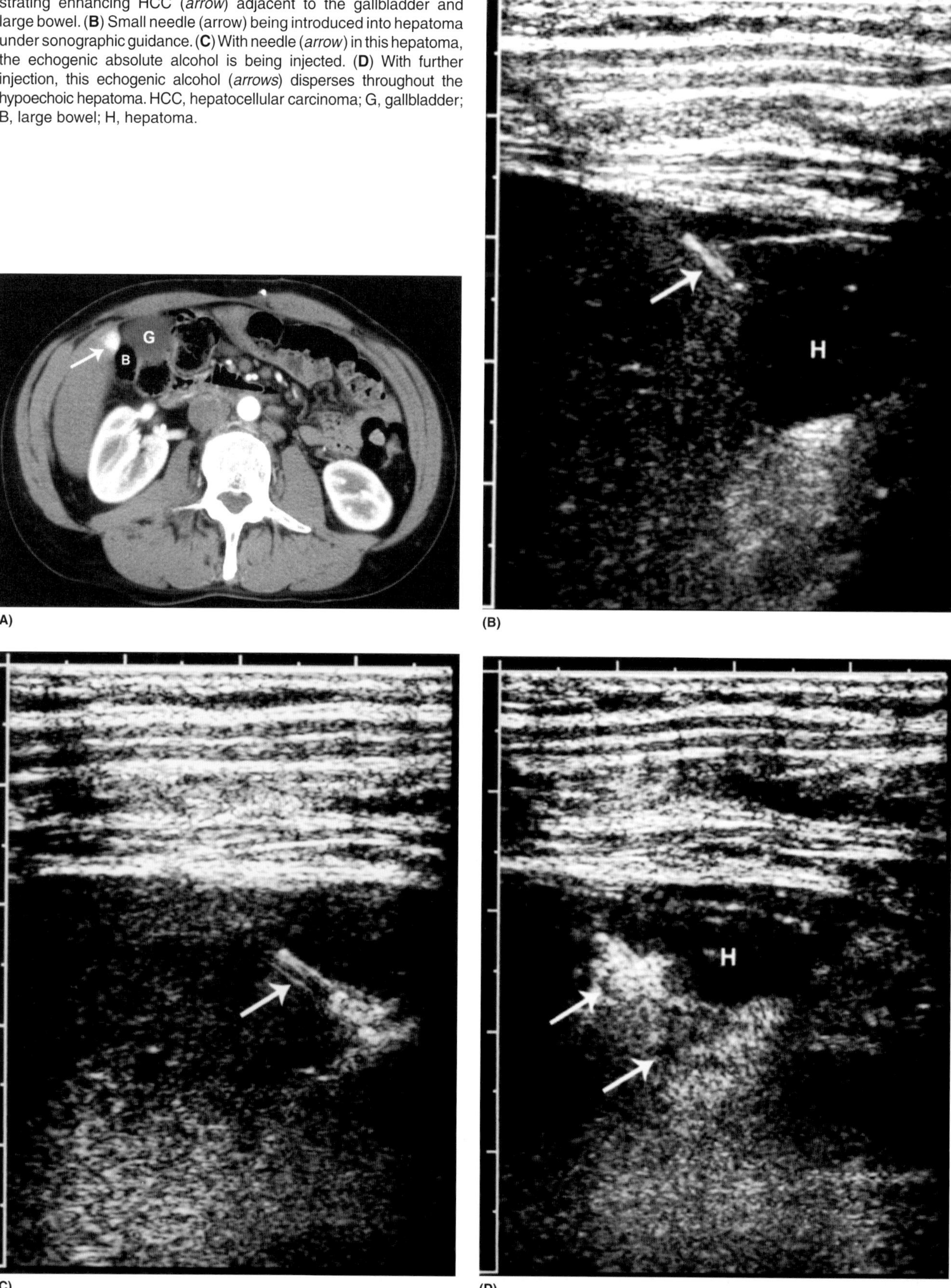

FIGURE 1 A–D ■ Ethanol ablation of the liver. (**A**) CT scan demonstrating enhancing HCC (*arrow*) adjacent to the gallbladder and large bowel. (**B**) Small needle (arrow) being introduced into hepatoma under sonographic guidance. (**C**) With needle (*arrow*) in this hepatoma, the echogenic absolute alcohol is being injected. (**D**) With further injection, this echogenic alcohol (*arrows*) disperses throughout the hypoechoic hepatoma. HCC, hepatocellular carcinoma; G, gallbladder; B, large bowel; H, hepatoma.

(A) (B) (C) (D)

4. If RF or microwave ablation is performed, this therapy may be monitored with US after needle placement.
5. For the placement of laser fibers for percutaneous interstitial hyperthermia, needles and trocars are placed percutaneously into the lesion by US. For Nd: YAG laser treatment, the trocar is withdrawn, and the bare or water-cooled fiberoptic cable is placed into the lesion in the appropriate position.
6. If a percutaneous cryoprobe is to be used after the Chiba needle is in place, a guide wire is placed into the tumor, and a dilator is passed over the wire, sequentially dilating the tract to a size appropriate to accept the percutaneously introduced probe. Newer probes with decreased diameter may allow trocar placement.
7. If interstitial radiotherapy is the chosen modality, large-bore needles (14 gauge) are percutaneously placed into the lesion, and iridium seeds are placed directly into the lesion. Alternatively, large afterloading catheters are placed under US control, and the introducing needles are withdrawn. The patient is subsequently placed in a shielded room or removed to the radiation oncology suite for afterloading of the interstitial catheters that were previously placed.

Procedure Notes

After completion of the therapy and confirmation of adequate tissue distribution of the destructive agent, the patient is monitored for both site-specific and systemic complications. Broad-spectrum antibiotics are continued for several days. Combination therapies with systemic or regional chemotherapy or radiotherapy can be considered at this point. Serum or urine biochemical tumor markers are periodically used to assess treatment. CT, magnetic resonance imaging (MRI), and less frequently, US may be used to evaluate the results of therapy. US-guided biopsy has proved definitive in assessing if viable tumor is still present.

PERCUTANEOUS ETHANOL INJECTION IN PRIMARY AND METASTATIC LIVER TUMORS

Method of Treatment

Percutaneous ethanol injection therapy (PEIT) for ablation of focal liver lesions was independently conceived at University of Chiba, Japan, and Vimercate Hospital in Italy. Alcohol causes tissue destruction by intracellular diffusion, dehydration of intracellular proteins, and consequently coagulation necrosis. Hepatocellular carcinomas (HCCs) are uniquely suited for PEIT, as these tumors are hypervascular and have softer consistency which facilitates uniform alcohol distribution. No universal agreement exists about the optimal method for performing percutaneous ethanol injection (PEI) for HCC. The greatest disagreement centers on the volume of ethanol needed for each treatment and the number of treatment sessions needed. For instance, in early work by the Italians, small volumes of ethanol (2–8 mL) were used that required multiple treatment sessions. For instance, Livraghi et al. (1–3) performed an average of 10 treatment sessions per tumor. Similarly, Borghetti et al. (4) performed 78 treatments on 14 HCC lesions, or 5.6 treatments per lesion. More recently, Livraghi et al. (5) treated 210 cirrhotic patients with HCC using both multiple treatment sessions and single treatment sessions with larger volumes of ethanol (>150 mL). Lesions <2 cm in size are treated with three to four sessions, those 2 to 3 cm in size in four to six sessions, and lesions 3 to 5 cm may require 6 to 10 sessions. Though the number of sessions needed is approximately twice the diameter of the tumor, the final volume of alcohol and the number of treatment depend on achieving complete necrosis as determined by CEUS. Although patients receiving the smaller doses were treated as outpatients, those with larger treatment volumes required general anesthesia and hospitalization. There was a higher complication rate with the use of higher dosages, including one death secondary to bleeding from esophageal varices.

Redvanly et al. (6) reviewed complications versus dosage of alcohol with PEI treatment of liver neoplasms. A number of complications were encountered that did not appear dose related, including pleural effusions, ascites, pneumothorax, decreased hematocrit, vasovagal reaction, and hypotension (6). Pain and fever, probably due in part to the tumor necrosis, were dose related. An analysis of complications related to ethanol dose showed a complication rate of 28% with less than 10 mL and a complication rate of 35% using 11 to 20 mL. With dosages of 21 to 30 mL, the complication rate increased to 73%, and it was 71% when using greater than 30 mL of ethanol. Therefore, patients who received 21 to 30 mL of ethanol had about twice the rate of side effects as those receiving 11 to 20 mL of ethanol.

Volume of Ethanol

Shiina et al. (7) proposed that the total amount of ethanol injected should be based on the total tumor volume plus a margin of safety of 0.5 cm in this calculation. Their volume calculated is as follows:

$$V = \frac{4}{3}\pi(r + 0.5)^3$$

where V is the volume in milliliters r is the radius of tumor in centimeters, and 0.5 is the value of the margin of safety.

This margin is provided to ensure that there is an adequate amount of ethanol diffusion into surrounding tissue to complete the tumor kill. Therefore, the number of sessions and the volume of ethanol injected at each session must be calculated against the volume of the tumor. For instance, using Shiina's formula, a 3-cm lesion requires 30 to 35 mL of ethanol. This could be injected in one session using this amount, in two sessions using 15 to 20 mL, or in multiple sessions using smaller amounts. When using multiple sessions, precise mapping of exactly where the ethanol diffuses must be performed with each session so that the entire tumor is treated.

Follow-up

Assessment of therapeutic response involves serial measurement of tumor markers such as α-fetoprotein supplanted with imaging studies. A number of different modalities have been advocated to follow up tumor necrosis or tumor recurrence after PEI. Imaging methods that have been used to evaluate therapy include US-guided biopsy (8), US (9), MRI (10), and contrast-enhanced CT (11). Of all these modalities, contrast-enhanced CT has been the most frequently used noninvasive technique to assess treatment success and to evaluate residual tumor (11). An increase in tumor markers also suggests local recurrence or development of new lesions. When there is doubt about possible areas of residual tumor, US-guided biopsy is more definitive (8).

Efficacy

Hepatocellular Carcinoma

Livraghi et al. (5,12,13) have published several large series regarding survival rates after treatment with PEI and HCC. Of 210 treated patients with HCC, the one-year, three-year, and five-year survival rates after PEI were 95%, 65%, and 41%, respectively, using the Kaplan-Meier method (5). These patients had Child's class A liver disease. In an Italian cooperative study that compared surgery with PEI and no treatment in patients with HCC, PEI did well. In this study, the three-year survival rates in the Child's class A group were 79% with surgery and 71% with PEI, compared with 26% with no treatment. There was no statistical difference between surgery and PEI, but there was statistical difference ($P < 0.001$) for both surgery and PEI compared with no treatment. Similarly, in the Child's class B group, the three-year survival rates were 40% for surgery and 41% for PEI, compared with 13% for no treatment. This was again statistically significant ($P < 0.01$) for surgery compared with no treatment, and $P < 0.001$ for PEI compared with no treatment (13). In these studies the main cause of death in Child's A patients was progression of the neoplastic disease while in Child's C mortality was related to hepatic insufficiency. As expected the incidence of local recurrence is dependent on the size of the HCC initially treated with PEIT. The incidence of new hepatic lesions has been reported to be around 70% in patients with solitary HCC, and in patients with multiple HCCs the incidence is approximately 98%.

Similarly, Castells et al. (14) compared survival rates in patients with solitary HCC lesions 4 cm or smaller who were treated with PEI, surgical resection, or liver transplantation. Despite poor liver functions, the one-year, two-year, three-year, and four-year survival rates of patients treated with PEI were 83%, 66%, 55%, and 34%, respectively, compared with those of surgically treated patients (81%, 73%, 44%, and 44%, respectively), which was not statistically different. The one-year and two-year survival rates of patients treated with liver transplantation were 81% and 66%, respectively. Therefore, these investigators thought that their data confirmed that PEI is a useful therapy for treatment of patients with solitary HCC lesions (14). At present PEIT can be considered in patients who are (*i*) not resectable, (*ii*) not candidates for liver transplantation based on the MELD (model for end-stage fever disease) criteria, or (*iii*) surgical candidates except for the presence of prohibitive comorbid conditions or advanced liver cirrhosis. We have also used PEI in patients in which we felt the heating or freezing of organs adjacent to the liver tumor mass potentially cause a problem. PEI might be chosen for an HCC adjacent to the gallbladder or bowel.

Metastatic Disease of the Liver

The results of PEI in liver metastases have been less favorable (15). Giovannini and Seitz reported their experience of 40 patients with 55 liver metastases, mostly of colorectal origin that was treated with PEI (16). Complete necrosis was noted in 58% and partial necrosis in 29% with an overall mean survival of 19 months. Giorgio et al. examined the efficacy of a single injection of a large volume of alcohol under general anesthesia for patients with liver metastases (17). They reported that complete necrosis was achieved in 30% with partial necrosis in 64% of the lesions. PEI was compared with laser interstitial thermal therapy (LITT) for colorectal metastasis performed under US guidance. Notably though, there were no major complications after LITT or PEI. Complete responses were obtained in 52% of the lesions treated with LITT but complete tumor necrosis was never achieved by PEI. These authors concluded that PEI is relatively ineffective for colorectal carcinoma (CRC) liver metastasis, as the complete necrosis rates are remarkably reduced compared with those obtained in HCC. This is probably due to presence of a more fibrous stroma in colorectal liver metastasis which prevents the diffusion into the metastases that is commonly seen with hepatio cellular carcinoma. In Giorgio's series, 70% of the metastatic colon lesions demonstrated residual tumor following the intervention. Livraghi reported the results of 14 patients with 21 liver metastasis of CRC treated with PEI (3). The diameter of these lesions ranges from 1 to 3 cm, and complete response was obtained only in those lesions that were 2 cm or smaller in diameter. One of the key difficulties in establishing the efficacy of such a treatment is the method used for assessing response. Follow-up is based on changes on US images, i.e., presence of a mixed echogenic pattern and tumor necrosis being represented by a characteristic posterior acoustic shadow. CT scans rely on the presence of hypodense lesions, and without enhancement after contrast injection. The disadvantage of such a method of follow-up was highlighted by Mazziotti et al. who reported the presence of viable tumor in liver resections in all patients with liver metastasis pretreated with PEI prior to surgery (18).

Another problem is that there is less optimal diffusion of ethanol with colon metastasis than with HCC. We attribute this to the different consistencies; many liver metastases are firmer than HCC. This firmness tends to prevent complete dispersion of ethanol. Therefore, other percutaneous methods may be more appropriate for treatment of metastatic liver disease.

Complications

Many complications or side effects of PEI are dose related, including pain and fever, which develop with tissue necrosis (6). Other complications associated with PEI include pleural effusions, pneumothorax, ascites, decreased hematocrit, vasovagal reaction, myoglobinuria, and transient hypotension (6). In addition, abscess formation (19), hemobilia (20), pleural seeding along the injection tract (21), and peritoneal bleeding (22) have been seen. Most studies have shown that necrosis occurs not only in the tumor but also in some of the adjacent liver. One case of massive liver necrosis has been reported that resulted in death (23).

OTHER PERCUTANEOUS LIQUIDS AND APPLICATIONS

Other Liquids for Percutaneous Injection

Other liquids can be injected as alternatives to alcohol for percutaneous US-guided tumor ablation. For instance, hot saline injection has been performed in patients with HCC. Honda et al. (24) reported that boiling saline was injected into needles placed in HCC lesions in 20 patients. Hot saline proved to be safe and without complications, and it showed a therapeutic effect in all patients. Veltri et al. (22) found hot saline to be useful in treatment of larger HCC lesions, with few side effects. Both groups thought that hot saline showed promise in treatment of HCC.

Ohnishi et al. (25) injected 50% acetic acid 82 times in patients with HCC without clinically significant complications. The one-year survival rate was 100%, and the two-year survival rate was 92%. Thus, acetic acid, hot saline, and other chemical agents may prove to be effective alternatives to PEI in treatment of HCC.

Hepatic and Renal Cysts

US can be used to guide percutaneous needle placement for therapeutic cyst ablation. US-guided puncture is performed as previously described. Usually, a small-bore catheter is left in place during the procedure. The cyst is completely aspirated, and up to 25% of the contents of the cyst is reinjected with absolute alcohol, taking care not to overinject the ethanol. The patient is usually maneuvered so that the walls of the cyst are coated. The cyst is again completely aspirated 20 to 30 minutes later, and the catheter is usually removed. In most patients, this treatment is effective for ablation of benign cysts (26). Cysts that recur or are multiloculated or are in any other way atypical in appearance should be evaluated for malignancy (27). Sclerosants, such as tetracycline, doxycycline, or others, may also be used for benign symptomatic cysts (27).

Parathyroid Ablation

Percutaneous ethanol ablation of enlarged parathyroid gland was one of the first US-guided tissue ablation techniques performed (28,29). Although this technique has been shown to be effective in treatment of primary and secondary hyperparathyroidism, it is reserved for nonoperative candidates. Problems include recurrent elevation of parathyroid hormone in secondary hyperparathyroidism, transient dysphonia, and permanent vocal cord paralysis. Surgeons reported increased tissue fibrosis surrounding the area of treatment when surgery was later performed. Care must be taken to inject only a small amount of ethanol, to avoid the posterior gland where the neurovascular bundle is present, and not to inject ethanol into the surrounding tissues. This technique is similar to other percutaneous ablation techniques. The enlarged parathyroid gland is visualized, the area is prepared and draped, and a high-resolution US probe is used. A small-gauge needle (22–25 gauge) is placed into the parathyroid tissue after administering local anesthesia. No more than 0.5 mL of ethanol is injected per 1 mL of gland volume. The gland usually becomes echogenic and similar in echo texture to the thyroid gland. The patient experiences pain for about one minute. After this, the needle is removed, and laboratory markers such as serum calcium and parathyroid hormone are followed (30,31).

INTERSTITIAL RADIOTHERAPY

Conventional, external beam radiation therapy has not gained wide acceptance in the treatment of liver metastases, primarily due to the radiosensitive nature of normal liver parenchyma which thus limits the total dose to 30 to 35 Gy (32). Therefore, approaches to deliver radiation therapy directly to the liver tumors have emerged. Systemic internal radiation therapy (SIRT) is a novel method of delivering a single dose of yttrium microspheres directly into the hepatic artery via a Port-A-Cath placed in the gastroduodenal artery. Placement of the hepatic artery port is not too dissimilar to the technique used for placing InFusaid pumps for hepatic artery infusion and involves preoperative assessment of hepatic artery anatomy and intraoperatively ligating all branches to the pancreas, stomach, and duodenum. To avoid adverse events, alternative access can also be achieved in a percutaneous manner via the femoral artery using the Seldinger technique. The yttrium resin microspheres (SIR-Spheres, Paragon Medical Ltd., Perth, Australia) are then infused over a 10-minute period to provide an average radiation dose of 200 to 300 Gy to the tumor with an average of 15 to 50 Gy to the normal liver parenchyma. At three months, 32 of 44 patients demonstrated reduction in tumor size, which was maintained in 23 patients at the six-month evaluation. These authors, however, did not use the standard Response Evaluation Criteria in Solid Tumors (RECIST) as developed by National Cancer Institute (NCI) Cancer Therapy Evaluation Program (CTEP) (33) for documenting response. Despite administering hepatic artery 5-flurouracil patients, over half of the group developed extrahepatic disease within six months of receiving SIRT. The median survival for the group from time of treatment was 9.8 months which is comparable or even somewhat inferior to the early reported series of patients treated with palliative chemotherapy alone. A 12% incidence of acute duodenal ulcers within the first two months, with one patient requiring emergency surgery for gastrointestinal bleeding, is concerning (34).

Koniaris et al. from Johns Hopkins evaluated the efficacy of a miniature, portable, hand-held photon radio surgery system that generates low energy, high-intensity photons in the 10 to 20 kev with a steep dose of dash-distance fall off (35). Lesion size varied with the duration of treatment and these lesions decreased in size over a six-month period. Histologic examination of the treated area at one month demonstrated well-circumscribed region of coagulative necrosis with multifocal hemorrhage surrounded by a dense lymphocytic infiltrate. Interestingly, the Photon Radiosurgery System (PRS) was able to ablate liver parenchyma in the vicinity of hepatic veins and the inferior vena cava (IVC) without evidence of late vascular thrombosis of stricture. However, when the same treatment was applied close to the portal structures, it reported hilar damage associated with arterial thrombosis and bile duct injury.

We have used placement of these 14-gauge needles in one patient using US guidance. US was used to place the needles in various sites within the tumor. These needles are hollow and serve as a port for placement of the iridium seeds. Computer planning is used to plan radiation treatment. Usually, these procedures are performed in a radiotherapy suite where US can be transported. Alternatively, if a CT scanner is in close proximity to the radiotherapy suite, the needles may be positioned under CT guidance and then the patient carefully transported with these needles in place (36,37).

INTERSTITIAL LASER THERAPY

Liver

In 1985, Hashimoto et al. (38) were the first to apply the concept of interstitial thermal injury clinically by using laser light. They recognized that light administered by the Nd:YAG laser could deliver light energy at the tip of an interstitially placed transmission fiber. Previous experimental work by others had established that the nature of such an injury was a spherical lesion at the tip of the fiber, which was visualized with real-time US. Since their report, others, including Hahl et al. (39), established that the technique is safe. As with alcohol injection, the laser fibers can be inserted through percutaneously placed needles introduced under ultrasonic guidance. The size of the fiber necessitates a 14-gauge needle with stylet for placement (39). More recent developments have included placement of fibers through a 19-gauge needle (40).

The extent of thermal injury is determined, as with all laser techniques, by the power in watts, exposure time, characteristics of light wavelength intensity, and absorption characteristics of the tissue. Using the Nd:YAG laser, applied power has ranged from 0 to 6 W, and exposure times have ranged from 500 to 1000 seconds. An advantage within the liver (especially with tumors located near major vascular structures that we wish to preserve) is the thermal conduction and protection afforded by blood flow, which saves major vessels from injury. Thus, the technique has potential application for lesions that are near structures that make them surgically unresectable. Heat, however, can cause bile duct injury, resulting in biliary obstruction or narrowing.

An additional danger is related to the power setting, as reported by Schroder et al. (41). With the Nd:YAG laser at low power settings in the range of 0.5 to 1.5 W, no cooling is needed. When 4 to 6 W of power is applied to decrease the exposure time, most investigators use coaxial gas flow in the range of 1 L/min to provide cooling and to avoid the vaporization that causes tissue disruption or vapor emboli. The application of heat and gas under pressure in a closed space has led to an instance of fatal air embolism. It appears that the lower power settings have the advantage of diminishing the risk of embolus, although it takes longer to create therapeutic heat injury. Alternative cooling techniques using water-cooled fibers are available.

To treat larger lesions, a pattern of fibers must be placed carefully such that the entire tumor is encompassed to ensure total ablation. A spread or pattern of laser fibers can achieve this effect. The major advantage of this technique is that the extent of necrosis can be monitored using real-time US and can be adjusted at the time of treatment (Figs. 2 and 3). The injury is predictably spherical, unlike the irregular lesions resulting from alcohol injection (43).

Amin et al. (40) showed that interstitial laser photocoagulation is more useful than PEI in treatment of liver metastasis. The technique requires only local anesthesia with intravenous sedation. Schroder et al. (41) also showed that laser photocoagulation is more effective in treatment of liver metastasis. A drawback of laser hyperthermia is that the lesions produced are most often about 1 cm in diameter (Fig. 6). For this reason, multiple fibers must be placed under US guidance to create effective tumor necrosis. Photocoagulation of this type is monitored by noting the increased echogenic focus surrounding the laser tip (43).

Vogl et al. treated 1259 patients with 3440 hepatic metastases with MRI guided LITT. The mean survival rate was 4.4 years and the median survival rate was 3.0 years (44). The procedure is always image guided and the preferred modality is MRI as part of preprocedure evaluation, during the procedure to monitor the progress of LITT, immediately after LITT to provide essential information about laser induced necrosis and possible complications, and finally, follow-up examination at regular intervals. Such an extensive use of resources is one of its drawbacks. More recently, intraoperative LITT combined with hepatic arterial occlusion has ablated lesions up to 8.6 cm (3) in diameter (45).

Although laser photocoagulation has proved more effective than PEI in treatment of liver metastasis, complete tumor necrosis is reported in only about half of lesions (40). Therefore, increased tissue destruction with lasers is necessary for greater applicability to therapeutic ablation (38–40,43).

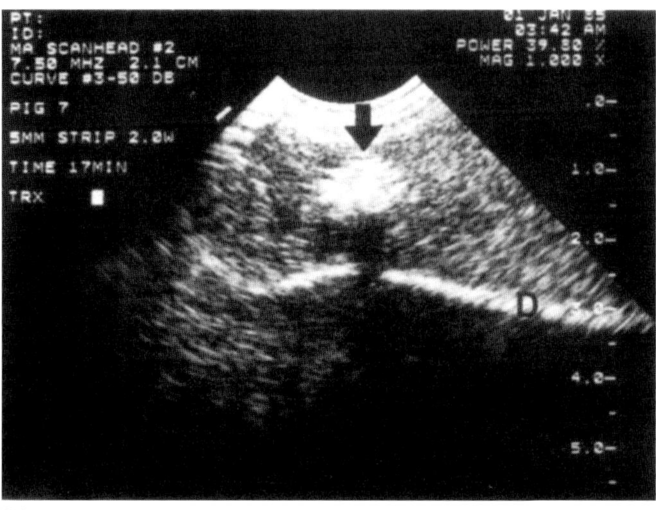

(A)

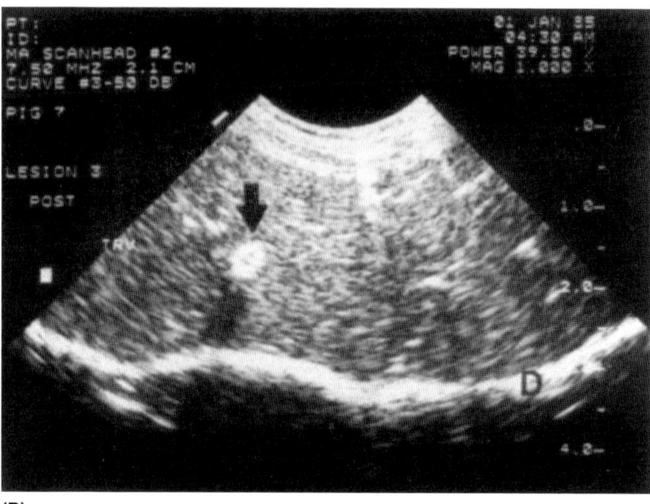

(B)

FIGURE 2 A AND B ■ Hepatic laser treatment. (**A**) Early during interstitial laser treatment of pig model, hyperechoic area is associated with posterior acoustic shadowing (*arrow*). (**B**) Slightly later, the lesion is smaller (*arrow*) and better defined. It has a central hypoechoic zone, a broad hyperechoic region, and a hypoechoic rim. The lesion zone is about 5 mm in diameter. *Source*: From Ref. 42.

Breast

Dowlatshahi et al. had reported their results of treating 36 patients with stereotactic guided laser therapy with subsequent resection for pathologic evaluation (46). Laser photocoagulation involves insertion of optical fibers into the tissues, which deliver laser light energy. Of these patients, 34 had invasive breast carcinoma, whereas the remaining two had in situ breast tumors. The mean tumor size recorded on prebiopsy mammogram and US was 12 mm, and with a laser energy ranging from 2500 to 10,000 J, they were able to achieve an 18 mm diameter of necrosis. They noted complete necrosis of tumor with negative margins in 24 patients with residual tumors noted in the remaining 12 patients. This group too felt that tumors with undefined borders such as that encountered with invasive lobular carcinoma and widespread microcalcification that indicates extensive ductal carcinoma in situ (DCIS) are unsuitable for this technique and furthermore tumors close to the skin surface (<1 cm) or the chest wall may result in skin burns or intractable skeletal pain, respectively.

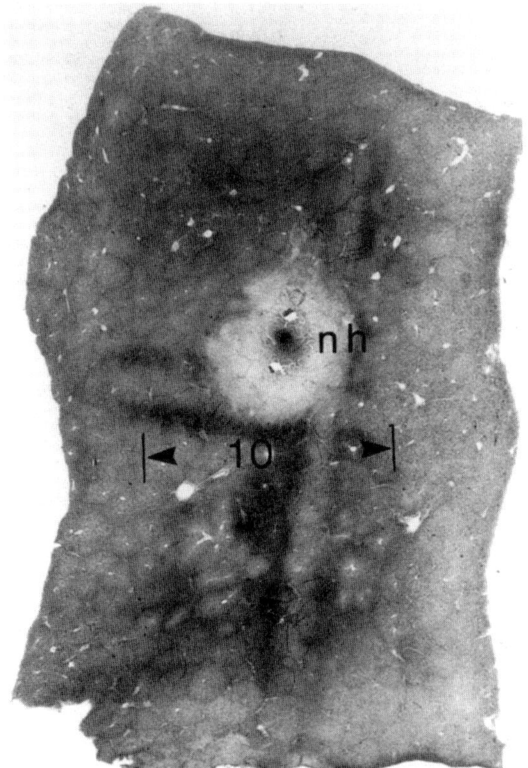

FIGURE 3 ■ Laser photocoagulation histology. Histologic section demonstrating central area of char surrounded by necrosis, which is surrounded by a narrow band of hemorrhage (H&E stain). n, necrosis; h, hemorrhage. *Source*: From Ref. 42.

Prostate

Laser photocoagulation has also been advocated in other areas, including the prostate. The laser fibers can be guided by transrectal US for either focal or more extensive prostate ablation (47).

RF ELECTROCAUTERY

Liver

In 1990, McGahan et al. (48) published a report on percutaneous ablation of liver tissue with RF electrocautery. This concept was novel because it proposed the use of focal application of RF electrocautery in the animal liver using US guidance. A monopolar electrocautery with an 18- to 20-gauge needle was placed deep in the liver parenchyma. The distal 1 cm of the needle tip was uninsulated and placed in the area of treatment. With gradual application of current, an elliptic echogenic focus was observed ultrasonographically (Fig. 4).

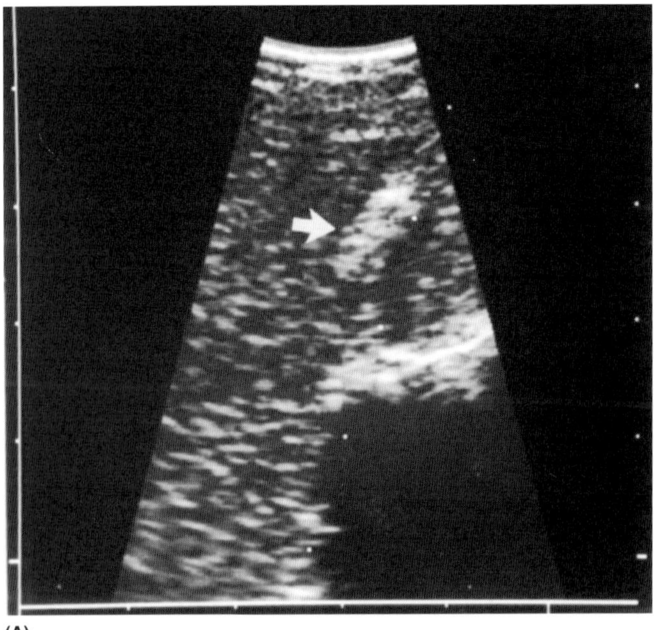

(A)

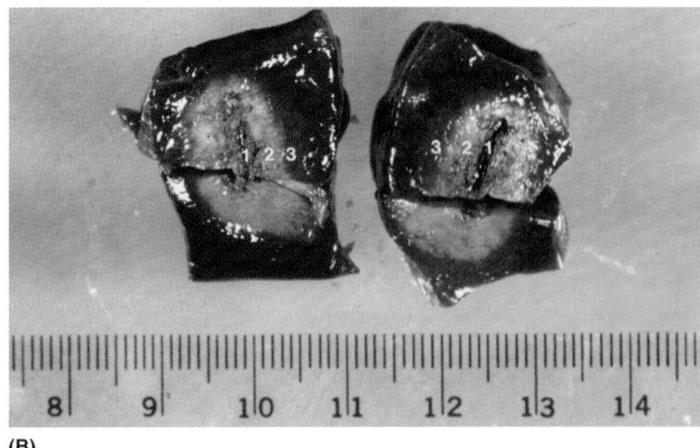

(B)

FIGURE 4 A AND B ■ Ultrasonographic and histologic correlation for radiofrequency coagulation. (**A**) Sonogram of monopolar radiofrequency lesion demonstrating hyperechoic regions surrounded by hypoechoic rim (*arrow*). (**B**) In vivo liver cut specimen demonstrates central area of char (1) surrounded by coagulation necrosis (2) and hyperemic rim (3). *Source*: From Ref. 49.

Pathologically, the echogenic lesion corresponded to an area of coagulation necrosis surrounded by a rim of partially destroyed tissue. The lesion size increased with added current. A larger volume of the liver could be destroyed by placing multiple needles for treatment. The authors believed that this percutaneous technique had great potential because (*i*) the lesion was well controlled, (*ii*) the technique allowed for retreatment, (*iii*) there appeared to be few complications, (*iv*) it could be performed without hospitalization, and (*v*) the technique could be combined with other therapeutic methods.

Initial research concentrated on the use of single or monopolar probe for RF tissue desiccation. These initial probes were needles that were insulated except for the tip, which was the unprotected portion of the needle where coagulation necrosis could occur. Using these simple designs, lesions similar in size to those produced with laser photocoagulation were produced (Fig. 5). While lesions appear similar to laser lesions, they are more echogenic than high-intensity focused US (HIFU) lesions (Fig. 6). Lesion size was usually 1 to 1.5 cm in diameter (43). Even given these initial size limitations, a

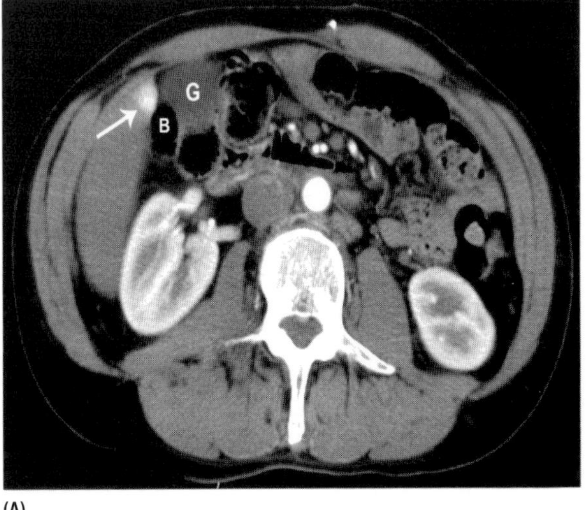

(A)

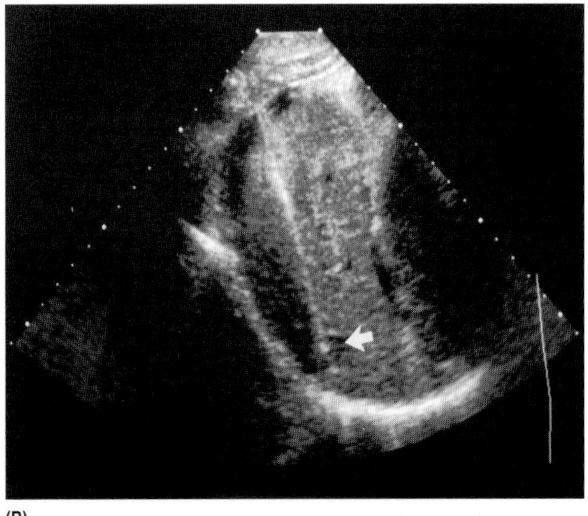

(B)

FIGURE 5 A–D ■ Hepatocellular carcinoma-radiofrequency ablation. (**A**) CT scan demonstrating enhancing mass in the dome of the liver (*arrow*). (**B**) With ultrasound, the small hepatoma is identified with the radiofrequency needle being placed into the hepatoma (*arrow*). (*Continued*)

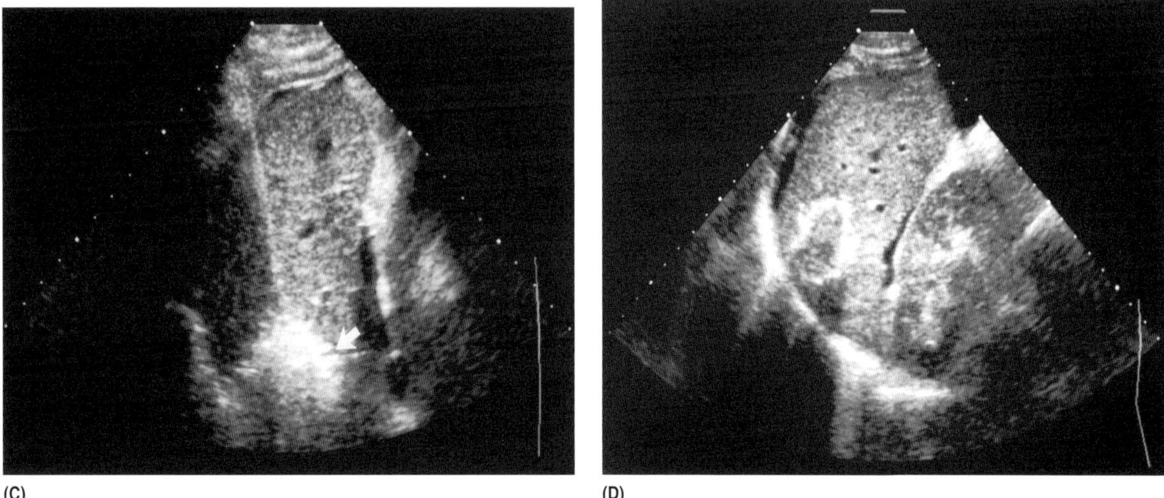

(C) (D)

FIGURE 5 A–D ■ (*Continued*) (**C**) Under ultrasound guidance, a needle is placed into the lesion and an echogenic region is observed (*arrow*). (**D**) Postablation image demonstrates area of ablation.

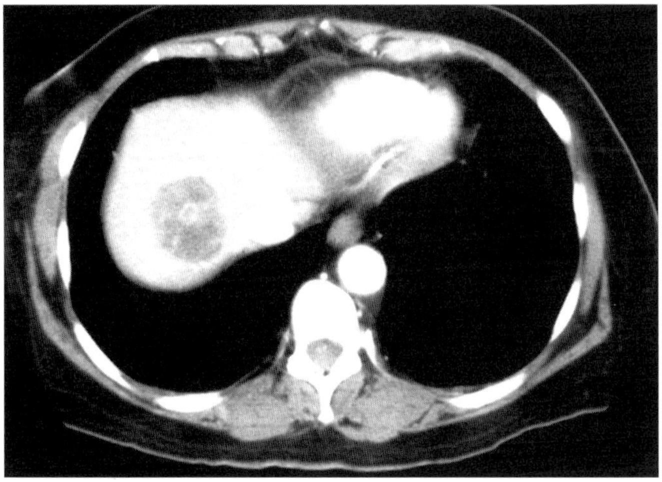

(A) 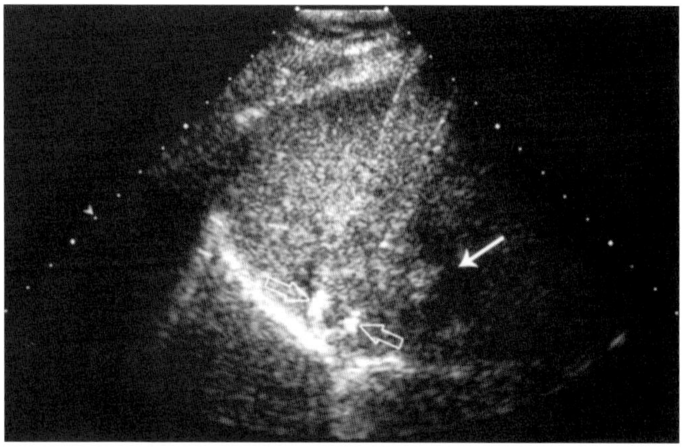 (B) 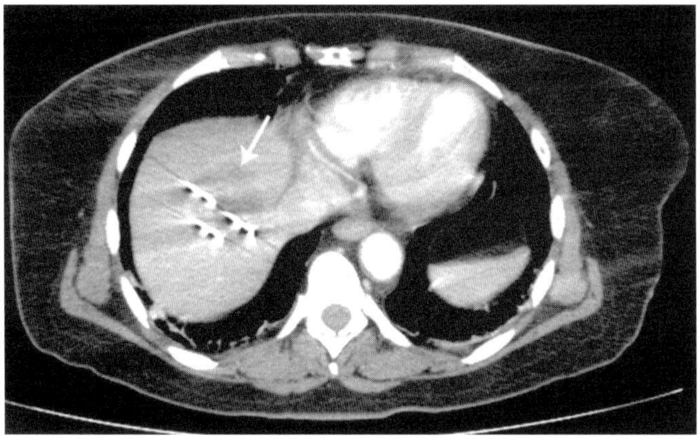 (C) 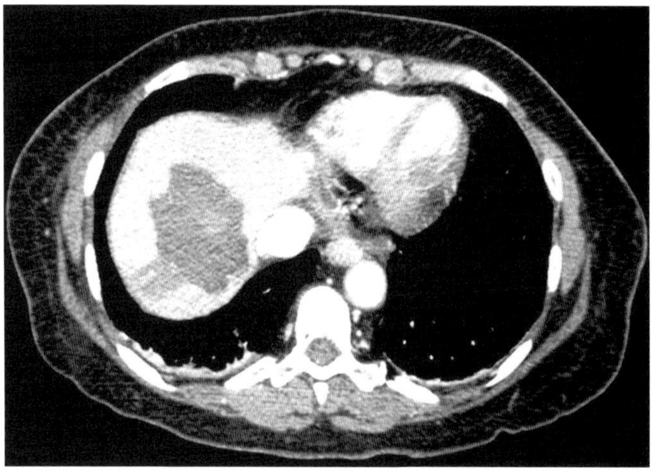 (D)

FIGURE 6 A–D ■ Metastatic colon cancer to the liver-radiofrequency ablation (RFA). (**A**) CT scan demonstrating low-density region seen within the dome of the liver corresponding to colon liver metastases (*arrow*). (**B**) Under ultrasound guidance, three radiofrequency (RF) needles are placed into the liver lesion. Two of the three needles are observed (*open arrow*). The needles are placed into a portion of the lesion, with the edges of the mass marked with an arrow. (**C**) After needle placement, CT demonstrating three of the needles within the lesion, pre-RFA. Also note needles placed in a portion of the lesion, with the edge of the mass marked with an arrow. (**D**) Postablation CT image demonstrates the large region of ablation zone after RFA. This was performed using two separate placements of the RF needles.

number of studies have demonstrated that RF electrocautery is useful in treatment of both HCC and liver metastases (50,51).

What is more promising with RF is that a number of investigators have shown novel methods of creating larger areas of tissue necrosis. For instance, Goldberg et al. (52) demonstrated that increased tissue destruction could be performed using multiple probes. Lorentzen (53) showed that different tip designs could increase the diameter of lesions using the monopolar RF. In a different experiment, McGahan et al. (50) showed that bipolar RF could be an effective method of causing increased tissue coagulation compared with the monopolar technique. In this method, two, instead of one, needles are placed into the tissue. One needle acts as a positive electrode, and the other acts as a negative electrode. Thus, tissue coagulation occurs between the two needles if parameters are optimized (50). New designs of monopolar RF or use of bipolar RF creating larger areas of tissue destruction may be helpful in treatment of liver metastasis or HCC in the near future.

A prospective nonrandomized study of radiofrequency ablation (RFA) for primary or metastatic hepatic malignancies that were deemed to be unresectable based on their number or location, proximity to major vascular structures precluding a margin negative resection, or limited hepatic reserve was reported by Curley et al. (54). Lesions that were >3 cm in diameter and located peripherally in the liver were treated percutaneously with RF under US guidance and the remainder were treated with RF during an open operative procedure (Fig. 7). During the open surgical procedure, vascular inflow occlusion was performed to increase the size of coagulative necrosis. Of the 123 patients treated, 49.6% had metastatic colorectal liver metastasis. At a median follow-up of 15 months, tumor recurrence at the RFA site occurred in 3 of the 169 treated tumors (1.8%) and these were either large (i.e., >6 cm in diameter) or located in a critical location between the right and middle hepatic veins near the IVC. Not surprisingly, as this is a purely local treatment, new intrahepatic and extrahepatic metastatic disease developed in 27.6% of the patients. There were no treatment-related deaths and the associated complication rate was 2.4%. This is in contrast to cryoablation that was associated with a death rate of 4% with an overall complication rate ranging from 15% to 50%.

Livraghi surveyed 41 Italian centers that were performing percutaneous RFA as part of a collaborative group to evaluate associate complication rates (55). A complete response was only achieved in 70% of all tumors (72% of HCCs and 68% of metastases). The mortality rate was 0.3% with a complication rate of 2.2%, and the most frequent of these included peritoneal hemorrhage, neoplastic seeding, intrahepatic abscesses, and intestinal perforation. Minor complications were observed in <5% of patients. As this trial included 2320 patients with 3554 lesions performed in a multicenter fashion, it attests to the notion that RFA is a relatively low-risk procedure for treatment of focal liver tumors.

A prospective nonrandomized study comparing RFA and cryoablation for treatment of unresectable malignant liver tumors was reported from MD Anderson Cancer Center (56). Cryoablation was used to treat 88 liver tumors in 54 patients, whereas RFA was performed on 138 tumors in 92 patients. The median greatest diameters of the tumors were comparable in the two groups (3.6 cm vs. 3.8 cm). At a median follow-up of 15 months, recurrence at the treated area occurred in 13.6% of cryoablated group and two-thirds of these were on or near a major hepatic blood vessel. In comparison, tumor recurred at the site of RFA in only 2.2% of the treated tumors. A retrospective review, with all of its limitations, was performed by Bilchik et al. to compare RFA versus cryosurgery for unresected hepatic malignant neoplasms (57). In this study, 308 patients underwent RFA, cryosurgery, or combination therapy with an underlying diagnosis of hepatoma, colorectal metastases, neuroendocrine metastases, and liver metastases from a variety of other primary neoplasms. The median lesion diameter in the cryosurgery group was larger than that in the RFA. They noted that when these two modalities were compared, cryosurgery was associated with a significantly longer, mean hospital stay, length of procedure, blood loss, thrombocythemia, pleural effusion, and intensive care unit stay. However, for hepatic lesions >3 cm in diameter, the duration of ablation and the number of ablations needed were significantly greater for RFA group. Such a comparison is limited, as there are only 13 patients within the RFA group which had lesions >3 cm in diameter. Conclusions from such comparisons have to be accepted with skepticism due to the heterogeneity of the treatment population.

An interesting cost-effective analysis of RFA treatment strategy compared with palliative care in the treatment of hepatocellular cancer and liver metastases was performed. In the analysis, rather than using a defined marginal median survival achieved by RFA treatment strategy, they instead used a more flexible strategy of using a range of marginal median survival between 1 and 60 months. They noted that RFA ablation would be required to generate a marginal median survival benefit of 6.14 months, 2.26 months, and 1.1 month to achieve strict ($20,000/life year gained), moderate ($50,000/life year gained), and generous ($100,000/life year gained) cost-effective thresholds, respectively. Despite the lack of long-term survival data, examining the available reports, they suggest that percutaneous RFA has likely already achieved the survival benefit required to meet even a strict cost-effectiveness criteria (58).

Kidney

While treatment of renal cell cancer is relatively new compared with RFA of hepatic malignancies, it has now been widely accepted in clinical practice. In a report of treatment of 100 renal tumors with RFA, 90 of the tumors showed complete necrosis. Best results were obtained for smaller tumors (<4 cm), which were exophytic. Most of these ablations were guided by CT. However, we have found using US for initial needle placement, followed by

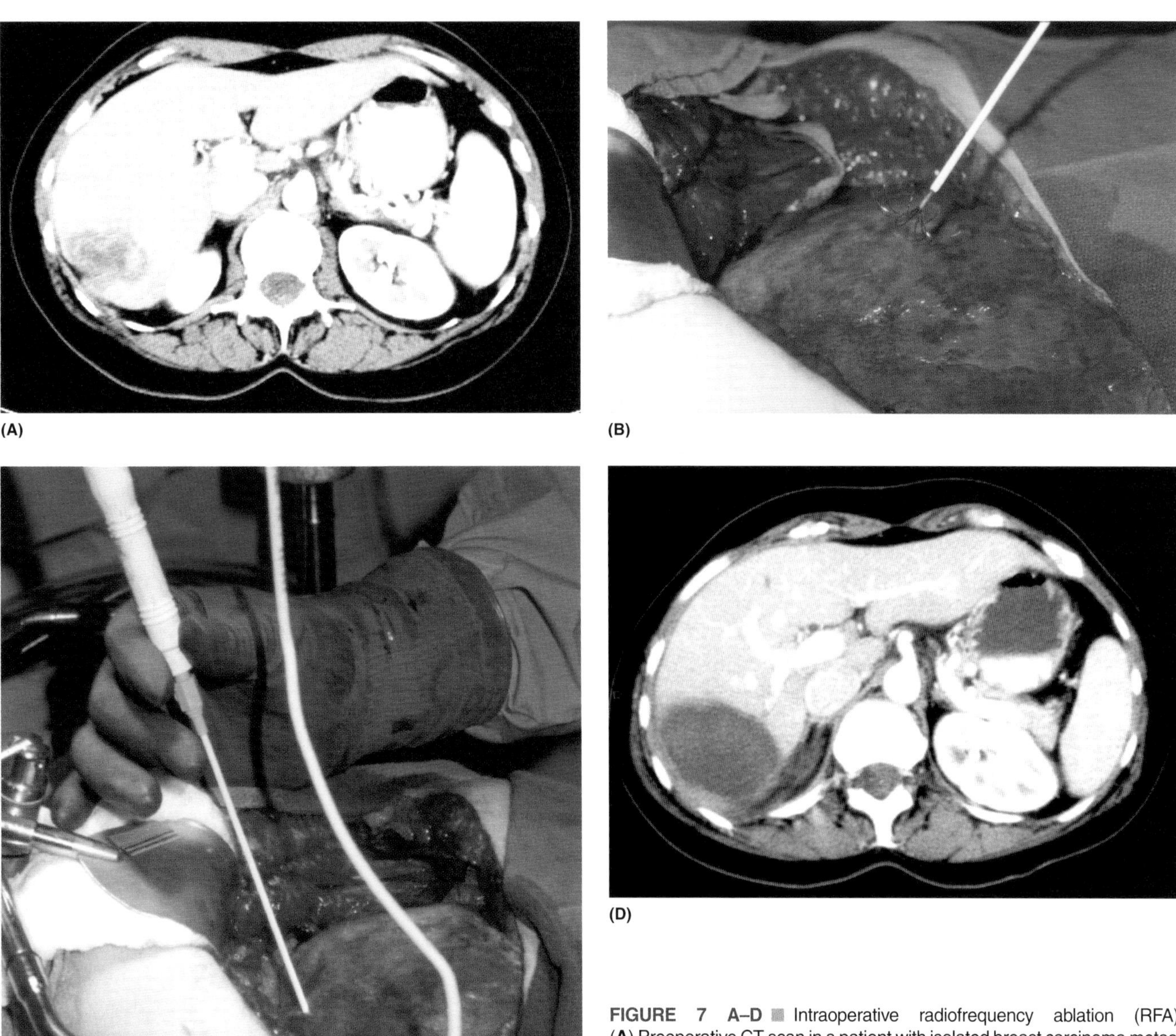

(A) (B) (C) (D)

FIGURE 7 A–D ■ Intraoperative radiofrequency ablation (RFA). (**A**) Preoperative CT scan in a patient with isolated breast carcinoma metastases to the liver. (**B**) During surgery, before insertion of the electrode, the tynes of the radiofrequency needle are deployed over the liver surface. (**C**) Then the tynes are pulled back into the needle and the needle is placed under ultrasound guidance into deep liver lesion. The tynes are then redeployed. (**D**) With two RFAs, using the Pringle maneuver, a large region of ablation is noted in the posterior sector of the right lobe of the liver.

CT to check final needle placement, utilizes the advantages of sonography for real-time needle placement without the use of radiation (Fig. 8). Complications with renal RFA including hemorrhage (5 patients), with ureteral injury (1 patient), ureteral strictures (2 patients), transient pain (2 patients), and grounding pad burns (1 patient) were reported in treatment of 100 renal tumors. RFA has shown to be a successful method of treatment of renal cell carcinoma without significant complications.

Breast

After various well-designed randomized trials demonstrated no survival difference between mastectomy and breast conservation therapy, in the last few decades, there has been a consistent trend toward less radical approaches to address local treatment of breast carcinoma. An animal study was conducted by McGahan et al. where both the acute the and chronic effects of RF electrocautery were evaluated in mammary tissue of three domestic swine (59). Our initial experimental results demonstrated that RFA was feasible in animal model and thus a phase II study was designed to determine the efficacy and safety of RFA of early human breast cancer. Khatri et al. (60) reported the results of this phase II study where 16 patients with biopsy-proven invasive breast cancer, ≤1.5 cm in diameter were enrolled. Under US guidance, the tumor

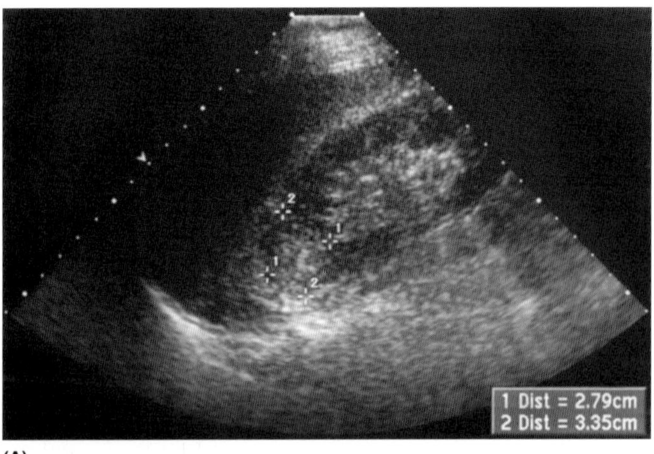

(A)

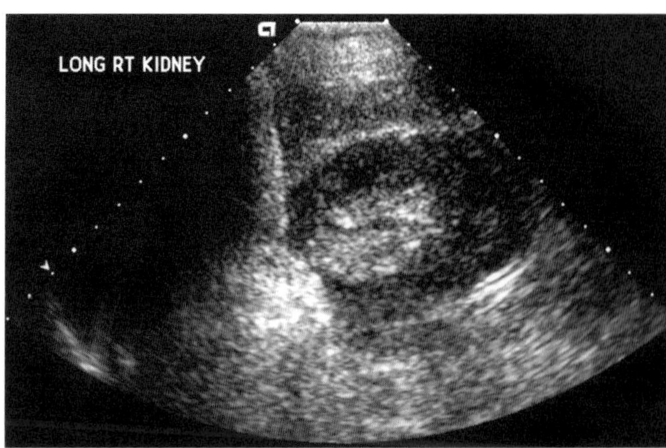

(B)

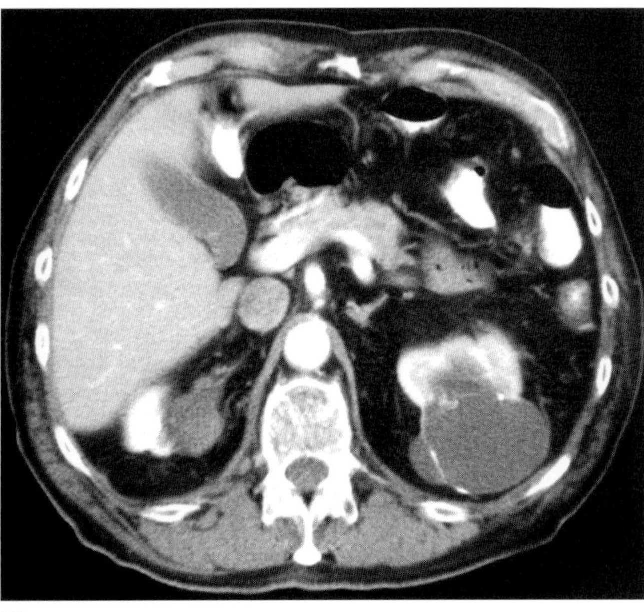

(C)

FIGURE 8 A–C ■ Radiofrequency ablation (RFA) of renal cell carcinoma. (**A**) Ultrasound demonstrating mass in the superior pole of the right kidney (*calipers*), which corresponds to renal cell carcinoma. (**B**) During RFA, the needle is identified and the mass becomes more echogenic. (**C**) Post-RFA CT scan shows nonenhancing region in the upper pole of the right kidney in region of ablation. Patient had an incidental cyst within the left kidney.

and a 5 mm margin of surrounding breast tissue were treated with RFA followed by immediate surgical resection (Fig. 9). In 13 of 14 patients (92.8%), the ablated tumor showed no evidence of viable malignant cells. In the pilot study by Izzo et al., coagulation necrosis was complete in 25 of 26 patients (96%) (61). Similar encouraging results were published from MD Anderson Cancer Center where sonography confirmed complete ablation of the targeted lesion in 93% (27/29) while the histological examination showed that 86% (25/29) of the primary tumors had been completely ablated (62).

Other Uses

RF is used in a number of other cases, including ablation of osteoid osteoma (63), the lung (64), and the prostate (65). Thus, tissue ablation with RF could easily be guided with US in areas such as the prostate for either needle tip placement or RF tissue ablation.

CRYOTHERAPY

Liver

In 1987, Ravikumar et al. (66) reported their surgical experience with hepatic cryosurgery for metastatic colon cancer to the liver. The development of 8- to 12-mm liquid nitrogen–cooled probes suitable for surgical placement within the liver marked the advent of interstitial therapy. Verification of the effectiveness of therapy was determined anatomically by the use of real-time US to measure the size of the increasing ice ball caused by freezing. Freezing and thawing for three cycles was an effective means of ensuring tumor necrosis. The average size of lesions treated in this series was less than 3 cm.

The disadvantage of cryotherapy appears to be that it requires an operation to place the large (8- and 12-mm) probes near the lesions. Thus, the surgical risks must be factored into the analysis of morbidity and mortality. The new smaller percutaneous probes will have risks

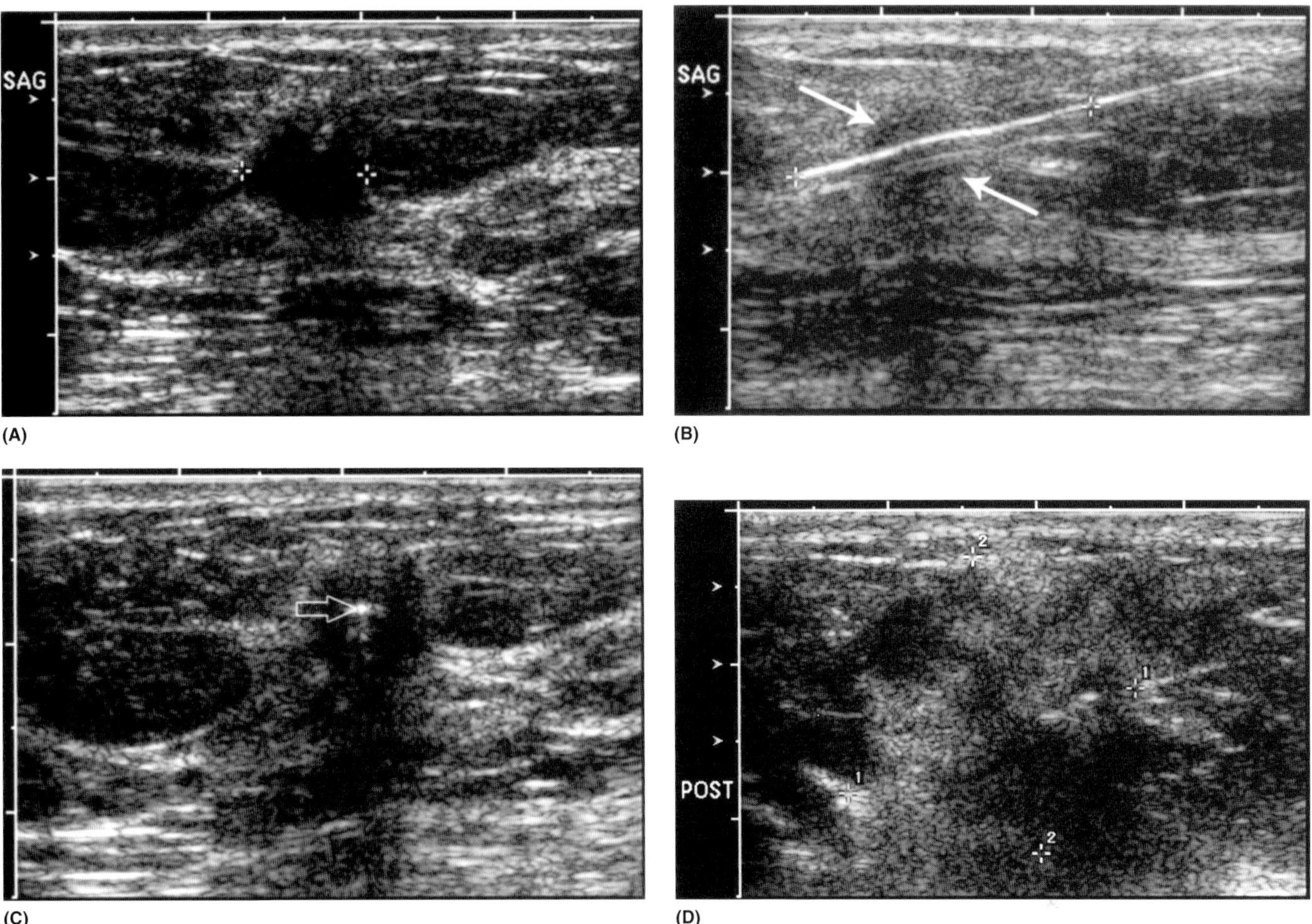

(A) (B) (C) (D)

FIGURE 9 A–D ■ Radiofrequency ablation (RFA) of the breast carcinoma. (**A**) Ultrasound of the breast demonstrated 8 mm hypoechoic breast carcinoma (*calipers*). (**B**) Under ultrasound guidance, a radiofrequency needle is inserted into the hypoechoic mass (*arrows*) with a 2 cm exposed tip, which is identified by calipers. (**C**) Moving the ultrasound probe 90° to scan transverse to the needle shaft shows the echogenic needle (*arrow*) located centrally within the hypoechoic breast carcinoma. (**D**) Post-RFA demonstrates an echogenic region within the breast, which corresponds to the RFA zone (*calipers*). Note the zone is much larger than the initial lesion.

that differ from those of surgical cryotherapy (67). US has been used to monitor the placement of the cryoprobes. Probes are placed on the liver capsule for superficial lesions or into the liver tissue under US guidance for deeper lesions. Probe placement should usually be in the center of the lesion to create a spherical lesion with freeze. When freezing, a very echogenic lesion may be observed with US (68). Usually, the freeze is continued beyond the margin of the tumor to ensure tumor kill.

Several alternatives to the usual protocol have been developed for hepatic cryotherapy, including the double-freeze cycle using laparoscopic surgery (69). The double freeze creates greater hepatic injury, which may help to achieve adequate destruction. Laparoscopic probe placement still requires surgery and anesthesia but is less invasive than open surgery.

Complications

Complications from cryosurgery include pleural effusions (70), "cracking" of the hepatic parenchyma (71), and death (72). There are a number of interesting imaging findings in patients who have had hepatic cryotherapy (70). These include air in the lesion (36%), hemorrhage in the lesion (93%), subcapsular hemorrhage (29%), peripheral fluid collections (43%), right-sided pleural effusions (93%), left-sided pleural effusions (64%), atelectasis (93%), and ascites (7%). Percutaneous techniques have resulted in thermal injury to the skin because effective insulation is difficult to achieve.

Results

In general, as with all treatment modalities, the results appear to be better for primary tumors, such as HCC, than for metastases. Onik et al. (67) believe the disease free rate of cryotherapy is comparable to other forms of therapy.

Breast

Another approach for less invasive treatment of breast cancer is to use freezing methods. However, cryoablation appears to be less effective due to incomplete freezing and a subsequent higher rate of residual disease and in a recent multi-center report, the technique was limited by the tumor size and also whether there was associated presence of DCIS (72). The efficacy of cryotherapy can be enhanced by increasing the cooling rates and by adding a double freeze/cycle. Interestingly, in an experimental murine model of breast carcinoma, a single freeze/cycle of breast tumor was associated with a local recurrence rate of 80%, and five freeze/cycles were needed to reduce the recurrence rates to an acceptable level of less than 5% (73). Furthermore, compared with normal tissue, malignant cells have been demonstrated to be more resistant to the lethal damage from freezing but most sensitive to hyperthermic energy (74). Cryotherapy has also been successfully applied as an office-based minimally invasive treatment for fibroadenomas (75).

Prostate

Cryosurgery of the prostate has been performed in a number of centers (73,74). A catheter is placed in the bladder and a urethral warming catheter is also placed. Thermal monitoring probes are also placed adjacent to the neurovascular bundle. Using a template, cryoprobes are placed percutaneously into the prostate under transrectal US guidance and cryotherapy is performed with a double freeze technique. Donnelly et al. have shown utility of this technique after failed radiation (73). Onik has advocated focal cryoablation for prostate cancer (75).

OTHER TREATMENTS

A number of other methods have been advocated for tissue destruction using US as a guidance method. For instance, Holm et al. (76) first proposed the use of transrectal US for guidance of implantation of radioactive seeds for treatment of prostate carcinoma. Seed placement guided by US has proved an effective method of treatment of prostate carcinoma, but initial results demonstrated a high incidence of complications, such as rectal fistulous. This method was initially abandoned by Holm, though it has experienced a recent resurgence in use.

High-Intensity Focused US

Several manufacturers have developed US probes that alternate imaging and therapy using HIFU (77–79). High-intensity US is focused to an area for potential tissue destruction (Fig. 10). This requires no needle placement as with RF or laser treatment. This method has shown limited success in tissue ablation of the prostate, but there has been some mixed results using this as an alternative to a transurethral resection of the prostate (81). We have tried HIFU ablation of other organs in our laboratory. Although HIFU successfully ablated the liver when the probe was placed directly on the liver, we have encountered problems with percutaneous ablation of the liver. Unfortunately, the liver moves with respiration, and there is no gating mechanism to ensure ablation of a focal area of the liver using HIFU. We have found that with increased power settings, thermal burns of the skin may occur.

However, better results for HIFU have also been reported for treatment of breast carcinomas. In a recent publication, Wu et al. randomized 78 women with biopsy- proven breast cancer into the experimental group treated with HIFU and compared with the control group where modified radical mastectomy was performed. In the 23 patients with a mean tumor diameter of 3.1 cm, the mean treatment time for HIFU was 1.3 hours (range, 45 minutes to 2.5 hours) (82).

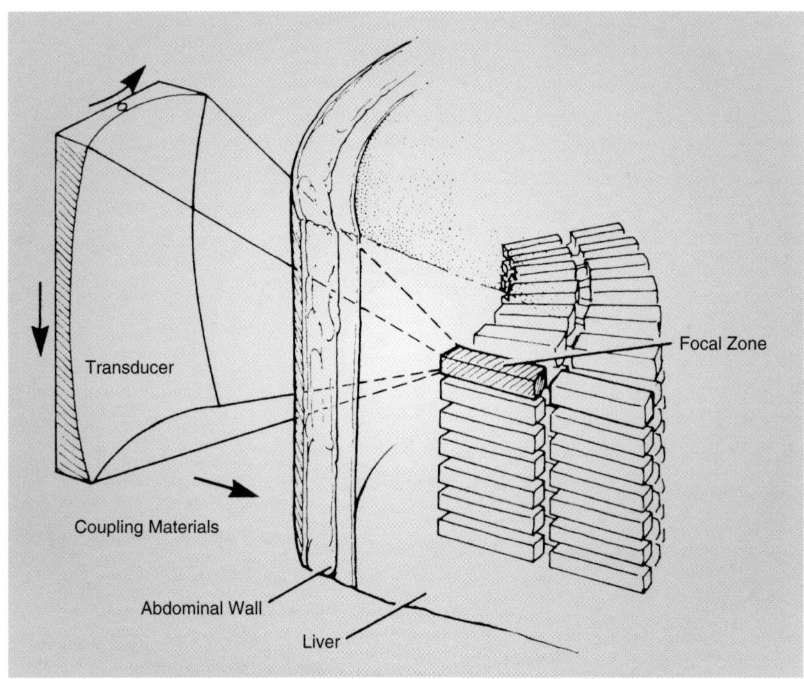

FIGURE 10 ■ Diagram of transcutaneous liver sonar ablation. With the transducer in the stationary position, only a single focal zone is treated. Within the stepping mode, however, multiple specific focal areas, labeled as focal zones, are treated within the liver. *Source*: From Ref. 80.

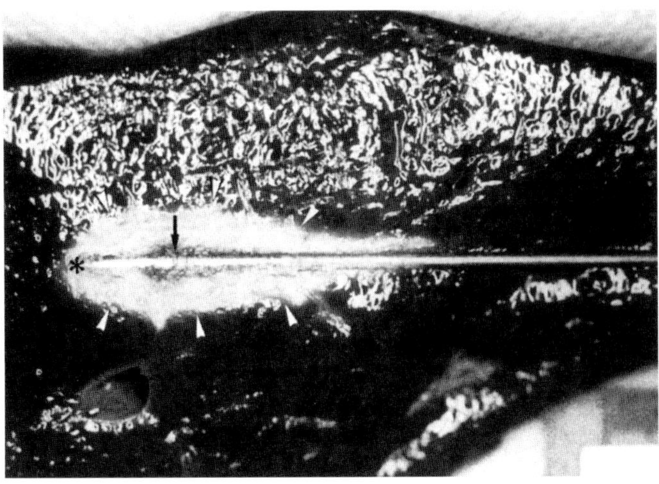

FIGURE 11 ■ Gross specimen of microwave coagulation. Appearance of a cut surface of a pig liver after microwave photocoagulation using a monopolar electrode (*arrow*). An area of coagulation necrosis surrounds the microwave tip (*arrowheads*). An asterisk marks the tip of the monopolar electrode. *Source*: From Ref. 83.

Microwave Coagulation Hyperthermia

Microwave coagulation is based on the principle of a high-frequency (2450 MHz) electromagnetic wave generated by magnetron and transmitted via a coaxial cable to an electrode tip that coagulates the target tissue. Not too dissimilar to RFA, the heat is generated due to vibration and intermolecular collision of polar molecules in the tissue exposed to the high frequency electromagnetic waves. Results demonstrate microwaves may be able to create ablation zones similar to, if not larger than, zones created by RFA (Figs. 11 and 12). This technique was first developed by Tabuse, in 1979, as an adjunct for hepatic surgery where it allows the surgeon to transect the liver parenchyma and coagulate the cut surface simultaneously (84).

Microwave hyperthermia is a method that may be used for US-guided tissue destruction (83). Most microwave therapy has been directed toward the treatment of benign prostatic hypertrophy. Although results have been mixed, some studies (85) indicated that transurethral microwave thermotherapy was successful in treatment of benign prostatic hypertrophy, while others (86) showed limited success with this technique.

Microwave hyperthermia has also been used to treat tumors in the liver (83,87). Seki et al. (87) treated 18 patients with small (<2 cm) HCC lesions. A microwave electrode is inserted into a tumor with US guidance (Fig. 13). The area became echogenic with microwave treatment similar to other percutaneous treatment modalities. Of the 18 patients, 17 remained alive 11 to 33 months after the treatment. Focal microwave hyperthermia may be another method of treatment of tumors.

A randomized study examined the efficacy of microwave ablation as a treatment modality for patients with multiple hepatic colorectal metastases with regard to survival and morbidity in comparison to standard hepatic resection (88). Inclusion criteria were patients with multiple but less than 10 metastatic tumor deposits, the largest tumor with a dimension of <8 cm, and no evidence of extra hepatic disease or cirrhosis. They noted no significant difference in the mean survival times (27 months in microwave group and 25 months in hepatectomy group) or the mean disease-free interval (11.3 months in the microwave group and 13.3 months in the hepatectomy group) between the two groups. Though there was no difference in the number of complications between the two groups, those patients who underwent microwave ablation had less blood loss and required significantly fewer blood transfusions. Microwave ablation has been shown to be an effective method of treatment of HCC (89). The results of percutaneous microwave and RF were similar in a recent report by Lu et al. (89). Microwave has also been successfully used in combined microwave and resection colorectal metastasis (90). High grade dysplastic liver nodules are also well treated with percutaneous microwave (91).

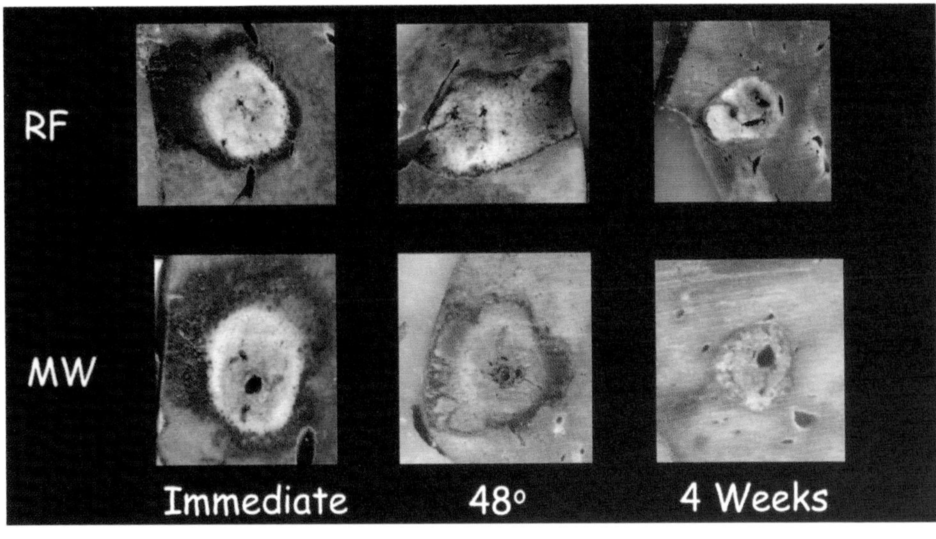

FIGURE 12 ■ Comparison of microwave and radiofrequency ablation of in vivo liver showing similar size of coagulation with a single probe immediately, at 48 hours, and at 4 weeks. *Source*: Courtesy of Drs. Thomas Winter and Fred Lee, University of Wisconsin Medical Center.

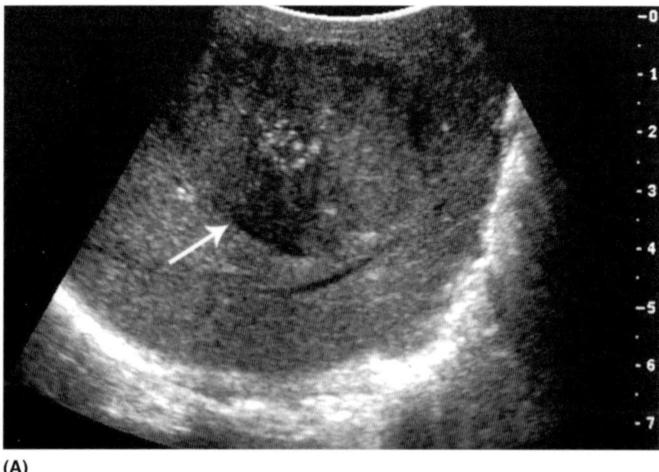

(A)

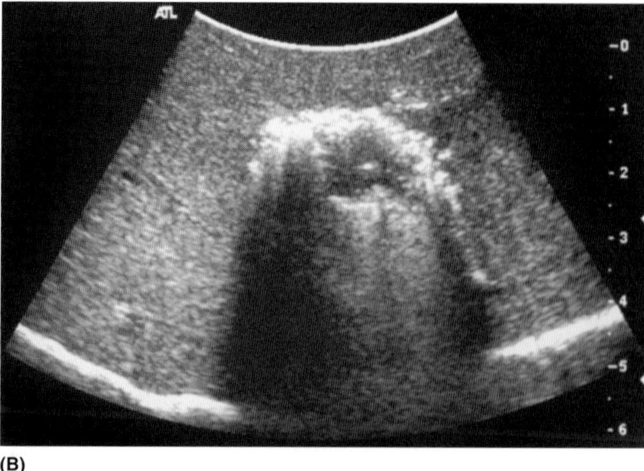

(B)

FIGURE 13 A AND B ■ (**A**) Intraoperative ultrasound showing hypoechoic metastatic colon cancer to the liver (with characteristic microcalcifications of mucinous subtype). (**B**) Intraoperative ultrasound performed after microwave application showing increased echogenicity with distal shadowing after treatment of metastatic colon cancer to the liver. *Source*: Courtesy of Drs. Thomas Winter and Fred Lee, University of Wisconsin Medical Center.

CONCLUSION

A number of these interstitial treatments cause reproducible tissue destruction and are well tolerated, with low risk to the patients. Interstitial techniques may replace hepatic resection in some instances in the future, particularly for lesions smaller than 3 cm. Combining therapies, such as transcatheter regional chemotherapy or systemic chemotherapy, with percutaneous ablative techniques may be worthwhile. Patients who are candidates for curative resection, but for whom surgical resection is not an option, should be offered participation in carefully conducted clinical trials using any of these interstitial techniques. This is an evolving technology-based clinical treatment with too little data on long-term results. We must proceed carefully and document our results meticulously.

REFERENCES

1. Livraghi T, Salmi A, Bolondi L, et al. Small hepatocellular carcinoma: percutaneous alcohol injection—results in 23 patients. Radiology 1988; 168(2):313–317.
2. Livraghi T, Vettori C. Percutaneous ethanol injection therapy of hepatoma. Cardiovasc Intervent Radiol 1990; 13(3):146–152.
3. Livraghi T, Vettori C, Lazzaroni S. Liver metastases: results of percutaneous ethanol injection in 14 patients. Radiology 1991; 179(3):709–712.
4. Borghetti M, Benelli G, Bonardi R. Treatment of small hepatocarcinomas by percutaneous ultrasound-guided alcohol injections. Personal experience in 14 lesions. Radiol Med (Torino) 1991; 81(4):502–509.
5. Livraghi T, Lazzaroni S, Meloni F, et al. Intralesional ethanol in the treatment of unresectable liver cancer. World J Surg 1995; 19(6):801–806.
6. Redvanly RD, Chezmar JL, Strauss RM, et al. Malignant hepatic tumors: safety of high-dose percutaneous ethanol ablation therapy. Radiology 1993; 188(1):283–285.
7. Shiina S, Tagawa K, Unuma T, et al. Percutaneous ethanol injection therapy of hepatocellular carcinoma: analysis of 77 patients. AJR Am J Roentgenol 1990; 155(6):1221–1226.
8. Yamashita Y, Matsukawa T, Arakawa A, et al. US-guided liver biopsy: predicting the effect of interventional treatment of hepatocellular carcinoma. Radiology 1995; 196(3):799–804.
9. Lencioni R, Caramella D, Bartolozzi C. Hepatocellular carcinoma: use of color Doppler US to evaluate response to treatment with percutaneous ethanol injection. Radiology 1995; 194(1):113–118.
10. Ito K, Honjo K, Fujita T, et al. Enhanced MR imaging of the liver after ethanol treatment of hepatocellular carcinoma: evaluation of areas of hyperperfusion adjacent to the tumor. AJR Am J Roentgenol 1995; 164(6):1413–1417.
11. Ebara M, Kita K, Sugiura N, et al. Therapeutic effect of percutaneous ethanol injection on small hepatocellular carcinoma: evaluation with CT. Radiology 1995; 195(2):371–377.
12. Livraghi T, Giorgio A, Marin G, et al. Hepatocellular carcinoma and cirrhosis in 746 patients: long-term results of percutaneous ethanol injection. Radiology 1995; 197(1):101–108.
13. Livraghi T, Bolondi L, Buscarini L, et al. No treatment, resection and ethanol injection in hepatocellular carcinoma: a retrospective analysis of survival in 391 patients with cirrhosis. Italian Cooperative HCC Study Group. J Hepatol 1995; 22(5):522–526.
14. Castells A, Bruix J, Bru C, et al. Treatment of small hepatocellular carcinoma in cirrhotic patients: a cohort study comparing surgical resection and percutaneous ethanol injection. Hepatology 1993; 18(5):1121–1126.
15. Bartolozzi C, Lencioni R. Ethanol injection for the treatment of hepatic tumours. Eur Radiol 1996; 6(5):682–696.
16. Giovannini M, Seitz JF. Ultrasound-guided percutaneous alcohol injection of small liver metastases. Results in 40 patients. Cancer 1994; 73(2):294–297.
17. Giorgio A, Tarantino L, Mariniello N, et al. Ultrasonography-guided percutaneous ethanol injection in large and/or multiple liver metastasis. Radiol Med (Torino) 1998; 96(3):238–242.
18. Mazziotti A, Grazi GL, Gardini A, et al. An appraisal of percutaneous treatment of liver metastases. Liver Transpl Surg 1998; 4(4): 271–275.
19. Solinas A, Erbella GS, Distrutti E, et al. Abscess formation in hepatocellular carcinoma: complications of percutaneous ultrasound-guided ethanol injection. J Clin Ultrasound 1993; 21(8):531–533.

20. de Sio I, Castellano L, Calandra M. Hemobilia following percutaneous ethanol injection for hepatocellular carcinoma in a cirrhotic patient. J Clin Ultrasound 1992; 20(9):621–623.
21. Zerbey AL, Mueller PR, Dawson SL, Hoover HC Jr. Pleural seeding from hepatocellular carcinoma: a complication of percutaneous alcohol ablation. Radiology 1994; 193(1):81–82.
22. Veltri A, Martina C, Bonenti G, et al. Therapy of malignant hepatic tumors using percutaneous hot saline injections. Feasibility study and preliminary results. Radiol Med (Torino) 1995; 90(4):463–469.
23. Taavitsainen M, Vehmas T, Kauppila R. Fatal liver necrosis following percutaneous ethanol injection for hepatocellular carcinoma. Abdom Imaging 1993; 18(4):357–359.
24. Honda N, Guo Q, Uchida H, et al. Percutaneous hot saline injection therapy for hepatic tumors: an alternative to percutaneous ethanol injection therapy. Radiology 1994; 190(1):53–57.
25. Ohnishi K, Ohyama N, Ito S, Fujiwara K. Small hepatocellular carcinoma: treatment with US-guided intratumoral injection of acetic acid. Radiology 1994; 193(3):747–752.
26. Montorsi M, Torzilli G, Fumagalli U, et al. Percutaneous alcohol sclerotherapy of simple hepatic cysts. Results from a multicentre survey in Italy. HPB Surg 1994; 8(2):89–94.
27. vanSonnenberg E, Wroblicka JT, D'Agostino HB, et al. Symptomatic hepatic cysts: percutaneous drainage and sclerosis. Radiology 1994; 190(2):387–392.
28. Solbiati L, Giangrande A, De Pra L, et al. Percutaneous ethanol injection of parathyroid tumors under US guidance: treatment for secondary hyperparathyroidism. Radiology 1985; 155(3):607–610.
29. Charboneau JW, Hay ID, van Heerden JA. Persistent primary hyperparathyroidism: successful ultrasound-guided percutaneous ethanol ablation of an occult adenoma. Mayo Clin Proc 1988; 63(9):913–917.
30. Giangrande A, Castiglioni A, Solbiati L, et al. Chemical parathyroidectomy for recurrence of secondary hyperparathyroidism. Am J Kidney Dis 1994; 24(3):421–426.
31. Karstrup S, Hegedus L, Holm HH. Ultrasonically guided chemical parathyroidectomy in patients with primary hyperparathyroidism: a follow-up study. Clin Endocrinol (Oxf) 1993; 38(5):523–530.
32. Malik U, Mohiuddin M. External-beam radiotherapy in the management of liver metastases. Semin Oncol 2002; 29:196–201.
33. http://ctep.cancer.gov/guidelines/recist.html.
34. Stubbs RS, Cannan RJ, Mitchell AW. Selective internal radiation therapy with 90 yttrium microspheres for extensive colorectal liver metastases. J Gastrointest Surg 2001; 5(3):294–302.
35. Koniaris LG, Chan DY, Magee C, et al. Focal hepatic ablation using interstitial photon radiation energy. J Am Coll Surg 2000; 191(2): 164–174.
36. Dritschilo A, Grant EG, Harter KW, et al. Interstitial radiation therapy for hepatic metastases: sonographic guidance for applicator placement. AJR Am J Roentgenol 1986; 147(2):275–278.
37. Holt RW, Nauta RJ, Lee TC, et al. Intraoperative interstitial radiation therapy for hepatic metastases from colorectal carcinomas. Am Surg 1988; 54(4):231–233.
38. Hashimoto D, Takami M, Idezuki Y. In depth radiation therapy Nd:YAG laser for malignant tumors of the liver under ultrasonic imaging. Gastroenterology 1985; 88:A1663.
39. Hahl J, Haapiainen R, Ovaska J, et al. Laser-induced hyperthermia in the treatment of liver tumors. Lasers Surg Med 1990; 10(4):319–321.
40. Amin Z, Bown SG, Lees WR. Local treatment of colorectal liver metastases: a comparison of interstitial laser photocoagulation (ILP) and percutaneous alcohol injection (PAI). Clin Radiol 1993; 48(3):166–171.
41. Schroder TM, Puolakkainen PA, Hahl J, Ramo OJ. Fatal air embolism as a complication of laser-induced hyperthermia. Lasers Surg Med 1989; 9(2):183–185.
42. Malone DE, Wyman DR, Moote DJ, et al. Sonographic changes during hepatic interstitial laser photocoagulation: an investigation of three optical fiber tips. Invest Radiol 1992; 27:804.
43. Bosman S, Phoa SS, Bosma A, van Gemert MJ. Effect of percutaneous interstitial thermal laser on normal liver of pigs: sonographic and histopathological correlations. Br J Surg 1991; 78(5):572–575.
44. Vogl TJ, Straub R, Zangos S, et al. MR-guided laser-induced thermotherapy (LITT) of liver tumours: experimental and clinical data. Int J Hyperthermia 2004; 20(7):713–724.
45. Veenendaal LM, de Jager A, Stapper G, et al. Multiple fiber laser-induced thermotherapy for ablation of large intrahepatic tumors. Photomed Laser Surg 2006; 24(1):3–9.
46. Dowlatshahi K, Fan M, Gould VE. Stereotactically guided laser therapy of occult breast tumors. Work in progress report. Arch Surg 2000; 135:1345–1352.
47. Mueller-Lisse UG, Heuck AF, Schneede P, et al. Postoperative MRI in patients undergoing interstitial laser coagulation thermotherapy of benign prostatic hyperplasia. J Comput Assist Tomogr 1996; 20(2):273–278.
48. McGahan JP, Browning PD, Brock JM, Tesluk H. Hepatic ablation using radiofrequency electrocautery. Invest Radiol 1990; 25(3):267–270.
49. McGahan JP, Brock JN, Tesluk H, et al. Hepatic ablation with use of radiofrequency electrocautery in the animal model. J Interven Radiol 1992; 3:291.
50. McGahan JP, Gu WZ, Brock JM, et al. Hepatic ablation using bipolar radiofrequency electrocautery. Acad Radiol 1996; 3(5):418–422.
51. Rossi S, Di Stasi M, Buscarini E, et al. Percutaneous radiofrequency interstitial thermal ablation in the treatment of small hepatocellular carcinoma. Cancer J Sci Am 1995; 1(1):73.
52. Goldberg SN, Gazelle GS, Dawson SL, et al. Tissue ablation with radiofrequency using multiprobe arrays. Acad Radiol 1995; 2(8):670–674.
53. Lorentzen T. A cooled needle electrode for radiofrequency tissue ablation: thermodynamic aspects of improved performance compared with conventional needle design. Acad Radiol 1996; 3(7):556–563.
54. Curley SA, Izzo F, Delrio P, et al. Radiofrequency ablation of unresectable primary and metastatic hepatic malignancies: results in 123 patients. Ann Surg 1999; 230(1):1–8.
55. Livraghi T, Solbiati L, Meloni MF, et al. Treatment of focal liver tumors with percutaneous radio-frequency ablation: complications encountered in a multicenter study. Radiology 2003; 226(2):441–451.
56. Pearson AS, Izzo F, Fleming RY, et al. Intraoperative radiofrequency ablation or cryoablation for hepatic malignancies. Am J Surg 1999; 178(6):592–599.
57. Bilchik AJ, Wood TF, Allegra D, et al. Cryosurgical ablation and radiofrequency ablation for unresectable hepatic malignant neoplasms: a proposed algorithm. Arch Surg 2000; 135(6):657–662; discussion 662–664.
58. Shetty SK, Rosen MP, Raptopoulos V, Goldberg SN. Cost-effectiveness of percutaneous radiofrequency ablation for malignant hepatic neoplasms. J Vasc Interv Radiol 2001; 12(7):823–833.
59. McGahan JP, Griffey SM, Schneider PD, et al. Radio-frequency electrocautery ablation of mammary tissue in swine. Radiology 2000; 217(2):471–476.
60. Khatri VP, McGahan JP, Ramsamoog R, et al. A Phase II trial of image-guided radiofrequency ablation of small (<1.5CM) breast cancers. Proceedings of the 66th Annual Meeting, Society of University Surgeons Nashville, Tennessee, 2005.
61. Izzo F, Thomas R, Delrio P, et al. Radiofrequency ablation in patients with primary breast carcinoma: a pilot study in 26 patients. Cancer 2001; 92(8):2036–2044.
62. Fornage BD, Sneige N, Ross MI, et al. Small (≤2 cm) breast cancer treated with US-guided radiofrequency ablation: feasibility study. Radiology 2004; 231(1):215–224.
63. Rosenthal DI, Springfield DS, Gebhardt MC, et al. Osteoid osteoma: percutaneous radio-frequency ablation. Radiology 1995; 197(2):451–454.
64. Goldberg SN, Gazelle GS, Compton CC, McLoud TC. Radiofrequency tissue ablation in the rabbit lung: efficacy and complications. Acad Radiol 1995; 2(9):776–784.
65. McGahan JP, Griffey SM, Budenz RW, Brock JM. Percutaneous ultrasound-guided radiofrequency electrocautery ablation of prostate tissue in dogs. Acad Radiol 1995; 2(1):61–65.
66. Ravikumar TS, Kane R, Cady B, et al. Hepatic cryosurgery with intraoperative ultrasound monitoring for metastatic colon carcinoma. Arch Surg 1987; 122(4):403–409.
67. Onik GM, Atkinson D, Zemel R, Weaver ML. Cryosurgery of liver cancer. Semin Surg Oncol 1993; 9(4):309–317.
68. Cuschieri A, Crosthwaite G, Shimi S, et al. Hepatic cryotherapy for liver tumors. Development and clinical evaluation of a high-effi-

ciency insulated multineedle probe system for open and laparoscopic use. Surg Endosc 1995; 9(5):483–489.
69. Stewart GJ, Preketes A, Horton M, et al. Hepatic cryotherapy: double-freeze cycles achieve greater hepatocellular injury in man. Cryobiology 1995; 32(3):215–219.
70. Kuszyk BS, Choti MA, Urban BA, et al. Hepatic tumors treated by cryosurgery: normal CT appearance. AJR Am J Roentgenol 1996; 166(2):363–368.
71. Ross WB, Horton M, Bertolino P, Morris DL. Cryotherapy of liver tumours—a practical guide. HPB Surg 1995; 8(3):167–173.
72. Polk W, Fong Y, Karpeh M, Blumgart LH. A technique for the use of cryosurgery to assist hepatic resection. J Am Coll Surg 1995; 180(2):171–176.
73. Donnelly BJ, Saliken JC, Ernst DS, et al. Role of transrectal ultrasound guided salvage cryosurgery for recurrent prostate carcinoma after radiotherapy. Prostate Cancer Prostatic Dis 2005; 8(3):235–242.
74. Prepelica KL, Okeke Z, Murphy A, Katz AE. Cryosurgical ablation of the prostate: high risk patient outcomes. Cancer 2005; 103(8):1625–1630.
75. Onik G. The male lumpectomy: rationale for a cancer targeted approach for prostate cryoablation. A review. Technol Cancer Res Treat 2004; 3(4):365–370.
76. Holm HH, Juul N, Pedersen JF, et al. Transperineal 125 iodine seed implantation in prostatic cancer guided by transrectal ultrasonography. J Urol 1983; 130(2):283–286.
77. Ebert T, Graefen M, Miller S, et al. High-intensity focused ultrasound (HIFU) in the treatment of benign prostatic hyperplasia (BPH). Keio J Med 1995; 44(4):146–149.
78. Gelet A, Chapelon JY, Margonari J, et al. Prostatic tissue destruction by high-intensity focused ultrasound: experimentation on canine prostate. J Endourol 1993; 7(3):249–253.
79. Prat F, Centarti M, Sibille A, et al. Extracorporeal high-intensity focused ultrasound for VX2 liver tumors in the rabbit. Hepatology 1995; 21(3):832–836.
80. Yang R, Sanghvi NT, Rescoria FJ, et al. Extracorporeal liver ablation using sonography-guided high-intensity focused ultrasound. Invest Radiol 1992; 27:796.
81. Foster RS, Bihrle R, Sanghvi NT, et al. High-intensity focused ultrasound in the treatment of prostatic disease. Eur Urol 1993; 23(suppl 1):29–33.
82. Wu F, Wang ZB, Cao YD, et al. A randomised clinical trial of high-intensity focused ultrasound ablation for the treatment of patients with localised breast cancer. Br J Cancer 2003; 89(12): 2227–2233.
83. Murakami R, Yoshimatsu S, Yamashita Y, et al. Treatment of hepatocellular carcinoma: value of percutaneous microwave coagulation. AJR Am J Roentgenol 1995; 164(5):1159–1164.
84. Tabuse K. A new operative procedure of hepatic surgery using a microwave tissue coagulator. Nippon Geka Hokan 1979; 48(2): 160–172.
85. Dahlstrand C, Walden M, Geirsson G, Pettersson S. Transurethral microwave thermotherapy versus transurethral resection for symptomatic benign prostatic obstruction: a prospective randomized study with a 2-year follow-up. Br J Urol 1995; 76(5):614–618.
86. Montorsi F, Guazzoni G, Rigatti P, et al. Is there a role for transrectal microwave hyperthermia in the treatment of benign prostatic hyperplasia? A critical review of a six-year experience. J Endourol 1995; 9(4):333–337.
87. Seki T, Wakabayashi M, Nakagawa T, et al. Ultrasonically guided percutaneous microwave coagulation therapy for small hepatocellular carcinoma. Cancer 1994; 74(3):817–825.
88. Shibata T, Niinobu T, Ogata N, Takami M. Microwave coagulation therapy for multiple hepatic metastases from colorectal carcinoma. Cancer 2000; 89(2):276–284.
89. Lu MD, Xu HX, Xie XY, et al. Percutaneous microwave and radiofrequency ablation for hepatocellular carcinoma: a retrospective comparative study. J Gastroenterol 2005; 40(11):1054–1060.
90. Tanaka K, Shimada H, Nagano Y, et al. Outcome after hepatic resection versus combined resection and microwave ablation for multiple bilobar colorectal metastases to the liver. Surgery 2006; 139(2):263–273.
91. Liang P, Dong B, Yu X, et al. Sonography-guided percutaneous microwave ablation of high-grade dysplastic nodules in cirrhotic liver. AJR Am J Roentgenol 2005; 184(5):1657–1660.

Breast • Catherine W. Piccoli and Annina N. Wilkes

9

NORMAL ANATOMY

The breast is composed of parenchymal and stromal structures. The parenchymal elements include glandular structures (acini and ducts). The stromal portions are the supporting structures made up of dense and loose connective tissue and fat. The amount and distribution of these structures are extremely variable among individual patients and change with age and hormonal status.

General Considerations

The parenchymal portion of the breast is composed of 15 to 25 lobes drained by separate collecting ducts that open onto the nipple. Just beneath the nipple, the duct dilates focally, a region referred to as the "lactiferous sinus." Each duct branches sequentially into numerous segmental, subsegmental, and terminal ducts. The terminal duct drains the acinar elements. The duct system is surrounded by stromal structures, or fibroadipose tissues, which constitute much of the bulk of the breast tissue in the nonpregnant, nonlactating woman.

The tissues forming the breast are divided into three layers (Fig. 1). The most superficial (subcutaneous) layer contains fat arranged in lobules surrounded and bound by supportive fibrous septa (Cooper's ligaments), which extend from the dermis to the superficial connective tissue of the middle layer. The fatty lobules are generally elliptical or polyhedral in shape. The middle (mammary) layer is bound by connective tissue on both its superficial and its deep aspects and contains the parenchymal tissue of the breast. The third (retromammary) layer, made up of fatty lobules, is bound anteriorly by the deep fascia of the mammary layer and posteriorly by the prepectoral fascia.

Morphologic Variations with Age and Hormonal Changes

There is tremendous variation among women in the amount and architecture of the different types of breast tissue and therefore in the imaging appearance of the breast. Variation with age and concomitant hormonal status also occurs within the individual. However, minimal changes of the breast parenchyma occur over the course of the menstrual cycle; these include formation of a dense cellular stroma, closed alveolar lumina, ductal proliferation during the follicular phase (days 7–14), and lobular enlargement due to alveolar dilation accompanied by hyperemia and edema during the luteal phase (days 15–20) (1). These proliferative changes regress after the luteal phase. Cyclic changes are, in general, not identifiable by ultrasound.

With the hormonal changes of pregnancy and lactation, there is a marked change of the parenchymal structures with proliferation of the ducts and acini. Concomitantly, the interlobular stroma regresses, and the fatty lobules of the subcutaneous and retromammary layers decrease (2). Postmenopausal involution involves a gradual regression of the lobular and ductal tissues and a variable proliferation of the stroma. The parenchyma may be replaced by predominantly fatty tissue containing few atrophic ducts and thin fibrous septa, or it may be replaced by coalescent dense connective tissue (2). The degree of either fatty or fibrous replacement

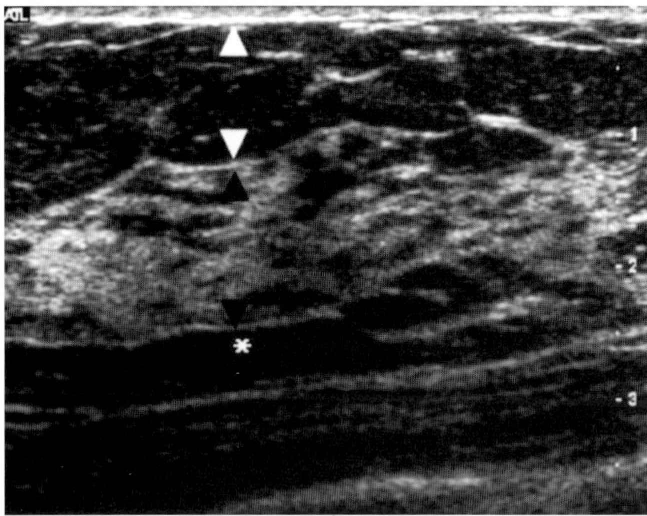

FIGURE 1 ■ Antiradial image showing the normal layers of the breast: subcutaneous layer (*white arrowheads*), mammary layer (*black arrowheads*), and retromammary layer (*asterisk*).

is highly variable among individual patients and within varying locations in the same breast.

Ultrasonographic Characteristics of the Normal Breast

The most superficial structure of the breast, the dermis, is an echogenic structure measuring about 2 mm in thickness, although the skin of the inferior breast and the areola may be slightly thicker. The fatty lobules of the subcutaneous and retromammary layers are of low echogenicity and contain a few moderately echogenic linear or punctate foci. The fibrous septa enveloping the fatty lobules are of high echogenicity. Fatty lobules may have an elliptical or polyhedral shape. The overall fatty lobular architecture produces a braided appearance on real-time imaging, in which one lobule flows into and conforms to the next. The tissue that makes up the mammary layer, a combination of closely associated parenchymal structures and connective tissue, is generally of intermediate-to-high echogenicity, although patches of hypoechoic fat may be interspersed within the field of fibroglandular tissue (Fig. 1). In the pregnant and lactating breast, the parenchyma is of intermediate echogenicity, with few hypoechoic areas corresponding to fat (Fig. 2). Hypoechoic, linear, branching structures coursing through this echogenic tissue represent ducts. The ducts can range in diameter from less than 1 mm to about 2 mm but are considered within the limits of normal if they are homogeneous in size, tapering as they course into the breast periphery without focal dilation (Fig. 3). The exception is the lactiferous sinus of each major duct, which is a focal dilation in the immediate retroareolar region (Fig. 4).

The chest wall at the level of the breast is made up of pectoralis major muscle overlying either the pectoralis minor muscle more superiorly or the serratus anterior muscle more inferiorly. These muscles overlie the ribs and intercostal muscles, which border the lung (Fig. 5).

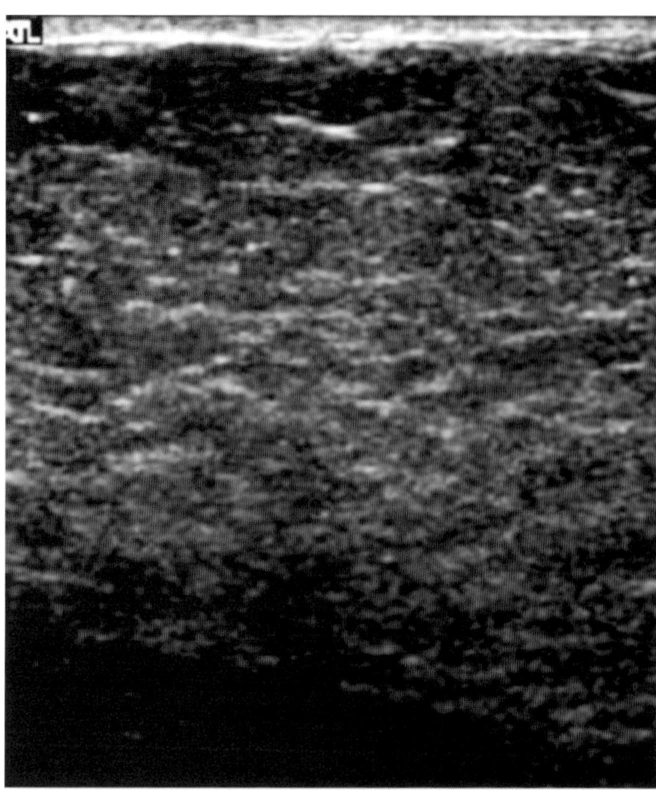

FIGURE 2 ■ Ultrasound image of the lactating breast shows a narrow subcutaneous layer of fat and a prominent mammary layer of intermediate echogenicity.

The Intact Breast Implant

Silicone gel and saline implants should also be considered in a discussion of breast imaging. The structure and manufacture of implants is diverse (Table 1). The implant shells are made of a silicone elastomer and may be smooth or textured. Older silicone implants may be coated with

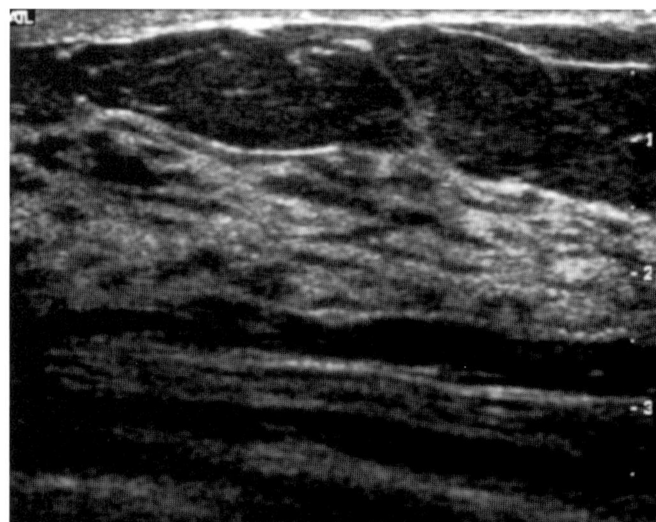

FIGURE 3 ■ Radial image showing normal hypoechoic linear ductal structures contained within hyperechoic fibroglandular tissue. The shorter hypoechoic structures are ducts coursing across the plane of imaging.

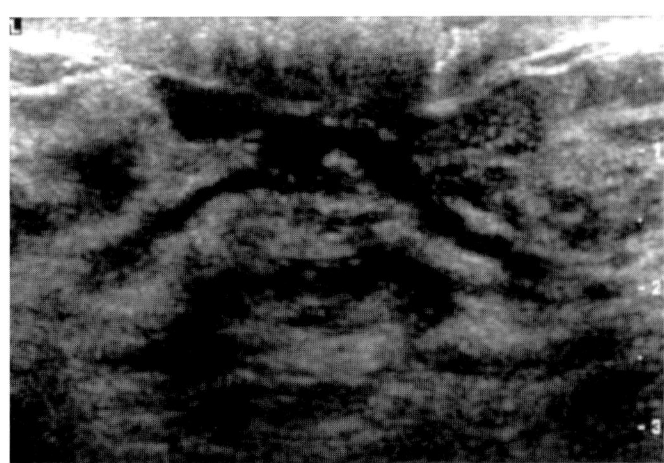

FIGURE 4 ■ Transverse image of the nipple and immediate retroareolar region shows prominent fluid filled ducts, the lactiferous sinus.

polyurethane. A fibrous capsule forms around virtually all implants in vivo. Significant contracture of the fibrous capsule may occur and the degree of contracture varies among patients and may differ between breasts of an individual patient. The surrounding capsule affects the degree of infolding of the implant casing, as does the amount of material filling the implant. Most implants have a single lumen, filled with silicone or saline. Double lumen implants have an inner chamber surrounded by an outer chamber. Most double lumen implants have a silicone chamber and a saline chamber. The silicone chamber is usually the inner lumen, but some implants have an inner chamber of saline and outer chamber of silicone. Expandable saline implants contain intraluminal valves for filling. Pericapsular seromas occur in some cases, particularly in the presence of polyurethane-covered or textured implants (3). When small, these seromas are of no clinical significance.

TABLE 1 ■ Common Types of Breast Implants

Single lumen
Matrix: silicone gel or saline
Double lumen
Most common: inner lumen silicone gel, outer lumen saline
Less common: outer lumen silicone gel, inner lumen saline
Implant casing
Smooth silicone elastomer
Textured
Polyurethane coated

On ultrasound evaluation of the intact single-lumen implant, a band of linear, striated reverberation echoes is seen at the anterior aspect of the implant. Below the reverberation band, the silicone gel or saline commonly appears anechoic (Fig. 6), but it may contain scattered echoes if the gain is set high. Occasional linear bands emanating from the implant margin represent infolding of the casing. Peri-implant seromas are generally anechoic but may contain low-level echoes that are of no significance in asymptomatic patients (Fig. 7).

ULTRASONOGRAPHIC PITFALLS

Technique

Errors in ultrasonographic diagnosis may result from lack of or poor visualization of an abnormality or mistaking normal for abnormal structures (Table 2). Optimal scanning technique is essential for accurate detection and diagnosis. A high-resolution transducer operating at 7.5 to 12 MHz is generally required for scanning most of the breast tissue, whereas a 5 MHz transducer may be

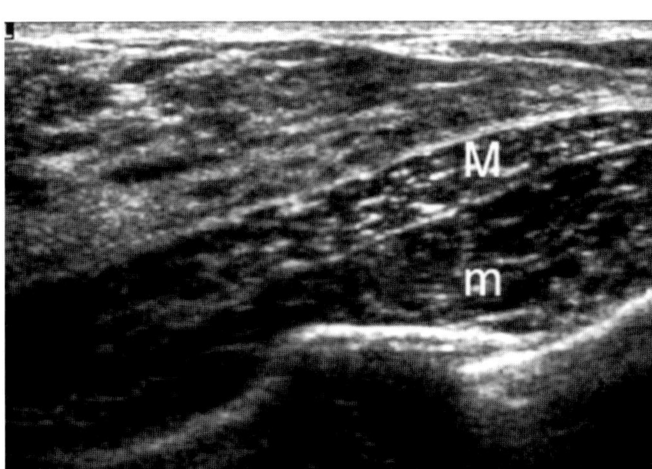

FIGURE 5 ■ Transverse image of the upper outer quadrant shows prominent pectoralis major (M) and minor muscles (m) overlying the chest wall.

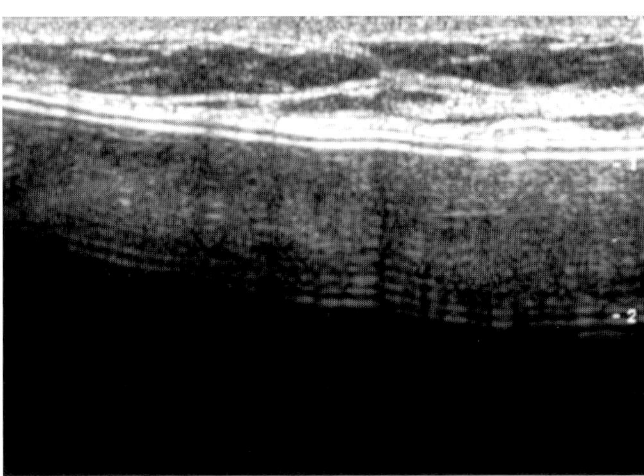

FIGURE 6 ■ This intact, textured silicone gel implant has an artifactual band of echoes due to reverberation, located deep to the implant shell. The shell, in this example, exhibits two parallel linear echogenic lines. The superficial line represents the top of the brush border of the textured shell; the deeper line is the surface of the shell.

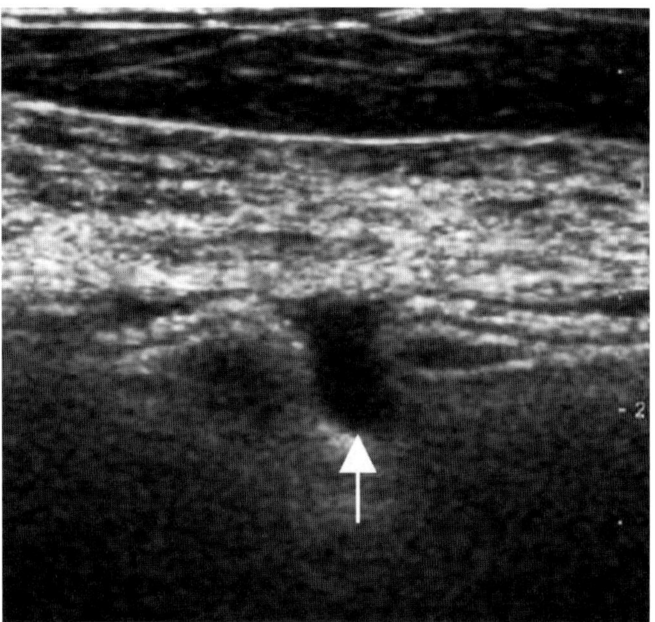

FIGURE 7 ■ Along the outer surface of a fold in the shell of this textured silicone gel implant is a small amount of peri-implant fluid (*arrow*) that contains scattered echoes, an insignificant finding in an asymptomatic patient.

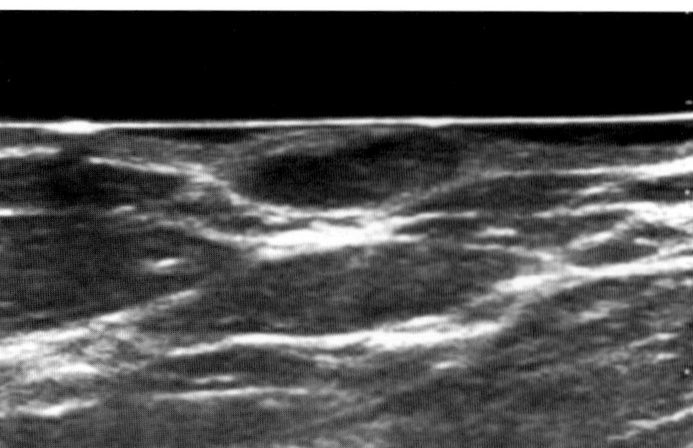

FIGURE 8 ■ Demonstration of the use of a stand-off pad to evaluate findings in the near-field. This is a case of a sebaceous cyst in the skin.

appropriate for the deep tissues of a large or fibrous breast. Superficial lesions in the immediate subcutaneous tissues may not be visible without the use of a stand-off gel pad or water path that optimizes focal depth (Fig. 8). Techniques such as harmonic imaging and compound imaging may help to improve conspicuity of a lesion or better resolve sonographic features such as margination, internal matrix, and effects on surrounding tissues.

Because the shape of fatty lobules may be elliptical, they may be confused with a mass (4). The converse problem is the mass that is isoechoic to and surrounded by fat. Such masses are highly visible on mammography but difficult to identify on ultrasound (Fig. 9). Real-time imaging is essential for differentiating a fatty lobule from true pathology as well as for the recognition of the isoechoic mass. Fatty lobules flow from one to another without mass effect, while a true mass interrupts the flowing braided appearance of fat, does not conform in shape to the surrounding structures, and may deform the adjacent fat lobule. Ribs can appear superficial in the small breast or at the medial aspect of the breast. Care must be taken to avoid mistaking a rib for a mass in the sagittal plane (Fig. 10). Note should be made of the location of the pectoralis major, which lies superficial to the rib cage. Additionally, ribs elongate in the transverse plane. All masses should be imaged in at least two planes.

Localization of the Lesion

Ultrasonographic evaluation of the breast is frequently performed in followup to an abnormal mammogram on

TABLE 2 ■ Ultrasonographic Pitfalls in Breast Mass Evaluation

Problems	Potential solutions
Inability to visualize lesion	–
Poor resolution	–
Inappropriate transducer	7.5 to 12 MHz transducer; 5 MHz for deep lesions in large breast
Suboptimal focal depth setting	Optimize focus setting; use water path for near-field imaging
Poor patient positioning	Position breast tissue evenly on chest wall with ipsilateral side of torso rotated anteriorly
	Changing patient position changes structural relationships, which may bring a mass into view
Location ambiguous on mammogram	Careful review of mammogram to understand relation of lesion location and mammographic projection
	Scan through fenestrated mammographic compression plate with lesion centered in fenestration
Mass isoechoic to surrounding fat	Note interruption of flowing pattern of fatty lobules by the mass
Fatty lobule mimicking mass	Note flowing pattern of fatty lobule
	Correlate with mammogram to exclude lipoma
Rib mimicking mass	Note location of pectoralis muscle; scan in two planes
Indeterminate cystic or solid differentiation	Requires followup if benign criteria are met or biopsy

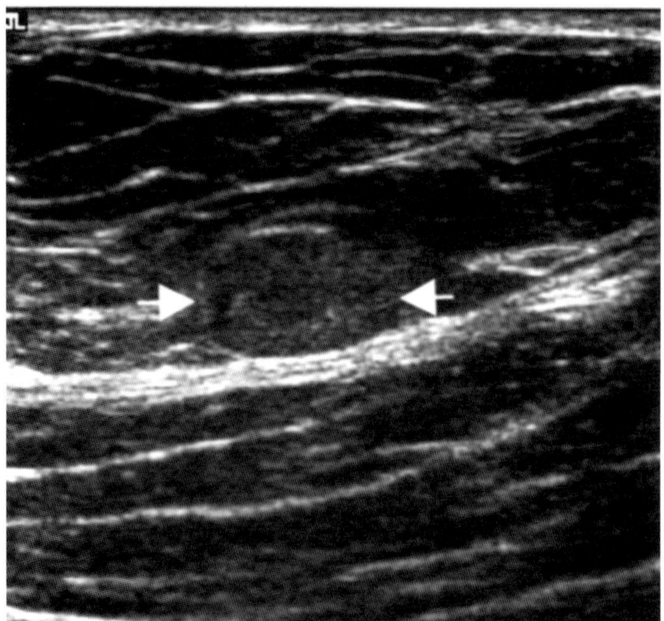

FIGURE 9 ■ This is a fibroadenoma (*arrows*) that is isoechoic to surrounding fat.

which a mass is visualized. An understanding of the location of a mass within the breast is essential before attempting to locate it on ultrasound. The location of a mass in the transverse axis as defined by the craniocaudal view of the mammogram is usually less difficult to project onto the breast during ultrasonographic evaluation than its location in the sagittal plane as suggested by the mediolateral oblique (MLO) mammographic view. Lesions that are lateral on the craniocaudal projection actually lie lower in the breast than suggested by their location on the MLO view. Lesions that are medial are located more superiorly than suggested by the MLO projection. If available, a 90° lateral (mediolateral) view of the breast can help to localize the mass in the sagittal plane if location is uncertain based on the MLO. Additionally, the mammogram is performed in only two or three projections with breast tissue pulled away from the chest wall, but ultrasonography allows a view of the breast from all projections and is generally performed with the patient supine and the breast flattened against the chest wall. Therefore, the depth of a lesion from the skin can be difficult to estimate. Masses that appear to be several centimeters from the chest wall on the mammogram may be located very close to the chest wall on ultrasound. Lesions that appear to be deep but peripheral on the mammogram may be superficial on ultrasonographic evaluation. Having the patient sit erect with the breast held in a position simulating the mammographic projection can help to localize a lesion otherwise difficult to identify. If prone and erect maneuvers fail, a fenestrated compression plate used for needle localizations can be used to perform a mammogram, with the lesion positioned within the fenestration (5). Using the location of the lesion in the fenestration on the mammographic image as guidance, the ultrasound transducer can be placed in the fenestration over the mass for ultrasonographic identification and evaluation.

Cysts

The conventional goal of breast ultrasound is the differentiation of a cyst from a solid mass. Simple cysts are usually not a diagnostic problem. Simple cysts are anechoic except for occasional artifact such as reverberation echoes. Benign breast cysts, however, are frequently not simple by ultrasound criteria. The American College of Radiology Breast Imaging and Reporting Data System (BIRADS) Lexicon for Breast Ultrasound has separated nonsimple cystic masses into two categories: complex and complicated (6).

Reverberation artifact may cause the appearance of septations or debris within a simple cyst (Fig. 11). On the

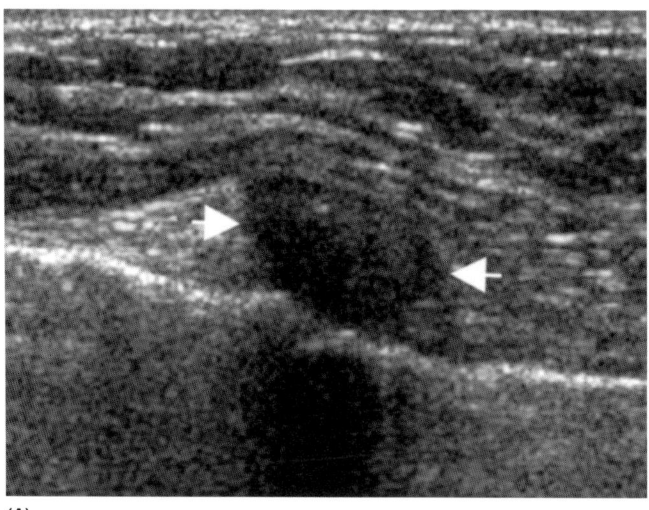

(A)

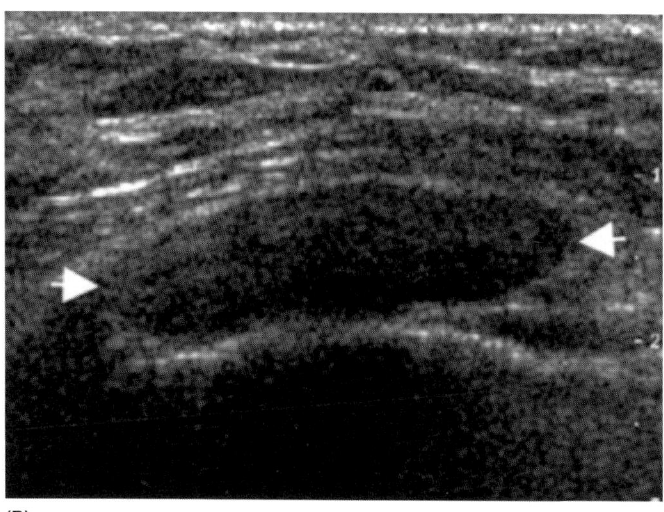

(B)

FIGURE 10 A AND B ■ (**A**) A rib (*arrows*) may be mistaken for a mass, particularly if palpable and the overlying muscle is thin. (**B**) Scanning in the orthogonal imaging plane should elucidate the nature of the finding as it becomes elongated (*arrows*).

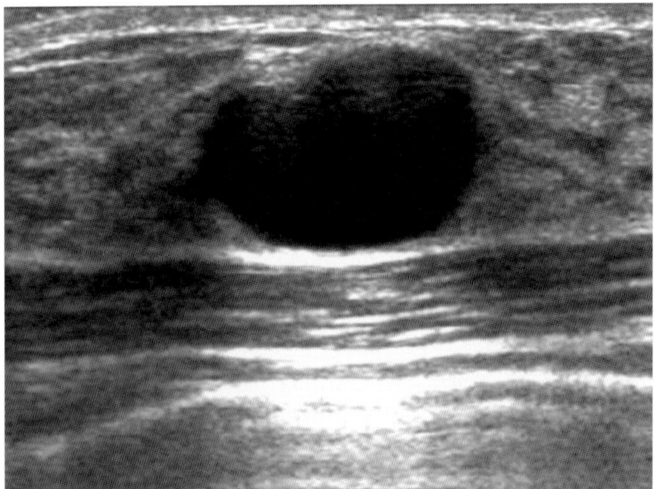

FIGURE 11 ■ Simple cyst. This is a lobulated, circumscribed anechoic mass. The echoes at the superficial aspect of the cyst represent artifact.

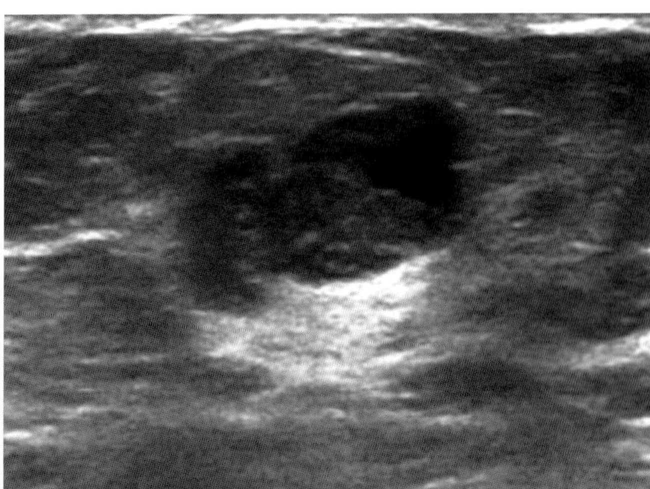

FIGURE 13 ■ Complex mass. This is an irregularly shaped, circumscribed mass with both solid and cystic components. Biopsy should be recommended.

other hand, true septations, low-level echoes, and floating debris are commonly found in benign complicated cysts, particularly in patients with multiple, long-standing cysts (Fig. 12). If a solid component is detected within a fluid-containing mass, the mass is referred to as complex (Figs. 13 and 14). Some benign cysts contain dense cellular debris and the echogenicity may be homogeneous or heterogeneous with or without posterior acoustic enhancement. Some benign debris-containing cysts may even exhibit shadowing (Fig. 15). Thus, a benign cyst may be difficult to distinguish from a solid neoplastic mass. This uncertainty commonly prompts biopsy. If fine-needle aspiration is performed, a small-gauge needle with no or minimal suction may not be sufficient to obtain obvious diagnostic material. An 18-gauge needle using a 20 mL syringe for suction may be required to obtain enough of the thick material contained in these cysts for diagnosis. If a core biopsy is performed, a nonspecific diagnosis of fibrocystic change may be reported and further workup (generally, excisional biopsy) may be necessary. An awareness of the phenomenon of solid-appearing benign cysts is beneficial when tissue sampling is deemed necessary for diagnosis.

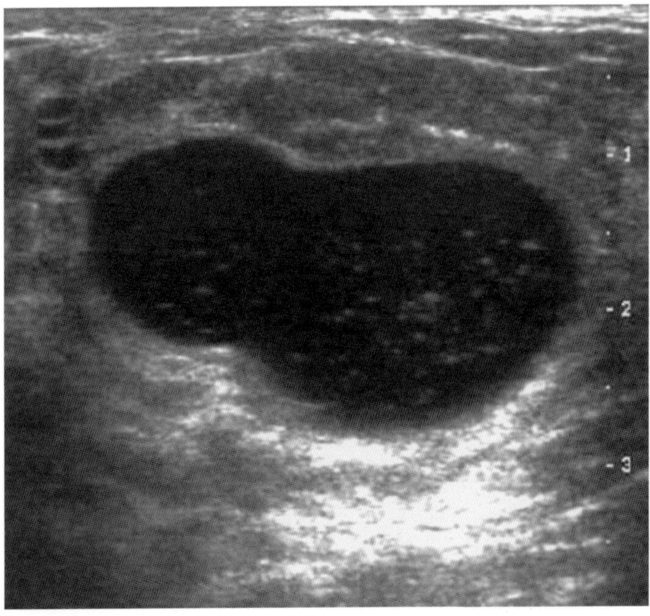

FIGURE 12 ■ Benign complicated cyst. This is a lobulated, circumscribed mass containing scattered echoes that swirled on real-time imaging.

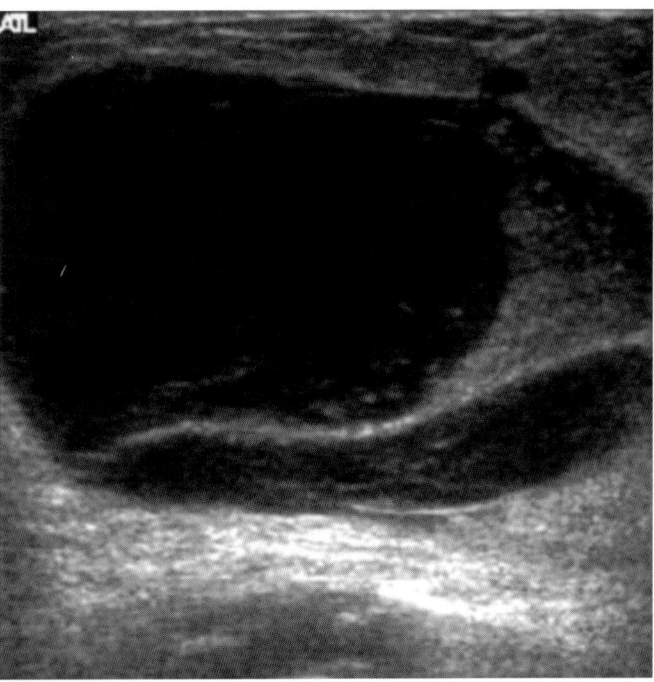

FIGURE 14 ■ Complex mass. This is a circumscribed, predominantly cystic mass with thick septations and internal echoes. The patient's history of recent surgery at this site is consistent with a diagnosis of hematoma.

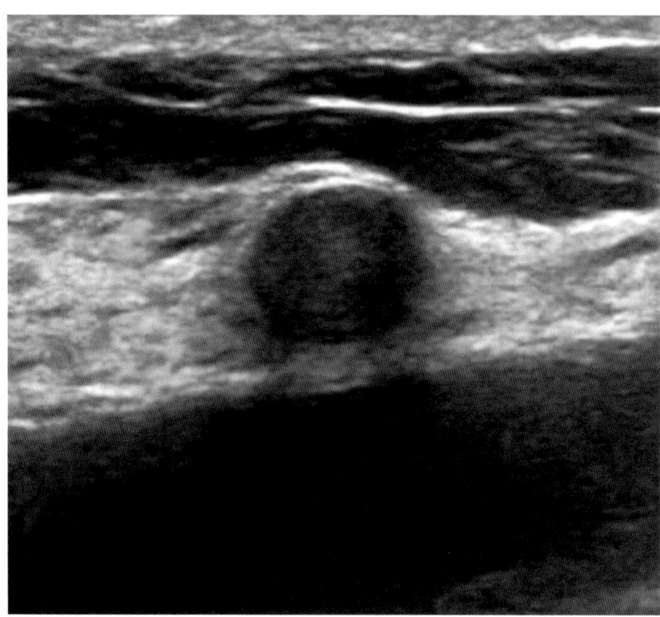

FIGURE 15 ■ Benign cyst containing thick debris causing the appearance of a solid mass with shadowing.

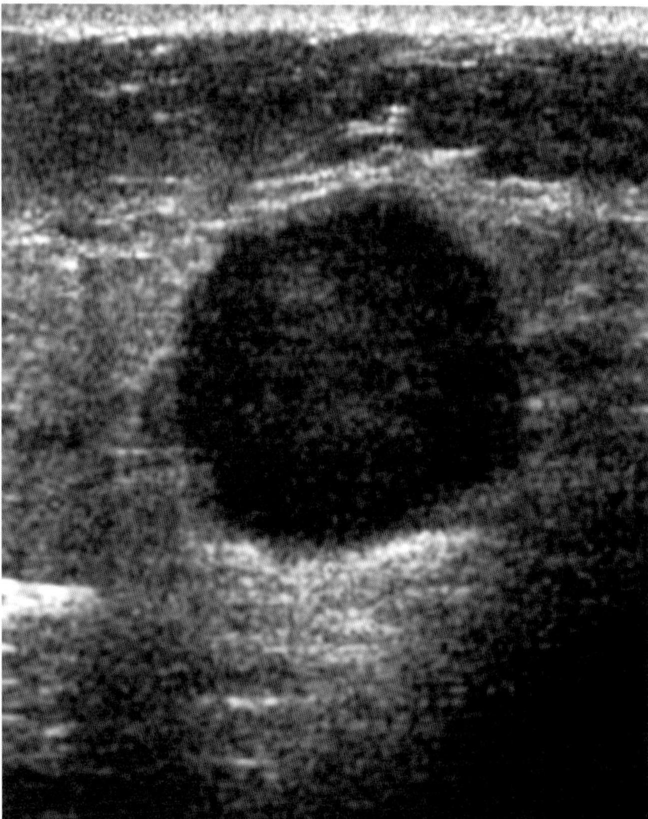

FIGURE 16 ■ Invasive ductal carcinoma. Despite posterior acoustic enhancement, this round, hypoechoic mass is suspicious because it has irregular margins and should not be mistaken for a benign, complicated cyst.

Solid Masses

Solid hypoechoic masses with posterior acoustic enhancement can be mistaken for cysts, particularly those that appear nearly anechoic. An important element in the ultrasonographic diagnosis of such lesions is the careful evaluation of the mass margins, the most significant factor in differentiating benign from malignant masses (7,8). Any irregularity of the margins should raise suspicion (Fig. 16). Although cystic malignancies are rare, a thick-walled cystic mass, although more likely an inflamed cyst or abscess, should undergo biopsy. Certain benign fibrotic lesions can mimic cancer if the shape is irregular or margins ill defined with or without architectural distortion (Fig. 17).

Doppler Technique

Investigation of Doppler technique for breast lesion evaluation has been ongoing for years but criteria have not yet been established and accepted for differentiation of benign from malignant disease. Studies using continuous wave, pulsed, color, or power (amplitude) Doppler indicate that the presence of detectable flow within a mass, with some regard for amount of vascularity and flow velocity, is suggestive of malignancy; but there is overlap between benign and malignant lesions (9–13). Doppler evaluation of a mass may be helpful if flow is demonstrated around or within the mass as an indication for biopsy. Vascularity detectable by Doppler techniques within a malignant lesion appears to indicate aggressive malignancy (14). Lack of demonstrable vascularity is nonspecific, however, and should not be used to indicate that a lesion is benign (15).

Implants

Although magnetic resonance imaging (MRI) has been shown to be more accurate than ultrasound for evaluation of silicone gel implant integrity (16,17), ultrasound is a less expensive and anxiety-provoking procedure than MRI and will continue to be used for initial implant evaluation for many patients. One of the problems in

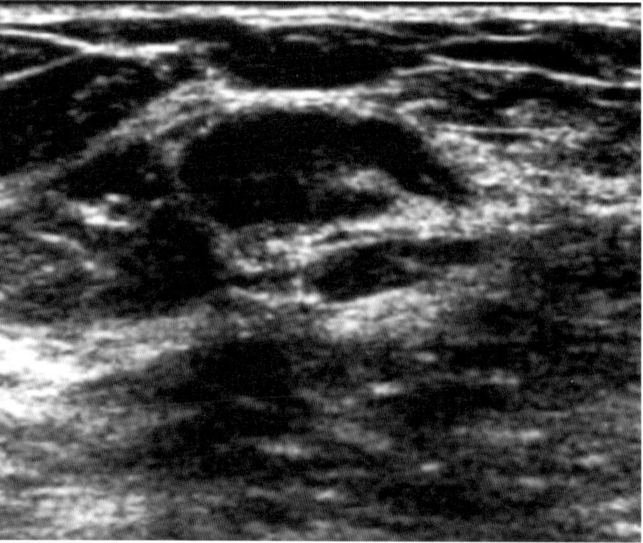

FIGURE 17 ■ Stromal fibrosis. The irregular shape of this mass prompted biopsy.

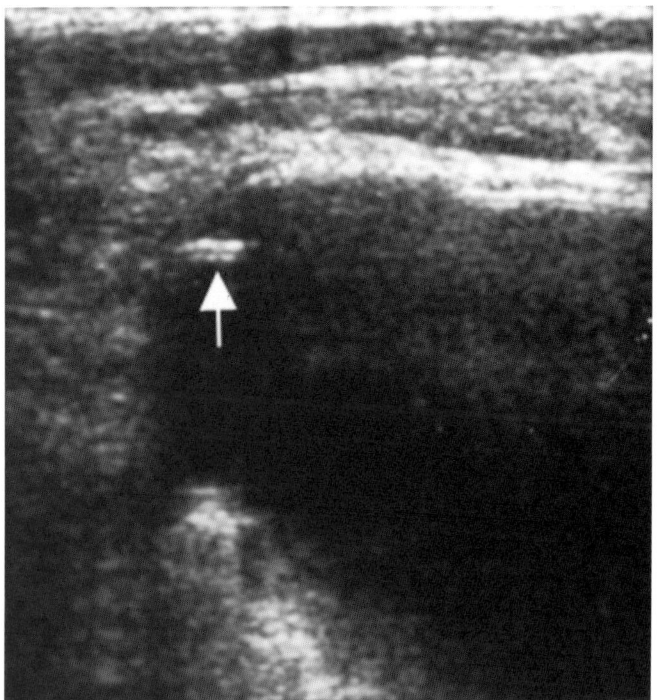

FIGURE 18 ■ Intact silicone gel implant. There is a normal fold of the implant shell extending toward the lumen of the implant (*arrow*).

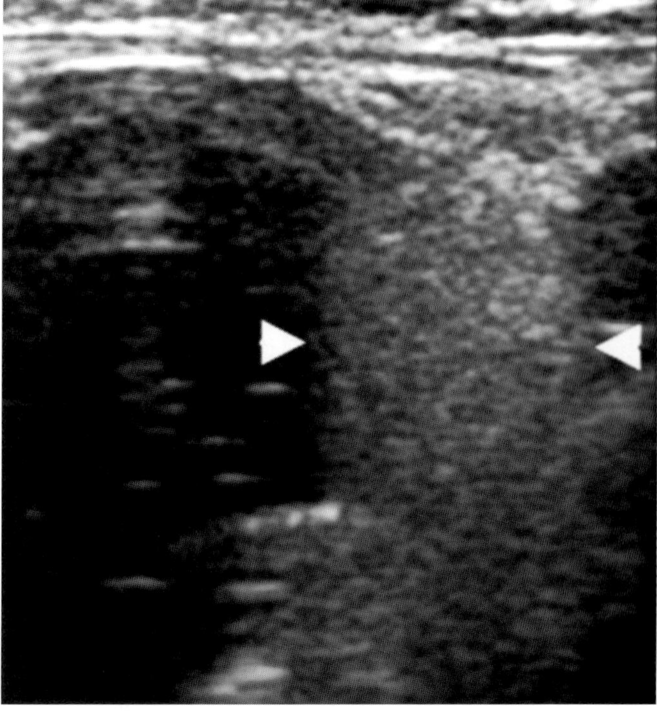

FIGURE 20 ■ Extracapsular rupture. There is free silicone in the soft tissues depicted as echogenic noise (*arrowheads*) contiguous with the ruptured implant.

evaluating silicone gel implants is the differentiation of normal infolding from rupture and collapse of the casing. Normal infolding is usually seen as a single linear structure that can be traced to the implant margin (Fig. 18). The presence of multiple overlapping layers of parallel lines representing intraluminal membranous debris should suggest rupture (Fig. 19) (18). The presence of echogenic noise within the soft tissues of the breast suggests extraluminal silicone (Fig. 20) (19). However, silicone in the soft tissues does not always correlate with rupture of the current implant. In a patient with previous rupture, silicone gel may have been left in the breast at the time of implant revision. Knowledge of the complete surgical history is necessary to avoid a misdiagnosis of extracapsular rupture of a second intact implant lying adjacent to free silicone from a prior ruptured implant. Additionally, small areas of echogenic noise located immediately at the margin of the implant may not indicate gross implant rupture. Despite the presence of this finding in several of our ultrasound cases, no evidence of rupture on MRI was appreciated, and the implants were visibly intact on explantation. Capsular calcification causes an irregular appearance of the capsule/implant surface but does not indicate rupture (Fig. 21).

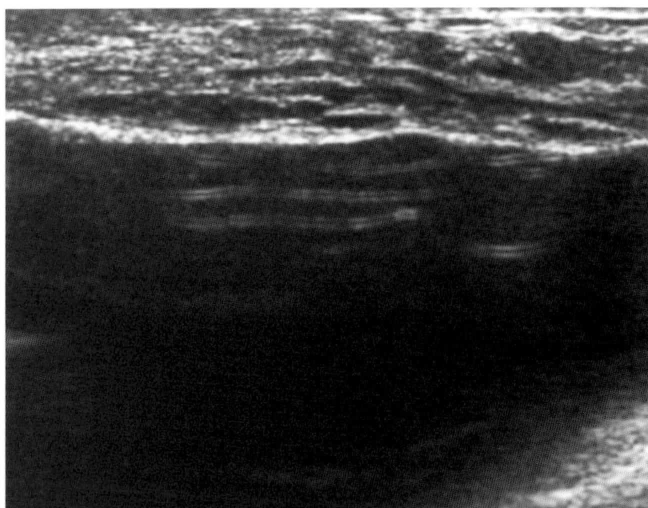

FIGURE 19 ■ Intracapsular silicone gel implant rupture. Multiple membranes overlap one another within the bed of the implant. These membranes represent the collapsed implant shell. The silicone contains diffuse low-level echoes.

ULTRASONOGRAPHIC ABNORMALITIES

Benign Cystic Masses

Fibrocystic dysplasia is the most common histopathologic change in the breast (Table 3). Microscopic epithelial cysts form in conjunction with fibrosis induced by the epithelial abnormality. Some cysts enlarge and are considered macroscopic if more than 2 mm in diameter (20). Macroscopic cysts visible on mammography or palpable on physical examination are common in women between the ages of 30 and 50 years, but these can occur in women of all ages.

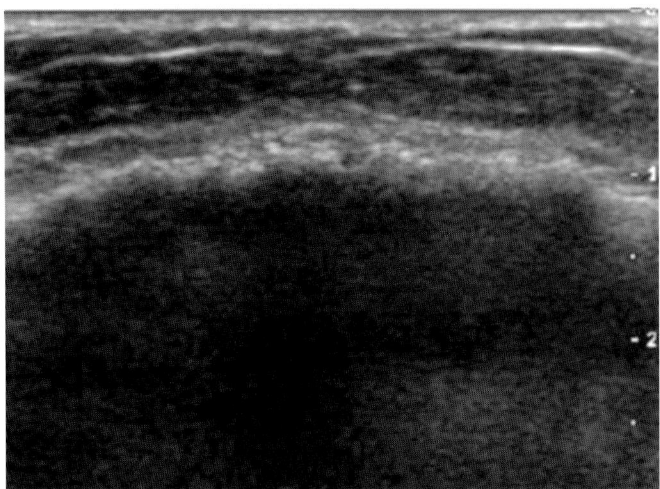

FIGURE 21 ■ Capsular calcification can give an irregular appearance to the soft tissue/capsule interface.

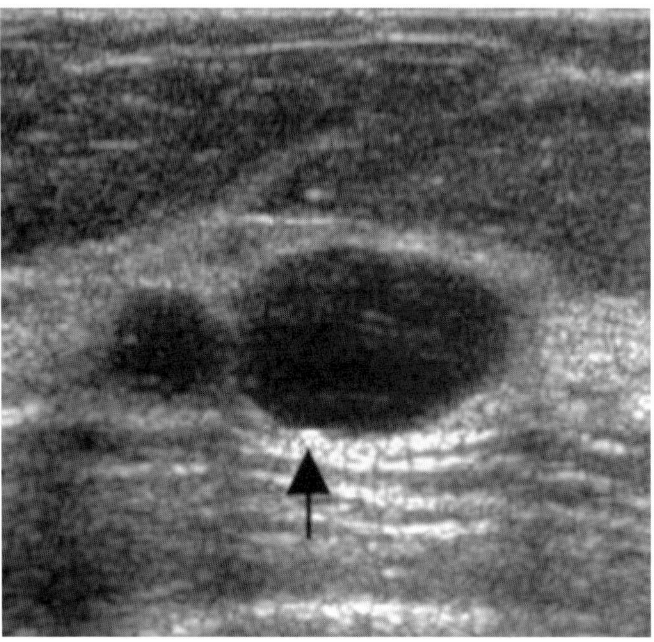

FIGURE 22 ■ Milk of calcium. The echogenic calcification (*arrow*) at the dependent aspect of this cyst visibly rolled when the patient changed position.

The uncomplicated cyst wall is thin, but it may thicken with fibrosis or inflammatory change. The cyst fluid content varies, ranging from clear and aqueous to opaque and turbid, and from nearly colorless to blue, green, or black. It may be rich in protein, hormones, and electrolytes with minimal to marked amounts of cellular debris. Calcifications may precipitate into the cyst fluid and can be visualized both mammographically and ultrasonographically as, respectively, radiodense or echogenic foci at the dependent aspect of the cyst ("milk-of-calcium") (Fig. 22). Clustered microcysts are defined as a group of tiny anechoic foci, each focus measuring 2 to 3 mm, with thin septations and no solid component. These are considered benign and may be followed up sonographically (21).

Ultrasound can diagnose uncomplicated cysts with nearly 100% accuracy (22). The diagnosis of a simple cyst can be made if there are sharp, well-circumscribed, and no internal echoes. Posterior acoustic enhancement may not be present if the mass is small (about 5 mm or less) or deep in location, particularly next to the chest wall. Occasionally, cysts may contain one or two thin septations, which do not suggest significant abnormality and should not be considered cause for intervention.

Although most complicated cystic masses represent benign epithelial cysts, other entities can have a similar appearance (Table 4). More ominous complex cystic masses with thickened, echogenic walls, indistinct margins or evaginations into the surrounding parenchyma, heterogeneous low-level echoes, thick septations or an intracystic solid component raise suspicion for malignancy (Figs. 23 and 24). Correlation with clinical presentation suggests the diagnosis of abscess, posttraumatic or postoperative hematoma, or galactocele. If the patient history does not suggest one of these entities, however, malignancy must be considered. Although most intracystic masses are benign papillomas, biopsy is generally performed to exclude malignant papilloma or intracystic carcinoma.

Some cysts have an ultrasonographic appearance similar to some solid masses. These require followup if benign in appearance or biopsy (fine-needle aspiration or core or excisional biopsy) if suspicious ultrasonographic characteristics are present.

TABLE 3 ■ Types of Cystic Breast Masses

Common—fibrocystic breasts
Simple cyst
Complicated cyst
Uncommon
Intracystic papilloma
Abscess
Galactocele
Intracystic carcinoma
Cystic carcinoma

Ductal Abnormalities

Ductal ectasia (periductal mastitis, plasma cell mastitis, secretory disease) is characterized by focal or segmental distention of one or multiple ducts and is associated with inflammation and periductal fibrosis (23). This is usually present in the retroareolar region but may occur along any ductal segment. The distended ducts are partially or completely filled with thick secretions and debris. Ultrasound provides excellent visualization of distended ducts and, unlike mammography, distinguishes them clearly from the surrounding parenchyma. Typically, one or more tubular structures radiate toward the nipple and are filled with low-level echoes (Fig. 25). When the intraductal debris

TABLE 4 ■ Ultrasonographic Characteristics of Masses: Differential Diagnosis

Anechoic masses	
Smooth margins (round, oval, or gently lobulated)	Cyst
Irregular margins	Malignant neoplasm; cyst
Hypoechoic or isoechoic masses	
Smooth margins (round, oval)	Common finding in: Cyst, complicated cyst, hemorrhagic cyst, periductal mastitis (ductal ectasia), fibroadenoma, other benign neoplasms, lymph node, oil cyst, lipoma
	Uncommon finding in: Stromal fibrosis, malignant neoplasm
Smooth margins (gently lobulated)	Common finding in: Fibroadonoma, other benign neoplasms
	Uncommon finding in: Malignant neoplasm
Ill-defined margins	Common finding in: Malignant neoplasm, radial scar, stromal fibrosis, abscess
Irregular margins, microlobulated	Malignant neoplasm, coalescence of microcysts
Homogeneous echogenic mass	Isolated fibroglandular tissue, lipoma, stromal fibrosis, fibroadenoma, hemangioma

appears tumefactive, resembling an intraductal mass, fine-needle aspiration yields a characteristic thick, whitish material with the consistency of toothpaste.

Ductal hyperplasia is epithelial proliferation perpendicular to the basement membrane (24). With practice, hyperplasia may be identified as a hypoechoic widening of the duct, more easily recognized when a thin, central echo-free line is present, representing fluid in the lumen (25). No indication for intervention or followup has been established for mild ductal widening (25). Irregular thickening, frond-like tissue, or masses within the duct, however, should encourage biopsy because these may represent intraductal carcinoma (Fig. 26) or papillomatosis, which carries a high risk of malignancy (26).

Solid Masses

The differentiation of benign from malignant solid masses is the leading focus of research in breast ultrasonography. With advancing technology and an increasingly cost-conscious health-care system, breast imaging has been challenged with not only the earlier identification of malignancy but also the reduction of the benign biopsy rate. Guidelines for B-mode ultrasonographic characterization of breast masses have been published (6,7). Limitations of breast ultrasonography must be recognized, however, and include the inability to visualize some solid masses owing to small size (particularly intraductal carcinomas) or isoechogenicity, the overlap in ultrasonographic appearance of some benign and malignant lesions, and the difficulty in identifying intraductal microcalcifications (which are readily depicted on mammography) in the absence of a mass (27). Nevertheless, an attempt should be made to characterize solid masses and to use this information in the management plan (Table 5).

Benign Solid Masses

Fibroadenomas are the most common benign solid breast tumors, occurring most frequently in women in their reproductive years. Multiplicity and bilaterality are common features at all ages. Fibroadenomas are composed of

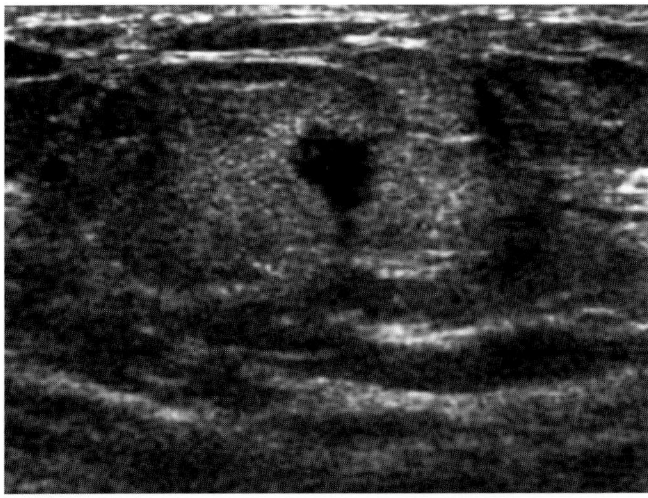

FIGURE 23 ■ Abscess. This irregularly shaped multiseptated cystic mass has the suggestion of an echogenic halo. The history of pain, swelling, and fever should suggest the diagnosis of abscess.

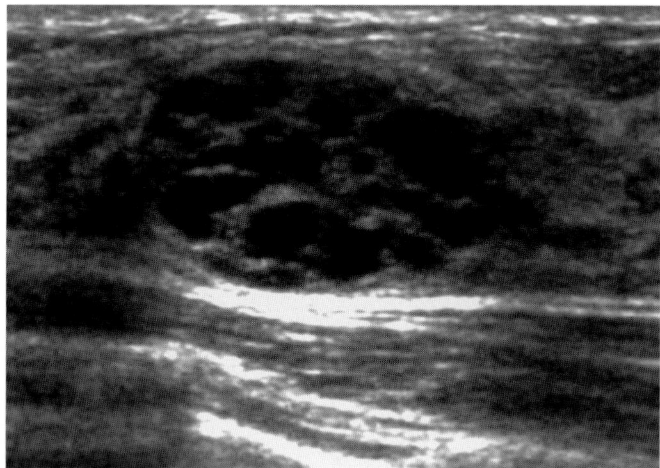

FIGURE 24 ■ Fibrocystic change. Although the appearance of this complex cystic mass is suggestive of a large cluster of cysts, the multiple thick septations should lead to a biopsy recommendation to exclude malignancy.

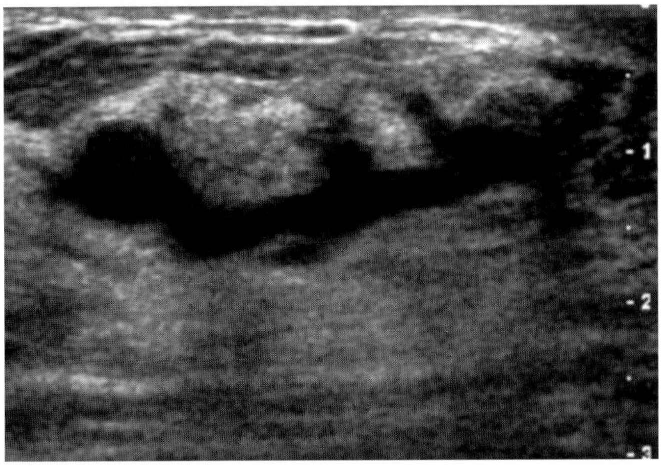

FIGURE 25 ■ Duct ectasia. This benign distended duct contains low-level echoes.

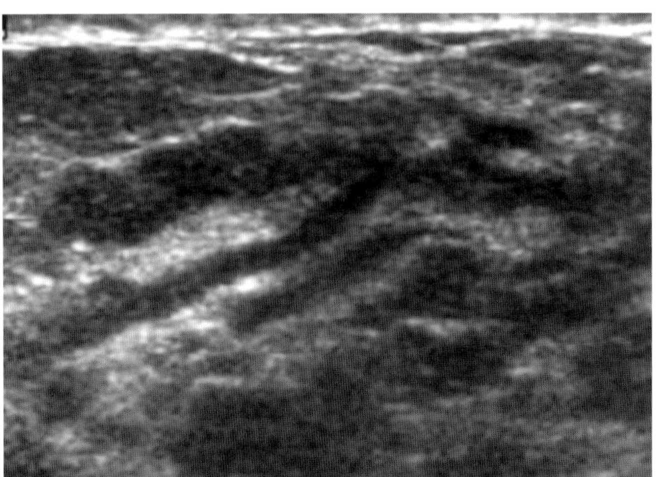

FIGURE 26 ■ Ductal carcinoma in situ. Multiple tubular structures representing distended ducts. Note the widest duct, which is irregular in contour and contains heterogeneous tissue.

fibrous stroma, proliferating ducts, and acinar tissue, evolving from proliferation of the lobules, which coalesce into nodules, enlarging centrally with continued epithelial and stromal proliferation and peripherally with addition of hyperplastic lobules (28). The epithelial and stromal components vary in amount. Some fibroadenomas are predominantly adenomatous; others contain stromal hypercellularity or extensive myxoid change. This range of histopathologic features accounts for some variation in the ultrasound appearance and should be taken into account when evaluating the cytopathology results of fine-needle aspiration and core biopsy of suspected fibroadenoma.

Ultrasonographically, fibroadenomas are sharply circumscribed masses that may be encapsulated. The long axis commonly lies parallel to the skin surface (29). The sharp margination of the mass is one of its most distinctive features by ultrasound and gross pathology (Fig. 27). The typical oval or gently lobulated shape of fibroadenomas is a characteristic rarely found in malignancy (7). Most fibroadenomas are homogeneously hypoechoic or isoechoic to fatty tissue (29). Posterior acoustic enhancement is associated with some fibroadenomas, whereas those that are hyalinized or calcified can exhibit shadowing (Fig. 28).

Papillomas are single formations of epithelial fronds supported by a fibrovascular stroma. They are most frequently located in the subareloar region within major ducts but also occur peripherally (26). Serous or serosanguineous nipple discharge is commonly present, and the involved duct is distended and occasionally cystic. Ultrasonographically, they generally appear hypoechoic to fibroglandular tissue. They may be a discrete well-marginated, gently lobulated or microlobulated mass or may conform to the shape of a duct and can be outlined by fluid if lying within a cyst or distended duct (Figs. 29 and 30).

Hamartomas are uncommon, sharply demarcated lesions made up of lobular units. They differ from fibroadenomas largely because of the presence of fat and thus are probably more easily recognized mammographically (23). They appear heterogeneous on ultrasound examination,

TABLE 5 ■ Management of Ultrasonographically Detected Breast Masses

Type of mass	Management options
Simple cyst	No further workup
Complicated cyst	No further workup
Indeterminate complicated cyst vs. solid	
Smoothly marginated, round, oval or gently lobulated, thin wall	Ultrasound follow-up at 6 mo and 1 yr or biopsy
Complex cyst	Biopsy
Solid	
Smoothly marginated, round, oval or gently lobulated	Ultrasound follow-up at 6 mo and 1 yr or biopsy
Ill defined or irregular margins or microlobulated	Biopsy

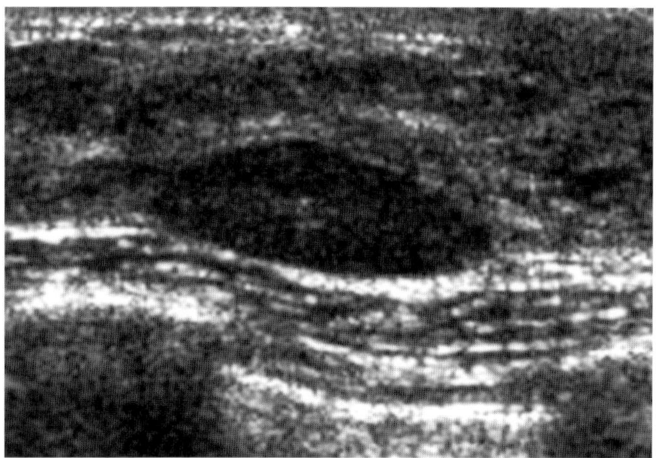

FIGURE 27 ■ Fibroadenoma. The typical fibroadenoma is well circumscribed, oval, or lobulated with a parallel orientation.

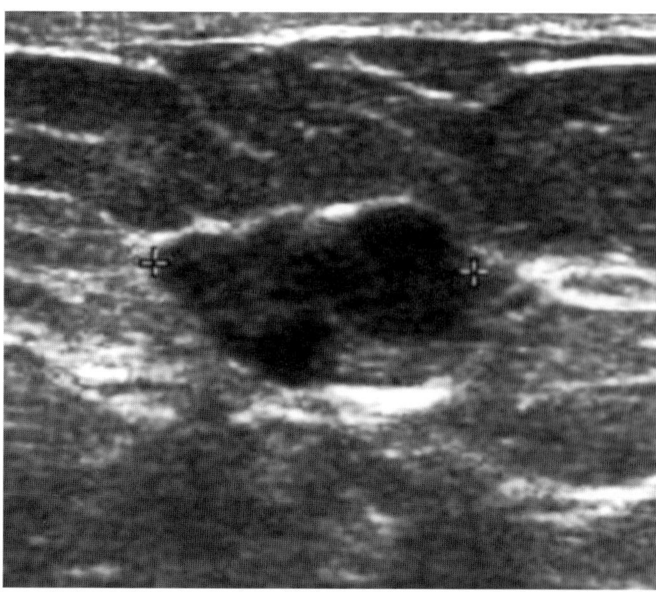

FIGURE 29 ■ Papilloma. This mass is gently lobulated and well circumscribed suggesting a benign diagnosis, but it also has an angular margin and is heterogeneous, which should prompt biopsy.

containing variable amounts of hypoechoic tissue (representing fat) and echogenic fibroglandular elements (Fig. 31). Other lesions containing fat include fat necrosis and lipomas. These may be mistaken for other neoplasms ultrasonographically but are readily diagnosed. Another benign entity, stromal fibrosis, is a frequent mimicker of both benign and malignant breast masses. Its ultrasonographic appearance ranges from ill-defined hyperechoic tissue to a well-defined hypoechoic mass.

Phyllodes tumors are usually indistinguishable from fibroadenomas on ultrasound evaluation, although they tend to be larger, 4 cm or greater, or exhibit rapid growth (Fig. 32) (30). Phyllodes tumors are described histologically as resembling intracanalicular fibroadenomas with increased stromal cellularity but heterogeneous. They differ from fibroadenomas, showing greater cellularity and the presence of mitotic activity. Benign phyllodes tumors contain few mitoses and minimal cellular overgrowth whereas malignant phyllodes tumors show marked hypercellularity and substantial mitotic activity. At our institution, because the risk of a well-circumscribed solid mass being a phyllodes tumor increases with lesion size, biopsy of a mass having the sonographic appearance

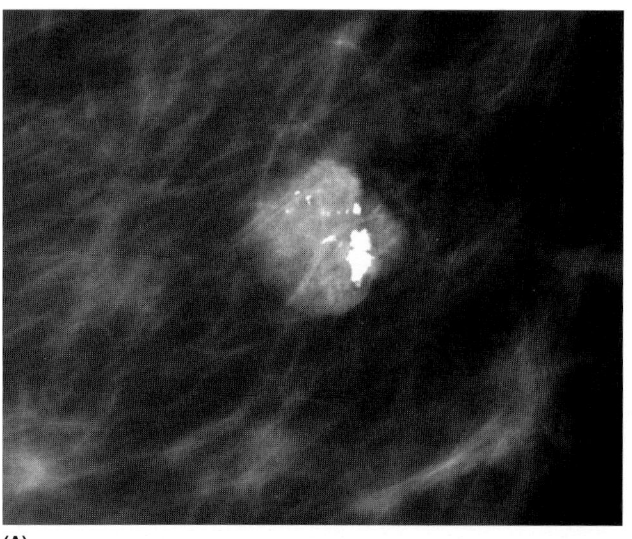

(A)

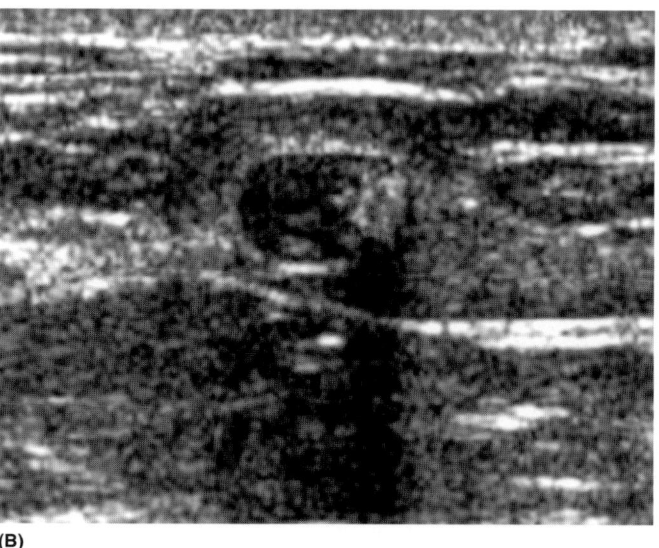

(B)

FIGURE 28 A AND B ■ Calcified fibroadenoma. (**A**) Mammographic image shows coarse calcification in a circumscribed mass, typical of a degenerating fibroadenoma. (**B**) Ultrasound image shows a well-circumscribed mass containing a shadowing echogenic calcification.

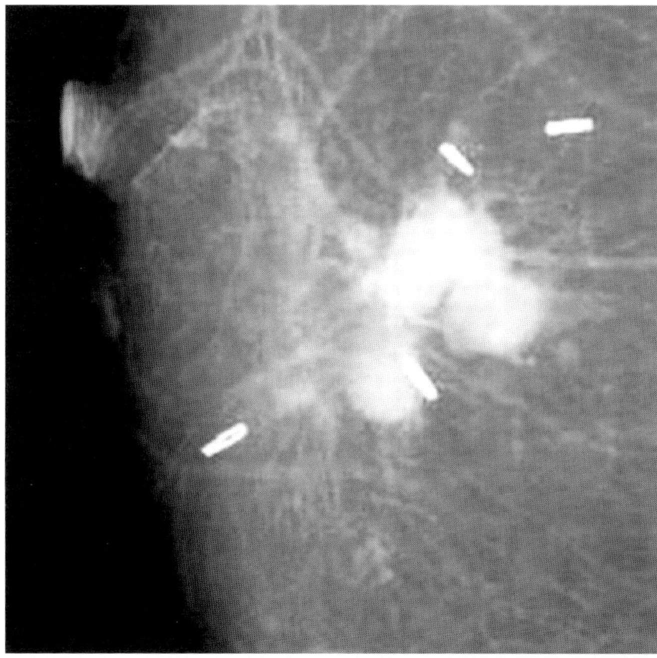

(A)

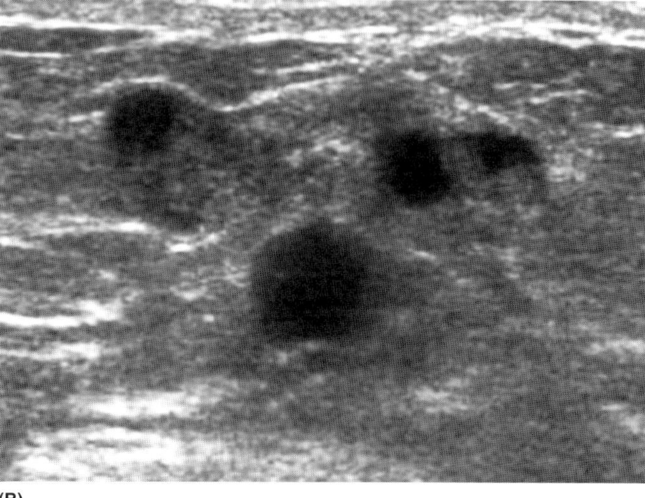

(B)

FIGURE 30 A AND B ■ Papillomatosis. (A) Mammographic image showing coalescent masses and a prominent duct extending from the masses toward the nipple. (B) Multiple heterogeneous, ill-defined round masses correlate with the mammogram. These masses were located in one ductal system.

of a fibroadenoma is performed when the mass is greater than 2 cm or has increased in size within a short follow-up interval.

Malignant Masses

Although mammography is the primary imaging modality for the early detection of breast cancer, ultrasound, used in conjunction with mammography, can further increase the cancer detection rate (31). The most common breast malignancies are of ductal epithelial origin and are either confined to the duct (in situ or intraductal) or infiltrative (invasive). Lobular and stromal cancers and metastases are less common (Table 6). The different histologic characteristics account for some variability in the ultrasound appearance. For example, although most invasive ductal carcinomas exhibit irregular or ill-defined margins related to infiltrative and fibrotic components (Fig. 33), carcinomas of uniform cell type or types that do not invade aggressively, may appear as well-circumscribed masses (Fig. 34) (32).

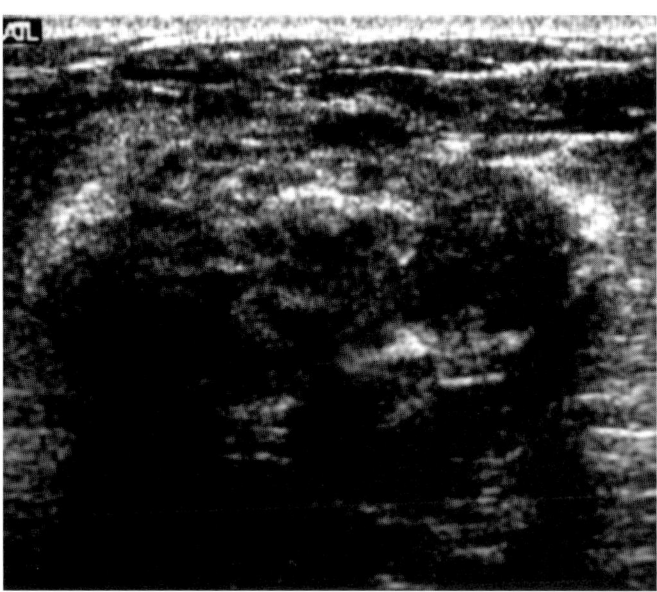

FIGURE 31 ■ Hamartoma. This heterogeneous mass with ill-defined margins is suspicious on ultrasound. Fatty elements and a partial capsule were present on the mammogram (not shown), which are helpful findings for making the diagnosis of a benign hamartoma without biopsy.

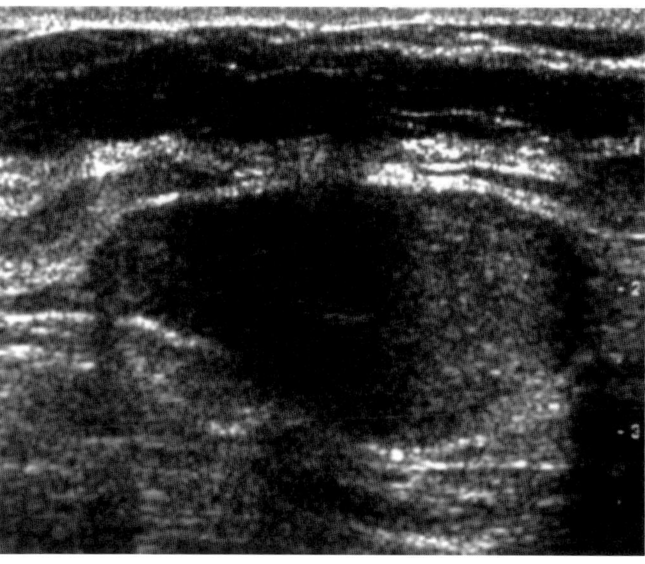

FIGURE 32 ■ Benign phyllodes tumor. This 3 cm oval, well-circumscribed mass has a similar appearance to a fibroadenoma. Biopsy was performed due to rapid growth.

TABLE 6 ■ Malignant Masses

- Intraductal carcinoma
- Invasive ductal carcinoma
- Medullary carcinoma
- Mucinous (colloid) carcinoma
- Tubular carcinoma
- Invasive lobular carcinoma
- Cystosarcoma phyllodes (varying malignant potential)
- Lymphoma
- Leukemia (chloroma)
- Myoepithelial lesions (varying malignant potential)
- Sarcomas

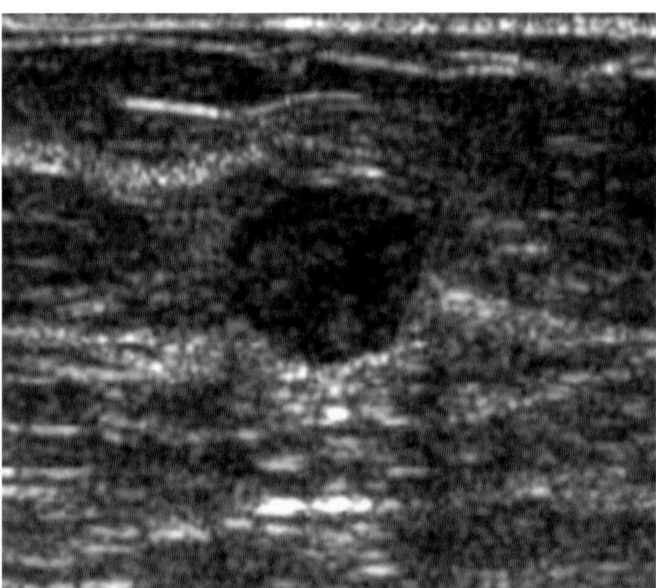

FIGURE 34 ■ Ductal carcinoma in situ. This solid, round mass has a sharp border, but on close analysis has subtle microlobulations for which biopsy is indicated.

Stavros et al. (7) reported a 98.4% sensitivity for diagnosis of malignant masses using ultrasonographic criteria for malignancy, including spiculation, angular margins, marked hypoechogenicity (relative to fat), shadowing, calcification, duct extension and branching pattern, and microlobulation. These results reflect the high resolution of state-of-the-art equipment and expanding skills of the radiologist. Suspicious masses identified on ultrasound, however, should always be correlated with mammography, which can depict extent and other sites of malignancy or reveal benign characteristics of the lesion in question, thus precluding unnecessary intervention.

The Ruptured Silicone Gel Implant

Several ultrasonographic signs of implant rupture have been described (Table 7) (18,19,33). The finding of multiple echogenic parallel lines ("stepladder" sign) within the implant lumen is highly suggestive of a broken and collapsed implant shell (Fig. 22) (17,18). Echogenic noise ("snowstorm" appearance) within the breast tissue correlates strongly with extraluminal or extracapsular silicone (17,19). Areas of moderate to marked homogeneous low-level echogenicity within the implant may be the most sensitive sign of rupture but is not highly specific (33). The cause for the latter two ultrasonographic findings of increased echogenicity of silicone gel is not known. Hypotheses include acoustic impedance mismatch between silicone gel microglobules in soft tissue (19), multiple scattering effects (34), and large silicone–protein complexes formed on contact of silicone gel with body tissues or fluid (35).

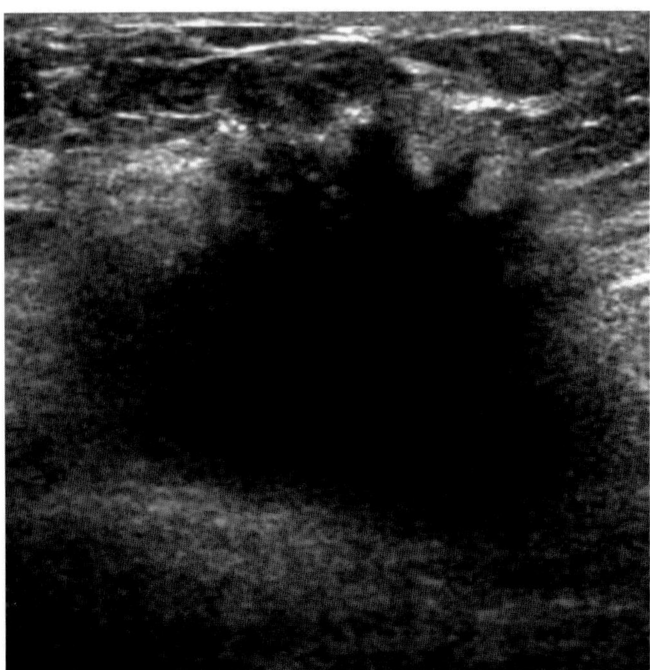

FIGURE 33 ■ Invasive ductal carcinoma. This irregularly shaped, ill-defined, and spiculated mass is highly suspicious for malignancy based on its ultrasound appearance.

TABLE 7 ■ Ultrasonographic Signs Suspicious for Implant Rupture

- Dense intraluminal echoes
- Multiple intraluminal parallel echoes
- Extracapsular extension of silicone
- Extraluminal echogenic noise

REFERENCES

1. Vogel PM, Georgiade NG, Fetter BF, et al. The correlation of histologic changes in the human breast with the menstrual cycle. Am J Pathol 1981; 104:23.
2. Cole-Beuglet CM, Goldberg BB, Patchefsky AS, et al. Normal breast structure and its ultrasound characteristics. In: Telles NC, ed. Atlas of Breast Ultrasound. Philadelphia: Thomas Jefferson University Hospital, 1980:38.

3. Berg WA, Caskey CI, Hamper UM, et al. Diagnosing breast implant rupture with MR imaging, US, and mammography. Radiographics 1993; 13:1323.
4. Spencer GM, Rubens DJ, Roach DJ. Hypoechoic fat: a sonographic pitfall. AJR Am J Roentgenol 1995; 164:1277.
5. Lunt LG, Peakman DJ, Young JR. Mammographically guided ultrasound: a new technique for assessment of impalpable breast lesions. Clin Radiol 1991; 44:85.
6. ACR BIRADS® Breast Imaging and Reporting Data System, American College of Radiology, 2003.
7. Stavros AT, Thickman D, Rapp CL, et al. Solid breast nodules: use of sonography to distinguish between benign and malignant lesions. Radiology 1995; 196:123.
8. Mendelson EB, Tobin CE, Merritt CB, et al. Marginal analysis of breast masses with high-resolution US [abstr]. Radiology 1994; 193(P):177.
9. Madjar H, Sauerbrei W, Münch S, et al. Continuous-wave and pulsed Doppler studies of the breast: clinical results and effect of transducer frequency. Ultrasound Med Biol 1991; 17:31.
10. Cosgrove DO, Bamber JC, Davey JB, et al. Color Doppler signals from breast tumors. Radiology 1990; 176:175.
11. McNicholas MMJ, Mercer PM, Miller JC. Color Doppler sonography in the evaluation of palpable breast masses. AJR Am J Roentgenol 1993; 161:765.
12. Birdwell RL, Ideda DM, Jeffrey SS, et al. Preliminary experience with power Doppler imaging of breast masses [abstr]. Radiology 1995; 197(P):269.
13. Raza S, Baum JK. Evaluation of solid breast lesions with Doppler power imaging [abstr]. Radiology 1995; 197(P):270.
14. Sohn C, Bastert G. Color-coded sonography of breast tumors with maximum entropy method technique: a new prognostic factor? [abstr]. Radiology 1995; 197(P):270.
15. Dock W, Grabenwöger F, Metz V, et al. Tumor vascularization: assessment with duplex sonography. Radiology 1991; 181:241.
16. Gorczyca DP, DeBruhl ND, Ahn CY, et al. Silicone breast implant ruptures in an animal model: comparison of mammography, MR imaging, US and CT. Radiology 1994; 190:227.
17. Berg WA, Caskey CI, Hamper UM, et al. Single- and double-lumen silicone breast implant integrity: prospective evaluation of MR and US criteria. Radiology 1995; 197:45.
18. Debruhl ND, Gorczyca DP, Ahn CY, et al. Sonographic evaluation of silicone breast implants. Radiology 1993; 189:95.
19. Harris KM, Ganott MA, Shestak KC, et al. Silicone implant rupture detection with US. Radiology 1993; 187:761.
20. Haagensen CD. Gross cystic disease. In: Diseases of the Breast. Philadelphia: WB Saunders, 1986:250.
21. Berg WA. Sonographically depicted breast clustered microcysts: is follow-up appropriate? AJR Am J Roentgenol 2005; 185:952–959.
22. Jackson VP. The role of US in breast imaging. Radiology 1990; 177:305.
23. Page DL, Simpson JF. Benign, high-risk, and premalignant lesions. In: Bland KI, Copeland EM, eds. The Breast: Comprehensive Management of Benign and Malignant Diseases. Philadelphia: WB Saunders, 1991:113.
24. Tavassoli FA. Intraductal hyperplasia, ordinary and atypical. In: Pathology of the Breast. Norwalk, CT: Appleton & Lange, 1992:155.
25. Teboul M, Halliwell M. Ductal echography: the correct ultrasonic approach to the breast. In: Atlas of Ultrasound and Ductal Echography of the Breast. Oxford: Blackwell Scientific, 1995:83.
26. Tavassoli FA. Papillary lesions. In: Pathology of the Breast. Norwalk, CT: Appleton & Lange, 1992:193.
27. Leucht WJ, Leucht D, Kiesel L. Sonographic demonstration and evaluation of microcalcifications in the breast. Breast Dis 1992; 5:105.
28. Tavassoli FA. Biphasic tumors. In: Pathology of the Breast. Norwalk, CT: Appleton & Lange, 1992:425.
29. Fornage BD, Lorigan JF, Andry E. Fibroadenomas of the breast: sonographic appearance. Radiology 1989; 172:671.
30. Rosen PP. Fibroepithelial neoplasms. In: Rosen's Breast Pathology. Philadelphia, PA: Lippincott Raven Publishers, 1997:155.
31. Gordon PB, Goldenberg SL. Malignant breast masses detected only by ultrasound. Cancer 1995; 79:626.
32. Pierson KK, Wilkinson EJ. Malignant neoplasia of the breast: infiltrating carcinomas. In: Bland KI, Copeland EM, eds. The Breast: Comprehensive Management of Benign and Malignant Diseases. Philadelphia: WB Saunders, 1991:193.
33. Caskey CI, Berg WA, Anderson N, et al. Breast implant rupture: diagnosis with ultrasonography. Radiology 1994; 190:819.
34. Rubin JM, Helvie MA, Adler RD, et al. US appearance of ruptured silicone implants (Letter). Radiology 1994; 190:583.
35. Forsberg F, Conant EF, Russell KM, et al. Quantitative ultrasonic diagnosis of silicone breast implant rupture: an in vitro feasibility study. Ultrasound Med Biol 1996; 22:53.

Diaphragm and Chest

William E. Brant

10

INTRODUCTION

Ultrasound (US) supplements plain film radiography and computed tomography (CT) of the chest by detecting and characterizing diseases of the diaphragm, pleural space, peripheral lung, and mediastinum (1,2). US is particularly helpful when radiographic findings are confusing or nonrevealing, such as when a hemithorax is totally opacified on a chest radiograph (3). US of the chest can be performed at the patient's bedside, quickly, reliably, and cheaply (4). US is preferable to CT in critically ill patients who are difficult to move. Patients can be examined in the upright position allowing layering of fluid to optimize visualization. US provides rapid and effective guidance of invasive procedures such as thoracentesis, pleural mass biopsy, empyema and abscess drainage, and biopsy of mediastinal and peripheral parenchymal masses. Any lesion that can be visualized with US can usually be aspirated or biopsied by US guidance.

US is excellent for evaluation of the diaphragm because of its capability to demonstrate motion of the diaphragm as well as the anatomic structures above and below the diaphragm (5). Examination of the chest in the normal patient is hindered by air in the lungs and the bony thorax and spine. However, diseases of the pleura, peripheral lung parenchyma, and mediastinum provide sonographic "windows" to the thorax. Pleural fluid is easily visualized via transabdominal and intercostal approaches. Lung consolidation allows visualization of more central tumors. Mediastinal masses widen the mediastinum allowing parasternal visualization.

It must be stressed that US is a "supplementary" technique for evaluation of the thorax. Sonographic findings must always be compared to findings on chest radiographs or chest CT scans to attain the highest accuracy for interpretation. The chest radiograph is a guide for sonography. Areas of abnormality on the chest X-ray are located and analyzed by US. Scanning may be done through the intercostal spaces by applying the transducer directly to the chest or by an abdominal approach using the liver and spleen as sonographic windows to the diaphragm and lower thorax. High frequency 5.0 or 7.5 MHz linear array, or 5.0 or 3.5 MHz sector or curved array transducers are used. Linear array transducers are preferred for examination of structures in the near field, whereas sector or curved array transducers are best for deeper structures.

This chapter discusses the use of US to evaluate the diaphragm, pleural space, lung parenchyma, and mediastinum. Pitfalls in US diagnosis are reviewed (Table 1).

THE DIAPHRAGM

Normal Anatomy

The diaphragm is a dome-shaped musculotendinous sheet that separates the thoracic and abdominal cavities (Fig. 1). It is composed of two parts: a large, strong, C-shaped, central tendinous portion and a peripheral muscular portion. The muscular portion is made up of bands of muscle fibers that converge radially toward the central tendon from their origins on the

TABLE 1 ■ US of the Chest: Pitfalls

Diaphragm
- Discontinuous diaphragm
- Diaphragmatic slip
- Diaphragmatic crura

Pleural space
- Mirror-image artifact
- Obscured near field

xiphoid process, the lower six ribs, and the upper lumbar vertebrae. The diaphragm is approximately 5 mm thick and is covered by pleura on its thoracic side and by peritoneum on its abdominal side. The central tendon is fused with the inferior surface of the fibrous pericardium. Motor nerve supply is entirely from the phrenic nerves, which arise from nerve roots C-3 through C-5.

Apertures in the diaphragm permit structures to pass between the abdomen and the thorax. The vena caval foramen pierces the right side of the central tendon at the level of T-8 vertebra. The aortic hiatus, at the level of T-12, is an archway formed by the two crura, which anchor the diaphragm to the spine and join in the midline to form the median arcuate ligament. The aortic hiatus transmits the aorta, thoracic duct, azygous vein, and hemiazygous veins. The esophageal hiatus, at the level of T-10, is anterior and cephalad to the aortic hiatus, and posterior and left of the vena caval foramen. Through it pass the esophagus, vagus nerves, and the esophageal branches of the left gastric artery and veins. Two embryonic foramina are sites for congenital diaphragmatic hernia. The small foramen of Morgani is anteromedial between muscle fibers arising from the sternum and muscle fibers arising from the seventh anterior rib. The internal mammary vessels pass through this foramen, which is normally filled with fat. The larger, posterior, foramen of Bochdalek is a remnant of the embryonic pleuroperitoneal canal between fibers arising from the posterior ribs.

Abnormal elevation of the diaphragm on chest X-ray is a sign of phrenic or juxtaphrenic disease (Fig. 2). Unilateral elevation of the diaphragm may be due to a variety of causes, most of which can be diagnosed by US (Table 2). On chest radiographs, the normal right dome of the diaphragm is at the level of the anterior end of the sixth rib. The normal left dome of the diaphragm is about half a rib interspace lower. However, a raised hemidiaphragm is a common normal variant.

On US scans of the abdomen, the diaphragm is recognized as a bright curving echogenic line defining the cephalad extent of the abdomen (Fig. 3A). This bright line is produced by strong sound wave reflection from the interface between the diaphragm and the air-filled lung above it. High-resolution US demonstrates a more complex three-layer appearance (Fig. 3B). The muscle of the diaphragm is seen as a thin hypoechoic line between a thin echogenic line representing the diaphragm/liver capsule interface on the abdominal side and a brighter thicker echogenic line representing the surface of the air-filled lung on the thoracic side. A third echogenic line that is sometimes seen on the thoracic side is a mirror-image artifact of the diaphragm/lung surface. When disease is present in the thorax, such as pleural effusion or tumor, the diaphragm is seen as a thin echogenic line.

Pitfalls

Discontinuous Diaphragm Artifact

When ascites is present in the perihepatic or perisplenic regions, the diaphragm may appear discontinuous (Fig. 4). This appearance of the diaphragm is an

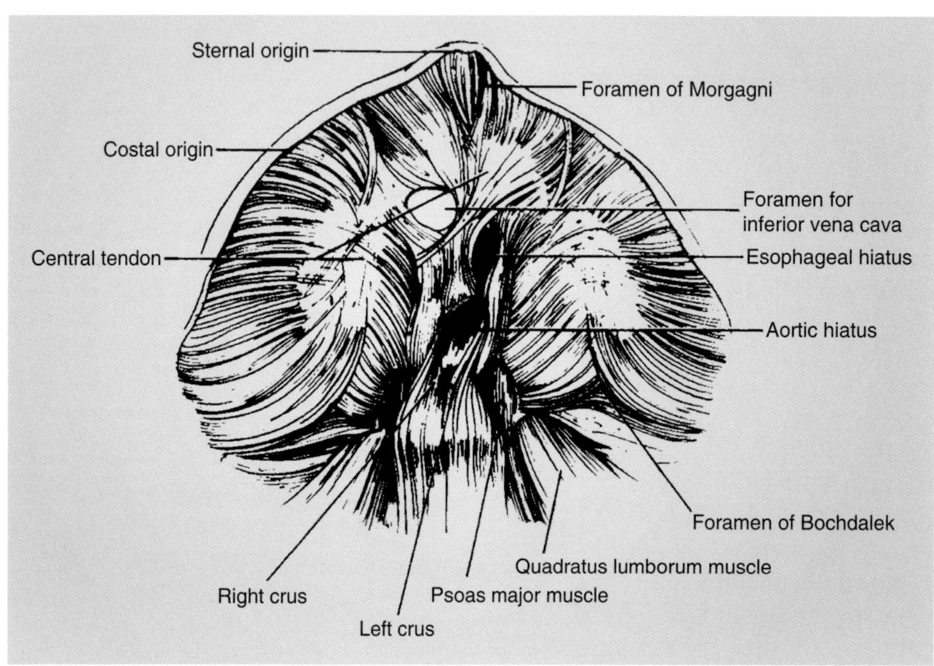

FIGURE 1 ■ Anatomy of the diaphragm viewed from the abdomen demonstrates the normal foramina and gaps in the diaphragm.

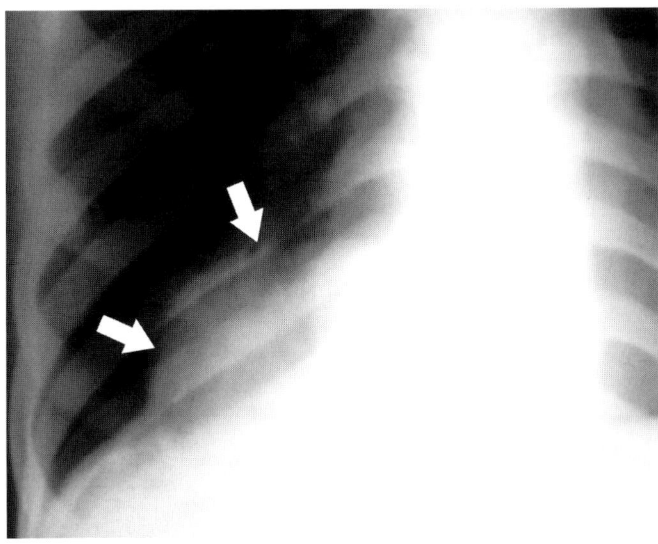

(A)

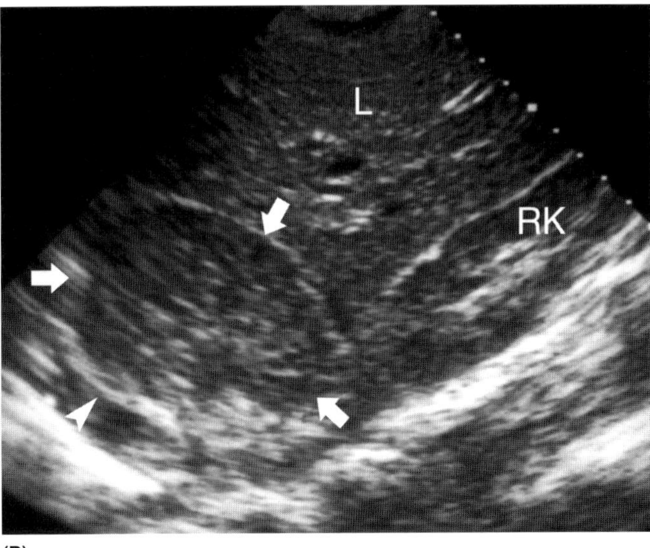

(B)

FIGURE 2 A AND B ■ Focal elevation of the diaphragm. (**A**) Cone-down view of a chest radiograph demonstrates abnormal focal elevation (*arrows*) of the posterior right hemidiaphragm. (**B**) Longitudinal US image of the abdomen reveals the cause of the bulging diaphragm (*arrowhead*) is a solid mass (*arrows*) of the right adrenal gland. The mass was a metastasis from an osteogenic sarcoma. RK, right kidney; L, liver.

artifact due to refraction of the sound beam at the interface between the liver and ascites or between the spleen and ascites. Refraction of the sound beam is due to differences in sound propagation speed in fluid compared to soft tissue and fat. Refraction causes misregistration of the location of a portion of the diaphragm on the US image.

TABLE 2 ■ Causes of Unilateral Elevation of the Diaphragm and Altered Motion of the Diaphragm

Normal variant	*Diaphragmatic hernia*
Phrenic nerve paralysis	Congenital
Lung tumor	Traumatic
Mediastinal tumor	Rupture of diaphragm
Trauma	*Diaphragmatic tumor*
Surgery	Metastasis
Infections	Mesothelioma
Idiopathic	Lipoma
Eventration of the diaphragm	Fibrosarcoma
Subpulmonic pleural effusion	*Diminished lung volume*
Subphrenic abscess	Lobectomy or lung resection
Postsurgical	Atelectasis
Ruptured viscus	Hypoplastic lung
Upper abdominal mass	
Hepatomegaly or liver mass	
Adrenal tumor	
Renal tumor	
Splenomegaly or splenic mass	
Ascites	
Bowel distension	

Diaphragmatic Slips

Diaphragmatic slips are prominent muscle bands that may simulate tumors in the liver or tumors on the peritoneal surface (6). Muscle bundles may form folds or strips on the inferior surface of the diaphragm, deeply indenting the liver and creating a mass (Fig. 5). They appear as highly echogenic nodules, which characteristically enlarge upon inspiration. The nodules have an average size of 1 to 2 cm and contain multiple linear echoes, which represent the folding of the diaphragm. Their presence causes a scalloped appearance to the diaphragm. They may be identified in 15% of normal individuals and increase in frequency with age.

Diaphragmatic Crura

The crura of the diaphragm have a variable size and shape and may be mistaken for lymphadenopathy or other pathology on US examination of the abdomen (Fig. 6). The crura have been noted to be normally hypertrophied in the newborn. The crura appear as hypoechoic nodules or bands on either side of the aorta. The right crus is broad and long, attaching on the L-3 vertebral body, whereas the left crus is narrower and shorter, attaching on the L-2 vertebral body. The crura characteristically thicken with inspiration.

Motion of the Diaphragm

The diaphragm functions as the chief muscle of respiration. Inspiration is attained by contraction of the muscles of the diaphragm, which causes the diaphragm to descend, increasing the volume of the thoracic cavity and decreasing the intrathoracic pressure, drawing air into the lungs. The descent of the diaphragm decreases the volume of the

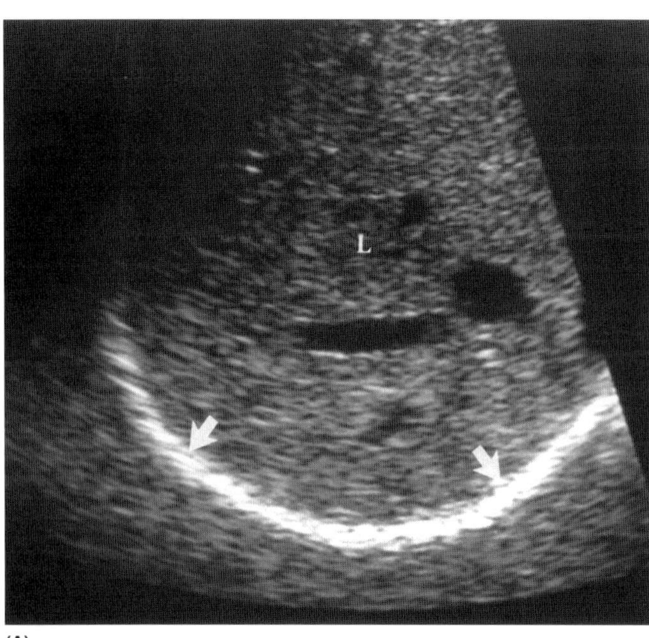

(A)

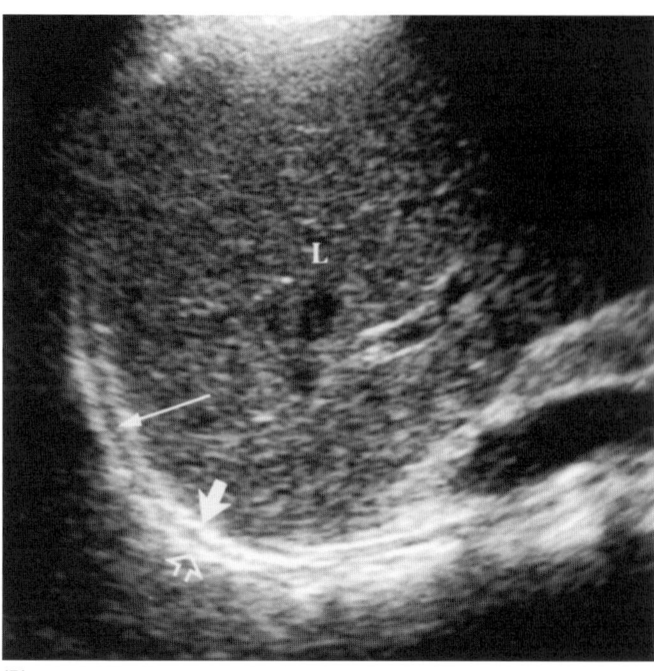

(B)

FIGURE 3 A AND B ■ Normal diaphragm. (**A**) Transverse US image through the liver (L) shows the diaphragm as a bright, curving, thick, echogenic line (*arrows*). (**B**) Longitudinal image through the liver shows the alternative "three-line" appearance of the diaphragm. The thin hypoechoic muscle of the diaphragm (*long arrow*) separates the echogenic line of the liver capsule/diaphragm interface (*short arrow*) from its mirror image (*open arrow*).

abdominal cavity and increases intra-abdominal pressure. The increased pressure compresses abdominal organs and promotes return of blood to the heart during inspiration. Expiration is largely passive. With muscle relaxation, the diaphragm expands and the dome rises. Abnormal diaphragm motion is a sign of phrenic or juxtaphrenic disease. The causes of abnormal motion of the diaphragm overlap with the causes of abnormal elevation of the diaphragm (Table 2). The two findings frequently coexist.

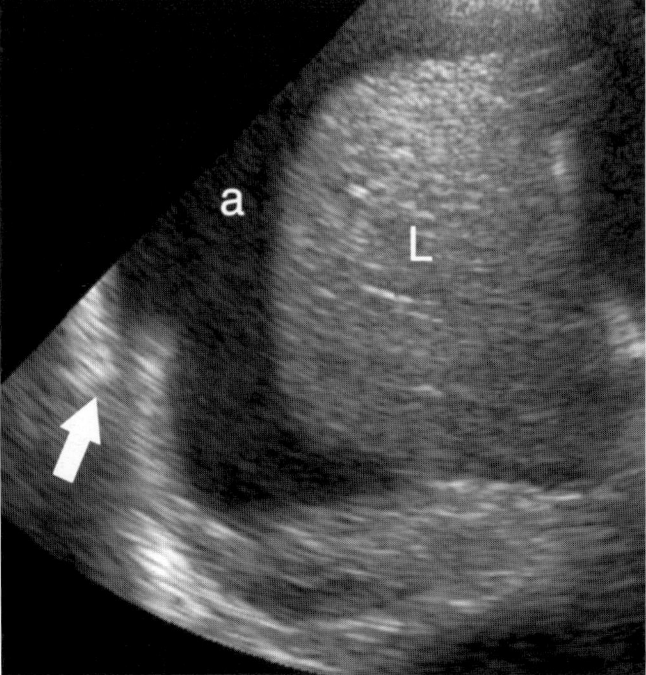

FIGURE 4 ■ Discontinuous diaphragm artifact. The diaphragm (*arrow*) appears discontinuous on this transverse image through the liver (L) in a patient with ascites (a). Differences in sound propagation speed between the liver and the adjacent fluid causes misregistration of the position of a portion of the diaphragm.

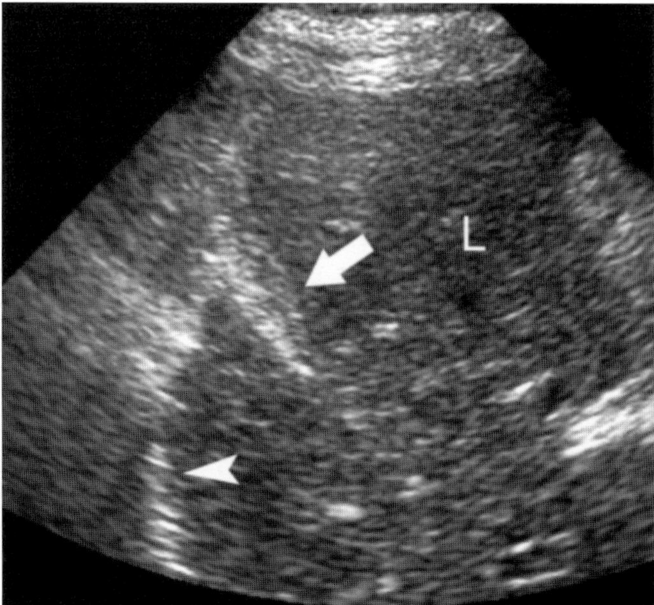

FIGURE 5 ■ Diaphragmatic slip. Oblique transverse US image of the liver (L) shows a bright fold (*arrow*) in the diaphragm indenting the liver parenchyma. The appearance is typical of diaphragmatic slip. The remainder of the diaphragm (*arrowhead*) has a somewhat wrinkled appearance of muscle laxity that comes with age.

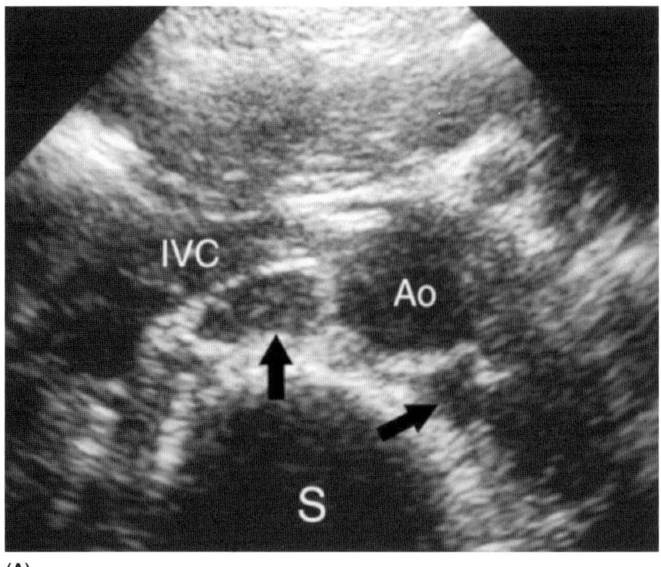

(A)

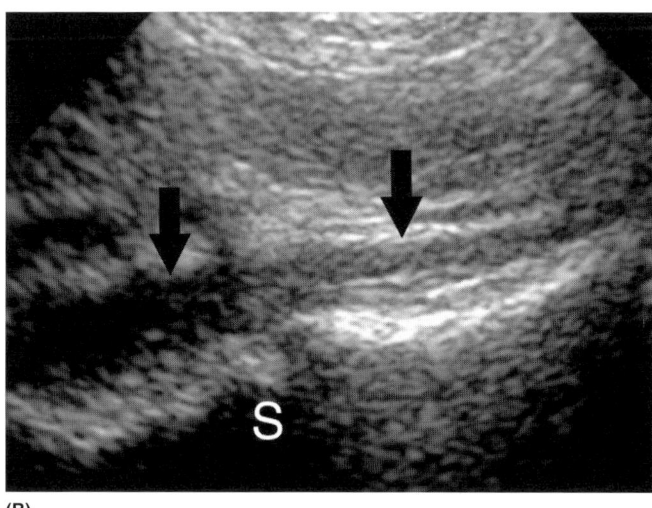

(B)

FIGURE 6 A AND B ■ Diaphragmatic crura. (**A**) The crura appear as hypoechoic nodules (*arrows*) on either side of the aorta (Ao) anterior to the shadow of the spine (S) on this transverse image of the upper abdomen. (**B**). Longitudinal image of the upper abdomen shows the right crus (*arrows*) as a tapering band of hypoechoic muscle anterior to the shadow of the spine. IVC, inferior vena cava.

US is the imaging method of choice to evaluate real-time motion of the diaphragm (7). Movement disorders of the diaphragm are commonly suspected from chest radiographs, which demonstrate abnormal elevation of the diaphragm. Mean excursion of the diaphragm between maximal inspiration and maximal expiration is 3.5 cm on the left and 3.3 cm on the right. However, the range of normal excursion is great, 0.8 to 8.1 cm. Minor asymmetry in excursion and uneven movement of portions of the diaphragm are common, normal findings (8). US assessment of diaphragm motion is best carried out in a longitudinal plane using the liver or spleen as a sonographic window (Fig. 7). A transverse, upward angled subxiphoid approach may allow simultaneous assessment of both

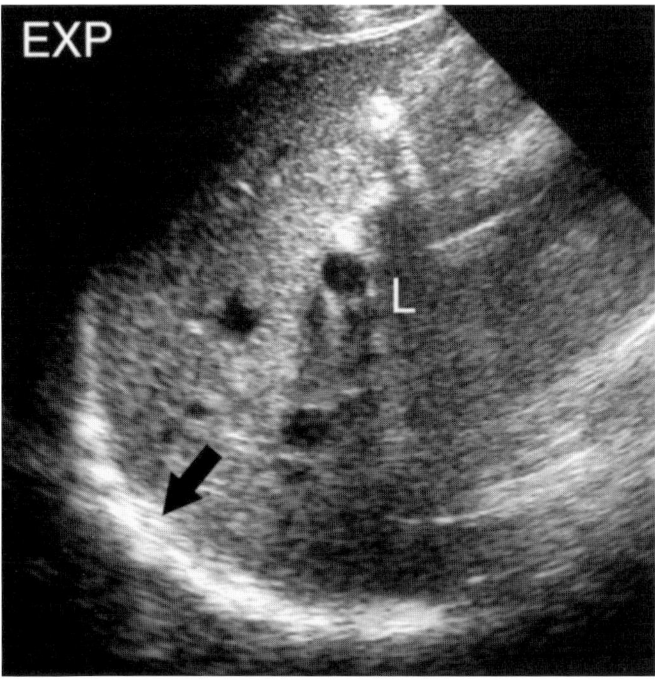

(A)

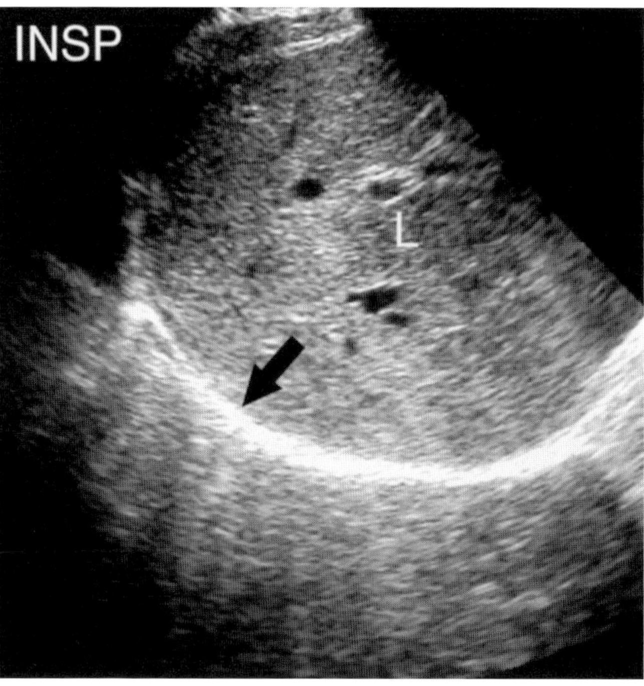

(B)

FIGURE 7 A AND B ■ Motion of the diaphragm. Longitudinal images of the diaphragm (*arrows*), through the liver (L), in expiration (**A**), and in inspiration (**B**), confirm normal motion of the diaphragm. Note the elongation of the posterior aspect of the diaphragm with inspiration.

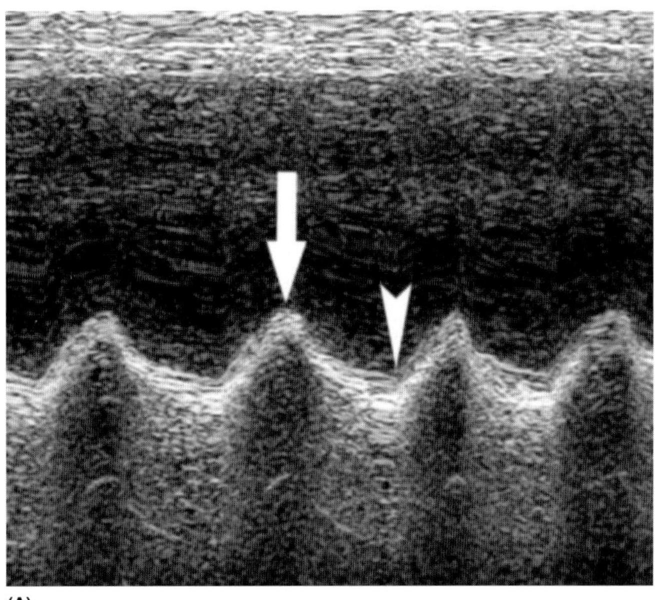

(A)

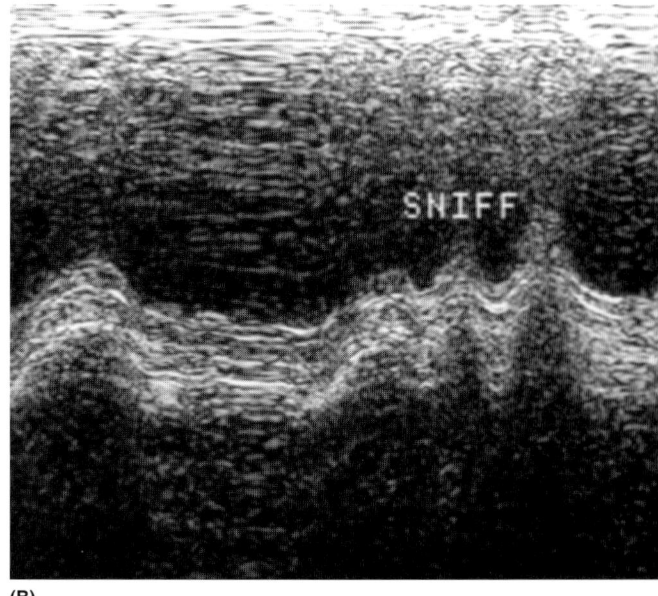

(B)

FIGURE 8 A AND B ■ Motion of the diaphragm—M-mode. M-mode documentation of motion of the diaphragm is illustrated during normal breathing (**A**), and during a sniff test (**B**). Diaphragmatic excursion is measured between inspiration (*arrow*) and expiration (*arrowhead*).

sides of the diaphragm. The dome and posterolateral diaphragm demonstrate maximal movement with respiration. Motion of the diaphragm can be measured utilizing M-mode US (Fig. 8). The posterolateral muscle fibers are the longest, providing the greatest amount of shortening with contraction. The peripheral attachments are fixed and do not move. The normal diaphragm descends with inspiration and ascends with expiration. Diaphragm motion may be assessed indirectly by measuring the craniocaudad displacement of branches of the left portal vein (9). The "sniff test" is used to exaggerate phrenic movement. The patient is asked to inhale suddenly through the nose with the mouth closed. Both sides of the diaphragm should descend rapidly. Unilateral passive upward movement is considered abnormal. However, it has been demonstrated that 6% of normal people have an abnormal sniff test.

Abnormal Excursion of the Diaphragm

Excursion of the diaphragm is considered abnormal when one side of the diaphragm moves twice the distance of the affected side of the diaphragm during maximal inspiration. This finding may, however, be observed in normal individuals and is therefore not an unequivocal sign of disease.

Paradoxical Motion

Paradoxical motion is a definitive sign of a diseased diaphragm (Fig. 9). It is defined as abnormal upward motion of the diaphragm during inspiration. This is usually a passive effect due to the increase in intra-abdominal pressure and the decrease in intrathoracic pressure produced by normal motion of the opposite side of the diaphragm. The differential diagnosis of paradoxical motion is paralysis, eventration, and diaphragmatic hernia.

Pathological Conditions

Diaphragm Paralysis

Paralysis of the diaphragm is suggested on chest radiographs by abnormal elevation of the diaphragm, paradoxical motion of the diaphragm (Fig. 9), and mediastinal shift toward the affected side. Common causes of phrenic nerve impairment are listed in Table 2. Paralysis of one side of the diaphragm commonly produces no symptoms

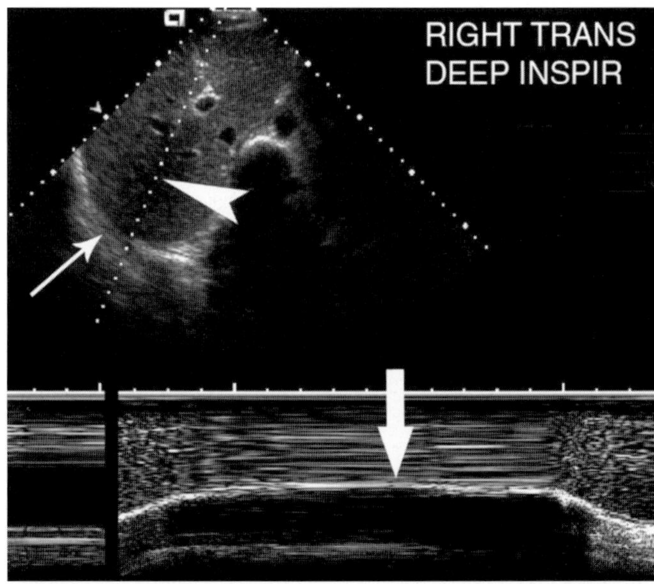

FIGURE 9 ■ Paralyzed diaphragm—paradoxical motion. Combined gray-scale and M-mode image demonstrates paradoxical upward motion (*thick arrow*) of the right hemidiaphragm during deep inspiration. The line of sight of the M-mode US beam through the liver to the diaphragm (*long thin arrow*) is indicated by the dotted line (*arrowhead*).

in adults and older children, but in infants, it causes major compromise of respiratory function. Infants have underdeveloped intercostal muscles, and ventilation is almost totally dependent on phrenic motion. US findings include absent or paradoxical motion of the affected side and exaggerated motion of the opposite side. Paralysis may be indistinguishable from eventration.

Eventration

Eventration refers to abnormal thinning or atrophy of all or a portion of the diaphragm (6). The musculature surrounding the eventration is normal. The thinned membranous eventration is elevated and moves abnormally. Most cases are asymptomatic and not clinically significant. The anterior aspect of the right hemidiaphragm is most commonly involved (Fig. 10). The area of eventration averages 4 to 7 cm in size. Liver commonly protrudes into the eventration pouch. Eventration may be congenital or acquired due to ischemia, infarction, or neuromuscular weakness. US demonstrates the protrusion of the intact diaphragm and the underlying abdominal structure, but the thinning of the diaphragm is generally not appreciated. The thinned portion demonstrates paradoxical motion or no motion during respiration.

Rupture/Perforation

Rupture of the diaphragm is most commonly caused by blunt or penetrating trauma of the abdomen (4). Ruptures due to blunt trauma usually involve the left hemidiaphragm (90%) and commonly exceed 10 cm in length. Knife injuries to the diaphragm are commonly abdominal wounds with an upward thrust into the diaphragm. Perforation of the diaphragm may occur with amebic or other hepatic abscesses. Chest radiograph findings include apparent elevation of the hemidiaphragm, pleural effusion, and density at the lung base. US findings include visualization of the defect in the diaphragm as a free edge outlined by fluid, fluid above and below the diaphragm, and liver or peristalsing bowel loops above the diaphragm.

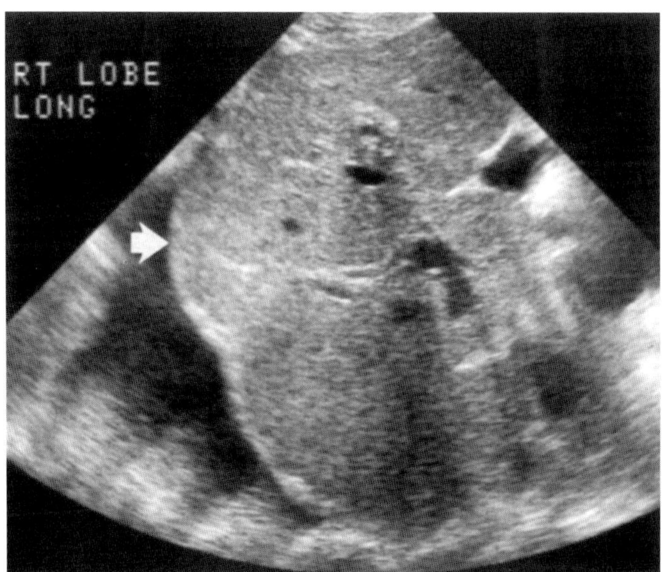

FIGURE 10 ■ Eventration. An eventration of the right hemidiaphragm (*arrow*) is outlined by fluid in the pleural space on this longitudinal image. Normal liver tissue protrudes into the eventration pouch.

Bochdalek Hernias

Bochdalek hernias are the most common congenital diaphragmatic hernias. Large hernias, containing bowel, stomach, spleen, or kidney are discovered on obstetric sonograms, or, in neonates, due to pulmonary compromise. Small hernias, containing abdominal fat, are asymptomatic and only detected as a mass on a chest radiograph or CT scan. The defect is posterior, at the site of pleuroperitoneal canal (Fig. 11). Bochdalek hernias are more common on the left (left:right = 2:1).

Morgagni Hernias

Morgagni hernias are rare. The defect is anteromedial near the sternum. Abdominal viscera or fat herniate into the thorax or pericardial sac. Morgagni hernias usually present in adults and are associated with obesity and trauma. Most patients are asymptomatic, and the hernia is discovered on a chest radiograph.

Diaphragm Inversion

Inversion of the diaphragm is seen with large pleural effusions and large thoracic masses (6). Inversion may involve the entire diaphragm or only a portion of the diaphragm. US demonstrates convexity of the diaphragm toward the abdomen rather than toward the thorax. With respiration, the inverted diaphragm shows little or no motion. Paradoxical motion is not observed.

Diaphragmatic Masses

The most common tumors of the diaphragm are metastases (Fig. 12), which implant on the pleural or peritoneal surfaces from tumors of the lung, colon, stomach, adrenal gland, or kidney. Mesothelioma may produce a sheet-like mass on the diaphragm. Primary tumors of the diaphragm are rare. Fibrosarcoma is the most common primary malignancy. Lipoma is the most common benign tumor. Lipomas are differentiated from hernias containing fat by the lack of a defect in the diaphragm. Other rare benign lesions include cysts, fibromas, schwannomas, and leiomyomas.

PLEURAL SPACE

Normal Anatomy

The pleural cavity is a thin, closed space containing a small volume of fluid between the visceral and the parietal pleura. The right and left pleural cavities are completely separate from each other. The visceral pleura is the closely adherent covering membrane of the lung. It invests the interlobar fissures and is continuous with the parietal pleura at the hila. The parietal pleura is the external wall of the pleural cavity, closely adherent to the ribs,

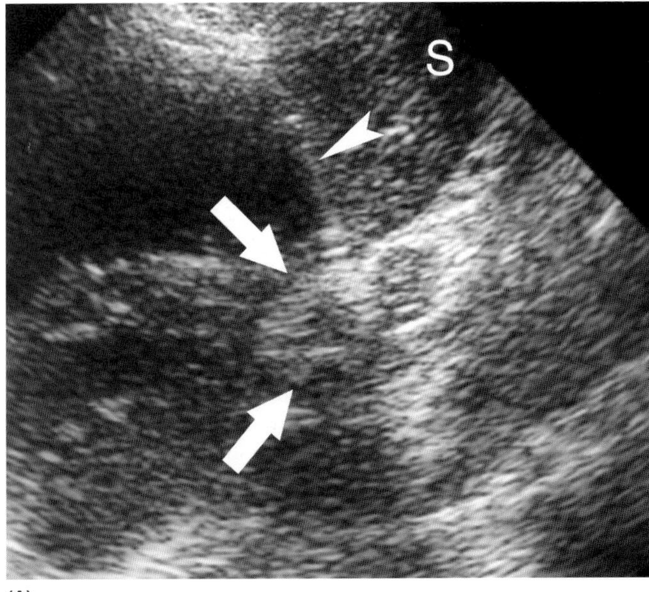

(A)

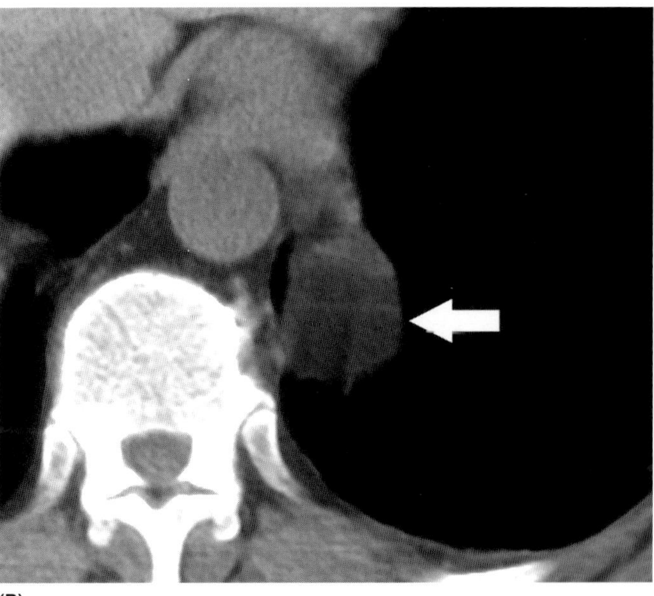

(B)

FIGURE 11 A AND B ■ Bochdalek hernia. (**A**) Coronal plane US image through the spleen (S) reveals a nodule of fat (*arrows*) herniating through the diaphragm (*arrowhead*) at the foramen of Bochdalek. (**B**) Axial plane CT image demonstrates the fat within the hernia (*arrow*).

intercostal muscles, sternum, mediastinum, and diaphragm. A double layer of pleura extends inferiorly from each hilum as the inferior pulmonary ligament, connecting the mediastinal pleura with the lung root and ending inferiorly as a free edge. The visceral pleura is supplied primarily by pulmonary arteries and veins and has lymphatic drainage to hilar lymph nodes. The parietal pleura is supplied by systemic arteries and veins and has lymphatic drainage toward the internal mammary and mediastinal lymph nodes. Pleural fluid lubricates the pleural surfaces and reduces friction between the visceral and the parietal pleura, promoting respiratory motion. One to 5 mL of pleural fluid occupies the normal pleural space. Approximately 10 mL of pleural fluid is produced each day, primarily by the parietal pleura. Lymphatic drainage of pleural fluid occurs mainly through the lymphatics of the parietal pleura.

FIGURE 12 ■ Diaphragmatic mass. A metastasis (M) from colon carcinoma is implanted on the peritoneal surface of the diaphragm (*arrow*). The mass is outlined by ascites (a) and causes a mass impression on the liver (L).

With a US transducer applied directly to the chest (intercostal scanning), the pleural space is most easily identified by observing the normal motion of the lung with respiration (Fig. 13). The air-filled lung surface totally reflects the US beam producing a bright echogenic line of sound reflection. Although transmission of the US beam deeper into the chest is blocked, the US image displays a characteristic pattern of bright echoes produced by reverberation artifact. This pattern should be recognized as normal for air-filled lung. The normal back and forth movement of the lung surface with respiration has been called the "gliding sign." With the transducer oriented perpendicular to the ribs, the ribs are displayed as rounded echogenic surfaces with prominent acoustic shadowing. The parietal pleura is located approximately 1 cm deep to the rib surface. Pleural fluid is visualized as the anechoic space between the parietal pleura and the highly reflective visceral pleura–lung interface (10).

Pitfalls

Mirror-Image Artifact

From an abdominal scanning approach, the curving diaphragm–lung interface acts as a specular (mirror-like)

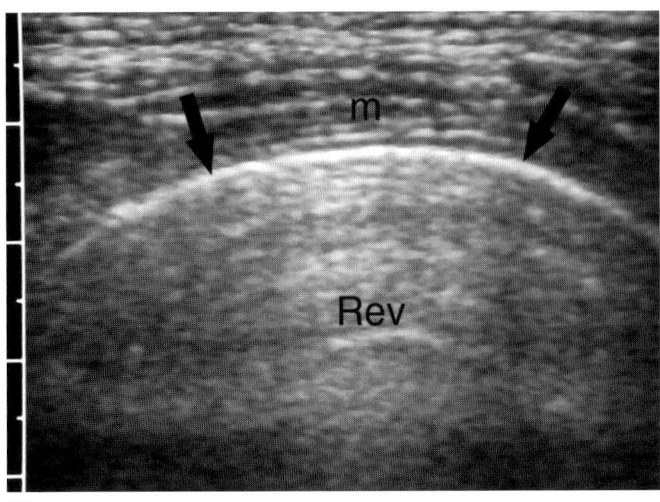

(A)

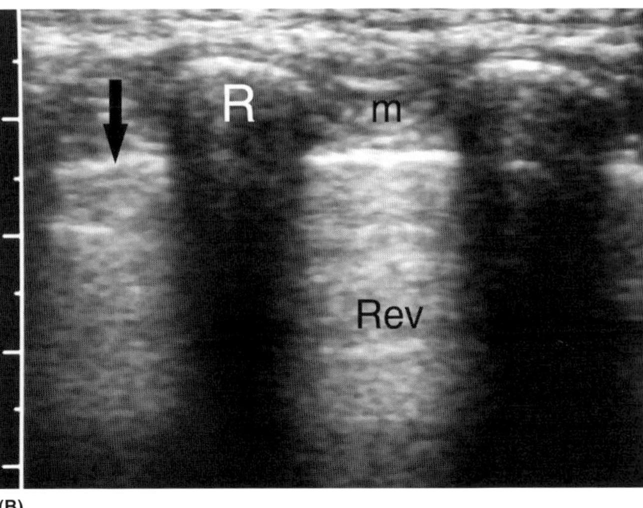

(B)

FIGURE 13 A AND B ■ Normal pleural space. Scans in intercostal (**A**) and longitudinal (**B**) planes, using a linear array transducer, reveal the normal pleural space. The visceral pleura/lung interface (*arrows*) is recognized by observing its gliding motion while the patient is breathing. Ribs (R) cast prominent acoustic shadows. The parietal pleura is 5 to 10 mm deep to the proximal surface of the ribs and is closely applied to the visceral pleura when no pleural effusion is present. Intercostal muscles (m) are seen between the ribs. The normal air-filled lung is totally reflective, resulting in bright reverberation artifact displayed on the US image in the location of the lung. Rev, reverberation artifact.

reflector producing an artifactual mirror image of the liver or spleen above the diaphragm (Fig. 14). This mirror-image artifact should be recognized as normal for air-filled lung.

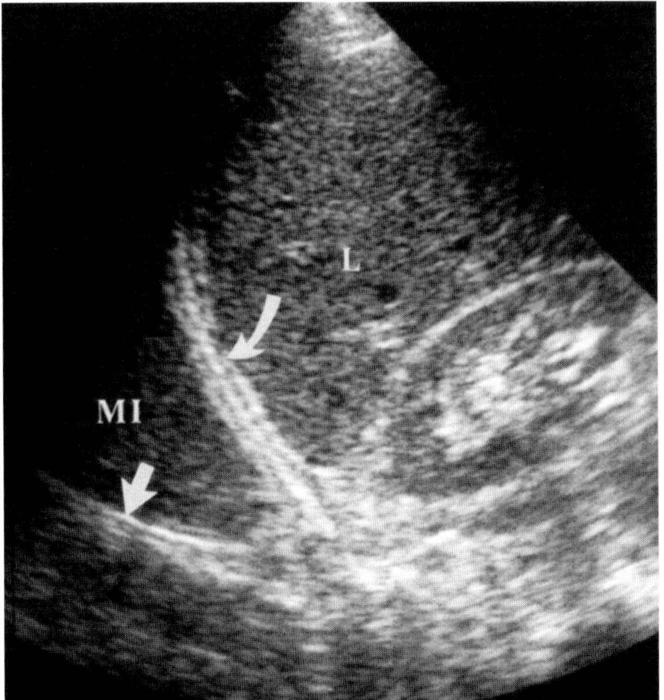

FIGURE 14 ■ Mirror image (MI) artifact. Longitudinal image demonstrates an MI artifact of the liver (L) above the diaphragm (*curved arrow*). An MI artifact (*straight arrow*) of the diaphragm is also seen above the MI artifact of the liver. Note the normal "three-line" appearance of the diaphragm. MI artifacts are produced only when air-filled lung is present above the diaphragm.

Obscured Near Field

The use of a sector or vector transducer for intercostal scanning may result in errors in diagnosis. The sector scanner has a narrow view in the near field that is usually obscured by near-field artifact. The superficial pleural space is poorly demonstrated; the ribs cannot be used as anatomic landmarks; and the liver or spleen may be misinterpreted as pleural fluid. Linear or broad, curved-array transducers are preferred for intercostal scanning. Sector or vector transducers are reserved for examination of deep structures and scanning using the abdominal approach.

Pathological Conditions

Disorders of the pleura are listed in Table 3.

Pleural Effusion

Pleural effusion is defined as an abnormal increased volume of fluid in the pleural space. On intercostal sonograms,

TABLE 3 ■ Differential Diagnosis of Pleural Abnormalities

Effusions
- Transudates
- Exudates

Empyema

Parapneumonic effusion

Pleural plaques

Pleural thickening

Tumors
- Localized fibrous tumor of the pleura
- Pleural metastases
- Mesothelioma

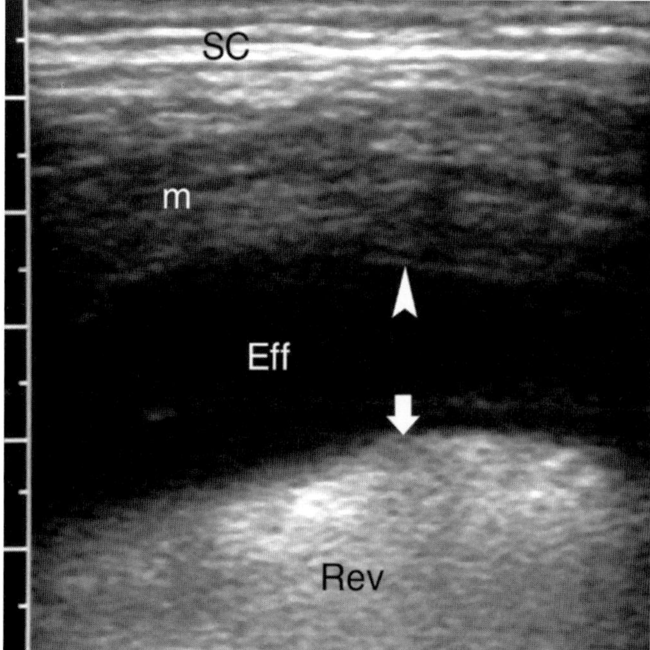

FIGURE 15 ■ Pleural effusion—intercostal scan. A linear array scan in an intercostal space reveals an anechoic pleural effusion. Fluid separates the parietal pleura (*arrowhead*) from the visceral pleura/lung surface (*arrow*). Beneath the skin is the fat-containing echogenic subcutaneous tissue (SC). The parietal pleura is applied to the deep surface of the intercostal muscle (m). Eff, pleural effusion; Rev, reverberation artifact form air in the lungs.

pleural effusions are diagnosed by increased separation of visceral and parietal pleura by fluid (Fig. 15). The fluid may be anechoic, echogenic, or may contain floating echogenic particles. Visualization of moving particulate matter or moving septations within the fluid confirms its liquid nature and provides differentiation from pleural thickening or pleural tumor. Stranding densities (septations) within pleural fluid are formed by fibrin and protein macroaggregates and reflect a high protein concentration within the fluid. On abdominal sonograms (Fig. 16), the signs of pleural effusion include (*i*) fluid, rather than mirror-image artifact, above the diaphragm and (*ii*) visualization of the ribs and posterior chest wall through the fluid (Table 4). Sonography has been shown to be highly accurate in the diagnosis of even small pleural effusions (11). The volume of pleural fluid present can be roughly estimated by measuring the separation of visceral and parietal pleura (Table 5). The sonographic measurement of pleural separation is made during maximum inspiration with the patient supine. The transducer is placed at posterolateral chest wall just cranial to the lung base. The maximum perpendicular distance from the posterior surface of the lung to the posterior chest wall is measured (12).

Transudative pleural effusions are ultrafiltrates of plasma and result from an increase in capillary hydrostatic pressure or a decrease in colloid osmotic pressure. Pleural membranes are usually normal. Treatment is

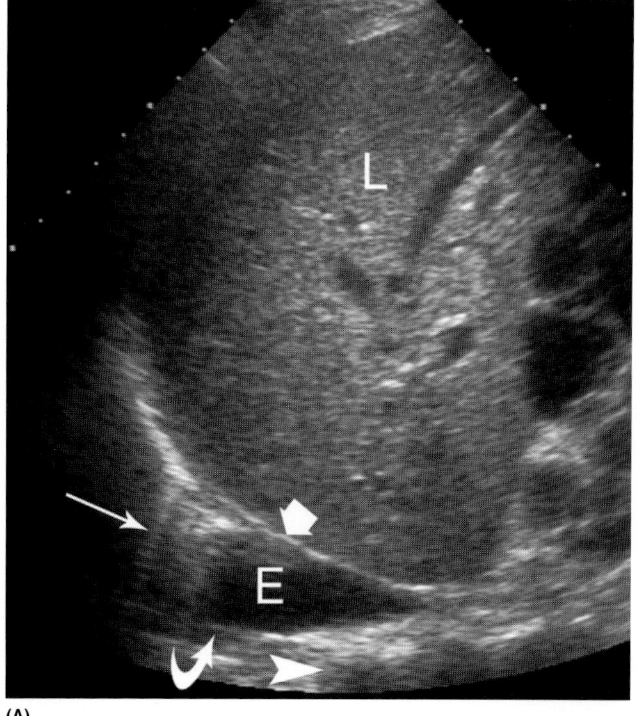

(A)

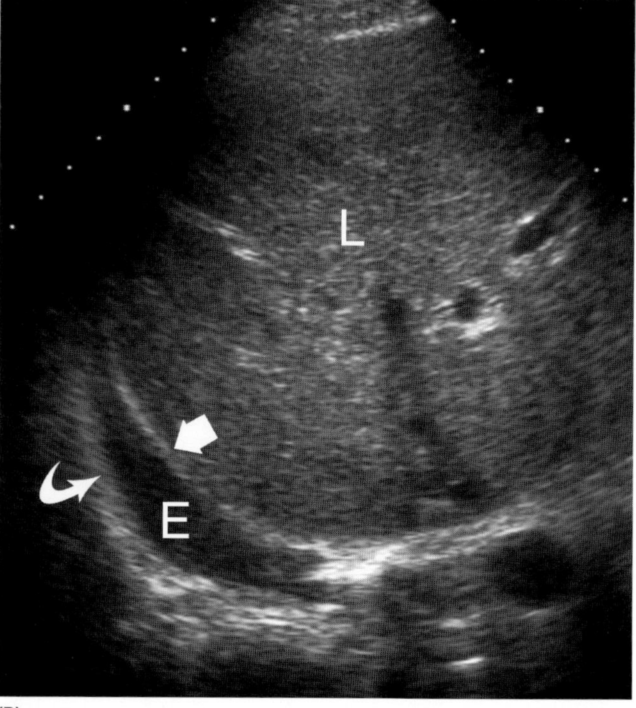

(B)

FIGURE 16 A AND B ■ Pleural effusion—abdominal scan. (**A**) Longitudinal scan through the liver (L) reveals a right pleural effusion (E), seen as echolucent fluid above the diaphragm (*thick arrow*). The ribs, marked by acoustic shadows (*arrowhead*), and chest wall (*curved arrow*) are visualized through the pleural fluid. The mirror-image artifact is absent. Air bubbles in collapsed lung produce a reverberation artifact (*thin arrow*). (**B**) Transverse scan in the same patient shows a right pleural effusion as a hypoechoic band of fluid between the diaphragm (*fat arrow*) and the chest wall (*curved arrow*). Acoustic shadows from the ribs (*arrowheads*) should be identified to ensure that the second echogenic line is the posterior chest wall and is not a mirror-image artifact.

TABLE 4 ■ Sonographic Signs of Pleural Effusion

Intercostal scan
- Anechoic to homogeneously hypoechoic space between visceral and parietal pleura
- Floating echodensities
- Moving septations
- Shape corresponding to pleural space
- Lung movement within fluid

Abdominal scan
- Anechoic or hypoechoic fluid above the diaphragm
- Absence of mirror-image reflection of liver or spleen above the diaphragm
- Visualization of the posterior wall of the thorax through the fluid collection

directed at the underlying disease, which is most commonly congestive heart failure (Table 6). Exudative pleural effusions have a high content of protein and other constituents of whole blood. They most commonly result from increased capillary permeability due to inflammatory or neoplastic processes that involve the pleura directly. The pleura itself is diseased. A pleural effusion is considered to be an exudate if at least one of the following criteria is met: (*i*) ratio of pleural fluid protein concentration to serum protein concentration greater than 0.5; (*ii*) ratio of pleural fluid lactate dehydrogenase (LDH) to serum LDH greater than 0.6; or (*iii*) pleural fluid LDH greater than two-thirds the upper limit of normal serum LDH. The sonographic signs that differentiate transudate from exudate are listed in Table 7. Anechoic pleural fluid may be either transudate or exudate. However, fluid that contains echogenic particulate matter, thick or thin fibrin septations (Fig. 17), or is associated with thickened pleura or pleural nodules is an exudate (13).

At times, it may be difficult to differentiate a small pleural effusion from pleural thickening. The "fluid color sign" may be helpful (14). In most (90%) pleural effusions, color signal will appear within pleural fluid during respiratory and cardiac cycles caused by motion of the pleural fluid. Pleural thickening does not show the fluid color sign.

TABLE 5 ■ Quantification of Pleural Effusion Volume

Thickness of effusion measured by US (mm)	Mean effusion volume (mL)	Range of effusion volume (mL)
0	5	0–90
5	80	20–170
10	170	50–300
15	260	90–420
20	380	150–660
30	550	210–1060
40	1,000	490–1670
50	1,420	650–1840

TABLE 6 ■ Causes of Pleural Effusion

Transudate	Exudate
Congestive heart failure	Parapneumonic effusion
Cirrhosis	Tuberculous pleurisy
Nephrotic syndrome	Collagen vascular diseases
Hypoalbuminemia	Empyema
Constrictive pericarditis	Hemothorax
Superior vena cava obstruction	Postpericardotomy syndrome
	Pulmonary infarction
	Intra-abdominal diseases
	Subphrenic abscess
	Pancreatitis
	Hepatic abscess
	Neoplasms
	Metastatic disease
	Bronchogenic carcinoma
	Lymphoma, leukemia
	Mesothelioma

Empyema and Parapneumonic Effusions

Empyema is defined as pus in the pleural cavity. Parapneumonic effusions are exudative pleural effusions associated with bacterial pneumonia or lung abscess. Image-guided or surgical placement of a pleural space drainage catheter is indicated for all cases of empyema and for those parapneumonic effusions with pH below 7.0 or pleural fluid glucose concentration below 40 mg/dL. Parapneumonic effusions accompany nearly 40% of bacterial pneumonias. Although most empyemas develop from parapneumonic effusions, most parapneumonic effusions do not develop into empyemas. Clinical criteria for the diagnosis of empyema include (*i*) grossly purulent pleural fluid; (*ii*) bacteria identified on pleural fluid Gram stain or culture; and (*iii*) pleural fluid white blood cell count greater than 15,000/mL. Additional causes of empyema include thoracic surgery, trauma, subphrenic abscess, and spinal osteomyelitis (Table 8).

There are no specific US findings of empyema or parapneumonic effusion requiring drainage. US demonstrates the findings associated with exudative pleural effusions (Table 7) (Fig. 18). Contrast enhancement of thickened

TABLE 7 ■ Sonographic Signs of Exudate and Transudate

Transudate	Exudate
Anechoic fluid	Anechoic fluid
	Echogenic fluid or floating echodensities
	Septations or fibrin strands
	Thickened pleura (>3 mm)
	Pleural nodules

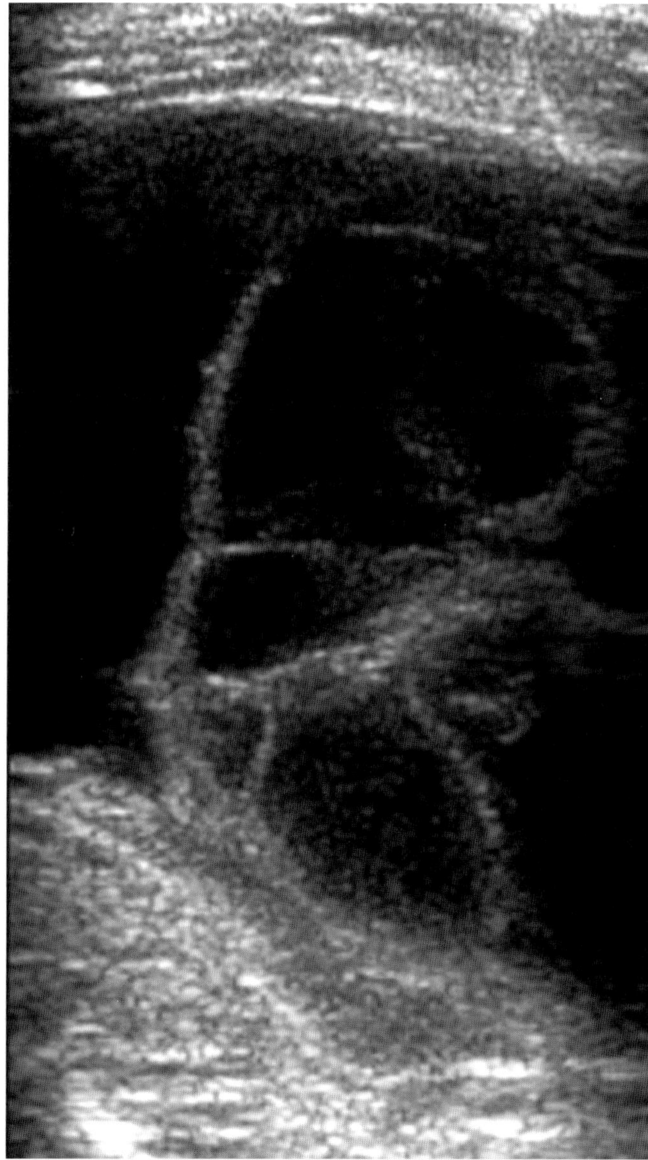

FIGURE 17 ■ Exudative pleural effusion. An intercostal scan reveals a network of thick septations that span the pleural place and produce loculations of echogenic pleural fluid in this patient with an exudative parapneumonic effusion.

visceral and parietal pleura on CT scan is suggestive. Diagnosis is made by thoracentesis, which may be guided by US. Extensive septations visualized by US within a known acute thoracic empyema may be an indication for early fibrinolytic therapy (15).

TABLE 8 ■ Causes of Empyema

- Bacterial pneumonia
- Lung abscess
- Thoracic surgery
- Trauma
- Subphrenic abscess
- Spinal osteomyelitis

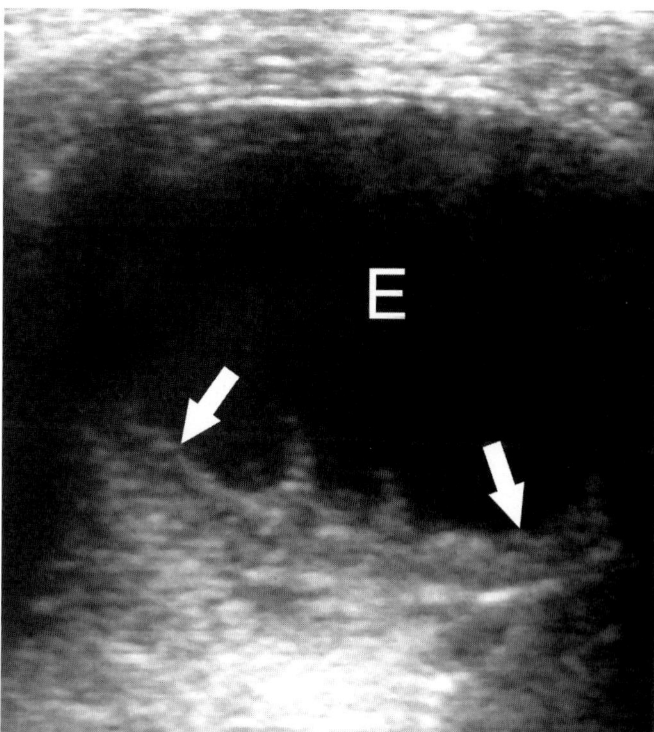

FIGURE 18 ■ Empyema. Loculation of a pleural effusion (E) is suggested, on this intercostal scan, by concavity of the lung surface (*arrows*) caused by mass effect of the pleural space fluid. The visceral pleura (*arrows*) is thickened and partial septations extend into the fluid. Thoracentesis revealed purulent fluid, confirming empyema.

Pleural Plaques

Pleural plaques are circumscribed collections of dense collagenous tissue. Pleural plaques or localized pleural thickening usually results from inflammatory disease of the pleural space or parenchyma, asbestos exposure, pulmonary infarction, or drug-related pleural disease. Plaques appear on US as smooth elliptical areas of echo-poor pleural tissue. Pleural plaques are hypoechoic compared with liver, spleen, and intercostal muscle. Visceral pleura plaques can be differentiated from parietal pleura plaques by real-time scanning during respiration showing movement of the plaques in association with gliding of visceral pleura. Calcified plaques, often caused by asbestos exposure, are echogenic and demonstrate acoustic shadowing or comet-tail artifacts (16).

Pleural Thickening

Diffuse pleural thickening may represent diffuse pleural fibrosis (fibrothorax and pleural peel) or pleural malignancy. Fibrothorax most commonly results from exudative pleural effusion, empyema, or hemothorax. Encasement of the entire lung restricts pulmonary ventilation. Pleural thickening appears on sonograms as irregular or lobulated, solid, thickening of the pleura (Fig. 19) that displaces air-filled lung away from the chest wall (Table 9).

Localized Fibrous Tumor of the Pleura

Localized fibrous tumor is a more appropriate term for the lesion that has previously been called benign

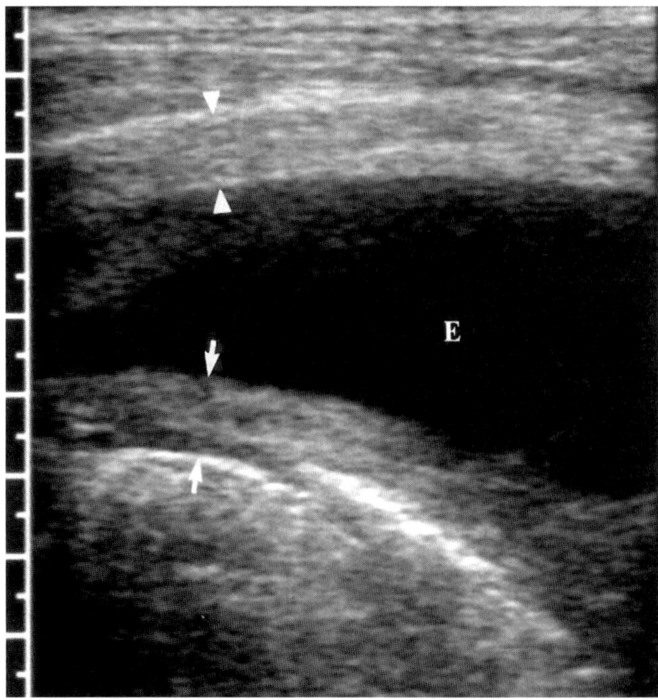

FIGURE 19 ■ Pleural thickening. Diffuse thickening of the parietal pleura (*arrowheads*) and visceral pleura (*arrows*) is caused, in this patient, by tuberculosis. An anechoic pleural effusion (E) separates the pleural surfaces.

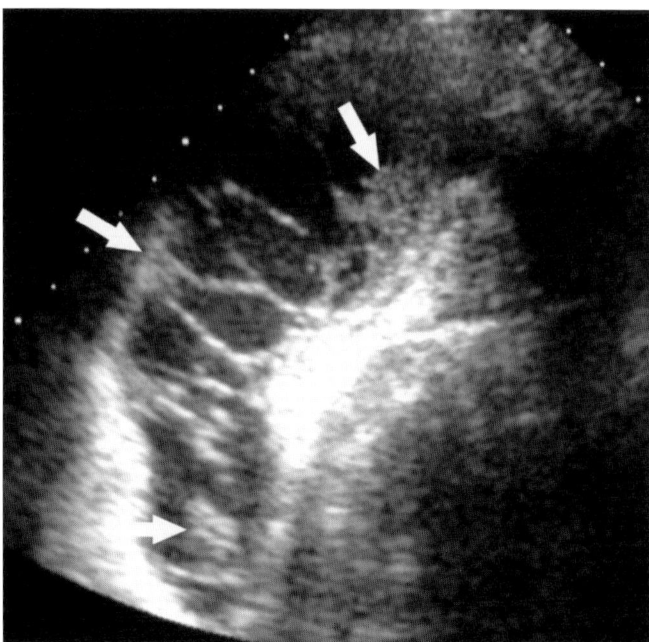

FIGURE 20 ■ Pleural metastasis. An intercostal scan of the pleural space reveals a complex pleural effusion with extensive irregular septations. Numerous nodules (*arrows*) are indicative of pleural metastases. Fine-needle aspiration confirmed metastatic adenocarcinoma of the colon.

mesothelioma (17). Microscopically, 40% of localized fibrous tumors are malignant, but most are curable by surgical resection. CT demonstrates smooth, sharply defined pleural masses with tapering edges (18). US reveals marked undulating hypoechoic soft-tissue thickening of the pleura.

Pleural Metastases

Metastatic disease is the second most common cause of pleural effusion in patients older than 50 years. Common primary tumors include lung and breast carcinoma, lymphoma, and ovarian and gastrointestinal malignancies (19). Pleural effusion is primarily caused by malignant infiltration of mediastinal lymph nodes, which drain the pleural space. Protein is removed from pleural fluid only by lymphatic drainage; therefore, malignant pleural effusions are characterized by high protein concentration. Tumor cells on, or just beneath, the pleural surface are the second major manifestation of pleural metastatic disease. Findings that favor malignant pleural disease include (*i*) circumferential pleural thickening, (*ii*) nodular pleural thickening, (*iii*) pleural thickening greater than 1 cm, and (*iv*) pleural thickening involving the mediastinal pleura. US can effectively demonstrate pleural metastases through pleural effusions as soft-tissue nodules (Fig. 20) studding the pleura or undulating sheet-like pleural thickening (20).

TABLE 9 ■ Sonographic Signs Pleural Effusion vs. Pleural Thickening

Pleural effusion	Pleural thickening
Changes shape with respiration	Thickened solid stripe (>3 mm)
Moving septations	Irregular or lobulated contour
Floating echodensities	Aerated lung displaced away from chest wall
Fluid color sign present	Fluid color sign absent

Mesothelioma

Most (80%) malignant mesotheliomas occur as a complication of asbestos exposure (21). The latency period is up to 35 years with a 10% lifetime risk in asbestos workers. The typical course is progressive deterioration to death with a mean survival of only 11 months. Sonography or CT demonstrates diffuse irregular or nodular thickened pleura (Fig. 21). Discrete pleural mass or pleural nodules are uncommon. Pleural effusion accompanies 75% of cases. Calcified pleural plaques, reflecting asbestos exposure, are found in 20%. Pleural biopsy is needed to confirm the diagnosis (22).

Pneumothorax

The normal surface of the aerated lung produces a highly echogenic line of US reflection that moves in concert with respiration. Pneumothorax produces a similar highly echogenic line of reflection but without visualization of respiratory movement (Table 10) (23,24). Reverberation artifact produces similar amorphous bright echoes deep to the hyperechogenic line in both normal lung and pneumothorax. The occurrence of pneumothorax can be recognized during US-guided procedures by the disappearance of lung lesions previously sonographically visualized (Fig. 22).

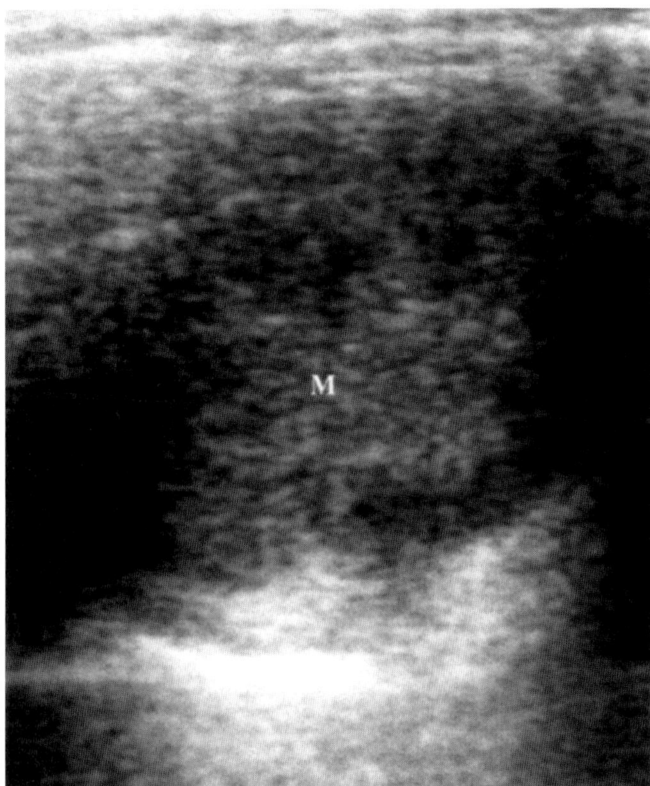

FIGURE 21 ■ Mesothelioma. Sonogram localizes a large pleural space soft-tissue mass (M) for guided percutaneous biopsy. Histology revealed malignant mesothelioma.

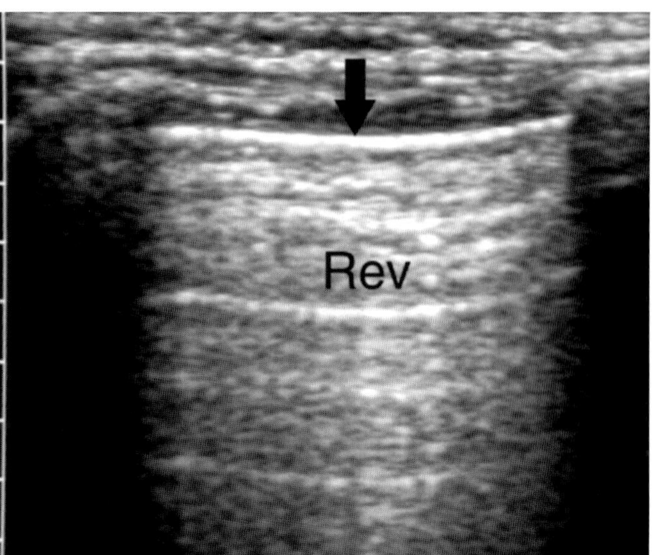

FIGURE 22 ■ Pneumothorax. During a US-guided biopsy of a peripheral lung mass, the lesion disappeared. A bright interface (*arrow*) was evident at the location of the pleural space. This interface did not move with respiration. Reverberation (Rev) artifact is displayed deeper in the image. This constellation of findings is indicative of development of a pneumothorax.

US-Guided Invasive Procedures

US can be used effectively to guide a number of diagnostic and therapeutic invasive procedures in the pleural space including diagnostic thoracentesis, therapeutic catheter drainage of symptomatic effusions, and empyema, pleurodesis, and pleural biopsy (25). US provides the advantages of real-time guidance, portability, and added safety. The incidence of pneumothorax is 18% for clinically guided thoracentesis versus 3% for sonographically guided thoracentesis.

LUNG PARENCHYMA

Normal Anatomy

The normal aerated lung parenchyma is not evaluated by US because the soft tissue–lung interface at the lung periphery causes total reflection of the US beam (Figs. 13 and 14). However, when the peripheral lung air spaces collapse or fill with fluid, a sonographic window to lung disease is created. The diseased lung parenchyma is examined directly through the intercostal spaces or via an abdominal approach through the liver or spleen. Correlation must be made with recent chest radiographs or CT scans to ensure that the proper area of the lung is examined.

TABLE 10 ■ Sonographic Signs of Pneumothorax

- Continuous hyperechoic line demonstrating reverberation artifact
- Absent respiratory movement of visceral pleura
- Absent comet-tail artifacts
- Disappearance of previously visualized lung lesion during ultrasound-guided procedures

Pathological Conditions

Disorders of the lung parenchyma are listed in Table 11.

Consolidation

Consolidation refers to inflammatory solidification of the lung. Alveolar air is replaced by fluid and inflammatory

TABLE 11 ■ Differential Diagnosis of Lung Parenchymal Abnormalities

Common
- Consolidation
- Atelectasis
- Lung mass:
  - Primary lung tumor
  - Metastasis
  - Infection
- Lung abscess

Rare
- Arteriovenous malformation
- Pulmonary sequestration

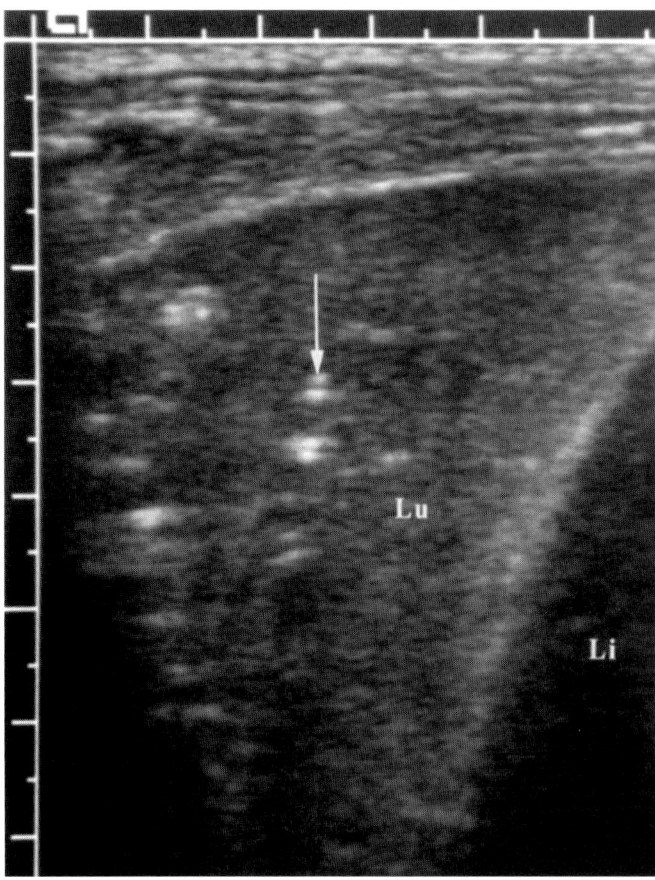

FIGURE 23 ■ Consolidation. Dense right middle lobe consolidation produces a solid tissue appearance to the lung (Lu), which is more echogenic than the liver (Li). Sonographic fluid bronchograms are evident (*arrow*).

cells. This process forms a firm, dense mass of lung tissue that transmits sound well (Fig. 23). The sonographic signs of lung consolidation are listed in Table 12. The consolidated lung becomes homogeneously hypoechoic due to increased fluid content. The diseased lung is wedge shaped and sharply defined peripherally by the visceral pleura. Centrally, consolidation tends to have irregular margins, whereas lung masses tend to have smooth margins. Islands of air-filled alveoli surrounded by consolidated lung produce globular echogenic foci called "sonographic air alveolograms." "Sonographic air bronchograms" and "sonographic fluid bronchograms" refer

TABLE 12 ■ Sonographic Signs of Pulmonary Consolidation

- Homogeneous hypoechoic lung
- Wedge shape
- Well defined peripherally by visceral pleura
- Ill defined centrally
- Sonographic air bronchograms
- Sonographic fluid bronchograms
- Sonographic air alveolograms
- Appropriate motion with respiration

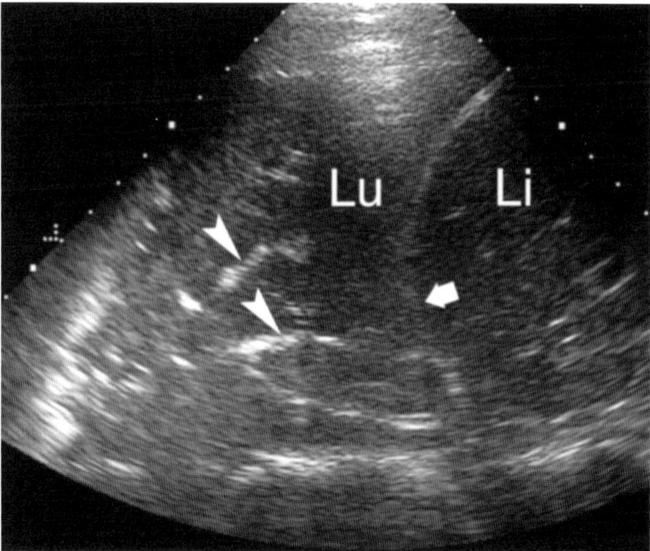

FIGURE 24 ■ Sonographic air bronchograms. Sonographic air bronchograms (*arrowheads*) appear as bright linear echoes within consolidated lung (Lu) in this patient with right lower lobe pneumonia. The liver (Li) is seen beneath the diaphragm (*arrow*).

to the US appearance of air or fluid within bronchi, which are surrounded by consolidated alveoli (Fig. 24). Fluid-filled bronchi appear as tubular structures with bright walls and anechoic interiors. Air-filled bronchi appear as strongly echogenic, nonpulsatile, branching linear structures converging toward the hilum through hypoechoic lung. Ring-down artifact and acoustic shadowing from the air collections are sometimes observed. Appropriate motion of the diseased tissue with respiration confirms lung origin. Multiple comet-tail artifacts seen over the surface of the lung are evidence of underlying diffuse parenchymal disease that remains mostly aerated (26,27).

Atelectasis

Atelectasis refers to an airless state of the lungs with collapse of alveoli in all, or a portion, of the lung. Atelectasis may be caused by obstruction of the bronchi or by compression of the alveoli by surrounding fluid or adjacent mass. Most large pleural effusions are accompanied by reflexive atelectasis of the lung within the fluid. Sonographic signs of atelectasis (Table 13) include visualization of a wedge-shaped mass of lung tissue (Fig. 25) sharply defined by its

TABLE 13 ■ Sonographic Signs of Pulmonary Atelectasis

- Wedge-shaped echogenic lung tissue
- Volume loss
- Crowding of fluid filled bronchi/vessels
- Sonographic fluid bronchograms
- No sonographic air bronchograms
- Appropriate motion with respiration

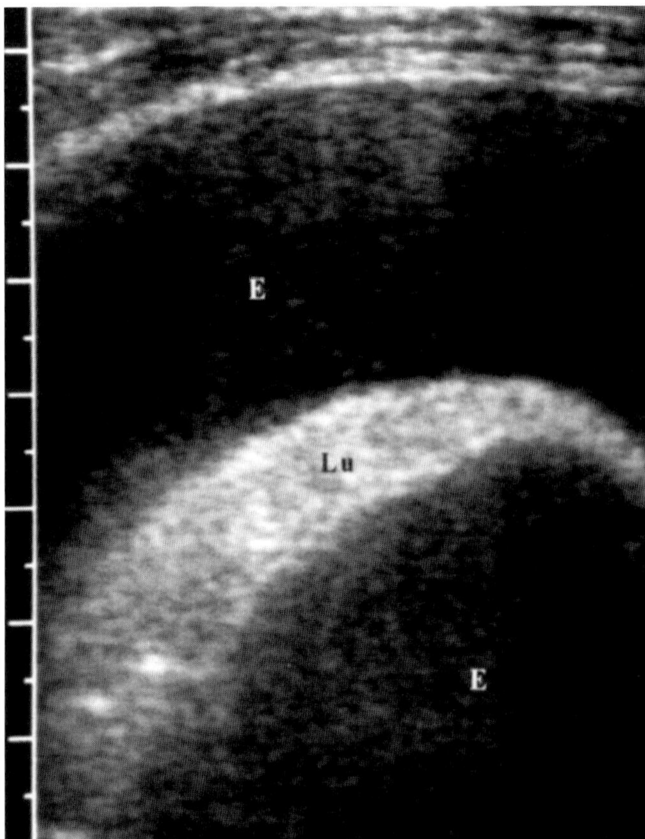

FIGURE 25 ■ Atelectasis. A tongue of collapsed lung (Lu) is suspended in a pleural effusion (E) and moves with respiration. The lung is echogenic and is sharply defined by its visceral pleura. Reflexive atelectasis accompanies all pleural effusions.

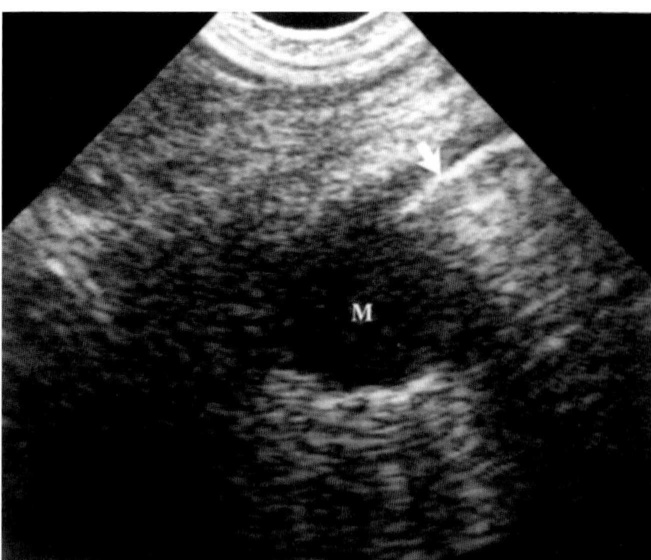

FIGURE 26 ■ Lung mass (M). A peripheral lung mass is localized by US for guided percutaneous biopsy. The mass is surrounded by echogenic, air-filled lung. Note the disappearance of the strong lung-surface echo (*arrow*) over the mass. No sonographic fluid or air bronchograms are seen within the mass favoring tumor over inflammation.

visceral pleura. Reduction of lung volume with crowding of visualized bronchi and pulmonary vessels is an essential feature of atelectasis. Sonographic air bronchograms are usually not evident. A tongue of atelectatic lung is commonly seen moving with respiration within pleural effusions.

Solid Lung Mass

Only lung masses that abut the pleura, or are surrounded by consolidated lung, can be visualized by US (Table 14). Lesions that abut the pleura are seen as hypoechoic masses (Figs. 26 and 27) surrounded by highly reflective air-filled lung. The strong lung surface echo, seen with normal lung, is absent over the aspect of the mass nearest the US transducer. The deeper aspect of the mass is relatively well defined compared to the irregular deep margin seen with consolidation. Sonographic air bronchograms are usually not seen in pulmonary tumors. The exception being bronchoalveolar carcinoma, which may masquerade clinically and radiographically as pneumonia. The lack of tapered edges helps to differentiate parenchymal masses from pleural masses. Central lung tumors near the hilum may be visualized when they are surrounded by consolidated lung (28). Tumors are usually hyperechoic compared to surrounding hypoechoic consolidation. Calcifications within a lung mass are seen on US as hyperechoic foci with acoustic shadowing. US identification of multiple pleural-based lung nodules suggests metastatic disease. Parenchymal nodules from infectious processes may also be considered within the differential diagnosis. Doppler identifies blood flow within pulmonary masses (29).

TABLE 14 ■ Sonographic Signs of Pulmonary Tumor

- Homogeneous hypoechoic mass within echogenic aerated lung
- Absent lung surface reflection echo
- Relatively well-defined deep margin
- Absence of tapered edges
- Absence of sonographic air bronchograms
- Homogeneous hyperechoic mass within hypoechoic consolidated lung

Lung Abscess

A lung abscess is an area of pulmonary necrosis, usually with cavitation. Lung abscesses may result from necrotizing pneumonia, aspiration, septic emboli, cavitated tuberculosis, pulmonary infarctions, or from necrotic cancers, infected lung cysts, or pulmonary sequestrations. Most lung abscesses abut the pleura and can be visualized by US (Fig. 28). The walls of the abscess form an irregular, thick hyperechoic ring that surrounds a central cavity, which may contain echogenic fluid and debris, air bubbles, air pockets, or air-fluid levels. Air within the cavity may produce reverberation or comet-tail artifacts and acoustic shadowing. Lung abscess is differentiated from

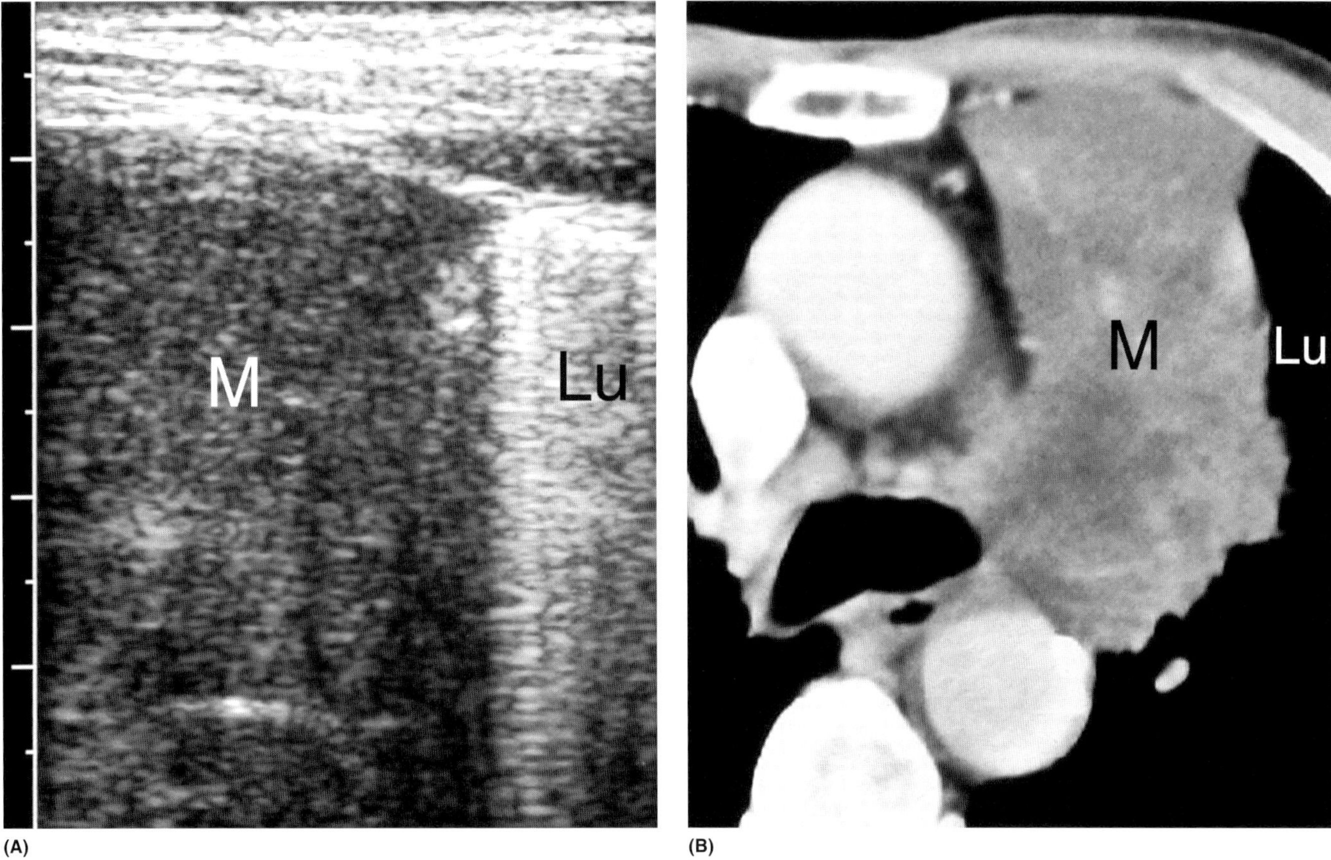

FIGURE 27 A AND B ■ Lung carcinoma. (**A**) US provides effective guidance for biopsy of a large lung mass (M) extending to the pleural surface. Avoidance of air-filled lung (Lu) is easy with US guidance. (**B**) Corresponding CT image showing the lung mass and adjacent air-filled lung. Biopsy provided a diagnosis of squamous-cell carcinoma.

empyema by real-time observation of wall motion (30). The entire circumference of the lung abscess walls will expand with inspiration, while only the wall adjacent to the lung (visceral pleura) shows slight movement with inspiration with empyema. Antibiotics and bronchoscopically aided drainage are the treatments of first choice. If noncurative, then lung resection or catheter drainage are the next options. US-guided percutaneous catheter drainage has been highly successful.

Pulmonary Arteriovenous Malformation

Most pulmonary vascular malformations are adjacent to the visceral pleura allowing noninvasive confirmation by US. Arteriovenous malformations are anomalous, direct connections between pulmonary arteries and pulmonary veins. Spectral and color-flow Doppler shows turbulent blood flow in the anomalous vessels. Flow velocities are high in diastole, reflecting low vascular resistance. Pulsations are usually not evident by real-time US, so Doppler evaluation is essential.

Pulmonary Sequestration

Pulmonary sequestrations are volumes of lung parenchyma that do not communicate with the tracheobronchial tree (31). Most are found at the lung bases. "Intralobar sequestrations" are contained within visceral pleura and have venous drainage via pulmonary veins. "Extralobar sequestrations" are contained within their own pleura and have venous drainage via systemic veins. All pulmonary sequestrations receive systemic blood supply. The goal of US diagnosis is to demonstrate the anomalous systemic arterial supply arising from the thoracic or abdominal aorta (Table 15). Color Doppler has proven effective in identifying the tortuous feeding vessel (32).

US-Guided Biopsy

Percutaneous biopsy of lung nodules is often performed under fluoroscopic or CT guidance. However, fluoroscopic visualization of lung nodules may be difficult when the nodules are at the lung apex, near the mediastinum or diaphragm, in the axilla, or are pleural based. US visualization is, by comparison, best in the very areas where fluoroscopic visualization is worst. Biopsy of peripheral nodules and masses by US guidance (Fig. 27) is usually quicker and safer than by CT guidance (33,34). Virtually any lung mass that can be visualized with US can be biopsied using US for guidance (35).

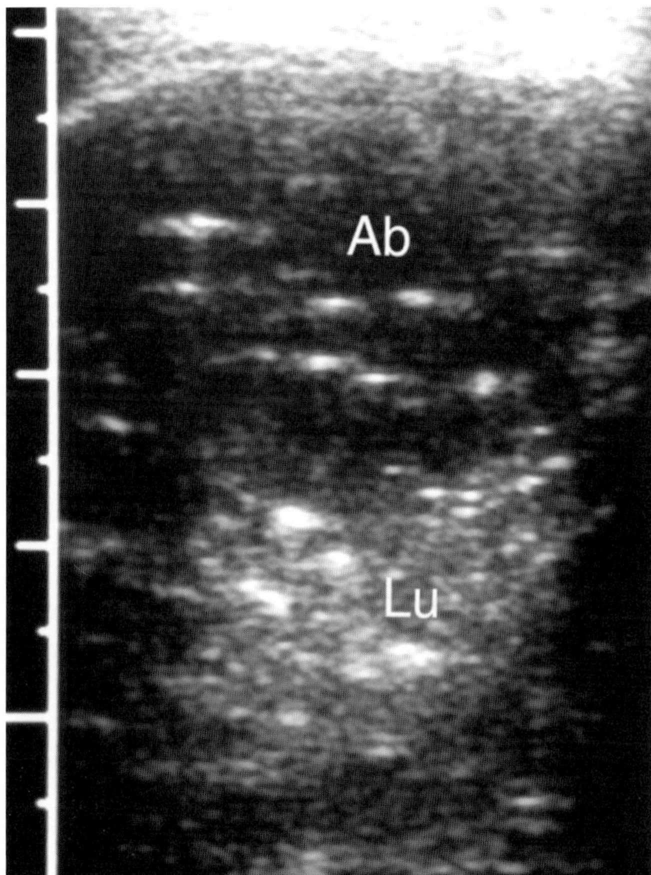

FIGURE 28 ■ Lung abscess (ab). Intercostal sonogram shows a lung abscess as a poorly marginated, markedly hypoechoic mass containing numerous bright air bubbles. The deep border of the abscess with consolidated lung (Lu) is ill defined. An empyema would have a well-marginated deep border with the visceral pleura covering the lung.

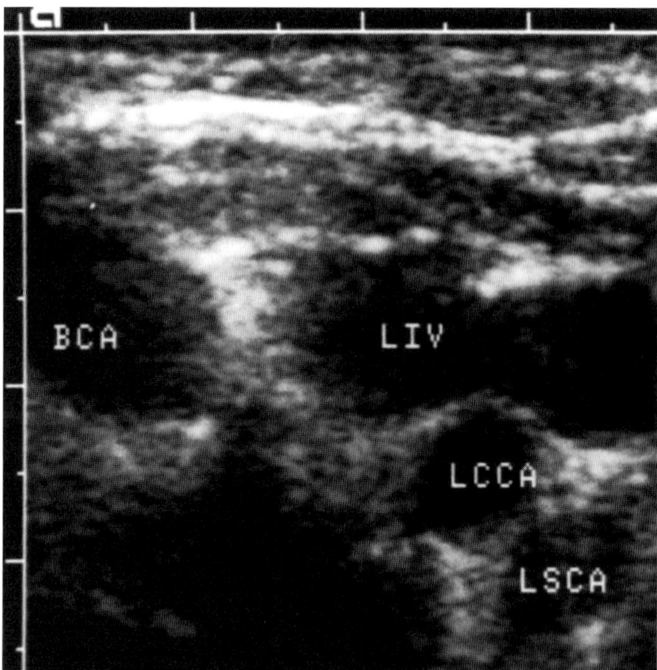

FIGURE 29 ■ Mediastinum—suprasternal approach. Image of the superior mediastinal vessels is obtained by angling the transducer transverse and downward into the mediastinum behind the sternum. Vessels are identified by location, pulsation, and Doppler characteristics. BCA, brachiocephalic artery; LIV, left innominate vein; LCCA, left common carotid artery; LSCA, left subclavian artery.

MEDIASTINUM

Normal Anatomy

The anterior and superior mediastinum are effectively evaluated by US. US is nearly equal to CT in characterizing lesions in the prevascular, pericardial, and supra-aortic regions. The paravertebral and retrotracheal regions are, however, poorly visualized by US, and CT or magnetic resonance (MR) are the imaging methods of choice for the posterior mediastinum. Doppler is used to identify and characterize vascular lesions and normal vascular structures.

TABLE 15 ■ Sonographic Signs of Pulmonary Sequestration

- Solid-appearing airless lung (fluid-filled cysts occasionally present)
- Conformation to shape of costophrenic angle
- No bronchi identified
- Feeding anomalous artery arising from aorta

The suprasternal approach is used to examine the upper mediastinum (Fig. 29). Patients are examined in supine position with a pillow placed beneath the shoulders and the neck extended. The transducer is placed just above the manubrium and is angled caudally to produce images in oblique sagittal and oblique coronal planes. The innominate and jugular veins, and the common carotid, brachiocephalic, and subclavian arteries are identified by their position and Doppler characteristics. Tortuous vessels, which cause widening of the upper mediastinum on chest radiographs, can easily be recognized. Substernal extension of goiter is readily documented. Mass lesions of the anterior mediastinum are characterized by location and by sonographic appearance as cystic, solid, vascular, or calcified (Tables 16–18).

The parasternal approach is used to examine the pericardial, precarinal, and subcarinal regions. Parasternal scanning is aided by placing the patient in lateral decubitus position, allowing gravity to enlarge the sonographic window by downward shift of the mediastinum. Large masses displace lung, creating their own sonographic windows for intercostal scanning. In children, the thymus provides an excellent sonographic window (Fig. 30).

Thymus

The normal thymus is a prominent sonographic landmark of the upper mediastinum in children up to the age of eight years (32). The thymus consists of two sharply

TABLE 16 ■ Sonographic Differentiation of Mediastinal Masses

Inflammatory adenopathy	Usually hypoechoic acutely; calcified if chronic
Malignant adenopathy	Hypoechoic, single or multiple; may calcify following therapy
Thymoma	Hypoechoic, sharply defined
Thymic lymphoma	Solid, variable echotexture; cyst formation common
Teratoma	Cystic or solid mass; calcification in 30%
Thyroid	Variable appearance; thyroid traced from the neck
Vascular mass	Color Doppler used to characterize
Cysts	Smooth walls, hypoechoic; may have layering echogenic debris

defined lobes that are triangular, or inverted teardrop, in shape with average dimensions of 1.4 cm anteroposterior and 2.5 to 2.9 cm in length. The parenchymal echogenicity is smooth and uniform, slightly less echogenic than the thyroid, and nearly equal in echogenicity to the liver. The normal gland is closely applied to the mediastinal vessels and may be seen to encircle the left innominate vein. In infants under two years, the normal thymus may extend from the upper portion of the heart to the lower cervical region. In children aged two to eight years, the thymus remains easily visualized by US, although it is less prominently seen on chest radiographs. Normal fatty replacement of the thymus in older children and adults makes the thymus isoechoic with mediastinum fat and not distinctly visible by US. A sonographically visible thymus in an adult suggests neoplastic infiltration.

Pathological Conditions

Lymphadenopathy

Normal mediastinal lymph nodes are not demonstrated sonographically. Every mediastinal lymph node seen by US (Fig. 31) should be considered to be abnormal due to a neoplastic or inflammatory process (36). Inflammatory lymph nodes, such as due to sarcoidosis or tuberculosis, are hypoechoic and become more echogenic with successful therapy (37). Calcified lymph nodes, usually the result of granulomatous disease, are highly echogenic and may cast acoustic shadows depending upon the extent of calcification. Small (<2 cm) neoplastic lymph nodes are hypoechoic, whereas larger neoplastic lymph nodes may be complex and septated due to necrosis. Lymphoma characteristically causes homogeneous hypoechoic lymph

TABLE 17 ■ Causes of Solid Anterior Mediastinal Masses

Thymic masses	*Thyroid masses*
■ Thymoma	■ Goiter
■ Thymolipoma	■ Adenoma
■ Thymic hyperplasia	■ Carcinoma
■ Thymic carcinoma	■ Adenomatous hyperplasia
■ Thymic lymphoma	■ Thyroiditis
Lymphadenopathy	*Ectopic parathyroid*
■ Lymphoma	■ Hyperplasia
■ Metastases	■ Adenoma
Germ-cell tumors	■ Carcinoma
■ Teratoma	
■ Seminoma	
■ Embryonal-cell carcinoma	
■ Choriocarcinoma	

TABLE 18 ■ Causes of Cystic Mediastinal Masses

Thymic masses
- Thymoma (cystic degeneration)
- Thymic cyst
- Thymic lymphoma (cystic degeneration)

Germ-cell tumors
- Dermoid cyst

Thyroid masses (cystic degeneration)
- Adenoma
- Carcinoma
- Adenomatous hyperplasia

Bronchogenic cysts

Pericardial cysts

Vascular masses
- Tortuous brachiocephalic artery
- Aortic aneurysm
- Double arch or right arch
- Enlarged pulmonary artery
- Dilated mediastinal veins

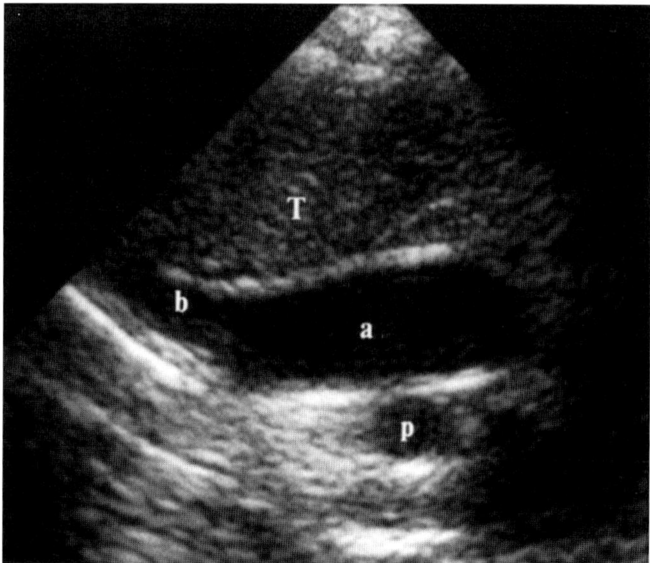

FIGURE 30 ■ Mediastinum—right parasternal approach. Longitudinal, right intercostal, parasternal image of the mediastinum in a child reveals normal thymus (T) and major vessels. a, ascending aorta; p, right pulmonary artery; b, brachiocephalic artery.

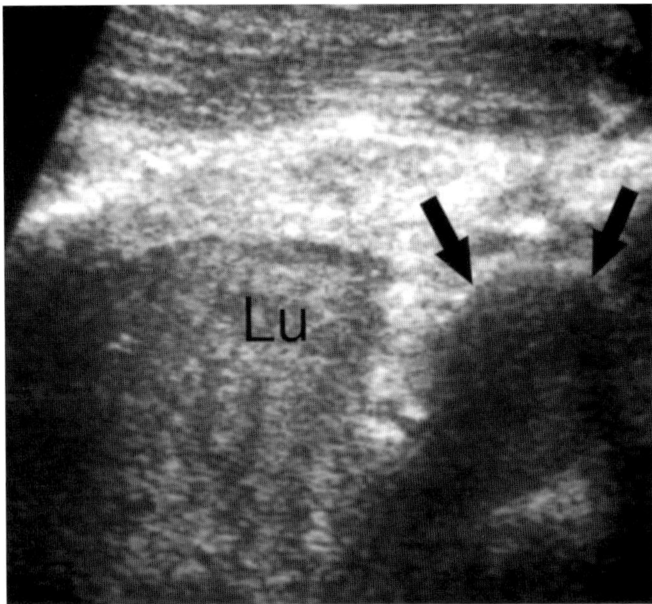

FIGURE 31 ■ Mediastinal adenopathy. Traverse right intercostal scan reveals an enlarged mediastinal lymph node (*arrows*). US visualization of the mediastinum is aided by consolidation of the right upper lobe of the lung (Lu) caused by a tumor occluding the right upper lobe bronchus. US-guided biopsy of the enlarged lymph node confirmed metastatic disease to the mediastinum.

node enlargement with coalescence of individual nodes into a larger mass (Fig. 32) (36). With successful treatment, the lymphomatous nodes shrink and become more echogenic.

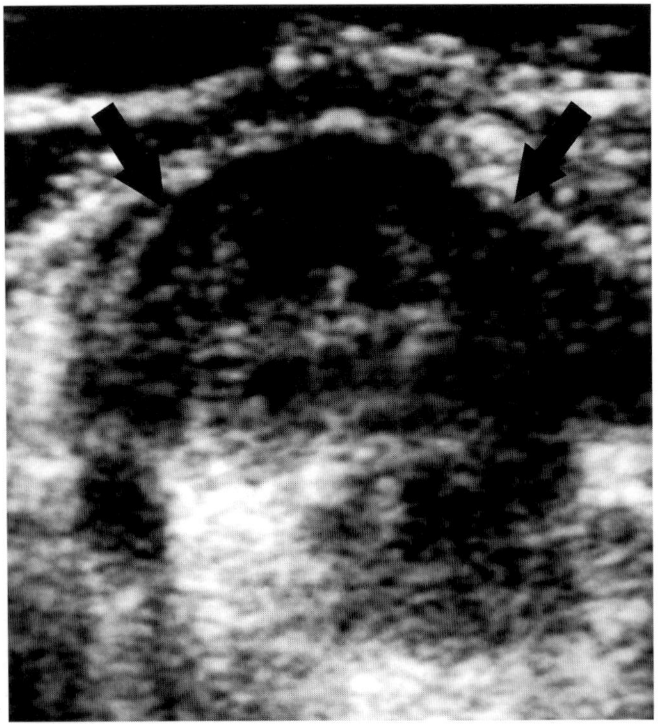

FIGURE 32 ■ Mediastinal lymphoma. Transverse image of the superior mediastinum from a suprasternal approach demonstrates a heterogeneous solid mass (*arrows*). US-guided percutaneous biopsy revealed non-Hodgkin's lymphoma.

Thymoma

Thymomas appear as round, oval, or lobulated, sharply defined, hypoechoic masses (36). Cystic components are rarely evident sonographically (38).

Thymic Lymphoma

Thymic involvement with lymphoma is suggested by thymic enlargement in an adult with lymphoma. The thymus appears as a nodular mass that may be hyperechoic, isoechoic, or hypoechoic. Cyst formation is common and typical. Adenopathy is usually seen elsewhere in the mediastinum.

Teratoma/Germ-Cell Tumors

Dermoid cysts (benign cystic teratomas) appear as well-defined cystic lesions with contents that are anechoic when serous or hyperechoic when containing fat, sebum, or hair (39). Echogenic floating spherule within a cystic mass is a characteristic finding of mature benign cystic teratoma (40). Calcification or bone formation is evident in one-third to one-half of cases. Benign solid teratomas are inhomogeneous solid masses with small cysts (38). Malignant teratomas tend to be large heterogeneous masses with poorly defined cystic areas of hemorrhage and necrosis.

Thyroid

Thyroid tissue extension into the mediastinum is easily demonstrated by US to be contiguous with thyroid tissue in the neck. Adenomatous goiter is characterized by multiple nodules, calcifications, and cystic degeneration.

Bronchogenic Cysts

Bronchogenic cysts are characteristically located near the carina or along the right wall of the trachea. Internal fluid is usually anechoic (32).

Pericardial Cysts

Cysts may arise from any portion of the pericardium (38). Most have anechoic fluid contents, but some have echogenic fluid due to hemorrhage.

Vascular Masses

Doppler is essential for the accurate characterization of mediastinal masses of vascular origin. A brachiocephalic artery made tortuous by atherosclerotic disease is a common cause of right upper mediastinal mass on chest X-ray. Mediastinal veins may be enlarged by venous obstruction or fluid overload. Aneurysm of the ascending aorta is confirmed by right parasternal scanning. Aneurysm or dissection involving the aortic arch is demonstrated by suprasternal or left parasternal US.

US-Guided Biopsy

US is the imaging method of choice for guidance of biopsy procedures for masses of the anterior mediastinum (41). Color-flow and spectral Doppler is used to exclude masses of vascular origin and to identify normal vascular structures to assure their avoidance (42). The primary indication for biopsy is to differentiate lymphoma from tumors that will require surgical excision. Core biopsy to obtain specimens for histological evaluation can be safely performed by sonographic identification of vascular structures and real-time guidance of cutting needles (43).

REFERENCES

1. Brant WE. Chest ultrasound. In: Brant WE, ed. The Core Curriculum - Ultrasound. Philadelphia: Lippincott Williams & Wilkins, 2001: 433–456.
2. Brant WE. The Thorax. In: Rumack CM, Wilson SR, Charboneau JW, eds. Diagnostic Ultrasound. St. Louis: Mosby, 2004:603–623.
3. Yuan A, Yang PC, Chang YC, et al. Value of chest sonography in the diagnosis and management of acute chest disease. J Clin Ultrasound 2001; 29:78–86.
4. Kim HH, Shin YR, Kim KJ, Hwang SS, et al. Blunt traumatic rupture of the diaphragm: sonographic diagnosis. J Ultrasound Med 1997; 16:593–598.
5. Tarver RD. The diaphragm: disorders. Radiologist 1994; 1:317–333.
6. Yeh H-C, Halton KP, Gray CE. Anatomic variations and abnormalities seen with US. Radiographics 1990; 10:1019–1030.
7. Gerscovich EO, Cronan M, McGahan JP, Jain K, Jones CD, McDonald C. Ultrasonic evaluation of diaphragmatic motion. J Ultrasound Med 2001; 20:597–604.
8. Kantarci F, Mihmanli I, Demirel MK, Harmanci K, et al. Normal diaphragmatic motion and the effects of body composition - determination with M-mode sonography. J Ultrasound Med 2004; 23:255–260.
9. Toledo NSG, Kodaira SK, Massarollo PCB, Pereira OI, Mies S. Right hemidiaphramatic mobility: assessment with US measurement of craniocaudad displacement of the left branches of the portal vein. Radiology 2003; 228:389–394.
10. Wernecke K. Sonographic features of pleural disease. AJR 1997; 168:1061–1066.
11. Kocijancic I, Vidmay K, Ivanovi-Herceg Z. Chest sonography versus lateral decubitus radiography in the diagnosis of small pleural effusions. J Clin Ultrasound 2003; 31:69–74.
12. Eibenberger KL, Dock WI, Ammann ME, et al. Quantification of pleural effusions: sonography versus radiography. Radiology 1994; 191:681–684.
13. Yang PC, Luh KT, Chang DB, et al. Value of sonography in determining the nature of pleural effusion: analysis of 320 cases. AJR Am J Roentgenol 1992; 159:29–33.
14. Wu RG, Yang PC, Kuo SH, Luh KT. Fluid color sign: a useful indicator for discrimination between pleural thickening and pleural effusion. J Ultrasound Med 1995; 14:767–769.
15. Chen KY, Liaw YS, Wang HC, et al. Sonographic septation: a useful prognostic indicator of acute thoracic empyema. J Ultrasound Med 2000; 19:837–843.
16. Morgan RA, Pickworth FE, Dubbins PA, McGavin CR. The ultrasound appearance of asbestos-related pleural plaques. Clin Radiol 1991; 44:413–416.
17. Rosado-de-Christenson ML, Abbott GF, McAdams HP, Franks TJ, Galvin JR. Localized fibrous tumors of the pleura. Radiographics 2003; 23:759–783.
18. Ferretti GR, Chiles C, Choplin RH, Coulomb M. Localized benign fibrous tumors of the pleura. AJR Am J Roentgenol 1997; 169:683–686.
19. Matthay RA, Coppage L, Shaw C, Filderman AE. Malignancies metastatic to the pleura. Invest Radiol 1990; 25:601–619.
20. Goerg C, Schwerk WB, Goerg K, Walters E. Pleural effusion: an "acoustic window" for sonography of pleural metastases. J Clin Ultrasound 1991; 19:93–97.
21. Miller BH, Rosado-de-Christenson ML, Mason AC, et al. Malignant pleural mesothelioma: radiologic-pathologic correlation. Radiographics 1996; 16:613–644.
22. Heilo A, Stenwig AE, Solheim OP. Malignant pleural mesothelioma: US-guided histologic core-needle biopsy. Radiology 1999; 211:657–659.
23. Targetta R, Bourgeois JM, Balmes P. Echography of pneumothorax. Rev Mal Respir 1990; 7:575–579.
24. Dulchavsky SA, Hamilton DR, Diebel LN, et al. Thoracic ultrasound diagnosis of pneumothorax. J Trauma 1999; 47:970–971.
25. Hsu W-H, Chiang C-D, Hsu J-Y, Chen ea, C-Y. Value of ultrasonically guided needle biopsy of pleural masses: an under-utilized technique. J Clin Ultrasound 1997; 25:119–125.
26. ReiBig A, Kroegel C. Transthoracic sonography of diffuse parenchymal lung disease - the role of comet tail artifacts. J Ultrasound Med 2003; 22:173–180.
27. Lim JH, Lee KS, Kim TS, Chung MP. Ring-down artifacts posterior to the right hemidiaphragm on abdominal sonography: sign of pulmonary parenchymal abnormalities. J Ultrasound Med 1999; 18:403–410.
28. Yang PC, Luh KT, Wu HD, et al. Lung tumors associated with obstructive pneumonitis: US studies. Radiology 1990; 174: 717–720.
29. Gorg C, Seifart U, Gorg K, Zugmaier G. Color Doppler sonographic mapping of pulmonary lesions - evidence of dual arterial supply by spectral analysis. J Ultrasound Med 2003; 22:1033–1039.
30. Yang PC, Luh KT, Lee YC, et al. Lung abscesses: US examination and US-guided transthoracic aspiration. Radiology 1991; 180: 171–175.
31. Ko SF, Ng SH, Lee TY, et al. Noninvasive imaging of bronchopulmonary sequestration. AJR Am J Roentgenol 2000; 175: 1005–1012.
32. Kim OH, Kim WS, Kim MJ, et al. US in the diagnosis of pediatric chest disease. Radiographics 2000; 20:653–671.
33. Liao W-Y, Chen M-Z, Chang Y-L, Wu HD, et al. US-guided transthoracic cutting biopsy for peripheral lesions less than 3 cm diameter. Radiology 2000; 217:685–691.
34. Sheth S, Hamper UM, Stanley DB, et al. US guidance for thoracic biopsy: a valuable alternative to CT. Radiology 1999; 210: 721–736.
35. Chen C-C, Hsu W-H, C-M H, Chen C-Y, et al. Ultrasound-guided fine-needle aspiration biopsy of solitary pulmonary nodules. J Clin Ultrasound 1995; 23:531–536.
36. Wernecke K, Diederich S. Sonographic features of mediastinal tumors. AJR Am J Roentgenol 1994; 163:1357–1364.
37. Asai S, Miyachi H, Suzuki K, Shimamura K, Ando Y. Ultrasonic differentiation between tuberculous lymphadenitis and malignant lymph nodes. J Ultrasound Med 2001; 20:533–538.
38. Jeung M-Y, Gasser B, Gangi A, Bogorin A, et al. Imaging of cystic masses of the mediastinum. Radiographics 2002; 22:S79–S93.
39. Wu T-T, Wang H-C, Chang Y-C, Lee Y-C, et al. Mature mediastinal teratoma - sonographic imaging patterns and pathologic correlation. J Ultrasound Med 2002; 21:759–765.
40. Shih J-Y, Wang H-C, Chang Y-L, Chang Y-C, et al. Echogenic floating spherules as a sonographic sign of cystic teratoma of the mediastinum. J Ultrasound Med 1996; 15:603–605.
41. Gupta S, Gulati M, Rajwanshi A, Gupta D, Suri S. Sonographically guided fine-needle aspiration biopsy of superior mediastinal lesions by the suprasternal route. AJR Am J Roentgenol 1998; 171:1303–1306.
42. Gorguner M, Misirlioglu F, Polat P, Kaynar H, et al. Color Doppler sonographically guided transthoracic needle aspiration of lung and mediastinal masses. J Ultrasound Med 2003; 22:703–708.
43. Rubens DJ, Strang JG, Fultz PJ, Gottlieb RH. Sonographic guidance of mediastinal biopsy: an effective alternative to CT guidance. AJR Am J Roentgenol 1997; 169:1605–1610.

Thyroid, Parathyroid, and Other Glands

Mary C. Frates

11

INTRODUCTION

High-frequency ultrasonography is now established as the optimal imaging modality for both screening and diagnostic evaluation of the thyroid and the parathyroid glands. Advantages of ultrasonography include its high resolution, short examination time, and low cost. Sonography is readily available, requires no patient preparation, and uses no ionizing radiation. The use of ultrasound (US) guidance for performance of interventional procedures such as fine-needle aspiration (FNA) of thyroid nodules and alcohol ablation of parathyroid adenomas has become widespread. Although other modalities such as nuclear medicine, thin-section computed tomography (CT), and magnetic resonance imaging (MRI) can provide imaging and functional information about the thyroid, none has the advantages of US. In addition to the thyroid and the parathyroid glands, lymph nodes and other neck masses can be evaluated with sonography and will be discussed in this chapter.

THYROID

Anatomy and Embryology

The thyroid gland is a butterfly-shaped structure in the lower anterior neck (Fig. 1A and B). The typically symmetrical right and left lobes are located laterally to the trachea and are joined across the midline by the isthmus, which crosses over the anterior trachea at the junction of the middle and the lower thirds of the gland. In some patients, a small midline pyramidal lobe can be identified arising from the isthmus and extending superiorly, anterior to the thyroid cartilage. The normal thyroid can vary significantly in size, but in adults, each lobe measures about 5 × 2 × 2 cm (1). Due to the wide variability of gland size, there are no definite measurements that can be used to diagnose enlargement; however, a gland greater than 5 cm in length is likely enlarged. In addition, the anterior surface of the gland is typically flat, so when an anterior bulge is seen, enlargement is likely (Fig. 2). Embryologically, the thyroid arises from the fourth pharyngeal pouch and migrates inferiorly from the base of the tongue (foramen cecum). The tract remaining between the base of the tongue and the top of the pyramidal lobe, if present, is the remnant thyroglossal duct, along which residual thyroid tissue is occasionally seen (see the section entitled Other Neck Masses). Descent beyond the normal location will result in mediastinal extension or presence of the gland.

The symmetrical strap muscles of the neck surround the thyroid gland. Anterior to the thyroid surface are the sternohyoid and the sternothyroid. Anterolaterally are the large sternocleidomastoid muscles. Immediately lateral to the thyroid is the carotid sheath, containing the common carotid artery medially and the jugular vein laterally. Posteriorly are the wedge-shaped longus colli muscles and cervical spine. In the midline, air-filled trachea is seen deep to the isthmus. The esophagus typically lies posterior to the left lobe of the thyroid, close to the spine. In the transverse plane, the esophagus can occasionally mimic a thyroid or a parathyroid lesion.

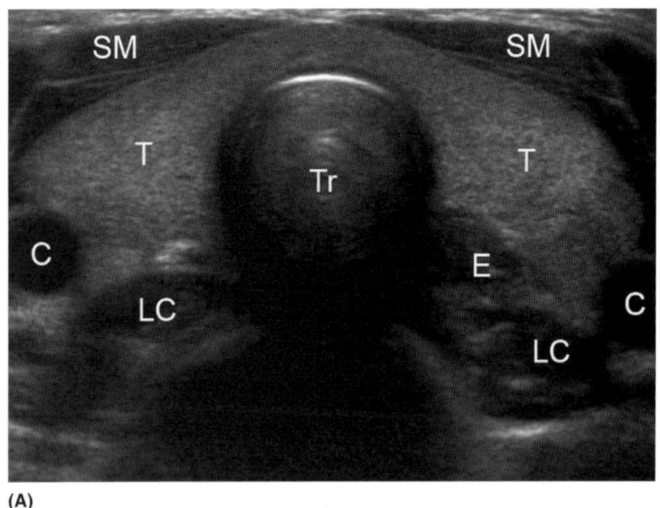

(A)

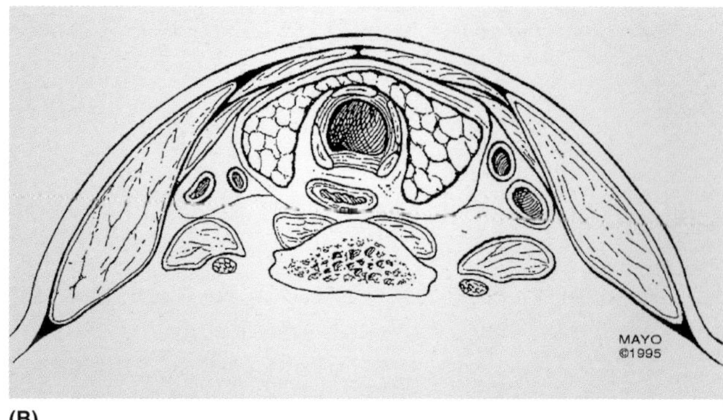

(B)

FIGURE 1 A AND B ■ Transverse image of the normal neck. (**A**) Transverse sonogram and (**B**) diagram of neck showing normal thyroid lobes (T) joined by midline isthmus. The trachea (Tr), esophagus (E), common carotid artery (C), anterior strap muscles (SM), and longus colli muscles (LC) are also visualized. *Source*: Courtesy of the Mayo Foundation.

US Technique

Sonography of the neck is performed with the patient supine and the neck in hyperextension (2). A towel or pad under the shoulders may aid in exposure of the anterior neck. High-frequency (7–15 MHz) linear transducers provide optimal spatial resolution and visualization in most patients. In obese patients with thick necks, the use of a 5 MHz transducer may be necessary to obtain adequate depth penetration. Rarely, a low-frequency (4–5 MHz) sector transducer may be necessary to fully evaluate glands that extend into a retrosternal location.

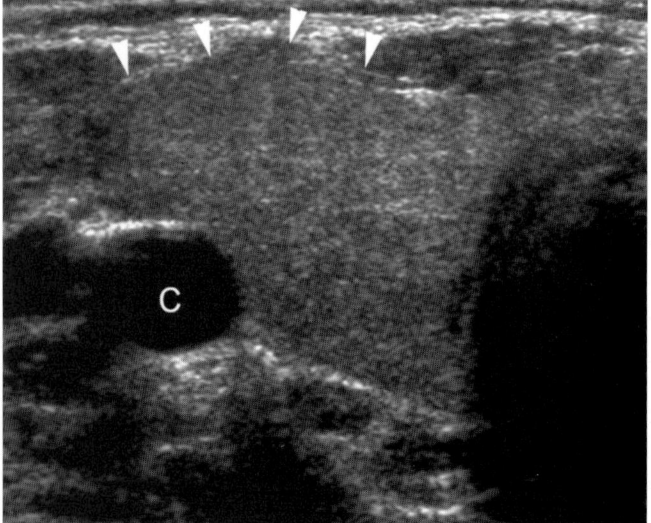

FIGURE 2 ■ Transverse image of the right lobe of the thyroid shows bulging anterior contour (*arrowheads*), confirming gland enlargement. The lobe extends over the anterior surface of the carotid artery (C).

In addition to standard sonography of the thyroid, researchers continue to search for improved methods of identifying thyroid pathology. Compound spatial sonography (3) and tissue harmonic imaging (4) each modify the standard gray-scale image and improve nodule conspicuity. These techniques have become widely used in the past several years. The value of elastography (5) and/or sonographic contrast agents (6,7) for the noninvasive differentiation of benign from malignant nodules remains unconfirmed.

Normal Thyroid and Imaging Pitfalls

The normal thyroid has a homogeneous echotexture that is more echogenic than the muscles of the neck. Small vessels may be seen, particularly in the periphery of the gland, but typically there are no other landmarks within the gland. Occasionally, an echogenic line or fold of the thyroid capsule can be identified in the right lower pole, which on transverse imaging may mimic a nodule but with longitudinal imaging correlation can be shown to be a pseudonodule (Fig. 3A and B). Color Doppler imaging of the normal thyroid demonstrates minimal background flow. Both right and left lobes should be measured in three dimensions and isthmic thickness determined. Transverse images of upper, mid and lower poles and longitudinal images of each lobe should be documented and evaluation made for focal or diffuse disease. All discrete nodules over 5 mm in diameter should be measured in three planes. The adjacent soft tissues should be examined for pathology, particularly lymphadenopathy (2,8). When imaging the thyroid, the main practical differentiation is between focal nodular and diffuse disease.

The thyroid gland may be partially or completely absent at birth. With absence of one lobe, there is compensatory hypertrophy of the remaining lobe (Fig. 4).

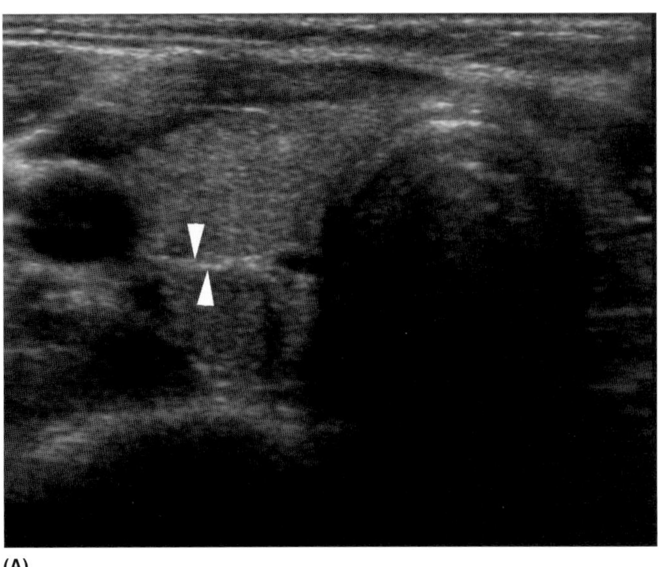
(A)

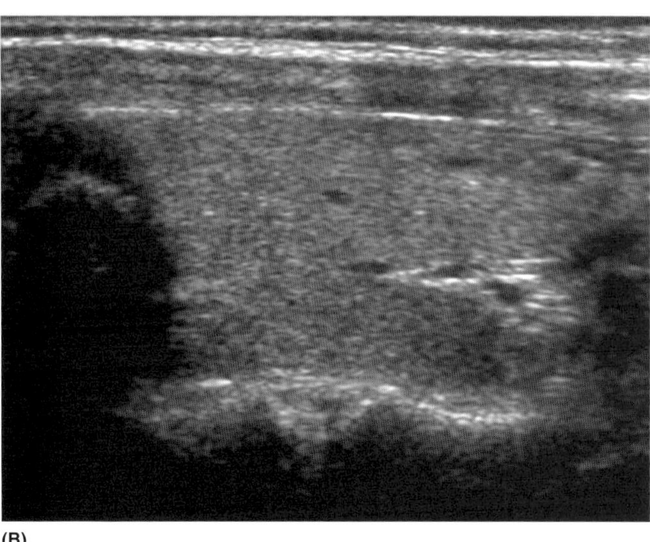
(B)

FIGURE 3 A AND B ■ Pseudonodule. (**A**) Transverse image of the right lower lobe of the thyroid shows an echogenic line (*arrowheads*), which suggests a solid isoechoic posterior nodule. (**B**) On the corresponding sagittal image of the right lobe, the echogenic line is shown to be a septation arising from the lower pole, and there is no nodule present.

In complete absence or thyroid agenesis, immediate diagnosis at birth is required to prevent the onset of cretinism. Early thyroid hormone supplementation is essential, and newborns are routinely screened for serum levels of thyroxine, thyroid-stimulating hormone (TSH), or both. Occasionally, the thyroid gland is located in an ectopic location such as a lingual gland (Fig. 5) (9,10).

Nodular Thyroid Disease

Nodular thyroid disease is extremely common. Palpable thyroid nodules are found in 4% to 7% of the adult population in the United States. Nodules are seen in up to 42% of glands at sonography (11–14), with a wide variety of sonographic appearances (Fig. 6A–C). At autopsy, up to 50% of glands demonstrate nodular disease (15). The role of US for the evaluation of thyroid nodules is proven, as sonography changed the clinical management in 63% of patients with thyroid nodular disease in one recent study (16). The majority of thyroid nodules are benign and represent hyperplastic nodules, adenomas, or colloid cysts. However, approximately 9.2% to 13.0% of thyroid nodules that undergo tissue sampling are malignant (17–21). The pathologic

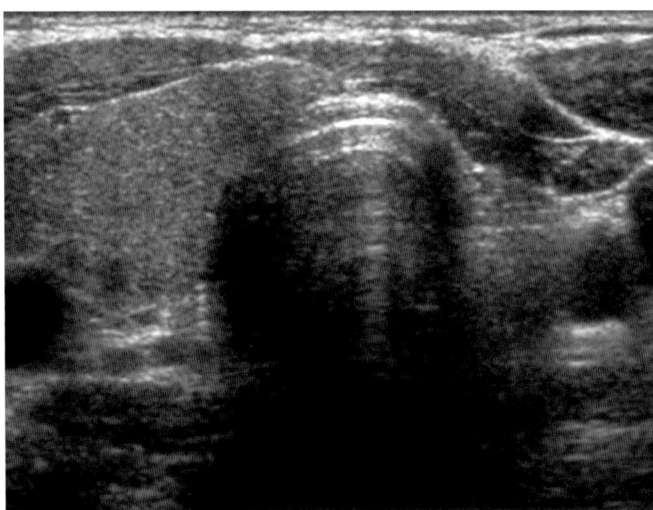
FIGURE 4 ■ Congenital absence of the left lobe, with an enlarged but otherwise normal right lobe.

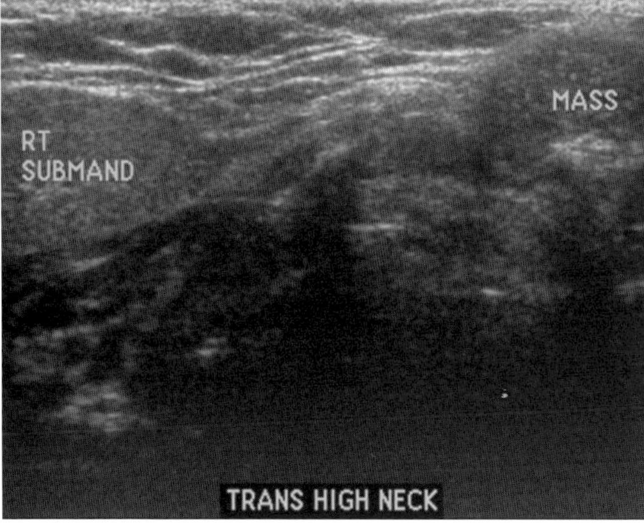

FIGURE 5 ■ Congenital absence of thyroid with high lingual thyroid. Transverse image of the upper neck at the level of the right submandibular gland. The homogeneous solid mass in the midline of the neck (*mass*) represents a lingual thyroid. There was no normal tissue in the thyroid bed.

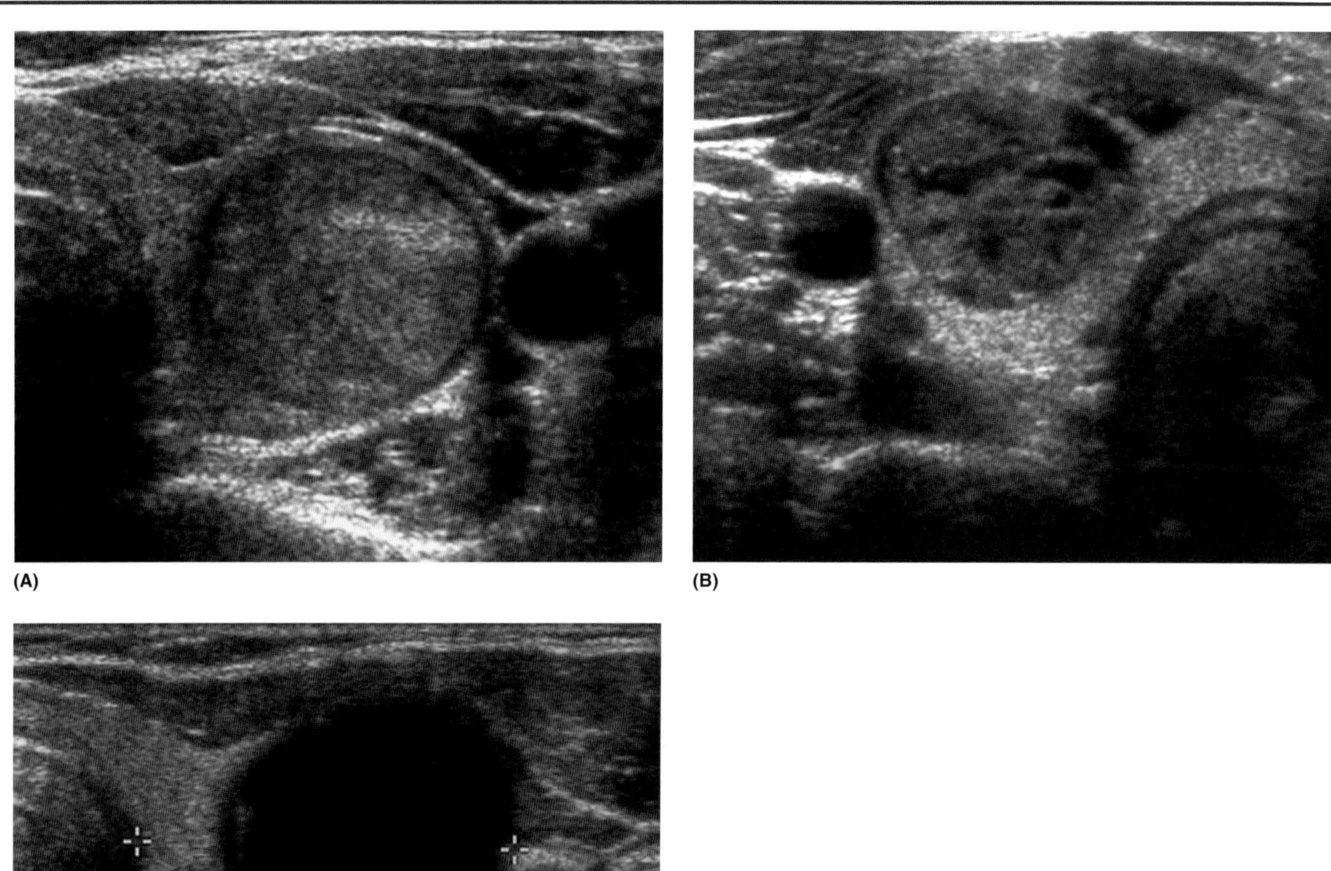

FIGURE 6 A–C ■ Variety of thyroid nodule appearances on sonography. (**A**) Transverse image of a solid mass in the left lobe of the thyroid with a well-defined hypoechoic halo at the periphery of the mass. (**B**) Transverse image of a mixed cystic and solid nodule in the right lobe of the thyroid. (**C**) Transverse image of a mostly cystic, left-sided thyroid nodule. A small amount of solid material is seen along the posterior wall of the nodule.

classification of benign and malignant thyroid nodules is shown in Table 1.

Benign Nodules

Colloid or Adenomatous Nodule ■ Many thyroid "nodules" are not true neoplasms but instead are benign growths caused by cycles of hyperplasia and involution of underlying thyroid tissue. These changes result in focal regions of colloid-filled follicles and parenchyma that form what are considered benign adenomatous or colloid nodules. As the nodule enlarges, cystic components may appear, due to hemorrhage or necrosis (22). Nodules are often multiple and usually hypofunctioning at radionuclide scanning. At cytology, benign follicular cells and colloid are found (23).

Adenomas ■ Follicular adenomas are true thyroid neoplasms (22). They are less common than colloid nodules, representing only 5% to 10% of all nodular diseases of the thyroid. An adenoma is surrounded by a fibrous capsule with a uniform histologic structure. It is a benign lesion that appears to arise from the follicular epithelium and is not believed to have malignant potential (24). However, at cytology, these lesions are indistinguishable from follicular carcinomas, because the differentiation is made by histologic criteria (wall invasion), indicating malignancy (25). Follicular adenomas must be considered surgical lesions and either removed or, rarely, ablated with alcohol injection. Although most adenomas are "cold" nodules on scintigraphy, demonstrating low radioiodine uptake and mimicking cancer, occasionally they will appear "hot" or functioning, and surgery can be avoided. Functioning adenomas that become insensitive to TSH are considered toxic and are usually treated with radioactive iodine, but they can be also treated with percutaneous injection of ethyl alcohol (ETOH) (see the section entitled Ultrasound-Guided Alcohol Ablation of Thyroid Cysts and Nodules). Similar to follicular adenomas are Hürthle-cell adenomas, benign lesions with uniform histologic structure. Hürthle cells are altered follicular cells, identified by abundant mitochondria. These adenomas are differentiated from Hürthle-cell carcinoma by evaluation of the capsule for invasion (25).

TABLE 1 ■ Pathologic Classification of Nodular Thyroid Disease

Classification	Associations
Benign	
Hyperplastic (adenomatous, colloid) nodule	The result of cycles of hyperplasia and involution of the thyroid parenchyma; no malignant potential
Adenoma (follicular or Hürthle cell)	Benign neoplasm arising from a single cell or group of cells
Cyst	Hemorrhagic cyst or adenoma or simple cyst. FNA often yields insufficient cells
Malignant	
Papillary	70–80% of all cases of thyroid cancer; multicentric; lymphatic spread; 5 yr survival rate, 95–99%
Follicular or Hürthle cell	10–20% of all cases of thyroid cancer; unifocal; hematogenous spread; 5 yr survival rate, 65%
Medullary	3–5% of all cases of thyroid cancer; unilateral (sporadic), bilateral (familial); lymphatic and hematogenous spread; 5 yr survival rate, 65%
Anaplastic	1–2% of all cases of thyroid cancer; aggressive local invasion; fatal in less than 36 mo
Other (metastases, lymphoma, etc.)	Rare, discrete or ill-defined

Abbreviation: FNA, fine-needle aspiration.

Cysts ■ Approximately 10% to 15% of thyroid nodules are cystic (21,23). These nodules may be hemorrhagic cysts, simple cysts, or hemorrhagic adenomas. A small percent may be cystic cancers. Attempts at FNA may be unsuccessful due to the inability to obtain sufficient cells.

Malignant Nodules

The four types of thyroid malignancy are papillary, follicular, medullary, and anaplastic. Although histologic tumor type is the most important prognostic factor, tumors with metastases or with mass fixation at presentation have a poorer prognosis. Stage at diagnosis particularly influences prognosis for follicular, medullary, and anaplastic cancers (26).

Papillary ■ Papillary cancer represents between 70% and 80% of the cases of thyroid cancer in the United States (26,27). Women are more commonly affected than men, at a ratio of approximately 2.5:1 (27) and most patients are between 30 and 50 years of age. The ultrasonographic appearance is variable but the nodule is often hypoechoic. Internal punctate shadowing calcifications (psammoma bodies) are a specific finding (28). The tumor is multicentric in 20% to 80% of patients (29) and these individual tumors appear to be independent (30). Papillary cancer spreads through the lymphatics, and ultrasonography can detect large or abnormal cervical nodes. Distant metastases (typically lungs) are rare (2–3% of patients) (29). Most patients with papillary thyroid cancer can be considered low risk, with a 99% survival rate at 10 years (26). Overall and disease-free survival may be improved with exogenous thyroid hormone sufficient to suppress TSH (31,32).

Follicular ■ Follicular cancer is a slow-growing type of malignancy that represents about 10% to 20% of cases of thyroid cancer (27). Because it is often isoechoic with the adjacent normal parenchyma, and often found in a multinodular gland, follicular cancer is the most difficult type to detect with ultrasonography (1). It is usually a single focus and encapsulated; however, capsular or vascular invasion seen microscopically distinguishes it from a benign follicular adenoma. The nodule may be homogeneous or may contain areas of hemorrhage, cysts, and necrosis. Hematogenous spread after vessel invasion is characteristic, both to the lungs and to the bones. Lymph-node involvement is uncommon (29). The five-year survival rate for follicular thyroid cancer is about 65%, and the prognosis is more dependent on stage at diagnosis than papillary cancer (22). Hürthle-cell neoplasm is similar to follicular neoplasm.

Medullary ■ Medullary cancer represents about 3% to 5% of cancer cases and arises from parafollicular neuroendocrine C cells (27,33). In 20% to 50% of cases, it may be part of the multiple endocrine neoplasia syndromes. Increased calcitonin levels (secreted in about 85% of medullary tumors) can help suggest the diagnosis even before imaging is performed and may be a marker of tumor recurrence postoperatively. At sonography, medullary carcinoma may present as a discrete tumor in one thyroid lobe (usually the sporadic type) or as numerous bilateral nodules (the more usual familial presentation). Focal hemorrhage or necrosis may occur. Coarsely calcified amyloid deposits and surrounding reactive fibrosis are often seen in both the primary and the metastatic tumor sites (34). Medullary cancer spreads through both lymphatic and hematogenous means to cervical nodes, liver, lungs, and bones. The five-year survival rate is about 65%.

Anaplastic ■ Anaplastic or undifferentiated carcinoma is a highly malignant fast-growing tumor that is typically found in elderly patients and makes up 1% to 2% of thyroid cancers (27). Patients may present with painful rapid enlargement of the thyroid, which can mimic thyroiditis.

(A)

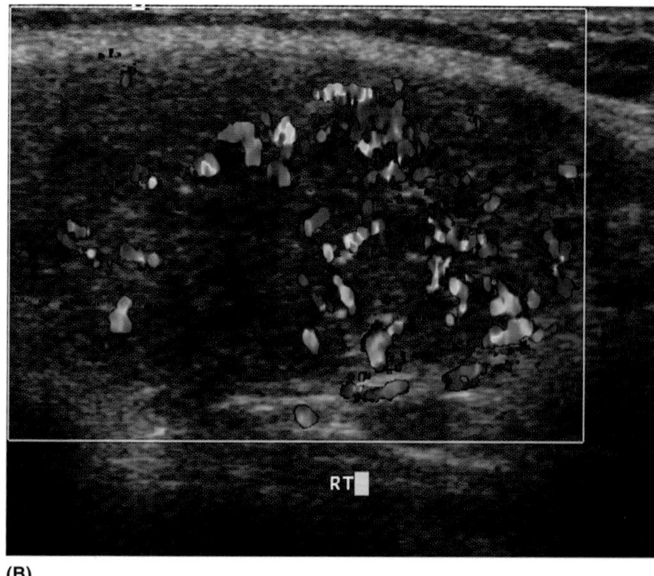

(B)

FIGURE 7 A AND B ■ Papillary cancer of the thyroid. (**A**) Sagittal image of an ill-defined, hypoechoic, solid nodule (*calipers*). (**B**) Color Doppler demonstrates prominent internal flow. This combination of characteristics increases the likelihood that a nodule may represent cancer.

Sonographically, anaplastic cancer appears as a poorly defined inhomogeneous, hypoechoic, solid mass that may invade local structures such as the jugular vein. The tumor is locally aggressive and frequently inoperable at the time of presentation. Average survival is less than one year (22).

Other ■ Thyroid lymphoma is extremely rare but may occur in the setting of chronic lymphocytic (Hashimoto's) thyroiditis (35). A dominant nodule in a patient with known Hashimoto's thyroiditis should undergo FNA. Primary sarcomas and squamous-cell carcinomas are both extremely rare. Metastases from other tumors are rarely found in the thyroid. Common primary malignancies include melanoma and renal cell, lung, and breast tumors (36,37).

Management of Thyroid Nodules

As stated above, between 9.2% and 13.0% of thyroid nodules that undergo tissue sampling are malignant (17–20). Although past teaching suggested a decreased risk of malignancy in patients with a multinodular gland (38), current research shows that a patient's overall rate of cancer in a multinodular gland is similar to the rate of a patient with a solitary nodule (19,20,39). In patients with multiple nodules, cancer is found in the largest nodule only 67% of the time, with one-third of cancers in smaller nodules (19). Clinical factors that increase the risk of thyroid cancer include age below 20 or above 60 years, history of irradiation to the neck, firmness on palpation, rapid growth, hoarseness or difficulty swallowing, or adenopathy (18,40).

Multiple studies have attempted to determine the sonographic characteristics that predict which thyroid nodule is malignant. Features that show increased risk of malignancy include a solid nature, hypoechoic echotexture, punctate or coarse calcification, and central hypervascularity (17,20,21,41–48). In particular, the combination of these findings within a single nodule is worrisome (Fig. 7A and B) (17,21,42). A hypoechoic mass with scattered hyperechoic foci may indicate the psammomatous calcifications of papillary cancer (Fig. 8) or the calcified amyloid deposits with surrounding fibrosis of medullary cancer. Direct invasion of adjacent tissues such as the jugular vein or esophagus is uncommon, but if present, it indicates a malignant lesion and raises concern in particular

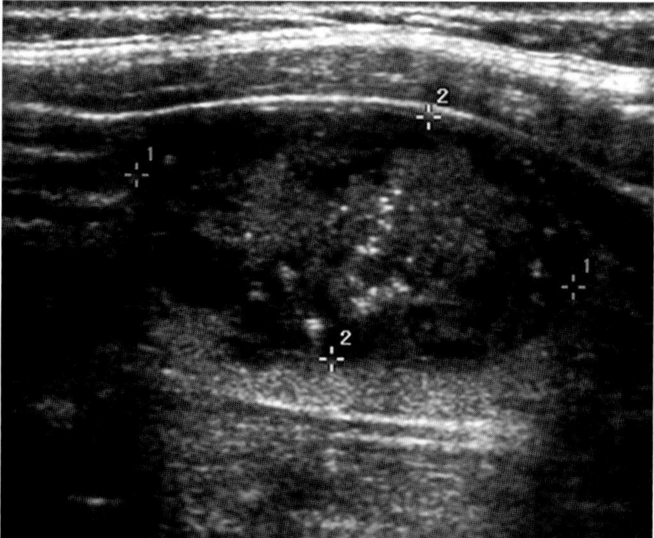

FIGURE 8 ■ Papillary cancer of the thyroid. Sagittal image shows a hypoechoic solid nodule (*calipers*) with scattered punctate calcifications. These psammomatous calcifications are highly suggestive of papillary carcinoma.

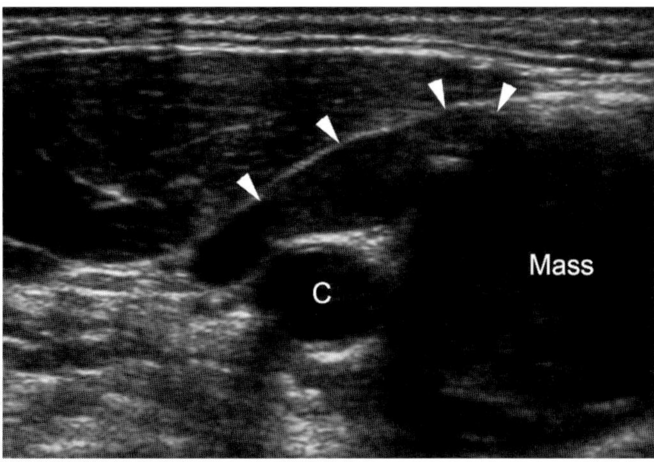

FIGURE 9 ■ Anaplastic thyroid cancer. Transverse ultrasound of the right thyroid that is replaced by a solid hypoechoic mass (*Mass*). The mass invades the jugular vein (*arrowheads*). C, carotid artery.

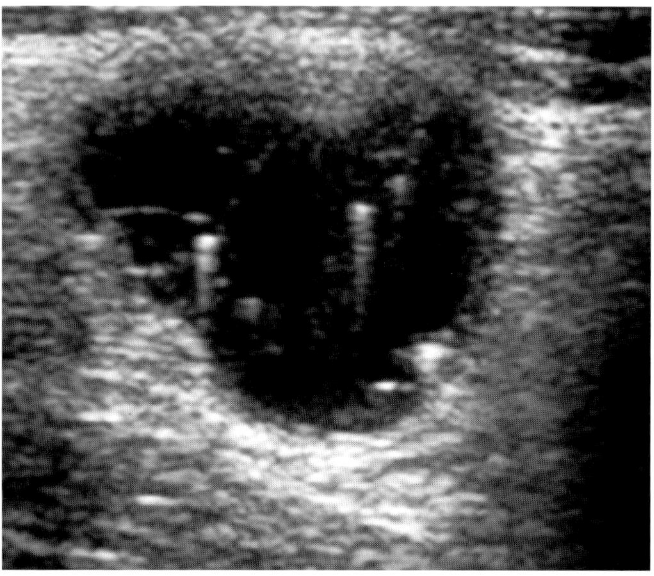

FIGURE 10 ■ Colloid crystals. Sagittal image of a mostly cystic nodule with punctate echogenicities that show posterior ring-down artifact, indicating colloid crystals and a high likelihood that the nodule is benign.

for anaplastic cancer (Fig. 9). Invasion of the trachea or the mediastinum is also uncommon and probably better imaged with CT. Thyroid gland fixation can at times be demonstrated sonographically by the lack of gland motion with swallowing or neck flexion and extension maneuvers. Adenopathy in the neck ipsilateral to the thyroid lesion, especially in the lower internal jugular (IJ) node chain, raises the suspicion of thyroid malignancy.

Conversely, nodules that are completely cystic, particularly those that contain the fine echogenicities with posterior comet-tail artifacts that correlate with colloid, have an extremely high likelihood of being benign (Fig. 10) (49). However, many benign nodules demonstrate at least one of the characteristics that have been associated with malignancy (50). Therefore, because no sonographic finding or combination of findings is absolutely predictive of malignancy, FNA with or without US guidance should be considered for most thyroid nodules (see the section entitled Biopsy and Ablation of Thyroid Lesions).

Which nodule requires FNA remains the subject of active debate. One school of thought recommends US-guided FNA of all nodules as small as 8 mm, as early diagnosis and treatment would seem to imply improved outcome. The opposing opinion is that as more FNAs are performed, the number of complications and unnecessary surgeries will increase for little benefit, due to the slow growing, nonaggressive nature of most thyroid cancers. Recently, the Society of Radiologists in Ultrasound (SRU) convened a consensus panel of experts in US, endocrinology, cytopathology, and thyroid surgery to discuss this issue (51). The panel utilized sonographic criteria to help select appropriate nodules for sampling. The recommended size cutoff is smaller for nodules with US features associated with malignancy, and larger size cutoffs are recommended for nodules with more benign features (Table 2). The lower limit in size of 10 mm reflected the concerns of the entire panel regarding the risk/benefit ratio of insufficient samples and FNA complications versus early diagnosis. The consensus panel recognized that highly suspicious nodules may require FNA at smaller sizes than 10 mm, and that for other patients, the need to obtain a tissue diagnosis might be less important. The statement produced by this group offers one means of approaching the decision regarding which nodule to sample.

Nodules that are identified incidentally with other imaging modalities have a similar rate of malignancy as nodules first identified at palpation and should undergo the same evaluation discussed above, regardless of whether the nodule is palpable (20,52,53).

Anywhere from 5% to 20% of thyroid nodule aspirations result in a nondiagnostic sample defined as containing a smaller number of cells than required for a benign diagnosis (54–56). Repeat FNA should be attempted in these patients, as the cancer rate at surgery in nodules with nondiagnostic results is 5% to 9% (57–59). It has been suggested that core-needle biopsy may have a role in definitive nonsurgical diagnosis for these nodules (60,61).

Some thyroid nodules that have undergone FNA with benign results at cytology undergo surgical resection for clinical symptoms such as pressure or difficulty swallowing, and some are removed for cosmetic reasons. Other nodules with indeterminate or atypical results at FNA are surgically resected as well. The remaining majority of benign nodules, when followed sonographically, appear to grow slowly over time, especially those with a solid composition (57,62,63). Rapid growth on followup may be due to interval hemorrhage, but additional evaluation with repeat FNA is likely indicated (57). Exactly how much and how quickly a benign nodule can grow has not been established. This deficiency in the thyroid nodule literature was identified by the SRU consensus panel as an important question that merits further research (51). Alternatives to surgery for either benign or malignant thyroid nodules include laser thermal ablation (64,65) and ETOH ablation (44,66–69).

TABLE 2 ■ Recommendations for Thyroid Nodules 1 cm or Larger in Maximum Diameter

Ultrasound features	Recommendation
Solitary nodule	
Microcalcifications	Strongly consider US-FNA if ≥ 1 cm
Solid (or almost entirely solid) or coarse calcifications	Strongly consider US-FNA if ≥ 1.5 cm
Mixed solid and cystic or almost entirely cystic with solid mural component	Consider US-FNA if ≥ 2 cm
None of the above but substantial growth since prior to US examination	Consider US-FNA
Almost entirely cystic and none of the above and no substantial growth (or no prior US)	US-FNA probably unnecessary
Multiple nodules	Consider US-FNA of one or more nodules with selection to be prioritized on basis of criteria (in order listed) for solitary nodule[a]

Note: FNA is likely unnecessary in diffusely enlarged gland with multiple nodules of similar US appearance without intervening parenchyma. Presence of abnormal lymph nodes overrides US features of the thyroid nodule(s) and should prompt US-FNA or biopsy of the lymph node and/or ipsilateral thyroid nodule.

[a]Panel had two opinions regarding selection of nodules for FNA. The majority opinion is stated here.

Abbreviations: FNA, fine-needle aspiration; US, ultrasound.

Source: From Ref. 51.

Postoperative Evaluation of the Neck

For patients who have undergone surgery for thyroid cancer, US in combination with serum thyroglobulin assay is the best way to evaluate for thyroid bed tumor recurrence and local metastases (70,71). Patients with all types of thyroid cancer should be followed up postoperatively, as approximately half of recurrences occur in low-risk patients (72). Ultrasonography is convenient for followup of patients who take thyroid-suppressing medications because radionuclide imaging may require that patients not take their medication for up to four weeks in preparation for the examination. Most patients with thyroid cancer undergo total or near-total thyroidectomy, frequently followed by radioactive iodine for ablation of any residual tissue or possible metastatic deposits. In these patients, the carotid and the jugular shift medially to the edge of the trachea, and there is no solid tissue seen in the thyroid bed. Rarely, a subtotal thyroidectomy is performed, and small amounts of normal thyroid tissue can be seen if ablation has not been performed.

In approximately 10% of patients, thyroid cancer may recur locally after operation or metastasize to the ipsilateral internal jugular (IJ) chain nodes (72). Recurrences and metastatic nodes generally appear as nodular masses of low echogenicity (see the section entitled Lymph Nodes). Solid, hypoechoic masses in the thyroid bed or inferior to the bed in the midline neck often represent abnormal lymph nodes, which slide into the potential space left by the absent gland and mimic local recurrence (Fig. 11). Papillary metastases may appear cystic due to central necrosis (73). US-guided FNA is commonly used to confirm suspected recurrence or local metastases. Whole-body iodine (^{131}I) scintigraphy may also be used to diagnose recurrence or metastases if tumor characteristics allow. Rarely, a hypoechoic mass in the postsurgical neck will represent granulomatous inflammation, a benign diagnosis that may be apparent at FNA (74).

Diffuse Thyroid Disease

Worldwide, the most common cause of diffuse thyroid hyperplasia with gland enlargement (goiter) is inadequate iodine ingestion, but this is unusual in the United

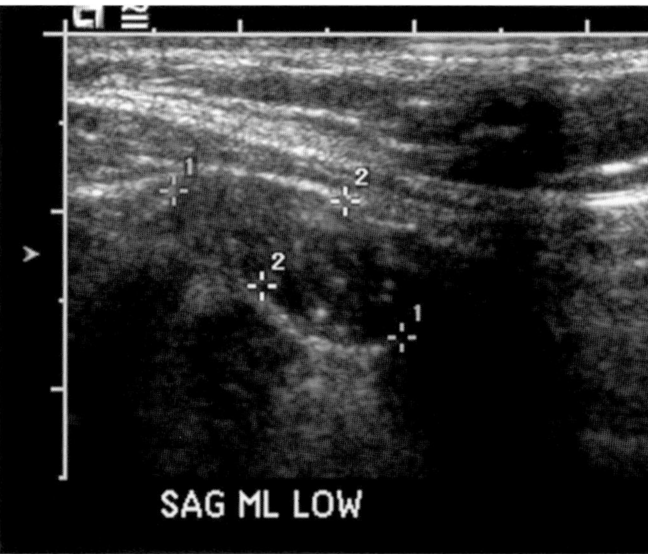

FIGURE 11 ■ Recurrent papillary cancer. Sagittal image of the midline low neck, in the region of the sternal notch. There is a hypoechoic solid mass with punctate calcifications that represented metastatic papillary cancer on pathology.

States. Here, the most commonly encountered diffuse thyroid diseases are chronic lymphocytic (Hashimoto's) thyroiditis and Graves' disease (diffuse toxic goiter); however, there are several other less common causes. Although laboratory values, clinical history, and physical examination results of these conditions are different, the US findings are relatively nonspecific. Ultrasonography is able to evaluate any possible increased volume of the thyroid gland, determine disease extent, and search for local adenopathy. Visualization of a thyroid isthmus thicker than a few millimeters suggests a diffusely enlarged gland. Ultrasonography is the most accurate method for calculating thyroid volume for the diagnosis of goiter and to determine the dose of ^{131}I-radionuclide to be administered in thyrotoxicosis. Sonography can be used to monitor disease progression and therapeutic response (8). An asymmetrically enlarged thyroid on palpation suggests a focal mass; US can help separate diffuse and focal disease.

Graves' Disease (Diffuse Toxic Goiter)

Graves' disease is an autoimmune disorder caused by antibodies against the TSH receptor sites on the thyroid follicles. The antibodies mimic TSH, thus stimulating thyroid cells to produce more thyroid hormone and resulting in thyrotoxicosis (75). It is the most frequent cause of hyperthyroidism as well as the most common autoimmune disorder in the United States, affecting primarily women between the ages of 40 and 60 years (76). On US, the thyroid affected by Graves' disease may have a normal appearance or be diffusely hypoechoic without palpable nodules (8,77). A characteristic increase in vascular flow in the thyroid during systole and diastole is present on color Doppler examination, termed the "thyroid inferno" by Ralls et al. (Fig. 12A and B) (78). Spectral Doppler examination demonstrates evidence of increased flow velocities (50–120 cm/sec) and arteriovenous shunts (1). Color and spectral Doppler have been proposed as means to both assess disease activity and predict relapse (79–81).

Thyroiditis

The various types of thyroiditis, or thyroid inflammation, include chronic lymphocytic thyroiditis, suppurative thyroiditis, painful subacute thyroiditis, postpartum thyroiditis, Riedel's thyroiditis and drug-induced thyroiditis. These may cause hyper- or hypothyroidism or both (82). Various sonographic manifestations will be discussed below.

Chronic Lymphocytic (Hashimoto's) Thyroiditis

Chronic lymphocytic (Hashimoto's) thyroiditis is the most common form of thyroiditis and the primary cause of clinical hypothyroidism in the United States. The typical clinical presentation is a painless, diffusely enlarged gland in a young or a middle-aged woman. Patients have elevated levels of antithyroid antibodies including those against thyroid peroxidase and thyroglobulin (82). There are several different sonographic manifestations of Hashimoto's thyroiditis. Most commonly seen are multiple ill-defined hypoechoic areas separated by thickened fibrous strands that create a coarsened echotexture, usually less echogenic than normal thyroid (Fig. 13). Although in some patients no normal parenchyma is identified, in others, the thyroiditis is patchy and ill-defined, with intervening more normal-appearing gland (Fig. 14). Both the thickened septae and the patchy appearance can create the suggestion of focal nodules. Imaging these areas in transverse and longitudinal planes confirms that the margins are not sufficiently well defined to be considered nodules. Typical for Hashimotos' thyroiditis is a thickened, heterogeneous isthmus. Another sonographic variant is micronodulation, with innumerable small hypoechoic nodules distributed throughout the gland (Fig. 15) (83). Discrete thyroid nodules are less typical, but adjacent adenopathy is common. Color-flow Doppler imaging is

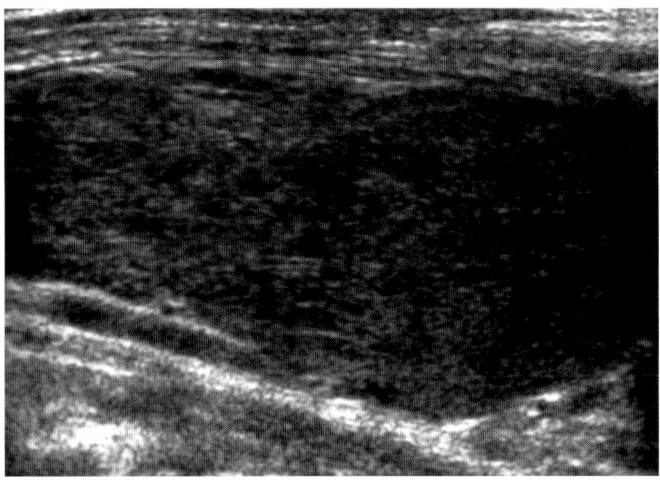
(A)

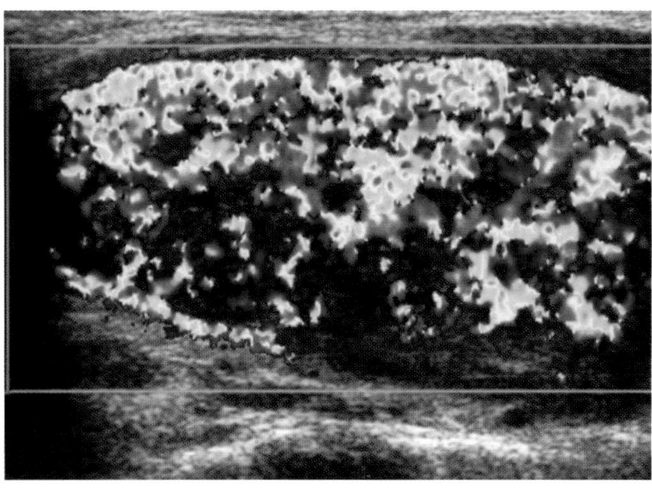
(B)

FIGURE 12 A AND B ■ Graves' disease. (**A**) Longitudinal image of a mildly enlarged, mildly heterogeneous thyroid lobe. (**B**) Addition of color Doppler shows marked increased vascularity typical for acute Graves' disease—the "thyroid inferno."

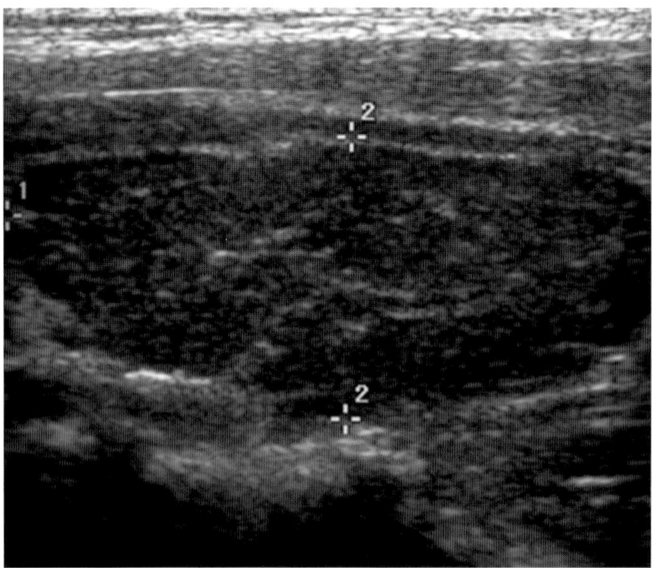

FIGURE 13 ■ Hashimoto's thyroiditis, diffuse. One of the most common appearances of Hashimoto's thyroiditis is a mildly enlarged heterogeneous gland without focal nodule.

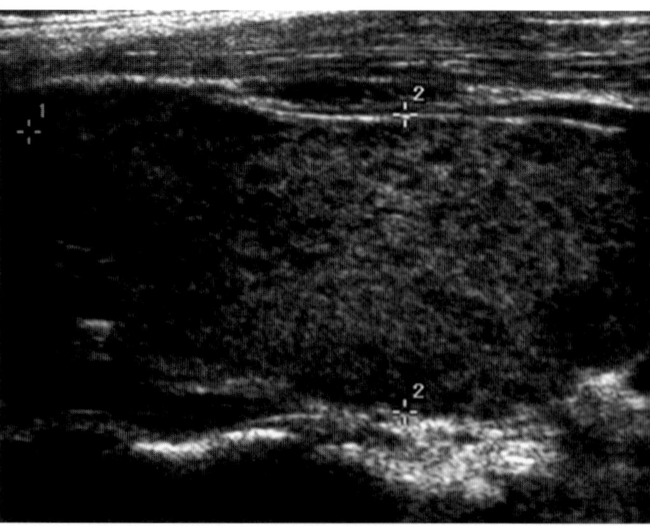

FIGURE 15 ■ Hashimoto's thyroiditis, micronodular variant. The thyroid lobe is replaced with innumerable tiny hypoechoic nodules, without a well-defined larger focal nodule.

variable and not extremely useful. End-stage disease may show a fibrotic gland that is small, ill-defined, and heterogeneous. Discrete thyroid nodules are occasionally seen in a background of heterogeneous Hashimoto's gland, and they should be evaluated with US-guided FNA to exclude primary thyroid cancer or lymphoma. Although rare, patients with Hashimoto's thyroiditis are at increased risk for primary thyroid lymphoma (35).

Acute Suppurative Thyroiditis

Acute suppurative thyroiditis usually is caused by a bacterial infection and presents as painful enlargement of the gland that may be focal or diffuse. Due to the vascular nature, high iodine content, and encapsulation of the thyroid gland, this type of thyroiditis is exceedingly rare (82). These patients are typically quite ill on presentation.

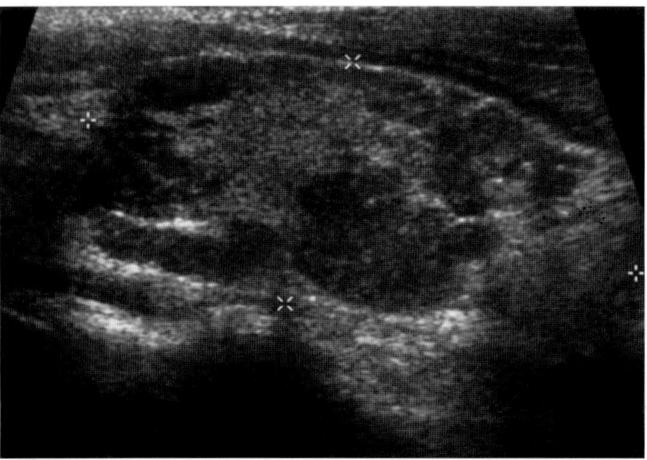

FIGURE 14 ■ Hashimoto's thyroiditis, focal. In this patient, the autoimmune process is affecting only portions of the lobe, particularly the periphery. This appearance can mimic focal nodules.

Ultrasonography demonstrates hypoechogenicity of the involved portion of the thyroid. US may also be used to detect the development of frank thyroid abscess or to guide sampling for Gram stain and culture.

Subacute (de Quervain's) Thyroiditis

Subacute granulomatous thyroiditis is a spontaneously remitting inflammatory disease that frequently follows an upper respiratory illness. Patients report pain and low-grade fever and classically have a markedly elevated erythrocyte sedimentation rate (82). During the active phase of subacute thyroiditis, either diffuse or focal poorly marginated areas of hypoechogenicity, sometimes called pseudonodules, are seen. These disappear completely with resolution of the symptoms (84). (Fig. 16A and B) There is no increase in vascularity with color Doppler (85). If there is confusion between a possible thyroid nodule and a subacute thyroiditis, a follow-up exam should be conducted in six to eight weeks.

Postpartum Thyroiditis

Postpartum thyroiditis is a lymphocytic infiltration of the gland that usually occurs within six months after delivery and is more common in patients with preexisting thyroiditis (82). US findings are nonspecific—mild enlargement of the thyroid, with some hypoechoic regions.

Riedel's Struma

Riedel's struma, or Riedel's thyroiditis, is a rare progressive fibrosis of the thyroid that affects primarily women and tends to progress to complete destruction of the thyroid gland. In the small number of patients who have been examined ultrasonographically, the gland is enlarged diffusely and has an inhomogeneous parenchymal echotexture, similar to the appearance of anaplastic thyroid carcinoma. Ultrasonography can be used to look for

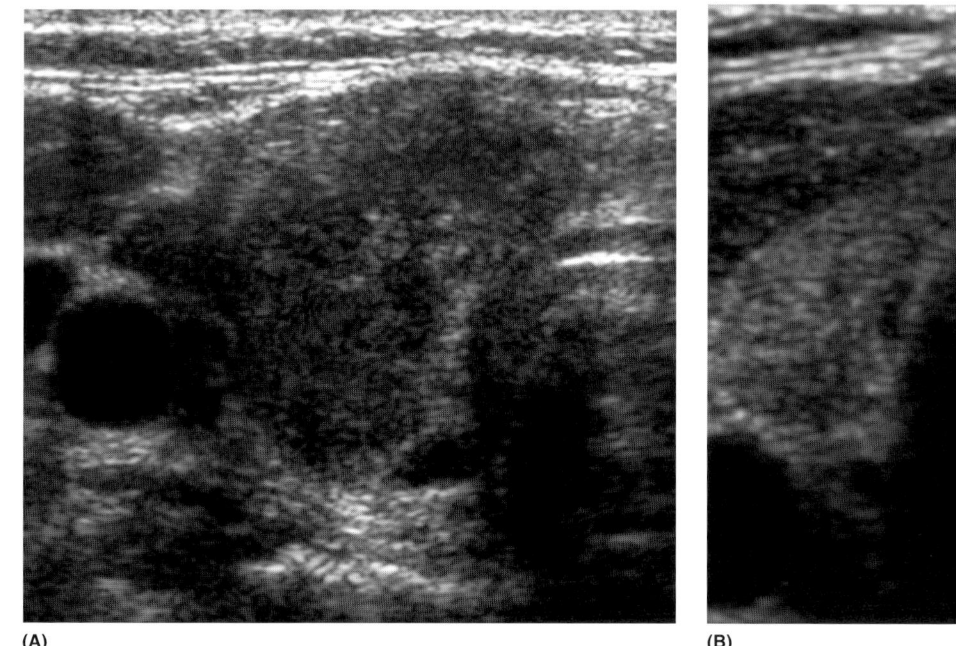
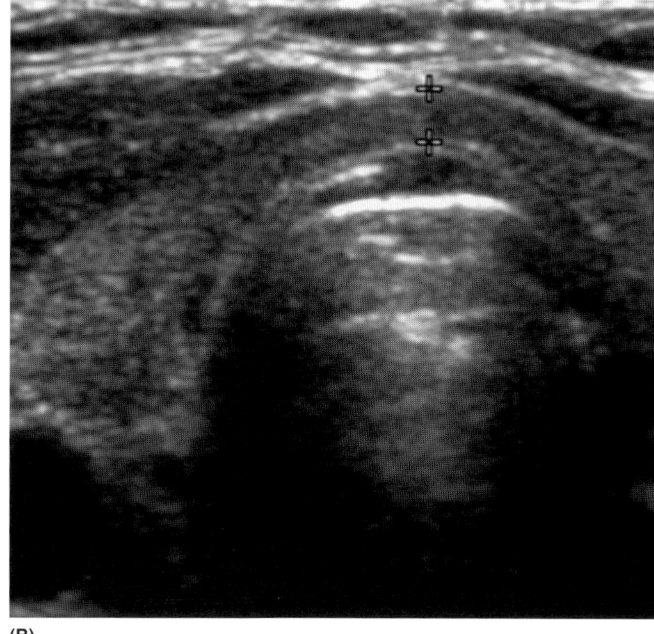

(A) (B)

FIGURE 16 A AND B ■ Subacute thyroiditis. (**A**) Transverse image of the right lobe shows a poorly defined hypoechoic process nearly replacing the lobe, which mimics a nodule. The patient reported low-grade fever and tenderness over the right neck. (**B**) Follow-up ultrasound performed three months later shows a normal gland, with complete resolution of the right-sided thyroiditis.

extrathyroidal extension of the inflammatory process, which may include encasement of adjacent vessels (77). Due to the fibrosis, FNA produces insufficient cells for diagnosis (25).

Amiodarone Thyroiditis

Two types of amiodarone thyroiditis are reported. With type I, there is synthesis and release of excess thyroid hormone. Type II is a destructive thyroiditis, with release of stored thyroid hormone from the damaged gland (82). Color Doppler US has been proposed as a noninvasive means of distinguishing the two types with varying results. Type I thyroiditis demonstrates normal or increased thyroid vascularity, while type II demonstrates absent vascularity (86). Others have found no difference in color Doppler appearance between the two types (87).

Biopsy and Ablation of Thyroid Lesions

FNA Biopsy

Because the nature of a thyroid nodule cannot be defined precisely on the basis of imaging features, and because FNA is highly accurate, palpation or US-guided aspiration biopsy is indicated for evaluation of thyroid nodules. FNA has been shown to be safe, inexpensive, and highly accurate (54,56). Complications are rare and usually minor, such as hematoma or pain. US guidance improves the diagnostic yield when compared to FNA by palpation alone (88). Performing FNA with US guidance confirms that the cytological sample is from the nodule in question and allows the needle to be directed into the solid portions of the nodule (55,89,90). While in some locations, immediate cytological analysis of the aspirated specimen is available, this practice increases procedure time without improving specimen adequacy, and it is probably unnecessary (91). In one practice, when FNA was used in thyroid nodule evaluation, the percentage of patients undergoing thyroidectomy decreased by 25%, the yield of carcinoma in patients who underwent surgery more than doubled (from 14% to 39%), and the overall cost of the evaluation for patients with thyroid nodules decreased by 25% (92). Thus, FNA increased the accuracy and decreased the cost of thyroid nodule evaluation. In this era of research in clinical outcomes, the efficacy of FNA is clear.

The possible results of FNA cytologic analysis are listed in Table 3. Two principles are noted in analysis of the cytology specimen. First, only a few malignant cells are needed to diagnose cancer; and second, at least six groups of 15 well-preserved normal cells are needed to make the diagnosis of negative or benign. Therefore, false-negative specimens are rare, but in 10% to 15% of patients, repeat US-guided FNA is necessary because of a nondiagnostic acellular or hypocellular biopsy specimen.

Biopsy Technique

We use a 5 to 8 MHz sector probe and a freehand biopsy method. The patient's neck is hyperextended, and the biopsy site is localized. The skin is cleansed with several alcohol swabs. A sterile transducer-covering sheath and sterile gel are not used. Infection is extremely rare with FNA of the thyroid due to the gland's highly vascular nature. Subcutaneous lidocaine is placed at the biopsy

TABLE 3 ■ Cytologic Results Obtained with Fine-Needle Aspiration Biopsy

Cytologic result	Pathologic features
Positive (malignant)	Papillary, medullary, anaplastic cancer
	Single or few malignant cells needed to make diagnosis
	98% of these cases are cancer at pathology[a]
Suspicious	Atypical cells or many tightly packed follicular cells
	Follicular neoplasm (cannot distinguish adenoma from carcinoma)
Atypical	Few atypical cells noted among mostly benign cells
	Repeat FNA indicated because of 11% cancer rate at pathology[a]
Negative (benign)	Requires six groups of 15–20 well-preserved normal cells to make diagnosis
	False-negative results are rare
	Cancer rate is 0.003%[a]
	Colloid, adenomatous, hyperplastic nodules
Nondiagnostic	Acellular or hypocellular specimen
	Approximately 1 in 15 FNAs or 7%[a]

[a]In our practice.
Abbreviation: FNA, fine-needle aspiration.

site. The probe is placed lateral to the thyroid gland, overlying the carotid artery, and the nodule is imaged in the transverse plane. The needle is inserted through the skin in a direct up and down plane medial to the transducer and within the image plane of the transducer, without the help of a guide. The sector probe allows localization of the needle while it is still in the subcutaneous tissue, which permits subtle adjustments to be made in needle position to direct the biopsy into the desired area (Fig. 17A and B).

The typical needle used to perform a thyroid FNA is a standard 1.5-inch, 25-gauge needle attached to a 10-mL syringe. Without suction, the needle is moved back and forth through the nodule several times. Capillary action causes cells to move into the needle as it is moved back and forth in the nodule. An ideal specimen for cytologic

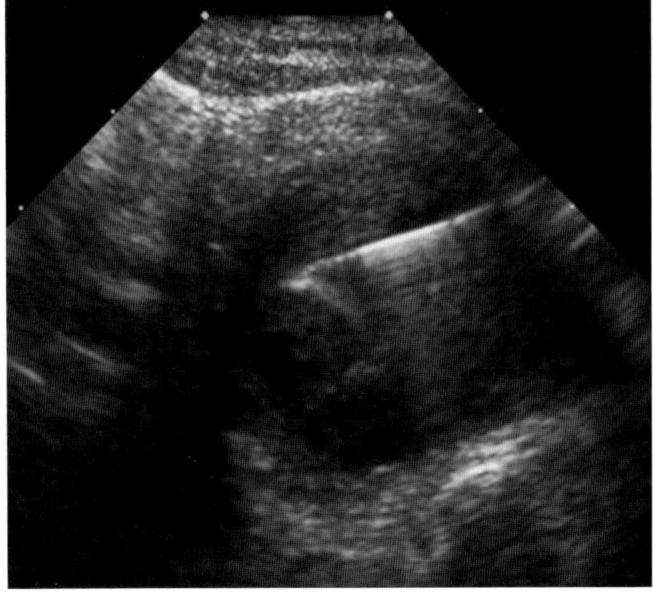

(A)

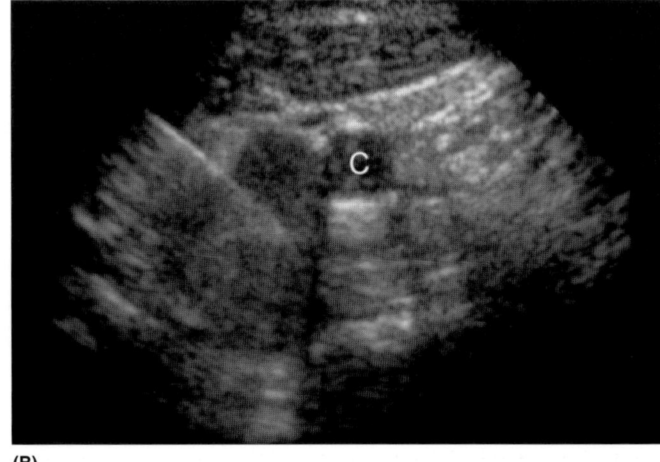

(B)

FIGURE 17 A AND B ■ Fine-needle aspiration. (**A**) Needle within a right-sided hypoechoic thyroid nodule. (**B**) Needle within a left-sided thyroid nodule. C, carotid artery.

analysis consists of one or two drops of blood-tinged fluid at the base of the needle. If the specimen contains too much blood, the specimen will be nondiagnostic. Three passes are made into each nodule.

US-Guided Alcohol Ablation of Thyroid Cysts and Nodules

In addition to guiding FNA, ultrasonography can be used to guide the injection of 95% ETOH for the ablation of recurrent thyroid cysts and thyroid nodules, by causing coagulative necrosis and small vessel thrombosis (93). After aspiration of a recurrent cyst, ETOH is injected at a volume of 30% to 60% of the aspirated fluid and left in place for a variable amount of time (1). Success rates of nearly 75% have been reported with this procedure, with rates somewhat lower for solid nodules (94). US-guided percutaneous injection of tetracycline has also been successful in sclerosing recurrent thyroid cystic masses (95). Reports of percutaneous US-guided alcohol ablation of autonomous hyperfunctioning thyroid nodules are encouraging, showing no recurrences and complete or partial long-term (greater than six months) cures in more than 90% of patients (66,67,96). With ETOH therapy, the incidence of treatment-induced hypothyroidism is less than 1%, as compared with 36% to 45% with radioactive iodine (97). Early results of alcohol ablation of cold thyroid nodules, as an alternative to surgical ablation, are also encouraging (98).

PARATHYROID GLANDS

Anatomy

The four parathyroid glands are typically located in the anterior neck, two on each side, closely related to the thyroid gland. These glands secrete parathyroid hormone, which regulates serum calcium. There are two superior and two inferior parathyroid glands, each measuring about 5 × 3 × 1 mm in adults. There are additional parathyroid glands in approximately 6% of the population and less than four in approximately 6% of adults (99). The glands normally are oval or bean shaped. The superior glands develop from the embryonic fourth pharyngeal pouch along with the thyroid gland and usually are located posterior to the upper pole or midportion of each thyroid lobe. Ectopic superior parathyroid tissue occurs at or above the superior thyroid pole, below the inferior thyroid artery, or posterior and medial to the esophagus. The inferior parathyroid glands develop in the superior aspect of the embryonic neck in the third pharyngeal pouch together with the thymus, and they are often more closely related to the thymus than the thyroid (100,101). During embryonic development, the inferior parathyroid glands usually migrate to a point at or just inferior to the posterior aspect of the lower thyroid poles, but they may fail to separate from the adjacent thymus and migrate with it caudally into the superior mediastinum. Because they begin their embryonic descent from the superior aspect of the neck, ectopic inferior parathyroid glands can be found anywhere from the superior thyroid pole (3% of patients) to the carotid artery bifurcation to the thymus and superior mediastinum (13% of patients) (34,102,103). A small percentage of both superior and inferior parathyroid glands are intrathyroidal. On initial operation, most parathyroidectomies do not require mediastinotomy. At reoperation, however, mediastinotomy is required for resection of about 19% of parathyroid glands (104).

US Technique

The normal parathyroid gland is not routinely identified at sonography but occasionally can be localized. The technique for imaging the parathyroid glands is similar to that for the thyroid gland, and attention to maximizing technical factors is imperative for imaging these generally small structures. A high-frequency (7–15 MHz) linear transducer is used. In obese patients or in those with large necks or enlarged thyroid glands, a 5-MHz transducer may be necessary to achieve adequate depth of penetration. On US examination, normal parathyroid glands are small and similar in echogenicity to the adjacent thyroid and surrounding tissues, making them difficult to visualize. The entire neck should be imaged, from high in the neck to as low as possible. The probe should be angled under the clavicles and the sternal notch. The common carotid artery sheath should be examined from the bifurcation to the clavicle (2,105).

Primary Hyperparathyroidism

Primary hyperparathyroidism is a common endocrine disorder, with an estimated prevalence of 100 to 200 per 100,000 population in the United States (22). Approximately 75% of primary hyperparathyroidism occurs in women, with an average age of 55 years (106). Laboratory values include increased serum levels of ionized calcium and parathyroid hormone as well as hypercalciuria. This results in increased rates of bone turnover as well as nephrocalcinosis or recurrent renal stones. In 85% of patients, primary hyperparathyroidism is caused by a solitary parathyroid adenoma that secretes parathyroid hormone; in 15%, it is caused by multiple-gland hyperplasia, multiple adenomas, or polyclonal hyperfunction; and in less than 1% of patients, it is caused by carcinoma (Table 4) (106).

Ultrasonographic examinations in patients with hyperparathyroidism may be unsuccessful with minimally enlarged parathyroid glands, adenomas displaced and obscured by an enlarged thyroid goiter, and ectopic adenomas (Table 5). Ectopic adenomas can occur in 1% to 3% of cases, and if the gland has migrated to the mediastinum, US is ineffective.

Structures in the neck that may result in a false-positive ultrasonographic diagnosis of an enlarged parathyroid are posterior exophytic thyroid nodules and cervical lymph nodes (Table 5) (107). Thyroid nodules can usually be shown to be within the confines of the gland and have mixed echogenicity, with possible cystic or calcified components. Color Doppler may be used to show the vascular supply to the nodule in question arises from within the thyroid gland itself (108). Lymph nodes are typically

TABLE 4 ■ Pathologic Classification of Primary Hyperparathyroidism

Pathologic classification	Appearance
Adenoma, enlargement of single gland	90% solitary Homogeneous, hypoechoic, well-marginated, oval shape Typical inferior adenoma located adjacent to caudal tip of lower pole of thyroid or in soft tissues of low neck Typical superior adenoma located posterior to the midportion of thyroid Variable size
Hyperplasia and multiple adenomas, enlargement of multiple glands	10% of patients have multiple-gland enlargement Primary hyperplasia involves all four parathyroid glands, but enlargement is usually asymmetric Multiple adenomas are rare, 20% of these are inherited
Carcinoma	Occurs in < 1% of patients Usually large, inhomogeneous echotexture Vascular invasion is pathognomonic but not commonly seen ultrasonographically Diagnosis usually is made intraoperatively (hard gland fixed to surrounding tissues by local invasion) or by presence of metastatic disease

more lateral in the neck along the IJ vein and contain a characteristic central echogenic hilum. However, small nodes are often found just inferior to the thyroid, mimicking an enlarged parathyroid. The collapsed esophagus should not be mistaken for a parathyroid lesion, as it lengthens on longitudinal scanning and air can be seen rushing through its central lumen if the patient is asked to swallow. Small veins surrounding the thyroid gland can be characterized as such with the addition of color Doppler.

Adenoma

On ultrasonography, parathyroid adenomas are oval, solid, and homogeneously hypoechoic (Fig. 18). The hypoechogenicity of parathyroid adenomas is due to their uniform hypercellularity, which leaves few interfaces for reflection of sound waves. This appearance can, at times, mimic a cyst, though without posterior through transmission. The shape of the adenoma can change as it enlarges, becoming more lobular. Most adenomas are solid, but some contain internal cystic components, and rarely do central fatty components create an echogenic appearance. Occasionally, color Doppler will demonstrate a peripheral vascular arc surrounding a portion of the parathyroid gland (109) distinguishing it from a lymph node that has

TABLE 5 ■ Causes of False-Positive and False-Negative Results Obtained with Ultrasonographic Imaging of Parathyroid Glands

False positive	False negative
Thyroid nodule	Small parathyroid adenoma size
Lymph node	Ectopic parathyroid location
Esophagus	Limited visualization due to large neck, obesity, or multinodular thyroid gland
Longus colli muscle	
Parathyroid vein	

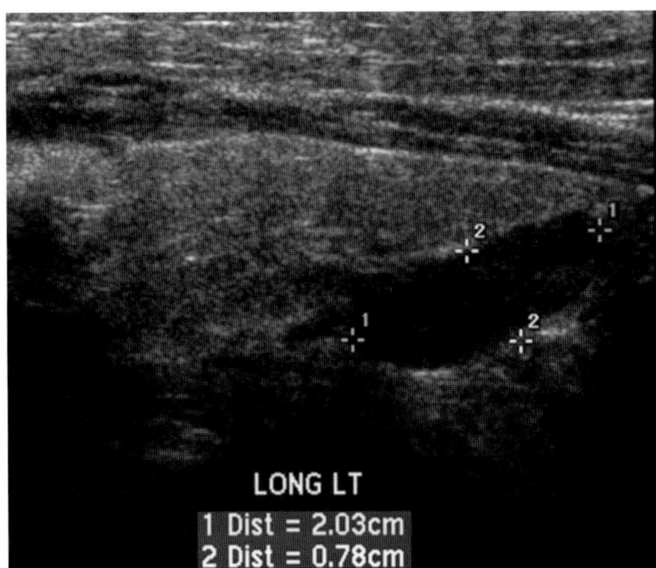

FIGURE 18 ■ Parathyroid adenoma. Sagittal image of the left lobe of the thyroid shows a well-defined, very hypoechoic mass (*calipers*) posterior to the lower pole of the normal thyroid, consistent with a parathyroid adenoma.

hilar flow. A plane of tissue separating the parathyroid adenoma from the adjacent thyroid can help distinguish parathyroid adenomas from thyroid masses. Small adenomas can be minimally enlarged glands that appear virtually normal on operation but are found to be hypercellular on pathologic examination. The largest adenomas can be 5 cm or more in length and weigh more than 10 g. On cytologic examination, suppressed normal parathyroid tissue can be demonstrated just external to the capsule of the adenoma, distinguishing it from generalized hyperplasia.

Most parathyroid adenomas have typical ultrasonographic features and lie in fairly typical locations. Superior parathyroid adenomas are usually posterior to the midportion of the thyroid gland. The location of inferior adenomas is more variable, but most commonly, they lie just inferior to the lower lobe of the thyroid or in the soft tissues of the low anterior neck. About 1% of adenomas are located within the thyroid gland, where they appear more homogeneous and hypoechoic than a typical thyroid nodule (Fig. 19). If there is only one nodule in the thyroid with the classic appearance of an intrathyroidal parathyroid, the diagnosis is straightforward. However, in many patients, the presence of true thyroid nodules complicates the matter, and FNA will be necessary to confidently localize the adenoma. The sensitivity of ultrasonography in localizing parathyroid adenomas in patients with primary hyperparathyroid varies, but with meticulous grayscale and color Doppler technique, it can reach 70% to 93% (108–110). In some institutions, localization of adenomas preoperatively is improved with the addition of nuclear medicine studies, specifically, technetium 99m sestamibi scintigraphy (111,112). US contrast agents have also been proposed to increase preoperative sensitivity (113). However, these agents are not approved for clinical use in the United States.

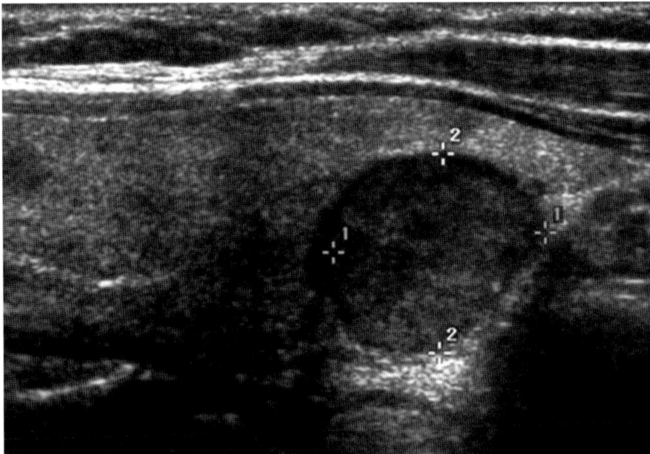

FIGURE 19 ■ Intrathyroidal parathyroid adenoma. Sagittal image of the thyroid shows a well-defined, very hypoechoic nodule (*calipers*) within the lower pole of the thyroid. No other nodules were seen in the thyroid gland, and the patient had an elevated parathyroid hormone level. At surgery, this mass was found to be an intrathyroidal parathyroid adenoma.

As preoperative localization techniques improve, many centers are now utilizing a minimally invasive surgical technique, where only the area identified on imaging is evaluated and resected, without exploration and identification of all four parathyroid glands. This procedure, in combination with rapid parathyroid hormone levels acquired intraoperatively, shortens surgical and anesthesia time and decreases both complications and costs (114). The minimally invasive approach following sonographic localization is reported to be successful in 65% to 85% of patients (114–116).

Enlargement of Multiple Parathyroid Glands

Of the patients with hyperparathyroidism, 10% have enlargement of multiple glands. The cause of parathyroid hyperplasia is not well understood. Although the hyperplasia involves all four glands, the glands are not involved equally, and the enlargement is always asymmetric. Pathologically, these glands are hyperplastic (multiple adenomas are rare). Approximately 20% of patients with hyperfunction of multiple glands have an inherited disorder such as multiple endocrine neoplasia type I, familial hypocalciuric hypercalcemia, neonatal severe primary hyperparathyroidism, or others (106). The sonologist must perform a complete and thorough search for multiple enlarged glands in all patients, resisting the temptation to stop once an adenoma is found.

Parathyroid Carcinoma

Parathyroid carcinoma is seen in less than 1% of patients with hyperparathyroidism. Clinically, the presentation is similar to that of other forms of primary hyperparathyroidism, with significantly elevated levels of serum calcium. The tumor on an average is larger and has a more heterogeneous appearance than typical parathyroid adenomas (Fig. 20), but there is no ultrasonographic criterion for reliably differentiating benign from malignant parathyroid disease (117). Internal calcifications are uncommon. Although vascular invasion by the lesion is also uncommon, it is diagnostic of malignancy. The criteria used to diagnose malignancy include metastatic disease, capsular invasion, and local recurrence after resection. Diagnosis of a tumor's malignant nature is not usually made until surgical resection. Metastases may be local, to the regional lymph nodes (22), or widely dispersed (118).

Parathyroid Cysts

True parathyroid cysts are rare. The majority arise from an inferior parathyroid gland and thus occur below the inferior edge of the thyroid gland (Fig. 21) (105). The appearance is that of a typical cyst on sonography—anechoic with enhanced through transmission. Most parathyroid cysts are nonfunctional (119). Aspiration yields a clear colorless liquid, thus aiding in differentiating it from a thyroid cyst aspirate, which is typically dark red or brown from prior hemorrhage. This fluid is high in parathyroid hormone and low in thyroglobulin. Treatment is repeated aspiration, surgery, or ablation.

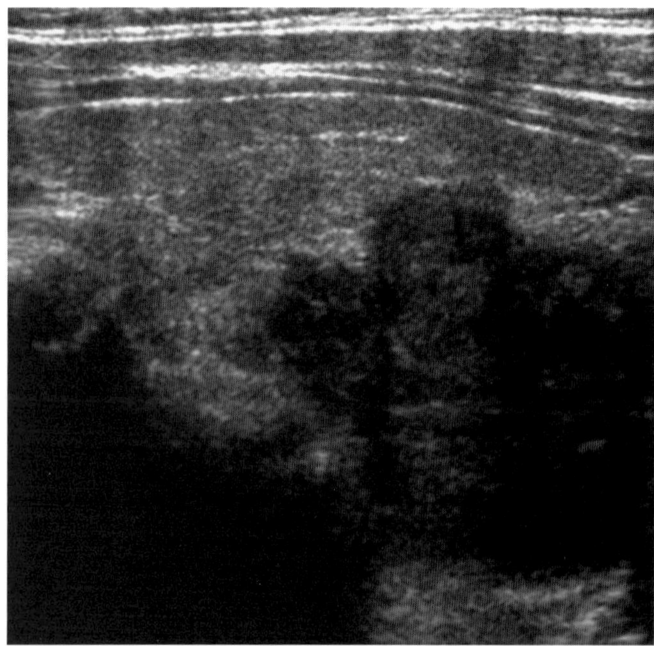

FIGURE 20 ■ Parathyroid carcinoma. Sagittal image of the right lobe of the thyroid in a 53-year-old man shows an irregular, very hypoechoic mass that appears to invade the lower pole of the thyroid. Fine-needle aspiration confirmed parathyroid carcinoma, which matched the biopsy of multiple liver metastases.

Secondary Hyperparathyroidism

The parathyroid glands may show compensatory enlargement and hypersecretion in patients with renal failure or vitamin D deficiency. This is secondary to end-organ resistance to the parathyroid hormone, leading to low serum levels of calcium. In secondary hyperparathyroidism, all parathyroid glands usually are affected, but individual glands may be spared. The parathyroid hormone levels generally return to normal if the underlying abnormalities are controlled. The term tertiary hyperparathyroidism is applied to those glands converting from secondary hyperplasia to autonomous hormone secretion. The imaging characteristics of the enlarged parathyroid glands in both secondary and tertiary hyperparathyroidism are similar to those of parathyroid adenomas.

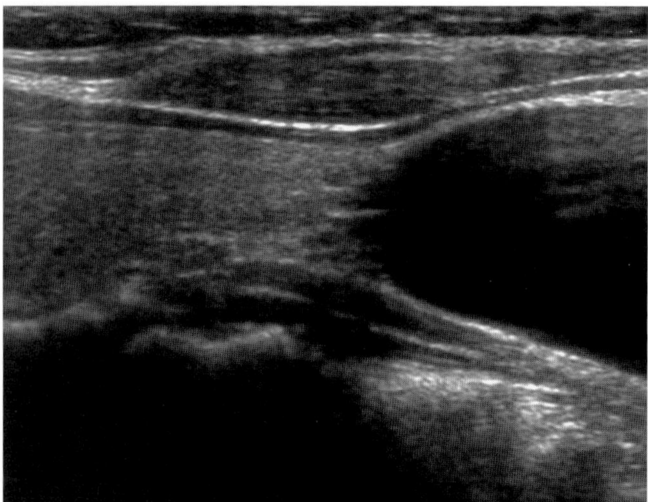

FIGURE 21 ■ Parathyroid cyst. Sagittal image of the thyroid shows an anechoic cyst extending inferiorly from just below the thyroid gland. Aspiration of this cyst resulted in clear fluid with a high parathyroid hormone level. The patient's serum parathyroid hormone level was normal.

US-Guided Biopsy and Therapy of Parathyroid Glands

Biopsy

If concern remains about the nature of a suspected parathyroid mass, ultrasonographically-guided percutaneous aspiration or biopsy, with the same technique described for FNA biopsy of thyroid nodules, can be used to differentiate suspected parathyroid adenomas from lymph nodes and thyroid nodules, although these latter entities are most likely in the presence of a normal serum calcium level. Specimens undergo cytologic analysis and parathyroid hormone assay, which is 100% specific (120–122). US is also used to guide percutaneous biopsy of suspected parathyroid adenomas in patients with postoperative persistent or recurrent hyperparathyroidism. Conclusive preoperative confirmation obtained with biopsy of a suspected parathyroid gland abnormality may have a role when patient or surgeon is undecided on treatment.

Alcohol Ablation

An outgrowth of the success of ultrasonographically-guided FNA of parathyroid adenomas is the use of ultrasonography to guide percutaneous injections of ETOH to ablate abnormal, enlarged parathyroid glands (123–126). ETOH ablation is most commonly used postoperatively in patients with recurrent or persistent hyperparathyroidism, who have an ultrasonographically visualized, FNA biopsy-proven parathyroid adenoma but who are not good candidates for reoperation. This technique also is used as alternative therapy for the small number of patients with primary hyperparathyroidism, who refuse surgical treatment, who are not good surgical candidates, or who present with emergent life-threatening malignant hypercalcemia. A small needle (22–25 gauge) is inserted into multiple regions of the mass, and 95% ETOH is injected (Fig. 21) (127). A volume equal to about half the volume of the mass is used. With real-time visualization, the tissue surrounding the needle tip becomes highly echogenic at the time of injection. This hyperechogenicity, which is probably due to microbubbles formed when the alcohol comes into contact with the soft tissues, slowly disappears during a period of about one minute. Injections are repeated every day or every other day until the serum level of calcium reaches the normal range. In most patients, two or three injections are necessary.

In uremic patients with secondary hyperparathyroidism, who are refractory to medical therapy, percutaneous injections of ETOH have been used to decrease gland mass so that medical therapy can be more effective (126). Decreased gland mass generally leads to decreased levels of parathyroid hormone and alkaline phosphates and improvement in bone lesions. In a series of 12 patients, parathyroid volume decreased 20% to 100% within six months of alcohol ablation (124).

A drawback of ETOH injection therapy is that ETOH seepage along the needle tract or spread along tissue planes adjacent to the parathyroid adenoma may damage the ipsilateral recurrent laryngeal nerve, leading to transient or, less commonly, permanent vocal cord paralysis. In one study, permanent unilateral vocal cord paralysis occurred in 2 of 32 patients receiving ETOH injections (123). ETOH injection can also induce a fibrotic reaction in the soft tissues immediately surrounding the parathyroid adenoma. If surgical resection of the adenoma is ultimately required, the fibrotic tissue may cause an added degree of difficulty. Because of these limitations, other percutaneous treatment methods, including electrocautery and laser therapy may have a role in the future for ablation of lesions in the neck and other superficial locations.

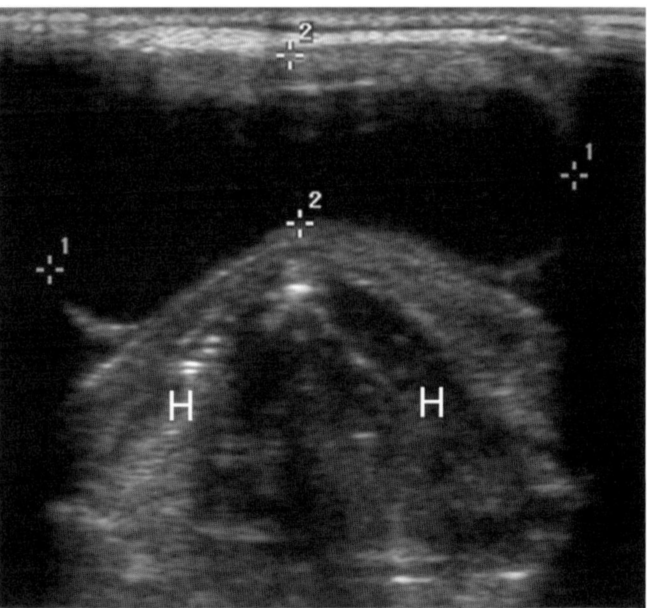

FIGURE 22 ■ Thyroglossal duct cyst. Transverse midline image of the neck, at the level of the hyoid cartilage (H). There is a simple cyst (*calipers*) anterior to the hyoid. Fine-needle aspiration shows follicular cells and surgical resection confirmed a thyroglossal duct cyst.

OTHER NECK MASSES

Congenital Neck Masses

General Embryology

Because of the complex embryology of the neck region, a wide variety of cystic lesions may result and subsequently be identified on sonography. Cystic hygroma, cavernous lymphangioma, and simple capillary lymphangioma are all malformations of the cervical thoracic lymphatic system (128–130). Branchial cleft cysts, thymic cysts, and parathyroid anomalies are anomalies of the branchial apparatus. Thyroglossal duct cysts are remnants of the thyroglossal duct. These masses usually have cystic internal components and a thin rim; however, their ultrasonographic characteristics can change markedly if the lesion becomes infected.

Ectopic thyroid tissue can occur anywhere between the tongue and the mediastinum. The most common variant is a lingual thyroid (Fig. 5), located at the foramen cecum in the posterior tongue and seen best with iodine scintigraphy. Most remnants are supernumerary to the normal thyroid gland and may be mistaken for lymph nodes of the anterior triangle or metastases.

Thyroglossal Duct Cyst

Thyroglossal duct cyst is a remnant of the thyroglossal duct that fails to regress in the embryo. Although these cysts can occur anywhere along the course of the duct from the foramen cecum at the base of the tongue to the pyramidal lobe of the thyroid gland, most are closely related to the hyoid bone in the midline (Fig. 22) (131). Approximately one quarter may be more lateral. Thyroglossal duct cyst appearance varies from completely anechoic in 25% to a cyst with homogeneous low-level internal echoes or even a heterogeneous solid mass. Posterior through transmission is common despite the internal echoes, and most lesions are not infected (131,132). In patients with a history of a fluctuating or gradually enlarging mass, superinfection may have occurred as the result of a patent duct extending from the base of the tongue. Cysts near the tongue have a squamous lining, while cysts closer to the thyroid may show thyroid epithelial cells. FNA of the cyst wall can demonstrate thyroid cells and confirm the diagnosis. Inflammatory changes may obliterate the mucosa entirely and convert it into an abscess cavity. Malignancy, primarily papillary carcinoma, can arise within thyroglossal duct cysts. When a possible thyroglossal duct cyst is identified sonographically, it is important to confirm the presence of a normally located thyroid gland, as an ectopic gland could masquerade as a thyroglossal duct cyst, and surgical resection would leave the patient permanently hypothyroid (133).

Branchial Cleft Cyst

Most branchial cleft cysts arise from the first or second branchial cleft (128). The cysts are located laterally in the neck, around the level of the carotid bifurcation (134), and anterior to the upper third of the sternocleidomastoid muscle (Fig. 23) (135). Larger cysts may extend posteriorly under the sternocleidomastoid muscle and displace the carotid sheath structures posteromedially. The cyst usually presents as a painless, smooth lateral neck mass, but it may become infected, painful, and tender, occasionally with a spontaneous draining sinus. A history of a recurring inflammatory mass at the same location in the anterior lateral neck suggests a second branchial cleft cyst. Most occur between the ages of 10 and 40 years. The cyst is lined with stratified squamous epithelium and contains

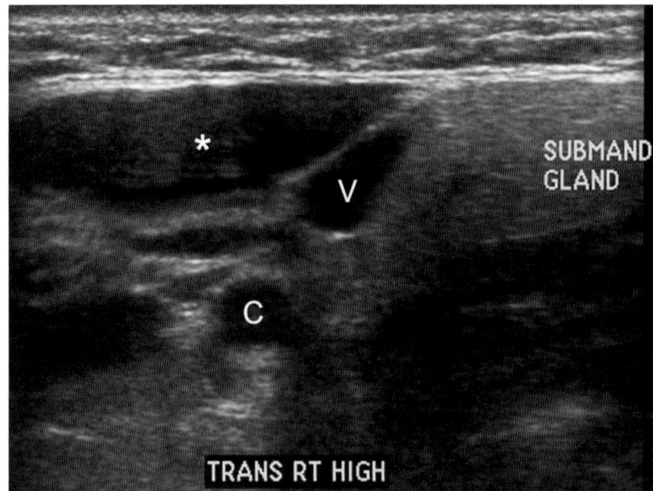

FIGURE 23 ■ Branchial cleft cyst. Transverse image of the right upper neck shows the carotid artery (C), jugular vein (V), submandibular gland, and a flattened, mostly simple cyst (*) in the superficial tissues of the right lateral neck, surgically proven to be a branchial cleft cyst.

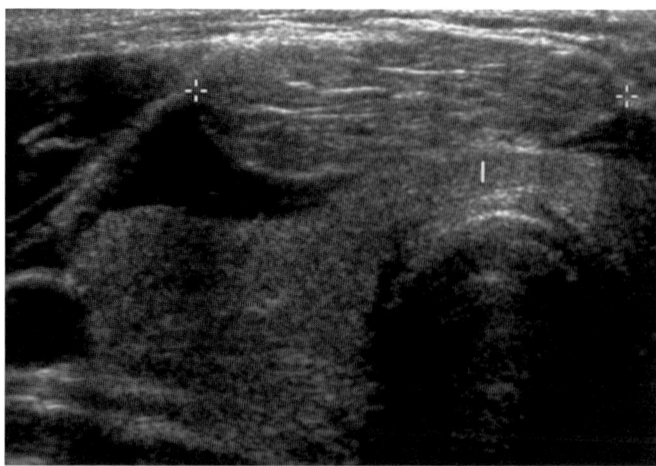

FIGURE 24 ■ Lipoma. Transverse image of the right neck just anterior to the thyroid isthmus (I) shows a heterogeneous, solid mass (*calipers*). The echotexture of the mass was indistinguishable from the subcutaneous fat, and the mass could be seen to move with swallowing.

turbid yellowish fluid. A noninfected cyst has a thin, uniform wall surrounding a homogeneous, usually fluid, core with fine internal echoes due to debris. With infection, the wall can become thick and the internal fluid more echogenic.

Cystic Hygroma

From 80% to 90% of congenital lymphatic malformations are detected by the age of two years (128), including some that are found at prenatal sonography. In up to 10% of patients, however, the malformations may not be discovered until adulthood. Cystic hygroma, the most common form of lymphangioma, consists of large dilated cystic lymphatic spaces. Of these malformations, 75% occur in the neck, particularly in the posterior compartment (130). A smaller percentage extend into the mediastinum. Cystic hygroma is differentiated from cavernous lymphangioma, capillary lymphangioma, and other lymphatic malformations on the basis of the size of its lymphatic spaces. All are composed of multicystic fluid-filled spaces, which are endothelial-lined lymphatic channels separated by connective tissue stroma. Cystic hygromas probably arise from sequestrations of primitive embryonic lymph sacs and enlarge either because of inadequate drainage of the central lymphatic channels into the IJ veins or because of excessive secretion from the lining cells. Most often, cystic hygromas are discovered as painless soft or semifirm masses in the posterior triangle of the neck. Sonographically, they are usually multiloculated homogeneous cystic masses, but a solitary cystic mass is found occasionally. The cyst wall typically is thin. Cystic hygromas are associated with Turner's syndrome (45XO).

TABLE 6 ■ Cystic Neck Masses

Common
- Thyroglossal duct cyst
- Branchial cleft cyst
- Lymphangioma (cystic hygroma)

Uncommon
- Abscess
- Necrotic lymphadenopathy
- Dermoid cyst
- Cervical bronchogenic cyst
- Cystic neuroma
- Aneurysm
- Seroma
- Thymic cyst
- Parathyroid cyst

Other Cystic Neck Masses

The differential diagnosis of a cystic neck mass also includes abscess, necrotic lymph nodes, dermoid cysts, rare cervical bronchogenic cysts, and cystic neuroma (Table 6) (128). Metastases, usually of pulmonary, genitourinary, or gastrointestinal origin, may also present as a cystic neck mass. Metastases from papillary thyroid cancer are usually solid but can be cystic.

Solid Neck Masses

Subcutaneous lipomas are typically hypoechoic and solid appearing but may be echolucent if they are large and have fewer cellular interfaces (Fig. 24) (Table 7). The

TABLE 7 ■ Solid Neck Masses

- Lymphadenopathy
- Parathyroid adenoma
- Hemangioma
- Lipoma
- Carotid body tumor
- Neurogenic tumor

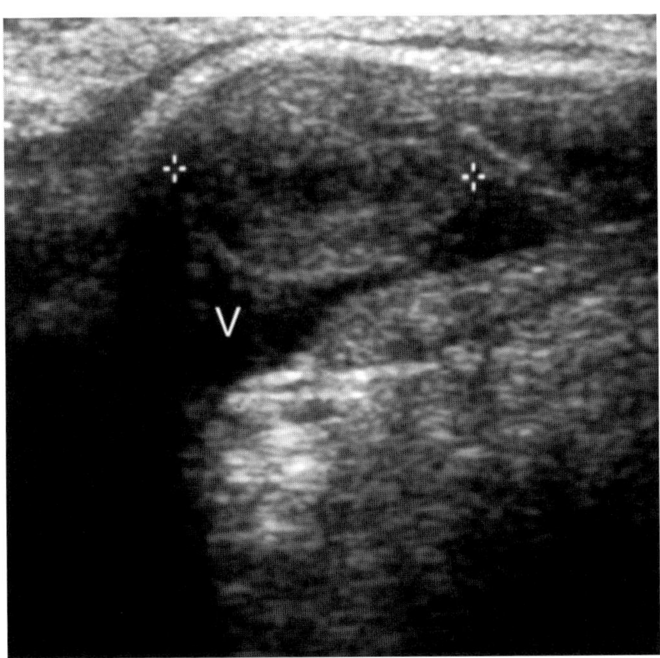

FIGURE 25 ■ Neurogenic tumor. Transverse magnified image of the right jugular vein (V) shows a hypoechoic mass (*calipers*) indenting the anterior aspect of the vein, surgically proven to be a schwannoma.

appearance of a lipoma depends on the relative amounts of fat and fibrous tissue (136). Occasionally, a lipoma is so similar in appearance to the surrounding subcutaneous fat that only real-time scanning will identify a lesion due to its mass effect. Hemangiomas and hemangiolymphangiomas usually are found in younger patients and are located in or around the parotid gland. Doppler examination should be helpful in demonstrating vascularity.

A carotid body tumor is a paraganglioma of the carotid body. These lesions are typically located high in the neck in the notch of the carotid bifurcation and are fed by the external carotid artery. Patients present with headache and a palpable neck mass. Carotid body tumors are highly vascular, and a high diastolic flow pattern in the external carotid artery may suggest their presence. FNA can lead to hemorrhage due to the high vascularity of the tumors (137). Neurogenic tumors such as neurofibromas or schwannomas are other solid masses that can occur in the neck, particularly in the posterior triangle (Fig. 25) (136). These lesions are typically hypoechoic and may be seen to be associated with a nerve. FNA is painful, which may be a clue to the diagnosis.

LYMPH NODES

Normal and Abnormal Shapes

US is an ideal modality for evaluation of the cervical lymph nodes (138). Most thyroid neoplasms spread locally to regional lymph nodes, as does parathyroid carcinoma. Most commonly, the lower half of the ipsilateral IJ chain is involved. The nodes in the superior submandibular region are commonly seen ultrasonographically in both normal and affected patients, but they are almost never involved by thyroid or parathyroid disease. Abnormal cervical lymph nodes may also be related to spread from other head and neck cancers as well as inflammatory or infectious processes. Reactive or inflammatory lymph nodes are commonly noted on sonography. Various size criteria have been proposed for inclusion in the US report (139); we use a transverse dimension of 7 mm or above for the middle and lower IJ chain.

Certain sonographic characteristics of lymph nodes may help to suggest benign or malignant disease, including size, shape, internal architecture, and Doppler findings (Table 8) (140). Most normal and inflammatory cervical lymph nodes have a flattened, elongated, oval shape, with the greatest dimension in the longitudinal axis (Fig. 26) (27). The ends of the node often point or taper. Color or power Doppler interrogation of a benign node shows flow entering the node at the hilum and branching radially toward the edge of the node (141).

In contrast to nodes with benign characteristics, the possibility of malignancy exists if the anteroposterior

TABLE 8 ■ Comparison of Ultrasonographic Features of Malignant and Benign Cervical Lymph Nodes

Ultrasonographic feature	Malignant node	Benign node
Shape	Round	Oval
	AP dimension/length ≥ 0.5	AP dimension/length < 0.5
Internal architecture	Inhomogeneous	Homogeneous
	Cystic component (worrisome if there is a history of papillary thyroid cancer)	
	Microcalcifications	
Central hilus	Absent (may be present, but if so, often distorted)	Present
Contour	Smooth or lobulated	Smooth

Abbreviation: AP, anteroposterior.

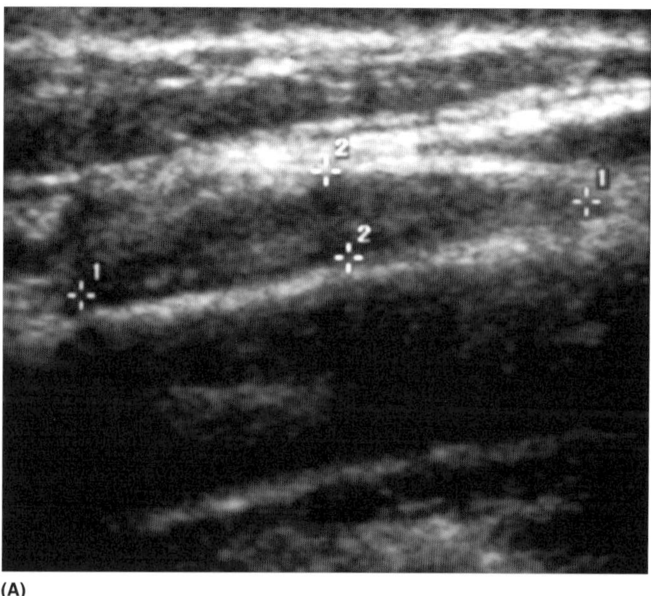

(A)

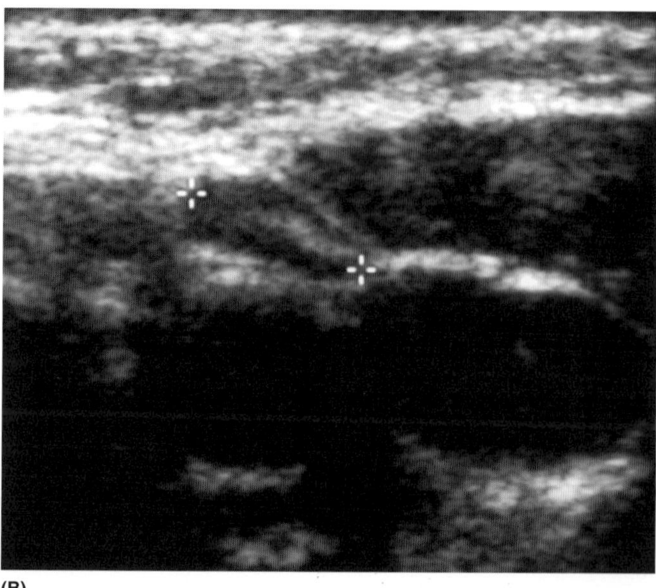

(B)

FIGURE 26 A AND B ■ Benign lymph node. (**A**) Longitudinal image of a normal, benign lymph node (*calipers*). The node is long and thin, with tapered ends. (**B**) Transverse image of the same node shows an echogenic fatty hilum.

dimension of a cervical lymph node is more than half the length of the node. In other words, the more rounded the node, the more likely it is to be malignant. Punctate psammomatous calcifications may be seen in nodal metastases from papillary cancer (Fig. 27). Both metastatic papillary cancer and squamous-cell carcinoma may cause central necrosis in a node, which results in a complex cystic appearance (136,138). In some young patients, the node can become completely cystic and mimic other cystic neck lesions (73). Large nodes involved with metastatic disease may show mass effect on adjacent structures such as vessels and, rarely, even invasion of those vessels (Fig. 28) (136). Abnormal patterns on color or power Doppler interrogation, where blood flow is seen to enter a node from the edges instead of through the hilum, are also worrisome (141–143). It should be noted that Doppler evaluation of a small structure such as a node is technically challenging and requires optimal

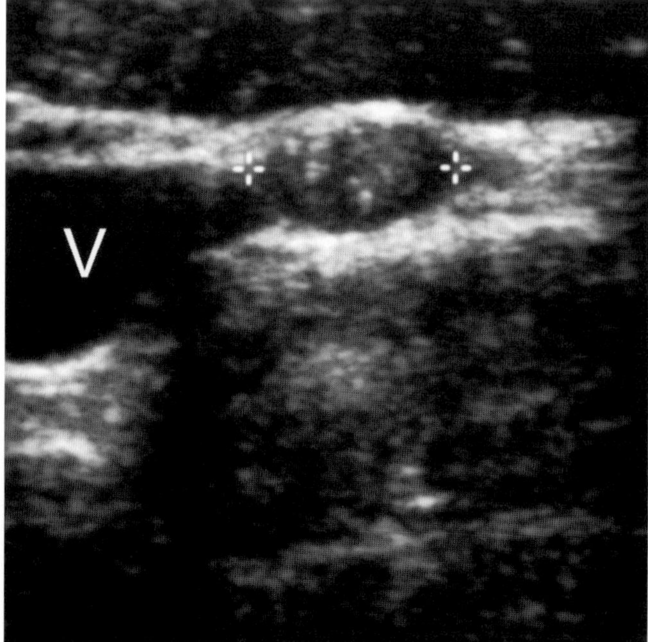

FIGURE 27 ■ Malignant lymph node. Transverse image of the left neck shows a solid, hypoechoic mass with punctate internal calcifications adjacent to the left internal jugular vein (V). Fine-needle aspiration and pathology showed metastatic papillary cancer to the node.

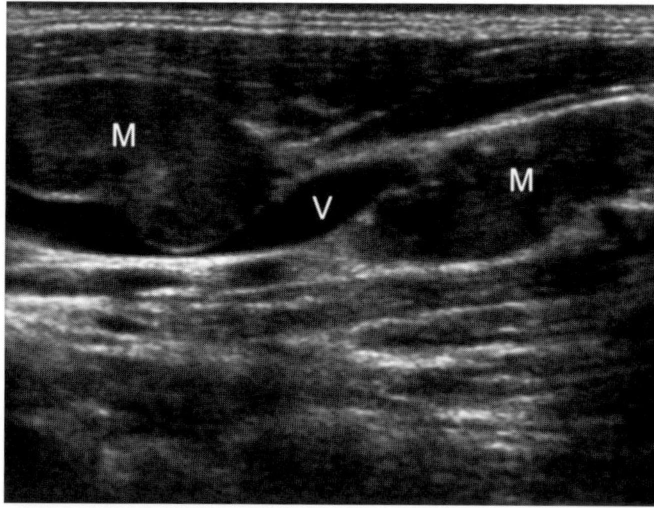

FIGURE 28 ■ Malignant lymph node. Longitudinal image of the right neck shows two large hypoechoic masses (M) indenting the anterior and posterior aspects of the right internal jugular vein (V). These masses are proven metastatic medullary carcinoma.

technique, patience, and practice. In addition, abnormal color Doppler findings most often appear in nodes that are already suspicious based on the gray-scale findings (136) and there is some overlap in color Doppler findings between benign and malignant nodes (144). The addition of sonographic contrast material may help improve identification of nodal metastases in the future (145).

In 2007, the evaluation of a postthyroidectomy patient for metastatic disease should include some knowledge of the type of cancer (aggressive vs. low risk), the side of malignancy, and the relevant blood work. Thyroglobulin levels are elevated in most patients with recurrent papillary cancer unless the patient has antibodies to thyroglobulin. Likewise, calcitonin is elevated in patients with recurrent medullary thyroid cancer. Although all patients with a history of thyroid cancer should undergo thorough sonographic evaluation of the neck, a rigorous approach is imperative in those patients with hematologic evidence of recurrent cancer, and lesions as small as 3 mm should be reported.

FNA of Nodes

Because of considerable overlap in the size and appearance of benign and malignant lymph nodes, percutaneous FNA of suspicious-appearing nodes is advocated, using the same techniques described earlier (see the section entitled Fine-Needle Aspiration Biopsy) (146–149). With meticulous technique, nodes as small as 3 mm in diameter can be safely and accurately sampled. Definitive tissue diagnosis is extremely useful for the patient and the surgeon when planning treatment options. ETOH injection for nonoperative treatment of metastatic nodes is another option for patients who are not surgical candidates (150).

Intraoperative Localization of Nodes

Surgical resection of metastatic nodes can be challenging, as it can be difficult to localize a tiny node at operation, particularly in patients with scarring from the primary thyroidectomy. Even if the radiologist is present in the operating room and scans the open neck, distortion of the tissues makes landmark localization difficult if not impossible, as the patient is intubated, the neck hyperextended, and sonographic landmarks gone. A technique for intraoperative needle localization of an abnormal node has been described (151). Our technique for localization of thyroid cancer recurrence has evolved to a simple and easy method. For patients with recurrent disease identified preoperatively and confirmed on FNA, we arrive with our US machine in the operating room immediately after the patient has been placed under anesthesia and the neck positioned by the surgeon. Before the patient is prepped and draped, the radiologist scans the neck, identifies the abnormal node or nodes as well as landmarks for localization, and the skin over the lesion is marked. The radiologist can then leave the room, and the surgeon can proceed with minimally invasive resection. This has proved successful and efficient for both imagers and surgeons in our busy institution.

REFERENCES

1. Solbiati L, Livraghi T, Ballarati E, Rizzatto G. Thyroid gland. In: Solbiati L, Rizzatto G, eds. Ultrasound of Superficial Structures: High Frequencies, Doppler and Interventional Procedures. New York: Churchill Livingstone, 1995:49–85.
2. AIUM practice guideline for the performance of a thyroid and parathyroid ultrasound examination. J Ultrasound Med 2003; 22:1126–1130.
3. Shapiro RS, Simpson WL, Rausch DL, Yeh HC. Compound spatial sonography of the thyroid gland: evaluation of freedom from artifacts and of nodule conspicuity. AJR Am J Roentgenol 2001; 177:1195–1198.
4. Szopinski K, Wysocki M, Pajk AM, Slapa RZ, Jakubowski W, Szopinska M. Tissue harmonic imaging of thyroid nodules. J Ultrasound Med 2003; 22:5–12.
5. Lyshchik A, Higashi T, Asato R, et al. Thyroid gland tumor diagnosis at US elastography. Radiology 2005; 237:202–211.
6. Spiezia S, Farian R, Cerbone G, et al. Analysis of color Doppler signal intensity variation after Levovist injection. J Ultrasound Med 2001; 20:223–231.
7. Calliada F, Pallavicini D, Pasamonti M, et al. Topical role and future perspectives of sonographic contrast agents in the differential diagnosis of solid thyroid lesions. Rays 2000; 25:191–197.
8. Kerr L. High-resolution thyroid ultrasound: the value of color Doppler. Ultrasound Q 1994; 12:21–43.
9. Ueda D, Mitamura R, Suzuki N, Yano K, Okuno A. Sonographic imaging of the thyroid gland in congenital hypothyroidism. Pediatr Radiol 1992; 22:102–105.
10. Muir A, Daneman D, Daneman A, Ehrlich R. Thyroid scanning, ultrasound and serum thyroglobulin in determining the origin of congenital hypothyroidism. Am J Dis Child 1988; 142:214–218.
11. Wiest PW, Hartshorne MF, Inskip PD, et al. Thyroid palpation versus high-resolution thyroid ultrasonography in the detection of nodules. J Ultrasound Med 1998; 17:487–496.
12. Carroll BA. Asymptomatic thyroid nodules: incidental sonographic detection. AJR Am J Roentgenol 1982; 133:499–501.
13. Brander A, Viikinkoski P, Nickels J, Kivisaari L. Thyroid gland: US screening in a random adult population. Radiology 1991; 181:683–687.
14. Bruneton JN, Balu-Maestro C, Marcy PY, Melia P, Mourou MY. Very high frequency (13 MHz) ultrasonographic examination of the normal neck: detection of normal lymph nodes and thyroid nodules. J Ultrasound Med 1994; 13:87–90.
15. Mortenson J, Woolner L, Bennett W. Gross and microscopic findings in clinically normal thyroid glands. J Clin Endocrinol Metab 1955; 15:1270–1280.
16. Marqusee E, Benson CB, Frates MC, et al. Usefulness of ultrasonography in the management of nodular thyroid disease. Ann Intern Med 2000; 133:696–700.
17. Papini E, Guglielmi R, Bianchini A, et al. Risk of malignancy in nonpalpable thyroid nodules: predictive value of ultrasound and color Doppler features. J Clin Endocrinol Metab 2002; 87:1941–1946.
18. Hegedus L, Bonema SJ, Bennedbaek FN. Management of simple nodular goiter: current status and future perspectives. Endocr Rev 2003; 24:102–132.
19. Kunreuther E, Orcutt J, Benson CB, et al. Prevalence and distribution of carcinoma in the uninodular and multinodular goiter. 76th Annual Meeting of the American Thyroid Association, Vancouver, BC, 2004.
20. Nam-Goong IS, Kim HY, Gong G, et al. Ultrasonography-guided fine-needle aspiration of thyroid incidentaloma: correlation with pathological findings. Clin Endocrinol 2004; 60:21–28.
21. Frates MC, Benson CB, Doubilet PM, et al. Likelihood of thyroid cancer based on sonographic assessment of nodule size and composition. Radiological Society of North America, RSNA, Inc., Chicago, IL, 2004.
22. DeLellis R. The endocrine system. In: Cotran RS, Kumar V, Robbins SL, eds. Robbins Pathologic Basis of Disease. Philadelphia: WB Saunders, 1989:1214–1284.
23. Mazzaferri EL. Management of a solitary thyroid nodule. N Engl J Med 1993; 328:553–559.

24. Murray D, Kovacs K, Asa SL. The thyroid gland. In: Kovacs K, ed. Functional Endocrine Pathology. Blackwell Scientific, 1991:293–374.
25. Cibas ES. Thyroid. In: Cibas ES, Ducatman BS, eds. Cytology: Diagnostic Principles and Clinical Correlates. New York: Saunders, 2003:247–272.
26. Gilliland FD, Hunt WC, Morris DM, Key CR. Prognostic factors for thyroid carcinoma: a population-based study of 15,698 cases from the surveillance, epidemiology and end results (SEER) program 1973–1991. Cancer 1997; 79:564–573.
27. Jemal A, Murray T, Ward E, Tiwari RC, Feuer EF, Thun MJ. Cancer statistics, 2005. CA Cancer J Clin 2005; 55:10–30.
28. Maitra A, Abbas AK. The endocrine system. In: Kumar V, Abbas A, Fausto N, eds. Robbins & Cotran Pathologic Basis of Disease. Philadelphia: Saunders, 1994:1155–1226.
29. Schlumberger MJ. Papillary and follicular thyroid carcinoma. N Engl J Med 1998; 338:297–306.
30. Shattuck TM, Westra WH, Ladenson PW, Arnold A. Independent clonal origins of distinct tumor foci in multifocal papillary thyroid carcinoma. N Engl J Med 2005; 352:2406–2412.
31. Cooper DS, Specker B, Ho M, et al. Thyrotropin suppression and disease progression in patients with differentiated thyroid cancer: results from the National Thyroid Cancer Treatment Cooperative Registry. Thyroid 1998; 8:737–744.
32. Pujol P, Daures J-P, Nsakala N, Baldet L, Bringer J, Jaffiol C. Degree of thyrotropin suppression as a prognostic determinant in differentiated thyroid cancer. J Clin Endocrinol Metab 1996; 81:4318–4323.
33. Gritzmann N, Koischwitz D, Rettenbacher T. Sonography of the thyroid and parathyroid glands. Radiol Clin North Am 2000; 38:1131–1145.
34. Gooding GA. Sonography of the thyroid and parathyroid. Radiol Clin North Am 1993; 31:967–989.
35. Holm LE, Blomgren H, Lowhagen T. Cancer risks in patients with chronic lymphocytic thyroiditis. N Engl J Med 1985; 312:601–604.
36. Pickhardt PJ, Pickard RH. Sonography of delayed thyroid metastasis from renal cell carcinoma with jugular vein extension. AJR Am J Roentgenol 2003; 181.
37. Tsou PL, Chang TC. Ultrasonographic and cytologic findings of metastatic cancer in the thyroid gland. J Formos Med Assoc 2001; 100:106–112.
38. Hermus AR. Clinical manifestations and treatment of nontoxic diffuse and nodular goiter. In: Braverman LE, ed. Werner & Ingbar's The Thyroid. A Fundamental and Clinical Text. Philadelphia, PA: Lippincott Williams & Wilkins, 2000:867.
39. Belfiore A, LaRosa GL, LaPorta GA, et al. Cancer risk in patients with cold thyroid nodules: relevance of iodine intake, sex, age, and multinodularity. Am J Med 1992; 93:363–369.
40. Sherman SI, Angelos P, Ball D, et al. Thyroid carcinoma. J Natl Comprehensive Canc Netw 2005; 3:404–457.
41. Khoo MLC, Asa SL, Witterick IJ, Freeman JL. Thyroid calcification and its association with thyroid carcinoma. Head Neck 2002; 24:651–655.
42. Peccin S, de Castro JAS, Furlanetto TW, Furtado APA, Brasil BA, Czepielewski MA. Ultrasonography: is it useful in the diagnosis of cancer in thyroid nodules? J Endocrinol Invest 2002; 25:39–43.
43. Chan BK, Desser TS, McDougall IR, Weigel RJ, Jeffrey RB. Common and uncommon sonographic features of papillary thyroid carcinoma. J Ultrasound Med 2003; 22:1083–1090.
44. Kim E-K, Park CS, Chung WY, et al. New sonographic criteria for recommending fine-needle aspiration biopsy of nonpalpable solid nodules of the thyroid. AJR Am J Roentgenol 2002; 178:687–691.
45. Iannuccilli JD, Cronan JJ, Monchik JM. Risk for malignancy of thyroid nodules as assessed by sonographic criteria. J Ultrasound Med 2004; 23:1455–1464.
46. Frates MC, Benson CB, Doubilet PM, Cibas ES, Marqusee E. Can color Doppler sonography aid in the prediction of malignancy of thyroid nodules? J Ultrasound Med 2003; 22:127–131.
47. Pacella CM, Guglielmi R, Fabbrini R, et al. Papillary carcinoma in small hypoechoic thyroid nodules: predictive value of echo color Doppler evaluation: preliminary results. J Exp Clin Cancer Res 1998; 17:127–128.
48. Holden A. The role of colour and duplex Doppler ultrasound in the assessment of thyroid nodules. Australas Radiol 1995; 39:343–349.
49. Ahuja A, Chick W, King W, Metreweli C. Clinical significance of the comet-tail artifact in thyroid ultrasound. J Clin Ultrasound 1996; 24:129–133.
50. Wienke JR, Chong WK, Fielding JR, Zou KH, Mittelstaedt CA. Sonographic features of benign thyroid nodules: interobserver reliability and overlap with malignancy. J Ultrasound Med 2003; 22:1027–1031.
51. Frates MC, Benson CB, Charboneau JW, et al. Management of thyroid nodules detected at US: Society of Radiologists in Ultrasound consensus conference statement. Radiology 2005; 237:794–800.
52. Liebeskind A, Sikora AG, Komisar A, Slavit D, Fried K. Rates of malignancy in incidentally discovered thyroid nodules evaluated with sonography and fine-needle aspiration. J Ultrasound Med 2005; 24:629–634.
53. Hagag P, Strauss S, Weiss M. Role of ultrasound-guided fine-needle aspiration biopsy in evaluation of nonpalpable thyroid nodules. Thyroid 1998; 8:989–995.
54. Gharib H, Goellner JR. Fine-needle aspiration biopsy of the thyroid: an appraisal. Ann Intern Med 1993; 118:282–289.
55. Court-Payen M, Nygaard B, Horn T, et al. US-guided fine-needle aspiration biopsy of thyroid nodules. Acta Radiol 2002; 43:131–140.
56. Cochand-Priollet B, Guillausseau P-J, Chagnon S, et al. The diagnostic value of fine-needle aspiration biopsy under ultrasonography in nonfunctional thyroid nodules: a prospective study comparing cytologic and histologic findings. Am J Med 1994; 97:152–157.
57. Alexander EK, Hurwitz S, Heering JP, et al. Natural history of benign solid and cystic thyroid nodules. Ann Intern Med 2003; 138:315–318.
58. McHenry CR, Walfish PG, Rosen IB. Non-diagnostic fine needle aspiration biopsy: a dilemma in management of nodular thyroid disease. Am Surg 1993; 59:415–419.
59. Chow LS, Gharib H, Goellner JR, van Heerden JA. Nondiagnostic thyroid fine-needle aspiration cytology: management dilemmas. Thyroid 2001; 11:1147–1151.
60. Screaton NJ, Berman LH, Grant JW. US-guided core-needle biopsy of the thyroid gland. Radiology 2003; 226:827–832.
61. Taki S, Kakuda K, Kakuma K, et al. Thyroid nodules: evaluation with US-guided core biopsy with an automated biopsy gun. Radiology 1997; 202:874–878.
62. Quadbeck B, Pruellage J, Roggenbuck U, et al. Long-term follow-up of thyroid nodule growth. Exp Clin Endocrinol Diabetes 2002; 110:348–354.
63. Brander AEE, Viikinkoski VP, Nickels JI, Kivisaari LM. Importance of thyroid abnormalities detected at US screening: a 5-year follow-up. Radiology 2000; 215:801–806.
64. Pacella CM, Bizzarri G, Spiezia S, et al. Thyroid tissue: US-guided percutaneous laser thermal ablation. Radiology 2004; 232:272–280.
65. Dossing H, Bennedbaek FN, Karstrup S, Legedus L. Benign solitary solid cold thyroid nodules: US-guided interstitial laser photocoagulation- initial experience. Radiology 2002; 225:53–57.
66. Livraghi T, Paracchi A, Ferrari C, et al. Treatment of autonomous thyroid nodules with percutaneous ethanol injection: preliminary results. Radiology 1990; 175:827–829.
67. Livraghi R, Paracchi A, Ferrari C, Reschini E, Macchi RM, Bonifacino A. Treatment of autonomous thyroid nodules with percutaneous ethanol injection: 4-year experience. Radiology 1994; 190:529–533.
68. Spiezia S, Cerbone G, Assanti AP, Colao A, Siciliani M, Lombardi G. Power Doppler ultrasonographic assistance in percutaneous ethanol injection of autonomously functioning thyroid nodules. J Ultrasound Med 2000; 19:39–46.
69. Lewis BD, Charboneau JW, Reading CC. Ultrasound-guided biopsy and ablation in the neck. Ultrasound Q 2002; 18:3–12.
70. Kouvaraki MA, Shapiro SE, Fornage BD, et al. Role of preoperative ultrasonography in the surgical management of patients with thyroid cancer. Surgery 2003; 134:946–955.
71. do Rosario PWS, Fagundes TA, Maia FFR, Franco ACHM, Figueireo MB, Purisch S. Sonography in the diagnosis of cervical recurrence in patients with differentiated thyroid carcinoma. J Ultrasound Med 2004; 23:915–920.

72. Frasoldati A, Pesenti M, Gallo M, Caroggio A, Salvo D, Valcavi R. Diagnosis of neck recurrences in patients with differentiated thyroid carcinoma. Cancer 2003; 97:90–96.
73. Wunderbaldinger P, Harisinghani MG, Hahn PF, et al. Cystic lymph node metastases in papillary thyroid carcinoma. AJR Am J Roentgenol 2002; 178:693–697.
74. Langer J, Luster E, Horii SC, Mandel SJ, Baloch ZW, Coleman BG. Chronic granulomatous lesions after thyroidectomy: imaging findings. AJR Am J Roentgenol 2005; 185:1350–1354.
75. Zakarija M, McKenzie JM, Banovac K. Clinical significance of assay of thyroid-stimulating antibody in Graves' disease. Ann Intern Med 1980; 93:28–32.
76. Weetman AP. Graves' disease. N Engl J Med 2000; 343:1236–1248.
77. James EM, Charboneau JW, Hay ID. The thyroid. In: Rumack CM, Wilson SR, Charboneau JW, eds. Diagnostic Ultrasound. Vol. 1. St. Louis: Mosby Year Book, 1991:507–523.
78. Ralls PW, Mayekawa DS, Lee KP, et al. Color-flow Doppler sonography in Graves' disease: "thyroid inferno." AJR Am J Roentgenol 1988; 150:781–784.
79. Castagnone D, Rivolta R, Rescalli S, Baldini MI, Tozzi R, Cantalamessa L. Color Doppler sonography in Graves' disease: value in assessing activity of disease and predicting outcome. AJR Am J Roentgenol 1996; 166:203–207.
80. Saleh A, Cohnen M, Furst G, Modder U, Feldkamp J. Prediction of relapse after antithyroid drug therapy of Graves' disease: value of color Doppler sonography. Exp Clin Endocrinol Diabetes 2004; 112:510–513.
81. Varsamidis K, Varsamidou E, Mavropoulos G. Doppler ultrasonography in predicting relapse of hyperthyroidism in Graves' disease. Acta Radiol 2000; 41:45–48.
82. Pearce EN, Farwell AP, Braverman LE. Thyroiditis. N Engl J Med 2003; 348:2646–2655.
83. Yeh HC, Futterweit W, Gilbert P. Micronodulation: ultrasonographic sign of Hashimoto thyroiditis. J Ultrasound Med 1996; 15:813–819.
84. Brander A. Ultrasound appearances in de Quervain's subacute thyroiditis with long-term follow-up. J Intern Med 1992; 232.
85. Hiromatsu Y, Ishibashi M, Miyake I, et al. Color Doppler ultrasonography in patients with subacute thyroiditis. Thyroid 1999; 9:1189–1193.
86. Bogazzi F, Martino E, Dell'Unto E, et al. Thyroid color flow Doppler sonography and radioiodine uptake in 55 consecutive patients with amiodarone-induced thyrotoxicosis. J Endocrinol Invest 2003; 26:635–640.
87. Sato K, Miyakawa M, Eto M, et al. Clinical characteristics of amiodarone-induced thyrotoxicosis and hypothyroidism in Japan. Endocr J 1999; 46:443–451.
88. Mittendorf EA, Tamarkin SW, McHenry CR. The results of ultrasound guided fine-needle aspiration biopsy for evaluation of nodular thyroid disease. Surgery 2002; 132:648–654.
89. Danese D, Sciacchitano S, Farsetti A, Andreoli M, Pontecorvi A. Diagnostic accuracy of conventional versus sonography-guided fine-needle aspiration biopsy of thyroid nodules. Thyroid 1998; 8:15–21.
90. Bellatone R, Lombardi CP, Raffaelli M, et al. Management of cystic or predominantly cystic thyroid nodules: the role of ultrasound-guided fine-needle aspiration biopsy. Thyroid 2004; 14: 43–47.
91. O'Malley ME, Weir MM, Hahn PF, Misdraji J, Wood BJ, Mueller PR. US-guided fine-needle aspiration biopsy of thyroid nodules: adequacy of cytologic material and procedure time with and without immediate cytologic analysis. Radiology 2002; 222:383–387.
92. Gharib H. Fine-needle aspiration biopsy of thyroid nodules: advantages, limitations, and effect. Mayo Clin Proc 1994;69:44–49.
93. Hegedus L. The thyroid nodule. N Engl J Med 2004; 351:1764–1771.
94. Kim JH, Lee HK, Lee JH, Ahn IM, Choi CG. Efficacy of sonographically guided percutaneous ethanol injection for treatment of thyroid cysts versus solid thyroid nodules. AJR Am J Roentgenol 2003; 180:1723–1726.
95. Goldfarb WB, Bigos ST, Nishiyama RH. Percutaneous tetracycline instillation for sclerosis of recurrent thyroid cysts. Surgery 1987; 102:1096–1100.
96. Ozdemir H, Ilget ET, Yucel C, et al. Treatment of autonomous thyroid nodules: safety and efficacy of sonographically guided percutaneous injection of ethanol. AJR Am J Roentgenol 1994; 163:929–932.
97. Reading CC. Ultrasound-guided percutaneous ethanol ablation of solid and cystic masses of the liver, kidney, thyroid and parathyroid. Ultrasound Q 1994; 12:67.
98. Goletti O, Monzani F, Lenziardi M. Cold thyroid nodules: a new application of percutaneous ethanol injection treatment. J Clin Ultrasound 1994; 22:175–178.
99. Gilmour J. The gross anatomy of the parathyroid glands. J Pathol Bacteriol 1938; 46:133.
100. Akerstrom G, Malmaeus J, Bergstrom R. Surgical anatomy of human parathyroid glands. Surgery 1984; 95:14–21.
101. Doppman JL, Shawker TH, Krudy AG, et al. Parathymic parathyroid: CT, US, and angiographic findings. Radiology 1985; 157:419–423.
102. Freitas JE, Freitas AE. Thyroid and parathyroid imaging. Semin Nucl Med 1994; 24:234–245.
103. Price DC. Radioisotopic evaluation of the thyroid and the parathyroids. Radiol Clin North Am 1993; 31:991–1015.
104. Wang CA. Parathyroid re-exploration: a clinical and pathological study of 112 cases. Ann Surg 1977; 186:140–145.
105. Meilstrup JW. Ultrasound examination of the parathyroid glands. Otolaryngol Clin N Am 2004; 37:763–778.
106. Marx SJ. Hyperparathyroid and hypoparathyroid disorders. N Engl J Med 2000; 343:1863–1875.
107. Frasoldati A, Pesenti M, Toschi E, Azzarito C, Zini M, Valcavi R. Detection and diagnosis of parathyroid incidentalomas during thyroid sonography. J Clin Ultrasound 1999; 27:492–498.
108. Reeder SB, Desser TS, Weigel RJ, Jeffrey RB. Sonography in primary hyperparathyroidism. J Ultrasound Med 2002; 21: 539–552.
109. Wolf RJ, Cronan JJ, Monchik JM. Color Doppler sonography: an adjunctive technique in assessment of parathyroid adenomas. J Ultrasound Med 1994; 13:303–308.
110. Lane MJ, Desser TS, Weigel RJ, Jeffrey RB. Use of color and power Doppler sonography to identify feeding arteries associated with parathyroid adenomas. AJR Am J Roentgenol 1998; 171:819–823.
111. Scheiner JD, Dupuy DE, Monchik JM, Noto RB, Cronan JJ. Preoperative localization of parathyroid adenomas: a comparison of power and colour Doppler ultrasonography with nuclear medicine scintigraphy. Clin Radiol 2001; 56:984–988.
112. De Feo ML, Colagrande S, Biagini C, et al. Parathyroid glands: combination of 99mTc MIBI scintigraphy and US for demonstration of parathyroid glands and nodules. Radiology 2000; 214: 393–402.
113. Mazzeo S, Caramella D, Marcocci C, et al. Contrast-enhanced color Doppler ultrasonography in suspected parathyroid lesions. Acta Radiol 2000; 41:412–416.
114. Gilat H, Cohen M, Feinmesser R, et al. Minimally invasive procedure for resection of a parathyroid adenoma: the role of preoperative high-resolution ultrasonography. J Clin Ultrasound 2005; 33: 283–287.
115. van Dalen A, Smit CP, van Vroonhoven TJMV, Burger H, de Lange EE. Minimally invasive surgery for solitary parathyroid adenomas in patients with primary hyperparathyroidism: role of US with supplemental CT. Radiology 2001; 220:631–639.
116. Siperstein A, Berber E, Mackey R, Alghoul M, Wagner K, Milas M. Prospective evaluation of sestamibi scan, ultrasonography, and rapid PTH to predict the success of limited exploration for sporadic primary hyperparathyroidism. Surgery 2004; 136: 872–880.
117. Edmonson GR, Charboneau JW, James EM, Reading CC, Grant CS. Parathyroid carcinoma: high frequency sonography features. Radiology 1986; 161:65–67.
118. Snell SB, Gaar EE, Stevens SP, Flynn MB. Parathyroid cancer, a continued diagnostic and therapeutic dilemma: report of four cases and review of the literature. Am Surg 2003; 69:711–716.
119. Jha BC, Nagarkar NM, Kochhart S, Mohan H, Dass A. Parathyroid cyst: a rare cause of an anterior neck mass. J Laryngol Otol 1999; 113:73–75.

120. Sacks BA, Pallotta JA, Cole A, Hurwitz J. Diagnosis of parathyroid adenomas: efficacy of measuring parathormone levels in needle aspirates of cervical masses. AJR Am J Roentgenol 1994; 163:1223–1226.
121. Karstrup S, Glenthoj A, Hainau B, Hegedus L, Torp-Pedersen S, Holm HH. Ultrasound-guided, histological, fine-needle biopsy from suspect parathyroid tumours: success-rate and reliability of histological diagnosis. Br J Radiol 1989; 62:981–985.
122. Bergenfelz A, Forsberg L, Hederstrom E, Ahren B. Preoperative localization of enlarged parathyroid glands with ultrasonically guided fine needle aspiration for parathyroid hormone assay. Acta Radiol 1991; 32:403–405.
123. Karstrup S, Hegedus L, Holm HH. Ultrasonically guided chemical parathyroidectomy in patients with primary hyperparathyroidism: a follow up study. Clin Endocrinol (Oxf) 1993; 38:523–530.
124. Solbiati L, Giangrande A, De Pra L. Percutaneous ethanol injection of parathyroid tumors under US guidance: treatment for secondary hyperparathyroidism. Radiology 1985; 155:607–610.
125. Karstrup S, Transbol I, Holm HH. Ultrasound-guided chemical parathyroidectomy in patients with primary hyperparathyroidism: a prospective study. Br J Radiol 1989; 62:1037–1042.
126. Kitaoka M, Fukagawa M, Ogata E. Reduction of functioning parathyroid cell mass by ethanol injection in chronic dialysis patients. Kidney Int 1994; 46:1110–1117.
127. Fugazzola C, Bergamo AI, Solbiati L. Parathyroid glands. In: Solbiati L, Rizzatto G, eds. Ultrasound of Superficial Structures. New York: Churchill Livingstone, 1995:87–97.
128. Som PM, Sacher M, Lanzieri CF, et al. Parenchymal cysts of the lower neck. Radiology 1985; 157:399–406.
129. Benson MT, Dalen K, Mancuso AA. Congenital anomalies of the branchial apparatus: embryology and pathologic anatomy. Radiographics 1992; 12:943–960.
130. Zadvinskis DP, Benson MT, Kerr HH, et al. Congenital malformations of the cervicothoracic lymphatic system: embryology and pathogenesis. Radiographics 1992; 12:1175–1189.
131. Ahuja AT, King AD, King W, Metreweli C. Thyroglossal duct cysts: sonographic appearances in adults. Am J Neuroradiol 1999; 20:579–582.
132. Wadsworth DT, Siegel MJ. Thyroglossal duct cysts: variability of sonographic findings. AJR Am J Roentgenol 1994; 163:1475–1477.
133. Lim-Dunham JE, Feinstein KA, Yousefzadeh DK, Ben-Ami T. Sonographic demonstration of a normal thyroid gland excludes ectopic thyroid in patients with thyroglossal duct cyst. AJR Am J Roentgenol 1995; 164:1489–1491.
134. Koischwitz D, Gritzmann N. Ultrasound of the neck. Radiol Clin North Am 2000; 38:1029–1045.
135. Remine WH. Branchial cleft cysts and sinuses: their embryologic development and surgical management. Surg Clin North Am 1963; 43:1033–1039.
136. Gritzmann N, Hollerweger A, Macheiner P, Rettenbacher T. Sonography of soft tissue masses of the neck. J Clin Ultrasound 2002; 30:356–373.
137. Zweibel WJ, Pellerito JS. Carotid occlusion, unusual carotid pathology and tricky carotid cases. In: Zweibel WJ, Pellerito JS, eds. Introduction to Vascular Sonography. New York: Elsevier Saunders, 2000:199–200.
138. Rosario PWS, de Faria S, Bicalho L, et al. Ultrasonographic differentiation between metastatic and benign lymph nodes in patients with papillary thyroid carcinoma. J Ultrasound Med 2005; 24:1385–1389.
139. Ying M, Ahuja A, Metreweli C. Diagnostic accuracy of sonographic criteria for evaluation of cervical lymphadenopathy. J Ultrasound Med 1998; 17:437–445.
140. Ahuja AT, Ying M. Sonographic evaluation of cervical lymph nodes. AJR Am J Roentgenol 2005; 184:1691–1699.
141. Tschammler A, Ott G, Schang T, Seelbach-Goebel B, Schwager K, Hahn D. Lymphadenopathy: differentiation of benign from malignant disease-color Doppler US assessment of intranodal angioarchitecture. Radiology 1998; 208:117–123.
142. Na DG, Lim HK, Byun HS, Kim HD, Ko YH, Baek JH. Differential diagnosis of cervical lymphadenopathy: usefulness of color Doppler sonography. AJR Am J Roentgenol 1997; 168:1311–1316.
143. Wu CH, Chang YL, Hsu WC, Ko JY, Sheen TS, Hsieh FJ. Usefulness of Doppler spectral analysis and power Doppler sonography in the differentiation of cervical lymphadenopathies. AJR Am J Roentgenol 1998; 171:503–509.
144. Chang DB, Yuan A, Yu CJ, Luh KT, Kuo SH, Yang PC. Differentiation of benign and malignant cervical lymph nodes with color Doppler sonography. AJR Am J Roentgenol 1994; 162:965–968.
145. Moritz JD, Ludwig A, Oestmann JW. Contrast-enhanced color Doppler sonography for evaluation of enlarged cervical lymph nodes in head and neck tumors. AJR Am J Roentgenol 2000; 174:1279–1284.
146. van den Brekel MW, Castelijns JA, Snow GB. Detection of lymph node metastases in the neck: radiologic criteria. Radiology 1994; 192:617–618.
147. Boland GW, Lee MJ, Mueller PR, Mayo-Smith W, Dawson SL, Simeone JF. Efficacy of sonographically guided biopsy of thyroid masses and cervical lymph nodes. AJR Am J Roentgenol 1993; 161:1053–1056.
148. Chang D, Yan P, Yu C. Ultrasonography and ultrasonographically guided fine-needle aspiration biopsy of impalpable cervical lymph nodes in patients with non-small cell lung cancer. Cancer 1992; 70:1111–1114.
149. Lee MJ, Ross DS, Muller PR. Fine-needle biopsy of cervical lymph nodes in patients with thyroid cancer: a prospective comparison of cytopathologic and tissue marker analysis. Radiology 1993; 187:851–854.
150. Lewis BD, Hay ID, Charboneau JW, McIver B, Reading CC, Goellner JR. Percutaneous ethanol injection for treatment of cervical lymph node metastases in patients with papillary thyroid carcinoma. AJR Am J Roentgenol 2002; 178:699–704.
151. Zimmerman P, DaSilva M, Izquierdo R, Cico L, Kort K, Numann P. Intraoperative needle localization during neck reexploration. Am J Surg 2004; 188:92–93.

Ultrasound and the Trauma Patient

John R. Richards and John P. McGahan

12

ABDOMINAL TRAUMA

Historical Perspective

The use of ultrasound for the detection of intra-abdominal injuries was first described more than 30 years ago (1). In a report published in 1976, the sensitivity of sonography for detection of splenic injury from blunt abdominal trauma was reported to be 80% (2). However, after these early reports, sonography was not routinely used for evaluation of blunt abdominal trauma, as the use of computed tomography (CT) for this indication became widespread. In the 1990s, sonography was utilized more frequently for screening patients with blunt abdominal trauma, as it could be performed during resuscitation (3,4). Thus, a new application for sonography was proposed, the focused abdominal sonography for trauma (FAST) examination. During this period, myriad studies were published reporting extremely high sensitivity and specificity for the FAST examination in detection of hemoperitoneum (5). Since then, more critical evaluations of FAST have appeared, especially regarding its high false-negative rate in stable trauma patients (6,7). Over time, a new role for FAST has evolved, in which its use in the evaluation of unstable, hypotensive trauma patients is emphasized (8). The utility of the FAST examination is now widely acknowledged, and FAST is being used in prehospital, combat, and veterinary settings as well as in outer space (9–12).

Anatomy

In the supine patient, the hepatorenal space is gravity dependent. Intraperitoneal free fluid may travel via the right paracolic gutter to or from this space. The left paracolic gutter is situated higher than the right, and the phrenicocolic ligament blocks flow to and from the splenorenal area; consequently, fluid tends to flow into the subphrenic area and not the splenorenal area (Fig. 1). This is significant because the subphrenic area may be difficult to visualize due to bowel and splenic flexure gas. Fluid in the pelvic region flows to the retrovesicular area in the male patient and to the pouch of Douglas in the female patient. These represent the most gravity-dependent areas of the pelvis. Given these anatomic relationships, the FAST examination has evolved from a single view of the hepatorenal fossa to multiple intraperitoneal views plus a cardiac view.

Procedure

The FAST examination has several procedural variants since its inception, which may partly be attributed to evolution of the procedure as well as different user and institutional preferences. The main focus of the FAST examination has been detection of free fluid within the abdomen of blunt trauma patients. One of the original studies on the use of sonography in trauma patients outlined a single view of the hepatorenal fossa, or Morison's pouch, to detect free fluid (3). However, the single view method has been abandoned in favor of a more comprehensive examination. At a

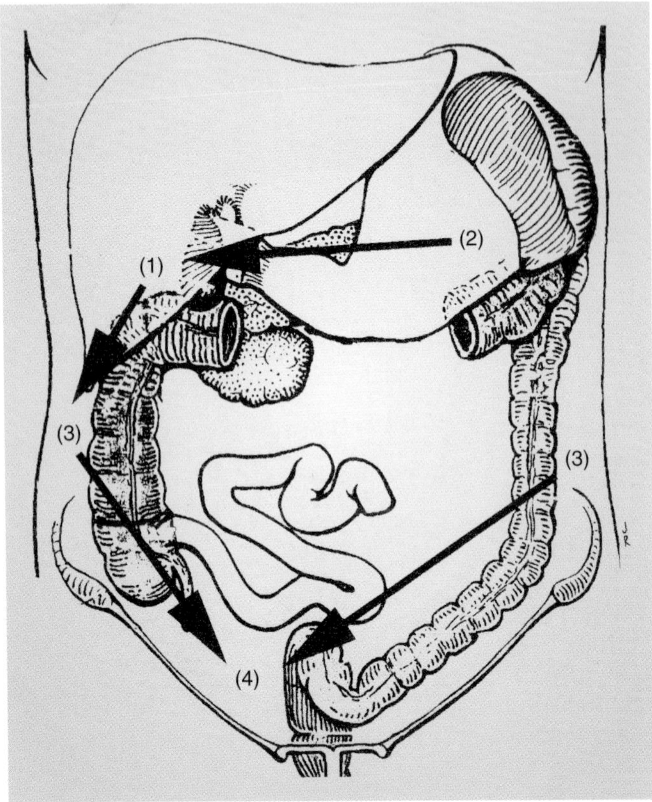

FIGURE 1 ■ Flow of intraperitoneal free fluid. The hepatorenal fossa (1), or Morison's pouch, receives fluid that originates from the splenorenal area (2). Flow continues down the paracolic gutters (3) and into the pelvis (4). The phrenicocolic ligament tends to obstruct flow from the splenorenal area to the left paracolic gutter.

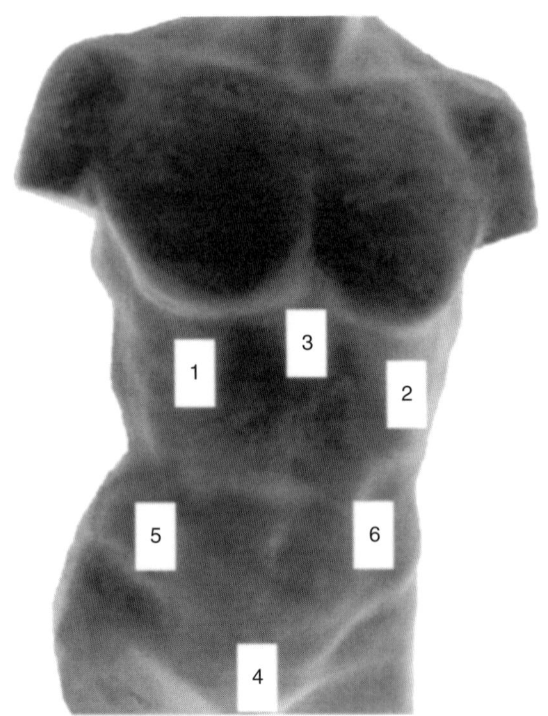

FIGURE 2 ■ The FAST (focused abdominal sonography for trauma) examination—common views. 1. hepatorenal area (Morison's pouch); 2. splenorenal area; 3. subcostal (subxiphoid); 4. pelvis; 5. right paracolic gutter; 6. left paracolic gutter. Additional views may include epigastric and parasternal depending on sonographer and institutional preference.

minimum, this involves scanning of the right upper quadrant, including the hepatorenal fossa and right chest; the left upper quadrant, including the perisplenic region and left chest; and longitudinal and transverse scans of the pelvis (Fig. 2). Further views include the right and left paracolic gutters, the epigastrium, and a subdiaphragmatic, parasternal, and/or intercostal view to assess for pericardial fluid. The FAST scan can be completed in less than five minutes. Although the bladder is not an intraperitoneal entity, a full bladder greatly enhances sonographic detection of free fluid within the pelvis by providing readily identifiable landmarks through an acoustic window and displacing overlying bowel. The paracolic gutter views are optional, and its inclusion in the FAST examination to improve accuracy has not been studied. Although the focus of the FAST examination is the detection of free fluid, additional scrutiny may be applied to the parenchyma of the spleen, liver, and kidneys for detection of solid organ injury.

Interpretation

The finding of free fluid during FAST in any location is considered a positive examination; however, one exception may be the visualization of small amounts of free fluid within the pelvis of women of childbearing age and children (Fig. 3). One study demonstrated a higher rate of intra-abdominal injury in female blunt trauma patients with pelvic free fluid, regardless of volume detected (14). It may thus be unwise to disregard the finding of minimal pelvic free fluid in the setting of trauma. The quantification of minimal pelvic free fluid has been studied. An average of 100 mL of pelvic free fluid was required to be visualized by FAST in one report (15). Quantification of free fluid has not been standardized and may be objectively measured in centimeters at its greatest width or subjectively described as small, moderate, and large. Free fluid will usually appear homogeneously hypoechoic but may be hypoechoic with a few internal echoes. At the site of the injured solid organ, there is often echogenic blood, which may be in the form of a subcapsular hematoma (Fig. 4). The echogenic fluid may be less obvious than the hypoechoic fluid but should not be overlooked, since it may pinpoint the site of injury. Free intraperitoneal fluid may also have mixed, swirling echogenicity representing active hemorrhage and clots (Fig. 5). It is otherwise difficult to distinguish ascites from intraperitoneal blood, and this is a common reason for false-positive scans. With regard to solid organs, aberrations of normally homogenous parenchymal architecture may be visualized, providing potential injury localization. Lacerations, hematomas, and contusions may be hyper- or hypoechoic, and the initial sonographic appearance may change over time.

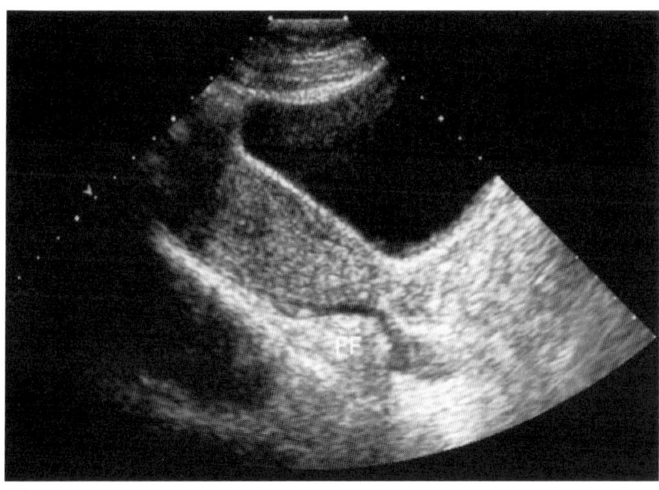

(A)

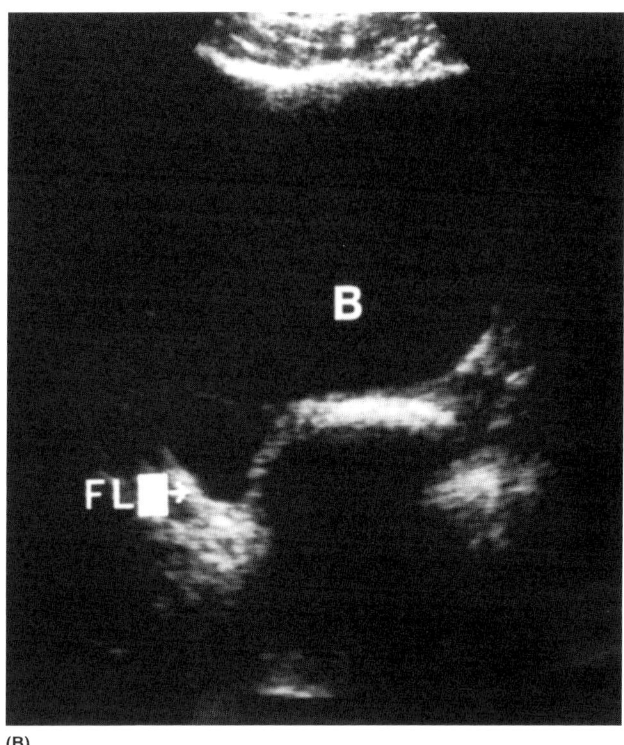

(B)

FIGURE 3 A AND B ■ Pelvic free fluid. (**A**) Longitudinal scan of the pelvis shows small amount of free fluid in the pouch of Douglas. The patient was later found to have a spleen laceration at laparotomy. (**B**) Transverse scan of the bladder reveals a small collection of free fluid (FL) inferior to the bladder (B). Ascending colon laceration was repaired at laparotomy. *Source*: From Ref. 13.

Free Fluid Scoring Methods

The first sonographic scoring method included a single view of Morison's pouch (Fig. 6). This was a simple all-or-none system for identification of a hypoechoic free fluid in the hepatorenal fossa. With this protocol, the authors reported a sensitivity of 82% (3). However, it became increasingly clear that a single view was insufficient. A later study demonstrated that when 400 mL of saline was infused in the peritoneal cavity during diagnostic peritoneal lavage with the patient in the Trendelenburg position, only 10% of patients had fluid identified in Morison's pouch (17). One liter of saline was necessary to identify fluid in Morison's pouch in 97% of cases. To develop a scoring

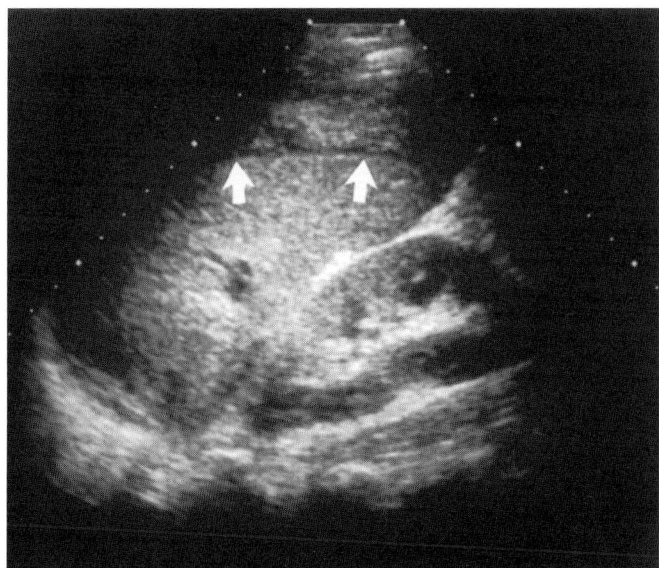

FIGURE 4 ■ Subcapsular spleen hematoma. Longitudinal scan of the left upper quadrant shows a hypoechoic crescent (*arrows*) representing a subcapsular hematoma. *Source*: From Ref. 16.

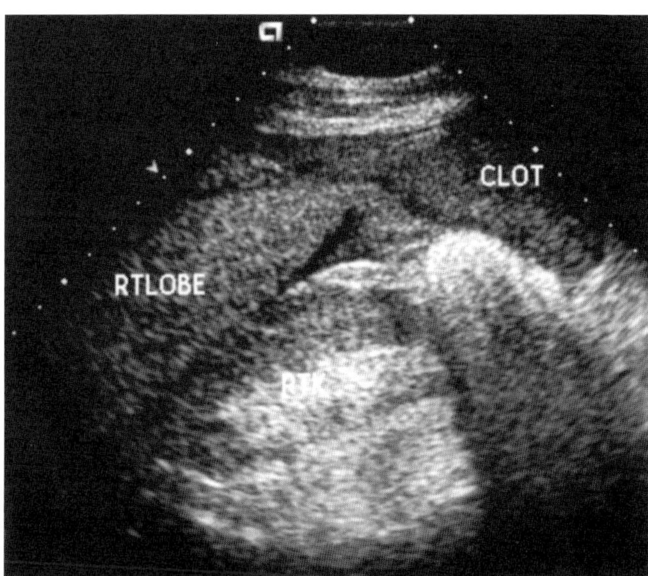

FIGURE 5 ■ Echogenic clot. Scan of the right upper quadrant reveals echogenic clot anterior and inferior to the right lobe of the liver. Note clot in the hepatorenal space.

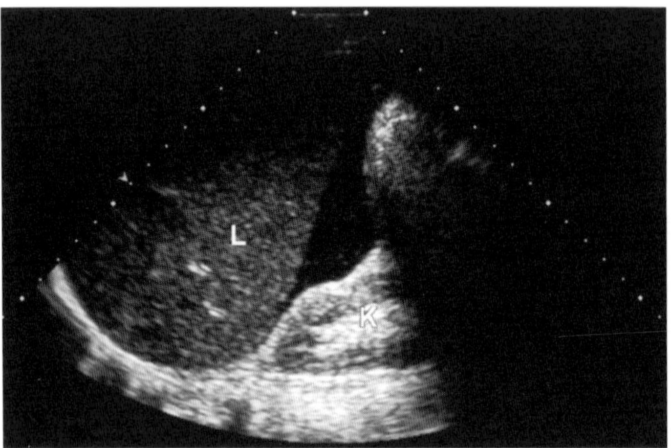

FIGURE 6 ■ Free fluid. Longitudinal scan of the right upper quadrant demonstrates a large amount of free fluid in Morison's pouch between the liver (L) and the kidney (K).

system for FAST that might predict injury, another research team determined each region or pocket of free fluid 2 mm or greater receive a score of 1 (18). Patients with three free fluid pockets, or a score of 3 or greater, proceeded to the operating room. Even with a score of less than 3, 38% of patients required surgery. In a subsequent study, another scoring system was proposed in which all vertical heights of intraperitoneal free fluid measured in centimeters were added (19). A score of greater than 3 was associated with an increased need for surgical intervention. The subphrenic, subhepatic, perisplenic, and pelvic locations represented the sites which would most often result in a need for surgery if fluid were isolated. Yet another group published two articles describing a novel scoring system (20,21). For each anatomic region in which fluid was detected, 1 point was given. With a score of 0, 1.4% of the patients had intra-abdominal injury; with a score of 1, 59% had injury; with a score of 2, 85% had injury; and with a score of 3, 83% had injury. Need for surgical intervention increased in parallel to patients' scores. From a practical standpoint, these myriad scoring methods have not found widespread recognition or use. However, there is a common theme between the systems. The increasing volume and number of locations of intraperitoneal free fluid detected by FAST directly correlates with likelihood of intra-abdominal injury.

Parenchymal Injury

The FAST examination was originally devised to detect intraperitoneal free fluid. However, sonography is well suited to detect abnormalities of solid organ parenchyma suggestive of injury. In 1983, a research team noted the appearance of blood in solid organs after fine-needle-aspiration biopsy (22). These hematomas appeared as linear echogenic foci within the parenchymal organs. Most research has not addressed this additional application of the FAST examination. One initial study had a 41% detection rate for solid organ injury, but other studies have not approached this figure (4). Although solid organ injury is infrequently identified during FAST, certain patterns become evident. A diffuse heterogeneous pattern is the predominant pattern visualized in splenic lacerations (Fig. 7), whereas a discrete hyperechoic pattern is shown most often in hepatic lacerations (Fig. 8) (16,23). For the spleen, subcapsular hematomas are detected as either hyperechoic or hypoechoic rims surrounding the parenchyma (Fig. 4). Splenic lacerations not detected by initial FAST tend to become hypoechoic over a few days. In kidneys, more severe injuries have mixed echogenicity and a disorganized pattern (Fig. 9) (24). Bladder hematomas may appear echogenic (Fig. 10).

Serial Examinations

The initial FAST examination represents an early snapshot in time. Serial FAST examinations performed as a part of a follow-up physical examination of the stable blunt trauma patient may be useful. Examination after stabilization allows the sonographer more time for a comprehensive examination. With active intraperitoneal hemorrhage, the amount of free fluid should increase with time and would be more amenable to sonographic detection. The value of serial sonography has not been fully investigated. One study group reported repeated FAST examinations in patients with deteriorating clinical status decreased the false-negative rate by 50% and increased the sensitivity for free fluid detection from 69% to 85% (25). A more recent study confirmed this trend, with sensitivity increasing from 31% to 72% (26). It should be emphasized these were stable blunt trauma patients, and the prevalence of false negatives is higher in this group than for unstable patients. Nevertheless, time and resources permitting, serial FAST examination may be a logical alternative for pregnant patients or those with low suspicion of intra-abdominal injury.

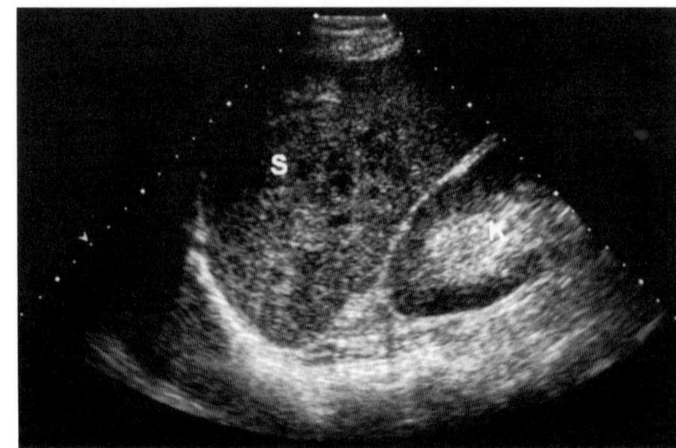

FIGURE 7 ■ Spleen laceration. Longitudinal scan of the left upper quadrant demonstrates a diffuse heterogenous parenchymal pattern of the spleen (S) but no free fluid.

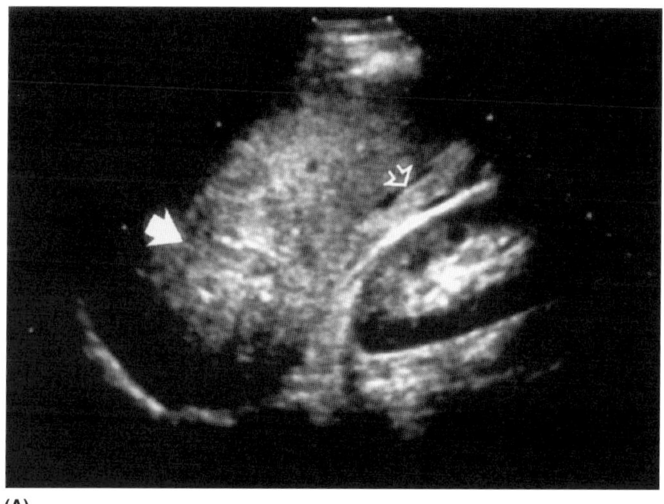
(A)

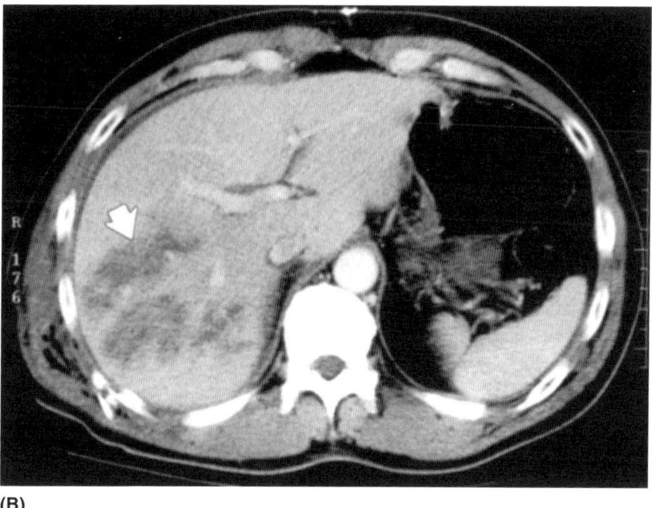
(B)

FIGURE 8 A AND B ■ Liver laceration. (**A**) The sonogram shows a diffuse hyperechoic pattern of liver parenchyma (*solid arrow*). There is also echogenic fluid and likely thrombus in the space (*open arrow*). (**B**) CT scan demonstrates a corresponding liver laceration. *Source*: From Ref. 23.

Pitfalls

Empty Bladder

There are several limitations with the FAST scan. One potential pitfall easily rectified is that in patients without a full bladder, hemoperitoneum and/or physiological free fluid in the pelvis may be missed (Fig. 11) (4).

Sensitivity of the FAST Scan

A number of articles have shown FAST may miss organ injuries requiring surgery, especially when used in hemodynamically stable trauma patients (6,7). A limitation in many published FAST studies has been the use of clinical observation to determine patient outcome, rather than CT. Patients discharged after negative FAST and no further imaging or procedures were considered to be true negatives. Some of these patients may have had minor injuries missed by FAST, and this would falsely elevate the calculated sensitivity and specificity. The treating physician's decision to clinically observe the patient, perform CT after FAST, or proceed to surgery is often arbitrary and subjective. In a study of the use of FAST in pediatric trauma patients, specificity and negative predictive value were high; however, sensitivity was moderate and improved slightly when parenchymal injury was sought (27). To avoid the aforementioned bias, patients who were observed clinically after FAST but did not undergo CT and/or laparotomy were excluded. The clinician must therefore retain elevated suspicion for intra-abdominal injury in the stable trauma patient with a negative FAST examination.

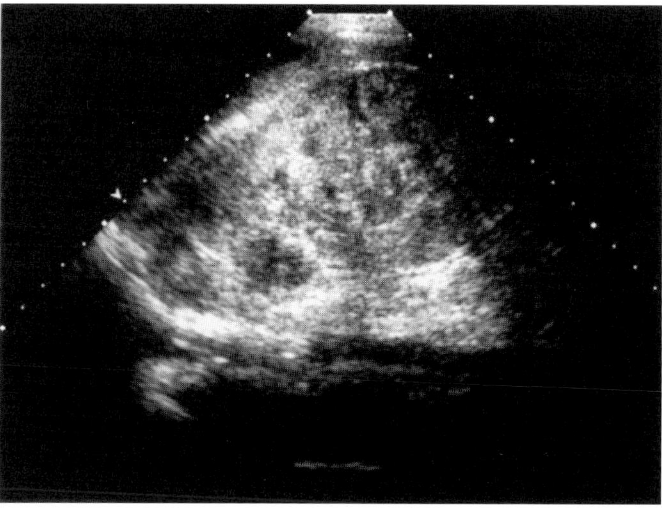
(A)

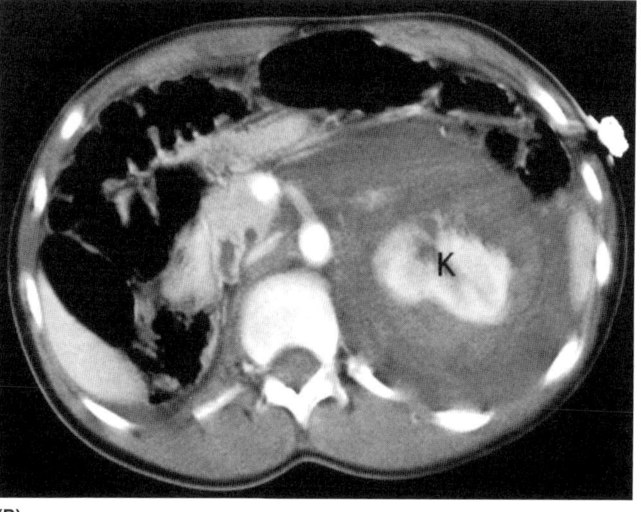

(B)

FIGURE 9 A AND B ■ Renal laceration. (**A**) Longitudinal sonogram of the left flank demonstrates disorganized pattern of renal parenchyma with mixed echogenicity. (**B**) CT scan demonstrates a severe renal laceration with surrounding hematoma. K, kidney.

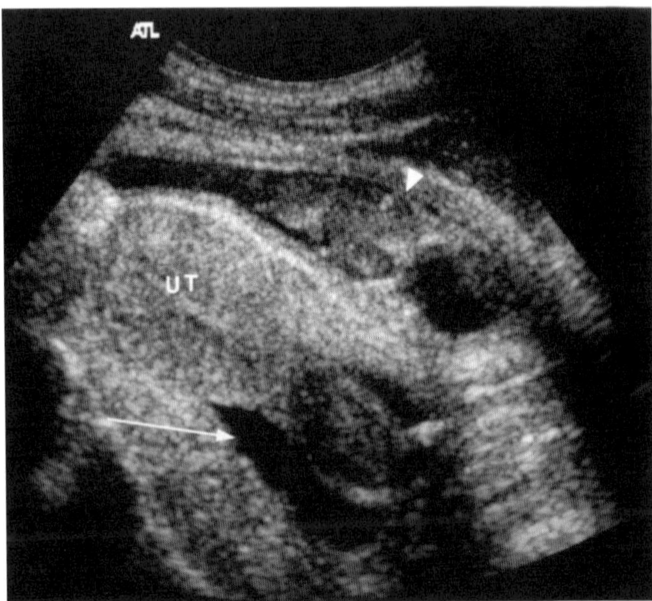

FIGURE 10 ■ Bladder hematoma. Longitudinal ultrasound of the female pelvis demonstrates free fluid (*arrow*) in the pelvis posterior to the uterus (UT). Note echogenic clot within the bladder (*arrowhead*).

Bowel vs. Free Fluid

Fluid-filled loops of bowel may be misinterpreted as free fluid. Free fluid usually forms acute angles between surrounding structures (Fig. 12). Bowel may also have peristalsis.

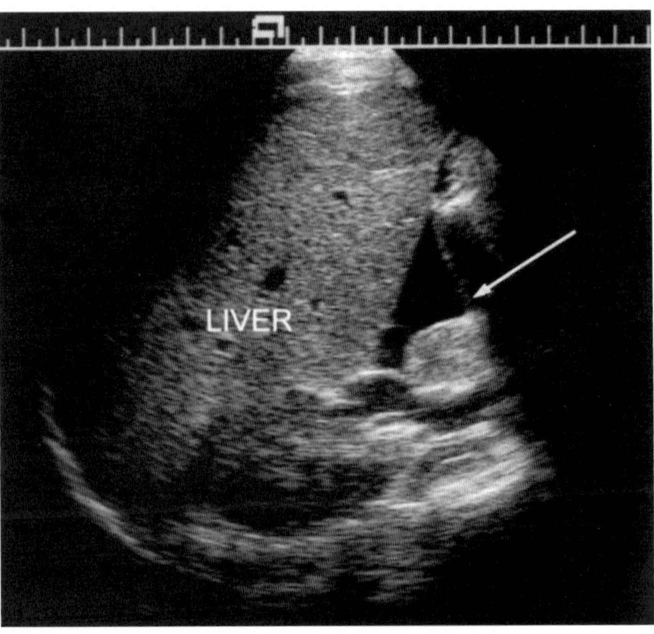

FIGURE 12 ■ Appearance of free fluid. In this patient with a splenic laceration, free fluid is noted caudal to liver. This fluid appears triangular in shape with borders with acute angles (*arrow*) and should not be misinterpreted as fluid-filled loops of bowels.

Other Limitations

Finally, sonography will be limited in showing or unable to show certain types of injuries. These include spinal and pelvic fractures, diaphragmatic ruptures, vascular injuries,

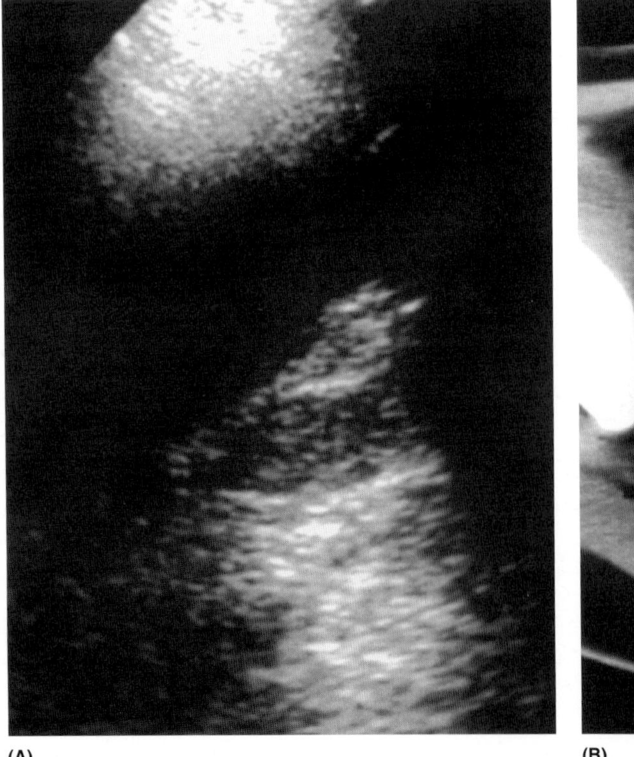

(A)

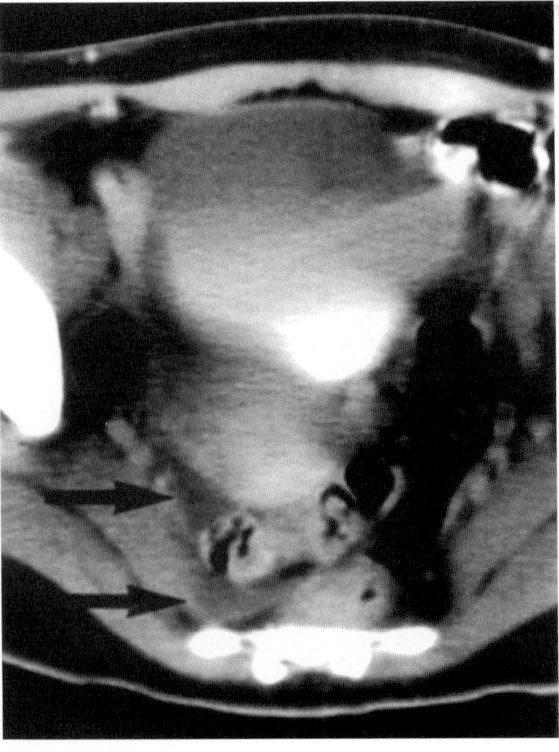

(B)

FIGURE 11 A AND B ■ Missed free fluid. (**A**) Longitudinal ultrasound through the pelvis with a partially filled bladder demonstrates no free fluid. (**B**) Corresponding CT demonstrates free fluid in the pelvis (*arrows*).

pancreatic injuries, adrenal injuries, and some bowel and mesenteric injuries (13). Initial FAST may be appropriate for these patients, but further evaluation with CT is warranted if these types of intra-abdominal injuries are suspected, or a patient with an initial negative FAST examination clinically deteriorates. We believe the role of the FAST examination has evolved such that its greatest utility at present is the triage of hemodynamically unstable blunt trauma patients to the operating room when positive. Conversely, a negative FAST examination in this patient subset may allow for further stabilization and diagnostic testing, such as peritoneal lavage or CT, to mitigate the possibility of unnecessary laparotomy.

THORACIC TRAUMA

Historical Perspective

Sonography was once considered to have limited application for respiratory disorders and trauma because air reflects sound waves. The first description of sonography in the diagnosis of pneumothorax was in 1986 in a study of horses (28). Since then, several prospective studies have demonstrated an overall sensitivity greater than 90% for ultrasound detection of pneumothorax (29–33). Sonography has been shown to be useful for diagnosing pleural effusions and pericardial effusions in addition to pneumothoraces (34–36). Cardiac lacerations or ruptures of the heart may also be detected with sonography (37).

Anatomy

The pericardium is a conical sac of fibrous tissue that surrounds the heart and roots of the great blood vessels and has two layers, the parietal and the visceral pericardium. The parietal pericardium is thick and tough, loosely cloaks the heart, and is attached to the central diaphragm and to the sternum. The visceral pericardium has two layers; one closely adheres to the epicardium while the other lines the inner surface of the parietal pericardium. In normal conditions, the intervening space contains a small volume of lubricating fluid. The amount and consistency of this fluid often changes with thoracic trauma and other pathological conditions. The parietal pleura is attached to the ribs and muscles of the thorax, whereas the visceral pleura is adherent to the lung. During inspiration and expiration, the visceral pleura slide back and forth adjacent to the parietal pleura. The bright echogenic line of the visceral pleura may be observed on real-time sonography and is a normal finding.

Procedure

Many examiners incorporate the subcostal or subxiphoid view of the heart as a portion of the FAST scan.

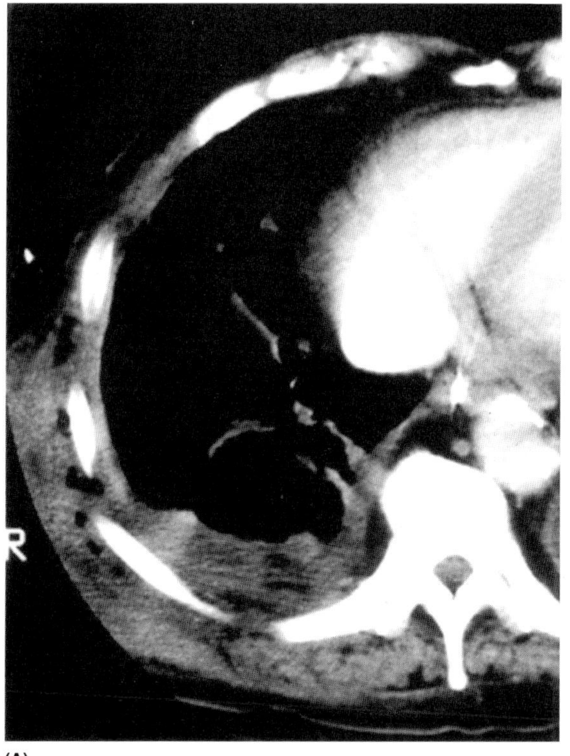

(A)

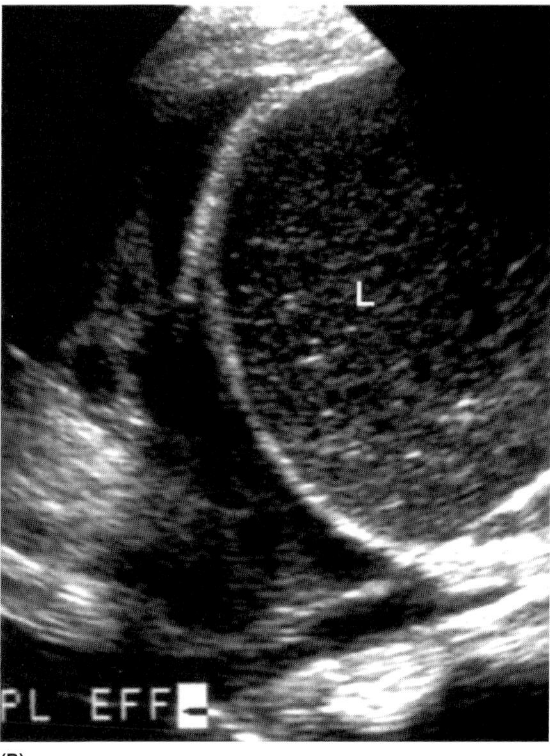

(B)

FIGURE 13 A AND B ■ Pleural effusion. (**A**) Axial CT in this trauma patient showing a pleural effusion. (**B**) Corresponding longitudinal ultrasound of the right chest shows pleural effusion. L, Liver.

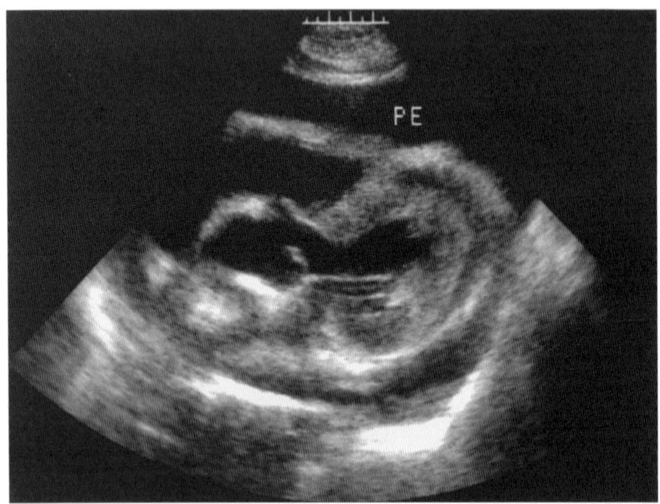

FIGURE 14 ■ PE. Ultrasound of the heart showing large pericardial effusion (PE).

This is useful in diagnosing pericardial effusion as well as global and regional mechanical dysfunction of the heart. Others include the parasternal or intercostal view. The parasternal view allows visualization of the aortic valve, ascending aorta, and posterior pericardium and is particularly helpful when the subcostal view is difficult to obtain. The subcostal view is obtained by placing the transducer at the left subcostal margin with the beam aimed at the left shoulder. The parasternal view is obtained by placing the transducer in the left parasternal area between the second and the fourth intercostal spaces. The plane of the beam is parallel to a line drawn from the right shoulder to the left hip. Several authors have suggested sonographic evaluation of the chest should supplement the FAST examination and, for an experienced sonographer, adds between two and four minutes to the entire evaluation. Diaphragmatic injuries may be detected with the

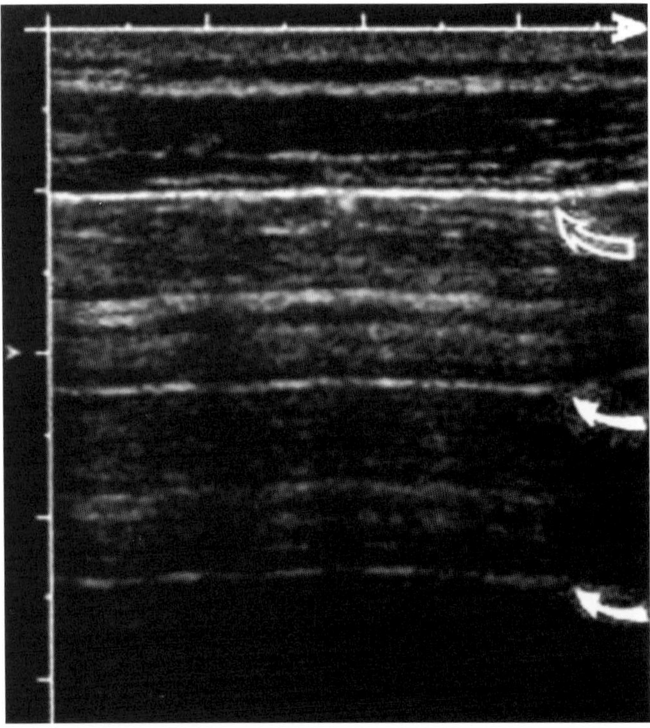

(A)

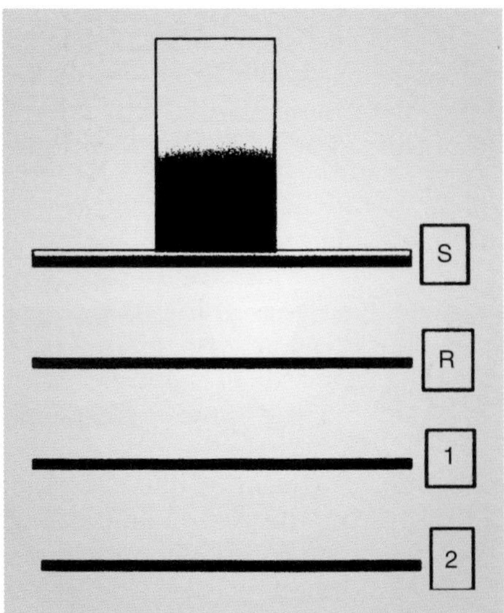

(B)

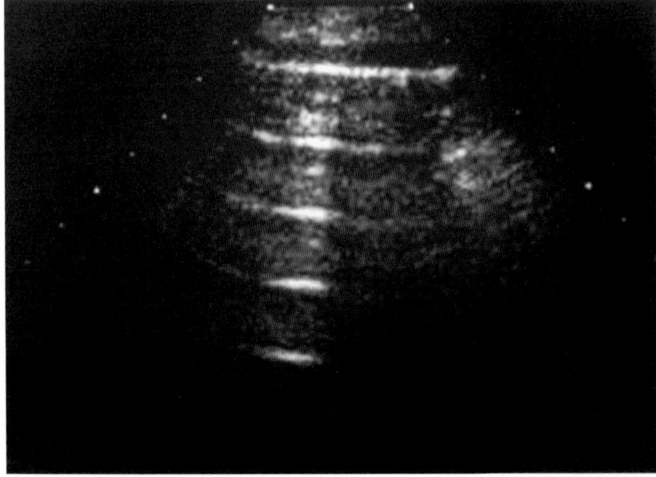

(C)

FIGURE 15 A–C ■ Normal lung. (**A**) Real-time examination with a linear array probe demonstrates the appearance of the normal lung. The first echogenic line (*open arrow*) corresponds to the interface between the parietal and the visceral pleura. Equally spaced parallel lines of decreasing echogenicity are observed posterior to this, which correspond to reverberation artifacts (*curved arrows*). (**B**) Reverberation artifact. The probe is placed on the skin surface (S). R refers to the interface between the parietal and the visceral pleura. Lines labeled as numbers 1 and 2, which are of decreasing echogenicity posterior to this, correspond to reverberation artifacts caused by the ultrasound beam "reverberating" or "bouncing" between the pleura and the transducer. (**C**) Similar pattern is seen with a sector scan of the lung in another patient. *Source*: From Ref. 41.

transducer directed through the diaphragm and may be confirmed by M-mode imaging (38,39). For detection of pneumothorax, either a curved array probe or, better yet, a linear array probe may be used. Free air within the thoracic cavity rises to the most nondependent portion, and the transducer should be placed in this area to check for pneumothorax. The lateral clavicular line in the third to fourth interspace is a good starting point. Confirmation of positive or negative findings should be undertaken for four to five respiratory cycles on both sides of the chest for comparison. The evaluation of lung sliding with power color Doppler may improve sensitivity (40).

Interpretation

Pleural effusion can be seen as a hypoechoic or an anechoic stripe in the dependent portion of the thorax when the right or left upper quadrant of the abdomen is examined (Fig. 13). Pericardial effusion is seen as a hypoechoic area bounded by the parietal and visceral pericardium (Fig. 14). With regard to the diaphragm, no or abnormal movement with concomitant respiratory effort suggests injury. The sliding motion of the visceral pleura against the parietal pleura observed in a normal patient is absent with pneumothorax. In a normal patient, a reverberation artifact usually is noted posterior to the parietal–visceral pleura interface (Fig. 15) and appears as equally spaced lines gradually decreasing in echogenicity. This represents the reverberation of the ultrasound beam as it strikes the parietal–visceral pleura interface and the air in the lung and is reflected back to the transducer, resulting in multiple, equally spaced echoes. According to a recent classification of such findings, these are also referred to as "A lines" (42). This reverberation artifact is not seen with pneumothorax, which may instead produce acoustic shadowing (Fig. 16).

The vertical "comet-tail" artifact, or "B line," has several characteristics. It arises from the pleural line, is well defined, spreads to the edge of the screen without fading, erases A lines, and moves with lung sliding. Several simultaneously visible B lines are labeled "lung rockets" and may indicate interstitial syndrome generated by pathologic conditions. The B lines can be isolated and do not possess precise pathologic significance. As B lines are generated by the visceral and not parietal pleura, it is expected these would no longer be visible in the case of pneumothorax; however, this is not always the case. Another kind of comet-tail artifact arises from the pleural line and is vertical like the B line but is otherwise different: It is ill defined, vanishes after a few centimeters, does not reach the screen limits, does not erase the A lines, and is independent of lung sliding. This is referred to as the "Z line" and may or may not be associated with pneumothorax. The area where normal lung findings disappear is known as the "lung point," a dynamic sign that corresponds to the edge of the pneumothorax (43). It is visible with respiratory excursion as the transducer is held in a fixed position on the patient's chest, but is only momentarily visualized.

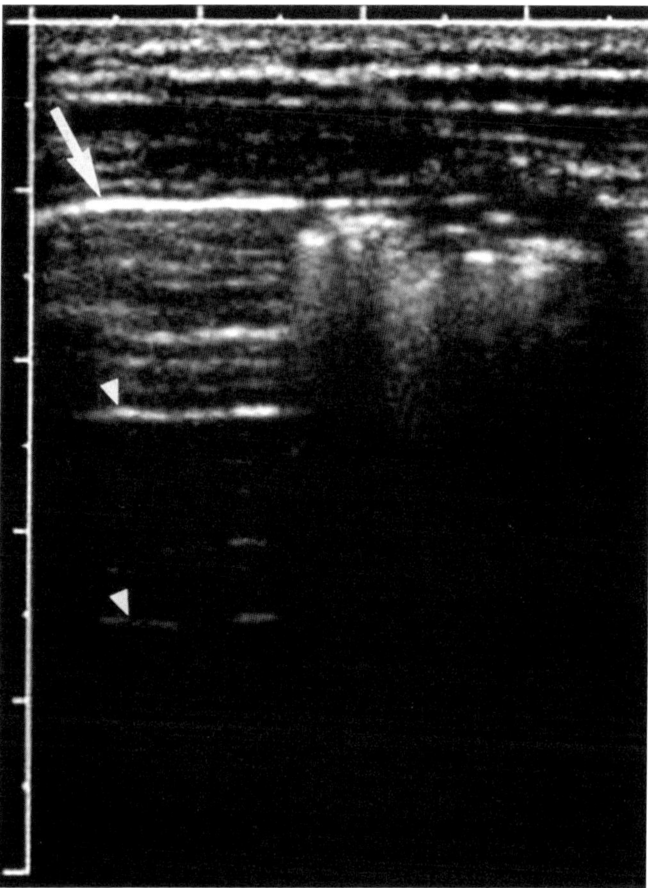

FIGURE 16 ■ Small pneumothorax. Real-time examination of a patient with a pneumothorax demonstrates the echogenic line that corresponds to the parietal and visceral pleura (*arrow*), which is noted on the left side of the image. Note more distal reverberation artifacts (*arrowheads*). To the right side of the image, there is loss of this pattern because of a pneumothorax. *Source*: From Ref. 41.

Pitfalls

Hypoechoic Myocardium

One study outlined the potential pitfalls of overdiagnosing pericardial effusions with ultrasound. Emergency medicine residents and fellows trained in sonography had trouble discerning the hypoechoic myocardium and epicardial fat from effusions (Fig. 17), and sonography had sensitivity of 73% and specificity of 44% (44).

Insufficient Gain

Absence or decrease of the reverberation artifact also may occur in a normal patient if the gain settings are set too low. As mentioned previously, the sole visualization of comet-tail artifacts to diagnose pneumothorax may be misleading, as there are variants of this pattern.

Underlying Lung Disease

False-positive ultrasonograms may occur in patients with underlying lung disease such as adult respiratory distress syndrome, congestive heart failure, lung fibrosis, and bullous disease (42).

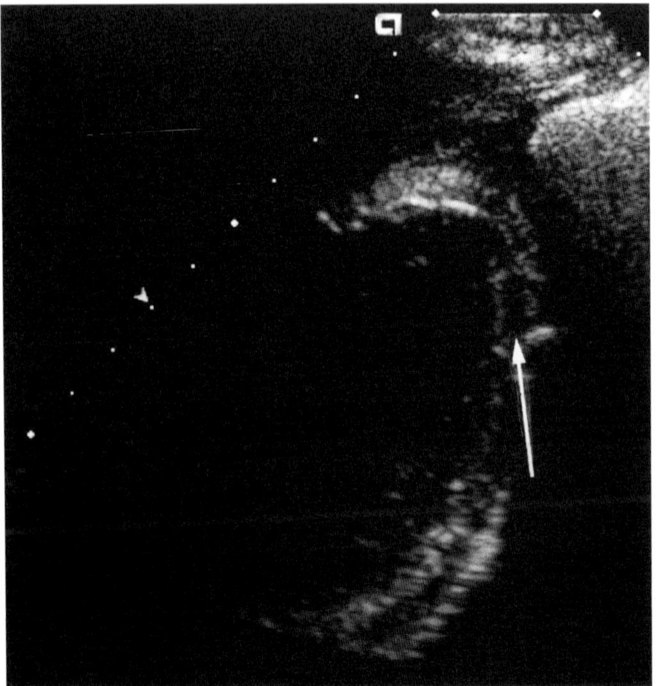

FIGURE 17 ■ Normal heart ultrasound. Ultrasound shows hypoechoic myocardium (*arrow*), which should not be misinterpreted as pericardial effusion.

FUTURE RESEARCH

The FAST examination is becoming more widespread in its application for the trauma patient. Ultrasound machines are becoming smaller and more portable, and hand-held units have performed well with regard to FAST (45,46). There has been interest in using FAST to triage penetrating injuries to the chest and abdomen, and initial results are equal or better than for blunt trauma (47,48). Based on several reports, the accuracy of the FAST examination improves with the addition of ultrasound contrast (Figs. 18 and 19) (49–51). The contrast agent consists of a suspension of microspheres of human serum albumin filled with octafluoropropane gas, which is rapidly eliminated through the lungs. Once injected into the venous system, the octafluoropropane microbubbles create an acoustic impedance different from blood. An echogenic effect is created, enhancing the images from solid organs, vessels, and soft tissue. The effective half-life is approximately five minutes. Other potential uses of ultrasound in trauma include ocular evaluation to detect globe rupture, retinal detachment, and retrobulbar hemorrhage. Musculoskeletal application has been proposed as well for evaluation of fractures and muscle, tendon, and ligament injuries (53,54).

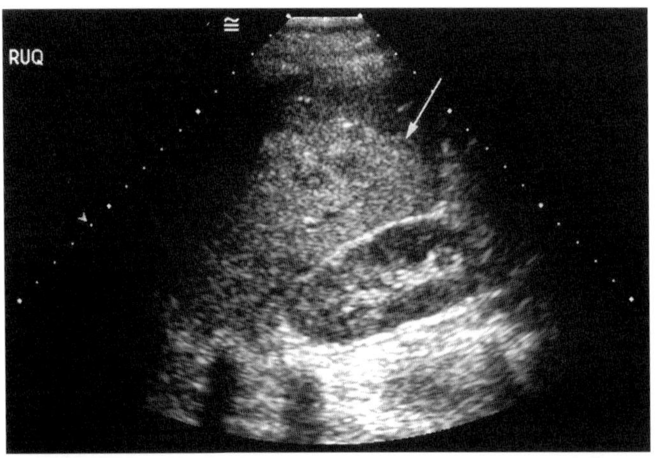

(A)

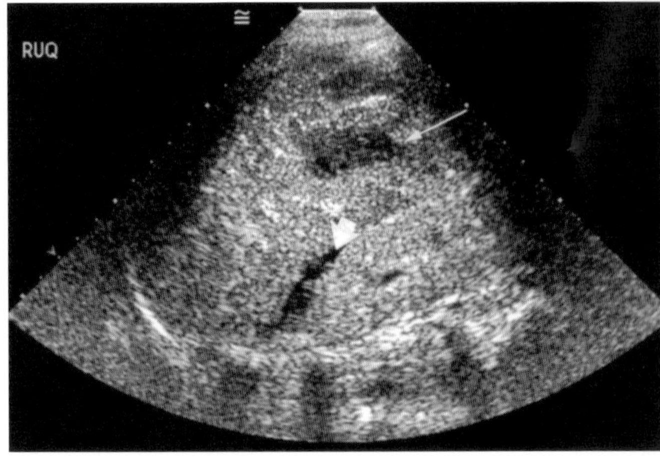

(B)

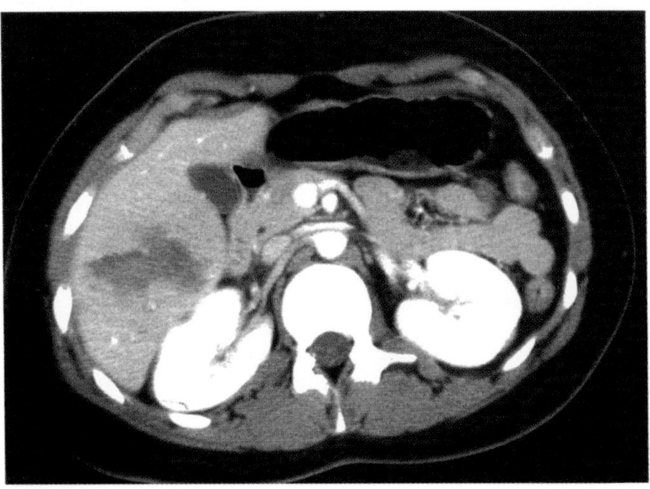

(C)

FIGURE 18 A–C ■ Contrast-enhanced liver laceration. (**A**) Base study prior to contrast. The appearance of the liver is extremely heterogeneous (*arrow*). (**B**) After contrast administration, vascularity was enhanced and appears echogenic, with central hypoechogenic region (*long arrow*) noted in the right lobe of the liver. Free fluid in Morison's pouch is now obvious (*short arrow*). (**C**) Corresponding CT demonstrates large liver laceration. *Abbreviation*: CT, computed tomography. *Source*: From Ref. 52.

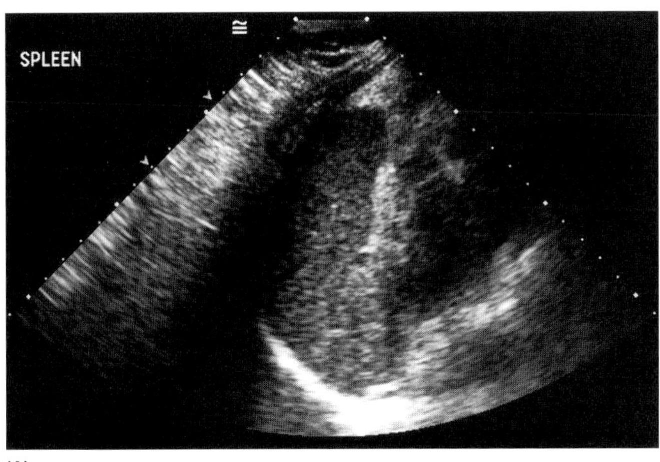

(A)

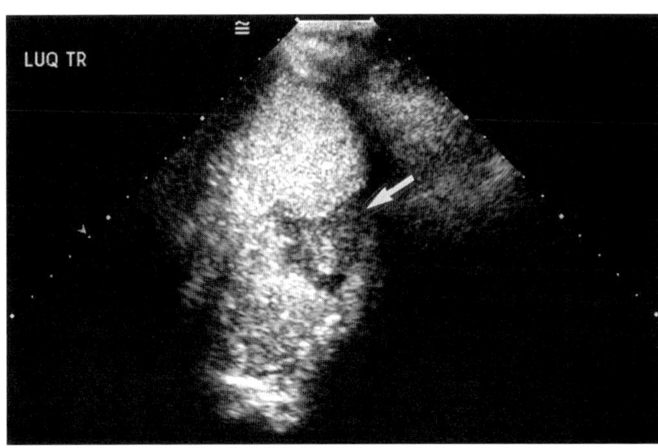

(B)

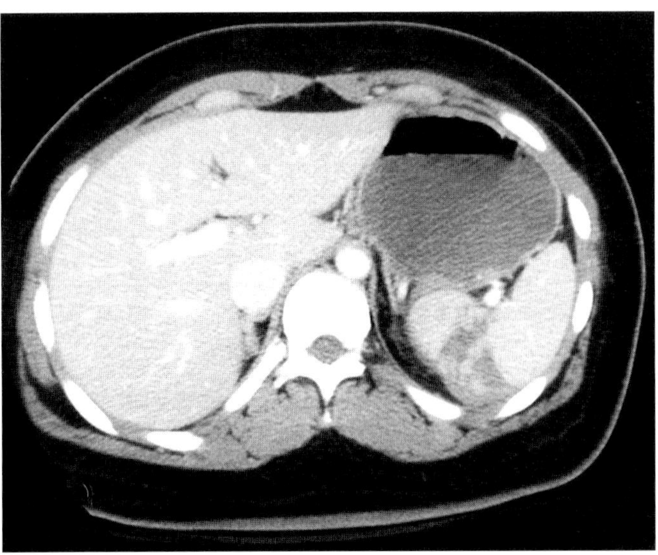
(C)

FIGURE 19 A–C ■ Contrast-enhanced splenic laceration. (**A**) Noncontrast ultrasound scan of the spleen, which appears normal. (**B**) Contrast-enhanced ultrasound showing well-defined nonperfused hypoechoic region in the spleen (*arrow*). This corresponded to a splenic laceration. (**C**) Corresponding CT scan of the spleen showing splenic laceration. *Source*: From Ref. 52.

REFERENCES

1. Kristensen JK, Buemann B, Kuehl E. Ultrasonic scanning in the diagnosis of splenic haematomas. Acta Chir Scand 1971; 137:653.
2. Asher WM, Parvin S, Virgilio RW, Haber K. Echographic evaluation of splenic injury after blunt trauma. Radiology 1976; 118:411.
3. Jehle D, Guarino J, Karamanoukian H. Emergency department ultrasound in the evaluation of blunt abdominal trauma. Am J Emerg Med 1993; 11:342.
4. McGahan JP, Rose J, Coates TL, Wisner DH, Newberry P. Use of sonography in the patient with acute abdominal trauma. J Ultrasound Med 1997; 16:653.
5. Pearl WS, Todd KH. Sonography for the initial evaluation of blunt abdominal trauma: a review of prospective trials. Ann Emerg Med 1996; 27:353.
6. Shanmuganathan K, Mirvis SE, Sherbourne CD, Chiu WC, Rodriguez A. Hemoperitoneum as the sole indicator of abdominal visceral injuries: a potential limitation of screening abdominal US for trauma. Radiology 1999; 212:423.
7. Miller MT, Pasquale MD, Bromberg WJ, Wasser TE, Cox J. Not so fast. J Trauma 2003; 54:52.
8. McGahan JP, Richards JR, Gillen M. The focused abdominal sonography for trauma scan: pearls and pitfalls. J Ultrasound Med 2002; 21:789.
9. Polk JD, Fallon WF Jr, Kovach B, Mancuso C, Stephens M, Malangoni MA. The "Airmedical F.A.S.T." for trauma patients—the initial report of a novel application for sonography. Aviat Space Environ Med 2001; 72:432.
10. Rozanski TA, Edmondson JM, Jones SB. Sonography in a forward-deployed military hospital. Mil Med 2005; 170:99.
11. Boysen SR, Rozanski EA, Tidwell AS, Holm JL, Shaw SP, Rush JE. Evaluation of a focused assessment with sonography for trauma protocol to detect free abdominal fluid in dogs involved in motor vehicle accidents. J Am Vet Med Assoc 2004; 225:1198.
12. Sargsyan AE, Hamilton DR, Jones JA, et al. FAST at MACH 20: clinical ultrasound aboard the international space station. J Trauma 2005; 58:35.
13. Richards JR, McGahan JP, Simpson JL, Tabar P. Bowel and mesenteric injury: evaluation with emergency abdominal US. Radiology 1999; 211:399.
14. Ormsby EL, Geng J, McGahan JP, Richards JR. Pelvic free fluid: clinical importance for reproductive age women with blunt abdominal trauma. Ultrasound Obstet Gynecol 2005; 26:271.
15. Jehle D, Stiller G, Wagner D. Sensitivity in detecting free intraperitoneal fluid with the pelvic views of the FAST exam. Am J Emerg Med 2003; 21:476.
16. Richards JR, McGahan JP, Jones CD, Zhan S, Gerscovich E. Ultrasound detection of blunt splenic injury. Injury 2001; 32:95.
17. Branney SW, Wolfe RE, Moore EE, et al. Quantitative sensitivity of ultrasound in detecting free intraperitoneal fluid. J Trauma 1995; 39:375.

18. Huang MS, Liu M, Wu JK, Shih HC, Ko TJ, Lee CH. Sonography for the evaluation of hemoperitoneum during resuscitation: a simple scoring system. J Trauma 1994; 36:173.
19. McKenney KL, McKenney MG, Cohn SM, et al. Hemoperitoneum score helps determine need for therapeutic laparotomy. J Trauma 2001; 50:650.
20. Sirlin CB, Casola G, Brown MA, Patel N, Bendavid EJ, Hoyt DB. Patterns of fluid accumulation on screening sonography for blunt abdominal trauma: comparison with site of injury. J Ultrasound Med 2001; 20:351.
21. Sirlin CB, Casola G, Brown MA, Patel N, Bendavid EJ, Hoyt DB. Quantification of fluid on screening sonography for blunt abdominal trauma: a simple scoring system to predict severity of injury. J Ultrasound Med 2001; 20:359.
22. vanSonnenberg E, Simeone JF, Mueller PR, Wittenberg J, Hall DA, Ferrucci JT Jr. Sonographic appearance of hematoma in liver, spleen, and kidney: a clinical, pathologic, and animal study. Radiology 1983; 147:507.
23. Richards JR, McGahan JP, Pali MJ, Bohnen PA. Sonographic detection of blunt hepatic trauma: hemoperitoneum and parenchymal patterns of injury. J Trauma 1999; 47:1092.
24. McGahan JP, Richards JR, Jones CD, Gerscovich EO. Use of sonography in the patient with acute renal trauma. J Ultrasound Med 1999; 18:207.
25. Nunes LW, Simmons S, Hallowell MJ, Kinback R, Trooskin S, Kozar R. Diagnostic performance of trauma US in identifying abdominal or pelvic free fluid and serious abdominal or pelvic injury. Acad Radiol 2001; 8:128.
26. Blackbourne LH, Soffer D, McKenney M, et al. Secondary ultrasound examination increases the sensitivity of the FAST exam in blunt trauma. J Trauma 2004; 57:934.
27. Richards JR, Knopf NA, Wang L, McGahan JP. Blunt abdominal trauma in children: evaluation with emergency US. Radiology 2002; 222:749.
28. Ranaten N. Diagnostic ultrasound: diseases of the thorax. Vet Clin N Am 1986; 2:49.
29. Dulchavsky SA, Schwarz KL, Kirkpatrick AW, et al. Prospective evaluation of thoracic ultrasound in the detection of pneumothorax. J Trauma 2001; 50:201.
30. Sargsyan AE, Hamilton DR, Nicolaou S, et al. Ultrasound evaluation of the magnitude of pneumothorax: a new concept. Am Surg 2001; 67:232.
31. Lichtenstein DA, Meziere G, Lascols N, et al. Ultrasound diagnosis of occult pneumothorax. Crit Care Med 2005; 33:1231.
32. Knudtson JL, Dort JM, Helmer SD, Smith SR. Surgeon-Performed ultrasound for pneumothorax in the trauma suite. J Trauma 2004; 56:527.
33. Blaivas M, Lyon M, Duggal S. A prospective comparison of supine chest radiography and bedside ultrasound for the diagnosis of traumatic pneumothorax. Acad Emerg Med 2005; 12:844.
34. Ma OJ, Mateer JR. Trauma ultrasound examination versus chest radiography in the detection of hemothorax. Ann Emerg Med 1997; 29:312.
35. Brooks A, Davies B, Smethhurst M, Connolly J. Emergency ultrasound in the acute assessment of haemothorax. Emerg Med J 2004; 21:44.
36. Chelly MR, Margulies DR, Mandavia D, et al. The evolving role of FAST scan for the diagnosis of pericardial fluid. J Trauma 2004; 56:915.
37. Symbas NP, Bongiorno PF, Symbas PN. Blunt cardiac rupture: the utility of emergency department ultrasound. Ann Thorac Surg 1999; 67:1274.
38. Blaivas M, Brannam L, Hawkins M, Lyon M, Sriram K. Bedside emergency ultrasonographic diagnosis of diaphragmatic rupture in blunt abdominal trauma. Am J Emerg Med 2004; 22:601.
39. Gerscovich EO, Cronan M, McGahan JP, Ultrasonographic evaluation of diaphragmatic motion. J Ultrasound Med 2001; 20:597.
40. Cunninghan J, Kirkpatrick AW, Nicolaou S, et al. Enhanced recognition of "lung sliding" with power color Doppler imaging in the diagnosis of pneumothorax. J Trauma 2002; 52:769.
41. Richards JR, McGahan JP, Fogata MC. Emergency ultrasound in trauma patients. Radiol Clin North Am 2004; 42:417–425.
42. Lichtenstein DA, Meziere G, Lascols N, et al. Ultrasound diagnosis of occult pneumothorax. Crit Care Med 2005; 33:1231.
43. Lichtenstein D, Meziere G, Biderman P, Gepner A. The "lung point": an ultrasound sign specific to pneumothorax. Intensive Care Med 2000; 26:1434.
44. Blaivas M, DeBehnke D, Phelan MB. Potential errors in the diagnosis of pericardial effusion on trauma ultrasound for penetrating injuries. Acad Emerg Med 2000; 7:1261.
45. Kirkpatrick AW, Sirois M, Laupland, KB, et al. Hand-held thoracic sonography for detecting post-traumatic pneumothoraces: the extended focused assessment with sonography for trauma (EFAST). J Trauma 2004; 57:288.
46. Kirkpatrick AW, Sirois M, Ball CG, et al. The hand-held ultrasound examination for penetrating abdominal trauma. Am J Surg 2004; 187:660.
47. Tayal VS, Beatty MA, Marx JA, Tomaszewski CA, Thomason MH. FAST (Focused assessment with sonography in trauma) accurate for cardiac and intraperitoneal injury in penetrating anterior chest trauma. J Ultrasound Med 2004; 23:467.
48. Aaland MO, Bryan FC III, Sherman R. Two-dimensional echocardiogram in hemodynamically stable victims of penetrating precordial trauma. Am Surg 1994; 60:412.
49. Catalano O, Lobianco R, Sandomenico F, Siani A. Splenic trauma: evaluation with contrast-specific sonography and a second-generation contrast medium: preliminary experience. J Ultrasound Med 2003; 22:467.
50. Blaivas M, Lyon M, Brannam L, Schwartz R, Duggal S. Feasibility of FAST examination performance with ultrasound contrast. J Emerg Med 2005; 29:307.
51. Catalano O, Lobianco R, Sandomenico F, Mattace Raso M, Siani A. Real-time, contrast-enhanced sonographic imaging in emergency radiology. Radiodiagnostics 2003; 108:454.
52. McGahan JP, Horton S, Gerscovich EO, et al. Appearance of solid organ injury with contrast-enhanced sonography in blunt abdominal trauma; preliminary experience. AJR 2006; 187:658.
53. Legome E, Pancu D. Future applications for emergency ultrasound. Emerg Med Clin North Am 2004; 28:337.
54. Cornejo CJ, Vaezy S, Jurkovich GJ, et al. High-intensity ultrasound treatment of blunt abdominal solid organ injury: an animal model. J Trauma 2004; 57:152.

Gastrointestinal Tract and Peritoneal Cavity

Matilde Nino-Murcia and R. Brooke Jeffrey

13

INTRODUCTION

This chapter focuses on clinical applications of transabdominal and endoluminal sonography to diseases of the gastrointestinal tract and peritoneal cavity. Emphasis will be placed on scanning technique, imaging findings, and correlative studies highlighting disease processes that are particularly well demonstrated by sonography.

GASTROINTESTINAL TRACT

Technical Aspects

The gastrointestinal tract may be studied either transabdominally or with endoluminal transducers. Most transabdominal techniques rely on linear- or curved-array technology using graded compression techniques. When using graded compression, the abdomen is scanned over the area of interest and compressed with gradually increasing pressure, in order to displace overlying loops of bowel so that the potentially abnormal region may be imaged. Furthermore, compression sonography is helpful to determine whether a loop of bowel has normal compressibility. Normally, the bowel wall compresses and collapses with gentle probe pressure. However, when there is inflammatory or neoplastic infiltration of the bowel wall, its compliance diminishes and is no longer readily compressible. The selection of transducer frequency should be carefully considered when scanning the gastrointestinal tract. In pediatric patients, a 7.5 MHz linear-array transducer is often the optimal frequency. Similar high-resolution transducers may be used to evaluate the newborn with projectile vomiting and suspected hypertrophic pyloric stenosis. Lower-frequency transducers in the range of 3.5 to 6 MHz are typically used to evaluate the gastrointestinal tract in adult patients.

Color and power Doppler interrogation of the gastrointestinal tract when optimized for low volume flow provides useful additional information when evaluating bowel wall thickening (1–3). Inflammatory conditions typically result in measurably increased blood flow, whereas ischemia or hemorrhagic conditions result in reduced flow (1–3). The normal bowel wall, which is only 2 to 3 mm thick, does not have demonstrable flow on color or power Doppler. Power Doppler imaging has been shown to improve visualization of intramural gastrointestinal vascularity compared to color Doppler, due to its increased sensitivity for low-volume flow (2).

Sonographic Features

Normal Bowel Wall

Histologically, the bowel wall is comprised of several distinct layers (Fig. 1 line drawing). These layers include (*i*) the mucous membrane, which is made up of the epithelium, lamina propria, and muscularis mucosa; (*ii*) the submucosa; (*iii*) the muscularis propria, which is made up of the inner circular layer and the outer longitudinal layer; and (*iv*) the serosa.

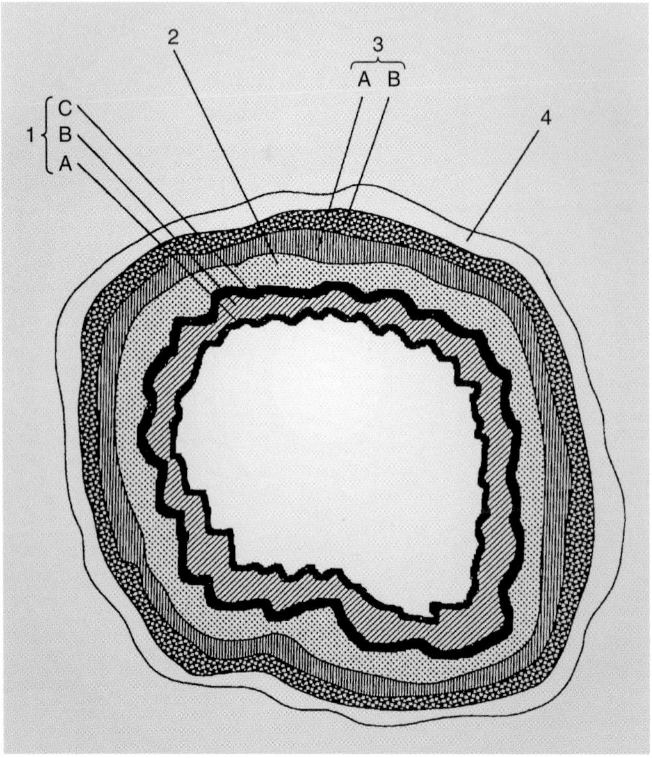

FIGURE 1 ■ Depiction of histologic layers of the gut wall.

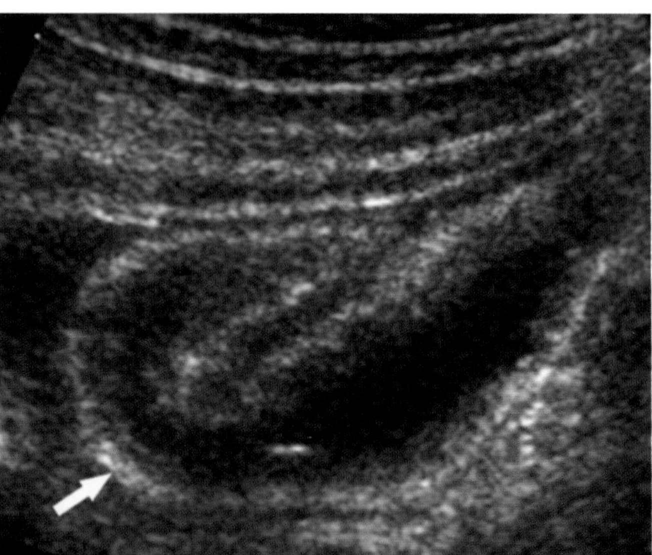

FIGURE 3 ■ Dilated loops of bowel in small bowel obstruction. Note distended fluid-filled bowel loops with echogenic walls (*arrow*) obstructed by adhesive band.

With high-resolution sonography, or endoluminal sonography, these distinct layers are often readily imaged (4). These include three echogenic layers and two hypoechoic layers (Fig. 2 line drawing). The different layers with their histologic correlations include (*i*) the echogenic superficial mucosa, including the luminal contents and the mucosal inner face; (*ii*) the hypoechoic, deep mucosa, which also includes the muscularis mucosa; (*iii*) the echogenic submucosa, which includes the interface between the submucosa and the muscularis propria; (*iv*) the hypoechoic muscularis propria; and (*v*) the echogenic serosa, which includes the serosal surface and the serosal fat. The normal gut wall has a variable thickness, depending on whether or not it is distended. In general, the normal wall should be no greater than 3 mm when distended but may be minimally thicker in appearance when nondistended (5,6).

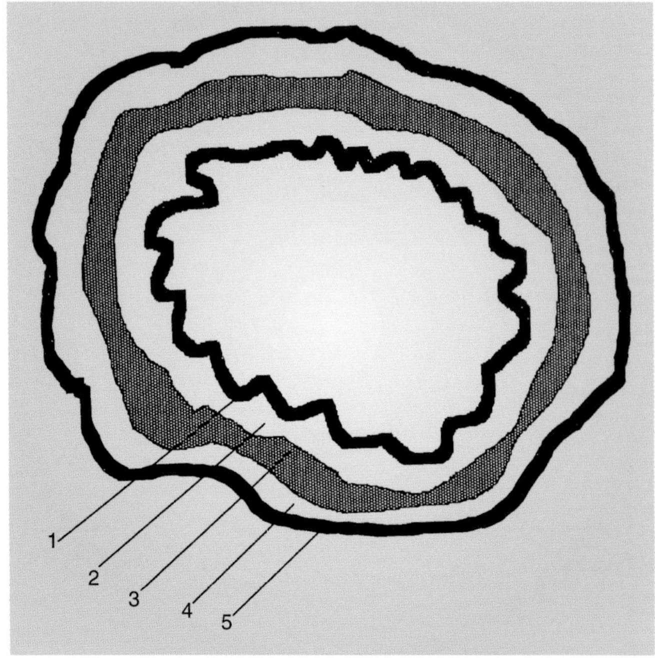

FIGURE 2 ■ Normal ultrasound: gut signature.

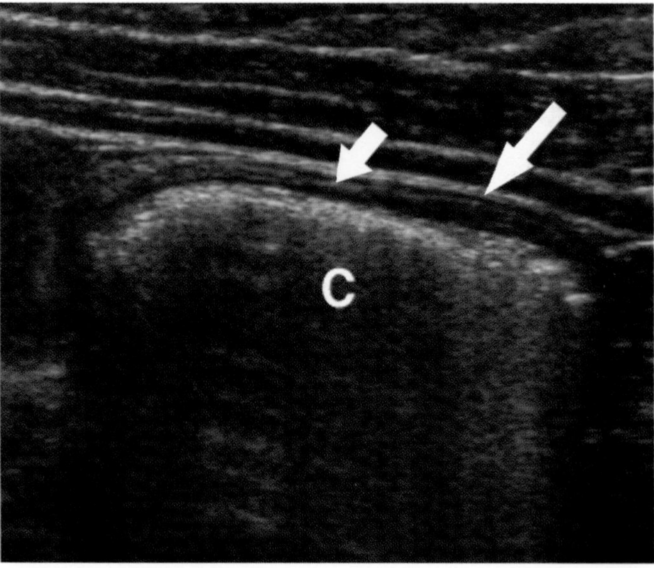

FIGURE 4 ■ Normal bowel wall of descending colon (C). Transverse scan of descending colon. Note thin echogenic line of submucosa (*short arrow*) and hypoechoic muscularis mucosa (*long arrow*).

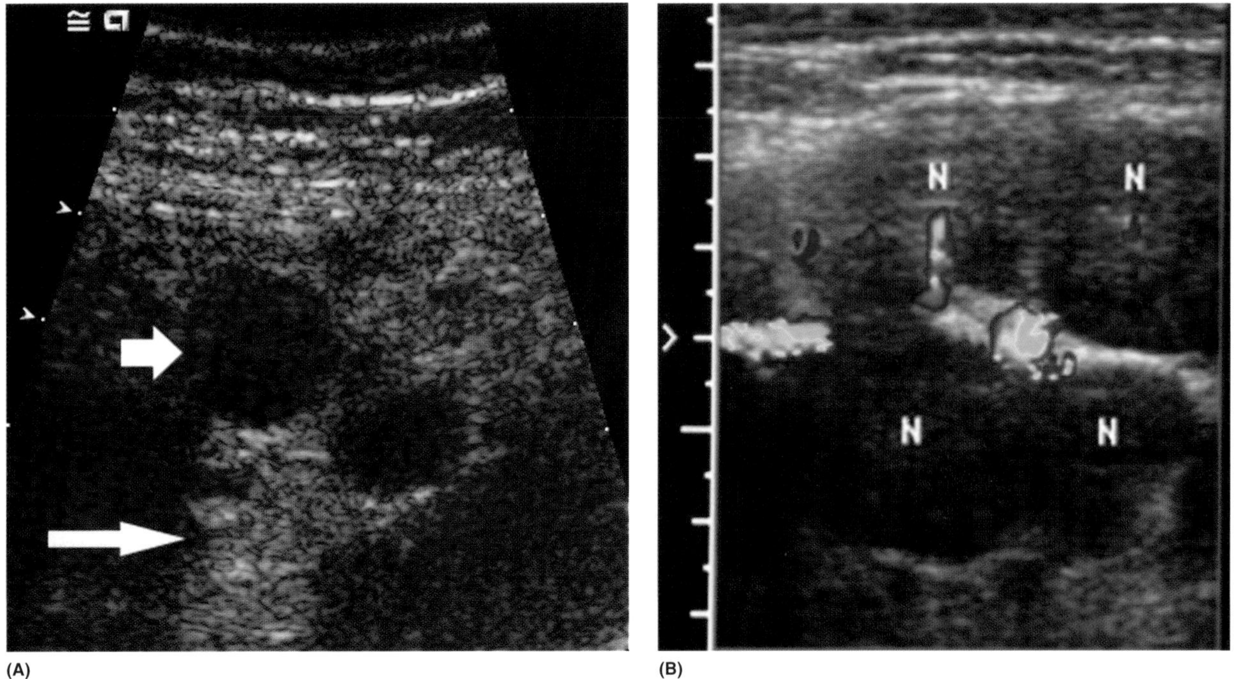

(A) (B)

FIGURE 5 A AND B ■ Mesenteric adenopathy. (**A**) Note the hypoechoic node (*short arrow*) with enhanced through sound transmission (*long arrow*) due to liquefied necrosis from mesenteric tuberculosis. (**B**) Enlarged mesenteric nodes (N) on color Doppler sonogram are identified as rounded hypoechoic structures due to lymphoma.

On routine transabdominal scanning, the normal bowel may appear as a collapsed structure with an echogenic center and a hypoechoic bowel wall surrounded by a more echogenic peripheral zone. However, this appearance varies, depending on which portion of the gastrointestinal tract is identified and whether the bowel is collapsed or fluid filled. When the bowel is fluid filled, it appears as an echogenic wall surrounding the central fluid-filled lumen (Fig. 3). Occasionally, discrete layers of the bowel wall may be identified on transabdominal scanning. However, with transducers in the 3.5 to 6 MHz range, the most prominent feature of the normal bowel is often the echogenic submucosal layer (Fig. 4). Not all hypoechoic structures in the abdomen are bowel loops, and enlarged mesenteric lymph nodes have a rounded hypoechoic appearance (Fig. 5).

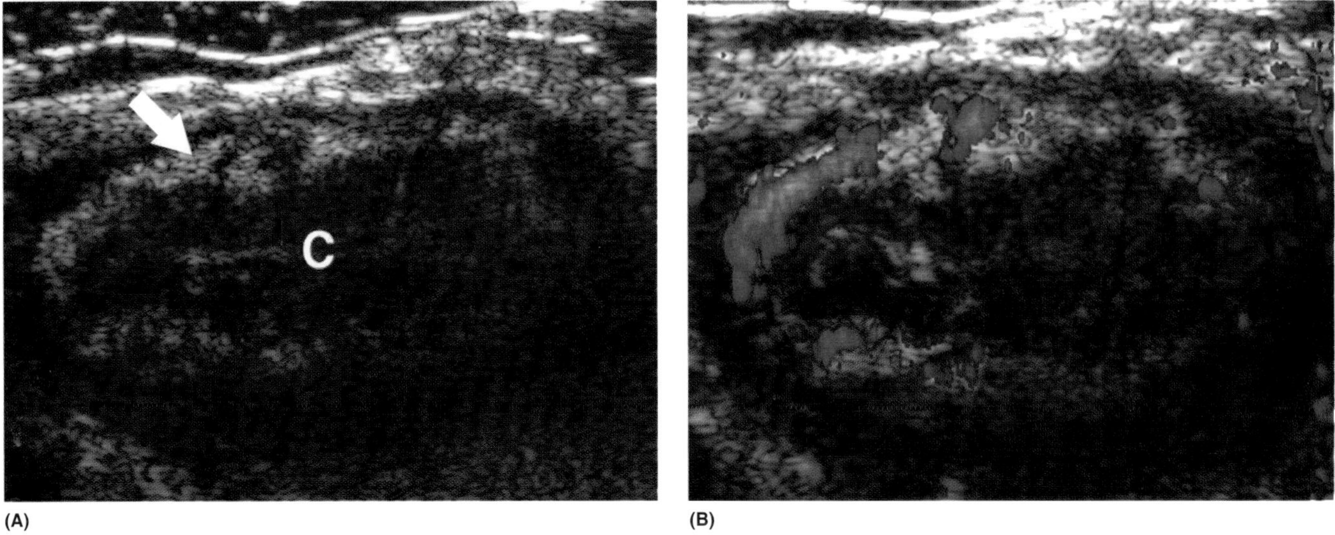

(A) (B)

FIGURE 6 A AND B ■ Mural thickening and hyperemia of the colon in colitis. (**A**) Note the mural thickening of the cecum (C) with prominence of the submucosal layer (*arrow*). (**B**) Power Doppler sonography demonstrates marked hyperemia of the cecum. Stool cultures were positive for *Campylobacter*.

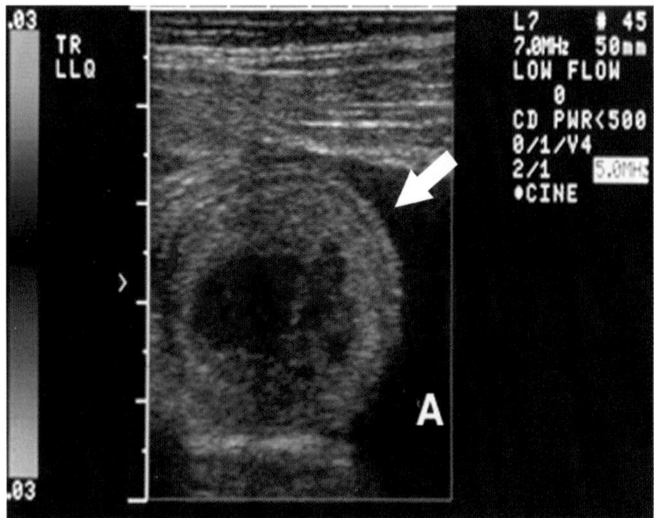

FIGURE 7 ■ Mural thickening due to bowel infarction on color Doppler sonography. Note thickened loop of bowel (*arrow*) with nearly absent flow on color Doppler. There are adjacent ascites (A).

Abnormal Bowel Wall

Most diseases of the gastrointestinal tract, regardless of etiology, typically result in thickening of the bowel wall. In hypertrophic pyloric stenosis, there usually is hypertrophy of the pyloric muscle, which may be measured by ultrasound both in the transverse and in the longitudinal scans of the pylorus (5,6). In addition, with inflammatory diseases of the gastrointestinal tract such as colitis or acute appendicitis, there is thickening of the wall with edema and inflammatory cells in conjunction with increased flow on color Doppler (Figs. 6–9). Mural thickening from a variety of focal abnormalities may result in a target pattern (Fig. 10) (7). The central mucosa and luminal contents appear echogenic and are surrounded by an enlarged hypoechoic region corresponding to an inflammatory or neoplastic involvement of the bowel wall. Thickened bowel may also appear as a "pseudokidney pattern" (Fig. 11) (8). The pseudokidney pattern occurs with oblique scanning and refers to the echogenic center, composed of mucosa and luminal contents surrounded by the hypoechoic thickened bowel wall. The echogenic mucosal surface appears similar to the renal hilar fat of the kidney. The abnormally thickened hypoechoic bowel wall mimics the sonographic appearance of the renal cortex. Both the target pattern and the pseudokidney pattern are nonspecific indicators of bowel wall disease. Identification of a thickened echogenic submucosal layer on sonography may be related to an acute gastrointestinal process such as submucosal edema or hemorrhage, while uniformly hypoechoic bowel wall thickening with loss of characteristic strata may represent subacute or chronic disease (Fig. 12) (9).

Color Doppler of the Gastrointestinal Tract

Color Doppler imaging is useful in evaluating patients with thickened bowel wall by demonstrating increased flow with inflammatory response and decreased-to-absent flow with ischemic necrosis of the gastrointestinal tract (1,3). Jeffrey et al. (1) reported increased mural flow in all 32 patients with gastrointestinal inflammatory

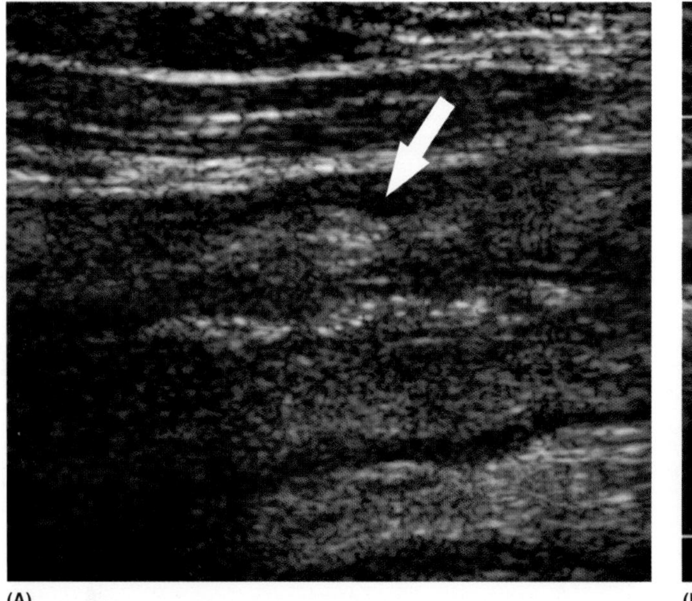

(A)

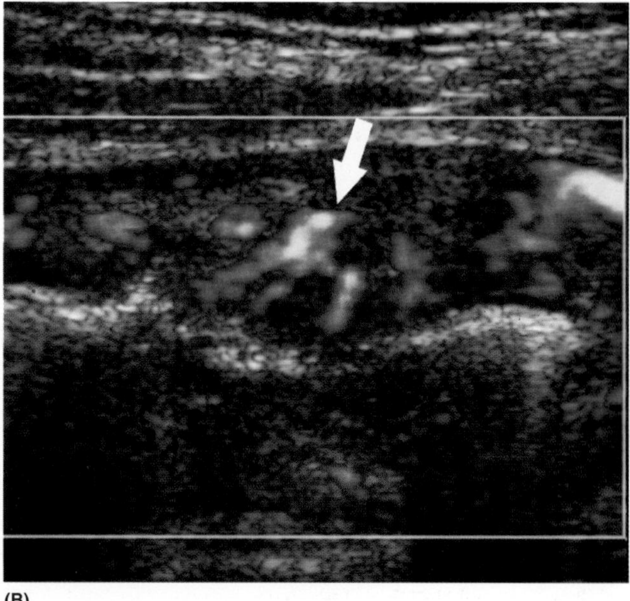

(B)

FIGURE 8 A AND B ■ Thickened bowel with mural hyperemia in Crohn's disease. (**A**) Longitudinal sonogram of a thickened terminal ileum (*arrow*). (**B**) Power Doppler sonogram of terminal ileum demonstrates increased mural flow indicating hyperemia (*arrow*).

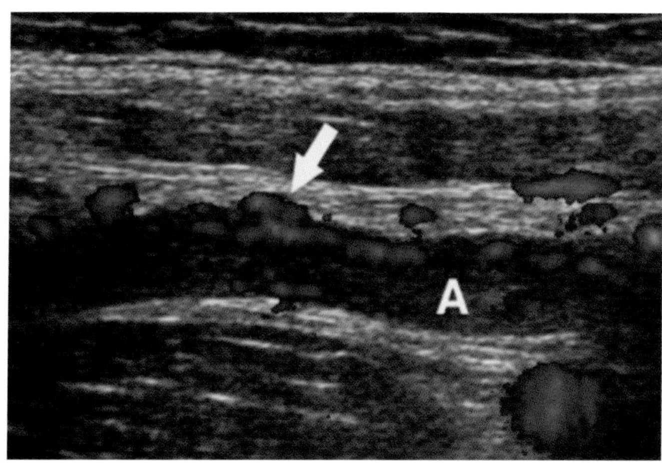

FIGURE 9 ■ Power Doppler sonogram in acute appendicitis. Longitudinal sonogram of appendix (A) demonstrates increased flow from hyperemia (*arrow*).

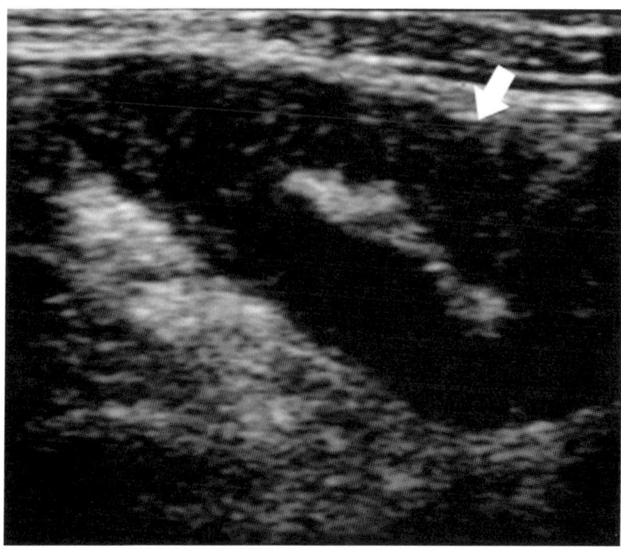

FIGURE 11 ■ Pseudokidney sign due to sigmoid colon cancer. Note diffuse hypoechoic thickening of the bowel wall (*arrow*) due to neoplastic infiltration with echogenic lumen mimicking the sonographic appearance of kidney.

disorders (Figs. 6–9), in seven of nine patients with neoplasms, and no mural flow in all four patients with small bowel infarction. Color Doppler sonography does not appear to be helpful in distinguishing inflammatory from neoplastic lesions. Teefey et al. (3) found in a study of 35 patients with inflammatory or ischemic bowel wall thickening that absence of or barely visible color Doppler flow and absence of an arterial signal were highly indicative of bowel wall ischemia (Fig. 7). They also found a resistive index less than 0.60 to be suggestive of inflammatory bowel wall thickening.

Clautice–Engle et al. (2) showed that power Doppler imaging was more sensitive than color Doppler imaging in detecting flow in gastrointestinal lesions (Figs. 8 and 9). Power Doppler imaging improved visualization of intramural gastrointestinal vascularity and improved confidence

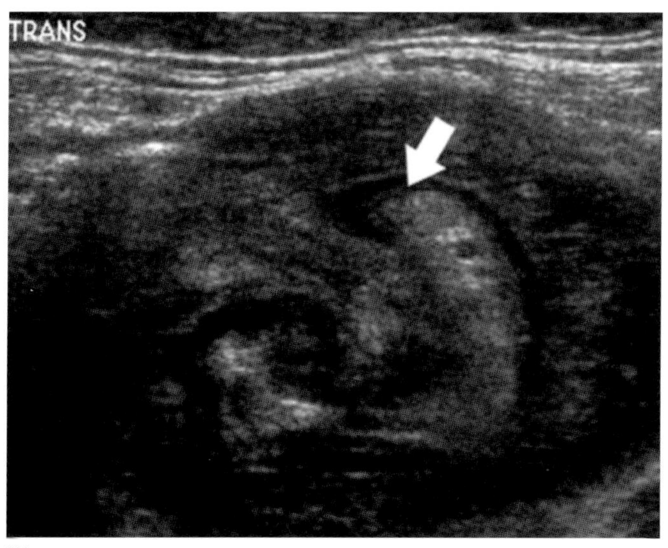

(A)

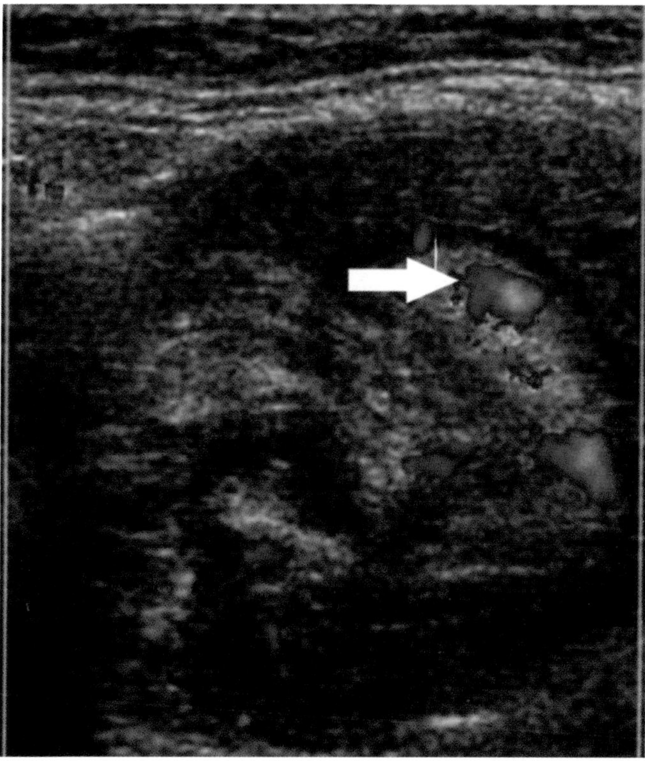

(B)

FIGURE 10 A AND B ■ Target pattern in colocolonic intussusception from colon cancer. (**A**) Transverse sonogram of the sigmoid colon demonstrating an echogenic center representing invaginating mass with its mesentery (*arrow*). The hypoechoic periphery is due to thickened colon wall. (**B**) Corresponding power Doppler sonogram demonstrating invaginated mesenteric vessels from intussusception (*arrow*).

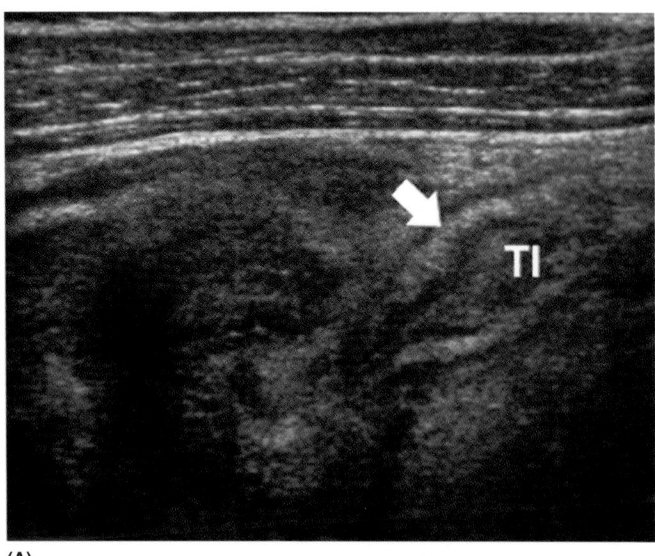

(A)

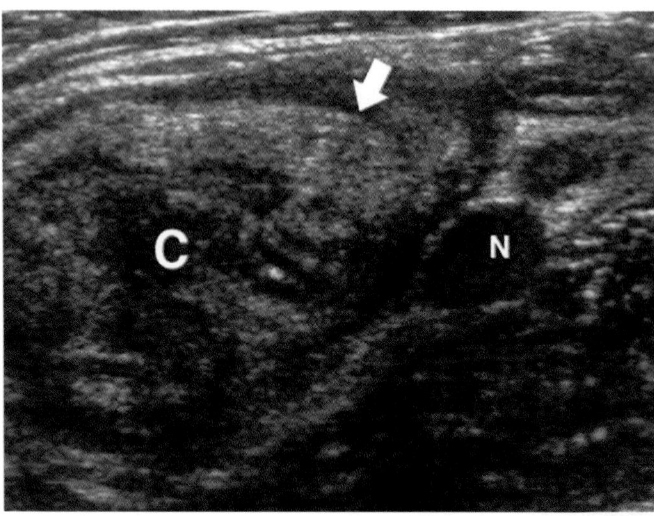

(B)

FIGURE 12 A AND B ■ Thickening of submucosal layer of bowel wall due to *Campylobacter ileocolitis*. (**A**) Transverse sonogram of the terminal ileum (TI) demonstrating thickened and enlarged submucosal layer (*arrow*). (**B**) Transverse sonogram of cecum (C). Note thickening of cecal submucosa (*arrow*) and adjacent lymph node (N).

in differentiating ischemic from nonischemic lesions. Thus, in the appropriate clinical setting of patients with focal bowel wall thickening, the absence of power Doppler signal suggests bowel ischemia.

DISEASE STATES

Acute Appendicitis

Both ultrasound and computed tomography (CT) have been shown to be reliable modalities in diagnosing acute appendicitis (10–16). Although in many instances, classic signs and symptoms permit clinicians to make the diagnosis of acute appendicitis, either ultrasound or CT may be a valuable technique for patients with atypical clinical findings. Ultrasound is more operator dependent than CT but has been shown to be useful in most studies in the evaluation of the patient with right lower quadrant pain, particularly in pediatric patients and in thin adults. Graded compression ultrasound of the right lower quadrant may be expedited with improved diagnostic accuracy if self-localization is added to the examination. It has been shown that when the patient points to the area of pain, this sonographic self-localization reduces the examination time and is a valuable addition to the standard graded compression ultrasound of the appendix (17). The examination of this area is performed by first obtaining scans of the right flank to identify the ascending colon. Once identified, the ascending colon is followed to the cecum. Although the location of the tip of the appendix is variable, the appendix always originates from the base of the cecum. Once the cecum is identified, graded compression is gradually applied in order to displace normal overlying bowel loops and to help identify the region of the appendix.

DIAGNOSTIC EXAMINATION

The sonographic examination is considered diagnostic if the cecum and the terminal ileum can be adequately visualized and adequately compressed to provide images of the periappendiceal and retrocecal regions. The psoas and iliac vessels are important landmarks to be identified during this portion of the examination (Fig. 13). The normal appendix may often be identified (18). Sonographic

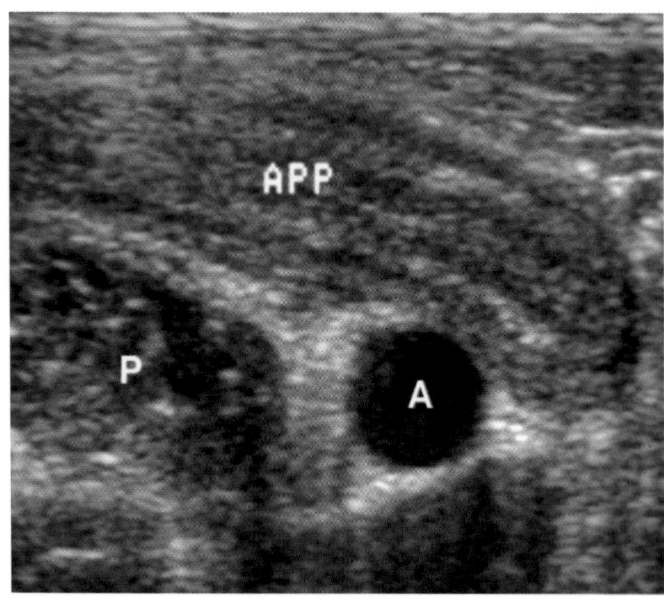

FIGURE 13 ■ Acute appendicitis. Sonographic landmarks in the right lower quadrant. Note enlarged noncompressible appendix (APP) with adjacent external iliac artery (A) and psoas muscle (P).

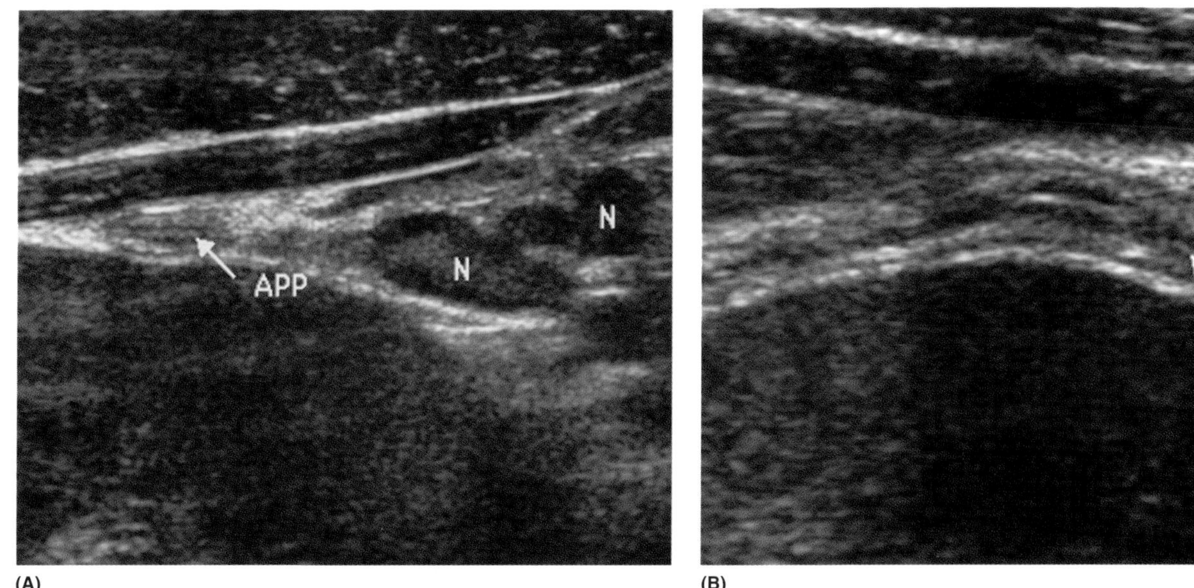

(A) (B)

FIGURE 14 A AND B ■ Normal appendix (APP) on graded compression sonography. (**A**) Note 4 mm appendix in short axis and adjacent mesenteric lymph nodes (N). (**B**) Longitudinal scan of normal appendix measuring 5 mm in outer diameter.

features of a normal appendix include (*i*) a maximum outer diameter of 6 mm or less; (*ii*) maximum wall thickness of 2 mm or less; (*iii*) demonstration that the appendix originates from the base of the cecum; (*iv*) demonstration of the inner echogenic submucosal ring and the outer hypoechoic ring; (*v*) no observable peristalsis; and (*vi*) termination in a blind pouch.

Although no specific measurement is completely conclusive of a normal appendix, some authors believe that 5 mm from outer wall to outer wall in the anteroposterior plane should be considered the upper limit of normal for the appendix (Fig. 14). A measurement of 7 mm or greater is considered positive for acute appendicitis. Thus, a measurement between 5 and 7 mm is inconclusive and warrants close scrutiny (19). Increased mural flow within the appendix may aid in suggesting appendicitis in patients where the appendix is borderline in size (5–7 mm).

Sonographic Criteria for Acute Appendicitis

Sonographic criteria for acute appendicitis include a noncompressible appendix with either an outer diameter of 7 mm or more, or wall thickness of 3 mm or greater (Fig. 15) (12). Color Doppler or power Doppler imaging may demonstrate increased flow with uncomplicated acute appendicitis; however, a perforated or necrotic appendix may demonstrate an absence of color flow (1,2).

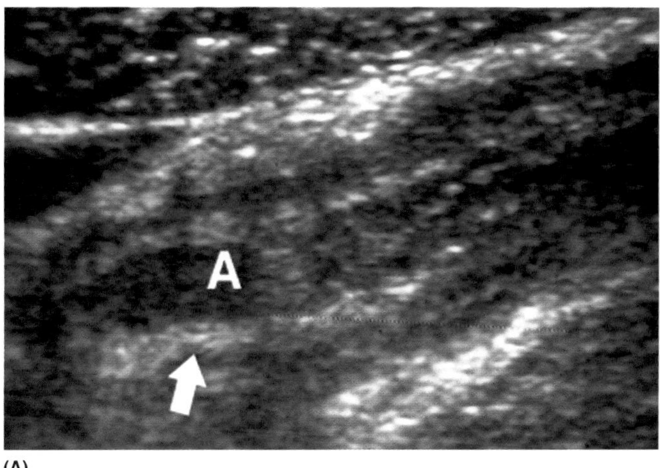

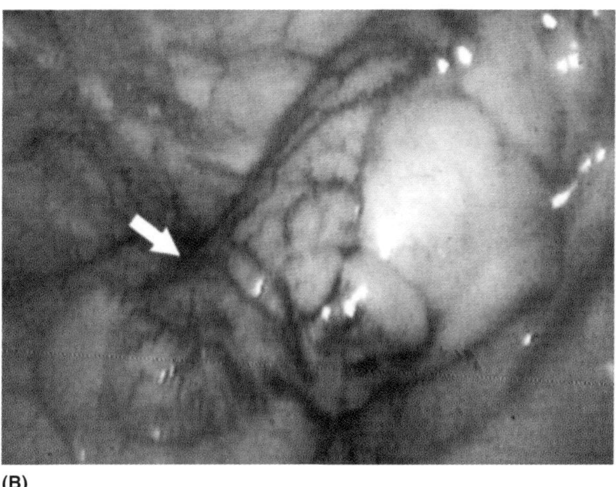

(A) (B)

FIGURE 15 A AND B ■ Acute appendicitis. (**A**) Longitudinal sonogram demonstrates enlarged noncompressible appendix (A) consistent with acute nonperforated appendicitis. Note preservation of echogenic submucosal layer (*arrow*). (**B**) Laparoscopic image of the inflamed appendix (*arrow*).

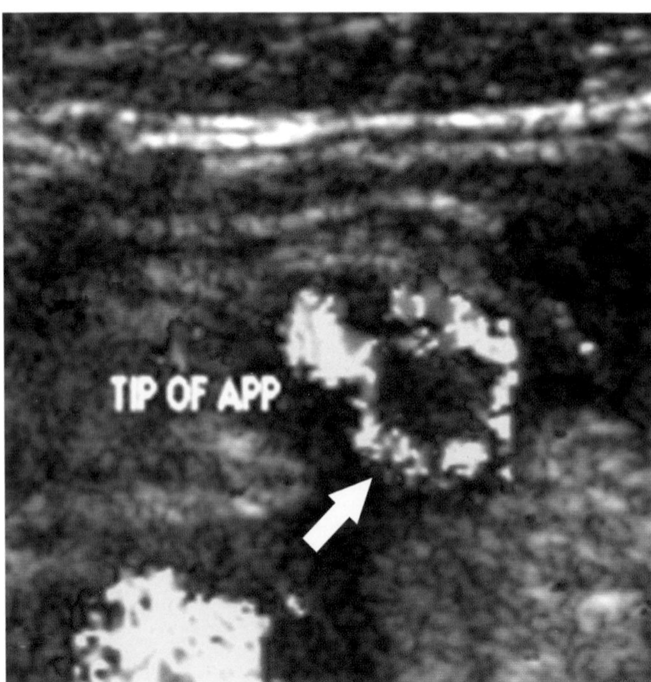

FIGURE 16 ■ Acute appendicitis at the tip. Transverse power Doppler scan of tip of appendix demonstrates hyperemia (*arrow*) consistent with acute appendicitis.

Pitfalls

There are several pitfalls in the diagnosis of appendicitis, including the following:

Appendicitis confined to the appendiceal tip. An early inflammatory response to the appendix may be confined to the more distal tip of the appendix. Thus, if examination is confined only to the base or proximal portion of the appendix, this early inflammatory response may be missed (Fig. 16).

TABLE 1 ■ Enlarged Appendix

- Acute appendicitis
- Resolving appendicitis
- Secondary inflamed appendix
  - Crohn's disease
  - Ulcerative colitis
  - Cecal diverticulitis
  - Salpingitis
- Appendiceal tumor

Retrocecal appendix. Whereas the base of the appendix originates from the cecum, the tip may lie in a variety of different locations. Most difficult to examine is the retrocecal appendix, which is tucked behind the cecum. Thus, graded compression sonography may be helpful in identifying this retrocecal area; images of the right iliac fossa using the lateral flank approach may also be helpful.

Perforated appendicitis. In patients with either gangrenous or perforated appendix, the characteristic sonographic features of an inflamed appendix may not be identified. The examiner, therefore, may be confused and believe that the examination results are normal since the appendix is not visualized; however, the appendix actually is either gangrenous or perforated (Figs. 17 and 18).

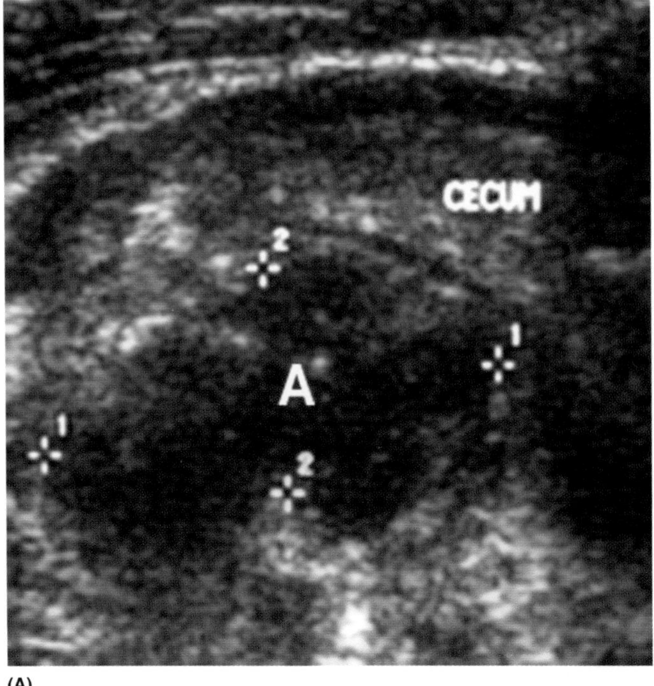

(A)

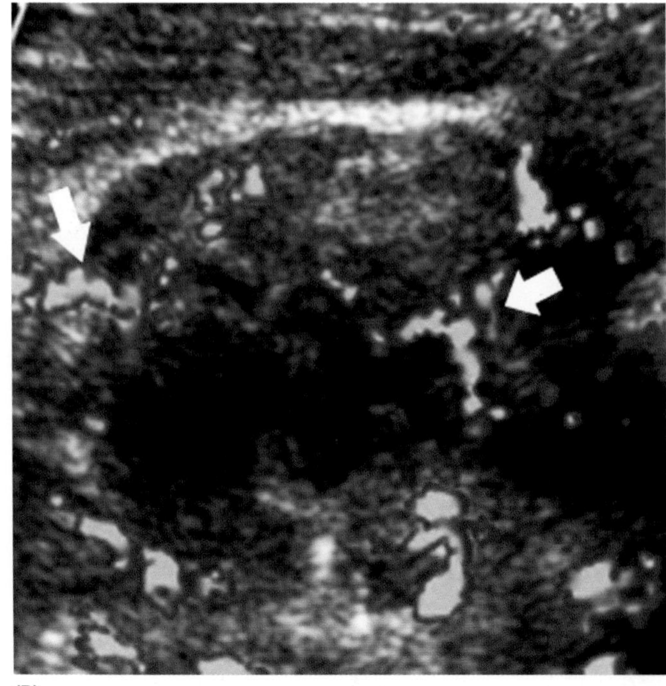

(B)

FIGURE 17 A AND B ■ Perforated appendicitis with retrocecal abscess. (**A**) Transverse gray-scale sonogram of cecum demonstrating irregular hypoechoic abscess cavity. (**B**) Power Doppler sonogram demonstrates marked adjacent hyperemia (*arrows*). A, abscess.

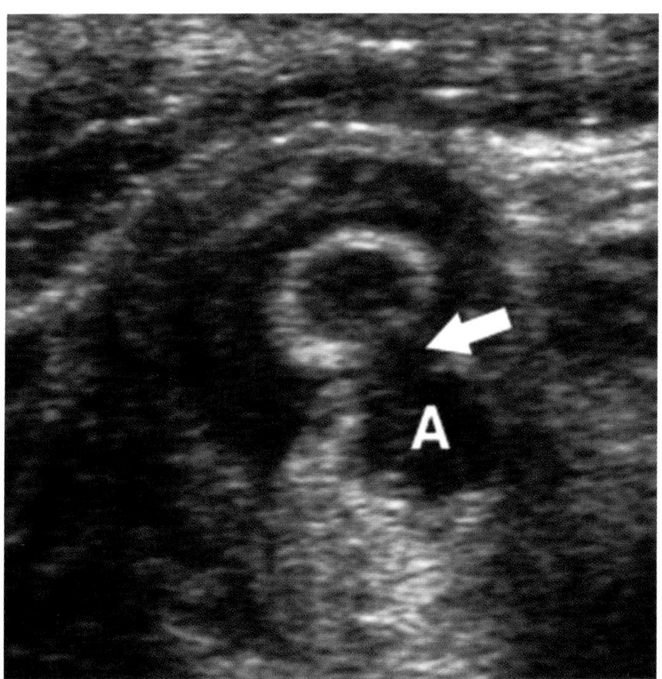

FIGURE 18 ■ Perforated appendicitis. Transverse sonogram of inflamed appendix demonstrates focal mural necrosis (*arrow*) with small adjacent abscess (A).

Gas-filled appendix. Rarely, gas may be present within the appendix as a result of gas-forming organisms. This acoustic shadowing may be difficult to interpret and may result in a false-negative diagnosis of appendicitis (19).

Spontaneous resolution of appendicitis. Ultrasound is a valuable method for documenting cases of appendicitis that spontaneously resolve. In approximately 10% of cases, there is an abortive clinical course that includes a rapid resolution of the patient's symptoms. However, findings of the ultrasound examination lag behind the clinical course; thus, though results of the ultrasound examination may show positive findings of an enlarged appendix, the patient has clinically improved (20).

Other causes of enlarged appendix (Table 1). Although acute appendicitis is the most common etiology for the enlarged noncompressible appendix, the appendix may enlarge due to several other etiologies. These include appendiceal tumors such as a carcinoid or adenocarcinoma of the appendix or secondary inflammation from surrounding disease such as Crohn's disease, ulcerative colitis, diverticulitis, or salpingitis (Fig. 19).

Other causes of right lower quadrant pain (Table 2). In addition to appendicitis, etiologies for right lower quadrant

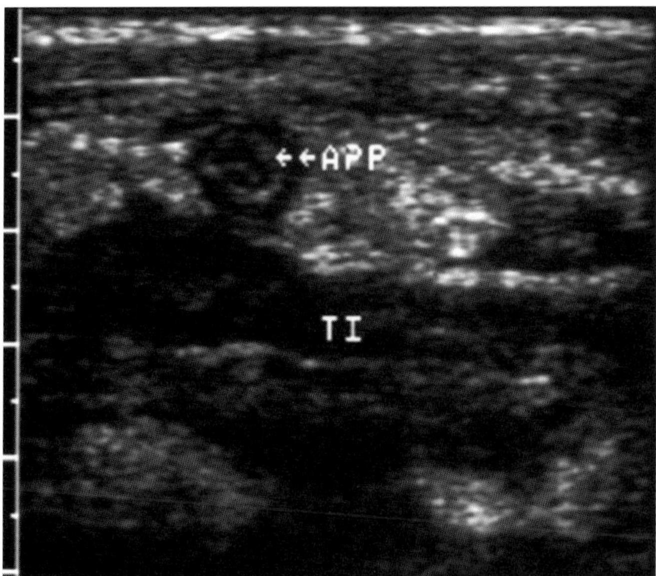

FIGURE 19 ■ Secondary enlargement of the appendix due to Crohn's disease. Note thickening of terminal ileum (TI) and enlargement of the appendix (APP).

TABLE 2 ■ Right Lower Quadrant Pain: Diagnostic Considerations

Gynecological
Ovarian cyst
Ectopic pregnancy
Ovarian torsion (Fig. 20)
Pyosalpinx/tubo-ovarian abscess (Figs. 21 and 22)
Endometriosis
Degenerating fibroids (Fig. 23)
Bowel disease
Diverticulitis (Figs. 24–26)
Infectious ileocecitis
Infectious colitis
Crohn's disease
Malignancy
Intussusception
Meckel's diverticulum
Ischemic colitis
Gallbladder
Cholecystitis
Perforation
Renal
Urolithiasis
Tumor
Mesentery
Mesenteric lymphadenitis
Right segmental omental infarction
Biliary
Liver abscess
Retroperitoneal
Tumor
Abscess
Appendix
Appendicitis
Secondary inflamed appendix
Tumor

Source: From Refs. 21, 22.

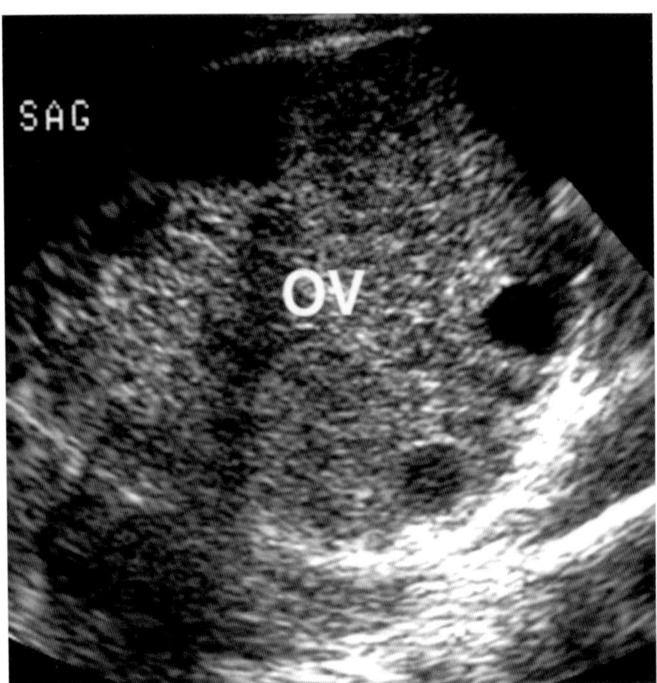

FIGURE 20 ■ Ovarian torsion mimicking appendicitis. Note enlarged echogenic right ovary (OV) on sagittal endovaginal scan.

pain include gynecologic abnormalities such as salpingitis and fibroids and bowel disease such as diverticulitis, infectious colitis, bowel malignancies, mesenteric lymphadenitis, cholecystitis, or urolithiasis (Figs. 20–23). Thus, when patients present with right lower quadrant symptoms and a normal appendix is identified, the sonographer should search for other causes of right lower quadrant pain (21).

Complications of Appendicitis

Acute appendicitis may resolve spontaneously in 10% of cases; however, if left untreated, acute appendicitis may progress to gangrenous appendicitis, periappendiceal phlegmon formation, or a periappendiceal abscess. These complications of appendicitis can be recognized sonographically. In some instances, gangrenous appendicitis may be recognized due to focal interruption of the echogenic submucosal layer of the appendix from necrosis (Fig. 18). The adjacent mesenteric fat is often thickened and echogenic due to inflammation from gangrenous appendicitis.

A periappendiceal phlegmon is an area of indurated soft-tissue inflammation that has not progressed to a periappendiceal abscess with liquefied pus. This phlegmon may be difficult to recognize sonographically because it is a poorly defined mass of mixed echogenicity. It can easily be overlooked if there has been a progression of acute appendicitis (23).

Finally, complex fluid collections surrounding or adjacent to the appendix are strongly suggestive of periappendiceal abscess (Figs. 17 and 18) (22). As described elsewhere within this text, sonography may be useful for either aspiration or drainage of these periappendiceal fluid collections.

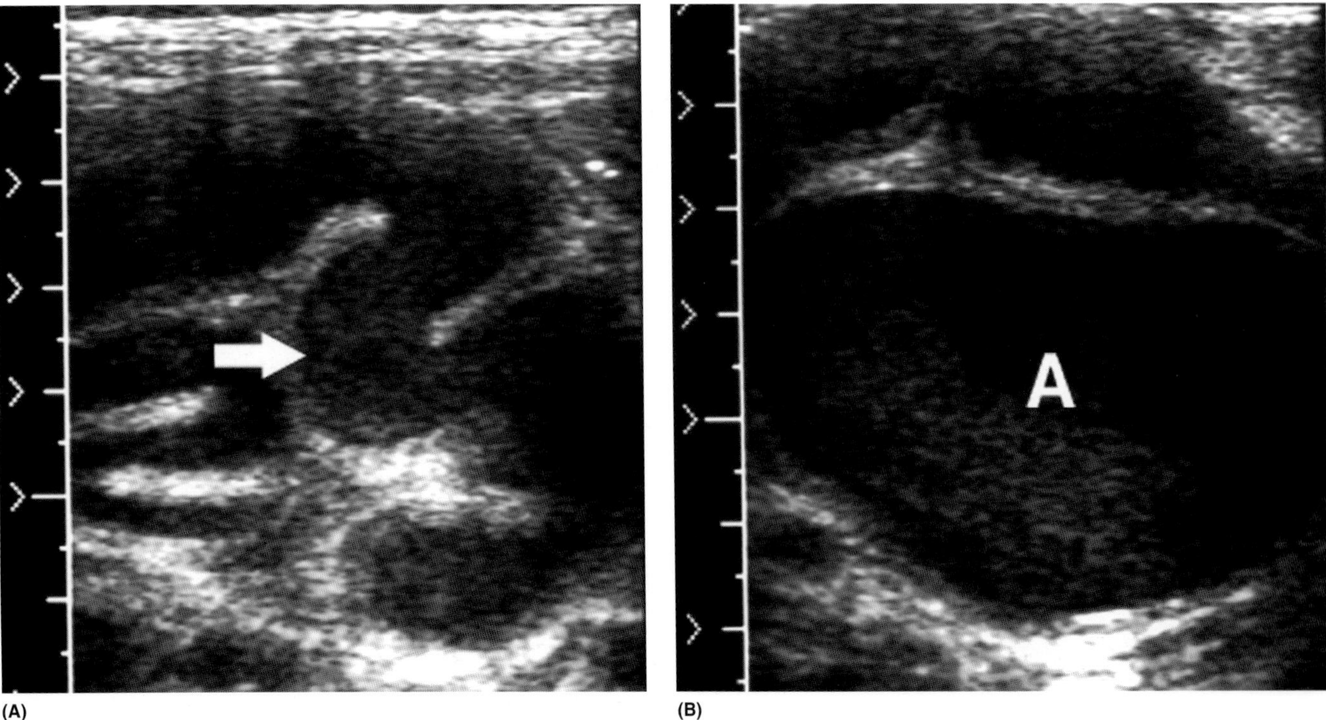

FIGURE 21 A AND B ■ Pyosalpinx with tubo-ovarian abscess (A). (**A**) Note dilated and tortuous fallopian tube (*arrow*) with low-level echoes consistent with pus. (**B**) Adjacent tubo-ovarian abscess is noted.

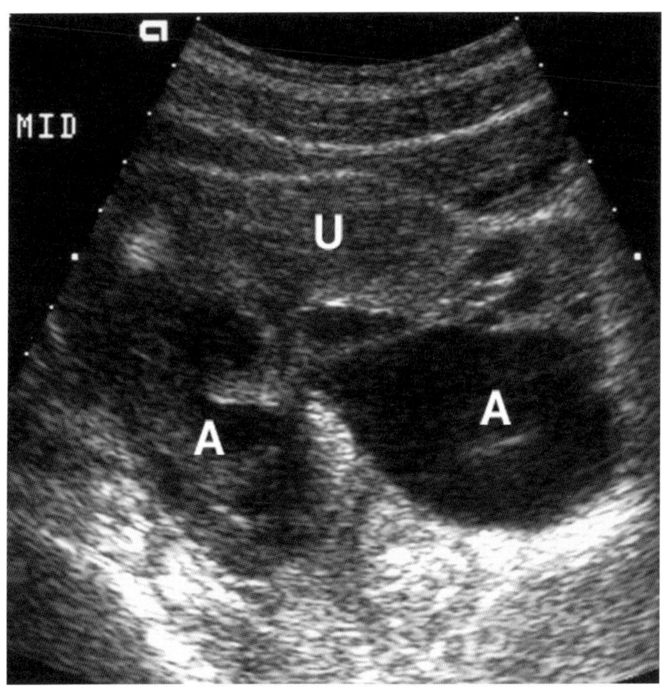

FIGURE 22 ■ Bilateral tubo-ovarian abscesses. Transverse scan of pelvis demonstrates bilateral complex fluid collections representing abscesses (A) posterior to the uterus (U).

Acute Diverticulitis

Patients with acute left-sided colonic diverticulitis typically present with left lower quadrant pain, fever, and leukocytosis. Prior to CT and sonography, diverticulitis was most often diagnosed with a barium enema, demonstrating thickening of the involved segment of bowel, fistula formation, or pericolonic abscesses (24). CT is most often the imaging method of choice and useful to identify changes associated with acute diverticulitis. These include thickened bowel, gas in perforated diverticula, pericolonic fistula formation, and associated abscesses (24). CT is superior to sonography in evaluating patients with diverticulitis, as it is not limited by patient body habitus or the overlying gas collections, and it may demonstrate the true extent of abscesses and fistulas (25–32).

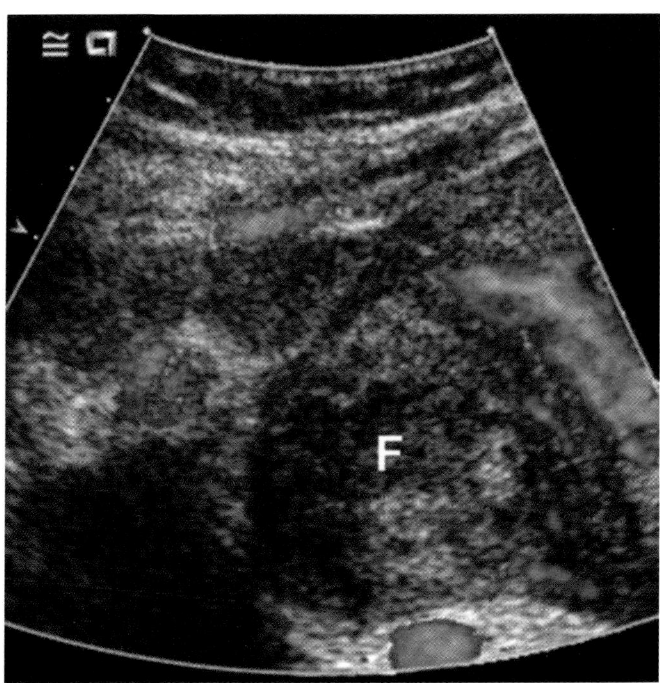

FIGURE 23 ■ Degenerating fibroid (F) mimicking appendicitis. Transverse power Doppler sonogram of right lower quadrant demonstrates avascular exophytic fibroid.

Sonographic features are often nonspecific and include the following:

Thickening of the involved segment of bowel. Muscular hypertrophy, inflammation, and edema cause segmental hypoechoic bowel wall thickening, a nonspecific sonographic finding that may occur with other etiologies such as neoplasms, Crohn's disease, or ulcerative colitis (26–28).

Identification of diverticula. Inflamed diverticula may be identified as hypoechoic, predominantly hyperechoic, hyperechoic with surrounding hypoechoic rim, or hyperechoic with acoustic shadowing, due to presence of air, fecal material, or enterolith within the diverticula (Figs. 24 and 25) (28,29). Inflamed diverticula are more frequently identified in patients with uncomplicated diverticulitis than those with complicated diverticulitis (29).

Changes in surrounding fat. Acute inflammatory changes of the pericolonic fat usually present as mass-like hyperechoic areas (Figs. 25 and 26) (31).

Abscess formation. Abscess collections may be identified as hypoechoic regions or loculated fluid collections surrounding the affected colonic segment. These fluid collections may contain air-producing echogenic foci, associated with dirty acoustic shadowing (31).

Associated fistula. Rarely, fistulous tracts may be identified as originating from the inflamed diverticula. These tracts are either fluid-filled and hypoechoic or gas-filled and echogenic with dirty acoustic shadowing.

Right-sided colonic diverticulitis is a less common entity than left-sided diverticulitis. It is more frequently seen in younger patients, often of Asian ethnicity, with symptoms similar to acute appendicitis (30). Imaging is therefore important in establishing the diagnosis, as surgery can be avoided in most patients with diverticulitis. Sonographically, right-sided diverticulitis presents with findings similar to left-sided diverticulitis. A definitive diagnosis can be established when an inflamed diverticulum is seen arising from the colon (30,32).

Color Doppler sonography (1) or power Doppler imaging (2) may be useful in demonstrating the increased Doppler flow in regions of inflammation from diverticulitis. Ultrasound may also be used to guide aspiration or drainage of fluid collections in these patients.

OTHER DISORDERS

Inflammatory Bowel Disease—Crohn's Disease

Crohn's disease most commonly affects the terminal ileum and the colon as a transmural granulomatous inflammatory process of the gut with associated fistula formation and, occasionally, abscess formation. Ultrasound may be helpful in the following:

Detection of bowel wall thickening. Thickened loops of bowel are the most frequent sonographic finding in Crohn's disease. The thickened wall may appear stratified with preservation of the wall layers or may have the appearance of a pseudokidney when the stratification of the layers is lost (33,34). Clinical disease activity appears to correlate with the degree of bowel wall thickening; however, correlation with wall echogenicity is controversial (35,36). Activity of the disease process correlates with hyperemia as demonstrated with the use of color Doppler (Fig. 27) (37,38).

Demonstration of a conglomerate mass. A conglomerate fibrofatty mass is often associated with Crohn's disease, representing matted bowel, inflamed mesentery, and thickened fat (Fig. 28).

Identification of a fistula. Fistula formation may be identified by ultrasound as a hypoechoic tract, or in some instances, a gas-filled fistulous tract may be identified (Fig. 27).

Identification of abscess formation. Ultrasound may also be used to identify associated abscess formation (Fig. 28) (33,34).

Mesenteric Adenitis

Mesenteric adenitis is a common cause of acute abdominal pain in pediatric patients (Fig. 29). This is one of the most frequent gastrointestinal causes of a missed diagnosis of acute appendicitis. Sonographic findings of mesenteric adenitis

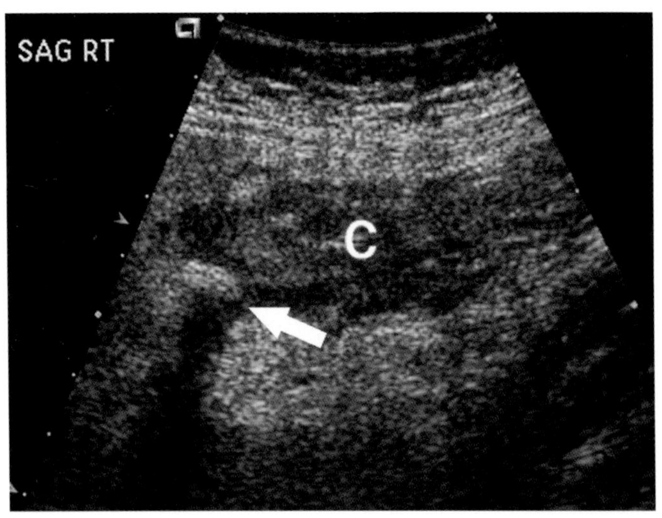

(A)

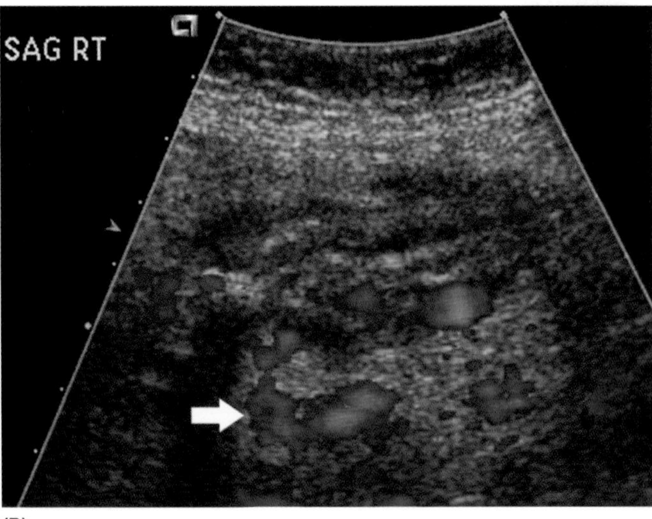

(B)

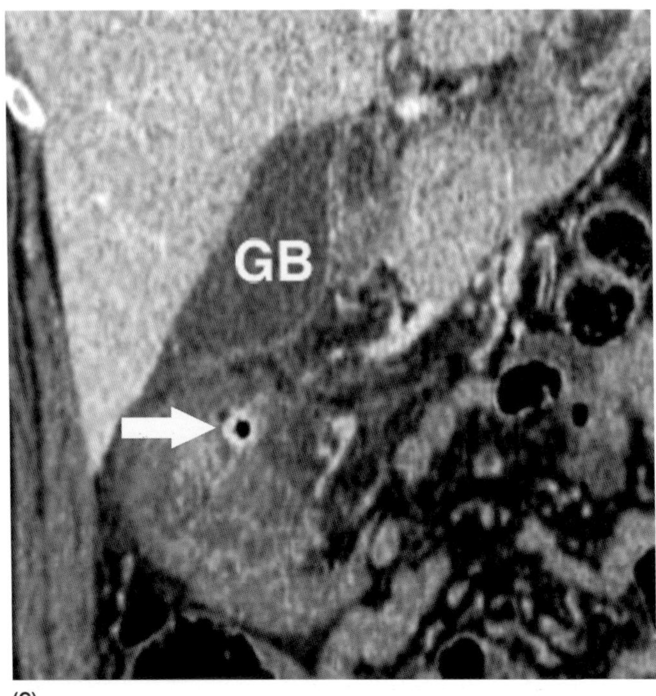

(C)

FIGURE 24 A–C ■ (**A**) Hepatic flexure diverticulitis diagnosed from a transverse sonogram of the right colon (C). Note acoustic shadowing from echogenic mural focus within diverticulum (*arrow*). (**B**) Note hyperemia within pericolonic fat on power Doppler sonogram (*arrow*). (**C**) Coronal reformation of a contrast CT demonstrating inflamed diverticulum (*arrow*) inferior to the gallbladder (GB).

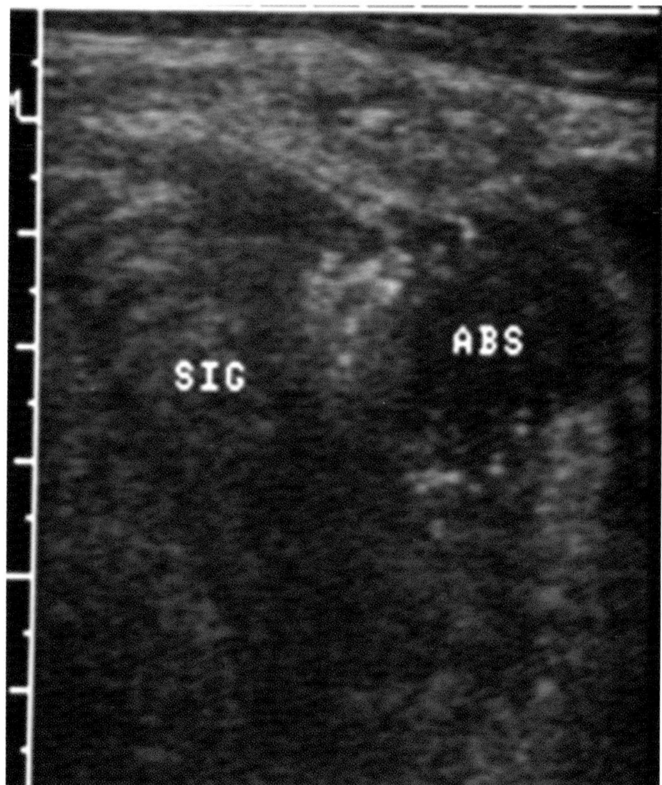

FIGURE 25 ■ Sigmoid diverticulitis with intramural abscess. On sagittal sonogram of sigmoid colon (sig), note hypoechoic intramural abscess (ABS).

include enlarged mesenteric lymph nodes, wall thickening of the terminal ileum, and a normal appendix (39).

Pneumatosis Intestinalis

Pneumatosis intestinalis may be an innocuous finding in an asymptomatic patient but in the appropriate clinical setting may be an ominous finding indicating either necrotic or ischemic bowel. Sonography may demonstrate a thickened loop of bowel with high-amplitude echoes representing gas within the bowel wall (Fig. 30) (40). Real-time imaging may demonstrate high-amplitude echoes within the portal vein and small discrete echoes noted within the periphery of the liver. These high-amplitude echoes represent air trapped within the more peripheral portal venous system; Doppler ultrasound of the portal vein usually demonstrates a highly disorganized Doppler flow pattern.

Ischemic Bowel Disease

Ischemic bowel disease demonstrates nonspecific findings on ultrasound, including thickening of the bowel wall (Fig. 30). However, color Doppler or power Doppler imaging may be helpful in diagnosing bowel ischemia, as normal color Doppler or power Doppler flow is absent in a thickened segment of ischemic or necrotic bowel (Fig. 7) (1–3,41).

Right-Sided Segmental Omental Infarction and Epiploic Appendagitis

Right-sided segmental omental infarction and epiploic appendagitis are uncommon conditions that may clinically mimic appendicitis, cholecystitis, or diverticulitis. Infarction of the omentum is usually segmental and characteristically involves the right side of the abdomen (Fig. 31). Epiploic appendages are small adipose tissue protrusions from the serosal layer of the colon that may spontaneously undergo infarction as a result of venous thrombosis or torsion (42). These benign, self-limiting conditions have a similar sonographic appearance characterized by moderately hyperechoic fatty tissue located at the area of maximal tenderness, directly under the

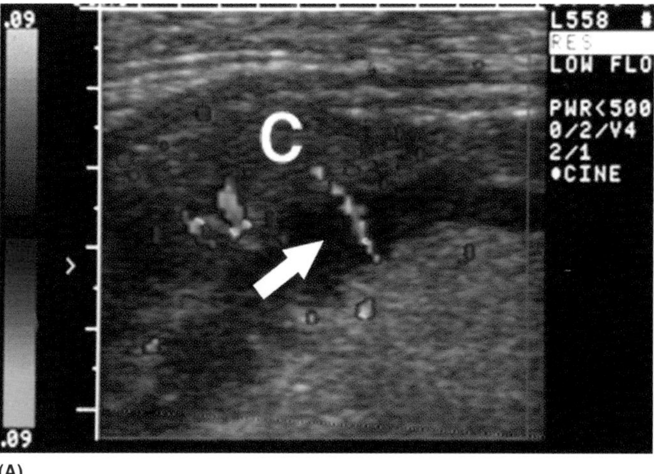

(A)

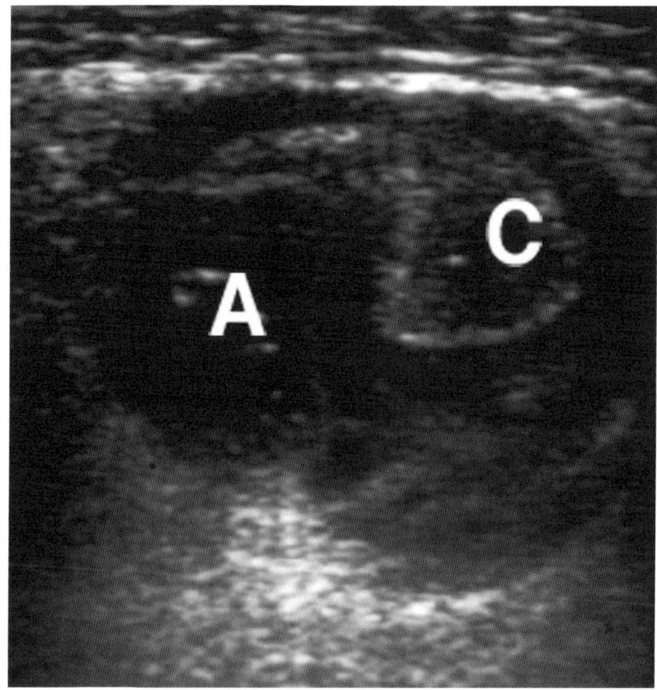

(B)

FIGURE 26 A AND B ■ Diverticular abscess with inflammatory changes in sigmoid mesentery. (**A**) Transverse color Doppler sonogram of sigmoid colon (C) demonstrates mural thickening and hyperemia (*arrow*) of sigmoid colon. Note increased echogenicity of sigmoid mesentery from inflammation (*open arrow*). (**B**) Note hypoechoic intramural abscess (A) involving sigmoid colon.

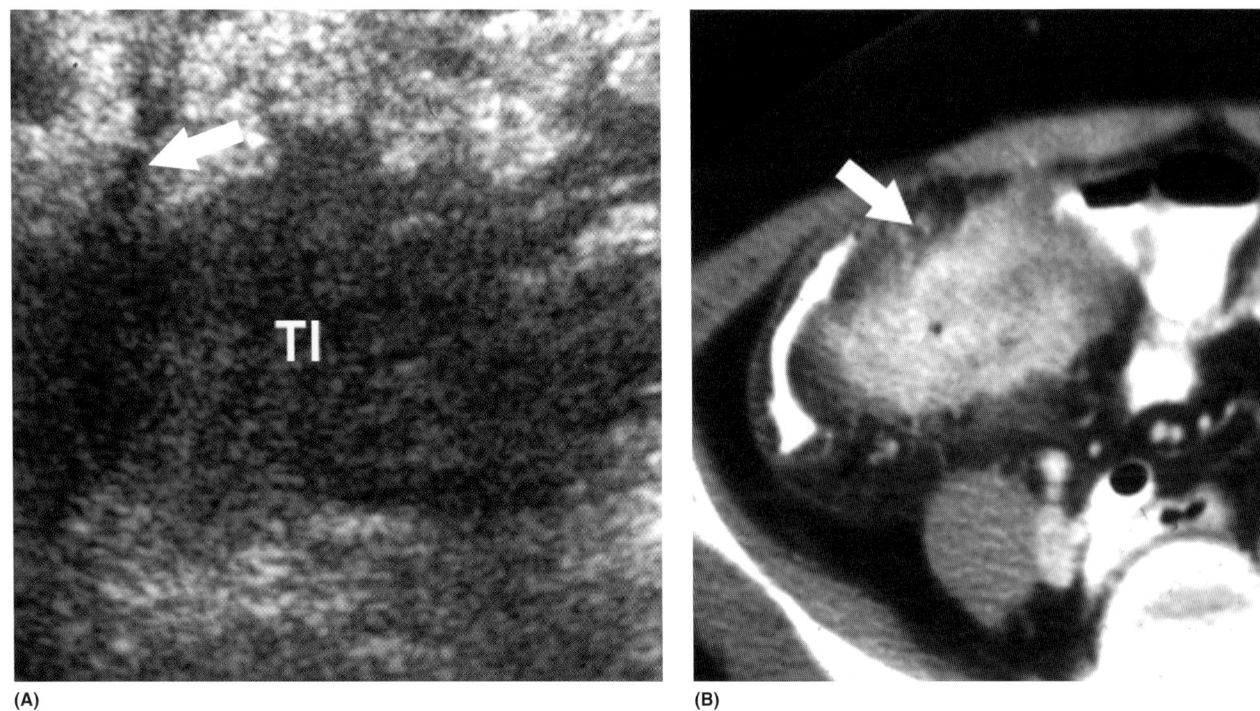

FIGURE 27 A AND B ■ Crohn's disease on sonography and CT. (**A**) Transverse sonogram of the terminal ileum (TI). Note marked hypoechoic thickening of the bowel wall and hypoechoic sinus tract extending into inflamed echogenic mesenteric fat (*arrow*). (**B**) Corresponding CT demonstrates mural thickening of ileum and extensive inflammatory changes surround terminal ileum (*arrow*).

abdominal wall and frequently adherent to the peritoneum. A peripheral hypoechoic rim may be seen surrounding the mass, with adjacent hypoechoic thickening of the involved segment of colon in cases of epiploic appendagitis (Fig. 32) (42–44).

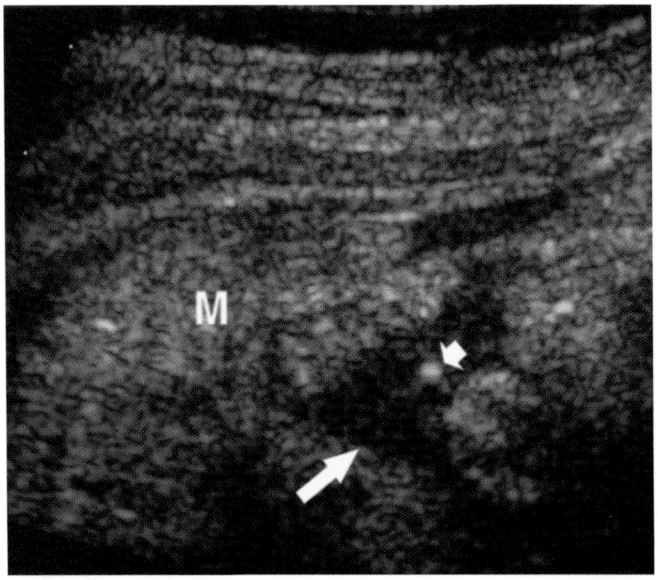

FIGURE 28 ■ Conglomerate fibrofatty mass (M) in Crohn's disease. Transverse sonogram of right lower quadrant demonstrates echogenic fibrofatty mass and adjacent hypoechoic abscess (*long arrow*) with central gas bubble (*short arrow*).

Enteritis or Colitis

Bacterial enteritis and colitis are characterized as mucosal thickening of the affected loop of bowel. Puylaert et al. (45,46) have shown ultrasound to be useful in establishing the diagnosis, which most commonly is bacterial enteritis (Fig. 33). The patient presents with right lower quadrant pain that may mimic appendicitis. Sonographic features include mucosal thickening of the ileum and the

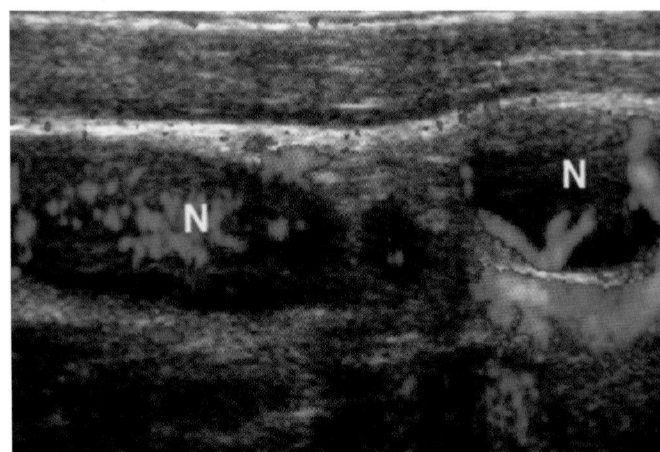

FIGURE 29 ■ Mesenteric adenitis. Transverse power Doppler sonogram of right lower quadrant demonstrates multiple enlarged hypoechoic mesenteric nodes (N).

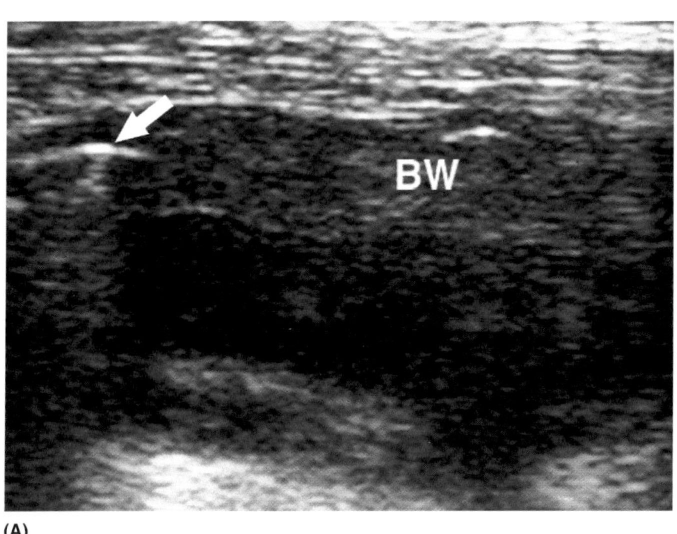

(A)

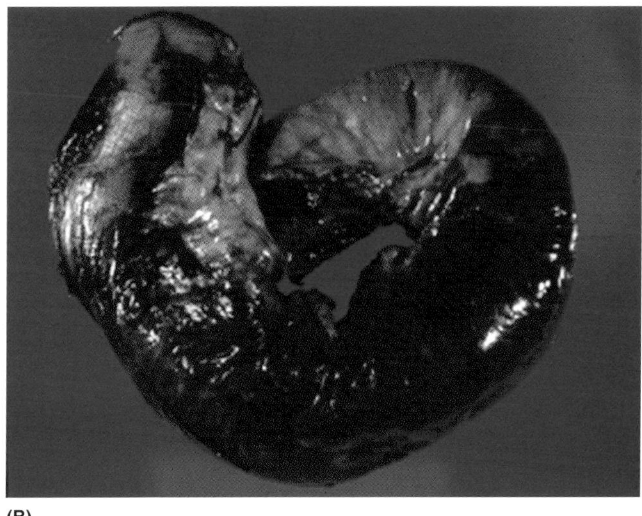

(B)

FIGURE 30 A AND B ■ Bowel infarction with pneumatosis. (**A**) Longitudinal sonogram of distal small bowel demonstrating air (*arrow*) within thickened bowel wall (BW). (**B**) Pathologic specimen of resected infarcted bowel.

cecum, with presence of enlarged mesenteric lymph nodes helping to make a more specific diagnosis (45,46).

Gastrointestinal Tract Tumors

Adenocarcinoma of the colon can be detected sonographically as a hypoechoic mass causing segmental concentric symmetric or asymmetric wall thickening (Fig. 34). This may appear as a nonspecific target or pseudokidney sign (Fig. 11) (7,8). Some tumors may have a more typical appearance than others, such as lymphoma, which appear as a bulky hypoechoic mass. Gastrointestinal stromal tumors may appear as well-marginated rounded masses of variable echogenicity, which may contain central cystic areas (Fig. 35). The tumor may be seen projecting into the bowel lumen or may appear as an exophytic mass. Malignant tumor masses of the gastrointestinal tract may have increased color Doppler or power Doppler compared

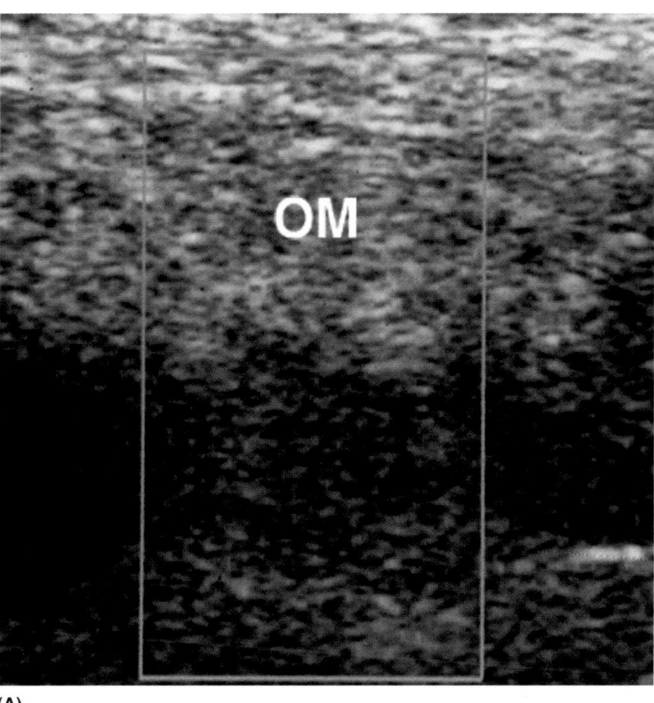

(A)

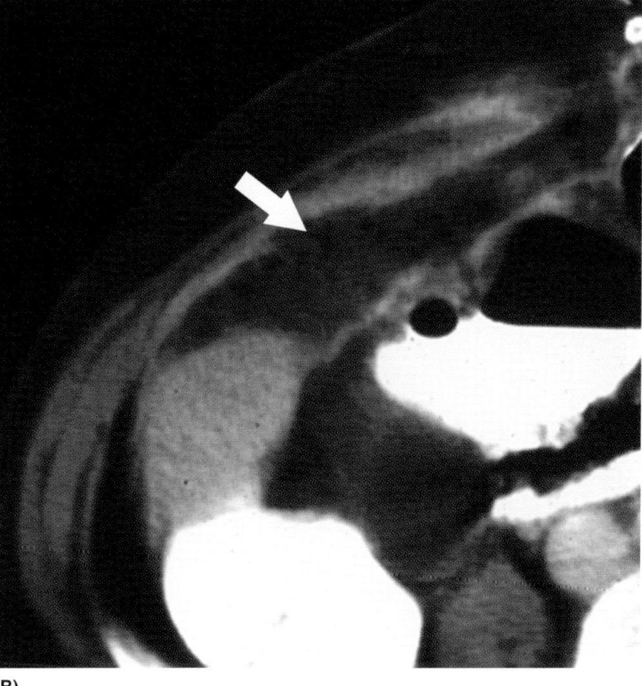

(B)

FIGURE 31 A AND B ■ Right-sided omental infarction on sonography and CT. (**A**) Transverse color Doppler sonogram of right lower quadrant demonstrating echogenic and avascular edematous omental fat (OM). (**B**) Corresponding CT demonstrates edema within omentum due to infarction (*arrow*).

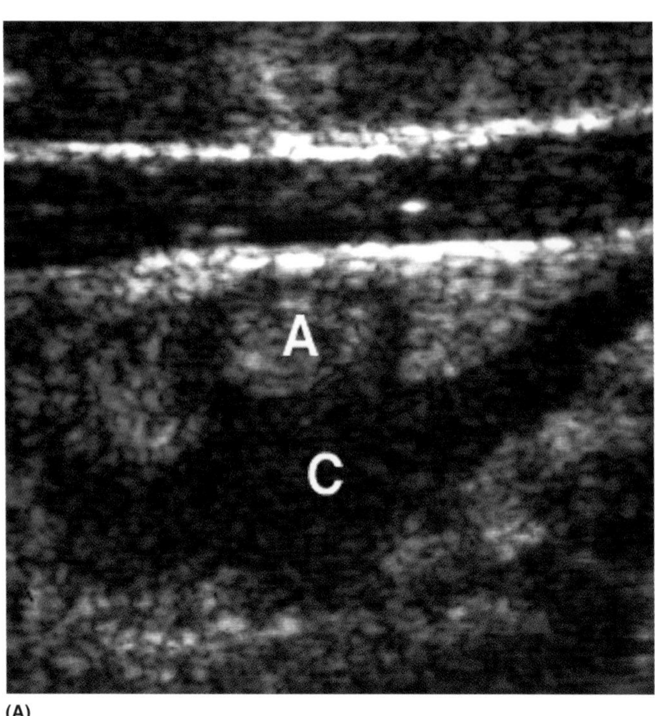

(A)

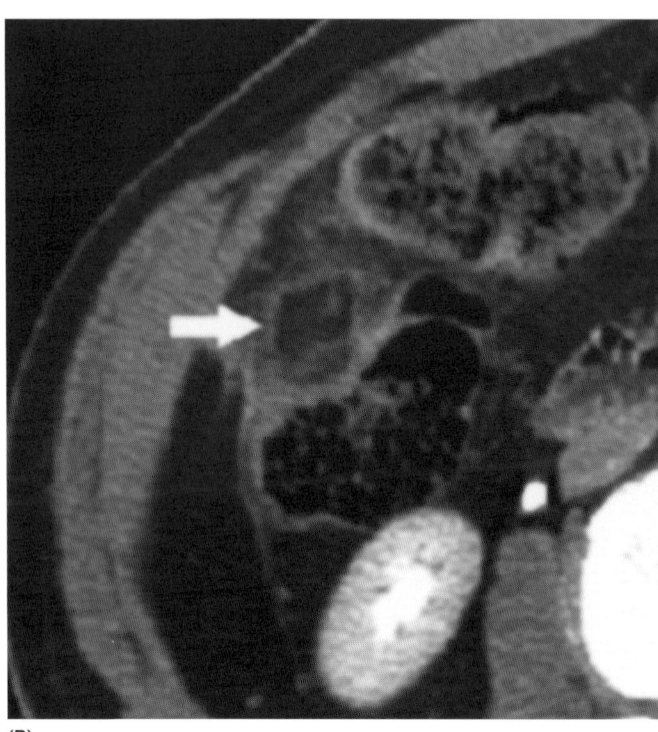

(B)

FIGURE 32 A AND B ■ Epiploic appendagitis on sonography and CT. (**A**) Transverse gray-scale sonogram of right colon demonstrating hypoechoic mural thickening of colonic (C) wall and echogenic mass representing edematous epiploic appendage (A). (**B**) Corresponding CT demonstrating inflamed fatty appendage (*arrow*).

with the normal bowel or be relatively hypovascular (1,2). Sonographic features such as asymmetric wall involvement, loss of stratification of the bowel wall, and involvement of a short segment are more frequently seen with malignancy than with benign gastrointestinal conditions.

Primary or metastatic small bowel tumors may occasionally be identified with ultrasound, particularly in patients with localized abdominal pain. Their appearance is variable, depending on whether they are intraluminal, intramural, or extramural tumors. Intraluminal tumors may appear as a mass surrounded by normal bowel, whereas intramural

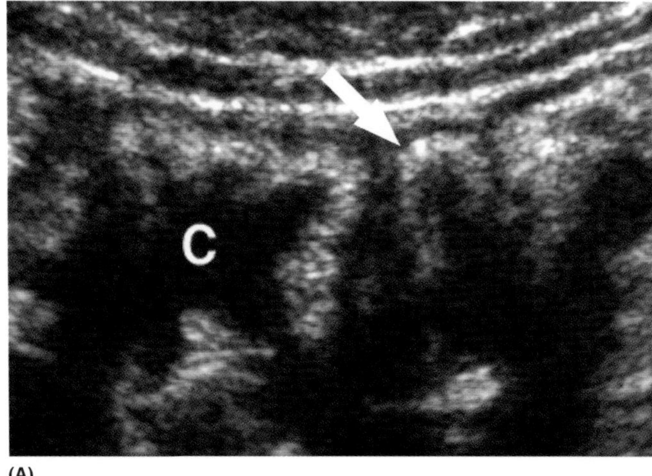

(A)

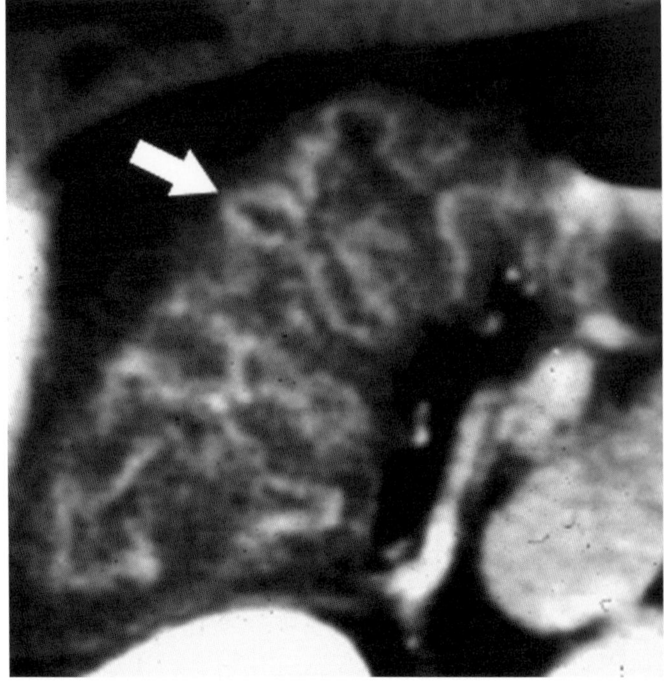

(B)

FIGURE 33 A AND B ■ Pseudomembranous colitis on sonography and CT. (**A**) Longitudinal scan of right colon (C) demonstrates mural thickening with prominence of echogenic submucosal layer (*arrow*). (**B**) Contrast CT in same patient demonstrates marked mucosal hyperemia of right colon consistent with pseudomembranous colitis (*arrow*).

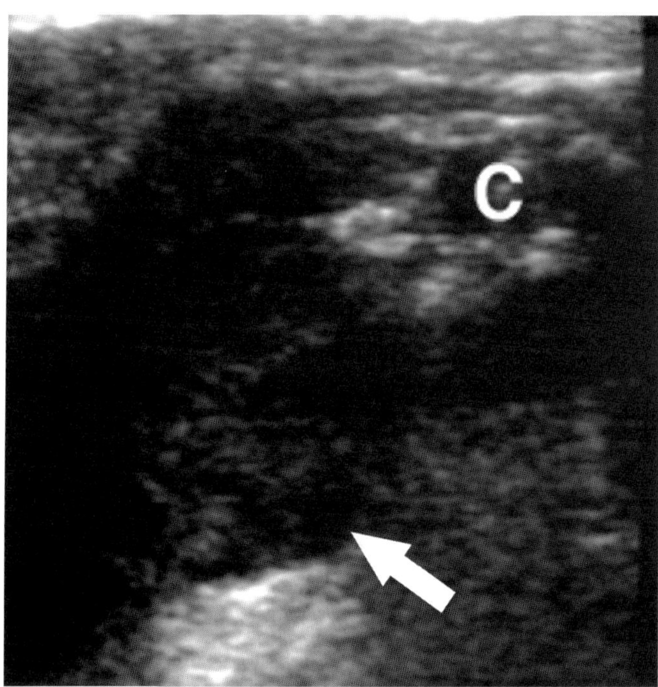

FIGURE 34 ■ Cecal carcinoma. Transverse sonogram of cecum (C) demonstrates large exophytic hypoechoic cecal mass (*arrow*) extending from cecum.

tumors have a pseudokidney or target appearance. Extraluminal tumors may have a dumbbell configuration or appear to be extrinsic to the bowel (47). Small-bowel neoplasms may be the lead point for intussusception (Fig. 36).

Gastrointestinal Obstruction

Ultrasound has a limited role to play in the patient with a clinically suspected bowel obstruction. CT has been increasingly used to evaluate these patients, supplanting plain films and barium studies as the imaging method of choice. The primary clinical questions to be answered are: (*i*) Is there a mechanical obstruction (i.e., a transition point from dilated to nondilated bowel) or merely a paralytic ileus? (*ii*) What is the likely etiology of the obstruction? (*iii*) What is the anatomic site of the obstruction? (*iv*) Is there associated strangulation or vascular compromise? Though CT is superior to sonography in addressing these clinical questions, one potential advantage of sonography is the real-time observation of increased peristalsis with early obstruction. Thus, in any patient with dilated bowel with fluid-filled hyperperistaltic loops, an effort should be made to identify a transition point indicating a mechanical obstruction (Fig. 3).

Intussusception

The clinical diagnosis of intussusception is suspected in pediatric patients presenting with abdominal pain, a palpable abdominal mass, and a currant jelly stool. Ultrasound, because of a sensitivity of nearly 100% (48), has been frequently utilized as a screening procedure in this clinical setting. The most commonly described sonographic feature of intussusception is the donut or pseudokidney sign. This entity is best understood in light of the mechanics of intussusception, where one segment of bowel (the intussusceptum) telescopes inside another segment of bowel (the intussuscipiens) (Figs. 10 and 36). Migrating internally with the intussusceptum are its associated blood vessels and mesenteric fat, which has a crescentic configuration. Although in pediatric patients a lead mass is often not identifiable, intussusception in adults is typically secondary to a benign or malignant lead mass (Figs. 10 and 36).

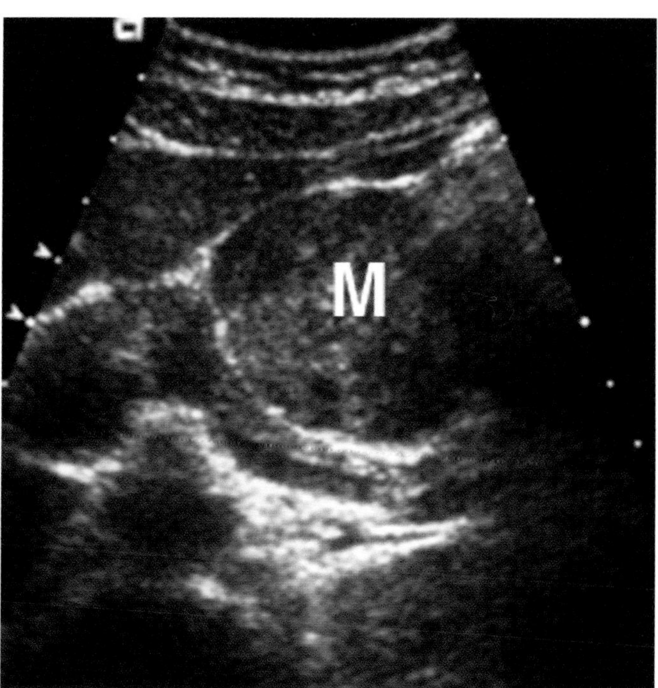

(A)

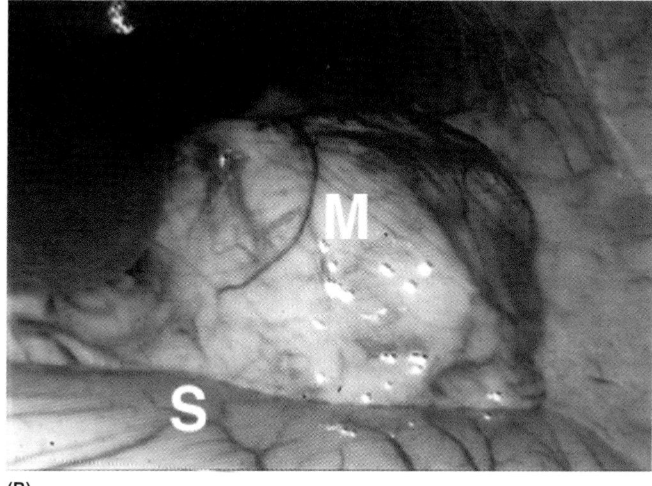

(B)

FIGURE 35 A AND B ■ Exophytic gastrointestinal stromal tumor arising from the stomach (S). (**A**) Note well-defined hypoechoic mass (M) extending medially from stomach. (**B**) Laparoscopic view demonstrates exophytic mass (M).

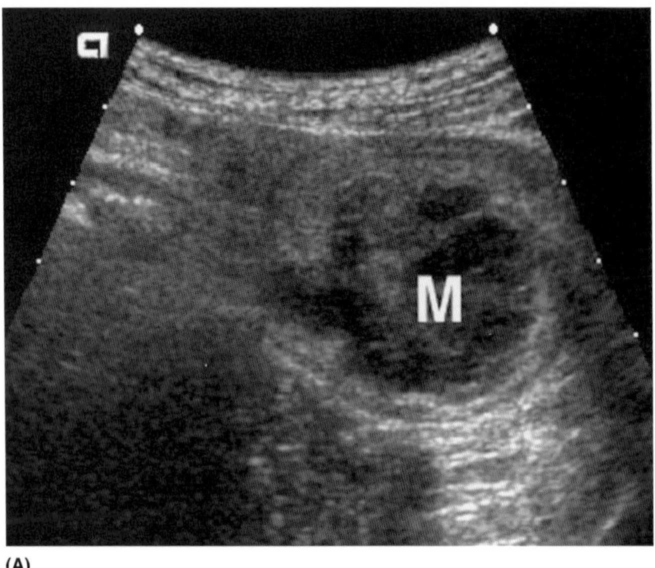

(A)

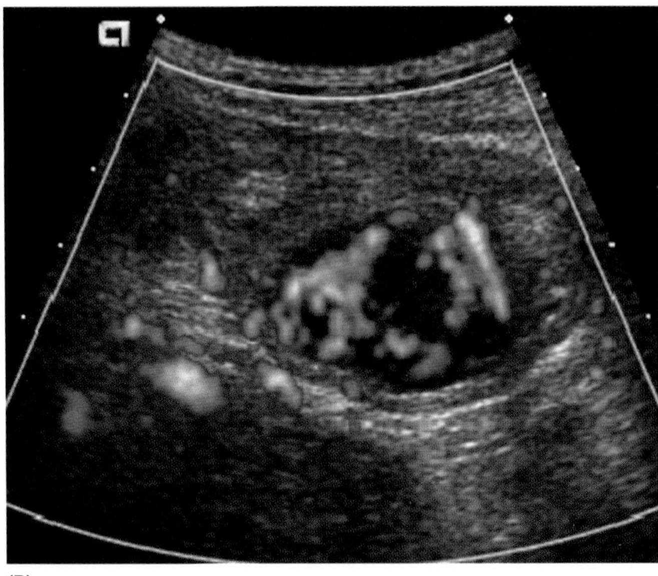

(B)

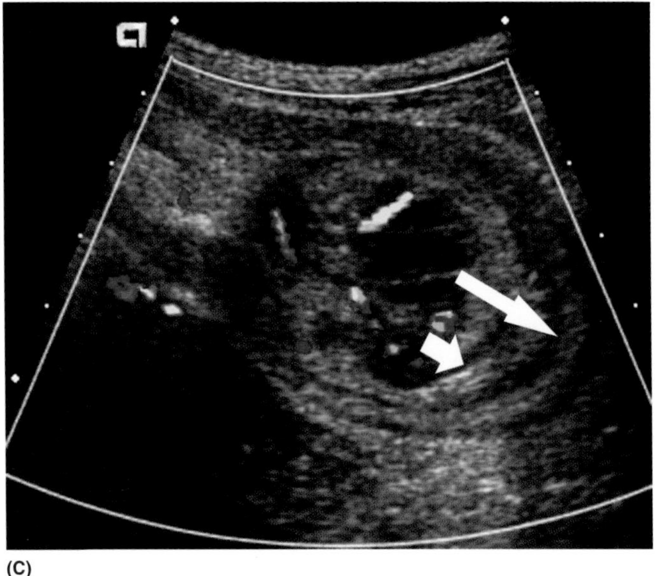

(C)

FIGURE 36 A–C ■ Metastatic melanoma to small bowel causing intussusception. (**A**) Transverse sonogram of small bowel demonstrates hypoechoic mass (M) involving small bowel. (**B**) Power Doppler image demonstrating the hypervascular nature of the mass. (**C**) Note concentric layers of submucosa of intussusceptum (*short arrow*) and intussuscipiens (*long arrow*).

Color Doppler sonography may be used to determine whether or not the intussusception is potentially reducible. Absence of color flow may be indicative of bowel wall necrosis and precludes vigorous attempts at reduction (49). Recently, sonography alone has been used to guide hydrostatic reduction without the need for fluoroscopy. Crystal et al. successfully reduced 88 of 99 cases (89%) using ultrasound guidance alone (48).

PERITONEAL CAVITY

Ultrasound Technique

The specific technique for ultrasound examination of the peritoneal cavity varies according to the clinical indication. When ultrasound is used to screen for abdominal fluid collections, a curved-array or curved-linear-array transducer with a frequency from 3.5 to 5 MHz is appropriate. Scanning must include visualization of all regions where fluid or abscesses may be located within the abdomen and the pelvis. Color Doppler or power Doppler imaging may be used to evaluate the vascularity of a particular area of interest. Although these color techniques are not helpful for evaluating possible ascites or abscesses, they may be helpful in evaluating the mesentery when there is increased vascularity from inflammation. In addition, color Doppler imaging may be used before performing interventional techniques such as paracentesis, abscess drainage, or peritoneal biopsy, in order to avoid vascular injury.

An understanding of the abnormalities of the peritoneal cavity has been aided by the pioneering anatomic work of Meyers (50). The peritoneal cavity may be divided into the abdomen proper, consisting of the upper abdominal peritoneal cavity (the greater sac) and the lesser

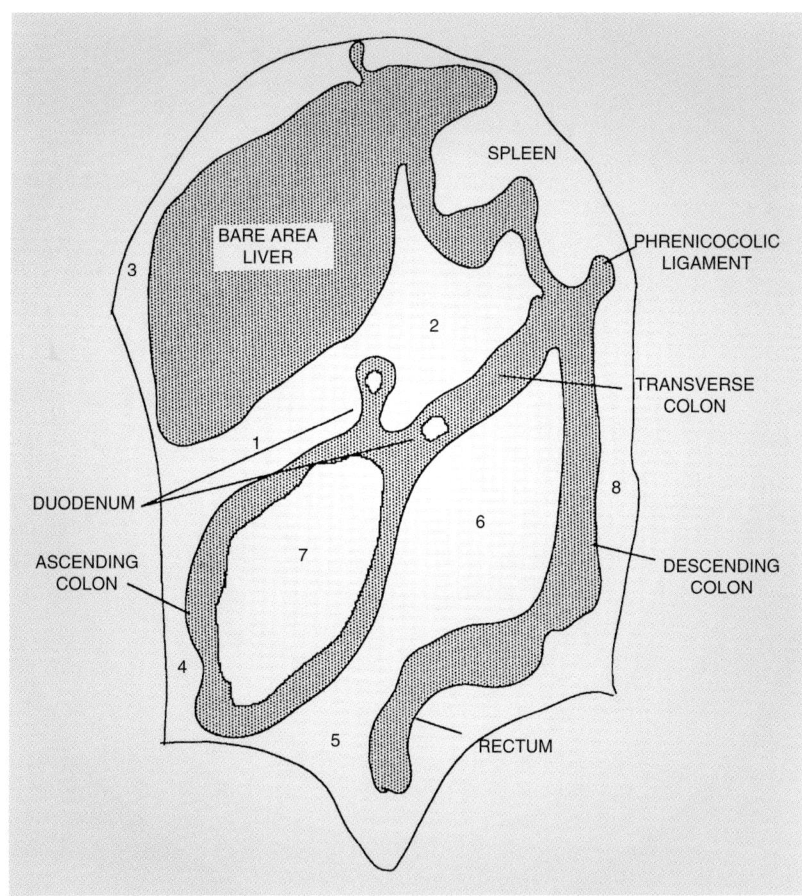

FIGURE 37 ■ Anatomic drawing of intraperitoneal spread of fluid.

peritoneal cavity (the lesser sac) (Fig. 37). The upper abdominal cavity freely communicates with the pelvis and the pelvic cul-de-sac. The cul-de-sac is the most dependent portion of the peritoneal cavity and may be the site for initial localization of fluid collections, hemorrhage in traumatized patients, or abscesses. The retroperitoneal space is usually subdivided into the anterior pararenal space, perirenal space, and posterior pararenal space. The retroperitoneum is not discussed in this chapter.

It is important to understand the compartmental anatomy of the abdomen when trying to determine where fluid collections, abscesses, or hematomas may be localized. The peritoneal compartments may be subdivided in relation to the transverse mesocolon. Four intraperitoneal spaces are located within the supramesocolic portion of the abdomen. The supramesocolic spaces lie between the diaphragm and the transverse mesocolon and include the right subhepatic space, lying between the right kidney and the liver, also called Morison's pouch; the lesser sac; the right suprahepatic space, also identified as the right subphrenic space; and the left subphrenic space. The infracolic portion of the peritoneal cavity is divided by the small bowel mesentery into the right inframesocolic space and the larger left inframesocolic space. These spaces then may communicate with the most dependent portion of the peritoneal cavity, the pelvic cul-de-sac. The intraperitoneal pelvic spaces communicate with the right paracolic gutter or the left paracolic gutter.

Although some of these spaces are contiguous, other spaces do not communicate, as they are separated by ligamentous attachments. For instance, fluid from the subhepatic space or Morison's pouch may communicate into the lesser sac through the foramen of Winslow. However, this fluid cannot communicate between the left subphrenic space and the left paracolic gutter due to the phrenicocolic ligament. Furthermore, fluid from the subhepatic space may pass into the right subphrenic space but not into the left subphrenic space, as it is blocked by the bare area of the liver. An understanding of the compartmental anatomy of the abdomen is important when identifying where ascitic fluid may collect and where abscesses are located.

Intraperitoneal Fluid Collections

Intraperitoneal fluid collections include ascites, bile, hemorrhage, lymph, urine, or pus (Table 3). Ascitic fluid may flow freely throughout the abdomen or may be loculated because of concurrent adhesions. Bile may be present within the peritoneal cavity after a bile leak from recent biliary or liver surgery. Urine may be present within the retroperitoneum but occasionally may be present within the abdomen, particularly in renal transplant patients. Other fluid collections secondary to disrupted lymphatics from previous surgery may localize as a lymphocele. Hematoma formation may result from trauma or

TABLE 3 ■ Intraperitoneal Fluid Collections

Collection	Location	Ultrasound features or acoustic characteristics
Bile	Within or adjacent to liver	Usually anechoic
Ascites	Most dependent portion of abdomen such as pelvis, "Morison's pouch," and paracolic gutters. May be localized to other areas in abdomen	Anechoic but may have internal echoes if malignant or infected
Abscess	Localizes to postsurgical site or dependent portion of abdomen such as pelvis, subphrenic, subhepatic, or paracolic gutters	Variable in appearance but usually hypoechoic with irregular margins. Septations often present, internal echoes frequent. Occasionally isoechoic within solid organs such as liver. May be echogenic with acoustic shadowing if containing gas
Hematoma	Near surgical site or independent portions of abdomen such as pelvis, "Morison's pouch," and paracolic gutters	Fresh blood is hypoechoic but may have echogenic areas throughout with occasional fluid interfaces. More chronic hematomas become more anechoic or isoechoic with adjacent solid organs
Urine	Usually retroperitoneal, but dependent on perforation site and will localize in more dependent portions of abdomen or pelvis	Anechoic unless infected; in this case, some internal debris will be present
Lymphocele	Adjacent to transplanted organs or in pelvis after radical surgery	Usually anechoic, occasionally with septations. Usually well demarcated

postsurgical bleeding. Finally, any fluid collection may become infected and present as an abdominal abscess. Each of these fluid collections is discussed separately.

Intraperitoneal Fluid

Many of the complex anatomic relations of the peritoneal cavity, such as the lesser sac and interloop compartments are better demonstrated with CT (51–53). However, ultrasound is excellent in detecting intraperitoneal fluid collections. In the upper abdomen, fluid is readily identified in the hepatorenal fossa and paracolic gutters. With increasing ascites, fluid is also noted in other spaces such as the subhepatic or subphrenic space. Only patients with a large amount of ascites demonstrate fluid within the interloop compartments. Ultrasound is an accurate technique in detecting fluid in the pelvis using the full bladder technique. However, small fluid collections within the pelvis are more clearly demonstrated with transvaginal rather than transabdominal ultrasound (54–57).

Ascitic fluid may be free flowing or loculated (Figs. 38 and 39). Free fluid may be detected in multiple intraperitoneal compartments, as discussed previously. Loculated ascites may be secondary to adhesions caused by peritonitis, prior surgery, or malignant seeding within the peritoneal cavity. In general, bowel loops in patients with loculated ascites do not float in the central abdomen as they do with free ascites. When free fluid or hemorrhage is detected, ultrasound is an excellent modality to demonstrate the communications between the different intra-abdominal compartments.

Serous ascitic fluid is generally hypoechoic. Peritoneal fluid containing septations, increased echoes, or debris may indicate concurrent infection or malignant implantation (Fig. 40). However, lower-level echoes in ascites in patients with coagulopathy may be secondary to hemorrhage. It is difficult to differentiate between hemorrhagic ascites and acute hemorrhage.

Intraperitoneal Hemorrhage

Acute intraperitoneal hemorrhage often results from blunt abdominal trauma, ruptured ectopic pregnancy, recent surgery, or interventional procedures. Ultrasound has become the modality of choice in evaluating patients with ectopic pregnancy and detecting hemorrhage within either the cul-de-sac or the other pelvic locations (58). Usually, transvaginal ultrasound is favored over transabdominal scanning in these patients (54–57). In addition,

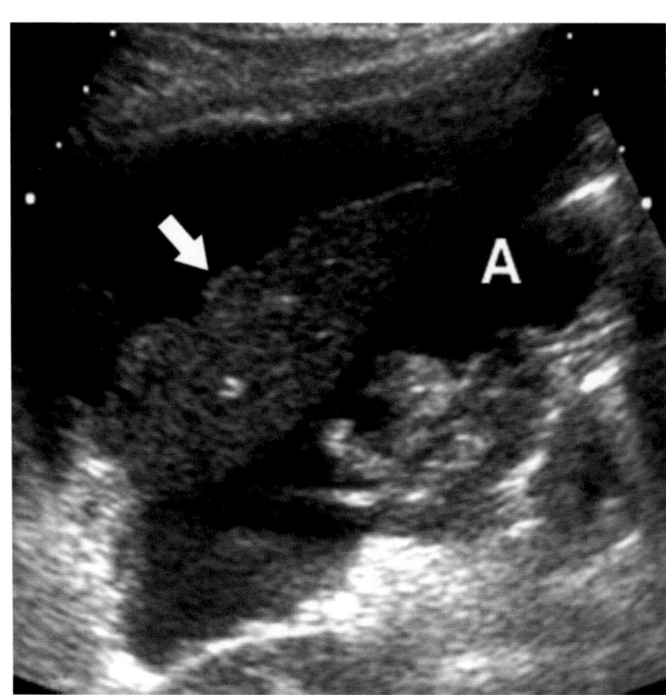

FIGURE 38 ■ Free-flowing massive ascites (A) from ovarian carcinomatosis. Sagittal sonogram of liver demonstrates extensive perihepatic ascites and tumor implants on the surface of the liver (*arrow*).

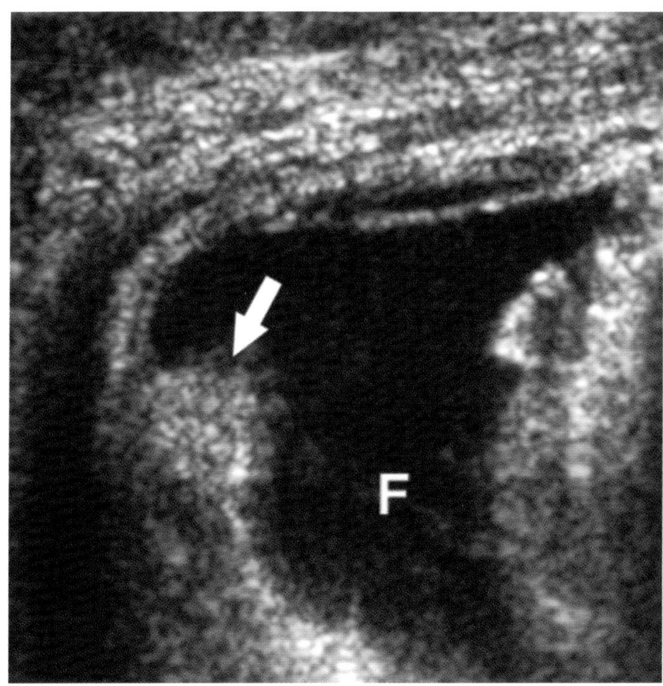

FIGURE 39 ■ Loculated ascites associated with peritoneal implants due to ovarian carcinoma. Transverse sonogram of right lower quadrant demonstrates echogenic free fluid (F) and implants (*arrow*) loculated in the right paracolic gutter.

several publications have reported the utility of ultrasound in evaluating patients with blunt abdominal trauma (59–61). Focused assessment with sonography for trauma (FAST), a limited screening technique to detect free intraperitoneal fluid, is gaining acceptance as a technique to evaluate patients with blunt abdominal trauma, replacing peritoneal lavage in many institutions (62). Many different protocols have been used; however, most include evaluation of parahepatic and parasplenic areas, including scans of both paracolic gutters and pelvis. Free fluid within the pelvis may be missed in trauma patients without an adequate acoustic window. In this respect, a full urinary bladder provides an optimal acoustic window. It is also valuable in the trauma patient to include a single view of the heart through the diaphragm for evaluation of possible pericardial hemorrhage.

The sonographic appearance of acute intraperitoneal hemorrhage is usually hypoechoic (Fig. 41) (59,60), and may also include mixed echoes within the fluid, isolated echogenic clot, or fluid–fluid interfaces (63). As clot formation occurs, the ultrasound appearance may vary, although the clot is usually isoechoic with solid organs; as the clot resolves, it appears more hypoechoic.

Intraperitoneal Abscesses

CT is often the diagnostic method of choice in detecting intra-abdominal abscesses. CT can readily differentiate loops of contrast-filled bowel from abscesses and is superior to sonography in identifying gas-containing abscesses. It may also be used to guide needle aspiration or drainage of abscesses (64). However, abscesses may also be readily detectible with ultrasound (65,66). Ultrasound is most helpful in situations in which the patient presents with a focal area of tenderness. For instance, in the patient who develops postsurgical pain, ultrasound may be helpful in identifying an abnormal fluid collection. Ultrasound may be used to guide aspiration and identify whether the fluid is bilious, serous, or infected. Nearly half of all intra-abdominal abscesses are postoperative and located in the

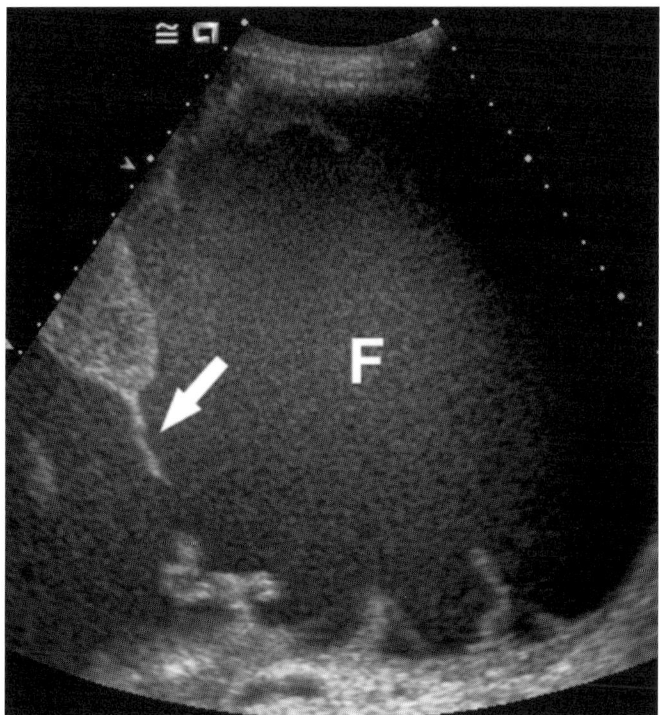

FIGURE 40 ■ Infected ascites in a patient with spontaneous bacterial peritonitis. Sagittal sonogram of mid-abdomen demonstrates echogenic fluid (F) with prominent septations and internal debris (*arrow*).

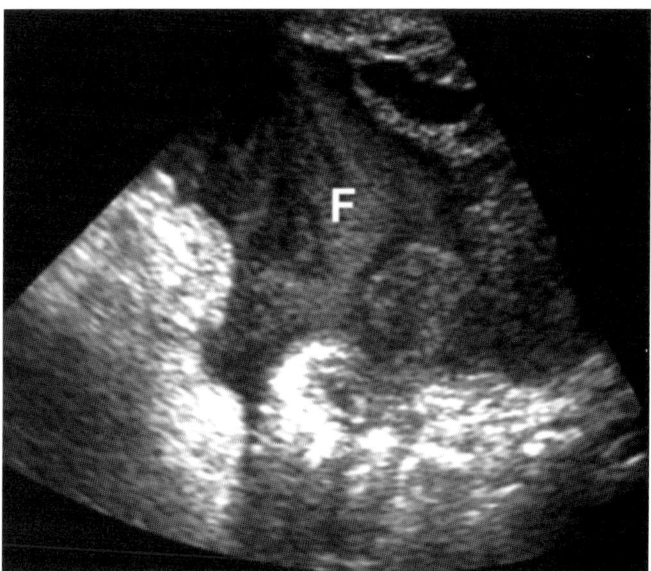

FIGURE 41 ■ Hemoperitoneum in a patient with a ruptured ectopic pregnancy. Note echogenic free fluid (F) in the pelvis on sagittal sonogram.

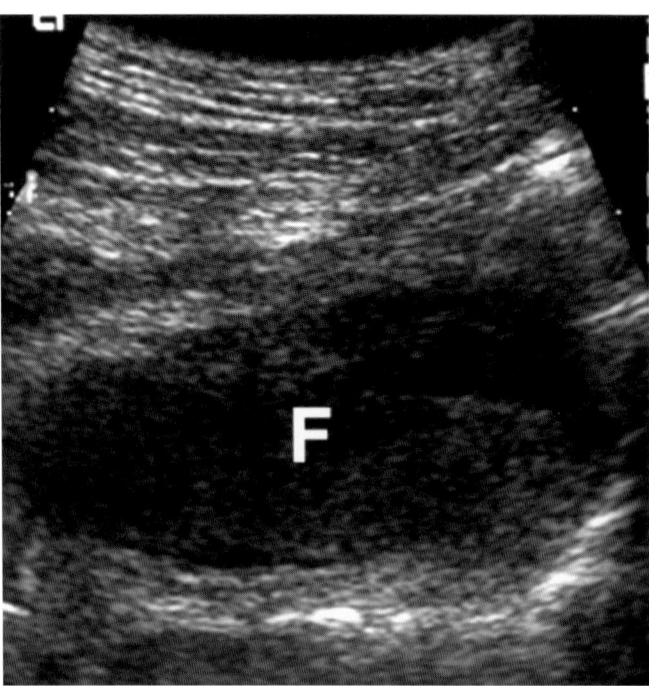

FIGURE 42 ■ Postoperative abscess on sonography. Note hypoechoic fluid (F) collection with internal echoes and fluid–fluid level (*arrow*) on sagittal sonogram of right lower quadrant.

subphrenic area. Common locations of intraperitoneal abscesses include the right and left subphrenic spaces, subhepatic space, the hepatorenal fossa, lesser sac, left and right paracolic gutter, and the pelvis. The pelvis should always be carefully evaluated, as abscesses often localize to the most dependent portion of the abdomen (i.e., the pelvic cul-de-sac). A typical example is a pelvic abscess from perforated appendicitis.

The lesser sac communicates directly with the rest of the intraperitoneal cavity through the foramen of Winslow. Lesser sac abscesses are commonly caused by perforation of a gastric ulcer or extension of a pancreatic abscess. Pancreatic fluid may dissect into the lesser sac and become loculated.

The sonographic appearance of abscesses is variable (66) and may be either hypoechoic or anechoic. Abscesses typically demonstrate complex fluid or septations with associate mass effect (Fig. 42). Gas-filled abscesses may be densely echogenic with acoustic shadowing (Fig. 43) (65). Reverberation artifact may occur with an air-fluid level within the abscess. This may be difficult to visualize and is a potential pitfall in the sonographic diagnosis of abdominal abscesses. Some abdominal abscesses may appear solid with minimal or no enhancement through sound transmission and can be misinterpreted as an intra-abdominal mass. Color Doppler imaging is of considerable value in differentiating avascular fluid collections from solid masses.

Boroujerdi-Rad et al. (67) demonstrated that CT and ultrasound may be helpful in diagnosing abdominal abscesses that occur in patients as a complication of peritonitis associated with ambulatory peritoneal dialysis. Prompt diagnosis was important in these patients who presented with abdominal pain, tenderness, fever, and nausea. Although peritonitis was common in these

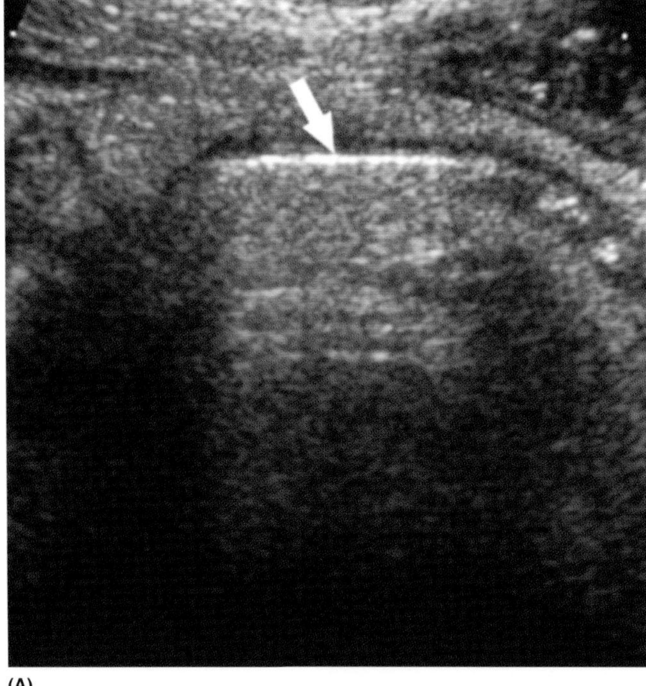

(A)

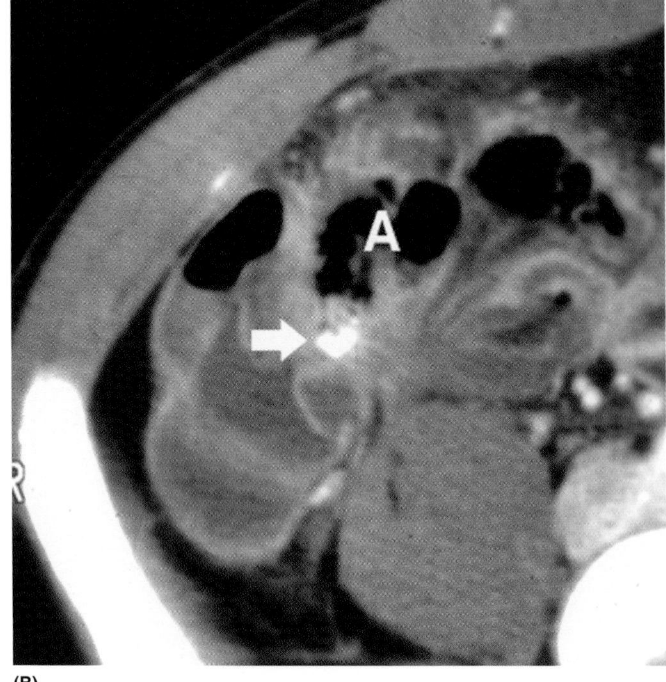

(B)

FIGURE 43 A AND B ■ Gas-containing abscess due to perforated appendicitis. (**A**) Transverse sonogram of right lower quadrant demonstrating linear reflections from gas (*arrow*) obscuring underlying abscess. (**B**) Contrast CT demonstrating air within abscess (A). Note calcified fecalith (*arrow*).

patients, abdominal abscesses were less common, occurring in only 0.7% of peritonitis episodes. These abscesses may then be aspirated or drained under ultrasound guidance.

As previously discussed, bowel perforation is an important etiology of abdominal abscesses. Diverticulitis with free pelvic perforation may be associated with intraabdominal abscesses (68). Burgard et al. (68) described an unusual case of perforation of a sigmoid diverticular abscess that caused gas in the portal vein and a liver abscess. Real-time ultrasound may be helpful to diagnose the diverticular abscess, identify gas within the portal vein, and aid in identification of the hepatic abscesses. Ultrasound may be helpful in diagnosing complications of Crohn's disease (69), such as abscesses and fistulous communications (Fig. 44). Moreover, Maconi et al. (69) found that ultrasound correctly identified the presence of abscesses caused by Crohn's disease in 83.3% of cases.

Ultrasound may also be useful in detecting nonbacterial abscesses such as tuberculous or parasitic infections. In a study by Kedar et al. (70), sonography was helpful in identifying the gastrointestinal and peritoneal findings in patients with tuberculosis. Lesions were encountered in the intestines in approximately 30% of cases, and in an extraintestinal site in approximately 40% of cases. Extraintestinal lesions included loculated ascites, adhesions, peritoneal thickening, lymphadenopathy, old abscesses, and, rarely, peritoneal nodules. The presence of fibrinous strands in the ascitic fluid, localized ascites, and either highly calcified or caseating lymph nodes were highly suspicious for tuberculosis in the appropriate setting. The sonographic signs of early abdominal tuberculosis found in the study of Jain et al. (71) included mesenteric thickness greater than 15 mm, increase in mesenteric echogenicity, and mesenteric lymphadenopathy. A recent report by Ghazinoor et al. (72) described the presence of hypoechoic mesenteric lymph nodes with increased through transmission, suggestive of caseating necrosis, in patients with abdominal tuberculosis (Fig. 5).

Parasitic infection such as amebiasis or Echinococcus infection may occasionally be identified within the peritoneal cavity. Although most commonly in the liver, hydatid cysts may also be loculated intraperitoneally and, at times, present as a multicystic mass (70).

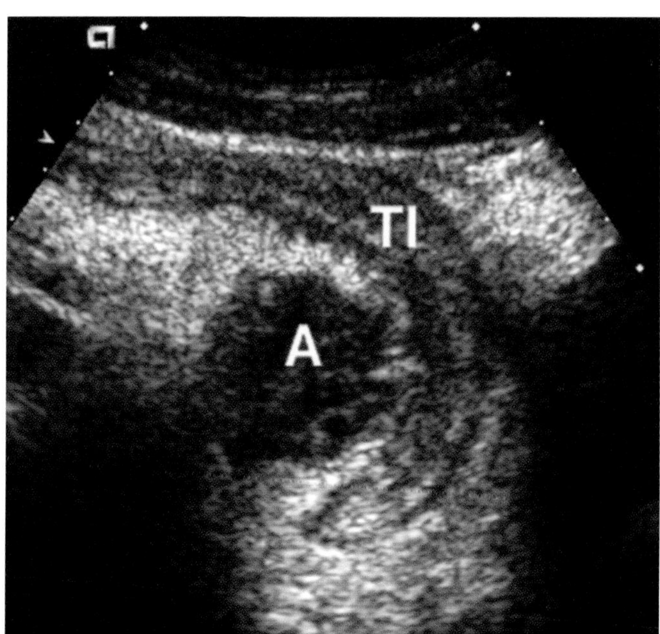

FIGURE 44 ■ Hypoechoic abscess (A) in Crohn's disease. Note echogenic fat surrounding hypoechoic abscess on sagittal sonogram of right lower quadrant. The abscess has minimal enhanced through sound transmission. TI, terminal ileum.

Peritoneal Inclusion Cysts

The physiologic fluid produced by the ovaries in premenopausal women is normally absorbed by the peritoneum. However, in patients with adhesions due to surgery, trauma, pelvic inflammatory disease, or inflammatory bowel disease, this fluid may not be absorbed by the peritoneum and be trapped by the adhesions, forming loculated fluid collections known as peritoneal fluid collections or benign encysted fluid. Peritoneal inclusion cysts may present as unilocular or multilocular cystic masses with ovoid or irregular contour and may contain internal echoes and septations. The key finding to establish the diagnosis is the demonstration of a normal ovary within or along the margin of the cyst (73,74).

PERITONEAL TUMORS

Metastatic tumors are more common than primary peritoneal tumors. Peritoneal metastases may result in peritoneal implants or cause diffuse infiltration of the omentum, appearing as an "omental cake" (Figs. 45 and 46). Mesenteric nodules and lymphadenopathy are also commonly observed features in peritoneal carcinomatosis. Ascites are also characteristic, and their presence facilitates the detection of small peritoneal metastases. Peritoneal implants within the intraperitoneal fluid appear as discrete hypoechoic nodules or masses (Fig. 46). Thickened septations may be observed within these peritoneal fluid collections. Omental caking characteristically appears as masses on sonography (75,76).

Primary peritoneal and mesenteric tumors are rare and vary in sonographic appearance. These tumors include mesothelioma, peritoneal serous papillary carcinoma, carcinoid tumors, desmoid tumors, and lymphoma. Mesothelioma may present with diffuse thickening of the peritoneum or peritoneal plaques, often seen as hypoechoic nodules; ascites are frequently present. Peritoneal serous papillary carcinoma is an entity similar to ovarian papillary serous carcinoma, with many of the same imaging characteristics. Patients usually present with a large quantity of ascites, diffuse peritoneal implants and omental caking (77,78). Most benign mesenteric tumors are focal, whereas other mesenteric tumors such as lymphomas are more diffuse. Lymphomas appear more hypoechoic than

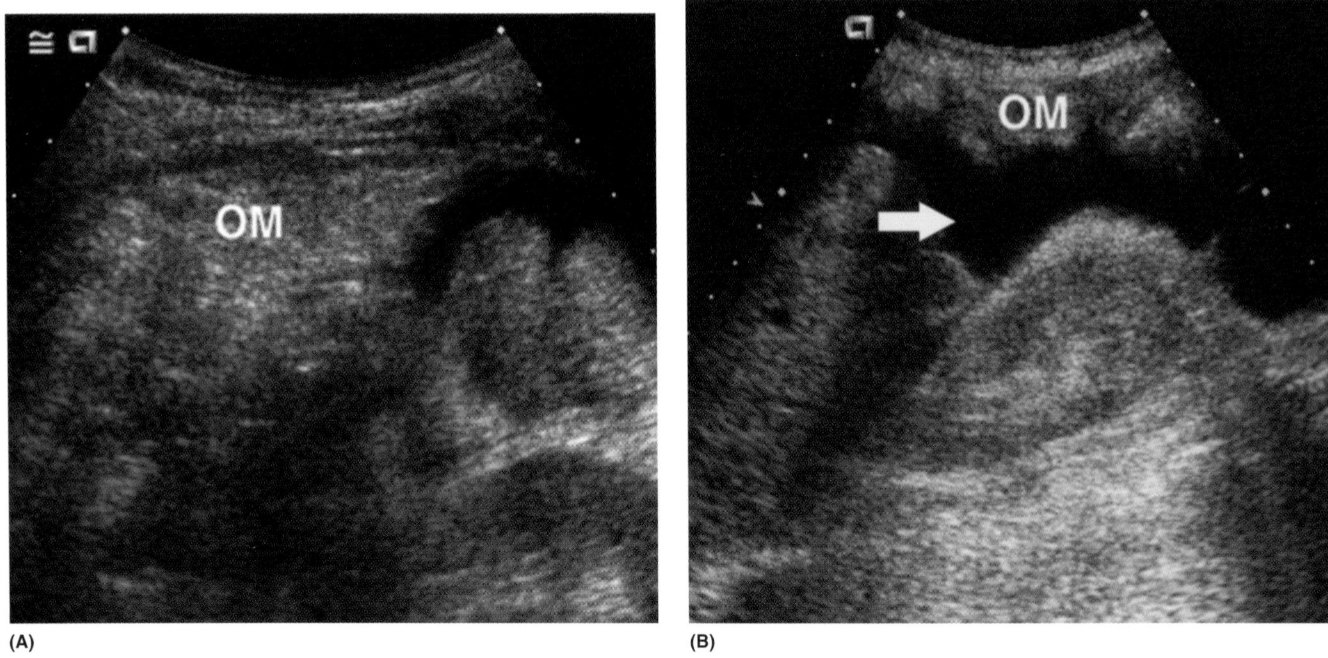

(A) (B)

FIGURE 45 A AND B ■ Peritoneal metastases ("omental cake") in two patients with ovarian carcinoma. (**A**) Note large echogenic mass within the omentum (OM) on transverse sonogram. (**B**) In another patient with ovarian carcinoma, note omental metastases (OM) and adjacent ascites (*arrow*) on sagittal sonogram.

metastatic tumors, which are typically more echogenic. Metastatic ovarian carcinoma may have echogenic calcified peritoneal implants unlike lymphoma, which is characteristically hypoechoic.

Pseudomyxoma peritonei is a rare disease characterized by the presence of mucinous ascites and multiple peritoneal implants that secrete large amounts of mucin. These tumors are produced by mucinous adenocarcinomas from the ovary, appendix, or colon. They are pathologically gelatinous, well-marginated masses with large septations. Although they may appear as a low attenuation mass on CT, these masses often contain echogenic

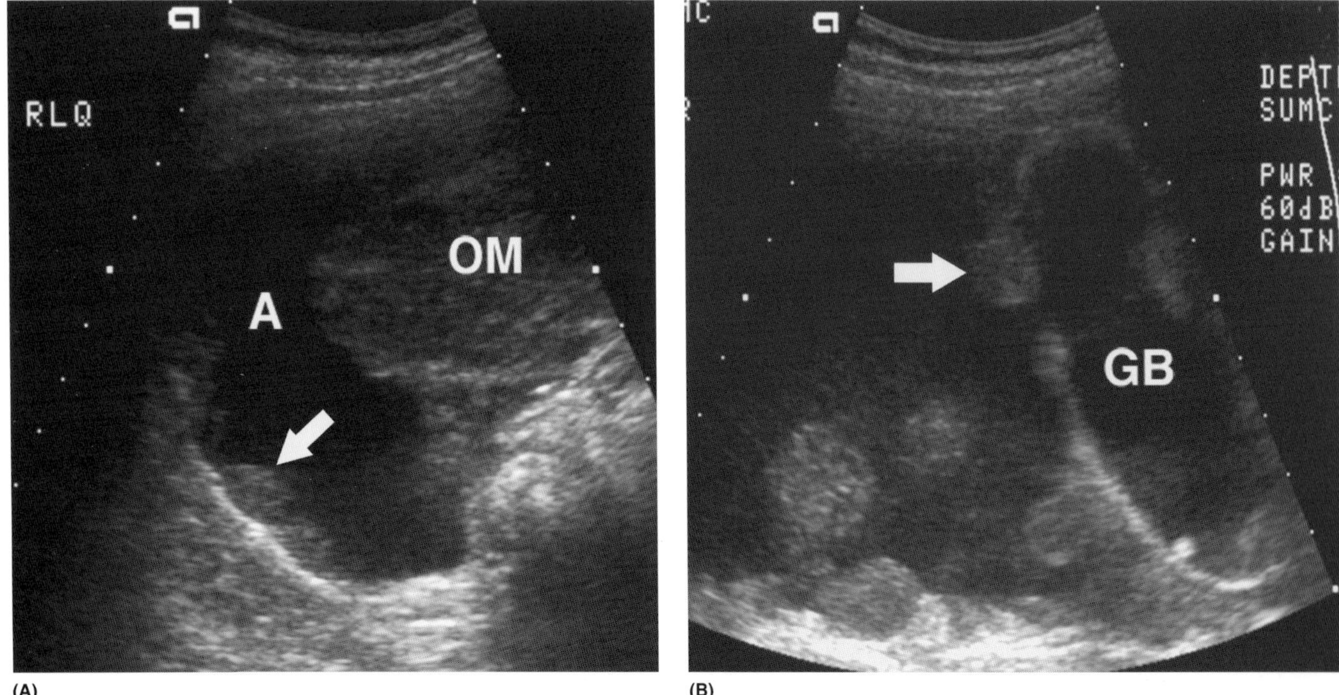

(A) (B)

FIGURE 46 A AND B ■ Peritoneal metastases from melanoma. (**A**) Transverse sonogram demonstrates omental cake (OM) and peritoneal implants (*open arrow*) adjacent to ascites (A). (**B**) Note peritoneal implants (*arrow*) on surface of gallbladder (GB).

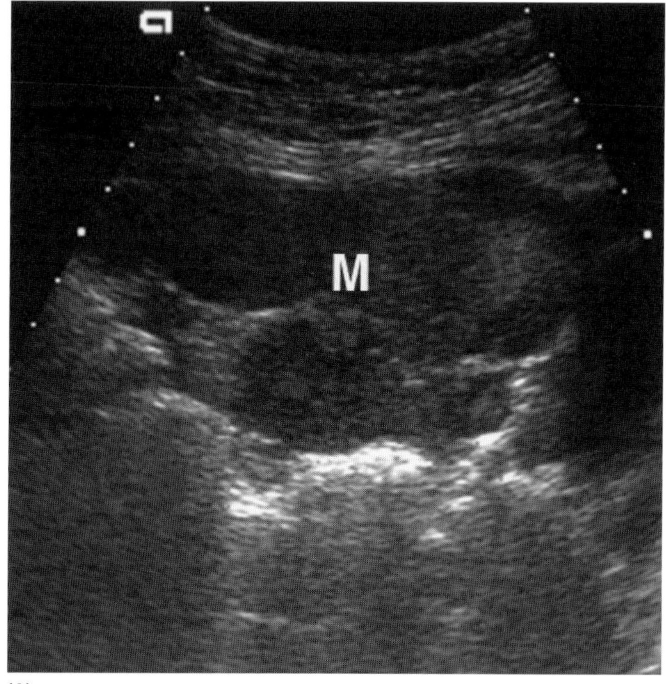

(A)

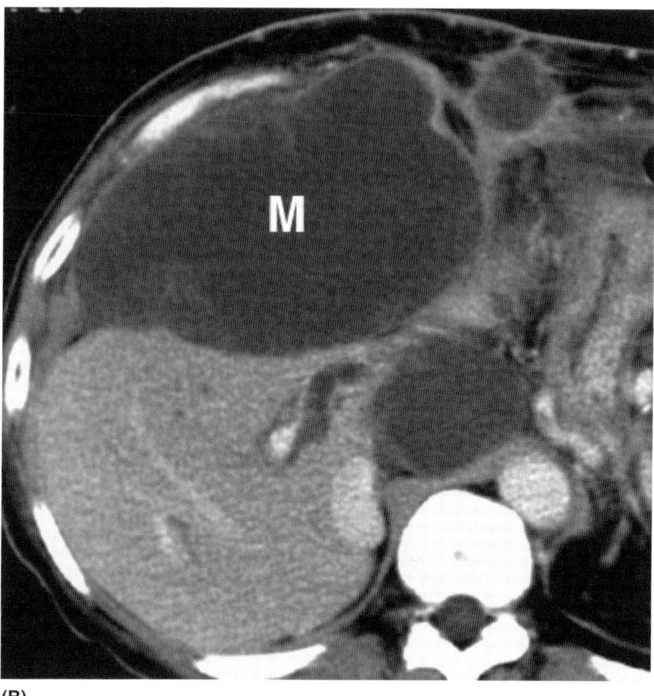

(B)

FIGURE 47 A AND B ■ Pseudomyxoma peritonei. (**A**) Note hypoechoic peritoneal mass (M) on transverse sonogram. (**B**) Corresponding CT demonstrates low attenuation mass compressing liver (M).

areas of mucinous debris on ultrasound (Fig. 47). Contour irregularity of the liver and spleen, described as scalloping, is a characteristic finding seen in pseudomyxoma peritonei (79,80). Graded compression technique with linear-array transducers is helpful in identifying these masses within the anterior abdomen.

REFERENCES

1. Jeffrey RB Jr, Sommer FG, Debatin JF. Color Doppler sonography of focal gastrointestinal lesions: initial clinical experience. J Ultrasound Med 1994; 13:473.
2. Clautice-Engle T, Jeffrey RB Jr, Li KC, et al. Power Doppler imaging of focal lesions of the gastrointestinal tract: comparison with conventional color Doppler imaging. J Ultrasound Med 1996; 15:63.
3. Teefey SA, Roarke MC, Brink JA, et al. Bowel wall thickening: differentiation of inflammation from ischemia with color Doppler and duplex US. Radiology 1996; 198:547–551.
4. Kimmey MB, Martin RW, Haggitt RC, et al. Histologic correlates of gastrointestinal ultrasound images. Gastroenterology 1989; 96:433–441.
5. Haller JO, Cohen HL. Hypertrophic pyloric stenosis: diagnosis using US. Radiology 1986; 161:335.
6. Strauss S, Itzchak Y, Manor A, et al. Sonography of hypertrophic pyloric stenosis. AJR Am J Roentgenol 1981; 136:1057.
7. Lutz H, Petzoldt R. Ultrasonic patterns of space occupying lesions of the stomach and the intestine. Ultrasound Med Biol 1976; 2:129.
8. Bluth EI, Merritt CR, Sullivan MA. Ultrasonic evaluation of the stomach, small bowel, and colon. Radiology 1979; 133:677.
9. Frisoli JK, Desser TS, Jeffrey RB Jr. Thickened submucosal layer: a sonographic sign of acute gastrointestinal abnormality representing submucosal edema or hemorrhage. AJR Am J Roentgenol 2000; 175:1595–1599.
10. Abu-Yousef MM, Bleicher JJ, Maher JW, et al. High-resolution sonography of acute appendicitis. AJR Am J Roentgenol 1987; 149:53.
11. Gaensler EHL, Jeffrey RB Jr, Laing FC, et al. Sonography in patients with suspected acute appendicitis: value in establishing alternative diagnoses. AJR Am J Roentgenol 1989; 152:49.
12. Jeffrey RB Jr, Laing FC, Townsend RR. Acute appendicitis: sonographic criteria based on 250 cases. Radiology 1988; 167:327.
13. Puylaert JB. Ultrasonography for diagnosing appendicitis. Br Med J 1988; 297:740.
14. Balthazar EJ, Birnbaum BA, Yee J, et al. Acute appendicitis: CT and US correlation in 100 patients. Radiology 1994; 190:31.
15. Malone AJ Jr, Wolf CR, Malmed AS, et al. Diagnosis of acute appendicitis: value of unenhanced CT. AJR Am J Roentgenol 1993; 160:763.
16. Birnbaum BA, Wilson SR. Appendicitis at the millennium. Radiology 2000; 215:337.
17. Chesbrough RM, Burkhard TK, Balsara ZN, et al. Self-localization in US of appendicitis: an addition to graded compression. Radiology 1993; 187:349.
18. Rioux M. Sonographic detection of the normal and abnormal appendix. AJR Am J Roentgenol 1992; 158:773.
19. Jeffrey RB, Jain KA, Nghiem HV. Sonographic diagnosis of acute appendicitis: interpretive pitfalls. AJR Am J Roentgenol 1994; 162:55.
20. Puylaert JB. When in doubt, sound it out. Radiology 1994; 191:320.
21. Yacoe ME, Jeffrey RB Jr. Sonography of appendicitis and diverticulitis. Radiol Clin North Am 1994; 32:899.
22. Jain KA, Ablin DS, Jeffrey RB, et al. Sonographic differential diagnosis of right lower quadrant pain other than appendicitis. Clin Imaging 1996; 20:12.
23. Borushok KF, Jeffrey RB Jr, Laing FC, et al. Sonographic diagnosis of perforation in patients with acute appendicitis. AJR Am J Roentgenol 1990; 154:275.

24. Johnson CD, Baker ME, Rice RP, et al. Diagnosis of acute colonic diverticulitis: comparison of barium enema and CT. AJR Am J Roentgenol 1987; 148:541.
25. Parulekar SG. Sonography of colonic diverticulitis. J Ultrasound Med 1985; 4:659.
26. Schwerk WB, Schwarz S, Rothmund M. Sonography in acute colonic diverticulitis: a prospective study. Dis Col Rectum 1992; 35:1077.
27. Verbanek J, Lanbrecht S, Rutgeerts L, et al. Can sonography diagnose acute colonic diverticulitis in patients with acute intestinal inflammation? a prospective study. J Clin Ultrasound 1989; 17:661.
28. Wilson SR, Toi A. The value of sonography in the diagnosis of acute diverticulitis of the colon. AJR Am J Roentgenol 1990; 154:1199.
29. Hollerweger A, Macheiner P, Rettenbacher T, Brunner W, Gritzman N. Colonic diverticulitis: diagnostic value and appearance of inflamed diverticula-sonographic evaluation. Eur Radiol 2001; 11:1956–1963.
30. Oudenhoven LF, Koumans RK, Puylaert JB. Right colonic diverticulitis: US and CT findings-new insights about frequency and natural history. Radiology 1998; 208:611–618.
31. O'Malley ME, Wilson SR. US of gastrointestinal tract abnormalities with CT correlation. Radiographics 2003; 23:59–72.
32. Chou YH, Chiou HJ, Tiu CM, et al. Sonography of acute right-sided colonic diverticulitis. Am J Surg 2001; 181:122–127.
33. Worlicek H, Lutz H, Heyder N, et al. Ultrasound findings in Crohn's disease and ulcerative colitis: a prospective study. J Clin Ultrasound 1987; 15:153.
34. Sarrazin J, Wilson SR. Manifestations of Crohn disease at US. Radiographics 1996; 16:499–520.
35. Haber HP, Busch A, Ziebach R, Dette S, Ruck P, Stern M. Ultrasonographic findings correspond to clinical, endoscopic and histologic findings in inflammatory bowel disease and other enterocolitides. J Ultrasound Med 2002; 21:375–382.
36. Maconi G, Parente F, Bollani S, et al. Abdominal ultrasound in the assessment of extent and activity of Crohn's disease: clinical significance and implication of bowel wall thickening. Am J Gastroenterol 1996; 91:1604–1609.
37. Esteban JM, Maldonado L, Sanchiz V, Minguez M, Benages A. Activity of Crohn's disease assessed by colour Doppler ultrasound analysis of the affected loops. Eur Radiol 2001; 11:1423–1428.
38. Spalinger J, Patriquin H, Miron MC, et al. Doppler US in patients with Crohn disease: vessel density in the diseased bowel reflects disease activity. Radiology 2000; 217:787–789.
39. Puylaert JB. Mesenteric adenitis and acute terminal ileitis: US evaluation using graded compression. Radiology 1986; 161:691.
40. Wilson SR, Burns PN, Wilkinson LM, Simpson DH, Muradali D. Gas at abdominal US: appearance, relevance, and analysis of artifacts. Radiology 1999; 210:113–123.
41. Danse EM, Van Beers BE, Jamart J, et al. Prognosis of ischemic colitis: comparison of color Doppler sonography with early clinical and laboratory findings. AJR Am J Roentgenol 2000; 175: 1151–1154.
42. Van Breda Vriesman AC, Lohle PN, Coerkamp EG, Puylaert JB. Infarction of omentum and epiploic appendage: diagnosis, epidemiology and natural history. Eur Radiol 1999; 9:1886–1892.
43. Puylaert JBCM. Right-sided segmental infarction of the omentum: clinical, US, and CT findings. Radiology 1992; 185:169.
44. Rioux M, Langis P. Primary epiploic appendagitis: clinical, US and CT findings in 14 cases. Radiology 1994; 191:523–526.
45. Puylaert JB, Lalisang RI, Van der Werf SDJ, et al. Campylobacter ileocolitis mimicking acute appendicitis: differentiation with graded-compression US. Radiology 1988; 166:737.
46. Puylaert JB, Vermeijden RJ, van der Werf SDJ, et al. Incidence and sonographic diagnosis of bacterial ileocaecitis masquerading as appendicitis. Lancet 1989; 2:84.
47. Bin W, Jianguo L, Baowei D. The sonographic appearances of small bowel tumours. Clin Radiol 1992; 46:30.
48. Daneman A, Navarro O. Intussusception. Part 1: a review of diagnostic approaches. Pediatr Radiol 2003; 33(2):79–85. Epub 2002.
49. Crystal P, Hertzanu Y, Farber B, et al. Sonographically guided hydrostatic reduction of intussusception in children. J Clin Ultrasound 2002; 30(6):343–348.
50. Meyers MA. The spread and location of acute intraperitoneal effusions. Radiology 1970; 95:547.
51. Federle MP, Crass RA, Jeffrey RB, et al. Computed tomography in blunt abdominal trauma. Arch Surg 1982; 117:645.
52. Federle MP, Jeffrey RB Jr. Hemoperitoneum studied by computed tomography. Radiology 1983; 148:187.
53. Siskind BN, Malat J, Hammers L, et al. CT features of hemorrhagic malignant liver tumors. J Comput Assist Tomogr 1987; 11:766.
54. Fleischer AC, Pennell RG, McKee MS, et al. Ectopic pregnancy: features at transvaginal sonography. Radiology 1990; 174:375.
55. Frates MC, Brown DL, Doubilet PM, et al. Tubal rupture in patients with ectopic pregnancy: diagnosis with transvaginal US. Radiology 1994; 191:769.
56. Nyberg DA, Hughes MP, Mack LA, Wang KY. Extrauterine findings of ectopic pregnancy at transvaginal US: importance of echogenic fluid. Radiology 1991; 178:823.
57. Thorsen MK, Lawson TL, Aiman EJ, et al. Diagnosis of ectopic pregnancy: endovaginal vs. transabdominal sonography. AJR Am J Roentgenol 1990; 155:307.
58. Sickler GK, Chen PC, Dubinsky TJ, Maklad N. Free echogenic pelvic fluid: correlation with hemoperitoneum. J Ultrasound Med 1998; 17:431–435.
59. Healey MA, Simons RK, Winchell RJ, et al. A prospective evaluation of abdominal ultrasound in blunt trauma: is it useful? J Trauma 1996; 40:875.
60. McKenney MG, Martin L, Lentz K, et al. 1000 Consecutive ultrasounds for blunt abdominal trauma. J Trauma 1996; 40:607.
61. Sirlin CB, Brown MA, Andrade-Barreto OA, et al. Blunt abdominal trauma: clinical value of negative screening US scans. Radiology 2004; 230:661–668.
62. Brown MA, Casola G, Sirlin CB, Patel NY, Hoyt DB. Blunt abdominal trauma: screening US in 2693 patients. Radiology 2001; 218:352–358.
63. Jeffrey RB, Laing FC. Echogenic clot: a useful sign of pelvic hemoperitoneum. Radiology 1982; 145:139.
64. Jeffrey RB Jr, Federle MP, Tolentino CS. Periappendiceal inflammatory masses: CT-directed management and clinical outcome in 70 patients. Radiology 1988; 167:13.
65. Kressel HY, Filly RA. Ultrasonographic appearance of gas-containing abscesses in the abdomen. AJR Am J Roentgenol 1978; 130:71.
66. Subramanyam BR, Balthazar EJ, Raghavendra BN, et al. Ultrasound analysis of solid-appearing abscesses. Radiology 1983; 146:487.
67. Boroujerdi-Rad H, Juergensen P, Mansourian V, et al. Abdominal abscesses complicating peritonitis in continuous ambulatory peritoneal dialysis patients. Am J Kidney Dis 1994; 23:717.
68. Burgard G, Cuilleron M, Cuilleret J. An unusual complication of perforated sigmoid diverticulitis: gas in the portal vein with biliary liver abscesses. J Chir 1993; 130:237.
69. Maconi G, Bollani S, Bianchi Porro G. Ultrasonographic detection of intestinal complications in Crohn's disease. Dig Dis Sci 1996; 41:1643.
70. Kedar RP, Shah PP, Shivde RS, et al. Sonographic findings in gastrointestinal and peritoneal tuberculosis. Clin Radiol 1994; 49:24.
71. Jain R, Sawhney S, Bhargava DK, Berry M. Diagnosis of abdominal tuberculosis: sonographic findings in patients with early disease. AJR Am J Roentgenol 1995; 165:1391–1395.
72. Ghazinoor S, Desser T, Jeffrey RB. Increase through-transmission in abdominal tuberculous lymphadenitis. J Ultrasound Med 2004; 23:837–841.
73. Sohaey R, Gardner TL, Woodward PJ, Peterson CM. Sonographic diagnosis of peritoneal inclusion cysts. J Ultrasound Med 1995; 14:913–917.

74. Kim JS, Lee HJ, Woo SK, et al. Peritoneal inclusion cysts and their relationship to the ovaries: evaluation with sonography. Radiology 1997; 204:481–484.
75. Yeh HC. Ultrasonography of peritoneal tumors. Radiology 1979; 133:419.
76. Yeh HC, Safer MK, Slater G, et al. Ultrasonography and computed tomography in pseudomyxoma peritonea. Radiology 1984; 153:507.
77. Furukawa T, Ueda J, Takahashi S, et al. Peritoneal serous papillary carcinoma: radiological appearance. Abdom Imaging 1999; 24:78–81.
78. Chopra S, Laurie LR, Chintapalli KN, Valente PT, Dodd GD III. Primary papillary serous carcinoma of the peritoneum: CT-pathologic correlation. J Comput Assist Tomogr 2000; 24:395–399.
79. Seshul MB, Coulam CM. Pseudomyxoma peritonei: computed tomography and sonography. AJR Am J Roentgenol 1981; 36:803–806.
80. Walensky RP, Venbrux AC, Prescott CA, Osterman FA Jr. Pseudomyxoma peritonei. AJR AM J Roentgenol 1996; 167:471–474.
81. Lim JH. Colorectal cancer: sonographic findings. AJR Am J Roentgenol 1996; 167:45–47.
82. Kaftori JK, Aharon M, Kleinhaus U. Sonographic features of gastrointestinal leiomyosarcoma. J Clin Ultrasound 1981; 9:11–15.
83. Truong M, Atri M, Bret PM, et al. Sonographic appearance of benign and malignant conditions of the colon. AJR Am J Roentgenol 1998; 170:1451–1455.
84. McGahan JP, Brown B, Jones CD, et al. Pelvic abscesses: transvaginal US-guided drainage with the trocar method. Radiology 1996; 200:579.

Endoscopic Ultrasound

Vasudha Dhar and Peter D. Stevens

14

(Continued)

INTRODUCTION

Since the first publications over a generation ago (1,2), almost 2000 articles have been published describing the diagnostic and therapeutic uses of endoscopic ultrasound (EUS). Advances in EUS have been discussed in books, monographs, supplements, and international symposia (3–11). One of the most potent procedures linked to EUS is fine-needle aspiration (FNA). With improvements in FNA techniques, EUS-guided fine needle aspiration (EUS-FNA) has now become the most important means of tissue sampling for gastrointestinal (GI) cancers and mediastinal lymph nodes.

OVERVIEW

High-Frequency Ultrasound and the GI Tract Wall

EUS uses high-frequency ultrasound (US) (≥5 MHz) for increased spatial resolution to produce uniquely detailed views of the gut wall and surrounding structures. With the higher frequency comes a shorter penetration depth and a more limited field of view. However, a limited field is acceptable with EUS because the transducer can be placed immediately adjacent to the area of interest. The images produced by EUS are unmatched by other imaging methods.

Using EUS at the most common frequencies (5–12 MHz), the wall of the GI tract can be imaged as a five-layer structure of alternating bright (hyperechoic and echogenic) and dark (hypoechoic) bands (Fig. 1). The generation of this US image is complex. The histologic correlates of the five layers were the object of intense in vitro and in vivo studies resulting in some controversies, which are now largely resolved (12). The first echogenic layer corresponds to the boundary echo plus the superficial mucosa; the second hypoechoic layer, the deep mucosa; the third hyperechoic layer, the submucosa and boundary echo; the fourth hypoechoic layer, the muscularis propria; the fifth hyperechoic layer, the serosa or adventitia and surrounding fat. Higher frequencies show even more detail, and seven-layer and nine-layer wall images have been produced.

The ability to image the wall of the GI tract as a series of definable layers corresponding to histologic features, rather than as a single entity, is the basis of most of the indications for EUS. Other indications have emerged from the ability of EUS to image structures in immediate proximity to the GI tract in greater detail; structures of principal interest for the gastroenterologist are the lymph nodes, the common bile duct (CBD), and the pancreas. Some indications are established on the basis of accumulated data, whereas others are potential indications that need further study. The indications for EUS can be divided into three main categories: (*i*) submucosal abnormalities; (*ii*) cancer staging; and (*iii*) pancreatobiliary disease (Table 1).

Submucosal Abnormalities

This category of indications involves the application of EUS not just to abnormalities in the submucosa but to any process below the normal

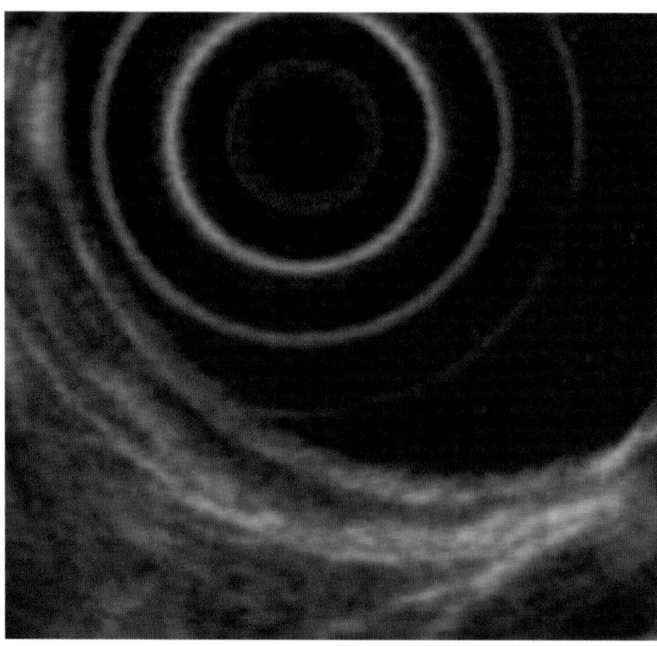

FIGURE 1 ■ Normal five-layer image of the gastric wall obtained with a radial echoendoscope.

mucosal lining of the GI tract. The first major distinction that can be made with EUS is whether an abnormality is extrinsic or intramural. Extrinsic processes that can be defined with EUS include contour abnormalities resulting from compression by normal organs or disease. The major sign of extrinsic compression is the finding on EUS of all five normal wall layers draped over the process that is causing the contour deformity.

Intramural tumors can be categorized on EUS according to the wall layer of origin and echogenicity. Basic distinctions can be made regarding whether the tumor is cystic, vascular, or solid. The size of the tumors can be measured accurately. Studies about differentiating between benign and

TABLE 1 ■ Indications for EUS

Established indications	Potential indications
Submucosal abnormalities	
Intramural versus extrinsic	Monitor variceal therapy
Tumor size and structure	Inflammatory bowel disease
Large gastric folds	Esophageal motility disease
Gastric varices	Benign ulcer healing
Gastrointestinal cancer staging	
Esophagus, stomach	Ulcer bleeding risk
Colorectal	Fine-needle aspiration
Pancreatobiliary disease	
Cancer staging	Cancer diagnosis/staging (including lung cancer)
Localize endocrine tumors	EUS-guided endoscopic mucosal resection
Detect common duct stones	Upper GI bleeding
Pancreatic pseudocyst drainage	EUS-guided antitumor injection therapy
Chronic pancreatitis	Future interventional indications
Celiac axis neurolysis	Posterior gastropexy
Achalasia: botulinum toxin injection	Gastrojejunal cruciate anastomosis

Abbreviations: EUS, endoscopic ultrasound; GI, gastrointestinal.

malignant tumors on EUS have shown that EUS can assist in revealing distinct differences in patterns, which can facilitate that distinction (13).

Of the intramural tumors, leiomyomas and gastrointestinal stromal tumors (GISTs) are amongst the most common. They usually arise from the fourth wall layer corresponding to the muscularis propria, and because they are relatively homogeneous with a tissue density similar to that of water, they appear as hypoechoic masses (Fig. 2). Chak et al. in their study of 35 GISTs found tumor size above 4 cm, irregular extraluminal border, echogenic foci, and cystic spaces were all independent factors associated with malignancy (14). In cases where two out of the three features were present, the sensitivity of EUS for detecting malignancy was as high as 80% to 100%. However, there was poor interobserver agreement in the interpretation of the above features. Palazzo et al., in a retrospective study of 56 benign and malignant GISTs, showed that the presence of cystic spaces and irregular extraluminal margins were independent predictors of malignancy. Size of 3 cm or less, homogeneous echo pattern, and regular margins were features associated with benign tumors. All three features combined had a specificity of 100% (15). Fat is highly echogenic on US imaging, and fatty tumors such as lipomas are distinguished by a bright echogenic appearance in the third layer (submucosa) (Fig. 3). Such distinction can be helpful in clinical management.

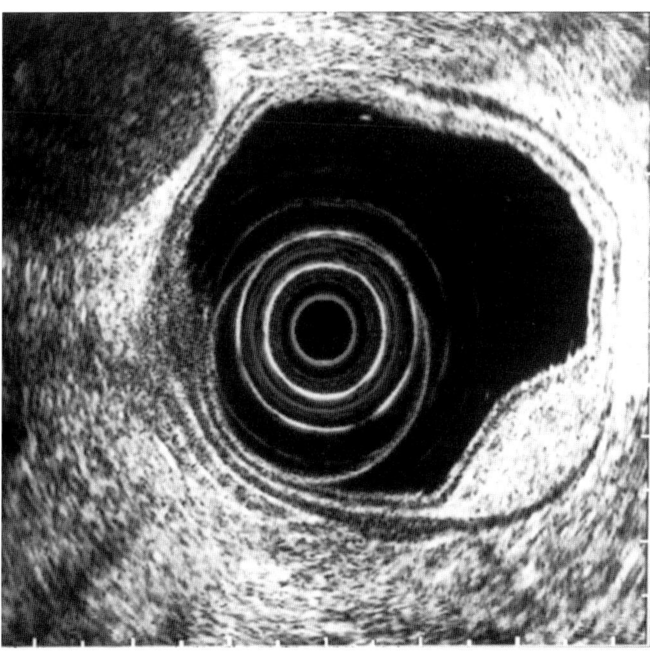

FIGURE 3 ■ Radial scanning image of a subepithelial gastric lesion showing a hypoechoic mass arising from the third layer of the gastric wall consistent with a lipoma.

Esophageal varices may be difficult to image with EUS because they are usually superficial and thin walled, and they may be compressed easily by larger dedicated US endoscopes. Newer, catheter-size probes have facilitated the imaging of esophageal varices. Gastric varices, which tend to be deeper in the submucosa, are routinely imaged in the water-filled stomach (Fig. 4). Monitoring the treatment of varices may be useful with EUS, but although some data exist in this regard, they are not yet established well enough to suggest the use of EUS for this purpose.

Extensive gastric varices may sometimes appear to the endoscopist as submucosal tumors or prominent gastric folds. Gastric varices can be readily distinguished by EUS, and potentially disastrous large or deep biopsies can be avoided. EUS provides a good approach to the evaluation of large gastric folds. If abnormalities are limited to the mucosal layers, jumbo biopsies should be diagnostic. Abnormalities showing wide infiltration and distortion of the third and fourth layers suggest malignant disease such as linitis plastica or infiltrating lymphoma. When results of standard endoscopic biopsies are

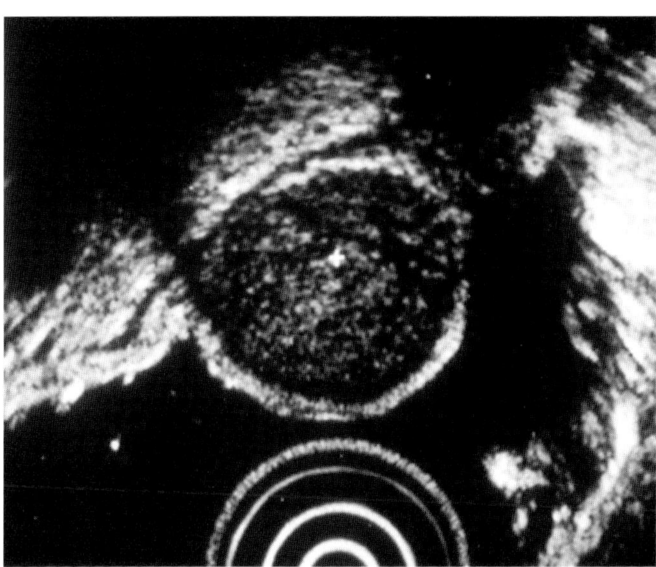

FIGURE 2 ■ Radial scanning image of a submucosal gastric lesion showing a hypoechoic mass arising from the fourth layer of the gastric wall consistent with a gastrointestinal stromal tumor.

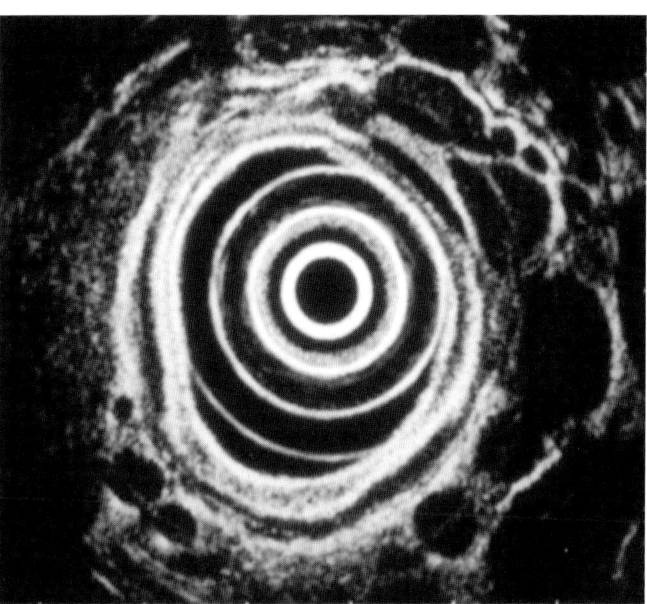

FIGURE 4 ■ Radial scanning image demonstrating fundal varices.

negative, other methods to sample these areas, such as needle aspiration or endoscopic mucosal resection (EMR), or even surgical exploration, may be indicated.

EUS has been proposed as a means to evaluate patients with achalasia and other esophageal motility disorders for evidence of thickening of the muscularis propria, but findings and utility remain controversial. EUS can be useful in newly diagnosed achalasia to determine the presence or absence of pseudoachalasia resulting from infiltrating tumor.

In the lower GI tract, EUS has been used in inflammatory bowel disease to differentiate superficial from transmural inflammation, and it has been used in Crohn's disease to map perirectal abscesses and fistulas. The clinical value of EUS in inflammatory bowel disease in general, however, has not yet been confirmed. To date, EUS criteria have not been established that can be used to differentiate ulcerative colitis from Crohn's disease (16). EUS has also been used to help define anal sphincter abnormalities form various causes.

GI Tumor Staging

Aside from detecting infiltrating gastric malignant disease, EUS seems to have little role in the diagnosis of GI cancer. Diagnosis depends primarily on histologic or cytologic evaluation of endoscopic biopsies. For example, EUS cannot be used reliably to differentiate benign from malignant ulcers, although some investigators have used EUS to predict benign gastric ulcer healing. On the other hand, EUS has been shown to be the most accurate method for the locoregional staging of cancer of the esophagus, stomach, colon, and rectum. EUS is also becoming a useful adjunct in lung cancer staging (17,18).

More studies have tested EUS for GI cancer staging than for any other indication. The ability of EUS to image the layers of the GI tract wall in detail enables highly accurate staging of the depth of the tumor (T stage). Regional lymph nodes can also be imaged in greater detail (N stage). On the other hand, high-frequency EUS has a short depth of field and, in general, is not a good test for staging distant metastases (M stage). Exceptions in esophageal cancer staging are lymph node metastases at the celiac axis, which are considered distant metastases (19).

The accuracy of EUS for staging depth of tumor invasion (T) is 85% compared with surgical pathology and 75% for the staging of regional lymph nodes (N) (20,21).

The improved locoregional staging provided by EUS helps in patient management, depending on the use of staging in determining therapy. Staging information provided by EUS can be factored into the total clinical equation in determining operative versus nonoperative management, in adding surgical adjuvant therapy, or in directing endoscopic therapy. EUS staging provides powerful prognostic information. Because the therapy of advanced GI cancer is notably unsatisfactory, EUS is helpful in patient selection for experimental treatment protocols.

EUS also appears to be sensitive for detecting recurrent upper GI cancer in the area of the surgical anastomosis. Specificity is lower because perianastomotic fibrosis and inflammation can mimic recurrent cancer. Similarly, EUS does not appear too reliable in assessing the response to radiation or chemotherapy because of an inability to differentiate residual tumor from treatment-related inflammation and fibrosis.

Pancreatobiliary Disease

EUS can be used from the stomach and duodenum to produce detailed images of the pancreas. These highly detailed images allow the detection of small pancreatic tumors, even those smaller than 1 cm. EUS has a high sensitivity and specificity for imaging focal pancreatic abnormalities and can be used when computed tomography (CT) scans and endoscopic retrograde cholangiopancreatography (ERCP) are equivocal. The differential diagnosis between pancreatic cancer and focal pancreatitis, however, remains difficult. There is an increasing recognition of an autoimmune form of pancreatitis; and EUS and FNA may play an important role in the diagnosis of this condition (22).

Echo-enhanced color and power Doppler has been shown to have a sensitivity of 94% and specificity of 100% for differentiating pancreatic carcinoma versus inflammatory changes (23). Contrast-enhanced power Doppler US also provides useful findings for differentiating pancreatic carcinoma from chronic focal pancreatitis (24). EUS is effective in localizing small, CT-negative endocrine tumors of the pancreas, with sensitivity in the range of 80% and a specificity of more than 90%. Tumors as small as 2 to 3 mm have been identified. Preoperative localization helps direct the surgeon using palpation and intraoperative US to detect and remove these tumors.

Locoregional staging of pancreatic and ampullary cancer can be done as accurately as in luminal GI cancer. In the evaluation of pancreatic cancer resectability, EUS appears to be among the most accurate methods to detect invasion of the portal venous system. This method also seems to be able to detect subtle changes of chronic pancreatitis not evident on other imaging tests.

The extrahepatic bile duct can be imaged with EUS in most patients with either the linear or the radial array endoscopes with equal ease. The bifurcation and liver hilum may be more easily imaged with linear EUS than radial. Bile duct cancer can be accurately staged and CBD stones accurately diagnosed. The sensitivity and specificity of EUS for detecting CBD stones are comparable to those of ERCP and are better than transabdominal US, CT, or magnetic resonance imaging (MRI). EUS has a much lower complication rate than ERCP and, therefore, can be considered a screening test for CBD stones before therapeutic ERCP when the probability of biliary stones is low or moderate. EUS is highly sensitive in detecting very small stones (sensitivity 100%; stone size 1–4 mm). Both magnetic resonance cholangiopancreatography (MRCP) and helical computed tomographic cholangiography (HCT-C) are less invasive than EUS. For stones above 5 mm, sensitivity has been shown to be comparable to EUS (100%) but falls to 67% for small stones less than 4 mm in diameter (25).

EUS-Guided FNA

The use of EUS-FNA for cytology has been developed in an effort to improve the differential diagnosis of submucosal lesions, lymph nodes, and pancreatic masses. The initial experience indicates that this may be helpful in cancer staging particularly in lymph node staging of non–small-cell lung cancer and in documenting pancreatic cancer.

EUS-guided puncture is also beginning to find therapeutic uses in celiac axis neurolysis for intractable pain in patients with abdominal malignant disease as well as in the injection of botulinum toxin into the lower esophageal sphincter of patients with achalasia. Celiac plexus block for chronic pancreatitis can also be performed (10). Phase II clinical trials in locally advanced pancreatic and esophageal cancer are under way with EUS-FNA guided delivery of antitumor agents (10).

Contraindications

The only contraindications to EUS (aside from those associated with endoscopy in general) are those related to the size and stiffness of currently available dedicated US endoscopes. The instruments used for upper GI examination have a large diameter up to 13 mm and a rigid distal tip to accommodate the US mechanism.

The optics is forward oblique or side viewing, and this property limits the view of the lumen in narrow areas. Because of the size, stiffness, and weight palpatory sense is diminished. Thus, passage of these instruments through narrow or irregular strictures must be approached with great caution.

US endoscopes may be difficult to guide past the cricopharyngeus in some patients, particularly elderly patients with abnormalities of the cervical vertebrae. If gentle attempts at passage fail in this setting, wire-guided or catheter-guided passage may help. If resistance persists, it may be prudent to abort the procedure rather than risk a pharyngeal tear.

The greatest risk of perforation involves passage of a US endoscope through a malignant esophageal stricture in an attempt to achieve accurate staging. If gentle pressure and careful angulation of the tip do not achieve passage, further efforts should cease. Rapid dilation of a narrow stricture followed by passage of the US endoscope has been associated with a 20% to 24% risk of perforation (26,27). However, dilation before EUS is considered not to be as dangerous by other investigators (28).

A prospective study done here in the United States also concluded that incremental, stepwise dilation of malignant strictures to 14 mm is safe and effective in permitting echoendoscope passage beyond the stenosis (29).

Complications

Overall, EUS is a safe procedure with a low complication rate comparable to that of diagnostic upper GI endoscopy. A study comparing monitored blood pressure, pulse, and oxygen saturation in 191 patients receiving esophagogastroduodenoscopy (EGD), EUS, and EGD plus EUS showed that procedures involving EUS took longer and required larger doses of sedative medication, but the rate of hypertension, hypotension, tachycardia, bradycardia, and desaturation were similar for all groups (30). Recorded abnormalities were all transient and required no intervention.

A retrospective survey of EUS procedures from 1985 to 1992 was carried out from 34 centers in the United States, Europe, and Japan (31). In upper GI EUS, 19 major complications occurred in 37,915 procedures (0.05%). These complications included 13 perforations associated with malignant (n = 11) or benign (n = 2) stenosis. One death occurred within 30 days (0.003%). Other complications were two pharyngeal perforations, one duodenal perforation, and two episodes of bleeding requiring transfusion. Among 4190 cases of lower GI EUS were two episodes of significant bleeding (0.05%) with no mortality.

EUS-FNA seems remarkably safe. The overall complication rate of EUS-FNA appears to be 1% to 2% (32). The major EUS-FNA complications reported are infections, bleeding, pancreatitis, and duodenal perforation (33). The greatest risk seems to be infection after aspiration of cystic lesions. In a multicenter prospective study of FNA biopsy involving 554 lesions in 435 patients, the complication rate for solid lesions was 0.5% and for cystic lesions it was 14% ($P < 0.001$) (34). There is one case report of tumor seeding to date secondary to EUS-guided FNA of a pancreatic mass (35). The number of EUS-FNA procedures performed for diagnosis of pancreatic adenocarcinoma is increasing and prospective studies of this potential complication are warranted.

Instruments

Endoscope-Based Probes

Two types of echoendoscopes are available for examination of the pancreas and the biliary tree: those with mechanically rotating transducers (7.5, 12, and 20 MHz scanning frequencies) and those with an electronic convex linear array (5, 7.5, 10, and 12 MHz scanning frequencies). For the upper GI tract, mostly oblique-viewing endoscopes are used, although recently, forward-viewing instruments have become available. For colorectal EUS, rigid probes for the rectum and a flexible forward-viewing echocolonoscope are available. The chief advantage of the rotating transducer is the 360° tomographic image produced by the US beam sweeping perpendicular to the insertion shaft that makes orientation easier. This is particularly relevant when imaging the retroperitoneum through the duodenum, where the anatomy is best appreciated by relating organs and structures to major blood vessels (36). The chief advantage of the electronic convex linear-array transducers, in which the US beam is directed parallel to the endoscope's accessory channel, is that needles and other accessories passed through the channel of the endoscope can be placed into a target area under real-time endosonographic guidance. This allows directed tissue and fluid sampling or therapeutic injection. A second advantage of the convex linear-array transducers is the availability of duplex and color Doppler techniques.

Catheter-Based Probes

Small, mechanically rotating transducers have been incorporated into catheter-size probes (7.5–30 MHz). These probes, designed initially for intravascular imaging, can be placed into the bile ducts by both percutaneous and transpapillary approaches and into the pancreas duct by the endoscopic retrograde method (37,38).

ESOPHAGUS CANCER STAGING

The great strength of EUS in staging esophageal cancer is the ability to define separate layers of the esophageal wall that correlate with histologic features. At the usual US frequencies of 5 and 12 MHz, five wall layers can be imaged. Tumors are usually imaged as a hypoechoic disruption of the normal wall. Thus, EUS becomes a powerful tool to distinguish depth of cancer invasion.

Technique

Most clinical experience for staging esophageal cancer has been with Olympus radial scanning instruments producing a 360° image with frequencies of 5 to 12 MHz. The water-filled balloon method is usually used for acoustic coupling. It may be difficult to image the first two layers with this technique, because they may be compressed by the balloon if filling is too great. With too little water in the balloon, the first two layers may be too close to the transducer to be in focus. Thus, a three-layer wall image is often obtained. To image five layers, the water in the balloon must be carefully adjusted, or small amounts of water must be injected into the esophagus itself.

The key to imaging small, early cancers confined to the mucosa or submucosa is to cover the tumor with a small quantity of water while maintaining the transducer in the water but off the lesion. This technique can be difficult with dedicated endoscopes, although the smaller tip on the latest instruments makes this easier than in the past. Using the water-filled balloon method, small lesions may become compressed and indistinguishable, or they may be pushed into the wall and appear artifactually deeper, resulting in an overstaging error.

High-frequency US (12 and 20 MHz) catheter-size probes used through a forward-viewing endoscope can be used to stage small lesions. Ideally, the patient is positioned so a small puddle of water remains over the lesion, and the probe is placed into the water under the endoscopic control.

The new EUS probes that operate at higher frequencies can visualize the esophageal wall as a series of seven or nine layers. Lymph nodes along the entire length of the esophagus may be imaged, including paratracheal, subcarinal, pericardial, and crural nodes. Important areas of intra-abdominal nodal drainage for cancer staging are the celiac axis, splenic artery, splenic hilum, hepatic artery, porta hepatis, and left gastric artery in the gastrohepatic ligament between the liver and the lesser curvature of the stomach (39).

Preoperative Staging

Many data are available regarding preoperative staging of esophageal cancer with EUS and for comparison of the results with postoperative surgical pathologic examination. In one review, 21 separate studies were identified, showing an average accuracy for staging T of 84% in 1154 patients and an average accuracy for staging N of 77% in 1035 patients (20). Accuracy for staging T1 and T2 cancers is less than that for T3 and T4 cancers (Figs. 5 and 6). Staging accuracy has been shown to be more than 90% for T3 disease (40).

In the staging classification of the American Joint Committee on Cancer (AJCC) and the International Union Against Cancer (UICC), a T1 esophageal cancer may invade the submucosa, but differentiating lesions confined only to the mucosa is critical when considering local treatment. Investigators estimate that lymph node metastases are uncommon in patients with mucosal tumors, but they can occur in up to 30% of patients who have submucosal invasion (41). The distinction between mucosal and submucosal cancer has been accomplished with EUS with an accuracy of 66% to 84% (42–46). Using high-frequency US probes, often called "mini probes," the accuracy of differentiating T1 and T2 lesions was 92% compared to 76% by EUS (47).

In patients with Barrett's esophagus, accurate staging of high-grade dysplasia and of early cancer is important in selecting patients for endoscopic therapy. Larghi et al. studied 48 consecutive patients with Barrett's esophagus

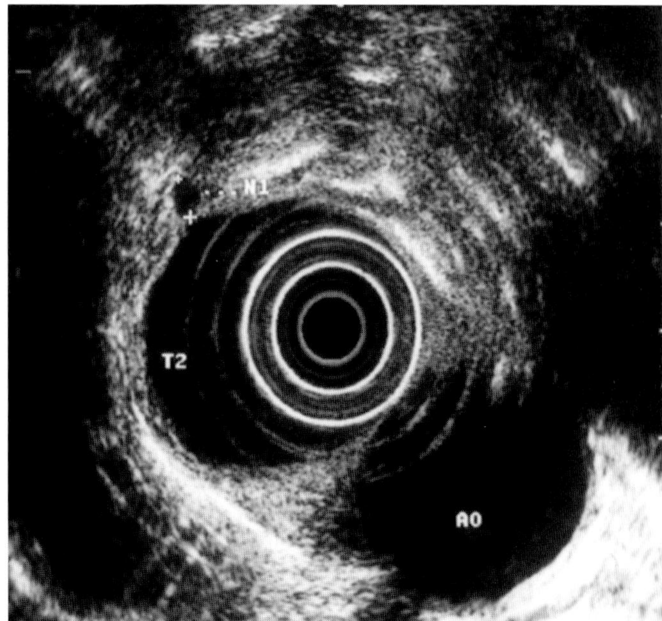

FIGURE 5 ■ Radial scanning image (Olympus GF UM-20) of a T2 N1 esophageal adenocarcinoma.

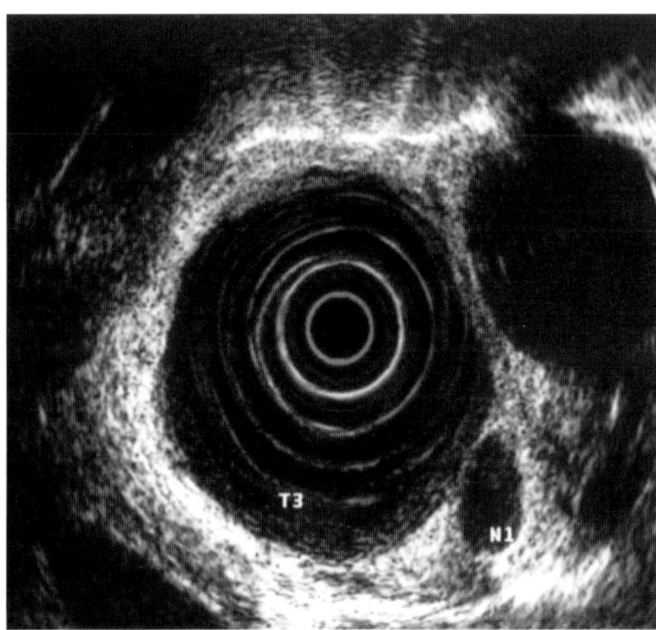

FIGURE 6 ■ Radial scanning image (Olympus GF UM-20) of a T3 N1 esophageal cancer.

and high-grade dysplasia with or without adenocarcinoma in focal nodular lesions or in flat lesions in short segment Barrett's. EUS was performed for initial staging (48). In patients with disease limited to the mucosa on EUS, cap-assisted EMR was performed. EUS provided accurate staging in 41/48 patients (85%) with one patient overstaged and six patients understaged compared with pathologic staging obtained by surgery or EMR. Of the 34 patients with mucosal disease after EMR, 29 were treated endoscopically and had no evidence of cancer after a mean followup of 22.9 months. The authors concluded that EMR provided pathologic staging information that, in addition, can be helpful after EUS if a stage-determined approach is used in the management of high-grade dysplasia and of early cancer in Barrett's esophagus.

The distinction between T2 cancers that invade into but not through the muscularis propria and T3 cancers that invade the adventitia can also be difficult. A roughened or irregular outer margin between the hypoechoic tumor and the surrounding hyperechoic fatty tissue has been used to indicate T3 disease, but this criterion is subjective. Invasion distance or tumor thickness has been proposed as a useful objective measurement (46). T4 invasion can be determined for the trachea, carina, aorta, pericardium, azygos vein, and diaphragm, usually by loss or irregularity of the bright tissue plane between the tumor and the adjacent structure. The invasion of the trachea and carina seems to be the most difficult to determine.

In esophageal cancer staging of regional lymph node metastases, the presence of metastases (N1) has been achieved with a greater accuracy of 89% (n = 343), compared with the absence of metastases (N0) at 69% (n = 231) (20). The sensitivity is greater than the specificity. The accuracy of N staging by conventional EUS was 79% in a meta-analysis done by Kelly et al. (49).

Comparison with CT

Ten studies available for review compare the results of locoregional staging with EUS with CT, using surgical pathologic examination as the ideal standard (20). For both T stage and N stage, EUS has a clear superiority in staging. Other studies comparing EUS with CT for evaluation of regional lymph node involvement have also demonstrated superiority of EUS to CT (20,49).

However, EUS cannot fully assess metastatic disease. The greatest overall staging accuracy is achieved by first obtaining a CT to stage for distant metastases (50). If distant metastases are present (M1), the patient has stage IV disease, and no further staging efforts are needed. If the patient is M0 on CT, EUS should be used for more accurate T and N staging. Compared with surgical pathologic examination, an overall 86% staging accuracy can be achieved with this algorithm.

LYMPH NODE DIFFERENTIAL DIAGNOSIS

Larger lymph nodes are more likely to be malignant, but nodal size, usually measured at its greatest diameter, can be misleading. Some investigators have concluded that malignant lymph nodes can be distinguished from benign nodes on the basis of EUS characteristics (8,51), whereas others believe that the criteria are too subjective and not useful (52). Diameter greater than 10 mm, uniform hypoechogenicity, a rounded shape, and nodes with sharp borders are some of the criteria for malignant nodes (53). Hyperplastic nodes can be large, usually elongated, and echogenic with a hazy outline, but exceptions are seen.

EUS-guided FNA improves the accuracy of EUS for N staging by providing cytologic material to confirm malignant involvement of lymph nodes. In a large prospective series, EUS-FNA sensitivity, specificity, and accuracy for evaluation of malignant lymph nodes was 92%, 93%, and 92%, respectively (54).

Limitations

Limitations of EUS accuracy in staging are understaging resulting from microscopic cancer invasion below the resolution of the US device and overstaging resulting from peritumor fibrosis and inflammation that cannot be distinguished from tumor. In the esophagus and gastric cardia, overstaging is associated with ulcerated lesions. Poor technique can also lead to errors, for example, oblique scanning or fold distortion by the water-filled balloon in the area of the esophagogastric junction.

Malignant Stenoses

An additional limitation of EUS staging of esophageal cancer is the inability to pass the dedicated US endoscope through a malignant stricture. Most, but not all, studies have shown that imaging the entire length of a tumor provides the greatest accuracy (20,26–28,55).

Most tumors large enough to obstruct the passage of the US endoscope are advanced, and most are likely to be stage T3. On the other hand, bulky T2 tumors are not rare and were found in 11% of patients with malignant strictures in one study (56). Detecting local invasion (T4) and celiac axis nodal metastases (M1) can have major repercussions regarding resectability for cure. To make these distinctions, the US probe must be passed into the stomach. Accuracy of EUS in establishing the T stage for nontraversable tumors is only slightly lower than that of traversable tumor (84% vs. 77%) (57,58). There was a more significant difference in accuracy: 92% in traversable cancers versus 46% in nontraversable cancer and in easily traversable tumors and stenosis that were difficult to pass (55).

Rapid dilation of a malignant esophageal stenosis to allow same-day passage of an US endoscope has an associated risk of perforation of up to 24% (26,27). However, a more gradual dilation has been reported to be safe (28). Incremental, stepwise dilation of malignant strictures to 14 mm has been shown prospectively to be effective in permitting echoendoscope passage beyond the stenosis (29).

Another approach is to use a specially designed wire-guided nonoptical probe, 7.9 mm in outer diameter, which seems safe and accurate in initial trials (57). Newer catheter-size probes or mini probes are able to pass tumor stenosis without dilation and provide more accurate T staging than low-frequency probes. They are however limited in their range.

EUS has already been shown to be superior to other imaging modalities for diagnosis and staging of esophageal cancer. Assessing impact of EUS–FNA on management and survival in these patients is being studied. Prospective trials evaluating the impact of EUS revealed that EUS staging changed the treatment plan in almost 75% of the cases with a tendency toward less-costly, less-risky, and less-invasive management. In evaluating the clinical impact of EUS-FNA, where a positive cytology result would change management, EUS-FNA was found to have a major impact in 13% of cases (59,60).

Harewood and Kumar in their study compared clinical outcomes of patients with esophageal carcinoma before and after the introduction of staging with EUS-FNA and demonstrated that EUS is associated with a recurrence-free survival advantage and an overall survival advantage. EUS staging of cancer led to appropriate use of preoperative neoadjuvant therapy (61).

Gress et al. found a relation of survival to T and N staging with EUS (62). Comparing surgery with nonoperative therapy, they found no survival benefit for surgery in patients with EUS stage T2, T3, T4, or N1 disease.

PORTAL HYPERTENSION

Esophageal varices may be difficult to image because they are usually superficial and thin walled, and they may be compressed easily by larger dedicated US endoscopes (63). Newer probes seem to make imaging of esophageal varices much easier. Gastric varices, which tend to occur deeper in the submucosa, are routinely imaged in the water-filled stomach (64).

The diameter of the portal vein (PV), splenic vein, and azygous vein can be measured to assess increase in portal hypertensive disease. Periesophageal and perigastric collateral vessels can be diagnosed and assessed. Gastric varices may be due to PV and splenic vein thrombosis, which can be detected with EUS (Fig. 4). The cause of splenic vein thrombosis, for example, cancer of the pancreatic tail may also be evident on EUS (65).

The effect of sclerotherapy can be demonstrated on EUS as hyperechoic mural thickening with a decrease or disappearance of submucosal varices (64). It may be useful to monitor the therapeutic eradication of varices, but although some data exist in this regard, clinical utility has not yet been firmly established (66). Doppler-guided manometry of esophageal varices is feasible and accurate but warrants further investigation to become a more reliable method for measuring variceal pressure (67).

STOMACH

Normal Anatomy

At the commonly used clinical frequencies of 5 and 12 MHz, EUS provides a characteristic five-layer image of the normal gastric wall. The five layers are an alternating series of bright and dark (hypoechoic) bands, which normally are 3 to 4 mm in total thickness. These layers are seen with greater clarity in the stomach than in any other part of the luminal GI tract. Using a combination of water-filled balloon and water in the stomach lumen for acoustical contact, the normal gastric folds appear as smooth, defined layers (Fig. 1).

The generation of this US image is complex, but a series of experiments has confirmed the relation to histologic features (12). The hyperechoic or echogenic bands consist in part of boundary echoes created as the US beam encounters a different medium. However, for clinical purposes, the first two layers correlate with the mucosa, the third layer with the submucosa, the fourth with the muscularis propria, and the fifth with the serosa plus the subserosa. Extremely large gastric folds may produce a confusing overlapping fold appearance on EUS. The folds can usually be made to float apart by filling the stomach with water and gently teasing the folds from the wall with the water-filled balloon.

The size ratio of layers 2, 3, and 4 is roughly 1:1:1, although the third layer with its boundary echo may often predominate slightly. In evaluating the use of EUS for enlarged gastric folds, Songur et al. studied the wall image in 16 presumably normal control subjects (68). Patients received an anticholinergic agent, and 300 to 800 mL water was instilled into the stomach. With a standard deviation of 0.1 mm, the mean thickness of the mucosa was 1.2 mm, the submucosa 1.4 mm, and the muscularis propria 0.8 mm. Full wall thickness was 3.9 mm, with a standard deviation of 0.6 mm. The major blood vessels around the stomach are also routinely imaged as well as lymphatic drainage areas along these vessels. These include most notably the celiac trunk, splenic artery, hepatic artery, and left gastric artery.

Pitfalls

When evaluating the gastric wall with EUS, scanning in areas of ulceration may lead to misinterpretation, because ulcers may focally involve deeper layers. Therefore, a focal disruption of layer 4 does not necessarily indicate the presence of a malignant process, but it may be related to inflammation and fibrosis around a benign ulcer. Infiltrating malignant disease causes a diffuse thickening and often a distortion of the normal fourth layer wall image.

Preoperative Staging of Gastric Cancer

EUS is fast becoming one of the routine methods in staging of gastric cancer. EUS has been shown to have a much higher accuracy for staging depths of tumor penetration (T) and regional lymph node metastases (N). Data from 22 centers revealed accuracy of EUS for T was 78% (n = 2263) and for N it was 70% (n = 1171) (20).

Comparing EUS locoregional staging with EUS for gastric cancer among 238 patients from three centers, EUS was superior for T (85% vs. 29%) and for N (83% vs. 43%) (69). In a recent study comparing EUS preoperative staging to histopathalogic staging, the overall accuracy of EUS for determination of the T stage was 80%, and for T1, T2, T3, and T4 was 100%, 71.4%, 87.5%, and 72.7%, respectively. For N stage, EUS had the accuracy of 68.6% with sensitivity and specificity of 66.7% and 73.7%, respectively. Resectability was predicted with sensitivity and specificity of 87.5% and 100%, respectively. The greatest overall staging accuracy results from using CT to screen for distant metastases. If these metastases are histologically confirmed, no further staging is usually required. If the patient is clinically M0, then EUS should be used to stage for T and N (Figs. 7–9) (70).

Limitations

Understanding the limitations of EUS staging of gastric cancer is important. Understaging occurs because of the inability to image micrometastases, whether in deeper wall layers or in lymph nodes. Overstaging is more common in gastric cancer than in esophageal cancer (20). Many gastric cancers are ulcerated, and inflammation and fibrosis may involve deeper wall layers than the malignant tumor itself (71). Large reactive lymph nodes may also be difficult to distinguish from metastatic lymph nodes.

A further problem is the inability to distinguish by EUS the subserosal fat from the actual serosa or visceral peritoneum, which may tent away from gastric wall, particularly at the curvatures of the stomach. Thus, in a patient with apparent disruption of the fifth layer on EUS on histologic section, one may see complete penetration of the muscularis propria by cancer with infiltration of the subserosa but without penetration through the serosa. As such, a tumor that is pathologically T2 may easily be overstaged by EUS as a T3 tumor. The presence of ascites may help the clinician to make a more accurate EUS diagnosis in such situations. This distinction is difficult for the pathologist as well, because the gastric serosa is only a few cells thick in some areas. Nonetheless, the accuracy of EUS for T2 stage gastric cancer is the most problematic.

Surgery remains the primary treatment of gastric cancer for both cure and palliation. Therefore, it can be argued that preoperative staging with EUS can have little benefit. However, EUS has been shown to be highly accurate in

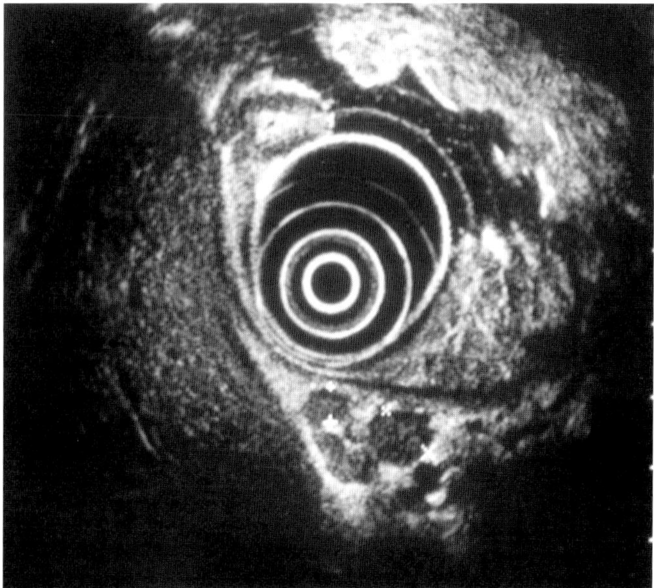

FIGURE 7 ■ Radial scanning image of gastric cancer. Also seen are malignant appearing gastrohepatic lymph nodes.

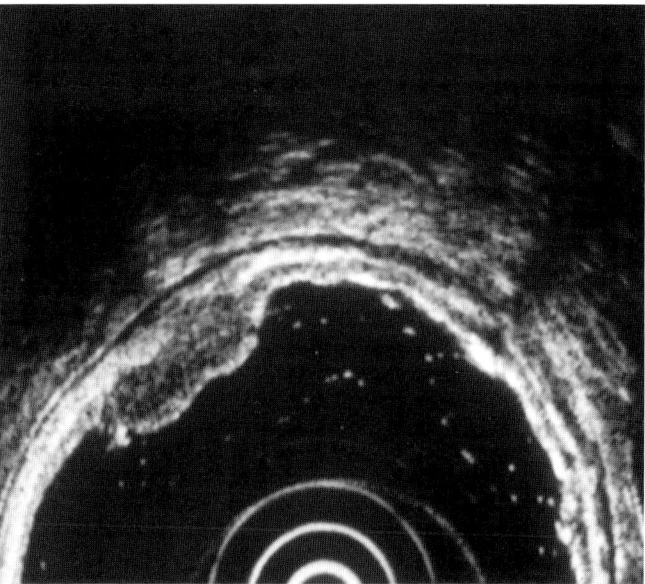

FIGURE 8 ■ Radial scanning image of a gastric cancer.

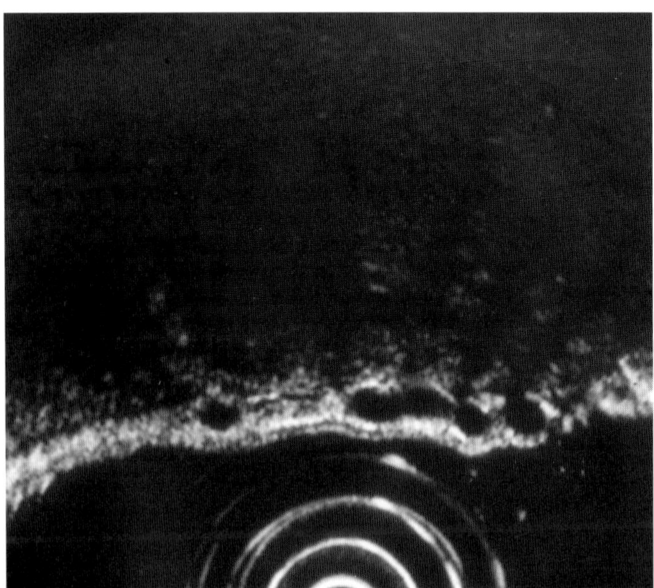

FIGURE 9 ■ Large gastric folds previously identified on computed tomography demonstrated to be varices on radial ultrasound exam.

distinguishing early (T1) from advanced (T2–T4) gastric cancer (20) and has provided an accurate guide to prognosis (72). Thus, in a patient at high risk for surgery and general anesthesia, EUS may help in choosing operative versus nonoperative management. EUS may also serve as a critical guide to the choice of endoscopic therapy for early cancer, such as laser therapy or mucosectomy (strip biopsy).

Early adenocarcinoma confined to the mucosa (T_1m) or submucosa (T_1sm) has a 95% five-year survival rate after resection (73). High-frequency (20 MHz) ultrasonic mini probes can be used with a standard endoscope to stage such small lesions with 92% accuracy. However, lesions over 2 cm are evaluated by standard echoendoscopes and are often overstaged, which decreases accuracy to 50% (74).

In conclusion, although limitations exist, EUS provides the most accurate means for locoregional staging of gastric cancer. The treatment of gastric cancer based on surgery alone for all stages is unsatisfactory. The staging accuracy afforded by EUS opens the way for new and better stage-directed therapy. Staging with EUS should help the clinician to select the best possible current management for the individual patient with gastric cancer and should help in carrying out clinical trials aimed at improving the treatment of this lethal disease.

Gastric Lymphoma Staging

Staging of gastric lymphoma has been accomplished with EUS in several small series with accuracy in the same range as that for the staging of gastric adenocarcinoma. Of a total of 44 patients from three centers with surgical pathology staged by the tumor node metastasis (TNM) classification for gastric cancer, the concordance of EUS for T was 93% and for N, 68% (75–77).

EUS is a valuable technique in assessing the extent and invasion of a lesion. By EUS, infiltrative carcinoma tends to show as a vertical growth in the gastric wall, whereas lymphoma tends to show mainly a horizontal extension (78,79).

It has been employed for accurate estimation of both the depth of invasion and the involvement of regional lymph nodes. In comparing EUS with US and CT in diagnostic staging of gastric lymphoma [mucosa-associated lymphoid tissue (MALT)], EUS was found superior to both US and CT (80). In assessing the diagnostic accuracy of EUS in the local staging of primary gastric lymphoma, comparing EUS with histopathalogic stage EUS correctly classified the lymphoma in 37 of 70 patients (53%). Sensitivity of EUS was as follows: Stage I_1, 67% [95% CI (38%, 88%); $P = 0.01$]; and stage I_2, 83% [95% CI (52%, 98%); $P = 0.001$]; stage II_1, 71% [95% CI (79%, 87%); $P = 0.02$].

EUS correctly visualized lymph node infiltration in 17 of 24 cases with stage II lymphoma, but 19 cases endosonographically staged as II_1 proved to be false positives when compared with histopathologic findings for tumor stage I (without lymph node involvement) and stage II_1 (with perigastric lymph node infiltration); the sensitivity of EUS was, respectively, 59%, 95%, CI (46%, 72%) and 71%; 95% CI (49%, 87%) $P = 0.02$ (81).

In the staging and followup of patients with MALT lymphoma treated conservatively, Pavlovic et al. studied the diagnostic importance of EUS by comparing EUS staging with histopathology and then also assessed EUS response to medical treatment (82).

Twenty-six patients with MALT lymphoma were investigated by EUS, six of them evaluated after the eradication of *Helicobacter pylori* infection and 20 after and during cyclophosphande/Mabtera and anti *H. pylori* treatment. Tumors were staged according to the 2000 TNM and modified Ann Arbor classification. Six patients were treated with anti-*H. pylori* eradication therapy. A full regression of lymphoma was seen in two of the six, which was endoscopically and histologically proven. EUS correlated with histology in all cases. In the other 20 patients, EUS revealed regression of lymphoma in 14 cases. Positive correlation with histology was found in 11 patients (11/14), i.e., 78%. In two cases, EUS showed thickened gastric wall, whereas biopsies were negative; six months later, histology revealed progressive lymphoma. Hence, it is not only sensitive for initial staging and assessing treatment response but also for detecting relapse early (82).

EUS has potential clinical utility in restaging of patients after radiation and chemotherapy. There is still a strong need to improve diagnostic accuracy and to also enhance the training of endosonographers to eliminate sources of error in diagnostic staging and monitoring of gastric lymphoma (81).

Enlarged Gastric Folds

Prominent gastric folds seen on barium contrast radiographs and a thickened gastric wall seen on CT scans are frequent indications for endoscopy. The usual concern is that such a finding may represent an infiltrating malignant disease such as linitis plastica or gastric lymphoma. On endoscopy, the appearance of the stomach usually makes it immediately clear that a malignant process is involved, but in a few cases, the endoscopist cannot be sure. If biopsy results show normal mucosa or nonspecific inflammation, the possibility persists of an infiltrating neoplasm below the mucosal folds (83–86). EUS provides a rational approach to this dilemma (68,87,88).

Differential Diagnosis

Enlarged gastric folds have been defined as those greater than 10 mm on barium contrast radiography and those that do not flatten with air insufflation at endoscopy. The differential diagnosis ranges from simple hyperrugosity (a normal variant) and gastritis to the serious malignancies of lymphoma and adenocarcinoma (89). Less-common causes include hypertrophic gastropathy or Menestrier's disease, Zollinger–Ellison syndrome, and infiltrative diseases such as amyloidosis, eosinophilic gastritis, and lymphoid hyperplasia. Infectious causes included histoplasmosis, secondary syphilis, and anisakiasis (90–92).

We reported results using EUS in 28 patients referred for enlarged gastric folds and concern for infiltrating malignancy (87). Patients with a gastric ulcer or localized mass were not included in this evaluation. In 17 patients, prior endoscopic biopsies were negative for cancer. On EUS, we found unsuspected gastric varices in four patients. The other patients all underwent biopsy with jumbo biopsy forceps.

Biopsy results in 16 patients with a thickened layer 2 showed normal mucosa (hyperrugosity) or gastritis (acute and chronic inflammation). These patients were followed for a mean of 35 months and none developed evidence of malignancy. In two other patients with layer 2 thickening, biopsy results were diagnostic of Menetrier's disease in one patient and lymphoma in the other. In six patients with thickening of layers 3 and 4, jumbo biopsy results were diagnostic of adenocarcinoma in two and lymphoma in one patient.

In three patients with thickening and distortion of layers 3 and 4, but with negative jumbo biopsy results, the EUS picture was believed to be so suggestive of malignancy that exploratory surgery was performed. All three had adenocarcinoma in linitis plastica distribution. A similar experience was reported by Andriulli et al. (93). Of our patients with a malignant cause of large gastric folds, layers 3 and 4 were enlarged in 86%.

Songur et al. had similar results in evaluating 35 patients in Japan (68). Again, one patient with Menetrier's disease had involvement of layer 2 only (10.1 mm thick). Patients with hyperrugosity showed layers 2 and 3 thickening, with average mucosal thickness of 2.3 mm and submucosal thickness of 5.5 mm. In this Japanese population, five patients had acute anisakiasis, a parasitic infestation associated with eating raw fish (68,92). Predominantly layer 3, the submucosa, was thickened to 5.5 mm in these patients.

In the series of Songur et al., all 15 patients with scirrhous carcinoma had thickening of layers 3 and 4. Of eight patients with lymphoma, six had thickening of layers 3 and 4 whereas two patients with lymphoma had thickening of layers 2 and 3 only. In gastric carcinoma, the five-layer wall imaged was well preserved in 10 patients, poorly preserved in two, and intermediate in three. In lymphoma, the wall image was preserved in five, poorly preserved in two, and intermediate in one (68).

Chen et al. performed EUS in 25 patients with giant gastric folds detected with upper GI X-ray or endoscopy. The final diagnoses in 25 patients were gastric varices in eight, gastric lymphangiectasis in one, gastritis in four, gastric carcinoma (scirrhous type) in six, and gastric lymphoma in six (94).

Some controversy has surrounded the possibility of differentiation of scirrhous carcinoma from infiltrating lymphoma using EUS (88,95–97). In the report by Songur et al., the mucosa was significantly thicker in lymphoma (average 3.9 mm) than in carcinoma (average 1.7 mm), whereas the submucosa was thicker in carcinoma (average 6.0 mm) than in lymphoma (average 3.1 mm) (68). However, the differentiation of infiltrating lymphoma from linitis plastica was not always possible.

EUS-guided needle-aspiration cytologic examination has been used in a few cases of large gastric folds (98). Whether specimens will be sufficiently diagnostic in scirrhous carcinoma or lymphoma is not clear, but this method could potentially be of use in sampling the submucosa and muscularis propria. Once the abnormality is determined not to be vascular, cautery and snare techniques may be used to obtain larger and deeper specimens for histologic analysis (99–101).

In conclusion, EUS provided a helpful approach to patients with large gastric folds with a concern of infiltrating malignancy. Gastric varices are easily identified, and a dangerous large biopsy of a varix can be avoided (Fig. 9). If only layer 2 (mucosa) is thickened, a strong likelihood exists that the disease is benign. Early cancer, particularly lymphoma, is a possibility, but jumbo biopsy should provide representative sampling of layer 2. Layer 3 thickening, symmetric and undistorted, may be seen in hyperrugosity, but diffuse layer 4 thickening, particularly with distortion of the normal smooth pattern of layers 3 and 4, is a strong indication of infiltrating malignant disease. If jumbo biopsy results are negative for malignancy in this setting, consideration should be given to deeper biopsy with needle, cautery, or snare techniques, or to exploratory surgery.

RECTUM AND ANUS

The wall layers of the rectum and the staging of rectal carcinoma are similar to those of the esophagus. The clinical utility of EUS for this disease lies in the stage-dependent treatment of rectal cancer, which is preoperative radiation and sensitizing chemotherapy for T4 and some T3 lesions (Fig. 10). In a meta-analysis for staging of rectal cancers, the overall accuracy of EUS for T stage was 83% and for N stage was 75% (102).

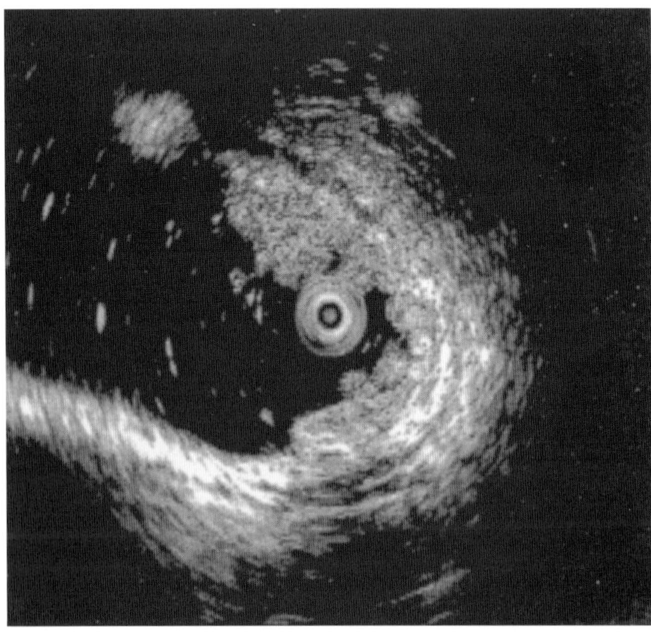
(A)

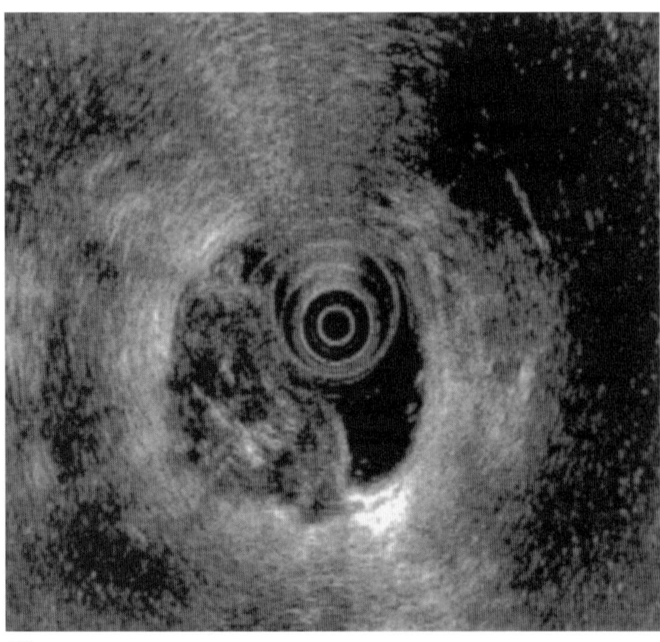
(B)

FIGURE 10 A AND B ■ (**A**) Radial scanning image obtained with the Olympus UM-3R probe, after instillation of deaerated water into the lumen, demonstrating a rectal villous adenoma. (**B**) Radial scanning image demonstrating a T3 rectal cancer (six to nine o'clock position).

EUS has little role in restaging patients after neoadjuvant therapy prior to surgery. EUS typically in this setting will overstage the tumor due to the difficulty in distinguishing post-radiation change from tumor (103–107).

Accuracy of EUS has been prospectively shown to be higher than CT (93–100% vs. 83–85%) (108,109). In detecting the recurrence of cancer, the addition of FNA improves the accuracy of EUS (110,111). EUS is being used for evaluation of perianal disease and for assessing sphincter injury. In a study by Orsoni et al. comparing rectal EUS, pelvic MRI, and examination under anesthesia in 22 patients with Crohn's perianal fistulas, rectal EUS was found to be the most sensitive modality for imaging perianal fistulas caused by Crohn's disease. The agreement of fistulas with rectal EUS and pelvic MRI when compared with the surgical findings were 82% and 50%, respectively (112). Endorectal US was found to be 100% sensitive in detecting internal or external anal sphincter defects in a prospective study where US findings were compared to operative findings in 44 patients undergoing pelvic floor repair (113).

PANCREATICOBILIARY SYSTEM

Normal Anatomy

The techniques for examining the biliary tree, pancreas, ampulla of Vater, and other retroperitoneal structures have been well described for both radial scanning (114) and linear-array probes (115,116). The pancreas appears as a generally homogeneous echogenic structure, with a granular echo pattern. Portions of the hypoechoic duct are seen as a 1 to 3 mm linear structure in the pancreatic body and tail. The bile duct is seen as a hypoechoic structure between the duodenum and the PV in 80% to 90% of anatomically normal patients, followed through the head of the pancreas to the ampulla in the second portion of the duodenum (Fig. 11).

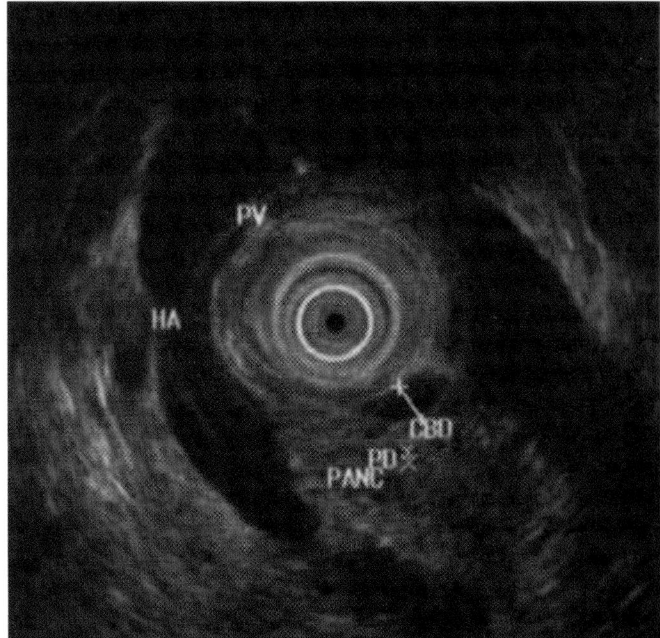

FIGURE 11 ■ Radial scanning image obtained with the Olympus UM-20 revealing a normal pancreatobiliary exam. PV, portal vein; HA, hepatic artery; CBD, common bile duct; PANC, pancreas.

A particularly confusing EUS characteristic of the pancreas is that the primitively ventral pancreas appears as a hypoechoic structure within the pancreas and can be misconstrued as focal pancreatitis or tumor (Fig. 12). In a well-illustrated report of their prospective experience in 100 patients undergoing EUS for various indications, Savides et al. (117) described this finding in 75% of anatomically normal subjects and in 40% of patients with suspected pancreatic disease.

Pancreatic Cancer

Detection

Abundant data indicate that EUS is the most sensitive method for detection of pancreatic tumors.

Multiple studies have shown the sensitivity of EUS for detecting pancreatic cancer to be in the range of 90% and above and is superior to abdominal US, CT, and MRI (118–122).

EUS is especially helpful for smaller lesions. EUS has an added advantage with its ability to perform FNA. The sensitivity of EUS-FNA for pancreatic masses is in the range of 85% to 90% and a specificity of virtually 100% (123–125).

Differential Diagnosis of Pancreatic Tumors

Most tumors are hypoechoic compared with pancreatic parenchyma, although the echo pattern becomes mixed and more variable the larger the size. Cancers tend to have an irregular margin, sometimes with extending pseudopodia, but malignant lesions smaller than 3.0 cm may have a smooth margin. Unfortunately, areas of focal inflammation can have a similar hypoechoic pattern, sometimes with an equally irregular margin of demarcation (126,127). Cystic tumors can be identified with regularity, but identifying which are malignant remains problematic, but FNA can now be used to detect malignancy.

The specificity of EUS for differentiating pancreatic cancer from focal pancreatitis has been reported to be about 70% (126,127). Echo-enhanced color and power Doppler has been shown to have a sensitivity of 94% and specificity of 100% for differentiating pancreatic carcinoma from inflammatory changes. Contrast-enhanced power Doppler US can also help differentiate pancreatic carcinoma from chronic focal pancreatitis.

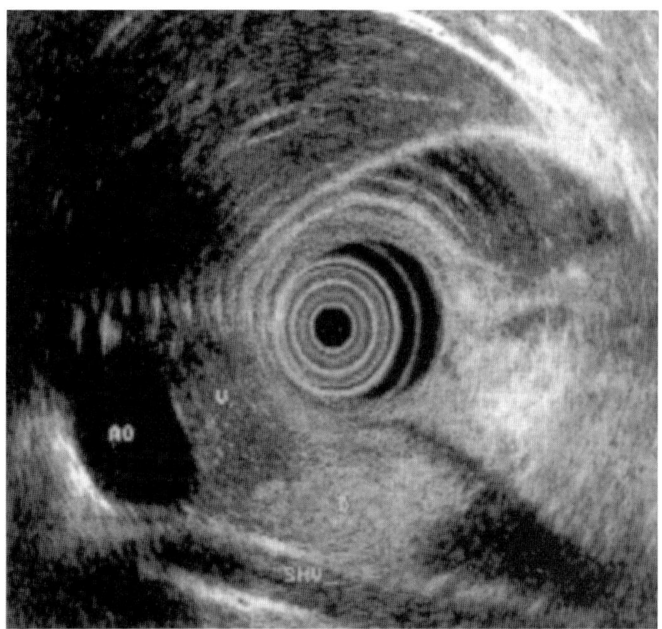

FIGURE 12 ■ Radial scanning image (Olympus GF UM-20, 7.5 MHz) showing the normal appearance of the pancreatic head from the second portion of the duodenum. The pancreatic parenchyma is surrounded by the aorta and SMV in this view, in which the primitively ventral pancreas can be distinguished from the more hyperechoic primitively dorsal pancreas. AO, aorta; SMV, superior mesenteric vein; V, ventral pancreas; D, dorsal pancreas.

Staging

The ability of EUS to define the parenchymal extent and size of a pancreatic cancer can provide potentially useful staging information. AJCC in 2002 modified the T staging system for pancreatic cancer to classify tumors invading the portal venous (superior mesenteric vein or PV) system as T3 (which previously were staged as T4). Tumors invading the celiac or superior mesenteric artery are now staged as T4. Accuracy of T staging for EUS ranges between 78% and 94% and N-stage accuracy ranges from 64% to 82% (119,127–129).

In another series of 89 patients where EUS was compared with surgical and histopathologic TNM staging, the overall accuracy of EUS for T staging was 69% and N staging was 54% (130).

With the advent of new helical CT scanners that can get thinner slices and improved image resolution, EUS has been shown to be still better for T stage accuracy for pancreatic tumors, especially in small tumors measuring less than 2 cm (131–134).

Hunt and Faigel in a recent review compared EUS and helical CT in the evaluation of pancreatic cancer and found that EUS detected more tumors (97% vs. 73%) and was more accurate for determining tumor resectability (91% vs. 83%). EUS was more sensitive for detecting vascular invasion (91% vs. 64%) (135). In two studies, EUS was found to be superior to helical CT in detecting vascular invasion (132,136). In two different reports, CT and EUS were found to be approximately equivalent in detecting the primary tumors (133,137).

EUS and helical CT are complementary for staging pancreatic cancer. EUS is more accurate for local T staging and assessing vascular invasion especially for small tumors, whereas helical CT is better for the evaluation of distant metastasis and for staging large tumors (Fig. 13).

Pancreatic Ductal Imaging

Using catheter-like probes, the clinician can image from within the pancreatic duct, but the clinical utility of this approach has not yet been established. Furukawa et al. (38) have used very high-frequency (30 MHz) catheter probes introduced into the pancreatic duct at ERCP in

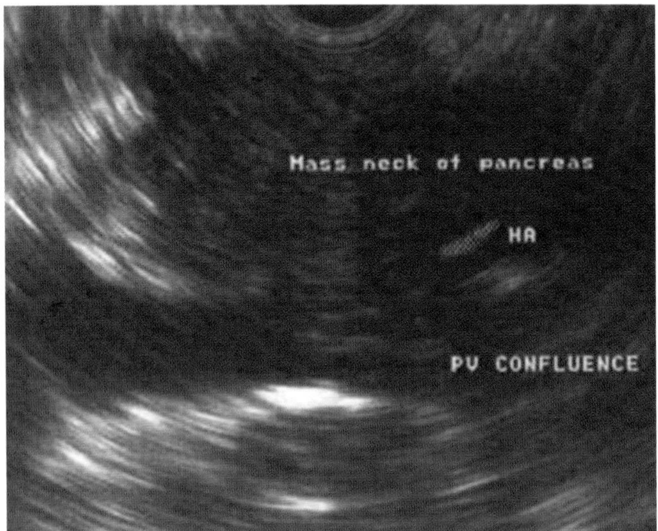

FIGURE 13 ■ Linear scanning image of a pancreatic mass in the neck with tumor encasing the hepatic artery. Presence of vessel confirmed with Doppler. HA, hepatic artery; PV, portal vein.

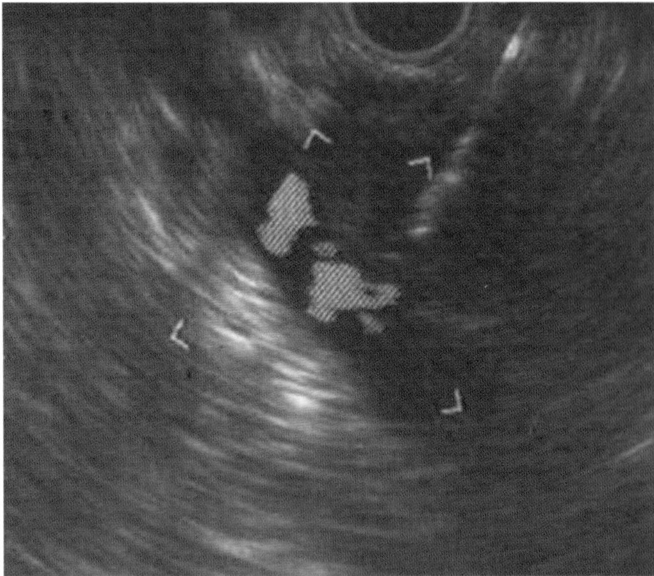

FIGURE 14 ■ Linear scanning image of a pancreatic adenocarcinoma with tumor invasion of the portal vein. An aspiration needle has been passed into the lesion for tissue sampling.

40 patients with pancreatic diseases, including 11 with adenocarcinoma and 15 with chronic pancreatitis. These investigators also examined surgical and autopsy specimens from these and other patients and were convinced that echo patterns obtained in this way can distinguish benign from malignant disease in most cases.

Pancreatic ductal imaging with catheter probes may have some utility in detecting early adenocarcinomas. Papillary neoplastic lesions confined to the wall of the pancreatic duct were described in four cases (one cancer and three adenomas). Complications were low; mild pancreatitis occurred in only one of the 40 cases. Prospective studies of high-frequency pancreatic duct imaging will be required to confirm these observations.

Clinical Utility for Pancreatic Lesions

Based on current data and our recent experience, we use EUS for pancreatic mass lesions as follows: For patients who have suspected pancreatic lesion on either CT or US, we perform EUS of the pancreas. EUS-FNA of suspicious lesions or nodes is conducted during the same examination. In this situation, we reserve ERCP for cases in which the EUS is inconclusive.

For patients with a potentially resectable pancreatic mass identified on CT or US for which biliary drainage is not required, we stage the tumor with EUS and perform EUS-FNA of imaged lesions, including celiac axis lymph nodes (Fig. 14). If biliary drainage is required, we initially perform ERCP with biliary and pancreatic stricture tissue sampling followed by biliary duct stenting. This procedure is followed, usually on a separate day in our institution, by EUS staging (including peripancreatic and celiac lymph node FNA). EUS-guided needle aspiration of the primary tumor is done only if ERCP tissue sampling was inadequate (Fig. 15).

Ampullary Cancer

The use of EUS is also helpful in the visualization of ampullary tumors. In patients with a common channel at the papilla, the ampulla can be visualized endosonographically as a hypoechoic, tubular structure into which the distal bile duct and pancreatic duct merge. The normal ampulla begins 2 mm upstream from the duodenal wall and endosonographically it may be seen partly inside and partly outside the fourth hypoechoic muscular layer (138). Tumors of the ampullary region appear as hypoechoic

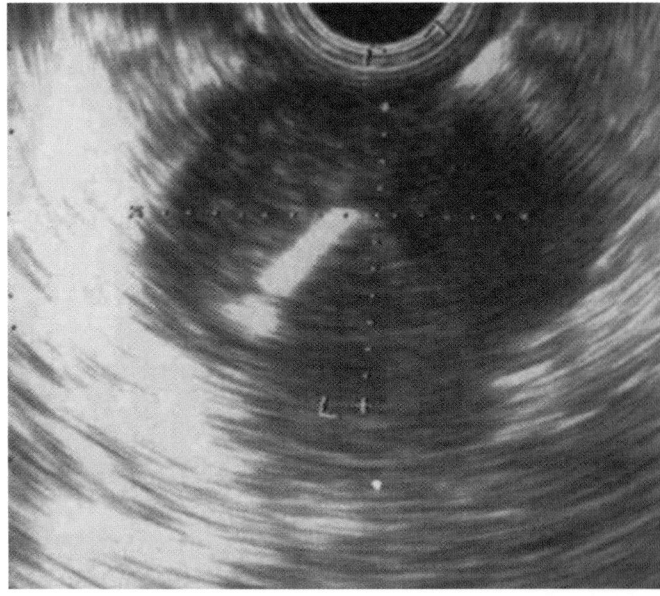

FIGURE 15 ■ Linear scanning image of a neoplasm in the tail of the pancreas. An aspiration needle passed into the lesion for tissue sampling can also be noted.

thickening in the area of the papilla of Vater (138,139). Most patients have dilated ducts that make tumor identification by EUS relatively easy. Many of these tumors are too small to be imaged by transabdominal US or CT. EUS is more effective and accurate in the preoperative staging and assessment of resectability of ampullary carcinomas than CT or US (138,140–144).

The use of EUS has some important limitations for ampullary lesions. As in other parts of the GI tract, in the absence of histologic diagnosis, one cannot determine the difference between a benign tumor and an early cancer. In advanced disease, distinguishing between a carcinoma of the head of the pancreas invading the ampulla and an ampullary cancer invading the pancreas may not be possible. In addition, in some patients, a swollen or inflamed papilla after stone passage or papillotomy cannot be distinguished from a small tumor by EUS.

High-frequency catheter probes may be useful in differential diagnosis of periampullary mass lesions and may help one to distinguish primary bile duct cancers from primary pancreatic cancers in some patients, but current experience is limited.

Ampullary adenocarcinomas are staged according to the TNM system. In this system, T1 tumors are limited to the papilla, T2 tumors invade the duodenal wall, and T3 lesions invade the pancreas. N1 designated the presence of regional lymph node involvement. The treatment for ampullary cancers is regional resection, and EUS staging is limited to cases in which the patient is elderly or otherwise a poor surgical candidate and local excision is contemplated. Moreover, for ampullary adenomas, it is prudent to stage the tumor as accurately as possible with EUS, with standard scope-based EUS and high-frequency catheter probes if available, before considering local resection of operative or endoscopic means.

In a retrospective analysis, DeFrain et al. have shown that EUS is accurate in the evaluation of suspected ampullary malignancies and EUS-guided FNA is effective in obtaining adequate diagnostic material. They had three false-negative results and no false-positive results. The diagnostic accuracy of EUS was 88.8% (145).

Pancreatic Endocrine Tumors

The diagnosis of pancreatic endocrine tumors is established by the clinical signs and laboratory tests. However, the preoperative localization of these tumors can still pose a problem. Noninvasive imaging tests such as US and CT fail in many cases, in approximately 20% of insulinomas and in up to 40% of gastrinomas, which have a high frequency of extrapancreatic sites, as opposed to insulinomas. The smaller the tumors are the lower is the detection rate. Although additional tumors are detected by palpation and intraoperative US, preoperative localization greatly facilitates the operative approach (Fig. 16).

In a cooperative study from six institutions (146), 82% of 39 pancreatic endocrine tumors not localized on CT were detected by EUS. The tumors were small (95% were less than 2.0 cm diameter, mean size 1.4 cm). The tumors included 31 insulinomas, seven gastonomas, and one

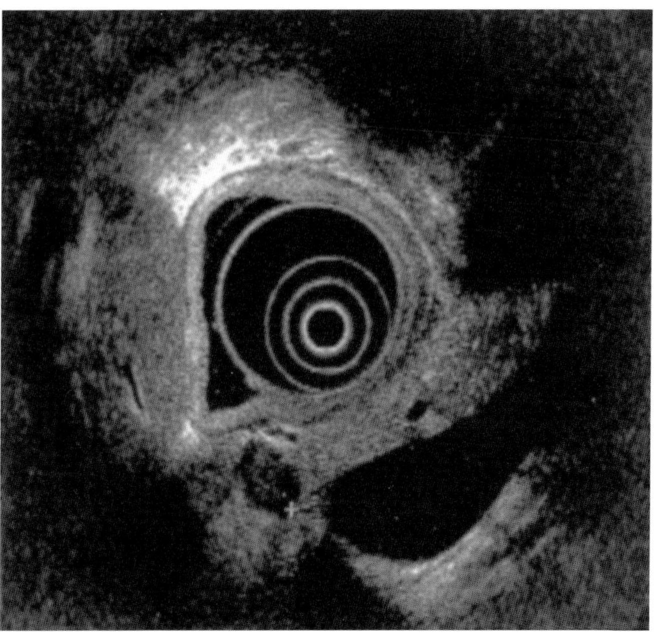

FIGURE 16 ■ Radial scanning image (12 MHz) of a pancreatic islet cell tumor measuring 12 mm (seven o'clock).

glucagonoma. In 19 patients thought to have endocrine tumors on initial workup but later found not to have such lesions, EUS was correctly negative in 18, for a 95% specificity. In 22 patients who had both EUS and angiography, EUS was significantly more sensitive in detecting and localizing the pancreatic endocrine tumors (82% vs. 27% $P < 0.05$).

Anderson et al. in their study of 82 patients with biochemical or clinical evidence of neuroendocrine tumors used EUS for diagnostic evaluation and showed that EUS had a sensitivity and accuracy of 93%. It has a specificity of 95% and was more accurate than angiography, US, and CT (147). It was not reliable though in localizing extrapancreatic tumors. EUS was found highly accurate in the localization of pancreatic neuroendocrine tumors and was found to be cost effective when used early in the preoperative localization strategy (148).

Pancreatitis

In the diagnosis of moderate and advanced forms of chronic pancreatitis, EUS is accurate. Both parenchymal and ductal changes indicative of chronic pancreatitis can be identified (149). Parenchymal changes include hyperechoic and hypoechoic foci scattered throughout the gland, enhancement of the lobular pattern, and hyperechoic duct and gland borders. These parenchymal changes can be detected even in patients with normal pancreatic ducts at ERCP.

EUS is fast becoming an important tool in the diagnosis of chronic pancreatitis but diagnosing "early or minimal change" disease still remains a controversy. EUS is as sensitive and effective as ERCP in detecting chronic pancreatitis especially when only mild disease is present; however, specificity of EUS is limited.

EUS-FNA with cytology can improve the negative predictive value (NPV). Hollerbach et al. studied 37 patients with chronic pancreatitis with six having normal findings at ERCP (150); EUS showed morphologic abnormalities in 33 patients. Sensitivity alone was 97% for morphologic abnormalities for chronic pancreatitis. The specificity was 60%, positive predictive value (PPV) was 94%, and NPV was 75%. EUS-FNA increased the NPV to 100% and the specificity to 67%. EUS results were in agreement as regards the severity of chronic pancreatitis: 5/8 with grade I disease, 11/13 in grade II, and 10/10 in grade III.

The major limitations of EUS for diagnosis of chronic pancreatitis are the lack of standard criteria or absence of gold standard and adequate training of endosonographers. Further improvements in tissue sampling are also necessary to support the use of FNA in patients with chronic pancreatitis.

EUS has also been used before endoscopic drainage of pancreatic pseudocysts through the stomach and duodenum. The relation of the cyst to the stomach or duodenal wall can be evaluated with particular attention to any large blood vessels in the area of proposed cystenterostomy (Fig. 17).

Bile Duct Cancer

In the detection of small bile duct tumors, EUS is equal to ERCP, but superior to US, CT, and angiography (151). Distal CBD tumors are usually easily imaged in a dilated duct, but more proximal tumors (e.g., Klatskin tumors) may be difficult to image because of limited penetration depth.

EUS can identify biliary strictures but tissue diagnosis is needed to differentiate malignant versus benign lesions. Fritscher-Ravens et al. evaluated the role of EUS-FNA in biliary strictures; in the 44 patients that they studied with hilar strictures, the accuracy of EUS-FNA was 91%, sensitivity was 89%, and specificity was 100%. EUS changed the surgical approach in 27/44 patients (152).

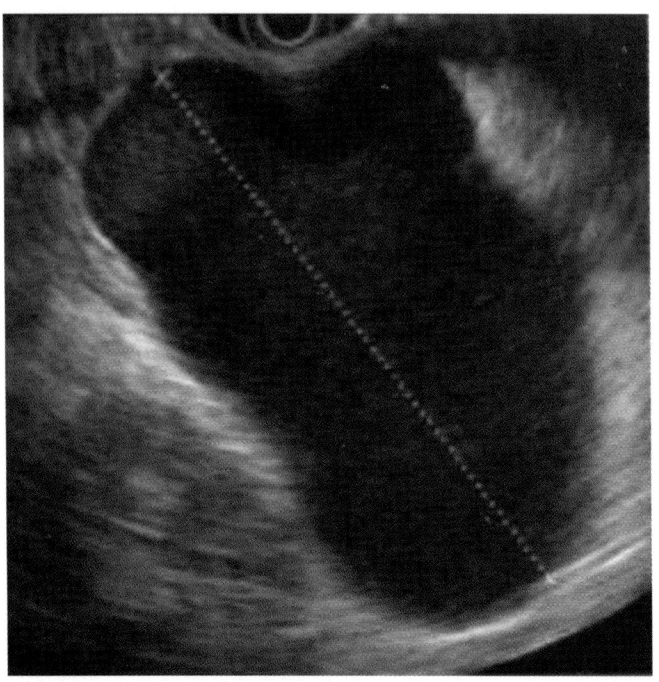

FIGURE 17 ■ Radial scanning image of a pancreatic pseudocyst.

Eloubeidi et al. studied 28 patients with previously failed tissue diagnosis who underwent EUS-FNA of biliary strictures. The sensitivity of EUS-FNA was 86% and specificity was 100%. PPV was 100%, NPV 57%, and accuracy was noted to be 88%. Of the patients, 84% were noted to have a positive impact in their management as in preventing surgery in patients with inoperable disease (n = 10), avoiding surgery in benign disease (n = 4), and facilitating surgery in patients with unidentifiable cancer by other modalities (n = 8) (153).

EUS is used for mid or distal bile duct lesions, but for hilar lesions not well visualized by standard EUS, intraductal ultrasound (IDUS) probes can be used. Menzel et al. reported the sensitivity, specificity, and accuracy of IDUS to be 91.1%, 80% and 89.1%, respectively (154). Tamada et al. compared IDUS with histological analysis of bile duct biopsy specimens obtained using percutaneous transhepatic cholangioscopy (PTCS) to assess the accuracy of IDUS in differentiating benign from malignant biliary strictures (155). Forty-two patients with bile duct strictures or filling defects that required PTCS were included. In 25/26 patients, malignancy was noted and IDUS showed disruption of bile duct wall structure. In three patients with cancer, no disruption was noted on IDUS. The specificity of IDUS was 50% inferior both to cytology and to PTCS and accuracy was lower than PTCS as well. The sensitivity however was 89% and negative productive value 100%. Combining IDUS and cytology, sensitivity increased to 96% and 100% for PTCS. IDUS however cannot distinguish between bile duct wall thickening and tumor versus inflammation and tissue diagnosis cannot be obtained.

IDUS is a valuable tool for characterization of biliary strictures in patients who present with painless jaundice in the absence of an abdominal mass on radiologic imaging. We studied 61 patients with painless jaundice and no mass on CT, who were found to have a biliary stricture on ERCP. Patients underwent IDUS with high-frequency (20 MHz), wire-guided probe and histopathological confirmation or clinical followup was used to establish the final diagnosis (156). Of the patients, 43 had malignant strictures and 18 had benign strictures. ERCP produced 25 false-negative diagnoses, 22 of which were identified as malignant by IDUS. IDUS provided seven false-negative and three false-positive diagnoses. IDUS when used in conjunction with ERCP increased the accuracy of ERCP from 58% to 90%.

In addition to staging and detecting malignant disease, IDUS has also been used to facilitate biliary interventions in critically ill patients when fluoroscopy cannot be used safely in the intensive care unit (ICU) setting. We described a novel nonfluoroscopic bedside ERCP technique using IDUS guidance in four critically ill patients in the ICU where cannulation was performed endoscopically at the bedside using a sphincter tome and a guide wire and IDUS rather than fluoroscopy was then used to confirm placement within the CBD prior to performing endoscopic sphincterotomy or stent placement. The technique was successful in all four patients (157).

Bile duct tumors are staged according to the TNM classification as follows: T1 tumors are limited to the bile duct wall (smooth outer margin); T2 tumors invade periductal tissue (interrupted outer margin); and T3 tumors invade adjacent structures (including major vessels). The use of EUS has allowed accurate staging of T and establishing of resectability in the 80% range (158,159).

Gallbladder Polyps

EUS can be used with transabdominal US to improve the differential diagnosis of gallbladder polyps (Fig. 18). Azuma et al. reviewed 89 patients with gallbladder polyps measuring less than 20 mm, who underwent US and EUS before surgery and then assessed the results of the differential diagnosis. About 86.5% of the polyps were correctly diagnosed by EUS compared to 51.7% by US.

Sensitivity, specificity, PPV, and NPV of EUS for the diagnosis of carcinoma were 91.7%, 87.7%, 75.9%, and 96.6%, respectively, compared to 54.2%, 53.8%, 54.2%, and 94.6%, respectively, for US (160).

Choi et al. presented a new method to predict neoplastic polyps of the gallbladder using a scoring system based on five EUS variables in a study of 132 patients with gallbladder polyps (161). Size was the most significant predictor in the reference group for the risk of neoplastic polyps. All polyps 5 mm or less were all non-neoplastic and majority of the polyps over 15 mm were neoplastic.

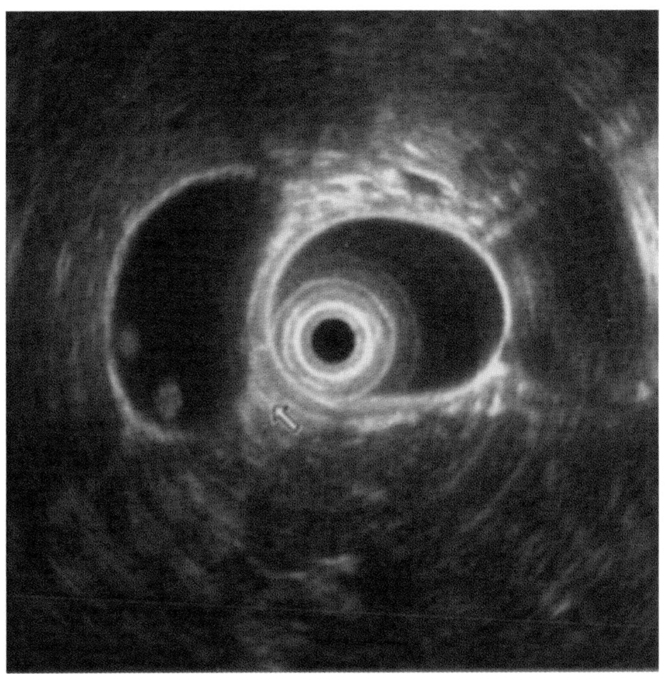

FIGURE 18 ■ Radial scanning image demonstrating gallbladder polyps.

With a cutoff EUS score of 6, the sensitivity, specificity, and accuracy for the risk of neoplastic polyps were 81%, 86%, and 83.7%, respectively. The authors noted that a score based on five EUS variables of neoplasia identified patients at risk when polyps were 5 to 15 mm in diameter. Hence, EUS can markedly improve the accuracy of differential diagnosis of gallbladder polyps and can help in playing an important role in deciding management strategies for gallbladder polyps.

Gallbladder Cancer

Gallbladder carcinoma presents as a polypoid intraluminal mass of varying echodensity and irregularity with progressive wall destruction. The endosonographic appearance of other mass lesions of the gallbladder has also been described (162). Adenomyomatosis shows thickening of muscular and serosal layers on EUS, with small cystic echoes corresponding to Rokitansky–Aschoff sinuses. Cholesterol polyps show a granular echo pattern with multiple hypoechoic spots. It can be difficult to differentiate biliary sludge without acoustic shadowing from intraluminal tumor growth.

The gallbladder and its wall structure can be very well delineated on US. EUS can help in staging gallbladder cancer.

In a study by Mizuguchi et al., the usefulness of EUS in differential diagnosis of gallbladder wall thickening with special reference to loss of multiple layer pattern in cancer patients was studied and compared with conventional US, CT, and MRI. EUS was found to be superior to US, CT, and MRI at demonstrating loss of multiple-layer patterns of the gallbladder wall, which was the most specific finding in diagnosing gallbladder cancer (163).

UICC defines T staging for gallbladder cancer as follows: "Tis, carcinoma in situ; T1a tumor invades lamina propria; T1b tumor invades muscle layer; T2 tumor invades perimuscular connective tissue, no extension beyond serosa or into liver; T3 tumor invades serosa (visceral peritoneum) or directly invades into one adjacent organ, or both (extension 2 cm or less into liver); T4 tumor extends more than 2 cm into liver and/or into two or more adjacent organs (stomach, duodenum, colon, pancreas, aventum, extrahepatic bile ducts, any involvement of liver)."

The accuracy of EUS in the staging of gallbladder cancer according to the TNM classification was assessed by Mitake et al. (164).

In 39 patients with gallbladder cancer, EUS was performed preoperatively and results were compared with histology. T1, T2, T3, and T4 carcinoma were correctly diagnosed by EUS in 87.5%, 66.7%, 71.4%, and 71.4% of cases, respectively. EUS was nondiagnostic in 13% of cases secondary to cholelithiasis and infiltration of the liver was correctly diagnosed as 71.4%. Accuracy for tumor invasion was 76.9%. The sensitivity of EUS for LNwas 81.8%, specificity was 92.9%, and accuracy was 89.7%. Hence, EUS is helpful for primary diagnosis and local staging of gallbladder cancer.

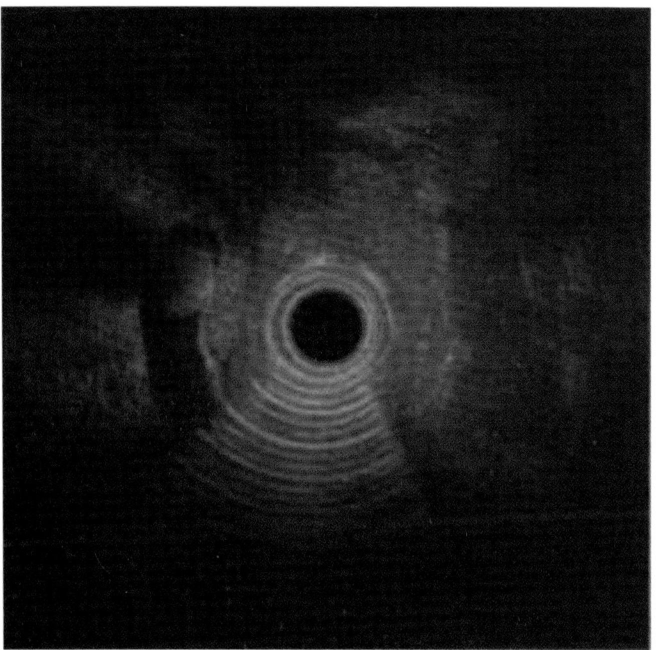

FIGURE 19 ■ Intraductal ultrasound image showing a large common bile duct stone. The hyperechoic stone casts a dense acoustic shadow.

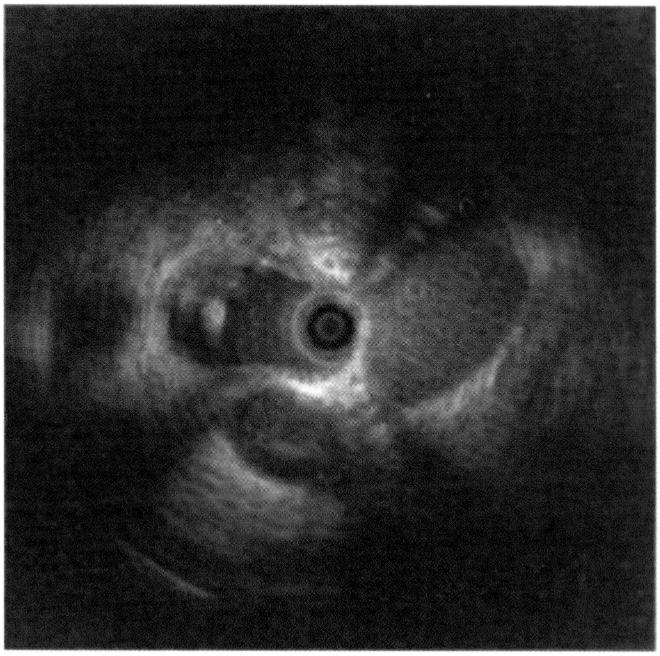

FIGURE 20 ■ Intraductal ultrasound image revealing minilithiasis in the common hepatic duct.

CBD Stones

EUS is a noninvasive method of evaluating for choledocholithiasis (Fig. 19). The accuracy of EUS in the diagnosis of choledocholithiasis in a prospective study was 100% (165). Several studies have been done comparing EUS with US and CT. Kondo et al. compared the diagnostic ability of EUS, MRCP, and HCT-C in patients with suspected choledocholithiasis (25). Of the patients with suspected CBD stones, 28 underwent EUS, MRCP, and HCT-C prior to ERCP (which served as the gold standard for comparison). ERCP in combination with IDUS detected CBD stones in 86% of cases. The sensitivity of EUS, MRCP, and HCT-C was 100%, 88% and 88%, respectively. EUS was superior in detecting stones smaller than 5 mm in diameter. The authors concluded that MRCP and HCT-C should be the first choice for examination of choledocholithiasis as they were less invasive than EUS; and if MRCP was negative, EUS was recommended.

In a prospective study of 62 consecutive patients using ERCP and intraoperative cholangiography as the standards, EUS had a sensitivity of 97% for diagnosis of CBD stones, significantly more sensitive than US (25%) and CT (75%) (166). Specificity for EUS was 100%. The NPV of EUS was 97%, significantly better than that of US (56%) and CT (78%). Two patients with stones noted on EUS but not on ERCP were subsequently shown to have stones. Other investigators have found comparable diagnostic accuracy for EUS compared with ERCP (167–172).

In three different studies comparing ERCP and EUS, the sensitivity of EUS was 88% to 100% and sensitivity of ERCP was 79% to 90%. False-negative results were more common with ERCP (168,173,174).

Comparing the accuracy of EUS and MRCP in the diagnosis of choledocholithiasis, de Ledinghen et al., in a prospective study of 32 patients, found the sensitivity, specificity, PPV, NPV, and accuracy to be 100%, 95.4%, 90.9%, 100%, and 96.9%, respectively. These numbers were true regardless of stone or CBD diameter. The corresponding values for MRCP were 100%, 72%, 62.5%, 100%, and 82.2%, respectively (175).

Although EUS has no therapeutic capacity, it does not have the 4% to 6% risk of pancreatitis associated with diagnostic ERCP. Moreover, EUS may evolve into the test of choice for screening for CBD stones, with ERCP reserved for when the clinical probability of a stone is high or for when EUS is positive.

Biliary Sludge

Biliary sludge, or microlithiasis, may be responsible for up to 60% of cases of idiopathic pancreatitis (Figs. 20 and 21) (176,177). Preliminary reports suggest that EUS can resolve small concentrations of sludge in vitro (178) and that EUS is more sensitive than US in patients with idiopathic pancreatitis (179).

Dill et al. (180) reported that the detection of biliary sludge by EUS may predict the response to cholecystectomy in patients with biliary-type pain from occult cholecystitis. If these studies are confirmed, EUS will come to occupy a pivotal role in the evaluation of patients with unexplained right upper quadrant pain or idiopathic pancreatitis.

EUS-GUIDED INVASIVE PROCEDURES

EUS over the last 20 years has evolved from a primarily diagnostic imaging modality to an interventional procedure. With the development of linear array echoendosonography

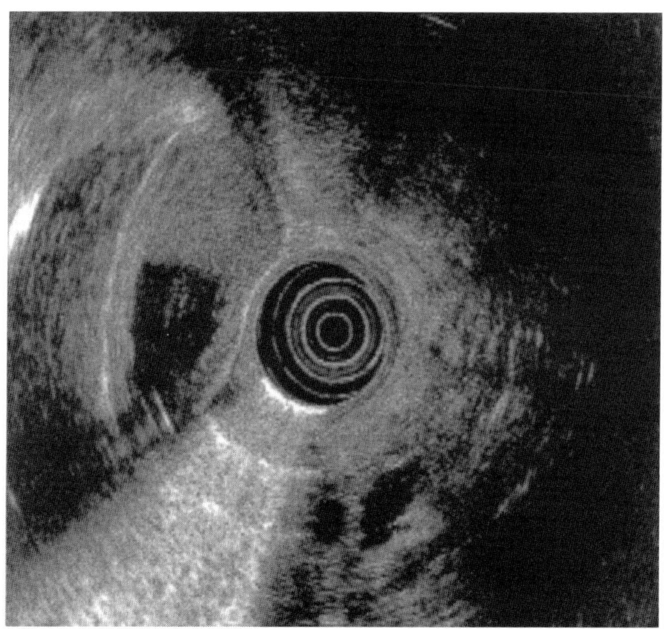

FIGURE 21 ■ Radial scanning image (Olympus GF UM-20, 7.5 MHz) showing a thick-walled gallbladder with layering sludge.

and EUS-guided FNA, the spectrum of applications of EUS is ever expanding. The ability to perform FNA in a noninvasive and safe manner for tissue biopsy or therapeutic injection has ushered in a new era for EUS.

Echoendoscopes

Both radial and linear endoscopes are now commercially available. The radial echoendoscopes generate a radial image of 360, perpendicular to the shaft axis of the scope. Although methods of FNA biopsy using the mechanical radial scanning echoendoscope have been described, this method does not allow continuous observation of the needle tip. The reason is that the US scanning plane of the radial scanning echoendoscope is perpendicular to the axis of the instrument channel of the endoscope—the needle is imaged in cross-section as a bright dot. Although this method can be useful for protuberant intramural submucosal masses, concern exists that it may be associated with an increased complication rate when used for lesions beyond the GI tract.

The linear-array endoscopes generate a linear-type image directed parallel to the shaft of the endoscope, which allows continuous observation of an accessory instrument passed into the beam. This allows for safe and effective EUS-guided FNA.

Needles

Various needles are now available commercially for FNA allowing for tissue diagnosis. Most commonly available are the 22-gauge needles; 19-gauge thicker needles and 25-gauge fine needles are also available.

The commercially available aspiration needle assembly includes four parts: (*i*) the needle is scored at the tip to be visible to US; (*ii*) a removable blunt stylet that, when fully inserted, protrudes just beyond the needle tip; (*iii*) a metal spiral housing sheath; and (*iv*) a handle that is luer locked to the scope at the instrument channel port.

Aspiration Technique

Once a lesion, such as a pancreatic mass or a mediastinal lymph node, is identified in or beyond the wall of the GI tract, the procedure for FNA is as follows: The scope is positioned so that the lesion is directly under the transducer, if possible; slight adjustments must be made so the needle will enter the lesion without passing through vascular structures or (in the case of lymph nodes) through tumor in the wall of the GI tract.

Once the lesion is positioned correctly in the US beam, the needle assembly is passed out of the scope until the stylet tip touches the wall of the bowel. Next, the blunt stylet is drawn back 1 cm to expose the tip of the needle. The needle is advanced slowly into the lesion; the stylet is first fully advanced (to clear the tip of the needle of epithelial debris) and then is completely withdrawn. A 10-mL syringe is attached to the needle, and the assistant aspirates with 6 to 8 mL of suction while the endoscopist moves the exposed needle in and out of the lesion. After 10 to 20 needle movements, the suction is released, and the needle is removed form the endoscope. The cytologic specimen is processed and evaluated immediately, if possible, by an on-call cytologist.

In a recent study by Annema et al. EUS-FNA prevented 70% of scheduled surgical procedures because of confirmation of lymph node metastasis. Sensitivity, specificity, and accuracy of EUS were 91%, 100%, and 93%, respectively (181).

Biopsy Techniques

Although aspiration needles are able to provide cytological specimen, core biopsy is required for pathological interpretation of tissue architecture. We tested the trucut needle biopsy device, which had been previously tested on animals, on humans with solid pancreatic lesions. Twenty-three consecutive patients with radiologically detected solid pancreatic lesions underwent EUS-guided trucut needle biopsy. Overall diagnostic accuracy was 61% and subgroup analysis of the 16 patients in whom EUS-guided trucut needle biopsy was successful and who were available for followup revealed a diagnostic accuracy of 87.5% (182).

CLINICAL APPLICATIONS OF FNA

Lymph Nodes

For patients with potentially resectable cancers, the information obtained from lymph node staging may be pivotal in deciding among available treatment options. EUS enables one to image small nodes (3–4 mm) adjacent to the GI tract. Although imaging alone cannot distinguish benign from malignant lymph nodes with certainty, EUS-FNA can provide tissue to increase the overall accuracy of the procedure for both benign and malignant conditions (183–192).

The usefulness of EUS-FNA for lymph node staging is not limited to GI tumors. Several groups have reported on the utility of EUS-FNA for the lymph node staging of non–small-cell lung caner (193,194). Mediastinal staging can affect the choice of treatment dramatically if contralateral lymph nodes are found to be positive.

Submucosal Lesions

Evaluation of submucosal lesions is an established indication for EUS imaging. Although needle aspiration of lesions often changes the diagnostic impression, aspiration samples of some tumors, such as leiomyomas, are frequently nondiagnostic. Diagnostic yield of FNA was studied in 101 patients by Mallery et al. with subepithelial intramural GI tract masses (195). The yield of EUS-FNA for solid, hypoechoic intramural tumors was 81% but yield of FNA for suspected lipomas or pancreatic rests was very low.

Pancreatic Lesions

Because EUS imaging is limited in its ability to differentiate benign from malignant lesions of the pancreas, EUS-FNA of pancreatic lesions has interested investigators worldwide. The sensitivity of EUS-FNA for pancreatic masses is in the range of 85% to 90% and a specificity of virtually 100% (123–125).

Although percutaneous FNA is often technically possible under sonographic or CT guidance, those imaging methods are limited by the inability to resolve small lesions. In addition, some concern exists about seeding of tumor along the line of puncture when the percutaneous approach is used (196). EUS-FNA can at least partially overcome the limitations of percutaneous puncture. With EUS, one is able to detect extremely small lesions, and given the short distance traveled by the needle during EUS-FNA compared with percutaneous techniques, the likelihood of tumor seeding is small. There is one case report of tumor seeding to date secondary to EUS-guided FNA of a pancreatic mass (35).

In a series of 44 patients studied by Chang et al., EUS-FNA had an accuracy rate of 95% for pancreatic lesions and 88% for lymph nodes (197). EUS-FNA can be used for confirmation of chronic pancreatitis.

EUS-FNA with cytology improves the NPV in detecting chronic pancreatitis.

Other Lesions

As experience with technique grows, applications will certainly expand. Potentially useful information may be obtained concerning adrenal masses, extrapancreatic retroperitoneal masses, and extrarectal pelvic masses. Hoffman et al. (198) reported making a definitive diagnosis of malignancy in five of eight patients with pelvic masses and a correct diagnosis of infectious or inflammatory lesions in the remaining three patients. The final diagnosis was confirmed by surgery or clinical followup, for diagnostic yield of 100%. The malignant lesions were one cervical carcinoma, one ovarian carcinoma, two adenocarcinomas, and one lymphoma. Two of these five patients with malignant lesions had previously undergone negative CT-guided aspiration.

Injection Techniques

As mentioned previously, precise placement of a needle assembly into a target beyond the GI wall allows not only tissue sampling but also directed diagnostic or therapeutic injection.

Cholangiopancreatography

Wiersema et al. first described EUS-guided ERCP (199). These investigators used a flexible needle catheter advanced into the US field of a convex linear-array echoendoscope to obtain pancreatic and bile duct ductograms after failed cannulation by ERCP. There are recent reports of therapeutic EUS-guided cholangiography/pancreatography with stent placement in patients with failed cannulation (200,201). These are still preliminary reports, and larger studies with longer followup are needed to ascertain safety.

Celiac Plexus Block

EUS-guided celiac plexus neurolysis has been useful for palliation of pain in patients with pancreatic cancer and less commonly chronic pancreatitis. Wiersema et al. (202) first described EUS-guided celiac plexus neurolysis in 30 patients with intra-abdominal malignant disease. Followup to this pilot study studied 58 patients with pain from inoperable pancreatic cancer, who underwent celiac plexus neurolysis (203). The pain scores were significantly lower two weeks after the procedure and the effect was sustained for 24 weeks after adjustment for morphine and adjuvant therapy. Of them, 78% reported a decrease in pain score but only 54% of patients had an improvement score of over 2 points using a standardized visual analog scale.

Gress et al. performed celiac plexus block in 90 patients affected from chronic pancreatitis. Of the patients, 55% reported an improvement in pain score, but this percentage decreased to 26% at 12 weeks and was only 10% at 24 weeks (204).

At the present time EUS-guided celiac plexus neurolysis for malignant disease can be offered as a safe and efficacious treatment option, but its use in chronic pancreatitis should still be considered investigational.

Botulinum Toxin Injection for Achalasia

Hoffman et al. (205) have described the use of EUS-guided puncture of the LES to inject botulinum toxin in seven patients with manometrically proven achalasia. Of the seven patients, six were tolerating a regular diet within 72 hours, and these six patients had no recurrence of symptoms after a follow-up period of 1 to 13 months.

Maiorana et al. in their study reported sustained responses after botulinum toxin injection (206). There is speculation though about whether EUS-guided injection is at all necessary.

FUTURE APPLICATIONS

Endoscopic Mucosal Resection

EMR is being used more frequently to remove superficial cancers. EUS is used to determine depth of penetration before EMR and it also helps to ascertain the relation of the lesion to vascular structures and adjacent organs. EUS-guided saline injection can theoretically confirm correct placement of injection needle into the appropriate layer and ensure complete separation of the lesion from normal tissue and after EUS confirms that the lesion is superficial, it can be removed endosurgically.

EUS and Upper GI Bleeding

Lee et al. studied 54 patients with gastric variceal bleeding and patients underwent biweekly EUS of the varices followed by injection of cyanoacrylate until the varices were obliterated. The rebleeding rate was lower compared to the non-EUS control group (207).

Lahoti et al. performed EUS-guided sclerotherapy in five patients with nonbleeding esophageal varices. Varices were obliterated in 2.2 sessions and no complications noted (208).

The use of EUS though for management of upper GI bleeding should still be considered investigational.

EUS-Guided Antitumor Injection Therapy

Puncture guided by EUS is a major force behind the transformation of EUS from a diagnostic imaging tool into an instrument with both diagnostic and therapeutic capabilities. Just as the introduction of hemostasis techniques, polypectomy, and sphincterotomy metamorphosed diagnostic endoscopic procedures into therapeutic procedures, EUS-guided puncture techniques ushered in the era of therapeutic endosonography.

There are different studies under way at the present time in different phases where antitumor injections are being given directly into tumors under EUS guidance. EUS-guided radiofrequency has also been reported.

The potential of future therapeutic indications with new and improved tools is large and intra and transluminal endosurgery with EUS playing a substantial role in these advances is going to expand in the next few years.

SUMMARY AND CONCLUSION

In a broad sense, EUS is following a classic progression within GI endoscopy. First is the development of imaging with visualization of normal and abnormal anatomy. Second is the obtaining of tissue by directed biopsy for analysis by a pathologist. Third is the introduction of endoscopically guided therapy.

The use of EUS represents a major advance in GI imaging. Its unique strength lies in depicting the gut wall as a series of layers correlating with histologic features and in showing detailed images of structures adjacent to the GI lumen, such as lymph nodes, the bile duct, and the pancreas. Newer instruments have been developed for improved imaging, including catheter-size probes that can be used by the operating channel of standard endoscopes. The use of FNA for cytologic examination under EUS guidance has been accomplished. Therapy, using precision EUS-controlled injection, has begun, and results are encouraging.

Current indications for EUS focus on improved definition of submucosal abnormalities, GI cancer staging, and pancreatobiliary disease, and even lung and mediastinal cancer staging. EUS has very low risk of complications.

Strong deterrents to the widespread use of EUS exist. US imaging is new for most GI endoscopists, the learning curve is steep, and the devices are costly. Yet, ample and accumulating evidence indicates that EUS in many cases achieves greater diagnostic accuracy than other imaging methods and offers new therapeutic opportunities. It seems likely that EUS will have a continuing and growing role in GI imaging.

REFERENCES

1. DiMagno EP, Buxton JL, Regan PT, et al. Ultrasonic endoscope. Lancet 1980; 1:629–631.
2. Strohm WD, Phillip J, Hagenmuller F, et al. Ultrasonic tomography by means of an ultrasonic fiberendoscope. Endoscopy 1980; 12:241–244.
3. Kawai K, ed. Endoscopic Ultrasonography in Gastroenterology. New York: Igaku-Shoin, 1998.
4. Sivak MV Jr, ed. Tenth international symposium on endoscopic ultrasonography. Gastrointest Endosc 1996; 43(suppl):S1.
5. Knox TA. Endoscopic ultrasound. Diagnostic and therapeutic uses. Surg Endosc1998; 12(8):1088–1090. Review.
6. Das A, Mourad W, Lightdale CJ, et al. An international survey of the clinical practice of EUS. Gastrointest Endosc 2004; 60(5):765–770.
7. Rosch T, ed. Endoscopic ultrasonography: state of the art 1995. Gastrointest Endosc Clin North Am 1995; 5:475.
8. Tio TL. Gastrointestinal TNM Cancer Staging by Endosonography. New York: Igaku-Shoin, 1995.
9. Dye CE, Waxman I. Endoscopic ultrasound. Gastroenterol Clin North Am 2002; 31(3):863–879. Review.
10. Klapman JB, Chang KJ. Endoscopic ultrasound-guided fine-needle injection. Gastrointest Endosc Clin N Am 2005; 15(1):169–177, x. Review.
11. Shami VM, Waxman I. Technology insight: current status of endoscopic ultrasonography. Nat Clin Pract Gastroenterol Hepatol 2005; 2(1):38–45. Review.
12. Kimmey MB, Martin RW, Haggitt RC, et al. Histologic correlates of gastrointestinal ultrasound images. Gastroenterology 1989; 96:433.
13. Kawamoto K, Yamada Y, Utsunomiya T, et al. Gastrointestinal submucosal tumors: evaluation with endoscopic US. Gastrointest Endosc 1997; 205:733–740.
14. Chak A, Canto MI, Rosch T, et al. Endosonographic differentiation of benign and malignant stromal cell tumors. Gastrointest Endosc 1997; 45:468–473.
15. Palazzo L, Landi B, Cellier C, et al. Endosonographic features predictive of benign and malignant gastrointestinal stromal cell tumors. Gut 2000; 46:88–92.

16. Lew RJ, Ginsberg GG. The role of endoscopic ultrasound in inflammatory bowel disease. Gastrointest Endosc Clin N Am 2002; 12:561–571.
17. Oh YS, Early DS, Azar RR. Clinical applications of endoscopic ultrasound to oncology. Oncology 2005; 68:526–537. Epub 2005.
18. Wallace MB, Woodward TA, Raimondo M. Endoscopic ultrasound and staging of non-small cell lung cancer. Gastrointest Endosc Clin N Am 2005; 15(1):157–167.
19. Beahrs OH, Henson DE, Hutter RVP, et al., eds. American Joint Committee on Cancer Manual for Staging of Cancer. 4th ed. Philadelphia: JP Lippincott, 1992:57.
20. Rosch T. Endosonographic staging of esophageal cancer: a review of literature results. Gastrointest Endosc Clin North Am 1995; 5:537.
21. Dancygier H, Lightdale CJ, eds. Endoscopic Sonography in Gastroenterology. Stuttgart (Germany): Thieme, 1999.
22. Farrell JJ, Gaber J, Sahani D, et al. EUS findings in patients with autoimmune pancreatitis. Gastrointest Endosc 2004; 60(6): 927–936.
23. Becker D, Strobel D, Bernatik T, Hahn EG. Echo-enhanced color- and power-Doppler EUS for the discrimination between focal pancreatitis and pancreatic carcinoma. Gastrointest Endosc 2001; 53:784–789.
24. Scialpi M, Midiri M, Bartolotta TV, et al. Pancreatic carcinoma versus chronic focal pancreatitis: contrast-enhanced power Doppler ultrasonography findings. Abdom Imaging 2005; 30:222–227.
25. Kondo S, Isayama H, Akahane M, et al. Detection of common bile duct stones: comparison between endoscopic ultrasonography, magnetic resonance cholangiography, and helical-computed-tomographic cholangiography. Eur J Radiol 2005; 54:271–275.
26. Van Dam J, Rice TW, Sivak MY, et al. Malignant esophageal stricture is predictive of tumor stage and a contraindication for endosonography using dedicated echoendoscopes. Cancer 1993; 71:2910.
27. Catalano MF, Van Dam J, Sivak MV Jr. Malignant esophageal strictures: staging accuracy of endoscopic ultrasonography. Gastrointest Endosc 1995; 41:535.
28. Kallimanis GE, Gupta PK, Al-Kawas FH, et al. Endoscopic ultrasound for staging esophageal cancer, with or without dilation, is clinically important and safe. Gastrointest Endosc 1995; 41:540.
29. Pfau PR, Ginsberg GG, Lew RJ, et al. Esophageal dilation for endosonographic evaluation of malignant esophageal strictures is safe and effective. Am J Gastroenterol 2000; 95:2813–2815.
30. Kallimanis G, Gupta PK, Kankaria A, et al. Complications of endoscopic ultrasonography (EUS) using conscious sedation at a university hospital [abstr]. Gastrointest Endosc 1994; 40:P27.
31. Rosch T, Oittler HJ, Fockens P, et al. Major complications of endoscopic ultrasonography: results of a survey of 42105 cases [abstr]. Gastrointest Endosc 1993; 39:341.
32. Bhutani MS. Endoscopic ultrasound guided fine needle aspiration of pancreas. In: Bhutani MS, ed. Interventional Endoscopic Ultrasonography. Amsterdam: Harwood Academic, 1999:65–72.
33. O'Toole D, Palazzo L, Arotcarena R, et al. Assessment of complications of EUS-guided fine-needle aspiration. Gastrointest Endosc 2001; 53:470–474.
34. Wiersema M, Vilmann P, Giovannini M, et al. Prospective multicenter evaluation of EUS guided fine needle aspiration biopsy (FNA): diagnostic accuracy and complication (cx) assessment [abstr]. Gastrointest Endosc 1996; 43:432.
35. Paquin SC, Gariepy G, Lepanto L, et al. A first report of tumor seeding because of EUS-guided FNA of a pancreatic adenocarcinoma. Gastrointest Endosc 2005; 61:610–611.
36. Snady H. Endoscopic ultrasonography images of the normal retroperitoneum. In: Lightdale CJ, ed. Endoscopic Ultrasonography. Gastrointest Endosc Clin North Am 1992; 2:637.
37. Yasusa K, Mukai H, Nakajima M, et al. Clinical application of ultrasonic probes in the biliary and pancreatic duct. Endoscopy 1992; 24(suppl 1):370.
38. Furukawa T, Tsukamota Y, Naitoh Y, et al. Differential diagnosis of pancreatic diseases with an intraductal ultrasound system. Gastrointestinal Endosc 1994; 40:213.
39. Botet JF, Lightdale CJ. Endoscopic sonography of the upper gastrointestinal tract. AJR Am J Roentgenol 1991; 156:63.
40. Rice TW, Blackstone EH, Adelstein DJ, et al. Role of clinically determined depth of tumor invasion in the treatment of esophageal carcinoma. J Thorac Cardiovasc Surg 2003; 125:1091–1102.
41. Holscher AH, Siewert JR, Fink U. Staging concepts for gastrointestinal malignancies: the importance of preoperative locoregional T- and N-staging. Gastrointest Endosc Clin N Am 1995; 5:529.
42. Murata Y, Suzuki S, Hashimoto H. Endoscopic ultrasonography of the upper gastrointestinal tract. Surg Endosc 1988; 2:180.
43. Souquet JC, Valette PJ, Burtin P, et al. Accuracy of endosonography in the diagnosis of superficial carcinoma in the stomach and esophagus [abstr]. Gastroenterology 1989; 96:483.
44. Takemoto T, Itoh T, Fukumoto Y, et al. Role of endoscopic ultrasonography in preoperative staging of esophageal cancer. In: Classen M, Oancygier H, eds. Fifth International Symposium on Endoscopic Ultrasonography, Demeter, Muniro. Z Gastroenterol 1989; 34(suppl).
45. Yoshikane H, Tsukamoto Y, Niwa Y, et al. Superficial esophageal carcinoma: evaluation by endoscopic ultrasonography. Am J Gastroenterol 1994; 89:702.
46. Brugge WR, Carey RW, Mathisen DJ, et al. What is the most accurate EUS method for tumor staging of esophageal cancer [abstr]. Gastrointest Endosc 1995; 41:299.
47. Hasegawa N, Niwa Y, Arisawa T, et al. Preoperative staging of superficial esophageal carcinoma: comparison of an ultrasound probe and standard endoscopic ultrasonography. Gastrointest Endosc 1996; 44:388–393.
48. Larghi A, Lightdale CJ, Memeo L, et al. EUS followed by EMR for staging of high-grade dysplasia and early cancer in Barrett's esophagus. Gastrointest Endosc 2005; 62(1):16–23.
49. Kelly S, Harris KM, Berry E, et al. A systematic review of the staging performance of endoscopic ultrasound in gastro-oesophageal carcinoma. Gut 2001; 49:534–539.
50. Botet JF, Lightdale CJ, Zauber AG, et al. Endoscopic ultrasonography in the preoperative staging of esophageal cancer: a comparative study with dynamic CT. Radiology 1991; 181:419.
51. Catalano MF, Sivak MV Jr, Rice T, et al. Endosonographic features predictive of lymph node metastases. Gastrointest Endosc 1994; 40:442.
52. Heintz A, Mildenberger P, Georg M, et al. In vitro studies of lymph node analysis. Gastrointest Endosc Clin N Am 1995; 5:577.
53. Tio TL, Coene PP, den Hartog Jager FC, et al. Preoperative TNM classification of esophageal carcinoma by endosonography. Hepatogastroenterology 1990; 37:376–381.
54. Wiersema MJ, Vilmann P, Giovannini M, et al. Endosonography-guided fine-needle aspiration biopsy: diagnostic accuracy and complication assessment. Gastroenterology 1997; 112:1087–1095.
55. Hordijk ML, Zander H, van Blankenstein M, et al. Influence of tumor stenosis on the accuracy of endosonography in the preoperative T staging of esophageal cancer. Endoscopy 1993; 25:171.
56. Binmoeller KF, Seifert H, Seitz U, et al. Ultrasonic esophagoprobe for TNM staging of highly stenosing esophageal carcinoma. Gastrointest Endosc 1995; 41:547.
57. Rosch T, Lorenz R, Zenker K, et al. Local staging and assessment of resectability in carcinoma of the esophagus, stomach, and duodenum by endoscopic ultrasonography. Gastrointest Endosc 1992; 38:460–467.
58. Dittler HJ, Siewert JR. Role of endoscopic ultrasonography in esophageal carcinoma. Endoscopy 1993; 25:156–161.
59. Nickl NJ, Bhutani MS, Catalano M, et al. Clinical implications of endoscopic ultrasound: the American Endosonography Club Study. Gastrointest Endosc 1996; 44(4):371–377.
60. Ainsworth AP, Mortensen MB, Durup J, et al. Clinical impact of endoscopic ultrasonography at a county hospital. Endoscopy 2002; 34(6):447–450.
61. Harewood GC, Kumar KS. Assessment of clinical impact of endoscopic ultrasound on esophageal cancer. J Gastroenterol Hepatol 2004; 19(4):433–439.
62. Gress F, Ikenberry S, Conces D, et al. Endoscopic ultrasound (EUS) staging in patients (pts) with esophageal cancer (ECa) is more accurate than CT and correlates with survival [abstr]. Gastrointest Endosc 1995; 41:349.

63. Burtin P, Cales P, Oberti F, et al. Endoscopic ultrasonographic signs of portal hypertension in cirrhosis. Gastrointest Endosc 1996; 44:257.
64. Caletti GC, Brocchi E, Baraldini M, et al. Assessment of portal hypertension by endoscopic ultrasonography. Gastrointest Endosc 1990; 36:S21.
65. Tio TL. Kimmings N, Rauws E, et al. Endosonography of gastroesophageal varices: evaluation and follow-up of 76 cases. Gastrointest Endosc 1995; 42:145.
66. Jaffe DL, Brugge WR. Endoscopic ultrasonography is useful in evaluating isolated gastric varices [abstr]. Gastrointest Endosc 1995; 41:306.
67. Pontes JM, Leitao MC, Portela F, et al. Endosonographic Doppler-guided manometry of esophageal varices: experimental validation and clinical feasibility. Endoscopy 2002; 34:966–972.
68. Songur Y, Okai T, Watanabe H, et al. Endosonographic evaluation of giant gastric folds. Gastrointest Endosc 1995; 41:468.
69. Rosch T, Classen M. Gastroenterologic Endosonography. Stuttgart: Thieme, 1992:71.
70. Botet JF, Lightdale CJ, Zauber AG, et al. Endoscopic ultrasonography in the preoperative staging of gastric cancer: a comparative study with dynamic CT. Radiology 1991; 181:426.
71. Fein J, Gerdes H, Karpeh M, et al. Overstaging of ulcerated gastric cancer by endoscopic ultrasonography. Gastrointest Endosc 1993; 39:274.
72. Smith JW, Brennan MF, Botet JF, et al. Preoperative endoscopic ultrasound can predict the risk of recurrence after operation for gastric carcinoma. J Clin Oncol 1993; 11:2380.
73. Yasuda K. Endoscopic ultrasonic probes and mucosectomy for early gastric carcinoma. Gastrointest Endosc 1996; 43:S29–S31.
74. Yanai H, Matsumoto Y, Harada T, et al. Endoscopic ultrasonography and endoscopy for staging depth of invasion in early gastric cancer: a pilot study. Gastrointest Endosc 1997; 46:212–216.
75. Caletti GC, Brocchi E, Gibilaro M, et al. Sensitivity, specificity, and predictive value of endoscopic ultrasonography in the diagnosis of gastric lymphoma [abstr]. Gastrointest Endosc 1990; 36:195.
76. Tio TL, den Hartog Jager FCA, Tytgat GNJ. Endoscopic ultrasonography in the evaluation of non-Hodgkin lymphoma of the stomach. Gastroenterology 1986; 91:401.
77. Fujishima H, Misawa T, Maruoka A, et al. Staging and follow-up of primary gastric lymphoma by endoscopic ultrasonography. Am J Gastroenterol 1991; 86:719.
78. Yucel C, Ozdemir H, Isik S. Role of endosonography in the evaluation of gastric malignancies. J Ultrasound Med 1999; 18:283–288.
79. Caletti G, Fusaroli P, Togliani T, et al. Endosonography in gastric lymphoma and large gastric folds. Eur J Ultrasound 2000; 11:31–40.
80. Hoepffner N, Lahme T, Gilly J, et al. Value of endosonography in diagnostic staging of primary gastric lymphoma (MALT type). Med Klin (Munich) 2003; 98:313–317.
81. Fischbach W, Goebeler-Kolve ME, Greiner A, et al. Diagnostic accuracy of EUS in the local staging of primary gastric lymphoma: results of a prospective, multicenter study comparing EUS with histopathologic stage. Gastrointest Endosc 2002; 56:696–700.
82. Pavlovic AR, Krstic M, Tomic D, et al. Endoscopic ultrasound (EUS) in initial assessment and follow-up of patients with MALT lymphoma treated drug therapy. Acta Chir Iugosl 2005; 52:83–89.
83. Winawer SJ, Posner G, Lightdale CJ, et al. Endoscopic diagnosis of advanced gastric cancer. Gastroenterology 1975; 69:1183.
84. Dworkin B, Lightdale CJ, Weingrad DN, et al. Primary gastric lymphoma: a review of 50 cases. Dig Dis Sci 1982; 27:986.
85. Fork F, Haglund U, Hostrom H, et al. Primary gastric lymphoma versus gastric cancer. Endoscopy 1985; 17:5.
86. Levine MS, Kong V, Rubesin SE, et al. Scirrhous carcinoma of the stomach: radiologic and endoscopic diagnosis. Radiology 1990; 175:151.
87. Mendis E, Gerdes H, Lightdale CJ, et al. Large gastric folds: a diagnostic approach using endoscopic ultrasonography. Gastrointest Endosc 1994; 40:437.
88. Tio L. Large gastric folds evaluated by endoscopic ultrasonography. Gastrointest Endosc Clin North Am 1995; 5:683.
89. Fujishima H, Misawa T, Chijiiwa Y, et al. Scirrhous carcinoma of the stomach versus hypertrophic gastritis: findings at endoscopic US. Radiology 1991; 181:197.
90. Fisher JR, Sanowski RA. Disseminated histoplasmosis producing hypertrophic gastric folds. Am J Dig Dis 1978; 23:282.
91. Morin ME, Tan A. Diffuse enlargement of gastric folds as a manifestation of secondary syphilis. Am J Gastroenterol 1980; 74:170.
92. Okai T, Mouri I, Yamaguchi Y, et al. Acute gastric anisakiasis: observations with endoscopic ultrasonography. Gastrointest Endosc 1993; 39:450.
93. Andriulli A, Recchia S, De Angelis C, et al. Endoscopic ultrasonographic evaluation of patients with biopsy negative gastric linitis plastica. Gastrointest Endosc 1990; 36:611.
94. Chen TK, Wu CH, Lee CL, et al. Endoscopic ultrasonography in the differential diagnosis of giant gastric folds. J Formos Med Assoc 1999; 98:261–264.
95. Suekane H, Iida M, Yao T, et al. Endoscopic ultrasonography in primary gastric lymphoma: correlation with endoscopic and histologic findings. Gastrointest Endosc 1993; 39(2):139–145.
96. Caletti GC, Lorena Z, Bolondi L, et al. Impact of endoscopic ultrasonography on diagnosis and treatment of primary gastric lymphoma. Surgery 1988; 103:315.
97. Bolondi L, Casanova P, Caletti GC, et al. Primary gastric lymphoma versus gastric carcinoma: endoscopic US evaluation. Radiology 1987; 165:821.
98. Chang K, Katz K, Durbin T, et al. Endoscopic ultrasound-guided fine-needle aspiration. Gastrointest Endosc 1994; 40:694.
99. Komorowski RA, Caya JG, Geenen JE. The morphologic spectrum of large gastric folds: utility of the snare biopsy. Gastrointest Endosc 1986; 32:190.
100. Martin TR, Onstad GR, Silvis SE, et al. Lift and cut biopsy technique for submucosal sampling. Gastrointest Endosc 1976; 23:29.
101. Karita M, Tada M. Endoscopic and histologic diagnosis of submucosal tumors of the gastrointestinal tract using combined strip biopsy and bite biopsy. Gastrointest Endosc 1994; 40:749.
102. Savides TJ, Master SS. EUS in rectal cancer. Gastrointest Endosc 2002; 56:S12–S18.
103. Kahn H, Alexander A, Rakinic J, et al. Preoperative staging of irradiated rectal cancers using digital rectal examination, computed tomography, endorectal ultrasound, and magnetic resonance imaging does not accurately predict T0, N0 pathology. Dis Colon Rectum 1997; 40:140–144.
104. Lindmark GE, Kraaz WG, Elvin PA, et al. Rectal cancer: evaluation of staging with endosonography. Radiology 1997; 204:533–538.
105. Rau B, Hunerbein M, Barth C, et al. Accuracy of endorectal ultrasound after preoperative radiochemotherapy in locally advanced rectal cancer. Surg Endosc 1999; 13:980–984.
106. Vanagunas A, Lin DE, Stryker SJ. Accuracy of endoscopic ultrasound for restaging rectal cancer following neoadjuvant chemoradiation therapy. Am J Gastroenterol 2004; 99:109–112.
107. Williamson PR, Hellinger MD, Larach SW, et al. Endorectal ultrasound of T3 and T4 rectal cancers after preoperative chemoradiation. Dis Colon Rectum 1996; 39:45–49.
108. Rotondano G, Esposito P, Pellecchia L, et al. Early detection of locally recurrent rectal cancer by endosonography. Br J Radiol 1997; 70:567–571.
109. Novell F, Pascual S, Viella P, et al. Endorectal ultrasonography in the follow-up of rectal cancer. Is it a better way to detect early local recurrence? Int J Colorectal Dis 1997; 12:78–81.
110. Lohnert MS, Doniec JM, Henne-Bruns D. Effectiveness of endoluminal sonography in the identification of occult local rectal cancer recurrences. Dis Colon Rectum 2000; 43:483–491.
111. Hunerbein M, Totkas S, Moesta KT, et al. The role of transrectal ultrasound-guided biopsy in the postoperative follow-up of patients with rectal cancer. Surgery 2001; 129:164–169.
112. Orsoni P, Barthet M, Portier F, et al. Prospective comparison of endosonography, magnetic resonance imaging and surgical findings in anorectal fistula and abscess complicating Crohn's disease. Br J Surg 1999; 86(3):360–364.
113. Deen K, Kumar D, Williams J, et al. Anal sphincter defects. Correlation between endoanal ultrasound and surgery. Ann Surg 1993; 218(2):201–205.
114. Rosch T, Classen M. Gastroenterologic Endosonography. Stuttgart: Thieme, 1992:14.

115. Hawes RH, Zaidi S. Endosonography of the pancreas. Gastrointest Endosc Clin North Am 1995; 5:61.
116. Chang KJ, Erickson RA. A primer on linear array endosonographic anatomy. Gastrointest Endosc 1996; 43:S43.
117. Savides TJ, Gress FG, Zaidi SA, et al. Detection of embryologic ventral pancreatic parenchyma with endoscopic ultrasound. Gastrointest Endosc 1996; 43:14.
118. Rosch T, Braig C, Gain T, et al. Staging of pancreatic and ampullary carcinoma by endoscopic ultrasonography. Comparison with conventional sonography, computed tomography, and angiography. Gastroenterology 1992; 102:188–199.
119. Palazzo L, Roseau G, Gayet B, et al. Endoscopic ultrasonography in the diagnosis and staging of pancreatic adenocarcinoma. Results of a prospective study with comparison to ultrasonography and CT scan. Endoscopy 1993; 25:143–150.
120. Tio TL, Tytgat GN, Cikot RJ, et al. Ampullopancreatic carcinoma: preoperative TNM classification with endosonography. Radiology 1990; 175:455–461.
121. Snady H, Cooperman A, Siegel J. Endoscopic ultrasonography compared with computed tomography with ERCP in patients with obstructive jaundice or small peri-pancreatic mass. Gastrointest Endosc 1992; 38:27–34.
122. Muller MF, Meyenberger C, Bertschinger P, et al. Pancreatic tumors: evaluation with endoscopic US, CT, and MR imaging. Radiology 1994; 190:745–751.
123. Eloubeidi MA, Jhala D, Chhieng DC, et al. Yield of endoscopic ultrasound-guided fine-needle aspiration biopsy in patients with suspected pancreatic carcinoma. Cancer 2003; 99:285–292.
124. Gress F, Gottlieb K, Sherman S, et al. Endoscopic ultrasonography-guided fine-needle aspiration biopsy of suspected pancreatic cancer. Ann Intern Med 2001; 134:459–464.
125. Harewood GC, Wiersema MJ. Endosonography-guided fine needle aspiration biopsy in the evaluation of pancreatic masses. Am J Gastroenterol 2002; 97:1386–1391.
126. Kaufman AR, Sivak MY. Endoscopic ultrasonography in the differential diagnosis of pancreatic disease. Gastrointest Endosc 1989; 35:214.
127. Rosch T, Lorenz R, Braig C, et al. Endoscopic ultrasound in pancreatic tumor diagnosis. Gastrointest Endosc 1991; 37:347.
128. Gress FG, Hawes RH, Savides TJ, et al. Role of EUS in the preoperative staging of pancreatic cancer: a large single-center experience. Gastrointest Endosc 1999; 50:786–791.
129. Yasuda K, Mukai H, Nakajima M, et al. Staging of pancreatic carcinoma by endoscopic ultrasonography. Endoscopy 1993; 25:151–155.
130. Ahmad NA, Lewis JD, Ginsberg GG, et al. EUS in preoperative staging of pancreatic cancer. Gastrointest Endosc 2000; 52:463–468.
131. Schwarz M, Pauls S, Sokiranski R, et al. Is a preoperative multidiagnostic approach to predict surgical resectability of periampullary tumors still effective? Am J Surg 2001; 182:243–249.
132. Mertz HR, Sechopoulos P, Delbeke D, et al. EUS, PET, and CT scanning for evaluation of pancreatic adenocarcinoma. Gastrointest Endosc 2000; 52:367–371.
133. Midwinter MJ, Beveridge CJ, Wilsdon JB, et al. Correlation between spiral computed tomography, endoscopic ultrasonography and findings at operation in pancreatic and ampullary tumours. Br J Surg 1999; 86:189–193.
134. Agarwal B, Abu-Hamda E, Molke KL, et al. Endoscopic ultrasound-guided fine needle aspiration and multidetector spiral CT in the diagnosis of pancreatic cancer. Am J Gastroenterol 2004; 99:844–850.
135. Hunt GC, Faigel DO. Assessment of EUS for diagnosing, staging, and determining resectability of pancreatic cancer: a review. Gastrointest Endosc 2002; 55:232–237.
136. Tierney WM, Francis IR, Eckhauser F, et al. The accuracy of EUS and helical CT in the assessment of vascular invasion by peripapillary malignancy. Gastrointest Endosc 2001; 53:182–188.
137. Legmann P, Vignaux O, Dousset B, et al. Pancreatic tumors: comparison of dual-phase helical CT and endoscopic sonography. AJR Am J Roentgenol 1998; 170:1315–1322.
138. Fockens P. The role of endoscopic ultrasonography in the biliary tract: ampullary tumors. Endoscopy 1994; 26:803.
139. Yasuda K, Mukai G, Fujimoto S, et al. The diagnosis of pancreatic cancer by endoscopic ultrasonography. Gastrointest Endosc 1988; 34:1.
140. Mukai H, Nakajima M, Yasuda K, et al. Evaluation of endoscopic ultrasonography in the pre-operative staging of carcinoma of the ampulla of Vater and common bile duct. Gastrointest Endosc 1992; 38:676–683.
141. Chen CH, Tseng LJ, Yang CC, et al. Preoperative evaluation of periampullary tumors by endoscopic sonography, transabdominal sonography, and computed tomography. J Clin Ultrasound 2001; 29:313–321.
142. Chen CH, Tseng LJ, Yang CC, et al. The accuracy of endoscopic ultrasound, endoscopic retrograde cholangiopancreatography, computed tomography, and transabdominal ultrasound in the detection and staging of primary ampullary tumors. Hepatogastroenterology 2001; 48:1750–1753.
143. Skordilis P, Mouzas IA, Dimoulios PD, et al. Is endosonography an effective method for detection and local staging of the ampullary carcinoma? a prospective study. BMC Surg 2002; 2:1–8.
144. Chang KJ, Katz KD, Durbin TE, et al. Endoscopic ultrasound-guided fine-needle aspiration. Gastrointest Endosc 1994; 40:694–699.
145. Defrain C, Chang CY, Srikureja W, et al. Cytologic features and diagnostic pitfalls of primary ampullary tumors by endoscopic ultrasound-guided fine-needle aspiration biopsy. Cancer 2005; 105:289–297.
146. Rosch T, Lightdale CJ, Botet JF, et al. Endosonographic localization of pancreatic endocrine tumors. N Engl J Med 1992; 326:1721.
147. Anderson MA, Carpenter S, Thompson NW, et al. Endoscopic ultrasound is highly accurate and directs management in patients with neuroendocrine tumors of the pancreas. Am J Gastroenterol 2000; 95:2271–2277.
148. Bansal R, Tierney W, Carpenter S, et al. Cost effectiveness of EUS for preoperative localization of pancreatic endocrine tumors. Gastrointest Endosc 1999; 49:19–25.
149. Zuccaro G, Sivak MV. Endoscopic ultrasonography in the diagnosis of chronic pancreatitis. Endoscopy 1992; 24(suppl):347.
150. Hollerbach S, Klamann A, Topalidis T, et al. Endoscopic ultrasonography (EUS) and fine-needle aspiration (FNA) cytology for diagnosis of chronic pancreatitis. Endoscopy 2001; 33:824–831.
151. Yasuda K, Nakajima M, Kawai K. Diseases of the biliary tract and the papilla of Vater. In: Kawai K, ed. Endoscopic Ultrasonography in Gastroenterology. New York: Igaku-Shoin, 1988:96.
152. Fritscher-Ravens A, Broering DC, Knoefel WT, et al. EUS-guided fine-needle aspiration of suspected hilar cholangiocarcinoma in potentially operable patients with negative brush cytology. Am J Gastroenterol 2004; 99:45–51.
153. Eloubeidi MA, Chen VK, Jhala NC, et al. Endoscopic ultrasound-guided fine needle aspiration biopsy of suspected cholangiocarcinoma. Clin Gastroenterol Hepatol 2004; 2:209–213.
154. Menzel J, Poremba C, Dietl KH, et al. Preoperative diagnosis of bile duct strictures–comparison of intraductal ultrasonography with conventional endosonography. Scand J Gastroenterol 2000; 35:77–82.
155. Tamada K, Ueno N, Tomiyama T, et al. Characterization of biliary strictures using intraductal ultrasonography: comparison with percutaneous cholangioscopic biopsy. Gastrointest Endosc 1998; 47:341–349.
156. Stavropoulos S, Larghi A, Verna E, et al. Intraductal ultrasound for the evaluation of patients with biliary strictures and no abdominal mass on computed tomography. Endoscopy 2005; 37(8):715–721.
157. Stavropoulos S, Larghi A, Verna E, et al. Therapeutic endoscopic retrograde cholangiopancreatography without fluoroscopy in four critically ill patients using wire-guided intraductal ultrasound. Endoscopy 2005; 37(4):389–392.
158. Tio TL. Endosonography in diagnosing and staging of pancreatic and ampullary tumors. Gastrointest Endosc Clin North Am 1992; 2:673.

159. Tio TL, Reeders JW, Sie LH, et al. Endosonography in the clinical staging of Klatskin tumor. Endoscopy 1993; 25:81.
160. Azuma T, Yoshikawa T, Araida T, et al. Differential diagnosis of polypoid lesions of the gallbladder by endoscopic ultrasonography. Am J Surg 2001; 181:65–70.
161. Choi WB, Lee SK, Kim MH, et al. A new strategy to predict the neoplastic polyps of the gallbladder based on a scoring system using EUS. Gastrointest Endosc 2000; 52:372–379.
162. Morita K, Nakazawa S, Kimoto E, et al. Gallbladder diseases. In: Kawai K, ed. Endoscopic Ultrasonography in Gastroenterology. New York: Igaku-Shoin, 1988:87.
163. Mizuguchi M, Kudo S, Fukahori T, et al. Endoscopic ultrasonography for demonstrating loss of multiple-layer pattern of the thickened gallbladder wall in the preoperative diagnosis of gallbladder cancer. Eur Radiol 1997; 7:1323–1327.
164. Mitake M, Nakazawa S, Naitoh Y, et al. Endoscopic ultrasonography in diagnosis of the extent of gallbladder carcinoma. Gastrointest Endosc 1990; 36:562–566.
165. Amouyal P, Palazzo L, Amouyal G, et al. Endosonography: promising method for diagnosis of extrahepatic cholestasis. Lancet 1989; 2:1195–1198.
166. Amouyal P, Amouyal G, Levy P, et al. Diagnosis of choledocholithiasis by endoscopic ultrasonography. Gastroenterology 1994; 106(4):1062–1067.
167. Edmundowicz SA, Neidich RL, Aliperti G, et al. A prospective comparison of endoscopic ultrasonography (EUS), ERCP and standard abdominal ultrasonography (US) for the detection of choledocholithiasis prior to laparoscopic cholecystectomy (LC) [abstr]. Gastrointest Endosc 1994; 40:P63.
168. Shim CS, Hoo JH, Park, et al. Effectiveness of endoscopic ultrasonography in the diagnosis of choledocholithiasis prior to laparoscopic cholecystectomy. Endoscopy 1995; 27:428.
169. Palazzo L, Girollet P, Salmeron M, et al. Value of endoscopic ultrasound in the diagnosis of common bile duct stones: comparison with surgical exploration and ERCP. Gastrointest Endosc 1995; 42:225.
170. Canto M, Chak A, Sivak MV Jr, et al. Endoscopic ultrasonography (EUS) versus cholangiography for diagnosing extrahepatic biliary stones: a prospective blinded study in pre- and post-cholecystectomy patients [abstr]. Gastrointest Endosc 1995; 41:391.
171. Stevens PD, Lightdale CJ, Chabot JA, et al. Endoscopic ultrasound in patients with suspected common bile duct stones before laparoscopic cholecystectomy [abstr]. Gastrointest Endosc 1995; 43:S52.
172. Prat F, Amouyal G, Amouyal P, et al. Prospective controlled study of endoscopic ultrasonography and endoscopic retrograde cholangiopancreatography in patients with suspected common-bile duct lithiasis. Lancet 1996; 347:75.
173. Burtin P, Palazzo L, Canard JM, et al. Diagnostic strategies for extrahepatic cholestasis of indefinite origin: endoscopic ultrasonography or retrograde cholangiography? results of a prospective study. Endoscopy 1997; 29:349–355.
174. Norton SA, Alderson D. Prospective comparison of endoscopic ultrasonography and endoscopic retrograde cholangiopancreatography in the detection of bile duct stones. Br J Surg 1997; 84:1366–1369.
175. de Ledinghen V, Lecesne R, Raymond JM, et al. Diagnosis of choledocholithiasis: EUS or magnetic resonance cholangiography? a prospective controlled study. Gastrointest Endosc 1999; 49: 26–31.
176. Ros E, Navarro S, Bru C, et al. Occult microlithiasis in "idiopathic" acute pancreatitis: prevention by cholecystectomy or ursodeoxycholic acid therapy. Gastroenterology 1991; 101:1701.
177. Lee SP, Nicholls JF, Park HZ. Biliary sludge as a cause of acute pancreatitis. N Engl J Med 1992; 326:589.
178. Stevens PD, Lightdale CJ, Saha SA, et al. In-vitro comparison of endoscope-based vs. catheter-based endoscopic ultrasound for the detection of biliary sludge [abstr]. Gastrointest Endosc 1996; 43:557.
179. Amouyal G, Amouyal P, Levy P, et al. Value of endoscopic ultrasonography in the diagnosis of idiopathic acute pancreatitis [abstr]. Gastroenterology 1994; 106:A283.
180. Dill JE, Hill S, Callis J, et al. Combined endoscopic ultrasound and stimulated biliary drainage in cholecystitis and microlithiasis: diagnoses and outcomes. Endoscopy 1995; 27:424.
181. Annema JT, Versteegh MI, Veselic M, et al. Endoscopic ultrasound-guided fine-needle aspiration in the diagnosis and staging of lung cancer and its impact on surgical staging. J Clin Oncol 2005; 23:8357–8361. Epub 2005.
182. Larghi A, Verna AC, Stavropoulos SN, et al. EUS-guided trucut needle biopsies in patients with solid pancreatic masses: a prospective study. Gastrointest Endosc 2004; 59(2):185–190.
183. Vilmann P, Jacobsen GK, Henriksen FW, et al. Endoscopic ultrasonography with guided fine-needle aspiration biopsy in pancreatic disease. Gastrointest Endsosc 1992; 38:172.
184. Vilmann P, Hancke S, Henriksen FW, et al. Endosonographically guided fine-needle aspiration biopsy of malignant lesions in the upper gastrointestinal tract. Endoscopy 1993; 25:523.
185. Wiersema MJ, Chak A. Real-time endoscopic ultrasound guided fine-needle aspiration of a mediastinal lymph node. Gastrointest Endosc 1993; 39:429.
186. Wegener M, Adamek RJ, Wedmann B, et al. Endosonographically guided fine-needle aspiration puncture of paraesophagogastric mass lesions: preliminary results. Endoscopy 1994; 26:586.
187. Wiersema MJ, Chak A, Wiersema LM. Mediastinal histoplasmosis: evaluation with endosonography and endoscopic fine-needle aspiration biopsy. Gastrointest Endosc 1994; 40:78.
188. Chang KJ, Katz KD, Durbin TE, et al. Endoscopic ultrasound-guided fine-needle aspiration biopsy. Gastrointest Endosc 1994; 40:649.
189. Wiersema MJ, Kochman ML, Cramer HM, et al. Endosonography-guided real-time fine-needle aspiration biopsy. Gastrointest Endsoc 1994; 40:700.
190. Wiersema MJ, Cramer HM. Preoperative staging of non-small cell lung cancer: transesophageal US-guided fine-needle aspiration biopsy of mediastinal lymph nodes. Radiology 1994; 190:239.
191. Giovannini M, Seitz JF, Monges G, et al. Fine-needle aspiration cytology guided by endoscopic ultrasonography: results in 141 patients. Endoscopy 1995; 27:171.
192. Vilmann P. Endoscopic ultrasonography-guided fine-needle aspiration biopsy of lymph nodes. Gastrointest Endosc 1996; 43:S24.
193. Gress F, Savides T, Ikenberry S, et al. A prospective cost-effective evaluation of EUS directed fine needle aspiration biopsy (EUS + FNA) of mediastinal lymphadenopathy in the preoperative staging of non—small cell lung cancer (NSCLCA). Gastrointest Endosc 1996; 43:A526.
194. Aabakken L, Silvestri G, Hawes R, et al. Cost effectiveness of endoscopic ultrasonography with fine needle aspiration vs. mediastinoscopy in the staging of patients with lung cancer. Gastrointest Endosc 1996; 43:495.
195. Mallery S, Lai R, Bardales R, et al. EUS guided needle aspiration in subepithelial intramural GI tract masses (SIGIM). Results in 105 lesions. Gastrointest Endosc 2004; 59(5):P234.
196. Warshaw AL. Implications of peritoneal cytology for staging of early pancreatic cancer. Am J Surg 1991; 161:26.
197. Chang KJ, Nguyen P, Erickson RA, et al. The clinical utility of endoscopic ultrasound-guided fine-needle aspiration in the diagnosis and staging of pancreatic carcinoma. Gastrointest Endosc 1997; 45:387–393.
198. Hoffman B, Bhutani M, Aabakken L, et al. Endoscopic ultrasound-guided fine needle aspiration in the evaluation of extrarectal pelvic masses. Gastrointest Endosc 1996; 43:532.
199. Wiersema MJ, Sandusky D, Carr R, et al. Endosonography-guided cholangiopancreatography. Gastrointest Endosc 1996; 43:102.
200. Burmester E, Niehaus J, Leineweber T, et al. EUS-cholangio-drainage of the bile duct: report of 4 cases. Gastrointest Endosc 2003; 57:246–251.
201. Kahaleh M, Yoshida C, Yeaton P, et al. EUS antegrade pancreatography with gastropancreatic duct stent placement: review of two cases. Gastrointest Endosc 2003; 58:919–923.
202. Wiersema M, Sandusky D, Carr R, et al. Endosonography guided celiac plexus neurolysis (EUS CPN) in patients with pain due to intra-abdominal (IA) malignancy. Gastrointest Endosc 1996; 43:553.

203. Gunaratnam NT, Sarma AV, Norton ID, et al. A prospective study of EUS-guided celiac plexus neurolysis for pancreatic cancer pain. Gastrointest Endosc 2001; 54:316–324.
204. Gress F, Schmitt C, Sherman S, et al. Endoscopic ultrasound-guided celiac plexus block for managing abdominal pain associated with chronic pancreatitis: a prospective single center experience. Am J Gastroenterol 2001; 96:409–416.
205. Hoffman B, Knapple W, Bhutani M, et al. EU5-guided injection of botulinum toxin for achalasia. Gastrointest Endosc 1996; 43:A534.
206. Maiorana A, Fiorentino E, Genova EG, et al. Echo-guided injection of botulinum toxin in patients with achalasia: initial experience. Endoscopy 1999; 31:S3–S4.
207. Lee YT, Chan FK, Ng EK, et al. EUS-guided injection of cyanoacrylate for bleeding gastric varices. Gastrointest Endosc 2000; 52:168–174.
208. Lahoti S, Catalano MF, Alcocer E, et al. Obliteration of esophageal varices using EUS-guided sclerotherapy with color Doppler. Gastrointest Endosc 2000; 51:331–333.

Ultrasound Evaluation of the Transplanted Liver, Kidney, and Pancreas

15

Myron A. Pozniak and Mitchell E. Tublin

INTRODUCTION

Approximately 25,000 transplant procedures are performed in the United States every year. Surgeons transplant approximately 16,000 kidneys, 6000 livers, 1400 pancreata, 2000 hearts, 1100 lungs, and 40 combined heart/lungs (1).

Graft and patient survival rates following solid organ transplantation continue to improve with refinements in surgical technique, advances in human leukocyte antigen (HLA) typing for recipient/donor matching (2), new and greatly improved immunosuppressive agents (3), widespread acceptance of the national coordinated organ sharing system, and advances in noninvasive transplant monitoring. The growing number of transplant recipients makes it imperative that practitioners in both transplant and nontransplant centers be familiar with the imaging appearance of transplants and their potentially correctable complications. The timely recognition of transplant dysfunction and identification of its etiology can significantly improve graft survival by guiding prompt medical or surgical intervention.

The objectives of this chapter are to

1. Review the surgical anatomy of liver, kidney, and pancreas transplantation as it impacts sonographic imaging, especially the variants
2. Review the many possible complications of organ transplantation and illustrate the sonographic and Doppler findings; assess the ability of ultrasound and Doppler to identify and differentiate the various complications
3. Provide a checklist for the basic organ transplant ultrasound examination and provide tables of differential diagnosis for the various imaging and Doppler findings

ULTRASONOGRAPHIC TRANSPLANT ANATOMY

Discussions of specific organ anatomy can be found in the chapters covering the liver, kidney, and pancreas. Descriptions of transplant anatomy are in the subsections of this chapter. It is mandatory for the sonographer and sonologist to understand the surgical anatomy of each transplanted organ prior to beginning its examination. Variations in the way a specific organ is transplanted may require a change in the imaging approach and will directly impact imaging findings. With the numerous variations of transplant surgical anatomy, documentation and communication of the surgical record is critical for perception and interpretation of imaging findings and Doppler flow profiles in organ transplantation. In addition to the written report, we encourage our transplant surgeons to make a drawing in the chart immediately after the transplant procedure. The drawing details the site and number of anastomoses, the orientation of the organ and its vasculature, and any other unusual anatomic information that may impact follow-up studies or procedures.

ULTRASONOGRAPHIC TECHNIQUE

Grayscale Technique

Sonographic evaluation of a transplanted organ can only be successful if image quality is optimized. This requires the use of newer, more advanced ultrasound equipment with adequate penetration for imaging and high sensitivity for Doppler. Improvements in scanner hardware often permit insonation of the transplant at higher frequencies (7 MHz). Recent software improvements—harmonic and compound imaging—may also improve inherent acoustic contrast.

Doppler Technique

The examiner must optimize the Doppler settings, since improper adjustment can result in slow flow being overlooked and thrombosis being incorrectly diagnosed. Two particularly important scanning factors that must be taken into account to ensure a successful examination of the transplant are optimizing the angle of insonation relative to vessel orientation of the transplant vascular pedicle and maintaining minimal transducer pressure.

Scale Setting (Pulse Repetition Frequency)

For the initial scan, the color and spectral Doppler scales should be set as low as possible. By doing so, the examiner will be able to localize the vessel in question with color Doppler and then demonstrate adequate excursion on the spectral Doppler tracing. If aliasing occurs, the examiner can always increase the scale setting until the optimal level for that particular vessel is achieved.

Doppler Gain

The gain should be set at the highest level possible without creating noise in the image or tracing.

Filtration Level

The Doppler filter reduces noise in both color and spectral modes. If the filtration level is set too high, it can eradicate the display of very slow flow in a vessel. Initially, filtration should be set at the lowest possible level and only increased incrementally when the low setting does not allow for an effective examination.

Optimizing Angle of Insonation Relative to Vessel Orientation

To ensure proper perception of flow by color Doppler or an accurate display of the spectral velocity, the angle of insonation should be less than 60°. Finding an appropriate angle can be especially problematic when examining the transplanted organ because its vessels may be extremely tortuous and, consequently, a committed search for a suitable Doppler window is required (4).

Minimizing Transducer Pressure

Often the imaging study is limited because intervening adipose tissue increases the distance from the patient's skin to the transplanted kidney or there is gas in the overlying bowel. By applying sufficient pressure, fat or bowel loops can be displaced. However, doing so will compromise the Doppler examination as the organ parenchyma also becomes compressed and inflow during diastole can be impeded (Fig. 1). This results in a perceived elevation of the resistive index (RI). Thus, care must be taken not to apply pressure to the transplant organ or its vessels, so that any diagnosis made on the basis of the RI or velocity measurement is more accurate (5).

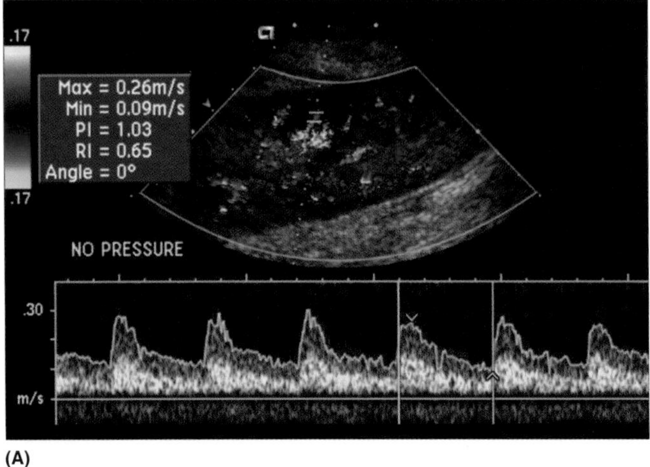

(A)

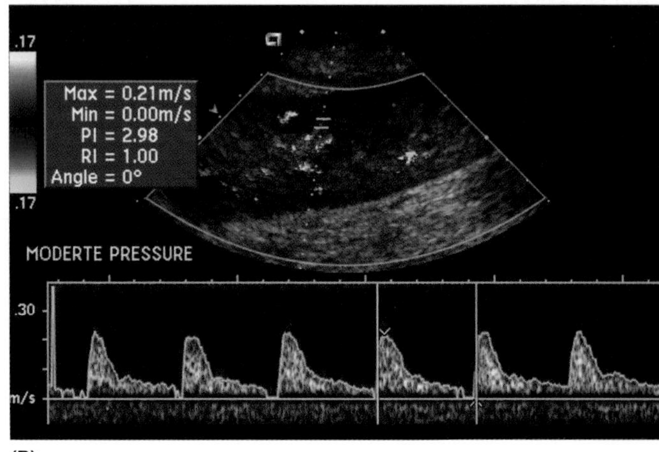

(B)

FIGURE 1 A AND B ■ (**A**) Renal transplant interlobar artery spectral Doppler tracing acquired with gentle transducer contact. Note the normal waveform and 65% resistive index. (**B**) When moderate pressure is applied by the transducer, the tracing of the same artery now exhibits an elevated resistive index of 100%. Transducer pressure alone is responsible for this increase in vascular impedance and resultant elevation of resistance.

LIVER TRANSPLANTATION

More than 28,000 liver transplants have been performed in the world since 1988. The waiting list for liver transplantation will continue to grow as a result of previously latent chronic hepatitis C and the increased incidence of nonalcoholic steatohepatitis. Acceptance of liver transplantation as the treatment of choice for limited hepatocellular carcinoma (HCC) will also increase the number of patients eligible for transplantation. Unfortunately, despite extensive outreach programs and the institution of living donor programs at several centers, the transplant donor pool has remained largely stagnant over the past several decades. Fortunately, graft and patient survival rates have continued to increase with improved surgical techniques, development of effective immunosuppressive medications, HLA typing for recipient matching, and establishment of coordinated transplant sharing. Graft survival statistics are further enhanced by prompt identification of liver transplant dysfunction and rapid intervention when appropriate. These advances are reflected in a current one-year graft survival rate in the United States of approximately 82.4% and a one-year patient survival rate of approximately 86% (6).

Preoperative Assessment

A complete sonographic examination of the liver transplant candidate should cover the points listed in Table 1.

The identification of a patient considered appropriate for liver transplantation is complex and involves clinical, surgical, radiological, and psychosocial evaluation. Preoperative imaging assessment consists of confirming vascular patency, mapping native vascular anatomy, quantification of diseased liver volume, identification of vascular collaterals secondary to portal hypertension, and a search for intra- or extrahepatic malignancy (Fig. 2). Much of this information may be obtained on either angiography or Doppler ultrasound, but optimized multidetector biphasic computed tomography (CT) is currently the primary screening imaging modality for adult liver transplantation.

Ultrasound may be used as a secondary screening examination for HCC, although the modality is probably not as sensitive as biphasic CT or magnetic resonance imaging (MRI). For HCC screening, the relatively low cost of sonography (and the lack of ionizing radiation) has prompted many groups to adopt surveillance protocols that alternate CT and ultrasound (7). Any solid lesion within a background of cirrhosis should be considered HCC until proven otherwise. Although CT and/or MRI are often performed to characterize these lesions (echogenic lesions within cirrhotic livers can be particularly problematic), ultimate confirmation of malignancy is usually made by ultrasound-guided biopsy.

TABLE 1 ■ Checklist for the Pre-Liver Transplantation Ultrasound Examination

- Confirm patency of the portal vein. Provide length and diameter measurements of the extrahepatic portal vein
- Identify any anatomic variation of the hepatic artery
- Confirm patency of the inferior vena cava
- Identify and describe collateralization from the portal to the systemic circulation
- Identify any hepatic mass that may represent hepatocellular carcinoma
- Quantify the amount of ascites
- Estimate the size of the diseased liver
- Provide a measurement of spleen size

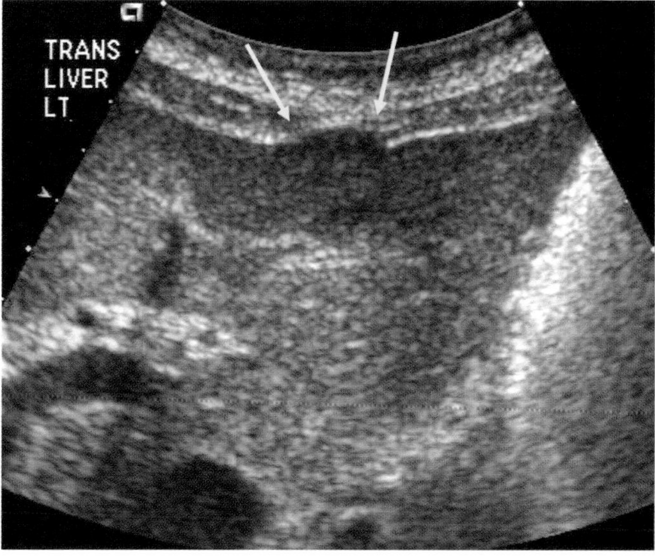

(A)

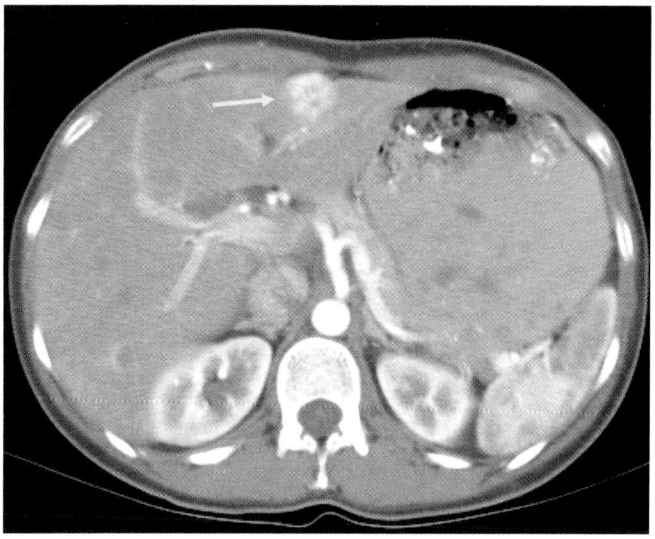

(B)

FIGURE 2 A AND B ■ (**A**) Transverse ultrasound image of the left lobe of the liver reveals a focal nodule making the capsular contour bulge (*arrows*). Ultrasound imaging alone cannot further characterize this lesion. (**B**) Arterial phase rapidly enhanced CT shows this lesion to be a hypervascular mass (*arrow*), most likely a hepatocellular carcinoma. With the addition of ultrasound contrast, some centers are able to use Doppler to identify malignancy during the transplant workup.

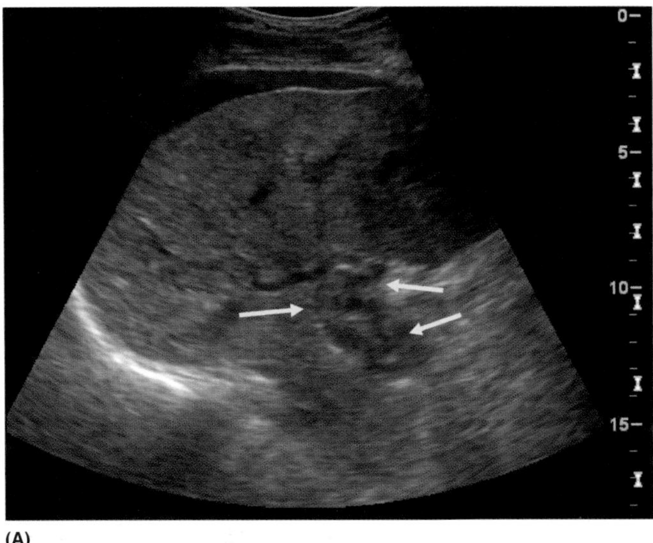

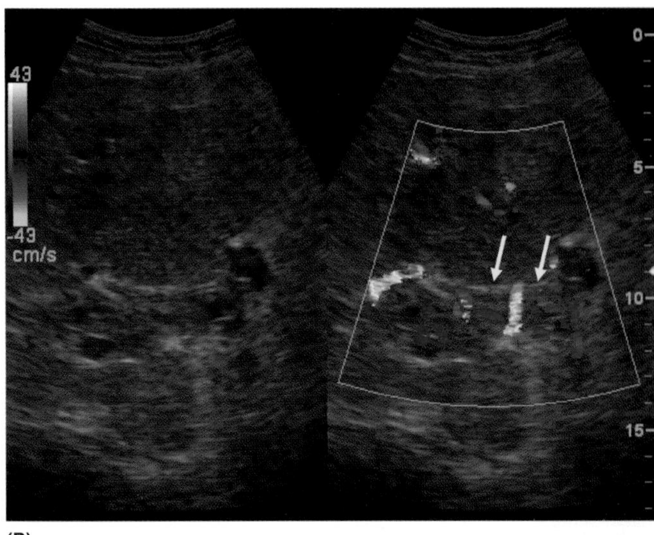

(A) (B)

FIGURE 3 A AND B ■ (**A**) Oblique ultrasound image of the liver and porta hepatis fails to identify the portal vein. Instead a tubular echo-filled structure (*arrows*) is seen. (**B**) Color Doppler image along the longitudinal axis of the portal vein reveals hepatopetal flow (*arrows*) coursing past an echogenic thrombus adherent to the portal vein walls.

Some centers rely on Doppler and MRI for assessment of hepatic vasculature, particularly within a pediatric candidate (8). Of patients with end-stage cirrhosis, 5% to 10% have portal vein thrombosis (9). This may complicate the transplant procedure and may necessitate either thrombectomy or complex venous jump grafts. In addition, portal vein thrombosis complicates the preoperative placement of a transjugular intrahepatic portovenous shunt. One additional benefit of Doppler ultrasound in the preoperative staging of the transplant candidate is the identification of vascular invasion by HCC. Differentiation between benign and malignant venous thrombus can be difficult, but the presence of a low-resistance arterial signal within expansile thrombus is diagnostic of vessel invasion (Fig. 3) (10). If a Doppler signal cannot be identified within the tissue plug and neoplasm is still strongly suspected, ultrasonographically guided needle biopsy can be performed (11).

Identification of portosystemic collateralization is an important component of the preoperative evaluation. If left unligated, these collateral pathways may persist after transplantation and divert portal blood flow away from the newly transplanted liver. This may contribute to transplant failure and actually require retransplantation. The most common collateral pathways include short gastric varices between the spleen and the greater curvature of the stomach, left gastric (coronary vein) varix behind the left lobe of the liver along the lesser curvature of the stomach, splenorenal mesenteric varices in the left flank, and a recanalized paraumbilical vein that drains from the left portal vein to the umbilicus (Fig. 4A–D). The recanalized

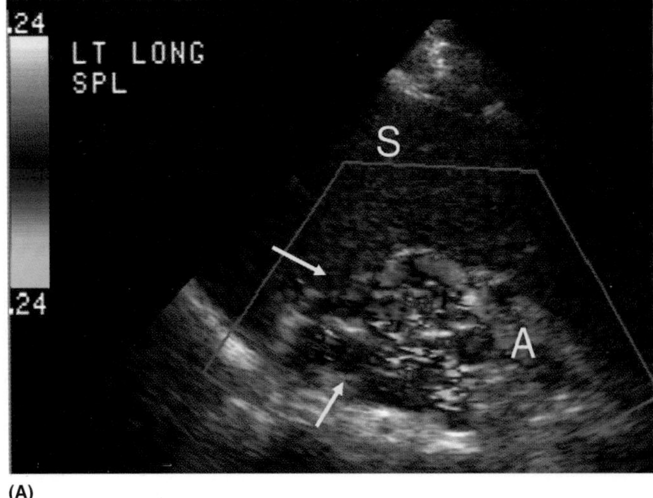

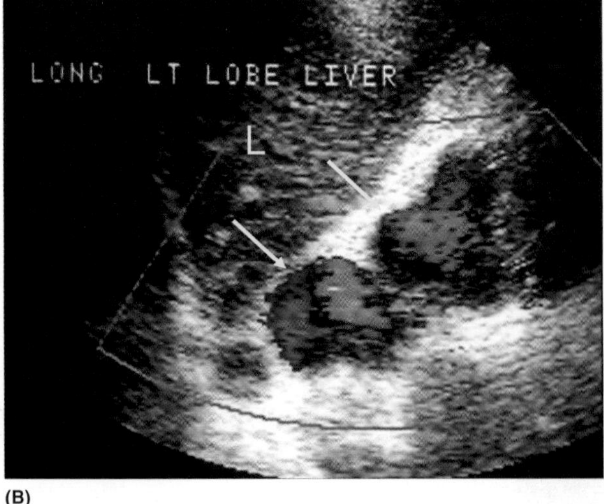

(A) (B)

FIGURE 4 A–F ■ (**A**) A longitudinal image through the enlarged spleen (S) shows numerous tortuous vessels (*arrows*) cephalad to the splenic hilum and the splenic artery (A). These are short gastric varices that course from the region of the splenic hilum, medially along the greater curvature of the stomach, and cephalad toward the gastroesophageal junction. (**B**) A longitudinal color image through the left lobe of the liver (L) reveals a large tortuous left gastric varix (*arrows*) coursing from the celiac axis region also to the gastroesophageal junction. (*Continued*)

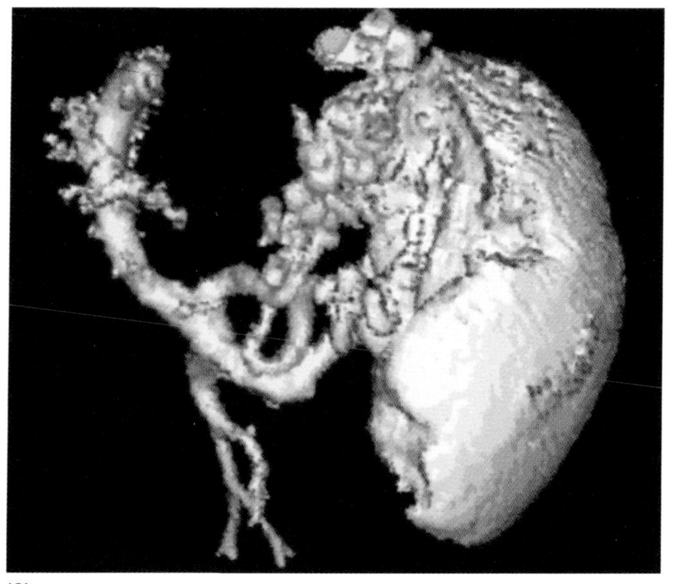

(C)

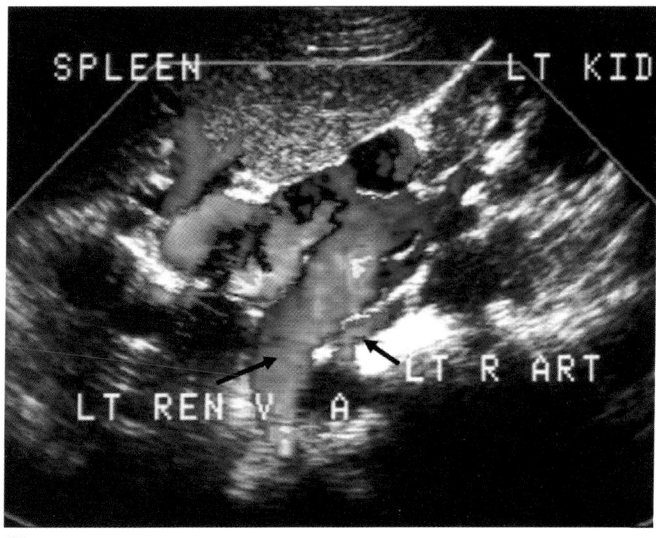

(D)

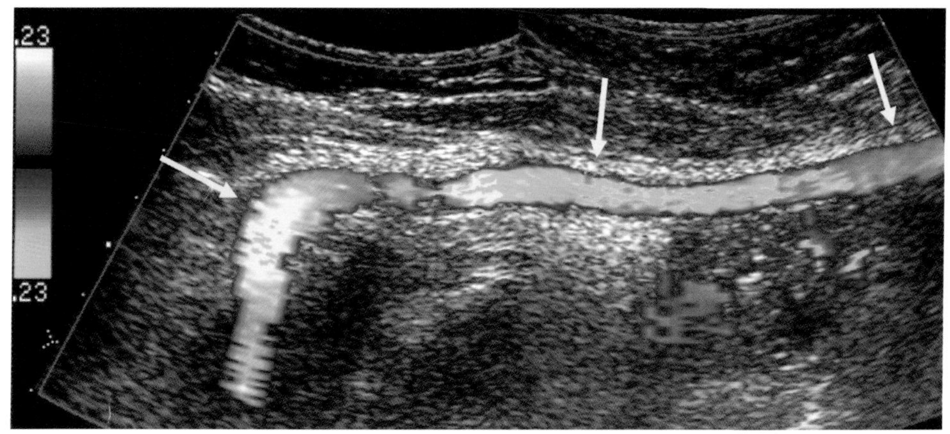

(E)

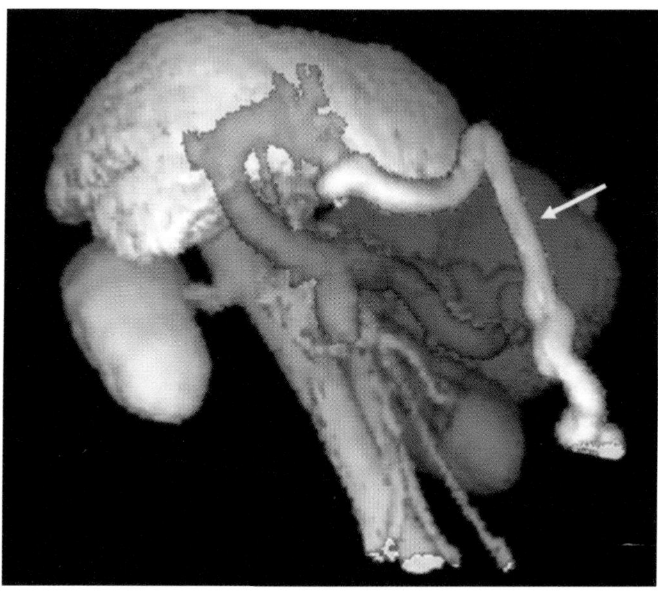

(F)

FIGURE 4 A–F ■ (*Continued*) (**C**) A 3D-rendered CT angiography image of the upper abdomen shows the portal system (*shaded pink*) and an enlarged spleen (*tan*). This patient has both short gastric varices (*shaded green*) and a large left gastric varix (*shaded red*). These varices surround the stomach and feed the esophageal varices. (**D**) A longitudinal color Doppler view of the left flank including spleen and kidney reveals a complex plexus of tortuous enlarged veins. These represent a splenorenal varix. Flow in these vessels passes from the splenic vein to the left renal vein (usually via the left gonadal vein) and subsequently back to the systemic circulation. (**E**) A composite longitudinal color Doppler image just to the right of midline reveals a large varix coursing out of the liver toward the umbilicus (*arrows*). This is a paraumbilical vein. (**F**) An oblique view of a 3D-rendered CT angiography image of the upper abdomen shows the portal system and paraumbilical vein (*shaded pink*). Note the varix (*arrow*) passing toward and then just deep to the anterior abdominal wall. From the umbilicus, this pathway usually continues via an inferior epigastric vein to the external iliac veins or via a caput medusa to the systemic circulation. LT REN V, left renal vein; LT R ART, left renal artery; LT KID, left kidney.

paraumbilical vein will be ligated with excision of the diseased liver; however, ligation of the other varices will occur only if the surgical team is made aware of their presence (12,13).

Hepatocyte transplantation is now performed at some centers as a temporizing bridge until a donor liver can be acquired for the candidate. Patients undergo intraportal infusion of cryopreserved, matched human allogenic hepatocytes. Portal vein thrombosis with liver failure and death has been reported as a complication of this treatment. Portal vein Doppler ultrasound during and after cell infusion is mandatory for these patients (14).

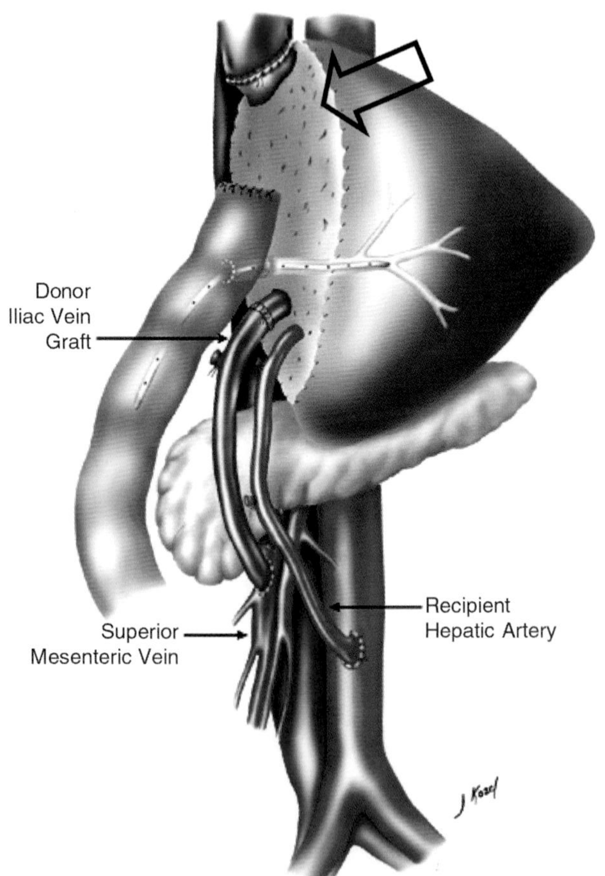

FIGURE 6 ■ Artist's rendering of a segmental liver transplant. The vascular anastomoses are similar except for the necessity to ligate the left lobe branches of the hepatic artery, portal vein, and bile duct (*arrows*). Note the cut edge (*open arrow*) of the liver. It is routinely cauterized but oozing from this surface often results in an adjacent hematoma.

Ultrasonographic Anatomy

Numerous variations of surgical technique are possible in liver transplantation. The imager must be aware of what variant is present since it will affect the ultrasound examination and findings. The most common procedure involves cadaveric orthotopic transplantation of the entire liver to the recipient (Fig. 5). Variations include segmental/lobar transplantation from a living related donor or segmental transplantation of a cadaveric liver (usually reduced for pediatric recipients) (Fig. 6) (15,16). Typically, five anastomoses are performed with liver transplantation. The inferior vena cava (IVC), because of its long intrahepatic segment, is transplanted along with the liver. The suprahepatic segment of the donor IVC is anastomosed to the recipient IVC approximately 2 cm from the right atrium. This is usually the first anastomosis performed. The caudal end of the IVC may then be anastomosed in line with the recipient IVC. The native intrahepatic IVC is excised with the resected diseased liver. If the recipient has congenital absence of the intrahepatic IVC as can be seen with biliary atresia, or if there is a marked size discrepancy between donor and recipient IVC caliber, the upper IVC anastomosis may be performed as an end-to-side anastomosis with the caudal end of the transplant IVC being oversewn (Fig. 7). Currently, surgeons at many centers are trending toward this variation (known as the "piggyback" technique) because of three major advantages: (*i*) Since recipient hepatectomy with this technique spares the native IVC, it continues to serve as a conduit for venous return from the lower torso; thus, the end hepatic phase of the procedure is more stable because of continued lower-body venous return; (*ii*) The procedure is faster since one less anastomosis is performed prior to releasing the clamps; and (*iii*) There is one less anastomotic site for potential complications (17).

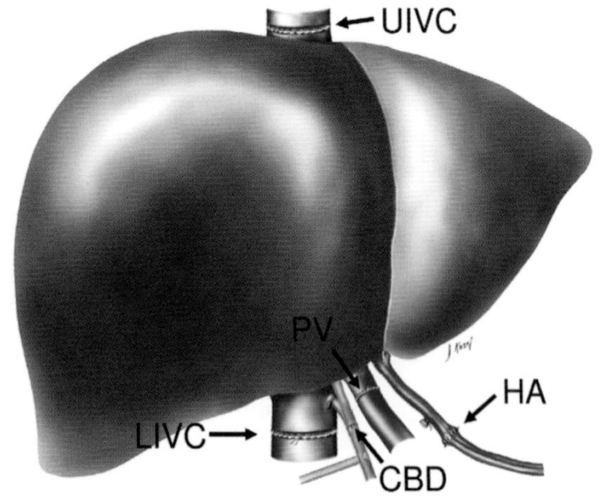

FIGURE 5 ■ Artist's rendering of a cadaveric orthotopic liver transplant with standard vascular anastomoses. UIVC, LIVC, HA, PV, and CBD over an indwelling t-tube. UIVC, upper inferior vena cava; LIVC, lower inferior vena cava; HA, hepatic artery Carrel patch; PV, portal vein anastomosis; CBD, biliary anastomosis.

The donor portal vein is usually anastomosed end-to-end to the recipient portal vein. If the recipient portal vein is thrombosed, hypoplastic, or of insufficient length, a graft may be placed from the recipient's superior mesenteric vein to the donor portal vein. This graft is typically created from the donor iliac vein (18,19).

The hepatic arterial anastomosis is technically the most difficult to perform because of its relatively small size and the thin and easily fractured intima. The donor liver arterial conduit usually incorporates the hepatic artery, celiac axis, and a small portion of aorta known as a

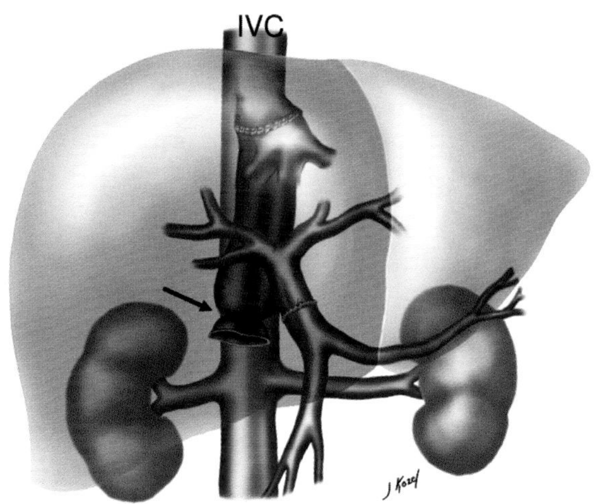

FIGURE 7 ■ Artist's rendering of a liver transplant anastomosed with a piggyback technique. The caudal end of the donor inferior vena cava (IVC) is oversewn (*arrow*). The upper anastomosis is performed end-to-side to the native unresected IVC.

TABLE 2 ■ Checklist for the Post-Liver Transplantation Ultrasound Examination

- Survey the liver parenchyma to rule out any focal abnormality, specifically fluid collections, areas of infarction, and possible neoplasm
- Survey any perihepatic recesses, lateral gutters, and pelvis to identify and quantify any hematoma or fluid collection
- Evaluate the biliary system, both intrahepatic and extrahepatic, to rule out obstruction, intraductal sludge, and stone formation
- Confirm the presence of both intrahepatic and extrahepatic artery flow and analyze the waveforms
- Confirm portal vein patency and analyze the Doppler waveform, particularly across the anastomosis
- Confirm patency of the three hepatic veins and evaluate their waveforms
- Evaluate flow in the inferior vena cava with attention to the anastomoses

Carrel patch. Variations of donor liver arterial anatomy complicate the procedure and often necessitate additional anastomoses, especially if there is dual arterial supply from the celiac axis and superior mesenteric artery (i.e., replaced left hepatic artery and replaced right hepatic artery, which occur in 12% and 15% of cases, respectively) (20). Variations of the recipient's hepatic arterial anatomy are less significant. The most common anastomosis is performed end-to-end in the subhepatic space from the donor Carrel patch to the recipient common hepatic artery (21). If this is not possible, then a jump graft may be necessary to connect the donor hepatic artery directly to the recipient's abdominal aorta. The graft is usually constructed from the donor iliac artery (22). Such creative vascularization must be properly documented since it is extremely difficult to perceive the presence or trace the course of variant surgical anatomy at the time of sonographic examination.

The biliary anastomosis is usually performed end-to-end from the donor to the recipient common bile ducts. At many centers, a T-tube or internal stent is placed across the anastomosis and left in place for several weeks. This stents the anastomosis during healing, allows monitoring of bile output, and provides a pathway for cholangiographic assessment of the biliary system. Those patients with preexisting biliary disease (i.e., primary sclerosing cholangitis) or in whom a direct bile-duct anastomosis is not possible, usually have a Roux-en-Y choledochojejunostomy created. An internal stent is left in place across the anastomosis. The stent typically falls out on its own and passes out of the patient via the bowel (23).

Postoperative Assessment

A complete posttransplant ultrasound requires evaluation of the liver parenchyma, biliary system, blood vessels, and surrounding spaces as detailed in Table 2.

Sonographic evaluation of the transplanted liver is usually performed several times within the first week of transplantation and prior to discharge of the patient. These early examinations reveal if the procedure was technically successful and, more importantly, serve as a baseline for future studies obtained at times of liver transplant dysfunction. The sonographic examination in the immediate post-op period is difficult due to overlying dressings, open wounds, and numerous drains. Scanning is performed as best as possible around these obstacles. The most optimal windows are typically along the anterior axillary line, over the right flank with an intercostal approach, or with a subxiphoid approach. Obviously, optimal scan windows will vary greatly from patient to patient. For purposes of Doppler interrogation, a lateral approach angling down the long axis of the porta hepatis is best to achieve an optimal angle of interrogation relative to the direction of flow in the main portal vein and hepatic artery. A subcostal transverse scan with cephalad angulation can interrogate the three hepatic veins, providing the liver extends below the costal margin. Asking the patient to take a deep breath in and hold it often helps to bring the liver down to the transducer.

The liver transplant ultrasound examination should include a general survey of the abdomen and pelvis in order to identify and quantify any hematomas or fluid collections. The liver parenchyma is then examined to rule out any focal abnormality; intrahepatic fluid collections are documented and measured; care should be taken to identify any hepatic lesions. Although infarcts, bilomas, recurrent tumor, and posttransplantation lymphoproliferative disorder (PTLD) may have a similar appearance, the differential diagnosis of these isolated or multiple hepatic lesions may be focused according to the patient's known clinical history. The biliary system should be evaluated to rule out obstruction or sludge/cast accumulation, especially in a patient with hepatic artery thrombosis. The intra- and extrahepatic arteries are checked to confirm patency and the waveforms are analyzed to rule out a more proximal stenosis (Fig. 8). Patency

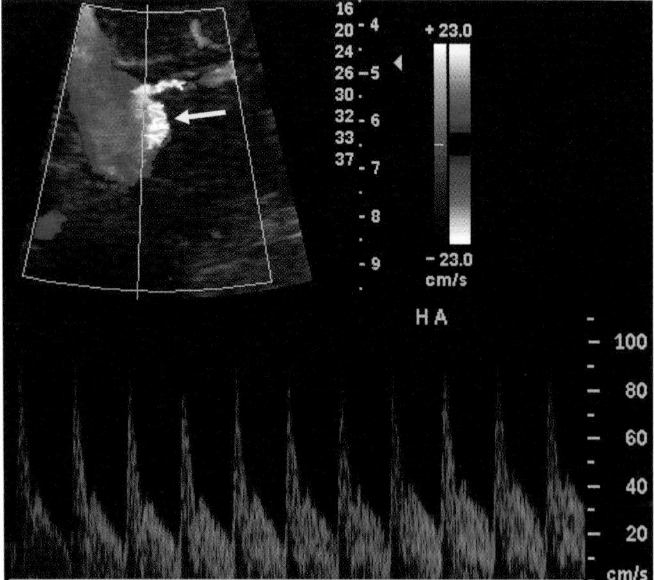

FIGURE 8 ■ Color and spectral Doppler of a normal hepatic artery. The artery (*arrow*) shows a higher color saturation corresponding to its higher velocity and is usually adjacent to the portal vein. The spectral tracing should show a brisk upstroke in systole. The resistive index should measure approximately 70%. HA, hepatic artery.

of the portal vein is confirmed and the Doppler waveform analyzed, particularly across the anastomosis (Fig. 9). Patency of the three hepatic veins is confirmed and their waveforms are evaluated. Finally, the IVC is checked with special attention to the upper anastomosis (Fig. 10).

Complications

The most common abnormal findings encountered in liver transplantation are listed in Table 3.

Perihepatic fluid collections are very common in the immediate postoperative period and may represent hematomas, seromas, or ascites (Fig. 11). Bilomas and abscesses are rare but obviously more significant. The presence or absence of septations or debris does not help specify the type of fluid collection. Fluid collections in the region of the portahepatis should be evaluated with Doppler to exclude a vascular complication such as pseudoaneurysm (PA) before intervention is considered. The sonographic identification of a complicated collection with varying degrees of internal echogenicity or debris should be correlated with clinical and laboratory findings and CT. Fluid collections increasing in size over a sequence of studies must be considered an active bleed in the immediate postoperative period. Clear rounded fluid collections occurring well after the transplant may represent bilomas or lymphoceles. The pressure they exert on adjacent structures may compromise organ perfusion (Fig. 12) (24).

Irregular echogenicity of the liver parenchyma should be considered an ominous finding in a transplant recipient. Compromise of hepatic artery flow from stenosis, thrombosis, or chronic rejection may result in segmental or subsegmental infarction (Fig. 13) (25). An ischemic or infarcted segment of liver may become infected and form an abscess (Fig. 14A and B). With chronic hepatic artery thrombosis, an irregular collection in the liver may also represent an intrahepatic bile leak secondary to breakdown of the biliary system (26). Immunosuppressed transplant

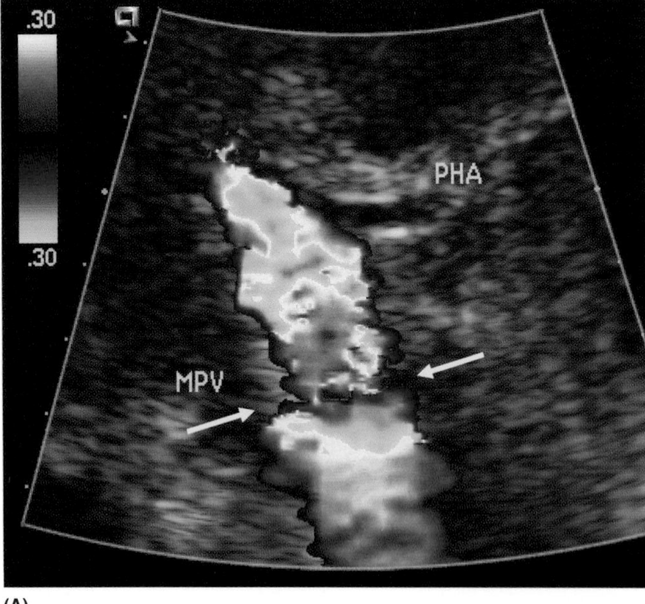

(A)

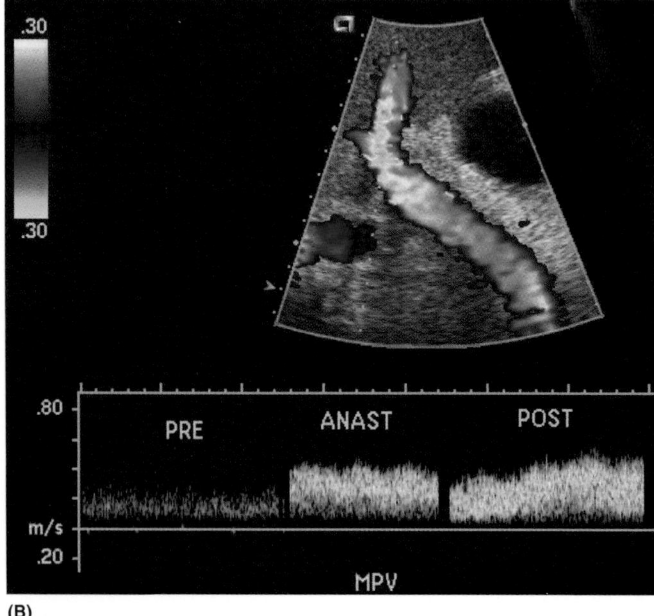

(B)

FIGURE 9 A AND B ■ (**A**) Color Doppler image of the porta hepatis. The anastomosis between donor and recipient portal vein is evident by the change in caliber, which causes the focal aliasing at that level (*arrows*). (**B**) Spectral Doppler tracing across the anastomosis and on either side reveals that velocity changes are relatively insignificant in this normal anastomosis. MPV, maximal peak velocity; PHA, proper hepatic artery.

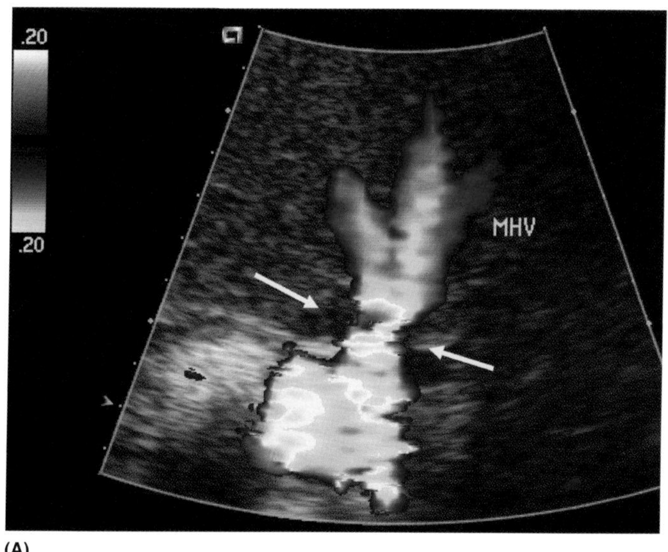

(A)

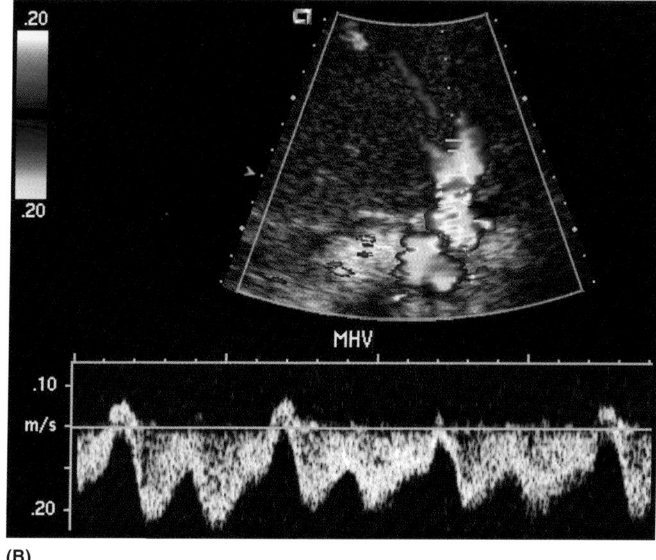

(B)

FIGURE 10 A AND B ■ (**A**) Transverse color Doppler image of the hepatic vein/inferior vena cava anastomosis. Three hepatic veins are indeed patent. Aliasing, however, is perceived at the caval anastomosis (*arrows*). (**B**) Spectral Doppler tracing reveals normal cardiac periodicity transmitting into the liver. Since this waveform must propagate against the direction of flow, its presence within the liver effectively rules out significant hepatic venous outflow obstruction. MHV, middle hepatic vein.

TABLE 3 ■ Differential Diagnosis of Ultrasound Findings in the Transplanted Liver

Diffusely irregular parenchymal echotexture
- Ischemia or necrosis secondary to hepatic artery stenosis or thrombosis
- Infection or abscess
- Recurrent hepatitis
- Posttransplantation lymphoproliferative disorder or lymphoma
- Geographic or diffuse fatty infiltration
- Hepatocellular carcinoma
- Diffusely metastatic neoplasm

Focal parenchymal abnormality
- Abscess
- Infarction
- Recurrent neoplasm
- Intraductal gas secondary to choledochojejunostomy or sphincterotomy
- Intraductal sludge or calculi

High-resistance flow in hepatic artery
- Preservation injury—common during the first few days after transplantation
- Organ compression by adjacent mass or fluid collection
- Hepatic venous outflow obstruction
- Severe hepatocellular disease

Low-resistance flow in hepatic artery
- Hepatic artery stenosis
- Severe aortoceliac atherosclerotic disease
- Diaphragmatic crus sling effect
- Intrahepatic arteriovenous fistula
- Arteriobiliary fistula

Flattening of hepatic vein waveform
- Hepatic parenchymal disease, including rejection
- Stenosis or kink of the upper inferior vena cava anastomosis

recipients may develop a lymphoma-like syndrome known as posttransplant lymphoproliferative disorder (PTLD). Its appearance on ultrasound is similar to non-Hodgkins lymphoma and may present as an infiltrating hepatic mass (27,28). Any mass identified in a patient treated with transplantation for HCC, cholangiocarcinoma, or any other malignancy should be suspect for recurrent or metastatic neoplasm (29). Finally, long-term administration of steroids as antirejection treatment may result in focal fatty infiltration with a geographic distribution. CT [potentially with CT angiography (CTA) if a hepatic arterial complication is suspected] is typically performed for any abnormal parenchymal pattern shown at sonography.

Hepatic Artery

The hepatic artery anastomosis is technically the most difficult to create and complications such as stenosis, thrombosis, and fistula formation may have a significant impact on liver transplant success as they predispose to infarction, intrahepatic abscess, biliary stricture, and biloma formation. Preservation of hepatic arterial inflow is crucial to graft function because biliary epithelium is exclusively supplied by arterial flow.

Within the first few days of transplantation, the hepatic artery tracing often shows a relatively high-resistance flow. This is a common manifestation of ischemic-reperfusion injury (the anoxia and traumatic insult sustained by the liver during recovery, handling, preservation, and surgery). It has been shown to be more common with older donor age and a prolonged period of ischemia (Fig. 15) (30). The high resistance is due to vasospasm and can be reversed with vasodilatory agents such as nifedipine. However, one must be cautious to ensure that the transplant recipient is stable enough to be given this drug as a

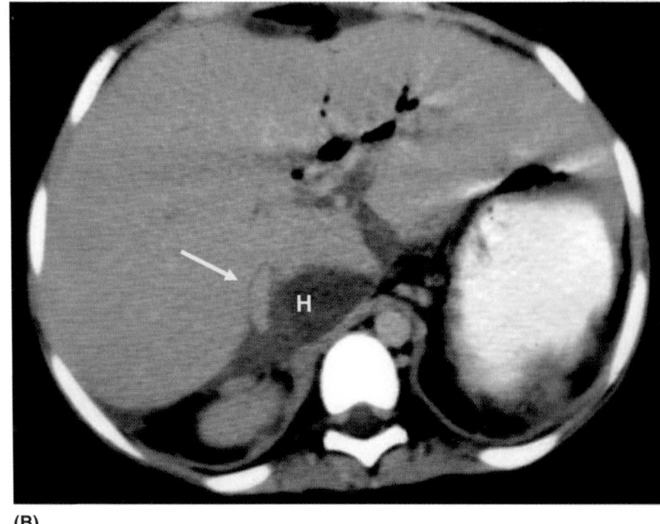

(A) (B)

FIGURE 11 A AND B ■ (**A**) Transverse ultrasound image of a cadaveric liver transplant reveals a fluid collection in the region of the bare area of the liver (*calipers*). This postoperative hematoma compresses the adjacent inferior vena cava (IVC) compromising venous return from the lower torso. (**B**) A CT image at a similar level confirms the compression on the adjacent IVC (*arrow*) by this bare area hematoma (H).

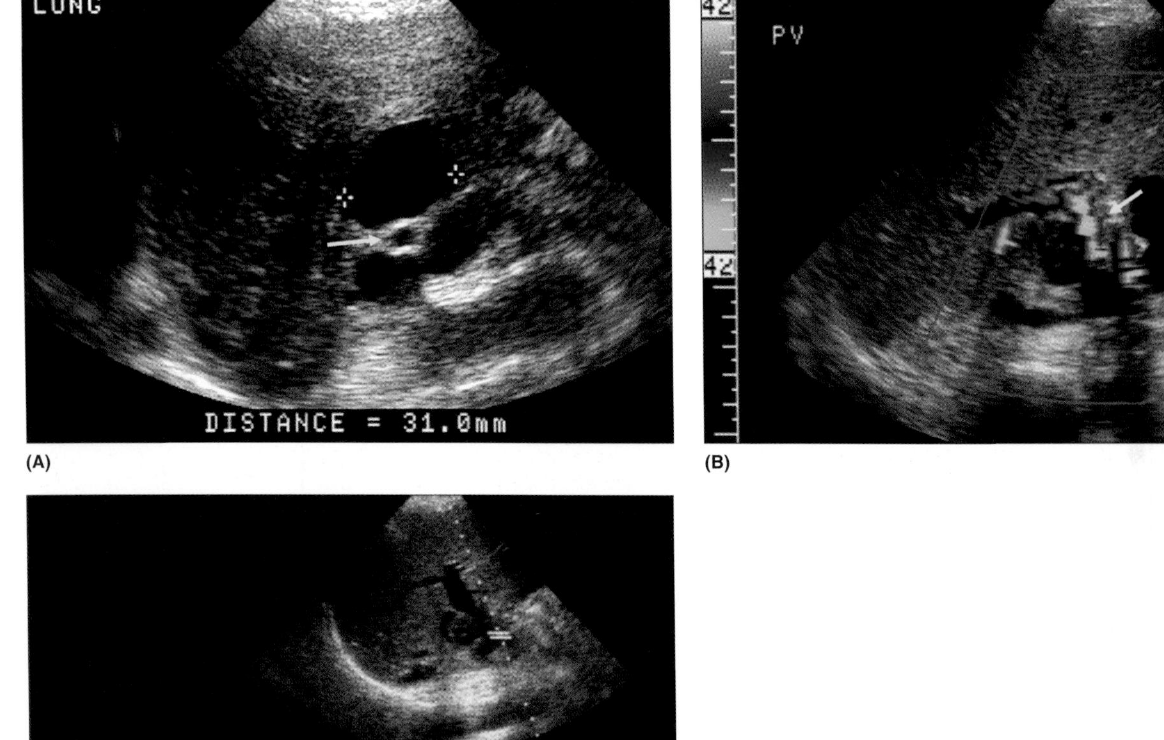

(A) (B)

(C)

FIGURE 12 A–C ■ (**A**) An ultrasound image at the level of the porta-hepatis shows rounded fluid collections (*calipers*) compressing the portal vein (PV) (*arrow*). (**B**) A color Doppler image along the portal vein confirms compression with aliasing (*arrow*). (**C**) A spectral Doppler tracing obtained above and below the area of compression shows a twofold velocity gradient.

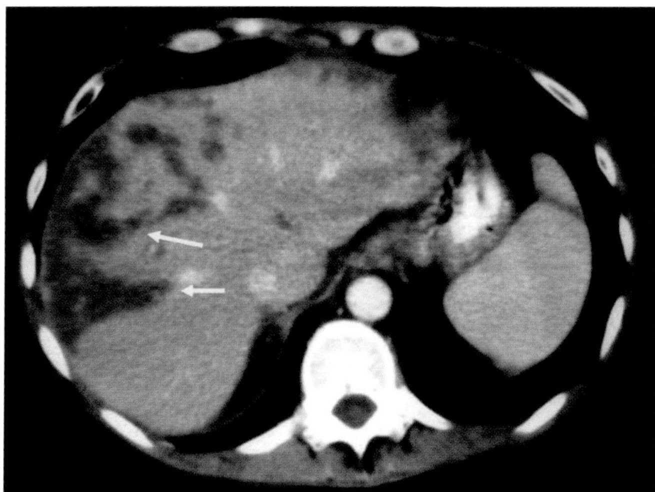

FIGURE 13 ■ A contrast-enhanced CT scan of a liver transplant recipient with known hepatic artery thrombosis. The ultrasound revealed nonspecific mottled echo texture of the liver that the CT identified as multiple peripheral wedge-shaped areas of nonenhancement consistent with infarcts (*arrows*).

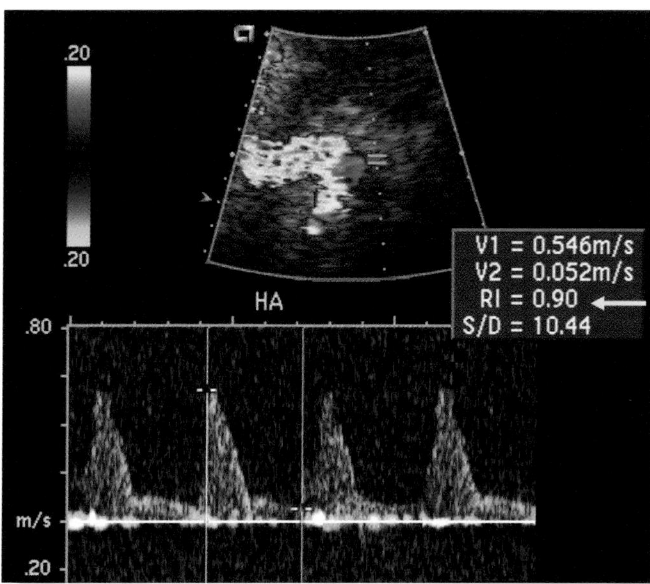

FIGURE 15 ■ Transverse spectral and color Doppler image within 24 hours of a liver transplant. Note the relatively high resistance to inflow with a measured resistive index of 90% (*arrow*). HA, hepatic artery.

diagnostic challenge. Augmenting the Doppler exam with this challenge, however, may obviate the need for an arteriogram if hepatic arterial inflow is compromised to the point where it appears to be occluded (Fig. 16). The spasm typically resolves within a few days of transplantation (31) and resistance returns to a normal range (32). A delayed finding of high resistance, beyond three to five days, is a poor prognostic indicator and some of these patients go on to develop arterial thrombosis (33); The exact cause of thrombosis is not always apparent and in numerous cases is presumed to be secondary to immunological causes and rejection. Care should be taken to examine patients after fasting, however. Markedly elevated hepatic arterial RIs are a normal finding after eating; diminished hepatic arterial flow is a physiologic response to elevated postprandial portal venous blood flow (the "buffer" response).

Hepatic arterial thrombosis typically occurs in the immediate postoperative period. The gray-scale manifestations of hepatic arterial stenosis/thrombosis are often subtle; the graft may appear normal despite severe hepatic dysfunction or biliary sepsis. Irregular biliary ductal dilatation (Fig. 17), biliary casts (Fig. 18), bile duct thickening, bilomas, and abscesses may be observed with the biliary ischemia that occurs after persistently diminished hepatic

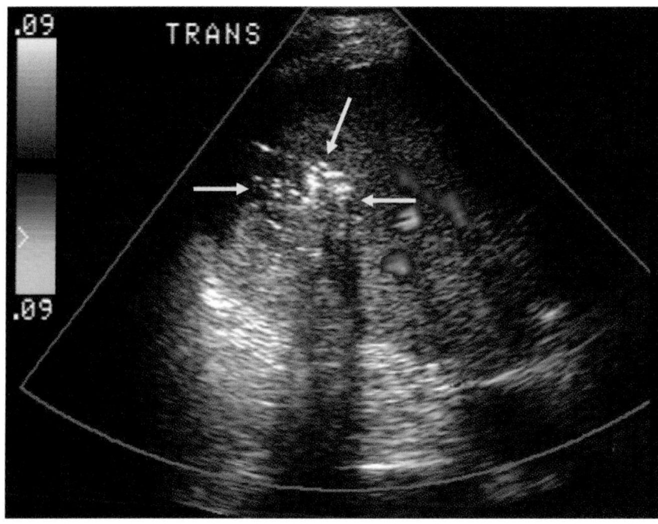

(A)

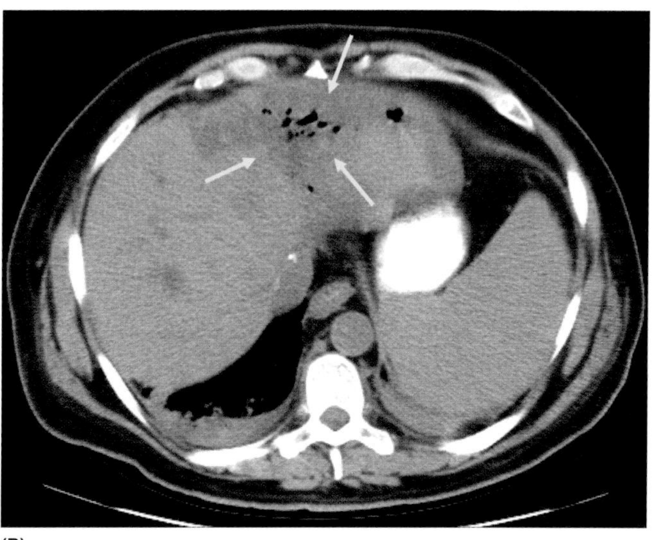

(B)

FIGURE 14 A AND B ■ (**A**) Transverse ultrasound image of a liver transplant in a patient with known hepatic artery stenosis. The area of irregular echogenicity in the lateral right lobe represents an intrahepatic abscess. Bright echogenic air collections with acoustic shadowing (*arrows*) are seen within the abscess. (**B**) CT scan through the abscess shows focal decreased perfusion and small air pockets within the abscess (*arrows*).

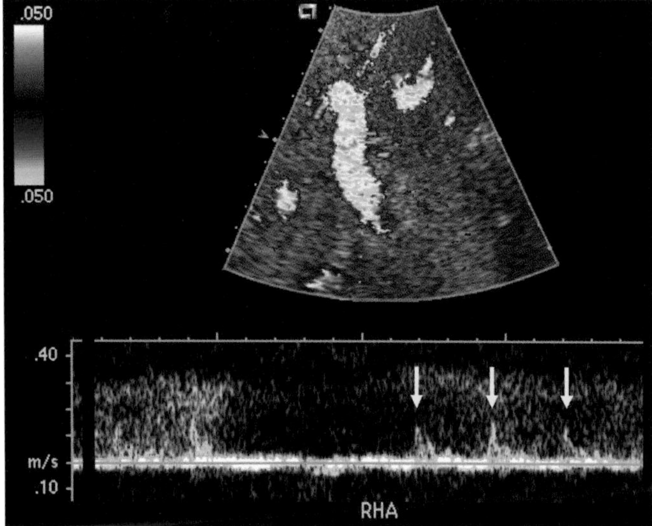

FIGURE 16 ■ Spectral Doppler tracing of the porta hepatis on the first postoperative day. The hepatic artery was extremely difficult to identify (*arrows*) because of the thready, high-resistance flow due to severe vasospasm. This patient may be considered a candidate for ultrasound contrast or a provocative test with vasodilating agents to confidently confirm arterial patency. RHA, right hepatic artery.

arterial flow. Thrombosis should be suspected if no intrahepatic flow is detected at Doppler despite technique optimization. False positive studies may occur in difficult-to-scan patients, in patients with severe hepatic edema, and in patients with high-grade, flow-limiting hepatic artery stenosis. If sufficient collateral flow develops after hepatic arterial occlusion, the arterial Doppler tracing may mimic the downstream findings of hepatic arterial stenosis.

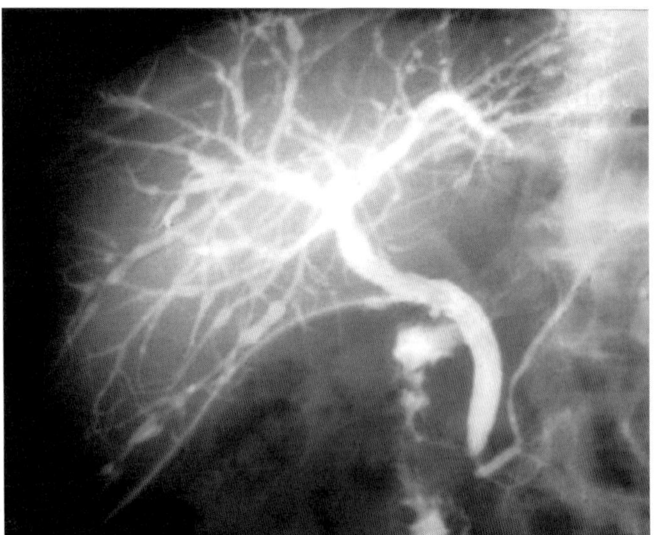

FIGURE 17 ■ This cholangiogram was performed in a patient with longstanding hepatic artery thrombosis. This grossly irregular intrahepatic biliary system has numerous strictures. Although collateralization reestablished hepatic arterial flow, the biliary system progressively deteriorated, as did liver function.

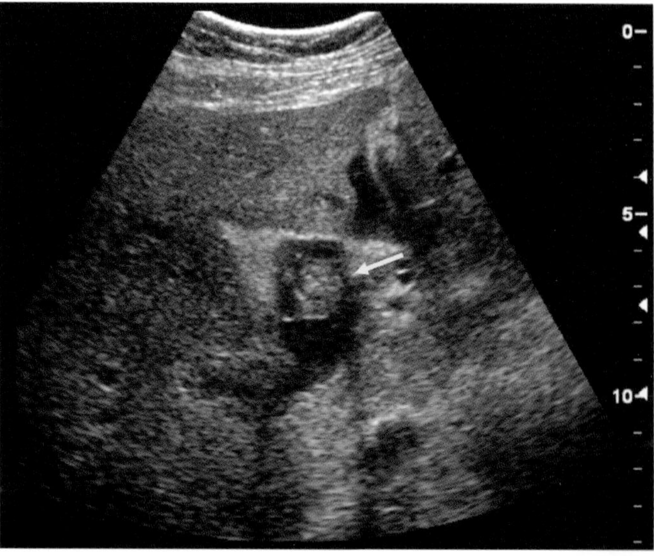

(A)

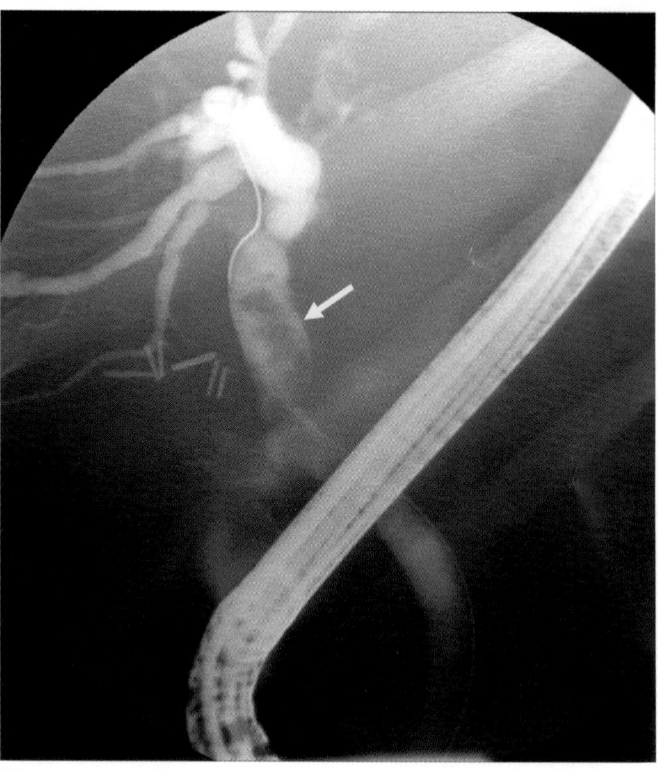

(B)

FIGURE 18 A AND B ■ (**A**) Transverse ultrasound of the porta hepatic. An echogenic clump of debris with acoustic shadowing fills and dilates the bile ducts (*arrow*). (**B**) The endoscopic retrograde cholangiopancreatography shows the plug of debris filling the common bile duct, a cast of sloughed mucosa, and sludge.

Absence of an arterial signal along the main portal vein and its branches on spectral and color Doppler ultrasound indicates hepatic artery thrombosis. Since this is a diagnosis based on the absence of flow, great care must be taken to ensure proper Doppler settings. Scanning by a second experienced sonologist is encouraged, since this ultrasound diagnosis routinely leads to either conventional arteriography or CTA. Use of ultrasound echo-enhancing agents has been recommended to improve perception of a weak arterial signal and decrease the rate of false positive diagnosis of hepatic artery thrombosis and reduce the frequency of hepatic artery arteriography (31,34).

In cases of hepatic artery thrombosis, which are treated conservatively, collaterals will develop and an intrahepatic arterial signal can be detected by Doppler ultrasound as early as two weeks after the thrombosis. This typically manifests as a thready tracing with a tardus-parvus appearance and can be seen in as many as 40% of patients with documented hepatic artery thrombosis; hepatic arterial collaterals rarely compensate for main hepatic arterial occlusion, although adequate inflow may ultimately be achieved particularly in pediatric liver transplant recipients (35).

Criteria that are employed at many centers for the diagnosis of hepatic artery stenosis include tardus-parvus intrahepatic arterial spectra, with a prolonged systolic upstroke (systolic acceleration time of >0.08 seconds) and a decreased hepatic arterial RI below 0.5. Rarely, the hepatic arterial stenosis may be directly shown as an area of color Doppler aliasing. Useful thresholds of significant stenosis include velocities within the main hepatic artery of greater than 200 cm/sec and a threefold velocity gradient (Fig. 19A and B) (36–38). One article suggests that in the pediatric donor population, the finding of hepatic arterial RI below 60% is highly predictive of impending hepatic artery thrombosis due to stenosis and thrombectomy and reanastomosis should be considered (39). Although an intrahepatic arterial tracing may be demonstrated, it should be remembered that a severe stenosis may still lead to biliary ischemia or may progress to complete thrombosis. CT hepatic arteriography is a useful confirmatory test in asymptomatic patients with Doppler findings suggestive of hepatic arterial stenoses/thromboses. Angiography should be performed in patients with unexplained graft dysfunction, relapsing biliary sepsis, and positive Doppler examinations. Therapeutic angioplasty can then be performed in the same setting.

Studies performed on patients with hepatic artery stenosis and thrombosis have identified certain factors that place patients at a higher risk and warrant more frequent Doppler screening. These factors include bench reconstruction of anatomical variants, the use of an interposition graft, and patients undergoing retransplantation (40).

At the time of implantation, there must be sufficient length of all of the vasculature to create the anastomoses. A longer pedicle is easier to work with, however; if the vessels are too long, a kink may occur as the liver is placed into the fossa and the abdominal wall is closed. Clinically the patient presents with liver dysfunction. A stenosis may be suspect on spectral Doppler. Color or power Doppler may reveal the tortuosity. Three-dimensional (3D) CTA may be performed to provide "the big picture" and determine if a stent of reoperation is the best treatment (Fig. 20).

Hepatic arterial PAs are rare complications of transplantation. Intrahepatic PAs are typically a result of post-biopsy arterial injuries. The appearance of an intrahepatic PA is similar to PAs elsewhere; color Doppler reveals swirling flow within an intrahepatic fluid collection. Pulsatile to and fro flow may be shown within the aneurysm neck. Intrahepatic PAs are usually asymptomatic and may be followed by sonography. On the other hand, extrahepatic PAs may be surgical (or angiographic) emergencies (41).

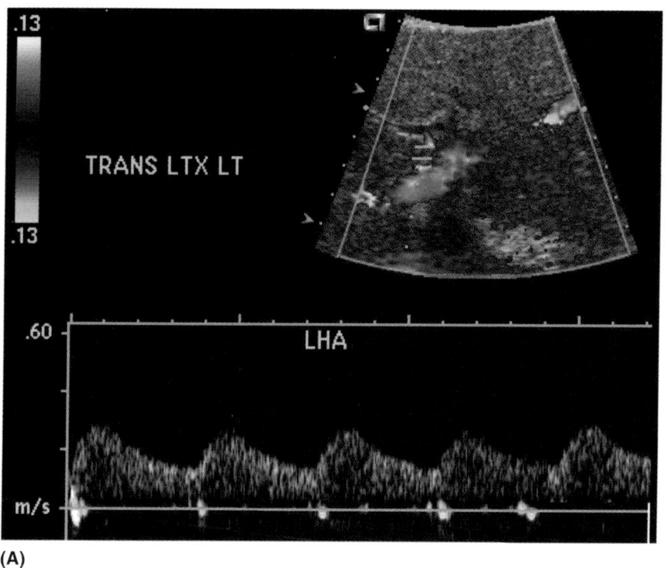

(A)

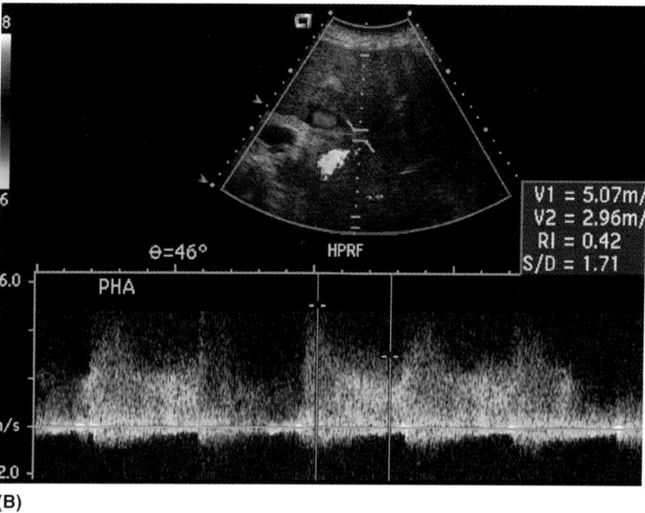

(B)

FIGURE 19 A AND B ■ (**A**) Color and spectral Doppler tracing of an intrahepatic arterial flow profile. Tardus-parvus pattern with a delayed upstroke in systole-rounded systolic curve and relatively low-resistance flow is indicative of insufficient hepatic arterial inflow and suggests stenosis. The examiner should carefully walk the sample volume down the hepatic artery and out of the liver looking for the anticipated point of stenosis. In this case, (**B**) a high-velocity jet measuring over 5 m/sec identified the point of stenosis in the subhepatic space. LHA, left hepatic artery; HPRF, high pulse repetition frequency; PHA, proper hepatic artery.

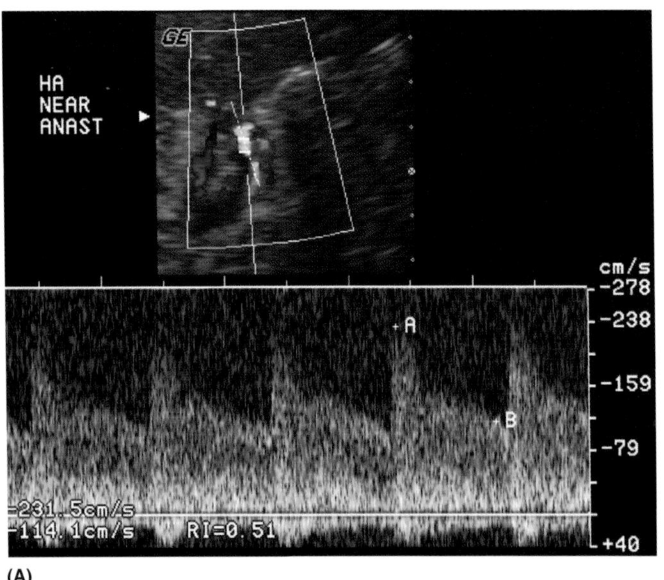

(A)

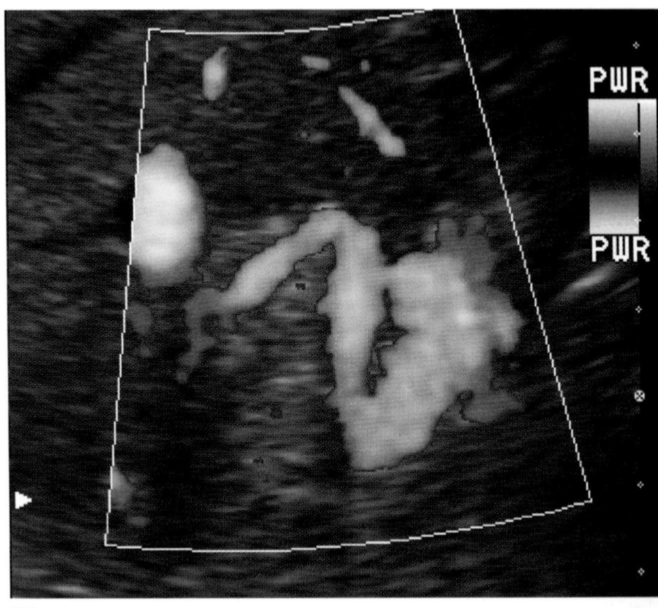

(B)

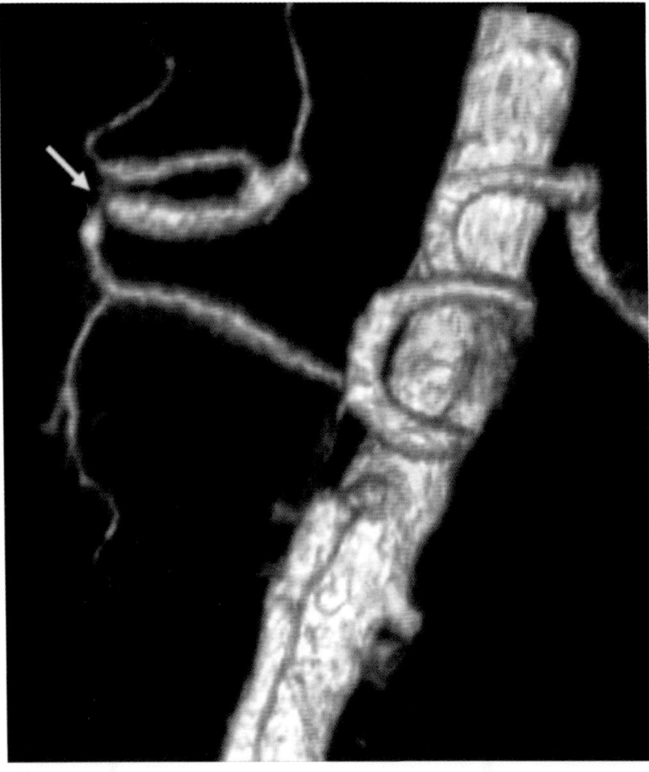

(C)

FIGURE 20 A–C ■ (**A**) Spectral Doppler tracing of the hepatic artery (HA) in the porta hepatis reveals a high-velocity jet, suggesting a stenosis. (**B**) Power Doppler image of the subhepatic space reveals a markedly tortuous hepatic artery. (**C**) The 3D rendering of the CT angiogram during the arterial phase reveals a kink (*arrow*) due to excessive vessel length in the subhepatic space.

An extrahepatic PA may erode into the adjacent portal vein, hepatic vein, or bile duct. If coil embolization fails, the PA should be surgically resected since it is likely to rupture.

Arteriovenous Fistulae

Arteriovenous or arteriobiliary fistulas are very rare and are most often the sequela of biopsy or other percutaneous intervention. Grayscale ultrasound imaging may not show an abnormality. A local flash artifact is seen on color Doppler at normal settings. When color Doppler settings are adjusted for the high velocities, the feeding artery and draining structure are better visualized. The spectral Doppler flow profile in the feeding artery manifests very low resistance with a high diastolic velocity (42,43).

Portal Vein

The donor portal vein is usually anastomosed end-to-end to the recipient portal vein. Variations may be required if the recipient portal vein is thrombosed, hypoplastic, or of insufficient length. Because the vessel is relatively large,

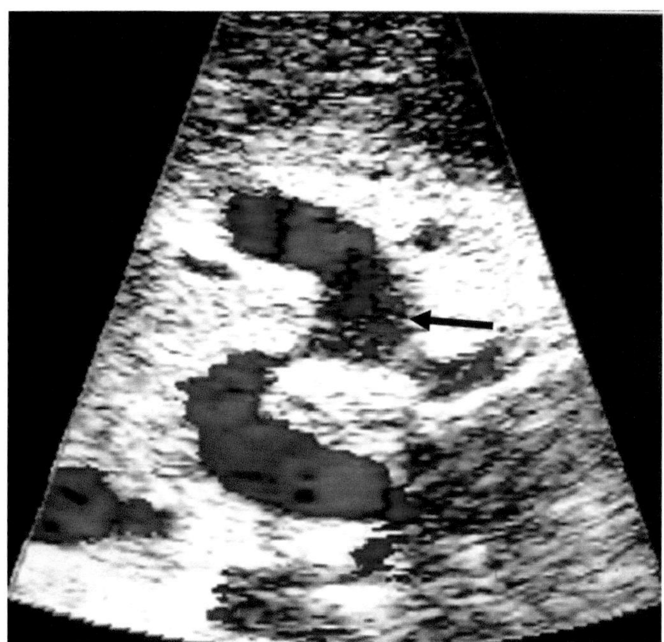

FIGURE 21 ■ Transverse color Doppler image of the porta hepatis. The portal vein (PV) is compressed under the transplant liver into an S-shaped kink. Doppler shows that the PV is still patent but note the aliasing just beyond the kink (*arrow*).

color Doppler findings can be rather striking (Fig. 9). Not all flow disturbances perceived by color Doppler are hemodynamically significant and compromise of portal vein flow is relatively rare. When it occurs, it may be due to faulty surgical technique, a mismatch between the diameter of the recipient and the donor portal veins, or an excessive length of vessel causing a kink (Fig. 21) (44). Clinical features of hemodynamically significant stenosis include persistent portal hypertension (ascites and varices) and graft dysfunction. Stenoses are manifested on color Doppler as an area of focal color aliasing. If a portal vein stenosis is suspected on color Doppler screening, the velocity gradient across the anastomosis should be measured by spectral Doppler; a velocity gradient of less than threefold is unlikely to be significant (Fig. 22A and B) (19). Clinically significant and Doppler-confirmed portal venous stenoses may be confirmed on CT venography. Percutaneous venoplasty (with or without stent placement) is often curative.

Posttransplantation portal vein thrombosis is quite rare and most often attributed to technical factors. Recipient donor size mismatch can lead to portal vein thrombosis. It is more likely to occur in the pediatric recipient, especially after split liver transplantation (44,45). Prompt detection with frequent Doppler evaluation and aggressive surgical treatment in selected cases are required to reduce the mortality and graft loss (Fig. 23). It can be treated by surgical thrombectomy, angioplasty, or thrombolytic infusion, but in some cases, retransplantation may be required (46).

If slow velocity is identified in the portal vein (<0.1 m/sec), it may be due to increased intrahepatic resistance from rejection or reduced inflow as can be seen with the collateral steal phenomenon. This occurs when large varices remain unligated, shunting blood from the portal system to the systemic circulation, bypassing the liver (47–49).

A pulsatile waveform in the portal vein may be observed within the first few weeks after transplantation,

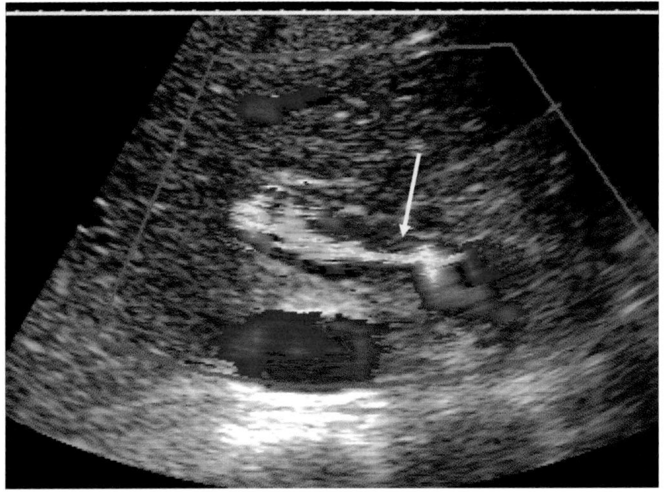

(A)

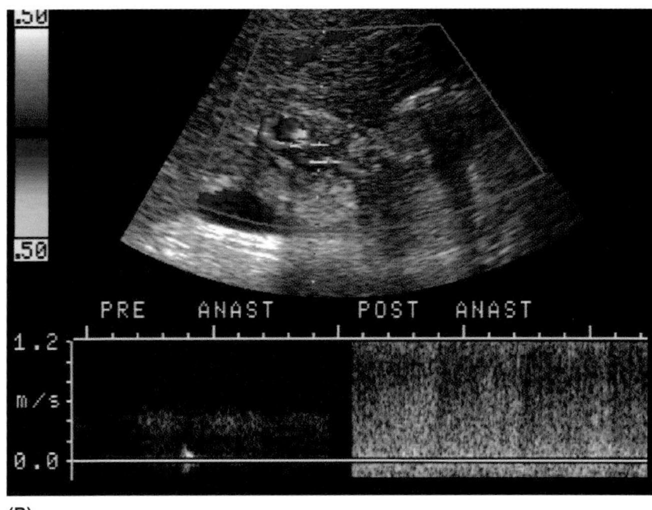

(B)

FIGURE 22 A AND B ■ (**A**) Color Doppler image of the portal vein in the region of the anastomosis. Note the area of relative narrowing at the point of anastomosis (*arrows*). A high-velocity jet with aliasing is seen shooting into the donor portal vein. (**B**) Spectral Doppler tracing on either side of this anastomosis had to be set low to project the relatively slow preanastomotic portal vein flow. As a result, the postanastomotic (post-stenotic) tracing shows a high degree of aliasing. This comparative velocity measurement on one tracing can be achieved by moving the sample volume across the anastomosis and allows an accurate comparison of pre- and postanastomotic velocities. Velocity gradients of less than fourfold are not likely to be clinically significant.

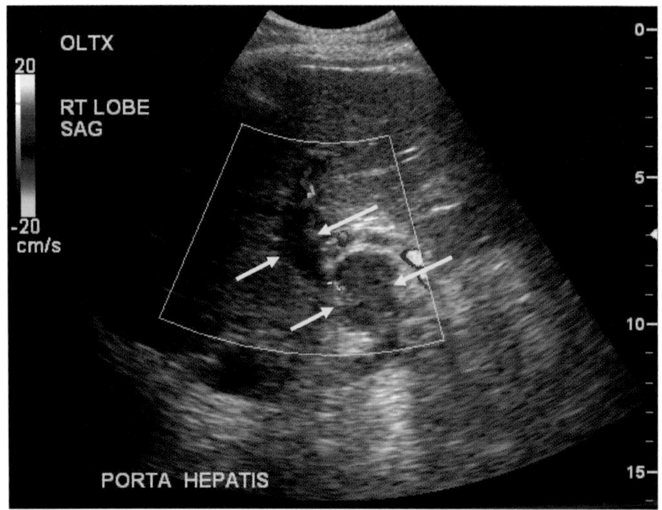

FIGURE 23 ■ Transverse color Doppler image of the porta hepatis. Instead of flow in the portal vein, ultrasound detects an echogenic complex, acute thrombus (*arrows*).

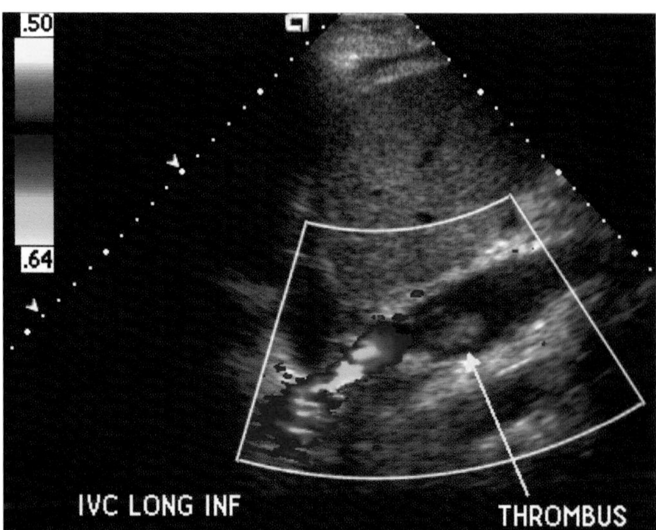

FIGURE 24 ■ Longitudinal color Doppler image of donor inferior vena cava. This liver is anastomosed with a piggyback technique; therefore, the flow within the cava is only a fraction of what it was previously. As a result, clot has formed, partially occluding the lumen (*arrow*).

especially in patients that received small grafts. This pulsatile flow often disappears without any treatment, although if it persists, the sonographer should take special care to search for an intrahepatic arterioportal shunt (50).

Inferior Vena Cava

The donor IVC has a long intra-hepatic course and is therefore transplanted along with the liver. The IVC may be inserted in-line with both supra- and infrahepatic anastomoses; the native intrahepatic IVC is excised with the diseased liver. The more common surgical technique retains the native IVC of the recipient in place and the upper end of the donor IVC is anastomosed end-to-side to the native IVC at the confluence of the hepatic veins of the explanted liver. The lower end of the donor IVC is oversewn, which functionally converts it into a hepatic vein. Relative flow volumes through this vessel are much less than when it served as the IVC; therefore clot may be seen partially filling the lumen (Fig. 24). This should not cause concern as long as some flow can be perceived. This type of anastomosis is commonly referred to as a "piggyback" (17). The incidence of hepatic venous complications in partial liver transplantation is more frequent than that in whole liver transplantation (51). Any compromise of the upper caval anastomosis, from either stenosis or kinking, may cause hepatic venous outflow obstruction. Ultrasound findings include marked damping, or complete flattening of the hepatic vein velocity profile with complete loss of periodicity, distension of the hepatic veins, and a high-velocity jet with turbulence just above the caval anastomosis (Fig. 25A–C). Hepatic vein or caval anastomotic stricture may be treated with balloon dilatation or endovascular stent placement. If these fail, then surgical intervention with a patch venoplasty of the anastomosis can be performed (51). Ideally, after a successful procedure, hepatic vein caliber should decrease and cardiac periodicity should return to the hepatic vein flow profile (52,53). Loss of periodicity may also be due to compression of the hepatic veins by the surrounding liver tissue by edema in the early postoperative period, typically due to preservation injury or by edema in the later postoperative period related to rejection (35,54). Due to the relatively large size of the IVC and the potential for a size mismatch between donor and recipient cava, a greater than fourfold velocity gradient at the anastomosis is required to confidently diagnose a hemodynamically significant stenosis. A persistent monophasic hepatic vein flow profile is highly suggestive of hepatic outflow obstruction, but it is not specific. On the other hand, the presence of periodicity within the hepatic vein tracing on Doppler ultrasound can confidently exclude the possibility of significant outflow obstruction (55).

In those patients with an in-line IVC, compromise of the lower anastomosis may present as lower extremity edema and renal failure. Ultrasound and color Doppler imaging of the anastomosis may reveal a kink or focal stenosis with a relatively high-velocity jet. As with a piggyback procedure, a size mismatch between donor and recipient vessels may produce a relatively high-velocity jet and a less than threefold velocity increase at the anastomosis is seldom clinically significant. A three- to fourfold gradient is likely to be significant and should be correlated with the clinical findings. A greater than fourfold gradient must be considered hemodynamically significant. We have found CT venography to be a useful noninvasive test in equivocal cases.

Thrombosis of the IVC in the transplant recipient is very rare and usually related to stenosis or an indwelling femoral venous catheter (56). Grayscale imaging may reveal an occlusive or partially occlusive plug of echogenic material. If the clot is relatively recent, it may be hypoechoic to the point that diagnosis is difficult by imaging

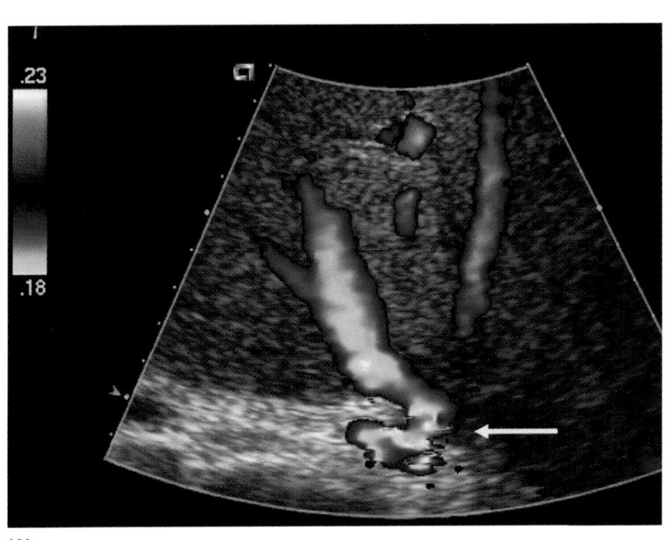

(A)

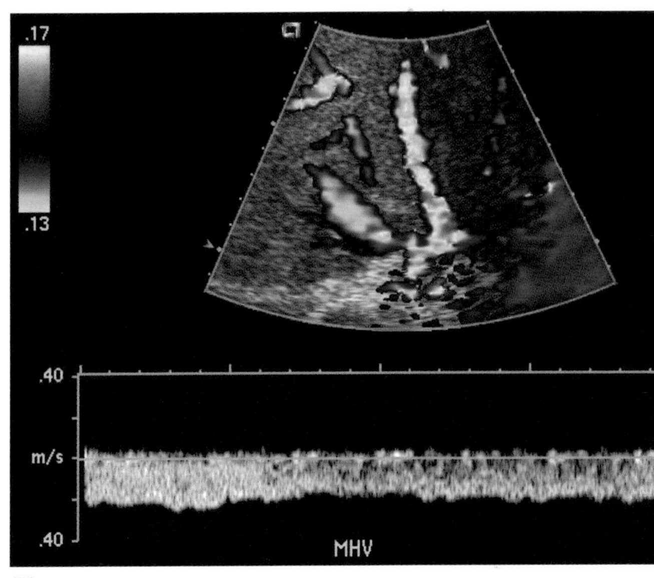

(B)

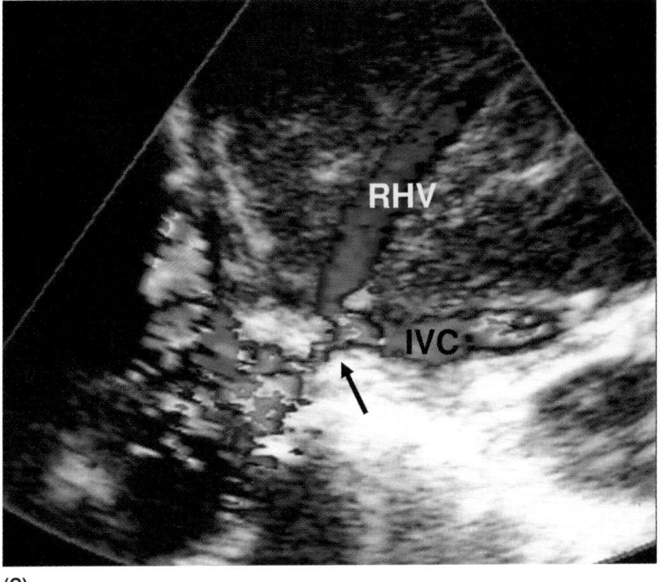

(C)

FIGURE 25 A–C ■ (**A**) Color Doppler image of the hepatic vein confluence with the inferior vena cava (IVC). Note the relatively distended hepatic veins and the color aliasing at the anastomosis (*arrow*). (**B**) Spectral Doppler tracing of the middle hepatic vein (MHV) shows complete absence of periodicity. Since this tracing is acquired within a few centimeters of the heart, one should expect to see normal hepatic vein flow periodicity. Its absence indicates hepatic venous outflow obstruction due to organ shift and kinking or stenosis due to fibrosis. (**C**) A longitudinal color Doppler image at the junction of the right hepatic vein (RHV) and IVC shows a distended hepatic vein with flow backed up behind a focal stenosis (*arrow*).

alone. Color Doppler evaluation augmented by a Valsalva maneuver will confirm absence of flow. Reversal of flow in the hepatic veins may be seen if the clot extends above the ostia of the hepatic veins. If only a single hepatic vein shows flow reversal, then compromise of that one vein must be assumed to be due to either clot or technical difficulty with construction of the venous cloaca. Finally, stagnant flow within the blind end of a piggyback anastamosis will often result in focal, nonocclusive, and functionally insignificant, clot within the oversewn donor caval segment.

Biliary System

Biliary complication can be seen in approximately 15% of liver transplant recipients (57). Ultrasound has a very limited role in the evaluation of suspect biliary complications; indeed it rarely identifies them. Strictures of the bile duct can develop at the anastomosis, but they can occur anywhere in the biliary system, especially after hepatic artery thrombosis and episodes of rejection or infection (58). In patients with a Roux-en-Y choledochojejunostomy, the biliary system should be completely decompressed since there is no sphincter to resist bile outflow. Therefore, the common bile duct should not measure greater than 4 mm and intrahepatic ductal dilatation should not be present. Patients undergoing an end-to-end anastomosis of the transplant common bile duct to the native duct still maintain drainage through the ampulla of Vater. Therefore, greater ductal prominence may be present (59). Biliary duct dilatation may be due to an ischemic stricture at the anastomosis or sphincter of Oddi dysfunction, a relatively common posttransplant functional obstruction. This is often successfully treated with endoscopic sphincterotomy (60,61).

The gallbladders of the recipient and transplant biliary systems are removed during the transplant procedure.

Small remnants of the native and donor cystic ducts remain. Since glands within the duct walls continue to produce mucus, these ducts can become quite distended if obstructed. The sonographic appearance is that of a sonolucent structure in the porta hepatis region without any internal flow on Doppler. These are known as mucoceles of the cystic duct remnant. They can exert a mass effect and extramural compression on the bile duct, resulting in biliary obstruction (62).

Biliary ischemia induced by hepatic arterial stenoses/thromboses may result in biliary sloughing and biliary casts (Figs. 17 and 18). Although the casts may be impressive at endoscopic retrograde cholangiopancreatography (ERCP), they are often missed on gray-scale examination since the echogenicity of the sludge is usually similar to the echogenicity of the adjacent liver parenchyma (63,64). Careful sonographic technique is needed to depict subtle periportal echogenicity in these cases.

Rejection

Several authors have studied the possibility of predicting acute liver transplant rejection by identifying changes in the hepatic vein waveform (65). During rejection, hepatocellular edema and inflammatory infiltration increase the pressure within the confining capsule of the liver. This reduces the compliance of the liver and results in a damped hepatic vein waveform. The theory is appropriate but other causes of hepatocellular edema, such as cholangitis, hepatitis, and upper IVC anastomotic stenosis, produce similar damping, thereby limiting the specificity of this finding. The diagnosis of rejection is best made by needle biopsy.

Liver Transplant Biopsy

Ultrasound guidance for liver transplant biopsy helps avoid complications and prevents inadvertent biopsy of adjacent organs. Ultrasound and Doppler guidance should be used to guide the biopsy needle into the liver but away from the large central vessels (66). Guidance should not consist of simply marking a spot but should be performed at the time of the biopsy procedure since variations in patient position and respiration can alter the relationship of the liver to the skin. Initial evaluation should rule out the presence of fluid in the area in which biopsy is being considered. The area of biopsy should also avoid major intrahepatic vasculature and bile ducts. We typically target the lateral segment of the left lobe of the liver via a subxiphoid approach. Immediately after the biopsy, the area is surveyed to rule out hemorrhage. Other complications such as arterial venous fistula, arterial biliary fistula, or PA formation are not shown immediately but may manifest within a few days of the biopsy (42,43).

RENAL TRANSPLANTATION

One-year renal allograft survival rates in the United States are approximately 89% for cadaveric and 95% for living-donor kidney transplants, with one-year patient survival rates at 94% for cadaveric recipients and 97% for living-related kidney recipients (67). When screening, laboratory test results indicate renal transplant dysfunction and imaging studies are often required to evaluate renal morphology and perfusion. Ultrasound is an ideal tool for this purpose—it is noninvasive, readily available, and has been shown to be the premier screening modality for the identification of renal transplant complications such as perinephric fluid collections and collecting system dilatation. With the addition of Doppler, vascular complications can be identified. Occasionally, ultrasound may also suggest functional problems such as rejection or acute tubular necrosis. Successful screening of the renal transplant, however, requires that the practitioner understand normal transplant anatomy, utilize optimized scan technique, and be familiar with the many potential complications of transplantation.

Ultrasonographic Technique

Representative sagittal and axial images of the transplant and bladder are obtained. The length of the transplant and the size of any perinephric fluid collections are measured. The degree of collecting system dilatation, if present, is then subjectively graded. Color Doppler is used to identify the renal vascular pedicle. Spectral Doppler is applied to the main renal artery, main renal vein, and intrarenal segmental or intralobar branches at the mid, upper, and lower poles. Segmental or intralobar arterial RIs (peak systolic velocity–end diastolic velocity/peak systolic velocity) are calculated. If any inflow compromise is suspected, then power Doppler can be applied to confirm uniform vascular perfusion throughout the kidney (Fig. 26). A complete sonographic examination of the renal transplant should cover the points listed in Table 4.

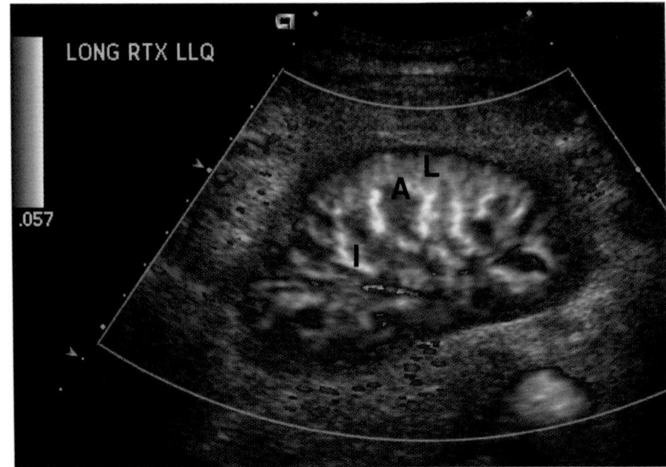

FIGURE 26 ■ Longitudinal power Doppler image of a normal renal transplant. With the setting set to a very sensitive level, flow can be perceived in the interlobar (I), arcuate (A), and intralobular (L) arteries all the way out to the capsular surface of the kidney. This is a normal finding and indicates good renal perfusion with normal resistance to inflow.

TABLE 4 ■ Renal Transplant Sonographic Examination Checklist

- Review any available prior imaging studies. Review the surgical record, especially with regard to the vasculature
- Evaluate the renal collecting system. If dilated, make certain that bladder outflow obstruction is not the underlying cause
- Measure the renal length. Record any change
- Rule out perinephric fluid collections. Record any change in size if previously present
- Rule out lymphocele
- Verify uniform parenchymal perfusion by color Doppler. Rule out tardus-parvus waveform by examining the interlobar or segmental arterial waveforms for resistance and delayed systolic upstroke
- Examine the main renal artery, particularly near its anastomosis (especially if a tardus-parvus waveform is observed within the transplanted kidney)
- Verify renal vein patency

Ultrasonographic Anatomy

In most cases, the transplant kidney is positioned retroperitoneally in the iliac fossa with an end-to-side anastomosis of the renal vasculature to the common or external iliac artery and vein. The transplanted ureter is implanted directly into the superior surface of the bladder or the native ureter (Fig. 27). In approximately 20% of transplants, multiple arterial or venous anastomoses may be required. Because numerous technical variations exist in the way kidneys are transplanted, it is very important that the sonologist and sonographer are familiar with the surgical technique common to their institution and the specific anatomic details of the patient being scanned (68,69).

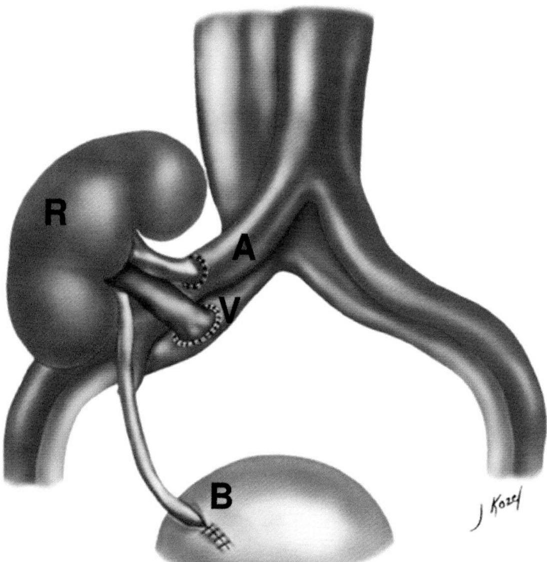

FIGURE 27 ■ Artist's rendering of a renal transplant (R) located in the right iliac fossa. The transplant renal artery is typically anastomosed to the common iliac artery (A). The transplant renal vein anastomosis is to the common iliac vein (V). The ureter is connected to the urinary bladder (B).

Ideally, if the transplant has variant vascular anatomy, a drawing is provided, which shows the orientation of the kidney and its vasculature, the number and location of anastomoses, and any other atypical anatomic information. Most renal transplants are placed within the right lower quadrant because the vascular dissection is technically easier. With simultaneous renal–pancreas transplants (SPK), however, the renal allograft is typically placed within the left lower quadrant.

Complications

The most common abnormal findings, which may be demonstrated, are listed in Table 5.

Functional Complications

Functional complications include hyperacute rejection, perioperative ischemia, acute tubular necrosis, acute rejection, chronic rejection, and drug toxicity (most commonly immunosuppressive agents) (70,71). Imaging techniques, including ultrasound with Doppler, are limited in their ability to identify and distinguish these functional complications (72).

With hyperacute rejection (humeral mediated rejection), graft failure occurs rapidly (within minutes of implantation), secondary to the presence of preformed circulating antibodies. This condition is typically observed in patients who have been sensitized by a previous transplant organ or a blood transfusion. The diagnosis of

TABLE 5 ■ Renal Transplant Sonographic Findings and Possible Causes

Increase in size of transplanted kidney
- Hypertrophy of the kidney
- Allograft rejection
- Postoperative infection
- Renal vein thrombosis

Reduction in size of transplanted kidney
- Ischemia
- Chronic rejection

Increased intrarenal arterial resistive index
- Compressive effect by transducer, adjacent mass, or fluid collection
- Infection
- Advanced stages of rejection
- High-grade obstruction
- Acute tubular necrosis

Decreased intrarenal arterial resistance index
- Renal artery stenosis
- Severe aortoiliac atherosclerosis
- Arteriovenous fistula

Renal collecting system dilatation
- Obstructive hydronephrosis
- Ureteral anastomosis stenosis
- Chronic distention of flaccid denervated system
- Sequela of prior obstructive episode
- Bladder outlet obstruction (neurogenic bladder)

hyperacute rejection is usually made in the operating suite, within minutes of unclamping the vascular pedicle. Since the renal transplant is so short lived, ultrasound has little role in the evaluation of this condition. Extremely high resistance to inflow can be expected.

Acute rejection is a cellular-mediated process, whereby the immune system attacks the foreign renal allograft. Acute rejection is controlled by the use of steroids, cyclosporine, tacrolimus, sirolimus, and other immunosuppressive agents. Occasional elevation in a transplant recipient's immune status (caused by viral illness or noncompliance with immunosuppressive drug therapy) can result in an acceleration of acute rejection to a critical level. The kidney becomes edematous and swollen, intracapsular pressure rises, and eventually vascular compliance is decreased (Fig. 28). Although early investigators proposed that RI elevation was useful in identifying acute rejection as the cause of kidney transplant dysfunction, subsequent laboratory and clinical studies have shown RI to be unreliable, and acute rejection remains a pathological diagnosis. Indeed, in a canine study, it has been found that RI actually decreases in the mild-to-moderate stages of acute rejection. During the early-to-mid stages of rejection, the physical effects of increased intrarenal pressure are counteracted by intrarenal hormonal autoregulatory mechanisms. Elevation of RI, therefore, does not manifest until the process of acute rejection is quite severe (73). Furthermore, several recent in-vitro and ex-vivo studies have shown that although the terms "renal vascular resistance" and "RI" were used interchangeably in the initial Doppler literature, the two are not intimately related. Rather, the RI is most affected by changes in tissue compliance and driving pulse pressures (74).

The RI is rarely affected in the mild-to-moderate stages of acute rejection and when it is, its specificity is low (75). It is not until acute rejection progresses to severe levels that the RI becomes consistently elevated. Elevation of RI, however, can also occur from many other causes such as hydronephrosis, acute tubular necrosis, infection, and compression of the kidney by an adjacent mass or fluid collection. Thus, specificity for the diagnosis of acute rejection by Doppler ultrasound is unacceptably low and

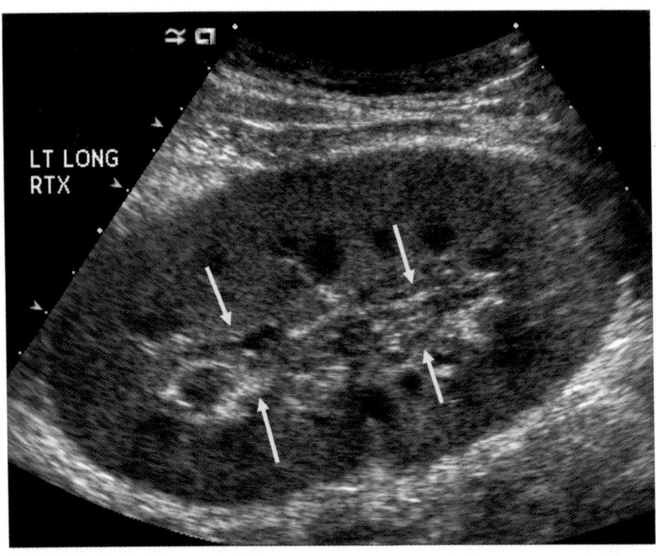

(A)

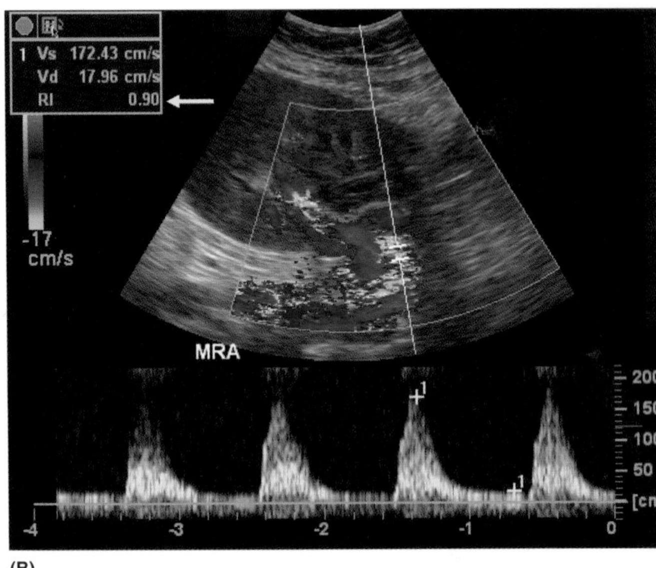

(B)

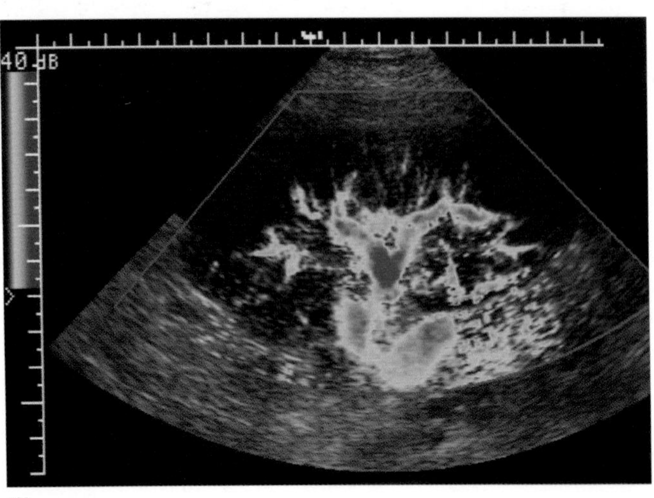

(C)

FIGURE 28 A–C ■ (**A**) Longitudinal gray-scale image of a transplanted kidney. Note the rounded globular configuration of the kidney. The central hilar space (*arrows*) is compressed due to edema and swelling; therefore, central hilar fat has been displaced. (**B**) Spectral Doppler tracing at the main renal artery level shows a resistive index of 90% (*arrow*). Biopsy confirmed severe acute rejection. (**C**) Power Doppler image of a severely rejecting renal transplant shows the main central vasculature and a few interlobar vessels but no flow can be seen out to the periphery of this rejecting kidney. The high resistance generated by the rejection process results in this color Doppler "pruned tree" appearance. Contrast this to the appearance of normal renal power Doppler flow in Fig. 26. MRA, main renal artery.

renal biopsy is still needed to establish the diagnosis (73–79). If a scan being performed in anticipation of transplant biopsy identifies the kidney to be edematous and swollen with loss of central sinus fat echo and very high RIs, thought should be given to deferring the biopsy. Puncturing the capsule of a tense rejecting kidney may cause it to rupture.

Chronic rejection is a multifactorial process including antibody-mediated rejection, and the pathophysiology is not entirely understood. Doppler indices rarely show any significant alteration in flow profiles with chronic rejection (78).

Perioperative ischemia can result in transient compromise of renal function, particularly at the level of the distal tubules, which are most sensitive to hypoxia. This condition is self-limiting and typically resolves within one to two weeks of transplantation. The kidney, and in particular, the renal medulla, appears edematous; Doppler studies will show an increase in the RI. Although the imaging and Doppler findings may suggest acute tubular necrosis, they are, once again, not specific (Fig. 29) (73,79).

Anatomical Complications

These include hematomas, seromas, urinomas, abscesses, lymphoceles, obstructive hydronephrosis, focal masses, arterial and venous stenosis or thrombosis, and intrarenal arteriovenous fistulae (AVFs) and PAs (70,71,79,80). Unlike functional complications, most anatomic complications are readily identified by ultrasound.

Perinephric fluid is a common sequela of renal transplantation and is not considered significant if it is crescentic in shape or decreases in size over time. Most fluid collections are hematomas or seromas, which result from oozing from the transplant bed; urinomas are relatively uncommon and usually are the result of breakdown at the ureteral anastomosis to the bladder. Doppler examination is of limited value in these cases. High-pressure collections such as hematoma after biopsy or organ rupture may exert mass effect upon the kidney and locally affect hemodynamics. In this case, Doppler may reveal a high-resistance spectral tracing in proximity to the fluid pocket (Fig. 30). A patient with a rounded, expansile collection with internal debris and associated signs of infection usually has an abscess. It is usually difficult to diagnose an abscess by sonography alone and CT is considered a better imaging study for this purpose, especially to determine its extent and the potential for percutaneous drainage. Occasionally, color Doppler may reveal hyperemia of the tissues surrounding the abscess.

Lymphoceles are usually shown six to eight weeks after transplantation and appear as rounded or lobulated collections near the vascular anastomoses (Fig. 31). They are the result of surgical disruption of lymphatic channels when the vascular anastomosis to the transplanted kidney is created. An expanding lymphocele may cause ureteric compression and hydronephrosis (81). If a lymphocele becomes large enough, it may compress or kink the renal vascular pedicle. In this situation, Doppler examination may show findings similar to arterial or venous stenosis (Fig. 32).

Transient dilatation of the collecting system as a result of ureteral anastomotic edema frequently occurs immediately

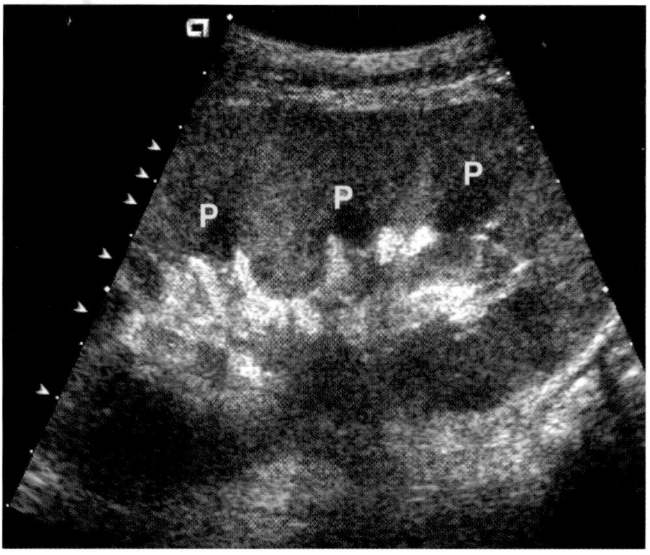

(A)

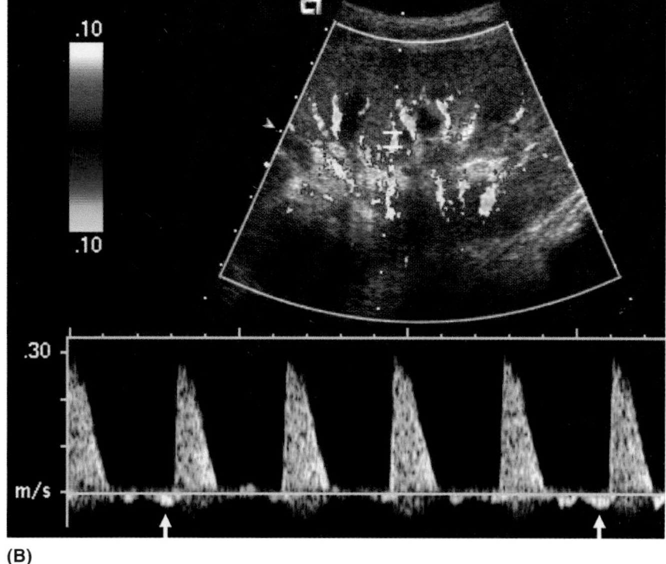

(B)

FIGURE 29 A AND B ■ (**A**) Longitudinal grayscale image obtained with 24 hours of implantation. This cadaver organ experienced prolonged ischemic time. Note that the kidney is not particularly rounded and the sinus fat is preserved. The medullary pyramids (P), however, are prominent, hypoechoic, and edematous. (**B**) Spectral and color Doppler image of the same kidney. The resistive index is elevated to over 100% since reversed flow can be perceived in diastole (*arrows*). This combination of findings in the appropriate clinical situation is consistent with acute tubular necrosis. This can be seen in the immediate post-op state but can also be caused by drug toxicity.

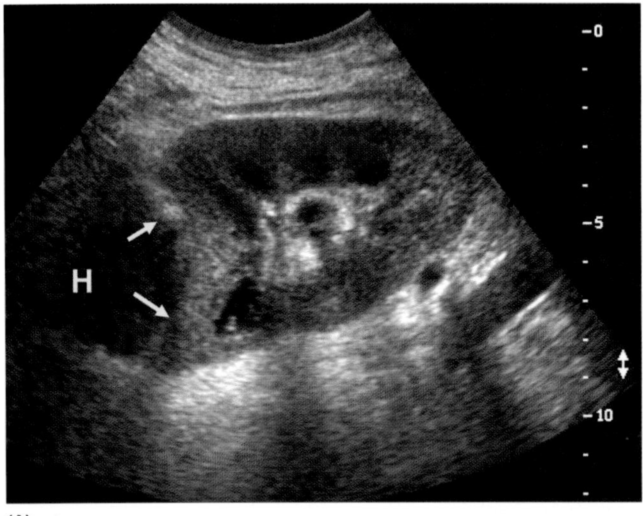

(A)

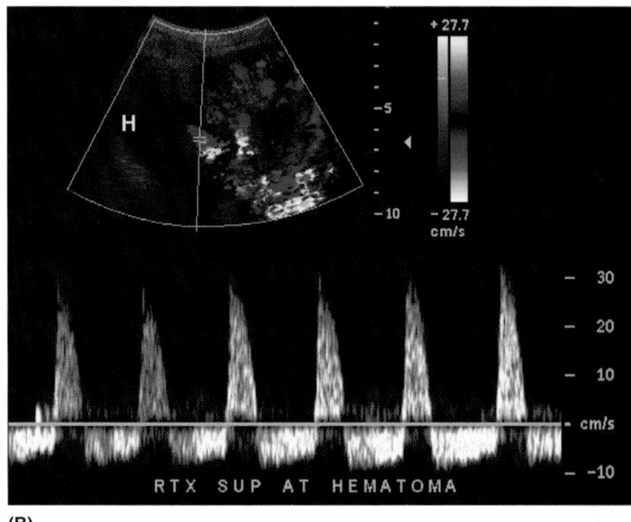

(B)

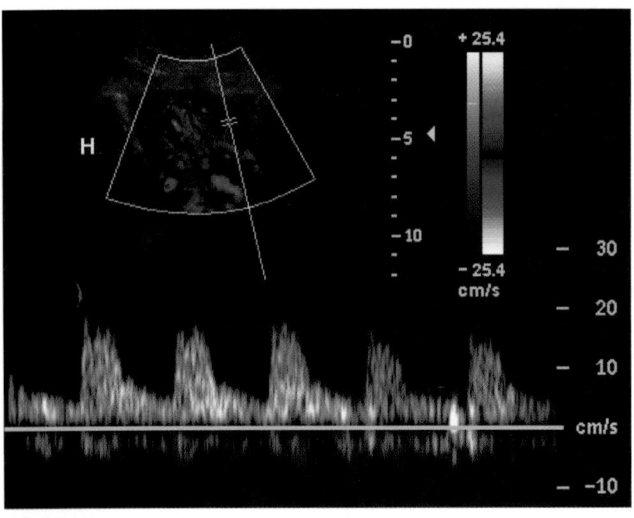

(C)

FIGURE 30 A–C ■ (**A**) Longitudinal gray-scale image of a renal transplant within 24 hours of an upper pole biopsy. The biopsy was complicated by hemorrhage (H). Blood accumulated in the subcapsular space and severely compressed the upper pole of this kidney (*arrows*). (**B**) Spectral Doppler tracing obtained of an interlobar artery just adjacent to the high pressure hematoma reveals extremely high resistive index with reverse flow in diastole. (**C**) Spectral Doppler tracing at the opposite (lower pole) of this same kidney shows a normal low resistance flow profile. The compressive hematoma exerts local mass effect and elevates resistance to flow.

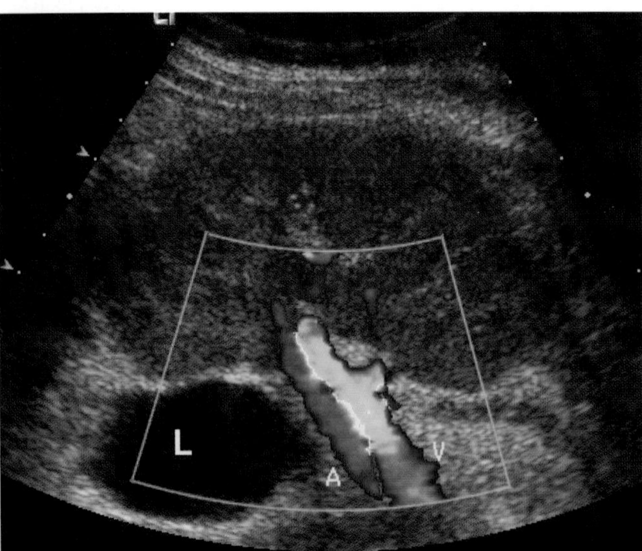

FIGURE 31 ■ Longitudinal color Doppler image of this renal transplant shows a large fluid collection medial to the kidney, immediately adjacent to the renal vascular pedicle. This is a simple lymphocele. L, lymphocele; A, renal artery; V, renal vein.

after renal transplantation or removal of the ureteral stent. The presence of a dilated transplant collecting system does not automatically signify an obstructed system under pressure, as the denervated, flaccid collecting system can become markedly dilated, particularly when the urinary bladder has been distended (80,82,83). This is common in diabetics who may develop a neurogenic bladder. In addition, reflux across an incompetent ureteroneocystostomy may result in varying degrees of collecting system dilatation. Improvement in collecting system dilatation after voiding is often helpful in differentiating these entities from true, obstructive pelvocaliectasis. Platt et al. proposed that the identification of an elevated RI was useful in distinguishing obstructive hydronephrosis from chronic, low-pressure dilatation of the transplant collecting system (82,83). Although this observation may be sensitive, its specificity is very poor because of the many other factors that similarly affect renal hemodynamics. The Whitaker test was the gold standard for the evaluation of upper urinary tract dilatation, but now most centers rely on the diuretic renogram.

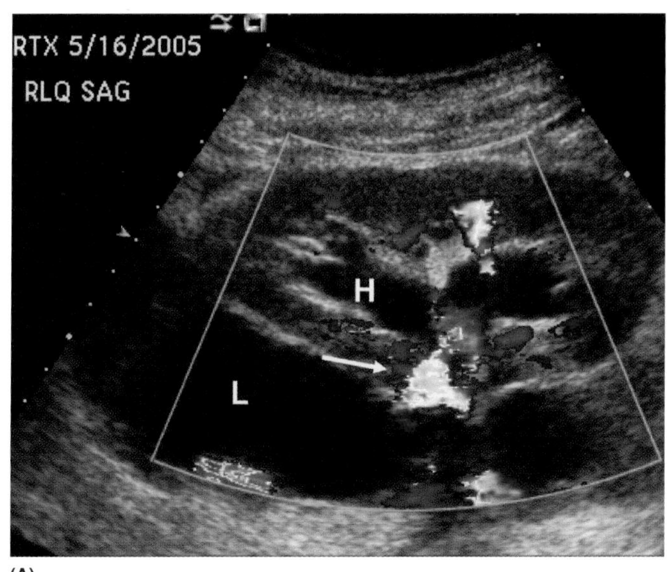

(A)

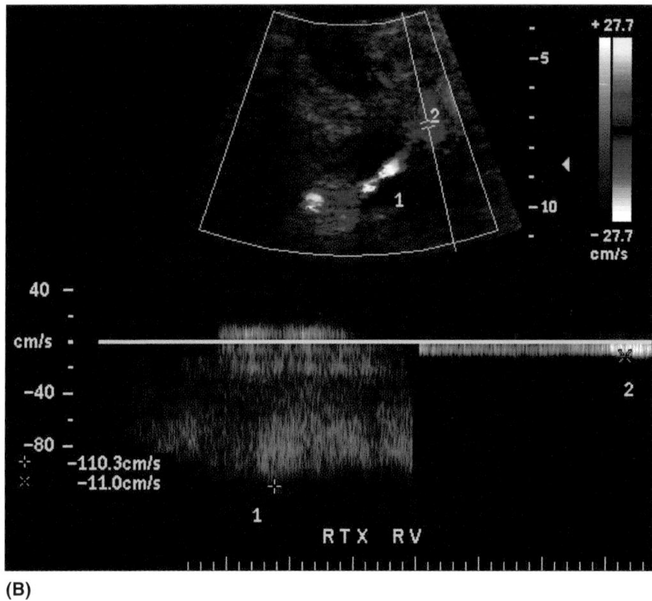

(B)

FIGURE 32 A AND B ■ (**A**) Longitudinal color Doppler image of this renal transplant shows a large fluid collection medial to the kidney, surrounding the renal vascular pedicle. This is a lymphocele (L) and it has caused distortion of the pedicle. Color aliasing can be seen in the renal artery (*arrow*). There is also obvious hydronephrosis (H) caused by compression of the ureter. (**B**) Spectral Doppler tracing of the renal vein shows marked compression where it courses past the lymphocele (1), the measured velocity at this area is 1.1 m/sec; whereas within the kidney [proximal to the lymphocele (2)], the velocity is only 0.1 m/sec. This 10-fold velocity gradient indicates that this is truly significant renal venous outflow obstruction.

Vascular Complications

Following renal transplantation, vascular complications are observed in less than 10% of recipients; however, when present, they are associated with high morbidity and mortality. Complications include renal artery or vein stenosis, compression, kinking, thrombosis, intrarenal AVFs, and PAs. If identified promptly, they can often be successfully repaired prior to transplant failure. Doppler sonography is a very effective, noninvasive screening modality for identifying significant vascular complications (84–86).

Intraperitoneal transplantation, as is common with combined pancreas transplantation, results in a more mobile kidney. Occasionally ptosis or rotation and torsion may occur of the kidney on its pedicle. This may cause compromised arterial inflow and venous outflow (Fig. 33) and even result in transplant infarction.

Renal Transplant Artery Stenosis

Arterial stenosis is usually observed within 1 to 2 cm of the anastomosis, usually as a result of vessel wall ischemia due to surgical disruption of the vasa vasorum. Patients typically present with severe hypertension and/or unexplained graft dysfunction. Fortunately, most stenoses are successfully treated with angioplasty and/or stent placement. A stenosis should be suspected if a tardus-parvus waveform and relatively low-resistance flow is noted in intrarenal branches. A tardus-parvus waveform is characterized by a delayed upstroke in systole (prolonged acceleration time >0.07 seconds), rounding of the systolic peak, and obliteration of the early systolic notch. A flow velocity greater than 2 m/sec with associated distal turbulence near the renal artery anastomosis is diagnostic of renal artery stenosis (Fig. 34). The examiner should conduct a thorough examination from the renal hilum to the iliac artery in search of a focal stenosis, if an intrarenal tardus-parvus waveform is observed (87–91). Occasionally, with severe renal artery stenosis, the intra-arterial waveforms become flattened to the point that it is very difficult to perceive the systolic–diastolic variation. Subtle pulsatile flow is enough to document the patency of the artery and avoid misdiagnosis of thrombosis. This should be further reinforced by the presence of constant outflow in the renal vein (Fig. 35). Angiography should be performed in those patients with direct findings of a stenosis and an appropriate clinical history. Magnetic resonance angiography (MRA) is a reasonable study for asymptomatic patients or for those patients with equivocal Doppler findings.

Approximately 20% of transplanted kidneys require more than one arterial anastomosis due to the presence of accessory arteries. If one of these vessels becomes compromised, then perfusion to the subtended segment of the kidney is decreased. Again, a tardus-parvus waveform may be seen, this time limited to the segments perfused by the affected artery. If thrombosis of this artery occurs, then the subtended area shows no flow on color or power Doppler and an arterial tracing will not be identified by spectral Doppler. The area affected will

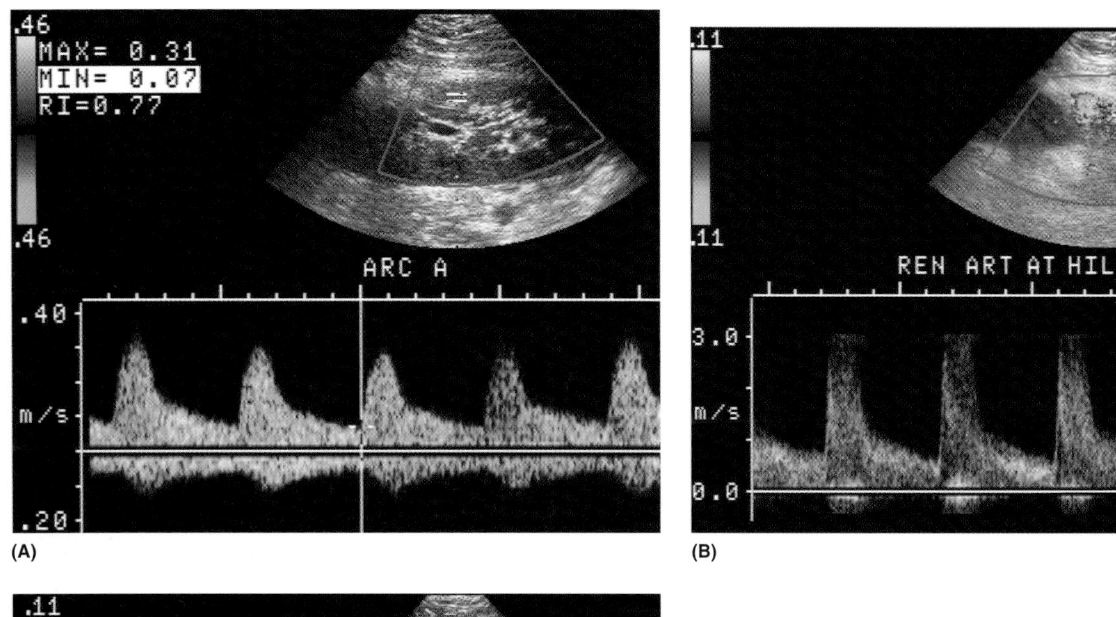

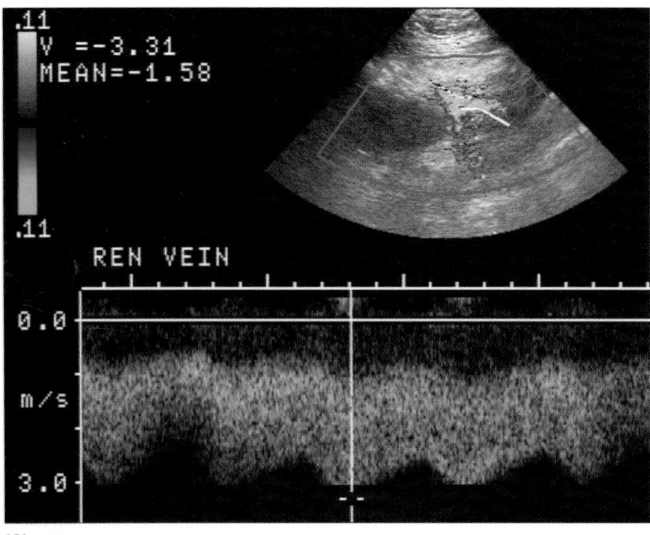

FIGURE 33 A–C ■ (**A**) Longitudinal color Doppler image along the long axis of an intraperitoneal renal transplant with a spectral Doppler tracing of an arcuate artery. The arterial waveform shows a tardus-parvus configuration, indicating arterial inflow compromise. (**B**) The main renal artery at the hilum reveals a high-velocity jet over 3 m/sec. (**C**) Immediately adjacent to the main renal artery, the main renal vein spectral Doppler tracing also shows turbulent high-velocity flow. This finding of high velocity, turbulent Doppler tracings in both artery and vein, is due to torsion of the renal vascular pedicle and resultant kink of the main artery and vein. Fortuitously, this was only partial torsion of the kidney and was corrected with nephropexy. Intraperitoneal torsion of a transplant kidney has been reported to result in infarction.

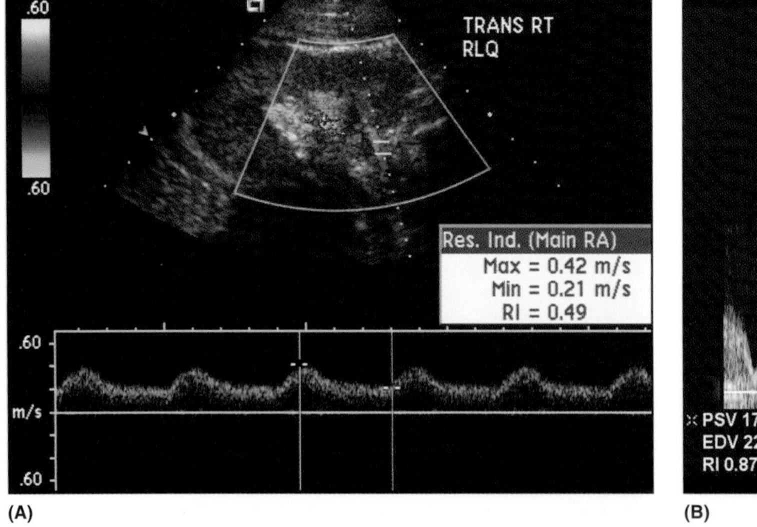

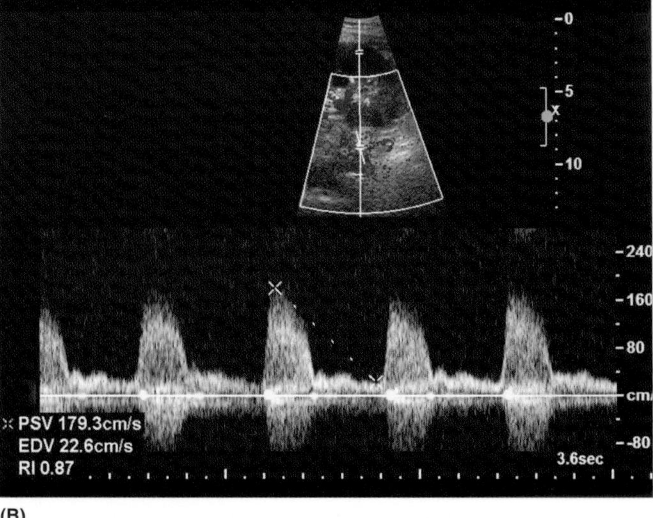

FIGURE 34 A–C ■ (**A**) Renal transplant arcuate artery spectral Doppler tracing in a hypertensive recipient with elevated serum creatinine. The renal arterial waveform manifests tardus-parvus waveform with a slow systolic upstroke, and a rounded systolic peak, relatively low resistance. These findings suggest a more proximal stenosis. (**B**) Spectral Doppler tracing just beyond the anastomosis of the main renal artery to the iliac artery. Note the high velocity (1.79 m/sec), turbulent flow characteristic of renal artery stenosis. (*Continued*)

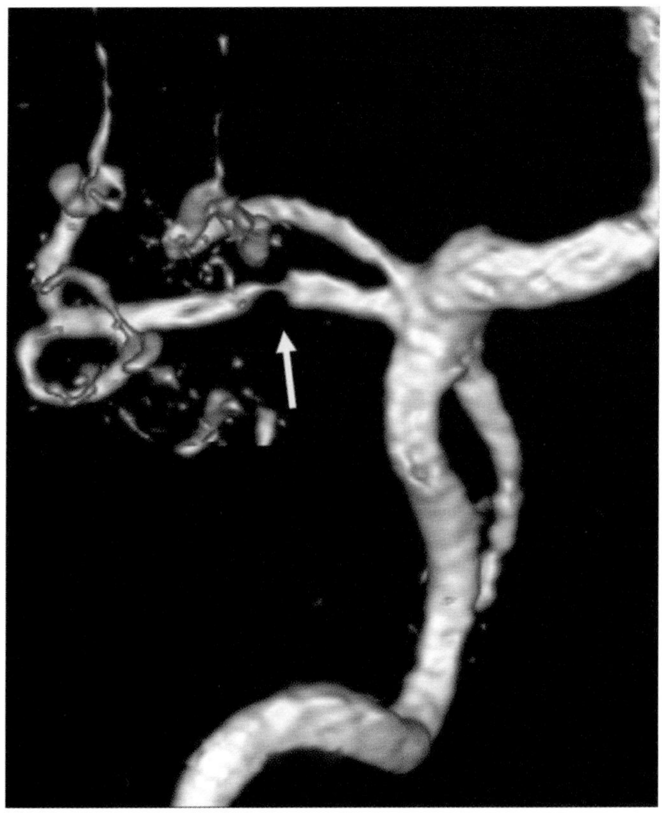

(C)

FIGURE 34 A–C ■ (*Continued*) (**C**) MR angiogram of this transplanted kidney actually revealed a double arterial anastomosis. The lower pole artery shows a high-grade stenosis (*arrow*) within 2 cm of its anastomosis.

vary depending on the anatomic vascular distribution (Fig. 36).

Renal parenchymal scarring secondary to chronic rejection may result in focal stenosis within branch arteries. This should be suspected if there is irregular distribution of flow on color Doppler through the kidney. Segmental or interlobar renal artery stenosis can be confirmed by the presence of intrarenal high-velocity flow. Because these lesions are typically multiple and distal, treatment options are limited (92).

A similar appearance can be seen with scarring after transplant biopsy. If the biopsy needle is guided centrally toward the renal hilum, there is a greater chance of vessel injury. Direct puncture of a major artery usually becomes immediately manifest as an area of turbulence on color Doppler, a rapidly expanding hematoma, or brisk hematuria due to an arterioureteral fistula (Fig. 37). Biopsy in close proximity to a major artery may present with delayed segmental perfusion as scarring results in progressive compromise of flow to that portion of kidney.

Renal Transplant Artery Thrombosis

Thrombosis of the main renal transplant artery is a rare event. It is typically due to a technical problem with the surgical anastomosis. Doppler fails to demonstrate any arterial flow. Rarely, severe acute rejection may cause microvascular thrombosis. Color and power Doppler show no flow within the kidney. Flow may still be present in the segmental or interlobar branches, but spectral Doppler shows very high resistance because the flow has

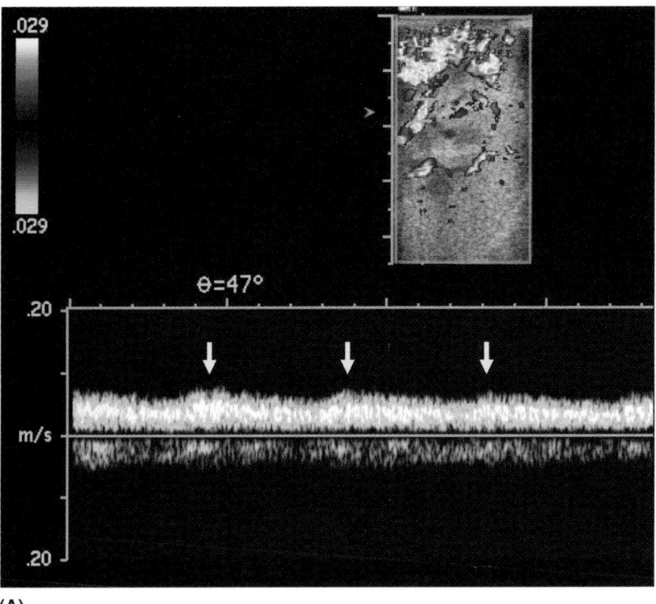

(A)

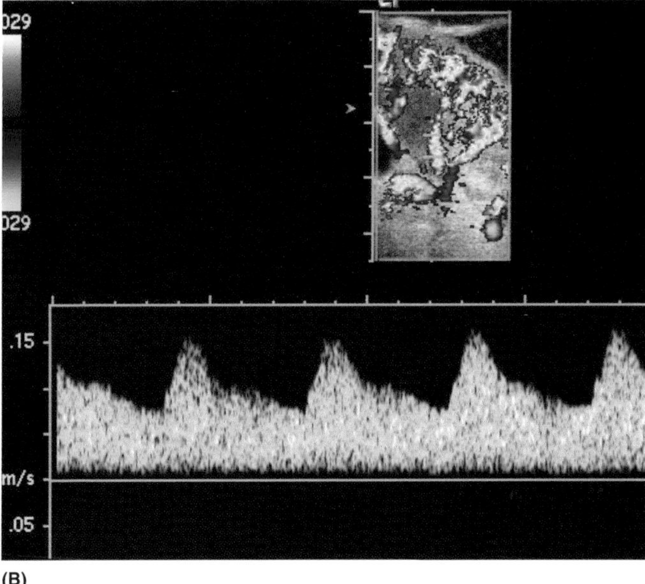

(B)

FIGURE 35 A AND B ■ (**A**) Intraoperative spectral and color Doppler ultrasound of a recent renal transplant recipient being reoperated because of nonfunction and a Doppler suggestion of arterial stenosis. This spectral Doppler tracing of a segmental artery and its adjacent vein shows only a very subtle undulation in the arterial waveform (toward the transducer) (*arrows*). The severe proximal stenosis almost completely wiped out the expected systolic velocity variation. The tracing below the baseline is not a mirror imaging of the tracing but venous outflow. (**B**) As the anastomosis was surgically manipulated, a sudden increase in arterial velocity with a more conspicuous arterial tracing became evident on spectral Doppler.

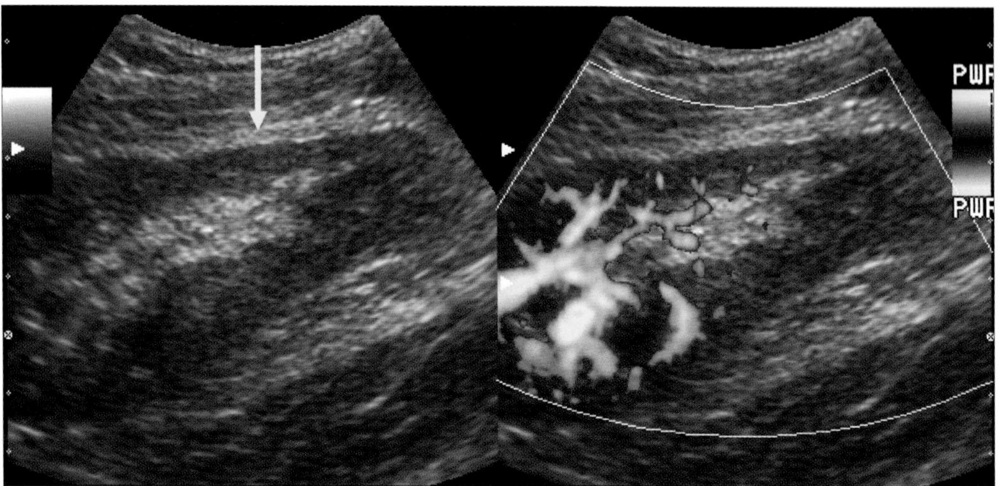

FIGURE 36 ■ Side-by-side longitudinal grayscale and power Doppler image of the low pole of a poorly functioning transplant kidney. Note the thin cortex (*arrow*) and complete absence of flow on power Doppler at the lower pole. This renal transplant required two arterial anastomoses. Thrombosis of the lower pole artery was suggested and was confirmed angiographically. Additionally, ultrasound-guided biopsy of the upper pole identified acute rejection.

nowhere to go (Fig. 38). It may be difficult to differentiate the two etiologies, but the nonrejecting kidney with arterial thrombosis is typically not as swollen and edematous as the acutely rejecting thrombosed kidney.

The spectral Doppler tracing of renal vein flow in microvascular thrombosis may be very confusing. The blood within the vein may be seen to slosh back and forth with cardiac periodicity transmitted down the IVC. This to-and-fro flow may mimic high-resistance arterial flow except for the fact that the upstroke is not brisk. In high-resistance arterial flow, the systole upstroke is brisk with a peak whereas venous to-and-fro flow has a rounded appearance.

Renal Transplant Vein Stenosis

Renal vein stenosis is an uncommon complication following kidney transplantation, but when present, it may be a significant cause of graft dysfunction. A venous stenosis may be seen as a focal narrowing with associated dilatation of the proximal vein. However, to confirm the diagnosis of a significant stenosis, there should be at least a fourfold velocity gradient across the lesion. If the gradient is less than fourfold, it is seldom considered clinically significant, even though it may have a dramatic appearance on Doppler examination (Figs. 32B and 39).

Renal Transplant Vein Thrombosis

Renal vein thrombosis is a rare posttransplantation complication. It is usually seen within the first week following surgery. Thrombosis is more likely to occur when there is technical difficulty with the venous anastomosis. It may occur with preservation injury, or it may evolve during an episode of severe acute allograft rejection. Doppler interrogation of segmental arteries shows reversed diastolic flow.

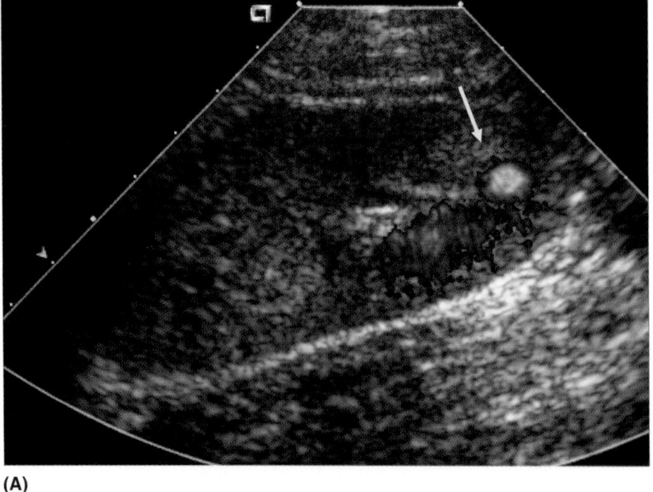

(A)

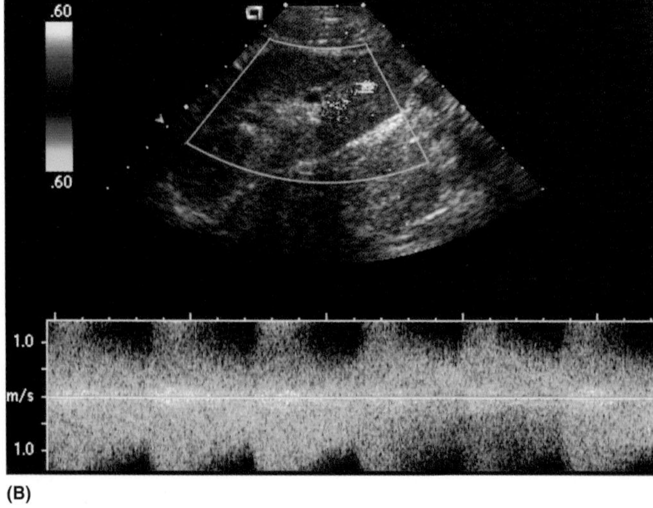

(B)

FIGURE 37 A AND B ■ (**A**) Power Doppler image of a renal transplant approximately two weeks after biopsy. A burst of color is seen overlying the lower pole (*arrow*). This flash artifact, due to tissue vibration, suggests an underlying arteriovenous fistula. (**B**) Spectral Doppler tracing obtained at the fistula site reveals a turbulent, high-velocity arterial waveform; that differentiates it from pseudoaneurysm that has to-and-fro flow.

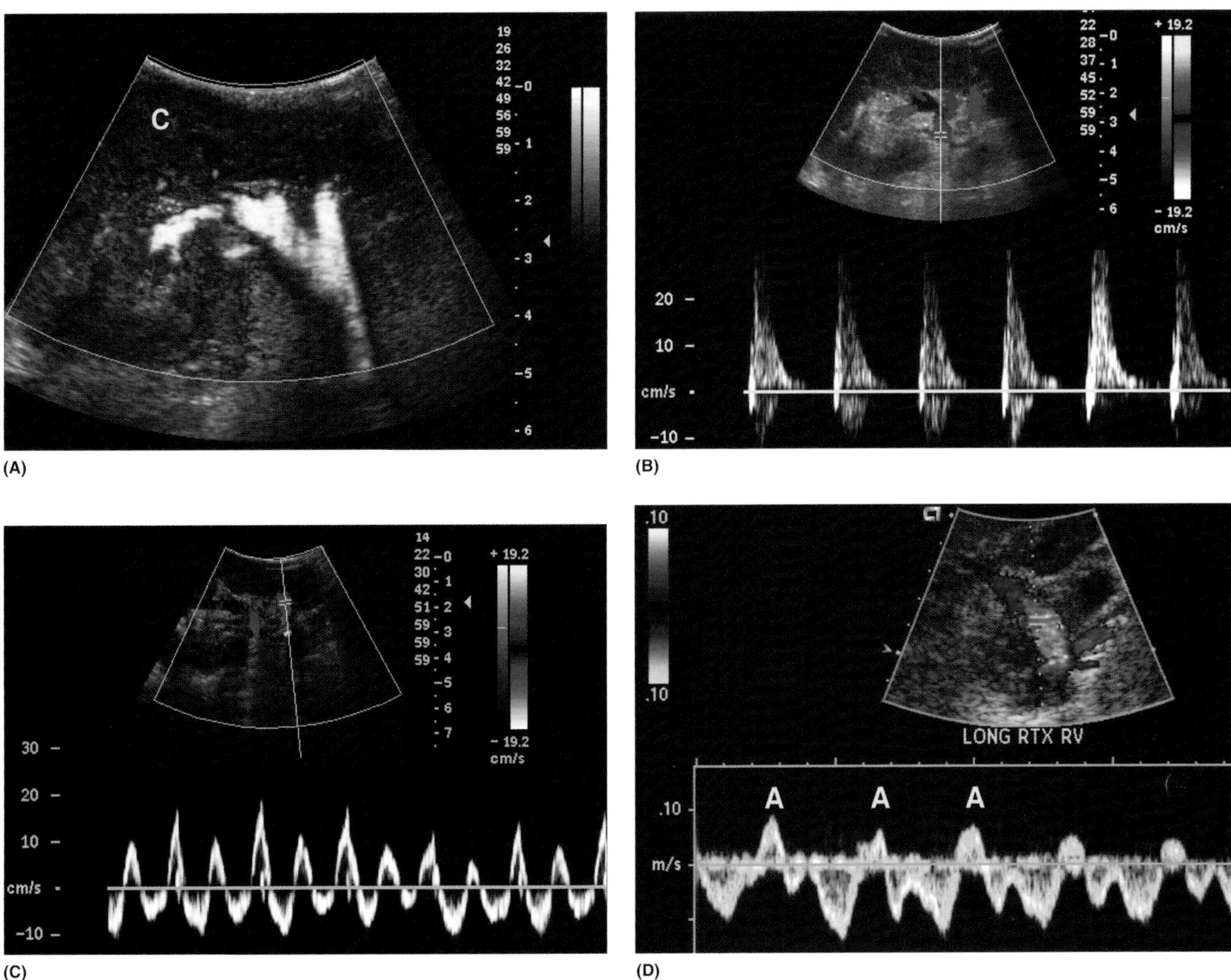

FIGURE 38 A–D ■ Longitudinal power, color, and spectral Doppler imaging of this renal transplant recipient with rapidly rising creatinine levels. (**A**) Power Doppler image shows central flow within the hilum of the kidney but no flow within the cortex (C) or medulla. Microthrombosis was suspect. (**B**) Spectral Doppler tracing of the artery shows a brisk spike in systole and essentially no flow during diastole. (**C**) The renal vein spectral Doppler waveform has an unusual to-and-fro pattern. In summating the area under the tracing above and below the baseline, it becomes evident that there is little total antegrade flow. Due to the microvascular thrombosis, the flow within the vein is simply stagnant moving to and fro responding to intrarenal pressure changes between systole and diastole and pressure changes in the inferior vena cava. Contrast this to a tracing of a normal renal vein. (**D**) The retrograde component of flow known as the a-wave occurs during atrial systole. But, note how relatively little reversed component of flow there is in comparison to the amount of flow below the baseline that is returning toward the heart.

This waveform is not entirely specific, however; reversed diastolic flow may also be shown with severe rejection, pyelonephritis, large perinephric and subcapsular fluid collections, and drug toxicity. Despite the imaging overlap, renal vein thrombosis should strongly be considered if renal venous flow is not identified despite prolonged interrogation (Fig. 40) (93). Prompt recognition of renal venous thrombus may allow for graft salvage after emergent thrombectomy. Usually, however, renal venous thrombus results in rapid graft failure.

Intrarenal AVFs and PAs

Both AVFs and PAs are typically the result of renal transplant biopsy. The true incidence of these complications varies from center to center depending on biopsy technique, but clinically insignificant arterial injuries after biopsy are extremely common. AVFs manifest as a flash of color, or "visible thrill," in the adjacent parenchyma when the kidney is examined at normal color Doppler settings. This phenomenon is caused by vibration of the surrounding tissues secondary to the rapidly flowing blood through the fistula. It is often possible to distinguish the feeding artery and the enlarged draining vein by increasing the pulse repetition frequency. Spectral Doppler tracings will demonstrate a high-velocity, low-resistance flow within the feeding artery. Turbulent, pulsatile (arterialized) flow will be present in the draining segmental vein. If the AVF is large enough, it may be

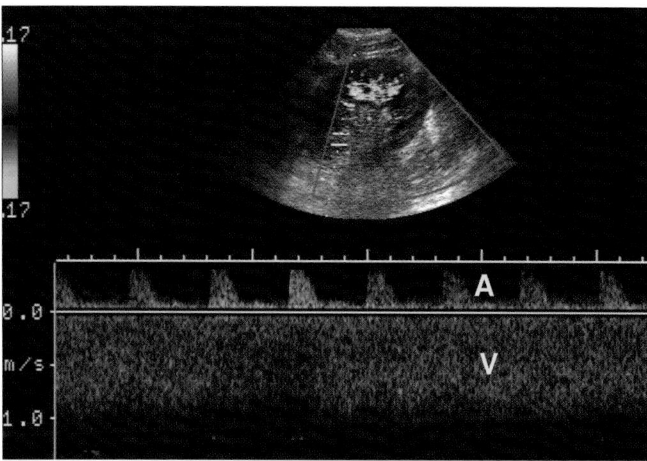

FIGURE 39 ■ Spectral Doppler tracing of the renal vascular pedicle incorporating both the arterial (A) and the venous (V) waveform. Note the high velocity in the vein approximating 1 m/sec. Note the corresponding high-resistance arterial waveform. A renal vein stenosis due to scarring was identified at surgery.

possible to observe pulsatile flow within the main renal vein (Fig. 37).

PAs are typically the result of a biopsy that captured partial thickness of an arterial wall. Therefore, they are extremely rare. They usually appear as a simple cystic structure or a small collection of paravascular fluid. Color Doppler, however, immediately reveals that the finding is not a simple cyst. Spectral Doppler tracings show to-and-fro blood flow at the neck of the PA and a distorted, turbulent, pulsatile waveform can be observed within the PA (Fig. 41). The vast majority of intrarenal AVFs and PAs resolve spontaneously, but if they increase in size over a period of time, angiographic embolization may be necessary (94,95).

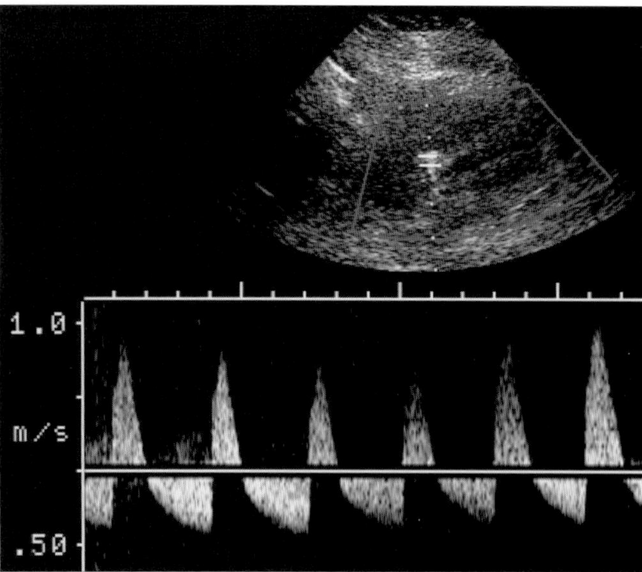

FIGURE 40 ■ Spectral Doppler tracing of the main renal transplant artery in a recent recipient with a rapidly rising creatinine. The arterial waveform reveals to-and-fro flow with the retrograde component being essentially equal to antegrade flow. The resistive index measures approximately 140%. No flow could be identified by spectral or color Doppler in the renal veins. Complete venous thrombosis was confirmed on angiography.

Renal Transplant Biopsy

When there is uncertainty as to the etiology of transplant dysfunction, biopsy is required. It is not without risk and ultrasound plays a significant role in decreasing the rate of complications. Ultrasound is first used to screen any obvious cause for transplant dysfunction, which could be investigated and treated without the need for biopsy. If the kidney appears swollen and edematous and the RI is high (over 100%), the risk of biopsy-induced renal rupture should be considered. Biopsy may be deferred and the kidney treated empirically with steroids until such time as the swelling decreases with a concomitant decrease in risk of transplant rupture. Biopsy guidance should focus on avoiding overlying bowel interposed between abdominal wall and kidney. Next, it should guide the needle away from the hilum and the major vessels. Finally, the path of the needle should aim for the cortex and not the medulla for two reasons: First, rejection primarily affects cortex. Second, the needle that gets to the medulla is also more likely to hit a major vessel with increased risk of bleeding or sequela of AVF.

PANCREAS TRANSPLANTATION

More than 16,000 pancreas transplants have been performed in the United States and more than 21,000 worldwide since 1978 (96). The recipient is typically a diabetic with severe, but not end-stage, complications that include retinopathy, neuropathy, nephropathy, and arteriopathy. Brittle diabetic patients who suffer multiple coma episodes are also considered as candidates for transplantation (97,98). Whole organ pancreaticoduodenal transplantation is the most reliable means of restoring normal glucose homeostasis—the ultimate goal in the treatment of type I diabetes mellitus. Some studies have suggested that the restoration of normoglycemia for extended periods of time have a beneficial effect on patient quality of life, recurrence of diabetic glomerulopathy, microangiopathy, and progression of peripheral and autonomic neuropathy.

The results of pancreas transplantation have steadily improved over the past 20 years; gains are largely due to the evolution of surgical techniques and more potent, selective immunosuppressive medications. In the United States, the current one-year pancreas graft survival rate (when combined with a renal transplant) is 89% (96). Despite the remarkable improvements made in the graft survival rates for all types of pancreatic transplantation, the high prevalence of graft loss caused by immunologic rejection and surgical complications continues to be a problem. Technical problems account for approximately 8% of transplant pancreas failure in the United States.

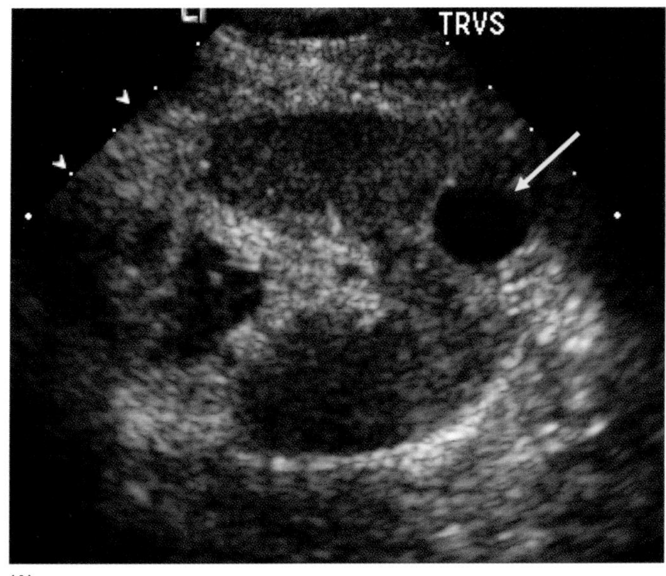

(A)

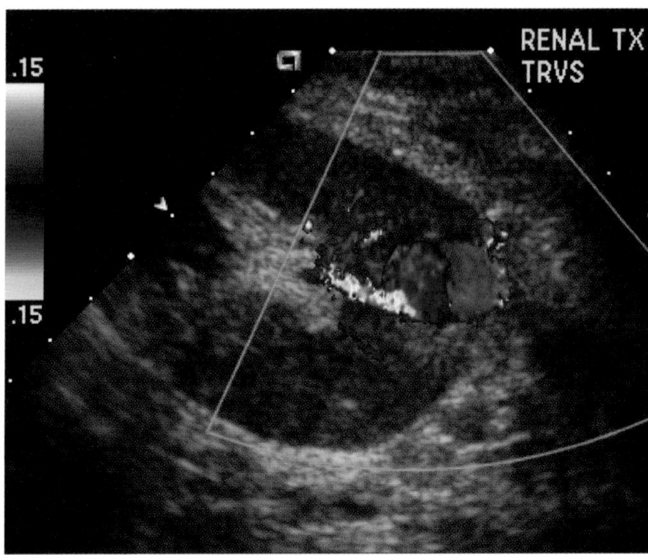

(B)

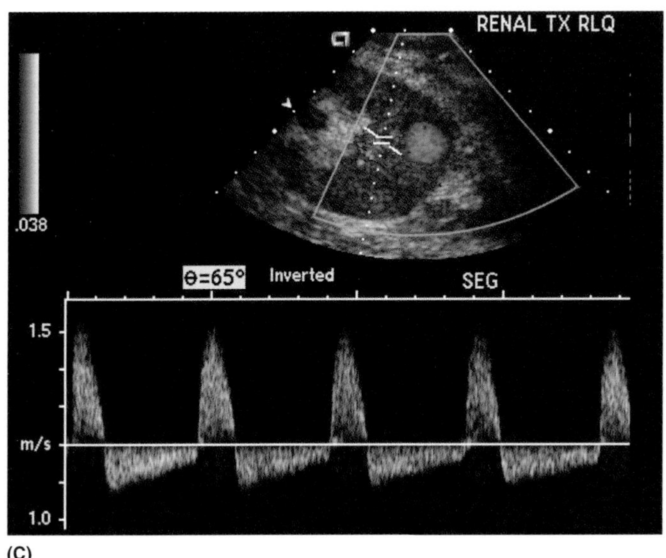

(C)

FIGURE 41 A–C ■ (**A**) Transverse image of the mid-renal transplant. An anechoic structure along the capsular surface mimics a cyst (*arrow*). (**B**) Color Doppler, however, shows flow within this "cyst." Note the swirling distribution of the color. (**C**) Spectral Doppler shows the classic "to and fro" pattern of a pseudoaneurysm. There is a higher likelihood of this complication with a more centrally directed biopsy. *Source*: Courtesy of Dr. Keyanoosh Hosseinzadeh.

These include thrombosis 6.4%, infection 1.1%, pancreatitis 0.3%, bleeding 0.3%, and anastomotic leak 0.7% (96).

The majority (78%) of pancreas transplants in the United States are performed simultaneously with a renal transplant (Fig 42). In this way, only one surgical procedure is required, a single immunosuppressive regimen successfully treats both organs, and a transplant rejection crisis can be more easily identified by monitoring of renal function rather than pancreas function alone.

A complete sonographic examination of the pancreas transplant recipient should cover the points listed in Table 6.

Ultrasonographic Anatomy

The transplanted pancreas is one of the more difficult organs to monitor by any imaging modality. Ultrasound evaluation of the pancreas transplant can be very difficult. Because the pancreas does not have a discrete investing capsule, it is difficult to define its margins with sonography. Taken out of its normal anatomic location, it becomes more difficult to perceive, especially when camouflaged among bowel loops. Furthermore, in the absence of an adjacent liver, determining its relative echogenicity is difficult. With inflammation of the pancreas and the associated edema of the adjacent tissues, the already hard-to-define pancreas becomes even more indistinct. The one intrinsic anatomic landmark helpful in determining that it is indeed the pancreas being imaged is the pancreatic duct, but it is not always conspicuous. Identification of the pancreas may be improved by use of color flow or power Doppler imaging. It identifies flow within the gland and the adjacent transplanted splenic artery and vein. This helps it stand out against background bowel loops (Fig. 43). The vascular pedicle to the transplant pancreas is probably the most conspicuous component of the organ. The splenic artery and vein are usually anastomosed to the distal aorta and IVC or the common iliac artery and vein.

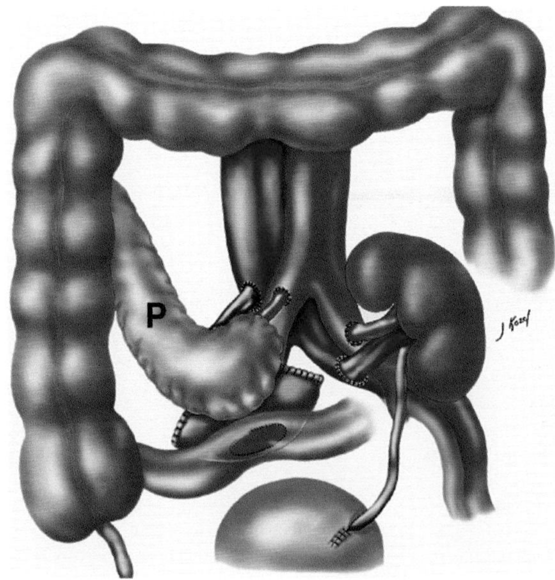

FIGURE 42 ■ Artist rendering of a combined renal pancreas transplant. Typically, the pancreas (P) is transplanted on the right with an interposed duodenal stump between pancreas and ileum. The splenic artery and vein, which serve as the vascular pedicle for the pancreas transplant, are anastomosed to the common iliac artery and vein.

The management of exocrine secretions is one of the most difficult aspects of pancreas transplantation and it continues to evolve. In the early 1980s, the technique of bladder drainage was developed; until recently, nearly all pancreas transplants had their exocrine drainage via a duodenal segment that was anastomosed to the urinary bladder. The two ends of the duodenum, harvested with the pancreas, are inverted and closed with a stapler (99–101). This technique also had numerous complications including hematuria 15.7%, duodenal segment leak 14.2%, reflux pancreatitis 11.4%, recurrent urinary tract infection 10.4%, urethritis 3.3%, and urethral stricture 2.8% (102). It was difficult to manage these complications medically and numerous recipients required enteric conversion (103–105). With the introduction of mycophenolate mofetil (Roche Laboratories, Nutley, New Jersey, U.S.A.), a dramatic decrease was seen in the incidence of acute pancreas transplant rejection (106). Because of the decrease in steroid use, the anastomotic integrity at the duodenoileal anastomosis is better maintained; this has decreased the incidence of multiple anastomotic complications (intra-abdominal infection, bowel obstruction, pancreatitis, and anastomotic mycotic PAs) previously highly associated with enteric drainage. More refined immunosuppression has thus largely accounted for the adoption of duodenal-ileal anastamosis as the primary exocrine drainage technique at most transplantation centers (Fig. 42).

TABLE 6 ■ Pancreas Transplant—Sonographic Examination Checklist

- Review the surgical record, especially with regard to the vasculature and drainage technique. Review any available prior imaging studies
- Evaluate organ echotexture. Make certain it is uniform throughout
- Rule out pancreatic duct dilatation
- Rule out peripancreatic fluid collections
- Rule out pseudocyst
- Examine the main artery to the transplant, particularly near its anastomosis
- Verify venous patency, particularly with high-resistance arterial inflow to the organ
- Verify uniform parenchymal perfusion by color and power Doppler

Up to 95% of multiorgan donors serve as both liver and pancreas donors. These organs are usually removed en bloc, minimizing the chances of injury to the hepatic blood supply. After a combined harvest, however, it may be necessary to reconstruct the pancreatic arterial blood supply with a donor iliac y-graft. The hypogastric artery is anastomosed to the splenic artery and external iliac artery to the superior mesenteric artery (107). Complex vascular reconstruction may confuse the sonographer, and therefore, an accurate description of the surgical anatomy is essential for successful ultrasound imaging and Doppler of the organ and its vascular supply.

Complications

Many sonographic patterns of pancreas transplant dysfunction have been described, including focal or diffuse inhomogeneity of the echo texture, increased or decreased overall echogenicity, and graft swelling. Unfortunately, none of these imaging findings is pathognomonic for any one complication of the pancreas transplant. In general, acute inflammatory changes tend to result in an edematous swollen pancreas and a chronic insult tends to result in a small echogenic gland. These characteristics, however, do not help in solving the immediate clinical dilemma, specifically, differentiation between pancreatitis, rejection, and vascular compromise.

Pancreas thrombosis results in rapid cessation of graft function. It usually occurs soon after transplantation. The graft becomes swollen and tender and graft necrosis ensues. The etiology is often unclear, but prolonged preservation time or graft injury is often implicated. Another factor is the relatively low flow state in the transplanted splenic artery (blind ending since the donor spleen has been removed). Twisting and kinking of the vascular pedicle must also be considered since these are intraperitoneal transplants. Nonvisualization of flow within the organ is an ominous finding (Fig. 44). If identified promptly, however, thrombolytic therapy alone, or in combination with surgical thrombectomy and/or organ detorsion, has been reported to succeed in restoring transplant perfusion. Early diagnosis of pancreas transplant vascular complications is thus of paramount importance for appropriate treatment and organ salvage (108).

The preferred screening modality for graft thrombosis is Doppler ultrasound (109,110). The sonologist, however, must optimize scan parameters for low-velocity flow. Since the examiner is asked to make a diagnosis of

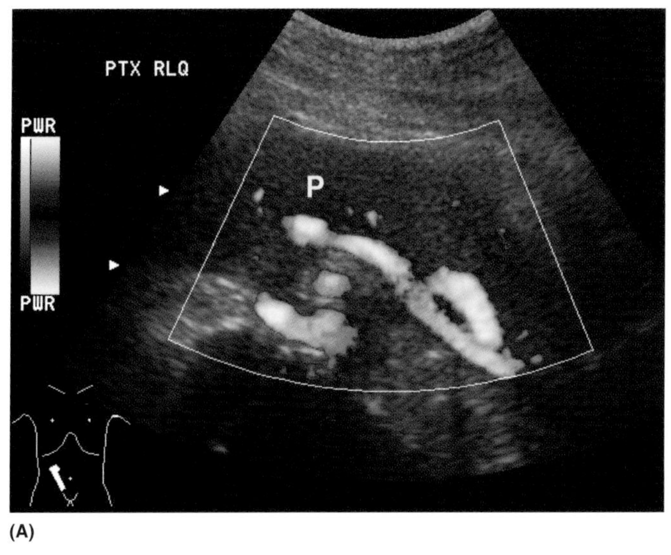

(A)

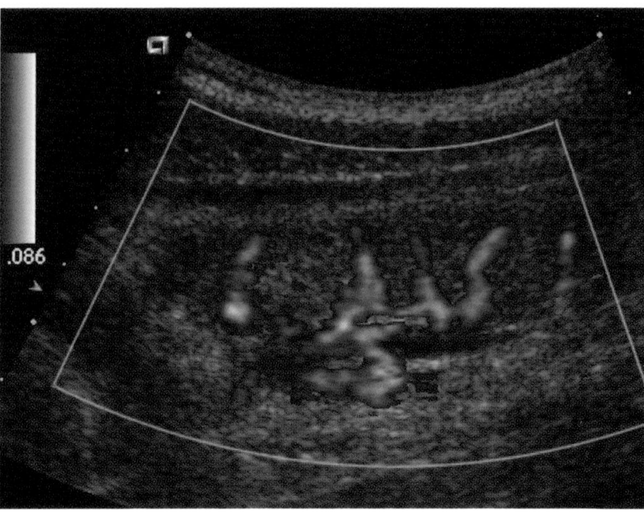

(B)

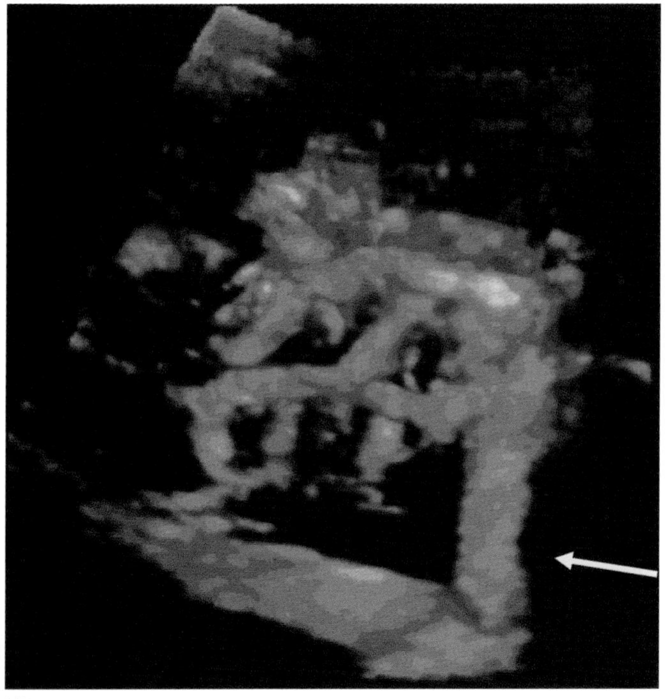

(C)

FIGURE 43 A–C ■ (**A**) Power Doppler image of the transplant pancreas (P). The vascular pedicle to the transplant pancreas is a prominent feature that helps to distinguish it from the surrounding bowel loops. (**B**) Setting scan parameters for slower velocities can depict branch vasculature within the pancreas transplant. This of course may be difficult when there is significant peristalsis in adjacent small bowel loops. (**C**) If a sufficient sonographic window is available, then a 3D rendering of the vascular pedicle (*arrow*) can document its integrity.

absent flow, inappropriate settings may result in a false positive diagnosis of thrombosis, leading to unnecessary angiography (111). Splenic vein thrombosis may be particularly difficult to confidently identify on Doppler examination. Clot is only rarely directly imaged, and the lack of flow within the splenic vein may be a result of severe venous stasis (secondary to rejection or transplantation pancreatitis). MRI/MRA is a useful diagnostic test in those patients with equivocal findings at Doppler examination.

Although ultrasound is excellent in identifying parapancreatic fluid collections, the finding is frequently nonspecific. Abscess, hematoma, complex pseudocyst, or liquefied phlegmon may all have similar ultrasound appearance of a complicated, debris-filled, irregular collection (Fig. 45). Since the pancreas is typically intraperitoneal, blood will track into the recesses of the pelvis and manifest as free intraperitoneal fluid with debris. The true extent of a fluid collection is better evaluated by CT in which bowel gas does not limit the field of view. Furthermore, follow-up CT examinations can be more reliably compared than ultrasound examinations. The source of a fluid collection is best evaluated by a contrast study or by aspiration. Postoperative infections can be very aggressive and difficult to treat (Fig. 46). Microbes, in combination with pancreatic fluids, can both digest and infect adjacent tissues. The patient has limited ability to contain the infection because of immunotherapy. Antibiotic therapy and percutaneous drainage of a peripancreatic abscess/phlegmon may resolve the infection but usually not until significant

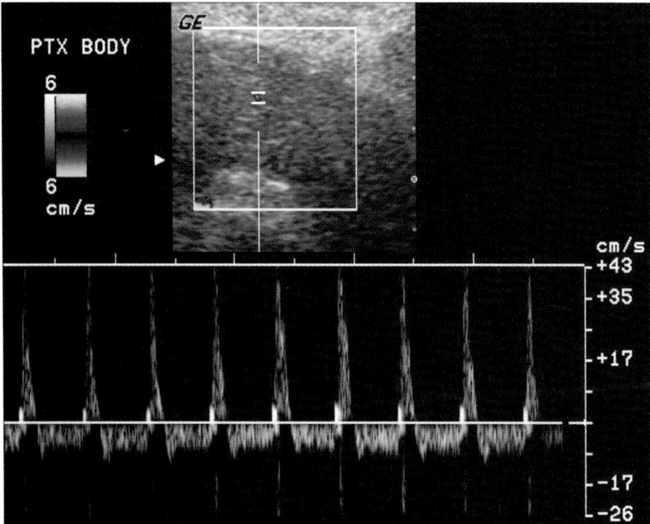

FIGURE 44 ■ Color and spectral Doppler image of the pancreas. No color flow can be identified within the gland. A spectral Doppler of the feeding artery shows extremely high resistance with spike of systolic inflow and reversed outflow throughout diastole.

loss of graft function, which eventually may require transplant pancreatectomy. CT is the most reliable technique for detecting an abscess, determining its extent, and guiding drainage.

Although the digestive enzymes are typically drained into the gut via the duodenal stump, some may leak around the pancreas vasculature predisposing to PA formation, especially in the region of the anastomosis. Arterial flow within a perianastomotic fluid collection, the presence of swirling blood on color Doppler, and a to-and-fro spectral Doppler waveform indicate a transplant associated PA (Fig. 32) (112). Rupture of transplant associated PA has been described and is a life-threatening event (113). The pancreas transplant, as any other transplanted organ, requires occasional biopsy and this increases the risk of developing an AVF. Doppler findings are similar to AVFs seen in other locations (Fig. 47).

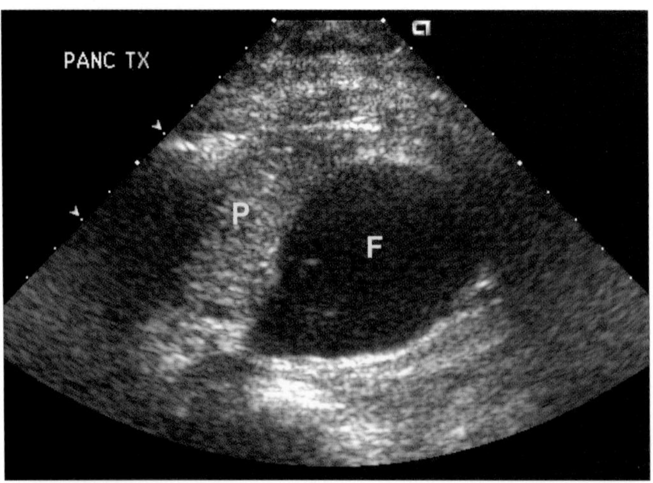

FIGURE 45 ■ Transverse right lower quadrant sonogram reveals a collection of fluid (F) with some debris adjacent to the pancreas transplant (P). With the clinical history and laboratory values, we were able to correctly suggest pseudocyst.

Rejection is the major cause of graft loss according to the International Pancreatic Transplant Registry (96). The overall rate has decreased steadily from 6% in the 1990s to 2.2% in the current era. In the setting of simultaneous pancreas kidney transplantation, the most sensitive marker for pancreas allograft rejection is the rise in serum creatinine that occurs with concurrent renal transplant rejection. In nearly 90% of rejection episodes, kidney dysfunction manifests before pancreas endocrine dysfunction. With isolated pancreas transplantation, or in the unusual episode of isolated pancreas rejection without kidney rejection, a drop in urinary amylase level is an indicator of pancreas transplant dysfunction (an important advantage of the bladder drainage technique). Studies by the University of Minnesota group have shown that mononuclear cell infiltration involves the pancreatic acinar tissues early in rejection (114). It is not until late in the rejection process that the islet cells are affected. Therefore, blood glucose levels do not become elevated until late in the course of rejection, after approximately 90% of the pancreas allograft has been destroyed. To date, there is no reliable serum assay for the evaluation of pancreas graft rejection. Imaging studies, including ultrasound, are limited in detecting or predicting rejection. Preliminary reports suggesting that RI elevation is a positive predictor of pancreas transplant rejection have not proven clinically effective. Many rejecting pancreas transplants have normal RIs (115,116).

Pancreas Transplant Biopsy

Finally, when all imaging alternatives fail, tissue diagnosis becomes necessary. Pancreas transplant biopsy is performed on a limited basis since complications though rare can be severe. Typically, biopsy of the bladder-drained pancreas is performed through a cystoscope advanced into the duodenal segment (117,118). The final orientation of the biopsy needle is guided by ultrasound. The enterically drained pancreas is biopsied percutaneously, again with sonographic guidance. Care must taken to avoid adjacent bowel and Doppler is helpful to avoid injury to major anastomoses and the splenic artery/vein (119).

POSTTRANSPLANTATION LYMPHOPROLIFERATIVE DISORDER

PTLD is a rare but serious complication following solid organ transplantation. The most commonly accepted theory for the pathophysiology of PTLD is that Epstein–Barr virus (EBV)-induced B-cell proliferation, unopposed by the pharmacologically suppressed immune system, causes plasma-cell hyperplasia, then premalignant polymorphic B-cell proliferation, and, eventually, malignant

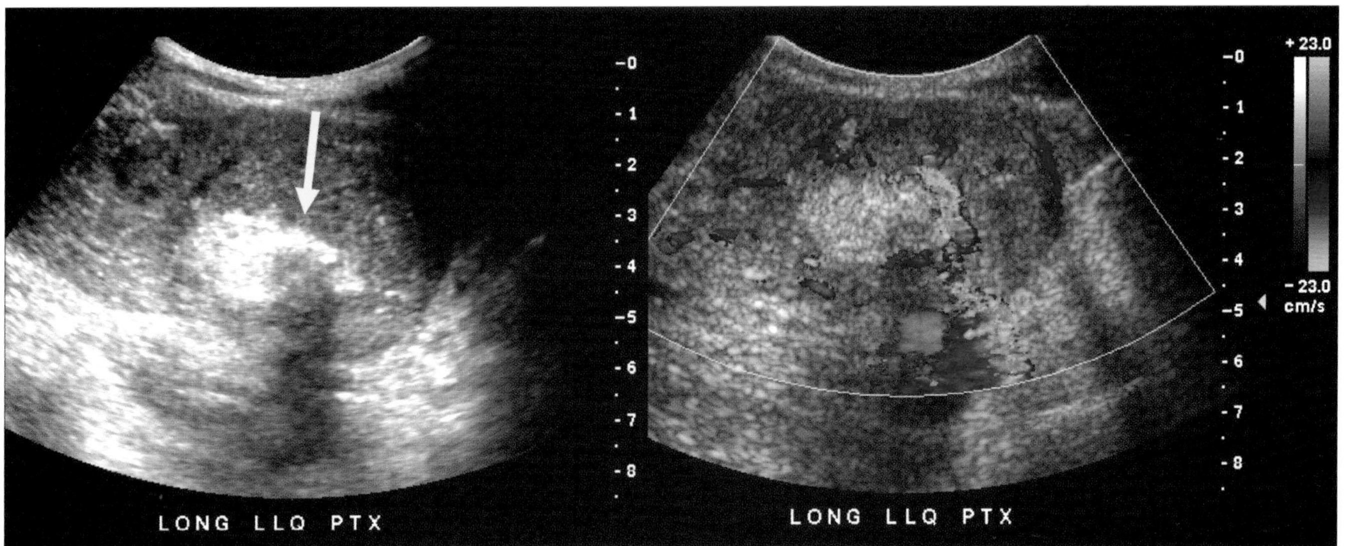

FIGURE 46 ■ Grayscale and color Doppler images of a pancreas transplant reveal an echogenic rounded area with shadowing from gas (*arrow*). Color Doppler shows some hyperemia immediately adjacent to this collection. This was a focal pancreatic abscess.

monoclonal lymphoma. If untreated, it can be fatal (73). Reduction or cessation of immunosuppression is the best treatment and usually results in tumor regression. Early diagnosis prior to the development of frank lymphoma is very important as these patients may have a much better response. A mass that does not decrease after alteration or suspension of immune suppression must be considered lymphoma, and biopsy should be performed (120).

In a large study of PTLD in renal transplant recipients, it occurred in 2% of 1383 patients and contributed to death in more than 50% of these cases (121). The incidence of PTLD has decreased over the past several years as most transplant centers have adopted protocols that minimize immunosuppression.

The liver is the organ most frequently involved in PTLD. It can appear as a focal mass, diffuse infiltration, or a periportal mass (122). PTLD can affect the transplanted kidney and may manifest as a focal renal mass or diffuse infiltration (123). The pancreas transplant may be involved and can present as diffuse enlargement of the allograft or as a focal mass that may be confused with pancreatitis or acute rejection (124).

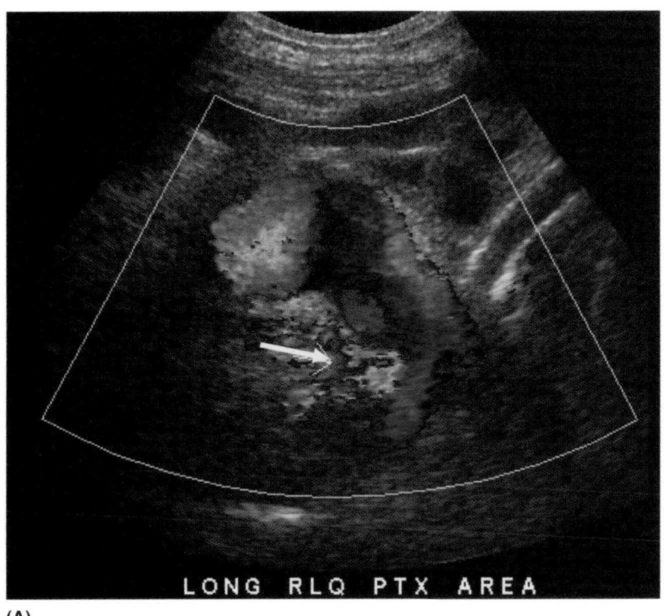

(A)

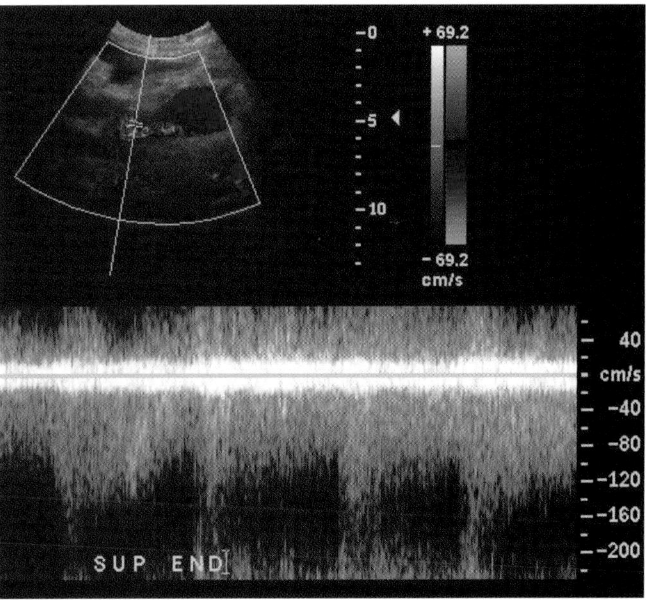

(B)

FIGURE 47 A AND B ■ Color (**A**) and spectral Doppler (**B**) images of a pancreas several days after a biopsy. High-velocity, turbulent, low-resistance arterial flow is present in an area of flash artifact (*arrow*). This was an arteriovenous fistula; a complication of the biopsy.

Since ultrasound is often the first imaging study performed when laboratory tests suggest transplant dysfunction, it plays an important role in the early diagnosis of PTLD. It may detect urinary or biliary obstruction associated with adenopathy or may perceive a new ill-defined, typically hypoechoic mass. Doppler may show vascular distortion by the adenopathy (78). Identification of adenopathy or bowel thickening during ultrasound evaluation of the renal, liver, or pancreas transplant should prompt additional imaging [CT, or CT-positron emission tomography (PET)] to document potential PTLD.

CONCLUSION

These are very rewarding times in the field of organ transplantation. Advances in organ procurement and preservation; better matching of donors and recipients; refined surgical techniques; availability of new, more effective immunosuppressive agents; and improved posttransplant monitoring of organ recipients have contributed to decreased patient morbidity and improved allograft survival. Although ultrasound with Doppler is only able to make a definitive diagnosis in a small percentage of cases, it is extremely useful as a screening tool in the management of transplant complications. All of these advances have allowed transplant recipients a greater opportunity to return to a more normal lifestyle after surgery (125,126).

ACKNOWLEDGMENTS

We would like to thank Joan Palmer for manuscript preparation, and Mike Ledwidge, RT, RDMS, for image preparation.

REFERENCES

1. US Department of Health and Human Services, Public Health Service, Annual report of the US Scientific Registry of Transplant Recipients and the Organ Procurement and Transplantation Network, 1995–2002 (2004 report, kidney transplant survivors): http://www.optn.org/AR2004/default.htm (accessed December 2005).
2. Takemoto SK. HLA matching in the new millennium. Clin Transpl 2003; 387–403.
3. Gabardi S, Cerio J. Future immunosuppressive agents in solid-organ transplantation. Prog Transplant 2004; 14(2):148–156.
4. Pozniak MA, Zagzebski J, Scanlan KA. Spectral and color Doppler artifacts. Radiographics 1992; 12(1):35–44.
5. Pozniak MA, Kelcz F, Stratta R, et al. Extraneous factors affecting resistive index. Invest Radiol 1988; 23(12):899–904.
6. US Department of Health and Human Services, Public Health Service, Annual report of the US Scientific Registry of Transplant Recipients and the Organ Procurement and Transplantation Network, 1995–2002 (2004 report, liver transplant survivors): http://www.optn.org/AR2004/default.htm (accessed December 2005).
7. Wernecke K, Rummeny E, Bongartz G, et al. Detection of hepatic masses in patients with carcinoma: comparative sensitivities of sonography, CT, and MR imaging. AJR Am J Roentgenol 1991; 157(4):731–739.
8. Ravindra KV, Guthrie JA, Woodley H, et al. Preoperative vascular imaging in pediatric liver transplantation. J Pediatr Surg 2005; 40(4):643–647.
9. LaMont J, Koff R, Isselbacker K. Cirrhosis. In: Petersdorf R, Adams R, Braunwald E, et al., eds. Harrison's Principles of Internal Medicine. 10th ed. New York: McGraw-Hill, 1983:1811.
10. Pozniak MA, Baus K. Hepatofugal arterial signal in the main portal vein: an indicator of intravascular tumor spread. Radiology 1991; 180(3):663–666.
11. Dusenbery D, Dodd GD III, Carr BI. Percutaneous fine-needle aspiration of portal vein thrombi as a staging technique for hepatocellular carcinoma: cytologic findings of 46 patients. Cancer 1995; 75(8):2057.
12. Ploeg RJ, Stegall MD, Sproat IA, et al. Effect of surgical and spontaneous portasystemic shunts on liver transplantation. Transplant Proc 1993; 25(2):1946.
13. Fujimoto M, Moriyasu F, Nada T, et al. Influence of spontaneous porotsystemic collateral pathways on portal hemodynamics in living-related liver transplantation in children: Doppler ultrasonographic study. Transplantation 1995; 60(1):41–45.
14. Baccarani U, Adani GL, Sanna A, et al. Portal vein thrombosis after intraportal hepatocytes transplantation in a liver transplant recipient. Transpl Int 2005; 18(6):750–754.
15. Neuhaus P, Platz KP. Liver transplantation: newer surgical approaches. Baillieres Clin Gastroenterol 1994; 8(3):481–493.
16. Houssin D, Boillot O, Soubrane O, et al. Controlled liver splitting for transplantation in two recipien technique, results and perspectives. Br J Surg 1993; 80(1):75–80.
17. Salizzoni M, Andorno E, Bossuto E, et al. Piggyback techniques versus classical technique in orthotopic liver transplantation: a review of 75 cases. Transplant Proc 1994; 26(6):3552–3553.
18. Figueras J, Torras J, Fabregat J, et al. Extra-anatomic venous grafts for portal thrombosis in liver transplantation. Transplant Proc 1995; 27(4):2311–2312.
19. Davidson BR, Gibson M, Dick R, Burroughs A, Rolles K. Incidence, risk factors, management, and outcome of portal vein abnormalities of orthotopic liver transplantation. Transplantation 1994; 57(8):1174–1177.
20. Soin AS, Friend PJ, Rasmussen A, et al. Donor arterial variations in liver transplantation: management and outcome of 527 consecutive grafts. Br J Surg 1996; 83(5):637–641.
21. Todo S, Makowka L, Tzakis AG, et al. Hepatic artery in liver transplantation. Transplant Proc 1987; 19(1 Pt 3):2406–2411.
22. Shaw BW, Iwatsuki S, Starzl TE. Alternative methods of arterialization of the hepatic graft. Surg Gynecol Obstet 1984; 159(5):490–493.
23. Dodd GD III, Orons PD, Campbell WL, et al. Imaging of hepatic transplantation. In: Taveras JM, Ferrucci JT, eds. Radiology: Diagnosis-Imaging-Intervention. Philadelphia: J. B. Lippincott, 1994:1–11.
24. Duncan KA, King SE, Radcliffe JF. Intraperitoneal fluid collections following liver transplantation in a pediatric population. Clin Radiol 1995; 50(1):40–43.
25. Abecassis JP, Pariente D, Hazebroucq V, Houssin D, Chapuis Y, Bonnin A. Subcapsular hepatic necrosis in liver transplantation: CT appearance. AJR Am J Roentgenol 1991; 156(5):981–983.
26. Bauman J, Campbell WL, Demetris AJ, et al. Intrahepatic cholangiographic abnormalities in liver transplan correlation with biopsy evidence of rejection and other disorders. AJR Am J Roentgenol 1989; 152(2):275–279.
27. McAlister V, Grant D, Roy A, Yilmaz Z, Ghent C, Wall W. Posttransplant lymphoproliferative disorders in liver recipients treated with OKT3 or ALG induction immunosuppression. Transplant Proc 1993; 25(1 Pt 2):1400–1401.
28. Moody AR, Wilson SR, Greig PD. Non-Hodgkin's lymphoma in the porta hepatis after orthotopic liver transplantation: sonographic findings. Radiology 1992; 182(3):867–870.

29. Bleday R, Lee E, Jessurun J, et al. Increased risk of early colorectal neoplasms after hepatic transplant in patients with inflammatory bowel disease. Dis Colon Rectum 1993; 36(10):908–912.
30. Garcia-Criado A, Gilabert R, Salmeron JM, et al. Significance of and contributing factors for a high resistive index on Doppler sonography of the hepatic artery immediately after surgery: prognostic implications for liver transplant recipients. AJR Am J Roentgenol 2003; 181(3):831–838.
31. Hall TR, McDiarmid SV, Grant EG, et al. False-negative duplex Doppler studies in children with hepatic artery thrombosis after liver transplantation. AJR Am J Roentgenol 1990; 154(3):573–575.
32. Stell D, Downey D, Marotta P, et al. Prospective evaluation of the role of quantitative Doppler ultrasound surveillance in liver transplantation. Liver Transpl 2004; 10(9):1183–1188.
33. Propeck PA, Scanlan KA. Reversed or absent hepatic arterial diastolic flow in liver transplants shown by duplex sonography: a poor predictor of subsequent hepatic artery thrombosis. AJR Am J Roentgenol 1992; 159(6):1199–1201.
34. Herold C, Reck T, Ott R, et al. Contrast-enhanced ultrasound improves hepatic vessel visualization after orthotopic liver transplantation. Abdom Imaging 2001; 26(6):597–600.
35. Kok T, Haagsma EB, Klompmaker IJ, et al. Doppler Ultrasound of the hepatic artery and vein performed daily in the first two weeks after orthotopic liver transplantation. Invest Radiol 1996; 31(3):173–179.
36. Dodd GD III, Memel DS, Zajko AB, et al. Hepatic artery stenosis and thrombosis in hepatic transplantation: Doppler diagnosis by use of the resistive index and systolic acceleration time. Radiology 1994; 192(3):657–661.
37. Platt JF, Yotzy GG, Bude RO, et al. Use of Doppler sonography for revealing hepatic artery stenosis in liver transplant recipients. AJR Am J Roentgenol 1997; 168(2):473–476..
38. Sidhu PS, Ellis SM, Karani JB, et al. Hepatic artery stenosis following liver transplantation: significance of the tardus parvus waveform and the role of microbubble contrast media in the detection of a focal stenosis. Clin Radiol 2002; 57(9):789–799.
39. Kaneko J, Sugawara Y, Akamatsu N, et al. Prediction of hepatic artery thrombosis by protocol Doppler ultrasonography in pediatric living donor liver transplantation. Abdom Imaging 2004; 29(5):603–605.
40. Vivarelli M, Cucchetti A, La Barba G, et al. Ischemic arterial complications after liver transplantation in the adult: multivariate analysis of risk factors. Arch Surg 2004; 139(10):1069–1074.
41. Worthy SA, Olliff JF, Olliff SP, Buckels JA. Color flow Doppler ultrasound diagnosis of a pseudoaneurysm of the hepatic artery following liver transplantation. J Clin Ultrasound 1994; 22(7):461–465.
42. Otobe Y, Hashimoto T, Shimizu Y, et al. Formation of a fatal arterioportal fistula following needle liver biopsy in a child with a living-related liver transplant: report of a case. Surg Today 1995; 25:916.
43. Jabbour N, Reyes J, Zajko A, et al. Arterioportal fistula following liver biopsy. Three cases occurring in liver transplant recipients. Dig Dis Sci 1995; 25(10):916–919.
44. Doria C, Marino IR. Acute portal vein thrombosis secondary to donor/recipient portal vein diameter mismatch after orthotopic liver transplantation: a case report. Int Surg 2003; 88(4):184–187.
45. Cheng YF, Chen CL, Huang TL, et al. Risk factors for intraoperative portal vein thrombosis in pediatric living donor liver transplantation. Clin Transplant 2004; 18(4):390–394.
46. Corno V, Torri E, Bertani A, et al. Early portal vein thrombosis after pediatric split liver transplantation with left lateral segment graft. Transplant Proc 2005; 37(2):1141–1142.
47. Durham JD, LaBerge JM, Kam I, et al. Portal vein thrombolysis and closure of competitive shunts following liver transplantation. J Vasc Interv Radiol 1994; 5(4):611–615.
48. Fujimoto M, Moriyasu F, Someda H, et al. Evaluation of portal hemodynamics with Doppler ultrasound in living related donor liver transplantation in children: implications for ligation of spontaneous portosystemic collateral pathways. Transplant Proc 1995; 27(1):1174–1176.
49. Nishida S, Kadono J, DeFaria W, et al. Gastroduodenal artery steal syndrome during liver transplantation: intraoperative diagnosis with Doppler ultrasound and management. Transpl Int 2005; 18(3):350–353.
50. Tang SS, Shimizu T, Kishimoto R, et al. Analysis of portal venous waveform after living-related liver transplantation with pulsed Doppler ultrasound. Clin Transplant 2001; 15(6):380–387.
51. Akamatsu N, Sugawara Y, Kaneko J, et al. Surgical repair for late-onset hepatic venous outflow block after living-donor liver transplantation. Transplantation 2004; 77:1768.
52. Carnevale FC, Borges MV, Pinto RA, et al. Endovascular treatment of stenosis between hepatic vein and inferior vena cava following liver transplantation in a child: a case report. Pediatr Transplant 2004; 77(11):1768–1770.
53. Totsuka E, Hakamada K, Narumi S, et al. Hepatic vein anastomotic stricture after living donor liver transplantation. Transplant Proc 2004; 36(8):2252–2254.
54. Rossi AR, Pozniak MA, Zarvan NP. Upper inferior vena caval anastomotic stenosis in liver transplant recipien Doppler US diagnosis. Radiology 1993; 187(2):387–389.
55. Ko EY, Kim TK, Kim PN, et al. Hepatic vein stenosis after living donor liver transplantation: evaluation with Doppler US. Radiology 2003; 229(3):806–810.
56. Kraus TW, Rohren T, Manner M, et al. Successful treatment of complete inferior vena cava thrombosis after liver transplantation by thrombolytic therapy. Br J Surg 1992; 79(6):568–569.
57. Yang MD, Wu CC, Chen HC, et al. Biliary complications in long-term recipients of reduced-size liver transplants. Transplant Proc 1996; 28(3):1680–1681.
58. Popescu I, Sheiner P, Mor E, et al. Biliary complications in 400 cases of liver transplantation. Mt Sinai J Med 1994; 61(1):57–62.
59. Campbell WL, Foster RG, Miller WJ, et al. Changes in extrahepatic bile duct caliber in liver transplant recipients without evidence of biliary obstruction. AJR Am J Roentgenol 1992; 158(5):997–1000.
60. Gholson CF, Zibari G, McDonald JC. Endoscopic diagnosis and management of biliary complications following orthotopic liver transplantation. Dig Dis Sci 1996; 41(6):1045–1053.
61. Colonna JO, Shaked A, Gomes AS, et al. Biliary strictures complicating liver transplantation: incidence, pathogenesis, management and outcome. Ann Surg 1992; 216(3):344–350.
62. Zajko AB, Bennett MJ, Campbell WL, et al. Mucocele of the cystic duct remnant in eight liver transplant recipien findings at cholangiography, CT, US. Radiology 1990; 177(3):691–693.
63. Barton P, Maier A, Steininger R, et al. Biliary sludge after liver transplantation: 1. Imaging findings and efficacy of various imaging procedures. AJR Am J Roentgenol 1995; 164(4):859–864.
64. Sheng R, Ramirez CB, Zajko AB, Campbell WL. Biliary stones and sludge in liver transplant patien 1 13-year experience. Radiology 1996; 198(1):243–247.
65. Jequier S, Jequier JC, Hanquinet S, et al. Orthotopic liver transplants in children: change in hepatic venous Doppler wave pattern as an indicator of acute rejection. Radiology 2003; 226(1):105–112.
66. Van Thiel DH, Gavaler JS, Wright H, Tzakis A. Liver biopsy. Its safety and complications as seen at a liver transplant center. Transplantation 1993; 55(5):1087–1090.
67. US Department of Health and Human Services, Public Health Service, Annual report of the US Scientific Registry of Transplant Recipients and the Organ Procurement and Transplantation Network, 1995–2002 (2004 report, kidney transplant survivors): http://www.optn.org/AR2004/default.htm (accessed July 2005).
68. Belzer FO. Transplantation of the right kidney: surgical technique revisited. Surgery 1991; 110(1):113–115.
69. Sollinger HW, Ploeg RJ, Eckhoff DE, et al. Two hundred consecutive simultaneous pancreas-kidney transplants with bladder drainage. Surgery 1993; 114(4):736–743.
70. Benoit G, Blanchet P, Moukarzel M, et al. Surgical complications in kidney transplantation. Transplant Proc 1994; 26(1):287–288.
71. Hashimoto Y, Nagano S, Ohsima S, et al. Surgical complications in kidney transplantation: experience from 1200 transplants performed

over 20 years at six hospitals in central Japan. Transplant Proc 1996; 28(3):1465–1467.

72. Drudi FM, Cascone F, Pretagostini R, et al. Role of color Doppler US in the evaluation of renal transplant. Radiol Med (Torino) 2001; 101(4):243–250. [Article in Italian].

73. Pozniak MA, Kelcz F, D'Alessandro A, et al. Sonography of renal transplan the effect of acute tubular necrosis, cyclosporine nephrotoxicity, and acute rejection on resistive index and renal length. AJR Am J Roentgenol 1992; 158(4):791–797.

74. Tublin ME, Bude RO, Platt JF. Review: the resistive index in renal Doppler sonography: where do we stand? AJR Am J Roentgenol 2003; 18 0(4):885–892.

75. Genkins SM et al. Duplex Doppler sonography of renal transplan lack of sensitivity and specificity in establishing pathologic diagnosis. AJR Am J Roentgenol 1989; 152(3):535–539.

76. Kelcz F, Pozniak MA, Pirsch JD, et al. Pyramidal appearance and resistive index: insensitive and nonspecific sonographic indicators of renal transplant rejection. AJR Am J Roentgenol 1990; 155(3):531–535.

77. Perrella RR, Duerincky AJ, Tessler FN, et al. Evaluation of renal transplant dysfunction by duplex Doppler sonography: a prospective study and review of the literature. Am J Kidney Dis 1990; 15(6):544–550.

78. Akiyama T, Ikegami M, Hara Y, et al. Hemodynamic study of renal transplant chronic rejection using power Doppler sonography. Transplant Proc 1996; 28(3):1458–1460.

79. Saarinen O. Diagnostic value of resistive index of renal transplants in the early postoperative period. Acta Radiologica 1991; 32(2):166–169.

80. Koga S, Tanabe K, Yagisawa TT, et al. Urological complications in renal transplantation. Transplant Proc 1996; 28(3):1472–1473.

81. Gruessner RW, Fasola C, Benedetti E, et al. Laparoscopic drainage of lymphoceles after kidney transplantation: indications and limitations. Surgery 1995; 117(3):288–295.

82. Platt JF, Rubin JM, Ellis JH. Distinction between obstructive and nonobstructive pyelocaliectasis with duplex Doppler sonography. AJR Am J Roentgenol 1989; 153(5):997–1000.

83. Platt JF, Ellis JH, Rublin JM. Renal transplant pyelocaliectasis: role of duplex Doppler US in evaluation. Radiology 1991; 179(2): 425–428.

84. Dodd GD, Tublin ME, Shah A, et al. Imaging of vascular complications associated with renal transplantation. AJR Am J Roentgenol 1991; 157(3):449–459.

85. Pozniak MA, Dodd GD, Kelcz F. Ultrasonographic evaluation of renal transplantation. Radiol Clin North Am 1992; 30(5): 1053–1066.

86. Grenier N, Douws C, Morel D, et al. Detection of vascular complications in renal allografts with color Doppler flow imaging. Radiology 1991; 178(1):217–223.

87. Baxter GM, Ireland H, Moss JG, et al. Colour Doppler ultrasound in renal transplant artery stenosis: which Doppler index? Clin Radiol 1995; 50(9):618–622.

88. Roberts JP, Ascher NL, Fryd DS, et al. Transplant renal artery stenosis. Transplantation 1989; 48(4):580–583.

89. Patriquin HB, Lafortune M, Jequier JC, et al. Stenosis of the renal artery: assessment of slowed systole in the downstream circulation with Doppler sonography. Radiology 1992; 184(2):479–485.

90. Saarinen O, Salmela K, Edgren J. Doppler ultrasound in the diagnosis of renal transplant artery stenosis - value of resistive index. Acta Radiol 1994; 35(6):586–589.

91. Handa N, Fukunaga R, Etani H, et al. Efficacy of echo-Doppler examination for the evaluation of renovascular disease. Ultrasound Med Biol 1988; 14(1):1–5.

92. Stavros AT, Parker SH, Yakes WF, et al. Segmental stenosis of the renal artery: pattern recognition of tardus and parvus abnormalities with duplex sonography. Radiology 1992; 184(2):487–492.

93. Kribs SW, Rankin RN. Doppler ultrasonography after renal transplantation: value of reversed diastolic flow in diagnosing renal vein obstruction. Can Assoc Radiol J 1993; 44(6):434–438.

94. Middleton WD, Kellman GM, Melson GL, et al. Postbiopsy renal transplant arteriovenous fistulas: color Doppler versus US characteristics. Radiology 1989; 171(1):253–257.

95. Hubsch PJS, Mostbeck G, Barton PP, et al. Evaluation of arteriovenous fistulas and pseudoaneurysms in renal allografts following percutaneous needle biopsy: color coded Doppler sonography vs. duplex Doppler sonography. J Ultrasound Med 1990; 9(2):95–100.

96. University of Minnesota, IPTR Annual Report 2003: http://www.med.umn.edu/IPTR/annual_reports/2003_annual.html (accessed 2006).

97. Stegall MD, Ploeg RJ, Pirsch JD, et al. Living-related kidney transplant or simultaneous pancreas-kidney for diabetic renal failure? Transplant Proc 1993; 25(1 Pt 1):230–232.

98. Pirsch JD, Andrews C, Hricik DE, et al. Pancreas transplantation for diabetes mellitus. Am J Kidney Dis 1996; 27(3):444–450.

99. Sollinger HW, Pirsch JD, D'Alessandro AM, et al. Advantages of bladder drainage in pancreas transplantation: a personal view. Clin Transplant 1990; 4(1):32–36.

100. Abouna GM, Kumar MS, Miller JL, et al. Combined kidney and pancreas transplantation for diabetes mellitus using modified bladder-drainage technique and employing pediatric donors. Transplant Proc 1993; 25(3):2232–2233.

101. Illner WD, Hofmann GO, Schneeberger H, et al. Experience with clinical pancreatic transplantation using the bladder drainage technique. Transplant Proc 1995; 27(6):2983.

102. Sollinger HW, Messing EM, Eckhoff DE, et al. Urological complications in 210 consecutive simultaneous pancreas-kidney transplants with bladder drainage. Ann Surg 1993; 218(4):561–568.

103. Sindhi R, Stratta RJ, Taylor RJ, et al. Experience with enteric conversion after pancreas transplantation with bladder drainage. Transplant Proc 1993; 27(6):3014–3015.

104. Ploeg RJ, D'Alessandro AM, Knechtle SJ, et al. Urological complications and enteric conversion after pancreas transplantation with bladder drainage. Transplant Proc 1994; 26(2):458–459.

105. Corry RJ, Egidi MJ, Shapiro R, et al. Enteric drainage of pancreas transplants revisited. Transplant Proc 1995; 27(6):3048–3049.

106. Anonymous. Mycophenolate mofetil—a new immunosuppressant for organ transplantation. Med Lett Drugs Ther 1995; 37(958): 84–86.

107. Sollinger HW. Current status of simultaneous pancreas-kidney transplantation. Transplant Proc 1994; 26(2):375–378.

108. Spiros D, Christos D, John B, et al. Vascular complications of pancreas transplantation. Pancreas 2004; 28(4):413–420.

109. Nikolaidis P, Amin RS, Hwang CM, et al. Role of sonography in pancreatic transplantation. Radiographics 2003; 23(4):939–949.

110. Foshager MC, Hedlund LJ, Troppmann C, et al. Venous thrombosis of pancreatic transplan diagnosis by duplex sonography. AJR Am J Roentgenol 1997; 169(5):1269–1273.

111. Finlay DE, Letourneau, JG, Longley DG. Assessment of vascular complications of renal, hepatic, and pancreatic transplantation. Radiographics 1992; 12(5):981–996.

112. Tobben PJ, Zajko AB, Sumkin JH, et al. Pseudoaneurysms complicating organ transplantation: roles of CT, duplex sonography, and angiography. Radiology 1988; 169(1):65–70.

113. Green BT, Tuttle-Newhall J, Suhocki P, et al. Massive gastrointestinal hemorrhage due to rupture of a donor pancreatic artery pseudoaneurysm in a pancreas transplant patient. Clin Transplant 2004; 18(1):108–111.

114. Sibley RK, Sutherland DE. Pancreas transplantation: an immunohistologic and histopathologic examination of 100 grafts. Am J Pathol 1987; 128(1):151–170.

115. Patel B, Wolverson MK, Mahanta B. Pancreatic transplant rejection: assessment with duplex US. Radiology 1989; 173(1):131–135.

116. Wong JJ, Klassen DK, Simon EM, et al. Sonographic evaluation of acute pancreatic transplant rejection: morphology-Doppler analysis versus guided percutaneous biopsy. AJR Am J Roentgenol 1996; 166(4):803–807.

117. Kuhr CS, Barr D, Perkins JD, et al. Use of ultrasound and cystoscopically guided pancreatic allograft biopsies and transabdominal

renal allograft biopsies: safety and efficacy in kidney-pancreas transplant recipients. J Urol 1995; 153(2):316–321.

118. Nelson NL, Lowell JA, Taylor RJ, et al. Pancreas transplan efficacy of US-guided cystoscopic biopsy. Radiology 1994; 191(1): 283–284.

119. Malek SK, Potdar S, Martin JA, et al. Percutaneous ultrasound guided pancreas allograft biopsy: a single-center experience. Transplantation Proc 2005; 37(10):4436–4437.

120. Garnier JL, Berger F, Martin X, et al. Post-transplant B-cell lymphomas–correlation of late stage B-cell differentiation and progression of disease: treatment with chimeric monoclonal antibody. Transplant Proc 1995; 27(2):1777.

121. Bates WD, Gray DWR, Dada MA, et al. Lymphoproliferative disorders in Oxford renal transplant recipients. J Clin Pathol 2003; 56(6):439–446.

122. Pickhardt PJ, Siegel MJ. Posttransplantation lymphoproliferative disorder of the abdomen: CT evaluation in 51 patients. Radiology 1999; 213(1):73–78.

123. Vrachliotis TG, Vaswani KK, Davies EA, et al. CT findings in posttransplantation lymphoproliferative disorder of renal transplants. AJR Am J Roentgenol 2000; 175(1):183–188.

124. Meador TL, Krebs TL, Cheong JJ, et al. Imaging features of posttransplantation lymphoproliferative disorder in pancreas transplant recipients. AJR Am J Roentgenol 2000; 174(1):121–124.

125. Lee HM. Quality of life after renal transplantation. Transplant Proc 1996; 28(3):1171.

126. Park IH, Yoo HJ, Han DJ, et al. Changes in the quality of life before and after renal transplantation and comparison of the quality of life between kidney transplant recipients, dialysis patients, and normal controls. Transplant Proc 1996; 28(3):1937–1938.

Liver ● *Suhas G. Parulekar and Robert L. Bree* 16

(*Continued*)

INTRODUCTION

The liver, the largest abdominal organ, occupies most of the right upper abdomen. Sonography of the liver is most frequently performed for evaluation of suspected focal or diffuse abnormalities. With the increasing availability of color Doppler ultrasound, sonography plays an important role in the evaluation of hepatic vascular abnormalities.

TECHNIQUE

Sonography of the liver is ideally performed when the patient has fasted for 8 to 12 hours before the examination, to avoid interference from bowel gas and residue. The examination is performed using 3.5- or 5-MHz sector or curved linear-array transducers. In obese patients, it is necessary to use 2.5-MHz transducers for adequate penetration of the right lobe. One can use 5- or 7.5-MHz linear-array transducers to evaluate the surface of the liver. The initial examination is performed with the patient in the supine position, followed by examination in the left posterior oblique position, which is specially useful for evaluation of the deeper posterior portions of the right lobe. Most of the liver is accessible by subcostal scanning. Cranial portions of the liver, especially the subdiaphragmatic portions of the right lobe, may be difficult to evaluate and are better seen by intercostal scanning with sector transducers. Electronic focusing, when available, should be adjusted throughout the examination to optimally evaluate both superficial and deep portions of the liver.

Duplex Doppler and color Doppler sonography can enable the clinician to differentiate blood vessels from bile ducts and to document vascular occlusions or thrombosis, collateral vessels, and flow within hepatic lesions.

NORMAL ANATOMY

Lobar and Segmental Anatomy

The liver is anatomically divided into right, left, and caudate lobes (Fig. 1). The right lobe is further subdivided into anterior and posterior segments, and the left lobe is subdivided into medial and lateral segments (Tables 1 and 2) (1). The right lobe, which is usually the largest lobe of the liver, is separated from the left lobe by the main lobar fissure. On the transverse view, the main lobar fissure is found in a line joining the gallbladder fossa with the inferior vena cava, but determining the plane of the line joining them may be difficult sonographically (Figs. 1 and 2) (1). Part of the main lobar fissure can be frequently seen as a hyperechoic linear structure that is anterior or cranial to the gallbladder on the transverse view and is between the right portal vein and the gallbladder on the sagittal view (Figs. 2 and 3). The middle hepatic vein courses within the cranial portion of the main lobar fissure and separates the anterior segment of the right lobe from

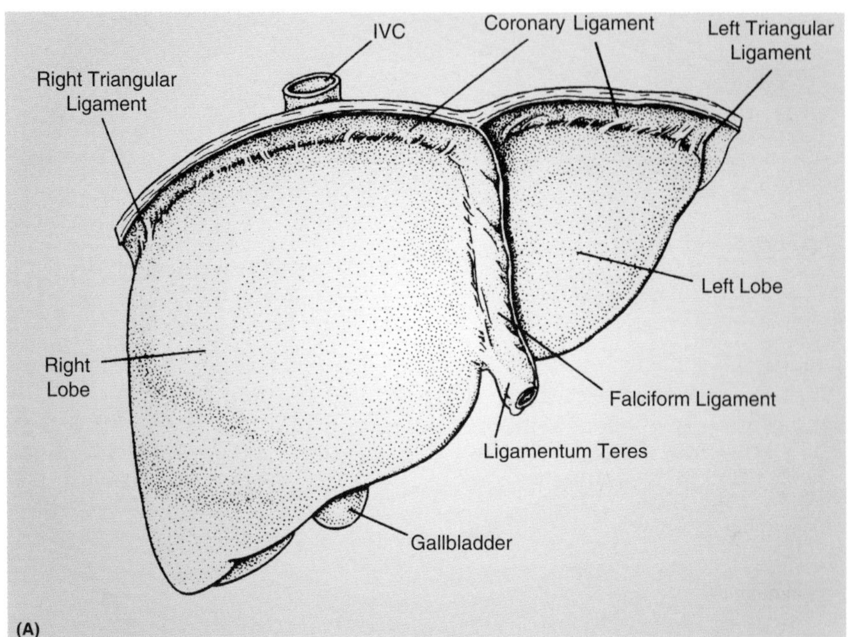

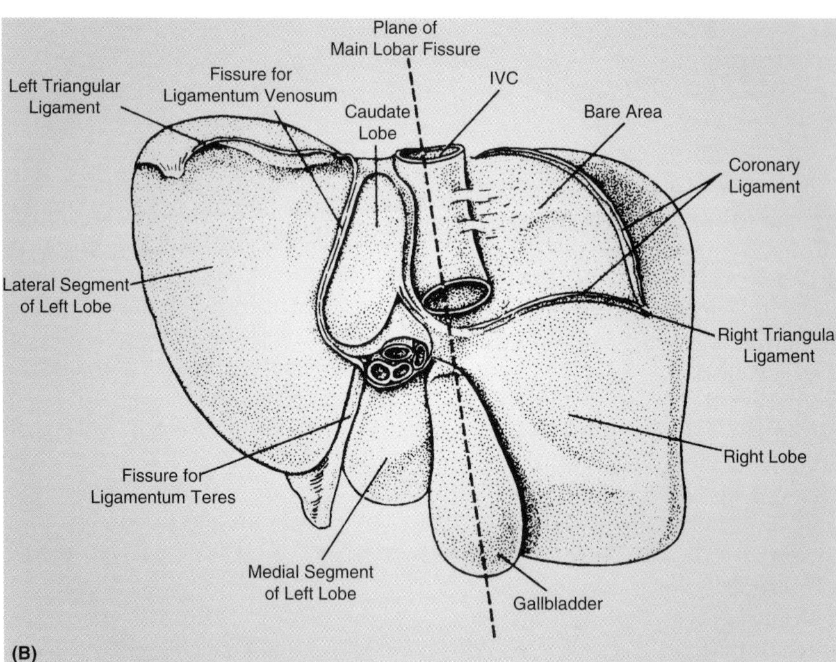

FIGURE 1 A AND B ■ Lobes, ligaments, and fissures of the liver. Diagrams of (**A**) the anterior surface and (**B**) the posterior surface of the liver.

the medial segment of the left lobe (Fig. 4). The right hepatic vein coursing through the right intersegmental fissure divides the right lobe into anterior and posterior segments (Fig. 4). In many persons, on sagittal view, a long, horizontal branch of the right hepatic vein is identified, separating the anterior and posterior segments of the right lobe (Fig. 5B). The anterior and posterior branches of the right portal vein course centrally in the anterior and posterior segments of the right lobe, respectively (Figs. 5 and 6A). The left lobe is divided into the medial segment (the quadrate lobe) and lateral segment by the left intersegmental fissure. The left intersegmental fissure can be divided into cranial, middle, and caudal thirds (1). The left hepatic vein courses within the cranial third (Fig. 4), the ascending portion of the left portal vein courses within the middle third (Fig. 6B), and the fissure for the

TABLE 1 ■ Anatomic Structures Useful for Separating and Identifying the Hepatic Segments

Structure	Location	Usefulness
Right hepatic vein	Right intersegmental fissure	Separates anterior and posterior segments of cephalic aspect of right lobe
Middle hepatic vein	Main lobar fissure	Separates cephalic aspects of right and left lobes
Left hepatic vein	Left intersegmental fissure	Separates medial and lateral segments of cephalic aspect of left lobe
Right portal vein (anterior branch)	Intrasegmental in anterior segment of right lobe	Courses centrally in anterior segment of right lobe
Right portal vein (posterior branch)	Intrasegmental in posterior segment of right lobe	Courses centrally in posterior segment of right lobe
Left portal vein (horizontal portion)	Courses anterior to caudate lobe	Separates caudate lobe from medial segment of left lobe
Left portal vein (ascending portion)	Turns anteriorly in left intersegmental fissure	Separates medial and lateral segments of left lobe
Gallbladder fossa	Main lobar fissure	Separates caudal aspects of right and left lobes
Ligamentum teres	Left intersegmental fissure	Separates medial and lateral segments of caudal aspect of left lobe
Fissure for ligamentum venosum	Left anterior margin of caudate lobe	Separates caudate lobe from lateral segment of left lobe

Source: Modified from Ref. 1.

ligamentum teres (Figs. 3A and 7) courses within the caudal third of the left intersegmental fissure. The falciform ligament also courses within the caudal third of this fissure. On the transverse view, the ligamentum teres is frequently seen as a rounded, hyperechoic structure within a fissure (Fig. 3A) (2).

The caudate lobe of the liver is anatomically distinct from both the right and the left hepatic lobes. It is interposed among the inferior vena cava posteriorly, the left hepatic lobe anteriorly and superiorly, and the main portal vein inferiorly (Fig. 8) (3). The proximal horizontal portion of the left portal vein (i.e., pars transversal) courses over the anterior margin of the inferior caudate lobe, separating it from the more anteriorly positioned medial segment of the left hepatic lobe (Fig. 6B). The left anterior margin of the caudate lobe is separated from the lateral segment of the left hepatic lobe by the fissure for the ligamentum venosum (Fig. 8). On the transverse view, the caudate lobe, between the inferior vena cava and the bifurcation of the portal vein, is contiguous with the right lobe. The right inferior margin of the caudate lobe extends in a tongue-like projection, known as the caudate process, between the inferior vena cava and the adjacent main portal vein and the medial portion of the right hepatic lobe. In most persons, the caudate process is small, permitting contact between the main portal vein and the inferior vena cava, and, thus, is not recognized sonographically. The papillary process is a small, ovoid prominence on the anteroinferior aspect of the caudate lobe. Both left and right portal triads give off portal-venous and hepatic-arterial branches to the caudate lobe and receive from it bile duct tributaries. The initial horizontal

TABLE 2 ■ Fissures of the Liver

Fissure	Usefulness	Structures within the Fissure
Main lobar	Separates right lobe from left lobe	Cephalic portion: middle hepatic vein
		Caudal portion: gallbladder fossa
Right intersegmental	Separates anterior and posterior segments of right lobe	Right hepatic vein
Left intersegmental	Separates medial and lateral segments of left lobe	Cranial third: left hepatic vein
		Middle third: ascending portion of left portal vein
		Caudal third: ligamentum teres
		Falciform ligament
Ligamentum teres	Separates medial and lateral segments of left lobe	Ligamentum teres
		Falciform ligament
Ligamentum venosum	Separates caudate lobe from lateral segment of left lobe	

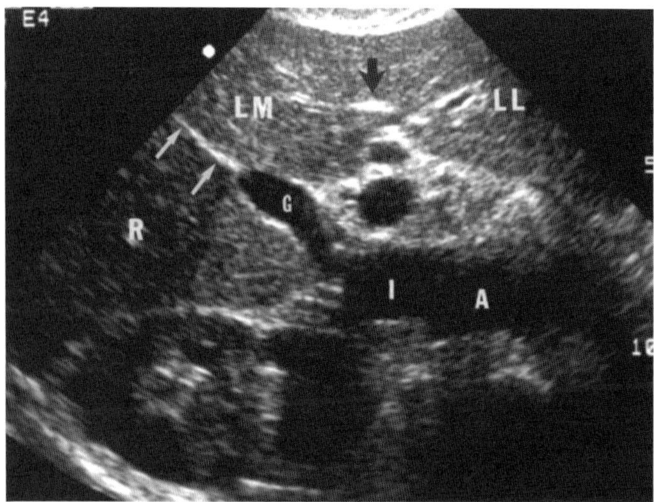

FIGURE 2 ■ Main lobar fissure. Transverse view shows the main lobar fissure (*white arrows*), which appears as a hyperechoic linear structure and is found in a line joining the gallbladder (G) with the inferior vena cava (I). *Black arrow*, ligamentum teres. R, right lobe; LM, medial segment of the left lobe; LL, lateral segment of the left lobe; A, aorta.

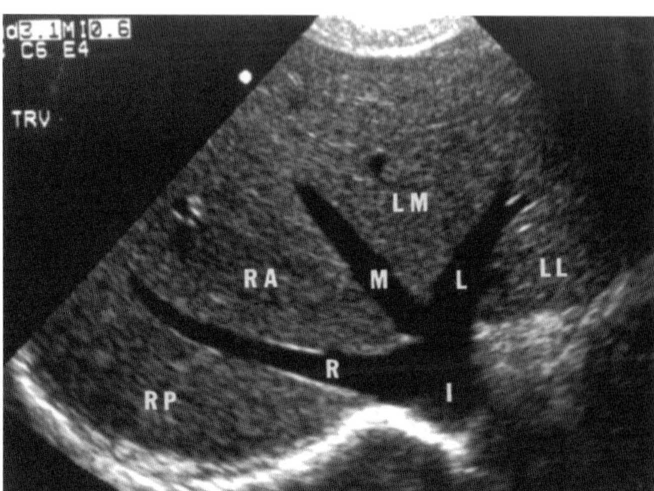

FIGURE 4 ■ Hepatic veins. Transverse view shows three major hepatic veins. The right hepatic vein (R), the middle hepatic vein (M), and the left hepatic vein (L) are seen draining into the inferior vena cava (I). The left and middle hepatic veins join together before entering the inferior vena cava. The right hepatic vein separates the anterior segment of the right lobe (RA) from the posterior segment of the right lobe (RP). The middle hepatic vein separates the anterior segment of the right lobe from the medial segment of the left lobe (LM). The left hepatic vein separates the medial segment of the left lobe from the lateral segment of the left lobe (LL). Note the echogenic walls of the proximal portion of the right hepatic vein and a branch of the left hepatic vein near its distal portion. Major hepatic veins and their larger branches frequently have echogenic walls similar to portal veins.

portion of the left portal vein gives off several branches to the caudate lobe (Fig. 6B). The caudate lobe is drained by a series of small, short, venous channels that extend directly from the posterior aspect of the caudate lobe into the inferior vena cava adjacent to the posterior margin of the caudate lobe. Three major anatomic landmarks—the fissure for the ligamentum venosum, the inferior vena cava, and the pars transversa of the left portal vein—permit sonographic localization of the caudate lobe (3).

The major hepatic veins are intersegmental and course between the hepatic lobes and segments, whereas the major portal vein branches are intrasegmental and course within the lobar segments (1). The only exception is the ascending portion of the left portal vein, which courses within the left intersegmental fissure, separating the medial and lateral segments of the left lobe.

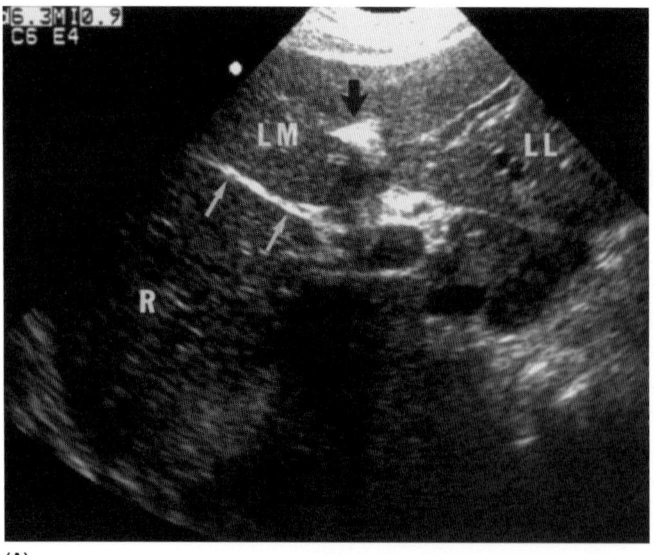

(A)

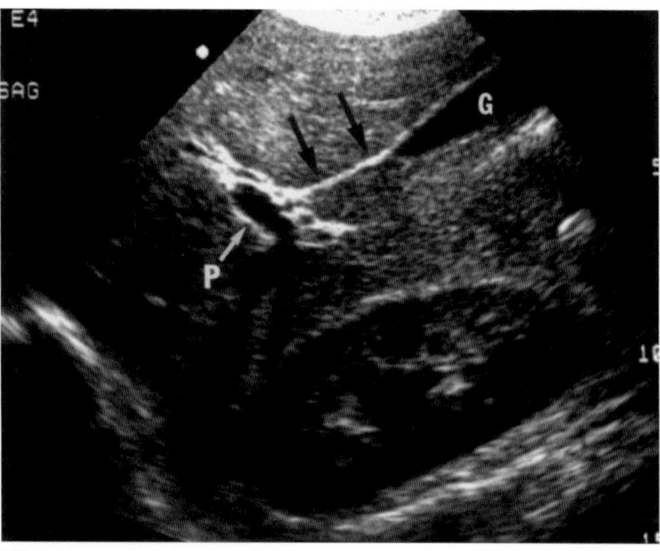

(B)

FIGURE 3 A AND B ■ Main lobar fissure on transverse and sagittal views. (**A**) Main lobar fissure is seen as a hyperechoic linear structure (*white arrows*) separating the right lobe (R) and the medial segment of the left lobe (LM). *Black arrow* indicates ligamentum teres, which appears as a hyperechoic structure with slight acoustic shadowing. (**B**) Sagittal view showing the main lobar fissure (*arrows*) as a linear hyperechoic structure between the right portal vein (P) and the gallbladder. LL, lateral segment of the left lobe.

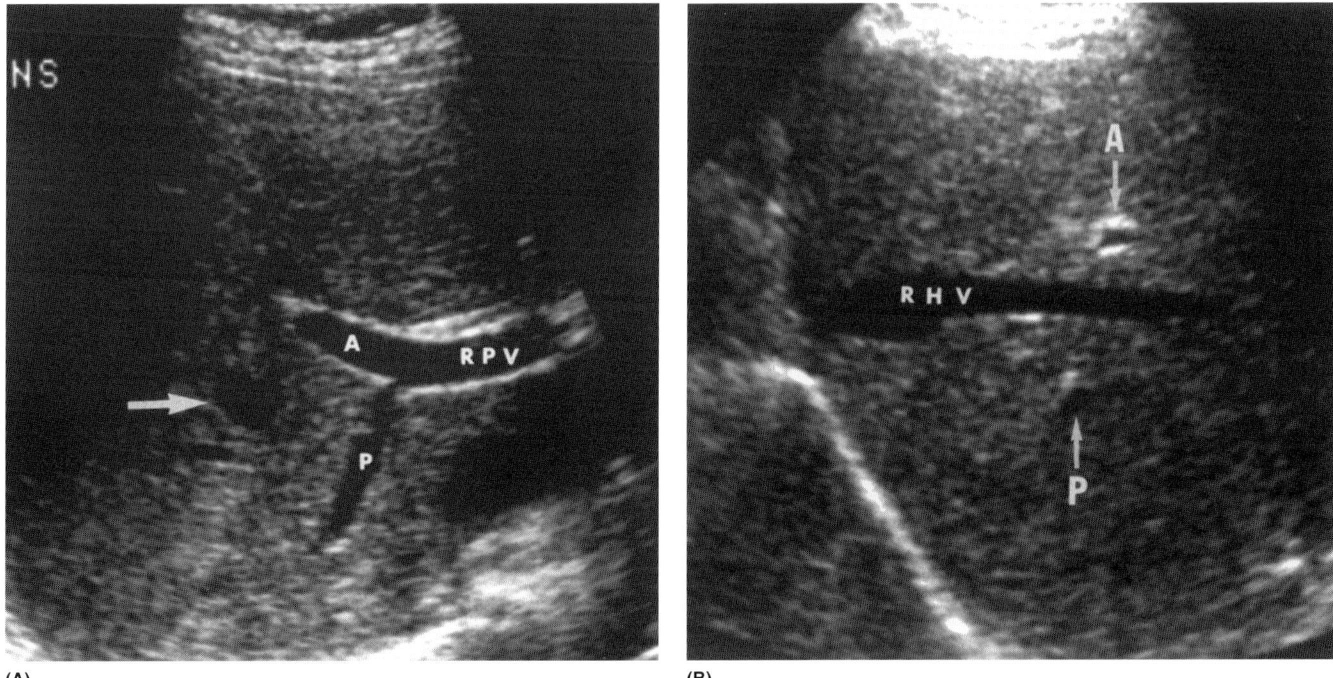

FIGURE 5 A AND B ■ A branch of the right hepatic vein (RHV) separating the right lobe into anterior and posterior segments. (**A**) Transverse view. A branch of the RHV (*arrow*) demarcates the plane of separation between the anterior and posterior segments of the right lobe. (**B**) Sagittal view. A long horizontally running branch of the RHV separates the anterior and posterior segments of the right lobe. Anterior and posterior branches of the right portal vein (RPV) are seen coursing centrally through the anterior and posterior segments of the right lobe. A, anterior branches of the right portal vein; P, posterior branches of the right portal vein.

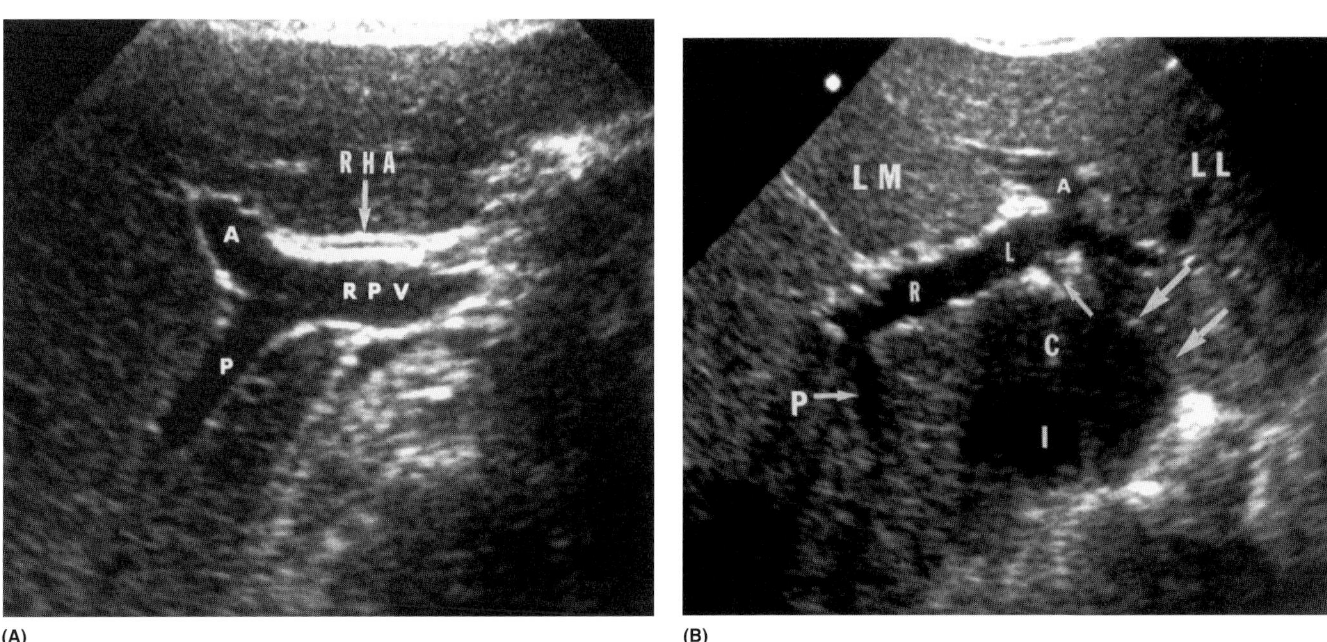

FIGURE 6 A AND B ■ Transverse views showing intrahepatic branches of the portal vein and their relationship to the hepatic lobes. (**A**) Anterior (A) and posterior (P) branches of the right portal vein (RPV) coursing centrally through the anterior and posterior segments of the right lobe. (**B**) Initial (*horizontal*) portion of the left portal vein (L) courses anterior to the caudate lobe (C). Ascending portion of the left portal vein coursing within the left intersegmental fissure separates the medial (LM) and lateral (LL) segments of the left lobe. *Small arrow*, branch of the left portal vein entering the caudate lobe. Note hypoechoic appearance of the caudate lobe secondary to shadowing from fibrous tissue and fat around the left portal vein and ligamentum venosum fissure (*large arrows*). RHA, right hepatic artery; I, inferior vena cava.

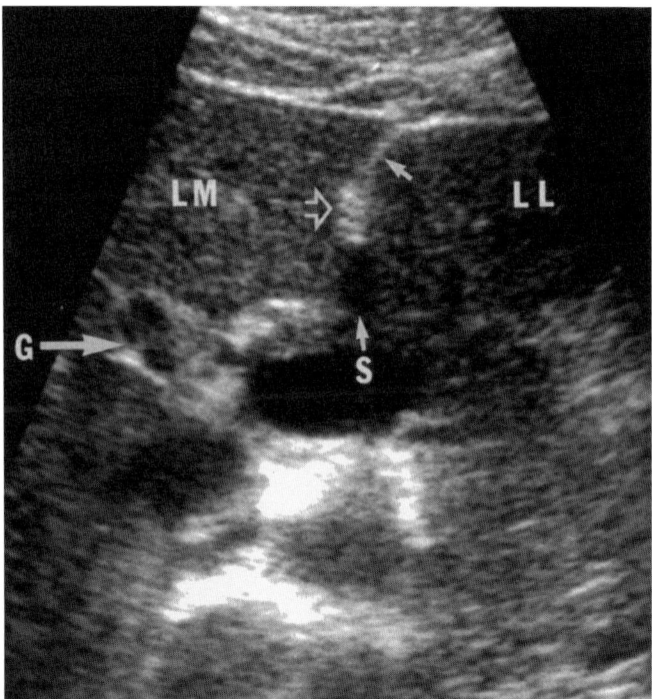

FIGURE 7 ■ Transverse view shows the fissure for the ligamentum teres (*open arrow*) coursing within the caudal third of the left intersegmental fissure (*solid and open arrows*) separating the medial segment of the left lobe (LM) from the lateral segment of the left lobe (LL). Ligamentum teres appears as a hyperechoic structure with acoustic shadowing (S). The falciform ligament (*solid arrow*) appears as a linear hyperechoic structure anterior to the ligamentum teres. G, gallbladder.

Functional Segmental Anatomy

To guide segmental and extended hepatic resections, the most commonly used functional segmental anatomy is based on the nomenclature of Couinaud (pronounced "kwee-NO") (4). This segmental anatomy is of importance during surgical segmental resection because each segment has its own blood supply and biliary drainage. Although the segmental location of tumors is not the sole criterion for determining resectability, such information is crucial for the preoperative planning of the type of resection. According to Couinaud, a segment is the smallest anatomic unit of the liver. The surgically relevant functional segmental anatomy described by Couinaud is a three-dimensional concept, based on the distribution of the portal and hepatic veins (Fig. 9) (5,6). Each segment has a branch of the portal vein at its center and a hepatic vein at

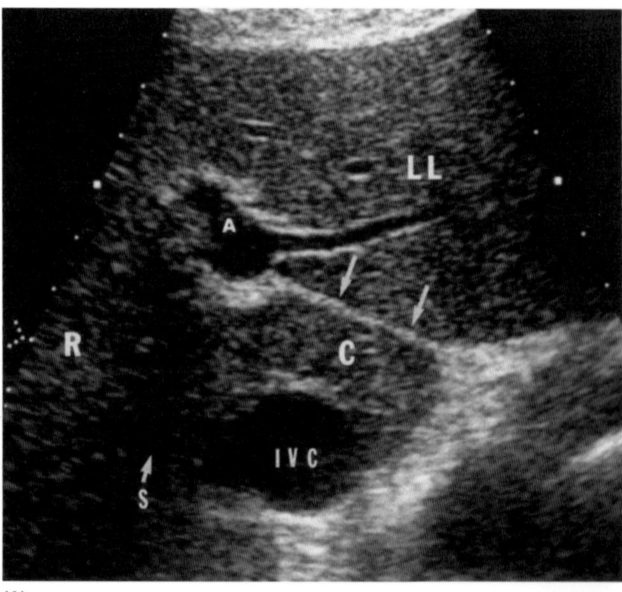

(A)

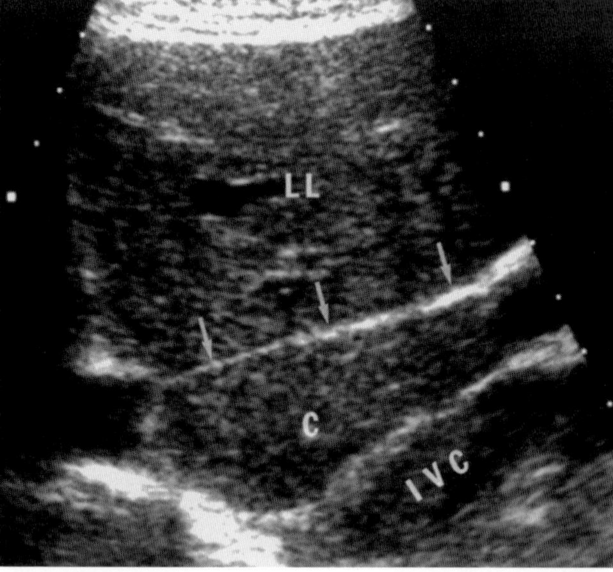

(B)

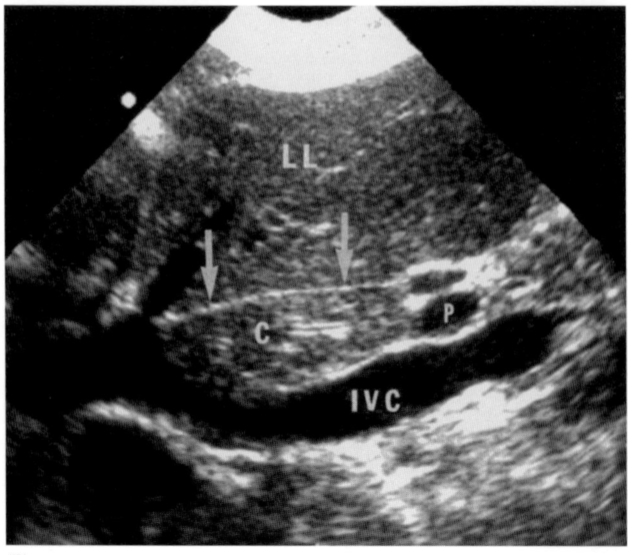

(C)

FIGURE 8 A–C ■ The caudate lobe. (**A**) Transverse and (**B** and **C**) sagittal views showing the caudate lobe (C) situated between the fissure for the ligamentum venosum (*arrows*) anteriorly and the inferior vena cava (IVC) posteriorly. The fissure for the ligamentum venosum seen as a linear hyperechoic structure (*arrows*) separates the caudate lobe from the lateral segment of the left lobe (LL). In **A**, the fissure for the ligamentum venosum (*arrows*) extends to the margin of the left portal vein (P) close to the origin of the ascending portion of the left portal vein. In **C**, the main portal vein is seen inferior (i.e., caudal) to the caudate lobe. A, ascending portion; R, right lobe; S, shadowing from fibrous tissue around left portal vein.

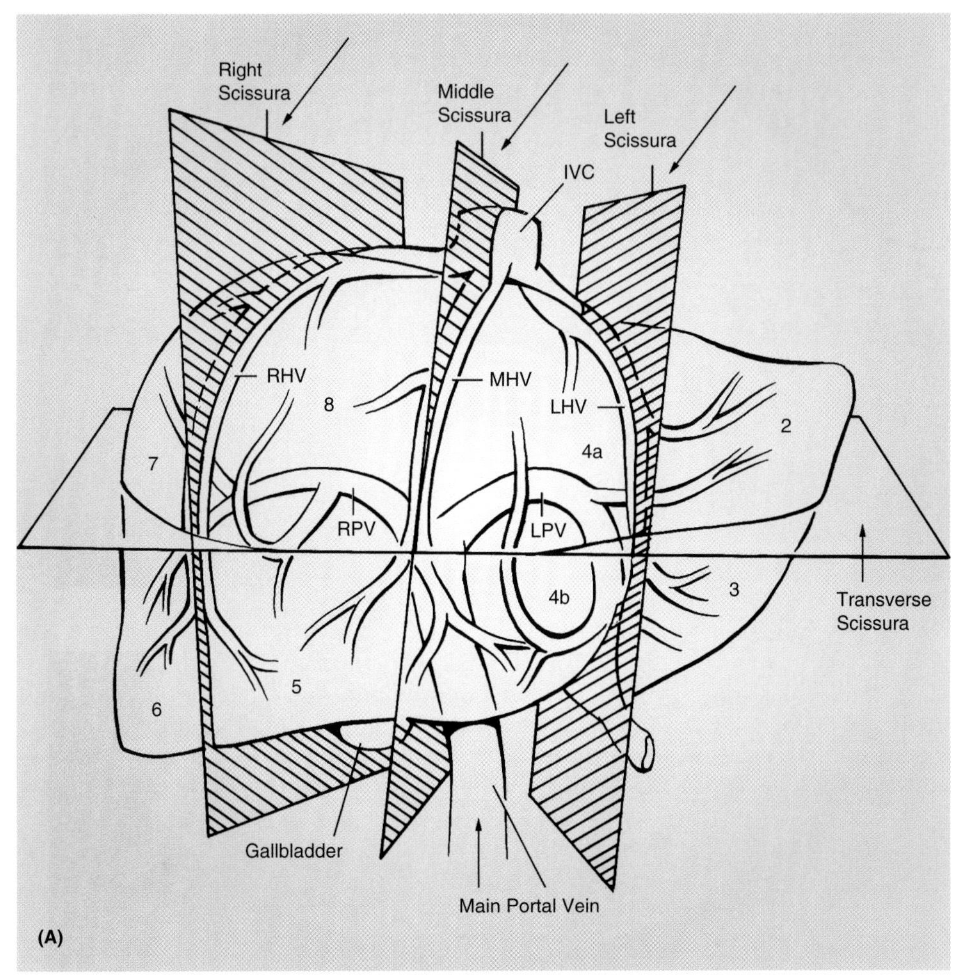

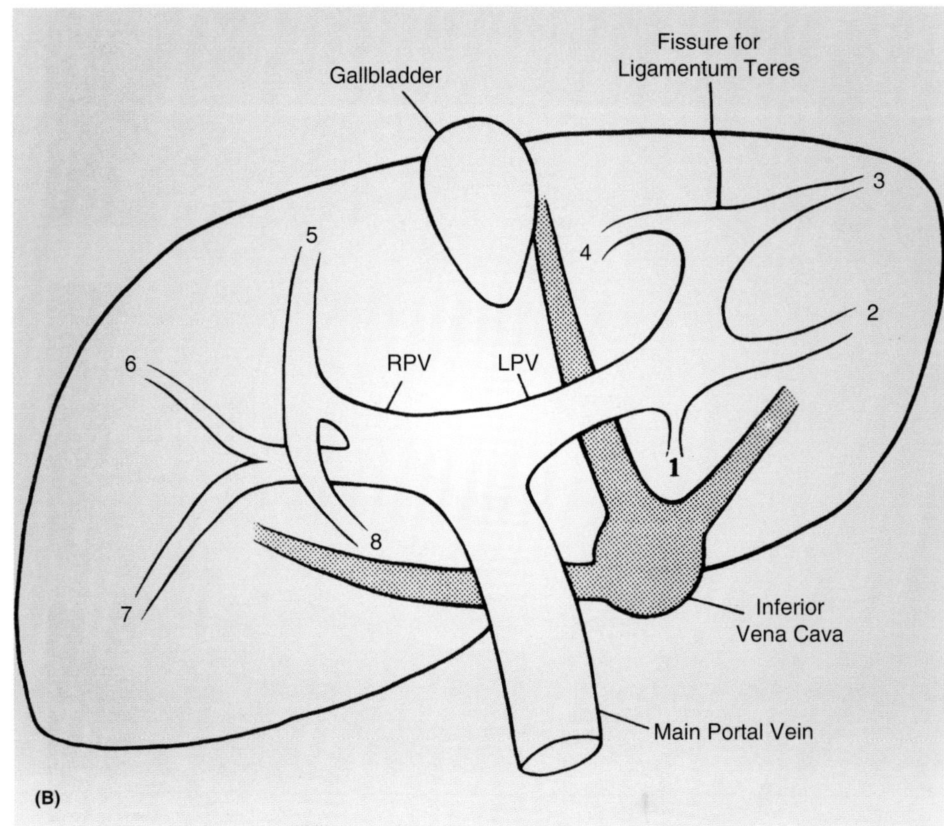

FIGURE 9 A AND B ■ Couinaud's segmental anatomy. (**A**) On this view, the segments are numbered clockwise. Longitudinal planes (scissurae) are defined by the three major hepatic veins (RHV, MHV, LHV). Transverse plane (scissura) is defined by the right (RPV) and left (LPV) divisions of the main portal vein. Segment 1 is the caudate lobe (*not shown*). (**B**) Couinaud's segmental anatomy: portal vein branches and their relationship to hepatic segments. In (B), the segments are numbered counterclockwise. Segment 1 is the caudate lobe. Segments 2, 3, and 4 are located around branches of the ascending portion of the LPV. Segments 5 and 8 are located around the branches of the anterior division of the RPV. Segments 6 and 7 are located around branches of the posterior division of the right portal vein. Shaded areas represent the inferior vena cava and the three major hepatic veins. *Key*: LPV, left portal vein; RPV, right portal vein; RHV, right hepatic vein; MHV, middle hepatic vein; LHV, left hepatic vein. *Source*: Modified from Refs. 5, 6.

TABLE 3 ■ Segmental Anatomy of the Liver: Anatomic Segments of the Liver and Corresponding Nomenclature

Anatomic Segment	Nomenclature		
	Couinaud	Bismuth	Goldsmith and Woodburne
Caudate lobe	1	1	Caudate lobe
Left lateral superior segment	2	2	Left lateral segment
Left lateral inferior segment	3	3	
Left medial superior segment	4	4a	Left medial segment
Left medial inferior segment	4	4b	
Right anterior inferior segment	5	5	Right anterior segment
Right anterior superior segment	8	8	
Right posterior inferior segment	6	6	Right posterior segment
Right posterior superior segment	7	7	

Source: Modified from Ref. 7.

its periphery. All hepatic segments except the caudate lobe are defined by three vertical scissurae (planes) and a single transverse scissura.

The three major hepatic veins divide the liver into four sections in the longitudinal plane (Fig. 9A). The lateral segment of the left lobe and the anterior and posterior segments of the right lobe are further subdivided into superior (cranial) and inferior (caudal) segments by a transverse plane defined by a line drawn through the right and left portal veins (Fig. 9A). Eight segments are recognized, as follows: 1, caudate lobe; 2 through 4, the left lobe; and 5 through 8, the right lobe (Fig. 9). Segment 4 may be further subdivided into superior (4a) and inferior (4b) subsegments. Comparison of various published nomenclatures of segmental anatomy is presented in Table 3 (7). The following description of the sonographic approach to Couinaud's segmental anatomy is based on the work by Lafortune et al. (5).

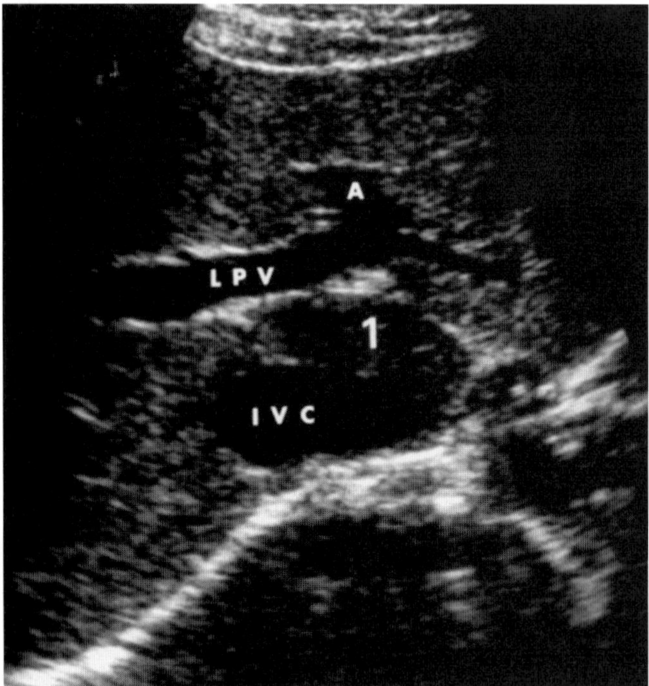

FIGURE 10 ■ Couinaud's segmental anatomy. Transverse view showing segment 1 (1), which is the caudate lobe. The horizontal portion of the left portal vein (LPV) is anterior to the caudate lobe. The inferior vena cava (IVC) is posterior to the caudate lobe. The caudate lobe is contiguous with the right lobe, between the IVC and the LPV. The caudate lobe appears hypoechoic because of shadowing from the ligamentum venosum fissure and fibrous tissue around the left portal vein. A, ascending portion of the left portal vein.

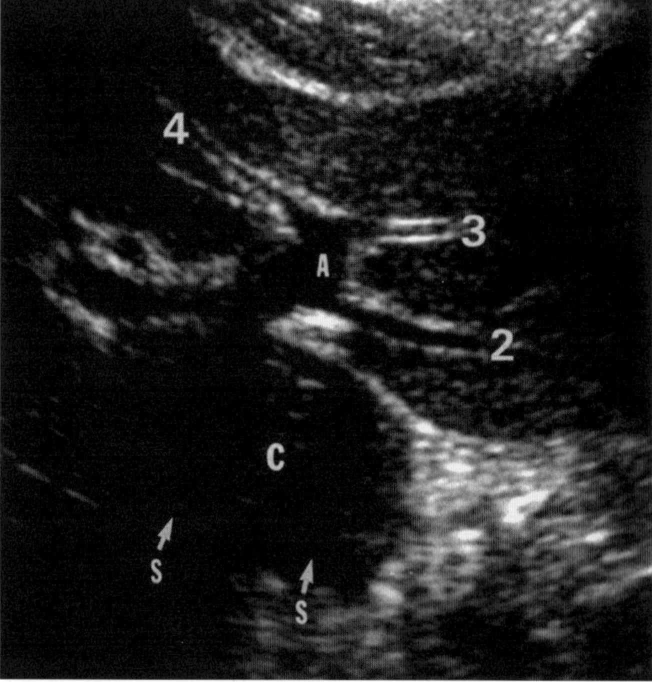

FIGURE 11 ■ Couinaud's segmental anatomy. Transverse view shows segments in the left lobe. Segments 2 and 3 are in the lateral segment of the left lobe and are located around the left posterior (2) and left anterior (3) branches of the ascending portion of the left portal vein. Segment 4 is located in the medial segment of the left lobe and is around the right branch of the ascending portion of left portal vein. Acoustic shadowing (S) within the caudate lobe (C) is caused by ligamentum venosum fissure and fibrous tissue around left portal vein.

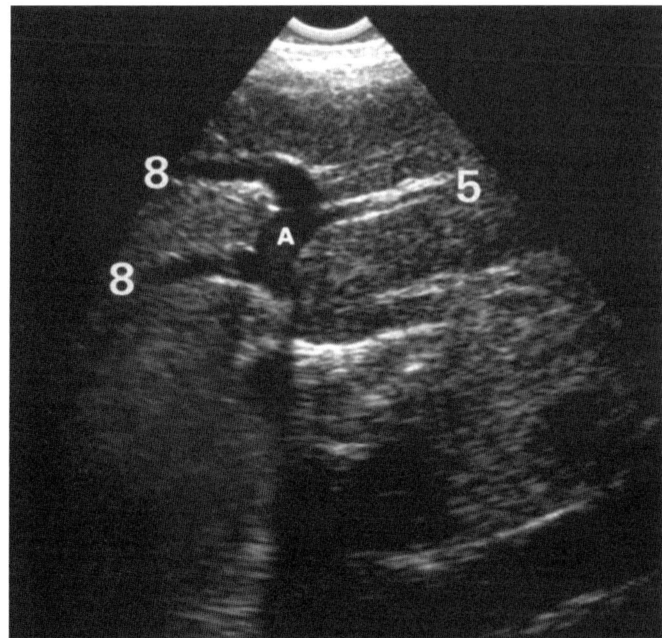

FIGURE 12 ■ Couinaud's segmental anatomy. Sagittal oblique view of the right lobe shows segments 5 and 8 around the branches of the anterior division of the right portal vein (A). *Source*: Courtesy of Michel LaFortune, MD, Montreal, Quebec, Canada.

Sonographically, use of hepatic veins for segmental anatomy is limited by three factors: (*i*) several segments are bordered by the same hepatic vein; (*ii*) the right hepatic vein and its branches are not always seen in the caudal portion of the right lobe; and (*iii*) the hepatic veins have abundant anatomic variations. Therefore, portal venous branches, which are at the center of the segments, are the key to the following description of the simplified version of Couinaud's segmental anatomy (Fig. 9B). Segment 1 is the caudate lobe (Fig. 10). Segment 2 is located around the left posterior branch of the left portal vein (which is usually a linear continuation of the horizontal portion of the left portal vein) and is located posteriorly (Fig. 11). Segment 3 is found around the left anterior branch of the ascending portion of the left portal vein and is located anteriorly (Fig. 11). The segment 4 is around the right branch of the ascending portion of the left portal vein (Fig. 11). Segments 5 through 8 are within the right lobe. Segments 5 and 8 are anteriorly situated (Fig. 12), and segments 6 and 7 are posteriorly situated (Fig. 13) around the branches of the anterior and posterior divisions of the right portal vein, respectively. For demonstration of segments 5 through 8, the right portal vein and its anterior and posterior branches are best seen with a sagittal or oblique, mid-axillary intercostal approach. The portal vein branches of segments 6 and 7 are obliquely oriented, and the transducer should be rotated slightly upward (cranially) for segment 7 and downward (caudally) in the direction of the right kidney for segment 6. Segments of the liver are frequently supplied by multiple branches arising from the right and left portal veins.

Hepatic Ligaments

The liver is surrounded by Glisson's capsule, which is a thin layer of connective tissue. The thin liver capsule is usually not visible sonographically. When the liver is surrounded by ascites and the ultrasound beam is perpendicular to the liver surface, a linear echo is frequently seen along the liver surface (Fig. 14). In addition, in the absence of ascites, when the liver is scanned with a 5- or 7.5-MHz linear-array transducer, a similar linear echo is seen along the liver surface. This linear echo may represent specular reflection from the liver

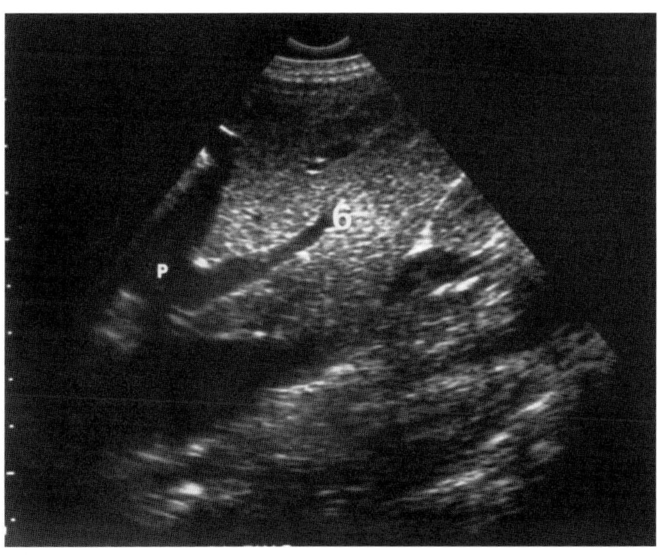

(A)

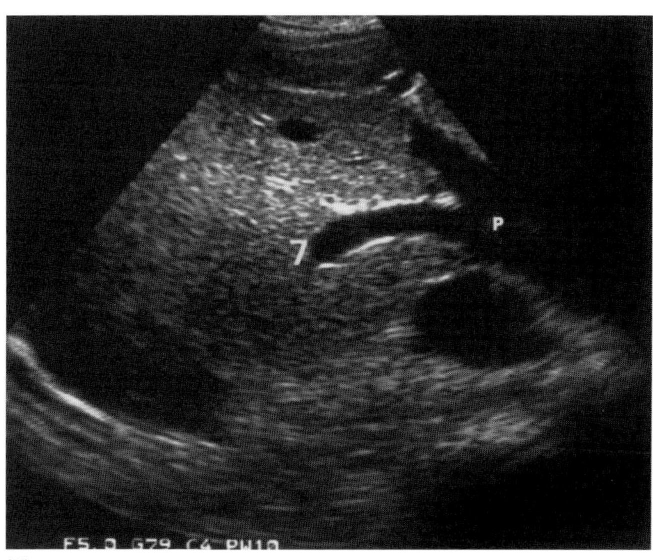

(B)

FIGURE 13 A AND B ■ Couinaud's segmental anatomy. Sagittal oblique views of the right lobe showing (**A**) segment 6 and (**B**) segment 7 around the branches of the posterior division of the right portal vein (P). *Source*: Courtesy of Michel LaFortune, MD, Montreal, Quebec, Canada.

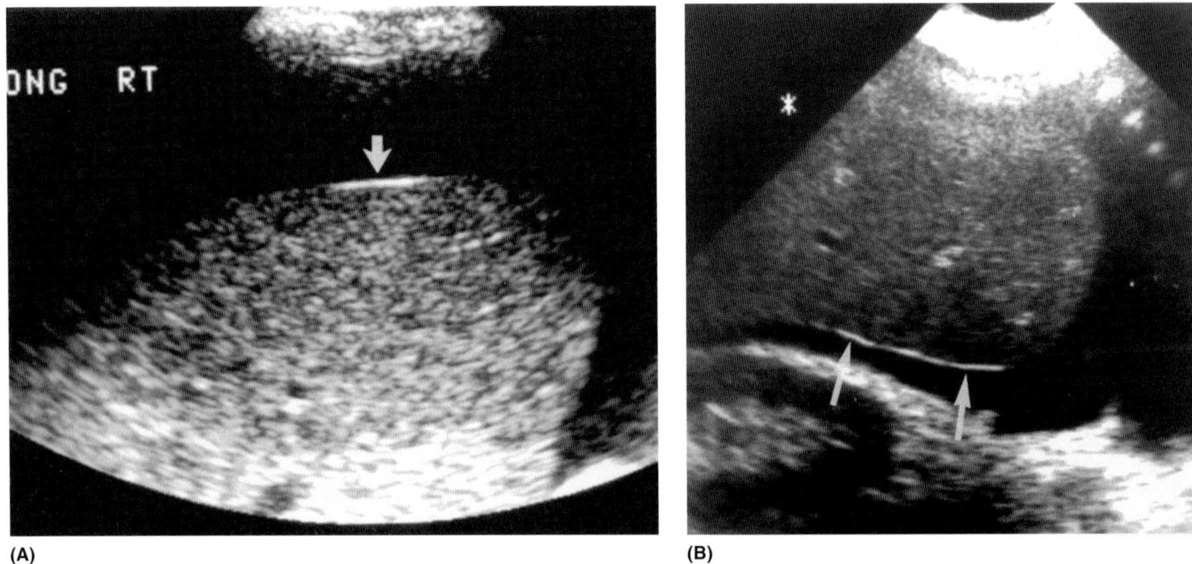

FIGURE 14 A AND B ■ Normal liver capsule. Longitudinal views of the liver surrounded by ascites show a thin, hyperechoic linear structure (*arrows*) seen only where the sound beam is perpendicular to the liver surface. This linear echo may represent specular reflection from the liver surface or the thin liver capsule (i.e., Glisson's capsule).

surface or the thin liver capsule. The falciform ligament is a sickle-shaped fold that courses over the anterior surface of the liver and connects the liver to the diaphragm and the anterior abdominal wall (Fig. 1). The falciform ligament is not visible unless it is surrounded by ascites (Fig. 15) or unless fibrofatty tissue is enclosed in the ligament (Fig. 7). When visible, the falciform ligament is a hyperechoic linear or band-like structure within the left intersegmental fissure (Fig. 7).

The ligamentum teres, which is the obliterated umbilical vein, runs in the posteroinferior free edge of the falciform ligament (Fig. 1). On the transverse view, the ligamentum teres can be seen as a rounded, hyperechoic structure within the fissure for the ligamentum

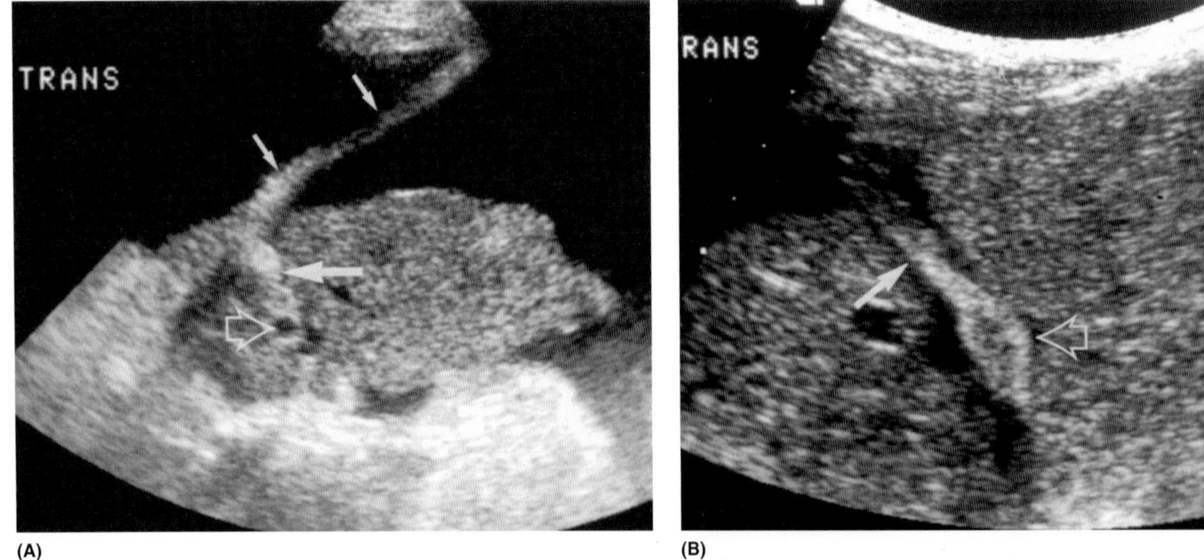

FIGURE 15 A AND B ■ Falciform ligament in ascites. (**A**) The falciform ligament (*small solid arrows*) surrounded by ascites is seen between the anterior abdominal wall and the anterior surface of the liver. The falciform ligament within the liver (*large solid arrow*) is seen as a hyperechoic band-like structure within the left intersegmental fissure, dividing the medial and lateral segments of the left lobe. *Open arrow*, dilated paraumbilical vein within the ligamentum teres along the posterior margin of the falciform ligament. (**B**) The falciform ligament (*solid arrow*) within the left intersegmental fissure is visible because of small amounts of ascites surrounding the falciform ligament within the fissure. *Open arrow*, ligamentum teres.

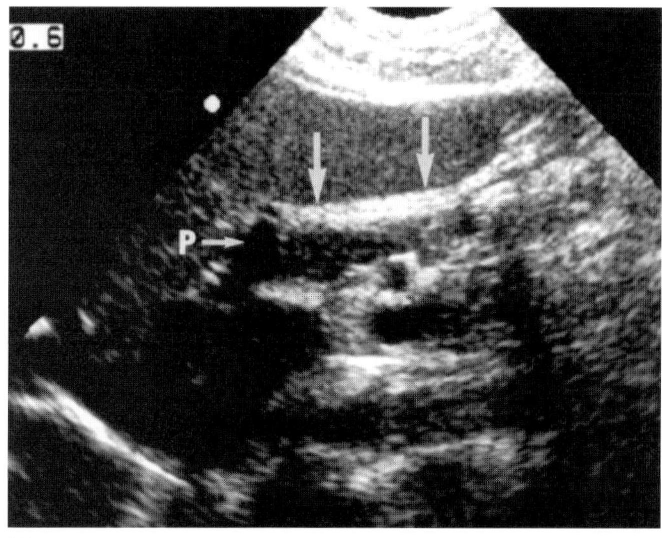

(A)

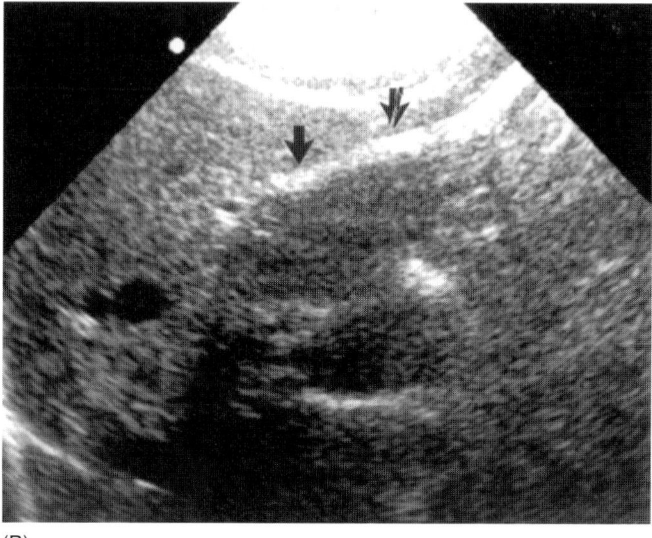

(B)

FIGURE 16 A AND B ■ Ligamentum teres fissure. (**A**) Sagittal view shows the fissure for the ligamentum teres (*arrows*) as a band-like hyperechoic structure extending caudally and inferiorly toward the anterior abdominal wall from the left portal vein (P). (**B**) Sagittal view in another patient shows prominent posterior acoustic shadowing from the ligamentum teres fissure (*arrows*).

teres, which divides the medial and lateral segments of the left lobe of the liver (Figs. 3A and 7). The ligamentum teres is occasionally prominent and variable in shape, and it may cause acoustic shadowing. On the sagittal view, the ligamentum teres is seen as a band-like hyperechoic structure extending caudally and anteriorly toward the anterior abdominal wall, from the ascending branch of the left portal vein (Fig. 16). The fissure for the ligamentum venosum, which contains the remnant of the ductus venosus, can be seen as a hyperechoic linear or band-like structure, separating the caudate lobe from the lateral segment of the left lobe (Fig. 8) (2). On the transverse view, the fissure for the ligamentum venosum extends to the posterior wall of the left portal vein, near the junction of the horizontal and ascending portions of the left portal vein (Figs. 8A and 11).

Some of the other ligaments of the liver (hepatoduodenal, hepatogastric, coronary, and right and left triangular ligaments) can only be seen when the liver is surrounded by ascites. The coronary ligament is formed by the reflection of the peritoneum from the diaphragm to the superior and posterior surfaces of the right lobe and consists of an upper and lower layers (Fig. 1). The two layers diverge widely to the left to enclose posteriorly a large triangular area of the right lobe that is not covered with peritoneum, termed the "bare area" (Fig. 1B). The upper layer is continuous with the right layer of the falciform ligament. The right triangular ligament is a short, V-shaped fold that connects the lateral part of the posterior aspect of the right lobe to the diaphragm (Fig. 1A). It constitutes the right limit of the upper and lower layers of the coronary ligament. The left triangular ligament, on the upper surface of the left lobe, consists of two closely applied layers of peritoneum (Fig. 1). The anterior layer is continuous with the left layer of the falciform ligament and the posterior layer with the anterior layer of the lesser omentum at the upper end of the fissure for the ligamentum venosum. The portion of the lesser omentum extending between the liver and the duodenum is named the hepatoduodenal ligament and that between the liver and the stomach is known as the hepatogastric ligament. From the upper border of the duodenum, the lesser omentum ascends to the porta hepatis, forming the hepatoduodenal ligament, which encloses the main portal vein, the main (proper) hepatic artery, and the common bile duct (8). The hepatogastric ligament consists of layers of lesser omentum ascending from the lesser curvature of the stomach to the bottom of the fissure for the ligamentum venosum (9).

Hepatic Vasculature

Hepatic Veins

Most people have three major hepatic veins—right, middle, and left—that enter the inferior vena cava (Fig. 4). Frequently, the middle and left hepatic veins join together before entering the inferior vena cava (Fig. 4). This distribution is seen in approximately 70% of the population. Variations in the distribution of the hepatic veins are common, and approximately 30% of the population has more than three hepatic veins. Absence of one of the major hepatic veins is uncommon. The accessory hepatic veins commonly seen include the right superior anterior segmental vein, which usually drains into the middle hepatic vein, and the right and left marginal veins, which drain into the right and left hepatic veins, respectively (Fig. 17) (10). Approximately 6% to 10% of the population has an accessory right hepatic vein, most commonly the inferior right hepatic vein, which enters the dorsal part of the inferior vena cava, usually caudal to the level of the major

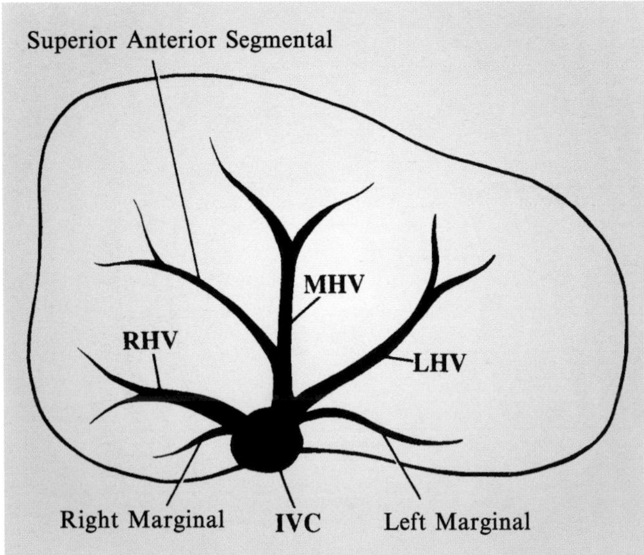

FIGURE 17 ■ Diagram of commonly seen accessory hepatic veins. The right superior anterior segmental vein drains into the MHV. The right and left marginal veins drain into the right RHVs and LHVs, respectively. RHV, right hepatic vein; MHV, middle hepatic vein; LHV, left hepatic vein; IVC, inferior vena cava. *Source*: Modified from Ref. 10.

hepatic veins (Fig. 18) (5,11). The inferior right hepatic vein is usually located posterior to the posterior branch of the right portal vein and is occasionally larger than the main right hepatic vein. Delineation of the inferior right hepatic vein is significant in hepatectomy, detection of tumor thrombus in hepatocellular carcinoma (HCC), and Budd–Chiari syndrome.

The major hepatic veins are intersegmental, separating different segments and lobes of the liver. The right hepatic vein separates the anterior and posterior segments of the right lobe, the middle hepatic vein separates the right and the left lobes, and the left hepatic vein separates the medial and lateral segments of the left lobe. The hepatic veins have no valves.

Portal Veins

The main portal vein ascends in the porta hepatis (Fig. 19), where it divides into right and left branches. The right portal vein divides into anterior and posterior branches (Fig. 6A). The initial horizontal portion of the left portal vein (i.e., pars transversa) gives branches to the caudate lobe of the liver and then enters the left lobe, coursing to the left along the anterior surface of the caudate lobe before abruptly turning anteriorly (Figs. 6B and 10). The ascending (anterior) portion of the left portal vein gives branches to the medial and lateral segments of the left lobe of the liver (Fig. 11). Variations in the intrahepatic portal venous branching are uncommon and include absence of the horizontal segment of the left portal vein and absence of the right portal vein (12). Congenital anomalies of the main portal vein, such as atresia or stricture, or absence of main portal vein are rare. Portal veins, like hepatic veins, do not have valves. Normally, the main portal vein is less than 13 mm in diameter when patients are examined in sagittal section in the left posterior-oblique position (13).

Hepatic Arteries

The celiac trunk, arising from the abdominal aorta, divides into three branches: (*i*) hepatic; (*ii*) splenic; and (*iii*) left gastric (Fig. 20). The hepatic artery is subdivided into the common hepatic artery, extending from the celiac trunk

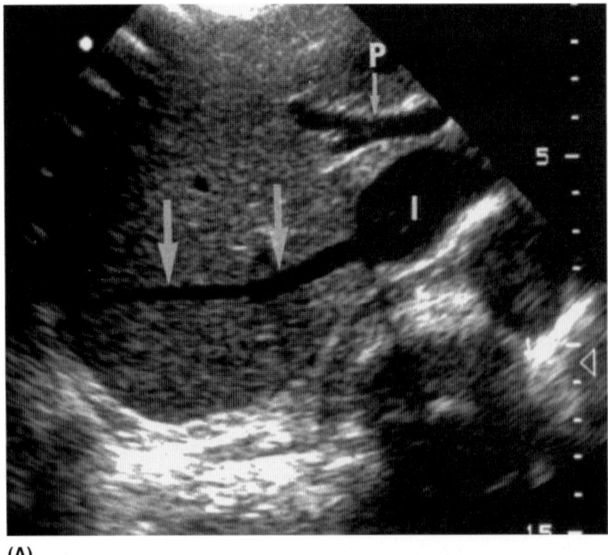

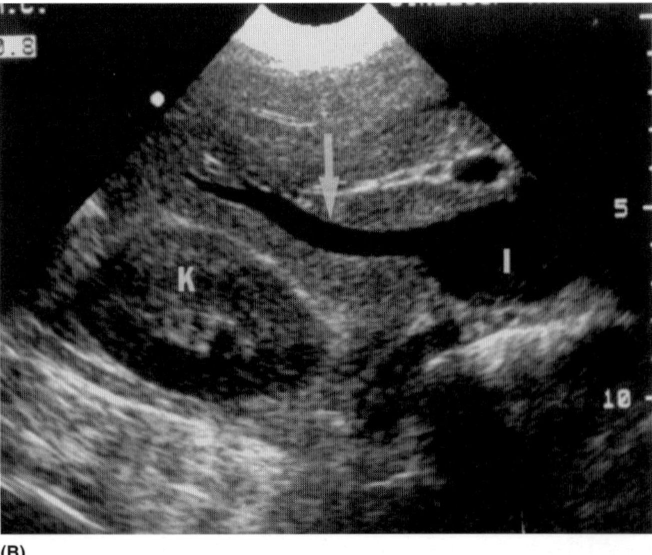

FIGURE 18 A AND B ■ The inferior right hepatic vein (IRHV). Transverse views. (**A**) The IRHV (*arrows*) is seen in the posterior portion of the right lobe entering the caudal portion of the inferior vena cava (I) on the right side. (**B**) The IRHV (*arrow*) is seen coursing in the posterior portion of the right lobe, anterior to the right kidney (K). P, right portal vein.

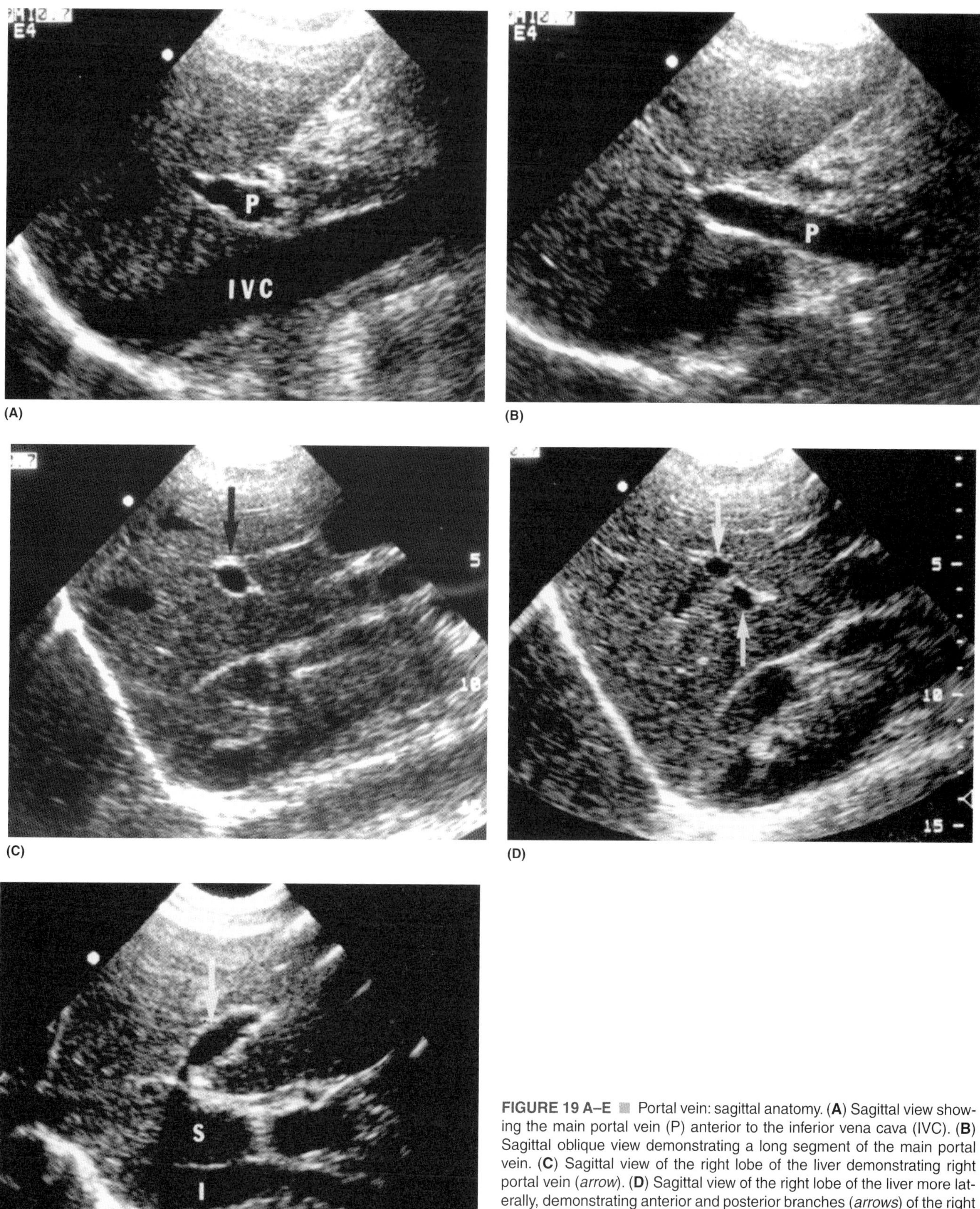

FIGURE 19 A–E ■ Portal vein: sagittal anatomy. (**A**) Sagittal view showing the main portal vein (P) anterior to the inferior vena cava (IVC). (**B**) Sagittal oblique view demonstrating a long segment of the main portal vein. (**C**) Sagittal view of the right lobe of the liver demonstrating right portal vein (*arrow*). (**D**) Sagittal view of the right lobe of the liver more laterally, demonstrating anterior and posterior branches (*arrows*) of the right portal vein. (**E**) Sagittal view of the left lobe of the liver demonstrating the ascending portion of the left portal vein (*arrow*). S, acoustic shadow from fibrofatty tissue within the ligamentum venosum fissure. The shadowing mimics a hypoechoic mass in the caudate lobe.

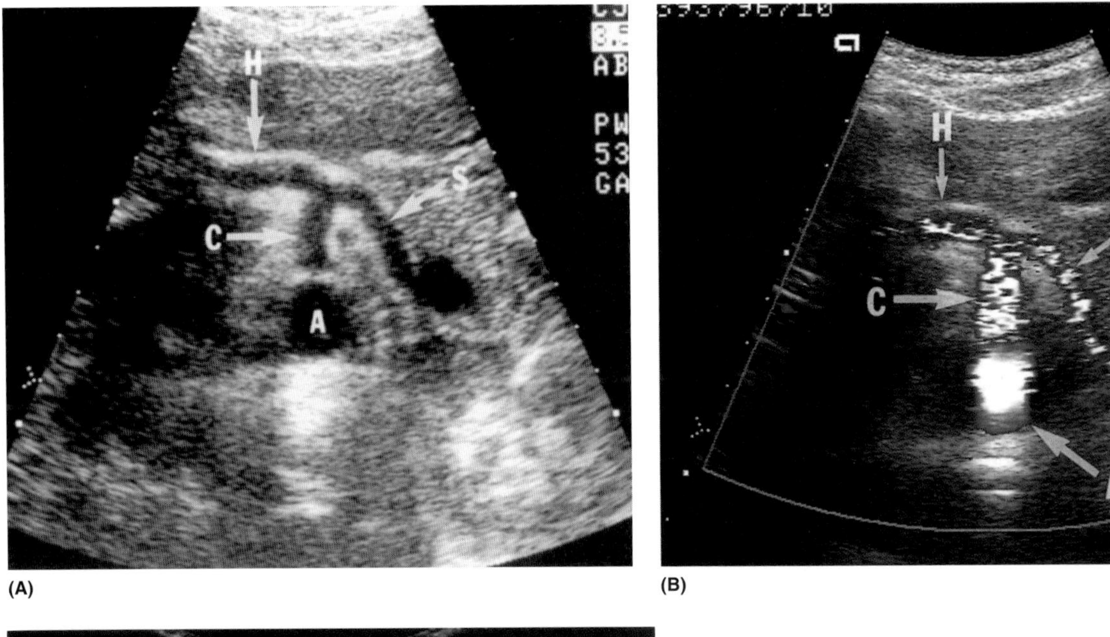

(A) (B)

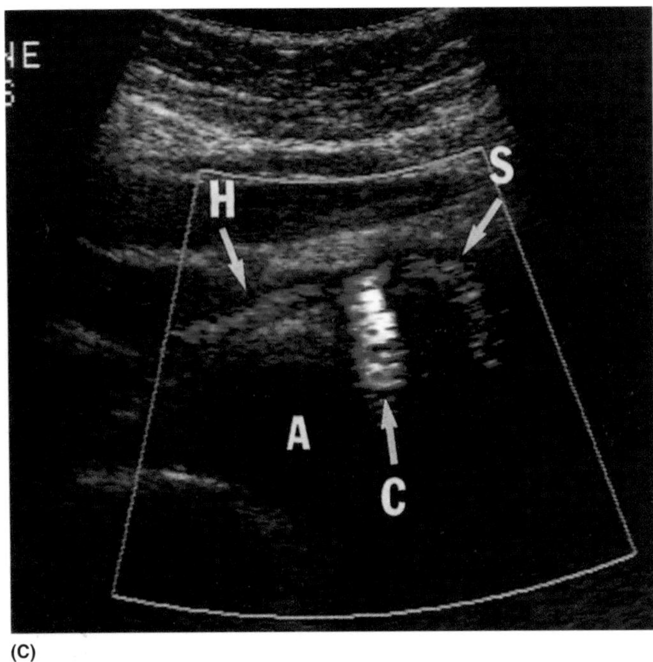

(C)

FIGURE 20 A–C ■ Celiac and hepatic arteries: transverse views. (**A**) Gray-scale and (**B** and **C**) color Doppler sonograms showing the celiac artery (C) arising from the abdominal aorta (A) and branching into the hepatic (H) and splenic (S) arteries.

to the origin of the gastroduodenal artery, and the hepatic artery proper, extending from that point to the bifurcation of the artery into its right and left branches (14).

The hepatic artery proper ascends into the porta hepatis, usually anterior to the main portal vein, before dividing into right and left hepatic arteries. Intrahepatic branches of the arteries accompany the portal veins. Sonographically, intrahepatic arteries are difficult to identify consistently because of their small size; however, they can be seen adjacent to the right and left branches of the main portal vein (Figs. 5 and 6A). Variations in the origin of the hepatic arteries occur in 45% of the population and are of surgical importance. When hepatic arteries with "anomalous" origin exist in conjunction with "normal" branches of the hepatic artery, they are called accessory hepatic arteries; on the other hand, when they replace the normal branches and constitute the sole supply to the appropriate parts of the liver, they are called replaced hepatic arteries (15). Variations include the following: (*i*) replaced right hepatic artery arising from the superior mesenteric artery (11%) (Fig. 21); (*ii*) replaced left hepatic artery arising from the left gastric artery (10%); and (*iii*) replaced common hepatic artery arising from the superior mesenteric artery (2%) (16). An aberrant (replaced or accessory) left hepatic artery is seen on the transverse view as a long, tubular, pulsatile channel within the fissure for the ligamentum venosum (Fig. 22). On the sagittal view, it is seen as a round, pulsatile, anechoic structure within the fissure (Fig. 22) (17).

The portal triad consists of the branches of the portal vein, hepatic artery, and bile ducts, which course

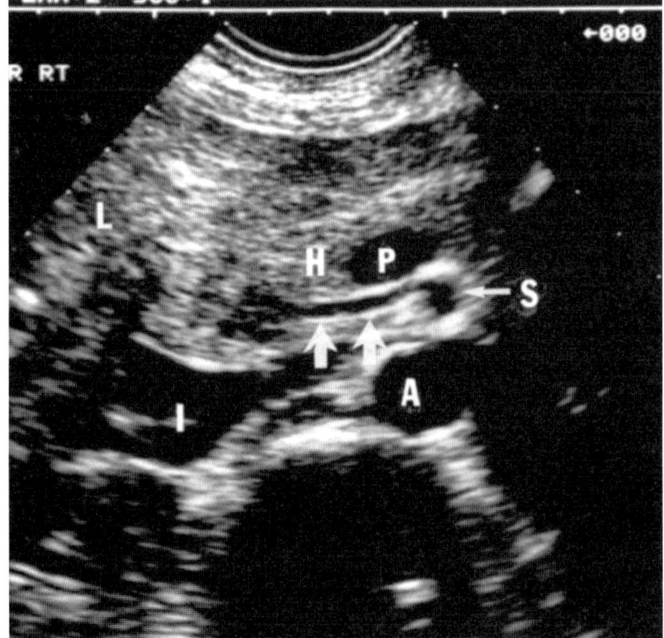

FIGURE 21 ■ Replaced right hepatic artery. Transverse view shows the replaced right hepatic artery (*arrows*) arising from the superior mesenteric artery (S). A, abdominal aorta; I, inferior vena cava; P, confluence of the splenic and superior mesenteric veins; H, head of the pancreas; L, liver.

together within the liver. In the porta hepatis, the common bile duct and the hepatic artery proper usually are located anterior to the main portal vein. Most commonly, the hepatic artery proper is medial to the common bile duct. Within the liver, the walls of the portal vein branches usually are more echogenic than the walls of the hepatic veins. However, this feature is not reliable for differentiating hepatic from portal veins because the major hepatic veins and their larger branches frequently have echogenic walls (Fig. 4).

The liver has a dual blood supply from the hepatic artery and the portal vein, and therefore, hepatic infarction is uncommon. The portal vein supplies 60% to 80% of the hepatic blood flow.

Duplex Doppler Evaluation of Normal Hepatic Vessels

The duplex Doppler examination of the hepatic vessels is ideally performed after a 6- to 12-hour fast while patients are holding their breath in the supine position (Fig. 23) (18).

Hepatic Artery ■ The normal hepatic artery, in a fasting person, is in a low-resistance system similar to the internal carotid and renal arteries. Therefore, the hepatic artery waveform demonstrates continuous flow throughout diastole (Fig. 23A). The velocity decreases at the end of systole, but it never reaches zero or flow reversal (19). In a healthy person with a normal liver, approximately 30 minutes after a meal, the diastolic flow in the hepatic artery decreases, with a corresponding increase in the hepatic arterial resistive index. The Doppler evaluation can be performed within the hepatic artery proper or intrahepatic arteries. The Doppler signal can be usually identified within the intrahepatic arterial branches adjacent to the right portal vein and the left portal vein, especially adjacent to the ascending portion of the left portal vein.

Main Portal Vein ■ The main portal vein is best evaluated in a sagittal oblique view demonstrating the vessels' longest axis. The normal mean velocity in the main portal vein is about 15 to 18 cm per second, but the normal range is wide (20). The normal portal vein flow is antegrade

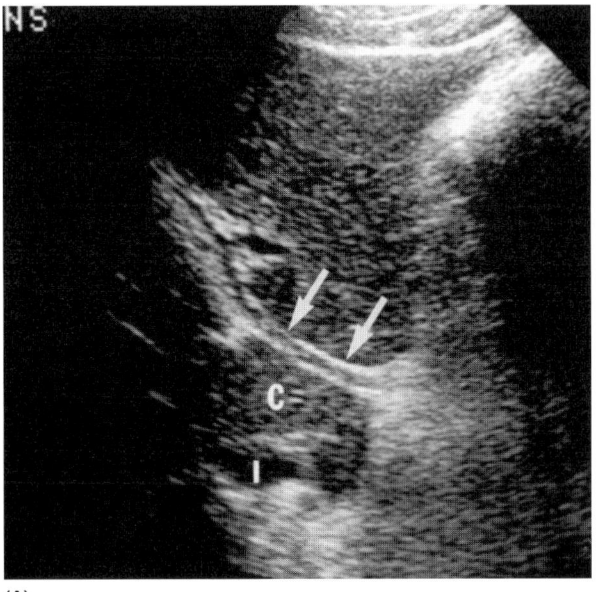

(A)

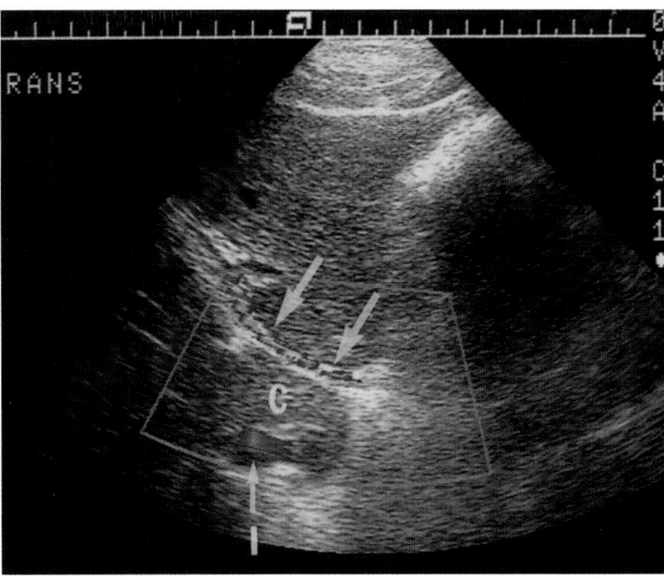

(B)

FIGURE 22 A–D ■ Replaced left hepatic artery. (**A**) Transverse view shows a replaced left hepatic artery (*arrows*) coursing through the ligamentum venosum fissure. (**B**) Transverse color Doppler sonogram shows hepatopetal color flow within the artery (*arrows*). (*Continued*)

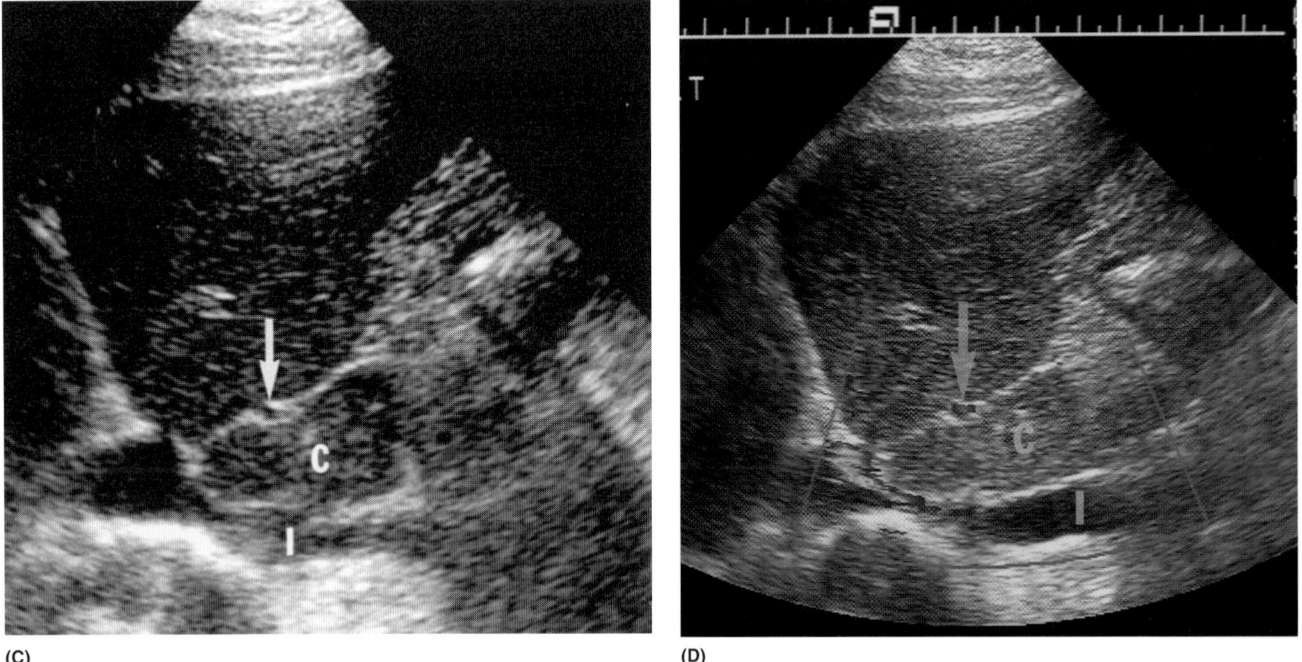

(C) (D)

FIGURE 22 A–D ■ (*Continued*) (**C** and **D**) Sagittal gray-scale and color Doppler sonograms demonstrate a replaced left hepatic artery (*arrow*) within the ligamentum venosum fissure. The artery appears as a rounded, anechoic structure within the fissure on the sagittal gray-scale sonogram. C, caudate lobe; I, inferior vena cava.

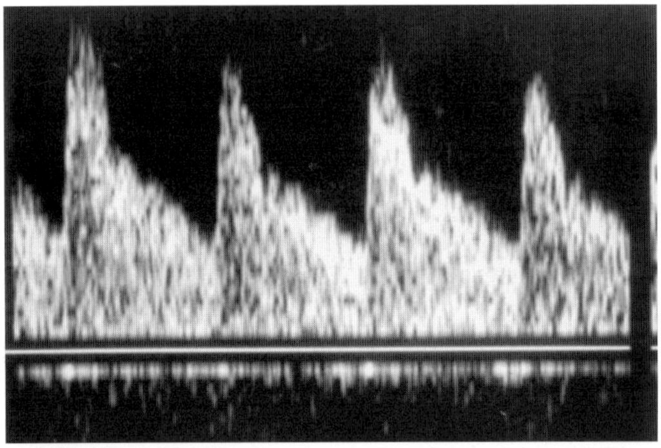

(A)

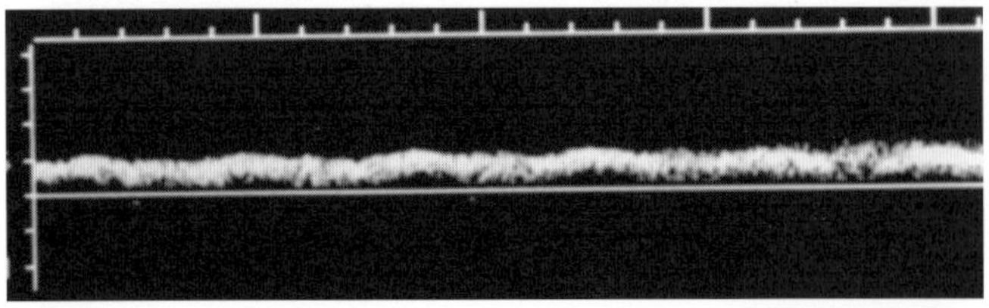

(B)

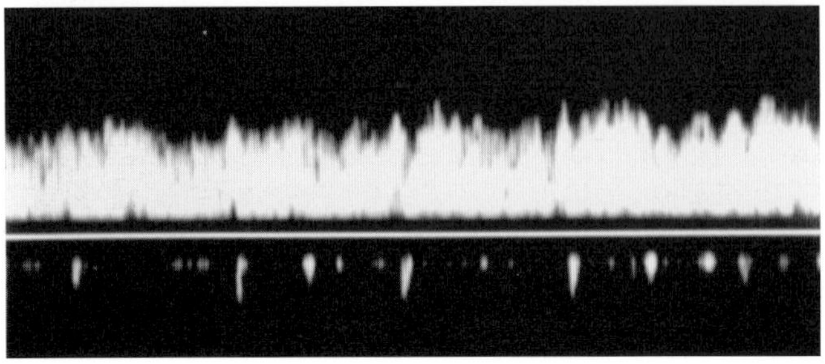

(C)

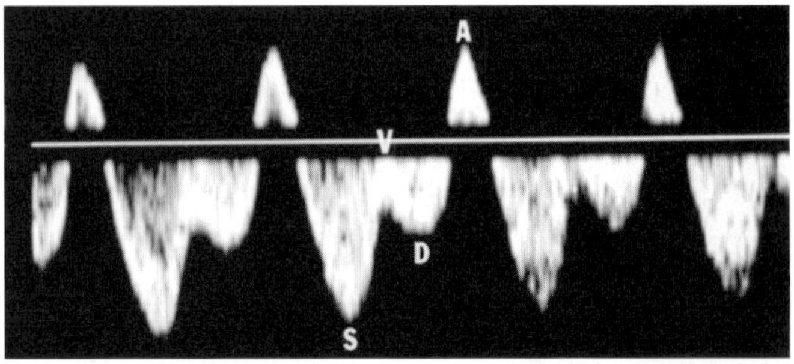

(D)

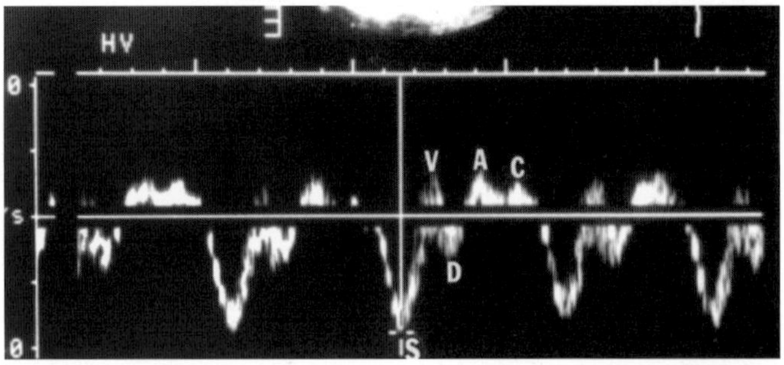

(E)

FIGURE 23 A–E ■ Normal duplex Doppler waveforms of hepatic vessels. (**A**) Normal hepatic artery waveform demonstrates low-resistance arterial flow signals with continuous forward flow in diastole. (**B** and **C**) Normal portal vein waveforms. Portal vein waveform is minimally phasic (**B**) or essentially nonpulsatile (**C**). The flow in the portal vein is continuous antegrade (hepatopetal). (**C**) A magnified recording of the Doppler waveform. (**D**) Normal hepatic vein waveform. The waveform is essentially triphasic with antegrade systolic and diastolic waves and a retrograde A-wave (A). The V-wave is seen just below the baseline. (**E**) Normal hepatic vein waveform in another patient shows a small retrograde V-wave (V) above the baseline and a small retrograde C-wave (C) above the baseline. (See text for complete discussion.) S, systolic; D, diastolic. *Source*: From Ref. 18.

hepatopetal throughout the entire cardiac cycle. The normal duplex Doppler waveform of the main portal vein is minimally phasic or almost nonpulsatile and continuously antegrade (Fig. 23B and C). One may see small pulsations that mirror the cardiac cycle (18).

Hepatic Veins ■ Hepatic veins can be evaluated in sagittal or transverse view. Hepatic venous waveforms are best sampled in the middle hepatic vein. The normal hepatic venous waveform is predominantly triphasic; however, in some patients, two additional waves (V and C waves) may be demonstrated (Fig. 23D and E). The normal hepatic vein waveform consists of waves in the following sequence: (*i*) a large antegrade systolic wave caused by the movement of the tricuspid annulus toward the cardiac apex; (*ii*) a small retrograde V-wave caused by right atrial overfilling; the V-wave is usually below the baseline but may be above the baseline; (*iii*) an antegrade diastolic wave caused by the opening of the tricuspid valve and flow of the blood from the right atrium to the right ventricle; (*iv*) a retrograde A-wave caused by right atrial contraction; and (*v*) a retrograde C-wave caused by the closure of the tricuspid valve at the beginning of systole, which may be seen in a few patients (18). In a study by Abu-Yousef, the normal mean systolic velocity in the hepatic veins was 29 cm per second, the normal mean diastolic velocity was 22 cm per second, and the normal mean ratio of systolic to diastolic velocities was 1.4 (18).

Normal hepatic vein and portal vein duplex Doppler waveforms show cyclic phasicity that is much more prominent in the hepatic vein (18). This phasicity is caused by changes in the right atrial pressure and hence is cardiac in origin rather than respiratory. The absolute and relative velocities of the various waves in both the hepatic and the portal veins are also influenced by different respiratory maneuvers (18).

Echo Pattern and Size of the Liver

The liver parenchyma normally has a homogeneous echo pattern interrupted only by vessels and fissures (Fig. 24). The echogenicity of the liver is usually greater than that

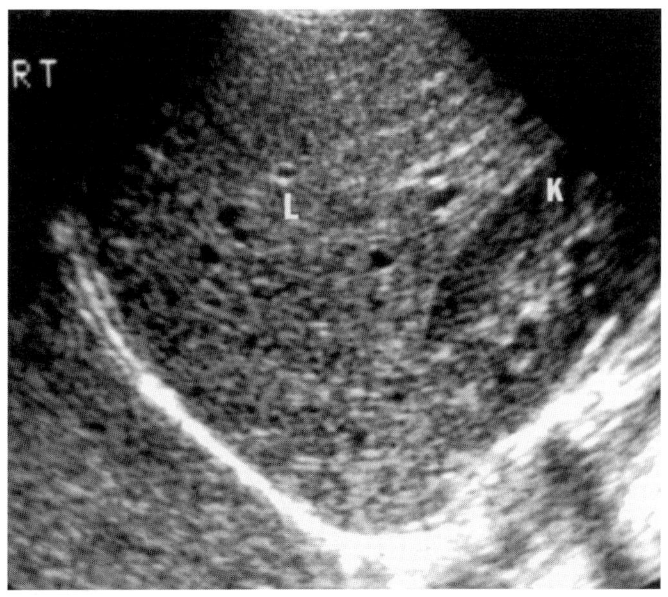

(A)

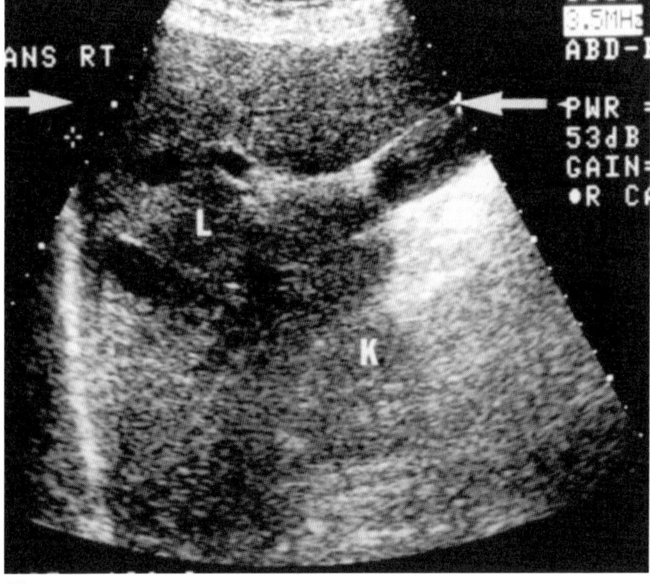

(B)

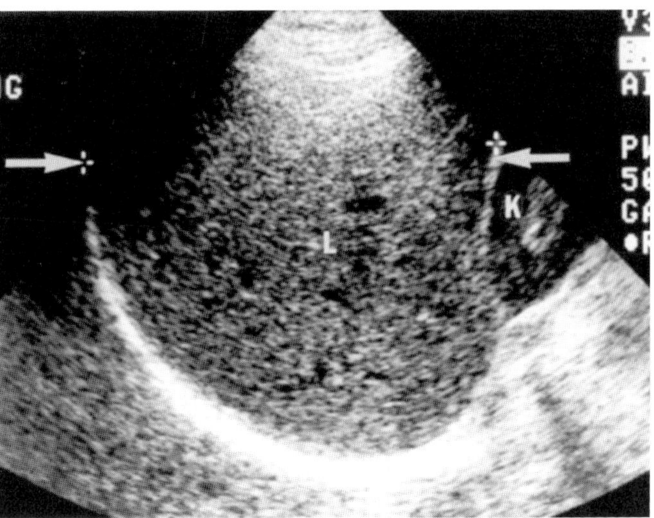

(C)

FIGURE 24 A–C ■ Normal liver echotexture and size measurement. (**A**) Sagittal view showing normal homogeneous echo pattern of the liver. The liver is more echogenic than the renal cortex (K). (**B** and **C**) Sagittal views in two different patients in the mid-clavicular line for measurement of the liver size. The length of the liver is measured in a straight line parallel to the anterior abdominal wall, in the longitudinal plane, from the diaphragm to the inferior (caudal) margin of the liver (*arrows*). K, Right kidney. In many persons, the right portal vein and gallbladder are visible in the mid-clavicular line (**B**); however, in some persons, a more lateral portion of the right lobe of the liver (**C**) is seen at this level.

TABLE 4 ■ Normal Liver Echogenicity

≥	Right renal cortex
≤	Pancreas
<	Spleen

of the adjacent right renal cortex (Table 4). Less commonly, the liver may be isoechoic with the renal cortex. The liver is usually less echogenic than the pancreas, but it may be isoechoic. The liver is normally less echogenic than the spleen. The size of the liver is difficult to measure accurately because of the limited field of view of available real-time ultrasound machines, especially when the liver is enlarged. The most widely used measurement is the length of the liver on the sagittal view in the mid-clavicular line, which usually corresponds to the mid-hepatic line (Fig. 24). If the liver exceeds 15 cm in length in the mid-clavicular line, a diagnosis of hepatomegaly should be considered (21,22). Indirect signs of hepatomegaly include extension of the right lobe below the lower pole of the right kidney (in the absence of a Reidel's lobe), rounding of the caudal margin of the liver on the sagittal view, and extension of the left lobe into the left upper quadrant above the spleen (23).

DEVELOPMENTAL ANOMALIES AND ANATOMIC VARIATIONS OF THE LOBES AND FISSURES

Riedel's lobe, a normal variation, more common in women, is a tongue-like projection of the right lobe that may extend to the iliac crest (Fig. 25). In situs inversus totalis, the liver is located in the left upper abdomen, with the "right" lobe on the left side and the "left" lobe across the midline within the right side of the abdomen. Variations in size of the left lobe are common. Agenesis of one of the lobes of the liver is rare. Accessory fissures of the liver are rare. The inferior accessory fissure is seen within the posterior segment of the right lobe as a thin, linear, hyperechoic structure extending caudally from the right portal vein and its posterior branch to the inferior (i.e., caudal) surface of the right lobe on the sagittal or coronal view (Fig. 26) (24).

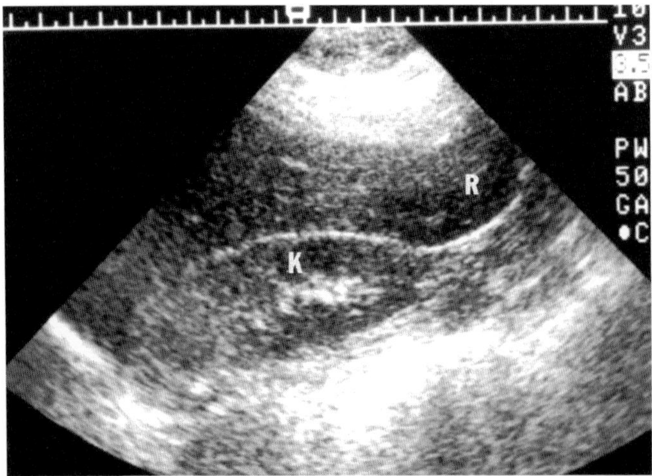

FIGURE 25 ■ Riedel's lobe. Riedel's lobe of the liver is seen as a tongue-like projection of the right lobe extending below (i.e., caudal to) the lower pole of the right kidney. R, liver; K, right kidney.

Pitfalls

A prominent ligamentum teres may mimic a hyperechoic mass (Fig. 3A); however, its location within the fissure for

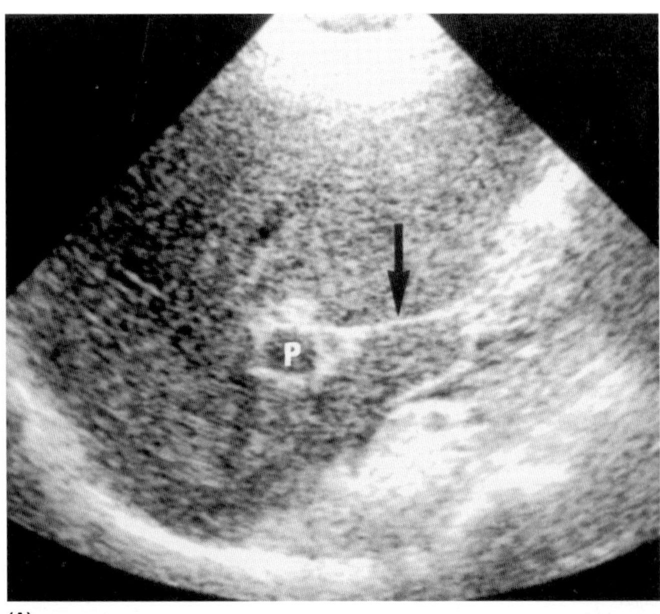

(A)

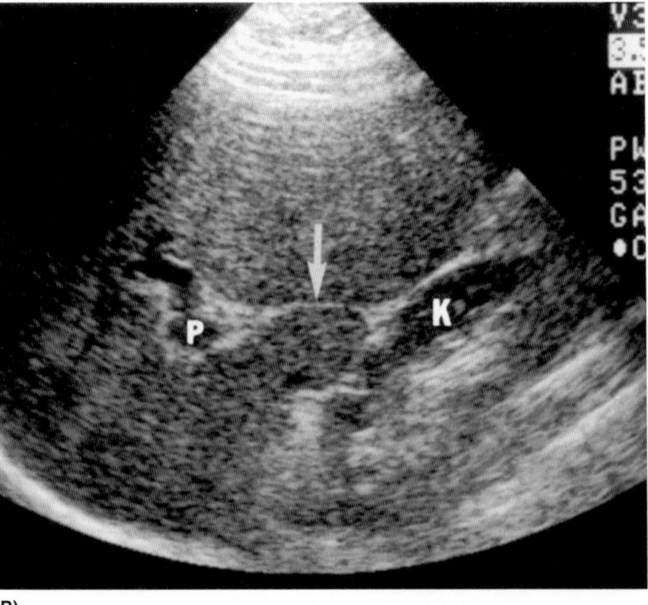

(B)

FIGURE 26 A AND B ■ Inferior accessory fissure. Sagittal views. (**A**) The inferior accessory fissure is seen as a thin, linear hyperechoic structure (*arrow*) extending from the right portal vein (P) to the inferior (caudal) surface of the liver. (**B**) More laterally, the inferior accessory fissure (*arrow*) is seen extending from the posterior branch (P) of the right portal vein to the inferior (caudal) margin of the right lobe of the liver and to the anterior margin of the right kidney (K).

TABLE 5 ■ Hepatic Pseudolesions

Mimic hyperechoic mass
- Prominent ligamentum teres
- Diaphragmatic slips
- Perihepatic or perinephric fat invaginating liver
- Focal fatty infiltration

Mimic hypoechoic mass
- Focal sparing in fatty liver
- Shadowing from fissure for ligamentum venosum causing hypoechoic appearance of caudate lobe
- Shadowing from other ligaments and fissures
- Shadowing from periportal fibrous tissue and fat

Mimic calcified mass
- Ligamentum teres with shadowing

the ligamentum teres and its band-like appearance on the sagittal view should confirm its origin (Table 5) (2). Papillary process, which is an ovoid prominence on the anteroinferior aspect of the caudate lobe, may appear separate from the liver on the transverse and sagittal views and may mimic an enlarged lymph node or pancreatic mass (Fig. 27). It is usually seen to the left of the inferior (caudal) end of the caudate lobe, posterior to the left lobe, above and anterior to the main hepatic artery, and close to the main portal vein and pancreatic isthmus (25). Usually, one sees a linear echogenic plane of separation between the papillary process posteriorly and the left lobe of the liver anteriorly. On the transverse and sagittal views, the papillary process appears separate from the liver because of the thinness of its junction with the superior (cranial) portion of the caudate lobe. It can be recognized primarily by its echo pattern, which is similar to that of the adjacent liver. Average dimensions of the papillary process in sagittal, transverse, and anteroposterior planes are 16, 17, and 8 mm, respectively (25). This process can be larger in patients with cirrhosis of the liver.

Invagination of the liver by diaphragmatic slip, created by diaphragmatic infolding, appears as a fissure-like, hyperechoic band within the cranial portion of the right lobe of the liver, best seen on the transverse view (Fig. 28) (26). When partially seen, usually on the sagittal view, diaphragmatic slip may mimic a hyperechoic mass in the liver (Fig. 28C). Less frequently, multiple diaphragmatic slips may mimic multiple hyperechoic masses. Scanning in multiple planes is necessary to demonstrate the origin of the pseudomass from the fissure created by the diaphragmatic slip.

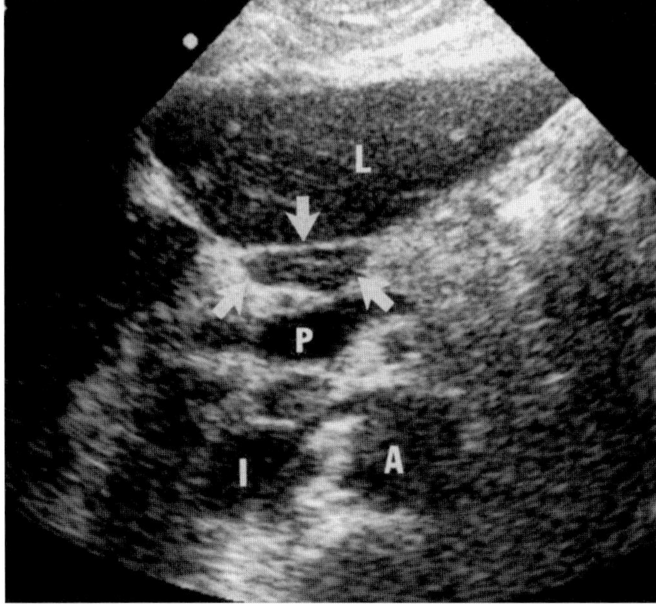

(A)

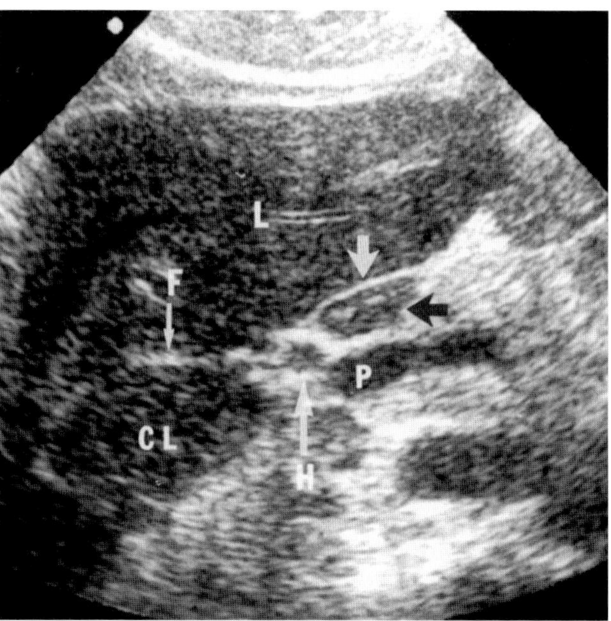

(B)

FIGURE 27 A AND B ■ Papillary process of the caudate lobe. (**A**) Transverse view shows the papillary process (*arrows*) posterior to and separated from the lateral segment of the left lobe (L) of the liver by a thin hyperechoic line. (**B**) Sagittal view shows the papillary process (*arrows*) posterior to and separated from the lateral segment of the left lobe (L) of the liver by a thin, hyperechoic line. On the sagittal view, the papillary process appears separate from the caudate lobe (CL) because of the thinness of its junction with the superior (cranial) portion of the caudate lobe. On both the transverse and the longitudinal views, the papillary process has echogenicity and an echo pattern similar to that of the adjacent left lobe of the liver. P, main portal vein near confluence of the splenic and superior mesenteric veins; I, inferior vena cava; A, aorta; H, hepatic artery; F, ligamentum venosum fissure.

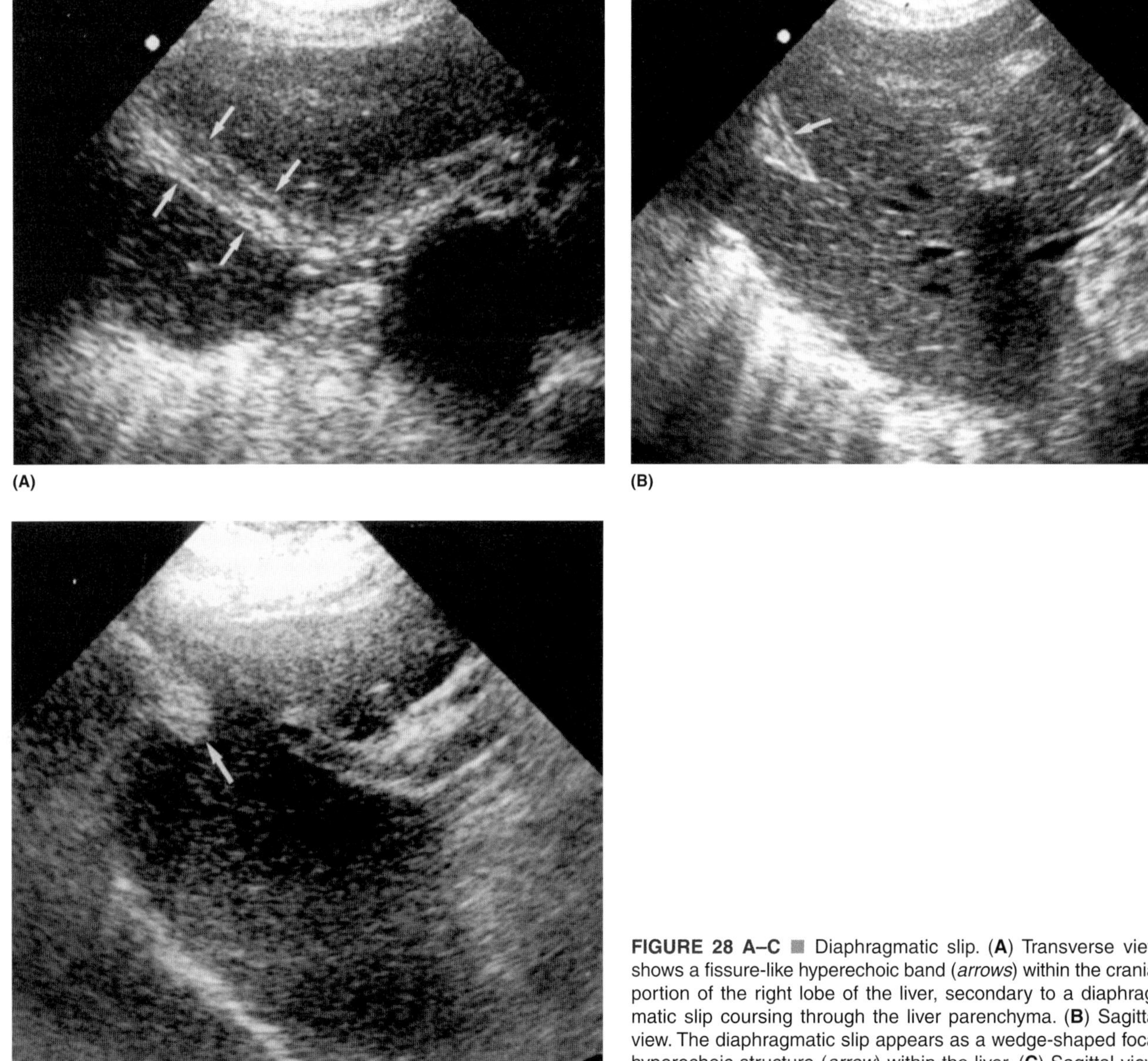

FIGURE 28 A–C ■ Diaphragmatic slip. (**A**) Transverse view shows a fissure-like hyperechoic band (*arrows*) within the cranial portion of the right lobe of the liver, secondary to a diaphragmatic slip coursing through the liver parenchyma. (**B**) Sagittal view. The diaphragmatic slip appears as a wedge-shaped focal hyperechoic structure (*arrow*) within the liver. (**C**) Sagittal view. In another patient, a thick diaphragmatic slip mimics a rounded, hyperechoic mass (*arrow*) in the liver.

ARTIFACTS

On the transverse view, the ligamentum teres may cause acoustic shadowing (Fig. 29) and may mimic a calcified mass; however, its location within the fissure for the ligamentum teres and its band-like appearance on the sagittal view should confirm its origin. On the sagittal view, the ligamentum teres may cause acoustic shadowing, so the liver parenchyma posterior to ligamentum teres may appear hypoechoic (Fig. 16B). The fissure for the ligamentum venosum may occasionally cause acoustic shadowing, so the caudate lobe may appear hypoechoic, mimicking a mass (Figs. 6B, 10, and 11). Scanning in multiple planes usually confirms the artifactual nature of this hypoechoic appearance. Similarly, acoustic shadowing of varying widths can be caused by prominent fibrous tissue and fat surrounding major branches of the portal veins (Figs. 8A, 11, and 30) (27). A large acoustic shadow may mimic a hypoechoic lesion within the liver (Figs. 16 and 30).

Mirror-image artifact is produced when a hepatic lesion, especially a hyperechoic or anechoic lesion, is located close to the diaphragm. Mirror-image artifact results in the supradiaphragmatic projection of an infradiaphragmatic mass, producing a mirror image of the lesion, outside and cranial to the liver (Fig. 31) (28). Mirror-image artifact may simulate acoustic enhancement from a hyperechoic lesion, especially hepatic hemangioma (Fig. 31B).

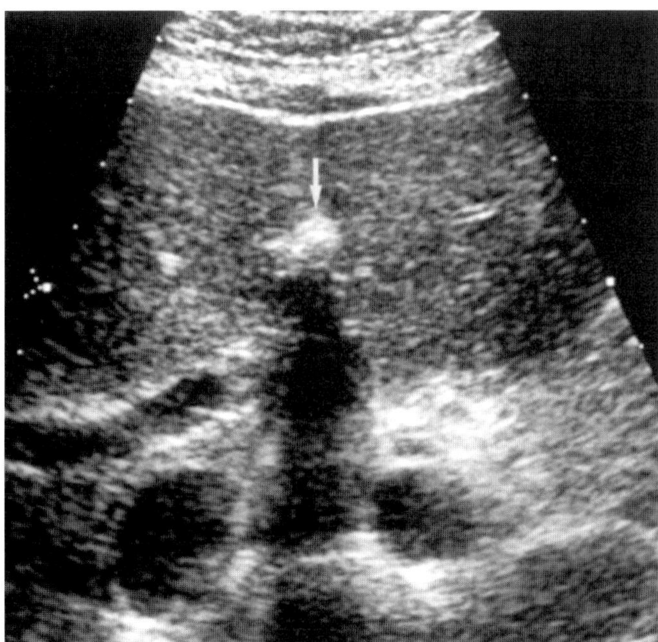

FIGURE 29 ■ Transverse view shows a prominent ligamentum teres (*arrow*) with a distal acoustic shadow.

Prominent hyperechoic fat around the upper pole of the right kidney may mimic a hyperechoic lesion in the liver (Fig. 32), usually on the transverse view (27). Scanning in different planes, especially the sagittal plane, confirms the artifactual nature of this pseudolesion.

FOCAL ABNORMALITIES

Focal liver abnormalities can be seen secondary to cysts, benign or malignant neoplasm, inflammatory or posttraumatic masses, and metabolic disorders or congenital abnormalities. With gray-scale and Doppler sonography, a specific diagnosis of hepatic neoplasms is frequently difficult due to overlapping sonographic features. Other imaging [computed tomography (CT) or magnetic resonance imaging (MRI)] or percutaneous biopsy is often needed for definitive diagnosis. Contrast-enhanced sonography may obviate the need for those other modalities, for characterization of some hepatic neoplasms (see Chapter 3).

Congenital Hepatic Cysts

Simple Hepatic Cysts

Simple hepatic cysts are frequent incidental findings during hepatic sonography, with an incidence of 2.5% to 4.6% of the population (Tables 6 and 7) (29,30). The cysts become increasingly common with age, and the incidence is higher after 40 years of age, reaching 7% in persons over 80 years old (30–32). Simple liver cysts are considered a congenital abnormality; however, whether all simple cysts are of congenital origin is uncertain (32), and the reason that they do not appear until middle age is unclear. The simple liver cysts have an epithelial lining, and the frequent presence of columnar epithelium suggests a biliary ductal origin, but the precise genesis is unclear (32). Hepatic cysts usually do not cause any symptoms. However, cysts that hemorrhage or larger

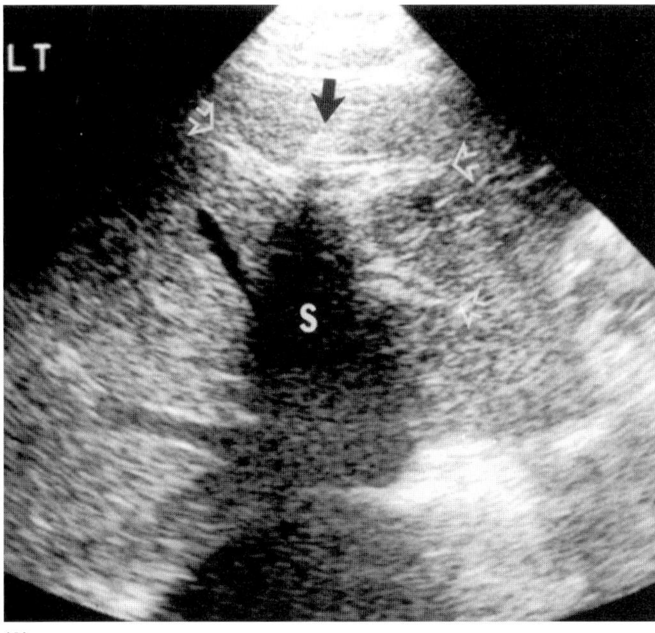

(A)

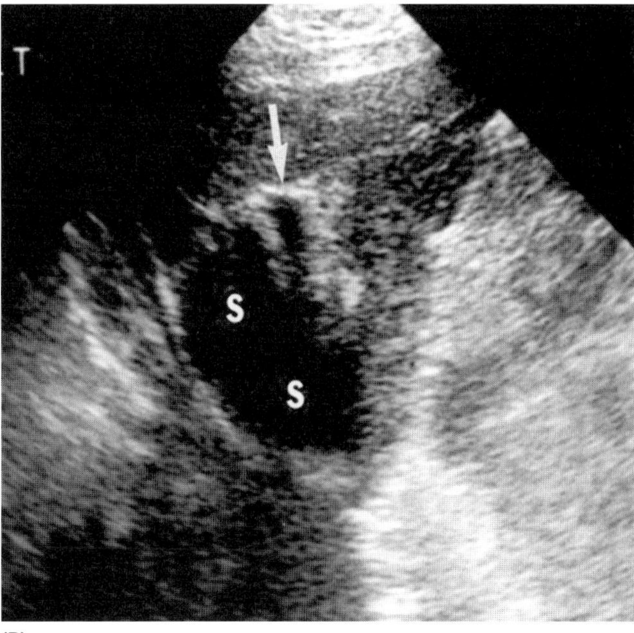

(B)

FIGURE 30 A AND B ■ Shadowing from fissure. Transverse (**A**) and sagittal (**B**) views of the left lobe of the liver demonstrate prominent acoustic shadowing (S) from fibrofatty tissue surrounding the ascending branch of the left portal vein (*solid arrow*) within the left intersegmental fissure. On the sagittal view, the shadow (S) mimics a hypoechoic mass within the liver. *Open arrows*, segmental branches of the left portal vein.

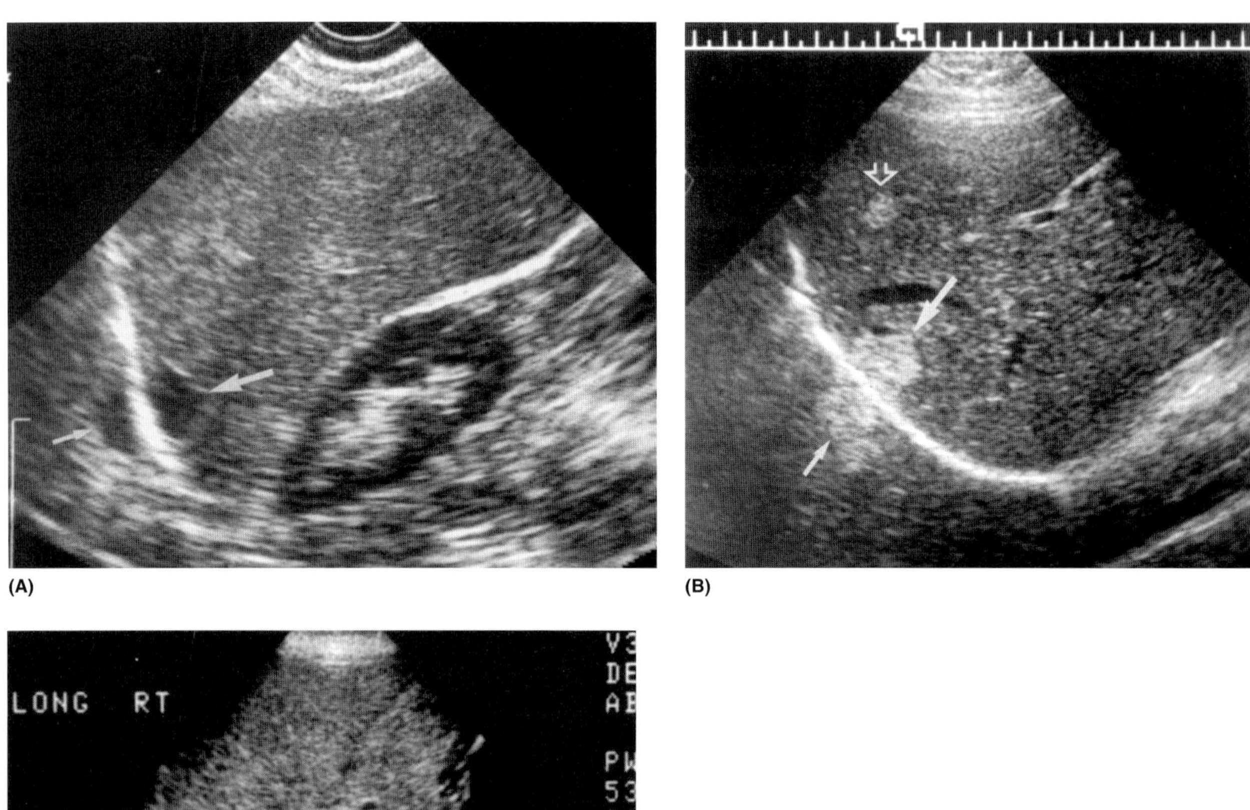

(A) (B)

(C)

FIGURE 31 A–C ■ Mirror-image artifact. Sagittal views. (**A**) A simple cyst (*large arrow*) adjacent to the diaphragm and a mirror-image artifact (*small arrow*) of the cyst outside the liver. (**B**) A hyperechoic hemangioma (*large arrow*) adjacent to the diaphragm and mirror image (*small arrow*) of the hemangioma outside the liver. The mirror image should not be mistaken for acoustic enhancement from the hemangioma. Another, smaller hyperechoic hemangioma (*open arrow*) is seen in the anterior portion of the liver. (**C**) A metastatic lesion with a target pattern (*solid arrow*) adjacent to the diaphragm and a mirror-image artifact (*open arrow*) of the metastatic lesion outside the liver.

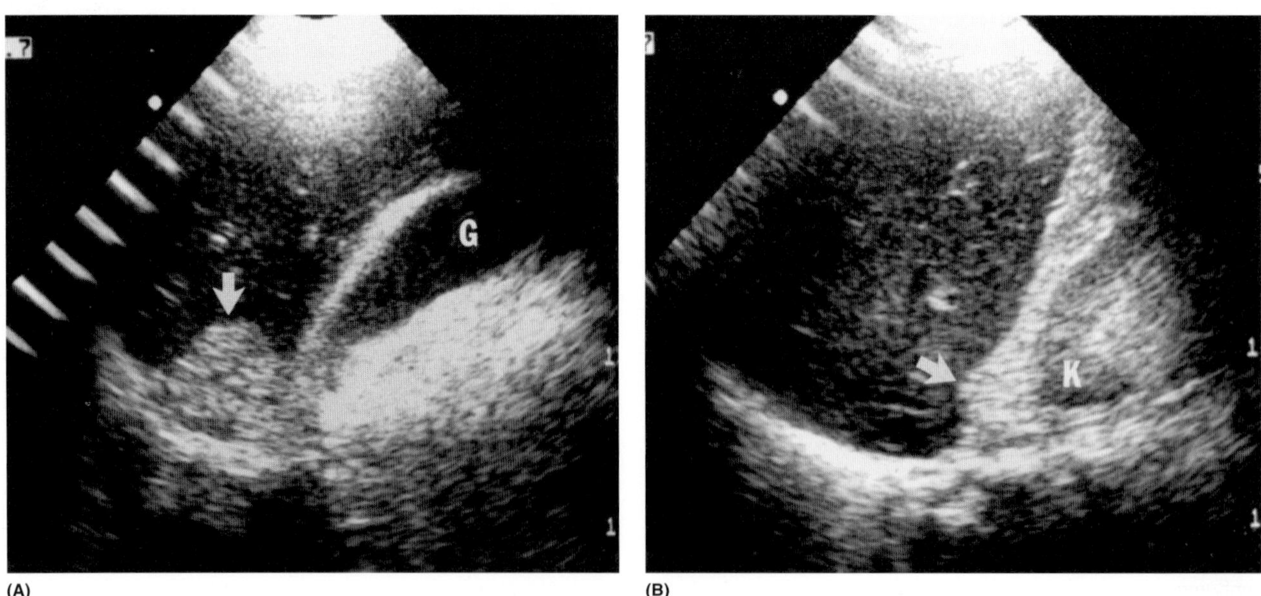

(A) (B)

FIGURE 32 A AND B ■ Perinephric fat mimicking a liver mass. (**A**) Transverse oblique view shows a hyperechoic structure (*arrow*) mimicking a mass within the posterior right lobe of the liver. (**B**) Sagittal view demonstrates the mass to be artifactual secondary to prominent perinephric fat (*arrow*) between the liver and the upper pole of the right kidney (K). G, gallbladder.

TABLE 6 ■ Cystic Liver Masses

Prevalence	Mass
Common	Simple cyst Polycystic liver disease Abscess Hematoma Hydatid cyst
Uncommon	Cystic metastasis Necrotic primary tumor Posttraumatic cyst Biloma
Rare	Caroli's disease Intrahepatic gallbladder Cavernous hemangioma Biliary cystadenoma or cystadenocarcinoma Mesenchymal hamartoma Angiosarcoma Cystic hepatoblastoma Hepatic artery aneurysm or pseudoaneurysm Congenital aneurysmal portosystemic venous shunt

cysts may cause abdominal pain. Sonographically, the cysts are anechoic, with well-defined imperceptible wall and distal acoustic enhancement proportionate to the size of the cyst (Fig. 33A). Slight focal irregularities of the wall are common (Fig. 33B). A thin septum or two may be occasionally present (Fig. 33B). The cysts are usually small (<5 cm in diameter), most frequently 1 to 2 cm in diameter; however, occasionally they are 20 cm or larger in diameter. They are more common in women, most common in the right lobe of the liver, and are occasionally (26%) multiple. Cysts that hemorrhage may have internal echoes or multiple septations and thickening of the wall (Fig. 33C,D). Symptomatic cysts can be treated with sonographically guided aspiration followed by alcohol injection (33). Aspiration alone without instillation of sclerosing agents results in cyst recurrence in most patients (34), although it may lead to temporary palliation of symptoms.

Polycystic Liver Disease

Patients with autosomal-dominant (adult) polycystic disease may have renal cysts only, liver cysts only, or variable degree of both kidney and liver involvement with multiple cysts (35). The frequency of liver cysts in autosomal-dominant polycystic kidney disease varies between 57% and 74% (35). It is generally believed that

TABLE 7 ■ Sonographic Features of Predominantly Solid Neoplasms

	Solitary	Multiple	Diffusely infiltrating	Hyper-echoic	Hypo-echoic	Mixed echo-genicity	Cystic areas	Calcifi-cations	Enhance-ment[a]	Shadowing[a]
Hemangioma	+P	+	–	+P	+	+	R	R	O	–
Adenoma	+P	+GSD	–	+	+	+	–	–	GSD	–
Focal nodular hyperplasia	+P	+	–	+	+	+	–	–	–	–
Infantile hemangio-endothelioma	+	+	–	+	+	+	+	+	–	–
Lipoma	+	R	–	+	–	–	–	–	–	+
Hepatocellular carcinoma	+	+	+	+	+	+	U	U	O	–
Fibrolamellar carcinoma	+	–	–	+	O	+	–	+	–	O
Peripheral cholangio-carcinoma	+P	+	R	+	+	+	–	O	–	–
Angiosarcoma	+	+P	–	–	–	+	+	–	–	–
Epithelioid hemangio-endothelioma	+	+	–	–	+	+	–	+	–	–
Hepatoblastoma	+	U	U	+P	O	+	O	+	–	–
Lymphoma	U	+P	–	R	+P	U	–	–	O	–

[a]Enhancement or shadowing not related to cystic areas or calcifications, respectively.

Abbreviations: P, predominantly; U, uncommonly; O, occasionally; R, rarely; GSD, adenoma in glycogen storage disease.

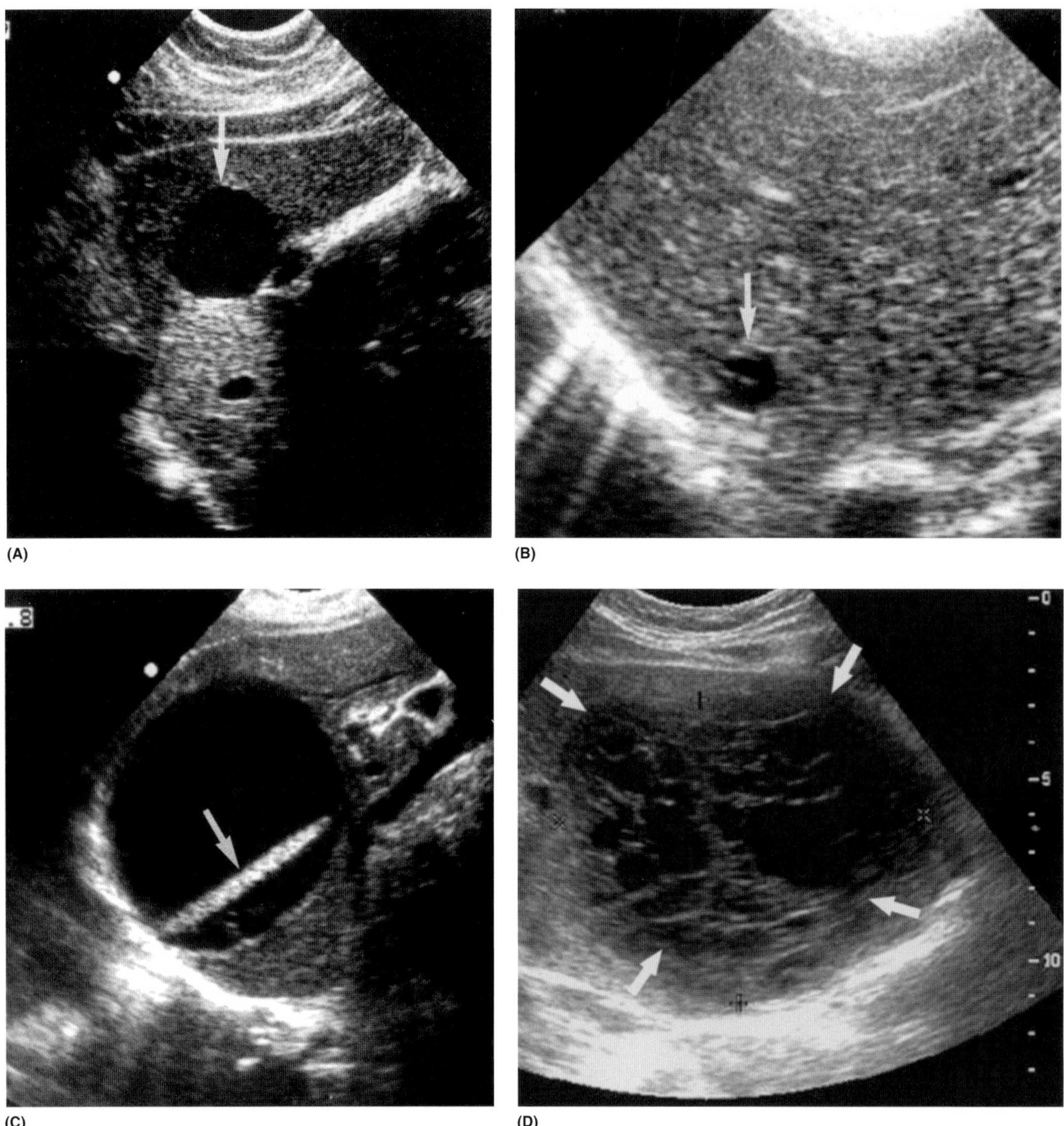

FIGURE 33 A–D ■ Hepatic cysts. (**A**) Sagittal view. A typical simple cyst (*arrow*) is seen as an anechoic mass with a sharp posterior wall and posterior acoustic enhancement. (**B**) Sagittal view. This cyst (*arrow*) has a thin septum and slight focal irregularities of the wall. (**C**) Transverse view. This cyst contains a hyperechoic layer of debris (*arrow*) secondary to hemorrhage within the lesion. (**D**) Cyst (*arrows*) with septa secondary to previous hemorrhage within the cyst.

the cysts develop from dilatation of aberrant bile ducts. The cysts, however, do not communicate with the biliary system. Complications such as cyst infection, hemorrhage within the cysts, jaundice, or portal hypertension are rare (35). The number and size of the cysts vary (Fig. 34). When liver involvement is extensive, the cysts may have irregular margins and an irregular or flattened shape. Occasionally, the flattened appearance of the cysts may be difficult to distinguish from dilated intrahepatic bile ducts.

Peribiliary Cysts

Peribiliary cysts that are believed to represent obstructed small periductal glands in the peribiliary tissues, primarily in association with severe liver disease, have been reported and may occasionally be seen by sonography (36). These cysts are primarily seen in porta hepatis, but less commonly may be seen in the peripheral portion of the liver parallel to the right or left portal veins and bile ducts. The cysts may appear as discrete

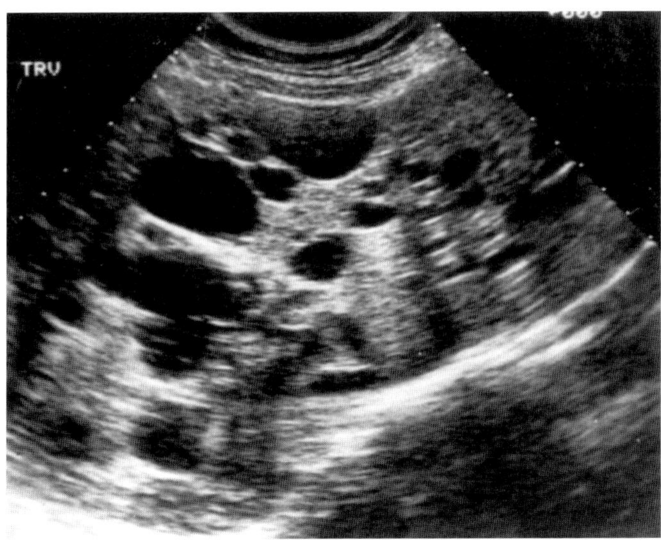

FIGURE 34 ■ Adult polycystic disease. Transverse view shows numerous cysts of varying size replacing most of the liver parenchyma.

cystic structures, clusters of cysts or tortuous tubular channel with thin septations. The appearances may mimic dilated bile ducts, cystic neoplasm, or abscess. These peribiliary cysts usually are small (<2.5 cm) and asymptomatic; however, rarely, larger cysts may cause biliary obstruction.

Benign Neoplasms

Cavernous Hemangioma

Cavernous hemangioma is the most common benign solid neoplasm of the liver, most frequently diagnosed incidentally during hepatic sonography. The incidence in autopsy series ranges from 0.4% to 7.4% (37). When all liver lesions are considered, hemangiomas are second only to hepatic metastases in frequency of occurrence (38). This lesion occurs at all ages but is commonest in adults and rare in young children (37). It occurs in women predominantly, with a reported female-to-male ratio of 4:1 to 6:1 (37). Most hemangiomas are small and asymptomatic. Large hemangiomas may occasionally produce symptoms secondary to hemorrhage within the mass, compression by the large mass, or, rarely, rupture with intraperitoneal hemorrhage. Hemangiomas may increase in size during pregnancy or after estrogen administration (37). However, most hemangiomas in adults do not change in size or appearance (39). No change in size or enlargement was seen in 90% and 99% of patients in two investigations with mean followup interval of 19 and 26 months, respectively (40,41). In one case, hemangioma was seen to decrease in size and then disappear. In a study of 36 giant hemangiomas with a mean follow-up period of 55 months, 32 of the 36 giant hemangiomas remained stable in size and there were only minor changes in 4 out of 36 giant hemangiomas (42). Pathologically, hemangioma is composed of many vascular channels of different sizes supported by fibrous septa. The vascular spaces may contain thrombi (37).

Sonographically, the classic appearance is that of a rounded, hyperechoic, homogeneous solid mass with well-defined margins (Fig. 35). Most hemangiomas are smaller than 3 cm in diameter. However, they can range in size from a few millimeters to more than 20 cm. When larger than 4 cm, they are termed giant hemangiomas. Hemangiomas are more commonly seen in the right lobe, especially the posterior segment, and frequently they are peripheral or subcapsular in location (Fig. 35A) (43,44). Most are solitary, but they are multiple in up to 10% of cases (Fig. 35A) (45). Occasionally, a variable degree of distal acoustic enhancement may be seen (Fig. 36), especially in lesions larger than 2.5 cm (46). Up to 23% have lobulated or irregular margins (Fig. 37) (43,46). A hyperechoic appearance may be secondary to numerous interspaces between the walls of the cavernous sinuses. Approximately 70% of hemangiomas are hyperechoic and homogeneous, and the remainder are hypoechoic, isoechoic, or of mixed echogenicity and rarely contain cystic areas (45). The heterogeneous appearance with central hypoechoic areas may be related to fibrosis, thrombosis, hemorrhage, or degeneration, and, in general, the echo pattern is more variable in larger (>4 cm) lesions (Fig. 37). In a study by Moody and Wilson, an echogenic border, seen as a thick echogenic rind or a thin echogenic rim (Fig. 38), was seen in 93% of atypical solid hemangiomas. This finding was considered suggestive of hemangioma (47). A typical hemangioma with hypoechoic areas may contain a single echogenic septum (Fig. 38A) or multiple septa (Fig. 37B) (44). A hypoechoic "halo" surrounding the periphery is rarely seen in a hemangioma. Hemangioma may appear hypoechoic when surrounded by diffusely fatty liver (45). Unlike hyperechoic metastasis or hyperechoic HCC, when hemangiomas are compressed during intraoperative ultrasound examination, they may become less echogenic and more isoechoic to normal liver, probably because of obliteration of cavernous sinuses within the hemangioma from direct scanning pressure (48). In one study, reduction of echogenicity during the ultrasound examination was seen in 41% of cavernous hemangioma after change in position, from supine to standing, for at least 30 minutes (49). This observation may be helpful to differentiate cavernous hemangioma from other tumors. Rarely, calcification is seen within the hemangioma (44).

With color Doppler sonography, internal color flow is rarely seen within a hemangioma (50,51). However, in one study, occasionally, presence of arterioportal shunts within the hemangioma was seen to influence color Doppler findings of hepatic hemangiomas with demonstration of large feeding artery, multiple intratumoral flows, and reversal of portal flow within or around the hemangioma, and these findings mimicked hypervascular tumors (52). When color Doppler flow is detected within a lesion that has the gray-scale appearance of a hemangioma, further evaluation is indicated (53). Two studies concluded that flow signals seen within hemangioma, with power Doppler sonography are artifactual, related to the architecture of the hemangioma (54,55). Therefore, the role of two-dimensional power Doppler remains controversial.

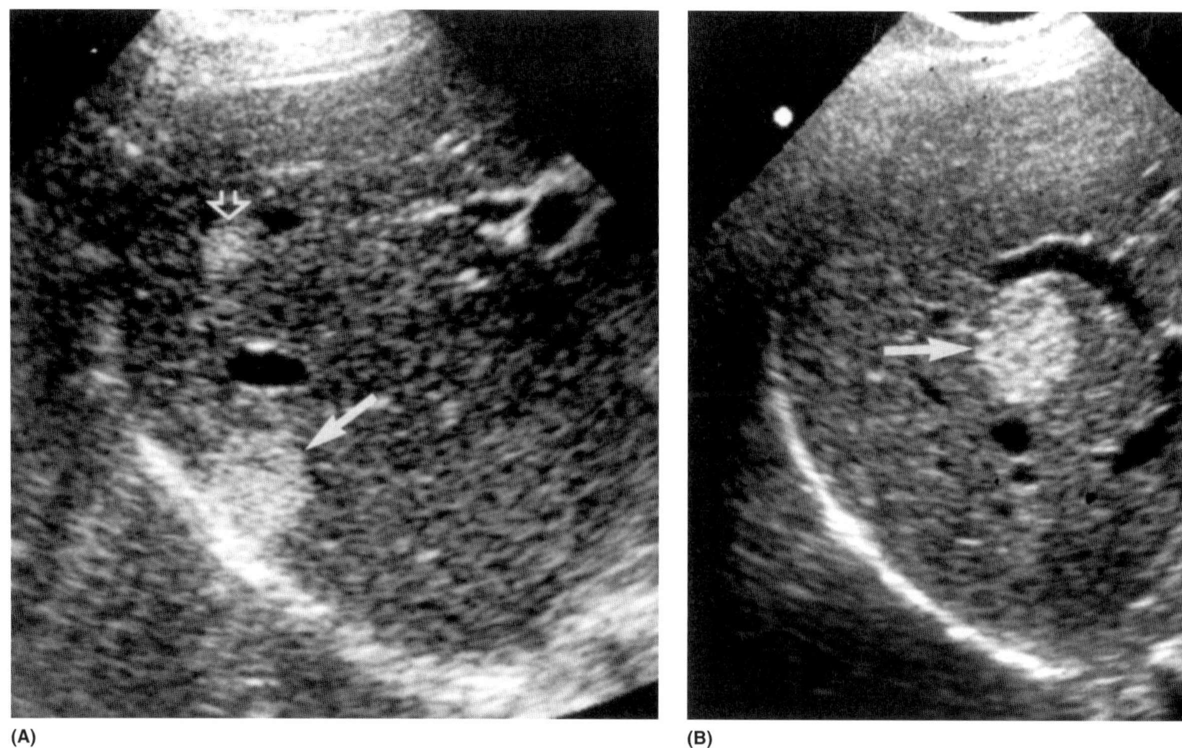

FIGURE 35 A AND B ■ Cavernous hemangioma. (**A**) Sagittal view. This typical hyperechoic hemangioma (*solid arrow*) is in a peripheral subcapsular location in the right lobe. Another smaller hemangioma (*open arrow*) is seen anteriorly. (**B**) Sagittal view. The hemangioma (*arrow*) is located centrally in the right lobe and is seen as a typical hyperechoic, relatively homogeneous solid mass with well-defined margins.

Diagnostic Workup of Sonographically Detected Hemangioma ■ In patients with symptoms related to the liver, abnormal liver function tests, or known malignant disease, and in patients with an atypical sonographic pattern of hemangioma, further evaluation by technetium-99 m–labeled red-blood-cell single photon emission computed tomography (RBC SPECT) scintigraphy or MRI is recommended. Dynamic contrast-enhanced CT is less specific than RBC SPECT scintigraphy or MRI.

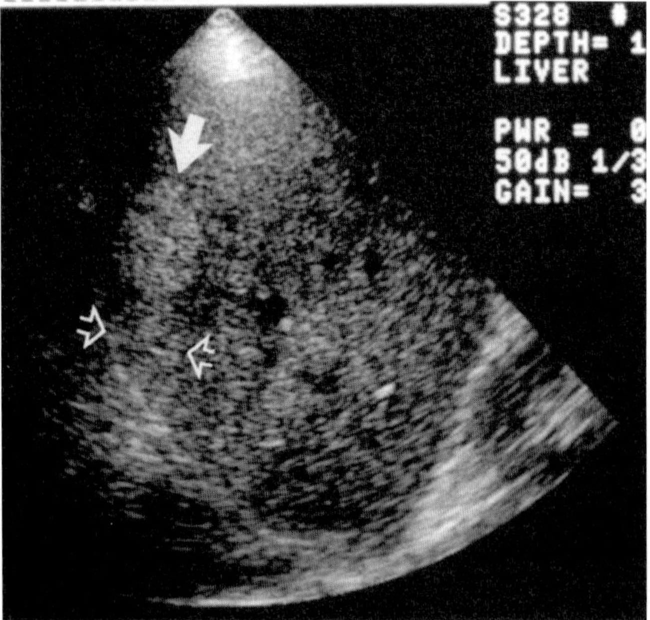

FIGURE 36 ■ Hemangioma (*solid arrow*) demonstrates minimal posterior acoustic enhancement (*open arrows*). *Source*: Courtesy of Philip W. Ralls, MD, Los Angeles, CA.

In asymptomatic patients with normal liver function tests and no known malignant disease, some clinicians consider that focal hepatic lesions demonstrating the classic or near-classic ultrasonic appearance of a hemangioma require no further workup, except perhaps follow-up imaging at three to six months. Other clinicians, however, prefer another confirmatory study (i.e., scintigraphy or MRI) for a specific diagnosis of hemangioma. Examination by RBC SPECT scintigraphy is recommended if the lesion is larger than 2.5 cm in diameter. However, MRI is recommended if the lesion is smaller than 2.5 cm or is adjacent to the heart or major hepatic vessels (56).

If the lesion has a classic appearance on the confirmatory RBC SPECT scintigraphy or MRI, no further workup is necessary. If neither scintigraphy nor MRI reveals classic features, percutaneous biopsy with a 20-gauge needle may be performed (45). Percutaneous fine-needle (22-gauge) aspiration or percutaneous biopsy with a 20-gauge Franseen needle is safe and effective in the diagnosis of hemangioma and is not associated with significant complications (57–59). In one study, no serious complications were found after 18-gauge core-needle biopsy of 47 liver hemangiomas (60).

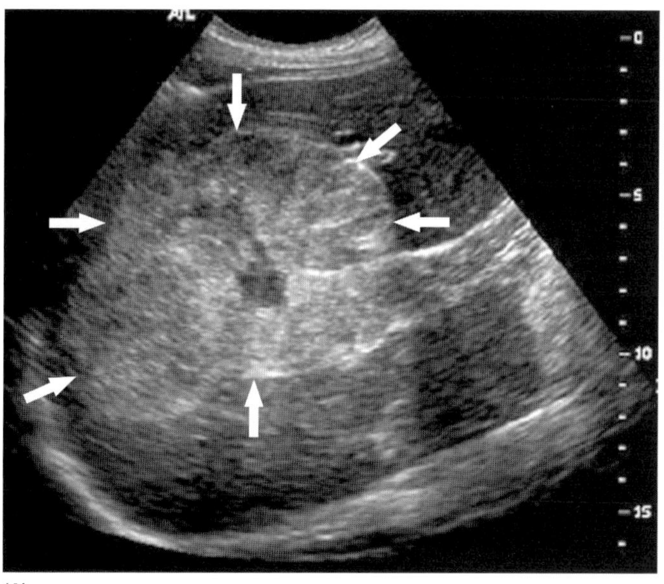

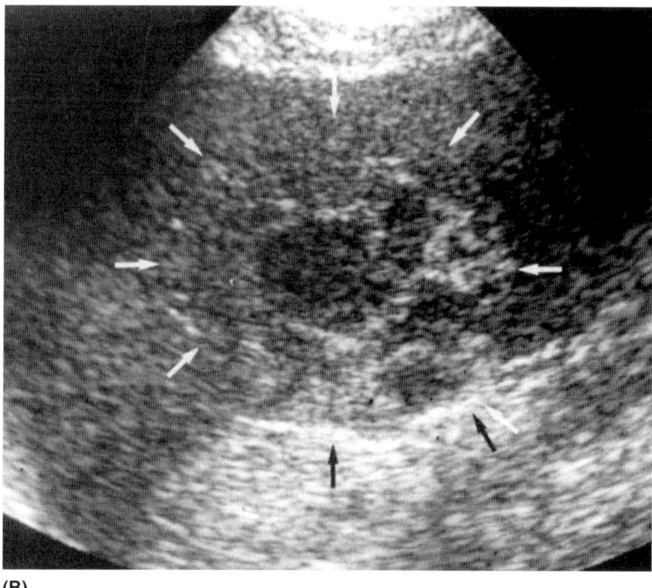

(A) (B)

FIGURE 37 A AND B ■ Large atypical hemangioma. (**A**) Sagittal view. This large hemangioma (*arrows*) has an inhomogeneous echo pattern and a slightly lobulated contour. (**B**) Large hemangioma (*arrows*), in another patient, shows hypoechoic areas and septations and distal acoustic enhancement.

Malignancies Mimicking Hemangioma

In a study of 1982 patients with newly diagnosed cirrhosis, 50% of the lesions with hemangioma-like appearance on the ultrasound examination were proven to be hyperechoic HCCs (61). In the same investigation, the probability of a diagnosis of HCC (or preneoplastic lesion) was 100% for hemangioma-like lesions detected during followup screening ultrasound in patients with cirrhosis, whose initial ultrasound scan depicted no lesions in the liver. Occasionally, hyperechoic hepatic metastasis may mimic a cavernous hemangioma (62). Therefore, in patients with cirrhosis of the liver or known malignancy, when ultrasound examination shows hemangioma-like lesion, other imaging studies or biopsy is suggested for confirmation of the diagnosis of hemangioma.

Hepatic Adenoma

Hepatic adenoma (liver-cell adenoma or hepatocellular adenoma) is a rare benign liver tumor, most commonly

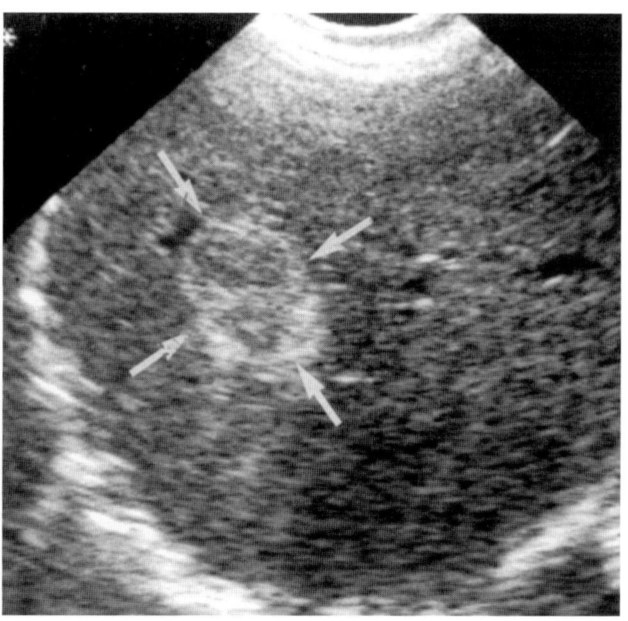

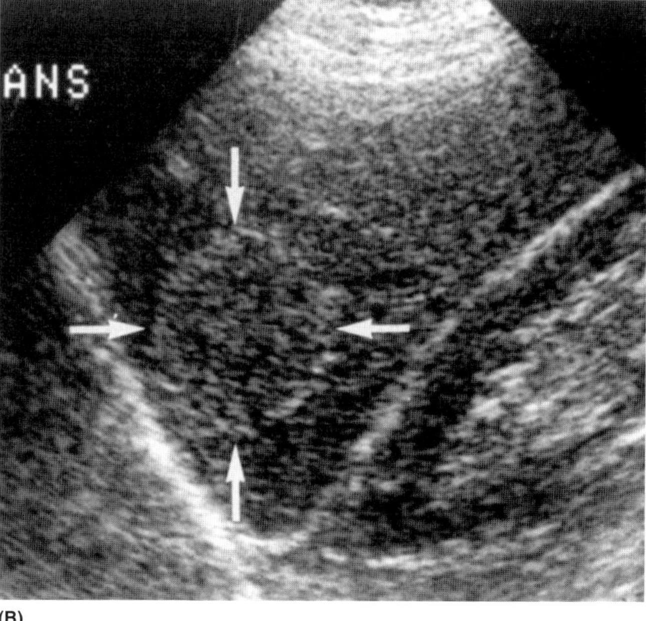

(A) (B)

FIGURE 38 A AND B ■ Atypical hemangioma with echogenic border. (**A**) Hemangioma (*arrows*) shows a thick, hyperechoic rim and a central echogenic septum. (**B**) Isoechoic hemangioma (*arrows*) with a thin echogenic rim.

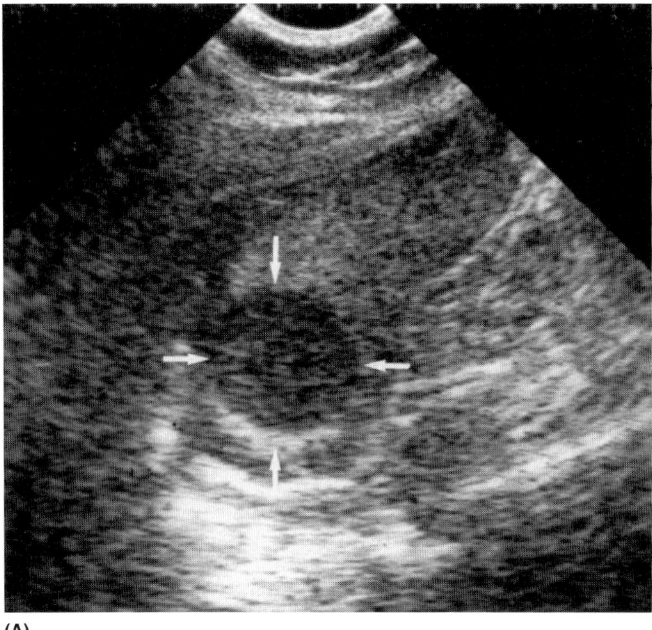
(A)

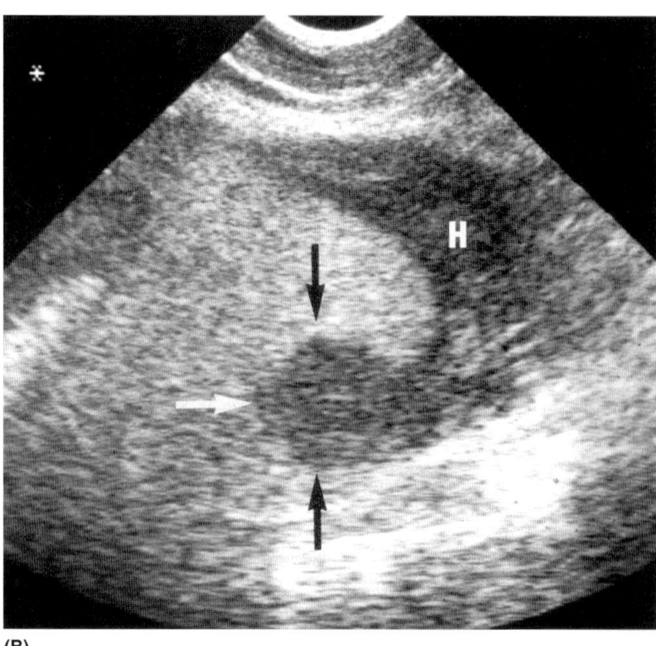

(B)

FIGURE 39 A AND B ■ Hepatic adenoma with hemorrhage. (**A**) Transverse view. The adenoma (*arrows*) is seen as a hypoechoic solid mass. (**B**) Sagittal view. This is a hypoechoic adenoma (*arrows*) with hemorrhage, resulting in a hematoma (H) surrounding the liver with posterior acoustic enhancement. One sees disruption of the inferior (caudal) margin of the liver at the site of hemorrhage.

related to oral contraceptive use and, therefore, most often seen in women of childbearing age. Anabolic steroid–induced hepatic adenoma is seen more commonly in young men (63). Adenomas associated with type I glycogen storage disease (von Gierke's disease) are multiple in about 50% of patients. Patients can present with a palpable mass, chronic abdominal pain, or acute abdominal pain caused by hemorrhage within the mass or into the peritoneal cavity. Because of the high incidence of hemorrhage or rupture, surgery is recommended whenever possible. Adenomas may undergo malignant transformation. Pathologically, hepatic adenoma usually occurs as a solitary, soft tumor that is sharply circumscribed and may or may not be encapsulated. Microscopically, the tumor is composed of sheets of normal-looking or slightly atypical hepatocytes, and it may mimic normal liver tissue. Kupffer cells are either markedly reduced in number or absent (35). Sonographically, adenomas appear as solid masses with variable echogenicity. Adenomas may be hypoechoic (20–40%) (Fig. 39) or hyperechoic (up to 30%) (Fig. 40), and the remainder are either isoechoic or of mixed echogenicity (64,65). Occasionally, hepatic adenomas contain abundant fat. The presence of fat in a hepatic adenoma may give it a hyperechoic appearance (Fig. 41) (66). When associated with glycogen storage disease, adenomas may be hyperechoic, with distal acoustic enhancement (67), or they may have variable echogenicity (68). Adenoma usually is solitary, but it may be multiple when associated with glycogen storage disease. In a study of adult patients with liver adenomatosis (more than 10 hepatic adenomas in each patient), 10 to 50 adenomas were found in each patient and the imaging features of individual adenomas were similar to those of solitary adenoma in young women taking oral contraceptive medication (69).

Most adenomas measure 8 to 15 cm in diameter, although they may range from 1 to 30 cm in diameter.

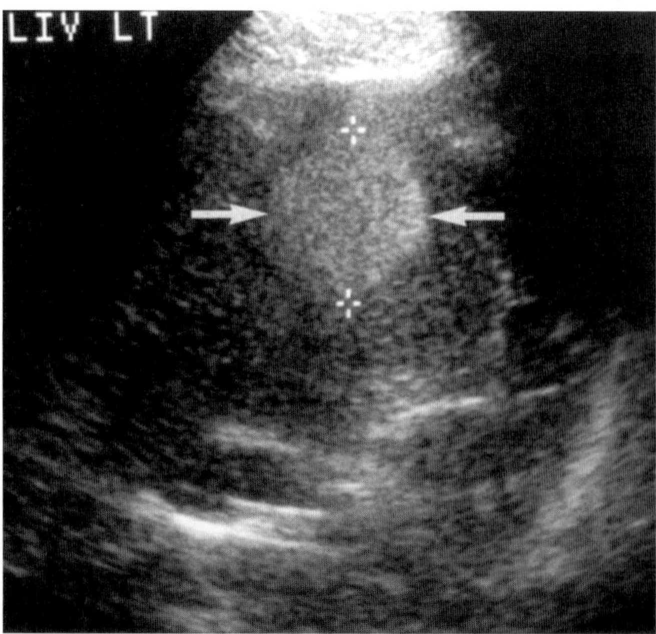

FIGURE 40 ■ Hepatic adenoma: hyperechoic pattern. Transverse view shows hyperechoic adenoma (*cursors, arrows*).

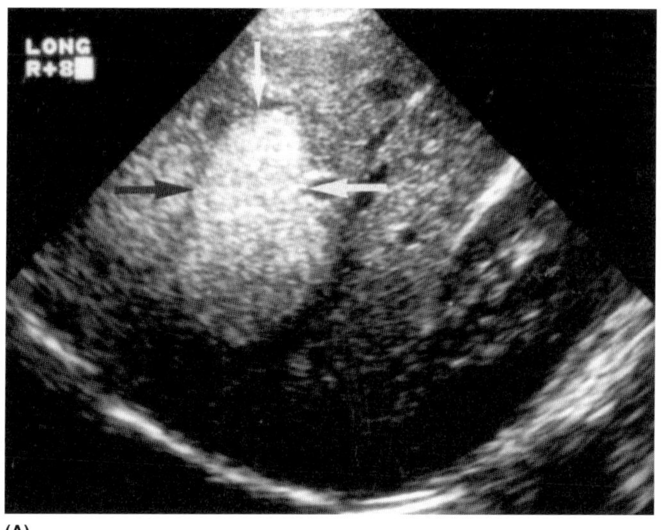

(A)

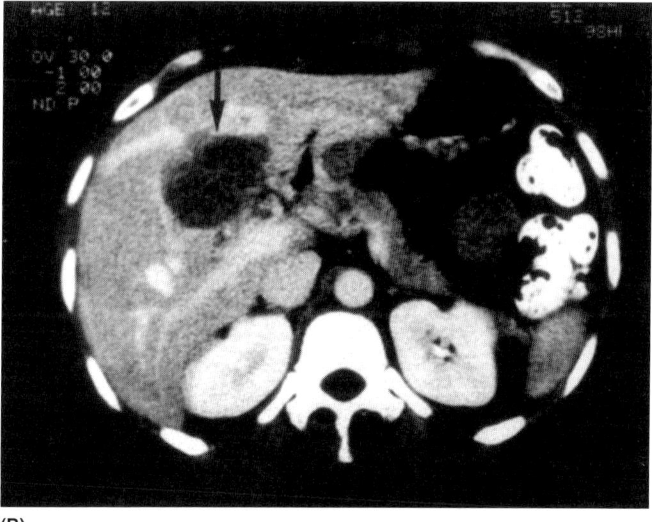

(B)

FIGURE 41 A AND B ■ Hepatic adenoma containing fat. (**A**) Sagittal sonogram shows a markedly hyperechoic adenoma (*arrows*) secondary to abundant fat content within this lesion. (**B**) CT scan demonstrates low attenuation within the mass (*arrow*) confirming the high fat content of the adenoma.

They are more common in the right lobe and usually are subcapsular and occasionally pedunculated. Hepatic adenoma usually appears as a photopenic defect on technetium-99 m sulfur colloid scintigraphy. However, uptake of the radiocolloid equal to or slightly less than surrounding normal liver has been reported in 23% of patients (70). The radiocolloid uptake is due to the presence of Kupffer cells in some adenomas, even though these cells are usually reduced in number.

Focal Nodular Hyperplasia

Focal nodular hyperplasia usually presents as a solitary mass, seen more commonly between the ages of 20 and 50 years and in women; however, the sex difference is less striking than in hepatic adenoma (71). Although a rare condition, focal nodular hyperplasia is more common than hepatic adenoma. Investigators are uncertain whether it represents a true neoplasm. Association with oral contraceptive use has been suggested, although in a review of 357 reported cases, only 11% of the women had a history of oral contraceptive use (71). Evidence does suggest, however, that this disorder may be hormone dependent because regression of the lesion after discontinuance of oral contraceptive agents has been reported (72). About 75% of patients are asymptomatic, and the mass is discovered incidentally. However, focal nodular hyperplasia in women taking oral contraceptive steroids is more likely to be symptomatic. The patient may complain of pain resulting from hemorrhage or necrosis within the mass. Hemorrhage is uncommon, however, and is seen much less frequently than in hepatic adenoma. Pathologically, focal nodular hyperplasia usually presents as a firm, coarsely nodular mass of variable size with a dense, central stellate scar and radiating fibrous septa that divide the lesion into lobules (72). Microscopically, the lesion closely resembles inactive cirrhosis. Hepatocytes appear normal, but they lack the normal cord arrangement. Kupffer cells are present, and the fibrous septa contain numerous bile ductules and vessels (72).

Sonographically, focal nodular hyperplasia appears as a solid mass of variable size and echogenicity (Fig. 42). The tumors often measure less than 3 cm, although lesions up to 20 cm in diameter have been reported (38). Lesions may be hypoechoic (33–36%) or hyperechoic (33%), and the remainder are either isoechoic or of mixed echogenicity (64,65). Focal nodular hyperplasia is usually solitary, but it may be multiple. It is usually located peripherally close to the liver capsule and may be pedunculated. The central scar may be seen as an echogenic linear or stellate structure within the central portion of the mass. However, demonstration of the central scar is infrequent. Moreover, central scar is a nonspecific finding that may be seen in other benign and malignant liver tumors (Table 8) (73). With color Doppler sonography, in addition to peripheral flow, centrifugal arterial flow originating from central portion of the tumor and, in some cases, radiating peripherally from a central vessel in a stellate configuration (Fig. 43) (76) has been reported (74–76). In a series of 269 hepatic neoplasms, both malignant and benign, this pattern was seen only in focal nodular hyperplasia (76). Even though this appearance cannot be considered specific for this lesion because of small number of reported cases, in patients clinically at low risk for malignant disease, this color flow pattern may suggest the diagnosis of focal nodular hyperplasia.

Characteristic angiographic findings include hypervascularity, prominent central artery with radiating branches (spoke-wheel sign), radiating septations, and intense capillary stain (65,71). "Scintigraphy," however, is most useful in the diagnostic workup of suspected focal nodular hyperplasia. Because of the presence of Kupffer cells, most (up to 70%) lesions show normal or

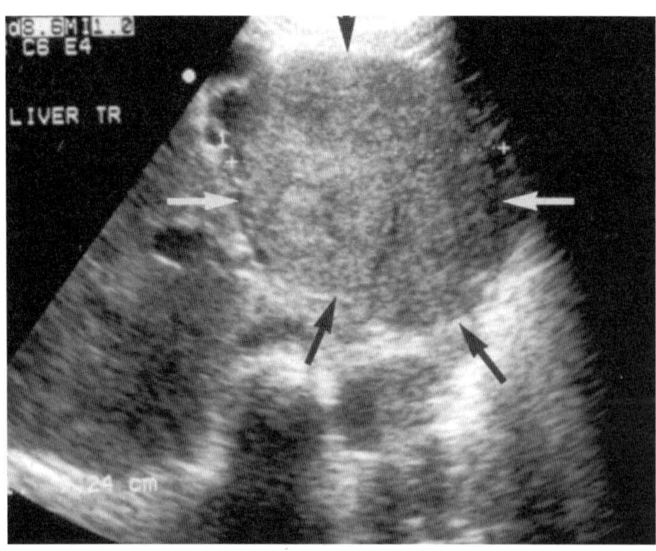

(A)

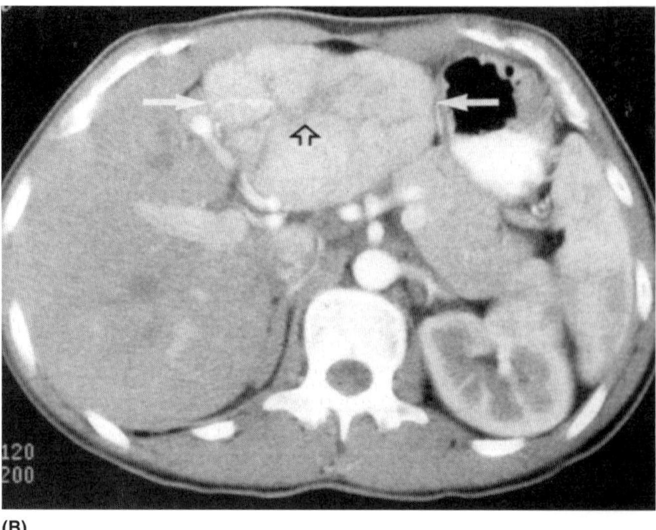

(B)

FIGURE 42 A AND B ■ Focal nodular hyperplasia. (**A**) Transverse view shows a large, predominantly slightly hyperechoic, inhomogeneous solid mass (*arrows*) within the left lobe of the liver. (**B**) CT scan with intravenous contrast. A stellate central scar (*open arrow*) is seen within the mass (*solid arrows*) in the left lobe of the liver. One sees slightly decreased attenuation in the central scar.

increased uptake of technetium-99m sulfur colloid (65). No other liver neoplasms have these scintigraphic characteristics, even though a study by Lubbers et al. (70) reported radiocolloid uptake equal to or slightly less than normal liver in 23% of hepatic adenomas. Increased uptake of the radiocolloid, however, may be a specific feature of focal nodular hyperplasia. A comparative study showed that MRI has higher sensitivity and specificity for diagnosis of focal nodular hyperplasia than ultrasonography or CT (77).

Lipoma

Hepatic lipomas are rare, usually asymptomatic, benign tumors measuring up to 6cm in diameter. They may be composed purely of fat cells, or they may be mixed with adenomatous, angiomatous, or myomatous tissue, resulting in lesions such as adenolipoma, angiomyolipoma, or myelolipoma (38). They are often associated with tuberous sclerosis and renal angiomyolipomas; however, most solitary lipomas are found as isolated entities (78). Lipomas range from 1 to 6cm in diameter. Sonographically, lipomas appear as solid, well-defined hyperechoic masses with a variable degree of distal acoustic shadowing (Fig. 44) (79). Focal displacement and discontinuity of the diaphragm deep to the lipoma may occur because of the slower speed of sound in fat compared with the normal liver and refraction of the ultrasound beam at the edge of the mass (Fig. 44) (79,80).

Sonographically, lipomas may appear similar to hemangiomas and hyperechoic metastases, which are the two most common causes of solid hyperechoic masses in the liver (Table 9). Hemangiomas may cause acoustic enhancement and rarely cause acoustic shadowing.

TABLE 8 ■ Central Scar within a Hepatic Mass

- Focal nodular hyperplasia
- Fibrolamellar carcinoma
- Hepatocellular carcinoma
- Giant hemangioma
- Hepatic adenoma

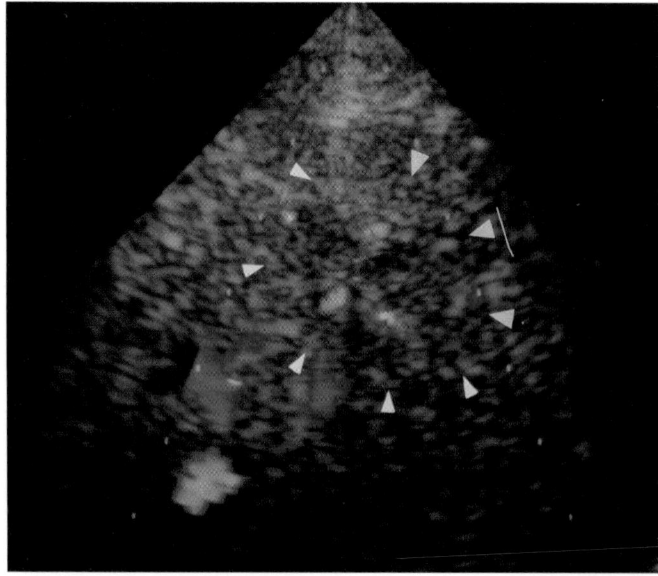

FIGURE 43 ■ Focal nodular hyperplasia. Color Doppler sonogram shows vessels radiating in a stellate configuration from the center of the mass (*arrowheads*). *Source*: From Ref. 76.

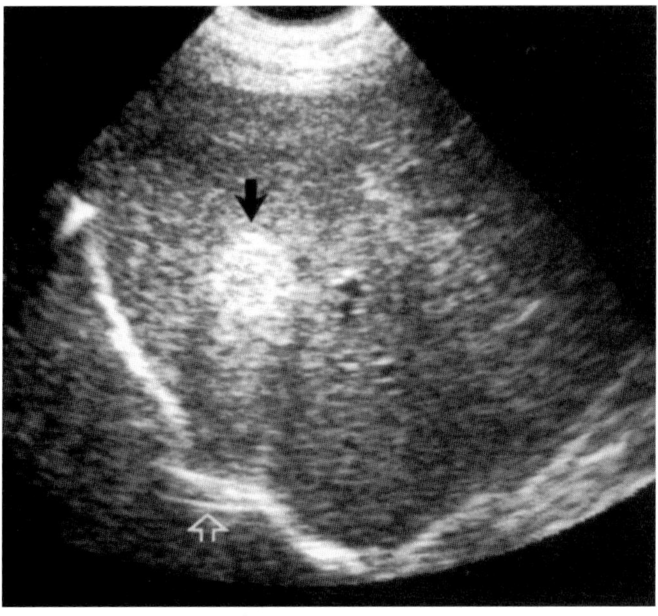

(A)

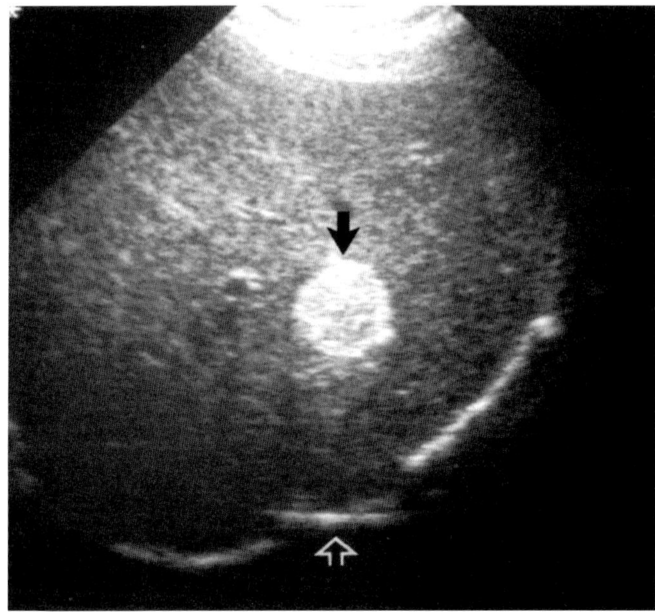

(B)

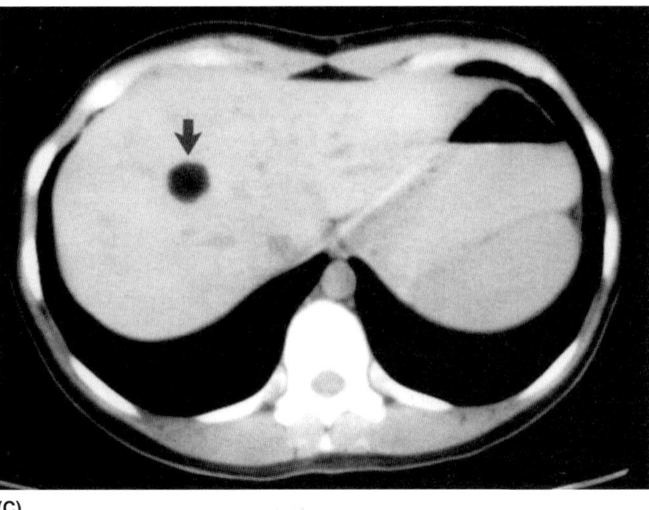

(C)

FIGURE 44 A–C ■ Hepatic lipoma. (**A** and **B**) Sagittal and transverse sonograms demonstrating lipoma (*solid arrow*) appearing as a hyperechoic solid mass with distal acoustic shadowing within the liver. Apparent displacement and discontinuity of the diaphragm (*open arrow*) deep to the mass is caused by slowed speed of sound in fat and by refraction of the ultrasound beam at the edge of the mass. (**C**) CT scan of the liver without intravenous contrast demonstrating a well-defined mass (*arrow*) of low attenuation (similar to that of fat) in the right lobe of the liver. *Source*: From Ref. 79.

Hyperechoic metastases are often inhomogeneous, are rarely solitary, and cause acoustic shadowing only when calcified. Moreover, hemangiomas and hyperechoic metastases do not cause artifactual displacement and discontinuity of the diaphragm deep to the mass. CT is helpful to confirm the diagnosis of lipoma, by demonstrating low density (−20 to −70 Hounsfield units) within the lesion, thus confirming the fatty nature of the tumor (81).

TABLE 9 ■ Hyperechoic Lesions

- Hemangioma (most common)
- Lipoma
- Hepatocellular carcinoma
- Metastases
- Other primary liver tumors
- Focal fatty infiltration

Biliary Cystadenoma and Cystadenocarcinoma

Biliary cystadenoma and cystadenocarcinoma are rare biliary tumors that arise in the liver or, less frequently, in the extrahepatic bile ducts (82). They are most commonly seen in middle-aged women. Pathologically, these lesions are well-encapsulated, multiloculated cystic masses with septations and varying degrees of mural and septal thickening and nodularity (83,84). Microscopically, the cysts are lined with a biliary type of epithelium supported by dense cellular fibrous stroma (82).

Sonographically, cystadenoma is a multilocular cystic mass, usually with thin septations (Fig. 45). Unilocular cystadenoma without septations is rare. Cystadenocarcinomas usually have thick septations, mural thickening, solid mural nodules, and papillary projections. Mural nodules are uncommon in benign cystadenoma. Calcifications may be seen within cystadenocarcinoma. However, cystadenoma and cystadenocarcinoma cannot be reliably differentiated on the

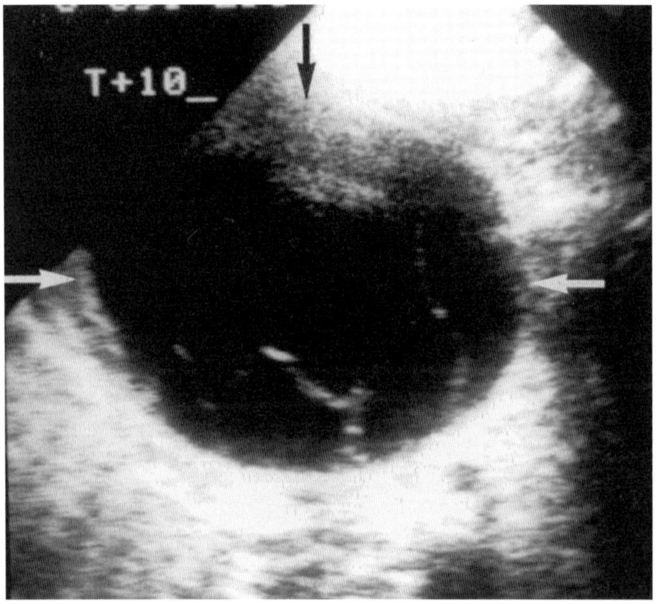

FIGURE 45 ■ Biliary cystadenoma. Benign biliary cystadenoma is seen as a large, cystic mass (*arrows*) with septations.

basis of imaging studies. Because benign cystadenomas may undergo malignant transformation, the therapeutic implication of the imaging distinction between cystadenoma and cystadenocarcinoma is minimal, and surgical excision is the preferred treatment for both lesions (38). Both tumors are usually solitary and large. Communication of these tumors with large intrahepatic bile ducts has been reported, but it is rare (84).

Infantile Hemangioendothelioma

Infantile hemangioendothelioma, although rare, is the most common symptomatic vascular liver tumor of infancy. More than 85% of the tumors present before six months of age (85). The female-to-male ratio is 2:1. The most common clinical presentation is hepatomegaly with or without a palpable mass. The tumor tends to grow rapidly after presentation and then regresses gradually over several months if the child survives. The incidence of congestive heart failure is high because of arteriovenous shunting within the mass, even though congestive heart failure is not as common as previously thought (85). Complications include anemia, thrombocytopenia, and hemorrhage. It is considered a benign tumor; however, rarely, distant metastases have been reported. Pathologically, the tumors are soft and spongy, and even though they have no true capsule, they are well demarcated. Central areas of large lesions may show infarction, hemorrhage, or calcification (85). Microscopically, the tumor is composed of anastomosing vascular channels lined by one or more layers of endothelial cells (86).

Sonographically, the appearance of these usually solid tumors is nonspecific. They may be hyperechoic, hypoechoic, or of mixed echogenicity, and they may contain cystic areas or calcifications. One may see a solitary mass, but frequently, the patient has multiple discrete masses throughout the liver (Fig. 46). Multiple hypoechoic or cystic lesions throughout the liver have been described (87). On sonography, a decreased caliber of the abdominal aorta distal to the origin of the celiac artery, a prominent celiac artery, and enlarged tortuous vascular structures adjacent to the mass within the liver may be seen (88).

Mesenchymal Hamartoma

Mesenchymal hamartoma of the liver is a rare cystic mass of infancy that probably is a developmental anomaly rather than a true neoplasm (72,89). It likely originates in the connective tissue along the portal tracts (89). Malignant transformation has not been reported. This lesion usually manifests before the age of two years and is extremely rare in adults (90). A slight male predominance has been reported. Clinically, patients present with diffuse abdominal enlargement or a palpable mass. Pathologically, the tumor consists of multiple cysts in an edematous stroma. Microscopically, it is characterized by an admixture of bile ducts in a prominent mesenchymal tissue stroma. Sonographically, it usually appears as a large, multiloculated cystic mass with multiple echogenic septa. Less commonly, the mass may be solid, containing multiple small cysts (Fig. 47). The size ranges from 5 to 20 cm, with an average diameter of 16 cm. It is commonly located in the right lobe. The mass is usually solitary and may be pedunculated. Calcification is rare (Fig. 47) (90).

Bile Duct Hamartomas (Von Meyenburg's Complex)

Multiple bile duct hamartomas are rare and are thought to represent developmental anomalies rather than true neoplasms (91). Association between multiple bile duct hamartomas and polycystic liver disease has been reported (91). The lesions are small and usually multiple. Pathologically, the lesion is composed of cystically dilated bile ducts lying in a fibrous tissue stroma, adjacent to the portal tracts (92). Sonographic appearance is variable and the lesions are usually hypoechoic or cystic but may be hyperechoic and solid (91,93). They usually range in size from 2 to 15 mm and may present as one or two discrete lesions or innumerable lesions uniformly or nonuniformly distributed throughout the liver (94). They may undergo malignant transformation into cholangiocarcinoma.

Focal Intrahepatic Extramedullary Hematopoiesis

Extramedullary hematopoiesis occurs most commonly secondary to myeloproliferative diseases. Other less common causes include aplastic anemia, marrow replacement syndromes, and multiple myeloma (95,96). This disorder may occur in liver, spleen, and lymph nodes, which may be enlarged. A focal mass within the liver secondary to extramedullary hematopoiesis is rare. Sonographically, a large, hypoechoic inhomogeneous mass in the liver has been described in two cases (95,96).

Other rare benign tumors of the liver include bile-duct adenoma, carcinoid tumor, fibroma, leiomyoma, benign mesenchymoma, and teratoma.

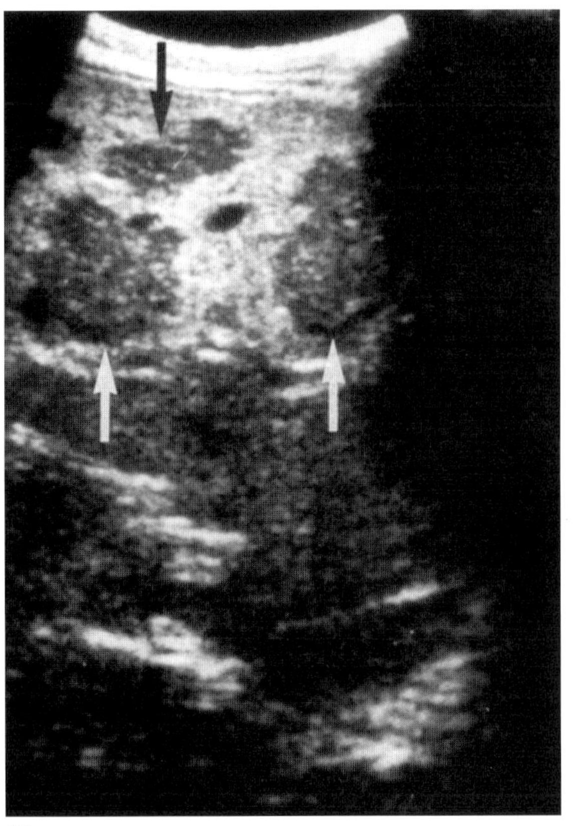

(A)

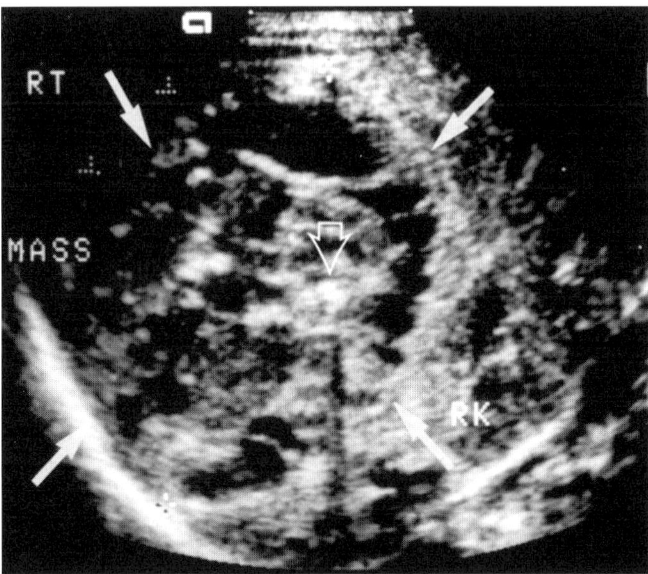

(B)

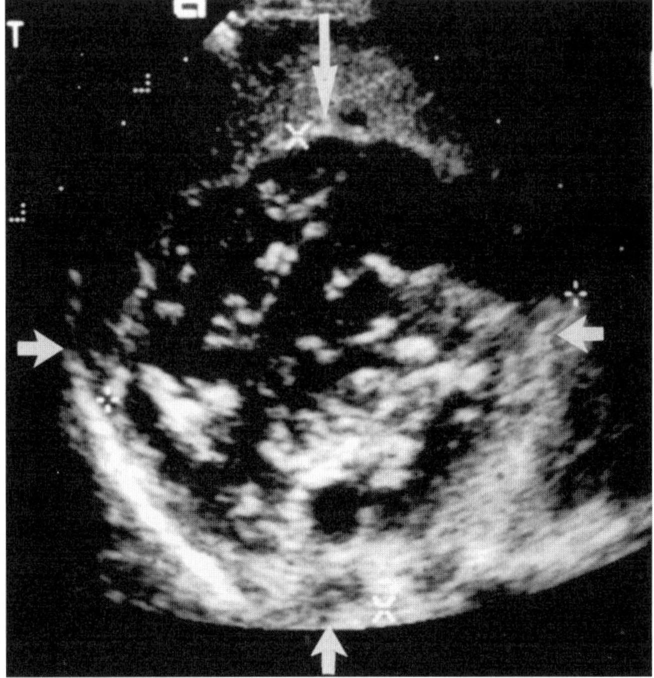

(C)

FIGURE 46 A–C ■ Infantile hemangioendothelioma. (**A**) Multiple discrete hypoechoic solid masses (*arrows*) are seen within the liver. (**B** and **C**) Sagittal and transverse sonograms in another patient demonstrate a large, solitary mixed solid and cystic mass (*solid arrows*) within the right lobe of the liver. Multiple small cystic areas are present within the mass. On the sagittal view (**B**), a calcification (*open arrow*) is seen as a hyperechoic focus with distal acoustic shadowing. RK, right kidney. *Source*: (**B** and **C**) Courtesy of Stuart C. Morrison, MD, Cleveland, OH.

Malignant Neoplasms

Hepatocellular Carcinoma

HCC is the commonest primary liver cancer. The incidence of HCC is much higher in certain parts of the world such as sub–Saharan Africa and the Far East than in the United States (97). The highest frequencies have been recorded in Mozambique, Taiwan, and southeast China. Moderately high incidences are encountered in Japan, southern Europe, Switzerland, and Bulgaria. The age of onset of HCC varies with geographic location (98). In sub-Saharan Africa, the tumor develops at a young age (third through fifth decades of life), whereas in populations with a low incidence, the elderly are affected predominantly (fifth through eighth decades of life). This tumor is rare in children and occurs between the ages of 5 and 15 years. It occurs predominantly in men, with male-to-female ratios ranging from 4:1 to 8:1 in high-incidence areas and 2.5:1 in the United States (99). Patients are usually asymptomatic in the early stages of the disease. The most common symptoms include abdominal pain and weight loss. This tumor usually occurs in association with chronic liver disease, most frequently cirrhosis, and is more commonly associated with nonalcoholic posthepatitic cirrhosis than with alcoholic micronodular cirrhosis (100). In low-incidence parts of the world, alcoholic cirrhosis seems to be the most common predisposing condition, whereas in high-incidence regions, the tumor is more frequently associated with hepatitis B virus and aflatoxins (99).

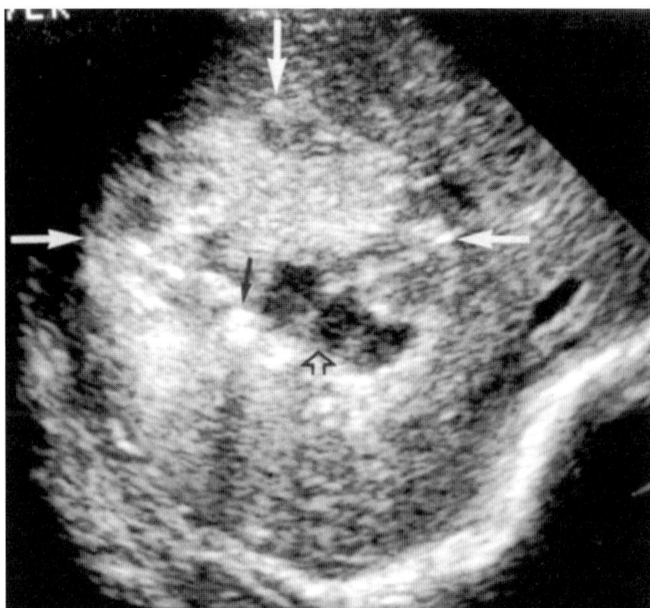

FIGURE 47 ■ Mesenchymal hamartoma. Transverse view shows a large predominantly hyperechoic, inhomogeneous solid mass (*large arrows*) containing cystic areas with debris (*open arrow*) and calcifications (*small black arrow*) with acoustic shadowing. More commonly, mesenchymal hamartoma appears as a multiloculated cystic mass with multiple septa (not shown).

Pathologically, three basic types of HCC are described: (*i*) nodular; (*ii*) massive; and (*iii*) diffuse (99). The nodular type is most common in cirrhotic livers. It consists of numerous nodules of varying sizes throughout the liver. The massive type is most common in noncirrhotic livers of younger patients and consists of a large, circumscribed mass occupying a significant proportion of the liver, often with smaller satellite nodules (99). The diffusely infiltrating type is rare, infiltrating a large portion of the liver with indistinct minute tumor nodules. Macroscopically, the tumor is usually soft and frequently contains areas of necrosis and hemorrhage. Microscopically, HCC can be divided into well-differentiated, moderately differentiated, and undifferentiated types. In approximately 4% of all hepatic carcinomas, histologic features of both HCC and cholangiocarcinoma are present in the same tumor (99).

Sonographically, the appearance of HCC is variable. The masses are usually solid and may be hypoechoic, hyperechoic, or of mixed echogenicity (Fig. 48) (101). Cystic areas within the tumor secondary to necrosis or hemorrhage are uncommon. Rarely, HCC may be seen as a multilocular cystic mass with solid component, mimicking cystadenocarcinoma (102). The masses may be solitary, multiple, or, less frequently (7–10%), diffusely infiltrating, thereby distorting of the liver architecture (Fig. 49) (103). This disorder is more frequently hyperechoic when tumors are multiple than when a tumor is solitary (101). The echogenicity of solitary tumors may also be related to the size of the tumors and to their stage of development. In a study by Sheu et al., 77% of the tumors smaller than 3 cm in diameter were hypoechoic (Fig. 50), and most small (<5 cm) HCCs evolved progressively from hypoechoic to isoechoic and then to inhomogeneously hyperechoic patterns as they grew (104). The hyperechoic pattern may be caused by either fatty metamorphosis or marked sinusoidal dilatation within the tumor (105). Small

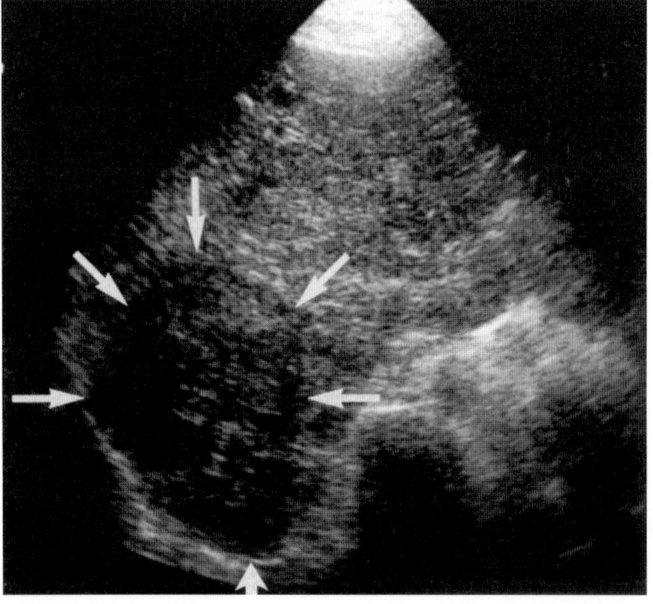

(A)

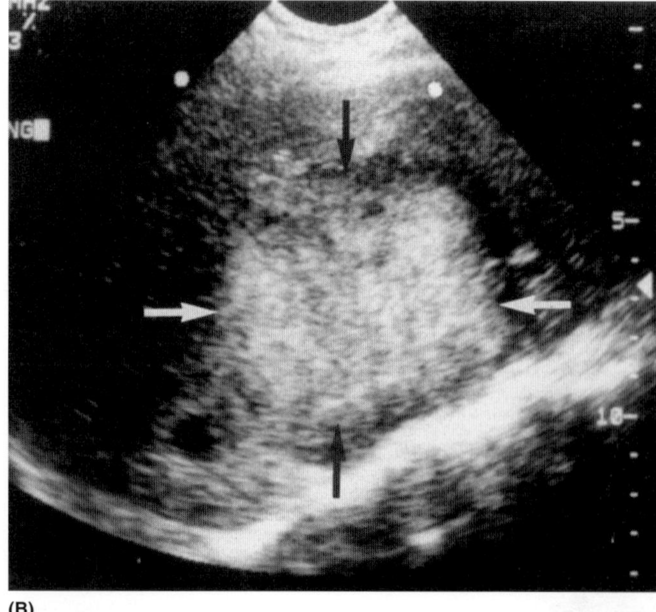

(B)

FIGURE 48 A AND B ■ Hepatocellular carcinoma. (**A**) Transverse view shows a large, hypoechoic solid mass (*arrows*) within the right lobe. (**B**) In another patient, sagittal view shows a large, predominantly hyperechoic, inhomogeneous mass (*arrows*) within the liver.

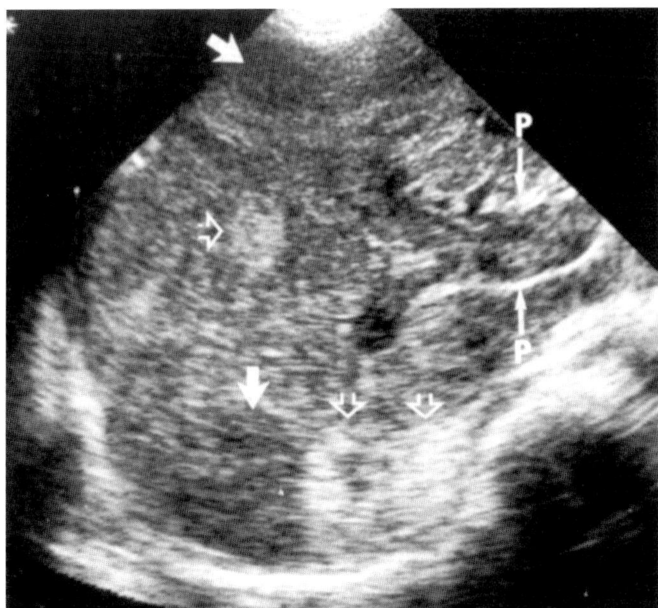

FIGURE 49 ■ Hepatocellular carcinoma: diffuse pattern. Transverse view shows hepatocellular carcinoma diffusely infiltrating the entire liver with hypoechoic (*solid arrows*) as well as hyperechoic (*open arrow*) solid areas within the liver. One sees tumor invasion, with tumor thrombus within the right portal vein (P) and its anterior and posterior branches.

HCCs with fatty metamorphosis may be seen as hyperechoic nodules resembling small hemangiomas (Fig. 51) (106). When the mass is diffusely hyperechoic, cavernous hemangioma, nodular focal fatty infiltration, lipomatous tumors (such as lipoma, angiomyolipoma, and myelolipoma), and adenoma containing fat should be considered in the differential diagnosis (Fig. 51).

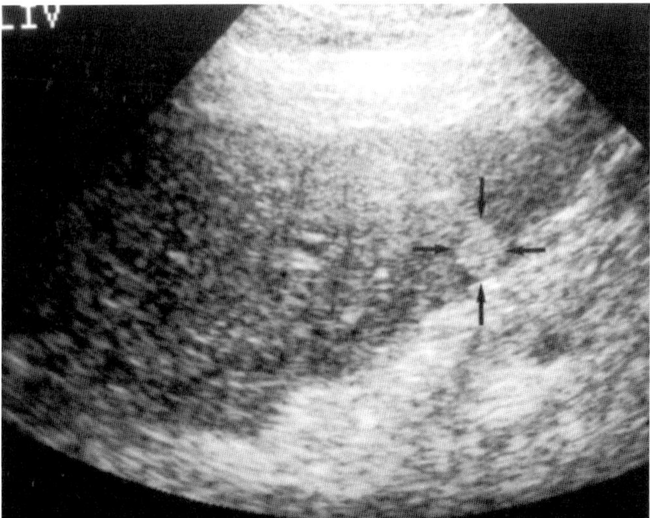

FIGURE 51 ■ Small hepatocellular carcinoma: hyperechoic pattern. Transverse view shows a small, hyperechoic mass (*arrows*) in the left lobe of the liver.

Although infrequent, calcification may occur in HCC (107). Distal acoustic enhancement may be seen in small (<5 cm) HCCs (108). These tumors frequently invade portal or hepatic veins. Portal vein invasion is much more common than hepatic vein involvement, and invasion of the intrahepatic portal veins is more common than extrahepatic portal vein involvement (Figs. 49 and 52) (109). Tumors invading the hepatic veins may extend into the inferior vena cava or the right atrium. Tumor invasion into the hepatic duct or common bile duct can be seen in 2% to 6% of advanced

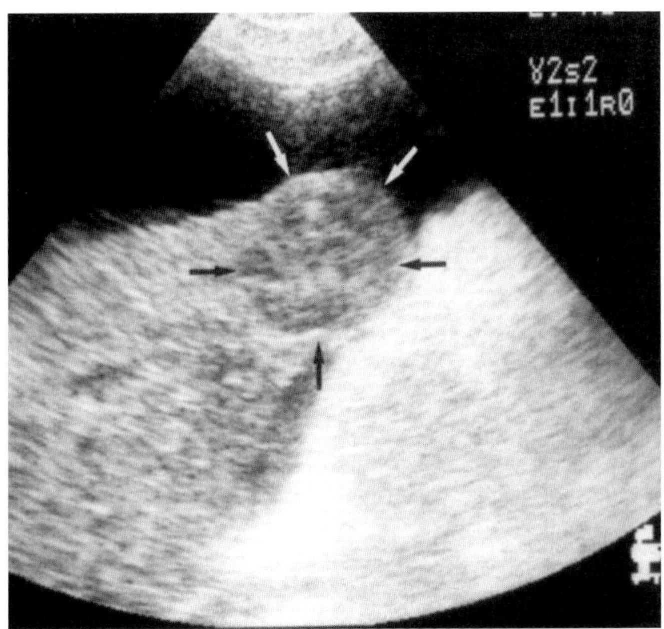

FIGURE 50 ■ Small hepatocellular carcinoma: hypoechoic pattern. Sagittal view shows a small, relatively hypoechoic mass (*arrows*) within a cirrhotic liver surrounded by ascites.

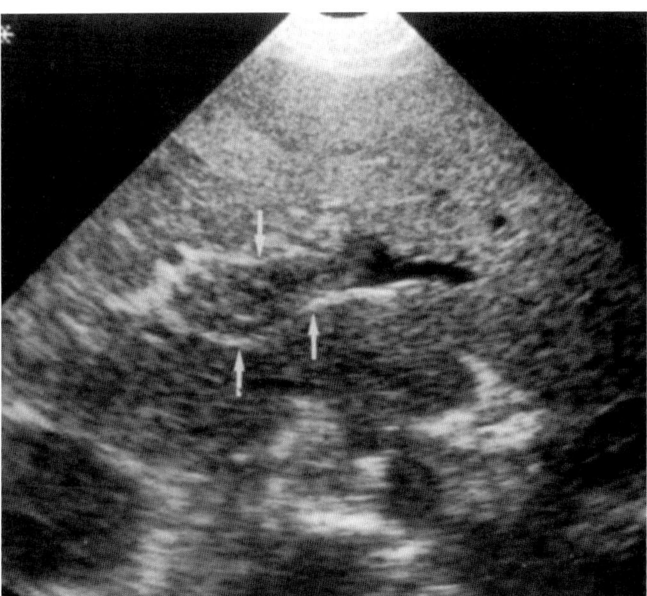

FIGURE 52 ■ Hepatocellular carcinoma invading the portal vein. Transverse view shows tumor thrombus within the right portal vein and part of the left portal vein (*arrows*). The right lobe of the liver is diffusely infiltrated with tumor.

HCCs (97). Obstructive jaundice can occur from direct invasion of the biliary tree or by compression by the tumor or lymph nodes.

Doppler Sonography ■ Because of arteriovenous shunting, which most commonly occurs at the periphery of the mass, duplex Doppler sonography frequently demonstrates high Doppler shifts at the periphery of HCC. In a study by Taylor et al., using a frequency of 3 MHz for both imaging and Doppler examination, Doppler shifts of 5 kHz or higher were considered specific for diagnosis of HCC (110). Because arterial portal shunting is either minor or absent in small HCCs, the value of duplex Doppler sonography in the diagnosis of these lesions is limited (111). Cirrhotic livers without malignant involvement also contain high-frequency shunts, further limiting the value of duplex Doppler for the diagnosis of HCC (112).

With color Doppler sonography, Tanaka et al. considered the basket pattern (a fine blood flow network surrounding the tumor nodule) and vessels within the tumor pattern (internal vascularity with blood flow running into and branching within the tumor) specific for HCC (113) (Fig. 53). However, using color Doppler techniques, internal vascularity and basket patterns similar to those seen in HCC have been described in focal nodular hyperplasia (74), and central vascularity with a venous signal has been seen in hepatic adenoma (114). Although most HCCs (76%) have internal vascularity on color Doppler sonography and most metastases (67%) do not, overlap between the color-flow findings in HCCs and metastases is significant (115). This overlap limits the usefulness of color Doppler sonography for distinguishing HCCs from metastatic tumors and other neoplasms.

Color Doppler sonography may be useful in determining the effectiveness of treatment of HCC after percutaneous ethanol injection or transcatheter arterial embolization by demonstrating a lack of color flow within the tumor after successful treatment and the presence of color flow within the tumor when residual tumor is present (116,117).

Screening ■ In those geographic regions where HCC is common, screening with serum α-fetoprotein determination and ultrasonography has been performed. When serum α-fetoprotein is increased (>500 ng/mL, by radioimmunoassay), the positive result almost always indicates the presence of HCC. In screening programs, the sensitivity of ultrasound to detect tumors less than 3 cm has been reported to be 84% (118), and for tumors of all sizes, it is 90% (119). However, in patients with end-stage cirrhotic livers, examined with ultrasound before hepatic

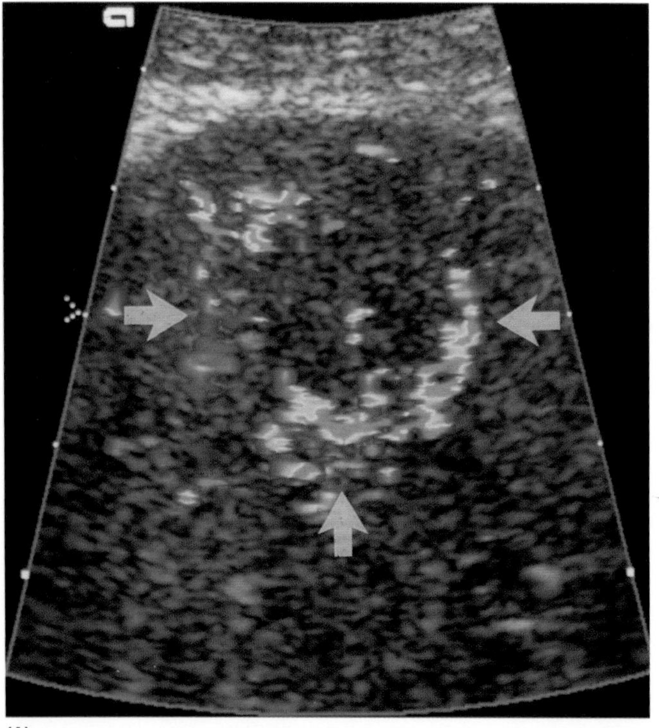

(A)

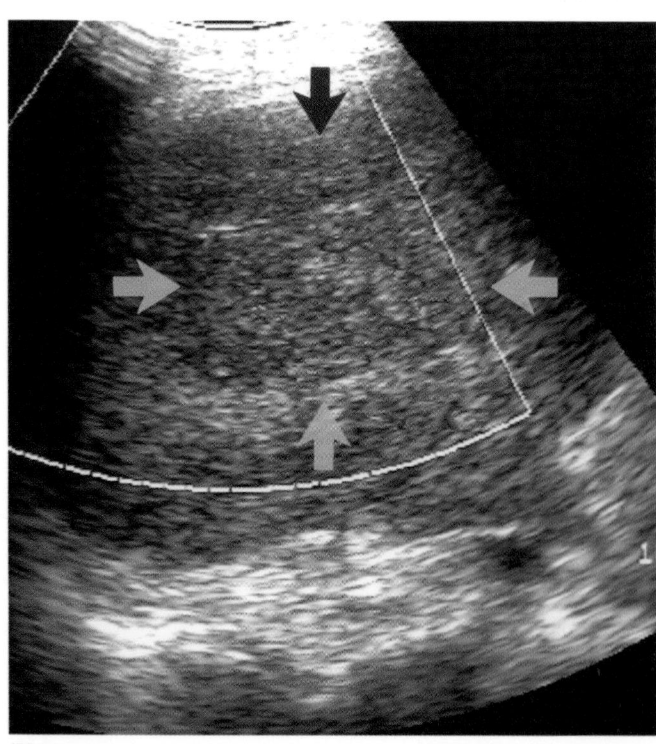

(B)

FIGURE 53 A AND B ■ Hepatocellular carcinoma: color Doppler sonography. (**A**) Increased color flow (*arrows*) is seen surrounding the tumor nodule (the "basket pattern"). (**B**) Abnormal vessels with increased color flow are seen within the tumor (*arrows*) ("vessels within the tumor" pattern), in another patient. *Source*: (**A**) Courtesy of Philip W. Ralls, MD, Los Angeles, CA.

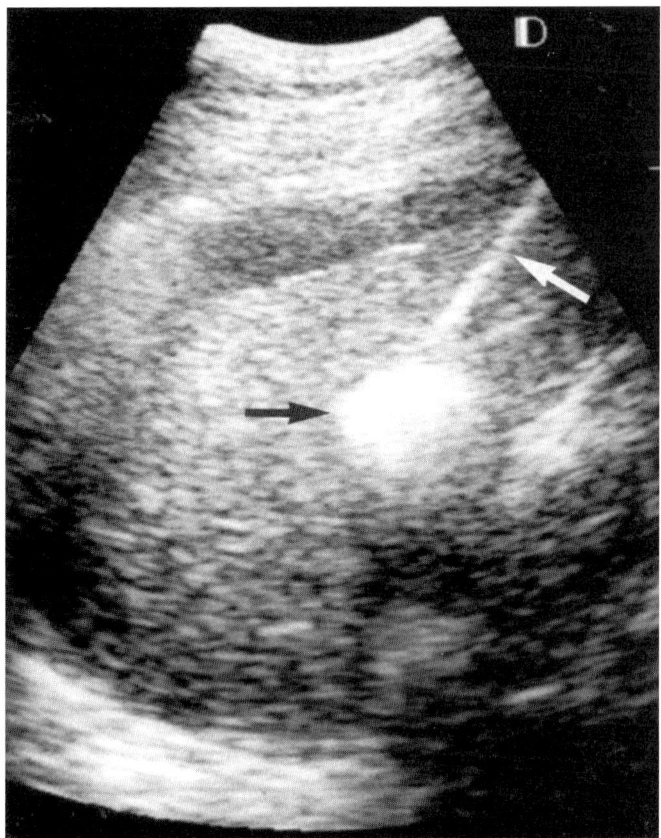

FIGURE 54 ■ Hepatocellular carcinoma: ethanol injection. Small hepatocellular carcinoma (*black arrow*) appears hyperechoic with acoustic shadowing, after therapeutic percutaneous ethanol injection into the mass. *White arrow*, needle.

transplantation, Dodd et al. reported a sensitivity of only 50% for detection of malignant tumors within the liver (120). In a study of screening for HCC in patients with advanced cirrhosis, in the United States, the sensitivity of CT scan (88%) was significantly higher than ultrasound (59%). Of patients with HCC, 63% had history of hepatitis C (121).

Treatment with Alcohol Injection ■ Patients with small HCC lesions (<4.5 cm) who are poor surgical risks may be treated with percutaneous injection of ethyl alcohol into the lesion, performed with ultrasound guidance (Fig. 54). No significant complications have been noted, and a one-year survival rate of 91.7% with no evidence of HCC at follow-up fine-needle biopsy has been reported (122).

Fibrolamellar Carcinoma

Fibrolamellar carcinoma, a variant of HCC, is mostly seen in adolescents and young adults without cirrhosis (63). It has an approximately equal sex distribution and is not associated with α-fetoprotein secretion. This tumor is more commonly resectable and less lethal than HCC (123). It is usually solitary and ranges in size from 8 to 15 cm. Sonographically, the mass is solid and has variable echogenicity. Most of the masses are predominantly

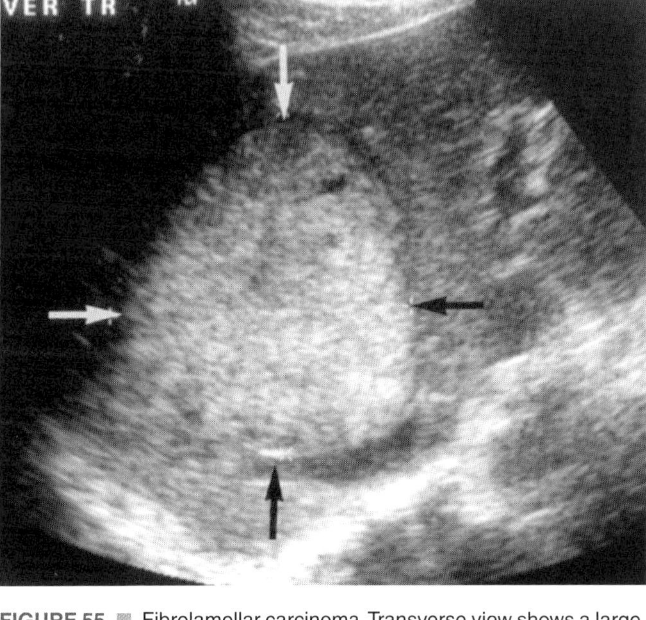

FIGURE 55 ■ Fibrolamellar carcinoma. Transverse view shows a large, predominantly hyperechoic mass (*arrows*) with a slightly inhomogeneous echo pattern.

hyperechoic (Fig. 55) or of mixed echogenicity, but they may be slightly hypoechoic (Fig. 56) or isoechoic. Focal calcifications (Fig. 56) as well as a central scar appearing as an echogenic band-like area can be seen within the mass (123–125).

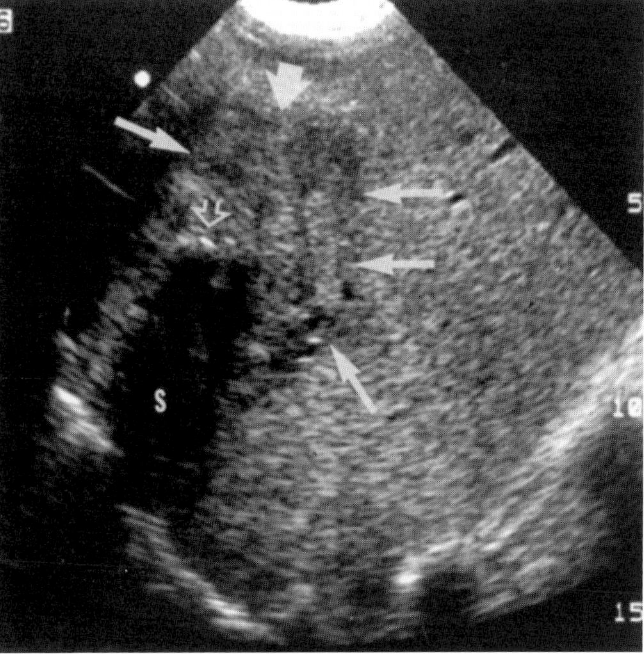

FIGURE 56 ■ Fibrolamellar carcinoma with calcification and shadowing. Sagittal view shows an inhomogeneous solid mass (*arrows*) containing hypoechoic and echogenic areas. Calcifications (*open arrow*) are seen as small, hyperechoic foci within the mass. Acoustic shadowing (S) is secondary to calcifications as well as fibrous tissue within the mass.

Peripheral Cholangiocarcinoma

Cholangiocarcinoma is a malignant tumor of the biliary epithelium. It may arise from either small peripheral intrahepatic bile ducts (i.e., peripheral cholangiocarcinoma) or large bile ducts, both the major intrahepatic bile ducts and extrahepatic bile ducts (i.e., hilar cholangiocarcinoma; see Chapter 17). It is 10 times more common in Japan than in the United States. Peripheral cholangiocarcinoma is considered to occur 10 times less frequently than HCC and accounts for 5% to 30% of primary liver cancer (126). It occurs in older persons and is rare before the age of 40 years. A higher incidence of cholangiocarcinoma has been associated with liver fluke infection, intrahepatic biliary calculi, ulcerative colitis, primary sclerosing cholangitis, cystic liver disease, congenital hepatic fibrosis, and exposure to thorium dioxide. Signs and symptoms of peripheral cholangiocarcinoma are similar to those of HCC, except that jaundice may be an earlier, more prominent, and more frequent feature (127). Pathologically, peripheral intrahepatic cholangiocarcinoma usually forms a large, solitary tumor, but a multinodular type may occur. Microscopically, it has acinar or tubular structures resembling those of other adenocarcinomas (127).

Sonographically, most masses are solid and may be hypoechoic or hyperechoic. Echogenicity, however, is variable, and the masses may also be isoechoic or of mixed echogenicity (Fig. 57) (128). Hypoechoic rim around the mass, calcification within the mass, or intrahepatic biliary dilatation peripheral to the mass may be seen. The size of the tumors ranges from 5 to 20 cm (126). It is usually solitary, but it may be multiple. Much less commonly, the tumor is an infiltrative type, demonstrating diffuse distortion of the liver parenchyma (128).

Angiosarcoma

Angiosarcoma (also known as hemangiosarcoma or malignant hemangioendothelioma) is an extremely rare hepatic tumor. It occurs in adults and is most frequently seen after 60 years of age. Men are affected four times more often than women (129). This tumor has been associated with exposure to the contrast agent Thorotrast, arsenic, and polyvinyl chloride. Rupture of the tumor with intraperitoneal bleeding is frequent. Angiosarcomas are usually multicentric and involve both lobes of the liver (129). The masses are usually mixed solid and cystic (130,131).

Epithelioid Hemangioendothelioma

Epithelioid hemangioendothelioma is a rare malignant neoplasm of vascular origin. It occurs in adults and is more common in women (132). Two types of hepatic lesions can be seen: (*i*) multiple nodules and (*ii*) large mass with or without calcifications. This tumor probably begins as multiple nodules that grow and coalesce, forming large, confluent masses (132,133). Sonographically, the masses are usually hypoechoic when multiple nodules are present and have variable echogenicity, with or without calcifications when larger masses are seen.

Hepatoblastoma

Hepatoblastoma, a malignant embryonal tumor of the liver, occurs almost exclusively in the first three years

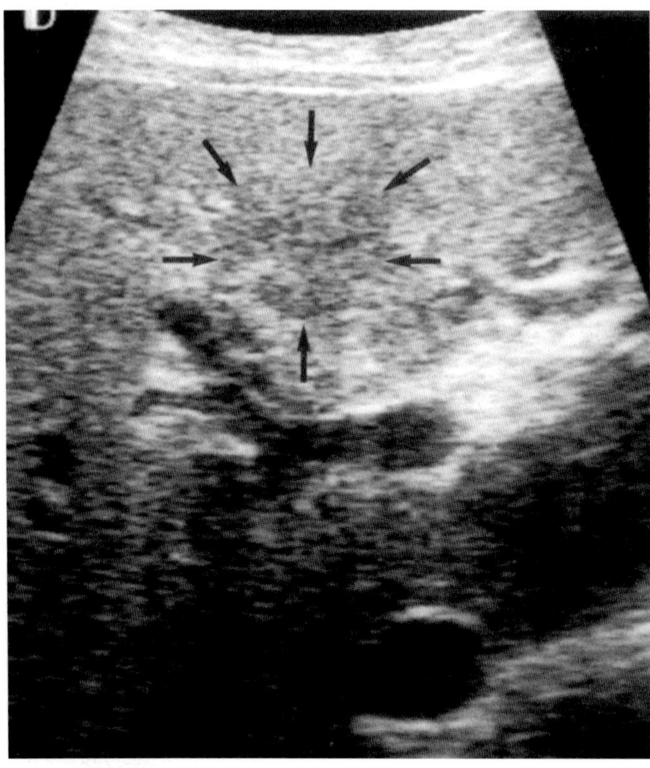

(A)

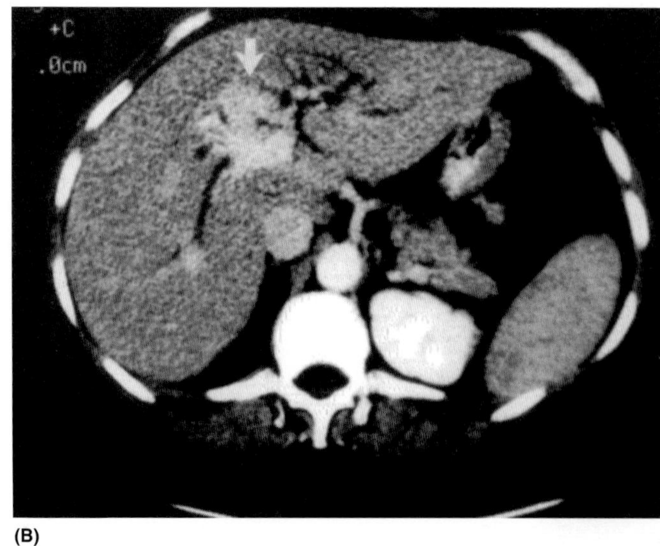

(B)

FIGURE 57 A AND B ■ Peripheral cholangiocarcinoma. (**A**) Transverse view shows a hypoechoic solid mass (*arrows*) in the liver. (**B**) Postcontrast CT demonstrates a high-attenuation mass (*arrow*) in the liver. Dilated intrahepatic bile ducts are seen adjacent to the mass.

of life and is the most common symptomatic liver tumor occurring under the age of five years (134,135). It is rare in adults. The tumor usually presents as a large, palpable mass. Serum α-fetoprotein levels are elevated in most patients. Sonographically, most hepatoblastomas are hyperechoic with an inhomogeneous echo pattern; they frequently contain internal calcifications and lobulation of the contour is often seen (Fig. 58) (135). Less commonly, tumors may be of mixed echogenicity or hypoechoic. Tumors occasionally contain cystic areas secondary to necrosis or hemorrhage. These tumors, which are usually solitary, range in size from 5 to 25 cm and are more common in the right lobe (134). The presence of multiple nodules or diffuse involvement of the liver is infrequent. Septations within the tumor may be seen on postcontrast CT. The tumors are usually hypervascular on angiography and may demonstrate a spoke-wheel pattern.

Cystic Hepatoblastoma

Benign cystic hepatoblastoma (more properly termed multilocular cyst of the liver) is thought to arise from aberrant bile ducts and may be potentially malignant. It occurs in children usually between one and four years of age (136). Sonographically, the mass is cystic and multilocular, and it contains multiple internal septations.

Kaposi's Sarcoma

In patients with acquired immunodeficiency syndrome (AIDS), Kaposi's sarcoma is rarely diagnosed during life, although it is seen in 34% of autopsy studies in these patients (137). Sonographically, Kaposi's sarcoma produces multiple, small (5–12 mm) hyperechoic nodules, and dense periportal bands may be seen within the liver. Prominent hyperechoic periportal bands have also been described in hepatic *Schistosoma mansoni* infection. The differential diagnosis includes angiomas, fungal microabscesses, and hepatic metastases.

Other rare malignant tumors of the liver include squamous carcinoma, mucoepidermoid carcinoma, embryonal sarcoma, fibrosarcoma, leiomyosarcoma, malignant mesenchymoma, mixed hepatic tumor, and carcinosarcoma.

Metastatic Disease

In Western countries, metastases are the most common cause of malignant focal liver lesions. Metastases are 18 to 20 times more common than primary malignant tumors. The most common primary sites causing liver metastases are colon, pancreas, stomach, breast, and lung. Metastases are most frequently multiple; however, solitary metastatic lesions can be seen. The sonographic appearance of liver metastases is variable, and no definite association exists between the histologic type of the tumor and the sonographic appearance. Tumors of the same primary origin may have different sonographic appearances (138). Because of the nonspecific appearance of the metastases, ultrasound-guided biopsy of the mass is frequently necessary for the diagnosis. Sonographic patterns of metastases include target pattern, hypoechoic, isoechoic, hyperechoic, calcified, cystic, and diffuse (Table 10).

The target pattern or bull's eye pattern is characterized by a central echogenic area and peripheral

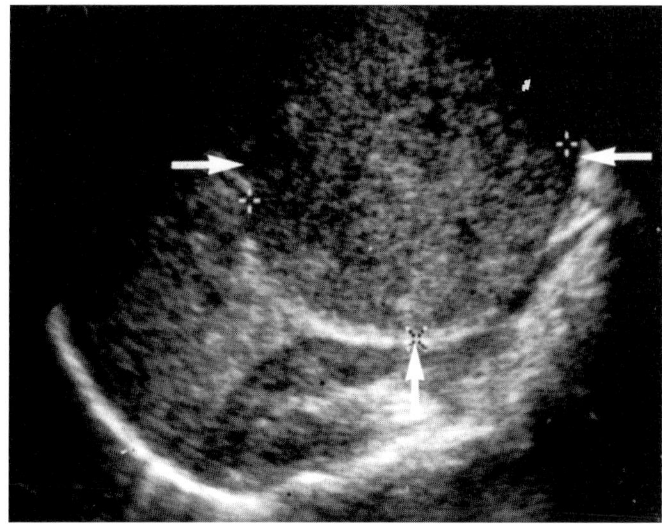

(A)

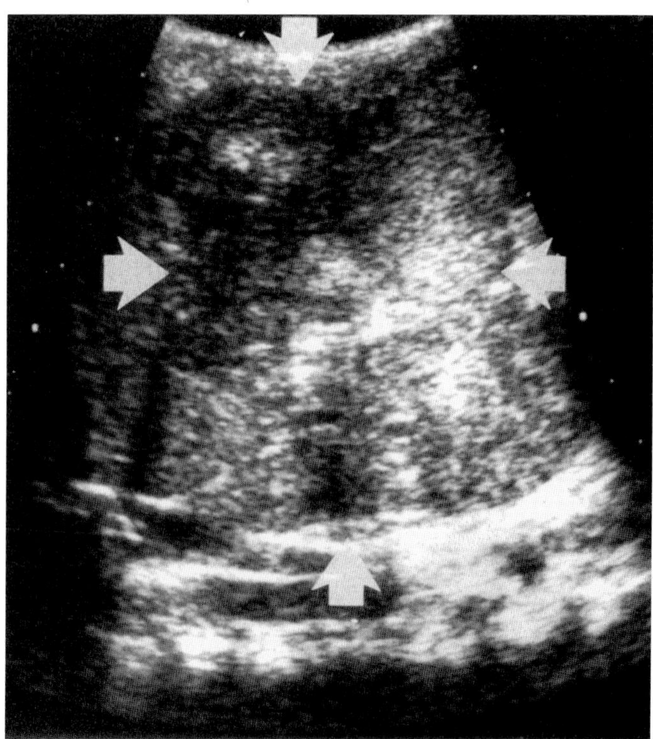

(B)

FIGURE 58 A AND B ■ Hepatoblastoma. (**A**) Sagittal view shows a large, solitary, predominantly echogenic mass (*arrows, cursors*) containing small hypoechoic areas. (**B**) Sagittal view of the left lobe in another patient shows a large, solitary, inhomogeneous mass (*arrows*) with hyperechoic as well as hypoechoic areas. *Source*: (**A**) Courtesy of Stuart C. Morrison, MD, Cleveland, OH. (**B**) Courtesy of Thomas L. Slovis, MD, Detroit, MI.

TABLE 10 ■ Echo Patterns of Hepatic Metastases

Pattern	Metastasis
Target pattern	Any primary malignant disease
Hypoechoic	Lymphoma (most common)
	Other primary malignant diseases (less common)
Hyperechoic	Colon carcinoma
	Other gastrointestinal malignant diseases
	Renal-cell carcinoma
	Islet-cell carcinoma of pancreas
	Carcinoid
	Choriocarcinoma
Calcified	Colon carcinoma (specially mucinous)
	Pseudomucinous cystadenocarcinoma of ovary
	Adenocarcinoma of stomach
	Islet-cell carcinoma of pancreas
	Leiomyosarcoma
	Osteosarcoma
	Neuroblastoma
	Adenocarcinoma of breast
	Melanoma
Cystic	Sarcomas: specially leiomyosarcoma of gastrointestinal origin
	Cystadenocarcinoma of ovary
	Cystadenocarcinoma of pancreas
	Mucinous carcinoma of colon
	Squamous-cell carcinoma

hypoechoic rim within the metastatic lesion (Figs. 31C and 59). Generally, when the peripheral hypoechoic rim is thin (<3 mm), the appearance has been described as the halo sign, and when the hypoechoic rim is thick (>3 mm), it is the target or bull's eye pattern. The hypoechoic peripheral rim may be caused by compressed normal liver parenchyma around the tumor (139) or by a zone of proliferating tumor in the periphery of the lesion (140). In a study of liver tumors in mice, the hypoechoic rim or halo around the tumors correlated with distended sinusoidal spaces, giving rise to new tumor-penetrating vessels (141). The halo or target pattern is not specific, but it is most often seen in malignant tumors, most commonly metastatic lesions in the liver, rather than benign tumors (Table 11) (142). In a study of 100 liver tumors, the target pattern was seen in 88% of malignant tumors and in only 14% of benign tumors (142). It is also occasionally seen in HCC. Hypoechoic metastases (Fig. 59B) can be seen secondary to lymphoma and, less commonly, to other primary malignant diseases. Isoechoic metastases (Fig. 59C) are uncommon and can only be detected if they are surrounded by a hypoechoic halo or if they displace adjacent vessels. Hyperechoic metastases frequently arise from gastrointestinal malignant tumors, most commonly from adenocarcinoma of the colon (Fig. 60). Less frequently, hyperechoic metastases are secondary to renal-cell carcinoma, islet-cell carcinoma of the pancreas, carcinoid, and choriocarcinoma. The echogenicity of the metastases may be related to their vascularity; most hypervascular lesions appear hyperechoic, and most hypovascular lesions are hypoechoic (143).

TABLE 11 ■ Target Lesions

- Metastases (most common)
- Hepatocellular carcinoma
- Candidiasis
- Lymphoma (uncommon)
- Benign hepatic tumors (rare)

Calcified metastases appear hyperechoic with distal acoustic shadowing (Fig. 61) (144,145). Calcification may be central within the mass, it may be peripheral around the mass, or the entire mass may be calcified. Calcified liver metastases are rare, most commonly seen secondary to carcinoma of the colon, especially the mucinous type as well as in patients with pseudomucinous cystadenocarcinoma of the ovary, adenocarcinoma of the stomach, islet-cell carcinoma of the pancreas, leiomyosarcoma, osteosarcoma, neuroblastoma, and, rarely, adenocarcinoma of the breast and melanoma (146,147).

Cystic metastases are uncommon and can occur secondary to metastatic sarcomas, most commonly leiomyosarcoma

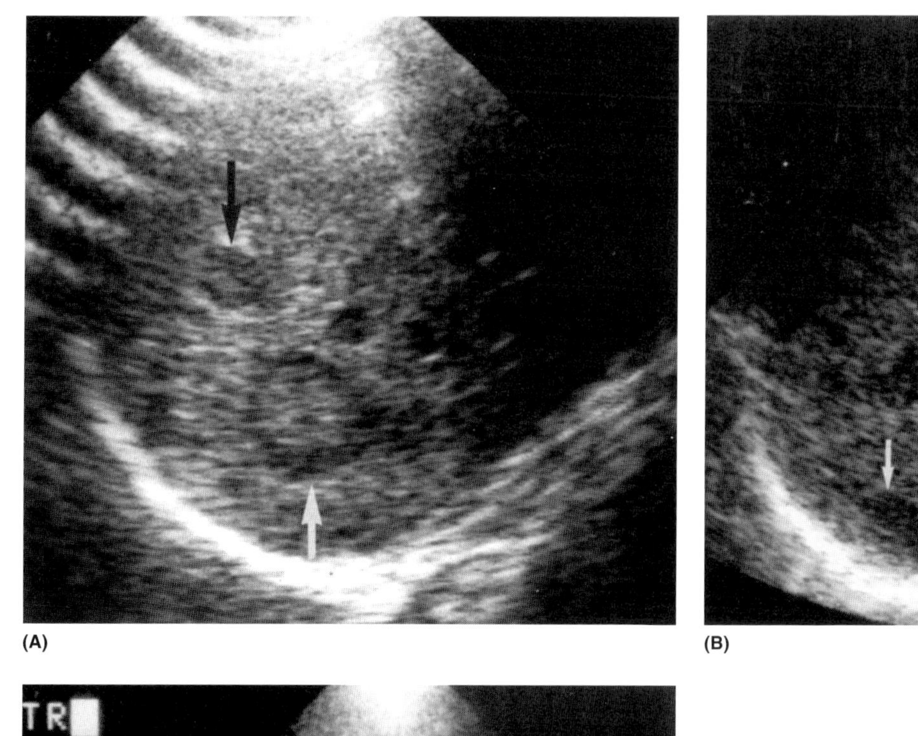
(A)

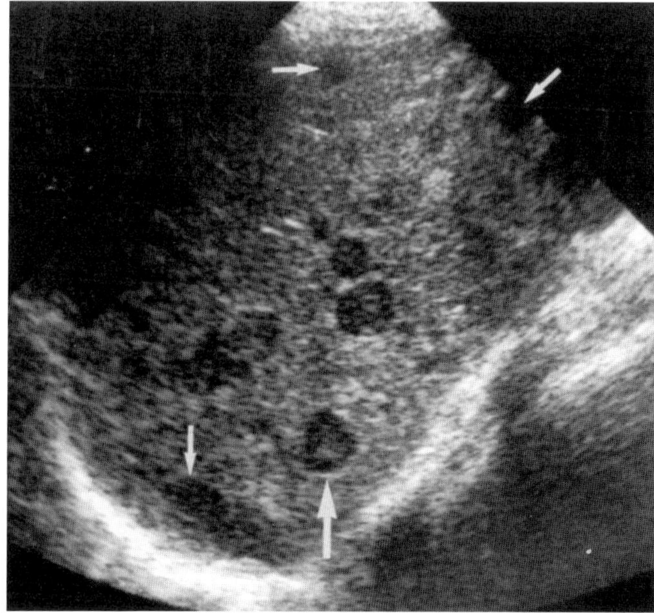
(B)

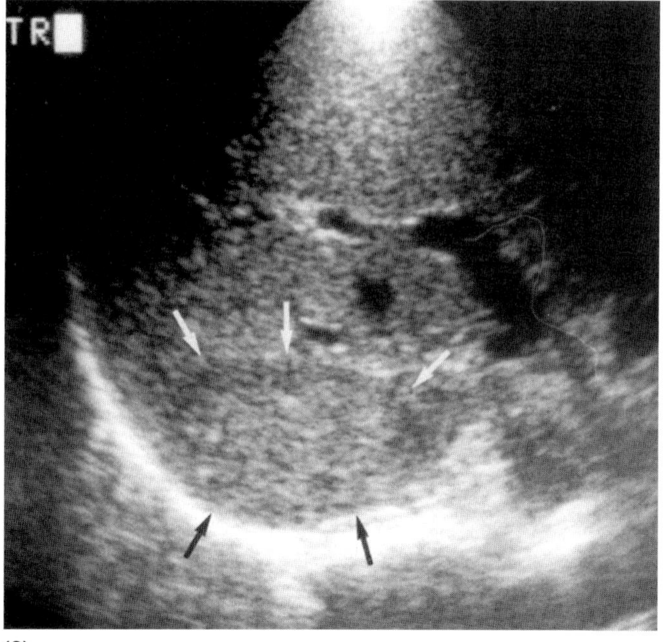

(C)

FIGURE 59 A–C ■ Metastases: target and halo pattern. (**A**) Target metastases from colon carcinoma. The metastases (*arrows*) have a peripheral hypoechoic rim and central echogenic areas of varying size. (**B**) Metastases from breast carcinoma show a target pattern (*large arrow*) as well as a hypoechoic pattern (*small arrows*). (**C**) Halo pattern around an isoechoic metastasis (*arrows*) from colon carcinoma. The isoechoic metastatic lesion can be recognized only because of a thin, hypoechoic halo (*white arrows*) around the mass.

of gastrointestinal origin. They can also occur secondary to other malignant diseases such as cystadenocarcinoma of the ovary and pancreas, mucinous carcinoma of the colon, and squamous-cell carcinoma (138,148). Cystic metastases can result from cystic primary tumors or from necrosis within the metastatic lesions. A portion of the mass or, less frequently, the entire mass may be cystic (Fig. 62). Unlike simple hepatic cysts, the cystic metastases usually have irregular margins, a thick wall, mural nodules, multiple septa, or a fluid–fluid level.

The diffuse type of metastatic disease distorts the parenchyma throughout the liver and sonographically produces a diffusely inhomogeneous echo pattern (Fig. 63). This disorder may be difficult to differentiate sonographically from cirrhosis, and CT or scintigraphy may be necessary for differentiation. Diffuse infiltration of the liver is frequently seen secondary to metastatic disease from breast carcinoma (149), but it can be secondary to other malignant tumors.

With color Doppler sonography, venous displacement around the lesion (the "detour sign") with no internal flow within the lesion has been described as characteristic of a metastatic lesion (Fig. 64) (113). However, even though most metastatic lesions are avascular as seen with color Doppler sonography, internal flow can be seen in 33% of metastatic lesions (115).

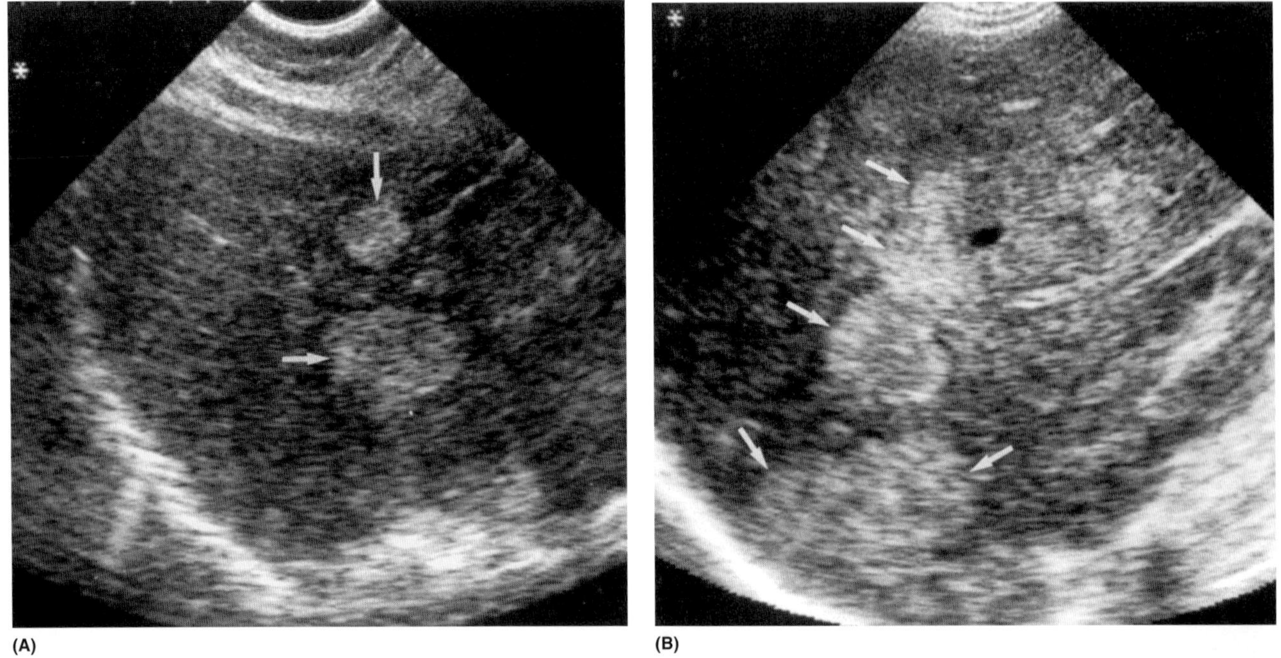

FIGURE 60 A AND B ■ Hyperechoic metastases. (**A**) Hyperechoic metastases (*arrows*) from colon carcinoma. (**B**) Hyperechoic metastases (*arrows*) from colon carcinoma in another patient.

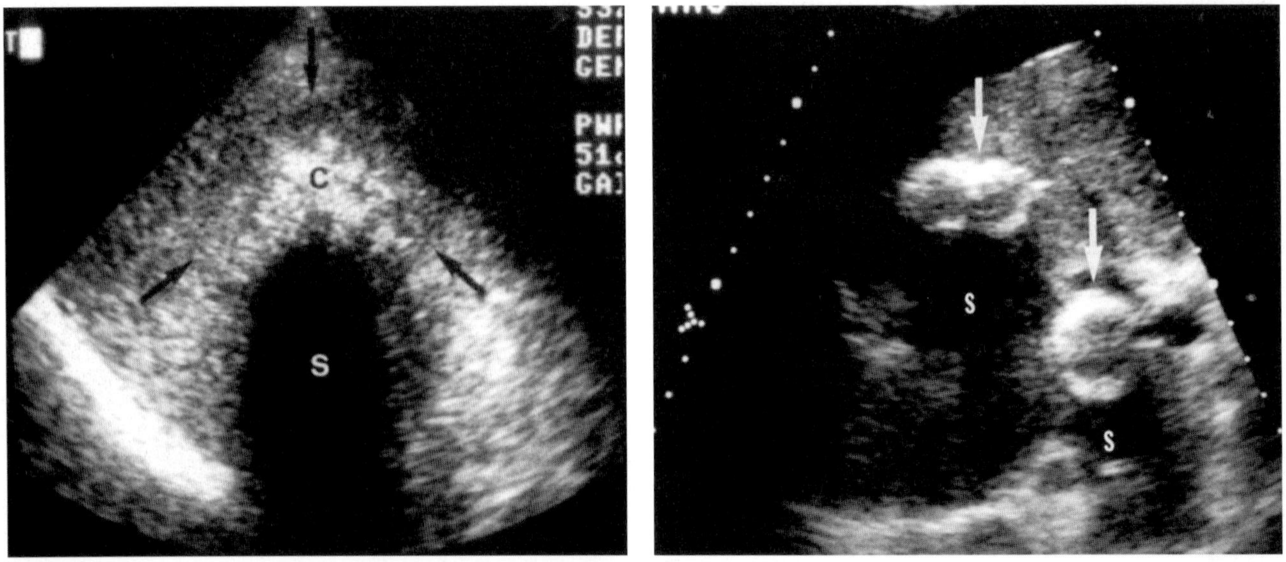

(A)

(B)

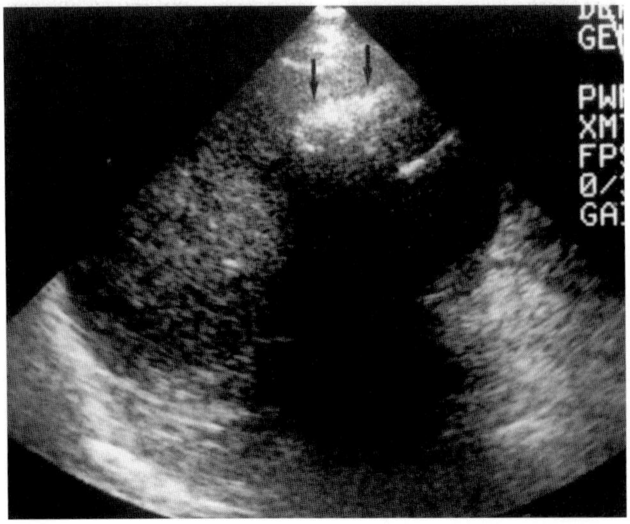

(C)

FIGURE 61 A–C ■ Calcified metastasis. (**A**) A hypoechoic metastatic mass (*arrows*) from primary colon carcinoma contains a central hyperechoic calcification (C) with distal acoustic shadowing (S). (**B**) In another patient, metastatic lesions (*arrows*) from a primary gastric carcinoma demonstrate peripheral calcification (*arrows*) with distal acoustic shadowing. (**C**) Entirely calcified metastasis (*arrows*) with prominent distal acoustic shadowing is from a primary colon carcinoma. *Source*: (**A** and **B**) From Refs. 144, 145.

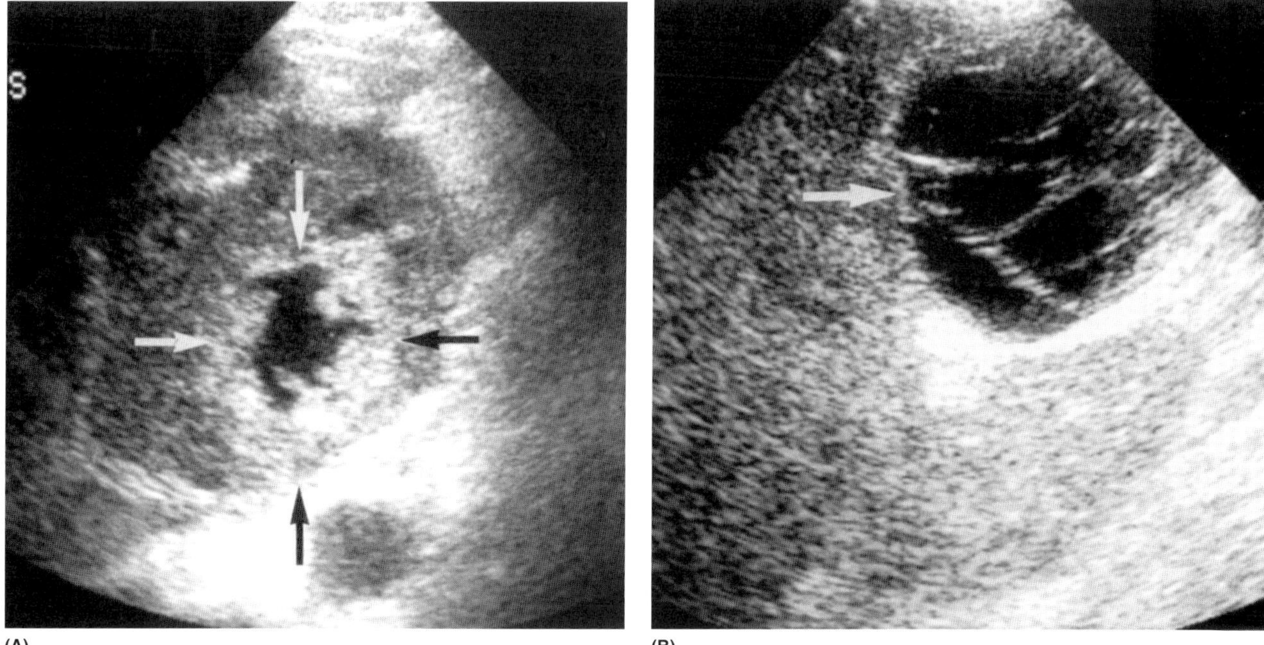

FIGURE 62 A AND B ■ Cystic metastases. (**A**) Transverse view shows cystic metastasis (*arrows*) in the left lobe of the liver from mucinous carcinoma of the colon. The cystic mass has a thick, irregular wall and small soft-tissue nodules projecting from the wall into the cystic area. Posterior acoustic enhancement is noted. (**B**) Sagittal view shows a cystic metastasis (*arrows*) from ovarian carcinoma. The large mass contains several septa, some thick and irregular. Considerable posterior acoustic enhancement is evident.

Lymphoma

The liver is often a secondary site of lymphomatous involvement on autopsy (150). Primary lymphoma of the liver is extremely rare. Diffusely infiltrative involvement of the liver cannot be recognized sonographically. Focal nodular lesions in the liver are more commonly seen secondary to non–Hodgkin's lymphoma compared with Hodgkin's lymphoma. Sonographically, the most common

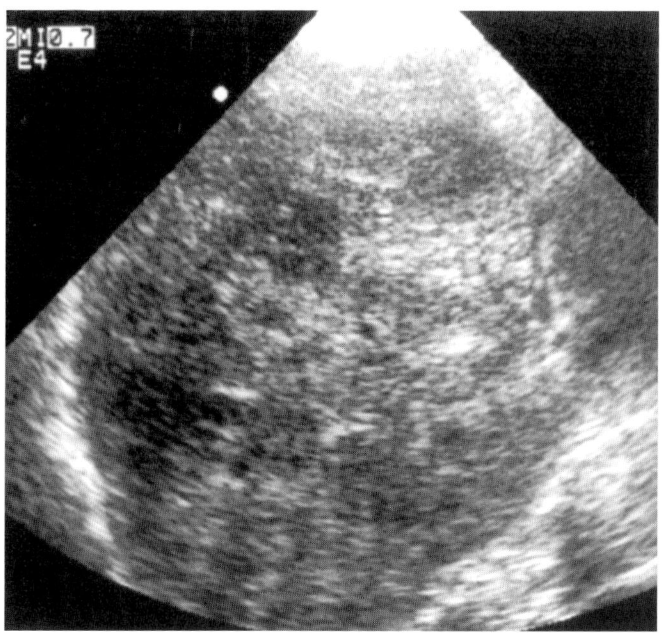

FIGURE 63 ■ Diffuse metastases from carcinoma of the pancreas. The liver has a diffusely inhomogeneous, disorganized echo pattern with scattered, poorly defined hypoechoic areas.

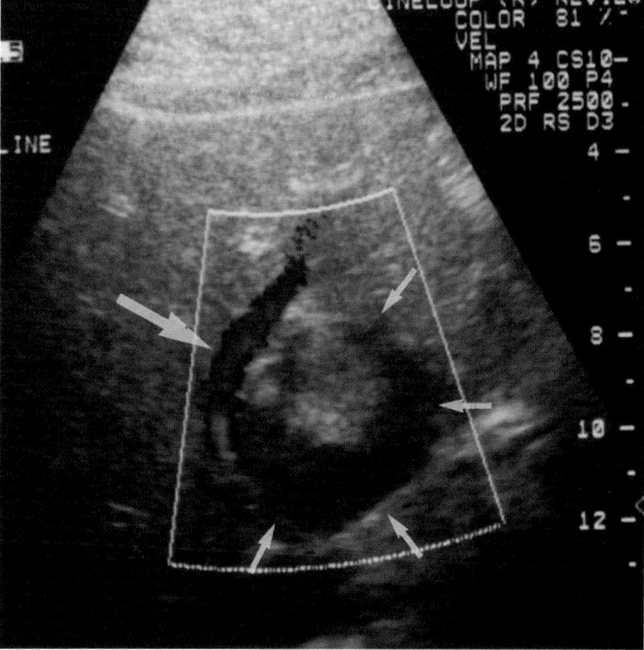

FIGURE 64 ■ Detour sign around a metastatic lesion. Color Doppler sonogram: transverse view shows the hepatic vein (*large arrow*) displaced around the metastatic lesion (*small arrows*). No internal flow is seen within the lesion.

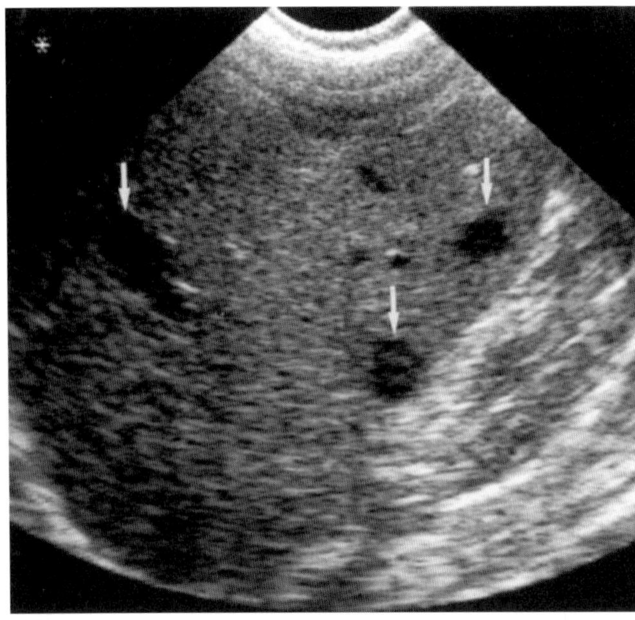

(A)

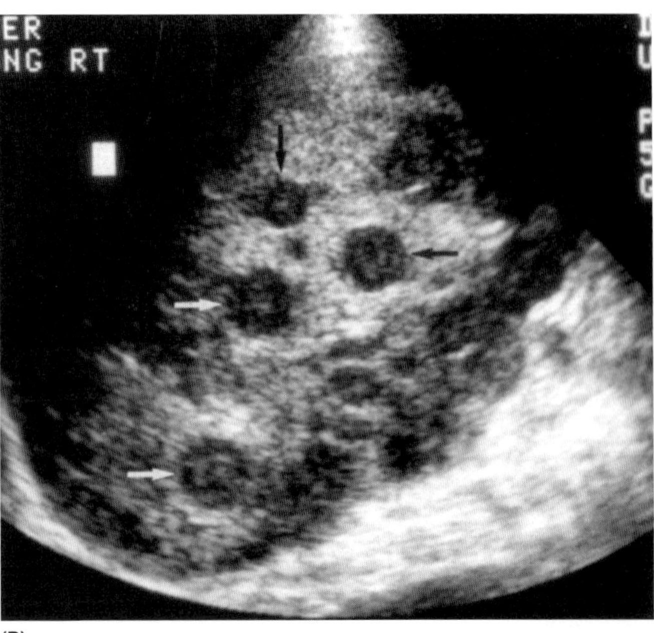

(B)

FIGURE 65 A AND B ■ Lymphoma. (**A**) Hypoechoic metastases (*arrows*) from non-Hodgkin's lymphoma. (**B**) Numerous hypoechoic metastases from non-Hodgkin's lymphoma, some with a target pattern (*arrows*). A target pattern is unusual in lymphoma.

pattern of secondary lymphoma is of multiple hypoechoic solid lesions, frequently with an irregular margin (Fig. 65) (151,152). Solitary lesions are less common (Fig. 66). Hyperechoic lesion and the target pattern (Fig. 65B) are unusual, but they can be seen in non–Hodgkin's lymphoma (153,154). Occasionally, the lesions may be nearly anechoic, with apparent septations and considerable distal acoustic enhancement mimicking a complex cystic mass (Figs. 66 and 67) (154). The size of the lesions ranges from 1 to 15 cm. In primary lymphoma of the liver, one usually sees a single large, poorly defined mass, rarely with calcifications (150).

Burkitt's Lymphoma

Burkitt's lymphoma, most common in central Africa, is rare in the United States. It is most commonly seen in children and young adults. It tends to involve sites other than the lymph nodes, unlike other lymphomas. Unlike the African variety, which frequently presents as easily visible painful facial (jaw) masses, the disorder seen in the United States presents as large abdominal masses that originate in the kidneys, ovaries, bowel, or mesentery (155). The large abdominal masses usually are hypoechoic or anechoic, with a homogeneous echo pattern. Hepatic involvement is uncommon but has been reported (156). Hepatic masses may be solitary or multiple and are usually hypoechoic or anechoic (Fig. 67).

Posttransplantation Lymphoma

Lymphoproliferative disorder is a known complication of organ and bone marrow transplantation. Immunosuppressive agents such as cyclosporine are associated with an increased incidence of non-Hodgkin's lymphoma resulting from lymphoproliferative disorder (157–159). When the liver is involved with lymphoma, sonographically, multiple hypoechoic solid masses may be seen (157).

Leukemia and Chloroma

Leukemic involvement of the liver is uncommon. It is usually seen in patients with acute myelogenous or lymphocytic leukemia causing microscopic infiltration that usually has no visible sonographic abnormality (160).

FIGURE 66 ■ Lymphoma: solitary mass, Non-Hodgkin's lymphoma. This large, solid mass (*arrows*) has anechoic as well as echogenic areas with considerable posterior acoustic enhancement. The appearance mimics that of a complex cystic mass.

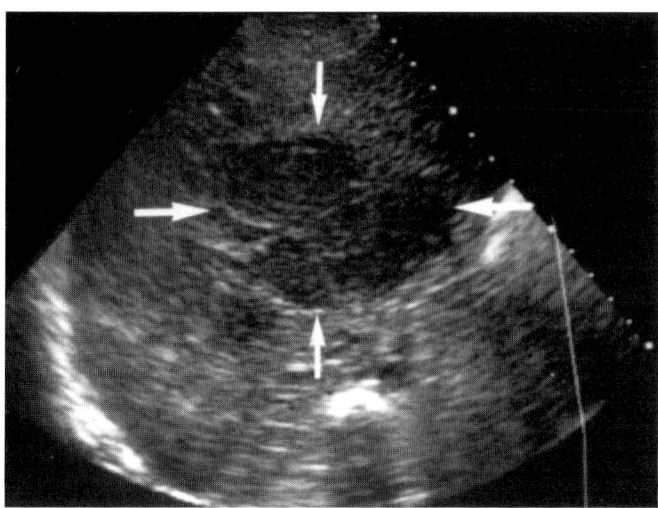

FIGURE 67 ■ Burkitt's lymphoma: transverse view shows a large, hypoechoic, almost anechoic solid mass (*arrows*) with apparent thin septations within the mass and minimal posterior acoustic enhancement. *Source*: Courtesy of William E. Brant, MD, Sacramento, CA.

"Chloromas" are localized myelogenous cell tumors within the liver in patients with myelogenous leukemia and may appear as multiple hypoechoic masses, some with the target pattern (160) or as multiple hyperechoic solid masses resembling hemangiomas (161).

Liver Lesions in Patients with Known Extrahepatic Malignancy

Sonography may be useful in cancer patients with average body habitus to characterize small (0.6–1.5 cm) indeterminate liver lesions detected on CT. In one study, 67% of lesions measuring 0.6 to 1.5 cm were detected on sonography versus only 19% of the lesions measuring 0.1 to 0.5 cm (162). Sonography characterized 93% of lesions detected by ultrasound as cysts, solid lesions/metastases, and hemangiomas (162).

Solitary solid liver lesion is often detected sonographically in cancer patients. In this series, hypoechoic nodules were almost always malignant (112 out of 128 lesions), whereas most hyperechoic lesions were benign cavernous hemangioma (155 out of 265 lesions) rather than metastasis (85 out of 265 lesions) (163). Abnormal liver function tests were found to have a very high predictive value for metastasis even in patients with solitary solid lesions in the liver (163).

INFECTIOUS DISEASES

Viral Hepatitis

Viral hepatitis is a systemic viral infection causing hepatic inflammation and hepatic cell necrosis. It is caused by at least five (A, B, C, D, E) and possibly six viral agents (164). Hepatitis A and E are transmitted enterically and by person-to-person contact. Hepatitis B, C, and D are transmitted by direct inoculation of human blood or its derivatives. Major sources of hepatitis B transmission include percutaneous spread resulting from parenteral drug abuse, contact spread resulting from heterosexual or homosexual activity, and maternal–neonatal transmission.

Viral hepatitis can be divided into acute and chronic types. Chronic viral hepatitis is further subdivided into chronic-persistent and chronic-active hepatitis. Serious sequelae of viral hepatitis include cirrhosis and HCC. Sonographically, in acute hepatitis, in most patients, no sonographic abnormalities are seen within the liver. Clearer visualization of the portal venous radicles and increased brightness of their walls, perhaps secondary to decreased echogenicity of the adjacent liver parenchyma, have been described in acute viral hepatitis (Fig. 68) (165, 166). However, in a study of 791 patients with acute viral hepatitis by Giorgio et al., these findings were seen in 32% of patients with acute hepatitis but also in 31% of normal control subjects, and therefore, they are not useful in the diagnosis of acute viral hepatitis (167). Rarely (2.4%), the echogenicity of the liver may be increased (the bright liver pattern), perhaps secondary to considerable vacuolar hepatocyte degeneration in acute hepatitis (167). In chronic viral hepatitis, the liver may have a coarse echo pattern. In addition, in patients with moderate-to-severe chronic hepatitis, visualization of the portal radicles may be decreased, with a corresponding decrease in the echogenicity of the liver walls (165).

Abnormal thickening of the gallbladder wall is seen in up to 98% of patients during the acute phase of viral hepatitis, usually within the first week of illness (168). Other less-frequent abnormalities of the gallbladder in acute hepatitis include decrease in size and abnormal luminal contents such as echogenic particles or sludge. Sonographic examination of the gallbladder after clinical recovery from acute hepatitis usually demonstrates complete resolution of the sonographic abnormalities.

Portal lymphadenopathy is frequently found in inflammatory liver diseases including patients with hepatitis C, especially when there is an increase of liver enzymes.

Pyogenic Abscess

Pyogenic liver abscess is a rare condition, with a reported prevalence at autopsy series of 0.3% to 1.5% (169). Worldwide, pyogenic liver abscess is much less common than amebic abscess, although in Western countries, pyogenic abscess is more frequent. Pyogenic abscess is most commonly caused by *Escherichia coli*; however, several other aerobic and anaerobic organisms can cause liver abscess. Most patients present with malaise, anorexia, nausea, weight loss, fever, and abdominal pain (169). This disorder usually occurs in middle-aged and older people, with an equal distribution among men and women. Pyogenic infection may be carried to the liver in hepatic arterial or portal venous blood and in bile. Biliary tract disease accounts

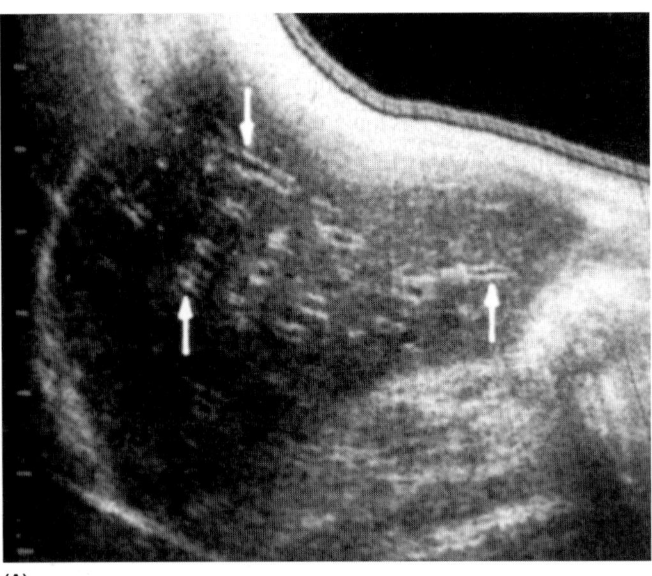
(A)

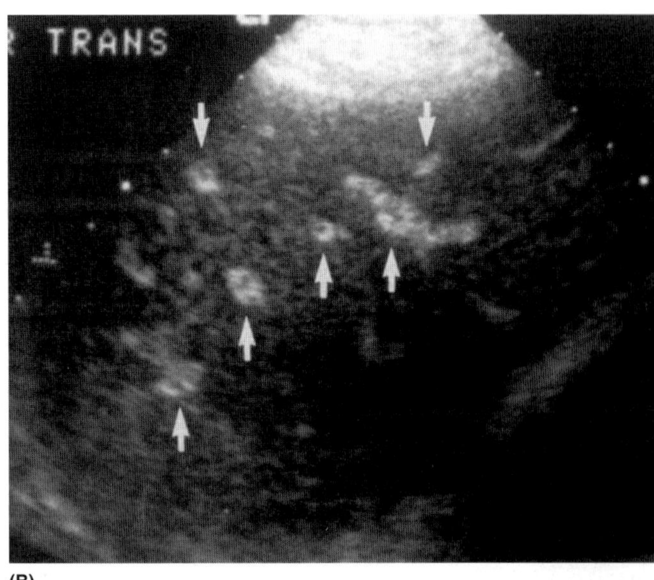

(B)

FIGURE 68 A AND B ■ Viral hepatitis. (**A**) Sagittal view shows overall decreased echogenicity of the liver parenchyma and increased brightness (accentuated echogenicity) of the walls of the portal vein radicles (*arrows*). (**B**) Transverse view demonstrates accentuated echogenicity (increased brightness) of the walls of the portal vein radicles (*arrows*) in another patient. *Source*: From Refs. 165, 166.

for the largest number of liver abscesses, with extrahepatic obstruction leading to cholangitis and abscess formation (170). Other causes of liver abscesses include the following: (*i*) direct extension of infection from contiguous organs such as cholecystitis, pyelonephritis, or perforated gastric ulcer; (*ii*) infection within a necrotic metastatic tumor; (*iii*) infected liver cyst; (*iv*) infection through the portal venous system secondary to appendicitis, diverticulitis, and other types of inflammatory bowel disease; and (*v*) liver trauma. In infancy and childhood, pyogenic abscesses occur most commonly secondary to umbilical infection or generalized septicemia. No cause is found for approximately 50% of hepatic abscesses. The abscesses may be solitary or multiple, and when solitary, they are most frequently seen in the right lobe. They range in size from less than 1 to 20 cm.

Sonographically, pyogenic abscesses have a variable appearance (171–173). Abscesses may appear cystic with an irregular, indistinct wall, a well-defined wall, or, less frequently, a thick wall (Fig. 69). Abscesses may contain echogenic debris, fluid–fluid interfaces, or septations (Fig. 70). In the early stage, abscesses may appear hypoechoic and solid (Fig. 71), usually with distal acoustic enhancement; they subsequently liquefy and become cystic and anechoic. Gas-containing abscesses appear hyperechoic, usually with distal acoustic shadowing and reverberation artifacts (Fig. 72) (174). Some gas-containing abscesses, however, may appear hyperechoic without distal acoustic shadowing, perhaps because of the presence of microbubbles of gas within the abscess (175,176). Pyogenic abscess, after diagnostic aspiration, can be treated by antibiotic therapy alone or in combination with percutaneous drainage guided by ultrasound or CT, although surgery remains essential in some cases (177). The differential diagnosis includes simple cyst with hemorrhage, necrotic tumor, echinococcal cyst, and hematoma (173).

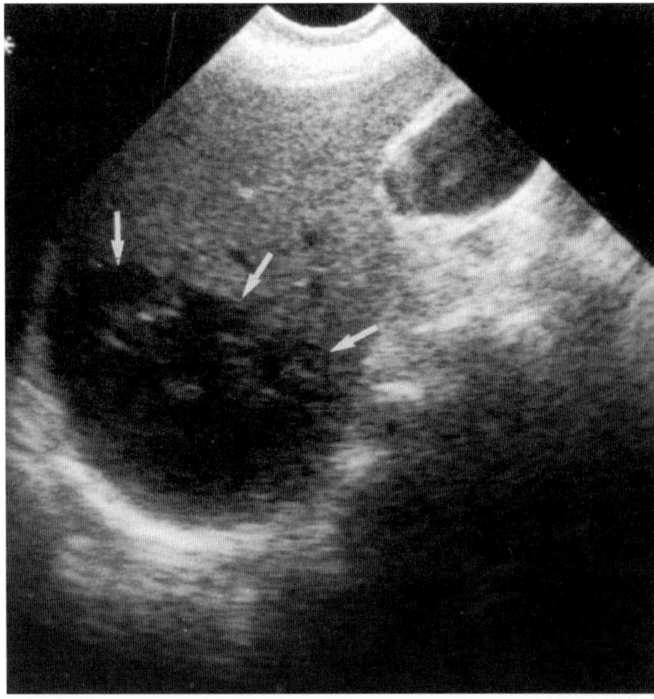

FIGURE 69 ■ Pyogenic abscess. Transverse view shows a large, anechoic cystic mass (*arrows*) with an indistinct wall, small echogenic solid areas anteriorly, and posterior acoustic enhancement.

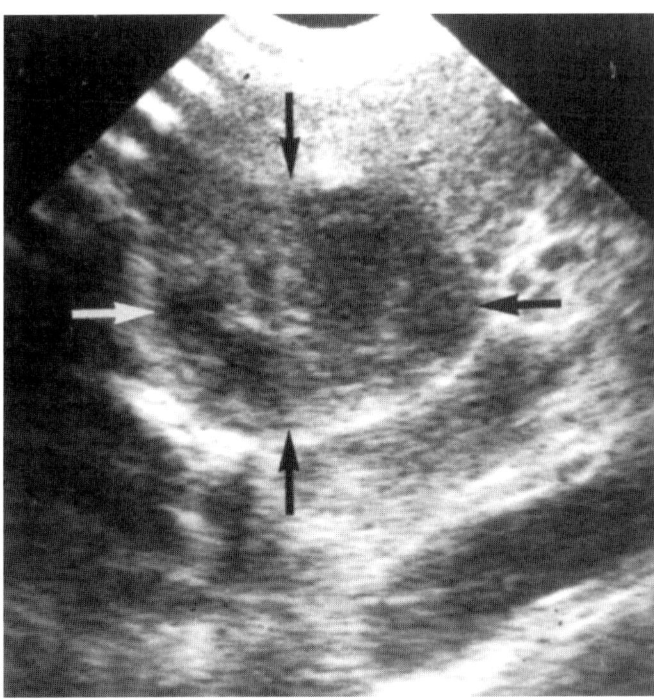

FIGURE 70 ■ Pyogenic abscess. Sagittal view shows a large mixed solid and cystic mass (*arrows*) in the left lobe of the liver.

Amebic Abscess

Amebiasis results from infection with the protozoan parasite *Entamoeba histolytica*. Amebiasis affects approximately one tenth of the world's population (178). In Western countries, amebic liver abscess is much less common than pyogenic abscess; however, worldwide, pyogenic liver abscess is much less common than amebic abscess. Symptoms include malaise, fever, anorexia, and abdominal pain. Infection occurs by the fecal–oral route. Amebas invade the colonic mucosa and are carried to the portal venous capillaries by the portal venous system, presumably accounting for the peripheral location of most amebic abscesses. The most common location for amebic abscess is near the dome of the right lobe of the liver.

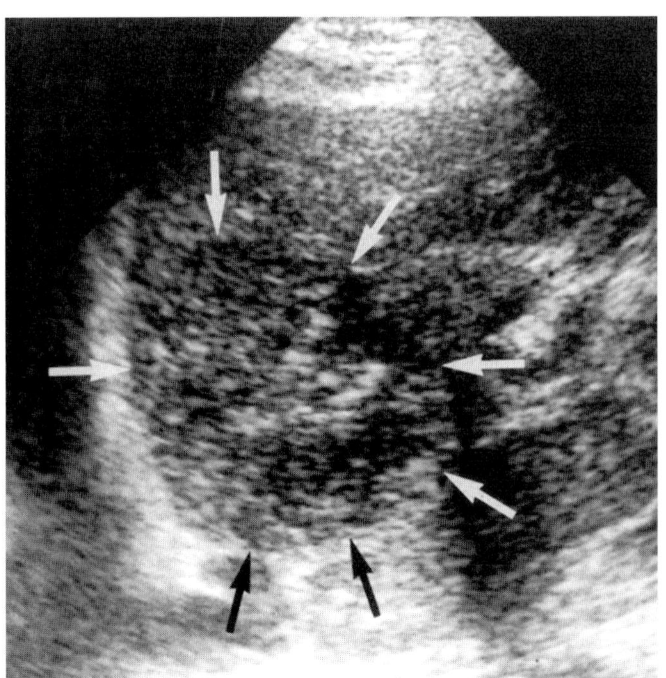

FIGURE 71 ■ Pyogenic abscess. Sagittal view of the left lobe shows a large, predominantly solid mass (*arrows*) with echogenic and hypoechoic areas. Posterior acoustic enhancement is evident.

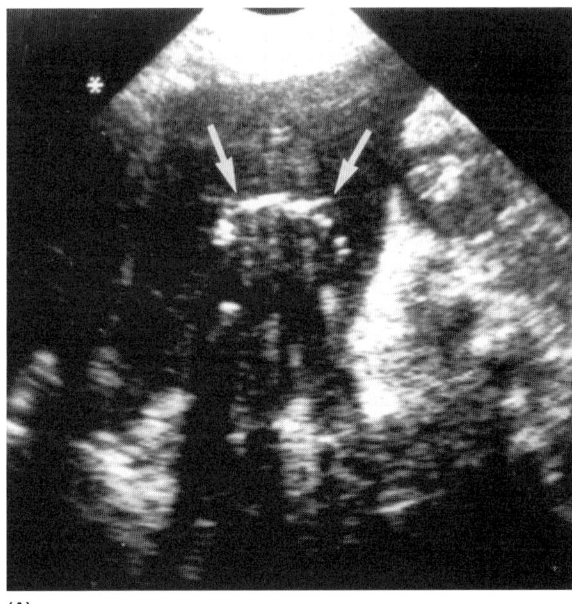

(A)

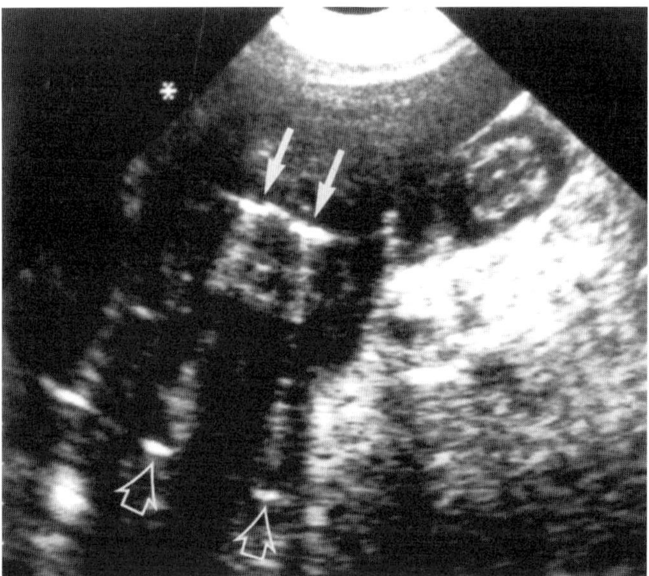

(B)

FIGURE 72 A AND B ■ Gas-containing abscess. Sagittal view shows a gas-containing abscess (*solid arrows*) within the left lobe of the liver. (**A**) A curvilinear hyperechoic area (*arrows*) secondary to reflection from gas within the abscess, associated with distal acoustic shadowing and comet tail (ring-down) artifacts. (**B**) Two large, hyperechoic foci (*solid arrows*) secondary to reflections from gas within the abscess are associated with reverberation artifacts (*open arrows*). Comet tail (ring-down) artifacts are also present.

Abscesses are usually solitary, but they can be multiple. The size varies from 3 to 40 cm (179,180).

Sonographically, approximately one-third of amebic abscesses demonstrate the following features: (*i*) round or oval shape; (*ii*) hypoechoic or anechoic mass with varying degrees of distal acoustic enhancement; (*iii*) absence of significant wall echoes (echo-poor wall); and (*iv*) contiguity with the liver capsule (181,182). These sonographic features, however, can also be seen with pyogenic abscesses. Two of these sonographic features, round or oval shape and hypoechoic appearance with fine homogeneous echoes throughout at high gain (Fig. 73), are more prevalent in hepatic amebic abscesses than in pyogenic liver abscesses (183). Occasionally (9%), amebic abscesses may have an irregular shape, a thick, echogenic wall, echogenic mural or internal solid nodules, or echogenic internal septa (180,181).

The diagnosis is made by clinical features and serologic testing. The commonest complication of hepatic amebic abscess is rupture into the chest, and the next most common complication is rupture into the peritoneal cavity. In most patients with amebic abscess, medical treatment with amebicidal agents alone is as effective as treatment with medical amebicidal therapy coupled with image-guided percutaneous therapeutic aspiration of the abscess (184). Image-guided therapeutic aspiration of the abscess is reserved for the following indications: (*i*) inability to differentiate pyogenic from amebic abscess; (*ii*) imminent rupture; (*iii*) poor response to medical therapy; (*iv*) location in the left lobe, especially a juxtacardiac location; and (*v*) pregnancy (185). Up to two years are required for resolution of the liver lesion, and some lesions stabilize with a persistent cyst. Therefore, the identification of a persistent lesion does not necessarily indicate failed therapy (186).

Echinococcal Cyst (Hydatid Disease)

Echinococcus granulosus

Hydatid cyst of the liver is secondary to parasitic infestation caused by the larval stage of the tapeworm *E. granulosus*. Hydatid disease resulting from *E. granulosus* is found most frequently in the Middle East, the countries of the Mediterranean area, Australia, and South America (187). It is also seen in some regions of North America (California, the Mississippi Valley, Utah, Arizona, and northern Canada) (188). Large-scale immigration has increased the prevalence of the disease in North America. The infection occurs through eating contaminated food. Even though hydatid cyst most commonly occurs in the liver, it can involve other organs such as lungs, spleen, kidneys, central nervous system, and bone (189). Patients with hydatid cyst present with low-grade fever and enlarged tender liver (190). Larger cysts can obstruct blood and bile flow, causing portal hypertension and jaundice, respectively. Cysts may rupture into the biliary tract and may lead to cholangitis; they may rupture through the diaphragm into the pleural or pericardial cavities, pulmonary

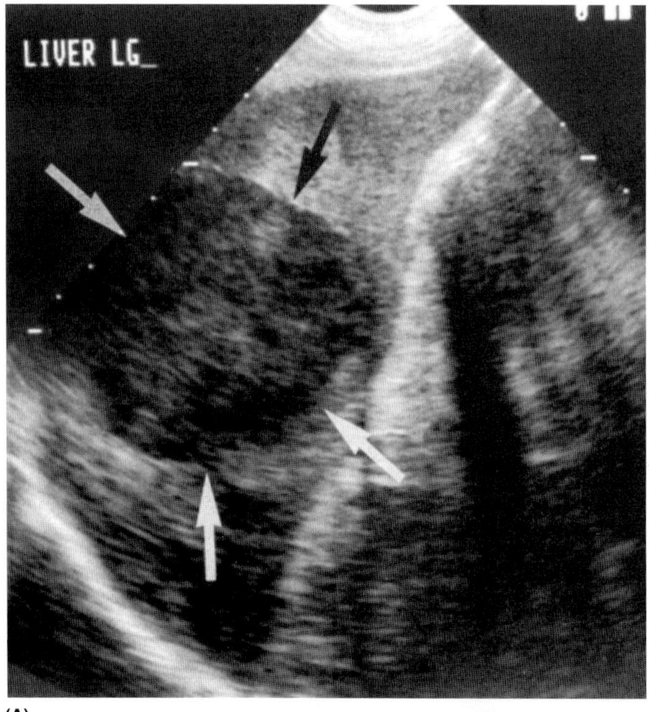

(A)

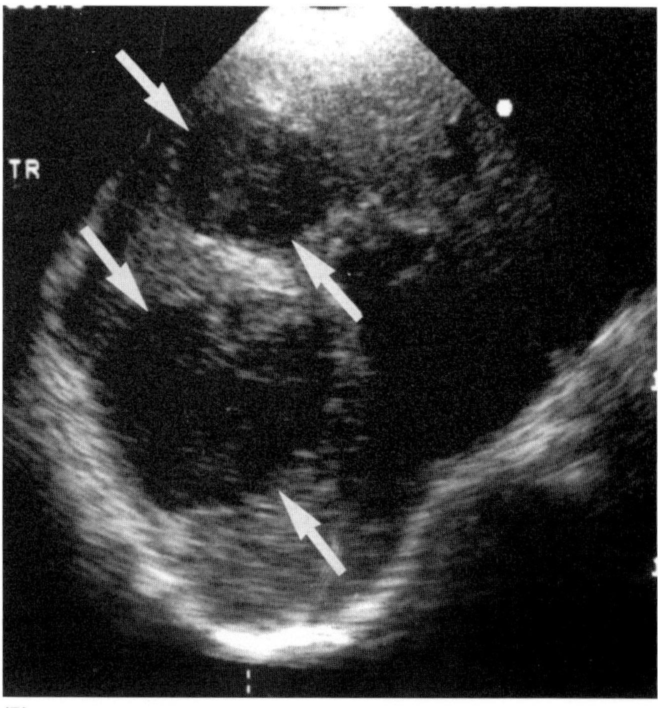

(B)

FIGURE 73 A AND B ■ Amebic abscess. (**A**) Sagittal view shows a well-defined, hypoechoic amebic abscess (*arrows*) containing diffuse internal echoes and posterior acoustic enhancement. (**B**) Transverse view in another patient shows two well-defined, hypoechoic amebic abscesses (*arrows*) containing low-level internal echoes. *Source*: Courtesy of Nagesh Ragavendra, MD, Los Angeles, CA.

parenchyma, or bronchi; or they may perforate the peritoneal cavity, the gastrointestinal tract, or the right kidney. Because the fluid in the cyst is highly antigenic, a rupture can produce anaphylactic shock and even death (189).

Morphologically, these cysts are made up of an ectocyst, composed of multilayered acellular wall and an endocyst, composed of a thin membrane. Pericyst is a dense connective tissue capsule around the entire cyst. Brood capsules and scoleces arising from the endocyst separate from the wall and form a fine sediment called hydatid sand, which settles into the dependent part of the cyst. Daughter cysts, when present, are considered pathognomonic for hydatid disease. The hydatid cysts can be solitary, but frequently they are multiple. The right lobe of the liver is more often affected than the left. The hydatid cyst can be as large as 30 cm in diameter.

The sonographic appearance of the hydatid cyst is variable, perhaps depending on the stage of evolution (191,192). The following sonographic patterns can be seen. First is a simple, fluid-filled anechoic cyst with well-defined borders and walls of variable thickness with distal acoustic enhancement. The cyst usually contains echogenic debris (hydatid sand), which may be visible only by rolling the patient during ultrasound scanning and enables the clinician to differentiate hydatid cyst from simple hepatic cyst (191). In addition, unilocular hydatid cyst frequently demonstrates two parallel echogenic lines along the wall of the cyst, representing the pericyst and the membrane of the endocyst (193). Second is a cystic mass containing undulating, free-floating membranes (the "water lily" sign) that represent a detached endocyst secondary to rupture. Third is a cystic mass containing daughter cysts with or without echogenic material (matrix) in between the daughter cysts (Fig. 74). The daughter cysts consist of one or more smaller cystic areas within the mass surrounded by usually thick and complete septa representing the walls of the daughter cysts. Fourth, dense calcifications appear as curvilinear hyperechoic areas with strong acoustic shadowing (Fig. 75). Thin, subtle calcifications in the wall of the cysts with or without acoustic shadowing may also be seen.

Cysts may contain multiple solid echogenic areas and thick irregular septations when infected. They may also appear as a predominantly solid mass of variable echogenicity, perhaps secondary to organization of the hydatid fluid within the cyst when multiple daughter cysts become deformed, collapsed, and crammed inside the hydatid cyst (Fig. 75B) (194).

The diagnosis is made by serologic testing. When patients with hydatid cysts are medically treated, follow-up ultrasound examinations during treatment may demonstrate progressive decrease in cyst size, detachment of the endocyst membrane, and progressive solidification of the mass (187). The conventional treatment of hydatid cyst is surgery. Percutaneous puncture or aspiration of the hydatid cyst has been contraindicated because of the risk of peritoneal spillage or anaphylaxis. However, both percutaneous diagnostic aspiration and percutaneous drainage with ultrasound guidance have been performed without significant complications (188,195).

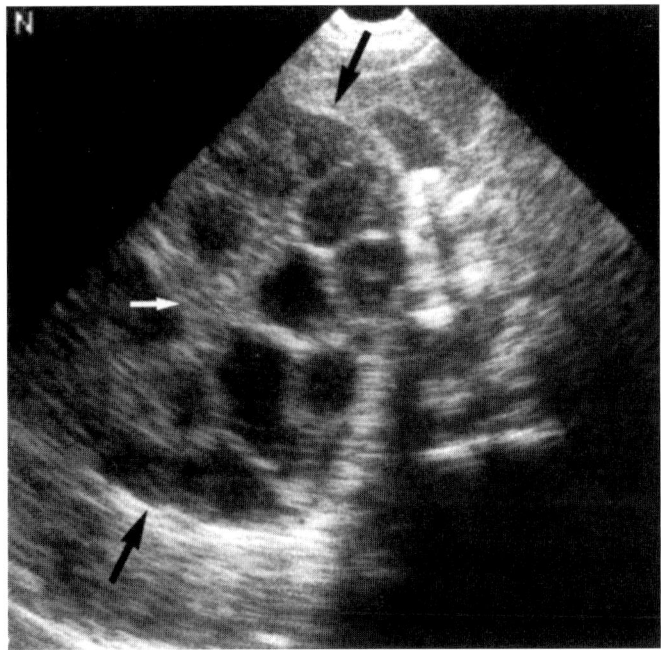

(A)

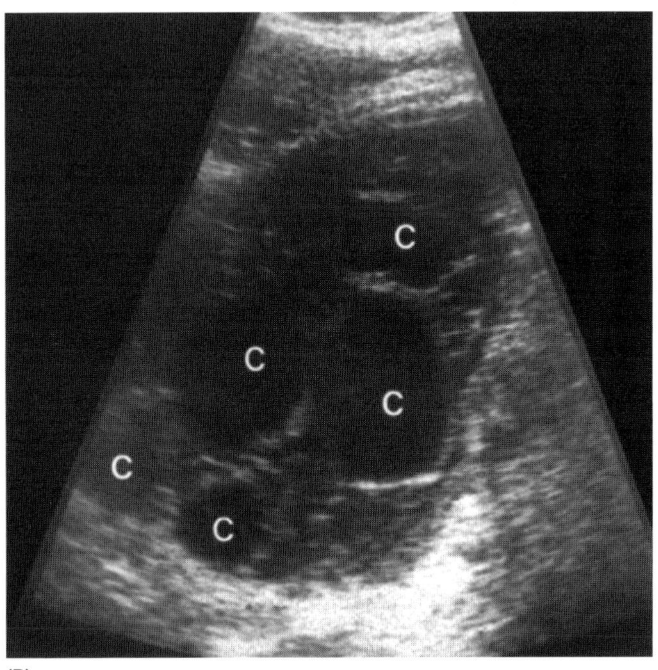

(B)

FIGURE 74 A AND B ■ Hydatid cyst containing daughter cysts. (**A**) Transverse view shows a large hydatid cyst (*large arrows*) containing numerous small daughter cysts with thick complete septa around the daughter cysts. In the center of the mass (*small arrow*), an echogenic matrix is seen in between the daughter cysts. (**B**) Large hydatid cyst containing several small daughter cysts (C) with thinner septa compared with (**A**). *Source*: (**A**) Courtesy of Bhaskara K. Rao, MD, Houston, TX and (**B**) courtesy of William E. Brant, MD, Sacramento, CA.

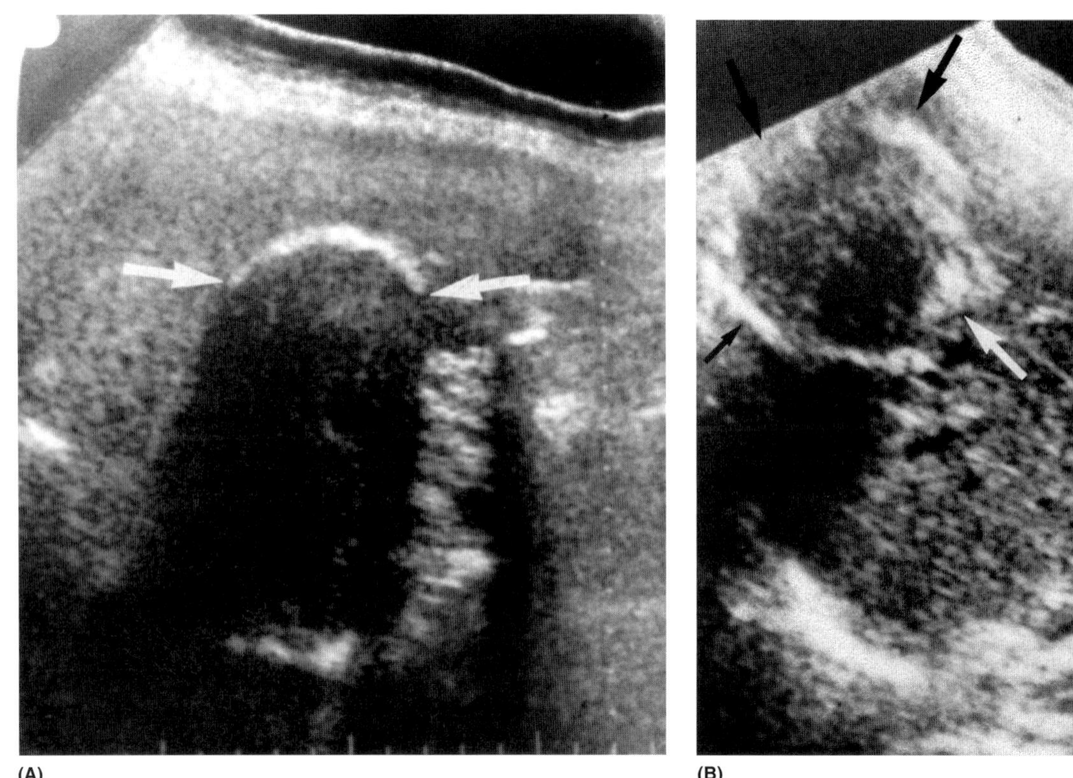

FIGURE 75 A AND B ■ Calcified hydatid cyst. (**A**) A large, hyperechoic curvilinear calcification (*arrows*) within the wall of the hydatid cyst causing posterior acoustic shadowing. (**B**) Hydatid cyst (*arrows*) with a hyperechoic calcified wall with posterior acoustic shadowing. Part of the cyst contains echogenic solid material secondary to organization of the hydatid fluid within the cyst. *Source*: Courtesy of William E. Brant, MD, Sacramento, CA.

Echinococcus multilocularis

Hepatic alveolar echinococcosis is a rare parasitic disease secondary to *E. multilocularis*. This organism is different from *E. granulosus*, which is involved in the common hydatid disease causing hydatid cyst of the liver (196). In infestation with *E. multilocularis*, the germinal membrane (endocyst) is not confined by a cyst wall within a single cyst. Scoleces develop in an uncontrolled manner, invading adjacent tissue (197).

Sonographically, three patterns can be seen: (*i*) a large, extensive solid mass with an inhomogeneous echo pattern, containing multiple echogenic and hyperechoic areas of varying size; (*ii*) a cystic, anechoic mass with irregular contours without a well-defined wall, containing peripheral echoes and echogenic debris; and (*iii*) a complex mass of mixed echogenicity, containing echogenic solid areas as well as multiple cystic regions (196). Calcifications are seen in 50% of the lesions. Intrahepatic biliary dilatation is commonly seen, secondary to narrowing of the intrahepatic bile ducts or hilar involvement causing common duct obstruction. Narrowing and obstruction of the intrahepatic portal venous branches may lead to portal hypertension. The diagnosis is made by serologic testing.

Schistosomiasis

Liver involvement with schistosomiasis is due to the helminthic parasites *S. mansoni* and *Schistosoma japonica*. *S. mansoni* has much larger geographic distribution than *S. japonica*. *S. mansoni* is prevalent in parts of Middle East and Africa and in Brazil and Venezuela. *S. japonica* is more common in Japan, China, the Philippines, Laos, and Cambodia. Schistosomiasis afflicts about 200 million people worldwide (198). The parasites (cercariae) penetrate the skin or mucosa, enter the circulation, and travel first to the lungs and subsequently to the liver (199). The parasites live in the portal venous system. The eggs entering the liver circulation elicit a severe granulomatous reaction, which causes marked periportal fibrosis leading to presinusoidal portal hypertension. Hematemesis from gastroesophageal varices is one of the most serious complications (200). Chronic schistosomiasis causes hepatosplenomegaly.

Sonographically, areas of increased echogenicity are seen around the walls of the major portal veins extending to involve the smaller intrahepatic branches, secondary to periportal fibrosis and thickening of the walls of the portal veins. Thickening of the walls of the portal veins can be considerable, up to 2 cm (198,201,202). Atrophy of the right hepatic lobe accompanied by hypertrophy of the left lobe is typical. The main portal vein, the splenic vein, and, to a lesser extent, the superior mesenteric vein are frequently dilated. Portal venous collaterals can be seen in patients with portal hypertension. Portal venous thrombosis is rare. Granulomas in the liver, caused by the parasites, may be rarely seen as rounded, solid nodules of increased echogenicity. Thickening of the gallbladder wall is a common finding.

Toxocariasis (Visceral Larva Migrans)

Toxocariasis is caused by the parasite *Toxocara canis*; infection is acquired by ingesting contaminated food or soil and occurs most commonly in children. Sonographically, multiple hypoechoic solid lesions (203) or multiple complex masses consisting of a central necrotic cystic area surrounded by thick echogenic walls (204) may be seen secondary to granulomatous lesions within the liver caused by the parasite.

Tuberculosis

In miliary tuberculosis, the liver is usually enlarged but has normal echogenicity. Occasionally, the liver may have increased echogenicity with increased attenuation of sound, resembling fatty infiltration of the liver (205). Macronodular tuberculosis of the liver is uncommon. Sonographic findings in macronodular tuberculosis include solitary or multiple hypoechoic, well-marginated solid masses with slight distal acoustic enhancement or densely calcified masses with acoustic shadowing (206). The masses are secondary to large tuberculous granulomas.

Candidiasis

Candidiasis of the liver or spleen is an unusual fungal infectious process that occurs usually in immunosuppressed patients with neoplastic disorders, most commonly leukemia and lymphoma, as well as in patients with renal transplants. Infection by *Candida albicans* causes multiple small abscesses in the liver and frequently the spleen that measure 3 to 10 mm in diameter (207), but these abscesses may measure up to 4 cm in diameter (208). Sonographically, four patterns can be seen (208): (*i*) the target or bull's eye appearance, which is classic for this diagnosis and consists of an anechoic cystic or hypoechoic mass containing a central, small, hyperechoic solid area (Fig. 76); (*ii*) the "wheel within a wheel" appearance, seen early in the course of the disease, consisting of a peripheral hypoechoic or anechoic zone with an inner echogenic wheel containing a central hypoechoic nidus (Fig. 77); (*iii*) the most common pattern, consisting of a uniformly hypoechoic lesion; and (*iv*) an echogenic or hyperechoic focus with a variable degree of acoustic shadowing. Lesions of pattern 4 are smaller (2–5 mm in diameter) than those of the other three patterns and are seen late in the course of the disease (208). The central hyperechoic nidus within the target pattern lesion probably consists of inflammatory cells rather than growing fungus or mycelial nidus (208–210).

The target lesions of candidiasis need to be differentiated from neoplastic (primary or secondary) lesions in the liver. In neoplastic lesions, the central hyperechoic area usually is much larger and the peripheral rim is hypoechoic, but it usually does not appear anechoic or cystic (209).

Pneumocystis carinii Infection

Extrapulmonary involvement by *P. carinii* in patients with AIDS is uncommon. When disseminated infection with *P. carinii* occurs, sonographically diffuse tiny hyperechoic foci without acoustic shadowing can be seen in the liver, spleen, kidneys, and thyroid (Fig. 78) (211,212). In the early stage of the disease, the tiny, hyperechoic nonshadowing foci may not be from calcifications; however, calcifications develop as the disease progresses, as demonstrated on CT examinations (211,212). Similar visceral hyperechoic foci

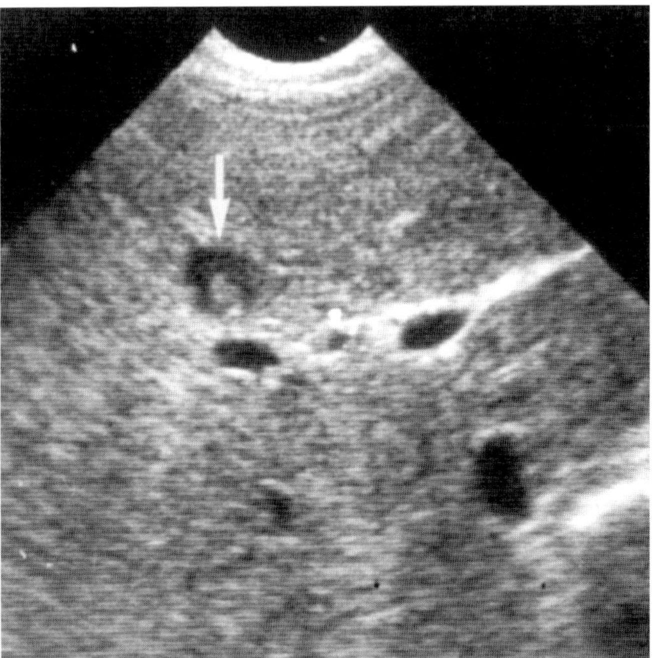

FIGURE 76 ■ Candidiasis: target pattern. A small, anechoic cystic abscess (*arrow*) contains a central hyperechoic solid area.

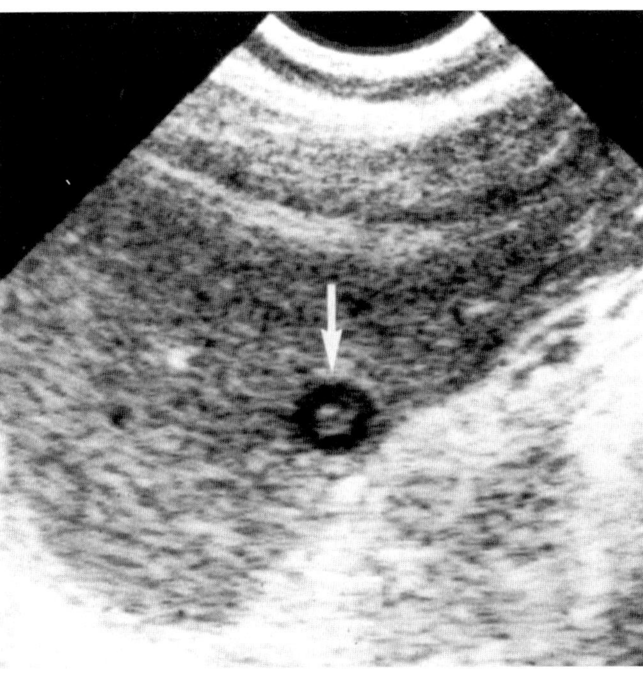

FIGURE 77 ■ Candidiasis: "wheel within a wheel" pattern. A small abscess (*arrow*) with a peripheral anechoic zone and an inner echogenic "wheel" is shown.

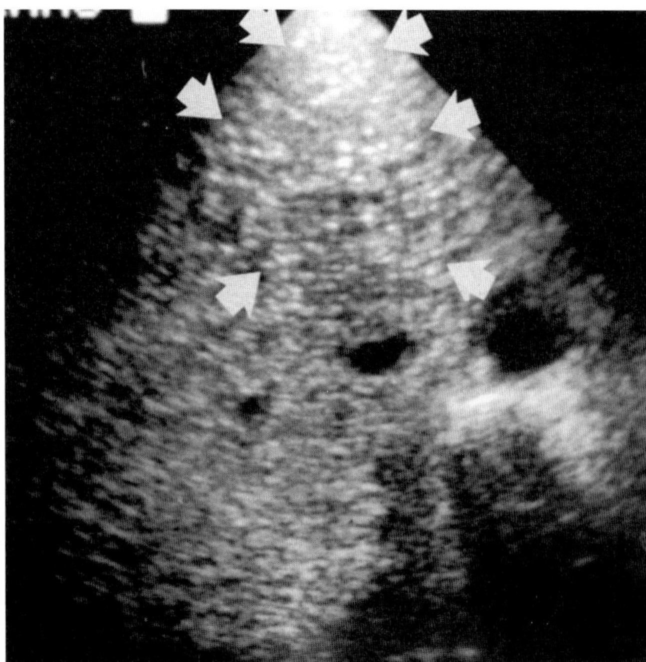

FIGURE 78 ■ *Pneumocystis carinii.* Numerous tiny hyperechoic foci without shadowing are seen in the anterior portions of the liver (*arrows*), secondary to involvement of the liver by *P. carinii* infection. *Source*: Courtesy of Nagesh Ragavendra, MD, Los Angeles, CA.

with or without calcifications have also been described secondary to cytomegalovirus and *Mycobacterium avium intracellulare* (213).

Chronic Granulomatous Disease

Chronic granulomatous disease is a familial disorder related to a congenital defect of leukocytes that causes recurrent infections in children. When the liver is involved, hypoechoic, poorly marginated solid masses secondary to hepatic granulomas or liver abscesses may be seen (214).

DIFFUSE LIVER DISEASE

Sonographic detection of diffuse liver disease may be difficult because diffuse liver disease does not always cause gray-scale abnormalities and when present, the abnormalities are frequently nonspecific.

Fatty Liver (Hepatic Steatosis)

Fatty liver results from accumulation of fat exceeding the normal 5% of liver weight. Fatty liver is caused by increased accumulation of triglycerides within the hepatocytes and is a reversible cellular response to various disease states and alterations in metabolism. Fatty liver is caused by numerous hepatocellular disorders including alcoholic liver disease, obesity, diabetes mellitus, starvation, gastrointestinal bypass surgery, endogenous and exogenous steroids, drug-induced liver disease, parenteral nutrition, severe hepatitis, glycogen storage disease, and cystic fibrosis (215,216).

TABLE 12 ■ Diffusely Increased Echogenicity of Liver ("Bright Liver")

Prevalence	Cause
Common	Fatty infiltration (most common)
	Cirrhosis
	Chronic hepatitis
Uncommon	Diffuse malignant infiltration
	Chronic right-sided heart failure
	Acute hepatitis (rare)
	AIDS
	Miliary tuberculosis
	Glycogen storage disease
	Wilson's disease
	Gaucher's disease

Sonographically the features of fatty liver include the following: (*i*) diffusely increased parenchymal echogenicity, often associated with unusually fine liver texture (Table 12); (*ii*) increased attenuation of the ultrasound beam causing poor visualization of the posterior portions of the liver; and (*iii*) decreased visualization of the portal and hepatic veins, probably secondary to compression by the surrounding fat-laden parenchyma as well as increased attenuation of sound and decreased contrast between echogenic fat and the walls of the vessels. The following grading of the degree of fatty infiltration has been proposed, using a 3.5-MHz (not a 2.5- or 5-MHz) transducer (Fig. 79) (217). In grade 1 (mild), echogenicity is slightly increased, with normal visualization of the diaphragm and the intrahepatic vessel borders. In grade 2 (moderate), echogenicity is moderately increased, with slightly impaired visualization of the diaphragm or intrahepatic vessels. In grade 3 (severe), echogenicity is markedly increased, with poor or no visualization of the diaphragm, the intrahepatic vessels, and posterior portion of the right lobe (217). Compared with CT (217) and liver biopsy (218), the overall accuracy of sonography in detecting fatty infiltration is 85% to 89%, and the specificity is 56% to 93%. The accuracy is particularly good for moderate and severe fatty infiltration. Quantitative methods for measuring liver echogenicity and attenuation and frequency-modulated sonography have been used in experimental settings for the diagnosis of diffuse parenchymal diseases of the liver; however, most of these methods are laborious and are not used in clinical ultrasound practice (215,219).

In acute fatty liver of pregnancy, the liver appears sonographically normal in most patients (220). Fatty infiltration can diffusely involve the entire liver, it may involve only a segment or a lobe, or it may involve scattered regions throughout the liver.

Focal Fatty Infiltration

Focal fatty infiltration appears as a hyperechoic area within normal or relatively normal liver parenchyma (Fig. 80). Areas of focal fatty infiltration may also be seen

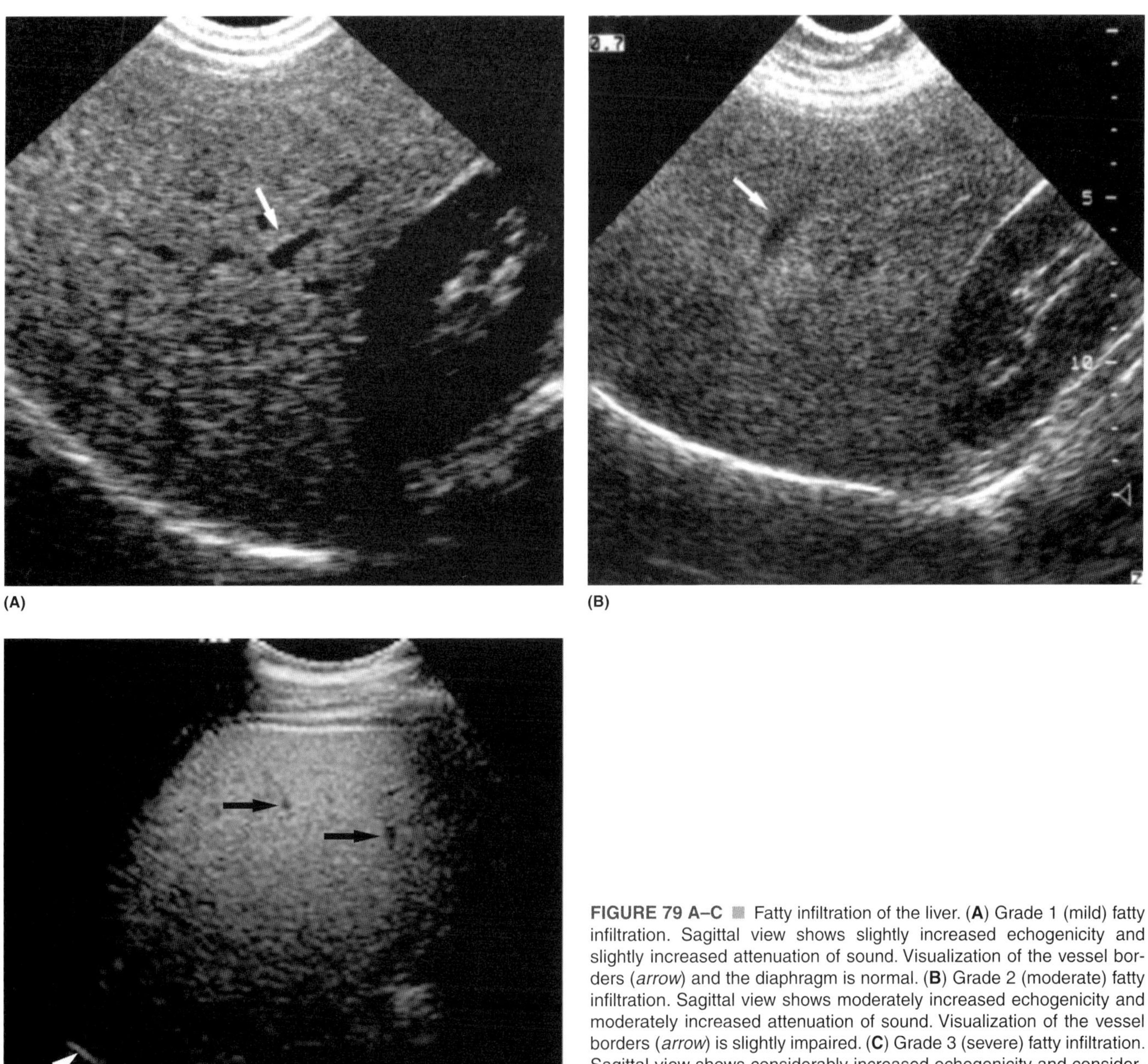

FIGURE 79 A–C ■ Fatty infiltration of the liver. (**A**) Grade 1 (mild) fatty infiltration. Sagittal view shows slightly increased echogenicity and slightly increased attenuation of sound. Visualization of the vessel borders (*arrow*) and the diaphragm is normal. (**B**) Grade 2 (moderate) fatty infiltration. Sagittal view shows moderately increased echogenicity and moderately increased attenuation of sound. Visualization of the vessel borders (*arrow*) is slightly impaired. (**C**) Grade 3 (severe) fatty infiltration. Sagittal view shows considerably increased echogenicity and considerably increased attenuation of sound. Parts of the diaphragm (*white arrows*) are poorly visualized, if at all, and visualization of the vessel borders (*black arrow*) is impaired.

within a liver, with scattered areas of patchy fatty infiltration and patchy focal sparing (Fig. 81). Areas of focal fatty infiltration can be recognized by their nonspheric shape, their straight, angulated, geometric margins, their wedge-shaped segmental or subsegmental distribution, the normal distribution (without displacement or distortion) of vessels within and around these lesions, and, occasionally, the interdigitation of normal and fatty tissue (221–223). However, focal fatty infiltration may appear as a rounded, hyperechoic area and may mimic a neoplasm (224,225). Such nodular-appearing focal fatty infiltration frequently occurs in the most anterior aspect of the medial segment of the left lobe, immediately adjacent to the falciform ligament (225). The clinician can usually confirm the fatty nature of these lesions with CT by demonstrating low attenuation in the corresponding regions. Because fatty infiltration is an intracellular accumulation of fat, and a normal array of Kupffer cells remains present, technetium-99 m sulfur colloid scintigraphy can be helpful by demonstrating no corresponding photon-deficient area, and xenon scintigraphy can be useful by demonstrating selective uptake and retention of xenon in the corresponding area. Follow-up ultrasound examinations may also be helpful because focal fatty infiltration can change in size or shape or disappear in a short time.

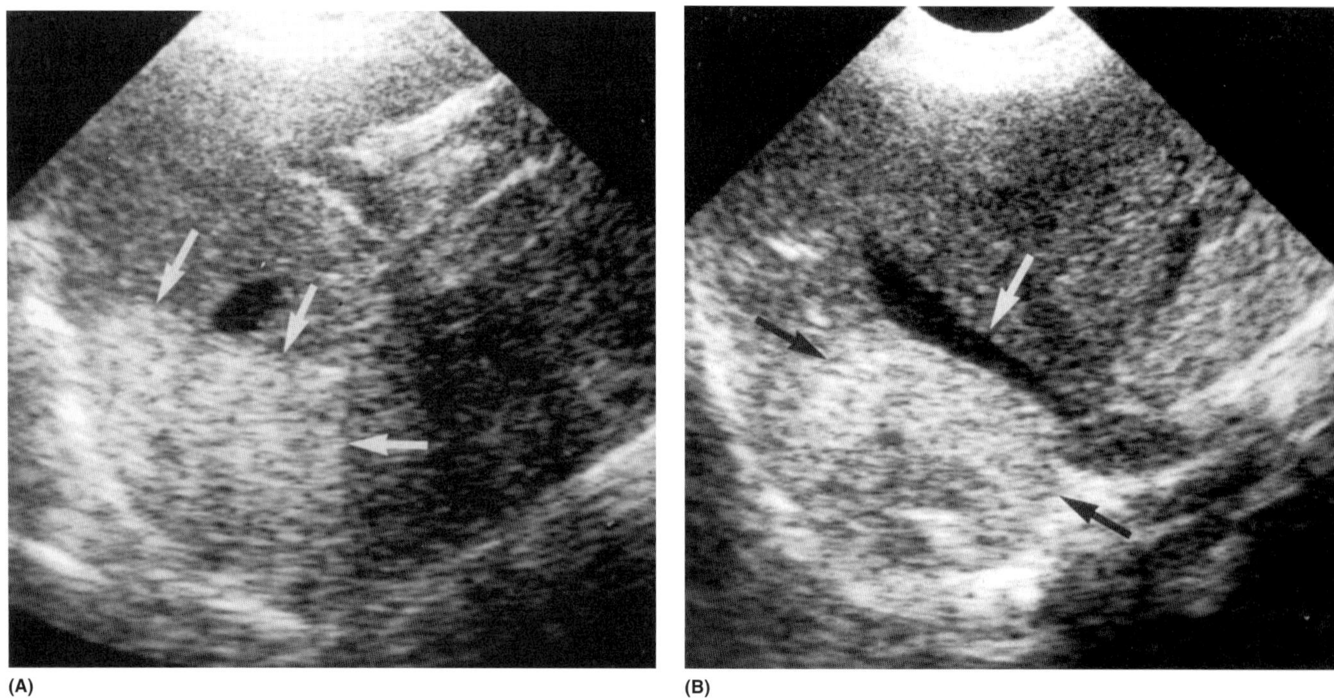

(A) (B)

FIGURE 80 A AND B ■ Focal fatty infiltration. (**A**) Sagittal view shows a typical hyperechoic area of focal fatty infiltration with long, straight margins (*arrows*). (**B**) Transverse view of the same area shows a hyperechoic region (*black arrows*) of focal fatty infiltration contiguous with but not displacing the hepatic vein (*white arrow*).

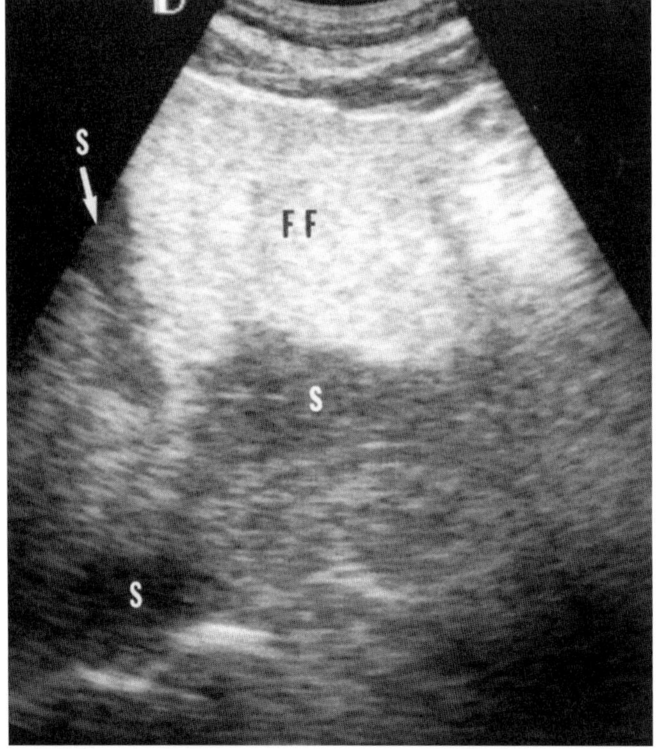

FIGURE 81 ■ Diffuse patchy pattern of fatty infiltration. A large, markedly hyperechoic area of focal fatty filtration (FF) with long, straight margins is seen anteriorly. Band-like hypoechoic areas (S) represent areas of focal sparing. Transverse view.

Focal Sparing

A diffusely fatty liver may have small areas of normal parenchyma, spared by fatty infiltration. The cause of focal sparing is unclear, but it may be related to decreased regional portal flow (226,227). This area of focal sparing usually is solitary, but it may be multiple. Focal sparing appears as a hypoechoic area with relatively distinct margins within hyperechoic fatty liver. Areas of focal sparing are most commonly located in the medial segment of the left lobe adjacent to the main lobar fissure (Fig. 82), anterior to the portal vein bifurcation, or medial and anterior to the neck and proximal body of the gallbladder (Fig. 83) (227–229). The shape is usually ovoid, but it varies from round to band-like (Figs. 81–83). It ranges in size from 1 to 8 cm. Rarely, areas of focal sparing are large and rounded, resembling a mass (230). One can usually confirm an area of normal parenchyma corresponding to the hypoechoic area within the fatty liver with CT. In larger (>3 cm) areas of focal sparing, technetium-99 m sulfur colloid scintigraphy may be performed to confirm the diagnosis by demonstrating normal radiocolloid uptake in the corresponding area. Occasionally, biopsy may be required to differentiate areas of focal fatty infiltration or focal sparing from neoplasm.

Hepatic Fibrosis

Hepatic fibrosis, by itself, has little or no effect on hepatic echogenicity. At most, hepatic fibrosis may increase

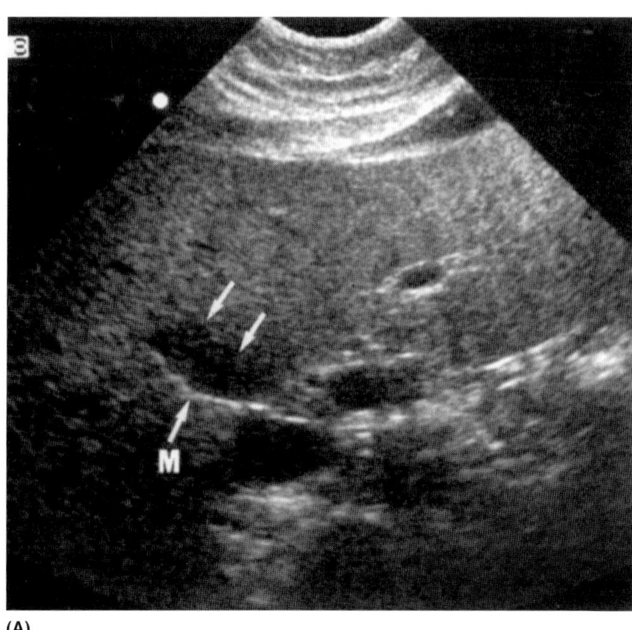

(A)

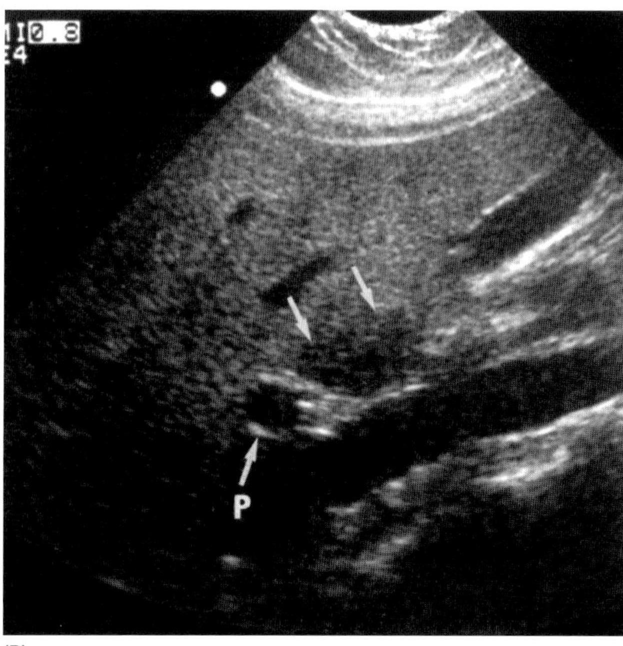

(B)

FIGURE 82 A AND B ■ Focal sparing in fatty liver. (**A**) Transverse view shows a hypoechoic, band-like area (*arrows*) of focal sparing contiguous with the main lobar fissure (M), within the medial segment of the left lobe of the liver. (**B**) Sagittal view of the same area shows an ovoid hypoechoic region (*arrows*) of focal sparing adjacent to the portal vein (P).

echogenicity slightly, and, in most cases, hepatic fibrosis cannot be detected by ultrasound examination (215).

Alcoholic Hepatitis

Alcoholic hepatitis is caused by inflammatory infiltrate and necrosis within the liver (231). The patient may be asymptomatic or may have clinical evidence of inflammation with low-grade fever and mild leukocytosis. Alcoholic hepatitis, however, is a histopathologic diagnosis and usually does not cause specific sonographic abnormalities, unless it is associated with fatty infiltration or cirrhosis.

FIGURE 83 ■ Focal sparing in fatty liver. Sagittal view shows a hypoechoic area (*arrow*) of focal sparing adjacent to the proximal body and neck of the gallbladder (G). A hyperechoic area of focal fatty infiltration (*arrowheads*) is also present adjacent to the area of focal sparing.

Chronic Hepatitis

In chronic hepatitis, hepatomegaly, inhomogeneous patchy echo pattern, or diffusely increased echogenicity may be seen, depending upon the degree of fatty infiltration and fibrosis present (232). In chronic active hepatitis, often alcohol related, enlarged hepatic arteries in the liver may be seen on color Doppler sonography due to increased arterial flow (232).

Cirrhosis

Cirrhosis is a chronic disease of the liver caused by parenchymal necrosis, scarring, fibrosis, and regeneration resulting in disorganization of the hepatic lobular and vascular architecture. Alcoholism accounts for 60% to 70% of all cases of cirrhosis in the Western world, whereas in Asia and Africa, viral hepatitis is the usual cause (233). Cirrhosis is among the 10 leading causes of death in the Western world and the sixth leading cause in the United States. Cirrhosis leads to two major potentially life-threatening complications: hepatocellular failure resulting from hepatocyte damage and portal venous hypertension (234). One-third of the deaths from cirrhosis are secondary to hemorrhage, usually from esophageal varices (234). The incidence of HCC is increased in patients with cirrhosis; this association is

TABLE 13 ■ Etiology of Cirrhosis

Alcohol-related disease
Viral hepatitis
Biliary disorders
- Chronic biliary obstruction
- Primary biliary cirrhosis
- Sclerosing cholangitis

Metabolic disorders
- Hemochromatosis
- Wilson's disease
- Type IV glycogen storage disease
- α_1-Antitrypsin deficiency
- Galactosemia
- Tyrosinemia

Cardiovascular disease
- Passive cardiac congestion
- Budd–Chiari syndrome
- Veno-occlusive disease

Drugs and toxins
Immunologic disorders ("lupoid" hepatitis)
Miscellaneous conditions
- Sarcoid
- Cryptogenic

TABLE 14 ■ Sonographic Signs of Cirrhosis

Coarse echo pattern
Diffusely inhomogeneous echo pattern
Increased echogenicity
Surface nodularity
Volume redistribution
- Enlarged caudate lobe and left lobe/small right lobe
- Caudate: right lobe ratio >0.65
- Right lobe: left lobe ratio <1.3
- Left portal vein diameter ≥right portal vein diameter

Signs of portal hypertension

stronger in patients with cirrhosis secondary to viral hepatitis than in those with cirrhosis secondary to alcoholism.

Cirrhosis can be classified morphologically as micronodular, macronodular, and mixed. In micronodular cirrhosis, the nodules are uniform in size and are usually less than 3 mm in diameter (235,236). This disorder is seen in chronic alcoholism, prolonged biliary obstruction, hemochromatosis, venous outflow obstruction, and small bowel bypass. In macronodular cirrhosis, the nodules vary in size; most nodules are larger than 3 mm in diameter and may measure several centimeters (235,236). Chronic viral hepatitis is the most common cause of macronodular cirrhosis, even though this disorder may be secondary to other forms of hepatitis. Other causes of cirrhosis include drug-induced hepatic injury, late stages of some parasitic diseases, and Wilson's disease (Table 13). Clinically, patients with cirrhosis may present with enlarged liver, jaundice, and ascites; however, only approximately 60% of patients with cirrhosis have signs and symptoms of liver disease (237).

Sonographic findings in cirrhosis (Table 14) include the following: A coarse echo pattern (Fig. 84) may range from a mildly grainy appearance to a diffusely inhomogeneous echo pattern in patients with advanced cirrhosis (Table 15). Increased echogenicity may be noted. The echogenicity and attenuation of sound in cirrhotic liver may be similar to normal liver, but when superimposed fatty infiltration is present, the echogenicity and attenuation may be increased (Fig. 85). Surface nodularity can be seen in cirrhosis and is most evident in the presence of ascites (Fig. 86) (238–240). In the absence of ascites, examination of the liver surface (usually the ventral left lobe), with 5- or 7.5-MHz linear-array transducers can detect early subtle nodularity. With this technique, for diagnosis of cirrhosis, demonstration of diffuse nodularity has reported a sensitivity of 88% and a specificity ranging from 81% to 95% (238,240). Ladenheim et al., however, found the evaluation of surface nodularity using a 5-MHz linear-array transducer to be useless because of its low positive predictive value (239). Therefore, even though detection of surface nodularity is generally considered a reliable sign of cirrhosis, further investigation is needed to determine the usefulness of the sonographic liver surface nodularity evaluation with 5- or 7.5-MHz linear-array transducers. Surface nodularity may also be seen secondary to subcapsular liver metastases. Volume redistribution is another sonographic finding in cirrhosis. In early stages of the disease, the liver may be enlarged; however, advanced cirrhosis may cause generalized shrinkage of the liver. Before cirrhosis becomes advanced, the right lobe often shrinks more than the other lobes, and one sees relative enlargement of the caudate lobe and the left lobe (Fig. 87).

The ratio of the caudate lobe to the right lobe, obtained by dividing the transverse dimension of the caudate lobe by the transverse dimension of the right lobe, may be useful in the diagnosis of cirrhosis (Fig. 88) (241). Measurements are obtained from transverse sonograms or CT scans, approximately at or less than 1 cm below the bifurcation of the main portal vein (Fig. 88). Measurements are easier to obtain from CT scans than from the sonograms, because of the reduced acoustic window of real-time ultrasound equipment. Cirrhosis can be diagnosed if the ratio of the caudate lobe to the right lobe exceeds 0.65, with a sensitivity ranging from 43% to 84% and a specificity of 100% (241–243). Subsequent studies have challenged the specificity of this ratio, and the caudate lobe may also be enlarged in patients with Budd–Chiari syndrome. Because of right lobe shrinkage and relative preservation and enlargement of the left lobe, the ratio of the right lobe to the left lobe may also be useful in the diagnosis of cirrhosis. The longitudinal dimensions (length) of the right and left lobes are measured on the sagittal scans obtained in the mid-clavicular line and the midline,

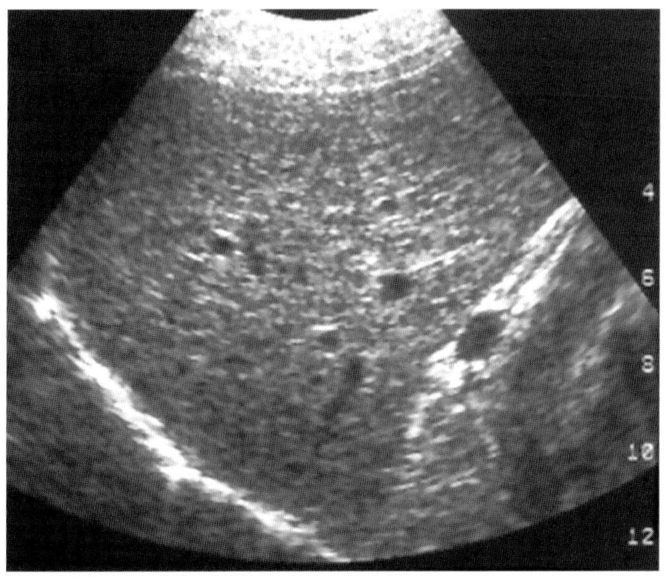

(A)

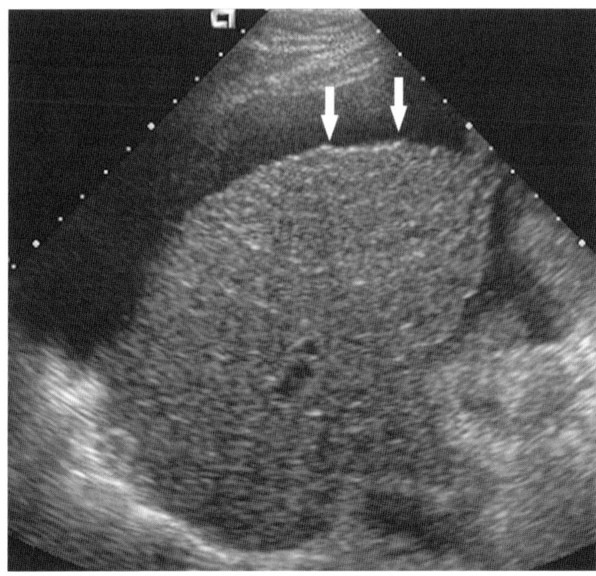

(B)

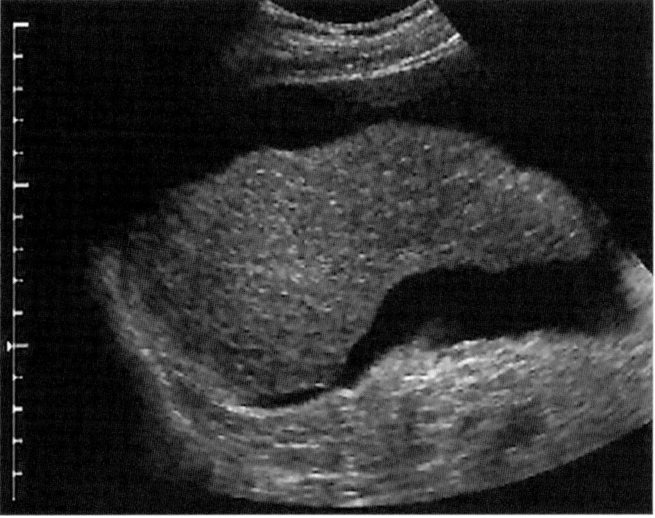

(C)

FIGURE 84 A–C ■ Cirrhosis: coarse echo pattern. (**A**) Longitudinal view shows coarse echo pattern. (**B, C**) Coarse slightly inhomogeneous echo pattern of the liver. The liver is surrounded by ascites. One sees slight nodularity of the anterior surface of the liver in (**B**) (*arrows*).

respectively. The ratio is obtained by dividing the longitudinal dimension of the right lobe by the longitudinal dimension of the left lobe. The normal ratio is 1.44 and is less than 1.3 in patients with cirrhosis (244). The ratio of 1.3 has a 74% sensitivity and a 100% specificity and 93% accuracy (244). The sensitivity is higher (83%) in hepatitis B virus (HBV)–related postnecrotic cirrhosis than in non-HBV related (alcoholic and other) cirrhosis (57%).

TABLE 15 ■ Diffusely Inhomogeneous Echo Pattern

- Cirrhosis
- Metastases
- Hepatocellular carcinoma
- Fatty infiltration (uncommon)
- Hepatoblastoma (uncommon)
- Peripheral cholangiocarcinoma (rare)

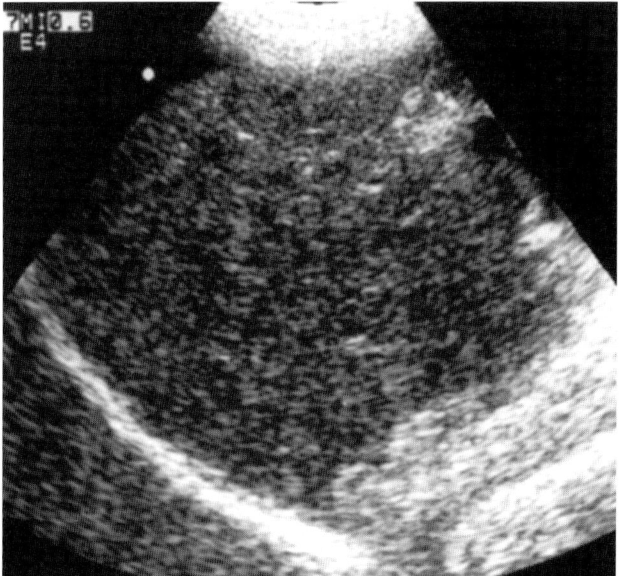

FIGURE 85 ■ Cirrhosis: coarse echo pattern. One also notes increased attenuation of sound secondary to superimposed fatty infiltration. Sagittal view.

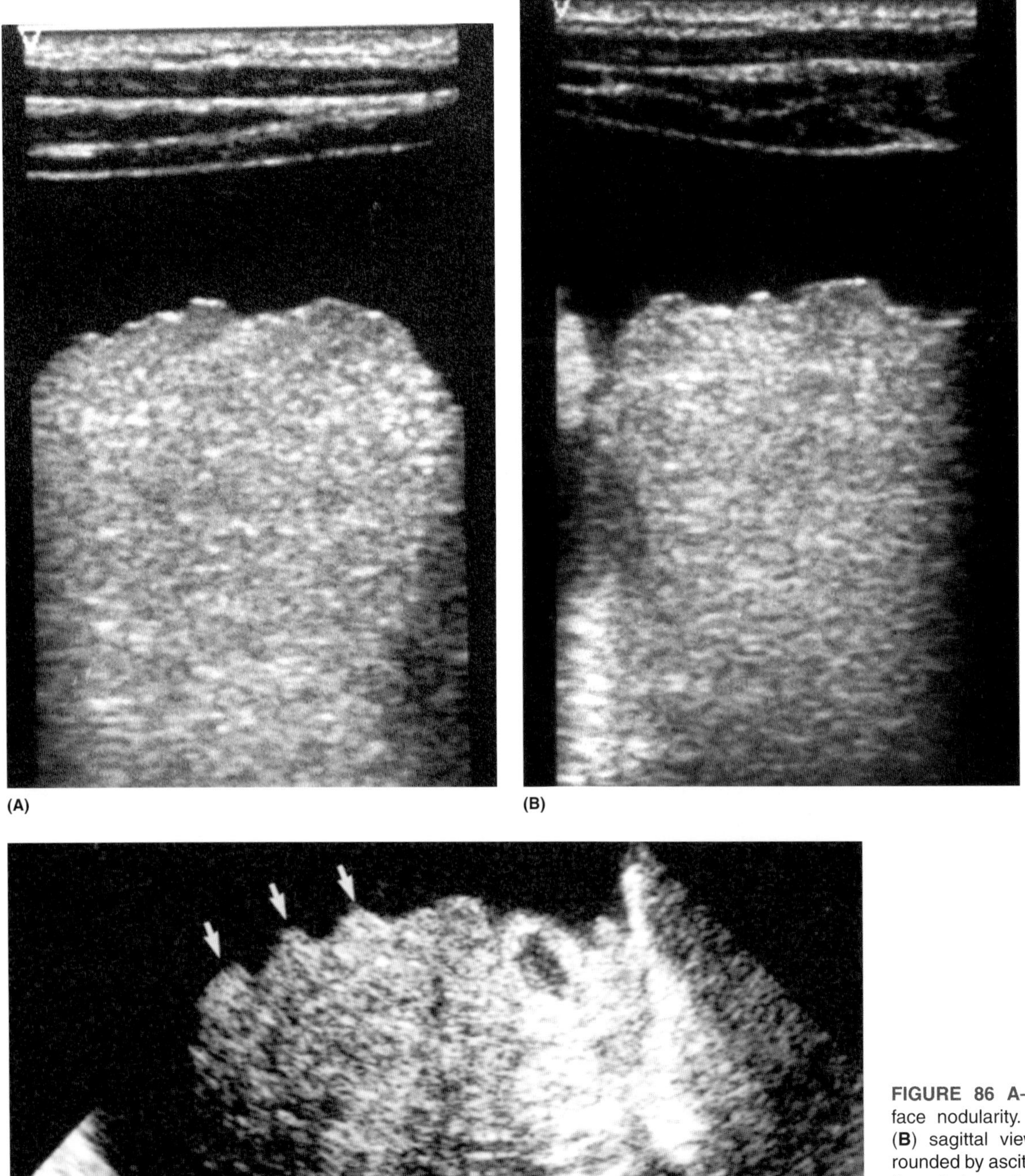

FIGURE 86 A–C ■ Cirrhosis: surface nodularity. (A) Transverse and (B) sagittal views of the liver surrounded by ascites show nodularity of the anterior surface of the cirrhotic liver. (C) Transverse view in another patient shows marked nodularity (*arrows*) of the anterior surface of the liver, surrounded by ascites. *Source*: Courtesy of Bhaskara K. Rao, MD, Houston, TX.

Another useful ratio is obtained by multiplying the longitudinal, transverse, and anteroposterior dimensions of the caudate lobe and dividing them by the transverse dimension of the right lobe. The mean ratio in patients with cirrhosis is 16.7, compared with 3.2 for normal livers. This ratio has sensitivity and specificity of 95% (245). In patients with cirrhosis, the ratio of the left to the right portal vein may be increased. Normally, the diameter of the right portal vein is greater than that of the left portal vein because the right lobe is larger than the left. When patients with cirrhosis have a relative increase in the size of the left lobe compared with the right lobe, the left portal vein diameter becomes equal to or greater than the right portal vein diameter. The anteroposterior diameter of the portal veins is measured on the transverse view, approximately 1 cm from the main portal vein bifurcation. Another feature of cirrhosis

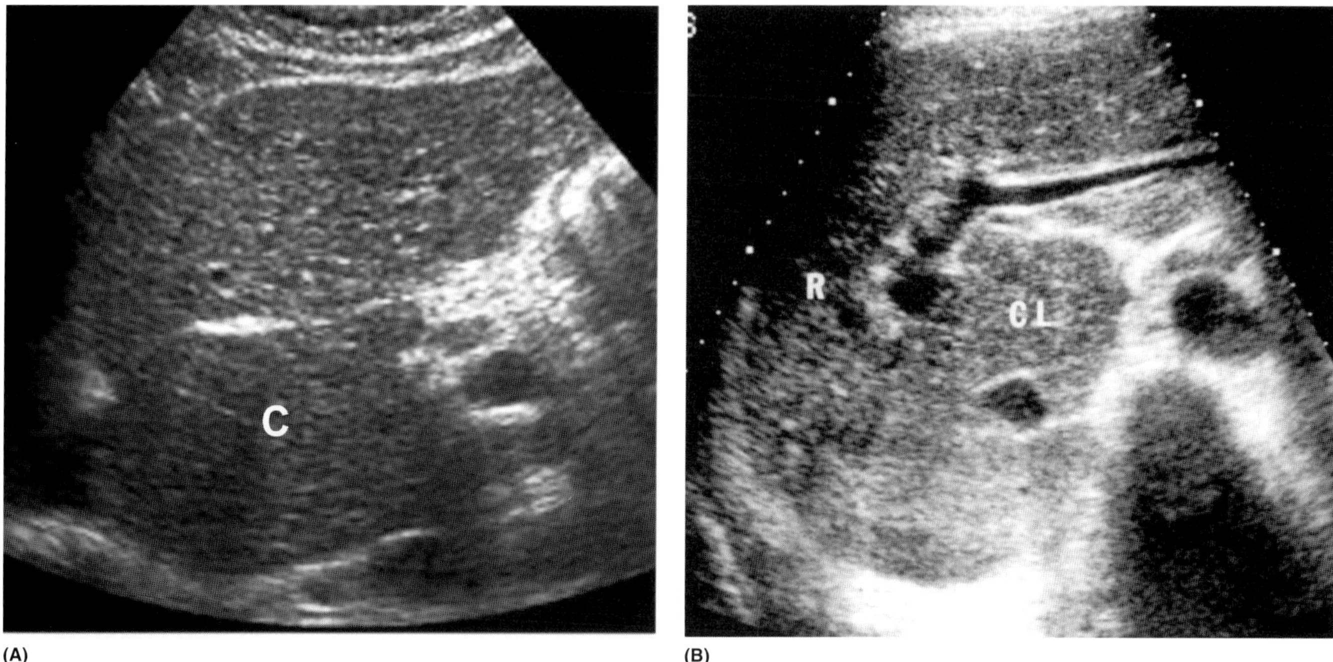

FIGURE 87 A AND B ■ Cirrhosis: enlarged caudate lobe. (**A**) Longitudinal view shows an enlarged caudate lobe (C). (**B**) Transverse view in another patient shows an enlarged caudate lobe (CL) and a small right lobe (R).

is portal hypertension. Sonographic findings associated with portal hypertension including portosystemic venous collaterals, ascites, and splenomegaly may be present.

In duplex Doppler imaging of hepatic veins of patients with cirrhosis of the liver, the normal triphasic pattern of the hepatic veins may be lost, probably because of decreased compliance of the veins secondary to fibrosis and steatosis in the parenchyma surrounding the hepatic veins (246). Changes in duplex

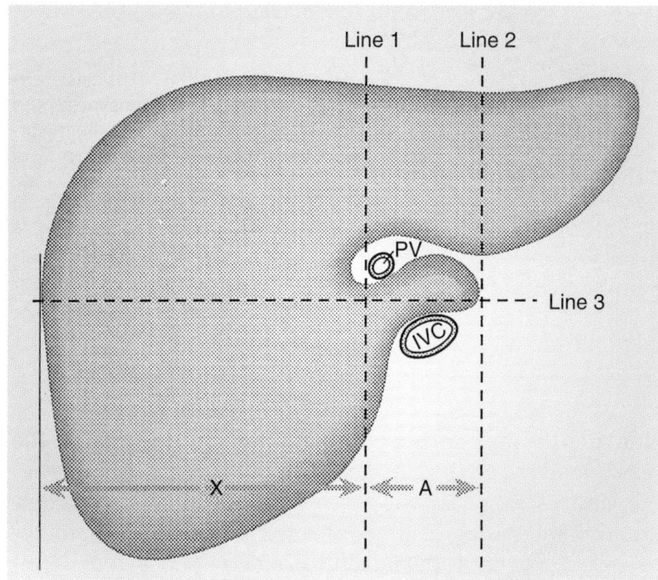

FIGURE 88 ■ Ratio of caudate lobe to right lobe. *Source*: Modified from Ref. 241.

Doppler waveform of hepatic veins in patients with cirrhosis, including (*i*) decreased amplitude of the basic oscillations without the short phase of the reverse flow in 31.7% of patients and (*ii*) completely flat waveform without any basic oscillation in 18.3% of patients have been reported (247). In a study of patients with well-compensated chronic liver disease and antibodies to hepatitis C virus, Colli et al. found flattening of the Doppler waveform of the hepatic veins to be an accurate sign of cirrhosis (246). Absent retrograde (hepatopetal) flow in the hepatic veins however may be seen, not only in patients with overt liver disease, but also in a few apparently liver-healthy patients (248).

Enlarged and tortuous hepatic arteries may be seen, with color Doppler sonography, in cirrhotic liver.

Regenerating Nodules

Cirrhotic livers contain numerous regenerating nodules (adenomatous hyperplastic nodules), most of which range from 5 mm to 1.5 cm (249). These small nodules, however, are rarely visualized by abdominal ultrasound examination (249). When seen, these nodules appear hypoechoic (Fig. 89), frequently with a thin echogenic rim. Large regenerating nodules (5–15 cm) are rarely encountered, and when seen, they may appear as an echogenic or inhomogeneous solid mass that cannot be differentiated from HCC or other neoplasms (250). Technetium-99 m sulfur colloid scintigraphy may detect regenerating nodules because they take up radionuclide, whereas neoplastic tissue has decreased or absent uptake (250). However, biopsy is often necessary for the diagnosis.

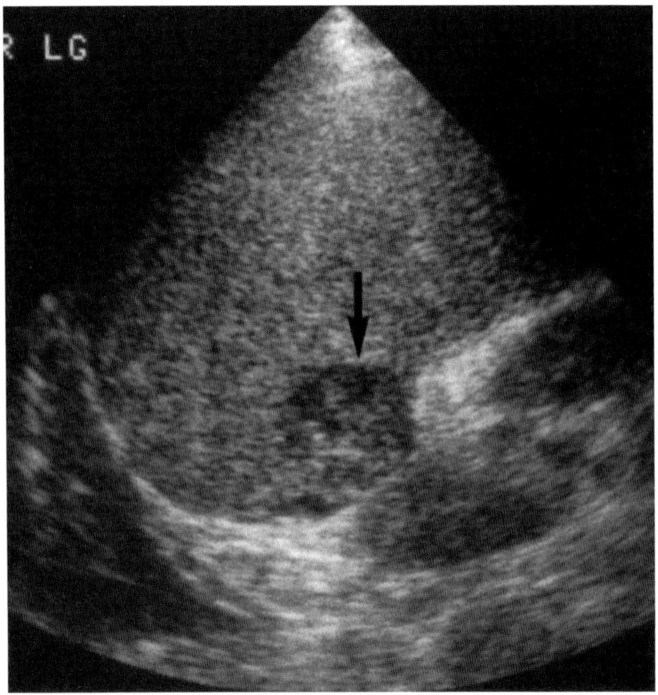

FIGURE 89 ■ Cirrhosis: regenerating nodule. Sagittal view shows a biopsy-proven, small, hypoechoic, solid, regenerating nodule (*arrow*) in a cirrhotic liver with a coarse echo pattern.

Biliary Cirrhosis

Primary biliary cirrhosis, a chronic progressive cholestatic liver disease of unknown cause, is characterized by inflammation and destruction of intrahepatic bile ducts (251). Although primary biliary cirrhosis occurs in all races worldwide, most patients are white. Of patients with primary biliary cirrhosis, 95% are women between the ages of 30 and 65 years. The liver is enlarged and smooth in early stages of the disease, but as the disease progresses, it may become finely nodular. Sonographic findings reflect abnormalities secondary to cirrhosis. Enlarged lymph nodes are frequently seen in the porta hepatis (252). Endoscopic retrograde cholangiopancreatography is the primary radiographic technique for establishing the diagnosis of primary biliary cirrhosis (253).

Secondary biliary cirrhosis results from long-standing biliary obstruction, cholangitis, and biliary atresia.

Other Diffuse Diseases

Other metabolic or storage diseases causing diffuse hepatic parenchymal abnormalities are occasionally encountered. Glycogen storage disease is an autosomal-recessive genetic disorder of glycogen metabolism that is manifested in the neonatal period by hypoglycemia, hepatomegaly, and nephromegaly. Of the several categories of glycogen storage disease, type I glycogen storage disease (Von Gierke's disease) is the most prevalent. Pathologically, one sees excessive glycogen deposition in the hepatocytes and proximal renal tubules. Type I glycogen storage disease causes hepatomegaly and may cause diffusely increased echogenicity secondary to concomitant fatty infiltration of the liver. The incidence of adenoma of the liver is increased in patients with type I glycogen storage disease (66,254,255).

Congenital generalized lipodystrophy is a rare hereditary disease that causes hepatomegaly and increased echogenicity and attenuation of sound secondary to fatty infiltration of the liver (256). In cystic fibrosis, diffusely increased echogenicity of the liver, inhomogeneous echo pattern, and increased periportal hyperechogenicity may be seen, along with small gallbladder containing sludge (257). In hemochromatosis, the sonographic abnormalities are related to fibrosis and cirrhosis of the liver. Parenchymal iron deposits in the liver usually do not cause any alteration of the liver echogenicity. Patients have hepatomegaly and, frequently, splenomegaly. In amyloidosis, the ultrasound shows nonspecific abnormalities. The liver is enlarged and may have an inhomogeneous echo pattern. Wilson's disease and Gaucher's disease also cause nonspecific sonographic abnormalities related to fatty infiltration and cirrhosis. Patients with AIDS may have hepatomegaly and increased echogenicity in the liver. Focal liver masses may be seen secondary to lymphoma, Kaposi's sarcoma, and pyogenic, fungal, or mycobacterial abscesses.

VASCULAR ABNORMALITIES AND DISORDERS

Portal Hypertension

Portal hypertension is defined as a portal vein pressure in excess of normal by 5 to 10 mm Hg (258). Portal hypertension results from increased resistance to portal venous blood flow. It can also be caused by increased flow into the portal system, so-called hyperkinetic portal hypertension. The causes of portal hypertension can be divided into three major groups, according to the level of obstruction or increased resistance to the portal venous blood flow: (*i*) prehepatic; (*ii*) intrahepatic; and (*iii*) posthepatic (Table 16) (259). Prehepatic portal hypertension can be caused by portal vein thrombosis, splenic vein thrombosis, splanchnic arteriovenous fistula, and splenomegaly. Intrahepatic portal hypertension can be caused by alcoholic cirrhosis, schistosomiasis, sarcoidosis, myeloproliferative diseases, malignant diseases of the liver, nodular regenerative hyperplasia, primary biliary cirrhosis, chronic active hepatitis, Wilson's disease, peliosis hepatis, Budd–Chiari syndrome (hepatic vein occlusion), veno-occlusive disease, and idiopathic portal hypertension. Posthepatic portal hypertension can be caused by inferior vena cava obstruction and cardiac disease (congestive heart failure, constrictive pericarditis).

Causes of portal hypertension can also be divided into presinusoidal, sinusoidal, and postsinusoidal categories (260). Portal hypertension is considered to be presinusoidal if the wedged hepatic venous pressure is normal or less than the portal pressure, sinusoidal if the wedged hepatic venous pressure is increased and equals the portal

TABLE 16 ■ Causes of Portal Hypertension

Origin	Disorder
Prehepatic	Portal vein thrombosis
	Splenic vein thrombosis
	Splanchnic arteriovenous fistula
Intrahepatic	Cirrhosis
	Schistosomiasis
	Sarcoidosis
	Myeloproliferative diseases
	Malignant diseases of the liver
	Nodular regenerative hyperplasia
	Peliosis hepatis
	Budd–Chiari syndrome (hepatic vein occlusion)
	Veno-occlusive disease
	Idiopathic portal hypertension
Posthepatic	Inferior vena cava obstruction
	Cardiac disease

pressure, and postsinusoidal if the site of obstruction to the flow is distal to the sinusoids (i.e., hepatic veins, heart). Unfortunately, patients with the same disease vary in whether they appear to have sinusoidal, presinusoidal, or mixed forms of portal hypertension, based on the wedged hepatic venous pressure (260).

Alcoholic cirrhosis is the most common cause of portal hypertension in Western nations, but hepatic vein occlusion, portal vein occlusion, and schistosomiasis are other frequent causes (20).

Sonographically, in patients with portal hypertension, ascites, splenomegaly, and portosystemic venous collaterals may be demonstrated (Table 17). Several parameters of gray-scale, duplex, and color Doppler sonography of the portal venous system and portosystemic collaterals can be helpful in the diagnosis of portal hypertension. These parameters are discussed in the following paragraphs.

Portal Vein Diameter

Main portal vein diameter larger than 13 mm indicates portal hypertension with a high degree of specificity (95–100%) but with low sensitivity (42%) (13,20,261). Although the diameter of the main portal vein may initially increase because of increasing portal venous pressure, later, as severe portal hypertension develops, the portal vein diameter may decrease, probably because more blood is diverted to portosystemic collaterals (262). The diameters are measured on the sagittal view during deep inspiration with the patient in supine position.

TABLE 17 ■ Sonographic Findings in Portal Hypertension

- Ascites
- Splenomegaly
- Portosystemic venous collaterals
- Hepatofugal (reversed) portal venous flow
- Portal vein diameter >13 mm
- Splenic and superior mesenteric vein diameters >10 mm
- Lack of normal respiratory variations in diameters of splenic and superior mesenteric veins
- Coronary vein diameter >5 mm

Splenic and Superior Mesenteric Vein Diameters

The diameter of the splenic vein (in the transverse view at the level of the superior mesenteric artery) and the diameter of the superior mesenteric vein (in the sagittal view close to the confluence with the splenic vein) are larger than 10 mm in 50% of patients with portal hypertension (13). The diameters are measured during deep inspiration with the patient in supine position.

Respiratory Variations in Venous Diameter

In healthy persons, the diameter of the splenic and superior mesenteric veins increases (about 50–100%) in inspiration compared with the diameter in expiration. Patients with portal hypertension lack normal diameter variation (<50% increase during deep inspiration). The lack of normal diameter variation has a sensitivity of 80% and a specificity of 95% to 100% for the diagnosis of portal hypertension (13,261).

Flow Direction in the Portal Vein

In healthy persons, the flow in the main portal vein is hepatopetal (toward the liver). Detection of hepatofugal (away from the liver) flow in the main portal vein is a specific sign of portal hypertension, but it occurs only in patients with advanced cases. Reversal of the direction of flow may also be seen in the splenic vein (20). To-and-fro flow in the main portal vein, another sign of portal hypertension, is best seen during active breathing. Inspiration draws blood toward the liver (hepatopetal flow), whereas expiration reverses it (hepatofugal flow). To-and-fro flow in the main portal vein may also be seen in patients with right-sided heart failure (262).

Portal Vein Velocity and Flow

In patients with portal hypertension, velocity and flow in the portal vein are usually decreased. The normal mean flow velocity in the main portal vein is about 15 to 18 cm per second, but the normal range is wide (20). Accurate determination of pressures and flow rates in portal veins, however, is difficult because of velocity variations with cardiac activity and respiration and because of flow variations with exercise and postural change (20,263). The normal respiratory variation in the duplex Doppler flow pattern of the portal vein may be attenuated or lost in patients with portal hypertension (264).

Coronary (Left Gastric) Vein Diameter

In patients with portal hypertension, the coronary vein may be dilated (Fig. 90). Sonographically, the presence

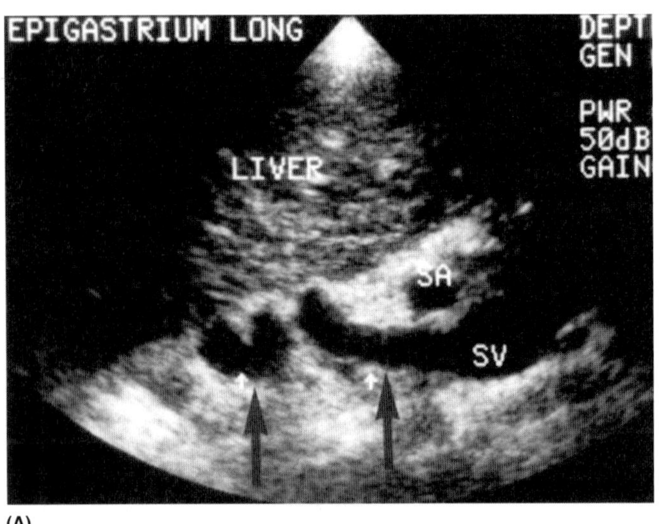

(A)

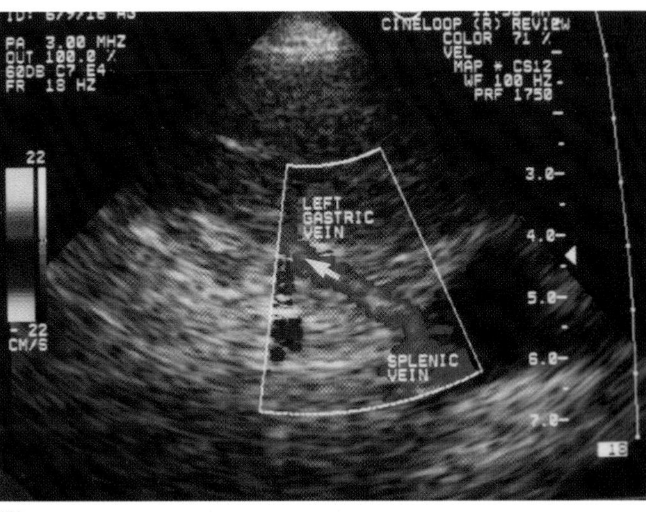

(B)

FIGURE 90 A AND B ■ Dilated coronary (i.e., left gastric) vein. (**A**) Longitudinal sonogram shows a large coronary vein (*arrows*) arising from the splenic vein. (**B**) Color Doppler sonogram in another patient demonstrates reversed flow direction within the coronary vein (left gastric vein). The flow within the coronary vein is away (*arrow*) from the splenic vein. *Source*: (**A**) From Ref. 265. (**B**) Courtesy of William D. Middleton, MD, St. Louis, MO.

of a coronary vein diameter of 5 mm or larger has a sensitivity of 80% in the diagnosis of portal hypertension (266). However, Wachsberg et al. found that 12% of healthy persons had a coronary vein diameter between 5 and 6 mm and therefore concluded that the coronary vein should be considered dilated only if it exceeds 6 mm in diameter (267). A coronary vein diameter larger than 7 mm, as measured on umbilicoportal venography, is associated with severe portal hypertension (262).

Portosystemic Venous Collaterals

In portal hypertension, numerous collateral veins can be seen that interconnect with the systemic circulation at different sites in the abdomen and pelvis (Fig. 91) (266). These collateral routes are formed when the resistance to portal venous flow exceeds the resistance to the flow in the communicating channels between the portal and the systemic circulations. Detection of portosystemic collateral veins is the most specific sign of portal hypertension. Color Doppler sonography is essential in detection of collateral veins and varices, because frequently these vessels are not apparent on gray-scale sonographic examination. The commonly seen collaterals are those of the paraumbilical vein, coronary vein, gastroesophageal vein, and splenorenal–gastrorenal vein.

The dilated paraumbilical vein courses in the fissure for the ligamentum teres and connects the left portal vein with the systemic veins around the umbilicus. On physical examination, it may cause a periumbilical venous hum (Cruveilhier–Baumgarten syndrome) (268). A dilated paraumbilical vein is seen on the transverse view as an anechoic, round structure within the ligamentum teres (Fig. 92) (266,269,270). Its origin from the left portal vein, its course posterior to the anterior abdominal wall, and its termination near the umbilicus are best seen in the longitudinal view (Figs. 92 and 93). In portal hypertension, color Doppler sonography demonstrates hepatofugal flow within the dilated paraumbilical vein (Fig. 93). A segment of remnant of the umbilical vein may be normally patent, and in 16% of healthy persons without portal hypertension, venous flow (hepatopetal or hepatofugal) can be seen in the ligamentum teres fissure by color Doppler sonography using a 5- or 7.5-MHz linear-array transducer (Fig. 94) (268,271). However, in healthy persons, flow extending anterior to the liver's surface is not seen with color Doppler sonography (271). Therefore, a paraumbilical vein should be considered diagnostic of portal hypertension only if the diameter of the vein is larger than 3 mm or if the hepatofugal venous flow has a velocity greater than 5 cm per second (268,270,271).

The dilated coronary vein can be seen posterior to the left lobe of the liver, extending cranially from the splenic vein near its confluence with the superior mesenteric vein, on the sagittal view (Fig. 90). In portal hypertension, color Doppler sonography may demonstrate reversal of flow direction (i.e., away from the splenic vein) within the coronary vein (Fig. 90). Reversal of flow direction within the coronary vein may be a more sensitive sonographic indicator of portal hypertension than coronary vein dilatation (267). Dilated gastroesophageal collateral veins may be seen near the gastroesophageal junction, posterior to the left lobe of the liver close to the diaphragm (Fig. 95). These are communications between the coronary and the short gastric veins and the systemic esophageal veins. One-third of the deaths from cirrhosis are secondary to hemorrhage, usually from esophageal varices (234). Dilated splenorenal (Figs. 95 and 96) and gastrorenal (Fig. 96) collateral veins can be seen as large, tortuous veins in the region of the splenic and left renal hila. Collateral veins may cause gallbladder wall varices and rarely common bile duct wall varices. Other less frequent

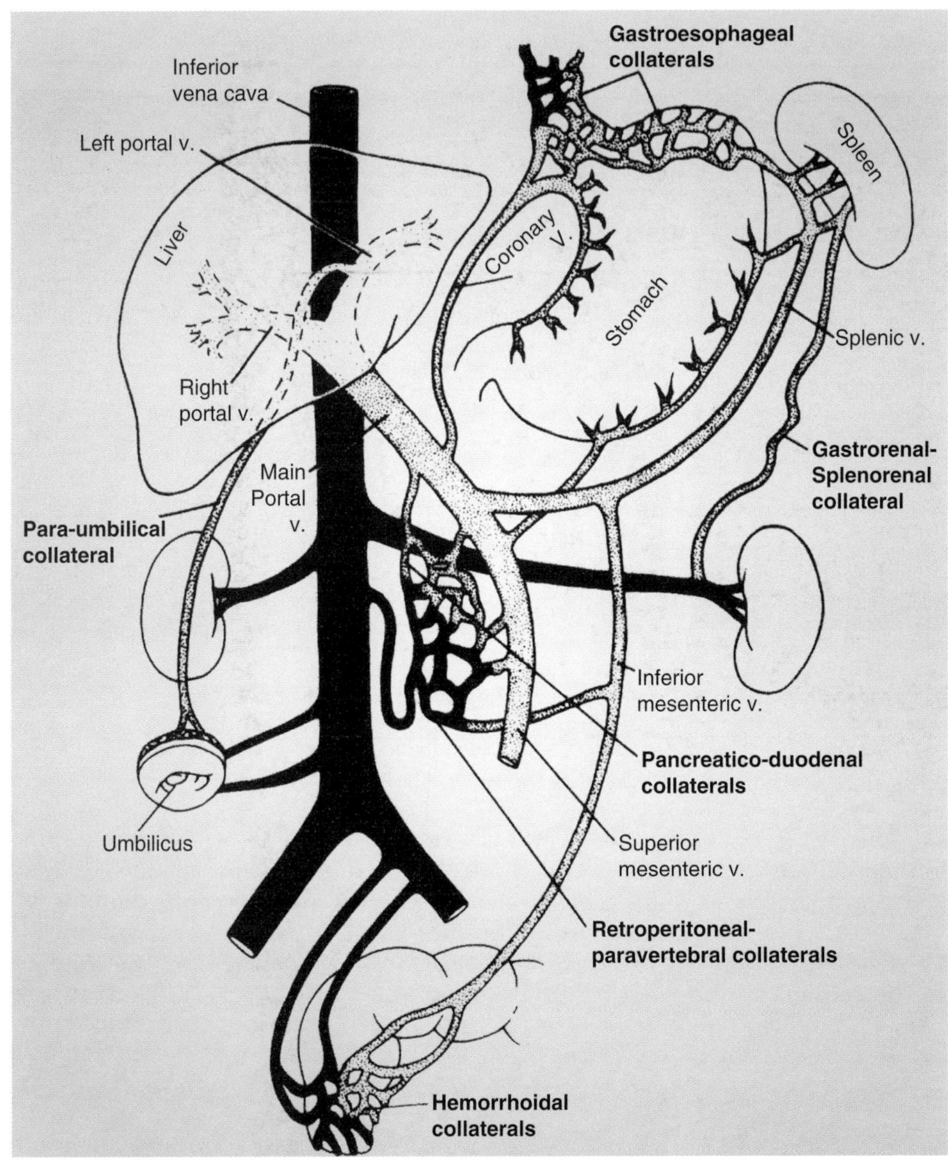

FIGURE 91 ■ Portal hypertension. Diagram of major portosystemic venous collaterals. *Source*: Modified from Ref. 266.

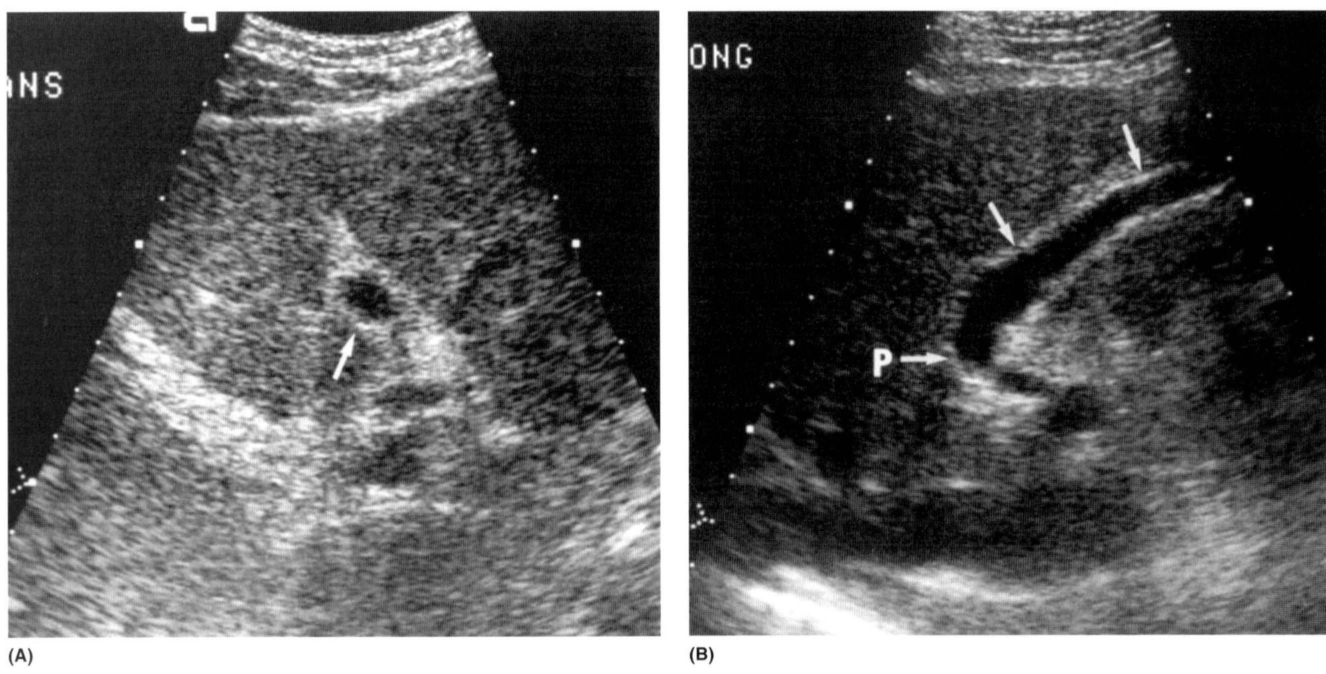

FIGURE 92 A AND B ■ Portal hypertension: paraumbilical vein collateral. (**A**) Transverse view shows a dilated paraumbilical vein (*arrow*) within the fissure for the ligamentum teres. (**B**) Sagittal view shows a dilated paraumbilical vein (*arrows*) arising from the left portal vein (P).

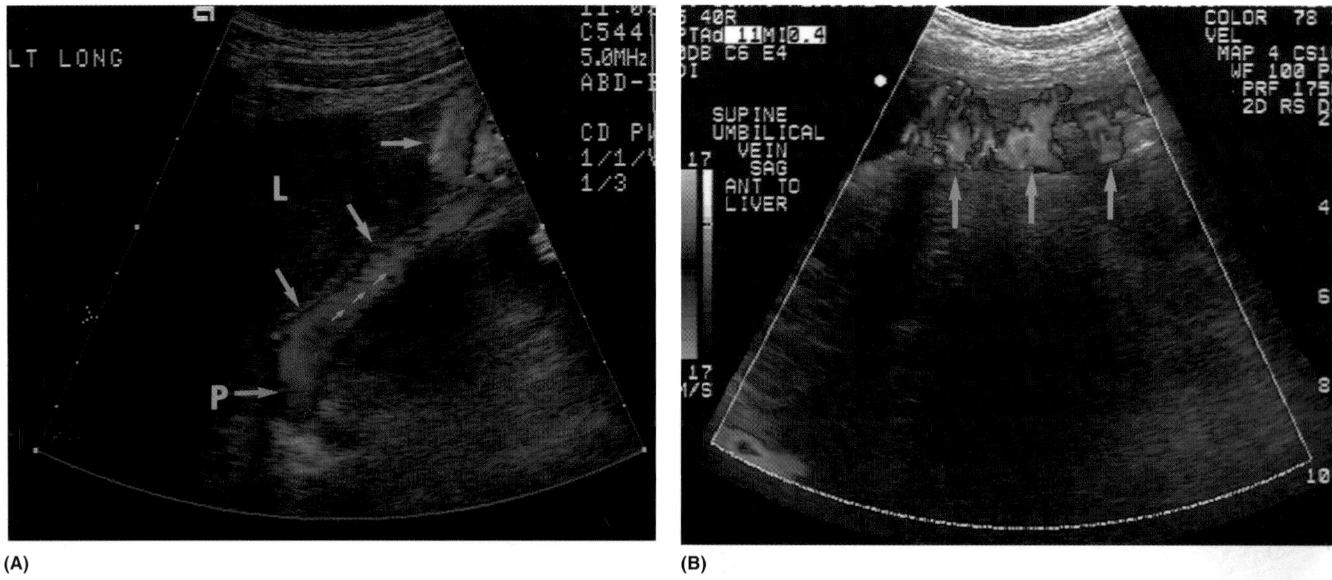

(A) (B)

FIGURE 93 A AND B ■ Portal hypertension. Dilated paraumbilical vein: color Doppler sonograms. (**A**) Sagittal view shows color flow in a dilated paraumbilical vein (*arrows*) within the fissure for the ligamentum teres. Flow is hepatofugal (*small arrows*). (**B**) Sagittal view shows color flow in a dilated tortuous paraumbilical vein (*arrows*) posterior to the anterior abdominal wall. P, left portal vein; L, liver.

collateral veins include pancreaticoduodenal, retroperitoneal-paravertebral, omental, and hemorrhoidal veins (Fig. 91) (266).

A comparative study showed that MR angiography was better than sonography for detecting varices and portal vein collaterals, assessing patency of existing portosystemic surgical shunts and diagnosing portal vein thrombosis (272). However, sonography continues to be used for initial screening because of cost considerations.

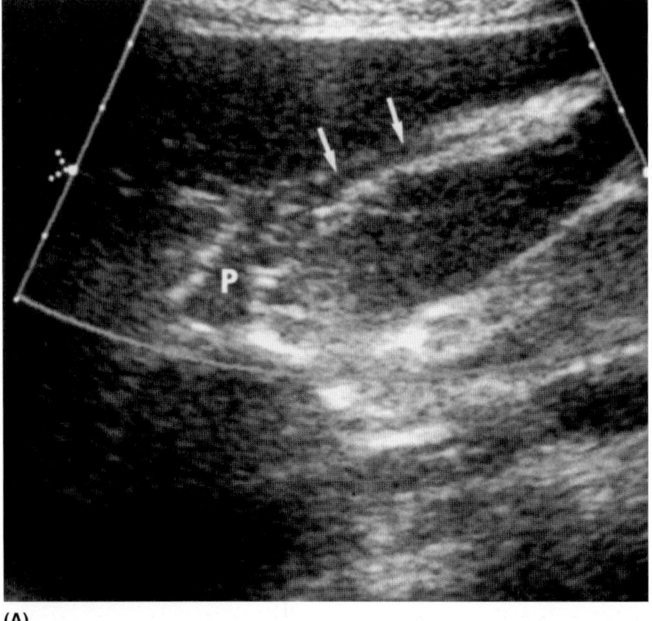

(A)

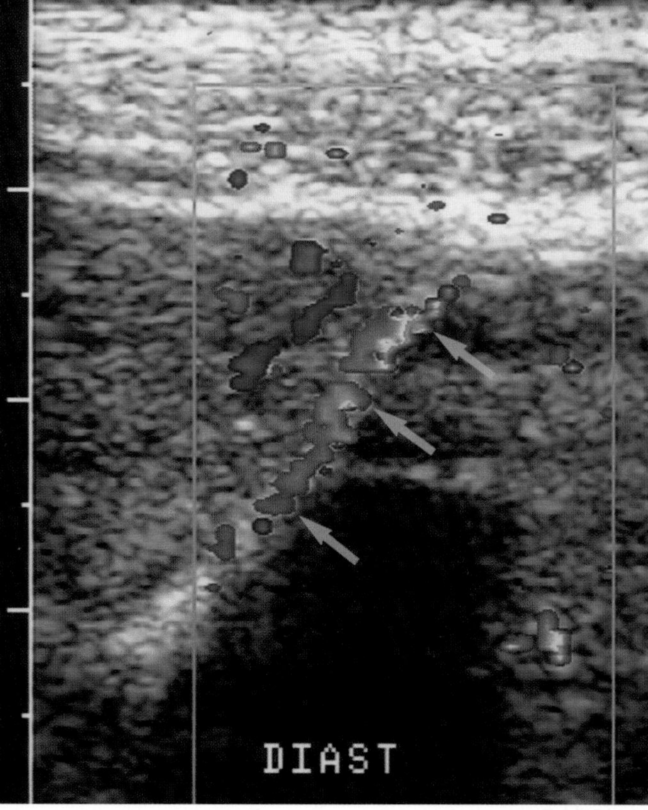

(B)

FIGURE 94 A AND B ■ Normal vein in the ligamentum teres fissure. (**A**) Sagittal gray-scale sonogram shows a short patent segment (*arrows*) of a normal vein within the ligamentum teres fissure. (**B**) Oblique color Doppler sonogram shows hepatofugal color flow within a patent short segment (*arrows*) of a normal vein (<2 mm in diameter) within the ligamentum teres fissure. P, left portal vein. *Source*: From Ref. 271.

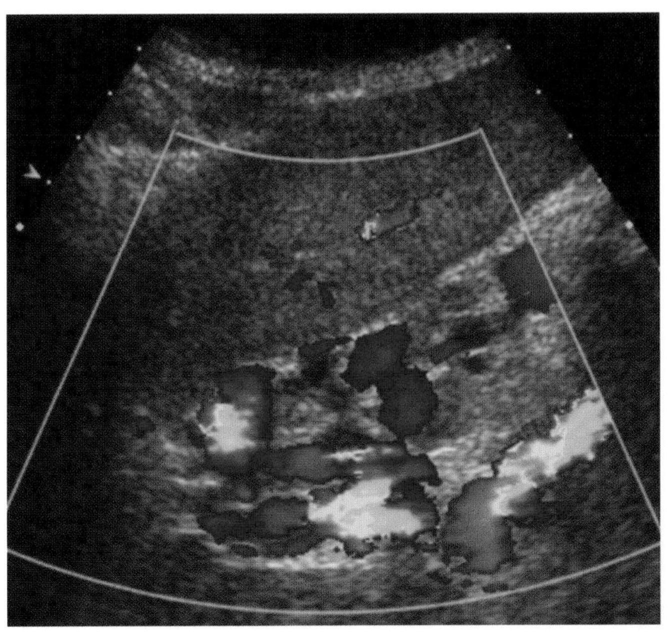

(A)

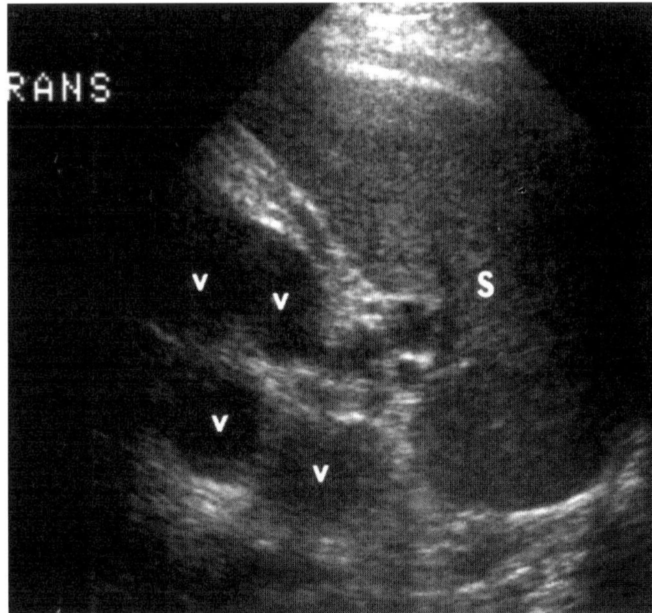

(B)

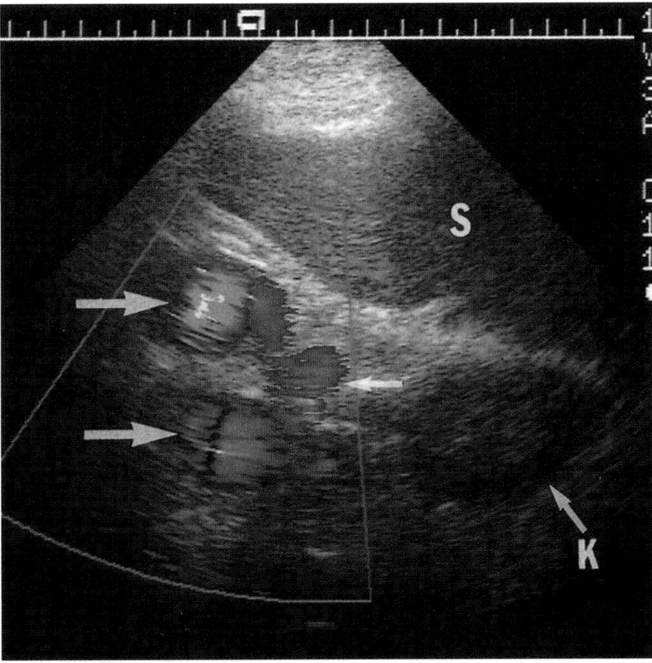

(C)

FIGURE 95 A–C ■ Portal hypertension: gastroesophageal and splenorenal collaterals. (**A**) Longitudinal color Doppler sonogram shows color flow within the gastroesophageal collateral veins, close to the diaphragm, posterior to the left lobe of the liver. (**B**) Transverse view shows large, rounded, cystic-appearing dilated splenorenal collateral veins (V) in the hilum of the spleen (S). (**C**) Transverse color Doppler sonogram shows color flow within the dilated rounded and tubular splenorenal collateral veins (*arrows*), coursing toward the left kidney (K). *Source*: (**A**) Courtesy of Philip W. Ralls, MD, Los Angeles, CA.

Portal Vein Thrombosis

Portal vein thrombosis can be bland, secondary to blood clot, or secondary to tumor thrombus from invasion by hepatic neoplasm. Bland portal venous thrombosis can be caused by pancreatitis, cirrhosis, intra-abdominal sepsis, gastrointestinal inflammatory diseases such as appendicitis and ulcerative colitis, hypercoagulable states (pregnancy, myelofibrosis, and tumors), dehydration, liver transplantation, portacaval shunting, or splenectomy, or it can be idiopathic. In children, portal vein thrombosis can be caused by umbilical sepsis and either local or systemic infection. Tumor thrombosis is most frequently seen secondary to HCC (in 30–70% of patients with HCC) or metastatic liver disease (in 5–8% of patients with diffuse liver metastases) (273). Sonographic findings in portal vein thrombosis include an echogenic thrombus within the portal vein (Figs. 49, 52, and 97), enlargement of the thrombosed portion of the vein, and cavernous transformation of the portal vein. Intraluminal echoes on grayscale images support but do not definitely establish the diagnosis of thrombus. Thrombus in the portal vein has variable echogenicity, and, if recently formed, it may be hypoechoic or anechoic (274). Color Doppler sonography is helpful to diagnose thrombus, by demonstrating absence of flow in the portal vein or by displaying flow around the thrombus, specially when the thrombus is hypoechoic or anechoic. Tumor thrombus within the portal vein can sometimes be differentiated from bland thrombus by demonstrating flow in the vessels within the tumor thrombus by color Doppler sonography (Fig. 97) and by demonstrating arterial waveforms, frequently in a hepatofugal direction, within the tumor thrombus by duplex Doppler (275–277). Pulsatile blood flow can however be seen in a very small percentage of benign portal vein thrombi. Continuous flow can be detected in benign and malignant portal vein thrombus and is thus not useful in differentiating between the two (278). Lack of color flow within the thrombus, however, does not entirely exclude the possibility of tumor thrombus.

Pitfalls

In cirrhotic patients without portal vein thrombosis, there may be absence of flow in the main portal vein on color Doppler, secondary to stagnant flow with very slow

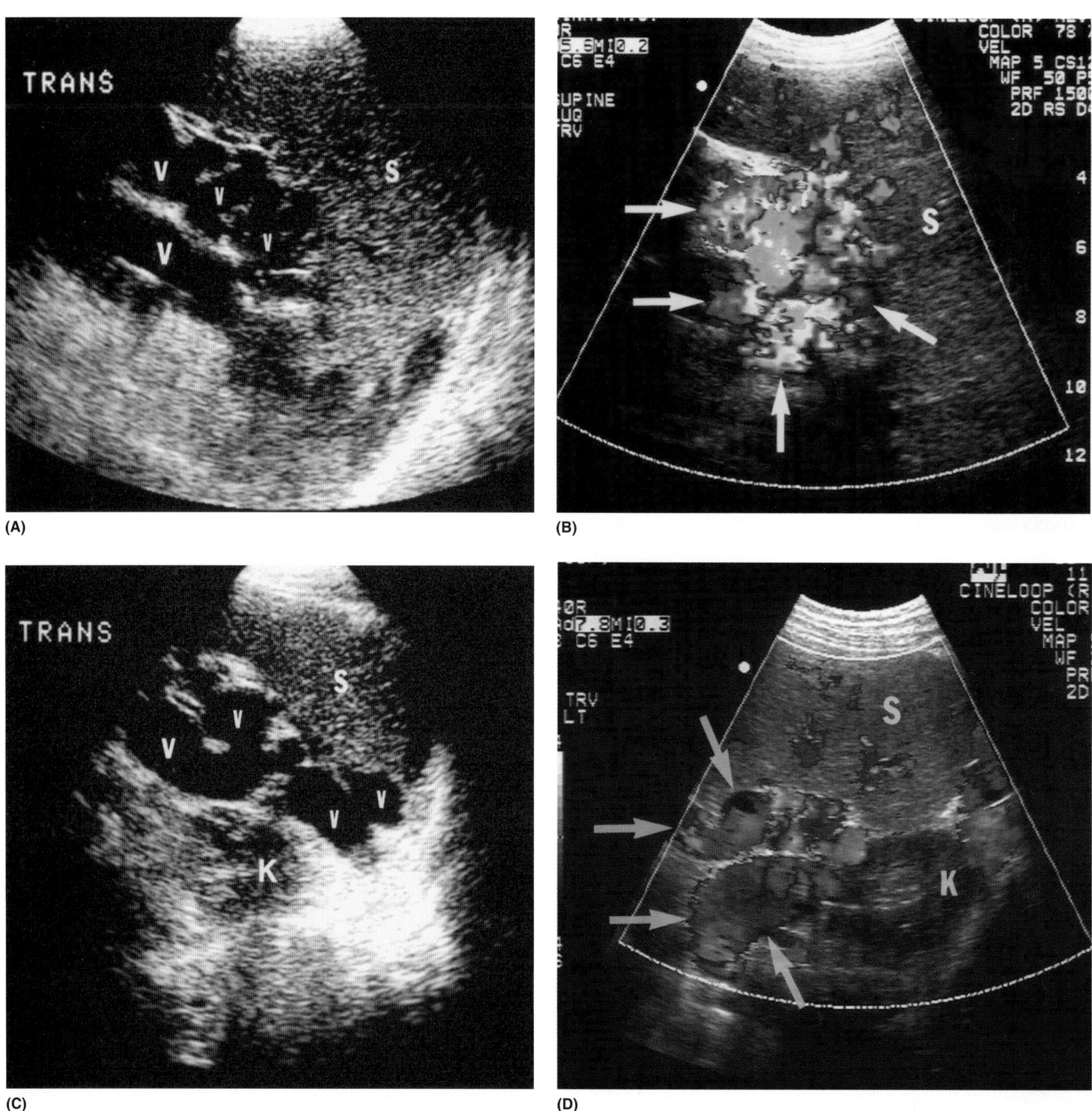

FIGURE 96 A–F ■ Portal hypertension: gastrorenal–splenorenal collateral veins. (**A**) Transverse view shows tortuous tubular dilated splenorenal collateral veins (V) in the region of the hilum of the spleen (S). (**B**) Transverse color Doppler sonogram demonstrates color flow within the collateral veins (*arrows*) in the hilum of the spleen. (**C**) Transverse view shows dilated tubular splenorenal collateral veins between the caudal portion of the spleen and the left kidney (K). (**D**) Transverse color Doppler sonogram demonstrates color flow within dilated splenorenal collateral veins (*arrows*) in the hilum of the left kidney. (*Continued*)

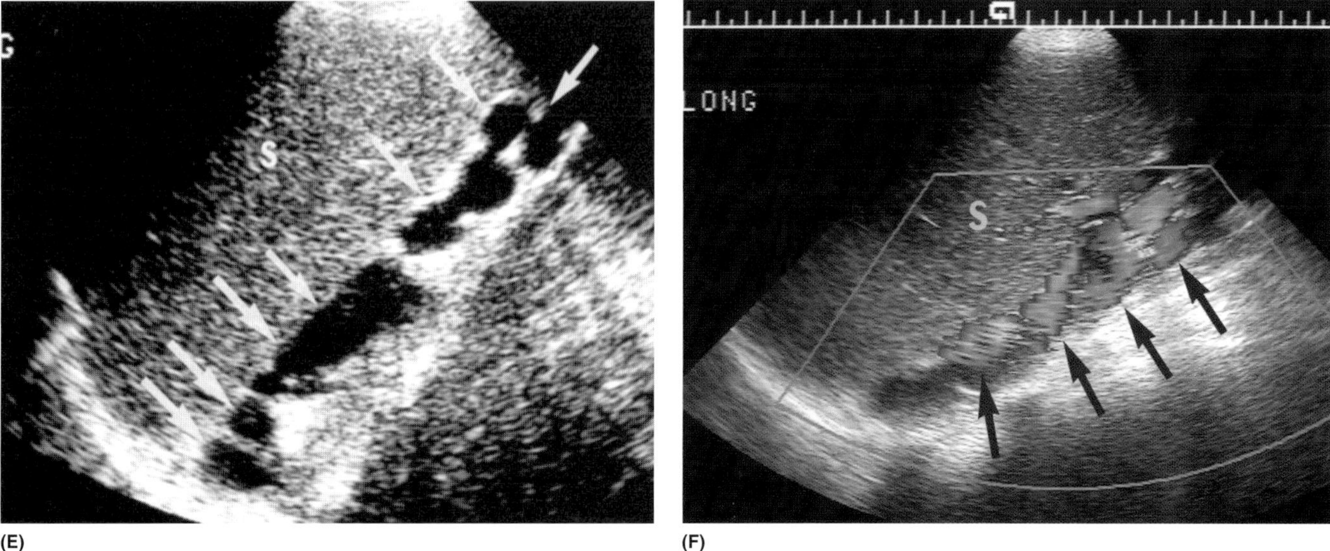

(E) (F)

FIGURE 96 A–F ■ (*Continued*) (**E**) Sagittal view demonstrates gastrorenal collateral veins close to the diaphragm and splenorenal collaterals posterior to the middle and caudal portions of the spleen. (**F**) Sagittal color Doppler sonogram corresponding to *E* demonstrates color flow within the collateral veins (*arrows*).

velocities (279). Because a color Doppler signal may not be detected in a patent portal vein with sluggish flow, in patients without visible thrombus (on gray-scale ultrasound), a lack of demonstrable color flow does not always indicate thrombosis. Other imaging studies should be performed for confirmation. Occasionally, portal vein thrombosis may be missed because of an apparently normal Doppler signal obtained from large collateral vessel around an occluded portal vein.

Cavernous Transformation of the Portal Vein

With long-standing occlusion of the main portal vein secondary to portal vein thrombosis, adjacent collateral

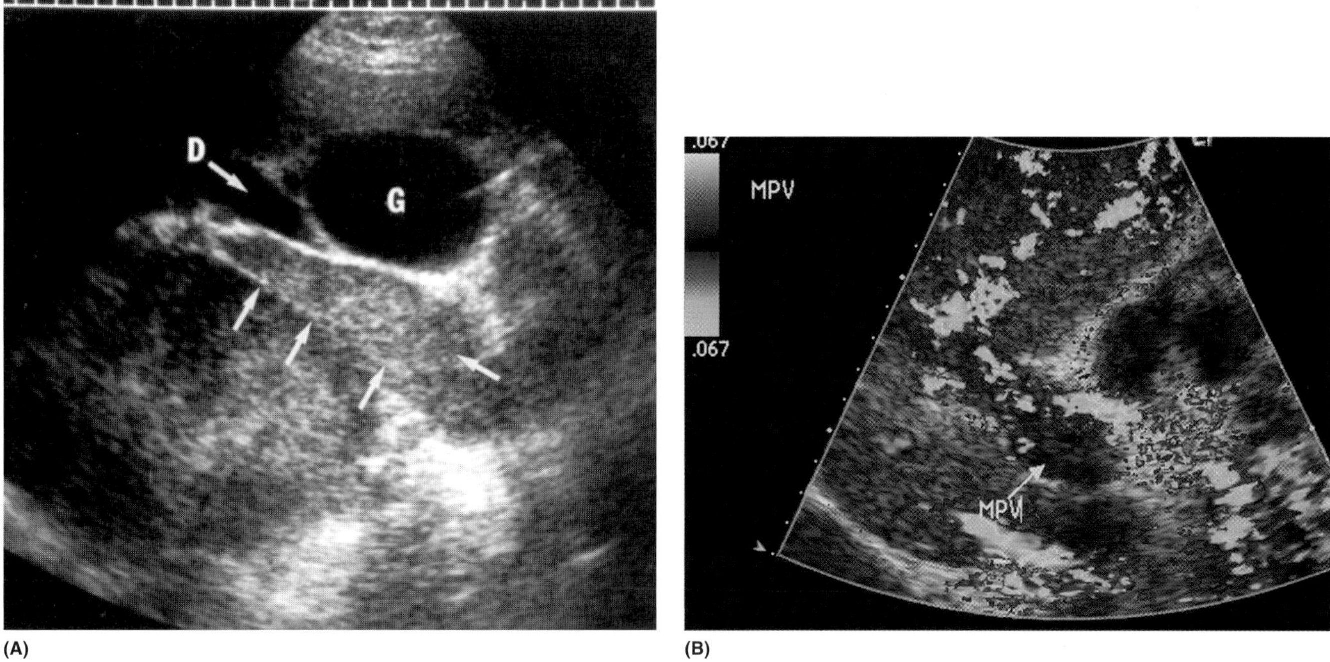

(A) (B)

FIGURE 97A–F ■ Portal vein thrombus. (**A**) Longitudinal view shows echogenic tumor thrombus filling almost the entire main portal vein (*arrows*) in a patient with pancreatic carcinoma with diffuse liver metastases. D, dilated common hepatic duct; G, gallbladder. (**B**) Color Doppler demonstrates vascularity within tumor thrombus in portal vein of a different patient. (*Continued*)

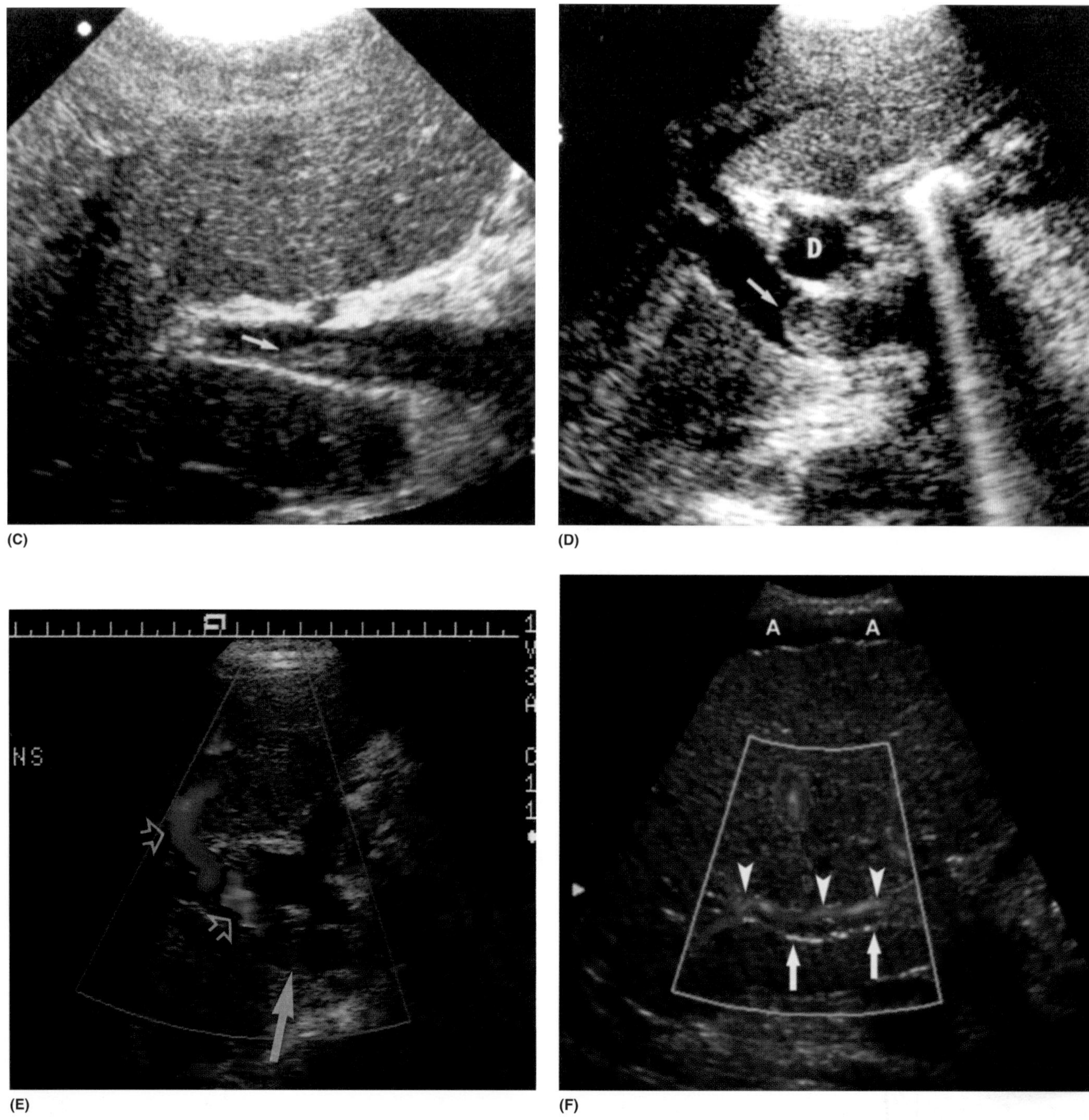

FIGURE 97 A–F ■ (*Continued*) (**C**) Longitudinal view shows an echogenic, bandlike thrombus (*arrow*) partially occluding the main portal vein. This was bland thrombus in a patient with pancreatitis. (**D**) Echogenic–hypoechoic thrombus with a sharp convex margin (*arrow*) within the main portal vein in a patient with pancreatic carcinoma. D, portion of dilated common bile duct. (**E**) Color Doppler sonogram corresponding to (**D**) shows turbulent color flow (*open arrows*) beyond the partially occluding thrombus (*solid arrow*). (**F**) Power Doppler sonogram of a completely thrombosed right portal vein (*arrows*) in a patient with a TIPS shunt (not shown). Flow is demonstrated in the adjacent hepatic artery (*arrow heads*). *Source*: (**B**) Courtesy of Monzer M. Abu-Yousef, MD, Iowa City, IA. (**F**) Courtesy of Daniel A. Merton, BS, RDMS, Philadelphia, PA.

veins enlarge to span the obstruction and permit continued hepatopetal flow of blood. These collateral channels represent the cavernous transformation of the portal vein (280). Because long-standing occlusion is required for the development of cavernous transformation, it is more likely to be caused by benign diseases. Sonography demonstrates multiple serpiginous, tortuous periportal collateral veins in the expected location of the main portal vein (Figs. 98 and 99) (281–283). The thrombosed main portal vein is usually not visible on gray-scale sonograms because of numerous periportal collateral veins in the expected location of the main portal vein. Color Doppler sonography demonstrates the absence of flow within the main portal

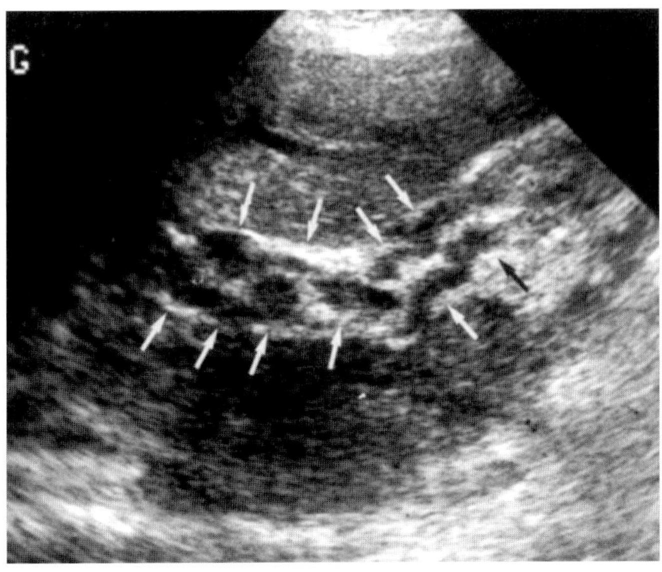

(A)

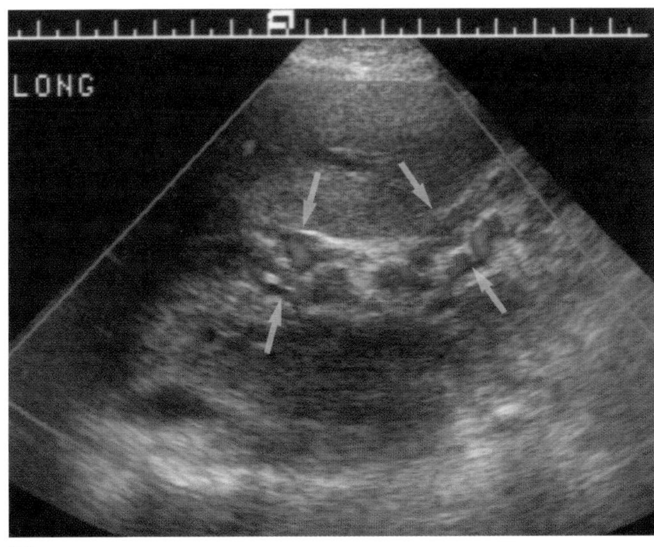

(B)

FIGURE 98 A AND B ■ Cavernous transformation of the portal vein. (**A**) Longitudinal view shows numerous tubular and rounded dilated collateral venous structures (*arrows*) in the expected location of the main portal vein. No normal portal vein is identified. (**B**) Color Doppler sonogram shows color flow within some of the collateral veins (*arrows*).

vein and color flow in the periportal collateral veins (Fig. 99). The flow in periportal collateral veins is in the hepatopetal direction and has a portal venous waveform.

Portal Vein Aneurysm

Portal vein aneurysms are rare. They can be either congenital or acquired secondary to portal hypertension. They can occur either at the junction of the splenic and superior mesenteric veins or more distally in the portal vein radicles (Fig. 100). They may be 3 cm or larger in diameter (284). Patients usually are asymptomatic, but, rarely, an aneurysm ruptures.

Budd–Chiari Syndrome

The Budd–Chiari syndrome is a rare disorder caused by obstruction to hepatic venous outflow. The causes of Budd–Chiari syndrome include occlusion of the major

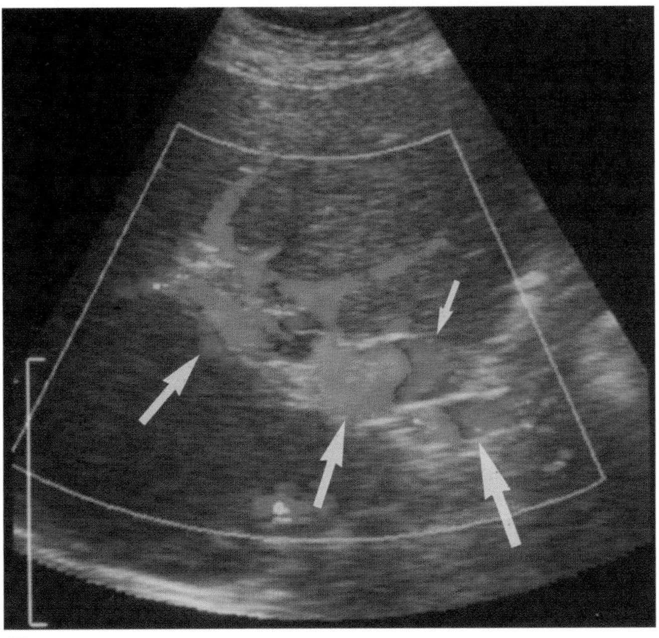

(A)

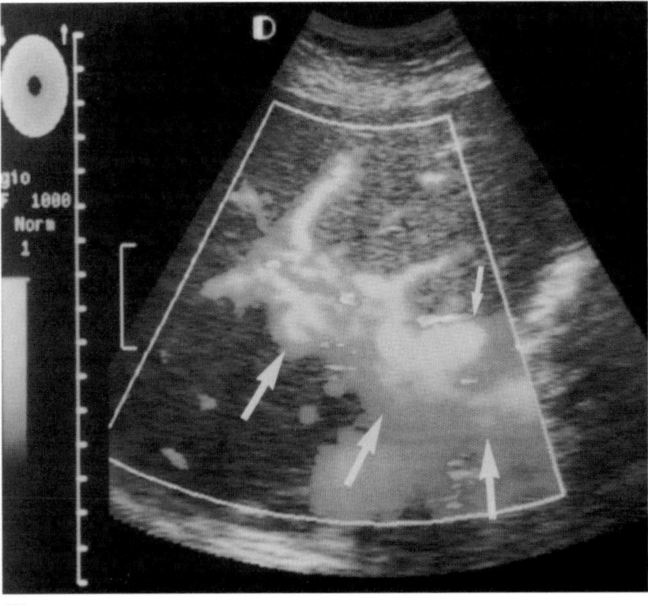

(B)

FIGURE 99 A AND B ■ Cavernous transformation of the portal vein: (**A**) color Doppler and (**B**) power Doppler sonograms. Longitudinal views show color flow within dilated periportal collateral veins (*arrows*) in the expected location of the main portal vein. No normal portal vein is identified.

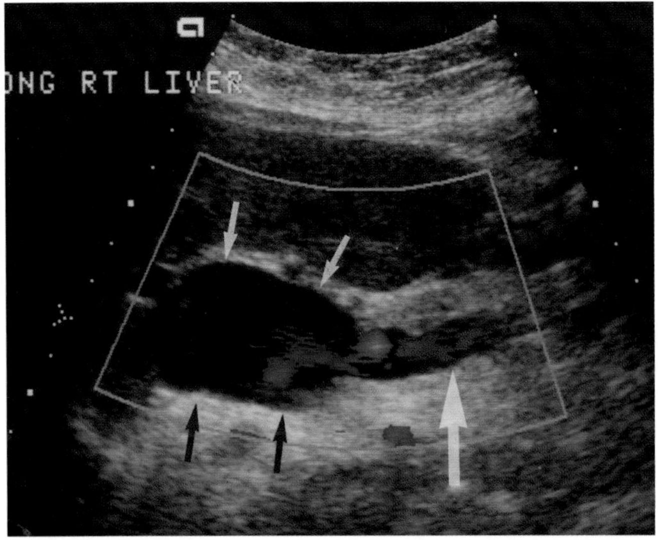

FIGURE 100 ■ Portal vein aneurysm. Longitudinal color Doppler sonogram shows a congenital aneurysm (*small arrows*) of the main portal vein. *Large arrow*, normal portion of the portal vein.

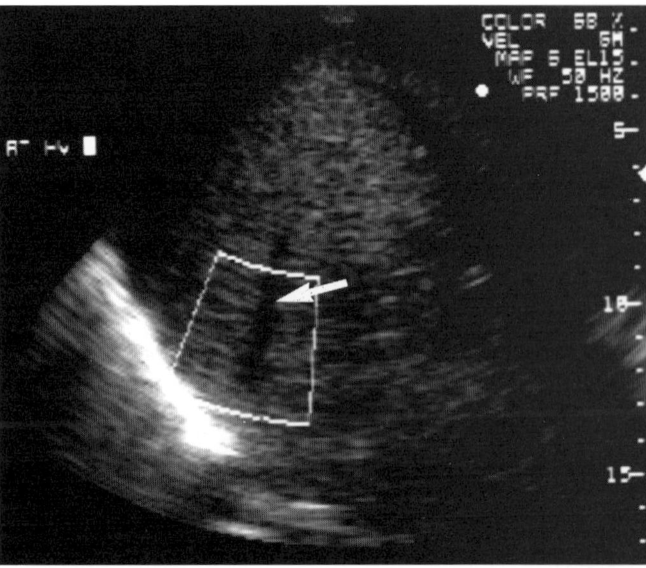

FIGURE 101 ■ Budd–Chiari syndrome: hepatic vein occlusion. Sagittal color Doppler sonogram shows occlusion of the right hepatic vein (*arrow*) secondary to thrombosis, as demonstrated by a lack of color flow within the vein. Similar findings were present in other two hepatic veins. *Source*: From Ref. 288.

hepatic veins and occlusion of the hepatic portion of the inferior vena cava. Patients with severe right-sided heart failure may present a clinical picture similar to that seen with hepatic venous occlusion. The most important clinical manifestations are abdominal pain, hepatomegaly, and ascites.

Hepatic Vein Occlusion

Causes of obstruction of the major hepatic veins include the following: (*i*) tumor invasion, most commonly from HCC; (*ii*) hepatic vein thrombosis secondary to hypercoagulable states, use of oral contraceptives, and abdominal trauma; and (*iii*) unexplained fibrous obliteration of the major hepatic veins (285,286). Sonographically, echogenic thrombus may be seen within the major hepatic veins, or one may fail to visualize one or more major hepatic veins. Nonvisualization of the hepatic veins by gray-scale sonography, however, is not diagnostic of occlusion because hepatic veins may be difficult to demonstrate when the liver is enlarged or when patients have cirrhosis. Color Doppler sonography is essential in demonstrating occlusion of hepatic veins and intrahepatic collaterals (287). Using this technique, hepatic venous findings include nonvisualization of the veins (Fig. 101) (288), narrowing, tortuosity, reversal of flow direction (Fig. 102), and intrahepatic hepatic venous collaterals (288–290). With color Doppler sonography, absence of detectable flow in the hepatic veins on gray-scale sonography, nonvisualization of the hepatic veins, and reversal of flow within the hepatic veins are the three most sensitive criteria. However, even with color Doppler sonography, one or more hepatic veins that are patent and not thrombosed may not be visible in a few patients with cirrhosis, thus reducing the specificity of this finding. Duplex Doppler examination may reveal absent, reversed, turbulent, or continuous flow within the nonoccluded portions of the hepatic veins (290). The flow in the portal vein may be slow or reversed. The caudate lobe is often enlarged in patients with Budd–Chiari syndrome.

Occlusion of the Inferior Vena Cava

Budd–Chiari syndrome secondary to occlusion of the hepatic portions of the inferior vena cava can be caused by neoplastic invasion, thrombosis from hypercoagulative states, and membranous obstruction. Membranous

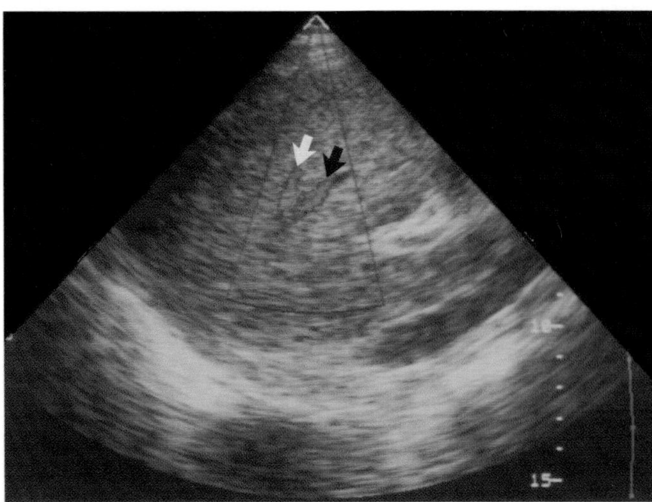

FIGURE 102 ■ Budd–Chiari syndrome: Hepatic vein occlusion. Sagittal color Doppler sonogram shows reversal of flow direction. Flow in one hepatic vein branch is directed normally (*white arrow*), whereas its counterpart is reversed (*black arrow*) and carries blood toward collaterals on the surface of the liver. *Source*: From Ref. 289.

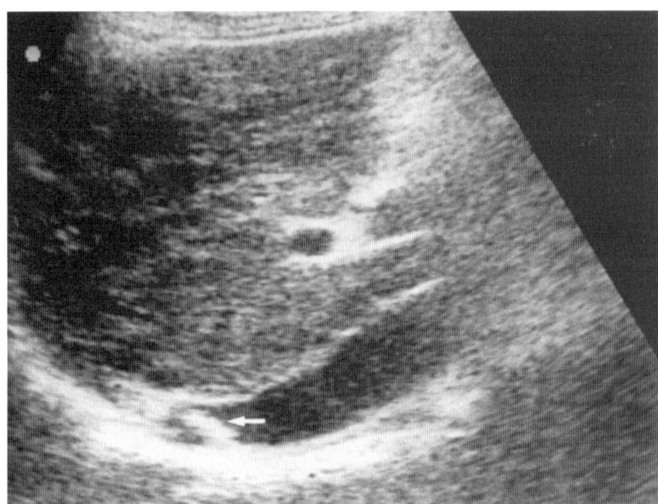

FIGURE 103 ■ Budd–Chiari syndrome: membranous obstruction of the inferior vena cava. Sagittal view shows obstruction of the inferior vena cava by a membranous web (*arrow*). The web appears as a hyperechoic, band-like structure within the inferior vena cava, near the diaphragm. *Source*: From Ref. 291.

obstruction of the inferior vena cava is rare in Western countries but is common in Asia, northern India, and South Africa. Membranous obstruction can be caused by a fibrous membrane or web within the inferior vena cava, at or just cranial to the entrance of the major hepatic veins, or by a segmental fibrous cord of variable length (2–5 cm long) (291–294). Sonographically, the web is detected as an echogenic membrane, with or without acoustic shadowing, within the inferior vena cava (Fig. 103) (291), and the segmental fibrous cord can be seen as an echogenic obliteration of the lumen involving a segment of the inferior vena cava 2 to 5 cm long.

In a study of 71 patients with Budd–Chiari syndrome, duplex Doppler ultrasound detected the site of occlusion in 80% of the patients (295). The obstruction was either in the hepatic vein or in the inferior vena cava (in some patients secondary to inferior vena cava membranes).

Hepatic Veno-Occlusive Disease

Hepatic veno-occlusive disease is secondary to nonthrombotic occlusion of small hepatic veins and terminal hepatic venules by connective tissue and collagen (296). Veno-occlusive disease can be caused by ingestion of plants containing pyrrolizidine alkaloids (acute bush tea disease), or it can occur secondary to cancer chemotherapy, hepatic radiation therapy, bone marrow and kidney transplantation, and arsphenamine and urethane therapy (296). In the United States, it is most commonly associated with chemotherapy and radiation therapy used before bone marrow transplantation. The clinical presentation of patients with veno-occlusive disease is usually more acute than with hepatic vein thrombosis, and the most common clinical features are jaundice, hepatomegaly, abdominal pain, and ascites (296). Although liver biopsy is usually diagnostic of veno-occlusive disease, biopsy cannot be performed because of coagulopathy in many patients (297).

Sonographically, the major hepatic veins are not involved, and they demonstrate normal hepatofugal flow direction. The inferior vena cava is patent with flow toward the heart. Decreased, reversed, or to-and-fro flow may be seen in the main portal vein (297,298); however, no significant correlation exists between abnormalities in portal flow and veno-occlusive disease (299). Significant elevation of the hepatic artery resistive index (>0.81) may be a sensitive sign of liver damage secondary to veno-occlusive disease (299). Doppler findings however are nonspecific and some authors have concluded that duplex sonography is of no value in the diagnosis of veno-occlusive disease after bone marrow transplantation (300). The gallbladder wall may be thickened.

Intrahepatic Portosystemic Venous Shunt

Intrahepatic portosystemic venous shunts are rare and may be congenital or secondary to portal hypertension. Congenital shunts between the branches of the portal and hepatic veins may be aneurysmal, presenting as a cystic mass communicating with branches of the portal and hepatic veins (Fig. 104). The second type is a complex mass of branching tubular venous channels that communicate with branches of the hepatic and portal veins (301–303). A shunt secondary to portal hypertension usually appear as a large, tubular shunt between the posterior branch of the right portal vein and the inferior vena cava and is considered a portosystemic collateral pathway. Intrahepatic portosystemic venous shunts may cause hepatic encephalopathy.

Hepatic Arterial–Portal Fistula

Intrahepatic arterial–portal fistula is usually secondary to trauma, primarily penetrating trauma or iatrogenic trauma secondary to liver biopsies, transhepatic cholangiography, and transhepatic catheterization of the bile ducts or portal veins. Extrahepatic fistula between the hepatic artery and the portal vein usually is secondary to rupture of a preexisting hepatic artery aneurysm into the portal vein (304). Hepatic arterial–portal fistula may cause life-threatening portal hypertension.

Hepatic Artery Aneurysm and Pseudoaneurysm

Hepatic artery aneurysm may be congenital or acquired. Of these aneurysms, 75% are extrahepatic, and 63% of these extrahepatic aneurysms involve the common hepatic artery (304). Pseudoaneurysms can also be extrahepatic or intrahepatic. Extrahepatic pseudoaneurysm of the hepatic artery can occur secondary to chronic pancreatitis. Intrahepatic arterial pseudoaneurysm can be secondary to trauma or can be iatrogenic secondary to liver biopsy. Sonography demonstrates a cystic mass that may

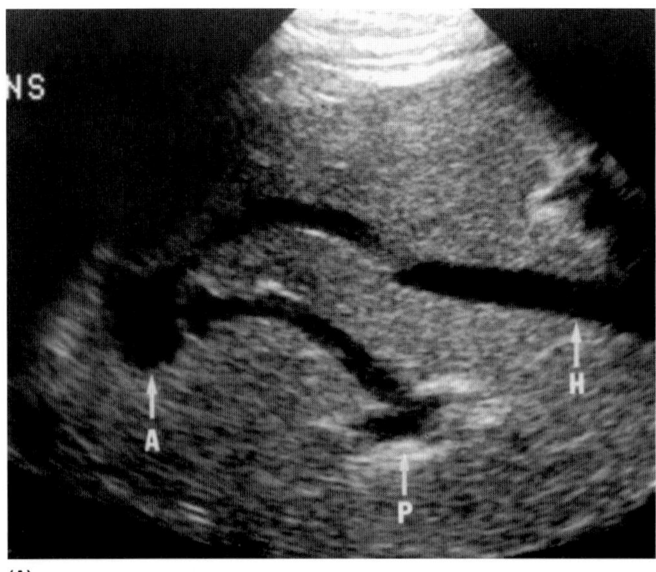

(A)

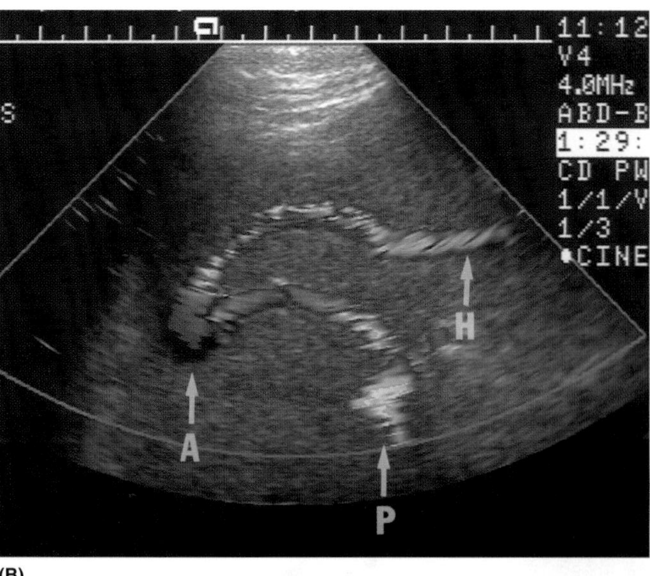

(B)

FIGURE 104 A AND B ■ Intrahepatic portosystemic venous shunt. (**A**) Transverse view shows a congenital portosystemic venous shunt presenting as an aneurysmal cystic mass (A) within the right lobe of the liver. Long venous channels are seen connecting the aneurysmal shunt to the portal vein (P) and the hepatic vein (H). (**B**) Color Doppler sonogram shows blood flowing from the portal vein into the aneurysmal shunt and from the shunt into the hepatic vein.

contain echogenic thrombus, communicating with the hepatic artery or its intrahepatic branch (Fig. 105). Color Doppler sonography demonstrates "swirling" turbulent flow within the pseudoaneurysm and to-and-fro flow in the neck of the pseudoaneurysm (Fig. 98) (305).

Hereditary Hemorrhagic Telangiectasia

Hereditary hemorrhagic telangiectasia or Osler–Weber–Rendu disease is an autosomal-dominant disorder that may involve virtually every organ. It is characterized by mucocutaneous and visceral vascular abnormalities including telangiectases, arteriovenous fistula, and aneurysms (306,307). Sonographic findings in arteriovenous malformations in the liver include large feeding arteries, prominent pulsations, the presence of ectatic vascular structures, and large draining veins (306). The dilated tubular vascular structures with serpiginous cords secondary to arteriovenous malformation may mimic dilated intrahepatic bile ducts. Color Doppler sonography demonstrates large arteriovenous malformations or tangled masses of enlarged tortuous arteries or multiple aneurysms of the hepatic arterial branches within the liver (307,308). One may see enlargement of the main hepatic and intrahepatic arteries and increased echogenicity from fatty infiltration or abnormal echo pattern from cirrhosis resulting from hereditary hemorrhagic telangiectasia.

Increased Hepatic Artery Flow: "Arterialization"

As portal venous flow to the liver decreases, hepatic arterial flow increases and may be pronounced in patients with a clot or surgical interruption of the main portal vein or when more blood exits the liver through the portal veins than enters it. This may result in considerably enlarged intrahepatic arteries with strikingly increased color flow shown by color Doppler sonography, referred to as "arterialization" of the hepatic blood supply. Arterialization is only occasionally observed in patients with advanced cirrhosis (309).

Effect of a Meal on Hepatic Artery Flow

When portal venous flow decreases, hepatic arterial flow increases, and when portal venous flow increases, hepatic arterial flow decreases (310). This reciprocal hemodynamic relationship has been called "the hepatic arterial buffer response." After a meal, portal venous blood flow increases, and hepatic arterial diastolic flow diminishes, with a corresponding increase in hepatic arterial resistive index in healthy persons with a normal liver (310). The normal marked increase in postprandial resistive index is generally not seen in patients with severe liver disease (311). Absence of the postprandial change in resistance of the hepatic artery, therefore, can signal abnormal liver function. In a study by Joynt et al., the mean postprandial increase in resistive index in healthy subjects was 42%, and in patients with liver disease, it was 7% (311). All normal subjects had a postprandial increase in resistive index of at least 20%, and a threshold value of 20% change after a meal was found useful for separating normal and abnormal livers (311). Examination of hepatic arterial flow after fasting is important because high resistance after a meal may be falsely interpreted as a sign of liver disease. Reduced or

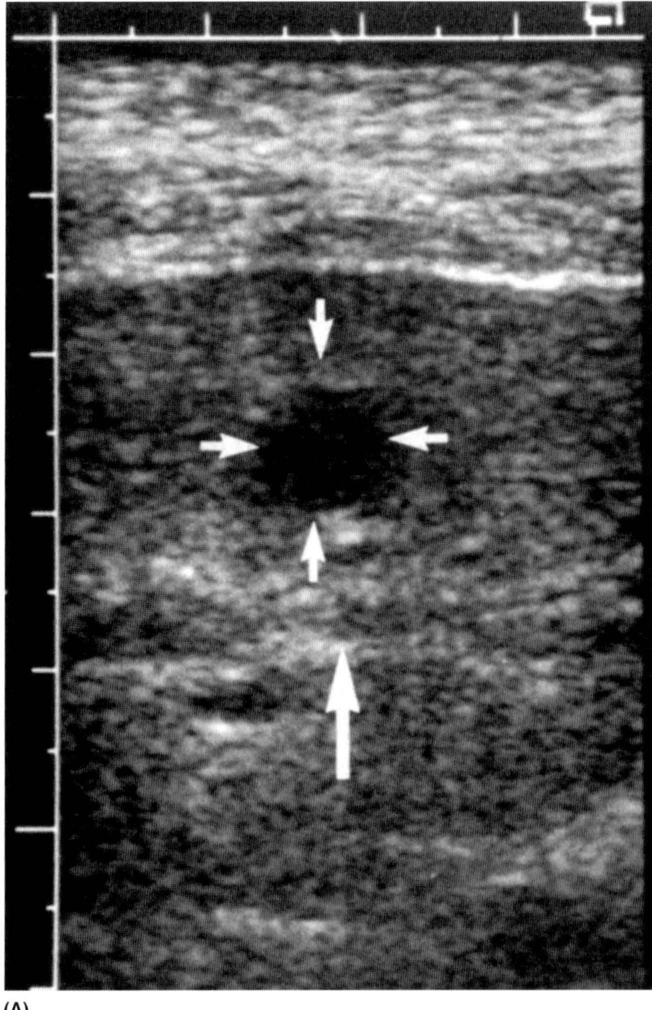

(A)

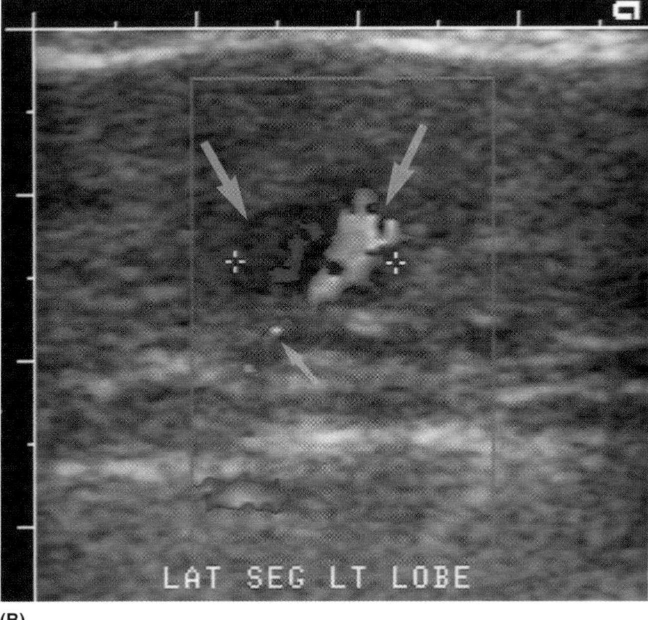

(B)

FIGURE 105 A AND B ■ Intrahepatic pseudoaneurysm after liver biopsy. (**A**) Transverse view shows a pseudoaneurysm appearing as a cystic mass (*small arrows*). The pseudoaneurysm arises from the lateral segment branch of the left hepatic artery, *large arrow*, lateral segmental branches of the left portal vein and left hepatic artery. (**B**) Transverse color Doppler sonogram demonstrates turbulent color flow within the pseudoaneurysm (*large arrows, cursors*). Color flow also is seen within the neck (*small arrow*) of the pseudoaneurysm, connecting the pseudoaneurysm with the hepatic artery (not shown).

absent diastolic flow with a high resistive index in the hepatic artery has been found in patients with hepatic veno-occlusive disease (310).

Liver in Cardiac Disease

Passive Congestion of the Liver

Passive congestion of the liver is a well-known complication of severe, acute, or chronic congestive heart failure and can be caused by all forms of heart disease, both acquired and congenital. Several factors have been postulated to be responsible including increased hepatic venous pressure producing central venous and sinusoidal stasis and decreased hepatic blood flow with reduction of the oxygen supply to the liver (312). The clinical picture is dominated by the signs and symptoms of severe heart failure; however, a mild, aching discomfort in the right upper quadrant may be caused by acute passive congestion of the liver. Hepatomegaly is present in most patients with significant right-sided congestive heart failure. Chronic passive congestion may progress to cardiac cirrhosis. Sonographically, hepatic enlargement and dilatation of the hepatic veins are seen in the early stages. The normal diameter of the major right hepatic vein is less than 6 mm, and in patients with congestive heart failure, the mean diameter is 9 mm (313). In patients with cardiac cirrhosis, the sonographic abnormalities in the liver are similar to those observed with cirrhosis from other causes.

Tricuspid Regurgitation

In patients with severe congestive heart failure and tricuspid regurgitation, duplex Doppler sonography often demonstrates abnormal Doppler waveforms in the hepatic and portal veins, best demonstrated with breath holding during inspiration. In tricuspid regurgitation, the hepatic vein waveform may demonstrate reversal of the systolic wave or a decrease in the size of the antegrade systolic wave (Fig. 106) (314) and a decrease in the systolic velocity with a systolic–diastolic flow velocity ratio of less than 0.6 (314). In patients with tricuspid regurgitation, the main portal vein waveform may become highly pulsatile (Fig. 107), with the minimum velocity dropping to or below zero (315). Retrograde flow below the baseline may be seen during part of the cardiac cycle (Fig. 107). Highly pulsatile portal venous waveform, however, may also be seen in some healthy persons without heart disease (316). Portal flow patterns suggestive of severe congestive heart failure

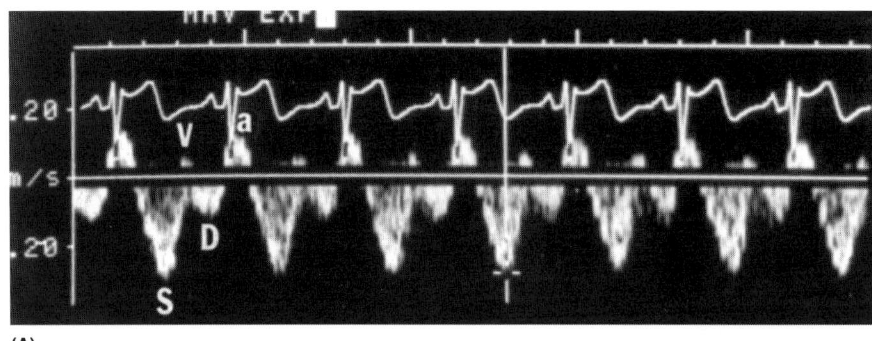

(A)

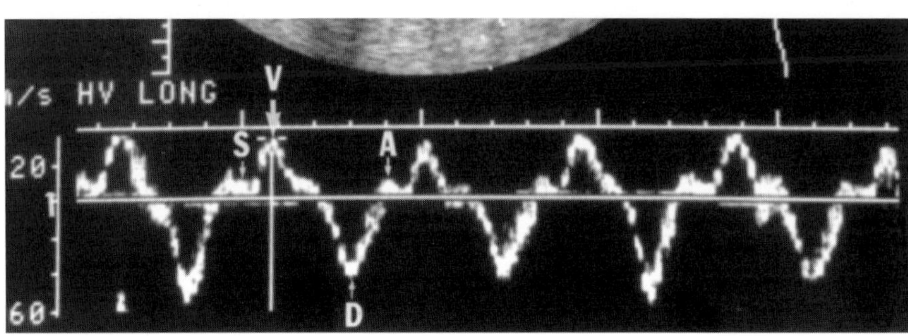

(B)

FIGURE 106 A AND B ■ Tricuspid regurgitation: hepatic vein duplex Doppler. (**A**) Normal hepatic vein waveform (*bottom*) with a simultaneous electrocardiographic tracing (*top*) shows the larger antegrade systolic wave (S) and the smaller antegrade diastolic wave (D). Note also the small retrograde V-wave (V) at end of systole and the retrograde A-wave (a) at end of diastole. (**B**) Abnormal hepatic vein waveform in tricuspid regurgitation shows a small retrograde systolic wave above the baseline and a large antegrade diastolic wave. The V-wave is now large. *Source*: From Ref. 314.

include the following: (*i*) a monophasic forward flow with peak velocity in ventricular diastole and gradual diminution of velocity throughout ventricular systole; (*ii*) a reversed flow in ventricular systole, and (*iii*) vena cava–like biphasic forward velocity peaks during each cardiac cycle (317).

Hepatic Infarction

Hepatic infarction is rare, probably because of the dual blood supply to the liver from the hepatic arterial and portal venous system. The portal vein supplies 60% to 80% of hepatic blood flow, and therefore, hepatic artery thrombosis resulting in infarction is uncommon in patients with an intact portal vein (318). Causes of hepatic infarction include hepatic artery occlusion due to arteriosclerosis, thrombosis, or embolism, hepatic artery aneurysm, polyarteritis nodosa, and sickle-cell disease. Infarction sometimes occurs without vascular occlusion in patients with shock, biliary disease, or complications of anesthesia (319). Clinically, these patients present with abdominal pain, fever, leukocytosis,

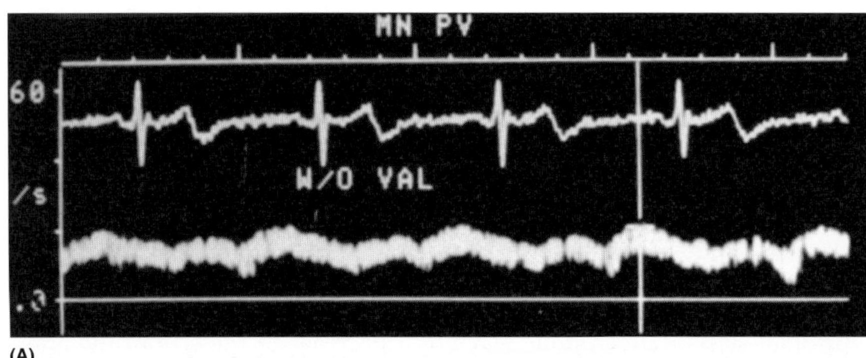

(A)

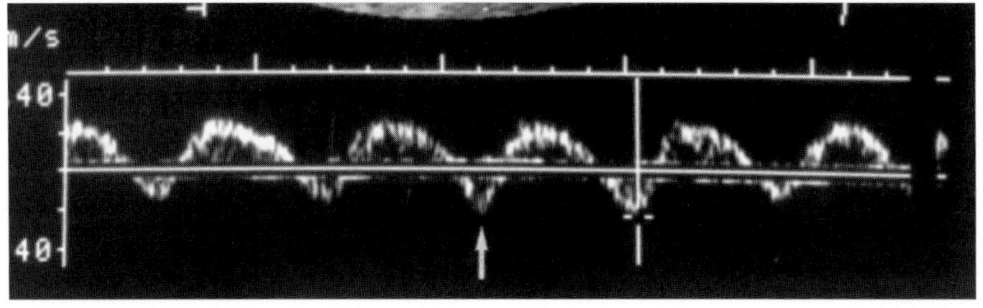

(B)

FIGURE 107 A AND B ■ Tricuspid regurgitation: main portal vein duplex Doppler. (**A**) In a normal duplex Doppler waveform (*bottom*) with simultaneous electrocardiographic tracing (*top*), flow is minimally phasic and constantly above the baseline (i.e., antegrade). (**B**) In tricuspid regurgitation, a highly pulsatile waveform is seen with retrograde flow below the baseline (*arrow*) during part of cardiac cycle. *Source*: From Ref. 315.

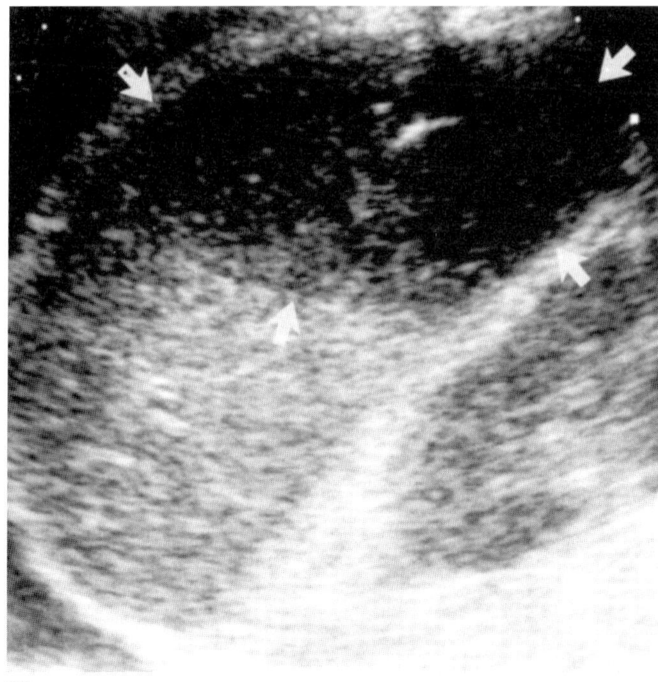

(A)

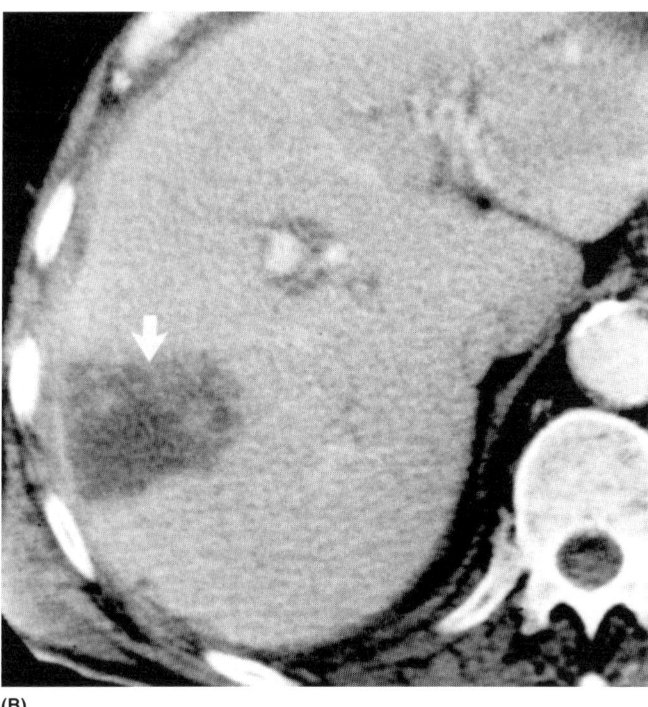

(B)

FIGURE 108 A AND B ■ Hepatic infarct. (**A**) Sagittal sonogram shows the wedge-shaped hypoechoic region of infarction (*arrows*) within the right lobe of the liver. Posterior acoustic enhancement is evident. (**B**) Contrast-enhanced CT image of the right lobe of the liver at the upper margin of the infarction shows a wedge-shaped area of low attenuation extending to the capsule (*arrow*). *Source*: From Ref. 320.

and abnormal liver function tests. The infarcts may appear wedge shaped and are frequently located in the periphery of the liver. However, the infarct can be centrally located within the liver and may be round or oval (319). Early infarcts appear hypoechoic on sonography (Fig. 108) and may have indistinct margins. In time, areas of infarction develop more distinct margins and may become anechoic and cystic. The cystic areas are frequently secondary to formation of a bile duct cyst or bile lake resulting from infarction (318,319,321). Gas formation within sterile hepatic infarcts has been described (319). It is difficult to differentiate hepatic infarcts from abscesses or necrotic tumors, and percutaneous aspiration is frequently required to exclude abscess or neoplasm.

Peliosis Hepatis

Peliosis hepatis is a rare condition characterized by the presence in the liver of multiple, blood-filled cystic spaces, which may or may not be lined with sinusoidal cells (322). The individual cysts or cavities usually are 1 mm to 1 cm in diameter, but they may be larger. In the past, this disorder was primarily associated with wasting diseases, such as tuberculosis, cancer, and chronic suppurative infection. It is seen most commonly now in association with the administration of anabolic steroids. It is also associated with AIDS and Hodgkin's disease. Sonographically, the liver may have a diffusely inhomogeneous echo pattern with scattered hypoechoic or nearly anechoic cystic areas within it. The differential diagnosis includes metastatic liver disease, multiple liver abscesses, and cirrhosis (323). Arteriography demonstrates multiple small accumulations of contrast material in the late arterial and capillary phases (324).

Portal Venous Gas

Portal venous gas may be detected in any patient with disruption of the gastrointestinal mucosa, markedly distended bowel, or sepsis with or without abscess (325). The most common causes of portal venous gas are necrotizing enterocolitis and infarcted bowel. Less common causes are intra-abdominal abscess, ulcerative colitis, and gastric ulcer. Sonographically, portal venous gas causes moving hyperechoic foci within the lumen of the main portal vein (Fig. 109) and portal vein branches in the liver, tiny hyperechoic foci or larger hyperechoic patches within the liver parenchyma (Fig. 109), and sharp bidirectional spikes superimposed on the usual Doppler tracing of the portal vein (326). Acoustic shadowings or reverberations may not be present and are not a constant feature of moving hyperechoic foci within the portal vein or hyperechoic patches within the liver parenchyma (326).

HEPATIC CALCIFICATIONS

Most common causes of hepatic calcifications are calcified granuloma (e.g., tuberculosis and histoplasmosis) and hydatid disease (Table 18) (327). Calcifications in histoplasmosis are usually 1 to 3 mm in diameter (Fig. 110).

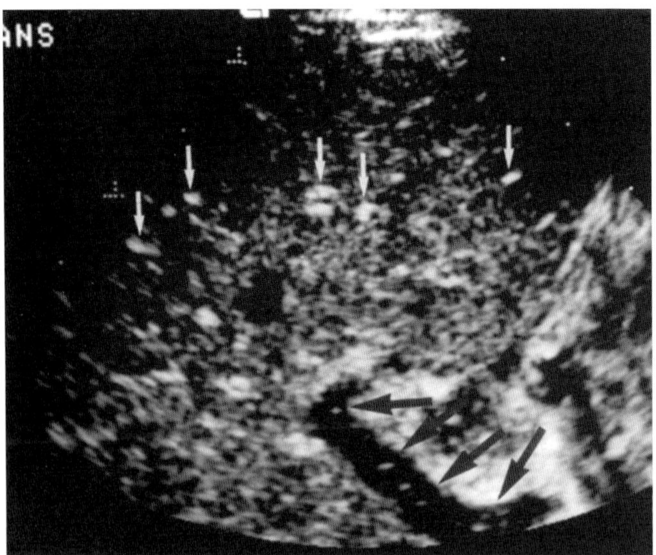

FIGURE 109 ■ Portal venous gas. In a patient with necrotizing enterocolitis, gas in the main portal vein is seen as multiple small hyperechoic foci (*large black arrows*) within main portal vein. These hyperechoic foci were seen to move during real-time examination. Gas within the portal vein radicles within the liver is seen as multiple larger hyperechoic foci (*small write arrows*) within the liver. *Source*: Courtesy of Stuart C. Morrison, MD, Cleveland, OH.

Calcifications secondary to tuberculosis are usually much larger. Calcifications may be caused by other infections and granulomatous disease of childhood. Hepatic calcifications may be seen in primary and metastatic neoplasms. Those occurring in HCC are rare in adults but common in children. Neonatal liver calcifications may be caused by congenital small focal infarcts secondary to vascular disruption phenomenon (328). Hepatic arterial calcifications may appear as hyperechoic, linear structures or multiple, small, hyperechoic foci with acoustic shadowing, adjacent to the portal veins and in the distribution of the portal triads (329). Calcification of the portal vein in adults is

TABLE 18 ■ Hepatic Calcifications

Cause	Disorders
Infection	Histoplasmosis
	Tuberculosis
	Hydatid cyst
	Old calcified abscess
Trauma	Old calcified hematoma
Tumor	Calcified metastases
	Fibrolamellar carcinoma
	Hepatoblastoma
	Infantile hemangioendothelioma
	Epithelioid hemangioendothelioma
	Hepatocellular carcinoma (uncommon)
	Peripheral cholangiocarcinoma (occasional)
	Mesenchymal hamartoma (rare)
	Cavernous hemangioma (rare)
Vascular disorders	Hepatic arterial calcifications
	Portal venous calcifications
Biliary disorders	Biliary calculi (usually not calcified)
	Ascariasis (calcified parasites)

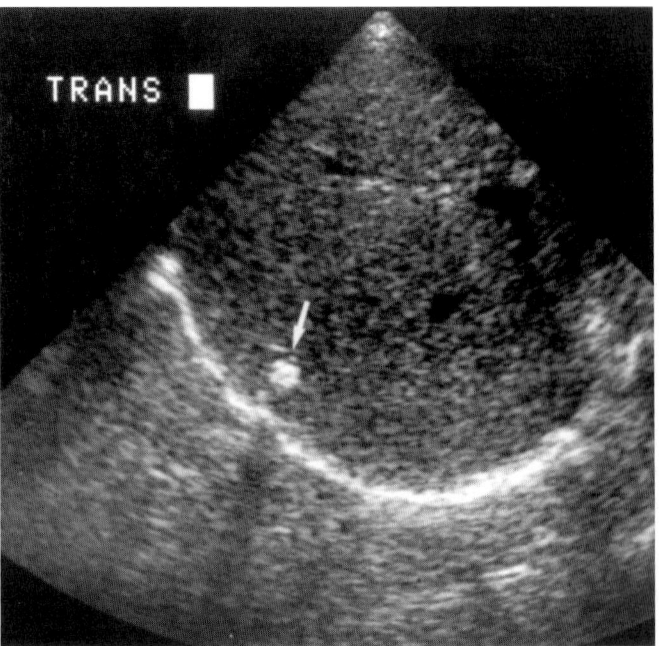

(A)

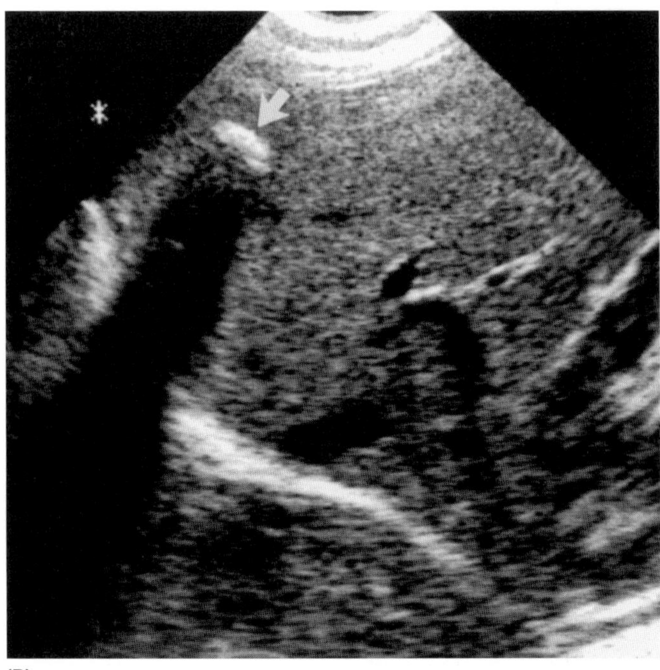

(B)

FIGURE 110 A AND B ■ Calcified granuloma. (**A**) Transverse view shows a small calcified granuloma (*arrow*) secondary to histoplasmosis, as a hyperechoic structure with acoustic shadowing. (**B**) Sagittal view shows a large calcified granuloma (*arrow*) with prominent distal acoustic shadowing.

an uncommon finding and occurs in a thrombus or within the vessel wall; it is seen in patients with long-standing portal hypertension. It is most commonly seen as hyperechoic, linear areas along the wall of the main portal vein, usually with acoustic shadowing or as hyperechoic, nodular material protruding into the lumen of the portal vein (330). The patient may have associated calcifications in the wall of the splenic, superior mesenteric, coronary, and peripancreatic veins. In infants, calcifications in the peripheral portions of the liver can be seen secondary to calcified portal vein thromboemboli, which are frequently associated with multiple anomalies (331). The differential diagnosis of liver calcifications includes intrahepatic biliary calculi, surgical clips, shotgun pellets, air in the intrahepatic biliary tract, and portal venous gas. Biliary calculi may be associated with dilated bile ducts or other biliary abnormalities. Surgical clips and shotgun pellets cause comet tail artifacts (Fig. 111). Air in the biliary tract usually is associated with reverberation artifacts, but small amounts of air, especially in the intrahepatic bile ducts, may produce acoustic shadowing without reverberation artifacts. Portal venous gas may produce hyperechoic foci, frequently without shadowing or reverberation artifacts.

HEPATIC TRAUMA

Hepatic injury is usually due to blunt trauma caused by motor vehicle accidents and falls or penetrating injuries from firearms and stabbings. Iatrogenic hepatic injuries are most frequently caused by liver biopsy, drainage procedures, or placement of catheters within the liver. Clinically, patients with hepatic trauma may present with right upper quadrant pain and tenderness, falling hematocrit, and hypotension. Hepatic injury may cause subcapsular or intraparenchymal hematoma, rupture of the liver and its capsule, fractures and tears of the liver parenchyma, and vascular injuries, most frequently hepatic venous injuries (332). The most common site of injury is the right hepatic lobe. Perivascular lacerations paralleling right and middle hepatic veins and the right portal vein branches are frequently seen (333). Ultrasound is not the primary imaging technique for evaluation of hepatic trauma. CT provides the most information of any single diagnostic imaging test commonly available (334).

Sonography can demonstrate subcapsular or intraparenchymal hematomas, parenchymal tears or contusions, hemoperitoneum, and bilomas (collections of bile secondary to bile leakage from biliary tract injury). A fresh hematoma may appear echogenic (335). A few days after the injury, the hematoma becomes hypoechoic and eventually becomes cystic (Fig. 112) (336). Septations and echogenic debris may be seen within the hematoma (Fig. 113). On follow-up sonograms, small residual abnormalities may persist for several months. Contusions may be seen as hypoechoic areas, and parenchymal tears or fractures may appear as irregular areas of abnormal echo pattern within the liver parenchyma (337). Bilomas, which are collections of bile within the peritoneal cavity or within the liver,

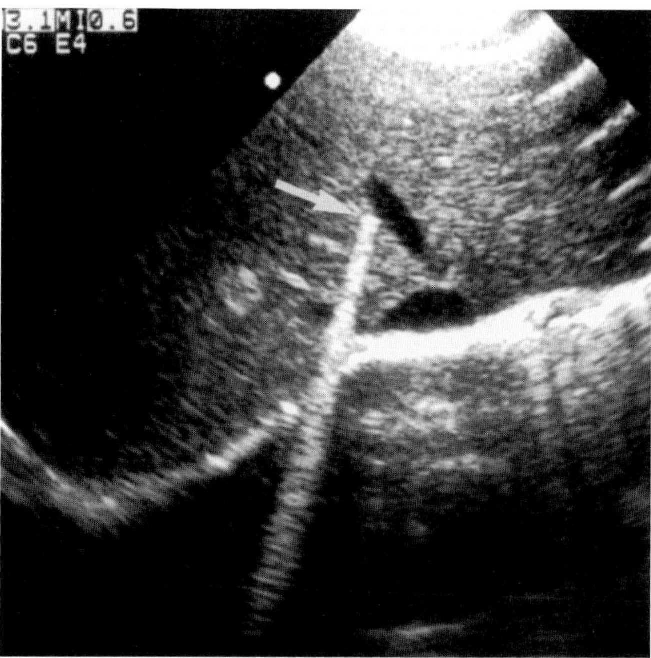

(A)

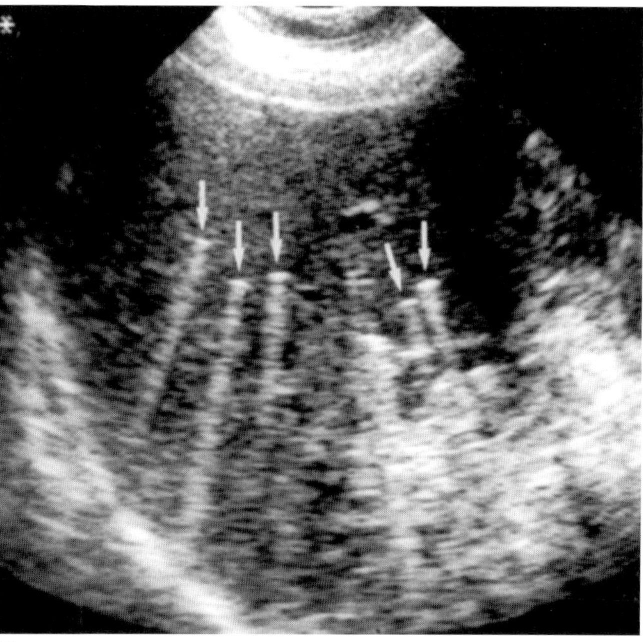

(B)

FIGURE 111 A AND B ■ Shotgun pellets. (**A**) Shotgun pellet in the liver appears as a hyperechoic structure (*arrow*) with associated comet tail reverberation artifacts. (**B**) Sagittal view in another patient shows multiple shotgun pellets within the liver appearing as multiple hyperechoic foci (*arrows*) associated with comet tail reverberation artifacts.

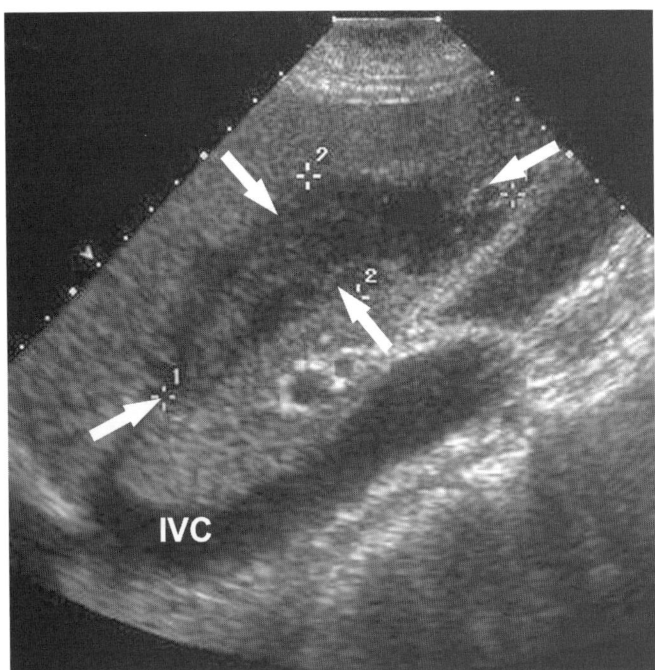

FIGURE 112 ■ Post-traumatic intraparenchymal hematoma. Sagittal view shows an intraparencnymal hematoma (*arrows*). IVC, inferior vena cava.

result from trauma to the biliary tract. Bilomas appear as cystic, anechoic masses with considerable distal acoustic enhancement, adjacent to the liver, occasionally within the liver, or in the peritoneal cavity in the upper abdomen. After initial evaluation with CT, ultrasound may be used for serially monitoring the hepatic injury, in selected hemodynamically stable patients who are treated conservatively. Operative exploration is necessary for patients who are in shock or for those who are hemodynamically unstable after abdominal injury (333).

SURGICAL PORTOSYSTEMIC SHUNTS

The principle of all portosystemic shunt operations is to reduce the pressure in the varices by diverting all or part of the portal venous blood into the systemic circulation. The most commonly performed surgical portosystemic shunts include mesocaval, distal splenorenal (Warren shunt), portacaval, and mesoatrial shunts (338). The shunts can be evaluated either by duplex Doppler or by color Doppler sonography (Fig. 114). Color Doppler sonography allows visualization of the shunt even when it is not apparent on real-time gray-scale imaging. Grant et al. reported 100% sensitivity and specificity for evaluating shunt patency using color Doppler techniques (339). Occlusion of the shunt can be diagnosed by demonstrating the absence of flow within the shunt veins or the shunt anastomosis. Thrombus within the veins or anastomosis or collateral vessels around the thrombosed veins may be seen secondary to occlusion of the shunt. Considerable turbulence as well as aliasing of the color flow secondary to higher velocities is common in the anastomotic regions of the shunt. Criteria for using increased velocity as a sign of shunt stenosis have not been well defined. Reversed flow (hepatofugal flow) in the intrahepatic portal veins and the main portal vein probably indicates a patent shunt (340). However, hepatopetal flow in the portal vein does not always indicate a thrombosed shunt and may be seen in patients with patent shunts (341).

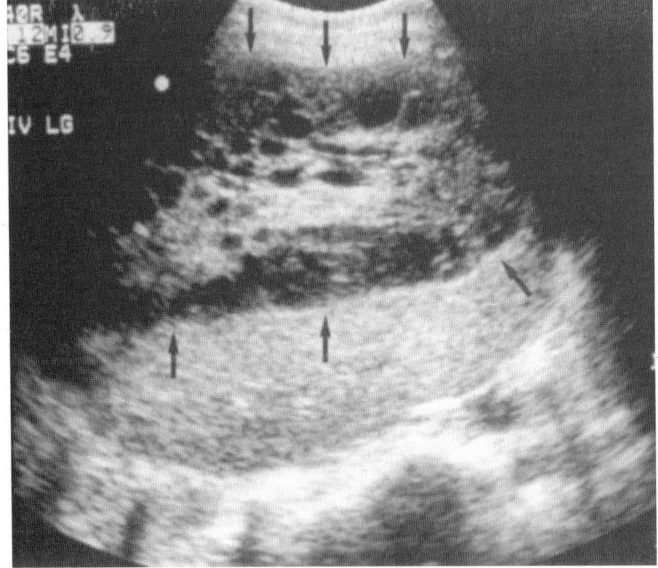

FIGURE 113 ■ Posttraumatic subcapsular hematoma. Sagittal view shows a large, mixed, solid cystic mass (*arrows*) compressing and deforming the edge of the liver (*posterior arrows*).

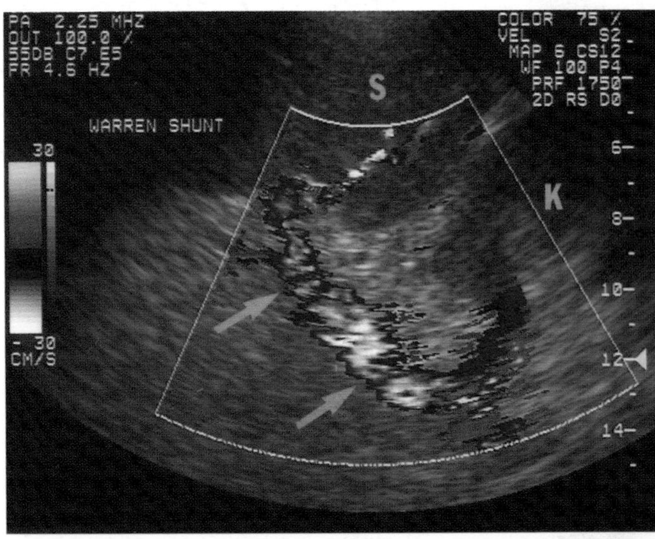

FIGURE 114 ■ Splenorenal (Warren) shunt. Color Doppler sonogram shows color flow within a patent shunt (*arrows*) between the splenic and left renal veins. S, spleen; K, kidney. *Source*: Courtesy of Nagesh Ragavendra, MD, Los Angeles, CA.

TRANSJUGULAR INTRAHEPATIC PORTOSYSTEMIC SHUNTS

Transjugular intrahepatic portosystemic shunts (TIPS) are more frequently being performed instead of surgically created shunts in the treatment of life-threatening sequelae of portal venous hypertension (342). TIPS are also performed for control of refractory ascites related to liver disease. Other indications include Budd–Chiari syndrome, refractory hydrothorax related to liver disease, and veno-occlusive disease. The TIPS procedure consists of placement of an expandable metallic stent, inserted through the internal jugular vein, into a track created in the liver between the intrahepatic portal vein and the hepatic vein. Blood is shunted from the portal circulation to the systemic circulation through the stent, thereby diverting blood away from the varices. The procedure is performed under fluoroscopic guidance. Real-time sonography can be used to provide direct visualization of the needle placement into the portal vein; however, sonography is not routinely used (342). Acute complications of TIPS procedure include puncture of the extrahepatic portion of the portal vein causing intraperitoneal hemorrhage, hepatic artery injury, arterial portal fistula, transient hemobilia, and subcapsular hematoma. Stents can retract or migrate even after successful placement. With gray-scale sonography, the shunt is seen as a tubular structure with hyperechoic walls connecting a portal vein and a branch of the hepatic vein. The walls of the shunt frequently have a corrugated appearance. Sonographically, the Palmaz stent appears straight, and the Wallstent appears curved. Color and duplex Doppler sonographic examinations soon after the shunt is created are recommended, so baseline flow velocity in the stent and flow direction in portal vein branches can be established, because a subsequent decrease in flow velocity in the stent or a change in direction of flow in a portal branch in the liver may indicate stent malfunction or occlusion. Hepatofugal flow in the portal vein branches is frequently seen after a successful TIPS procedure. Patent, well-functioning shunts are characterized by high-velocity (75–200 cm/sec) turbulent flow (343). A velocity gradient between portal and hepatic venous side of a TIPS may be a normal finding (with mean peak velocity on the portal venous side considerably less than at the hepatic venous side); however, this remains controversial (344). Peak systolic velocity in TIPS is substantially altered by the respiratory state of the patient at the time of the measurement but not by the patient position, with peak velocities in the mid stent averaging 22 cm per second greater in quiet respiration than in deep inspiration (345). Mean peak velocities in the main portal vein are significantly increased after a successful TIPS procedure (343). Base line flow velocities in the main portal vein in patients with 12 mm diameter stents exceed those in patients with 10 mm stents, although neither maximum nor minimum flow velocities in the stent differ between these two groups of patients (346).

TIPS have a limited patency and therefore routine surveillance and percutaneous intervention are continuously required to maintain TIPS patency. Trans-shunt venography is the gold standard technique for TIPS evaluation. Doppler ultrasound however is the routinely used noninvasive tool for evaluation for TIPS patency (347).

Color Doppler and, particularly, power Doppler are effective in demonstrating shunt patency (Fig. 115). Absence of flow indicates complete occlusion of the

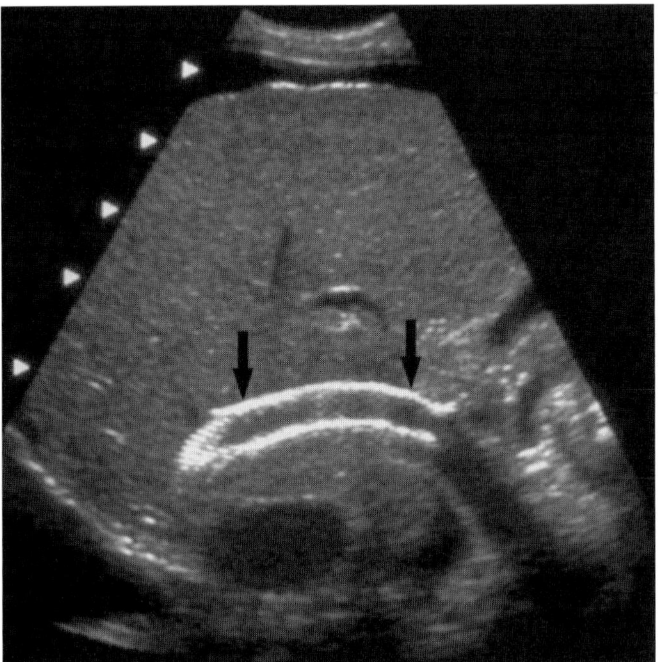
(A)

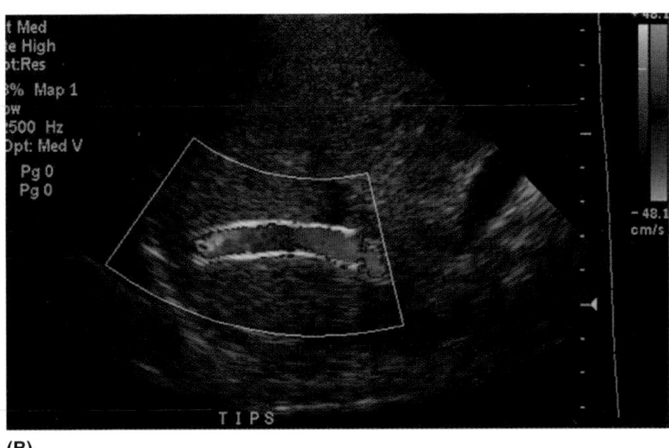

(B)

FIGURE 115 A AND B ■ Patent transjugular intrahepatic portosystemic shunt (TIPS). (**A**) The walls of the stent appear hyperechoic (*arrows*). (**B**) Color Doppler sonogram shows color flow within a patent TIPS stent. *Source*: Courtesy of Vikram S. Dogra, MD, Rochester, NY.

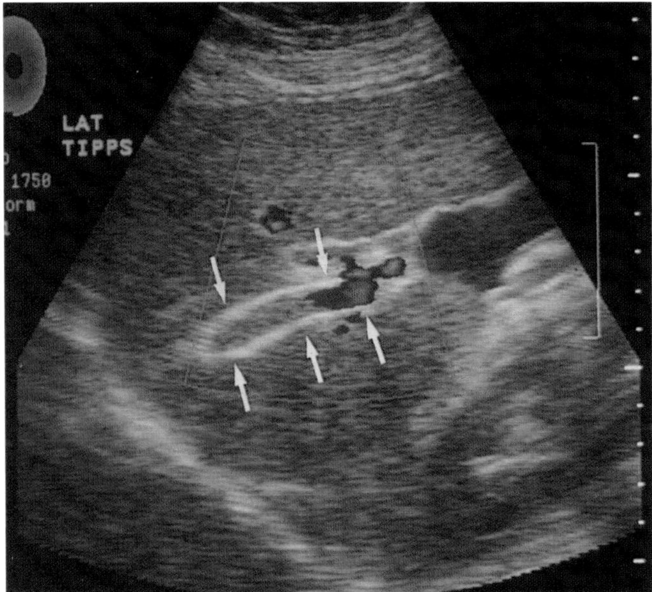

FIGURE 116 ■ Occluded transjugular intrahepatic portosystemic shunt (TIPS). Power Doppler sonogram shows the absence of flow within the occluded TIPS stent (*arrows*). The walls of the stent appear hyperechoic.

shunt secondary to thrombosis (Fig. 116). Echogenicity of the stent lumen on gray-scale is not a useful means of detecting thrombosis. Pseudointimal hyperplasia can be seen as early as a few weeks after TIPS procedure and can cause stenosis and occlusion of the shunt. Pseudointimal hyperplasia may be manifested by incomplete filling of the stent lumen on color Doppler studies. Color and duplex Doppler sonographic techniques can be used for detecting shunt stenosis (342,348). There is yet no consensus on the appropriate Doppler parameters to measure or on the best criteria for diagnosing shunt malfunction. However, good results have been obtained at multiple centers using a variety of Doppler parameters (349–353). The following are the criteria for diagnosing TIPS malfunction due to significant stenosis suggested in one of these investigations (350):

1. Peak stent velocity of less than 90 or greater than 190 cm per second, in the mid and distal (hepatic vein side) portions of the stent
2. Change in peak stent velocity over baseline
   A. Decrease in velocity of greater than 40 cm per second
   B. Increase in velocity of greater than 60 cm per second
3. Main portal vein velocity of less than 30 cm per second
4. Temporal change in flow direction from hepatofugal to hepatopetal, in right or left portal vein

The combined analysis of multiple parameters is found to be better than any individual parameter in detection of TIPS malfunction (354).

Because of low sensitivity of Doppler criteria, some investigators have suggested that it would seem prudent to monitor patients after TIPS with ultrasound at frequent intervals, supplemented by regular (although less frequent) invasive pressure measurements and venography (347).

INTRAOPERATIVE ULTRASOUND

Intraoperative ultrasound is performed by using 5- to 7.5-mHz transducers placed directly over the surgically exposed surface of the liver, before surgical resection of hepatic neoplasms, especially metastatic lesions. Intraoperative ultrasound is the most sensitive indicator of the number of lesions present in the liver (355–357). In a study by Clarke et al., intraoperative ultrasound showed 25% to 35% additional lesions compared with preoperative ultrasound and CT, and 40% of the lesions demonstrated by intraoperative ultrasound were neither visible nor palpable at surgery (355). Intraoperative ultrasound is also helpful in determining the segmental location of the lesions and in determining the involvement of hepatic and portal veins. A survey of the published literature reported that intraoperative ultrasonography influences surgical strategy in up to 50% of liver resections for malignancy and intraoperative ultrasonography is the single most sensitive technique for the detection of occult liver metastases (358). Therefore, intraoperative ultrasound is considered essential in all patients in whom resection of hepatic neoplasms, especially metastatic lesions, is planned. However in a recent study, the authors concluded that preoperative contrast-enhanced MRI is as sensitive as intraoperative ultrasound in detecting liver lesions before hepatic resection (359).

CONTRAST-ENHANCED SONOGRAPHY OF LIVER MASSES

Gray-scale appearance of liver masses is frequently nonspecific because of considerable overlap of the gray-scale sonographic features. Similarly, the role of color and duplex Doppler sonography in distinguishing HCC from metastasis and malignant from benign hepatic lesions is limited due to overlapping color flow and duplex Doppler findings. Therefore, ultrasound contrast agents are being increasingly used for evaluation of liver masses. Contrast-enhanced sonography of liver masses has been shown to be helpful in characterization and detection of liver masses and may obviate the need for additional (i.e., computed tomographic or magnetic resonance) imaging for characterization of certain liver masses (please see Chapter 3).

REFERENCES

1. Marks WM, Filly RA, Callen PW. Ultrasonic anatomy of the liver: a review with new applications. J Clin Ultrasound 1979; 7:137.
2. Parulekar SG. Ligaments and fissures of the liver: sonographic anatomy. Radiology 1979; 130:409.

3. Brown BM, Filly RA, Callen PW. Ultrasonographic anatomy of the caudate lobe. J Ultrasound Med 1982; 1:189.
4. Dodd G III. An American's guide to Couinaud's numbering system. AJR Am J Roentgenol 1993; 161:574.
5. Lafortune M, Madore F, Patriquin H, et al. Segmental anatomy of the liver: a sonographic approach to the Couinaud nomenclature. Radiology 1991; 181:443.
6. Sugarbaker P. En bloc resection of hepatic segments 4B, 5 and 6 by transverse hepatectomy. Surg Gynecol Obstet 1990; 170:250.
7. Soyer P. Segmental anatomy of the liver: utility of a nomenclature accepted worldwide. AJR Am J Roentgenol 1993; 161:572.
8. Warwick R, Williams PL, eds. The peritoneum. Gray's Anatomy, British ed 35. Philadelphia: WB Saunders, 1973:1265.
9. Warwick R, Williams PL, eds. The peritoneum. Gray's anatomy, British ed 35. Philadelphia: WB Saunders, 1973:1259.
10. Cosgrove DO, Arger PH, Coleman BG. Ultrasonic anatomy of hepatic veins. J Clin Ultrasound 1987; 15:231.
11. Makuuchi M, Hasegawa H, Yamazaki S, et al. The inferior right hepatic vein: ultrasonic demonstration. Radiology 1983; 148:213.
12. Fraser-Hill MA, Atri M, Bret PM, et al. Intrahepatic portal venous system: variations demonstrated with duplex and color Doppler US. Radiology 1990; 177:523.
13. Bolondi L, Gandolfi L, Arienti V, et al. Ultrasonography in the diagnosis of portal hypertension: diminished response of portal vessels to respiration. Radiology 1982; 142:167.
14. Warwick R, Williams PL, eds. Angiology. Gray's anatomy, British ed 35. Philadelphia: WB Saunders, 1973:661.
15. Warwick R, Williams PL, eds. Angiology. Gray's anatomy, British ed 35. Philadelphia: WB Saunders, 1973:663.
16. Michels NA. Newer anatomy of the liver: variant blood supply and collateral circulation. JAMA 1960; 172:125.
17. Nichols DM, Cooperberg PL. Sonographic demonstration of the aberrant left hepatic artery. J Ultrasound Med 1984; 3:219.
18. Abu-Yousef MM. Normal and respiratory variations of the hepatic and portal venous duplex Doppler waveforms with simultaneous electrocardiographic correlation. J Ultrasound Med 1992; 11:263.
19. LaFortune M, Patriquin H. Doppler sonography of the liver and splanchnic veins. Semin Intervent Radiol 1990; 7:27.
20. Zwiebel WJ. The liver: diffuse disease and vascular disorders. Semin Ultrasound 1995; 16:34.
21. Wolson AH. Liver. In: Goldberg BB, Kurtz AB, eds. Atlas of Ultrasound Measurements. Chicago: Year Book, 1990:100.
22. Gosink BB, Leymaster CE. Ultrasonic determination of hepatomegaly. J Clin Ultrasound 1981; 9:37.
23. Kurtz, AB, Middleton WD, eds. Liver. Ultrasound: the Requisites. St Louis: Mosby-Year Book, 1996:5.
24. Lim JH, Ko YT, Han MC, et al. The inferior accessory hepatic fissure: sonographic appearance. AJR Am J Roentgenol 1987; 149:495.
25. Donoso L, Martinez-Noguera A, Zidan A, et al. Papillary process of the caudate lobe of the liver: sonographic appearance. Radiology 1989; 173:631.
26. Auh YH, Rubenstein WA, Zirinsky K, et al. Accessory fissures of the liver: CT and sonographic appearance. AJR Am J Roentgenol 1984; 143:565.
27. Prando A, Goldstein H, Bernadine M, et al. Ultrasound pseudolesions of the liver. Radiology 1979; 130:403.
28. Laing FC. Commonly encountered artifacts in clinical ultrasound. Semin Ultrasound 1983; 4:27.
29. Gaines PA, Sampson MA. The prevalence and characterization of simple hepatic cysts by ultrasound examination. Br J Radiol 1989; 62:335.
30. Caremani M, Vincenti A, Benci A, et al. Echographic epidemiology of non-parasitic hepatic cysts. J Clin Ultrasound 1993; 21:115.
31. Chang CS, Lin KC, Hwang SL, et al. Nonparasitic hepatic cysts detected in ultrasonographic examination: analysis of 95 cases. Taiwan I Hsueh Hui Tsa Chih 1989; 88:394.
32. Witzleben CL. Cystic diseases of the liver. In: Zakim D, Boyer TD, eds. Hepatology: A Textbook of Liver Disease. Philadelphia: WB Saunders, 1990:1396.
33. Bean WJ, Rodan BA. Hepatic cysts: treatment with alcohol. AJR Am J Roentgenol 1985; 144:237.
34. Saini S, Mueller PR, Ferrucci JT Jr, et al. Percutaneous aspiration of hepatic cysts does not provide definitive therapy. AJR Am J Roentgenol 1983; 141:559.
35. Levine E, Cook LT, Granthem JJ. Liver cysts in autosomal-dominant polycystic kidney disease: clinical and computed tomographic study. AJR Am J Roentgenol 1985; 145:229.
36. Baron RL, Campbell WL, Dodd GD III. Peribiliary cysts associated with severe liver disease: imaging-pathologic correlation. AJR Am J Roentgenol 1994; 162:631.
37. Kew MC. Tumors of the liver. In: Zakim D, Boyer TD, eds. Hepatology: A Textbook of Liver Disease. Philadelphia: WB Saunders, 1990:1230.
38. Vassiliades VG, Bree RL, Korobkin M. Focal and diffuse benign hepatic disease: correlative imaging. Semin Ultrasound 1992; 13:313.
39. Gibney RG, Hendin AP, Cooperberg PL. Sonographically detected hemangiomas: absence of change over time. AJR Am J Roentgenol 1987; 149:953.
40. Okano H, Shiraki K, Inoue H, et al. Natural course of cavernous hepatic hemangioma. Oncol Rep 2001; 8:411.
41. Mungovan JA, Cronan JJ, Vacarro J. Hepatic cavernous hemangiomas: lack of enlargement over time. Radiology 1994; 191:111.
42. Pietrabissa A, Giulianotti P, Campatelli A, et al. Management and follow-up of 78 giant haemangiomas of the liver. Br J Surg 1996; 83:915.
43. Bree RL, Schwab RE, Neiman HL. Solitary echogenic spot in the liver: is it diagnostic of a hemangioma? AJR Am J Roentgenol 1983; 140:41.
44. Wiener SN, Paurlekar SG. Scintigraphy and ultrasonography of hepatic hemangioma. Radiology 1979; 132:149.
45. Nelson RC, Chezmar JL. Diagnostic approach to hepatic hemangiomas. Radiology 1990; 176:11.
46. Taboury J, Porcel A, Tubiana JM, et al. Cavernous hemangiomas of the liver studied by ultrasound. Radiology 1983; 149:781.
47. Moody AR, Wilson SR. Atypical hepatic hemangioma: a suggestive sonographic morphology. Radiology 1993; 188:413.
48. Choji K, Shinohara M, Nojima T, et al. Significant reduction of the echogenicity of the compressed cavernous hemangioma. Acta Radiol 1988; 29:317.
49. Okano H, Shiraki K, Inoue H, et al. "Variable echo sign" (ultrasonographical alteration of echogenicity) in cavernous hepatic hemangioma. Int J Oncol 2001; 19:337.
50. Perkins AB, Imam K, Smith WJ, et al. Color and power Doppler sonography of liver hemangiomas: a dream unfulfilled? J Clin Ultrasound 2000; 28:159.
51. Wachsberg RH, Jilani M. Duplex Doppler sonography of small (<3 cm diameter) liver tumours: intralesional arterial flow does not exclude cavernous haemangioma. Clin Radiol 1999; 54:103.
52. Naganuma H, Ishida H, Konno K, et al. Hepatic hemangioma with arterioportal shunts. Abdom Imaging 1999; 24:42.
53. Jeffrey RB, Ralls PW, eds. The liver. Sonography of the Abdomen. New York: Raven Press, 1995:79.
54. Kim TK, Han JK, Kim AY, et al. Signal from hepatic hemangiomas on power Doppler US: real or artefactual? Ultrasound Med Biol 1999; 25:1055.
55. Young LK, Yang WT, Chan KW, et al. Hepatic hemangioma: quantitative color power US angiography-facts and fallacies. Radiology 1998; 207:51.
56. Birnbaum BA, Weinreb JC, Megibow AJ, et al. Definitive diagnosis of hepatic hemangiomas: magnetic resonance imaging versus Tc-99 m–labeled red blood cell SPECT. Radiology 1990; 176:95.
57. Caturelli E, Rapaccini GL, Sabelli C, et al. Ultrasound guided fine needle aspiration biopsy in the diagnosis of hepatic hemangioma. Liver 1986; 6:326.
58. Solbiati L, Livraghi T, DePra L, et al. Fine needle biopsy of hepatic hemangioma with sonographic guidance. AJR Am J Roentgenol 1985; 144:471.
59. Cronan JJ, Esparza AR, Dorfman GS, et al. Cavernous hemangioma of the liver: role of percutaneous biopsy. Radiology 1988; 166:135.

60. Heilo A, Stenwig AE. Liver hemangioma: US-guided 18-gauge core-needle biopsy. Radiology 1997; 204:719.
61. Caturelli E, Pompili M, Bartolucci F, et al. Hemangioma-like lesions in chronic liver disease: diagnostic evaluation in patients. Radiology 2001; 220:337.
62. Kurtaran A, Raderer M, Muller C, et al. Vasoactive intestinal peptide and somatostatin receptor scintigraphy for differential diagnosis of hepatic carcinoid metastasis. J Nucl Med 1997; 38:880.
63. Okuda K, Kojiro M, Okuda H. Neoplasms of the liver: benign tumors of the liver. In: Schiff L, Schiff E, eds. Diseases of the Liver. Philadelphia: JB Lippincott, 1993:1236.
64. Mathieu D, Bruneton JN, Drouillard J, et al. Hepatic adenomas and focal nodular hyperplasia: dynamic computed tomography study. Radiology 1986; 160:53.
65. Welch TJ, Sheedy PF, Johnson CM, et al. Focal nodular hyperplasia and hepatic adenoma: comparison of angiography, computed tomography, ultrasound and scintigraphy. Radiology 1985; 156:595.
66. Goodman ZD, Mikel UV, Lubbers PR, et al. Kupffer cells in hepatocellular adenomas. Am J Surg Pathol 1987; 11:191.
67. Bowerman RA, Samuels BI, Silver TM. Ultrasonographic features of hepatic adenomas in type I glycogen storage disease. J Ultrasound Med 1983; 2:51.
68. Sandler MA, Petrocelli RD, Marks DS, et al. Ultrasonic features and radionuclide correlation in liver cell adenoma and focal nodular hyperplasia. Radiology 1980; 135:393.
69. Grazioli L, Federle MP, Ichikawa T, et al. Liver adenomatosis: clinical, histopathologic, and imaging findings in 15 patients. Radiology 2000; 216:395.
70. Lubbers PR, Ros PR, Goodman ZD, et al. Accumulation of technetium-99 m sulfur colloid by hepatocellular adenoma: scintigraphic-pathologic correlation. AJR Am J Roentgenol 1987; 148:1105.
71. Rogers JY, Mack LA, Freenyu PC, et al. Hepatic focal nodular hyperplasia: angiography, computed tomography, sonography, and scintigraphy. AJR Am J Roentgenol 1981; 137:983.
72. Kew MC. Tumors of the liver. In: Zakim D, Boyer TD, eds. Hepatology: A Textbook of Liver Disease. Philadelphia: WB Saunders, 1990:1234.
73. Rummeny E, Weissleder R, Sironi S, et al. Central scars in primary liver tumors: MR features, specificity, and pathologic correlation. Radiology 1989; 171:323.
74. Golli M, Mathieu D, Anglade M, et al. Focal nodular hyperplasia of the liver: value of color Doppler US in association with MR imaging. Radiology 1993; 187:113.
75. Learch TJ, Ralls PW, Johnson MB, et al. Hepatic focal nodular hyperplasia: findings with color Doppler sonography. J Ultrasound Med 1993; 12:541.
76. Kudo M, Tomita S, Minowa K, et al. Color Doppler flow imaging of hepatic focal nodular hyperplasia. J Ultrasound Med 1992; 11:553.
77. Hussain SM, Terkivatan T, Zondervan PE, et al. Focal nodular hyperplasia: findings at state-of-the-art MR imaging, US, CT, and pathologic analysis. Radiographics 2004; 24:3.
78. Roberts JL, Fishman E, Hartman DS, et al. Lipomatous tumors of the liver: evaluation with computed tomography and ultrasound. Radiology 1986; 158:613.
79. Reading CC, Charboneau JW. Case of the day. Ultrasound. Hepatic lipoma. Radiographics 1990; 10:511.
80. Marti-Bonmati L, Menor F, Vizcaino I, et al. Lipoma of the liver: US, CT and MRI appearance. Gastrointest Radiol 1989; 14:155.
81. Bruneton JN, Kerboul, Drouillard J, et al. Hepatic lipomas: ultrasound and computed tomographic findings. Gastrointest Radiol 1987; 12:299.
82. Kew MC. Tumors of the liver: benign hepatic tumors. In: Zakim D, Boyer TD, eds. Hepatology: A Textbook of Liver Disease. Philadelphia: WB Saunders, 1990:1233.
83. Korobkin M, Stephens DH, Lee JKT. Biliary cystadenoma and cystadenocarcinoma: CT and sonographic findings. AJR Am J Roentgenol 1989; 153:507.
84. Choi BI, Lim JH, Han MC, et al. Biliary cystoadenoma and cystadenocarcinoma: CT and sonographic findings. Radiology 1989; 171:57.
85. Dachman AH, Lichtenstein JE, Friedman AC, et al. Infantile hemandioendothelioma of the liver: a radiologic-pathologic-clinical correlation. AJR Am J Roentgenol 1983; 140:1091.
86. Kew MC. Tumors of the liver: benign hepatic tumors. In: Zakim D, Boyer TD, eds. Hepatology: A Textbook of Liver Disease. Philadelphia: WB Saunders, 1990:1232.
87. Pardes JG, Bryan PJ, Gauderer MWL. Spontaneous regression of infantile hemangioendotheliomatosis of the liver: demonstration by ultrasound. J Ultrasound Med 1982; 1:349.
88. Abramson S, Lack E, Teele R. Benign vascular tumors of the liver in infants: sonographic appearance. AJR Am J Roentgenol 1982; 138:629.
89. Ros PR, Goodman ZD, Ishak KG, et al. Meschenchymal hamartoma of the liver: radiologic–pathologic correlation. Radiology 1986; 158:619.
90. Megremis S, Sfakianaki E, Voludaki A, et al. The ultrasonographic appearance of a cystic mesenchymal hamartoma of the liver observed in a middle-aged woman. J Clin Ultrasound 1994; 22:338.
91. Bravo SM, Laing FC. Multiple bile duct hamartomas: von Meyenburg complexes detected on sonography and CT scanning. J Ultrasound Med 1994; 13:649.
92. Kew MC. Tumors of the liver: tumor-like lesions. In: Zakim D, Boyer TD, eds. Hepatology: A Textbook of Liver Disease. Philadelphia: WB Saunders, 1990:1235.
93. Salo J, Bru C, Vilella A, et al. Bile-duct hamartomas presenting as multiple focal lesions on hepatic ultrasonography. Am J Gastroenterol 1992; 87:221.
94. Lev-Toaff AS, Bach AM, Wechsler RJ, et al. The radiologic and pathologic spectrum of biliary hamartomas. AJR Am J Roentgenol 1995; 165:309.
95. Wiener MD, Halvorsen RA Jr, Vollmer RT, et al. Focal intrahepatic hematopoiesis mimicking neoplasm. AJR Am J Roentgenol 1987; 149:1171.
96. Park JH. Sonography of extramedullary hematopoiesis of the liver. AJR Am J Roentgenol 1990; 154:900.
97. Okuda K, Kojiro M, Okuda H. Neoplasms of the liver: primary malignant epithelial tumors. In: Schiff L, Schiff ER, eds. Diseases of the Liver. Philadelphia: JB Lippincott, 1993:1243.
98. Kew MC. Tumors of the liver: primary malignant tumors. In: Zakim D, Boyer TD, eds. Hepatology: A Text-Book of Liver Disease. Philadelphia: WB Saunders, 1990:1206.
99. Kew MC. Tumors of the liver: primary malignant tumors. In: Zakim D, Boyer TD, eds. Hepatology: A Text-Book of Liver Disease. Philadelphia: WB Saunders, 1990:1207.
100. Okuda K, Kojiro M, Okuda H. Neoplasms of the liver: hepatocellular carcinoma. In: Schiff L, Schiff ER, eds. Diseases of The Liver. Philadelphia: JB Lippincott, 1993:1245.
101. Sharma SS, Yasseen I, el-Desoky I, et al. Primary hepatocellular carcinoma: clinical, ultrasonic and pathologic patterns and correlations. Cancer Detect Prev 1986; 9:227.
102. Heywood G, Van Buren SF, Smyrk T, et al. Multilocular cystic hepatocellular carcinoma (CHCC) mimicking mucinous cystadenocarcinoma. Hepatogastroenterology 2003; 50:368.
103. Teefey SA, Stephens DH, James EM, et al. Computed tomography and ultrasonography of hepatoma. Clin Radiol 1986; 37:339.
104. Sheu J-C, Chen D-S, Sung J-L, et al. Hepatocellular carcinoma: ultrasound evaluation in the early stage. Radiology 1985; 155:463.
105. Tanaka S, Kitamura T, Imaoka S, et al. Hepatocellular carcinoma: sonographic and histologic correlation. AJR Am J Roentgenol 1983; 140:701.
106. Yoshikawa J, Matsui O, Takashima T, et al. Fatty metamorphosis in hepatocellular carcinoma: radiologic features in 10 cases. AJR Am J Roentgenol 1988; 151:171.
107. Teefey SA, Stephens DH, Weiland LH. Calcification in hepatocellular carcinoma: not always an indicator of fibromellar histology. AJR Am J Roentgenol 1987; 149:1173.

108. Makuuchi M, Hasegawa H, Yamazaki S, et al. Ultrasonic characteristics of the small hepatocellular carcinoma. Ultrasound Med Biol 1983; (suppl 2):489.
109. Subramanyam BR, Balthazar EJ, Hilton S, et al. Hepatocellular carcinoma with venous invasion: sonographic–angiographic correlation. Radiology 1984; 150:793.
110. Taylor KJW, Ramos I, Morse SS, et al. Focal liver masses: differential diagnosis with pulsed Doppler ultrasound. Radiology 1987; 164:643.
111. Ohnishi K, Nomura F. Ultrasonic Doppler studies of hepatocellular carcinoma and comparison with other hepatic focal lesions. Gastroenterology 1989; 97:1489.
112. Marn CS, Rubin JM, Platt JF, et al. Arteriovenous shunts in cirrhosis: pitfalls in the Doppler evaluation of focal hepatic lesions. Abstract 420. In: Scientific Program of the 7th Scientific Assembly and Annual Meeting of Radiological Society of North America, Chicago, 1990:156.
113. Tanaka S, Kitamura T, Fujita M, et al. Color Doppler flow imaging of liver tumors. AJR Am J Roentgenol 1990; 154:509.
114. Golli M, Van Nhieu JT, Mathieu D, et al. Hepatocellular adenoma: color Doppler US and pathologic correlations. Radiology 1994; 190:741.
115. Nino-Murcia M, Ralls PW, Jeffrey RB Jr, et al. Color Doppler characterization of focal hepatic lesions. AJR Am J Roentgenol 1992; 159:1195.
116. Lencioni R, Caramella D, Bartolozzi C. Hepatocellular carcinoma: use of color Doppler US to evaluate response to treatment with percutaneous ethanol injection. Radiology 1995; 194:113.
117. Tanaka K, Inoue S, Numata K, et al. Color Doppler sonography of hepatocellular carcinoma before and after treatment by transcatheter arterial embolization. AJR Am J Roentgenol 1992; 158:541.
118. Takayasu K, Moriyama N, Muramatsu Y, et al. The diagnosis of small hepatocellular carcinomas: efficacy of various imaging procedures in 100 patients. AJR Am J Roentgenol 1990; 155:49.
119. Maringhini A, Cottone M, Sciarrino E, et al. Ultrasonography and alpha-fetoprotein in diagnosis of hepatocellular carcinoma in cirrhosis. Dig Dis Sci 1988; 33:47.
120. Dodd GD III, Miller WJ, Baron RL, et al. Detection of malignant tumors in end-stage cirrhotic livers: efficacy of sonography as a screening technique. AJR Am J Roentgenol 1992; 159:727.
121. Chalasani N, Horlander JC Sr, Said A, et al. Screening for hepatocellular carcinoma in patients with advanced cirrhosis. Am J Gastroenterol 1999; 94:2988.
122. Livraghi T, Salmi A, Bolondi L, et al. Small hepatocellular carcinoma: percutaneous alcohol injection. Results in 23 patients. Radiology 1988; 168:133.
123. Brandt DJ, Johnson CD, Stephens DH, et al. Imaging of fibrolamellar hepatocellular carcinoma. AJR Am J Roentgenol 1988; 151:295.
124. Bedi DG, Kumar R, Morettin LB, et al. Fibrolamellar carcinoma of the liver: CT, ultrasound and angiography. Case report. Eur J Radiol 1988; 8:109.
125. Titelbaum DS, Burke DR, Meranze SG, et al. Fibrolamellar hepatocellular carcinoma: pitfalls in nonoperative diagnosis. Radiology 1988; 167:25.
126. Ros PR, Buck JL, Goodman ZD, et al. Intrahepatic cholangiocarcinoma: radiologic-pathologic correlation. Radiology 1988; 167:689.
127. Kew M. Tumors of the liver: primary malignant tumors. In: Zakim D, Boyer TD, eds. Hepatology: A Text-Book of Liver Disease. Philadelphia: WB Saunders, 1990:1222.
128. Wibulpolprasert B, Dhiensiri T. Peripherals cholangiocarcinoma: sonographic evaluation. J Clin Ultrasound 1992; 20:303.
129. Kew M. Tumors of the liver: primary malignant tumors. In: Zakim D, Boyer TD, eds. Hepatology: A Text-Book of Liver Disease. Philadelphia: WB Saunders, 1990:1224.
130. Mahony B, Jeffrey RB, Federle MP. Spontaneous rupture of hepatic and splenic angiosarcoma demonstrated by computed tomography. AJR Am J Roentgenol 1982; 138:965.
131. Bruneton JN, Drouillard J, Fenart D, et al. Echography in hepatic angiomas. Ultrasound Med Biol 1983; 2:485.
132. Radin R, Craig JR, Colletti PM, et al. Hepatic epithelioid hemangioendothelioma. Radiology 1988; 169:145.
133. Furui S, Itai Y, Ohtomo D, et al. Hepatic epithelioid hemangioendothelioma: report of five cases. Radiology 1989; 171:63.
134. Kew M. Tumors of the liver: primary malignant tumors. In: Zakim D, Boyer TD, eds. Hepatology: A Textbook of Liver Disease. Philadelphia: WB Saunders, 1990:1223.
135. Dachman AH, Parker RL, Ros PR, et al. Hepatoblastoma: radiologic–pathologic correlation in 50 cases. Radiology 1987; 164:15.
136. Miller JH. The ultrasonographic appearance of cystic hepatoblastoma. Radiology 1981; 138:141.
137. Luburich P, Bru C, Ayuso MC, et al. Hepatic Kaposi sarcoma in AIDS: US and CT findings. Radiology 1990; 175:172.
138. Wooten WB, Green B, Goldstein HM. Ultrasonography of necrotic hepatic metastases. Radiology 1978; 128:447.
139. Marchal GJ, Pylyser K, Tshibwabwa-Tumba EA. Anechoic halo in solid liver tumors: sonographic, microangiographic, and histologic correlation. Radiology 1985; 156:479.
140. Wernecke K, Henke L, Vassallo P, et al. Pathologic explanation for hypoechoic halo seen on sonograms of malignant liver tumors: an in vitro correlative study. AJR Am J Roentgenol 1992; 159:1011.
141. Kruskal JB, Thomas P, Nasser I, et al. Hepatic colon cancer metastases in mice: dynamic in vivo correlation with hypoechoic rims visible at US. Radiology 2000; 215:852.
142. Wernecke K, Vassallo P, Bick U, et al. The distinction between benign and malignant liver tumors on sonography: value of a hypoechoic halo. AJR Am J Roentgenol 1992; 159:1005.
143. Rubaltelli L, Del Mashio A, Candiani F, et al. The role of vascularization in the formation of echographic patterns of hepatic metastases: microangiographic and echographic study. Br J Radiol 1980; 53:1166.
144. Kurtz AB, Middleton WD, eds. The liver. Ultrasound: the Requisites. St Louis: Mosby–Year Book, 1996:7.
145. Jeffrey RB, Ralls, PW, eds. The liver. Sonography of the Abdomen. New York: Raven Press, 1995:104.
146. Bruneton JN, Ladree D, Caramella E, et al. Ultrasonographic study of calcified hepatic metastases: a report of 13 cases. Gastrointest Radiol 1982; 7:61.
147. Katrugadda CS, Goldstein HM, Green B. Gray scale ultrasonography of calcified liver metastases. AJR Am J Roentgenol 1977; 129:591.
148. Federle MP, Filly RA, Moss AA. Cystic hepatic neoplasm: complementary roles of computed tomography and sonography. AJR Am J Roentgenol 1981; 136:345.
149. Martinez A, Sanchez M, Rosello R, et al. Ultrasonic patterns observed in hepatic metastases from breast carcinoma: diagnosis and evolution. Gastrointest Radiol 1989; 14:49.
150. Sanders LM, Botet JF, Straus DJ, et al. Computed tomography of primary lymphoma of the liver. AJR Am J Roentgenol 1989; 152:973.
151. Soyer P, Van Beers B, Teillet-Thiebaud F, et al. Hodgkin's and non–Hodgkin's hepatic lymphoma: sonographic findings. Abdom Imaging 1993; 18:339.
152. Gorg C, Schwerk WB, Gorg K, et al. Focal involvement of malignant lymphoma in the liver. Bildgebung 1991; 58:67.
153. Ginaldi S, Bernardino ME, Jing BS, et al. Ultrasonographic patterns of hepatic lymphoma. Radiology 1980; 136:427.
154. Townsend RR, Laing FC, Jeffrey RB, et al. Abdominal lymphoma in AIDS: evaluation with ultrasound. Radiology 1989; 171:719.
155. Shawker TH, Dunnick NR, Head GL, et al. Ultrasound evaluation of American Burkitt's lymphoma. J Clin Ultrasound 1979; 7:279.
156. Siegal MJ, Melson GL. Sonographic demonstration of hepatic Burkitt's lymphoma. Pediatr Radiol 1981; 11:166.
157. Honda H, Franken EA Jr, Barloon TJ, et al. Hepatic lymphoma in cyclosporine-treated transplant recipients: sonographic and computed tomography findings. AJR Am J Roentgenol 1989; 152:501.
158. Mulvihill DM, Munden MM, Edell D. Lymphoproliferative disorder involving the liver following transplantation: CT appearance. J Comput Assist Tomogr 1994; 18:47.

159. Harris KM, Schwartz ML, Slasky BS, et al. Post-transplantation cyclosporine-induced lymphoproliferative disorders: clinical and radiologic manifestations. Radiology 1987; 162:697.
160. Lepke R, Pagani JJ. Sonography of hepatic chloromas. AJR Am J Roentgenol 1982; 138:1176.
161. Jeffrey RB, Ralls PW, eds. The liver. Sonography of the Abdomen. New York: Raven Press, 1995:133.
162. Eberhardt SC, Choi PH, Bach AM, et al. Utility of sonography for small hepatic lesions found on computed tomography in patients with cancer. J Ultrasound Med 2003; 22:335.
163. Bruneton JN, Raffaelli C, Balu-Maestro C, et al. Sonographic diagnosis of solitary solid liver nodules in cancer patients. Eur Radiol 1996; 6:439.
164. Koss RS. Viral hepatitis. In: Schiff L, Schiff, ER, eds. Diseases of the Liver. Philadelphia: JB Lippincott, 1993:492.
165. Kurtz AB, Rubin CS, Cooper HC. Ultrasound findings in hepatitis. Radiology 1980; 136:717.
166. Kurtz AB, Middleton WD, eds. The liver. Ultrasound: the Requisites. St Louis: Mosby–Year Book, 1996:16.
167. Giorgio A, Ambroso P, Fico P, et al. Ultrasound evaluation of uncomplicated and complicated acute viral hepatitis. J Clin Ultrasound 1986; 14:675.
168. Sharma MP, Dasarath S. Gallbladder abnormalities in acute viral hepatitis: a prospective ultrasound evaluation. J Clin Gastroenterol 1991; 13:697.
169. DeCock KM, Reynolds TB. Amebic and pyogenic liver abscess: pyogenic liver abscess. In: Schiff L, Schiff ER, eds. Diseases of the Liver. Philadelphia: JB Lippincott, 1993:1327.
170. Brandborg LL, Goldman IS. Bacterial and miscellaneous infections of the liver: pyogenic abscess of the liver. In: Zakim D, Boyer TD, eds. Hepatology: A Textbook of Liver Disease. Philadelphia: WB Saunders, 1990:1086.
171. Newlin N, Silver TM, Stuck KJ, et al. Ultrasonic features of pyogenic liver abscess. Radiology 1981; 139:155.
172. Kuligowska E, Noble J. Sonography of hepatic abscesses. In: Raymond HW, Zwiebel WJ, eds. Semin Ultrasound 1983, 4:102.
173. Kuligowska E, Connors SK, Shapiro JH. Liver abscess: sonography in diagnosis and treatment. AJR Am J Roentgenol 1982; 138:253.
174. Samad SA, Zulfiger MA, Maimunah A. Gas-containing liver abscesses: assessment by ultrasound (US) and computed tomography (CT). Med J Malaysia 1993; 48:33.
175. Kressel HY, Filly RA. Ultrasonographic appearance of gas-containing abscesses in the abdomen. AJR Am J Roentgenol 1978; 130:71.
176. Conrad MR, Bregman R, Kilman WJ. Ultrasonic recognition of parenchymal gas. AJR Am J Roentgenol 1979; 132:395.
177. DeCock KM, Reynolds TB. Amebic and pyogenic liver abscess: treatment. In: Schiff L, Schiff ER eds. Diseases of the Liver. Philadelphia: JB Lippincott, 1993:1333.
178. DeCock KM, Reynolds TB. Amebic and pyogenic liver abscess: amebic liver abscess. In: Schiff L, Schiff ER, eds. Diseases of the Liver. Philadelphia: JB Lippincott, 1993:1320.
179. Sukov RJ, Cohen LJ, Sample WF. Sonography of hepatic amebic abscesses. AJR Am J Roentgenol 1980; 134:911.
180. Berry M, Bazaz R, Bhargava S. Amebic liver abscess: sonographic diagnosis and management. J Clin Ultrasound 1986; 14:239.
181. Ralls PW, Colletti PM, Quinn MF, et al. Sonographic findings in hepatic amebic abscess. Radiology 1982; 145:123.
182. Widjaya P, Bilic A, Babic Z, et al. Amebic liver abscess: ultrasonographic characteristics and results of different therapeutic approaches. Acta Med Yugosl 1991; 45:15.
183. Ralls PW, Barnes PF, Radin DR, et al. Sonographic features of amebic and pyogenic liver abscesses: a blinded comparison. AJR Am J Roentgenol 1987; 149:499.
184. Van Allan RJ, Katz M, Johnson MB, et al. Uncomplicated amebic liver abscess: prospective evaluation of percutaneous therapeutic aspiration. Radiology 1992; 183:827.
185. vanSonnenberg E, Mueller PR, Schiffman HR, et al. Intrahepatic amebic abscesses: indications for and results of percutaneous catheter drainage. Radiology 1985; 156:631.
186. Ralls PW, Quinn MF, Boswell WD Jr, et al. Patterns of resolution in successfully treated hepatic amebic abscess. Radiology 1983; 149:541.
187. Bezzi M, Teggi A, De Rosa F, et al. Abdominal hydatid disease: ultrasound findings during medical treatment. Radiology 1987; 162:91.
188. Bret PM, Fond A, Bretagnolle M, et al. Percutaneous aspiration and drainage of hydatid cysts in the liver. Radiology 1988; 168:617.
189. Goldman IS, Brandborg LL. Parasitic diseases of the liver: helminthic infestations. In: Zakim D, Boyer TD, eds. Hepatology: A Textbook Of Liver Disease. Philadelphia: WB Saunders, 1990:1074.
190. Farid Z, Kilpatrick ME, Chiodini PL. Parasitic diseases of the liver: protozoal infections. In: Schiff L, Schiff ER, eds. Diseases of the Liver. Philadelphia: JB Lippincott, 1993:1338.
191. Lewall DB, McCorkell SJ. Hepatic echinococcal cysts: sonographic appearance and classification. Radiology 1985; 155:773.
192. Gharbi HA, Hassine W, Brauner MW. Ultrasound examination of the hydatid liver. Radiology 1981; 139:459.
193. Esfahani F, Rooholamini SA, Vessal K. Ultrasonography of hepatic hydatid cyst: new diagnostic signs. J Ultrasound Med 1988; 7:443.
194. Barriga P, Cruz F, Lepe V, et al. An ultrasonographically solid tumor-like appearance of echinococcal cysts in the liver. J Ultrasound Med 1983; 2:123.
195. Khuroo MS, Zargar SA, Mahajan R. *Echinococcus granulosus* cysts in the liver: management with percutaneous drainage. Radiology 1991; 180:141.
196. Didier D, Wieler S, Rohmer P, et al. Hepatic alveolar echinococcosis: correlative US and CT study. Radiology 1985; 154:179.
197. Goldman IS, Brandborg LL. Parasitic diseases of the Liver: helminthic infestations. In: Zakim D, Boyer TD, eds. Hepatology: A Textbook of Liver Disease. Philadelphia: WB Saunders, 1990:1076.
198. Cerri GG, Alves VAF, Magalhaes A. Hepatosplenic schistosomiasis mansoni: ultrasound manifestations. Radiology 1984; 153:777.
199. Goldman IS, Brandborg LL. Parasitic diseases of the Liver: helminthic infestations. In: Zakim D, Boyer TD, eds. Hepatology: A Textbook of Liver Disease. Philadelphia: WB Saunders, 1990:1072.
200. Farid Z, Kilpatrick ME, Chiodini PL. Parasitic diseases of the liver: trematodes. In: Schiff L, Schiff ER, eds. Diseases of the Liver. Philadelphia: JB Lippincott, 1993:1346.
201. Abdel-Wahab MF, Esmat G, Farrag A, et al. Grading of hepatic schistosomiasis by the use of ultrasonography. Am J Trop Med Hyg 1992; 46:403.
202. Abdel-Rahim IM, Ali QM, Kardorff R, et al. Sonographical morphometrical findings of the liver and spleen in Sudanese patients with Schistosoma mansoni induced periportal fibrosis. East Afr Med J 1994; 71:311.
203. Clarke HM, Hinde FR, Manns RA. Case report: hepatic ultrasound findings in a case of toxocariasis. Clin Radiol 1992; 46:135.
204. Jain R, Sawhney S, Bhargava DK, et al. Hepatic granulomas due to visceral larva migrans in adults: appearance on US and MRI. Abdom Imaging 1994; 19:253.
205. Andrew WK, Thomas RG, Gollach BL. Miliary tuberculosis of the liver: another cause of the 'bright liver' on ultrasound examination. S Afr Med J 1982; 62:808.
206. Brauner M, Buffard MD, Jeanitis V, et al. Sonography and computed tomography of macroscopic tuberculosis of the liver. J Clin Ultrasound 1989; 17:563.
207. Callen PW, Filly FA, Marcus FS. Ultrasonography and computed tomography in the evaluation of hepatic microabscesses in the immunosuppressed patient. Radiology 1980; 136:433.
208. Pastakia B, Shawker TH, Thaler M, et al. Hepatosplenic candidiasis: wheels within wheels. Radiology 1988; 166:417.
209. Ho B, Cooperberg PL, Li DKB, et al. Ultrasonography and computed tomography of hepatic candidiasis in immunosuppressed patients. J Ultrasound Med 1982; 1:157.

210. Miller JH, Greenfield LD, Wald BR. Candidiasis of the liver and spleen in childhood. Radiology 1982; 142:375.
211. Radin DR, Baker EL, Klatt EC, et al. Visceral and nodal calcification in patients with AIDS-related *Pneumocystis carinii* infection. AJR Am J Roentgenol 1990; 154:27.
212. Spouge AR, Wilson SR, Gopinath N, et al. Extrapulmonary *Pneumocystis carinii* in patients with AIDS: sonographic findings. AJR Am J Roentgenol 1990; 155:76.
213. Towers MJ, Withers CE, Hamilton PA, et al. Visceral calcification in patients with AIDS may not always be due to *Pneumocystis carinii*. AJR Am J Roentgenol 1991; 156:745.
214. Garel LA, Pariente DM, Nezelop C, et al. Liver involvement in chronic granulomatous disease: the role of ultrasound in diagnosis and treatment. Radiology 1984; 153:117.
215. Ralls PW, Johnson MB, Kanel G, et al. FM sonography in diffuse liver disease: prospective assessment and blinded analysis. Radiology 1986; 161:451.
216. Marn CS, Bree RL, Silver TM. Ultrasonography of liver: technique and focal and diffuse disease. Radiol Clin North Am 1991; 29:1151.
217. Scatarige JC, Scott WE, Donovan PJ, et al. Fatty infiltration of the liver: ultrasonographic and computed tomographic correlation. J Ultrasound Med 1984; 3:9.
218. Joseph AE, Saverymuttu SH, al-Sam S, et al. Comparison of liver histology with ultrasonography in assessing diffuse parenchymal liver disease. Clin Radiol 1991; 43:26.
219. Taylor KJW, Riely CA, Hammers L, et al. Quantitative ultrasound attenuation in normal liver and in patients with diffuse liver disease: importance of fat. Radiology 1986; 160:65.
220. Van Le L, Podrasky A. Computed tomographic and ultrasonographic findings in women with acute fatty liver of pregnancy. J Reprod Med 1990; 35:815.
221. Quinn SF, Gosink BB. Characteristic sonographic signs of hepatic fatty infiltration. AJR Am J Roentgenol 1985; 145:753.
222. Wang S-S, Chiang J-H, Tsai Y-T, et al. Focal hepatic fatty infiltration as a cause of pseudotumors: ultrasonographic patterns and clinical differentiation. J Clin Ultrasound 1990; 18:401.
223. Baker MK, Wenker JC, Cockerill EM, et al. Focal infiltration of the liver: diagnostic imaging. Radiographics 1985; 5:923.
224. Yates CK, Streight RA. Focal fatty infiltration of the liver simulating metastatic disease. Radiology 1986; 159:83.
225. Yoshikawa J, Matsui O, Takashima T, et al. Focal fatty change of the liver adjacent to the falciform ligament: computed tomography and sonographic findings in five surgically confirmed cases. AJR Am J Roentgenol 1987; 149:491.
226. Arai K, Matsui O, Takashima T, et al. Focal spared areas in fatty liver caused by regional decreased blood flow. AJR Am J Roentgenol 1988; 151:300.
227. Sauerbrei EE, Lopez M. Pseudotumor of the quadrate lobe in hepatic sonography: a sign of generalized fatty infiltration. AJR Am J Roentgenol 1986; 147:923.
228. White EM, Simeone JF, Mueller PR, et al. Focal periportal sparing in hepatic fatty infiltration: a cause of hepatic pseudomass on ultrasound. Radiology 1987; 162:57.
229. Berland LL. Focal areas of decreased echogenicity in the liver at the porta hepatis. J Ultrasound Med 1986; 5:157.
230. Scott WW, Sanders RC, Siegelman SS. Irregular fatty infiltration of the liver: diagnosis dilemmas. AJR Am J Roentgenol 1980; 135:67.
231. Mendenhal CL. Alcoholic hepatitis: pathology and pathogenesis. In: Schiff L, Schiff ER, eds. Diseases of the Liver. Philadelphia: JB Lippincott, 1993:856.
232. Tchelepi H, Ralls PW, Radin R, et al. Sonography of diffuse liver disease. J Ultrasound Med 2002; 21:1023.
233. Conn HO, Atterbury CE. Cirrhosis: definition and history. In: Schiff L, Schiff ER, eds. Diseases of the Liver. Philadelphia: JB Lippincott, 1993:875.
234. Gore RM. Diffuse liver disease. In: Gore RM, Levine MS, Laufer I, eds. Textbook of Gastrointestinal Radiology. Philadelphia: WB Saunders, 1994:1968.
235. Conn HO, Atterbury CE. Cirrhosis: definition and history. In: Schiff L, Schiff ER, eds. Diseases of the Liver. Philadelphia: JB Lippincott, 1993:876.
236. Lefkowitch JH. Pathologic diagnosis of liver disease: major pathologic forms of liver disease. In: Zakim D, Boyer TD, eds. Hepatology: A Textbook of Liver Disease. Philadelphia: WB Saunders, 1990:729.
237. Zakim D, Boyer TD, Montgomery C. Alcoholic liver disease: clinical features of alcoholic liver disease. In: Zakim D, Boyer TD, eds. Hepatology: A Textbook of Liver Disease. Philadelphia: WB Saunders, 1990; 850.
238. Di Lelio A, Cestari C, Lomazzi A, et al. Cirrhosis: diagnosis with sonographic study of the liver surface. Radiology 1989; 172:389.
239. Ladenheim JA, Luba DG, Yao F, et al. Limitations of liver surface US in the diagnosis of cirrhosis. Radiology 1992; 185:21.
240. Ferral H, Male R, Cardiel M, et al. Cirrhosis: diagnosis by liver surface analysis with high-frequency ultrasound. Gastrointest Radiol 1992; 17:74.
241. Harbin WP, Robert NJ, Ferrucci JT. Diagnosis of cirrhosis based on regional changes in hepatic morphology. Radiology 1980; 135:273.
242. Giorgio A, Amoroso P, Lettiri G, et al. Cirrhosis: value of caudate to right lobe ratio in diagnosis with ultrasound. Radiology 1986; 161:443.
243. Hess CF, Schmiedl U, Koelbel G, et al. Diagnosis of liver cirrhosis with ultrasound: receiver-operating characteristic analysis of multidimensional caudate lobe indexes. Radiology 1989; 171:349.
244. Goyal AK, Pokharna DS, Sharma SK. Ultrasonic diagnosis of cirrhosis: reference of quantitative measurements of hepatic dimensions. Gastrointest Radiol 1990; 15:32.
245. Gore RM. Diffuse liver disease. In: Gore RM, Levine MS, Laufer I, eds. Textbook of Gastrointestinal Radiology. Philadelphia: WB Saunders, 1994:1995.
246. Colli A, Cocciolo M, Riva C, et al. Abnormalities of Doppler waveform of the hepatic veins in patients with chronic liver disease: correlation with histologic findings. AJR Am J Roentgenol 1994; 162:833.
247. Bolondi L, Bassi SL, Gaiani S, et al. Liver cirrhosis: changes of Doppler waveform of hepatic veins. Radiology 1991; 178:513.
248. Pedersen JF, Dakhil AZ, Jensen DB, et al. Abnormal hepatic vein Doppler waveform in patients without liver disease. Br J Radiol 2005; 78:242.
249. Freeman MP, Vick GW, Taylor KJW, et al. Regenerating nodules in cirrhosis: sonographic appearance with anatomic correlation. AJR Am J Roentgenol 1986; 146:533.
250. Laing FC, Jeffrey RB, Federle MP, et al. Noninvasive imaging of unusual regenerating nodules in the cirrhotic liver. Gastrointest Radiol 1992; 7:245.
251. Kaplan MM. Primary biliary cirrhosis: incidence, epidemiology and genetics. In: Schiff L, Schiff ER, eds. Diseases of the Liver. Philadelphia: JB Lippincott, 1993:377.
252. Kaplan MM. Primary biliary cirrhosis: pathology. In: Schiff L, Schiff ER, eds. Diseases of the Liver. Philadelphia: JB Lippincott, 1993:378.
253. Gore RM. Diffuse liver disease. In: Gore RM, Levine MS, Laufer I, eds. Textbook of Gastrointestinal Radiology. Philadelphia: WB Saunders, 1994:1983.
254. Grossman H, Ram PC, Coleman RA, et al. Hepatic ultrasonography in type I glycogen storage disease (von Gierke disease). Radiology 1981; 141:753.
255. Lee P, Mather S, Owens C, et al. Hepatic ultrasound findings in the glycogen storage diseases. Br J Radiol 1994; 67:1062.
256. Smevik B, Swensen T, Kolbenstvedt A, et al. Computed tomography and ultrasonography of the abdomen in congenital generalized lipodystrophy. Radiology 1982; 142:687.
257. Quillin SP, Siegel MJ, Rothbaum R. Hepatobiliary sonography in cystic fibrosis. Pediatr Radiol 1993; 23:533.
258. Genecin P, Groszmann RJ. Portal hypertension. Pathogenesis: resistance and flow. In: Schiff L, Schiff ER, eds. Diseases of the Liver. Philadelphia: JB Lippincott, 1993:935.
259. Genecin P, Groszmann RJ. Portal hypertension: classification of portal hypertensive states. In: Schiff L, Schiff ER, eds. Diseases of the Liver. Philadelphia: JB Lippincott, 1993:946.

260. Boyer TD. Portal hypertension. In: Zakim D, Boyer TD, eds. Hepatology: A Textbook of Liver Disease. Philadelphia: WB Saunders, 1990:584.
261. Cottone M, D' Amico G, Marginghini A, et al. Predictive value of ultrasonography in the screening of non-ascitic cirrhotic patients with large varices. J Ultrasound Med 1986; 5:189.
262. Lafortune M, Marleau D, Breton G, et al. Portal venous system measurements in portal hypertension. Radiology 1984; 151:27.
263. Ohnishi K, Saito M, Nakayama T, et al. Portal venous hemodynamics in chronic liver disease: effects of posture change and exercise. Radiology 1985; 155:757.
264. Gore RM. Normal anatomy and examination techniques. In: Gore RM, Levine MS, Laufer I, eds. Text-Book of Gastrointestinal Radiology. Philadelphia: WB Saunders, 1994:1801.
265. Diagnostic Ultrasonography: Test and Syllabus. Reston, VA, American College of Radiology, 1994:69.
266. Subramanyam BR, Balthazar EJ, Madamba MR, et al. Sonography of portosystemic venous collaterals in portal hypertension. Radiology 1983; 146:161.
267. Wachsberg RH, Simmons MZ. Coronary vein diameter and flow direction in patients with portal hypertension: evaluation with duplex sonography and correlation with variceal bleeding. AJR Am J Roentgenol 1994; 162:637.
268. Lafortune M, Constantin A, Breton G, et al. The recanalized umbilical vein in portal hypertension: a myth. AJR Am J Roentgenol 1985; 144:549.
269. Glazer GM, Laing FC, Brown TW, et al. Sonographic demonstration of portal hypertension: the patent umbilical vein. Radiology 1980; 136:161.
270. Saddekni S, Hutchinson DE, Cooperberg PL. The sonographically patent umbilical vein in portal hypertension. Radiology 1982; 145:441.
271. Wachsberg RH, Obolevich AT. Blood flow characteristics of vessels in the ligamentum teres fissure at color Doppler sonography: findings in healthy volunteers and in patients with portal hypertension. AJR Am J Roentgenol 1995; 164:1403.
272. Finn JP, Kane RA, Edelman RR, et al. Imaging of the portal venous system in patients with cirrhosis: MR angiography vs duplex Doppler sonography. AJR Am J Roentgenol 1993; 161:989.
273. Atri M, deStempel J, Bret PM, et al. Incidence of portal vein thrombosis complicating liver metastasis as detected by duplex ultrasound. J Ultrasound Med 1990; 9:285.
274. Parvey HR, Raval B, Sandler CM. Portal vein thrombosis: imaging findings. AJR Am J Roentgenol 1994; 162:77.
275. Wang L-Y, Lin Z-Y, Chang W-Y, et al. Duplex pulsed Doppler sonography of portal vein thrombosis in hepatocellular carcinoma. J Ultrasound Med 1991; 10:265.
276. Pozniak MA, Baus KM. Hepatofugal arterial signal in the main portal vein: an indicator of intravascular tumor spread. Radiology 1991; 180:663.
277. Furuse J, Matsutani S, Yoshikawa M, et al. Diagnosis of portal vein tumor thrombus by pulsed Doppler ultrasonography. J Clin Ultrasound 1992; 20:439.
278. Dodd GD III, Memel DS, Baron RL, et al. Portal vein thrombosis in patients with cirrhosis: does sonographic detection of intrathrombus flow allow differentiation of benign and malignant thrombus? AJR Am J Roentgenol 1995; 165:573.
279. Görg C, Riera-Knorrenschild J, Dietrich J. Colour Doppler ultrasound flow patterns in the portal venous system. Br J Radiol 2002; 75:919.
280. Marx M, Scheible W. Cavernous transformation of the portal vein. J Ultrasound Med 1982; 1:167.
281. Van Gansbeke D, Avni EF, Delcour C, et al. Sonographic features of portal vein thrombosis. AJR Am J Roentgenol 1985; 144:749.
282. Niron EA, Ozer H. Ultrasound appearances of liver hydatid disease. Br J Radiol 1981; 54:335.
283. Frider B, Marin AM, Goldberg A. Ultrasonographic diagnosis of portal vein cavernous transformation in children. J Ultrasound Med 1989; 8:445.
284. Vine HS, Sequira JC, Widrich WC, et al. Portal vein aneurysm. AJR Am J Roentgenol 1979; 132:557.
285. Reynolds TB. Budd–Chiari syndrome. In: Schiff L, Schiff ER, eds. Diseases of the Liver. Philadelphia: JB Lippincott, 1993:1091.
286. Boyer TD. Portal hypertension and bleeding esophageal varices: portal hypertension. In: Zakim D, Boyer TD, eds. Hepatology: A Textbook of Liver Disease. Philadelphia: WB Saunders, 1990:589.
287. Ralls PW, Johnson MB, Radin DR, et al. Budd–Chiari syndrome: detection with color Doppler sonography. AJR Am J Roentgenol 1992; 159:113.
288. Millener P, Grant EG, Rose S, et al. Color Doppler imaging findings in patients with Budd–Chiari syndrome: correlation with venographic findings. AJR Am J Roentgenol 1993; 161:307.
289. Grant EG, Perrella R, Tessler FN, et al. Budd–Chiari syndrome: the results of duplex and color Doppler imaging. AJR Am J Roentgenol 1989; 152:377.
290. Hosoki T, Kuroda C, Tokunaga K, et al. Hepatic venous outflow obstruction: evaluation with pulsed Duplex sonography. Radiology 1989; 170:733.
291. Lee DH, Ko YT, Yoon Y, et al. Sonography and color Doppler imaging of Budd–Chiari syndrome of membranous obstruction of the inferior vena cava. J Ultrasound Med 1994; 13:159.
292. Makuuchi M, Hasegawa H, Yamazaki S, et al. Primary Budd–Chiari syndrome: ultrasonic demonstration. Radiology 1984; 152:775.
293. Park JH, Lee JB, Han MC, et al. Sonographic evaluation of inferior vena caval obstruction: correlative study with vena cavography. AJR Am J Roentgenol 1985; 145:757.
294. Sakugawa H, Higashionna A, Oyakawa T, et al. Ultrasound study in the diagnosis of primary Budd–Chiari syndrome (obstruction of the inferior vena cava). Gastroenterol Jpn 1992; 27:69.
295. Singh V, Sinha SK, Nain CK, et al. Budd-Chiari syndrome: our experience of 71 patients. J Gastroenterol Hepatol 2000; 15:550.
296. Boyer TD. Portal hypertension and bleeding esophageal varices: portal hypertension. In: Zakim D, Boyer TD, eds. Hepatology: A Textbook of Liver Disease. Philadelphia: WB Saunders, 1990:592.
297. Brown BP, Abu-Youssef M, Farner R, et al. Doppler sonography: a non-invasive method for evaluation of hepatic venocclusive disease. AJR Am J Roentgenol 1990; 154:721.
298. Kriegshauser SJ, Charboneau JW, Letendre L. Hepatic venocclusive disease after bone marrow transplantation: diagnosis with duplex sonography. AJR Am J Roentgenol 1988; 150:289.
299. Herbetko J, Grigg AP, Buckley AR, et al. Veno-occlusive liver disease after bone marrow transplantation: findings at duplex sonography. AJR Am J Roentgenol 1992; 158:1001.
300. Teefey SA, Brink JA, Borson RA, et al. Diagnosis of veno-occlusive disease of the liver after bone marrow transplantation: value of duplex sonography. AJR Am J Roentgenol 1995; 164:1397.
301. Chagnon SF, Vallee CA, Barge J, et al. Aneurysmal portohepatic venous fistula: report of two cases. Radiology 1986; 159:693.
302. Kudo M, Tomita S, Tochio H, et al. Intrahepatic portosystemic venous shunt: diagnosis by color Doppler imaging. Am J Gastroenterol 1993; 88:723.
303. Mori H, Hayashi K, Fukuda T, et al. Intrahepatic portosystemic venous shunt: occurrence in patients with and without liver cirrhosis. AJR Am J Roentgenol 1987; 149:711.
304. Ramchandani P, Goldenberg NJ, Soulen RL, et al. Isobutyl 2-cyanoacrylate embolization of a hepatoportal fistula. AJR Am J Roentgenol 1983; 140:137.
305. Falkoff GE, Taylor KJW, Morse S. Hepatic artery pseudoaneurysm: diagnosis with real-time and pulsed Doppler ultrasound. Radiology 1986; 158:55.
306. Cloogman HM, DiCapo RD. Hereditary hemorrhagic telangiectasis: sonographic findings in the liver. Radiology 1984; 150:521.
307. Ralls PW, Johnson MB, Radin DR, et al. Hereditary hemorrhagic telangiectasis: findings in the liver with color Doppler sonography. AJR Am J Roentgenol 1992; 159:59.

308. Pompili M, Rapaccini GL, Marzano MA, et al. Doppler ultrasound findings in Osler–Weber–Rendu disease with hepatic involvement: a case report. Ital J Gastroenterol 1994; 26:83.
309. Jeffrey RB, Ralls PW, eds. The liver. Sonography of the Abdomen. New York: Raven Press, 1995:168.
310. Lafortune M, Dauzat M, Pomier-Layrargues G, et al. Hepatic artery: effect of a meal in healthy persons and transplant recipients. Radiology 1993; 187:391.
311. Joynt LK, Platt JF, Rubin JM, et al. Hepatic artery resistance before and after standard meal in subjects with diseased and healthy livers. Radiology 1995; 196:489.
312. Cello JP, Grendell JH. The liver in systemic conditions: liver dysfunction in heart disease. In: Zakim D, Boyer TD, eds. Hepatology: A Textbook of Liver Disease. Philadelphia: WB Saunders, 1990:1416.
313. Gore RM. Vascular disorders of the liver and splanchnic circulation. In: Gore RM, Levine MS, Laufer I, eds. Textbook of Gastrointestinal Radiology. Philadelphia: WB Saunders, 1994:2026.
314. Abu-Yousef MM. Duplex Doppler sonography of the hepatic vein in tricuspid regurgitation. AJR Am J Roentgenol 1991; 156:79.
315. Abu-Yousef MM, Milam SG, Farner RM. Pulsatile portal vein flow: a sign of tricuspid regurgitation on duplex Doppler sonography. AJR Am J Roentgenol 1990; 155:785.
316. Wachsberg RH, Needleman L, Wilson D. Portal vein pulsatility in normal and cirrhotic adults without cardiac disease. J Clin Ultrasound 1995; 23:3.
317. Hosoki T, Arisawa J, Marukawa T, et al. Portal blood flow in congestive heart failure: pulsed duplex sonographic findings. Radiology 1990; 174:733.
318. Peterson IM, Neumann CH. Focal hepatic infarction with bile lake formation. AJR Am J Roentgenol 1984; 142:115.
319. Lev-Toaff AS, Friedman AC, Cohen LM. Hepatic infarcts: new observations by CT and sonography. AJR Am J Roentgenol 1987; 149:87.
320. Wachsberg RH, Cho KC, Raina S. Liver infarction following unrecognized right hepatic artery ligation at laparoscopic cholecystectomy. Abdom Imaging 1994; 19:53.
321. Doppman JL, Dunnick NR, Girton M, et al. Bile duct cysts secondary to liver infarction: report of a case and experimental production by small vessel hepatic artery occlusion. Radiology 1979; 130:1.
322. Witzleben CL. Cystic diseases of the liver: polycystic liver disease. In: Zakim D, Boyer TD, eds. Hepatology: A Textbook of Liver Disease. Philadelphia: WB Saunders, 1990:1401.
323. Lloyd RL, Lyons EA, Levi CS, et al. The sonographic appearance of peliosis hepatis. J Ultrasound Med 1982; 1:293.
324. Pliskin M. Peliosis hepatis. Radiology 1975; 114:29.
325. Dennis MA, Pretorius D, Manco-Johnson ML, et al. CT detection of portal venous gas associated with suppurative cholangitis and cholecystitis. AJR Am J Roentgenol 1985; 145:1017.
326. Merritt CRB, Goldsmith JP, Sharp MJ. Sonographic detection of portal venous gas in infants with necrotizing enterocolitis. AJR Am J Roentgenol 1984; 143:1059.
327. Darlak JJ, Moskowitz M, Kattan KR. Calcifications in the liver. Radiol Clin North Am 1980; 18:209.
328. Avni EF, Rypens F, Donner C, et al. Hepatic cysts and hyperechogenicities: perinatal assessment and unifying theory on their origin. Pediatr Radiol 1994; 24:569.
329. White LM, Wilson SR. Hepatic arterial calcification: a potential pitfall in the sonographic diagnosis of intrahepatic biliary calculi. J Ultrasound Med 1994; 13:141.
330. Ayuso C, Luburich P, Vilana R, et al. Calcifications in the portal venous system: comparison of plain films, sonography and CT. AJR Am J Roentgenol 1992; 159:321.
331. Friedman AP, Haller JO, Boyer B, et al. Calcified portal vein thromboemboli in infants: radiography and ultrasonography. Radiology 1981; 140:381.
332. Gore RM, Nahrwold DL. Hepatic trauma and surgery. In: Gore RM, Levine MS, Laufer I, eds. Textbook of Gastrointestinal Radiology. Philadelphia: WB Saunders, 1994:2052.
333. Foley WD, Cates JD, Kellman GM, et al. Treatment of blunt hepatic injuries: role of computed tomography. Radiology 1987; 164:635.
334. Kaufman RA, Towbin R, Babcock DS, et al. Upper abdominal trauma in children: imaging evaluation. AJR Am J Roentgenol 1984; 142:449.
335. vanSonnenberg E, Simeone JF, Mueller PR, et al. Sonographic appearance of hematoma in the liver, spleen and kidney: a clinical, pathologic and animal study. Radiology 1983; 147:507.
336. Lam AH, Shulman L. Ultrasonography in the management of liver trauma in children. J Ultrasound Med 1984; 3:199.
337. Gore RM, Nahrwold DL. Hepatic trauma and surgery. In: Gore RM, Levine MS, Laufer I, eds. Textbook of Gastrointestinal Radiology. Philadelphia: WB Saunders, 1994:2055.
338. Boyer TD. Portal hypertension. In: Zakim D, Boyer TD, eds. Hepatology: A Textbook of Liver Disease. Philadelphia: WB Saunders, 1990:602.
339. Grant EG, Tessler FN, Gomes AS, et al. Color Doppler imaging of portosystemic shunts. AJR Am J Roentgenol 1990; 154:393.
340. Lafortune M, Patriquin H, Pomier G, et al. Hemodynamic changes in portal circulation after portosystemic shunts: use of duplex carotid sonography in 43 patients. AJR Am J Roentgenol 1987; 149:701.
341. Rice S, Lee KP, Johnson MB, et al. Portal venous system after portosystemic shunts or endoscopic sclerotherapy: evaluation and Doppler sonography. AJR Am J Roentgenol 1991; 156:85.
342. Foshager MC, Ferral H, Finlay DE, et al. Color Doppler sonography of transjugular intrahepatic portosystemic shunts (TIPS). AJR Am J Roentgenol 1994; 163:105.
343. Surratt RS, Middleton WD, Darcy MD, et al. Morphologic and hemodynamic findings at sonography before and after creation of a transjugular intrahepatic portosystemic shunt. AJR Am J Roentgenol 1993; 160:627.
344. Bodner G, Peer S, Fries D, et al. Color and pulsed Doppler ultrasound findings in normally functioning transjugular intrahepatic portosystemic shunts. Eur J Ultrasound 2000; 12:131.
345. Kliewer MA, Hertzberg BS, Heneghan JP, et al. Transjugular intrahepatic portosystemic shunts (TIPS): effects of respiratory state and patient position on the measurement of Doppler velocities. AJR Am J Roentgenol 2000; 175:149.
346. Lin EC, Middleton WD, Darcy MD, et al. Hemodynamics revealed by Doppler sonography in patients who have undergone creation of transjugular intrahepatic portosystemic shunts: comparison of 10- and 12-mm metallic stents. AJR Am J Roentgenol 1999; 172:1245.
347. Benito A, Bilbao J, Hernández T, et al. Doppler ultrasound for TIPS: does it work? Abdom Imaging 2004; 29:45.
348. Dodd GD, Zajko AB, Orons PD, et al. Detection of transjugular intrahepatic portosystemic shunt dysfunction: value of duplex Doppler sonography. AJR Am J Roentgenol 1995; 164:1119.
349. Feldstein VA, Patel MD, LaBerge JM. TIPS shunts: accuracy of Doppler US in determination of patency and detection of stenoses. Radiology 1996; 201:141.
350. Kanterman RY, Darcy MD, Middleton WD, et al. Doppler sonography findings associated with transjugular intrahepatic portosystemic shunt malfunction. AJR Am J Roentgenol 1997; 168:467.
351. Murphy TP, Beecham RP, Kim HM, et al. Long-term follow-up after TIPS: use of Doppler velocity criteria for detecting elevation of the portosystemic gradient. J Vasc Interv Radiol 1998; 9:275.
352. Zizka J, Elias P, Krajina A, et al. Value of Doppler sonography in revealing transjugular intrahepatic portosystemic shunt malfunction: a 5-year experience in 216 patients. AJR Am J Roentgenol 2000; 175:141.
353. Haskal ZJ, Carroll JW, Jacobs JE, et al. Sonography of transjugular intrahepatic portosystemic shunts: detection of elevated portosystemic gradients and loss of shunt function. J Vasc Interv Radiol 1997; 8:549.
354. Middleton WD, Teefey SA, Darcy MD. Doppler evaluation of transjugular intrahepatic portosystemic shunts. Ultrasound Q 2003; 19:56.
355. Clarke MP, Kane RA, Steele G Jr, et al. Prospective comparison of preoperative imaging and intraoperative ultrasonography in the detection of liver tumors. Surgery 1989; 106:849.

356. Parker GA, Lawrence W Jr, Horsley JS III, et al. Intraoperative ultrasound of the liver affects operative decision making. Ann Surg 1989; 209:596.
357. Rifkin MD, Rosato FE, Branch HM, et al. Intraoperative ultrasound of the liver: an important adjunctive tool for decision making in the operating room. Ann Surg 1987; 205:466.
358. Luck AJ, Maddern GJ. Intraoperative abdominal ultrasonography. Br J Surg 1999; 86:5.
359. Sahani DV, Kalva SP, Tanabe KK, et al. Intraoperative US in patients undergoing surgery for liver neoplasms: comparison with MR imaging. Radiology 2004; 232:810.

Gallbladder and Bile Ducts

Suhas G. Parulekar

17

INTRODUCTION

Ultrasound remains the primary imaging modality in the evaluation of the gallbladder and bile ducts. The most common indications include suspected gallstones, cholecystitis, and biliary obstruction.

GALLBLADDER

Normal Anatomy

The gallbladder is partly contained in a fossa on the inferior surface of the right hepatic lobe, extending from near the right extremity of the porta hepatis to the inferior (caudal) border of the liver. Sonographically, on the transverse view, the gallbladder is located posterior to or partly within the main lobar fissure, between the right lobe and the medial segment of the left lobe (Fig. 1). On the longitudinal view, the linear hyperechoic main lobar fissure can be seen between the gallbladder caudally and the right portal vein cranially in many persons (nearly 70%) (Fig. 1) (1). Recognition of this relation of the gallbladder to the main lobar fissure is important, especially when the gallbladder is contracted, contains no fluid (bile), or is completely filled with stones or sludge. The gallbladder is divided into fundus, body, and neck (Fig. 2). The fundus is the expanded distal end, and the neck is the narrow proximal end continuous with the cystic duct. The mucous membrane lining the interior of the neck and the cystic duct has a series of crescentic folds, presenting an appearance of a spiral valve (Heister's valves; Fig. 2). From the right wall of the neck of the gallbladder, a small pouch (Hartmanns's pouch) may project toward the duodenum; however, it is not sonographically discernible (2). Sonographically, the gallbladder is an anechoic, fluid-filled, pear-shaped or ellipsoid structure, widest at the fundus and narrowest at the neck. The wall of the normal gallbladder is predominantly hyperechoic and sharply defined, and it measures 3 mm or less in thickness. Measurements are most accurate when the anterior wall of the gallbladder is measured in the long-axis view of the gallbladder, with the sound beam perpendicular to the wall of the gallbladder. Minor angulation of the transducer or decentering can cause pseudothickening of the gallbladder wall. The normal gallbladder is 8 to 12 cm in length. The anteroposterior diameter, as measured on long-axis view of the gallbladder, and the transverse diameter are normally less than 4 cm in adults (3).

The normal gallbladder in children is less than 3.5 cm in transverse diameter and less than 7.5 cm in length (4). The mean normal transverse diameter ranges from 1 cm at one year to 2 cm at 12 to 16 years of age (4). The thickness of the wall of the normal gallbladder in children is less than 3 mm (4). The normal gallbladder in the newborn and in infants under one year is less than 3 cm in length (with a range of 1.5–3 cm) and less than 1 cm in transverse diameter (3,4).

The shape of the gallbladder can vary because of its folds. The folds are caused by infolding of the gallbladder wall and do not represent true septations within the gallbladder. The most common fold (the junctional fold)

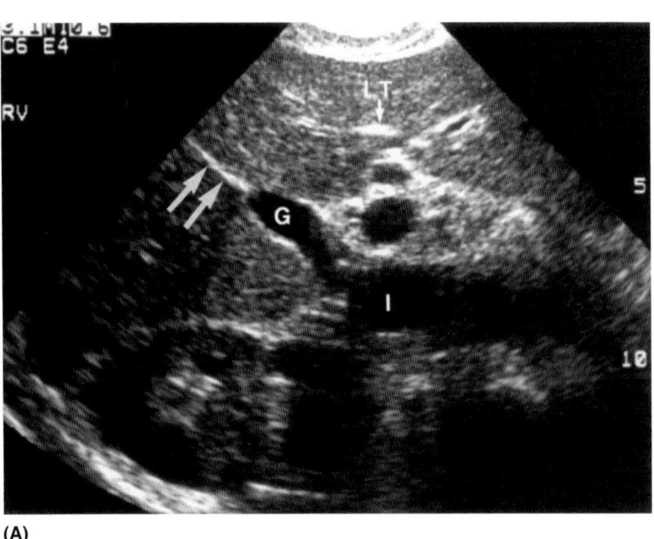

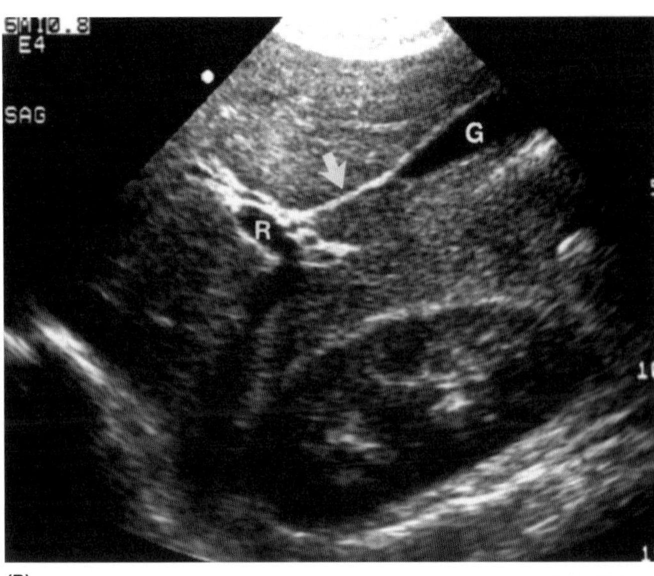

(A) (B)

FIGURE 1 A AND B ■ Relation of the gallbladder to the main lobar fissure. (**A**) Transverse view shows the gallbladder (G) posterior/linear to the hyperechoic main lobar fissure (*arrows*). (**B**) Longitudinal view shows a linear echo from the main lobar fissure (*arrow*) between the right portal vein and the gallbladder. LT, ligamentum teres; I, inferior vena cava; R, right portal vein.

is seen at the junction of the neck and the body of the gallbladder (Fig. 3). Less commonly, folds can occur in the mid-body or distal body of the gallbladder, and multiple folds can give the gallbladder a sigmoid (S) shape (Fig. 3). A "phrygian cap" deformity is caused by folding of the fundus over the body of the gallbladder and is seen in approximately 4% of healthy persons (Fig. 3) (5). A phrygian cap deformity results when a mucosal fold partially subdivides the lumen of the gallbladder. Occasionally, prominent folds may cause acoustic shadowing (6). When only a part of the fold is visualized, it may mimic a polyp or a stone.

The normal gallbladder has a capacity of 30 to 50 mL (2). However, sonographic volume measurements are difficult to perform, and reported values (17–27 mL) for fasting volunteers vary widely (3).

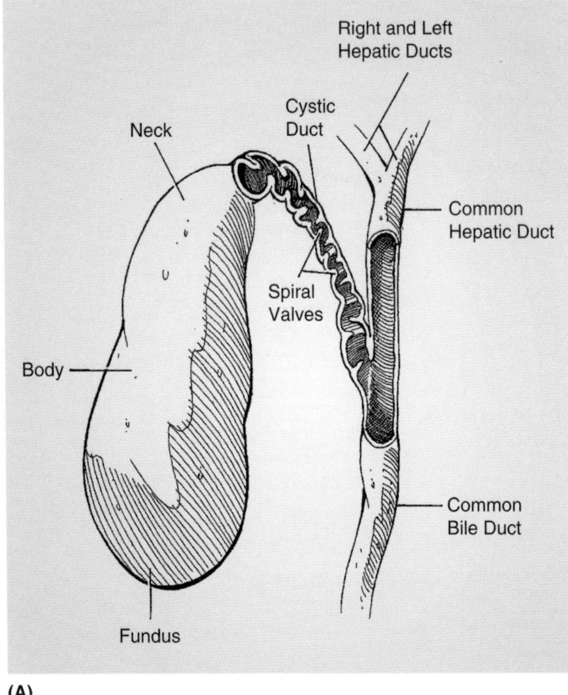

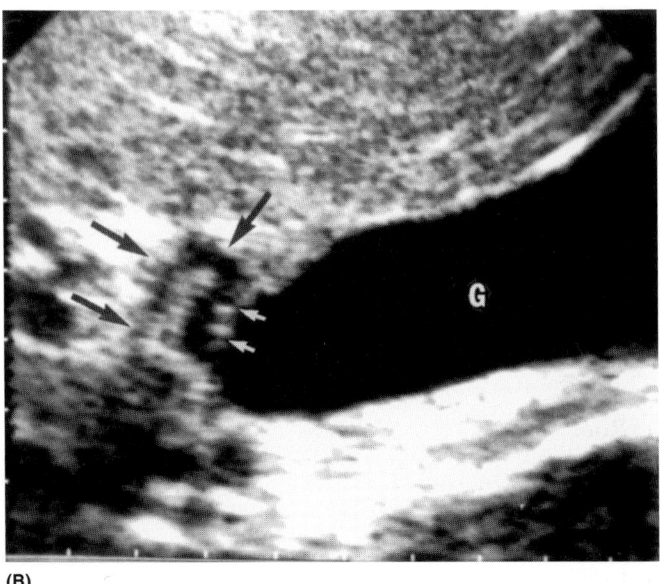

(A) (B)

FIGURE 2 A AND B ■ (**A**) Diagram of the normal biliary tree. (**B**) Gallbladder neck (G) and proximal cystic duct: longitudinal view demonstrating neck and slightly dilated proximal cystic duct (*arrows*). The serrated appearance of the walls of the cystic duct is secondary to valves of Heister.

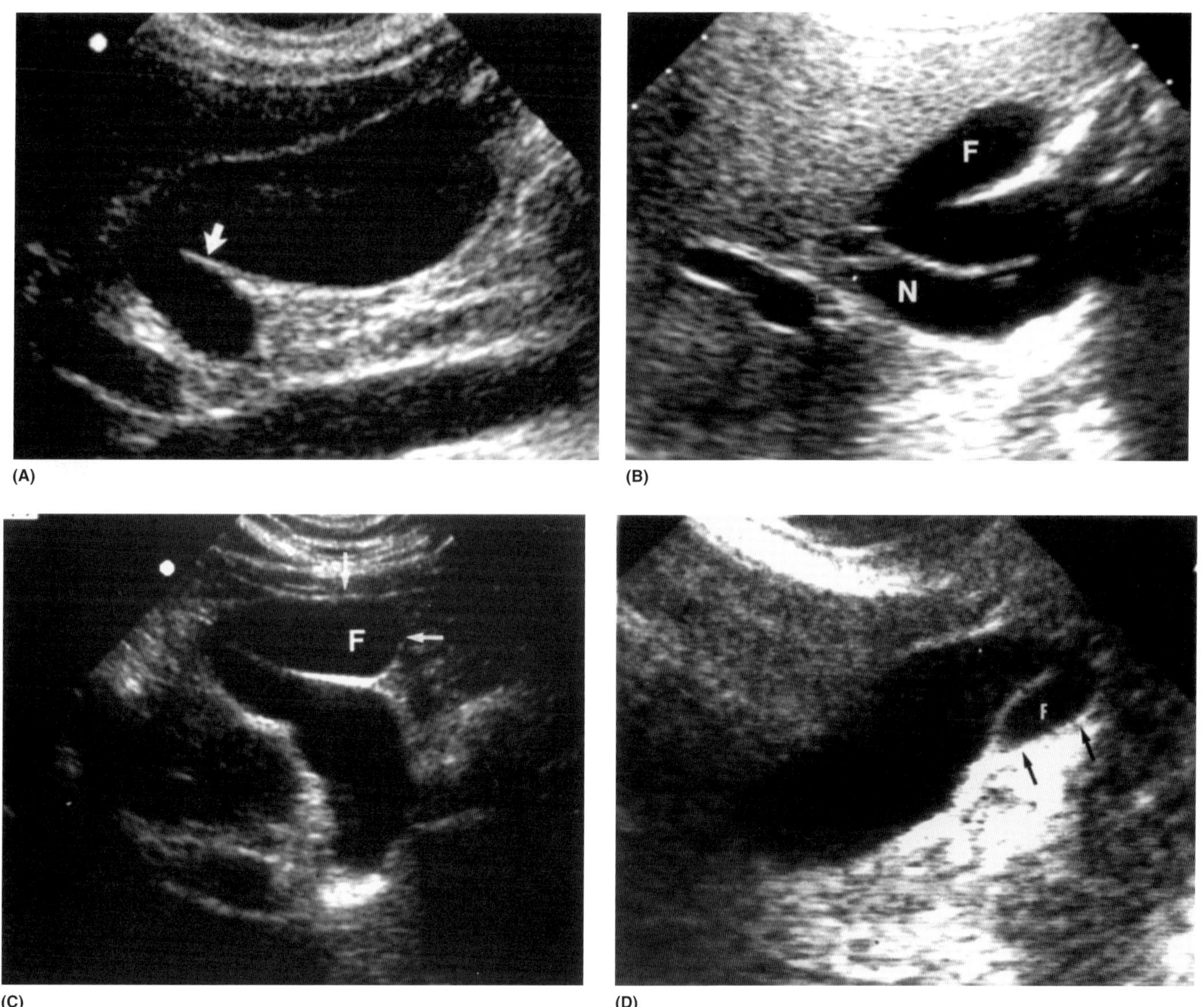

FIGURE 3 A–D ■ Gallbladder folds. (**A**) Longitudinal view showing the junctional fold (*arrow*) between the neck and the body of the gallbladder. (**B**) Longitudinal view showing a sigmoid gallbladder secondary to multiple folds. (**C** and **D**) Phrygian cap. Longitudinal views show a phrygian cap deformity (*arrows*) caused by folding of the fundus over the body of the gallbladder. N, neck; F, fundus of the gallbladder.

Scanning Technique

Sonography of the gallbladder is ideally performed with the patient fasting for 8 to 12 hours before the examination. However, in emergency situations, the gallbladder can be examined without the patient's fasting. The examination is usually performed using a 3.5 to 5MHz transducer. Routine examination includes scanning subcostally in supine and left posterior oblique positions. Scanning may be performed intercostally, if there is shadowing from bowel gas. Additionally, examination in either the erect or the prone position, preferably the prone position, is often helpful (7). The prone view is obtained by scanning in transverse and coronal planes, with the transducer placed in the right lateral intercostal spaces at the right mid-axillary line with the patient in the prone position and using the liver as an acoustic window (7). The prone view is useful for demonstrating the mobility of the stones, for avoiding reverberation artifacts in anteriorly placed gallbladders (Fig. 4), for avoiding shadowing from bowel gas, and for demonstrating stones hidden in the neck of the gallbladder. Occasionally, stones or sludge in the gallbladder can be demonstrated exclusively on prone views.

In a study of patients with completely contracted gallbladders after overnight fasting, reexamination with ultrasound 30 minutes after fatty meal demonstrated distended gallbladders containing stones (8). Therefore, the authors of this study concluded that in patients whose gallbladders are completely contracted after overnight fasting and cannot be adequately evaluated on sonography, reexamination after a fatty meal may be helpful (8).

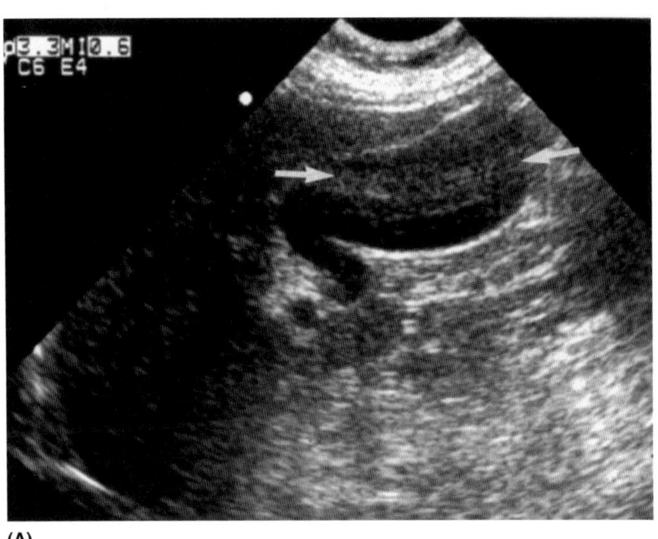

(A)

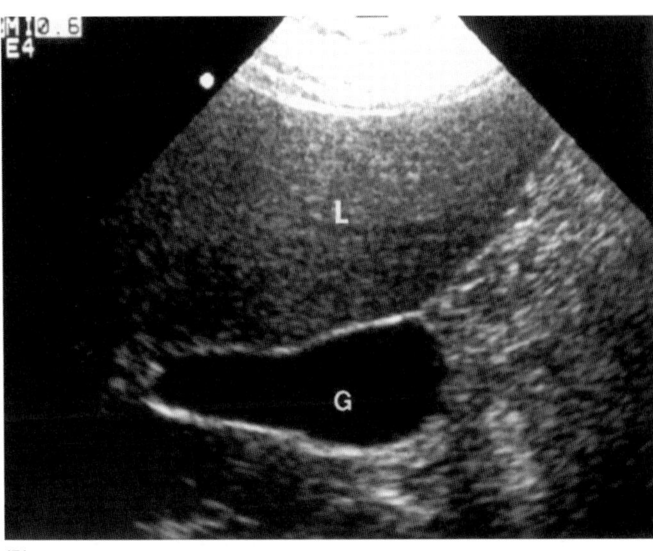

(B)

FIGURE 4 A AND B ■ Prone view. (**A**) Reverberation artifacts (*arrows*) obscure part of the anteriorly located gallbladder on the supine view. (**B**) On the prone view, the gallbladder is clearly seen without reverberation artifacts. No reverberations occur within the gallbladder because of the larger volume of the liver between the transducer and the gallbladder on the prone view. G, gallbladder; L, liver.

Pitfalls

A hepatic cyst or a renal cyst, located near the gallbladder fossa, or a choledochal cyst may mimic a gallbladder. The relation of the cystic structure to the main lobar fissure and the shape of the cystic structure help to distinguish these from the true gallbladder. The choledochal cyst can be distinguished from the gallbladder by its continuity with the common bile duct.

Congenital Abnormalities

Congenital abnormalities of the gallbladder include agenesis, ectopic location, duplication, multiseptate gallbladder, and diverticulum of the gallbladder (Table 1).

Agenesis of the Gallbladder

Agenesis of the gallbladder is a rare anomaly, with a reported incidence of 0.01% to 0.04% (9–11). The diagnosis may be suggested by sonographic nonvisualization of the gallbladder, but it must be confirmed by other imaging modalities, and only operative findings including cholangiography can be considered diagnostic.

Ectopic Location

The most common ectopic or anomalous locations of the gallbladder are (*i*) on the left side (posterior to the left lobe), (*ii*) intrahepatic, followed by (*iii*) suprahepatic (between the right lobe of the liver and the diaphragm), and (*iv*) retrohepatic (posterior to the right lobe of the liver) (Fig. 5). Other reported ectopic sites include the gallbladder in the retroperitoneum posterior to the right kidney, lateral to the right lobe of the liver, within the falciform ligament, within the anterior abdominal wall, and in the lesser peritoneal sac (11–14).

Duplication of the Gallbladder

Duplication is a rare anomaly, with an incidence of one in 3000 to 4000 (15–17). Sonography demonstrates either two contiguous cystic structures with a septum dividing the entire length of the two cavities, or two cystic structures slightly separated from each other (Fig. 6). Definitive diagnosis of double gallbladder requires demonstration, which is difficult sonographically, of two separate cystic

TABLE 1 ■ Congenital Abnormalities of the Gallbladder

Abnormality	Ultrasound features
Agenesis of the gallbladder	Nonvisualization of the gallbladder
	Confirmation with other tests
Ectopic gallbladder location	Abnormal locations
	Posterior to left lobe
	Intrahepatic
	Suprahepatic
	Posterior to right lobe
	Others (much rarer)
Duplication of the gallbladder	Either two separate cystic structures or contiguous cystic structures with septum
	Triple or quadruple gallbladders (very rare)
Multiseptate gallbladder	Multiple septa
	Septa traversing entire lumen
	Honeycomb appearance
Gallbladder diverticulum	Outpouchings of lumen
	Any location in gallbladder

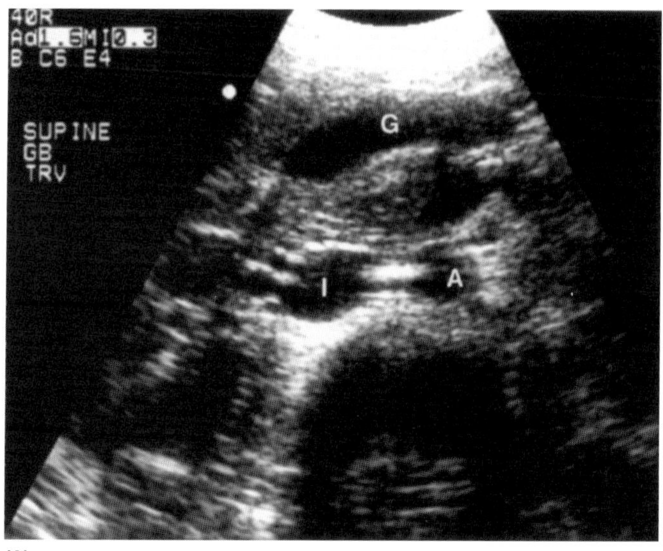

(A)

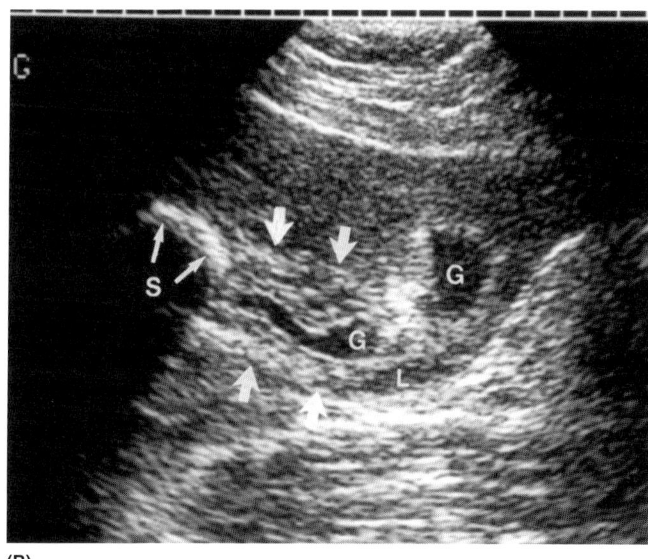

(B)

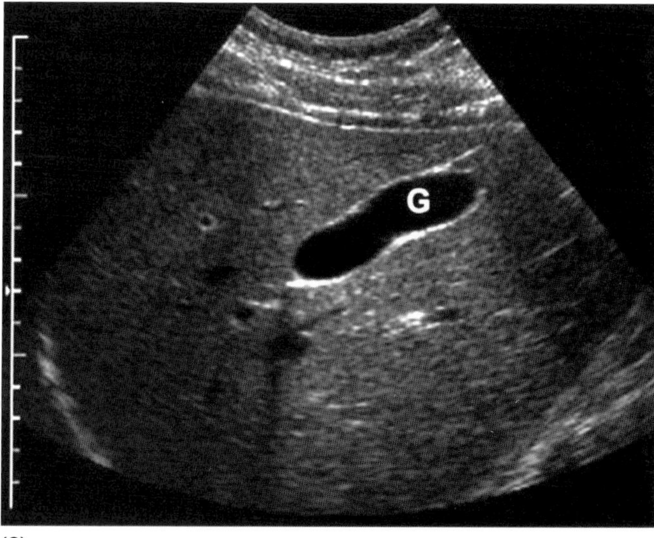

(C)

FIGURE 5 A–C ■ Ectopic location of the gallbladder. (**A**) Transverse view showing a transversely oriented gallbladder located anteriorly in the midline and extending into the left abdomen. (**B**) Intrahepatic gallbladder: longitudinal view showing the entire gallbladder located within the liver surrounded by liver parenchyma. The patient has acute cholecystitis with a thick gallbladder wall (*large arrows*) and a stone in the neck of the gallbladder with distal shadowing. (**C**) Intrahepatic gallbladder: longitudinal view of the right lobe in a different patient showing the entire gallbladder located within the liver surrounded by liver parenchyma. G, gallbladder; I, inferior vena cava; A, aorta; S, stone; L, posterior margin of the liver. *Source*: (**C**) Courtesy of Oksana Baltarowich, MD, Philadelphia, PA.

ducts. Less commonly, the gallbladder may be bilobed with a single cystic duct. Triple and quadruple gallbladders have also been reported.

Multiseptate Gallbladder

Multiseptate gallbladder is a rare anomaly manifested by multiple septations within the entire gallbladder or part of the gallbladder. Sonographically, multiple thin septa are seen within the gallbladder, most of them traversing the entire gallbladder lumen and sometimes producing a honeycomb appearance (18–20). The differential diagnosis includes intraluminal membranes in gangrenous cholecystitis and polypoid cholesterolosis. The clinical setting of acute cholecystitis differentiates intraluminal membranes from multiseptate gallbladder. In polypoid cholesterolosis, the polyps projecting from the wall are more bulbous and do not traverse the entire lumen of the gallbladder.

Diverticulum

True diverticulum of the gallbladder is an extreme rarity (Fig. 7) (21). It can occur anywhere in the gallbladder, is

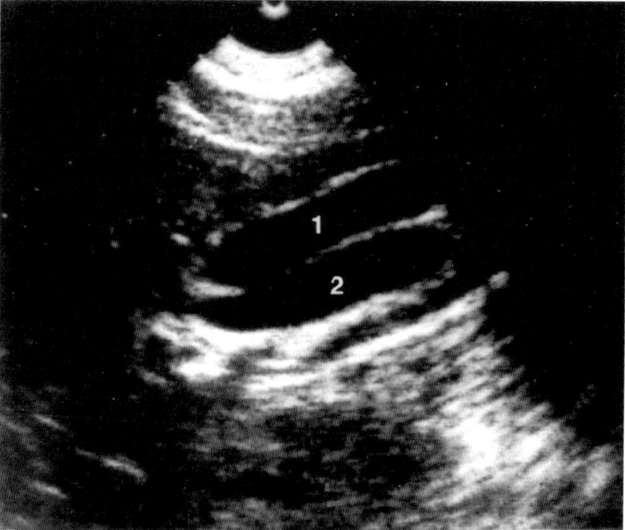

FIGURE 6 ■ Duplication of the gallbladder. Two gallbladders (1, 2) are seen on the longitudinal view. *Source*: Courtesy of Jerome A. Adell, RDMS, Cleveland, OH.

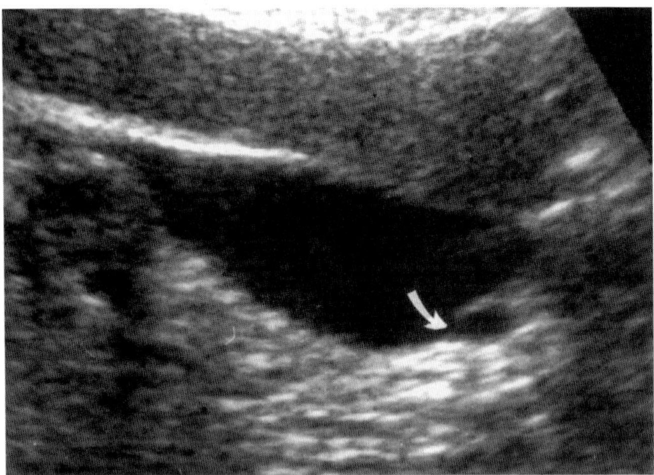

FIGURE 7 ■ A small diverticulum (*arrow*) of the gallbladder is seen protruding from the wall of the gallbladder.

usually single, and varies greatly in size. Pseudodiverticula can be seen in adenomyomatosis. Traction diverticula from adjacent adhesions may also occur.

Abnormalities of Size

Enlarged Gallbladder

The gallbladder is considered distended when the anteroposterior diameter on the long-axis view or the transverse diameter exceeds 4 cm (in adults). Numerous causes of gallbladder distension are known, including acute cholecystitis, cystic duct or common bile duct obstruction, hyperalimentation, prolonged fasting, postsurgical distension, and diabetes mellitus. In children, gallbladder distension can be seen secondary to Kawasaki's disease (mucocutaneous lymph node syndrome) (22–26). Hydrops of the gallbladder in infants and children has also been reported to be associated with total parenteral nutrition and, less commonly, with upper respiratory infections, gastroenteritis, scarlet fever, and leptospirosis (22–27).

Small Gallbladder

The gallbladder is considered abnormally contracted if the diameter (in adults) is less than 2 cm despite adequate fasting (28). Causes of small or contracted gallbladder include postprandial examination, chronic cholecystitis, acute viral hepatitis, cystic fibrosis, and congenital hypoplasia (Fig. 8).

Cholelithiasis

Symptomatic gallbladder disease secondary to gallstones accounts for substantial morbidity and mortality. Approximately 10% to 15% of the population may be affected by cholelithiasis (29). The incidence of gallstones increases with age, and specific risk factors include obesity, rapid weight reduction, ileal disease or resection, hyperalimentation, elevated triglyceride levels, and ethnic background (highest in Pima Indians) (30). Patients treated with ceftriaxone (parenteral cephalosporin) have an increased incidence of gallstones and sludge that resolve and disappear spontaneously with discontinuation of the drug (31). The gallstones may be composed of cholesterol, pigment (calcium bilirubinate), or calcium carbonate. Ninety percent of gallstones have mixed composition. Pure cholesterol stones represent 10% of all stones, and pure calcium carbonate stones are rare.

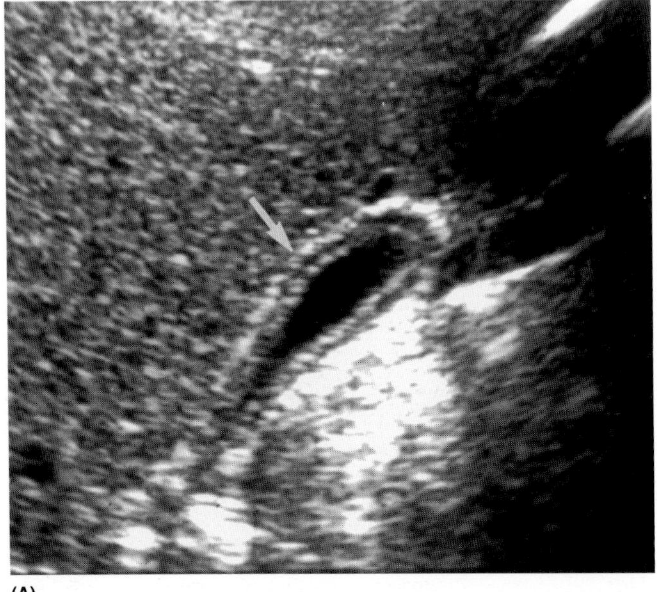

(A)

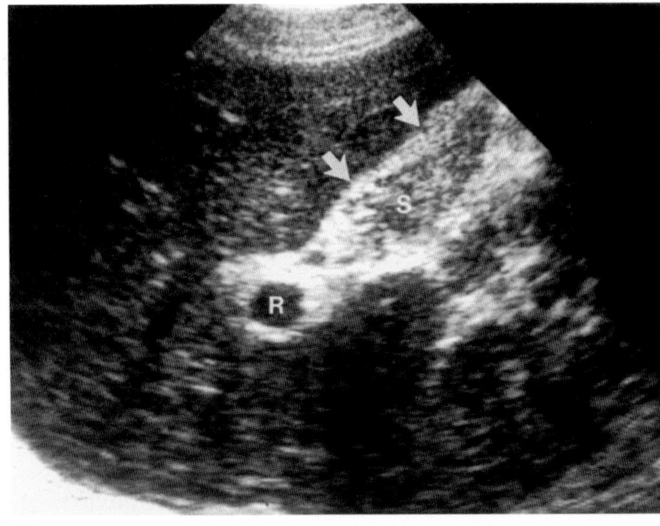

(B)

FIGURE 8 A AND B ■ Contracted gallbladder. (**A**) Small gallbladder secondary to postprandial physiologic contraction. The wall (*arrow*) appears prominent but is less than 3 mm thick. (**B**) Longitudinal view showing a thick-walled, contracted gallbladder (*arrows*) filled with sludge (S) secondary to acute viral hepatitis. R, right portal vein.

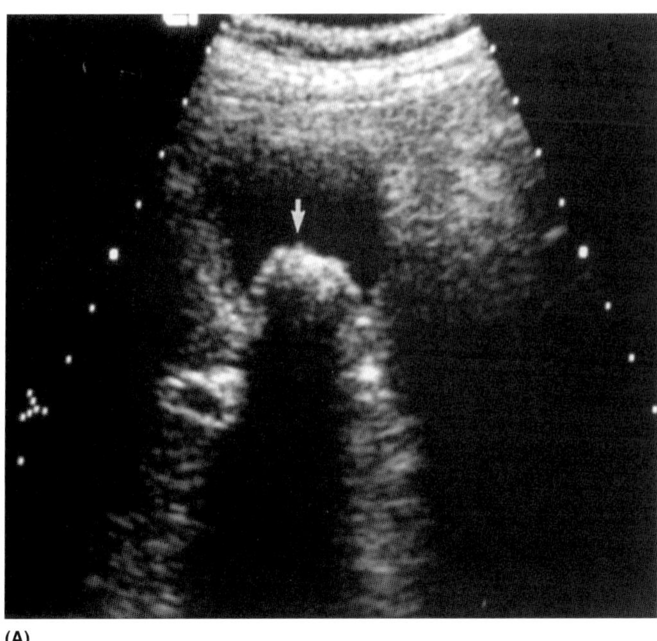
(A)

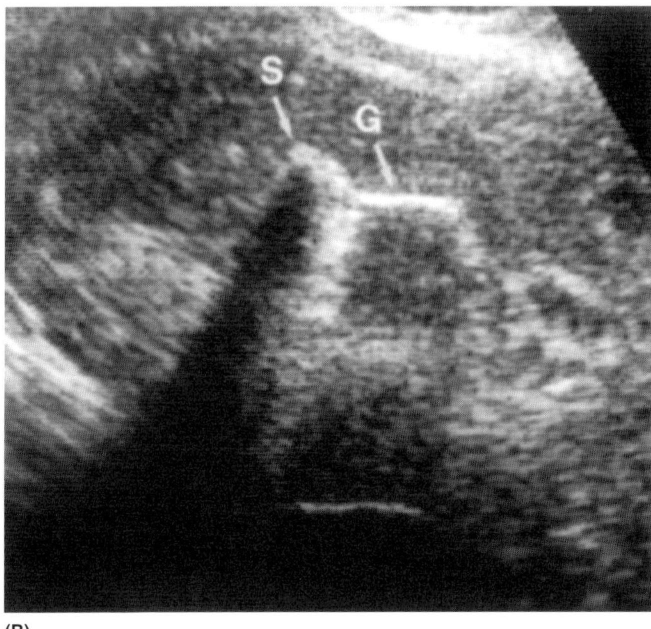

(B)

FIGURE 9 A AND B ■ Gallstone shadowing. (**A**) Gallstone (*arrow*) with a typical clean shadow. (**B**) Transverse view showing a clean shadow distal to a stone (S) within a contracted gallbladder. Adjacent gas in the bowel (G) produces dirty shadow and reverberation artifacts.

Only 20% (reported range of 10–40%) of gallstones are sufficiently calcified to be radiopaque on plain abdominal films. Most (up to 78%) of the patients with gallstones are asymptomatic (30). Gallstones may give rise to vague abdominal symptoms, but the most suggestive clinical finding is right upper quadrant abdominal pain secondary to postprandial biliary colic. Once symptomatic, patients have a 1% to 2% per year risk of developing acute cholecystitis or other complications (30). A residual gallbladder containing stones may be seen with abdominal ultrasound in patients with right upper quadrant pain after laparoscopic cholecystectomy, secondary to incomplete gallbladder resection (32).

Sonographically, an echogenic structure within the gallbladder lumen that causes distal acoustic shadowing and moves with gravity (change in patient position) is virtually 100% diagnostic of gallstone (Fig. 9). Accuracy of sonography in the diagnosis of gallstones is high, up to 96% (29,33). However, gallstone size and number cannot be estimated accurately by ultrasound examination (34,35). Most gallstones typically produce a clean acoustic shadow (i.e., a shadow with distinct margins and no echoes or reverberations within the shadow) (Fig. 9). In contrast, the bowel gas adjacent to the gallbladder typically produces a dirty shadow that has indistinct margins and contains echoes within the shadow as well as frequent reverberation artifacts within the shadow (Fig. 9). Most gallstones produce a clean shadow without reverberations because the attenuation of sound by most gallstones is caused primarily by absorption within the stone. Only 20% to 30% of the incident ultrasound is reflected by gallstones (36). In contrast, almost 99% of the incident ultrasound is reflected from the bowel gas, thus producing reverberations and backscattered echoes (dirty shadow). Some gallstones however may produce a dirty shadow (Fig. 10), secondary to low-level backscatter echoes within the shadow, which may be related to the surface characteristic of the stones; the stones with a smooth surface produce a dirty shadow, and those with a rough surface produce a clean shadow (37).

Reverberation artifacts may be caused by calcified stones, pure cholesterol stones, and fissured stones containing gas within the fissures. Typically, calcified gallstones produce a

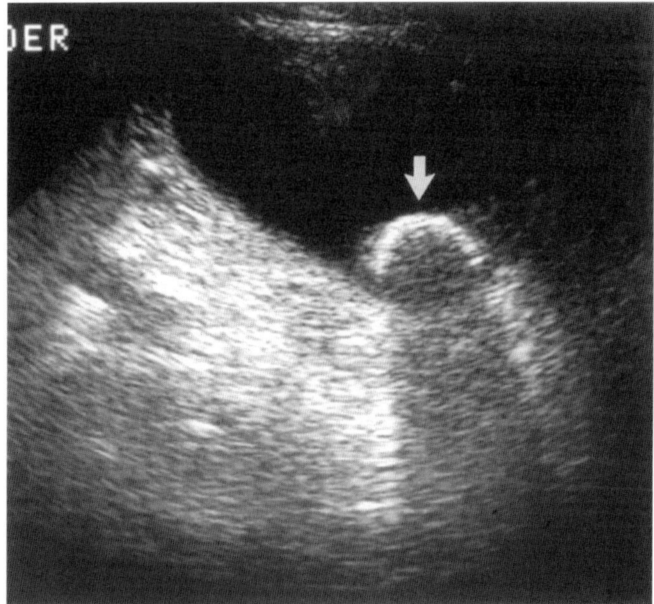

FIGURE 10 ■ Gallstone (*arrow*) producing a dirty shadow.

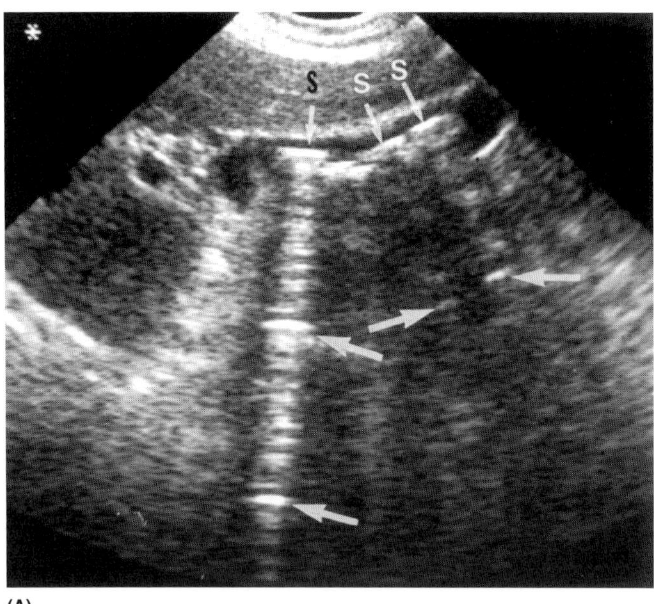

(A)

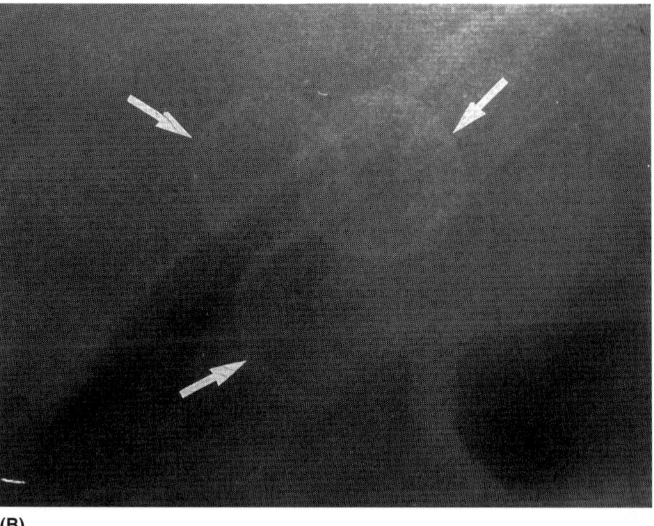

(B)

FIGURE 11 A AND B ■ Calcified gallstones. (**A**) Calcified gallstones produce (S) reverberation artifacts (*arrows*) within the shadows. The stone with heavier calcification (black S) produces more prominent reverberations and comet-tail artifacts. (**B**) Abdominal radiograph showing multiple stones (*arrows*) with varying degrees of calcification.

strong acoustic shadow containing predominantly widely spaced (at transducer-stone distance) reverberations and occasionally comet-tail artifacts (closely spaced reverberations) (Fig. 11) (38). In contrast, (purely or predominantly) cholesterol stones produce predominantly comet-tail artifacts (39). Particles of sludge or small fragments of stones (after biliary lithotripsy) containing cholesterol crystals may produce comet-tail artifacts without associated acoustic shadow (Fig. 12) (40).

Distal acoustic shadows are best seen when the stone lies within the focal zone of the transducer, is in the center of the beam, and is large in comparison with the beam width or wavelength (41). It is easier to demonstrate an acoustic shadow with a higher-frequency transducer or with a more nearly focused transducer, both of which situations narrow the width of the beam (Fig. 13) (42). High-gain settings may obscure the acoustic shadow by minimizing the difference between the shadow and the adjacent tissue. The acoustic shadow is likely to be stronger when the sound beam is perpendicular to the surface of the stone and weak or absent when the sound beam is largely tangential to the stone surface. Therefore, when an echogenic structure, especially small (less than 5 mm), is identified within the gallbladder lumen, but no shadow is seen, (*i*) reducing the overall or far gain, (*ii*) changing the angle between the transducer and the stone by slight alterations in transducer position or scanning the patient in different position, and (*iii*) scanning with a higher frequency transducer (5 MHz instead of 3.5 MHz) may produce a shadow and thereby indicate that a stone is present (41–44). Despite optimal technique, small (less than 3 mm) stones may not demonstrate acoustic shadowing. The shadowing effect of multiple small stones is cumulative and, therefore, is much easier to detect when multiple stones collect together within the gallbladder than when they are dispersed (Fig. 14).

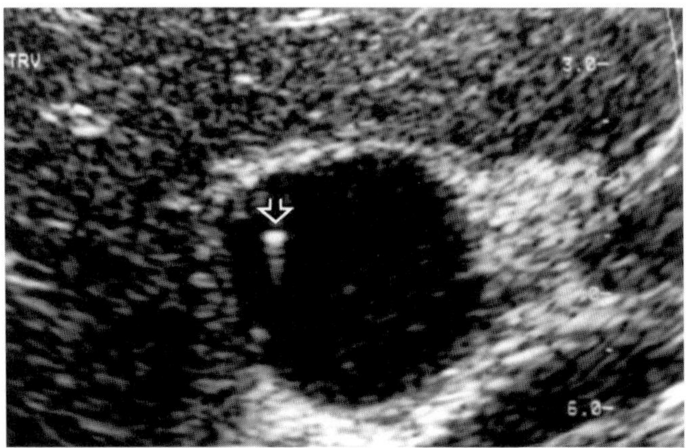

FIGURE 12 ■ Small (2 mm) intraluminal particle (*arrow*) containing cholesterol crystals produces a comet-tail artifact.

Wall-Echo-Shadow or Double Arc–Shadow Sign

When the gallbladder is completely filled with stones, a hyperechoic structure with distal acoustic shadowing is seen within the gallbladder fossa, and a fluid-filled gallbladder cannot be identified (Fig. 15). In these situations, it is essential to demonstrate the constant relation of the hyperechoic structures causing acoustic shadowing to the anatomic location of the gallbladder fossa in different patient positions, to confirm the origin of the shadow from within the gallbladder. The demonstration of a wall-echo-shadow (WES) or double arc–shadow sign, which consists of two parallel arcuate hyperechoic lines separated by a thin hypoechoic space and distal acoustic shadowing,

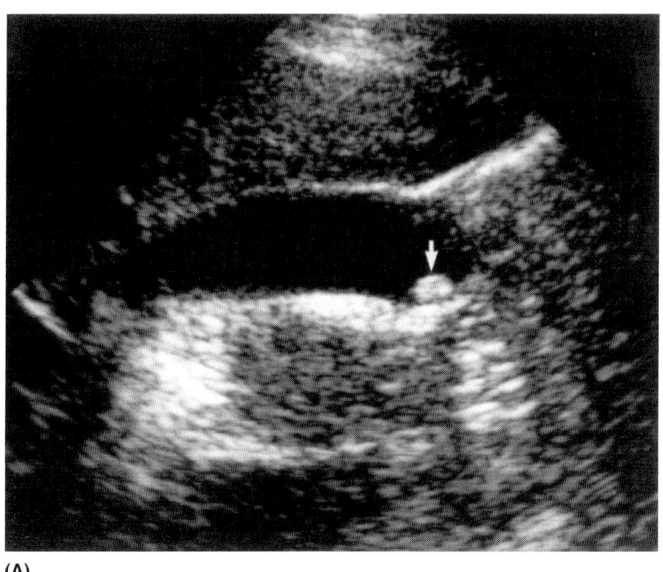

(A)

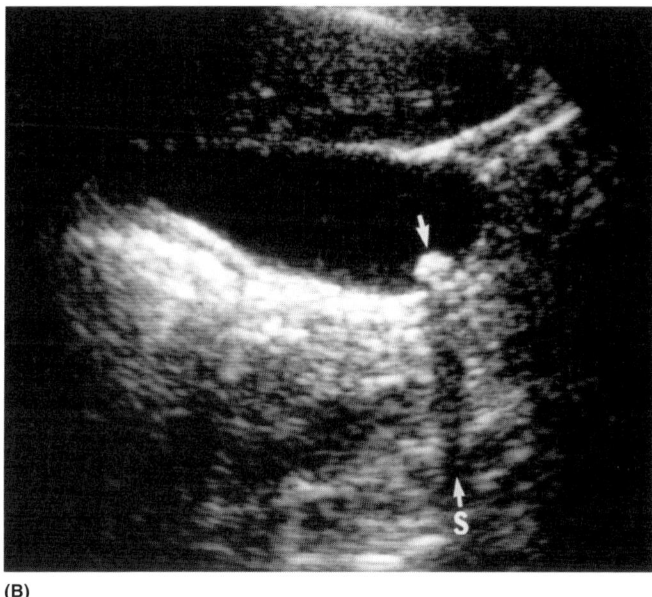

(B)

FIGURE 13 A AND B ■ Dependence of gallstone shadowing on transducer frequency. (**A**) No definite shadow is seen distal to the stone (*arrow*) with a 3.5 MHz transducer. (**B**) Definite acoustic shadowing (s) is seen distal to the stone (*arrow*) with a 5 MHz transducer.

confirms the diagnosis of gallstones (Fig. 15) (45–47). The proximal hyperechoic arc represents the wall of the gallbladder, the distal hyperechoic arc represents the reflections from gallstones, and the hypoechoic space in between represents either a small sliver of bile between the wall of the gallbladder and the gallstones or a hypoechoic portion of the wall of the gallbladder. This sign can be seen in approximately 80% of patients whose gallbladders are completely filled with stones. Gallstones usually produce a clean shadow without reverberation artifacts. Shadowing from the gallbladder fossa may also be caused by porcelain gallbladder (i.e., calcified wall of the gallbladder) or gas in the gallbladder in patients with acute emphysematous cholecystitis (Table 2). When double arc–shadow sign is absent or when shadowing is associated with reverberation artifacts, abdominal radiography or computed tomography should be obtained to exclude porcelain gallbladder or gas in the gallbladder.

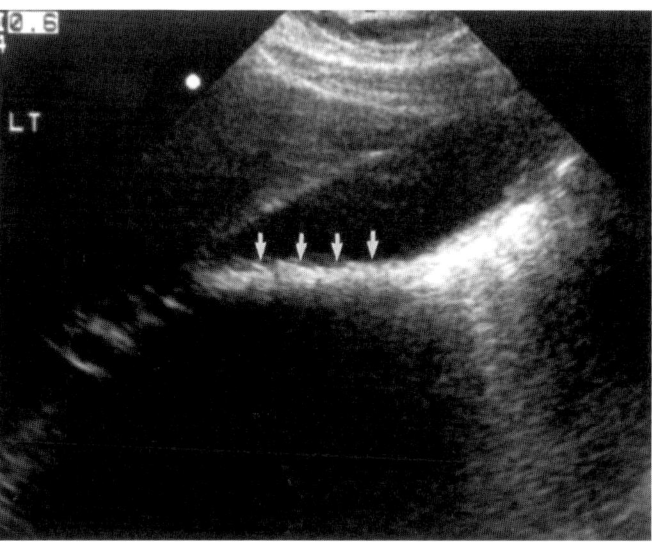

(A)

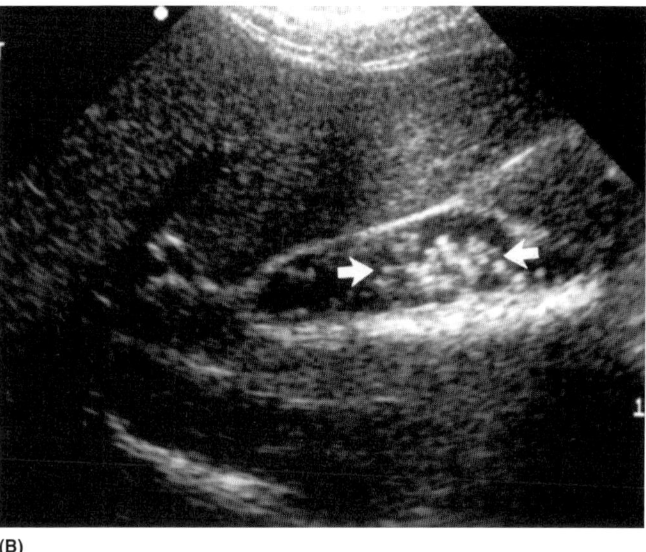

(B)

FIGURE 14 A AND B ■ (**A**) Multiple small stones layered together (*arrows*) produce acoustic shadowing. (**B**) When the small stones are dispersed within the gallbladder lumen (*arrows*), the small individual stones do not produce acoustic shadowing. The shadowing effect of multiple small stones is cumulative.

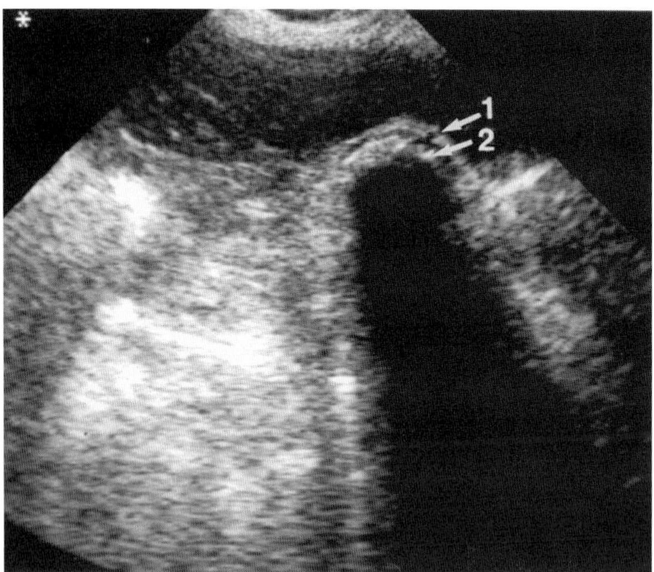

FIGURE 15 ■ Wall-echo-shadow (WES) or double arc–shadow sign. Two parallel arcuate hyperechoic lines (1, 2) are separated by a thin anechoic space with posterior acoustic shadowing, secondary to a contracted gallbladder filled with stones.

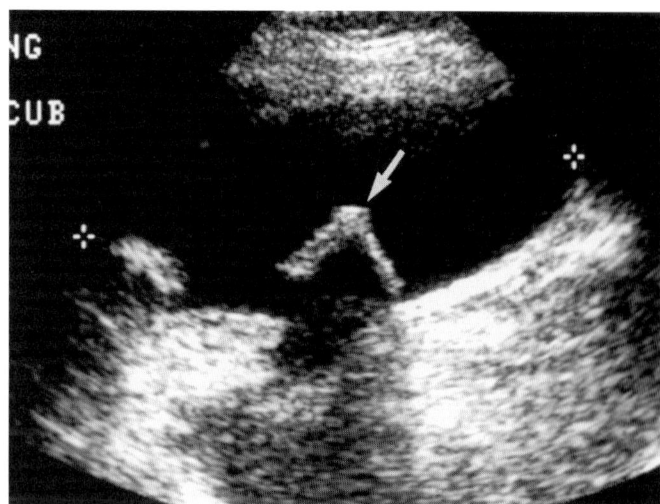

FIGURE 16 ■ Gallstone with a pyramidal shape (*arrow*).

Pyramidal Stones

Gallstones usually have a round or slightly faceted shape. However, occasionally, gallstones have flat surfaces with straight edges of equal length, producing unusual pyramidal shape on sonograms (Fig. 16) (48). Acoustic shadowing from pyramidal stones is often not as prominent as would be expected for their size.

Floating and Fissured Gallstones

Sonographically, most gallstones are seen in the dependent portion of the gallbladder because the specific gravity of the stones usually is greater than that of the bile. Stones, especially cholesterol stones, may float within the gallbladder when sonography is performed after ingestion of contrast material for oral cholecystography (49,50). The contrast material raises the specific gravity of the bile within the gallbladder, causing the stones to float. In the absence of contrast material, it is rare to find floating stones with sonography except when the specific gravity of the bile is raised because of biliary sludge or extrahepatic biliary obstruction (49–51). Another exception is gas-containing fissured stones, which may float even in the absence of contrast material within the gallbladder (Figs. 17 and 18) (52,53). The fissures most commonly are arranged in a triradiate pattern (Fig. 17); however, less commonly, gas-containing stones may have a large, rounded gas bubble surrounded by thin rim of solid material. If a large amount of gas is present within the stones, they may be associated with reverberations or comet-tail artifacts (Fig. 17). Fissured stones may also appear as two parallel linear echoes (double echo sign), probably secondary to reflections from the anterior surface of the stone and the gas within the stone (Fig. 18) (53). Gas-containing stones are rarely recognized on sonographic examination, even though gas has been noted by computed tomography in 4% of patients with visible stones (53).

TABLE 2 ■ Shadowing from Gallbladder Fossa

	Distinguishing features[a]			
Causes	Double arc–shadow or wall-echo-shadow sign	Shadow	Reverberations or comet-tail artifacts	Abdominal radiography or CT
Contracted gallbladder filled with stones	+	Clean	–	–
Porcelain gallbladder	–	Clean	–	Calcified wall
Gas in the gallbladder wall or lumen	–	Dirty	+	Gas in the gallbladder

Note: Occasionally, a small amount of gas in the gallbladder may produce shadow without reverberations. Calcified gallstones or heavily calcified wall of the gallbladder may produce reverberations.

[a]Double arc–shadow sign may be absent in contracted gallbladder filled with stones and rarely present in porcelain gallbladder.

Cholelithiasis in Children

Cholelithiasis in children is uncommon and has been associated with cystic fibrosis, hemolytic anemia (sickle-cell anemia, hereditary spherocytosis, and thalassemia), total parenteral nutrition, furosemide therapy, malabsorption, and bowel resection (54–56). In sickle-cell disease, sludge and stones can be seen in 20% to 30% of patients (56). In cystic fibrosis, a 12% incidence of gallstones has been reported (54). Reversible biliary sludge or cholelithiasis can be seen in children on ceftriaxone therapy (57).

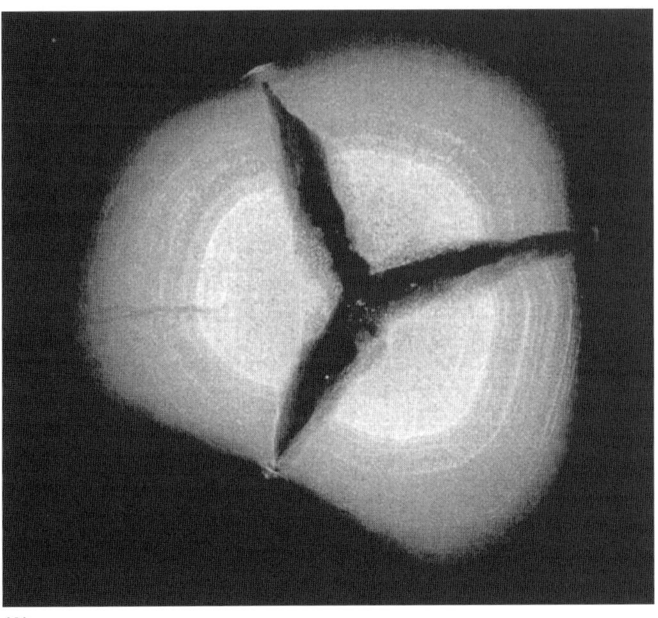

(A)

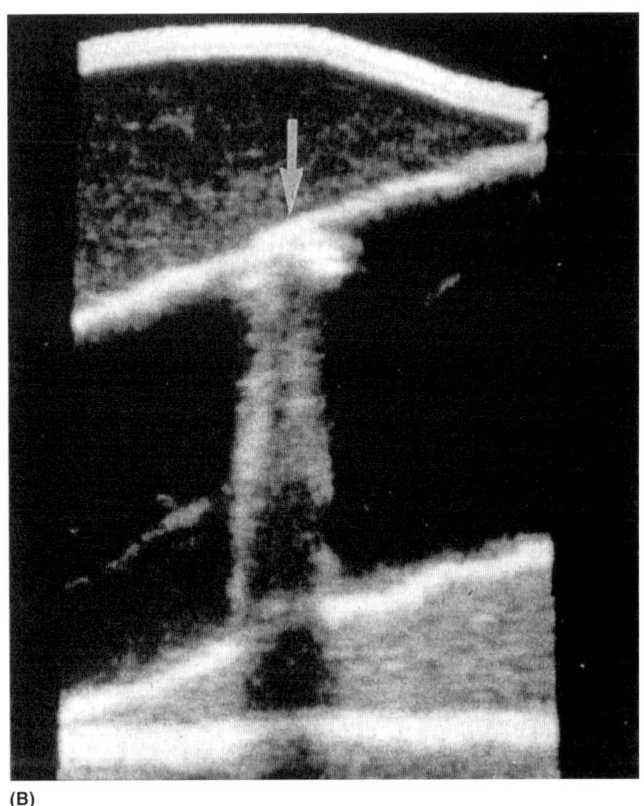

(B)

FIGURE 17 A AND B ■ Fissured stones. (**A**) In vitro radiograph of the fissured stone showing wide, gas-containing fissures within the stone. (**B**) In vitro sonogram showing a floating fissured stone (*arrow*) with associated comet-tail artifacts. *Source*: From Ref. 52.

Fetal Gallstones

Fetal gallstones are uncommon if not rare. The echogenic material in the fetal gallbladder may appear as typical stones with distal shadowing, echogenic foci without acoustic shadowing, echogenic sludge partially or completely filling the gallbladder, or, rarely, hyperechoic foci along the wall of the gallbladder with associated comet-tail reverberations (58–60). Most fetal gallstones are seen in the third trimester (58). In most reported cases, follow-up sonographic examinations performed between 1 and 12 months after birth demonstrated spontaneous resolution and disappearance of the gallstones (58–62). Therefore, in the absence of biliary obstruction or clinical sequelae, infants with gallstones diagnosed prenatally can be treated

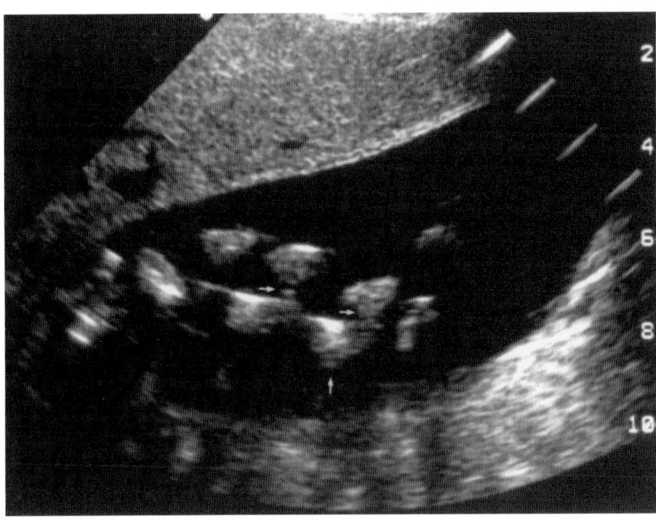

(A)

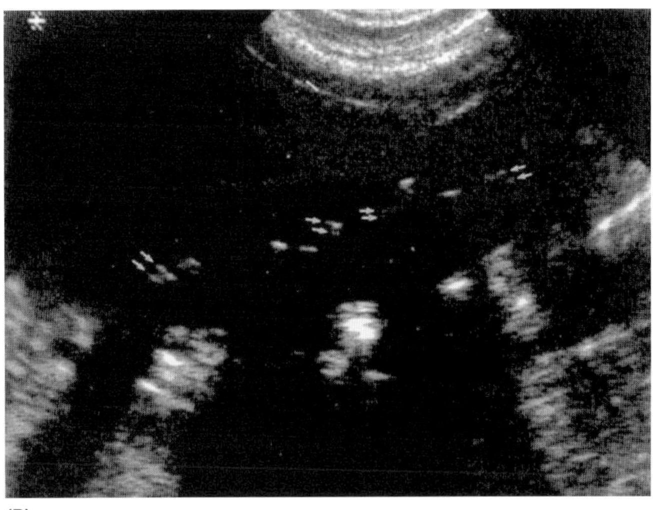

(B)

FIGURE 18 A AND B ■ Floating fissured stones. (**A**) Several fissured stones are seen floating within the gallbladder. Some of the stones are associated with short comet-tail artifacts (*arrows*). (**B**) "Double echo" sign: several small, floating, fissured stones with two parallel echoes (*arrows*) are seen in a nondependent position within the gallbladder.

TABLE 3 ■ Mobile Shadowing Echogenicities in the Gallbladder

Causes	Distinguishing features[a]
Gallstones	Clean shadow
Intraluminal gas bubbles	Reverberations or comet-tail artifacts
Calcified parasites (Clonorchis, Ascaris)	Clinical history and findings

[a]Calcified or cholesterol gallstones may produce reverberations, and occasionally, small gas bubbles may produce clean shadow without reverberations.

TABLE 4 ■ Nonmobile Shadowing Echogenicities in the Gallbladder

Causes	Distinguishing features
Partially seen fold	Contiguity with the rest of the fold
Gallstone impacted in neck	Acute cholecystitis; biliary colic
Gallstone adherent to wall	Strong shadow
Cholesterol polyp[a]	Weak, subtle shadow
Focal intramural gas in acute emphysematous cholecystitis	Reverberations
Adenomyomatosis with stone in Rokitansky–Aschoff sinus	Presence of other echogenic foci in the wall with comet-tail artifacts

[a]Shadowing from a cholesterol polyp is rare.

conservatively. Whether these stones dissolve or are passed through the biliary tract into the duodenum is uncertain.

Pitfalls in Diagnosis

Mobile Shadowing Echogenicities ■ Intraluminal gas bubbles and, rarely, calcified parasites may cause shadowing and mimic gallstones (Table 3). Gas bubbles frequently are associated with reverberation or comet-tail artifacts. Gas bubbles, however, may be seen as echogenic foci without shadowing or reverberations. Calcified parasites may be suspected in the appropriate clinical setting and geographic location.

Nonmobile Shadowing Echogenicities ■ Folds in the gallbladder when partially visible may produce echoes occasionally associated with acoustic shadowing (Fig. 19) (Table 4). These can be distinguished from stones by demonstrating their contiguity with the rest of the fold by scanning in different planes. Occasionally, gallstones may adhere to the wall of the gallbladder. Rarely, cholesterol polyps may cause shadowing, although the shadow is usually subtle. Focal intramural gas in acute emphysematous cholecystitis may mimic stone; however, it is usually associated with reverberations or comet-tail artifact.

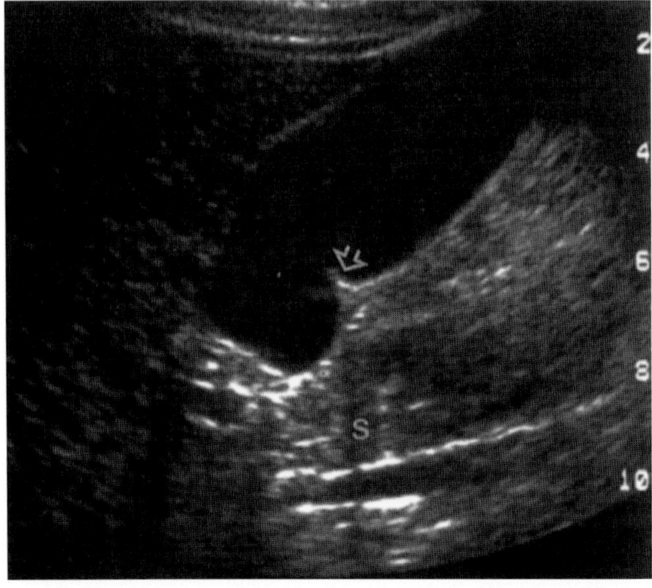

FIGURE 19 ■ Part of a fold (*arrow*) within the gallbladder producing an acoustic shadow (S).

Mobile Nonshadowing Echogenicities ■ Small (less than 3 mm) gallstones may not cause acoustic shadow (Table 5). Amorphous aggregated material containing sludge may present as a mobile intraluminal nonshadowing echogenic mass (sludge ball) (Fig. 20) (63). On follow-up sonograms, sludge balls usually change in appearance or disappear. Blood clots or aggregated material containing infectious debris or pus can usually be recognized from the patient's clinical history (i.e., cause for hemobilia or evidence of sepsis). Parasites (Ascaris, Clonorchis, and Fasciola) in the gallbladder can be suspected from the clinical history and occasionally can be recognized by the spontaneous movement of living worms.

Adjacent Bowel ■ Residue in the bowel contiguous with and indenting the posterior wall of the gallbladder may appear hyperechoic, with relatively clean distal shadowing, and may mimic gallstone (Fig. 21). This artifact can be recognized by scanning the patient in different positions, a method that usually moves the bowel away from the gallbladder.

Edge Refraction Shadow ■ Edge refraction shadow near the neck on the longitudinal section can be differentiated

TABLE 5 ■ Mobile Nonshadowing Echogenicities in the Gallbladder

Causes	Distinguishing features
Small gallstones (<3 mm)	Symptoms, persistence over time
Sludge balls	Change in appearance over time
Blood clots	Clinical evidence of hemobilia; change in appearance over time
Infectious debris; pus	Sepsis
Parasites (Ascaris, Clonorchis, Fasciola)	Clinical history and findings; spontaneous movements of living worms

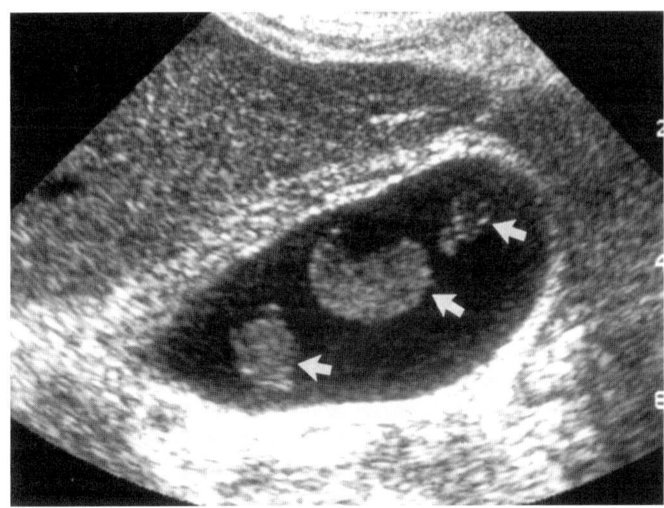

FIGURE 20 ■ Sludgeballs (*arrows*) within the gallbladder appearing as nonshadowing echogenic structures.

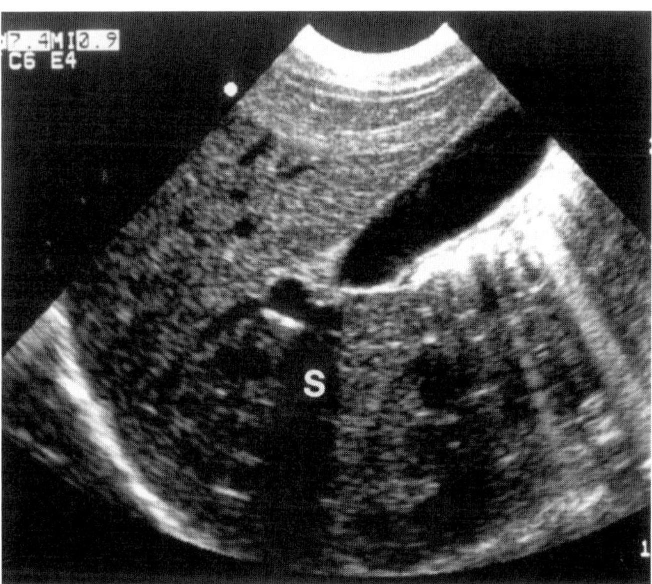

FIGURE 22 ■ Pitfall. Edge refraction shadow (S) produced from the neck of the gallbladder mimics shadowing produced by a gallstone.

from a stone by scanning in different positions and by the absence of visible stone at the origin of the shadow (Fig. 22).

Extracorporeal Shock Wave Lithotripsy

Extracorporeal shock wave lithotripsy (ESWL) is used for fragmentation of stones within the gallbladder. With the advent of laparoscopic cholecystectomy, ESWL is rarely used in the United States. Sonography is used for targeting during lithotripsy. Performance of gallbladder ESWL requires a thorough knowledge of sonographic anatomy and technique to localize gallstones and their fragments rapidly during the procedure (64). The criteria for patient eligibility include the presence of fewer than three stones within the gallbladder, stone size of less than 3 cm, the absence of calcification within the stone on abdominal radiograph, and the presence of gallbladder function by oral cholecystography (65). For determining the number of stones, oral cholecystography is better than sonography. Measurement of the size of the stones, especially large stones, may be less accurate with sonography than with oral cholecystography. The smaller the fragments after ESWL, the faster the patient becomes stone free. ESWL results are best with noncalcified single stones no larger than 2 cm (66). Stone-free rates after ESWL range from 20% to 41% of patients at six months (65). Various degrees of gallbladder wall thickening and pericholecystic fluid are commonly seen early after treatment and usually resolve promptly without clinical sequelae.

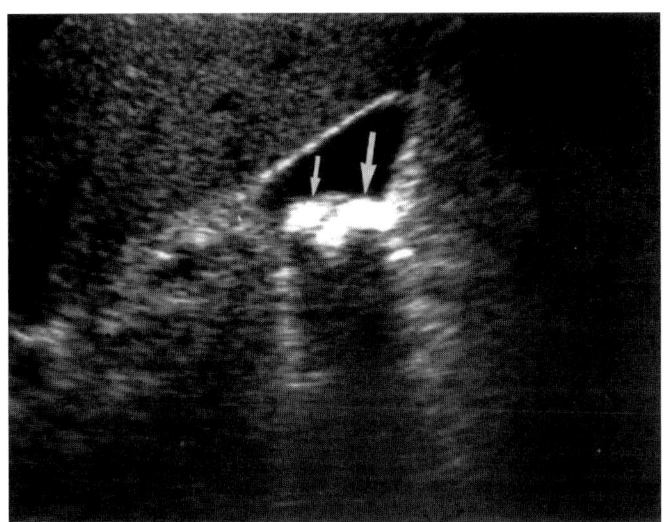

FIGURE 21 ■ Pitfall. Residue in the bowel indenting the posterior wall of the gallbladder mimics gallstones (*arrows*) with distal acoustic shadowing.

Gallbladder Sludge

Gallbladder sludge or echogenic bile is most often seen in patients with prolonged fasting, with extrahepatic bile duct obstruction, with various intrinsic disorders of the gallbladder, and with sickle-cell disease or other causes of hemolysis. The sludge usually consists of bilirubinate granules and cholesterol crystals embedded in a gel matrix of mucous glycoproteins (67,68). Biliary sludge can develop within five to seven days in fasting patients after gastrointestinal surgery, in patients in intensive care units, and in trauma patients receiving total parenteral nutrition (69–71). Sludge often has a fluctuating course, including frequent disappearance and reappearance over several months or years, and it may be an intermediate step in the formation of stones. In a follow-up ultrasound study of 96 patients, 8% of the patients with sludge developed asymptomatic gallstones (72). Sonographically, the sludge produces nonshadowing, low-amplitude echoes that tend to layer in the most dependent portion of the gallbladder (Fig. 23) and move slowly when the patient changes position. Occasionally, the sludge can be

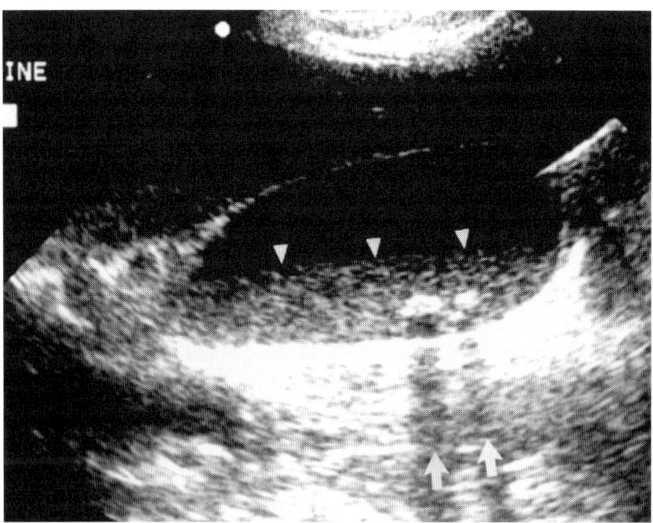

FIGURE 23 ■ Sludge (*arrowheads*) is seen as nonshadowing echogenic material layering in the dependent portion of the gallbladder. Two small stones with distal acoustic shadowing (*arrows*) are seen within the sludge.

TABLE 6 ■ Dependent Debris in the Gallbladder

Dependent debris	Sonographic findings
Sludge	Nonshadowing; dependent or entire gallbladder; mild to highly echogenic
Blood	Nonshadowing; dependent or entire gallbladder; variable echogenicity; associated with hemobilia
Pus	Associated findings of acute cholecystitis; nonshadowing echogenic debris throughout gallbladder
Multiple small gallstones	Echogenic layer with acoustic shadowing; occasionally, separate small stones
Pseudosludge	Artifactual; disappears with different transducer and patient positions
Milk of calcium bile	Flat echogenic layer with acoustic shadowing

highly echogenic. Other less common causes of echogenic debris within the gallbladder, indistinguishable from sludge, include blood, pus, or inflammatory debris within the gallbladder; however, these may be differentiated by the clinical findings (Table 6). Aggregated sludge may present as a mobile nonshadowing echogenic mass (sludge ball) (Fig. 20), or it may appear as a nonshadowing polypoid mass (tumefactive sludge) in the dependent portion of the gallbladder (Fig. 24) (63,73,74). Tumefactive sludge usually moves slowly with changes in patient position, but it may be nonmobile. Change in appearance or disappearance on follow-up sonograms (in several days or weeks) differentiates sludge ball or tumefactive sludge from a stone or neoplasm. Gallbladder entirely filled with sludge may be isoechoic with adjacent liver (sonographic hepatization of the gallbladder) and therefore difficult to identify (Fig. 24).

Pitfalls: Pseudosludge

Artifactual echoes mimicking sludge within the gallbladder, most commonly seen along the posterior surface of the gallbladder, can be produced secondary to slice-thickness artifact causing "partial-volume effect" or secondary to sidelobe artifacts (Fig. 25). These artifactual echoes usually disappear when the patient is scanned in different

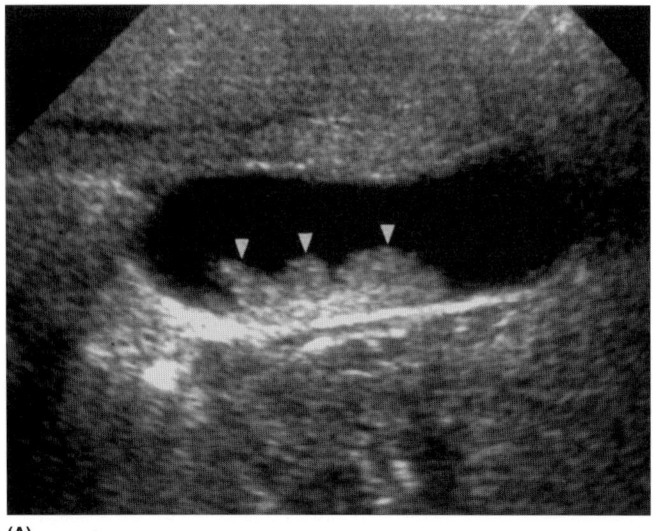

(A)

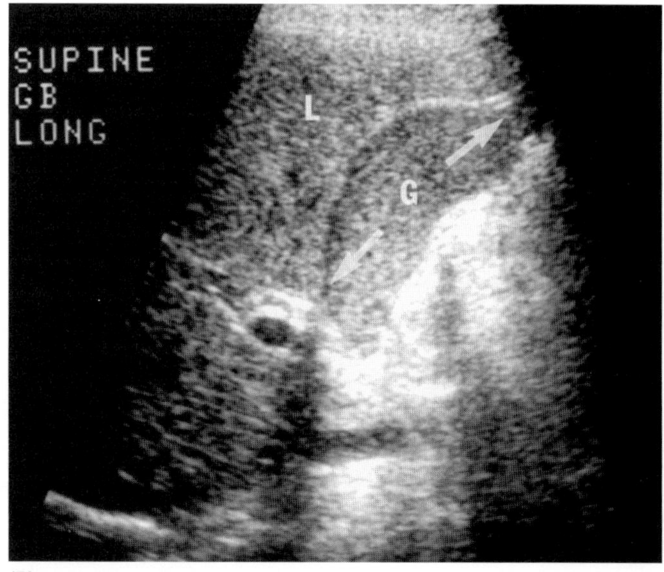

(B)

FIGURE 24 A AND B ■ Pitfalls. (**A**) Tumefactive sludge (*arrowheads*) appears as a polypoid mass within the gallbladder. (**B**) The gallbladder (G) (*arrows*) entirely filled with sludge is isoechoic with adjacent liver parenchyma (L).

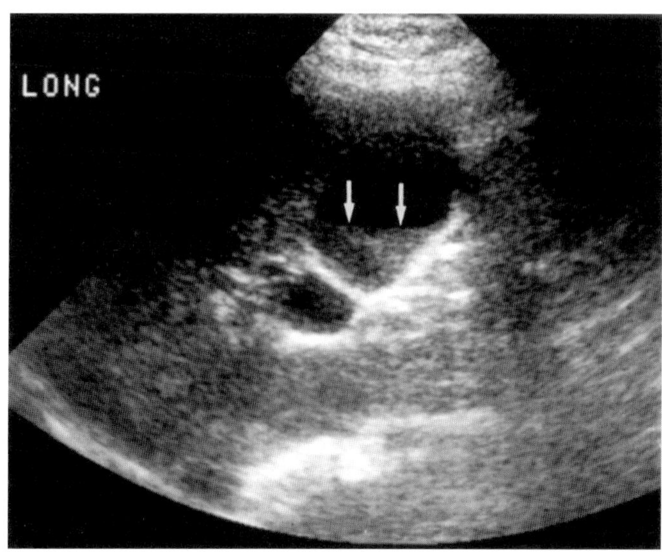

(A)

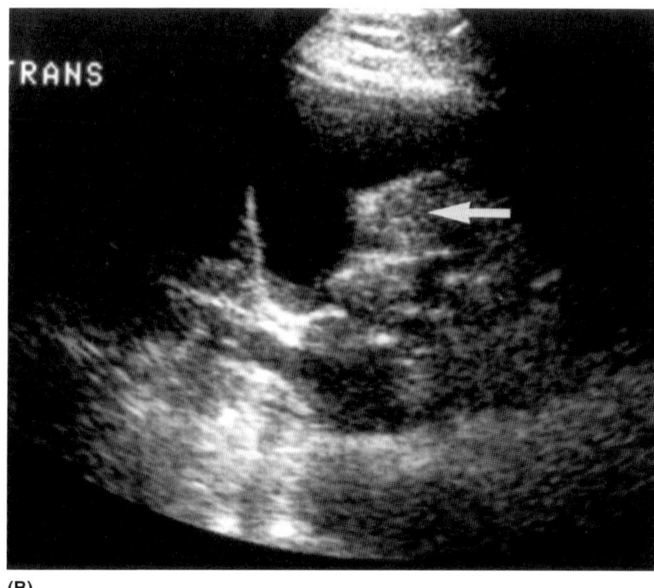

(B)

FIGURE 25 A AND B ■ Pitfall: pseudosludge. (**A**) Longitudinal view showing artifactual echoes appearing as layering sludge (*arrows*) within the gallbladder. (**B**) Transverse view showing residue in the bowel (*arrow*) indenting the medial wall of the gallbladder responsible for a partial-volume effect, causing artifactual echoes within the gallbladder on the longitudinal view.

positions, by changing the angulation of the transducer, and when the central portion of the gallbladder is scanned (75–77). Moreover, artifactual echoes do not layer with changes in patient position. Nondependence of the height of the debris on the receiver gain and lack of change in height of the debris between transverse and longitudinal scans are important characteristics of true sludge and help to differentiate true sludge from artifactual echoes (75).

Hemobilia

In patients with hemobilia, the blood may appear as echogenic or hyperechoic sludge within the gallbladder in the initial stage, and in the later stage, an echogenic, hyperechoic, or hypoechoic nonshadowing mobile mass (blood clot) may be seen within the gallbladder (Fig. 26) (Table 5) (78–81). Occasionally, the mass (i.e., hematoma) may be nonmobile and may mimic a polyp, carcinoma, or tumefactive

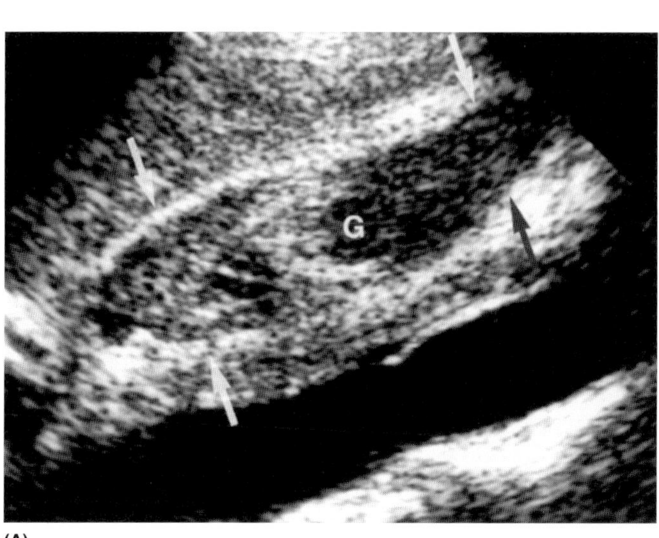

(A)

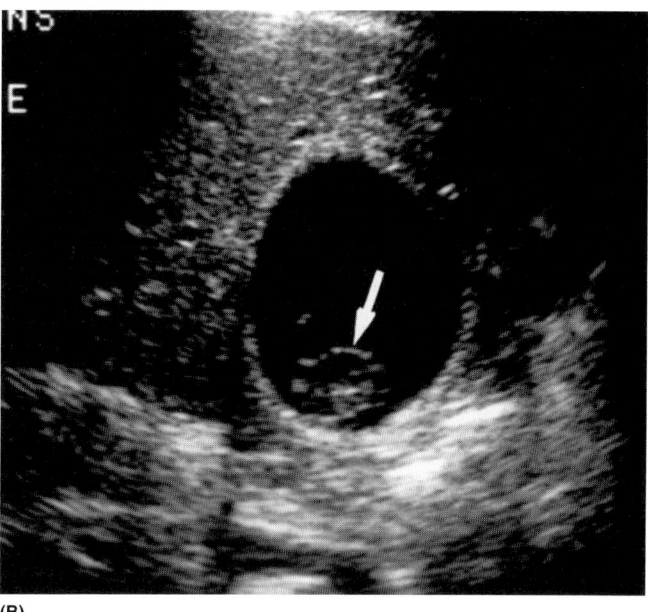

(B)

FIGURE 26 A AND B ■ Hemobilia. (**A**) Clotted blood filling the entire gallbladder (G) (*arrows*) has variable echogenicity. (**B**) Blood clot appearing as mobile, nonshadowing, hypoechoic structure (*arrow*) within the gallbladder.

sludge. Follow-up sonograms in a few days or weeks usually reveal a change in size or appearance, thus excluding a polyp or carcinoma. Causes of blood clot within the gallbladder secondary to hemobilia include liver trauma, most commonly liver biopsy or other invasive procedures, rupture of an aneurysm of the hepatic artery, cholecystitis, especially hemorrhagic cholecystitis, blood dyscrasias, biliary tumors, and vascular abnormalities.

Milk of Calcium Bile

Milk of calcium bile or limy bile is an uncommon disorder manifested by markedly thickened bile with high calcium content, usually calcium carbonate, within the gallbladder. It may be associated with chronic intermittent cystic duct obstruction by a stone, although it can be associated with chronic cholecystitis without obstruction at the neck of the gallbladder (82–84). Milk of calcium bile results in radiographic opacity of the gallbladder. Sonographic findings include echogenic or hyperechoic layering material with a flat fluid–fluid level, a convex meniscus, or an unusually shaped area within the gallbladder, all usually associated with acoustic shadowing (Fig. 27). Milk of calcium bile may produce a weak reverberation artifact (38). Diagnosis of milk of calcium bile can be confirmed by abdominal radiography or computed tomography.

Acute Cholecystitis

Acute cholecystitis complicates the course of symptomatic gallstones in 10% to 20% of patients (29). The cause of acute cholecystitis is not well understood, but it may result from bacterial infection or ischemia. Most of the cases are caused by obstruction of the cystic duct, usually by a gallstone, resulting in inflammation of the gallbladder wall. Clinically, patients most commonly present with constant pain that localizes in the right subcostal region, although epigastric pain may predominate in early stages. Physical findings are variable; right upper quadrant tenderness with involuntary guarding is common. Leukocytosis is also common, and abnormalities of liver function tests can occur. The differential diagnosis of acute cholecystitis includes acute appendicitis, acute pancreatitis, perforated gastroduodenal ulcers, right-sided nephroureterolithiasis, acute hepatitis, and hepatic congestion from right-sided cardiac failure (29). Sonographic findings that are nonspecific but suggestive of acute cholecystitis include gallstones, sludge, gallbladder distension, thickened gallbladder wall, especially hypoechoic or anechoic zone within the thickened wall, pericholecystic fluid, intraluminal membranes, positive sonographic Murphy's sign, and increased flow with color Doppler sonography (CDS) (Table 7) (85–89). By themselves, none of the sonographic findings are pathognomonic for acute cholecystitis; however, multiple positive sonographic findings yield greater accuracy in the sonographic diagnosis of acute cholecystitis. Sonography using multiple positive

TABLE 7 ■ Sonographic Findings Associated with Acute Cholecystitis

Gallstones
Gallbladder sludge
Gallbladder distension
Thickened gallbladder wall (especially hypoechoic zone)
Pericholecystic fluid
Intraluminal membranes
Positive sonographic Murphy's sign
Positive color Doppler (increased flow)

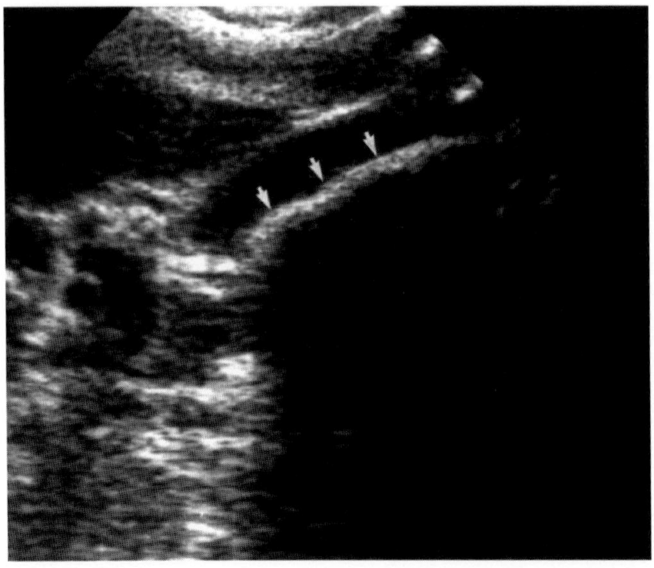

(A)

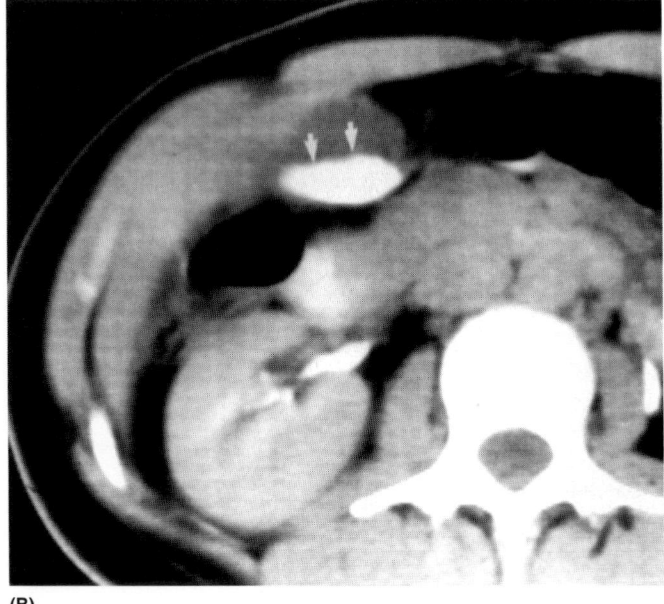

(B)

FIGURE 27 A AND B ■ Milk of calcium bile. (**A**) Milk of calcium bile appears as layering echogenic material (*arrows*) in the dependent portion of the gallbladder with associated acoustic shadowing. (**B**) Computed tomography showing layering milk of calcium bile (*arrows*) within the dependent portion of the gallbladder.

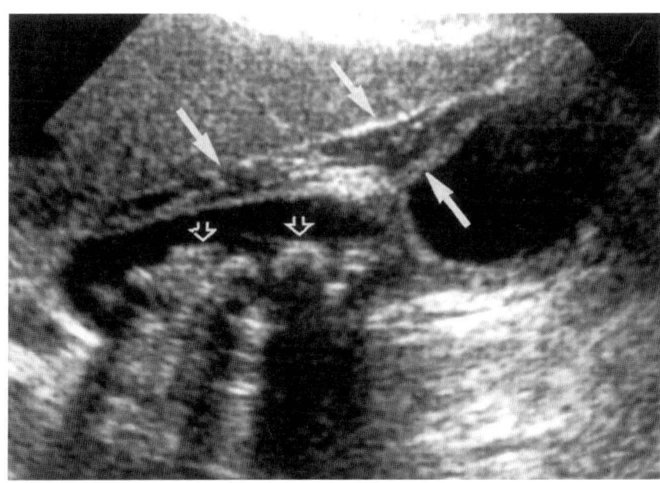

FIGURE 28 ■ Acute cholecystitis. Predominantly hypoechoic thickening of the gallbladder wall (*solid arrows*) is seen in a patient with acute cholecystitis. Multiple gallstones (*open arrows*) are present.

findings can be definitive in nearly 80% of patients with suspected acute cholecystitis.

Gallbladder wall thickening (Figs. 5B and 28) occurs in the majority (50–75%) of patients with acute cholecystitis; however, it is nonspecific, and several other nonbiliary causes of wall thickening are recognized. Occasionally, sonography can detect stone impacted in the neck of the gallbladder or cystic duct, causing obstruction and acute cholecystitis (Fig. 29). Multiple views, including left posterior oblique view and prone views, are helpful to diagnose stones impacted in the neck of the gallbladder (7).

A positive sonographic Murphy's sign, defined as the presence of maximal tenderness elicited by direct pressure of the transducer over a sonographically localized gallbladder, is present in most patients with acute cholecystitis. The sonographic Murphy's sign is different from surgical Murphy's sign, which consists of arrest of inspiration caused by pain from an inflamed gallbladder when the examiner's hand is placed on the patient's subcostal right upper quadrant (90,91). The positive predictive value of sonographic Murphy's sign alone for diagnosis of acute cholecystitis has been reported to be as low as 43% and as high as 73% (90,91). This wide range of results for sonographic Murphy's sign may be secondary to significant operator-specific variability and the inability of some patients to localize the area of maximal tenderness. Sonographic Murphy's sign may be negative in up to 70% of patients with gangrenous cholecystitis. Sonographic Murphy's sign is also difficult to elicit in patients on ventilator support or with altered mentation due to severe illness. The positive predictive value of sonographic Murphy's sign combined with the presence of gallstones is higher and reported to be 77% to 92% (90,92).

CDS of the cystic artery flow in the anterior wall of the gallbladder has been used to diagnose acute cholecystitis by demonstrating increased color flow in patients with acute cholecystitis (93–95). CDS of the gallbladder in the long-axis view (i.e., longitudinal or oblique view) is performed with a 5 MHz transducer, with the color Doppler parameters optimized for low-volume, slow-flow sensitivity. Normally, the color flow is visible only in the neck and proximal body of the gallbladder and can be seen in up to 24% to 40% of healthy persons (93–95). Jeffrey et al. reported increased color flow with visualization of cystic artery length, greater than half of the anterior gallbladder wall length, in 26% of patients with acute cholecystitis compared with only 2% of normal gallbladders (Fig. 30) (94). However, increased color flow can also be seen in patients with chronic cholecystitis as well as in patients with gallbladder wall thickening from causes other than cholecystitis (93,95). Moreover, many patients with acute cholecystitis have no detectable color flow or

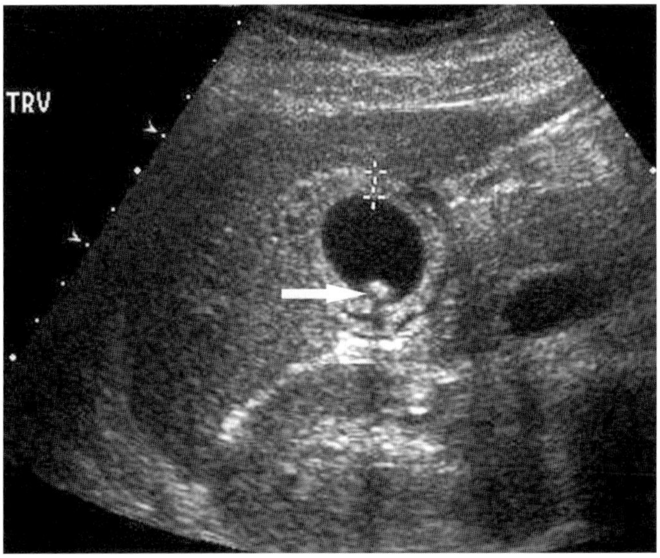

FIGURE 29 ■ Acute cholecystitis. A stone (*arrow*) in the gallbladder is seen with distal acoustic shadowing. The abnormally thick gallbladder wall (between *calipers*) measures approximately 7 mm. *Source*: Courtesy of Daniel A. Merton, BS, RDMS, Philadelphia, PA.

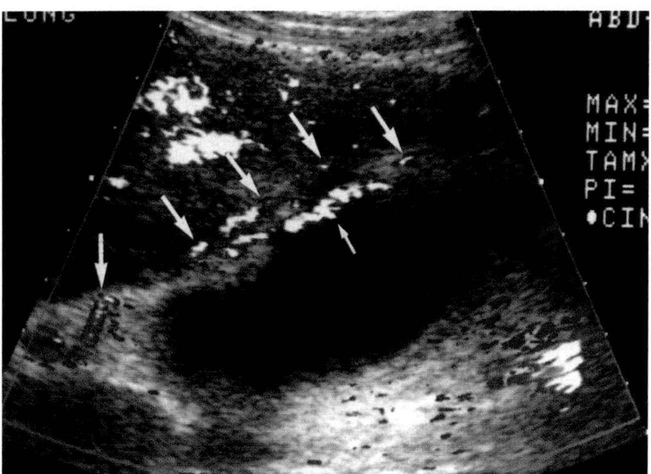

FIGURE 30 ■ Acute cholecystitis. Longitudinal view. Color Doppler sonography demonstrating increased vascularity in the gallbladder wall (*arrows*) in a patient with acute cholecystitis.

have normal color flow patterns. Therefore, even though increased color flow in appropriate clinical setting is suggestive of acute cholecystitis, the usefulness of CDS in the diagnosis of acute cholecystitis is limited by its low sensitivity (40%) and low positive predictive value (24%) (93).

Sonography, using multiple positive findings, can be definitive in nearly 80% of patients with suspected acute cholecystitis (92). However, because cholescintigraphy is highly accurate in the diagnosis of acute cholecystitis, with sensitivities greater than 95% and specificities as high as 100%, there continues to be a debate regarding the use of cholescintigraphy versus sonography in the diagnosis of acute cholecystitis (96–101). Sonography should be the screening test of choice in acute cholecystitis because it is less expensive, can be performed more quickly, and is better at detecting other abdominal disorders that may mimic acute cholecystitis. Acute cholecystitis is present in only 13% to 34% of patients who present with acute upper abdominal pain and tenderness (85). If sonographic findings are equivocal and diagnosis remains uncertain, cholescintigraphy may be performed for further evaluation.

Preoperative sonography can be helpful to determine which patients should have conventional cholecystectomy (i.e., with laparotomy) rather than laparoscopic cholecystectomy. In one study, authors concluded that gallbladder wall thickening is the most sensitive indicator and pericholecystic fluid is the most specific indicator of technical difficulties during laparoscopic cholecystectomy. Such difficulties may require conversion to laparotomy (102).

Complications

Complications of acute cholecystitis include empyema, gangrenous cholecystitis, perforation and pericholecystic abscess, hemorrhagic cholecystitis, acute emphysematous cholecystitis, and chronic perforation resulting in biliary–enteric fistula.

Empyema ■ Suppurative cholecystitis or empyema of the gallbladder occurs in a small percentage of patients with acute cholecystitis and may be more common in diabetic patients. The gallbladder is distended and filled with pus. Sonographically, pus within the gallbladder resembles sludge. Pus may appear as diffuse echogenicity within the gallbladder, secondary to nonlayering debris (Fig. 31) (103). Although empyema of the gallbladder has no specific sonographic or clinical findings, it may behave like an intraabdominal abscess with rapid progression of symptoms (29). If clinically suspected, the diagnosis may be established by sonographically guided percutaneous needle aspiration of the gallbladder.

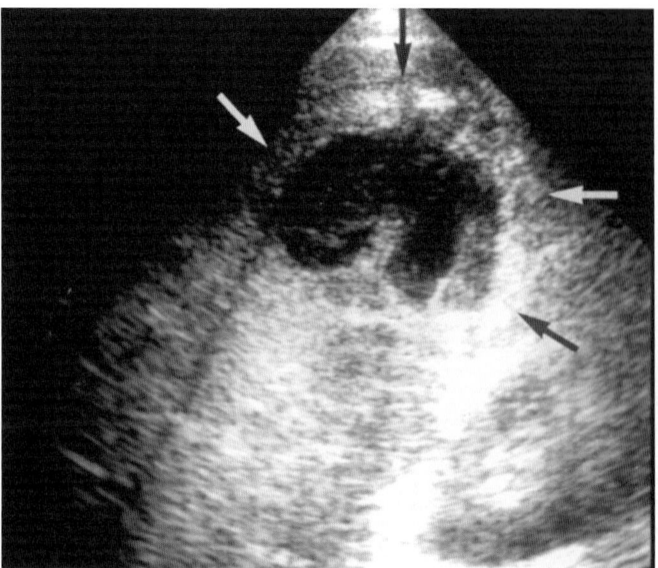

FIGURE 31 ■ Empyema of the gallbladder. The gallbladder wall is thickened (*arrows*). Multiple small echoes are seen within the gallbladder lumen secondary to nonlayering debris (i.e., pus). *Source*: From Ref. 103.

Gangrenous Cholecystitis ■ Gangrenous cholecystitis is a major complication of acute cholecystitis and is associated with significantly increased morbidity and mortality, requiring emergency cholecystectomy. The pathologic features include hemorrhage, necrosis, and microabscesses within the wall of the gallbladder, mucosal ulcers as well as strands of fibrinous exudate, and purulent debris within the gallbladder (104). The incidence of gangrenous cholecystitis has been reported to be between 2% and 38% of all patients with acute cholecystitis (104). Perforation of the gallbladder can occur in up to 10% of cases of acute cholecystitis, frequently a sequela of gangrenous cholecystitis. Clinical findings are variable, and it is difficult to diagnose gangrenous cholecystitis clinically. The disorder has no specific diagnostic sonographic findings. However, in the clinical setting of acute cholecystitis, se1veral sonographic features suggest gangrenous cholecystitis, including striated thickening of the wall, intraluminal membranes (Fig. 32),

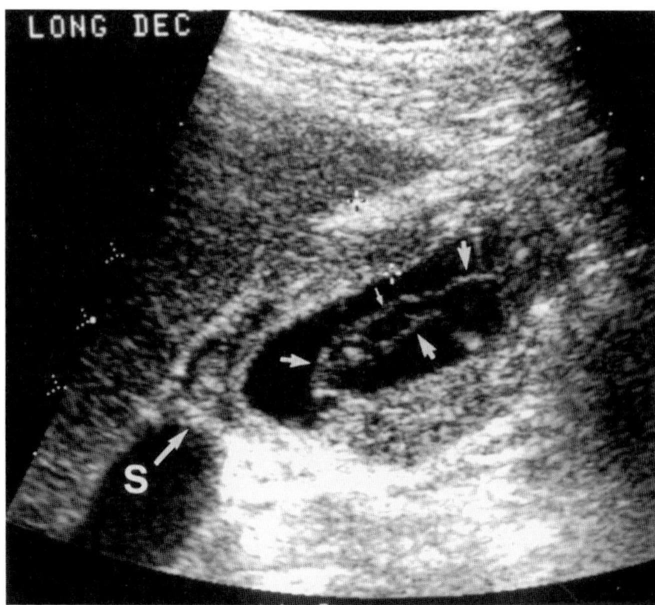

FIGURE 32 ■ Gangrenous cholecystitis: intraluminal membranes. Linear echogenic intraluminal membranes (*arrows*) are seen secondary to strands of fibrinous exudate and desquamated mucosa. Diffuse thickening of the gallbladder wall is also visible. S, stone in the neck of the gallbladder with distal shadowing. *Source*: Courtesy of Cyndi Peterson, RDMS, Canton, OH.

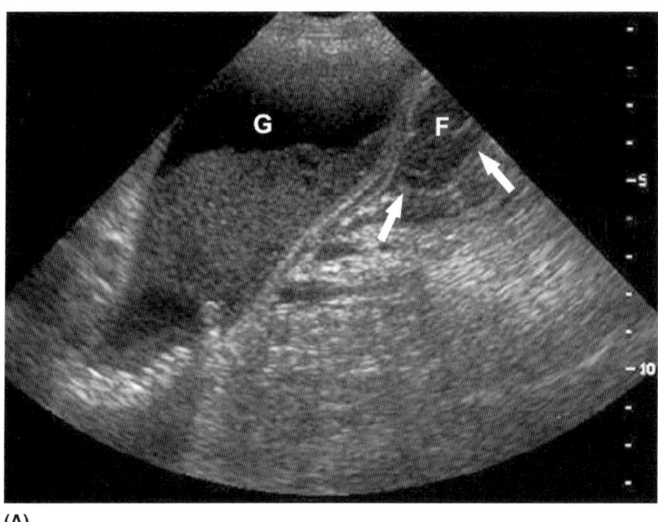

(A)

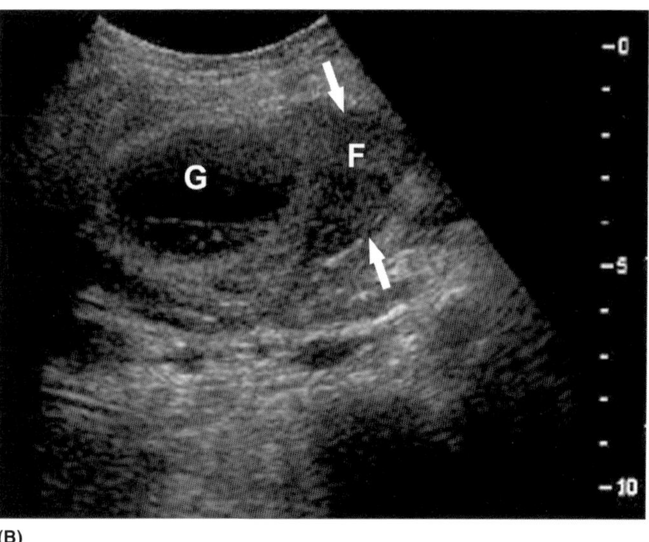

(B)

FIGURE 33 A AND B ■ Gangrenous cholecystitis with localized pericholecystic fluid collection (*arrows*). (**A**) Longitudinal view. (**B**) Transverse view. G, gallbladder with sludge; F, pericholecystic fluid. *Source*: Courtesy of Oksana Baltarowich, MD, Philadelphia, PA.

marked asymmetry of the gallbladder wall causing focal irregularities or mass-like intraluminal protrusions from the wall, nonlayering echogenic debris within the gallbladder, and loculated pericholecystic fluid collections containing debris (Fig. 33) (104–107). Sonographic Murphy's sign may be negative in up to 70% of patients with gangrenous cholecystitis, possibly because of denervation of the gallbladder wall by gangrenous changes (108).

Intraluminal membranes may be related to strands of fibrinous exudate as well as desquamated mucosa (Fig. 32) (86,104). Marked asymmetry of the wall is caused by intramural hemorrhage or microabscess formation. Coarse intraluminal echoes probably result from fibrinous and mucosal debris within the gallbladder. Complex pericholecystic fluid collections are usually the result of perforation of the gallbladder wall.

Perforation and Pericholecystic Abscess ■ Perforation of the gallbladder occurs in 5% to 10% of patients with acute cholecystitis and is more common after gangrenous cholecystitis. The fundus of the gallbladder is the most common site of perforation because of its poor vascular supply. The predisposing factors for gallbladder perforation include cholelithiasis, infection, malignancy, trauma, steroid use, and impaired vascular supply (109). Gallbladder perforations can be divided into three types: acute, subacute, and chronic. The acute type consists of perforations of the gallbladder into the free peritoneal cavity, causing generalized peritonitis. The subacute perforation results in a pericholecystic abscess that is sealed off by adhesions from the peritoneal cavity. Chronic perforation may lead to a fistulous communication between the gallbladder and adjacent viscera or the formation of an internal biliary fistula. It is difficult to discriminate clinically between patients with perforated gallbladders and those with uncomplicated acute cholecystitis. Perforation and abscess formation should be suspected in those patients with acute cholecystitis, whose conditions deteriorate rapidly or who become increasingly toxic for unexplained reasons. Sonographically, in patients with perforation, pericholecystic fluid collections and abscesses have varying appearances, ranging from anechoic to complex fluid collections (Figs. 34 and 35). Pericholecystic abscess may appear as a hypoechoic mass surrounding the gallbladder secondary to debris within the abscess (Fig. 34). The gallbladder frequently has irregular indistinct outline (110,111). Occasionally, the site of perforation of the gallbladder wall may be demonstrated as a focal

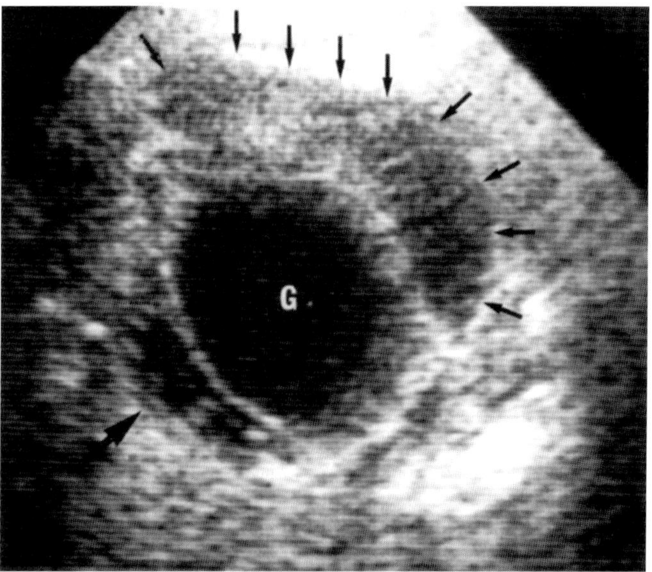

FIGURE 34 ■ Pericholecystic abscess. Transverse view showing hypoechoic, echogenic, pericholecystic abscess (*small arrows*). The wall of the gallbladder (G) adjacent to the abscess has an irregular, indistinct outline. *Large arrow*, pericholecystic fluid.

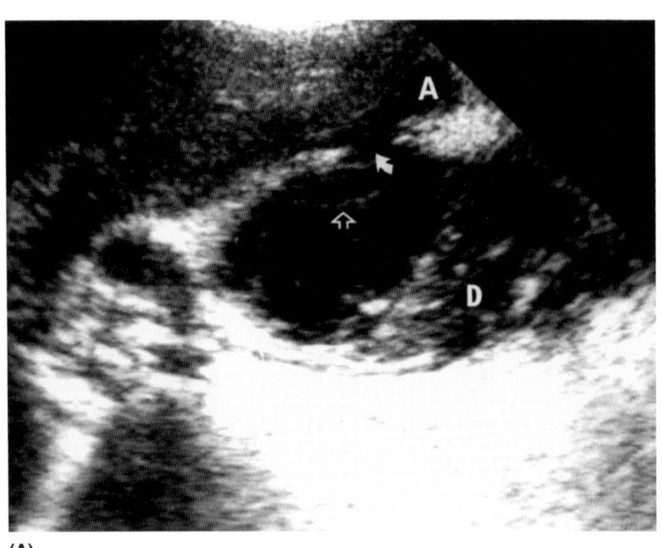

(A)

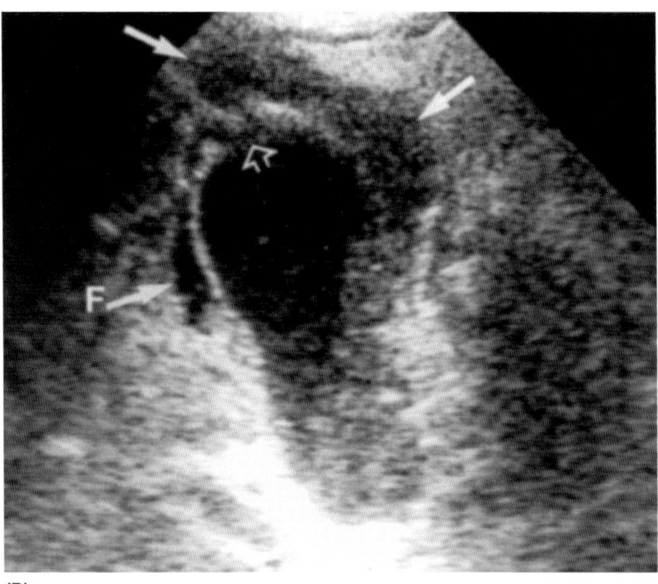

(B)

FIGURE 35 A AND B ■ Perforation of the gallbladder and pericholecystic abscess. (**A**) Focal interruption of the anterior wall of the gallbladder (*curved arrow*) indicates the site of perforation. Hypoechoic area (A) anterior to the fundus of the gallbladder represents a pericholecystic abscess. Intraluminal membrane (*open arrow*) is seen secondary to desquamated mucosa. Coarse intraluminal echoes secondary to inflammatory debris (D) are also present within the gallbladder. (**B**) In another patient, the site of perforation (*open arrow*) is seen as a focal area of disruption in the wall of the fundus of the gallbladder. A hypoechoic–echogenic area (*solid arrows*) around the fundus of the gallbladder represents a pericholecystic abscess. A localized pericholecystic fluid (F) collection is also visible. Sludge and inflammatory debris fill most of the gallbladder lumen.

interruption of the gallbladder wall (i.e., the hole sign) (Fig. 35) (112). The residual gallbladder lumen or calculi may be identified within or peripheral to the pericholecystic abscess (109,113). Prominent echogenic areas around or adjacent to the abscess may be seen because of inflamed omental and pericholecystic fat. The abscess may involve the adjacent liver (114), or it may be located in the peritoneal cavity adjacent to the gallbladder.

Pericholecystic fluid collections simulating gallbladder perforation may be seen secondary to ascites, peritonitis, pancreatitis, and perforated peptic ulcer (115,116). Scanning in decubitus, prone, or upright position may be helpful to demonstrate displacement of the ascitic fluid from the gallbladder region.

Hemorrhagic Cholecystitis ■ Hemorrhagic cholecystitis frequently coexists with gangrenous cholecystitis and is an earlier and less severe complication of acute cholecystitis. Clinical presentation is similar to that of acute cholecystitis, and overt gastrointestinal bleeding is an uncommon presentation of hemorrhagic cholecystitis (117). Sonographic findings in hemorrhagic cholecystitis are similar to those in gangrenous cholecystitis and include coarse, nonshadowing nonmobile intraluminal echoes, intraluminal membranes, and focal asymmetric gallbladder wall thickening (117,118). Computed tomography may be helpful in confirming the diagnosis of hemorrhage within the gallbladder.

Acute Emphysematous Cholecystitis ■ Acute emphysematous cholecystitis is a rare, rapidly progressive, and often fatal disease, in which gas is present within the lumen or the wall of the gallbladder. Gas-forming organisms are most commonly Clostridium and *Escherichia coli.* Thirty percent of cases of emphysematous cholecystitis are acalculous (29). In patients with acute emphysematous cholecystitis, 38% are diabetic, cholelithiasis does not seem to be a major pathogenic factor, gangrene is common, and the incidence of perforation is five times higher than in acute cholecystitis (119,120). Therefore, this condition is usually treated as a surgical emergency. Sonographically, the gas in the gallbladder lumen typically produces hyperechoic reflection in the nondependent position associated with reverberations or comet-tail (or ring-down) artifacts within an acoustic shadow (Fig. 36) (120). The acoustic shadow is usually dirty. Occasionally, reverberation artifacts may be difficult to demonstrate or absent within the dirty shadow produced by the gas in the gallbladder. If the entire gallbladder lumen is filled with gas, a dense, hyperechoic band outlining the anterior margin of the gallbladder is seen, with associated shadowing containing reverberations. A double arc–shadow or WES sign is usually absent. Gas within the wall of the gallbladder is usually seen as a hyperechoic ring around the fluid-filled gallbladder, with or without associated reverberations (121). Rarely, gas bubbles may be seen as small, echogenic foci rising from the dependent portion of the gallbladder (Fig. 36C) (122). The differential diagnosis includes a contracted gallbladder filled with stones and calcified wall of the gallbladder (porcelain gallbladder) (Table 2). Gas within the gallbladder lumen can also be seen secondary to biliary–enteric anastomosis or fistula. Even though a characteristic

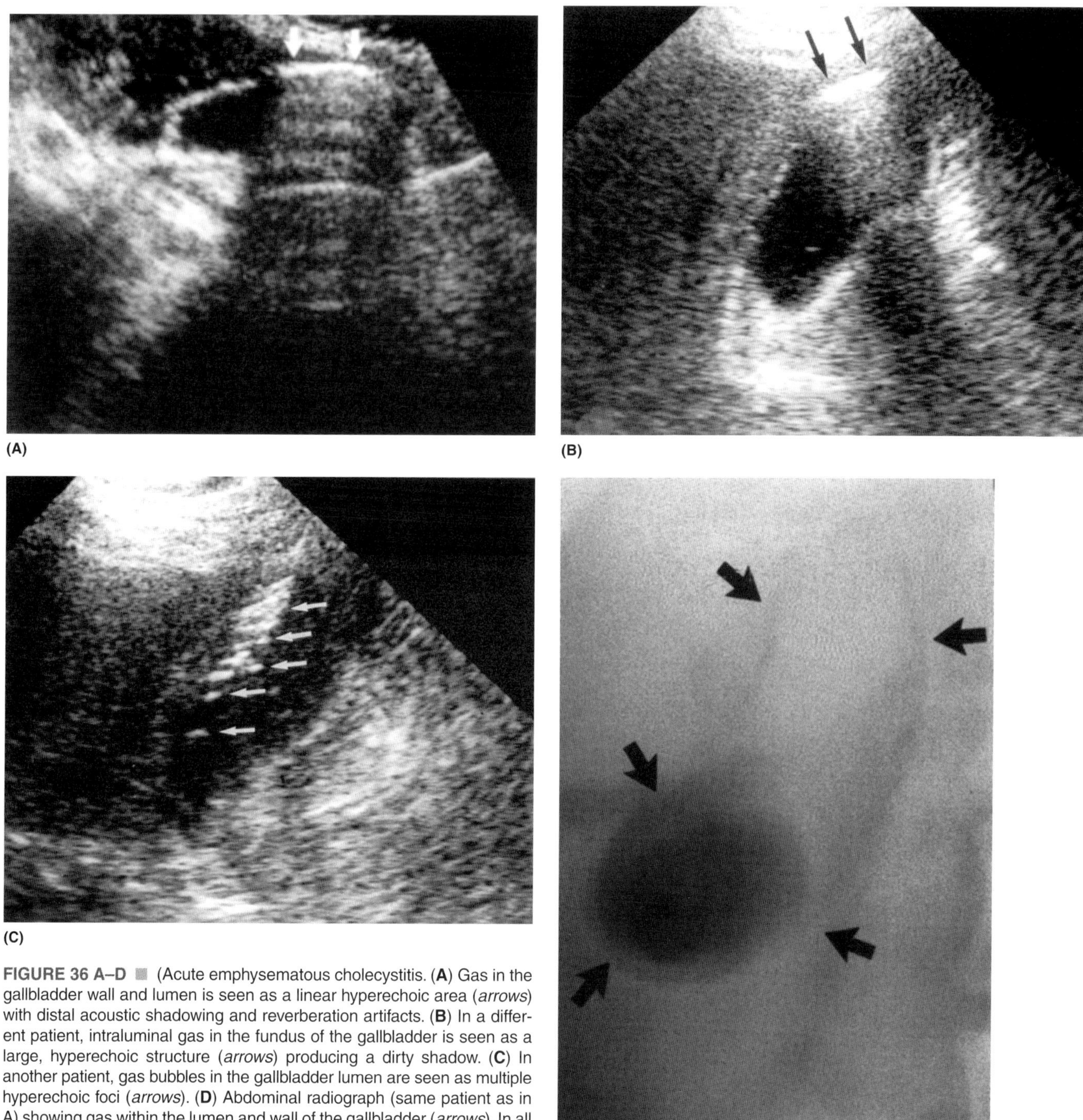

FIGURE 36 A–D ■ (Acute emphysematous cholecystitis. (**A**) Gas in the gallbladder wall and lumen is seen as a linear hyperechoic area (*arrows*) with distal acoustic shadowing and reverberation artifacts. (**B**) In a different patient, intraluminal gas in the fundus of the gallbladder is seen as a large, hyperechoic structure (*arrows*) producing a dirty shadow. (**C**) In another patient, gas bubbles in the gallbladder lumen are seen as multiple hyperechoic foci (*arrows*). (**D**) Abdominal radiograph (same patient as in A) showing gas within the lumen and wall of the gallbladder (*arrows*). In all sonograms, the gas is in the most anterior (nondependent) portion of the gallbladder. *Source*: (**A**) and (**D**), from Ref. 120.

shadow containing reverberations in the absence of biliary–enteric anastomosis or fistula strongly suggests acute emphysematous cholecystitis, the diagnosis should be confirmed by correlation with abdominal radiographs or computed tomography.

Biliary–Enteric Fistulae ■ Chronic perforation of the gallbladder resulting in biliary–enteric fistula occurs in approximately 15% to 20% of patients with gallbladder perforation (29,112). Biliary–enteric fistulae usually result from repeated attacks of cholecystitis when the gallbladder becomes adherent to a surrounding viscus as a result of inflammation. Nearly 90% of fistulae arise from the gallbladder and the rest from the common bile duct secondary to choledocholithiasis. Commonly, the fistulae are cholecystoduodenal (75%), cholecystocolic (15%), and cholecystogastric (5%). Most biliary–enteric fistulae are not diagnosed preoperatively. Cholangitis is unusual in patients with fistulae in the upper gastrointestinal tract, but it complicates about 50% of cases of cholecystocolic fistula. Intestinal obstruction from gallstones or *gallstone ileus* is the presenting sign in about 15% of patients with biliary–enteric fistula. Sonography may demonstrate air in the biliary tree or, rarely, stones within obstructed dilated fluid-filled loops of small bowel (112,123,124). Computed tomography followed by plane X ray of the abdomen are more sensitive in demonstrating pneumobilia, dilated bowel loops, and ectopic stone (125). Barium contrast studies of the gastrointestinal tract, hepatobiliary scintigraphy, and endoscopic retrograde cholangiography may be helpful in confirming the diagnosis.

Acute Acalculous Cholecystitis

Acute acalculous cholecystitis (AAC) is acute gallbladder wall inflammation in the absence of gallstones and accounts for 5% to 15% of all cases of acute cholecystitis and 47% of cases of postoperative cholecystitis (126). About 50% of children with acute cholecystitis have acalculous disease (29). It is most likely to occur in adults who are critically ill or who have recently undergone stress in the form of severe trauma, burns, or major surgery. It has also been associated with hyperalimentation, sepsis, diabetes, cardiac arrest, arteriosclerosis, and prolonged fasting. Gallbladder wall necrosis occurs in about 60% of cases, gangrene and perforation are common, and the mortality rate is as high as 30% to 50% (29,127). Pathogenesis is not clear; however, it most likely results from a gradual increase in bile viscosity due to prolonged stasis that leads to a functional obstruction of the cystic duct (128). Other factors implicated in the pathogenesis include gallbladder ischemia, infection, direct chemical toxicity, and activation of Hageman factor (factor XII), which directly damages gallbladder blood vessels. Pathologically and clinically, AAC is indistinguishable from the calculous disorder. Clinical diagnosis is exceedingly difficult, and AAC should be considered in the differential diagnosis of every patient with sepsis in the postoperative or posttraumatic period. Sonographically, distension of the gallbladder and sludge are nonspecific findings, especially because these are frequently present in critically ill patients. Sonographic abnormalities more indicative of AAC include gallbladder wall thickening, especially with hypoechoic regions within the wall (in the absence of new onset of heart failure, hepatic failure, fluid overload, or hypoalbuminemia), pericholecystic fluid, diffuse echogenicity within the gallbladder secondary to pus or hemorrhage, intraluminal membranes, and a positive sonographic Murphy's sign (129,130). A sonographic Murphy's sign, however, is difficult to elicit in patients on ventilator support or with altered mentation due to severe illness. In a review article, the authors found that gallbladder wall thickening and pericholecystic fluid were the two most reliable criteria for diagnosis of AAC (131).

Imaging diagnosis of AAC can be difficult. In patients with inconclusive initial sonograms, follow-up sonography within 24 hours may be helpful in demonstrating gallbladder abnormalities (132). Because of considerable variability in gallbladder response, lack of contraction of the gallbladder after injection of cholecystokinin cannot be considered a major criterion in the diagnosis of AAC (127). The results of studies comparing sonography and cholescintigraphy for diagnosing AAC are conflicting. Cholescintigraphy may have low specificity, because prolonged parenteral alimentation, prolonged fasting, hepatocellular dysfunction, and severe nonbiliary intercurrent illness are known to produce false-positive results and are also commonly found in patients at high risk for developing AAC. In one study, sonography and computed tomography had sensitivity equivalent to and specificity superior to cholescintigraphy in the diagnosis of AAC (128). However, in another study of critically ill trauma patients, the authors found that for diagnosis of AAC, ultrasound had a low sensitivity of 30% and a specificity of 93%, whereas cholescintigraphy had a sensitivity of 100% and a specificity of 88% (133). Computed tomography, because of its superior ability in assessing pericholecystic inflammation, may provide additional diagnostic information even after a thorough sonographic study (134). Diagnostic percutaneous aspiration of bile from the gallbladder may be a valuable method for confirming the diagnosis of AAC, but a sterile specimen without leukocytes cannot be used reliably to exclude the diagnosis (128).

Xanthogranulomatous Cholecystitis

Xanthogranulomatous cholecystitis (XGC) is a rare inflammatory disease of the gallbladder characterized histologically by the infiltration of round cells, lipid-laden histiocytes, and multiple nucleated giant cells, and the proliferation of fibroblasts in the muscle layer (135–137). The cause is probably similar to that of xanthogranulomatous pyelonephritis, which is a chronic infection associated with the formation of calculi. Gallstones are present in most patients with XGC.

XGC is uncommon, although the incidence in cholecystectomy specimens ranges from 0.7% to 13% (138). Sonographic findings are nonspecific and include marked thickening of the gallbladder wall, which may be lobulated and irregular, and the border between the gallbladder and the adjacent liver may be indistinct. Hypoechoic nodules may be seen within the gallbladder wall. The sonographic appearance may be indistinguishable from that of gallbladder carcinoma.

Torsion

Torsion of the gallbladder is rare and occurs predominantly in gallbladders that are mobile ("floating gallbladder") because they are suspended from the liver by a mesentery. Floating gallbladder with a mesentery is seen in 4% to 5% of autopsy cases. Loss of connective tissue with aging leads to elongation of the mesentery, a factor that may explain the higher incidence of torsion of the gallbladder in the elderly population (139). Clinical features are nonspecific, and the clinical presentation usually includes right upper quadrant pain, nausea, and vomiting. Complete torsion produces gangrene and eventually perforation. Gallstones are infrequent, occurring in only 20% to 33% of cases (140,141). Sonographic findings are nonspecific; however, the most suggestive finding is unusual location of the gallbladder, outside the gallbladder fossa, inferior (caudal) or lateral to the liver, or anterior to the lower pole of the right kidney close to the anterior abdominal wall (140,142). The gallbladder frequently has an unusual transverse orientation, and one may see an echogenic conical structure connecting the gallbladder to the liver, which represents the twisted pedicle.

Chronic Cholecystitis

Clinically, patients with chronic cholecystitis have symptoms of recurrent biliary colic, most commonly (90%) associated with gallstones. The diagnosis is based on clinical findings, even though clinically, it is frequently difficult to distinguish between symptoms of chronic and acute cholecystitis. Secondary to long-standing chronic inflammation, the gallbladder wall may become thickened with muscular hypertrophy and fibrotic reaction, and dilatation of the Rokitansky–Aschoff sinuses and hyperplastic cholecystopathy may result (143). In symptomatic patients, sonographic findings of gallbladder wall thickening and gallstones are suggestive, but nonspecific.

Chronic Acalculous Cholecystitis

Chronic acalculous cholecystitis is a poorly understood entity that may be associated with right upper quadrant pain similar to that seen in biliary colic. An incidence of 7% to 13% in surgically removed gallbladders has been reported (144,145). Sonographically, diffuse gallbladder wall thickening and nonshadowing particles within the gallbladder may be seen. None of the different tests including sonography, oral cholecystography, and cholescintigraphy provide any specific diagnostic sign for chronic acalculous cholecystitis. Biliary scintigraphy may be the most sensitive technique (145). Symptoms are often resolved with cholecystectomy.

Abnormalities of the Gallbladder Wall

Thickening

The normal gallbladder wall measures 3 mm or less. Measurements are most accurate when the anterior wall of the gallbladder is scanned in the long-axis view, with the sound beam perpendicular to the wall of the gallbladder (146). Minor angulations of the transducer or decentering can cause pseudothickening of the gallbladder wall. *Diffuse* gallbladder wall thickening is a nonspecific finding caused by numerous disorders including acute and chronic cholecystitis, viral hepatitis, hypoalbuminemia, cirrhosis, congestive heart failure, AIDS, pancreatitis, and renal disease (Table 8) (147–150). Rarely, obstruction of the lymphatic drainage of the gallbladder may cause diffuse hypoechoic wall thickening (151). *Asymmetric* or *focal* thickening of the gallbladder wall may be caused by gangrenous or hemorrhagic cholecystitis, XGC, adenomyomatosis, carcinoma, or, rarely, metastases to the wall of the gallbladder (Table 9). Sonographically, diffuse gallbladder wall thickening has the following variable nonspecific echo patterns: (*i*) a uniformly echogenic pattern (Fig. 37); (*ii*) a diffusely hypoechoic pattern (Fig. 38), frequently appearing as a single central hypoechoic zone separated by two echogenic layers (Fig. 29); and (*iii*) a striated pattern consisting of multiple alternating hyperechoic and hypoechoic or anechoic layers (Fig. 39).

The *striated* wall pattern is not specific for acute cholecystitis; however, when seen in the clinical setting of acute cholecystitis, it suggests gangrenous changes in the gallbladder (107,152). Striated wall pattern can also be seen secondary to other causes, including acute viral hepatitis, hypoproteinemia, cirrhosis, and congestive heart failure. In patients with acute viral hepatitis, wall thickening (Fig. 40) and diffuse intraluminal echoes (Fig. 8B) are seen in up to 98% of patients, most commonly within one week of illness, with resolution of these abnormalities on clinical recovery (153). The gallbladder is often contracted (154,155). The pathogenesis of gallbladder wall thickening in viral hepatitis is uncertain, but it probably is secondary to an inflammatory process. The cause of wall thickening in patients with AIDS is unknown, although in some of these patients, opportunistic organisms have been found in the gallbladder (156). The wall thickening in patients with ascites is most likely secondary to underlying disease (such as alcoholic liver disease or hypoalbuminemia), rather than

TABLE 8 ■ Causes of Diffuse Gallbladder Wall Thickening

Common
- Acute cholecystitis
- Chronic cholecystitis
- Viral hepatitis
- Hypoproteinemia
- Cirrhosis
- Congestive heart failure
- AIDS
- Pancreatitis
- Renal failure

Uncommon
- Adenomyomatosis
- Gallbladder carcinoma
- Lymphatic obstruction
- Gallbladder wall varices
- Xanthogranulomatous cholecystitis
- Multiple myeloma
- Sclerosing cholangitis
- Schistosomiasis

TABLE 9 ■ Causes of Focal Gallbladder Wall Thickening

- Gangrenous or hemorrhagic cholecystitis
- Adenomyomatosis
- Polyp
- Carcinoma of gallbladder
- Metastasis to gallbladder wall

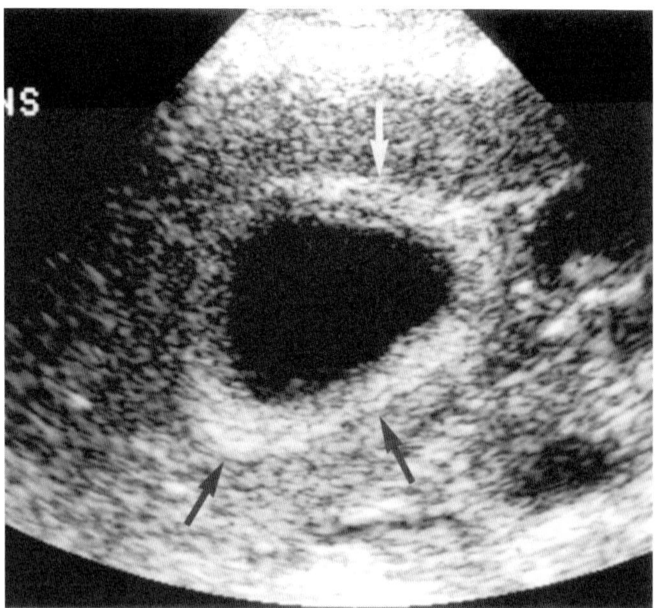

FIGURE 37 ■ Gallbladder wall thickening: echogenic pattern. Diffuse echogenic thickening of the wall (*arrows*) in a patient with chronic cholecystitis.

secondary to ascites itself (Fig. 39D) (146). In patients with malignant ascites, the gallbladder wall is usually normal in thickness, whereas a thick wall in patients with ascites is usually associated with benign disease (157). In a study by Huang et al., the normal thickness of the gallbladder wall in patients with ascites had a sensitivity of 81% and specificity of 94% for prediction of malignant ascites (158). The gallbladder wall may appear prominent after physiologic contraction of the gallbladder (i.e., after a meal); however, the wall usually remains less than 3 mm thick (Fig. 8A) (149). In a physiologically contracted gallbladder, three components of the wall can be recognized: (*i*) a strongly hyperechoic outer contour (serosa); (*ii*) a less hyperechoic inner contour (mucosa); and (*iii*) a hypoechoic area (muscularis) in between (159).

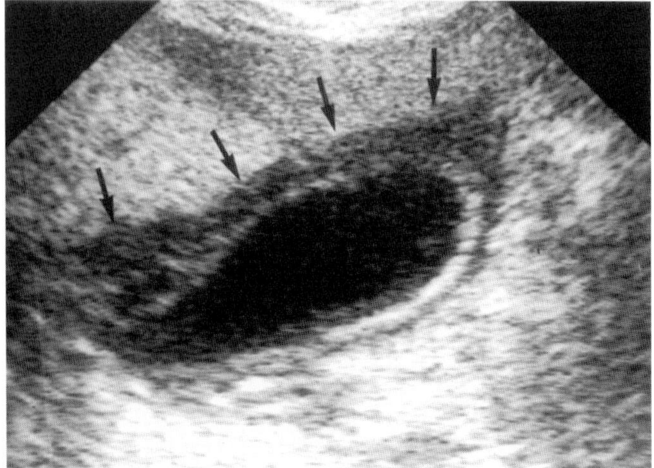

FIGURE 38 ■ Gallbladder wall thickening: hypoechoic pattern. Diffusely hypoechoic thickening of the wall (*arrows*) in a patient with cirrhosis of the liver.

Varices

Gallbladder wall varices can be seen secondary to portal hypertension in patients with cirrhosis or secondary to portal vein thrombosis (160). Gallbladder wall varices rarely cause hemobilia and gastrointestinal bleeding. Sonographically, varices may appear as numerous tortuous vascular structures within and around the wall of the gallbladder (Fig. 41) (161), small cystic areas within the wall of the gallbladder (Fig. 42), or irregular thickening of the wall of the gallbladder without anechoic spaces (162–164). CDS is the most sensitive and specific noninvasive imaging modality for the diagnosis of portal collateral veins causing gallbladder wall varices. The venous nature of these dilated vessels however should be confirmed by duplex ultrasound, because increased arterial color flow can be seen within the gallbladder wall in patients with wall thickening secondary to acute cholecystitis or other causes.

Porcelain Gallbladder

Calcification of the gallbladder wall (porcelain gallbladder) is an uncommon manifestation of chronic cholecystitis, resulting from chronic inflammation of the gallbladder wall. It has a characteristic appearance on plain radiographs of the abdomen. The term "porcelain gallbladder" indicates the brittle consistency and bluish discoloration of the wall. The wall is calcified in two patterns: (*i*) broad, continuous calcification of the muscularis; and (*ii*) multiple punctate calcifications that occur in the glandular spaces of the mucosa. Gallstones are almost always present and often cause cystic duct obstruction, leading to hydrops of the gallbladder (143). The incidence of porcelain gallbladder is low, ranging between 0.06% and 0.8% of cholecystectomy specimens (165). It is much more common in women, and the mean age of patients is 54 years. A high incidence (11–33%) of gallbladder carcinoma is associated with porcelain gallbladder (165). Therefore, some clinicians advocate prophylactic cholecystectomy in patients with porcelain gallbladder, even when they have few or no gallbladder symptoms. Sonographically, three distinct patterns of calcified wall are identified: (*i*) a hyperechoic linear or semilunar structure with acoustic shadowing; (*ii*) a biconvex, curvilinear hyperechoic structure with variable acoustic shadowing; and (*iii*) an irregular clump of echoes with acoustic shadowing (Fig. 43) (166). Only a part of the wall or the entire wall of the gallbladder may be calcified. Porcelain gallbladder usually produces a clean shadow; however, occasionally, a heavily calcified gallbladder wall may produce reverberations or dirty shadow. A double arc–shadow or WES sign is usually absent. Contracted gallbladder filled with stones and acute emphysematous cholecystitis should be considered in the differential diagnosis (Table 2). The sonographic diagnosis of porcelain gallbladder should be confirmed by either abdominal radiography or computed tomography.

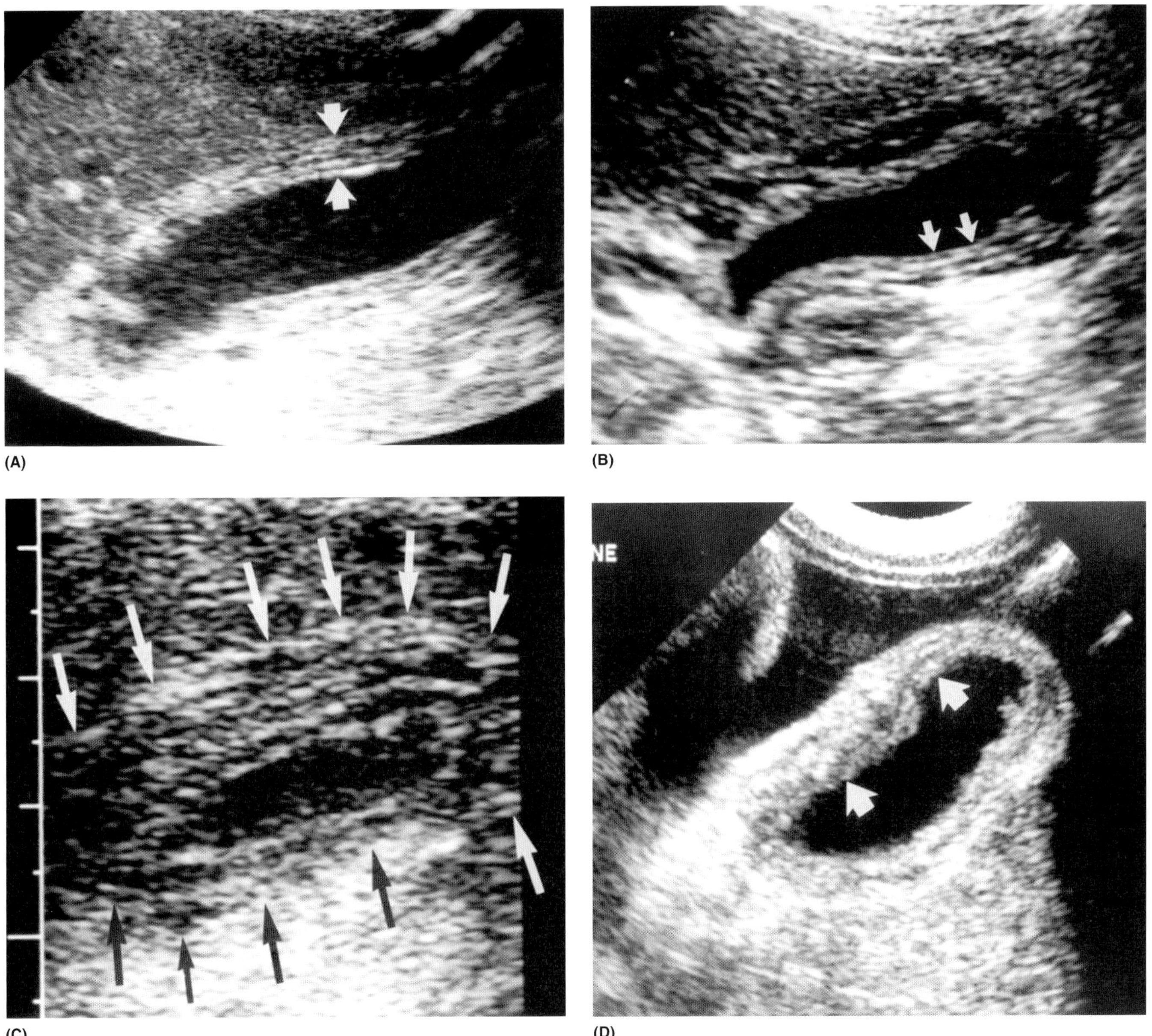

(A) (B) (C) (D)

FIGURE 39 A–D ■ Gallbladder wall thickening: striated pattern. (**A**) Diffuse wall thickening with striated pattern (*arrows*) in acute cholecystitis. The striated pattern consists of multiple alternating hyperechoic and hypoechoic or anechoic layers. (**B**) Diffuse wall thickening with striated pattern (*arrows*) in a patient with hypoproteinemia. (**C**) Considerable wall thickening (*arrows*) in a patient with congestive heart failure. A striated pattern is seen in the anterior wall of the gallbladder. (**D**) Diffuse wall thickening in a patient with cirrhosis and ascites. A striated pattern is seen in the anterior wall (*arrows*).

Hyperplastic Cholecystoses

The term "hyperplastic cholecystoses" encompasses a diverse group of benign, nonneoplastic, noninflammatory gallbladder abnormalities, thought to be characterized by hyperplasia of gallbladder wall. The two most common abnormalities of the gallbladder, other than cholelithiasis, are the two pathologic forms of the hyperplastic cholecystoses known as adenomyomatosis and cholesterolosis. The incidence is difficult to determine, but these disorders occur in 5% to 25% of surgically removed gallbladders (167). Adenomyomatosis has been reported in 5% of oral cholecystograms. In the presence of substantial symptoms for which no other cause is apparent, surgery appears to be justifiable if one of the hyperplastic cholecystoses is found (29).

Adenomyomatosis

Adenomyomatosis is characterized by epithelial proliferation, with muscular hypertrophy and mucosal diverticula called Rokitansky–Aschoff sinuses. Three types of adenomyomatosis have been described: diffuse, segmental, and localized (168).

1. The *diffuse* type is relatively rare, involving the entire gallbladder, with diffuse wall thickening that may be

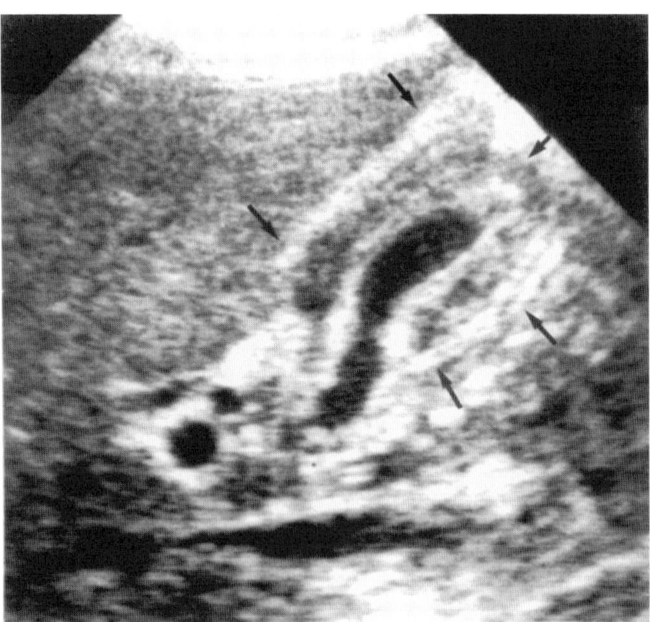

FIGURE 40 ■ Acute viral hepatitis. Contracted gallbladder with diffuse wall thickening (*arrows*).

difficult to distinguish from other causes of gallbladder wall thickening.

2. The *segmental* type also is rare, usually involving the mid-body of the gallbladder; segmental thickening of the wall of the body of the gallbladder may cause an "hour-glass" configuration of the gallbladder (Fig. 44).
3. The *localized* form is the most common, nearly always confined to the fundus of the gallbladder and causing circumferential wall thickening. Localized wall thickening in the fundus may appear as a solid mass and may mimic carcinoma (Fig. 45) (169). Sonographically, fundal adenomyomatosis may be indistinguishable from gallbladder carcinoma.

The *intramural diverticula (Rokitansky–Aschoff sinuses)* may be seen as small, anechoic spaces within the thick wall when they contain bile, or, much more commonly, as small, nonshadowing, hyperechoic foci within the wall of the gallbladder associated with comet-tail reverberation artifacts with or without wall thickening (Fig. 46) (170,171). The cause of reverberation artifacts is uncertain, but they may result from cholesterol crystals or, less likely, frond-like mucosal projections within the intramural diverticulum (170,171). The hyperechoic foci most likely represent cholesterol crystals or tiny cholesterol stones within the intramural diverticula. Occasionally, larger stones within the diverticula may cause acoustic shadowing. Oral cholecystography typically demonstrates contrast accumulation within the Rokitansky–Aschoff sinuses and may be helpful in confirming the diagnosis when sonographic findings are not definitive.

Cholesterolosis

Cholesterolosis is the result of deposits of cholesterol esters in the submucosal macrophages in the lamina propria. The macroscopic mucosal excrescences create a yellow reticular pattern on the gallbladder mucosa. Two

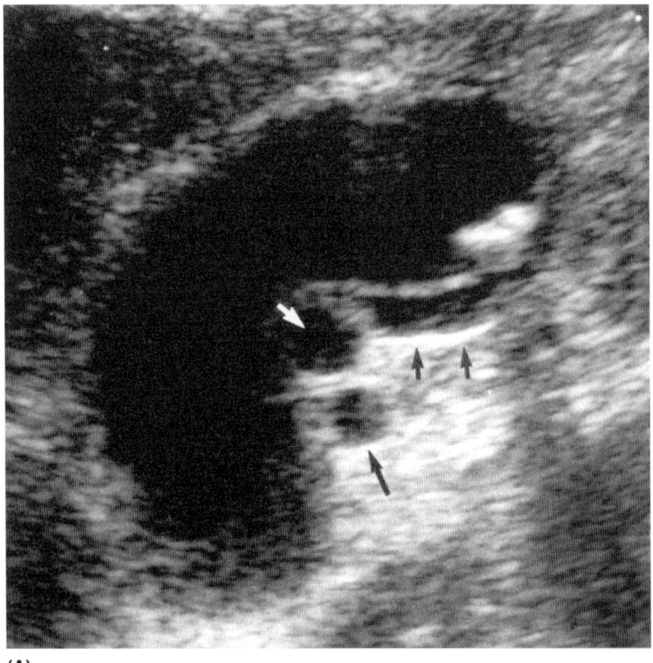

(A)

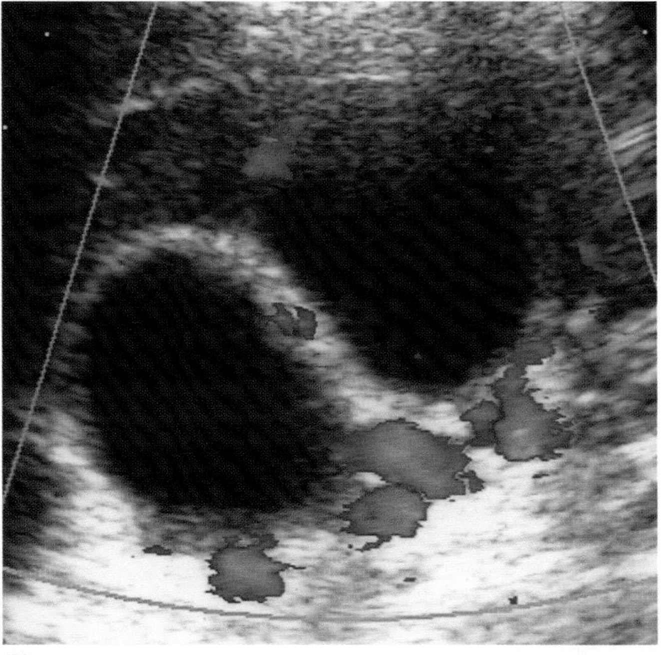

(B)

FIGURE 41 A AND B ■ Gallbladder wall varices. (**A**) Longitudinal sonogram showing large, rounded, and tubular anechoic vascular structures (*arrows*) along the posterior wall of the gallbladder. (**B**) Transverse color Doppler sonogram showing tubular and rounded cystic structures to be pericholecystic varices. *Source*: From Ref. 161.

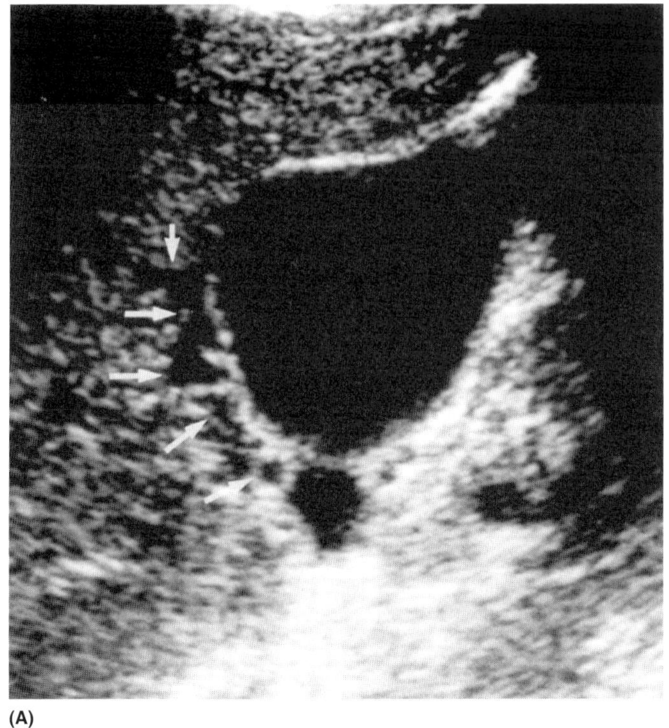

(A)

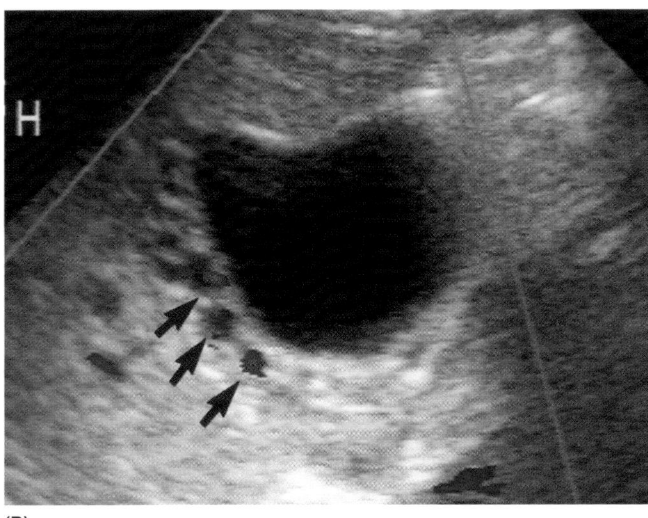

(B)

FIGURE 42 A AND B ■ Gallbladder wall varices. (**A**) Smaller varices appear as small, rounded, and tubular anechoic structures (*arrows*) along the wall of the gallbladder. (**B**) Color Doppler sonogram showing flow (*arrows*) in some of the varices.

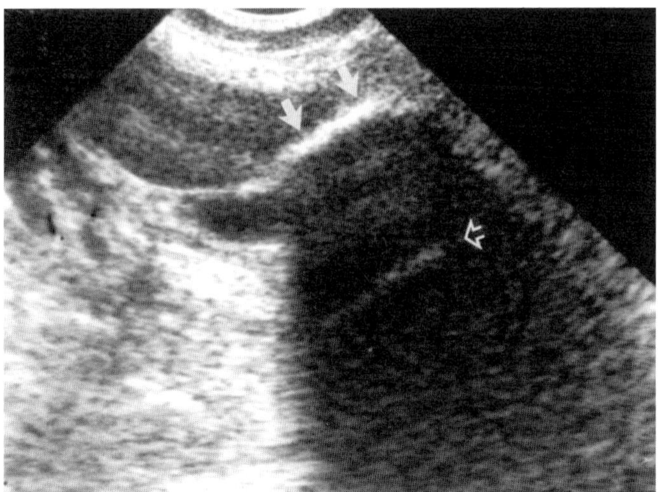

(A)

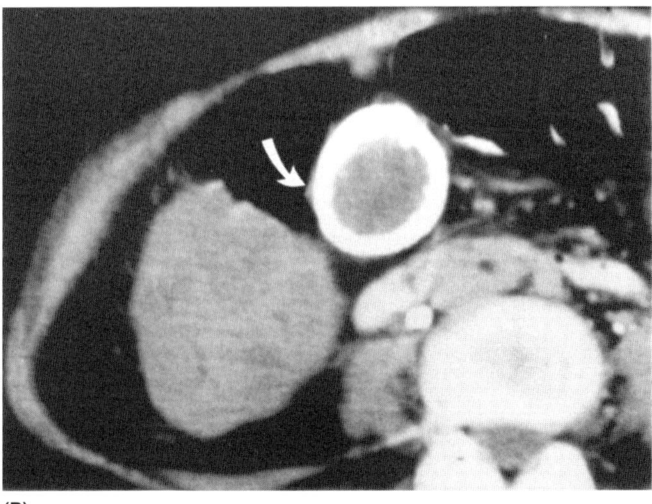

(B)

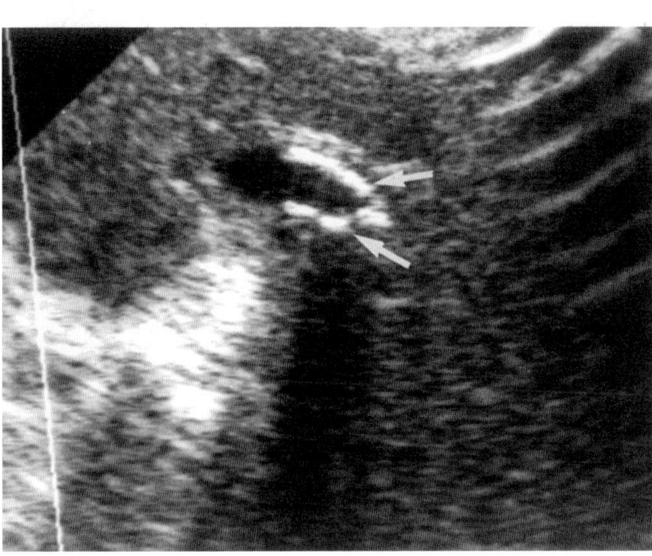

(C)

FIGURE 43 A–C ■ Porcelain gallbladder. (**A**) Longitudinal view showing a thick linear hyperechoic area (*solid arrows*) with acoustic shadowing secondary to calcification in the wall of the distal body and fundus of the gallbladder. A weak reverberation artifact (*open arrow*) is noted within the shadow. (**B**) Computed tomography of the same patient as in (**A**) demonstrating a calcified wall of the gallbladder (*arrow*). (**C**) In another patient, calcification in the anterior and posterior wall of part of the gallbladder appears as a biconvex, curvilinear hyperechoic area (*arrows*) with clean acoustic shadowing.

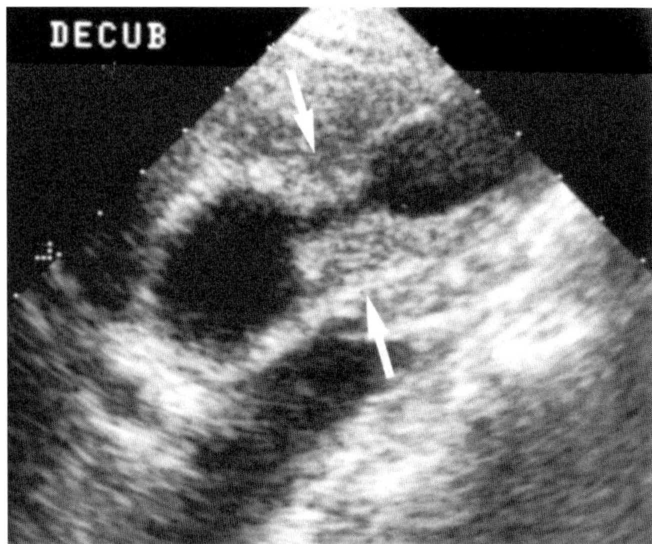

FIGURE 44 ■ Adenomyomatosis: segmental. Segmental adenomyomatosis seen as focal thickening of the anterior and posterior wall of the mid-body of the gallbladder (*arrows*), causing an "hourglass" configuration of the gallbladder. *Source*: Courtesy of Andrew H. Myers, MD, Cleveland, OH.

forms of cholesterolosis can be seen: diffuse planar type and polypoid type. The diffuse form of cholesterolosis cannot be appreciated sonographically. However, cholesterol polyps occur in about 20% of cases of cholesterolosis and can be seen sonographically as nonmobile, nonshadowing echogenic structures attached to the wall of the gallbladder (Fig. 47). Cholesterol polyps are usually less than 1 cm in size and are frequently multiple (172,173). Rarely, a cholesterol polyp may produce subtle acoustic shadowing; however, it can be distinguished from a stone by its lack of mobility (174). Multiple polyps usually are secondary to cholesterolosis; however, a solitary cholesterol polyp cannot be differentiated from an adenomatous polyp.

Benign Neoplasms

Adenomatous Polyp

The most common benign neoplasm of the gallbladder is an adenoma presenting as a polyp. Adenomatous polyps are uncommon, and cholesterol polyps account for most gallbladder polyps (172). In a large sonographic screening study involving 2739 men, the overall prevalence of all gallbladder polyps was 5.3% (175). In another pathologic study of cholecystectomy specimens of 2145 patients, the incidence of adenomatous polyps was 0.4% (176). Most patients with gallbladder polyps are asymptomatic. Most adenomatous polyps are sessile; however, they may be pedunculated. Most adenomatous polyps are less than 1 cm in size. Malignancy should be considered when the polyp exceeds 1 cm in diameter or when rapid growth of the polyp is seen on sonographic follow-up examinations (177). In polyps larger than 1 cm, the incidence of malignancy is higher in sessile polyps than in pedunculated polyps (178). Sonographically, an adenomatous polyp appears as a solitary, echogenic, nonmobile, nonshadowing structure protruding from the wall of the gallbladder (Fig. 48). It is difficult to distinguish from the more common cholesterol polyp, although cholesterol polyps are more often multiple.

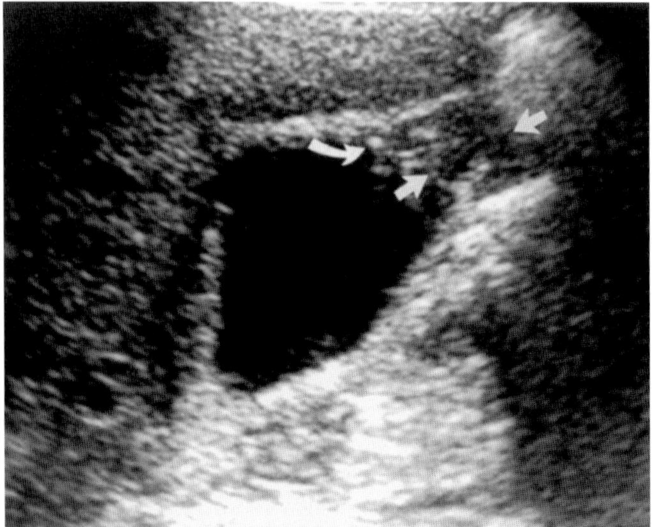

(A)

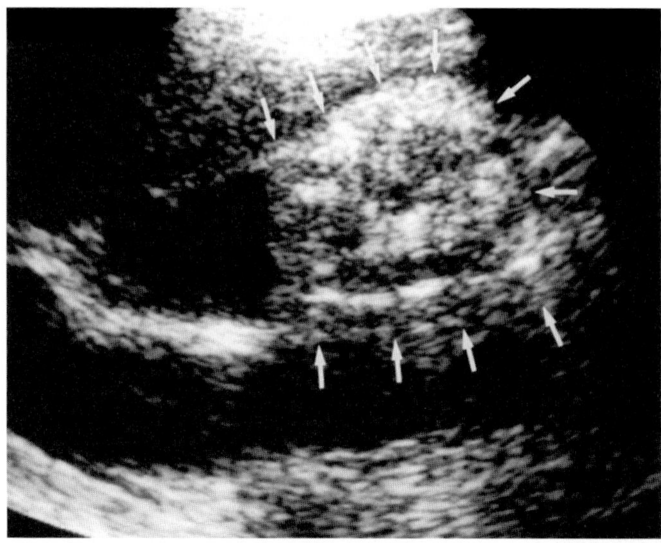

(B)

FIGURE 45 A AND B ■ Adenomyomatosis: localized (fundal). (**A**) Localized type of adenomyomatosis causing wall thickening of the fundus of the gallbladder appearing as a focal mass (*straight arrows*) within the fundus of the gallbladder. One (*curved arrow*) of the many hyperechoic foci representing cholesterol crystals in Rokitansky–Aschoff sinuses. (**B**) Another patient with fundal adenomyomatosis. Longitudinal view showing a hypoechoic–echogenic solid mass (*arrows*) in the fundus and the distal body of the gallbladder secondary to circumferential wall thickening. The mass mimics carcinoma of the gallbladder.

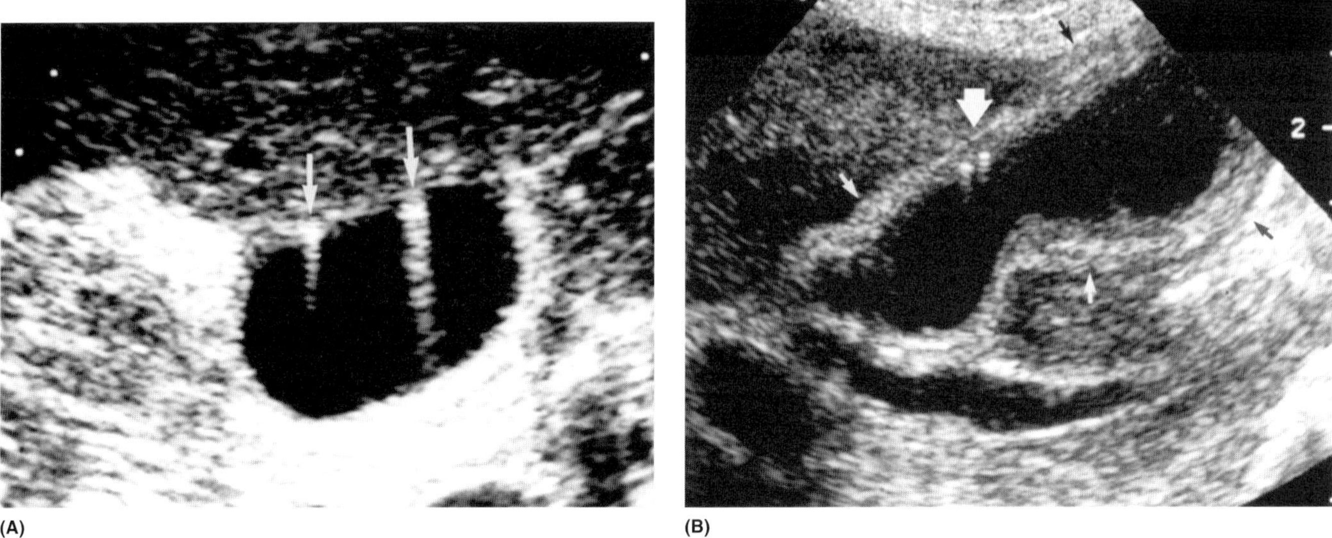

(A) (B)

FIGURE 46 A AND B ■ Adenomyomatosis: comet-tail artifacts. (**A**) Hyperechoic foci within the anterior wall of the gallbladder (*arrows*) producing comet-tail artifacts. These are most likely secondary to cholesterol crystals within Rokitansky–Aschoff sinuses in the gallbladder wall. (**B**) Diffuse wall thickening (*small arrows*) is seen in another patient with adenomyomatosis. *Large arrow*, comet-tail artifacts from hyperechoic foci within the anterior wall.

Management of Gallbladder Polyps ■ A major concern regarding gallbladder polyps is the differentiation of benign from malignant polyps. The majority of gallbladder polyps are cholesterol polyps and, therefore, the gallbladder polyps have a low malignant potential overall. Most polyps do not change significantly in size over time (179). Therefore, increase in size of a polyp over time raises the possibility of malignancy.

Although there are no firm guidelines, cholecystectomy for patients with polyp >10 mm seems warranted. Authors of a review article (179) suggested the following strategy for management of gallbladder polyps: all patients with gallbladder polyps who are symptomatic (compatible symptoms, including biliary type pain and dyspepsia), or have polyp greater than 10 mm in diameter or have factors that increase the risk of malignancy (i.e., age over 50 years, concurrent gallstones, or polyp growth) should undergo resection (i.e., cholecystectomy). All others should be followed every three to six months with repeat abdominal ultrasound (180). The frequency of ultrasound examinations

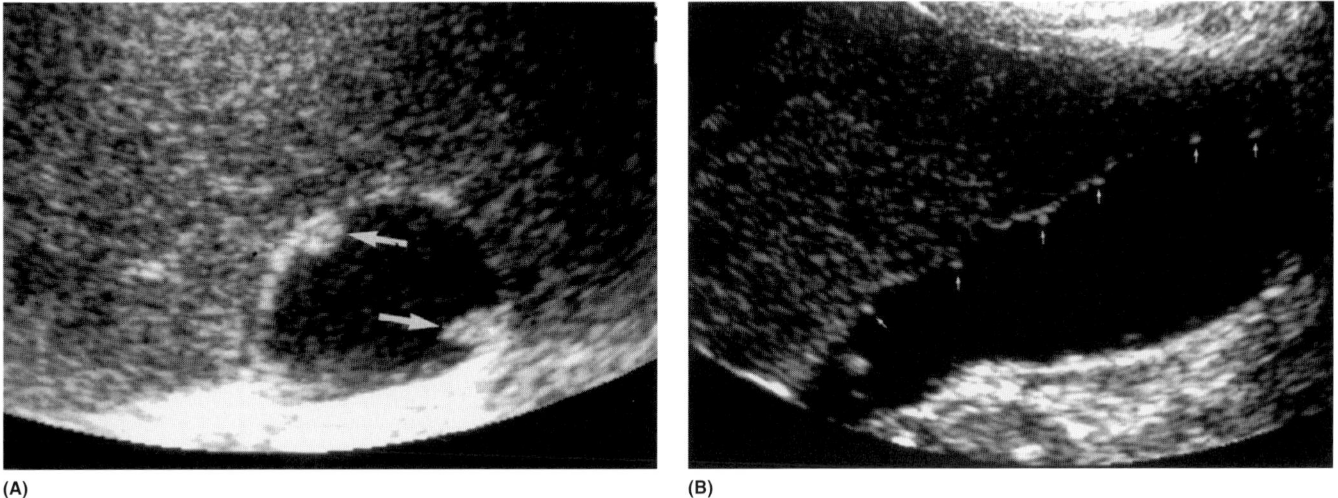

(A) (B)

FIGURE 47 A AND B ■ Cholesterolosis. (**A**) Two cholesterol polyps (*arrows*) measuring 6 and 7 mm each are seen as nonshadowing echogenic structures along the wall of the gallbladder. Several other polyps (not shown) were present within the gallbladder. (**B**) Another patient with numerous smaller (2–3 mm) cholesterol polyps (*arrows*) along the anterior wall of the gallbladder. Polyps were also present along the posterior wall (not shown).

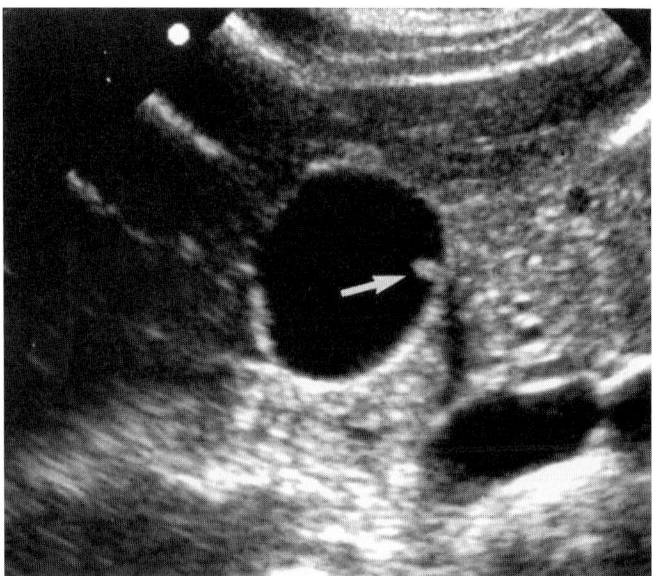

FIGURE 48 ■ Adenomatous polyp is seen as a 4 mm nonshadowing echogenic structure (*arrow*) along the wall in the nondependent portion of the gallbladder.

after stability over two serial six-month ultrasound examinations should be determined on a case by case basis depending on existing risk factors (179). Patients demonstrating growth of polyps on serial ultrasound examinations should undergo cholecystectomy (179).

Whether asymptomatic patients over the age of 50 years who have a solitary polyp or multiple polyps <10 mm in diameter should have cholecystectomy or be followed by ultrasound remains controversial.

Other Benign Neoplasms

Other causes of benign polypoid lesions in the gallbladder include inflammatory polyp (181), heterotopic gastric or pancreatic tissue, and rare benign neoplasms of the gallbladder including cystadenoma, hemangioma, lipoma, and leiomyoma (182).

Malignant Neoplasms

Carcinoma

Gallbladder carcinoma is the fifth most common malignant tumor of the gastrointestinal tract. The average age at diagnosis is 70 years in the United States. It is three times more common in women than in men, and the incidence increases with age and with gallstones larger than 3 cm in diameter (29). About 70% to 80% of gallbladder carcinomas are associated with gallstones. The incidence of carcinoma in calcified (porcelain) gallbladders is high (11–33%) (165). Other, less frequent associations include inflammatory bowel disease and familial colonic polyposis. Most gallbladder cancers are adenocarcinoma. Clinical features are often nonspecific and may include right upper quadrant pain, anorexia, weight loss, and jaundice.

Four sonographic patterns are seen: (*i*) a subhepatic mass replacing most or all of the gallbladder (40–65% of all carcinomas); (*ii*) an intraluminal polypoid mass, usually larger than 2 cm (15–25%); (*iii*) focal or diffuse thickening of the gallbladder wall without associated mass (less common); and (*iv*) focal mucosal thickening (least common) (183–187). Associated sonographic findings include gallstones, porcelain gallbladder, invasion of the liver and other adjacent structures, common bile duct obstruction, and metastatic lymph nodes around the common bile duct or in the region of the head of the pancreas (113,188). Replacement of most or all of the gallbladder by a mass is the most common form of gallbladder cancer (Figs. 49A and 50). The masses are solid, have variable echogenicity, and may be homogeneous or inhomogeneous. Sonographically, the mass may be difficult to separate from the liver, especially when carcinoma invades the liver; however, the absence of normal gallbladder and the presence of gallstones within the subhepatic mass can be helpful clues to the diagnosis. Carcinoma manifesting as *focal or diffuse thickening* of the gallbladder wall without associated mass is the type most likely to be missed sonographically (Fig. 49B). Focal wall thickening may be obscured by shadowing from overlying gallstones or may be missed because of its small size (73). Diffuse wall thickening may be difficult to differentiate from acute or chronic cholecystitis, although the wall infiltrated by cancer is typically thicker and more irregular than wall thickened by inflammation. *Intraluminal polypoid carcinoma* may present as solitary or multiple polypoid solid masses (Fig. 49C and D). Polypoid masses are larger than 1 cm and most frequently are larger than 2 cm.

Authors of a study of arterial flow velocity in the gallbladder wall (primarily the anterior wall of the gallbladder) reported that when the velocity was greater than 30 cm/sec, gallbladder cancer could be diagnosed with 100% sensitivity and 96% specificity, irrespective of the location of the cancer within the gallbladder (189). With CDS, an abnormally high velocity arterial blood flow signal within the mass and in the gallbladder wall is a significant feature of primary gallbladder cancer; however, this area needs further investigation (190). CDS may be useful in differentiating carcinoma of the gallbladder from sludge filling the entire gallbladder or tumefactive sludge, by demonstrating intrinsic vascularity within the mass (i.e., carcinoma) (Fig. 50). Lack of color flow, however, does not completely exclude carcinoma.

Sonographic diagnosis of gallbladder carcinoma is difficult, especially when no focal mass can be demonstrated. In one study, in 71% of the patients with gallbladder cancer, ultrasound examination revealed only cholecystitis (191).

Pitfalls ■ Tumefactive sludge or gallbladder entirely filled with sludge may be mistaken for a solid mass or carcinoma of the gallbladder (63,74). A change in appearance or disappearance of the sludge on follow-up sonograms (in several days or weeks) confirms the diagnosis of sludge and excludes neoplasm. Demonstration of color flow within the mass may be helpful in distinguishing carcinoma from tumefactive sludge. Focal circumferential wall thickening in the fundus of the gallbladder secondary

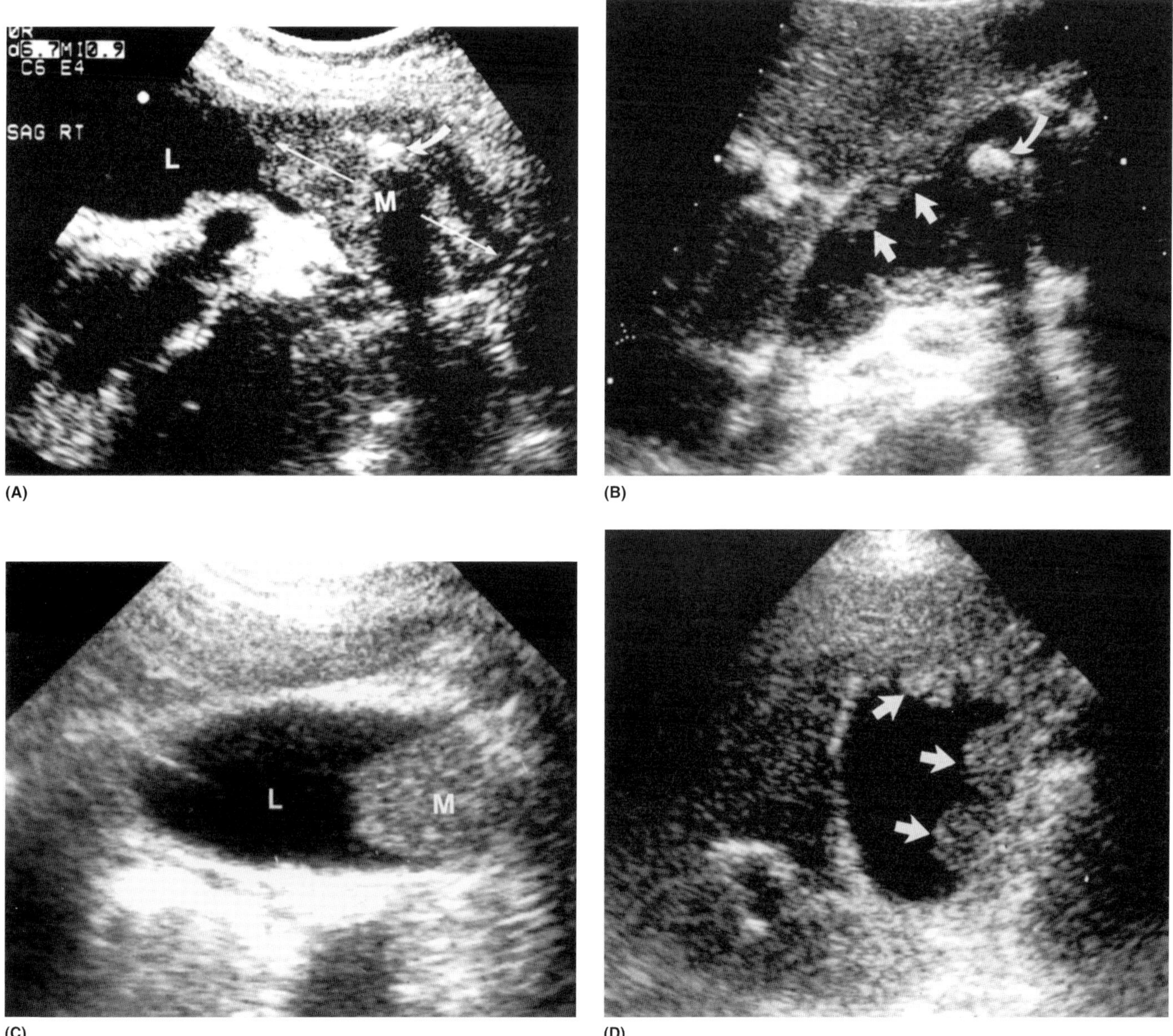

(A) (B) (C) (D)

FIGURE 49 A–D ■ Carcinoma of the gallbladder. (**A**) Carcinoma appears as an echogenic mass (*arrows*) replacing the distal body and fundus of the gallbladder. A stone (*curved arrow*) with distal acoustic shadowing is present within the mass. (**B**) Focal irregular thickening of the anterior wall of the gallbladder (*arrows*) secondary to carcinoma. Gallstones are also present (*curved arrow*). (**C**) Carcinoma appearing as a 2 cm polypoid mass in the fundus of the gallbladder. (**D**) Carcinoma appearing as multiple polypoid masses (*arrows*) measuring 11 to 15 mm each. Other polypoid masses, some larger than 15 mm, were present in the gallbladder (not shown). M, mass; L, gallbladder lumen.

to localized fundal adenomyomatosis may be difficult to differentiate from carcinoma. Irregular, nodular wall thickening in XGC may also be indistinguishable from gallbladder carcinoma.

Other Malignant Neoplasms

Primary malignant gallbladder neoplasms other than carcinoma are rare and include carcinoid tumors, lymphomas, and sarcomas (182). Hematogenous metastases to the gallbladder are rare; metastatic malignant melanoma is the most common. Sonographically, both metastatic and other primary tumors of the gallbladder may appear as focal wall thickening or one or more polypoid masses, or, rarely, they may even replace the entire gallbladder with tumor and thus may be indistinguishable from primary carcinoma.

Nonvisualization of the Gallbladder

Nonvisualization of the gallbladder as a fluid-filled structure by ultrasound in a fasting patient is most common secondary to contracted gallbladder filled with stones

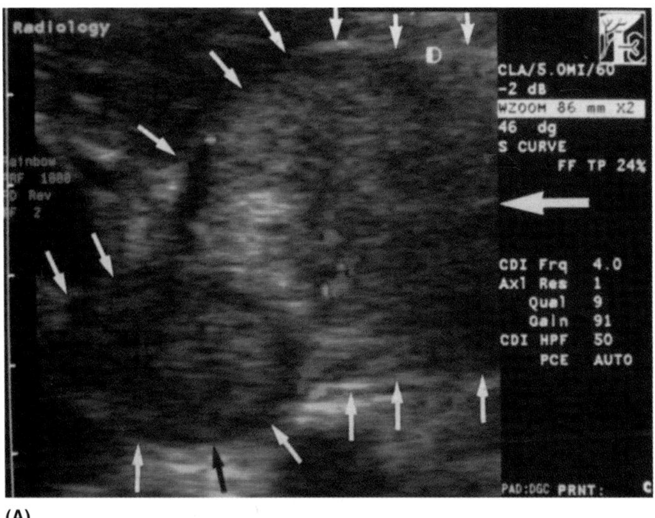

(A)

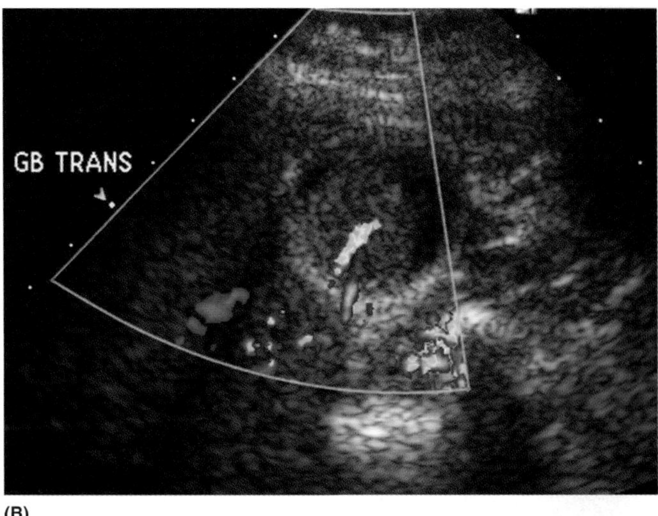

(B)

FIGURE 50 A AND B ■ Color Doppler sonography of gallbladder carcinoma. (**A**) Intrinsic vascularity confirms the diagnosis of carcinoma replacing almost the entire gallbladder (*arrows*) and differentiates carcinoma from sludge filling the gallbladder. (**B**) Intrinsic vascularity is seen in a polypoid mass secondary to gallbladder carcinoma. *Source*: (**A**) Courtesy of Philip W. Ralls, MD, Los Angeles, CA. (**B**) Courtesy of Monzer M. Abu-Yousef, MD, Iowa City, IA.

(Table 10). However, certain other conditions may produce nonvisualization or nonrecognition of the gallbladder. These conditions include the following: (*i*) congenital anomalies such as agenesis of the gallbladder, which is extremely rare, ectopic gallbladder, and biliary atresia; (*ii*) contracted gallbladder secondary to postprandial examination, viral hepatitis, cystic fibrosis, or marked biliary obstruction proximal to the cystic duct insertion; (*iii*) calcification in the wall of the gallbladder or air within the gallbladder or gallbladder wall causing acoustic shadowing; (*iv*) gallbladder completely filled with sludge, appearing as a solid structure (sonographic hepatization of the gallbladder); and (*v*) gallbladder carcinoma entirely filling the gallbladder. Demonstration of the relation of the abnormal structure to the main lobar fissure, demonstration of the gallbladder wall separating the solid structure from the liver, understanding of sonographic features of specific abnormalities, and correlation with abdominal radiography or computed tomography and clinical history are helpful in the diagnosis of gallbladder abnormalities in these situations (11,192).

TABLE 10 ■ Nonvisualization of the Gallbladder

After cholecystectomy
Agenesis of gallbladder
Ectopic gallbladder
Biliary atresia
Contracted gallbladder
■ Postprandial contraction
■ Viral hepatitis
■ Cystic fibrosis
Contracted gallbladder filled with stones
Porcelain gallbladder with shadowing
Gas in the gallbladder lumen or wall with shadowing
Sludge completely filling the gallbladder
Gallbladder carcinoma completely filling the gallbladder

INTRAHEPATIC BILE DUCTS

Normal Anatomy

The intrahepatic bile ducts run parallel to the portal veins and hepatic arteries (the portal triads). The relation of the intrahepatic bile ducts to the portal veins is variable, and the bile ducts may be anterior, posterior, or interlaced (tortuous) relative to the portal vein branches (193,194). Because of their small size, normal intrahepatic bile ducts are difficult to demonstrate reliably by ultrasound examination. However, small (<2 mm in diameter) tubular structures representing either normal hepatic arteries or bile ducts can be frequently seen adjacent to the portal veins, especially the right and left branches of the main portal vein and the portal vein branches in the lateral segment of the left lobe (Fig. 51) (195).

Intrahepatic Biliary Dilatation

In the past, "the parallel channel sign," consisting of two parallel tubular structures in the distribution of intrahepatic portal venous branches, was considered to be diagnostic of biliary dilatation (196,197). However, parallel tubular structures cannot be considered to be diagnostic of biliary dilatation unless the tubular structures adjacent to the portal veins are larger than 2 mm in diameter or they are more than 40% of the diameter of the adjacent portal vein (195). In minimal biliary dilatation, it is essential to confirm the biliary origin of these tubular structures by

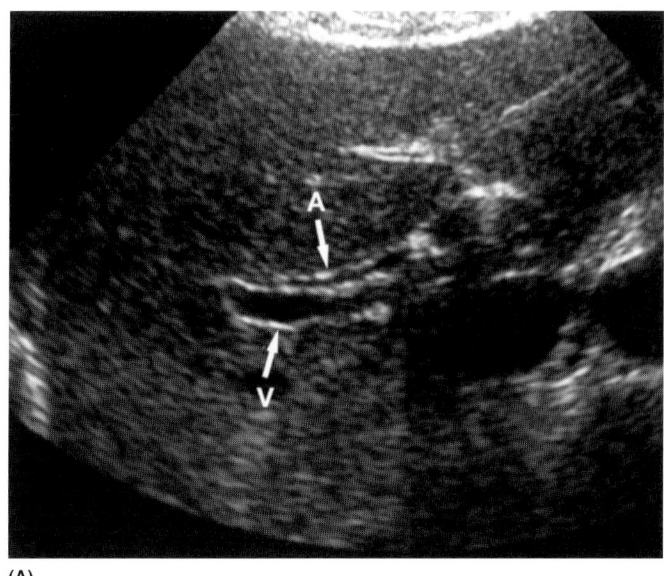

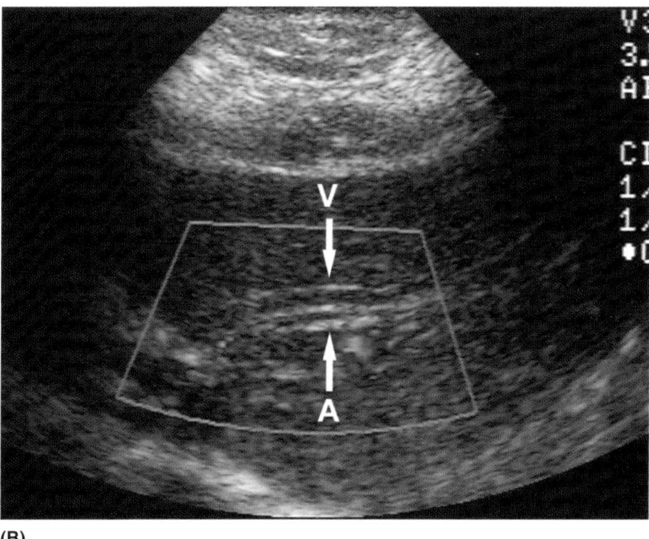

(A) (B)

FIGURE 51 A AND B ■ Normal parallel channels within the liver. (**A**) Transverse view showing right hepatic artery (A) anterior to the right portal vein (V). (**B**) Transverse view showing branches of the portal vein and hepatic artery within the lateral segment of the left lobe of the liver as two parallel tubular structures. Color Doppler sonography demonstrates hepatopetal flow in both vascular structures.

demonstrating the lack of color flow by CDS (Fig. 52) (198). Duplex Doppler evaluation is technically difficult and tedious because of the small size of the tubular structures. Important sonographic criteria for diagnosis of biliary dilatation and for differentiation between bile ducts and portal veins include (*i*) alteration of the normal anatomic pattern of the portal triads (Figs. 53 and 54), (*ii*) irregularity of the walls of the bile ducts secondary to tortuosity (Figs. 53 and 54A), (*iii*) stellate confluence of the dilated tubular ducts (Fig. 54), and (*iv*) acoustic enhancement behind the dilated bile ducts (Fig. 55) (199). Acoustic enhancement is frequently seen behind dilated bile ducts and is usually not seen behind portal veins. The most reliable differentiating feature is detection of an alteration in the normal appearance of the portal triads (199). With biliary dilatation, two or more tubular structures are visible in the expected position of the portal vein; this is best seen on the transverse

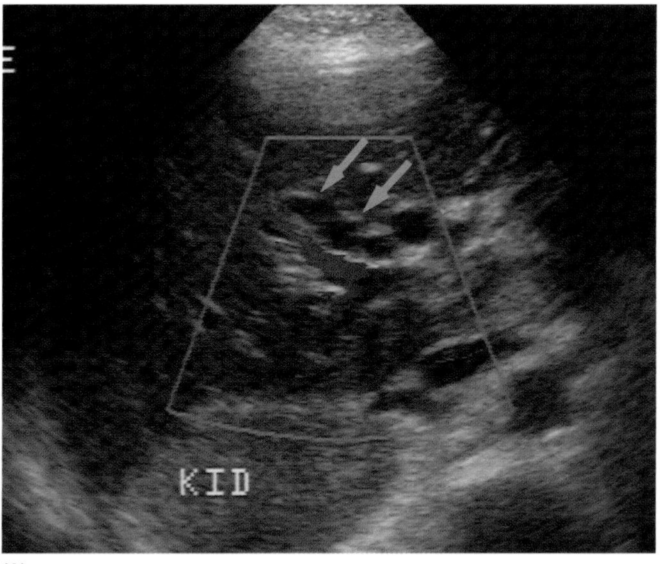

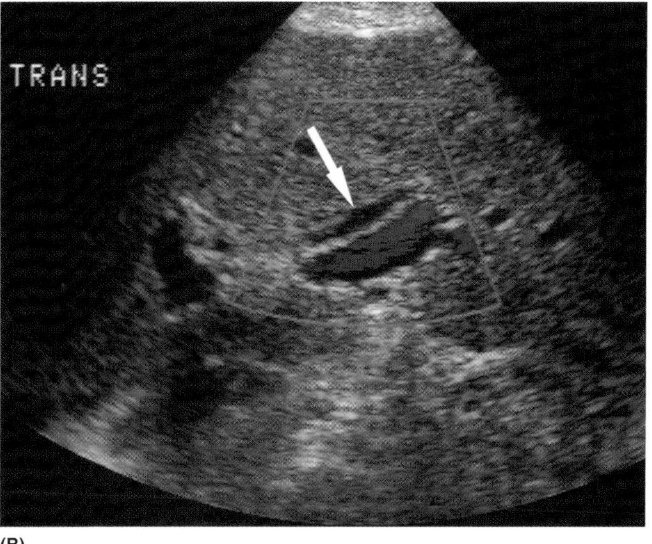

(A) (B)

FIGURE 52 A AND B ■ Dilated intrahepatic bile ducts: color Doppler. Transverse color Doppler sonograms confirming minimal intrahepatic biliary dilatation by demonstrating the absence of flow signals in the dilated bile duct (*arrows*) within the right (**A**) and the left (**B**) lobe of the liver. Color signals appear in the adjacent portal veins.

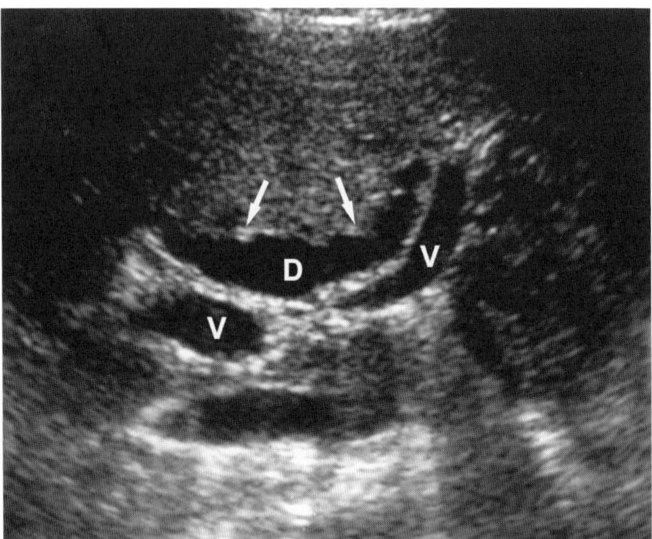

FIGURE 53 ■ Dilated intrahepatic bile ducts: irregular wall. Transverse view showing dilated right and left intrahepatic bile ducts (D) (*arrows*) anterior to the right and left portal veins (V). The wall of the dilated bile ducts has an irregular contour (*arrows*).

view, adjacent to the right and left branches of the main portal vein, around the anterior and posterior branches of the right portal vein and segmental branches of the left portal vein. A longitudinal view at the level of the right portal vein is also helpful in demonstrating multiple dilated tubular structures.

Pitfalls

Dilated Hepatic Arteries ■ Dilated hepatic arteries in the liver, seen most often in patients with cirrhosis and portal hypertension, may mimic dilated bile ducts (Fig. 56) (200). These structures, however, can be easily distinguished by CDS.

Focal Biliary Obstruction ■ Focal segmental biliary dilatation can occur secondary to neoplasm, strictures, calculi, or Caroli's disease and requires thorough examination of the portal triads throughout the entire liver for its detection.

Postoperative Dilatation ■ With sonography, it is not possible to distinguish persistent postoperative biliary dilatation without obstruction, which can occur in some patients with biliary–enteric anastomosis, from dilatation secondary to obstruction. In these patients, hepatobiliary scintigraphy is helpful in distinguishing obstructive from nonobstructive dilatation of the bile ducts (201).

Debris in Ducts ■ Dilated bile ducts may not be recognized if they contain blood clot, pus, or sludge. Blood clots, pus, or sludge in the bile ducts may be isoechoic with the adjacent liver parenchyma and thus may obscure the dilated bile ducts.

Pneumobilia ■ In patients with pneumobilia, shadowing from air in the bile ducts frequently obscures the lumen of the dilated bile ducts. Pneumobilia can be caused by surgical biliary–enteric anastomosis, biliary–enteric fistula complicating surgery, incompetent sphincter of Oddi, erosion of a gallstone into the gastrointestinal tract, peptic ulcer erosion into the common bile duct, and, uncommonly, acute emphysematous cholecystitis with a patent cystic duct and cholangitis due to gas-forming organisms (202). With the patient in the supine position,

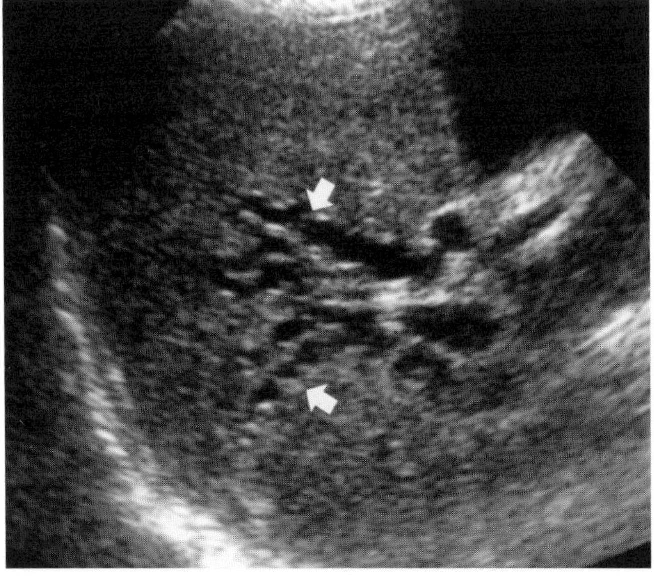

(A)

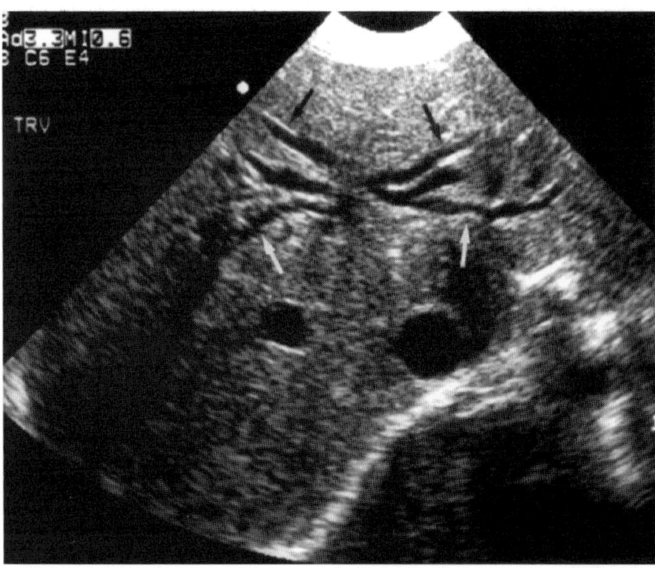

(B)

FIGURE 54 A AND B ■ Dilated intrahepatic bile ducts: stellate appearance. (**A**) Longitudinal view of the right lobe of the liver demonstrating stellate confluence of dilated bile ducts (*arrows*). The walls of the bile ducts are irregular (*arrows*). (**B**) Transverse view demonstrating stellate confluence of dilated intrahepatic ducts (*arrows*).

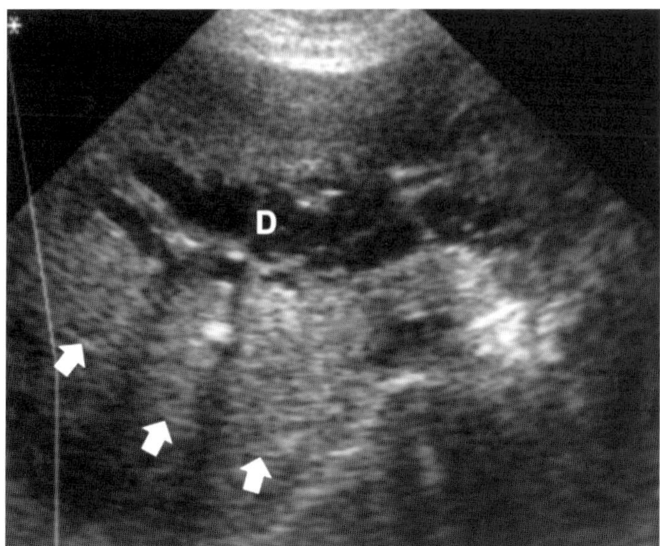

FIGURE 55 ■ Dilated intrahepatic bile ducts (D): acoustic enhancement. Transverse view showing acoustic enhancement (*arrows*) posterior to the dilated bile ducts in the right lobe of the liver.

the gas preferentially fills the anteriorly located left hepatic bile ducts. Sonographically, pneumobilia is characterized by echogenic foci, either short or linear, in the distribution of the bile ducts (Fig. 57). The echogenic foci may cast an acoustic shadow and frequently produce reverberations and comet-tail artifacts (Fig. 57). Motion of the air bubbles within the bile ducts may be recognized by rapidly moving reverberations, frequently seen in patients with surgical biliary–enteric anastomosis. A small amount of air in the bile ducts may produce clean shadow without reverberations and may mimic biliary calculi or liver calcifications (Fig. 58).

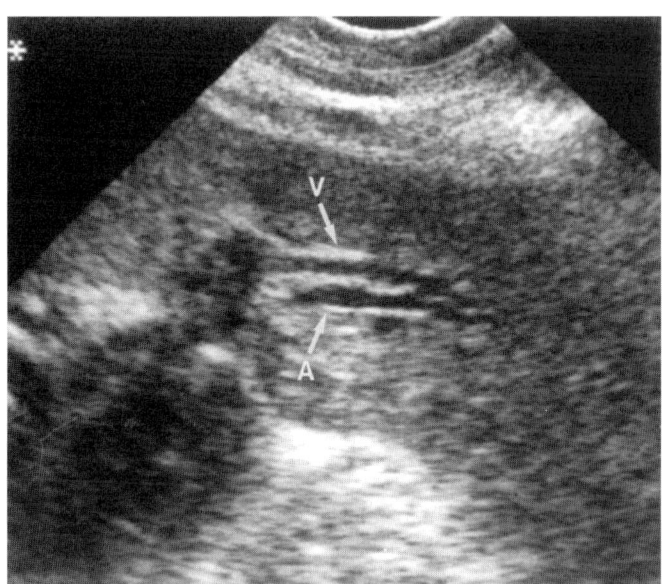

FIGURE 56 ■ Pitfall. Dilated hepatic artery (A) posterior to the portal vein (V) mimics a dilated bile duct in the lateral segment of the left lobe of the liver.

Cholangitis

Bacterial Cholangitis

Bacterial cholangitis is almost always associated with biliary obstruction causing bacterial infection secondary to bile stasis. Benign causes of obstruction are much more likely to cause bacterial cholangitis than malignant causes (203). Cholangitis can also occur in up to 18% of patients with biliary–enteric anastomosis (201). Patients present clinically with right upper quadrant abdominal pain, chills, fever, and jaundice. Sonography in most patients demonstrates significant ductal dilatation and identifies the cause and

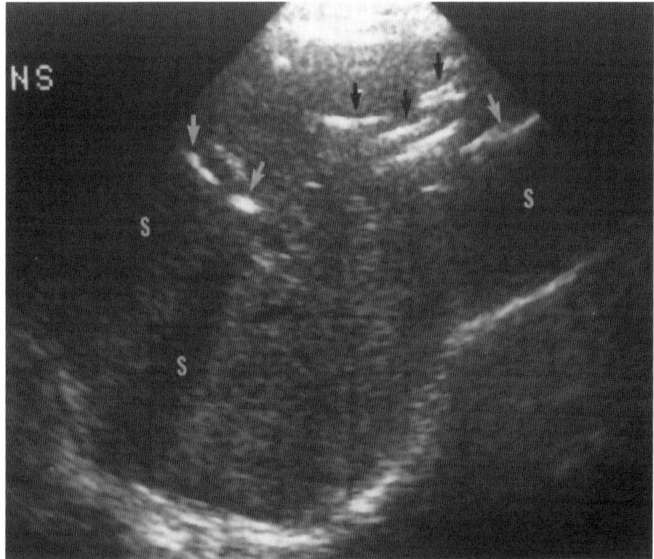

(A)

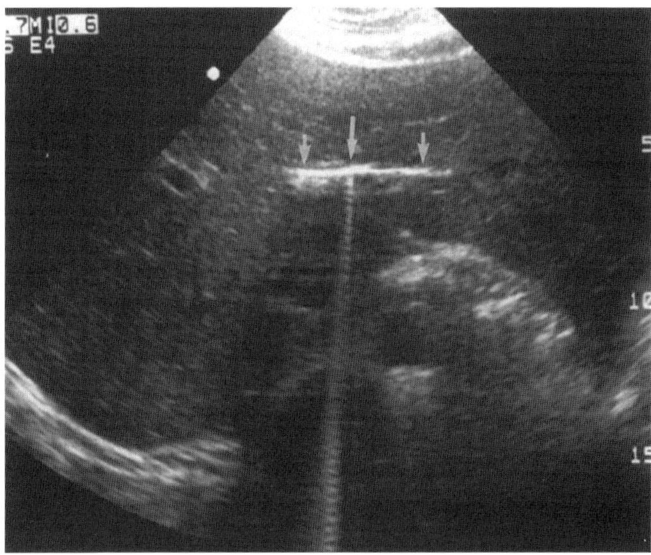

(B)

FIGURE 57 A AND B ■ Pneumobilia. (**A**) Transverse view demonstrating air within the intrahepatic bile ducts appearing as multiple linear or bandlike hyperechoic areas (*arrows*), some associated with distal acoustic shadowing. (**B**) Transverse view demonstrating air within the bile duct in the left lobe of the liver appearing as a linear hyperechoic structure (*arrows*). Comet-tail or ring-down artifact (*long arrow*) is produced by air bubbles within the bile duct.

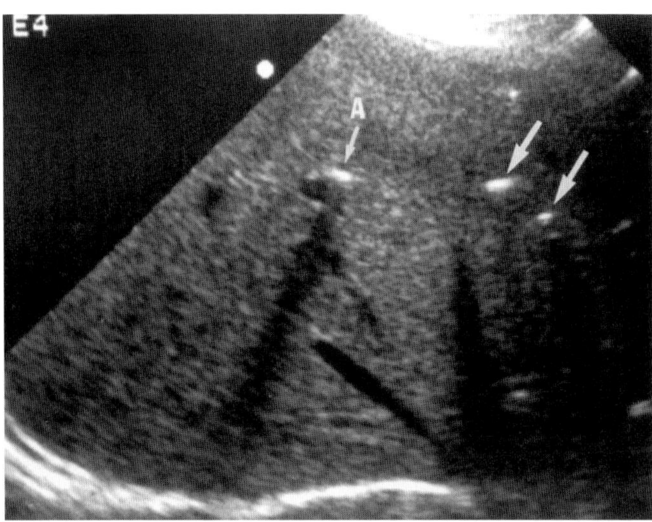

FIGURE 58 ■ Pneumobilia mimicking calcifications. Transverse view of the liver. Air in the bile duct appears as a hyperechoic focus (A) with distal clean acoustic shadowing. Other hyperechoic foci (*arrows*) secondary to air in the bile ducts are seen with less obvious acoustic shadowing.

level of obstruction. In acute ascending cholangitis, purulent bile may be identified as intraluminal echogenic material within the dilated bile ducts. Hepatic abscesses not uncommonly complicate bacterial cholangitis. Prompt biliary drainage is mandatory, and sonography may be valuable in guiding percutaneous biliary drainage. Chronic obstructive cholangitis with repeated infections may cause ductal strictures, intrahepatic or extrahepatic ductal wall thickening (Fig. 59) (Table 11), peripheral narrowing of intrahepatic bile ducts, and biliary cirrhosis.

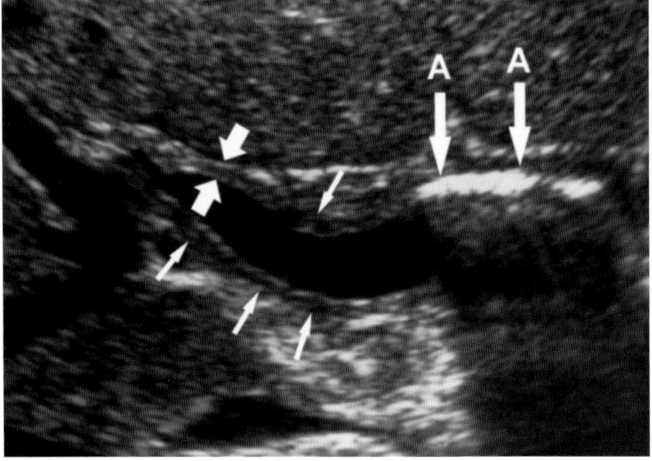

FIGURE 59 ■ Bacterial cholangitis. Longitudinal view demonstrating a dilated common bile duct with diffuse wall thickening (*large and small arrows*) in a patient with chronic bacterial cholangitis. A hypoechoic central layer is seen between the hyperechoic serosa and mucosa of the duct wall (*large arrows*). The thick, bandlike hyperechoic area (A) with acoustic shadowing represents air within the common duct secondary to biliary–enteric anastomosis.

TABLE 11 ■ Causes of Bile Duct (Intrahepatic or Extrahepatic) Wall Thickening

Disorder	Intrahepatic bile ducts	Common duct
Cholangitis		
■ Chronic bacterial cholangitis	✓	✓
■ Primary sclerosing cholangitis	✓	✓
■ AIDS cholangitis	✓	✓
■ Recurrent pyogenic cholangitis	✓	✓
Choledocholithiasis		✓
Pancreatitis		✓
Parasites (clonorchiasis)	✓	
Cholangiocarcinoma (unusual)		✓

Primary Sclerosing Cholangitis

Primary sclerosing cholangitis is a chronic cholestatic disease of unknown origin that is characterized by diffuse fibrosing inflammation of the intrahepatic and extrahepatic bile ducts, resulting in biliary cirrhosis and hepatic failure. The term "primary" is used to distinguish this disease from the biliary strictures that may result from operative injury or choledocholithiasis. It is associated, in nearly 75% of cases, with ulcerative colitis, and approximately 70% of patients are male and younger than 45 years of age. Clinical features include fatigue, pruritus, right upper quadrant pain, jaundice, and hepatosplenomegaly. Most characteristic imaging findings are seen on cholangiography and include multiple short segmental strictures, beading, pruning, diverticula, and mural thickening of the bile ducts. These findings are difficult to demonstrate sonographically unless the patient has biliary dilatation. The walls of the common bile duct and intrahepatic bile ducts may be thickened in a smooth or irregular fashion (Fig. 60) (204). Gallbladder abnormalities occur in 40% of patients, including gallbladder wall thickening and increased incidence of gallstones and gallbladder neoplasms such as adenoma and carcinoma. Enlarged lymph nodes may be seen in porta hepatis. Cholangiocarcinoma complicates primary sclerosing cholangitis in about 15% of patients, and sonographic differentiation may be difficult unless an associated mass lesion is present. Markedly dilated intrahepatic bile ducts also raise the possibility of complicating cholangiocarcinoma.

AIDS-Related Cholangitis

Cholangitis related to AIDS causes intrahepatic and extrahepatic bile duct changes identical to those seen in sclerosing cholangitis (strictures, focal dilatation, and thickened duct walls) (Fig. 61) (205). An additional finding is a dilated common bile duct with a hyperechoic nodule in the distal end of the common bile duct probably caused by edema of the papilla of Vater, with thickening of the adjacent common bile duct wall (206). The combination of papillary stenosis and intrahepatic ductal strictures appears to be unique to AIDS-related cholangitis. Associated findings include thickening of the gallbladder wall and, in children, abnormal hepatic echotexture (207). The abnormalities are

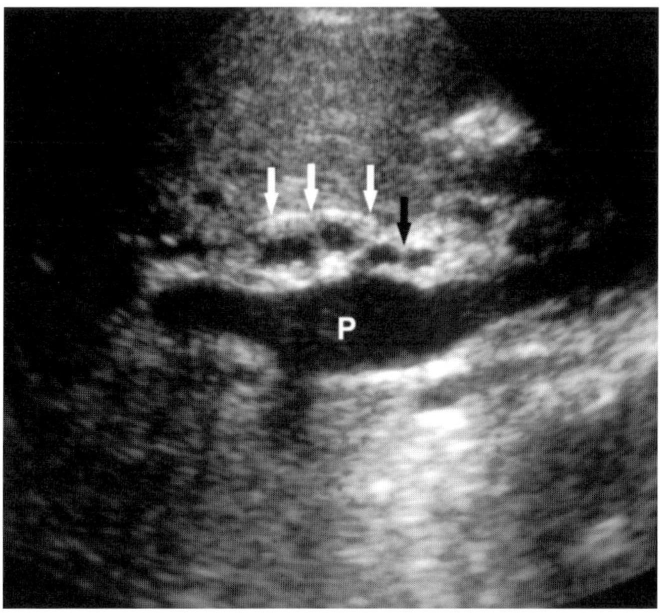

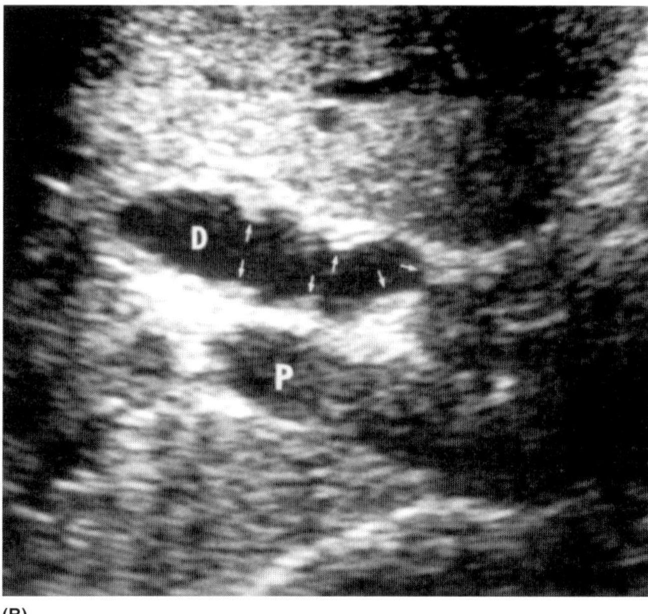

(A) (B)

FIGURE 60 A AND B ■ Sclerosing cholangitis. (**A**) Transverse view demonstrating irregular wall thickening of a dilated right intrahepatic bile duct (*arrows*). Echogenic septations within the bile duct are secondary to several annular strictures within the duct. P, right portal vein. (**B**) Longitudinal oblique view showing irregular thickening (*arrows*) of the wall of the dilated proximal common hepatic duct (D). *Source*: Courtesy of Bhaskara K. Rao, MD, Houston, TX.

probably caused by cytomegalovirus or Cryptosporidium infection (205,208).

Recurrent Pyogenic Cholangitis

Recurrent pyogenic cholangitis, commonly known as Oriental cholangiohepatitis, is endemic in Southeast Asia and is characterized by recurrent attacks of abdominal pain, fever, and jaundice. Pathologically, the intrahepatic and extrahepatic ducts are dilated and contain soft, pigmented stones and pus (209). The pathologic changes are most marked in the intrahepatic ducts, with patchy stenosis and dilatation of the bile ducts secondary to fibrosis; secondary biliary cirrhosis may develop after repeated infections. The cause of this disease is unknown, but parasitic infestation (clonorchiasis and ascariasis), malnutrition, portal bacteremia, and intrahepatic calculi secondary to congenital biliary strictures have been etiologically implicated. Sonographic findings include intrahepatic or extrahepatic duct stones, dilatation of the common bile duct and right and left hepatic ducts with relatively mild or no dilatation of the peripheral intrahepatic ducts, localized dilatation of the lobar or segmental bile ducts especially left lobe, bile duct wall thickening, increased periportal echogenicity, segmental hepatic atrophy, and gallstones. The gallbladder is distended and palpable in about 30% of cases (210). Recurrent pyogenic cholangitis is most commonly associated with pigment stones that may be soft and mudlike in consistency and that may form a cast of the biliary tree (Fig. 62A). The stones are usually of medium echogenicity, with variable degrees of acoustic shadowing (Fig. 62), and they may be difficult to demonstrate in the absence of acoustic shadowing. Computed tomography is helpful in demonstrating the full extent of ductal abnormalities.

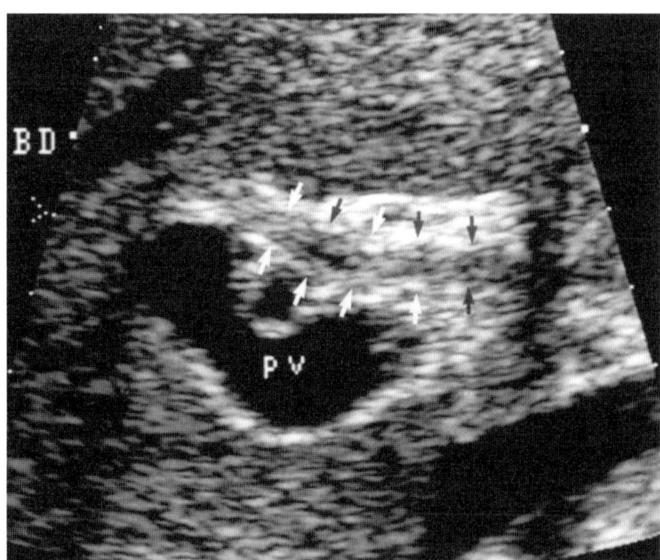

FIGURE 61 ■ AIDS cholangitis. Longitudinal view demonstrating considerable echogenic thickening of the walls of the common bile duct (*arrows*) almost completely obliterating the lumen of the duct. PV, main portal vein. *Source*: Courtesy of Ronald H. Wachsberg, MD, Newark, NJ.

Intrahepatic Biliary Calculi

Intrahepatic biliary calculi are uncommon in patients with gallstones, but they frequently occur in patients with

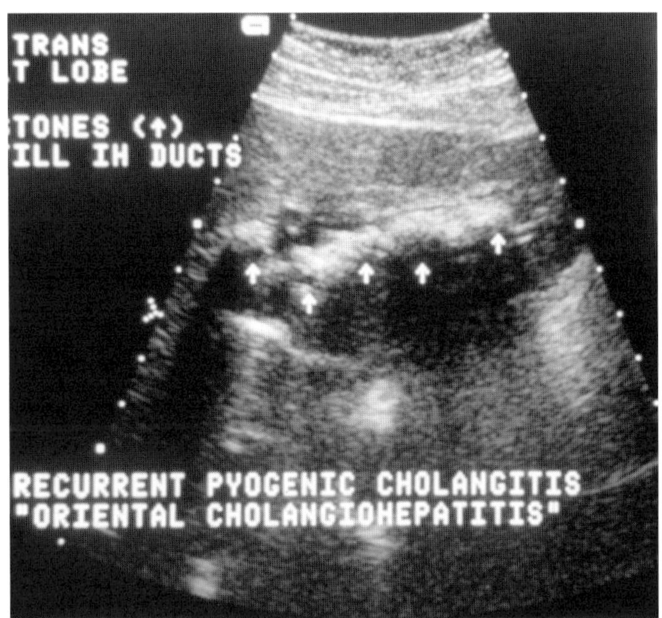

(A)

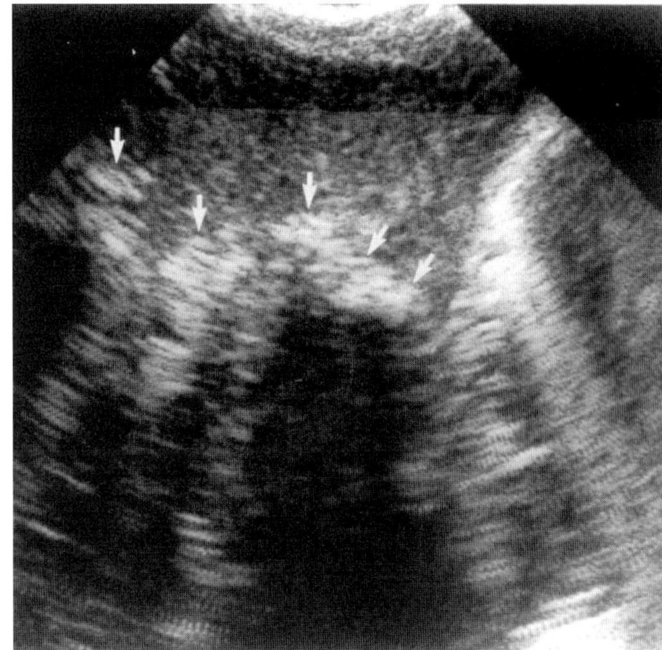

(B)

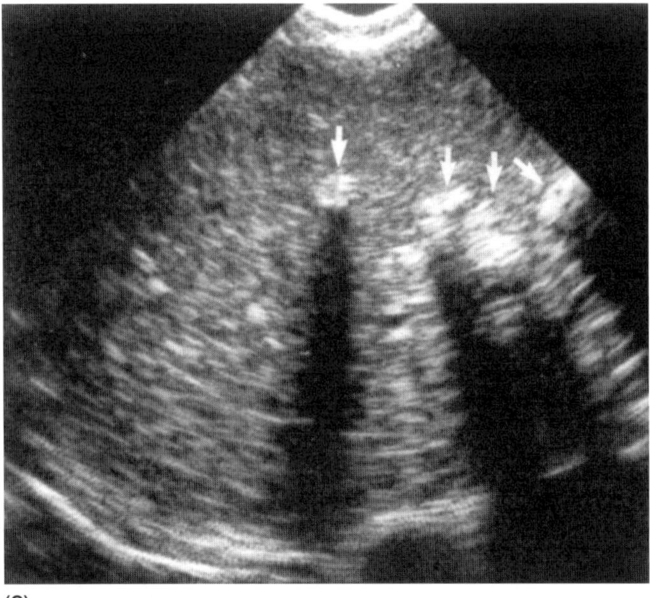

(C)

FIGURE 62 A–C ■ Recurrent pyogenic cholangitis, with intrahepatic biliary calculi. (**A**) Transverse view demonstrating multiple stones (*arrows*) completely filling the bile duct within the lateral segment of the left lobe of the liver. Stones produce distal acoustic shadowing. (**B**) Transverse view and (**C**) longitudinal view, in another patient, showing multiple intrahepatic biliary calculi (*arrows*) with distal acoustic shadowing. *Source*: (**A**) Courtesy of Philip W. Ralls, MD, Los Angeles, CA. (**B**, **C**) Courtesy of Bhaskara K. Rao, MD, Houston, TX.

recurrent pyogenic cholangitis. They may also be associated with benign or malignant biliary strictures, Caroli's disease, or other causes of intrahepatic biliary stasis. Sonographically, biliary calculi are seen as focal hyperechoic structures, usually with clean distal shadowing and are located adjacent to the portal vein branches (Fig. 63). Associated bile duct dilatation is frequently seen.

Pitfalls

Calcified Arteries ■ Intrahepatic arterial wall calcifications also occur adjacent to the portal venous branches, and when associated with acoustic shadowing, they may mimic intrahepatic biliary calculi (211). Computed tomography in these patients is helpful in demonstrating arterial calcifications.

Other Calcifications or Clips ■ Other intrahepatic calcifications such as calcified granulomas or surgical clips, if located close to the portal triads, may also mimic stones. Surgical clips frequently are associated with comet-tail reverberation.

Pneumobilia ■ Air within the bile ducts may cause shadowing without reverberations and may mimic stones (Fig. 58).

Caroli's Disease

Caroli's disease is a rare congenital malformation causing nonobstructive multifocal saccular dilatation of intrahepatic segmental bile ducts, and is frequently associated with

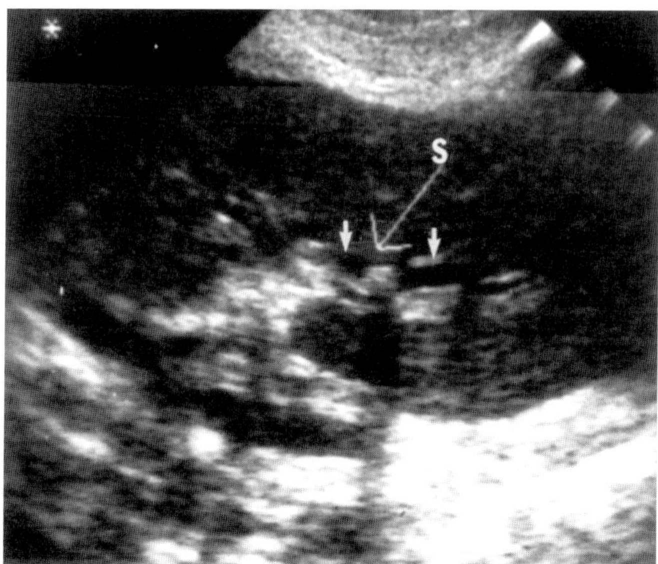

FIGURE 63 ■ Transverse view demonstrating a stone (S) with distal acoustic shadowing, within a dilated intrahepatic bile duct (*arrows*) in the lateral segment of the left lobe of the liver. The patient had gallstones as well as stones in the common bile duct (not shown).

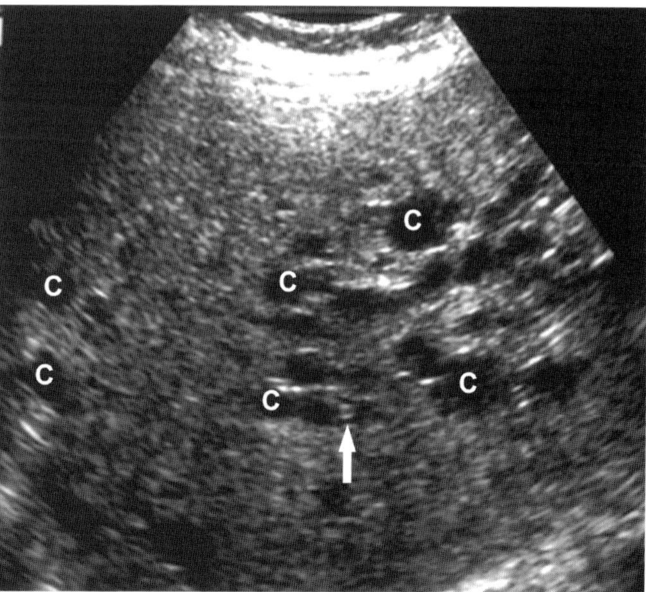

FIGURE 64 ■ Caroli's disease. Transverse view showing multiple areas of cystic dilatation of the intrahepatic bile ducts. The portal radicle is seen as a small hyperechoic structure (*arrow*) protruding from the wall of one of the cystic areas (the "central dot" sign). C, cystic dilatation. *Source*: Courtesy of Oksana Baltarowich, MD, Philadelphia, PA.

infantile autosomal recessive polycystic kidney disease and congenital hepatic fibrosis. Caroli's disease is likely to be present at birth, but it usually remains asymptomatic for the first 5 to 20 years of life. Most common complications are recurrent bacterial cholangitis, which may be complicated by liver abscess and formation of intracystic pigment stones (212). Association of cholangiocarcinoma and hepatocellular carcinoma has been reported with Caroli's disease (212). Sonographically, cysts of varying sizes are seen scattered throughout the liver or are confined to part of the liver (Fig. 64) (213). Tubular or saccular dilatation of the segmental bile ducts may be associated with the cysts (Fig. 65). Marchal et al. described sonographic findings that are suggestive of Caroli's disease including (*i*) intraluminal bulbar protrusions, (*ii*) bridge formation across dilated bile ducts resembling internal septa within the dilated bile ducts, and (*iii*) portal radicles partially or completely surrounded by dilated bile ducts (215). Sonographically, portal radicles partially or completely surrounded by dilated bile ducts may appear as tiny, hyperechoic structures centrally or protruding from the wall of the dilated cystic-appearing bile ducts ("central dot" sign) (Figs. 64 and 65) (216). Color Doppler signals within the septations or central dots in the dilated bile ducts may be other helpful diagnostic criteria (Fig. 65) (217,218). Computed tomography may demonstrate tiny dots within dilated bile ducts that enhance after intravenous contrast, corresponding to intraluminal portal venous radicles. Demonstration of communication between the cysts and the bile ducts is necessary to distinguish Caroli's disease from polycystic liver disease or multiple simple liver cysts. When the biliary communication is not obvious on sonography, hepatobiliary scintigraphy or endoscopic retrograde cholangiopancreatography may be performed.

EXTRAHEPATIC BILE DUCTS

Normal Anatomy

The right and left hepatic ducts join to form the common hepatic duct, which is located anterior to the right and main portal veins. Approximately 3 cm from the confluence of the right and left hepatic ducts, the distal cystic duct joins the common hepatic duct to form the common bile duct (2). In the porta hepatis, the common hepatic and the common bile ducts are located anterior to the main portal vein. The main (proper) hepatic artery is also located anterior to the main portal vein, but it is usually medial to the common bile duct (Fig. 66). From the porta hepatis, the common bile duct, along with the main portal vein and the main (proper) hepatic artery, descends within the hepatoduodenal ligament. The distal common bile duct passes behind the duodenum and then runs in a groove on the upper and lateral part of the posterior surface of the head of the pancreas, anterior to the inferior vena cava. The common bile duct and the pancreatic duct usually join together to form the ampulla (of Vater) in the descending part of the duodenum. The common hepatic duct is approximately 3 cm long, and the common bile duct is about 7.5 cm long.

Common Duct

Because sonographically, the junction of the distal cystic duct and the common hepatic duct cannot be seen in everyone, the term "common duct" is used to describe both the common hepatic and common bile ducts. The common duct can be divided into the proximal and the distal segments. The proximal or hilar (i.e., porta hepatis) segment is anterior to the main portal vein. The distal

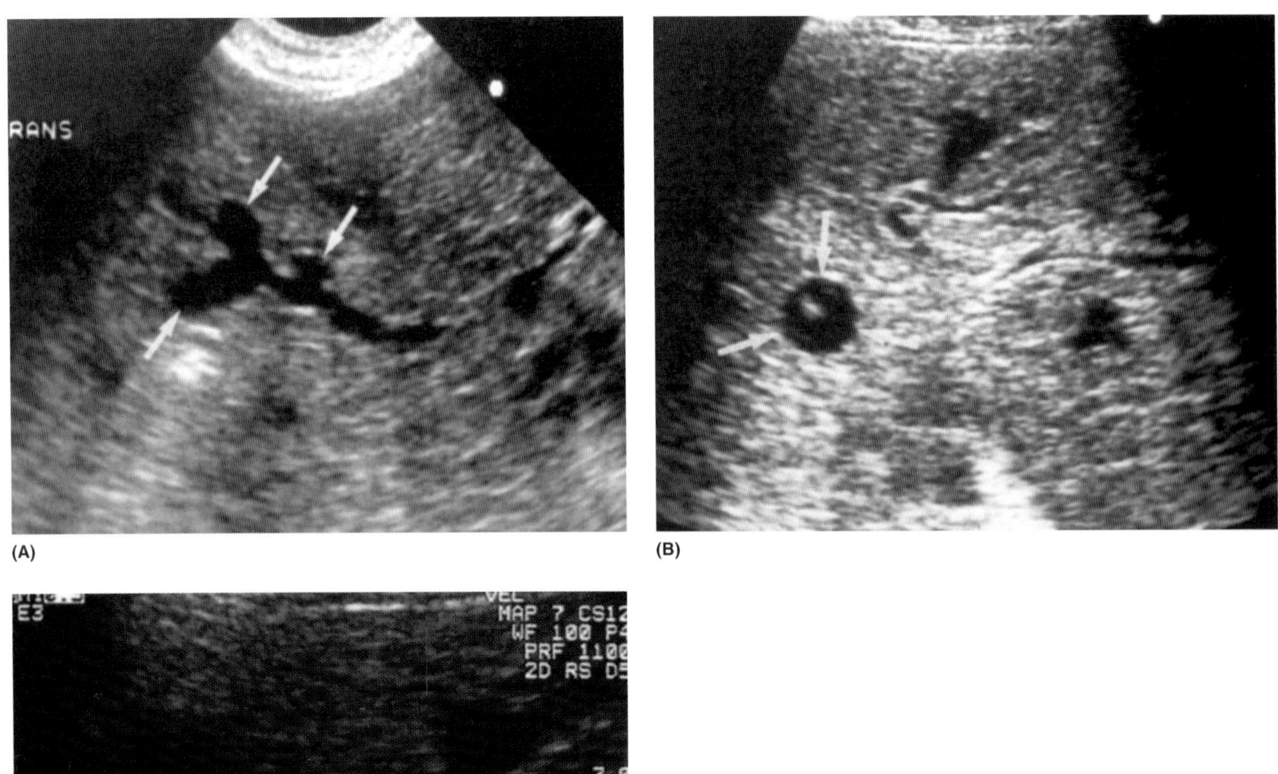

FIGURE 65 A–C ■ Caroli's disease. (**A**) Transverse view demonstrating dilated intrahepatic bile duct with several areas of saccular dilatation (*arrows*). (**B**) Longitudinal view demonstrating cystic dilatation of the intrahepatic bile duct (*arrow*). A central echogenic focus is present (the "central dot" sign). (**C**) Color Doppler showing flow within the central dot, confirming its vascular nature. *Source*: From Ref. 214.

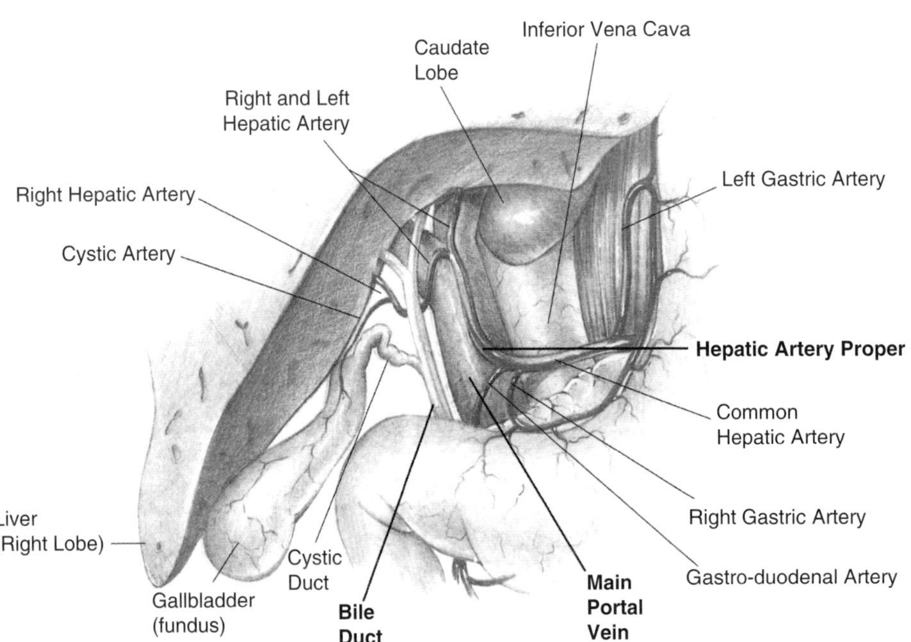

FIGURE 66 ■ Diagram. Porta hepatis: relation of common bile duct, main portal vein, and main (proper) hepatic artery (labeled in bold letters). *Source*: From Ref. 2.

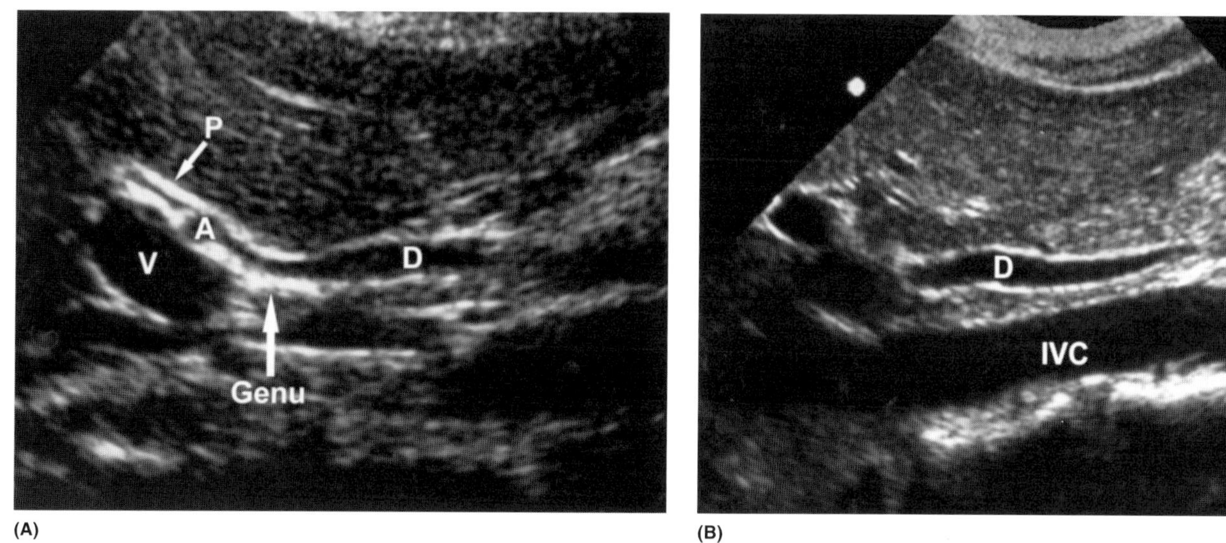

FIGURE 67 A AND B ■ Normal common duct. Longitudinal views. (**A**) The proximal segment (P) of the common duct is seen parallel to the main portal vein (V). Dorsal angle (Genu) is seen between the proximal and distal (D) segments of the common duct. (**B**) The distal (suprapancreatic) common duct (D) is seen parallel to the inferior vena cava (IVC).

segment can be further divided into suprapancreatic and pancreatic portions. The suprapancreatic portion is between the porta hepatis and the pancreatic head. The pancreatic portion is at the level of the head of the pancreas. Sonographically, on the longitudinal view, the *proximal segment* is seen anterior to the right and main portal veins and runs parallel to the main portal vein (Fig. 67). Most of the *distal segment* runs almost parallel to the plane of the inferior vena cava in the sagittal axis (Fig. 67). Most persons have a dorsal bend or angle between the proximal and distal segments (Fig. 67). This angle is designated the *genu of the common duct* (Fig. 67) (219). At the level of the pancreatic head, the common duct is seen posterior to the head on the longitudinal view and posterolateral to the head on the transverse view (Fig. 68) (214).

The right hepatic artery appears as a rounded, anechoic structure between the common duct and the portal

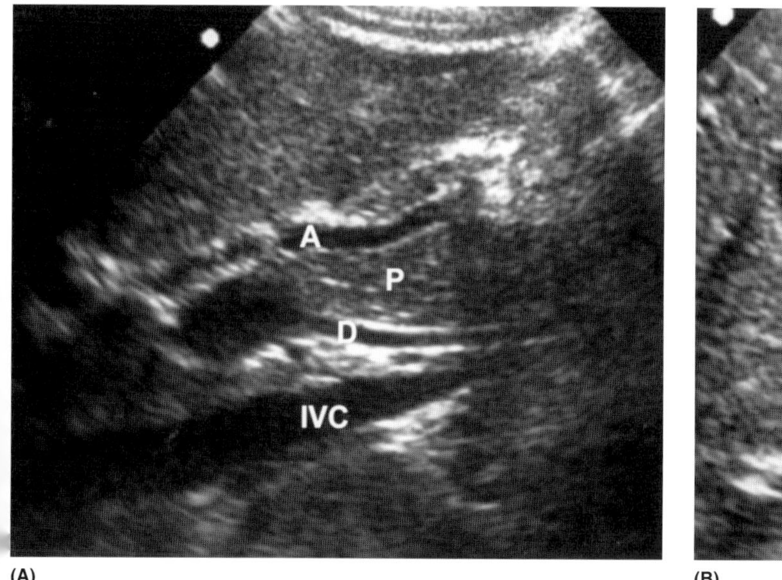

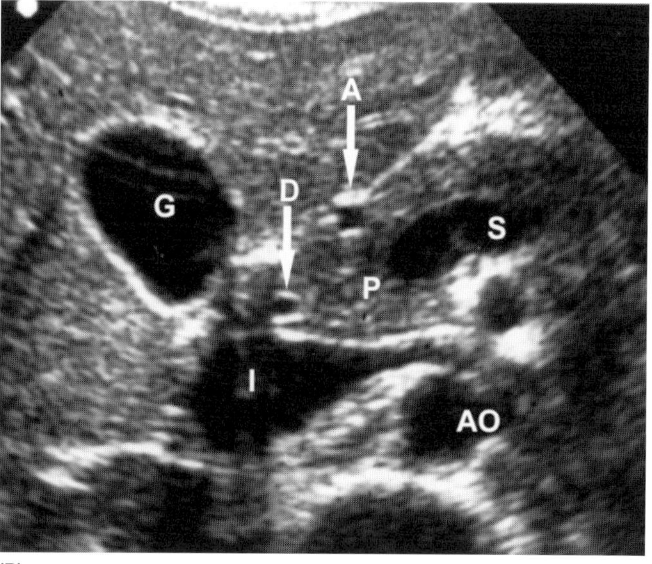

FIGURE 68 A AND B ■ Normal distal common duct: pancreatic portion. (**A**) Longitudinal view showing distal common duct (D) posterior to the head of the pancreas (P). (**B**) Transverse view showing the distal common duct (D) along the posterior and lateral margin of the head of the pancreas (P). Gastroduodenal artery is seen anterior to the head of the pancreas. A, gastroduodenal artery; IVC or I, inferior vena cava; G, gallbladder; S, splenic vein; AO, aorta.

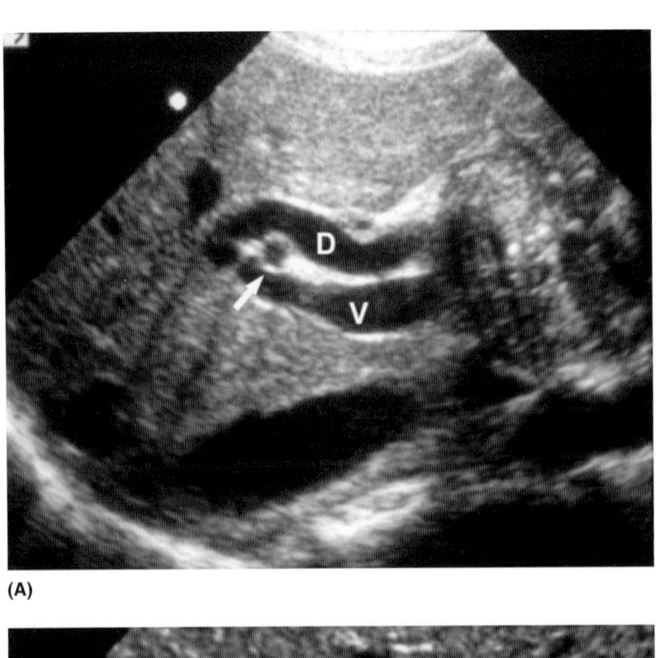

(A)

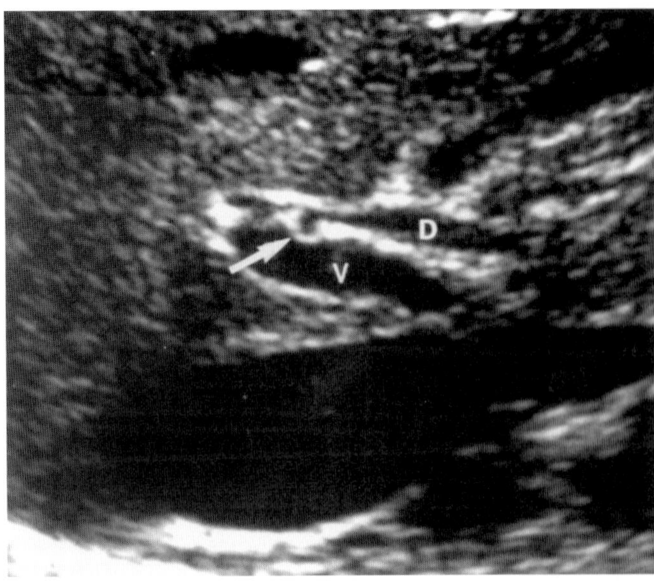

(B)

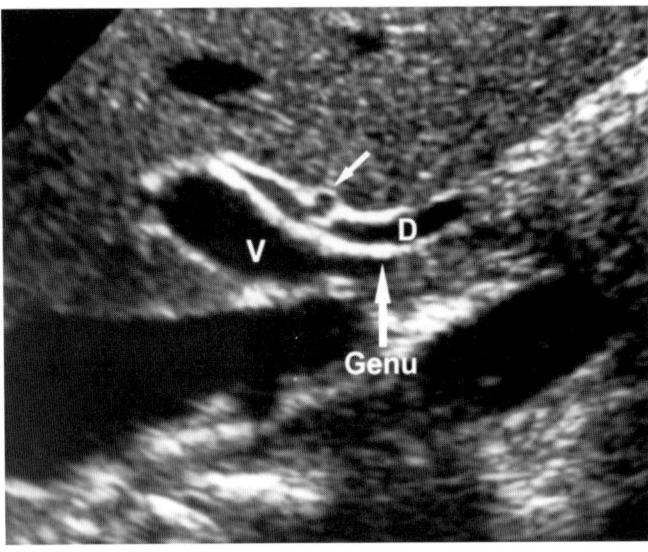

(C)

FIGURE 69 A–C ■ Relation of the right hepatic artery to the common duct on longitudinal views. (**A**, **B**) Right hepatic artery (*arrow*) is seen as a rounded anechoic structure posterior to the common duct, between the common duct and the main portal vein. The common duct is slightly dilated in **A** and is of normal size in **B**. (**C**) Right hepatic artery (*arrow*) is seen anterior to the common duct. Dorsal angle (Genu) is seen between the proximal and distal segments of the common duct. D, common duct; V, main portal vein.

vein in approximately 85% of patients and is seen anterior to the common duct in approximately 15% (Fig. 69) (220). The right hepatic artery forms an indentation, frequently prominent, on the wall of the common duct.

Common Duct Size

The size of the normal common duct has been reported to be as small as 4 mm or as large as 8 mm (219,221–223). These discrepancies are primarily related to the location of the common duct measurement and also are possibly related to respiratory phase. The distal portions of the common duct are usually larger than the proximal portion. A few persons may have an increase in ductal diameter (1 mm or more) after deep inspiration compared with the diameter measured in expiration (224).

In adults, the average (mean) diameter of the normal common duct is 4 mm (219). Generally, a common duct diameter of 6 mm or less is considered to be normal, 7 mm is considered equivocal, and more than 7 mm is considered dilated (219,225). These measurements are maximal internal luminal diameters of the *proximal segment* of the common duct (Fig. 67) anterior and parallel to the main portal vein, close to the genu of the common duct, in *longitudinal view*, in deep inspiration. The lumen of the common duct is measured from the inside of the near wall to the inside of the far wall.

Common Duct Size and Age

The common duct diameter has been reported to increase with age (226–228). In the study by Wu et al. (226), the upper limit of the normal diameter of the common duct is reported to be 10 mm in elderly persons (older than age 60 years). However, in this study, only 29 individuals were older than 60 years. Also, the diameter of the common duct was measured at its widest point, which was usually in its most distal portions. However, the most commonly used published sonographic measurements are of the proximal portion or midportion of the common duct anterior to the main portal vein. This is because the most consistently visualized portion of the common duct is anterior to the main portal vein. In a study of patients 20 years and older, Bachar et al. reported that the mean common duct size was 3.128 ± 0.862 mm in patients younger than 50 years and 4.19 ± 1.15 mm in patients older than 50 years (229). They found that the common duct gradually dilated by 0.04 mm/yr and suggested that the upper normal limit of the common duct in elderly persons be set at 8.5 mm (229).

However, two studies of US populations concluded that overall, there was no significant increase in size of the common duct with age (227,230). A study by Horrow et al. concluded that there was no increase in the size of the extrahepatic bile duct with age in an adult population (230). Another study by Perret et al. (227) evaluated the diameter of the common duct in 1018 patients between the ages of 60 and 96 years. Unlike those in other studies, the individuals in this study were not examined after overnight fasting. Instead, they were examined at varying, uncontrolled time intervals after meals. The authors state that the potential effect of this uncontrolled variable should be negligible because of the large sample (1018 patients). The results of this study demonstrated a statistically significant, but small, increase in the diameter of the common duct with increasing age (60-years-old or younger with mean diameter of 3.6 ± 0.26 mm vs. 85-years-old or older with mean diameter of 4 ± 0.25 mm). These authors concluded that although the common duct did increase slightly in size with aging, 98% of all ducts remained smaller than 6 mm. Also, 99% of all ducts remained smaller than 7 mm, which is the commonly accepted normal upper range for adults.

Common Duct Size in Children

A common duct diameter larger than 2 mm is considered abnormal and suggests obstruction in neonates (231). The upper limit of normal diameter of the distal segment of the common duct has been reported to be 2 mm in infants and 3 mm in children under 13 years of age (232).

Common Duct Size after Cholecystectomy

Considerable controversy also exists regarding dilatation of the unobstructed common duct in asymptomatic patients after cholecystectomy (219,222,223,233–235). Some studies report no or minimal dilatation and some report significant dilatation (219,222,228,233–239). In all studies reporting lack of common duct dilatation or minimal common duct dilatation, the maximum interval after cholecystectomy was 24 months, except for two studies with five-year intervals (233,234,238,239). Perhaps patients with increasing time intervals (five years or more) after cholecystectomy may have increasing diameters of the common duct. In our experience, many persons who are asymptomatic after cholecystectomy, and who have no evidence of obstruction, have dilated common ducts (219). In a study of 67 patients who were asymptomatic after cholecystectomy, a significant minority (16%) of patients had dilated common ducts up to 10 mm in diameter (233). After cholecystectomy and in patients with previous common bile duct surgery, a common duct diameter of 10 mm or larger in asymptomatic patients with normal liver function tests and 7 mm or larger in symptomatic patients or in patients with abnormal liver function tests should warrant further investigation (240).

Sonographic bile duct diameter may be significantly larger immediately after endoscopic retrograde cholangiopancreatography, especially in patients after cholecystectomy (241).

The sonographic measurements of the common duct are smaller than measurements obtained from radiographic procedures such as intravenous cholangiography and endoscopic retrograde cholangiopancreatography. This finding is most likely secondary to measurements obtained at two different (noncorresponding) levels by the two techniques, even though radiographic magnification, choleretic effect, and distending effects of radiographic procedures may be responsible to a lesser extent (242,243). Sonographic measurements are most frequently obtained in the proximal segment of the common duct, anterior to the main portal vein, whereas radiographic measurements are obtained at the widest point of the common duct, which is usually in the distal segment of the common duct.

Pitfalls

Mistaken Hepatic Artery ■ The main (proper) hepatic artery is generally located anterior to the main portal vein and medial to the common duct (Fig. 66). On the transverse view of the porta hepatis, this configuration produces the typical "Mickey Mouse" appearance: the portal vein forms the head, the hepatic artery forms one ear, and the bile duct forms the other ear (Fig. 70). However, on the longitudinal view, the main hepatic artery may be mistaken for a normal common duct or, when prominent, for a dilated common duct (Fig. 71). With color Doppler and duplex Doppler sonography, the artery can be easily distinguished from the common duct. The differences in the orientation and course of these two structures are also helpful in differentiation. The hepatic artery courses anteriorly and may be traced toward its origin from the celiac artery, whereas the common duct courses posteriorly toward the head of the pancreas (244).

Transverse Common Duct ■ Occasionally, the distal common duct, especially when dilated, may have a long transverse segment reaching to or extending beyond midline that is best seen in transverse cross sections and may be mistaken for a vascular structure (245).

Distal Cystic Duct

The junction of the distal cystic duct and the common hepatic duct is usually situated immediately below the porta hepatis (Fig. 2A), but it may be at a considerably lower (distal) level. Anomalies of cystic duct insertion include (*i*) absent cystic duct, (*ii*) low insertion into the common duct, (*iii*) long conjoined segment with common duct, (*iv*) insertion into right hepatic duct, and (*v*) proximal insertion at the confluence of the right and left

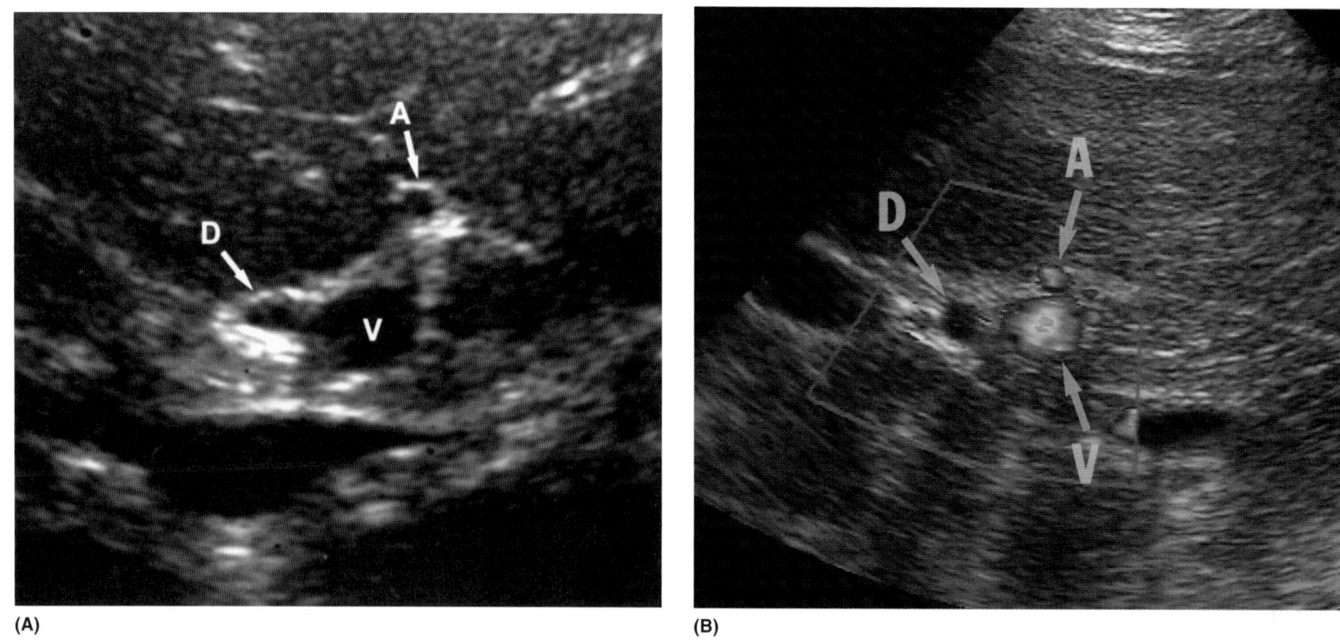

FIGURE 70 A AND B ■ Transverse ("Mickey Mouse") view of the porta hepatis showing the relation of the main hepatic artery and the common duct to the main portal vein. (**A** and **B**) The main hepatic artery is located anterior and medial to the main portal vein. The common duct is located anterior and lateral to the main portal vein. This configuration produces the typical "Mickey Mouse" appearance: the portal vein forms the head, and the hepatic artery and bile duct form the ears. (**B**) Color Doppler sonogram showing flow in the portal vein and hepatic artery and absence of flow in the bile duct. D, common duct; V, main portal vein; A, hepatic artery.

hepatic ducts (Fig. 72) (246). The distal cystic duct runs parallel to and adheres to the common hepatic duct for a short distance before entering it (Fig. 73). Occasionally, a long segment of the distal cystic duct may run parallel to and contiguous with the common hepatic duct (Fig. 73C). Sonographically, the normal distal cystic duct (Fig. 73) can be seen in 51% of healthy persons and has an average (mean) diameter of 1.8 mm (247). The distal cystic duct is seen much more frequently when it is dilated (Fig. 73B). In 95% of patients, the distal cystic duct is

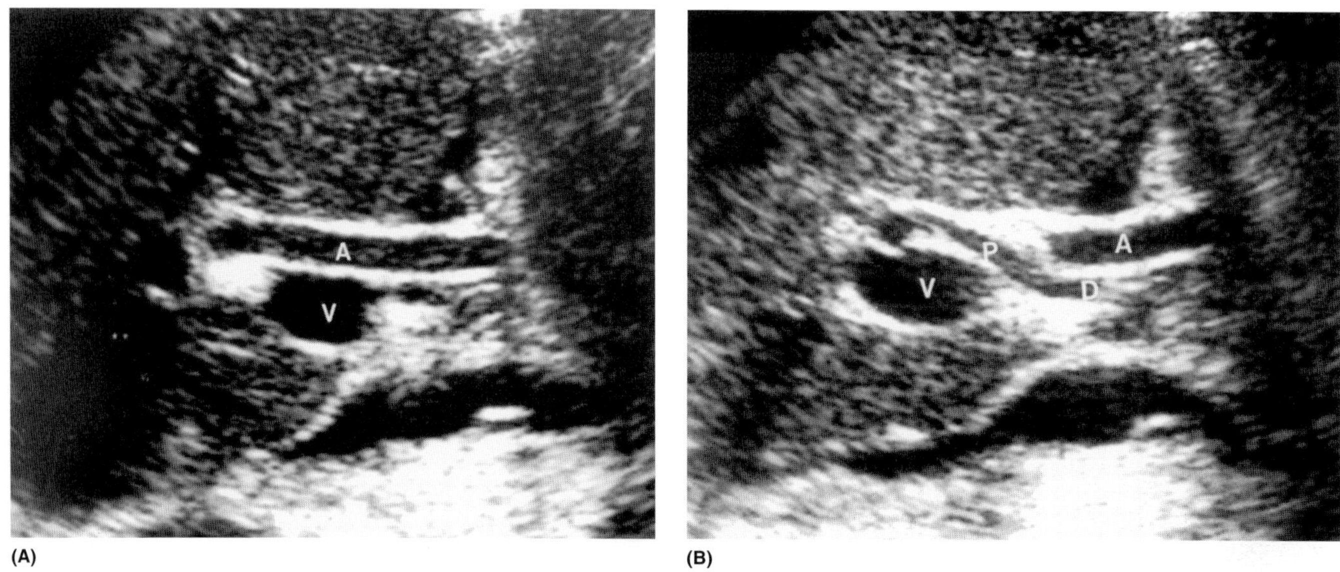

FIGURE 71 A AND B ■ Pitfall: longitudinal views. (**A**) The prominent main hepatic artery mimicking a dilated common duct anterior to the portal vein. (**B**) In the same patient, a longitudinal oblique view shows the normal proximal common duct anterior to the portal vein. The distal common duct is seen to course posteriorly. The main hepatic artery courses more anteriorly before joining the celiac artery (not shown). D, distal common duct; V, main portal vein; A, hepatic artery; P, proximal common duct.

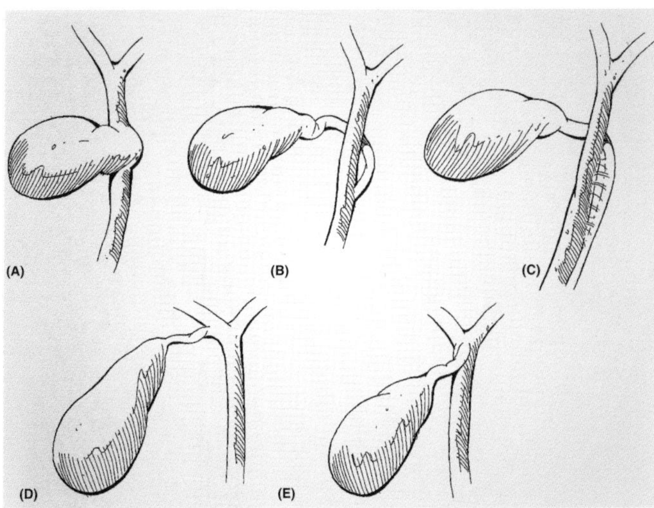

FIGURE 72 A–E ■ Diagram of anomalies of the cystic duct insertion. (**A**) Absent cystic duct. (**B**) Low insertion into common duct. (**C**) Long, conjoined segment with common duct. (**D**) Insertion into right hepatic duct. (**E**) Insertion at confluence of right and left hepatic ducts. *Source*: From Ref. 246.

located posterior to the common duct, and in 5%, it is anterior to the common duct.

Scanning Technique

The *proximal* common duct is examined by sagittal scans with the patient in the supine as well as in the left posterior oblique position (219,223). The scanning is started in the sagittal plane, in the mid-clavicular line subcostally, and is continued using slight changes in position of the transducer and varying angulations of the sound beam, until the main portal vein and the common duct are identified. The common duct is frequently best seen by scanning in the sagittal oblique plane, with the transducer angled to the left and cranially. In most patients, the distal common duct can also be demonstrated using this technique; however, it is located more medially and is better seen with the patient in the supine position rather than in the left posterior oblique position. The distal common duct, especially the pancreatic portion of the duct, is frequently better seen by transverse scans, with the patient in an erect right posterior oblique position (248). If the distal common duct is obscured by shadowing from bowel gas, patients can be examined in the erect position after they have ingested water, using the fluid-filled stomach as an acoustic window (249). If the proximal common duct is obscured by shadowing from bowel gas, intercostal scanning, using liver as an acoustic window, is often helpful.

The distal cystic duct is best seen by sagittal or sagittal oblique scanning with the patient in the supine or the left posterior oblique position. It may also be demonstrated by transverse scanning.

Congenital Abnormalities

Biliary Atresia

The cause of biliary atresia remains uncertain. It was previously thought to be a congenital anomaly; however, it may be secondary to an infectious process of viral origin, and it has its onset in the prenatal period or shortly after birth (250). Pathologically, one sees progressive obliteration of the extrahepatic bile ducts and, in many instances, the gallbladder. This obliteration extends into the proximal intrahepatic ductal system, near the hilum of the liver (250). Clinically, there is persistent neonatal jaundice. Sonographically, the gallbladder in patients with biliary atresia is usually small (less than 1.5 cm long) or absent (251). However, a normal-sized gallbladder is present in 10% to 20% of patients with biliary atresia (252,253). Investigators have suggested that if the gallbladder contracts after an oral feeding, the diagnosis of biliary atresia

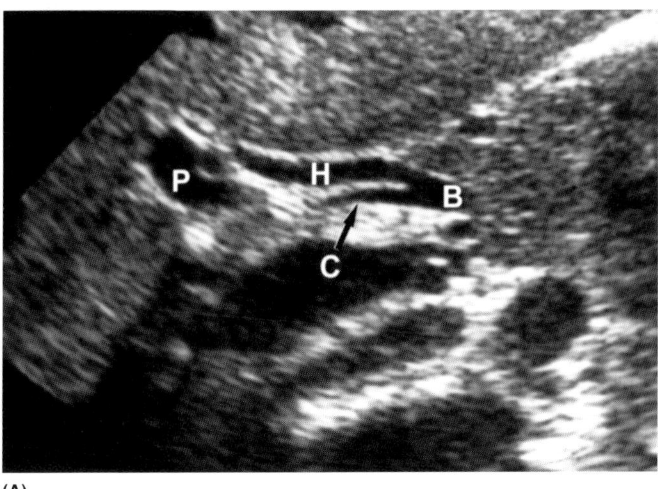

(A)

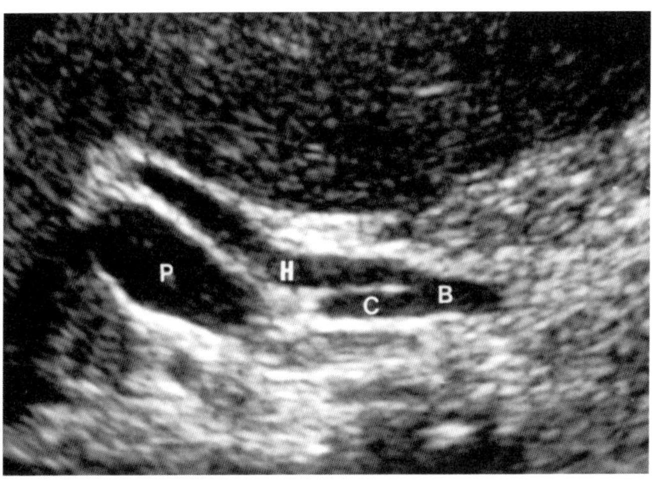

(B)

FIGURE 73 A–D ■ The distal cystic duct. (**A**) Longitudinal view showing normal distal cystic duct entering the common duct posteriorly. (**B**) Longitudinal view showing slightly dilated distal cystic duct measuring 4 mm in diameter. (*Continued*)

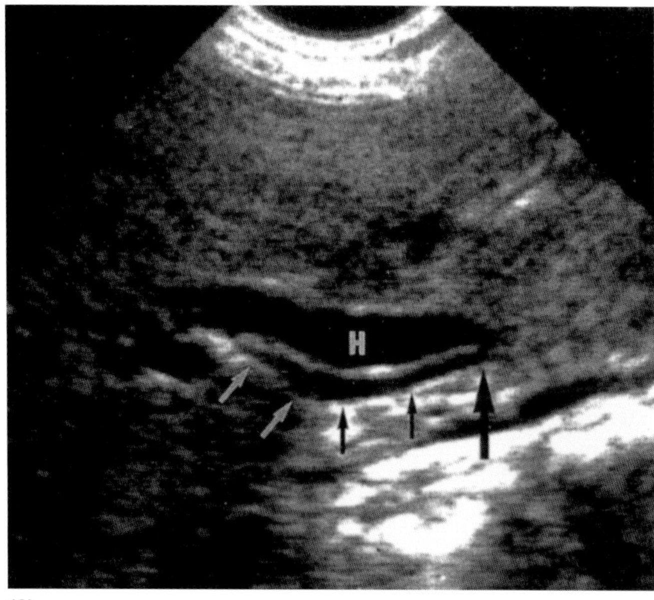

(C)

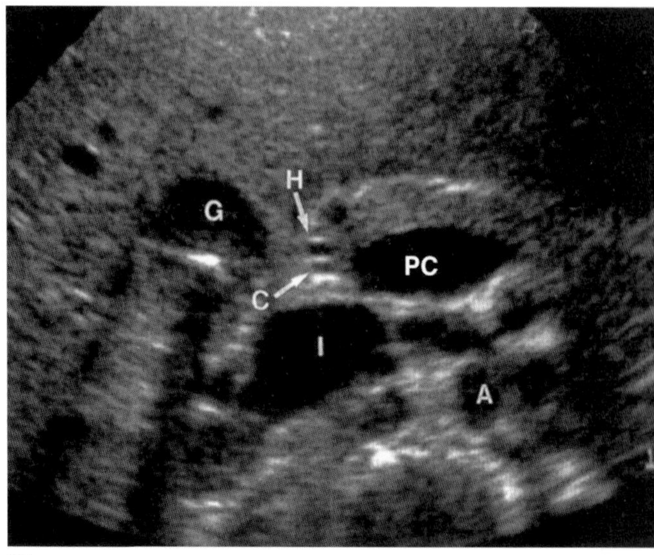

(D)

FIGURE 73 A–D ■ (*Continued*) (**C**) Longitudinal view demonstrating a long segment of the distal cystic duct (*arrows*) running parallel to and contiguous with the common hepatic duct. (**D**) Transverse view showing distal cystic duct posterior to the distal common hepatic duct. H, common hepatic duct; B, common bile duct; P, portal vein; C, cystic duct. PC, portal confluence between the superior mesenteric vein and the splenic vein; G, gallbladder; I, inferior vena cava; A, aorta.

is unlikely (250). However, occasionally, gallbladder contraction after oral feeding can occur in patients with biliary atresia (254). Associated findings include polysplenia, preduodenal portal vein, and anomalies of intestinal rotation.

Biliary atresia must be distinguished from neonatal hepatitis, because biliary atresia can be treated surgically, and surgical results are best when performed before the patient reaches two months of age. Patients with neonatal hepatitis usually have a normal-sized (greater than 1.5 cm in length) gallbladder that contracts after oral feeding. However, it may be small or non-visualized (251). Most patients with neonatal hepatitis have a sonographically visible common hepatic duct, whereas patients with biliary atresia frequently have no visible common hepatic duct anterior to the portal vein (250).

Because sonographic findings are nonspecific, hepatobiliary scintigraphy is performed for further evaluation and is usually helpful in differentiating biliary atresia and neonatal hepatitis in the first three months of life. Patients with biliary atresia have normal hepatic extraction of tracer with no excretion into the gastrointestinal tract. Patients with neonatal hepatitis demonstrate normal hepatic extraction of the tracer and delayed tracer excretion into the gastrointestinal tract. If the patient has neonatal hepatitis with severe hepatocellular damage, the hepatic extraction of tracer activity is decreased, and excretion may be delayed or absent (251). Liver biopsy and cholangiography are usually required for final diagnosis.

Choledochal Cyst

Choledochal cysts are an uncommon anomaly of the biliary system that are manifested by cystic dilatation of the extrahepatic or intrahepatic biliary tree or both. They most commonly involve the common duct. There is a 3:1 female predominance, and 60% of cases present before the age of 10 years, although choledochal cysts can present from birth to old age (246). The clinical picture varies from absence of symptoms to the classic clinical triad of pain, jaundice, and abdominal mass (255). The cause may be an anomalous union between the common bile duct and the main pancreatic duct at a high position, forming an abnormally long common channel, which weakens the wall of the common bile duct secondary to free reflux of enzymes into the bile duct (256). Choledochal cysts can be classified into five types (Fig. 74) (257).

1. The type 1 cyst is most common, accounting for 80% to 90% of cases. It is divided into type 1A, cystic dilatation of the common duct; type 1B, focal segmental common duct dilatation; and type 1C, fusiform dilatation of the common bile duct.
2. The type 2 cyst accounts for about 2% of cases and consists of a true diverticulum arising from the common duct.
3. The type 3 cyst, accounting for 1% to 5% of cases, consists of a choledochocele, and involves only the intraduodenal portion of the duct.
4. The type 4 cyst is divided into type 4A, multiple intrahepatic cysts and an extrahepatic cyst, which accounts for 19% of cases, and type 4B, multiple extrahepatic cysts, which are much less common.
5. The type 5 cyst, or Caroli's disease, consists of single or multiple intrahepatic biliary cysts. Approximately two-thirds of patients with Caroli's disease also have extrahepatic disease.

Classification schemes vary, however, and definitions of types 4 and 5 are controversial.

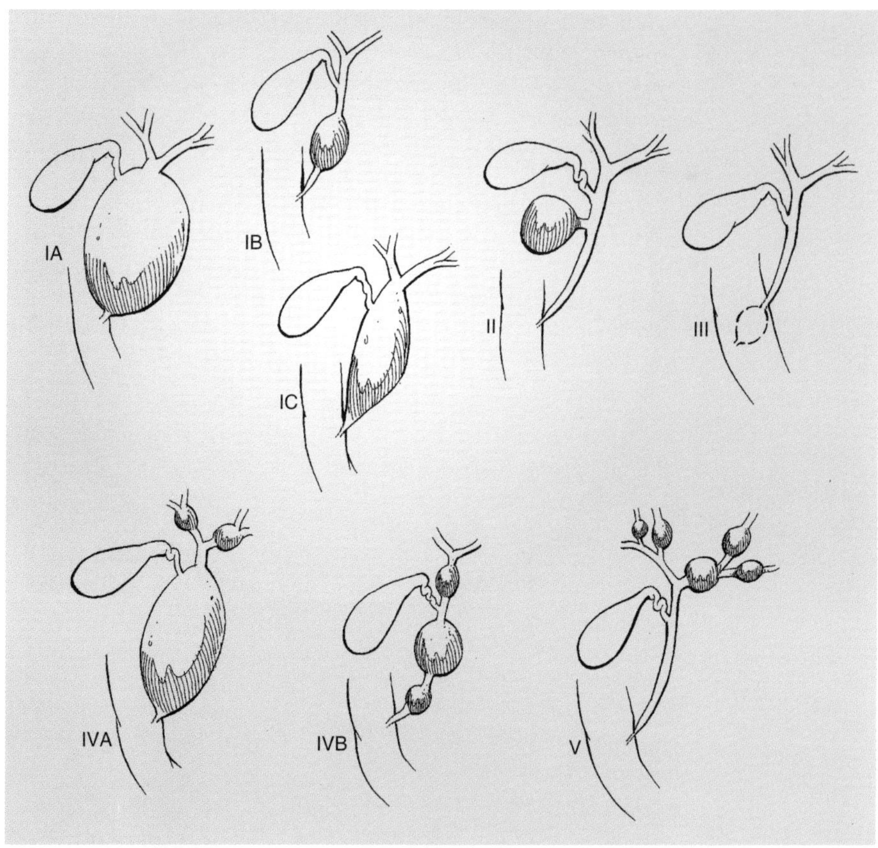

FIGURE 74 ■ Diagram of the classification of choledochal cysts. (IA) Cystic dilatation of common duct. (IB) Focal segmental dilatation of common duct. (IC) Fusiform dilatation of common duct. (II) True diverticulum arising from common duct. (III) Choledochocele. (IVA) Multiple intrahepatic cysts and an extrahepatic cyst. (IVB) Multiple extrahepatic cysts. (V) Caoli's disease (intrahepatic cysts). *Source*: From Ref. 257.

Sonographically, the most common type of cyst, type 1, appears as an anechoic cystic mass in continuity with the common bile duct and is separated from the gallbladder (Fig. 75). The choledochal cysts communicate with the common duct, and larger cysts may occasionally contain sludge (Fig. 75A). The differential diagnosis includes hepatic cysts, pancreatic pseudocysts (Fig. 76), and hepatic artery aneurysm. Occasionally, massive dilatation of the common bile duct secondary to obstruction by a stone or stricture may mimic a choledochal cyst (258). Complications

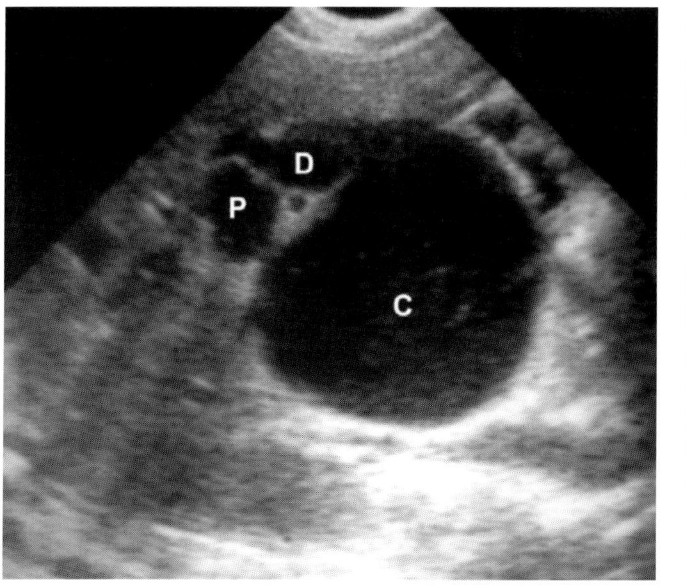

(A)

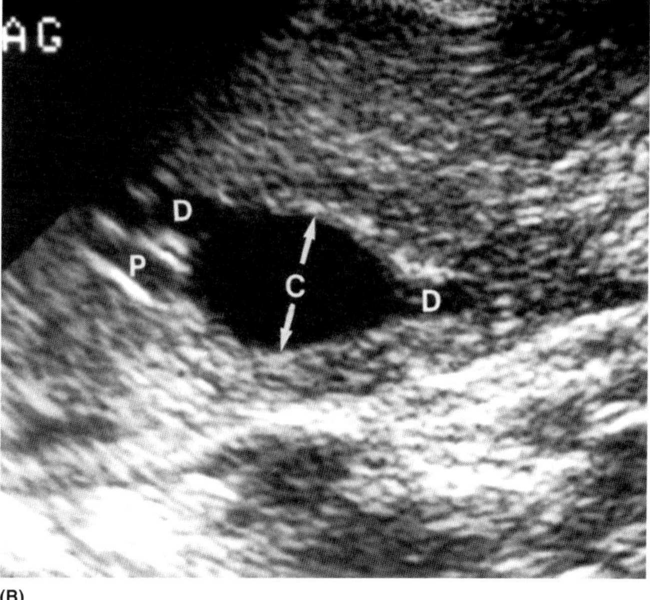

(B)

FIGURE 75 A–C ■ Choledochal cyst: longitudinal views. (**A**) Type 1A. Longitudinal view demonstrating a large area of cystic dilatation in the common duct. Sludge is present within the dependent portion of the choledochal cyst (C). D, proximal common hepatic duct; P, main portal vein. (**B**) Type 1B. A small (2 cm) choledochal cyst is seen as a focal segmental dilatation of the common duct. (*Continued*)

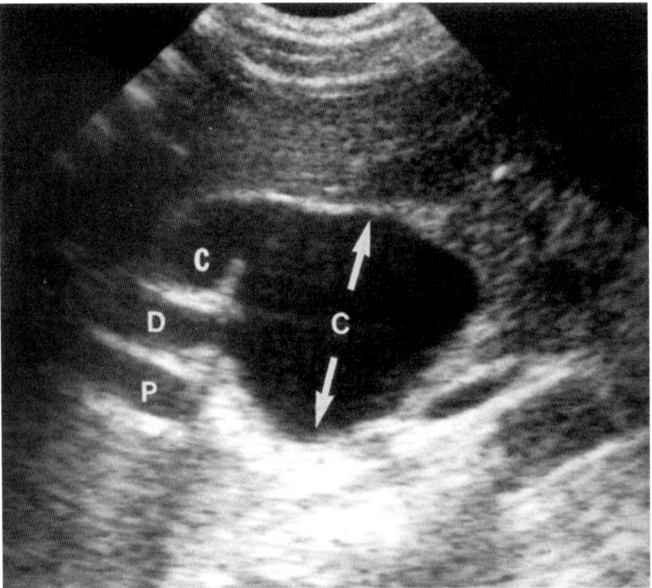

(C)

FIGURE 75 A–C ■ (*Continued*) (C) A large (5 cm) choledochal cyst is seen as a lobulated diverticulum-like cystic mass arising from the common duct.

in adults include calculus formation within the cyst, secondary infection, rupture with bile peritonitis, pancreatitis, and portal vein thrombosis. The incidence of cholangiocarcinoma within the choledochal cyst is high.

Biliary Obstruction

Ultrasound remains the initial screening modality of choice for evaluating the bile ducts because of its capability of differentiating between nonobstructive and obstructive jaundice in more than 90% of cases (Fig. 77) (259). It can also be used to determine the level and cause of biliary obstruction (Fig. 78) (Table 12) (260–262). Although the results of some of the earlier studies were disappointing (263,264), more recent studies suggest that the level of obstruction can be correctly identified in 92% to 95% of patients, and the cause of obstruction can be correctly diagnosed in 71% to 88% of patients by sonographic examination (259,265). The level of obstruction can be defined as (*i*) hilar or porta hepatis, (*ii*) suprapancreatic, or (*iii*) pancreatic (259).

1. Obstruction at the hilar or porta hepatis level is most commonly secondary to a neoplasm, most frequently cholangiocarcinoma, and less commonly metastatic adenopathy.

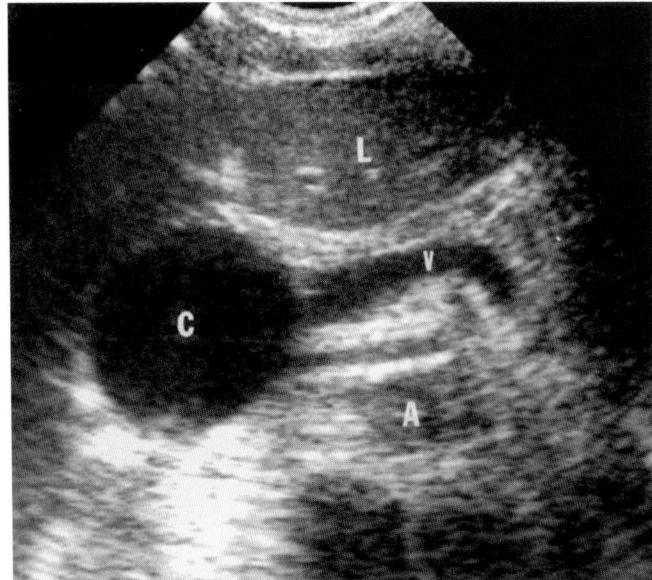

FIGURE 76 ■ Transverse view. Choledochal cyst mimicking a pseudocyst in the head of the pancreas. C, choledochal cyst; V, splenic vein; A, aorta; L, left lobe of the liver.

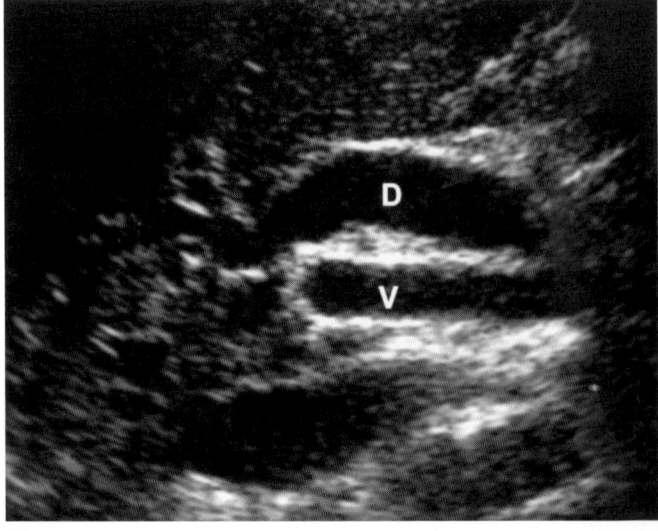

(A)

(B)

FIGURE 77 A AND B ■ Dilated common bile ducts. (A) A long axis demonstrating the dilated common bile duct anterior to the main portal vein. (B) An oblique view in a different patient demonstrating a common bile duct (*arrow*) measuring approximately 12 mm anterior to the main portal vein. D, common bile duct; V, portal vein. *Source*: (B) Courtesy of Oksana Baltarowich, MD, Philadelphia, PA.

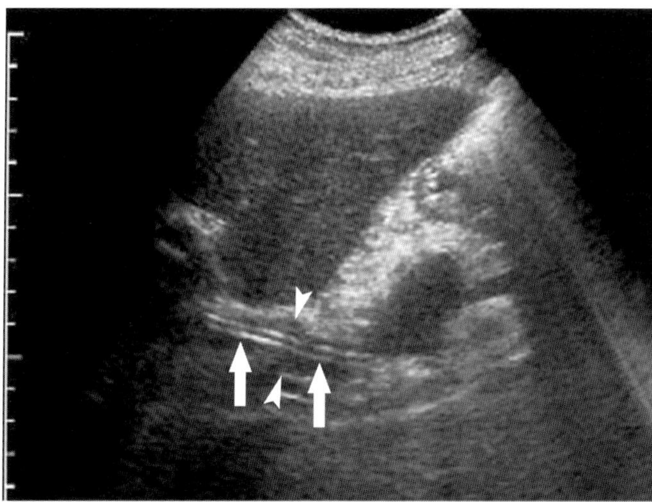

FIGURE 78 ■ Longitudinal view of a dilated distal common duct (*arrowheads*). The tubular structure with hyperechoic walls within the duct represents a stent (*arrows*). *Source*: Courtesy of Oksana Baltarowich, MD, Philadelphia, PA.

2. *Suprapancreatic* level is defined as obstruction between the pancreas and the porta hepatis; it is most commonly caused by primary or metastatic neoplasm and less commonly by calculi or inflammatory strictures (259).
3. *Pancreatic* level is usually the most common site of biliary obstruction and is caused by choledocholithiasis, neoplastic, or inflammatory masses in the head of the pancreas and benign strictures or neoplasms of the distal common duct. Benign strictures are usually secondary to inflammatory processes (i.e., cholangitis) or previous biliary surgery. Sonographically, the stricture usually is not visible, and the dilated common duct usually terminates abruptly at the level of the stricture. When the obstruction is caused by an extrinsic mass, the dilated common duct terminates at the level of the mass.

Special Features of Biliary Dilatation

Anicteric Biliary Dilatation with Obstruction ■ Sonographically, dilatation of the intrahepatic and extrahepatic bile ducts can be seen in patients without jaundice and with normal serum bilirubin level (266–269). Anicteric dilatation of the biliary tree can be caused by partial or intermittent obstruction from common duct stones, partially obstructing masses, or partial obstruction secondary to either bile duct stricture or papillary stenosis (266,267). Anicteric intrahepatic biliary dilatation can be caused by obstruction of only one hepatic duct.

Anicteric Biliary Dilatation without Obstruction ■ Anicteric dilatation of the common duct without obstruction can result from aging, remote cholecystectomy, previous inflammation and obstruction, previous biliary surgery, and intestinal hypomotility. Intestinal hypomotility secondary to recent major abdominal surgery or paralytic ileus resulting from miscellaneous abdominal and thoracic inflammatory processes or trauma may cause persistent contraction of the sphincter of Oddi, resulting in common duct dilatation (270).

Obstruction without Biliary Dilatation ■ Some patients with obstructive jaundice may have no sonographic evidence for intrahepatic or extrahepatic biliary dilatation (271). This condition is usually seen in patients with partial biliary obstruction and with intermittent common duct obstruction by choledocholithiasis. Moreover, in the earlier phases of biliary obstruction, the bile ducts may not be dilated. Hepatobiliary scintigraphy is highly sensitive and is likely to show abnormal biliary drainage at the earliest phases of such obstruction (272).

Disparate Dilatation of the Bile Ducts ■ Bile ducts usually dilate centrifugally from the point of obstruction. Therefore, with early or partial distal common duct obstruction, the common duct may be dilated several days before the intrahepatic bile ducts (268). In some patients, initially the distal common duct may be dilated, whereas the proximal common duct may be normal in size (Fig. 79).

TABLE 12 ■ Biliary Obstruction in Adults

Malignant disease
■ Pancreatic carcinoma
■ Periampullary carcinoma
■ Cholangiocarcinoma
■ Metastatic disease
Benign disease
■ Calculi
■ Pancreatitis
■ Sclerosing cholangitis
■ Postoperative stricture

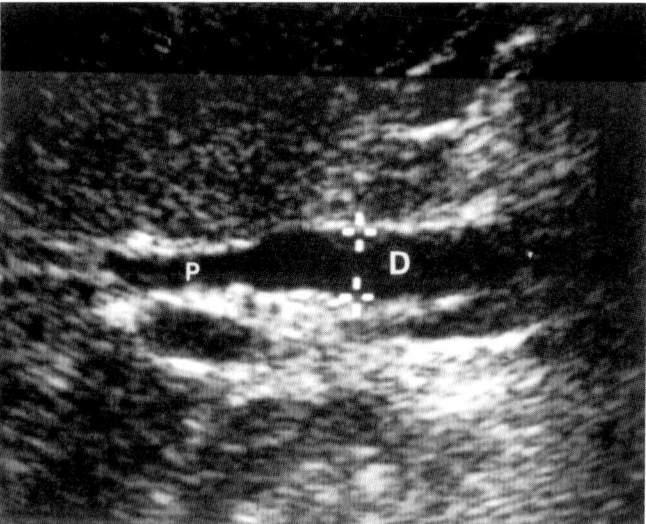

FIGURE 79 ■ Disparate dilatation of the common duct. The proximal common duct is normal in caliber (5 mm), whereas the distal common duct is dilated (9 mm). P, proximal common duct; D, distal common duct.

Rapid Change in Bile Duct Caliber ■ The extrahepatic bile ducts are capable of substantial acute distension over a short time. Changes in duct size (increase or decrease) can occur over a short period, often within several hours or days (273,274). Rapid decrease in size of dilated common duct, within several minutes, during sonographic examination has also been reported (275). In some patients, rapid change in bile duct caliber may explain discordant measurements of bile duct diameter on successive examinations with different diagnostic modalities.

Ductal Response to Fatty Meal

Sonography after fatty meal stimulation may be useful for differentiating obstructive from nonobstructive dilatation of the common duct, when no cause of obstruction is obvious on the sonographic examination. It is particularly useful in patients with either a dilated common duct and normal liver function tests or a common duct of normal size and abnormal liver function tests (273,276). It is also helpful in asymptomatic patients with mild common duct dilatation, especially after previous cholecystectomy.

Common duct diameter is measured before a fatty meal and at 45 minutes after the fatty meal. The measurement should be taken at the same location and in the same phase of respiration. Ingestion of a fatty meal stimulates cholecystokinin release and causes gallbladder contraction, increased bile flow in the liver, and relaxation of the sphincter of Oddi.

The significance of various common duct responses to fatty meal stimulation is as follows:

1. Asymptomatic healthy persons with a common duct of normal size have either a decrease or no change in duct size 45 minutes after fatty meal ingestion.
2. A decrease in duct size after a fatty meal indicates normal biliary dynamics and virtually excludes obstruction, regardless of whether the duct was dilated or normal before the fatty meal.
3. An increase in duct size of greater than 1 mm (preferably 2 mm or more) after a fatty meal is an abnormal response and strongly indicates underlying duct obstruction, regardless of whether the duct was dilated or of normal size before the fatty meal.
4. In normal, healthy persons, no change in the size of a normal-sized duct is a normal response to a fatty meal. A dilated duct that does not decrease in size after a fatty meal is not a specific indicator of obstruction. In a study by Willson et al., 84% of patients with dilated common ducts without change in size after a fatty meal had no evidence of common duct obstruction (277,278).

In a study by Darweesh et al., fatty meal sonography had a 74% sensitivity and 100% specificity for detecting partial common duct obstruction (279). The use of fatty meal stimulation is unlikely to be helpful if the duct wall is rigid or fibrotic and unable to change in caliber. Fatty meal sonography may not be useful in critically ill patients because of failure of gallbladder contraction in these patients after fatty meal ingestion or intravenous cholecystokinin administration (28).

Ductal Response to Valsalva Maneuver

The effect of Valsalva maneuver on the diameter of the common duct may be useful in differentiating obstructed from nonobstructed ducts (280). The diameter of the proximal segment of the common duct anterior to the main portal vein is measured during quiet respiration and at maximal Valsalva maneuver. A normal response is defined as a decrease in the diameter of greater than 1 mm after Valsalva maneuver and is seen in nonobstructed ducts. This normal response to the Valsalva maneuver is absent in patients with obstructed ducts. In a study by Quinn et al., the sensitivity and specificity of the response in predicting extrahepatic biliary obstruction were 100% and 92%, respectively (280).

Pitfalls in the Diagnosis of Common Duct Dilatation

Gallbladder Neck ■ Elongation or folding of the gallbladder neck can mimic a dilated common duct (Fig. 80) (281). In such cases, scanning in different planes is necessary to demonstrate the contiguity of the neck with the rest of the gallbladder and to visualize the true common duct separate from the neck of the gallbladder.

Hepatic Artery ■ A dilated main or aberrant hepatic artery, anterior to the main portal vein, may be mistaken for a dilated common duct (244). However, a hepatic artery can be easily distinguished from a common duct by CDS.

Debris in Duct ■ Sludge or blood clot in the common duct may obscure the duct partially or entirely. In patients with hemobilia, blood clot in the common duct may be diffusely echogenic, rendering the duct imperceptible as a discrete structure. When the echogenic clot fills most of the lumen of a long segment of a dilated common duct, only the residual lumen may be visible and may be mistaken for a normal-sized common duct (282). The blood clot may appear as a rounded, echogenic soft tissue mass within the duct or the gallbladder. A fresh blood clot within the common duct or gallbladder may be highly echogenic (i.e., hyperechoic), and a residual clot may persist for weeks. Hemobilia occurs in 14% of patients with percutaneous biliary drainage and also may occur after liver biopsy and transhepatic cholangiography (282).

Choledocholithiasis

Choledocholithiasis occurs in approximately 15% of patients with gallstones (283). In Western countries, most common duct stones are secondary stones, originating from the gallbladder. In the United States, only 5% of common duct stones are of the primary type (i.e., forming de novo in the common duct) (143). Parasites such as Ascaris and *Clonorchis sinensis* are major causes of primary duct stones in Asia. Common bile duct stone caused by migration of a surgical clip into the common bile duct following laparoscopic cholecystectomy as well as migration of a fishbone into the common bile

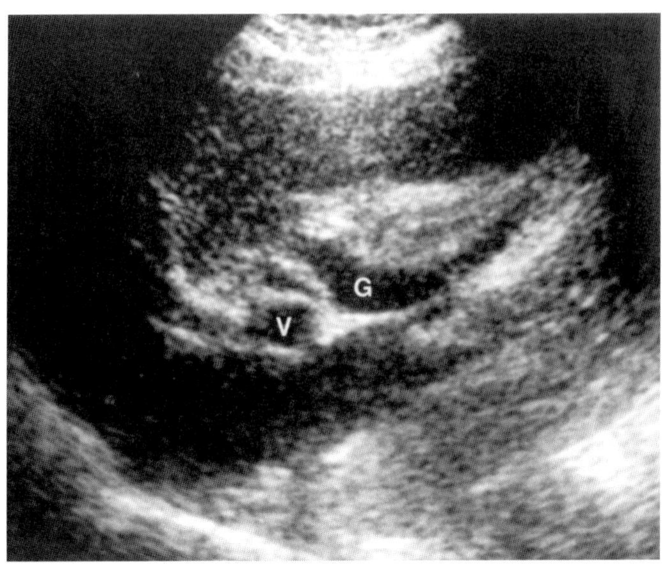

(A)

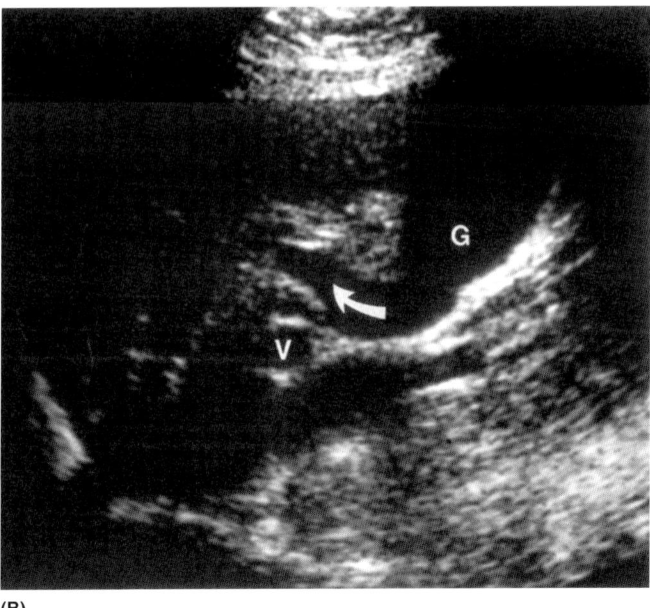

(B)

FIGURE 80 A AND B ■ Pitfall: longitudinal views. (**A**) Elongated neck of the gallbladder mimics a dilated common duct anterior to the right portal vein. (**B**) Scanning in a different plane demonstrates the continuity of the elongated, folded neck of the gallbladder (*arrow*) with the rest of the gallbladder. G, gallbladder; V, right portal vein.

duct has been reported (284,285). Reported sensitivities for sonographic detection of stones in the common duct range from 25% to 75% (248,249,286,287). The newer, higher-resolution ultrasound machines and improved techniques are partly responsible for the higher sensitivities reported in more recent studies. Most stones are seen in the distal common duct near its pancreatic portion. In addition to scanning in supine and left posterior oblique positions, transverse scanning over the distal duct at the level of the pancreatic head with the patient in the erect position may be helpful in detecting calculi in the distal common duct. Using a gastric window after ingestion of water may also be helpful in detecting calculi in the distal common duct. Sonographically, common duct stones appear as hyperechoic structures with distal acoustic shadowing similar to stones within the gallbladder (Figs. 81 and 82). Shadowing from common duct stones may be difficult to demonstrate, especially when the duct is not dilated or the stone is small. It is more difficult to demonstrate stones in a normal-sized common duct than in a dilated common duct. However, sonographically, stones can be detected in a normal-sized common bile duct, and therefore, a normal size of the common bile duct does not necessarily exclude the possibility of stones within it (288).

Pitfalls

Several possible sources of confusion exist in the diagnosis of common duct stones (289,290).

Adjacent Bowel ■ Air or residue in the adjacent bowel may mimic a common duct stone, but this artifact can be recognized by scanning the patient in different positions.

Pneumobilia ■ Air in the common duct may mimic a stone, although reverberation artifacts usually are associated with air bubbles. Air bubbles, however, may be seen without shadowing or reverberations (Fig. 83).

Adjacent Artery or Cystic Duct ■ The right hepatic artery indentation or distal cystic duct insertion may produce an echo within the common duct mimicking a stone (Fig. 84). However, no associated acoustic shadowing is noted, and scanning in different planes demonstrates the origin of the echo from the wall of the hepatic artery or the cystic duct.

Surgical Clips ■ After cholecystectomy, surgical clips close to the common duct may mimic stones; however, these are usually associated with comet-tail reverberations (Fig. 85).

Tortuous Common Duct ■ Rarely, in a tortuous dilated common duct, folds secondary to tortuosity may be associated with distal shadowing and may mimic stones (Fig. 86).

Pancreatic Calcification ■ Occasionally, it may be difficult to differentiate calcification within the head of the pancreas adjacent to the distal common duct from a stone within the common duct.

Ultrasound of the Common Bile Duct Before Laparoscopic Cholecystectomy

A preoperatively dilated common duct on ultrasonography has a high chance of containing stones (291). The frequency of stones in the common duct increases with

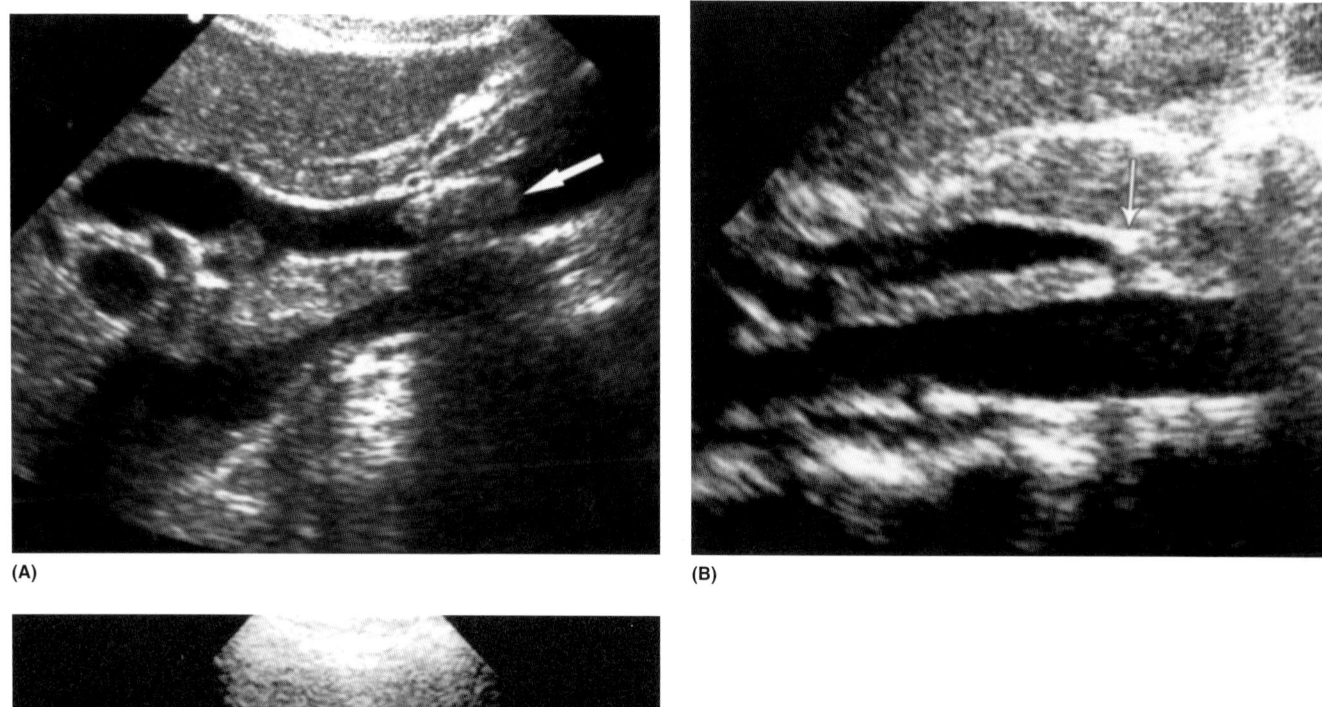

(A)

(B)

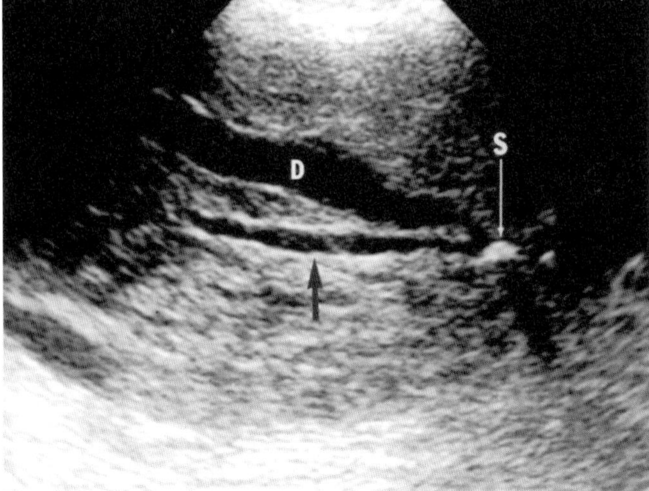

(C)

FIGURE 81 A–C ■ Choledocholithiasis: longitudinal views. (**A**) A large stone (*arrow*) with distal acoustic shadowing is seen within a dilated common duct. (**B**) A small stone (*arrow*) with subtle acoustic shadowing is seen within the distal common duct near the head of the pancreas. (**C**) Small stone with posterior shadowing in the distal common bile duct, causing obstruction of the common bile duct and the distal cystic duct (*black arrow*), with low insertion into the common duct. S, stone; D, common bile duct.

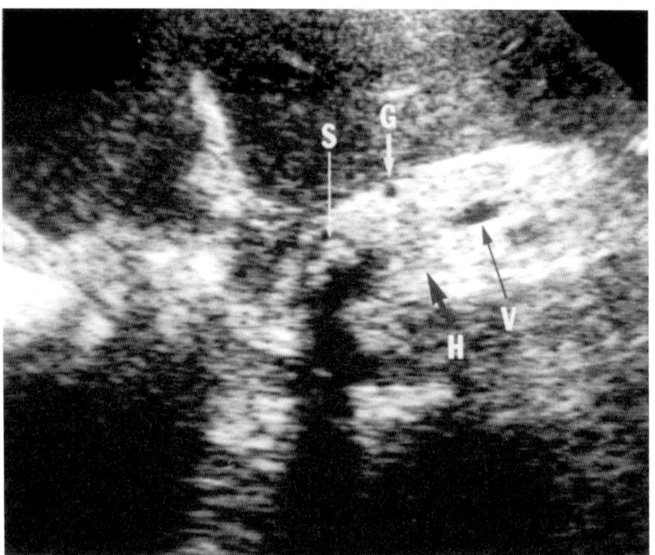

FIGURE 82 ■ Transverse view showing a stone with a posterior acoustic shadowing within the distal common bile duct. S, stone; H, head of the pancreas; V, superior mesenteric vein at the portal confluence; G, gastroduodenal artery.

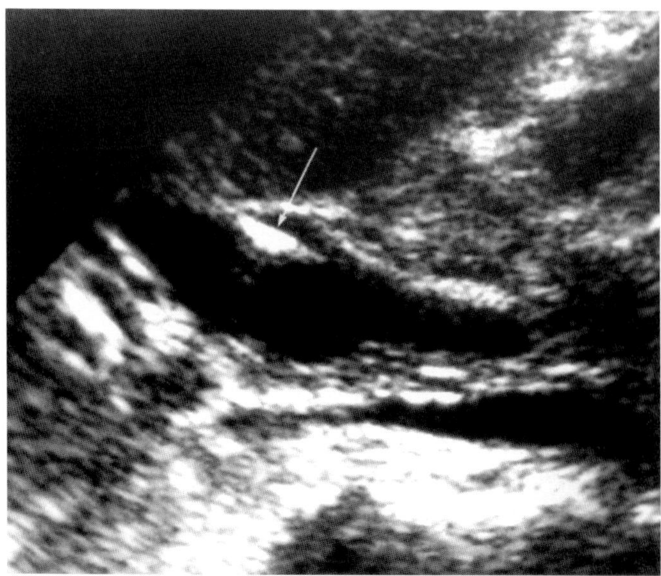

FIGURE 83 ■ Pitfall: air bubble mimicking a stone. Large air bubble (*arrow*) within dilated common duct causing subtle acoustic shadowing and a subtle comet-tail artifact.

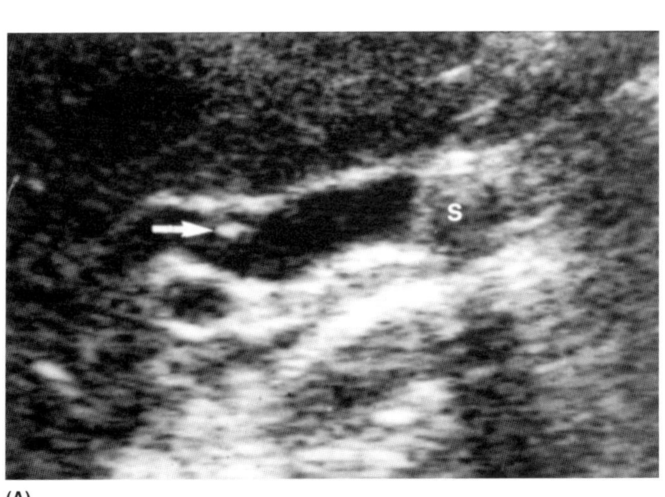

(A)

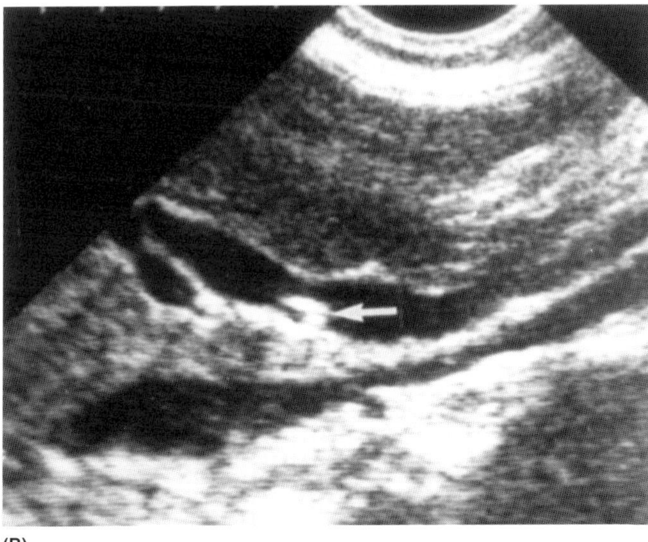

(B)

FIGURE 84 A AND B ■ Pitfall: longitudinal views. (**A**) Prominent indentation by the anterior right hepatic artery produces an echogenic focus (*arrow*) within the common duct mimicking a stone (S). However, no acoustic shadowing is present. (**B**) A large echo (*arrow*) within the common duct, produced by insertion of the distal cystic duct, mimics a stone. However, no acoustic shadowing is present.

increasing size (diameter) of the common duct. However, stones can occur in a small but significant portion of patients with normal-sized common ducts. Even though a dilated common bile duct on preoperative transabdominal ultrasound is a useful predictor of common bile duct stones, preoperative abdominal sonography alone cannot reliably select patients who require exploration of common bile duct or select patients for operative cholangiography.

Distal Cystic Duct Stones

Because of its small size, it is difficult to demonstrate stones within the distal cystic duct. However, when the distal cystic duct is dilated, stones or sludge may be

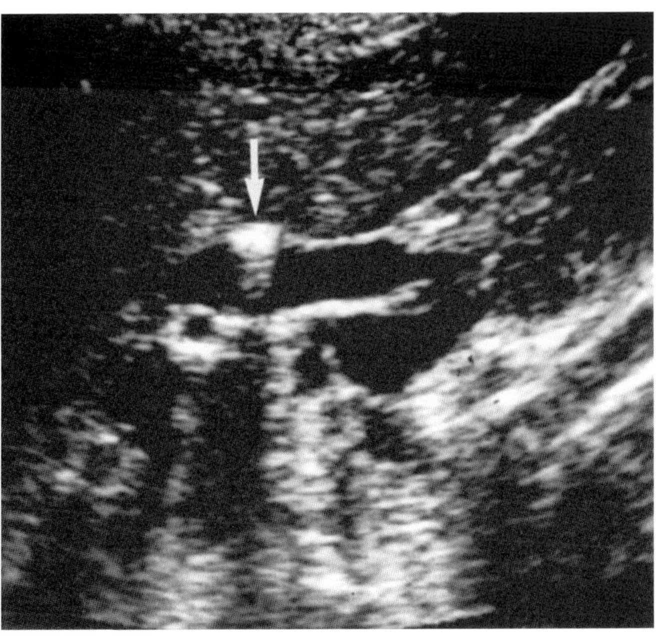

(A)

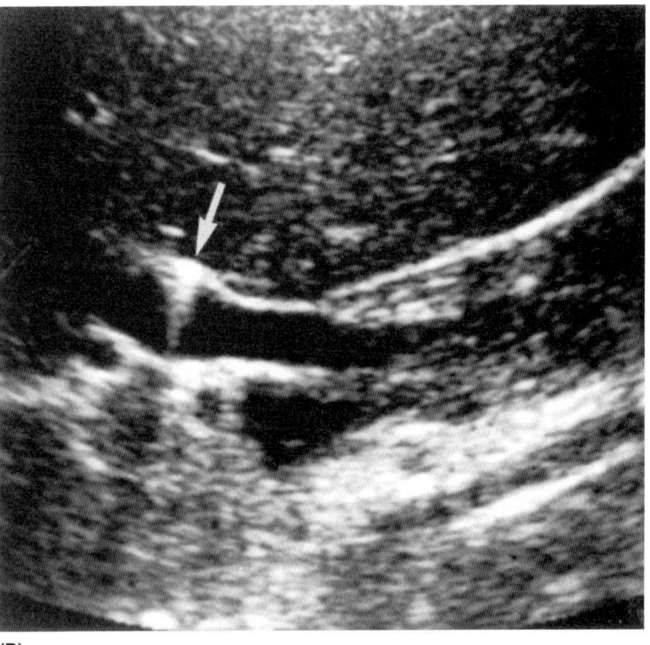

(B)

FIGURE 85 A AND B ■ Pitfall. (**A**) A surgical clip in a patient with remote cholecystectomy produces a large echo (*arrow*) within the common duct near the anterior wall of the duct. Subtle acoustic shadowing mimics a stone. A subtle comet-tail artifact is seen distal to the echogenic focus. (**B**) Scanning in a slightly different plane demonstrates an obvious comet-tail artifact typically seen distal to the echo produced by the surgical clip (*arrow*).

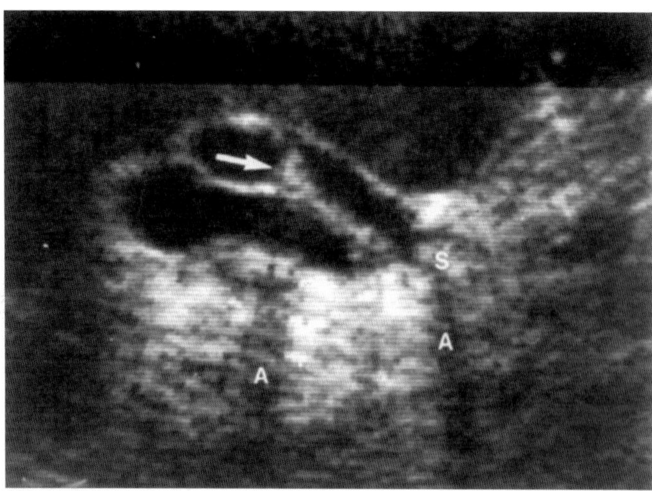

FIGURE 86 ■ Pitfall. Longitudinal view shows a prominent echo (*arrow*) with distal acoustic shadowing (A) within the common duct. This echo is produced by a prominent fold within a tortuous dilated common duct. There is a stone (S) in the distal common duct with acoustic shadowing (A).

visible. In patients who have undergone cholecystectomy, the cystic duct remnant may be dilated and may contain stones (Fig. 87) (247,292). Even though it is common surgical practice to leave behind a cystic duct stump of about 1 cm or shorter, cystic duct remnants may measure between 1 and 6 cm in length, especially in patients with low cystic duct insertion with a long segment of the cystic duct running parallel to the common duct.

Mirizzi's Syndrome

Mirizzi's syndrome is a rare, but surgically correctable, cause of extrahepatic biliary obstruction. It is caused by an impacted cystic duct stone, leading to extrinsic compression or inflammatory stricture of the common duct, which results in obstructive jaundice. The features of Mirizzi's syndrome include: (*i*) the presence of an impacted stone in the cystic duct, cystic duct remnant, or gallbladder neck, (*ii*) the partial mechanical obstruction of the common hepatic duct by compression from cystic duct stone or by the resulting inflammatory reaction around the impacted cystic duct stone, and (*iii*) sequelae of jaundice, recurrent cholangitis, or formation of cholecystobiliary fistula (293). The most common sites for the impacted stone include the proximal cystic duct near the neck of the gallbladder and the distal cystic duct near its insertion into the common duct. Sonographic features include: (*i*) a gallstone impacted in the distal cystic duct (Fig. 87) or the gallbladder neck (Fig. 88), (*ii*) dilatation of the biliary system including the common hepatic duct, and (*iii*) an abrupt change of the dilated common hepatic duct to normal diameter below the level of the cystic duct

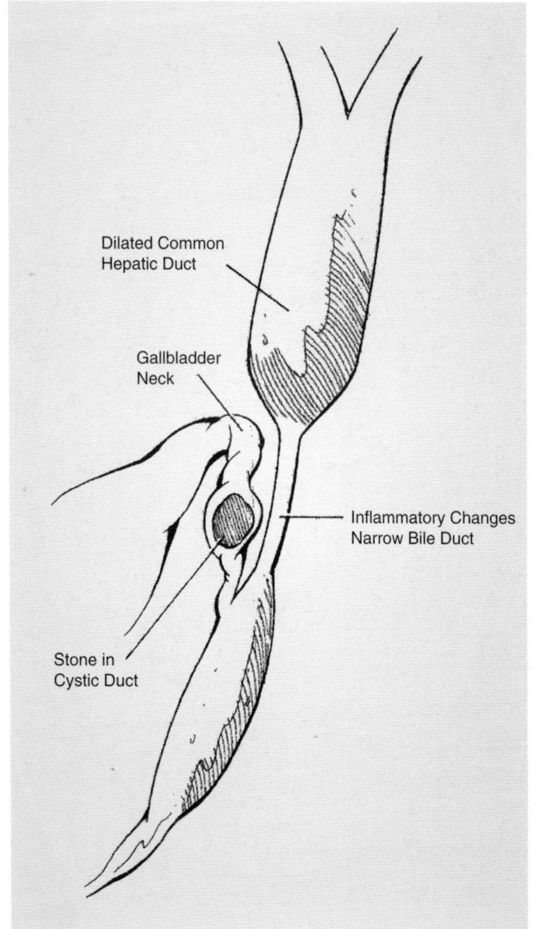

(A)

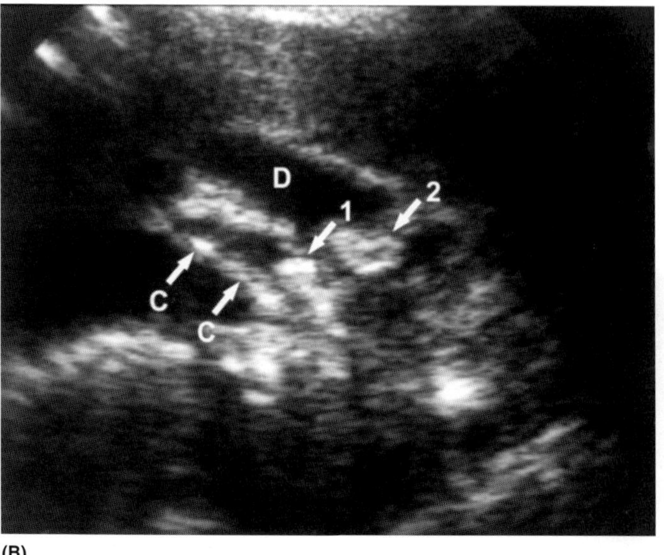

(B)

FIGURE 87 A AND B ■ Mirizzi's syndrome: distal cystic duct stone. (**A**) Diagram. (**B**) Longitudinal view showing a stone (1) with distal shadowing, within the dilated cystic duct remnant (C) in a patient with remote cholecystectomy. A second, larger stone (2) with shadowing is seen within the distal cystic duct insertion into the common duct. Dilatation of the common hepatic duct (D) is caused by extrinsic compression by the larger stone and surrounding inflammation, at the cystic duct insertion (Mirizzi's syndrome). *Source*: (**A**) From Ref. 292.

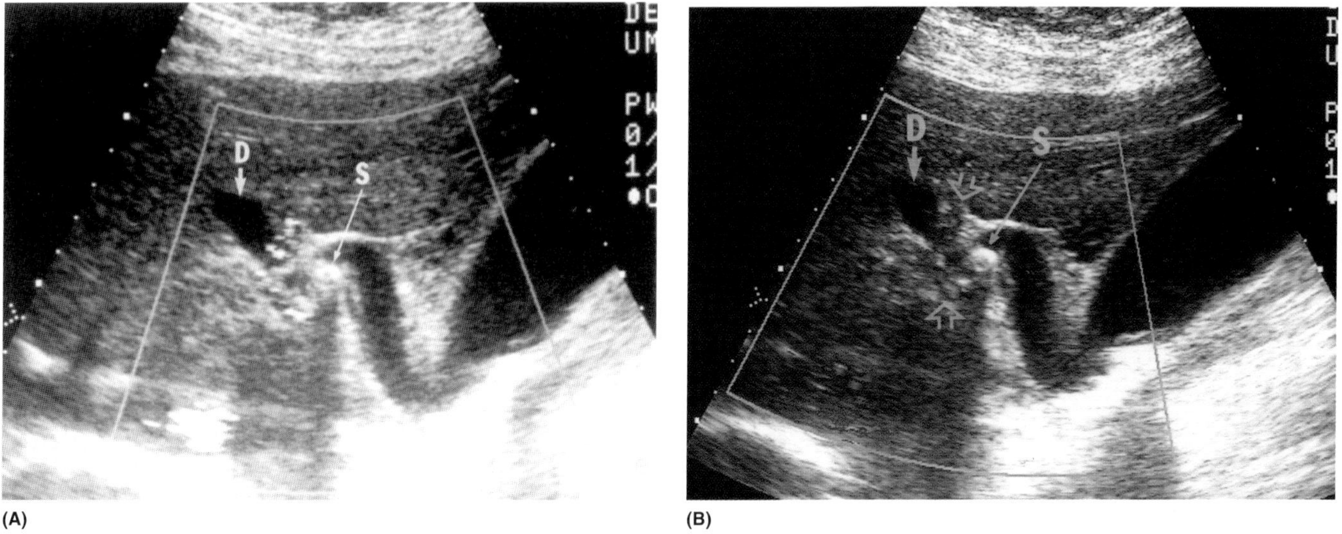

(A) (B)

FIGURE 88 A AND B ■ Mirizzi's syndrome: gallbladder neck stone. (**A** and **B**) Longitudinal color Doppler sonograms (**A** reproduced in black and white) demonstrating a dilated proximal common hepatic duct (D) secondary to extrinsic compression and surrounding inflammation caused by the stone (S) impacted in the neck of the gallbladder. Color signals (**B**) indicate flow in the hepatic artery (*open arrows*), and color flow signals are absent in the common hepatic duct. *Source*: From Ref. 161.

stone (294). A low cystic duct insertion, associated with a parallel course shared by the long distal cystic duct and the adjacent common hepatic duct, frequently forms the setting in which Mirizzi's syndrome can occur (295). However, the syndrome has no uniform appearance, and one or more of its typical features may be absent. Moreover, the stone in the distal cystic duct may be difficult to distinguish from the stone in the common duct (Fig. 87B). Therefore, Mirizzi's syndrome cannot be detected routinely on sonography, and when suspected, computed tomography and cholangiography should be performed.

Common Duct Sludge

Sludge in the common duct is an uncommon finding. The sludge appears as echogenic material without shadowing, occasionally demonstrating layering within the common duct (Fig. 89). Echogenic sludge may have a

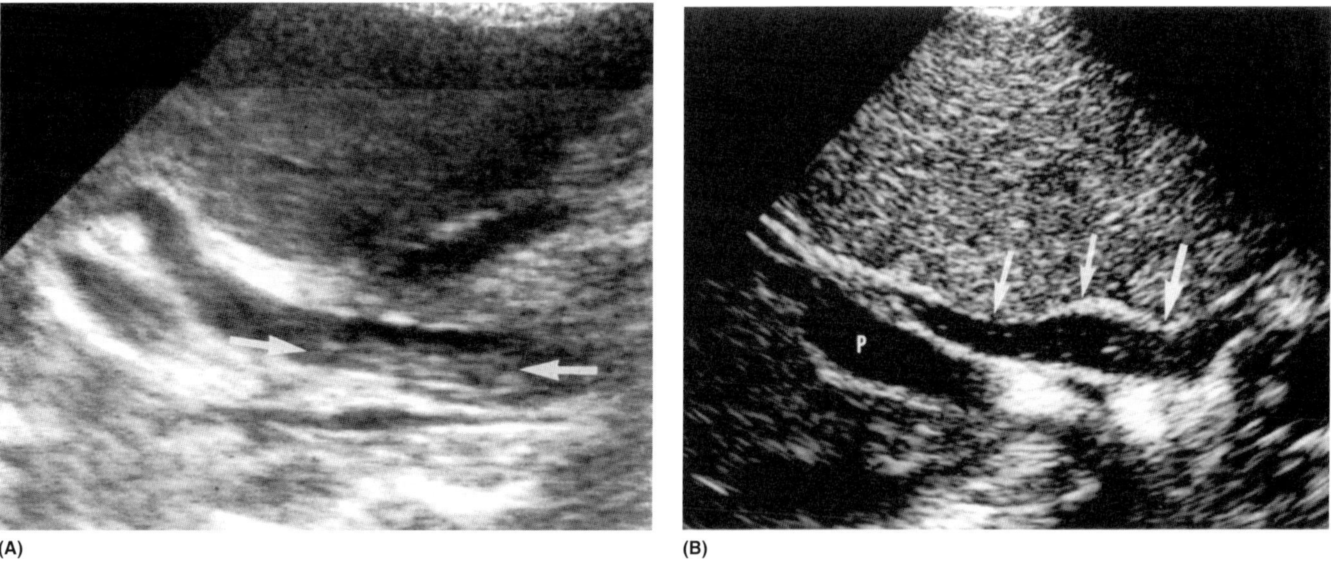

(A) (B)

FIGURE 89 A AND B ■ Common duct sludge. (**A**) Longitudinal view showing layering echogenic sludge (*arrows*) within the distal common duct. (**B**) Longitudinal view demonstrating sludge within the common duct appearing as echogenic debris (*large arrow*) and small echogenic particles (*small arrows*). P, main portal vein.

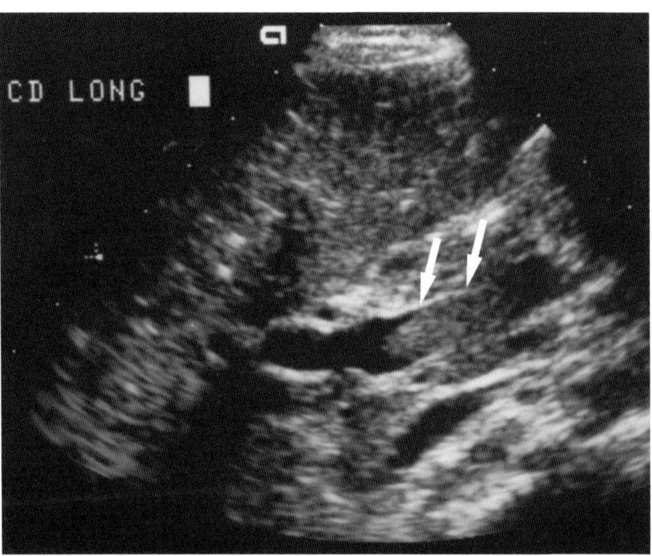

FIGURE 90 ■ Pitfall. Sludge within the common duct (*arrows*) has a pluglike appearance. This appearance can be mistaken for a tumor within the common duct. *Source*: Courtesy of Stuart C. Morrison, MD, Cleveland, OH.

pluglike appearance (Fig. 90) (296). In a study of patients with biliary acute pancreatis, sludge in the common bile duct was found by sonography in 25 out of 45 patients (297). Biliary sludge, leading to biliary obstruction and ascending cholangitis, is a life-threatening complication of liver transplantation and is seen in 10% to 29% of these patients (296). A hydatid cyst may rupture into the biliary tree and may cause obstruction secondary to the entrance of hydatid debris and daughter cysts into the bile ducts, resembling sludge (298,299). The diagnosis may be suggested when dilated bile ducts are seen in contiguity with the hydatid cyst within the liver.

The bile-plug syndrome is defined as extrahepatic obstruction of the common bile duct by sludge in full-term infants without anatomic abnormalities, congenital chemical defects of bile, or hepatocellular lesions (300). Bile-plug syndrome is rare and has been associated with total parenteral nutrition and cystic fibrosis. Sonographically, echogenic sludge without acoustic shadowing is seen within a dilated common bile duct (301).

Biliary Parasites

Ascariasis

Ascariasis is caused by the roundworm *Ascaris lumbricoides*. Ascariasis is the most common helminthic parasitic human infection, infecting approximately 25% of the world population, especially in the Far East, Latin America, and Africa. The infection occurs through ingestion of contaminated food or water, and children are especially susceptible. The adult worm is 15 to 50 cm long and 3 to 6 mm thick and lives mainly in the jejunum. However, the worms frequently enter the biliary tree through the common bile duct. Sonographically, adult roundworms can be seen in the common bile duct as nonshadowing, tubular echogenic structures containing a central anechoic line or as nonshadowing echogenic strips (Fig. 91) (302,303). Multiple worms in the common duct can appear as multiple echogenic strips, giving a spaghetti-like appearance (304). The worms can also be present in the gallbladder, causing acute cholecystitis, and in the intrahepatic biliary tree, causing cholangitis and liver abscess. In the gallbladder, the worms can appear as echogenic strips (Fig. 92), as echogenic coils, or less commonly as echogenic amorphous fragments, all without acoustic shadowing (303,305–308). Living worms sometimes display slow, spontaneous movements (309).

Clonorchiasis

Clonorchiasis is a disease caused by the parasite *C. sinensis* within the intrahepatic bile ducts, and it occurs after ingestion of raw or incompletely cooked fresh water fish. It is prevalent in the Far East including Japan, South Korea, Taiwan, China, and Vietnam. *C. sinensis* is a flat, leaf-shaped, transparent fluke, 10 to 25 mm long, 3 to 5 mm broad, and about 1 mm thick. The mature flukes live in the intrahepatic bile ducts, pancreatic ducts, and, occasionally, the gallbladder. They cause mechanical obstruction of the intrahepatic bile ducts, cholangitis, and periductal fibrosis, leading to thickening of the walls of the bile ducts. The incidence of recurrent pyogenic (Oriental) cholangitis and of cholangiocarcinoma is increased in patients with clonorchiasis (310). Sonographically, one sees diffuse, uniform dilatation of the small intrahepatic bile ducts with no or minimal dilatation of the large intrahepatic and extrahepatic bile ducts (310,311). The diffuse thickening of the bile duct walls is seen as echogenic bands along the bile ducts when the bile ducts are seen in their long axis and as echogenic nodules with a small, anechoic center representing the dilated duct when the bile ducts are seen in their short axis (310). The living flukes can be seen as rapidly moving linear echoes within the dilated intrahepatic bile ducts. The flukes in the gallbladder appear as fusiform, discrete, echogenic, nonshadowing foci measuring 3 to 6 mm in diameter. These echogenic foci may move and float spontaneously, suggesting living worms. The wall of the gallbladder may be thickened. Calcified dead flukes may mimic gallstones.

Bile Duct Wall Thickening

The wall of the normal common bile duct is less than 1 mm thick (312). It appears as a single echogenic line. The thickening of the wall may appear as two peripheral echogenic lines containing a central hypoechoic stripe. The thick wall may also appear predominantly echogenic or predominantly hypoechoic.

Marked, concentric hypoechoic thickening of the walls of the common duct may mimic a dilated common duct (Fig. 93) (313). Demonstration of a thin, linear, hyperechoic reflection in the center of the common duct, representing the interface between the coapted luminal surfaces of the thick hypoechoic wall of the duct, is helpful in making the correct diagnosis (Fig. 93).

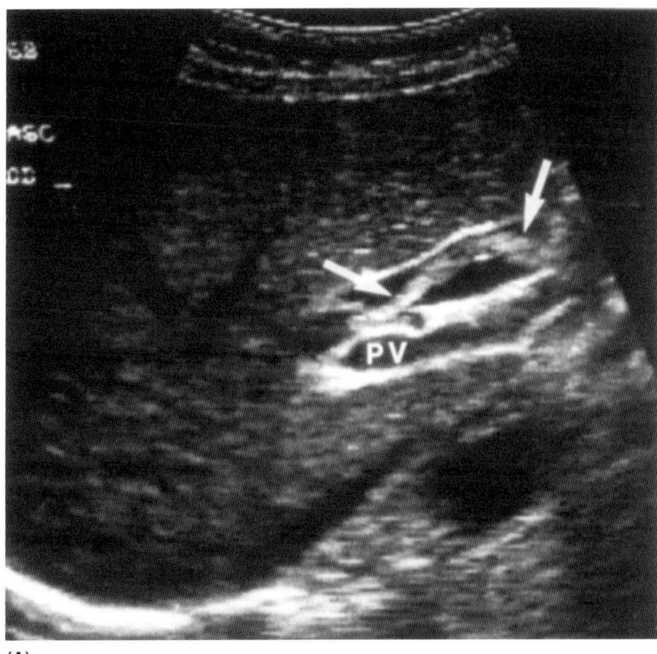

(A)

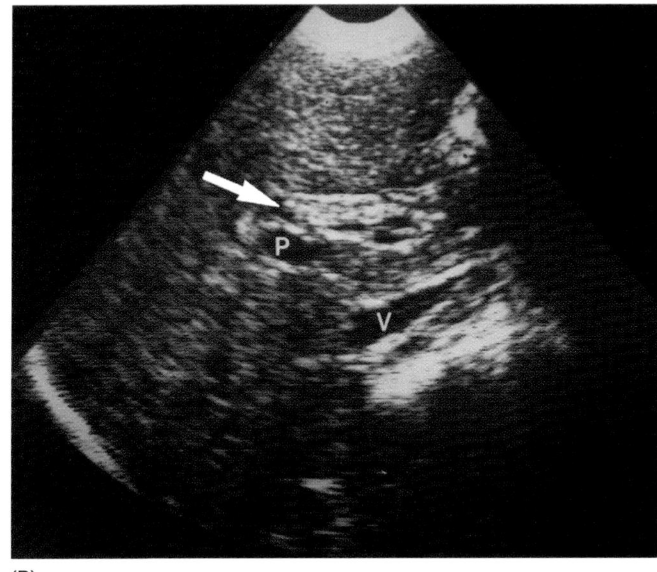

(B)

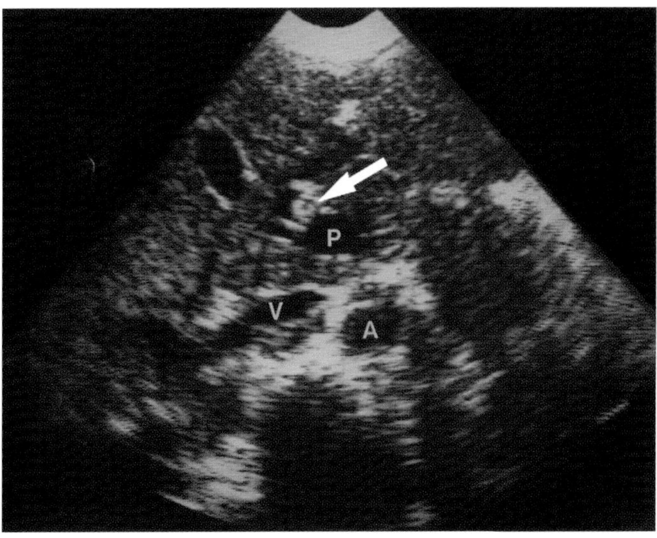

(C)

FIGURE 91 A–C ■ Biliary parasites. (**A**) Longitudinal view demonstrating Ascaris (roundworm), appearing as an echogenic strip (*arrows*) within a dilated common bile duct. (**B**) Longitudinal and (**C**) transverse views in another patient demonstrating Ascaris (roundworm) within the common bile duct. On the longitudinal view, the worm appears as a bandlike echogenic strip (*arrow*), and on the transverse view, as a rounded echogenic structure (*arrow*) within the common bile duct. On the transverse view, the small central anechoic area within the worm probably corresponds to the parasite's intestinal tract. PV, portal vein; () V, inferior vena cava; A, aorta. *Source*: Courtesy of William E. Brant, MD, Sacramento, CA.

Thickening of the wall of the common duct can be caused by cholangitis, choledocholithiasis, pancreatitis, and, rarely, cholangiocarcinoma. Thickening of the wall of the intrahepatic bile ducts can be caused by cholangitis or parasites (clonorchiasis). Thickening of the wall of the common duct rarely can be caused by varices in the wall, secondary to portal vein thrombosis.

Common Bile Duct Varices

Common bile duct varices are not a well-recognized feature of portal venous obstruction. They are rare and can be seen in patients with cavernous transformation of the portal vein secondary to portal vein thrombosis. They can be located around and/or within the wall of the common duct. When they are located within the wall of the common duct, transabdominal sonography may reveal thickening of the wall, and CDS may be necessary to demonstrate dilated veins within the wall (Fig. 94) (314). Pericholedochal varices may be seen by transabdominal sonography as tortuous, anechoic structures contiguous with the wall of the common duct. Endoscopic ultrasound is much more sensitive in diagnosing common bile duct varices compared with transabdominal sonography. Common bile duct varices have also been demonstrated by intraductal sonography. Although they are mainly asymptomatic, they may cause compression of the common duct and obstructive jaundice and have been treated by portosystemic shunting or biliary endoprosthesis (i.e., stent) (315,316).

Biliary Neoplasms

Cholangiocarcinoma

Almost all cholangiocarcinomas are adenocarcinomas arising from the bile duct epithelium. There is an increased frequency of cholangiocarcinoma in primary sclerosing

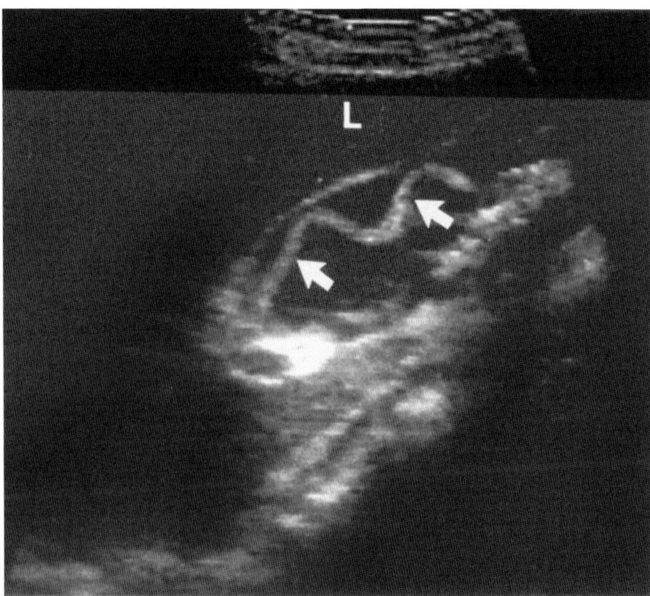

FIGURE 92 ■ Ascaris (roundworm) in the gallbladder. The worm (*arrows*) is seen as a serpiginous echogenic strip within the gallbladder. L, liver. *Source*: Courtesy of William E. Brant, MD, Sacramento, CA.

cholangitis, choledochal cysts, ulcerative colitis, Crohn's disease, familial polyposis, liver fluke infection (*C. sinensis*), and Caroli's disease. The average age of onset is approximately 60 years. Cholangiocarcinoma may be (*i*) intrahepatic, peripheral to the liver hilus (Chapter 16); (*ii*) hilar (Klatskin tumor); or (*iii*) distal, involving the distal common hepatic duct or common bile duct. Morphologic tumor types include (*i*) exophytic intrahepatic masses (19%), (*ii*) scirrhous infiltrating neoplasms causing stricture of the common duct (69%), and (*iii*) polypoid neoplasms of the duct wall bulging into the duct lumen (12%) (317–319).

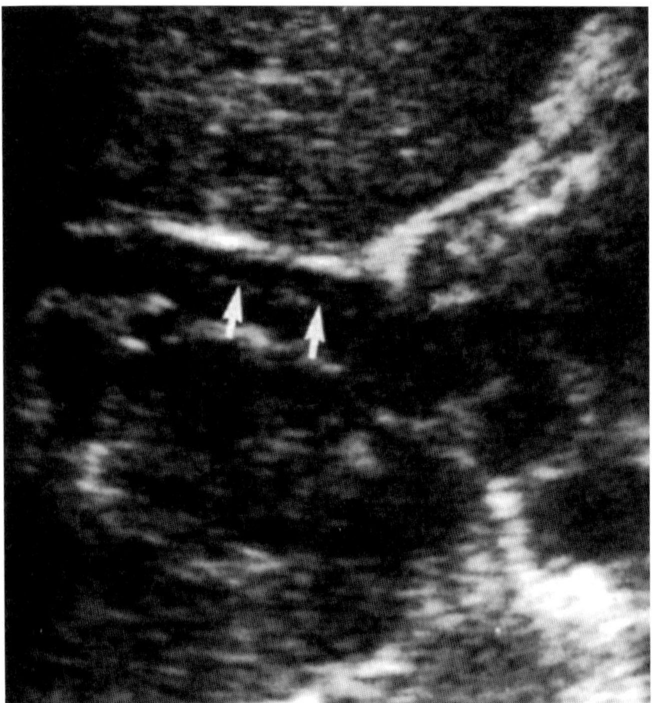

FIGURE 93 ■ Longitudinal view demonstrating marked concentric hypoechoic wall thickening of the common bile duct. The interface between the coapted luminal surfaces of the thick hypoechoic wall of the duct is seen as a thin linear hyperechoic reflection (*arrows*) in the center of the common duct. *Source*: From Ref. 313.

Hilar-Type Cholangiocarcinoma (Klatskin Tumor) ■ Hilar cholangiocarcinoma most often occurs at the confluence of the right and left hepatic ducts and the proximal common hepatic duct, and it is usually of the scirrhous type. Tumors at this location, at the bifurcation of the common hepatic duct, are referred to as Klatskin tumors. Sonographic findings in hilar tumors include dilatation of the intrahepatic bile ducts, but not the extrahepatic duct, nonunion of the dilated right and left hepatic ducts, and small, solid masses at the hepatic hilus (Figs. 95 and 96) (320). When masses are present, they are detected by sonography 21% to 47% of the time and by computed tomography 40% to 69% of the time, whereas cholangiography demonstrates almost all the tumors (318,319). Cholangiography is necessary to evaluate the extent of the hilar cholangiocarcinoma completely. Frequently, the hilar mass is not visible sonographically, but when seen, it is usually echogenic, reflecting the scirrhous nature of the tumor, and poorly defined. Hepatic lobar or segmental atrophy can occur after obstruction of the ipsilateral portal vein by hilar cholangiocarcinoma (321). The tumor can infiltrate the wall of the portal vein, causing portal vein thrombosis, which is much less common than hepatocellular carcinoma (322). Hepatic invasion or lymphadenopathy may occur.

Distal-Type Cholangiocarcinoma ■ Cholangiocarcinomas of the distal common hepatic or common bile duct are usually small and have a better prognosis than the hilar type. Sonographically, the tumor, when polypoid, may be seen as an echogenic or hypoechoic solid mass within the common duct or in contiguity with the common duct (Fig. 97) (323). Sonographically, the mass frequently is not visible, but the dilated common duct is abruptly terminated (324). Cholangiography is necessary to confirm the diagnosis. The differential diagnosis of common duct cholangiocarcinoma includes benign stricture, primary sclerosing cholangitis, metastases or lymphoma in the porta hepatis, benign neoplasms of the common duct, and, rarely, hepatocellular carcinoma invading the common duct.

Pitfalls ■ Sludge within the common duct can appear echogenic and may mimic intraductal soft tissue mass (Fig. 90) (Table 13). The clinical presentation and change in appearance or resolution of the sludge on follow-up examinations are helpful in the differentiation.

Other Malignant Neoplasms

In adults, cholangiocarcinoma and biliary cystadenoma and cystadenocarcinomas (Chapter 16) account for most bile duct neoplasms. Other malignant neoplasms of the

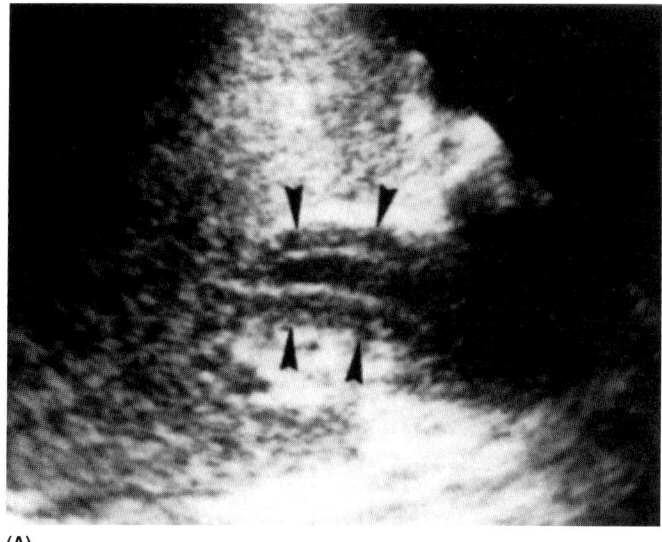
(A)

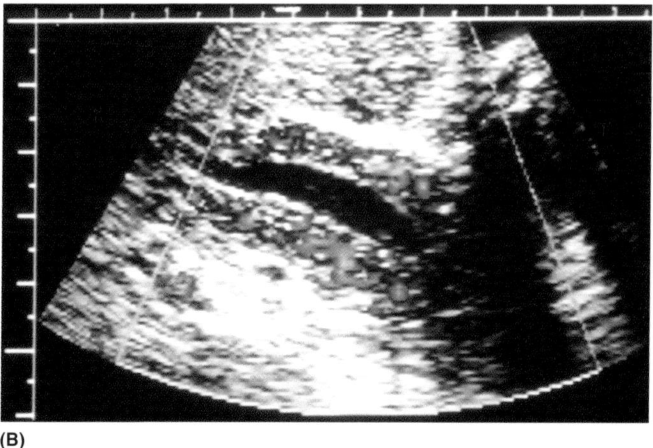
(B)

FIGURE 94 A AND B ■ Common duct wall varices. (**A**) Longitudinal sonogram of porta hepatis showing thickened wall of common bile duct (*arrowheads*). The portal vein is not visible. (**B**) Color Doppler sonogram of porta hepatis at the same level as (**A**) shows a network of small hepatopetal vessels within the wall of the common bile duct. *Source*: From Ref. 314.

bile duct are rare and include lymphoma, leiomyosarcoma, carcinoid tumors, and metastases.

Rhabdomyosarcoma ■ Rhabdomyosarcoma of the biliary tract is rare, but it is the most common pediatric biliary neoplasm (325). Typically, patients are between one and five years of age and present with progressive obstructive jaundice (326). Sonographically, solid masses containing hypoechoic areas secondary to rhabdomyosarcoma of the bile ducts within the liver, as well as in the porta hepatis, involving the cystic duct, have been described (327).

Periampullary Carcinoma ■ Periampullary carcinoma includes a group of neoplasms arising from the bile duct, pancreas, or duodenum. The origin of the tumor is often unclear on histologic examination. Periampullary carcinoma causes obstruction of the distal common duct at the ampulla of Vater. When the lesions are small, they are difficult to demonstrate by sonography. Sonographically, periampullary carcinoma may appear as a polypoid intraluminal mass in the distal common duct, or it may appear as a small (less than 2 cm) mass contiguous with the distal end of the obstructed common duct (Fig. 98) (328,329).

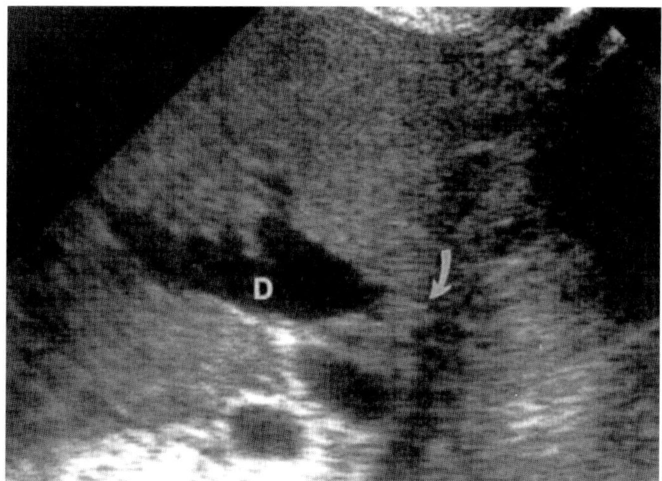

FIGURE 95 ■ Hilar cholangiocarcinoma: Klatskin tumor. Transverse oblique view showing a dilated right hepatic bile duct (D) obstructed by hilar cholangiocarcinoma (*arrow*) at the confluence of the right and the left hepatic bile ducts (not shown). Part of the echogenic mass (*arrow*) is protruding into the bile duct. The left hepatic bile ducts were also dilated (not shown).

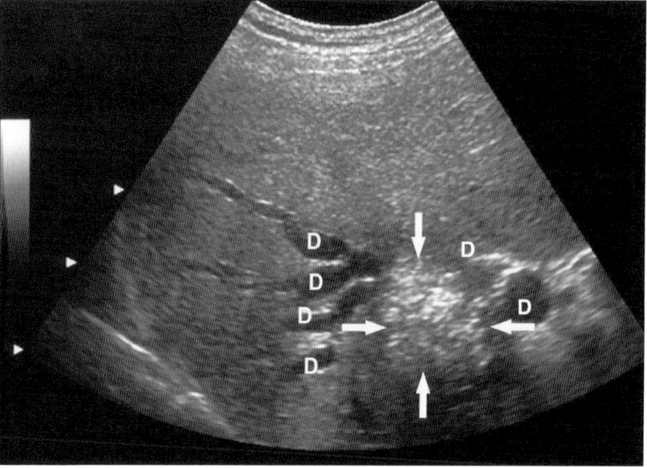

FIGURE 96 ■ Hilar cholangiocarcinoma: Klatskin tumor. Transverse view demonstrating dilated intrahepatic bile ducts (D). No communication exists between these dilated ducts because of the presence of a central hyperechoic mass (*arrows*). *Source*: Courtesy of Oksana Baltarowich, MD, Philadelphia, PA.

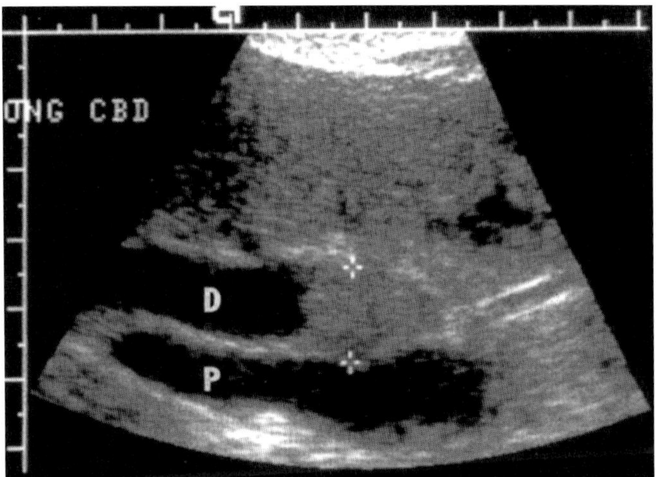

FIGURE 97 ■ Cholangiocarcinoma: the distal type. Longitudinal view demonstrating an echogenic solid mass (*cursors*) within the dilated common bile duct (D). P, main portal vein. *Source*: Courtesy of Robert L. Bree, MD, Ann Arbor, MI.

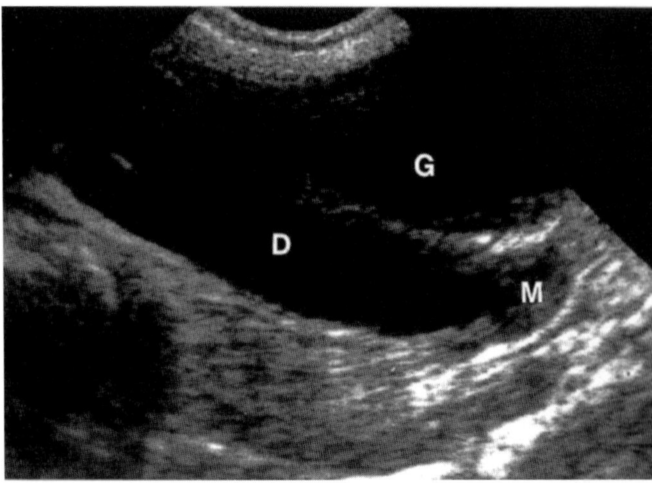

FIGURE 98 ■ Periampullary carcinoma. Longitudinal view showing a considerably dilated common duct obstructed by a small, hypoechoic mass secondary to periampullary carcinoma. G, distended gallbladder; D, common duct; M, mass.

Hepatocellular Carcinoma Invading the Common Duct ■ Hepatocellular carcinoma rarely extends into the lumen of the proximal extrahepatic bile ducts and common hepatic duct, causing common duct obstruction (330–333). Sonographically, it may resemble echogenic sludge filling the common duct, or a solid mass may be seen within the lumen of the common duct.

Benign Neoplasms

Benign neoplasms of the bile ducts are rare and include adenomas, which are the most common, granular cell tumors, hamartomas, fibromas, neuromas, lipomas, and heterotopic gastric or pancreatic mucosal rests (334). Most adenomas are asymptomatic; they are found incidentally at surgery and appear as polyps in the extrahepatic bile ducts.

TABLE 13 ■ Echogenicities in Bile Ducts

Calculi
Sludge
Air bubbles
Blood clots
Neoplasm
■ Cholangiocarcinoma
■ Hepatoma
■ Benign mesenchymal tumors
■ Metastatic tumors
Mirizzi's syndrome
Parasites
■ *Ascaris lumbricoides*
■ Liver flukes
■ Hydatid cyst debris
Artifacts
■ Compression from adjacent structures

Biloma

Biloma is a localized collection of bile within the peritoneal cavity or within the liver secondary to complication of biliary surgery, blunt or penetrating trauma, or, rarely, spontaneous rupture of biliary tree. Spontaneous perforation of the extrahepatic bile ducts in infancy is a rare cause of biloma and occurs most frequently between the ages of 4 and 12 weeks (325). It usually occurs at the junction of the common duct and the cystic duct. Bilomas are usually located in the right upper abdomen adjacent to the liver or biliary tree; however, they can also be found in the left upper abdomen or lower abdomen. Bilomas usually conform to the shape and surface of the adjacent organ, but they may displace the adjacent organs (335). Sonographic features of the biloma include an anechoic mass with prominent distal acoustic enhancement, a sharp, well-defined margin, and loculation (Fig. 99). Occasionally, internal echoes or debris and septations may be seen within the biloma (336). Intrahepatic bilomas appear as cystic masses within the liver (336). The differential diagnosis includes hematoma and abscess, both of which usually have more internal echoes and less pronounced distal acoustic enhancement compared with biloma. Accumula-tion of fluid in the gallbladder fossa is a common finding in the first week after cholecystectomy or after bile duct exploration and should not be mistaken for a biloma. These fluid collections are usually small and self-limiting and resolve spontaneously (337). The diagnosis of biloma can be confirmed by hepatobiliary scintigraphy (338) and percutaneous aspiration. Biloma can be treated by percutaneous catheter drainage (339).

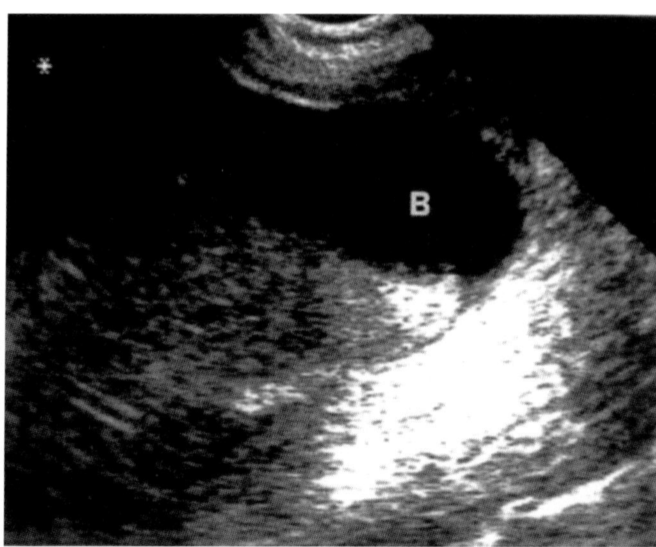

FIGURE 99 ■ Biloma. Longitudinal view of the right lobe of the liver showing a cystic mass (B) contiguous with the liver, with considerable distal acoustic enhancement. The mass is secondary to leakage of bile within the peritoneal cavity after biliary surgery.

Laparoscopic Ultrasound and Endoscopic Ultrasound of the Common Bile Duct

Laparoscopic sonography has been reported to be as accurate as laparoscopic video fluoroscopic cholangiography in visualizing the common bile duct and in detecting common duct stones (340). Endoscopic ultrasonography has also been reported to be highly accurate in detection of stones within the common bile duct (accuracy of 96%) (341). The sensitivity of endoscopic ultrasound in detection of common duct stones has been reported to be similar to or better than endoscopic retrograde cholangiopancreatography (341). Endoscopic ultrasound is also valuable in the diagnosis and staging of ampullary tumors, especially infiltration of the tumor into the pancreas.

Intraductal Sonography and Three-Dimensional Ultrasound of the Common Bile Duct

Intraductal sonography (i.e., images obtained by placing an ultrasound probe within the lumen of the common duct) is an evolving technique. It may be useful in the diagnosis and evaluation of common duct tumors, varices in the wall of the common duct, and other common duct pathology. Three-dimensional ultrasound, by demonstrating the common duct in different planes, may be helpful for more accurate determination of the diameter of the common duct and better demonstration of common duct abnormalities (342).

REFERENCES

1. Callen PW, Filly RA. Ultrasonographic localization of the gallbladder. Radiology 1979; 133:687.
2. Pancreas and liver. In: Warwick R, Williams PL, eds. Gray's Anatomy. 35th ed. Philadelphia: WB Saunders 1973:1299.
3. Wolson AH. Ultrasound measurements of the gallbladder. In: Goldberg BB, Kurtz AB, eds. Atlas of Ultrasound Measurements. Chicago: Year Book, 1990:108.
4. McGahan JP, Phillips HE, Cox KL. Sonography of the normal pediatric gallbladder and biliary tree. Radiology 1982; 144:873.
5. Edell S. A comparison of the "phrygian cap" deformity with bistable and grayscale ultrasound. JCU J Clin Ultrasound 1978; 6:34.
6. Sukov RJ, Sample WF, Sarti DA, et al. Cholecystosonography: the junctional fold. Radiology 1979; 133:435.
7. Parulekar SG. Evaluation of the prone view for cholecystosonography. J Ultrasound Med 1986; 5:617.
8. Samovsky M, Loberant N. Postprandial dilatation of the gallbladder in cholelithiasis. J Clin Ultrasound 2001; 29:513.
9. Jackson RJ, McClellan D. Agenesis of the gallbladder. Am Surg 1989; 55:36.
10. Wilson JE, Deitrick JE. Agenesis of the gallbladder. Surgery 1986; 99:106.
11. Hammond DI. Unusual causes of sonographic nonvisualization or nonrecognition of the gallbladder: a review. JCU J Clin Ultrasound 1988; 16:77.
12. McLoughlin MJ, Fanti JE, Kura ML. Ectopic gallbladder: sonographic and scintigraphic diagnosis. JCU J Clin Ultrasound 1987; 15:198.
13. Youngwirth LD, Peters JC, Perry MC. The suprahepatic gallbladder, an unusual anatomic variant. Radiology 1983; 149:57.
14. Pradeep VM, Ramachandran K, Sasidharan K. Anomalous position of the gallbladder: ultrasonographic and scintigraphic demonstration in four cases. JCU J Clin Ultrasound 1992; 20:593.
15. Garfield HD, Lyons EA, Levi CS. Double gallbladder. J Ultrasound Med 1988; 7:589.
16. Gupta S, Kumar A, Gautam A. Preoperative sonographic diagnosis of gallbladder duplication: importance of challenge with fatty meal. JCU J Clin Ultrasound 1993; 21:399.
17. Cunningham JJ. Empyema of a duplicated gallbladder: echographic findings. JCU J Clin Ultrasound 1980; 8:511.
18. Strauss S, Starinsky R, Alon Z. Partial multiseptate gallbladder: sonographic appearance. J Ultrasound Med 1993; 12:201.
19. Lev-Toaff AS, Friedman AC, Rindsberg SN, et al. Multiseptate gallbladder: incidental diagnosis on sonography. AJR Am J Roentgenol 1987; 148:1119.
20. Pery M, Kaftori JK, Marvan H, et al. Multiseptate gallbladder: report of a case with coexisting choledochal cyst. JCU J Clin Ultrasound 1985; 13:570.
21. Chin NW, Chapman I. Carcinoma in a true diverticulum of the gallbladder. Am J Gastroenterol 1988; 83:667.
22. Bradford BF, Reid BS, Weinstein BJ, et al. Ultrasonographic evaluation of the gallbladder in mucocutaneous lymph node syndrome. Radiology 1982; 142:381.
23. Koss JC, Coleman BG, Mulhern CG, et al. Mucocutaneous lymph node syndrome with hydrops of the gallbladder diagnosed by ultrasound. J Chin Ultrasound 1981; 9:477.
24. Choi YS, Sharma B. Gallbladder hydrops in mucocutaneous lymph node syndrome. South Med J 1989; 82:397.
25. Suddelson EA, Reid B, Woolley MM, et al. Hydrops of the gallbladder associated with Kawasaki syndrome. J Pediatr Surg 1987; 22:956.
26. Grisoni E, Fisher R, Izant R. Kawasaki syndrome: report of four cases with acute gallbladder hydrops. J Pediatr Surg 1984; 19:9.
27. Barth RA, Brasch RC, Filly RA. Abdominal pseudotumor in childhood: distended gallbladder with parenteral hyperalimentation. AJR Am J Roentgenol 1981; 136:341.
28. Laing F. The gallbladder and bile ducts. In: Rumack CM, Wilson SR, Charboneau JW, eds. Diagnostic Ultrasound. Vol. 1. St Louis: Mosby-Year Book, 1991:106.
29. Barie PS, Jacobson IM. Epidemiology of gallstones. In: Zakim D, Boyer TD, eds. Hepatology: A Textbook of Liver Disease. Vol. 2. 2nd ed. Philadelphia: WB Saunders, 1990:1516.
30. Zeman R. Cholelithiasis and cholecystitis. In: Gore RM, Levine MS, Laufer I, eds. Gastrointestinal Radiolology. Philadelphia: WB Saunders, 1994:1636.

31. Kirejcyzk WM, Crowe HM, Mackay IM, et al. Disappearing gallstones: biliary pseudolithiasis complicating ceftriaxone therapy. AJR Am J Roentgenol 1992; 159:329.
32. Hellmig S, Katsoulis S, Folsch U. Symptomatic cholecystolithiasis after laparoscopic cholecystectomy. Surg Endosc 2004; 18:347.
33. Zeman R. Cholelithiasis and cholecystitis. In: Gore RM, Levine MS, Laufer I, eds. Gastrointestinal Radiolology. Philadelphia: WB Saunders, 1994:1657.
34. Brink JA, Simeone JF, Mueller PR, et al. Routine sonographic techniques fail to quantify gallstone size and number: a retrospective study of surgically proved cases. AJR Am J Roentgenol 1989; 153:6.
35. Brakel K, Lameris JS, Nijs HG, et al. Accuracy of ultrasound and oral cholecystography in assessing the number and size of gallstones: implications for nonsurgical therapy. Br J Radiol 1992; 65:779.
36. Sommer FG, Taylor KJW. Differentiation of acoustic shadowing due to calculi and gas collections. Radiology 1980; 135:399.
37. Rubin JM, Adler RS, Bude RO, et al. Clean and dirty shadowing: a reappraisal. Radiology 1991; 181:231.
38. Parulekar SG. Ultrasonic detection of calcification in gallstones: "the reverberation shadow." J Ultrasound Med 1984; 3:123.
39. Cover KL, Slasky BS, Skolnick ML. Sonography of cholesterol in the biliary system. J Ultrasound Med 1985; 4:647.
40. Shapiro RS, Winsberg F. Comet-tail artifact from cholesterol crystal: observations in the postlithotripsy gallbladder and an in-vitro model. Radiology 1990; 177:153.
41. Taylor KJW, Jacobson P, Jaffee CC. Lack of an acoustic shadow on scans of gallstones: a possible artifact. Radiology 1979; 131:463.
42. Filly RA, Moss AA, Way LW. In vitro investigation of gallstone shadowing with ultrasound tomography. JCU J Clin Ultrasound 1979; 7:255.
43. Carroll BA. Gallstones: in vitro comparison of physical radiographic and ultrasonic characteristics. AJR Am J Roentgenol 1978; 131:223.
44. Simeone JF, Mueller PR, Ferrucci JT, et al. Significance of nonshadowing focal opacities at cholecystosonography. Radiology 1980; 137:181.
45. Laing FC, Gooding GAW, Herzog KA. Gallstones preventing ultrasonographic visualization of the gallbladder. Gastrointest Radiol 1977; 1:301.
46. MacDonald FR, Cooperberg PL, Cohen MM. The WES triad: a specific sonographic sign of gallstones in the contracted gallbladder. Gastrointest Radiol 1981; 6:39.
47. Raptopoulos V, D'Orsi C, Smith E, et al. Dynamic cholecystosonography of the contracted gallbladder: the double-arc-shadow sign. AJR Am J Roentgenol 1982; 138:275.
48. Wall DT, Cooperberg PL, Mathieson JR. An unusual sonographic appearance: the pyramidal gallstone. J Ultrasound Med 1992; 11:521.
49. Strijk SP, Boetes C, Rosenbusch G. Floating stones in nonopacified gallbladder: ultrasonographic sign of gascontaining gallstones. Gastrointest Radiol 1981; 6:261.
50. Scheske GA, Cooperberg PL, Cohen MM. Floating gallstones: the role of contrast material. JCU J Clin Ultrasound 1980; 8:227.
51. Yeh HC, Goodman J, Rabinowitz JG. Floating gallstones in bile without added contrast material. AJR Am J Roentgenol 1986; 146:49.
52. Rubaltelli L, Talenti E, Rizzatto G, et al. Gas-containing gallstones: their influence on ultrasound images. JCU J Clin Ultrasound 1984; 12:279.
53. Mitchell DG, Needleman L, Frauenhoffer S, et al. Gas containing gallstones: the sonographic "double echo sign." J Ultrasound Med 1988; 7:39.
54. Henschke CI, Teele RL. Cholelithiasis in children: recent observations. J Ultrasound Med 1983; 2:481.
55. Callahan J, Haller JO, Cacciarelli AA, et al. Cholelithiasis in infants: association with total parenteral nutrition and furosemide. Radiology 1982; 143:437.
56. Cunningham JJ, Houlihan SM, Altay C. Cholecystosonography in children with sickle cell disease: technical approach and clinical results. JCU J Clin Ultrasound 1981; 9:231.
57. Bor O, Dinleyici EC, Kebapci M, et al. Ceftriaxone-associated biliary sludge and pseudocholelithiasis during childhood: a prospective study. Pediatr Int 2004; 46:322.
58. Brown DL, Teele RL, Doubilet PM, et al. Echogenic material in the fetal gallbladder: sonographic and clinical observations. Radiology 1992; 182:73.
59. Devonald KJ, Ellwood DA, Colditz PB. The variable appearances of fetal gallstones. J Ultrasound Med 1992; 11:579.
60. Suchet IB, Labatte MF, Dyck CS, et al. Fetal cholelithiasis: a case report and review of the literature. JCU J Clin Ultrasound 1993; 21:198.
61. Klingensmith WC III, Cloffi-Ragan DT. Fetal gallstones. Radiology 1988; 167:143.
62. Abbitt PL, McIlhenny J. Prenatal detection of gallstone. JCU J Clin Ultrasound 1990; 18:202.
63. Jeanty P, Ammann W, Cooperberg P, et al. Mobile intraluminal masses of the gallbladder. J Ultrasound Med 1983; 2:65.
64. Torres WE, Zeman RK. Treatment of gallstones. In: Gore RM, Levine MS, Laufer I, eds. Gastrointestinal Radiology. Philadelphia: WB Saunders, 1994:1678.
65. Ferrucci JT. Biliary lithotripsy. AJR Am J Roentgenol 1989; 153:15.
66. Torres WE, Zeman RK. Treatment of gallstones. In: Gore RM, Levine MS, Laufer I, eds. Gastrointestinal Radiology. Philadelphia: WB Saunders, 1994:1680.
67. Filly RA, Allen B, Minton MJ, et al. In vitro investigation of the origin of echoes within biliary sludge. JCU J Clin Ultrasound 1980; 8:193.
68. Angelico M, De Santis A, Capocaccia L. Biliary sludge: a critical update. J Clin Gastroenterol 1990; 12:656.
69. Murray FE, Stinchcombe SJ, Hawkey CJ. Development of biliary sludge in patients on intensive care units: results of a prospective ultrasonographic study. Gut 1992; 33:1123.
70. Bolondi L, Gaiani S, Testa S, et al. Gallbladder sludge formation during prolonged fasting after gastrointestinal tract surgery. Gut 1985; 26:734.
71. Toursarkissian B, Kearney PA, Holley DT, et al. Biliary sludging in critically ill trauma patients. South Med J 1995; 88:420.
72. Lee SP, Maher K, Nicholls JF. Origin and fate of biliary sludge. Gastroenterology 1988; 94:170.
73. Kuo YC, Liu JY, Sheen IS, et al. Ultrasonographic difficulties and pitfalls in diagnosing primary carcinoma of the gallbladder. JCU J Clin Ultrasound 1990; 18:639.
74. Fakhry J. Sonography of tumefactive biliary sludge. AJR Am J Roentgenol 1982; 139:717.
75. Goldstein A, Madrazo BL. Slice thickness artifacts in grayscale ultrasound. JCU J Clin Ultrasound 1981; 9:365.
76. Fiske CE, Filly RA. Pseudo-sludge: a spurious ultrasound appearance within the gallbladder. Radiology 1982; 144:631.
77. Laing FC, Kurtz AB. The importance of ultrasonic sidelobe artifacts. Radiology 1982; 145:763.
78. Marchal G, Fevery J, Snowball S, et al. The sonographic aspects of hemobilia: clinical and experimental study. Eur J Radiol 1985; 5:211.
79. Grant EG, Smirniotopoulos JC. Intraluminal gallbladder hematoma: sonographic evidence of hemobilia. JCU J Clin Ultrasound 1983; 11:507.
80. Kauzlaric D, Barmeir E. Sonography of intraluminal gallbladder hematoma. JCU J Clin Ultrasound 1985; 13:291.
81. Scharling ES, Geisinger KR. Case of the day. Hemobilia: intraluminal gallbladder hematoma. J Ultrasound Med 1993; 12:244.
82. Gya D, Sali A, Vivetta L, et al. Limy bile cholecystitis; an in vitro study and a case report. Aust N Z J Surg 1990; 60:998.
83. Love MB. Sonographic features of milk of calcium bile. J Ultrasound Med 1982; 1:325.
84. Childress MC. Sonographic features of milk of calcium cholecystitis. JCU J Clin Ultrasound 1986; 14:312.
85. Laing FC, Federle MP, Jeffrey RB, et al. Ultrasonic evaluation of patients with acute right upper quadrant pain. Radiology 1981; 140:449.
86. Wales LR. Desquamated gallbladder mucosa: unusal sign of cholecystitis. AJR Am J Roentgenol 1982; 139:810.

87. Handler SJ. Ultrasound of gallbladder wall thickening and its relation to cholecystitis. AJR Am J Roentgenol 1979; 132:581.
88. Raghavendka BN, Feiner HD, Subramanyam BR, et al. Acute cholecystitis: sonographic-pathologic analysis. AJR Am J Roentgenol 1981; 137:327.
89. Marchal GJF, Casaer M, Baert AL, et al. Gallbladder wall sonolucency in acute cholecystitis. Radiology 1979; 133:429.
90. Bree RL. Further observations on the usefulness of the sonographic Murphy sign in the evaluation of suspected acute cholecystitis. JCU J Clin Ultrasound 1995; 23:169.
91. Ralls PW, Halls J, Lapin SA, et al. Prospective evaluation of the sonographic Murphy sign in suspected acute cholecystitis. JCU J Clin Ultrasound 1982; 10:113.
92. Ralls PW, Colletti PM, Lapin SA, et al. Real-time sonography in suspected acute cholecystitis. Radiology 1985; 155:767.
93. Parulekar SG, Hillier SA, Adell JA, et al. Color Doppler sonography of the gallbladder wall. J Ultrasound Med 1995; 14(suppl):S21.
94. Jeffrey RB Jr, Nino-Murcia M, Ralls PW, et al. Color Doppler sonography of the cystic artery: comparison of normal controls and patients with acute cholecystitis. J Ultrasound Med 1995; 14:33.
95. Paulson EK, Kliewer MA, Hertzberg BS, et al. Diagnosis of acute cholecystitis with color Doppler sonography: significance of arterial flow in thickened gallbladder wall. AJR Am J Roentgenol 1994; 162:1105.
96. Shuman WP, Mack LA, Rudd TG, et al. Evaluation of acute right upper quadrant pain: sonography and 99mTc-PIPIDA cholescintigraphy. AJR Am J Roentgenol 1982; 139:61.
97. Weissman HS, Frank MS, Bernstein LH, et al. Rapid and accurate diagnosis of acute cholecystitis with 99mTc-HIDA cholescintigraphy. AJR Am J Roentgenol 1979; 132:523.
98. Ralls PW, Colletti PM, Halls JM, et al. Prospective evaluation of 99mTc-IDA cholescintigraphy and gray-scale ultrasound in the diagnosis of acute cholecystitis. Radiology 1982; 144:369.
99. Samuels BI, Freitas JE, Bree RL, et al. A comparison of radionuclide hepatobiliary imaging and real-time ultrasound for the detection of acute cholecystitis. Radiology 1983; 147:207.
100. Mauro MA, McCartney WH, Melmed JR. Hepatobiliary scanning with 99mTc-PIPIDA in acute cholecystitis. Radiology 1982; 142:193.
101. Fink-Bennett D, Freitas JE, Ripley SD, et al. The sensitivity of hepatobiliary imaging and real-time ultrasonography in the detection of acute cholecystitis. Arch Surg 1985; 120:904.
102. Hinkel HP, Kraus S, Heimbucher J, et al. Sonography for selecting candidates for laparoscopic cholecystectomy: a prospective study. AJR Am J Roentgenol 2000; 174:1433.
103. Bree RL. Gallbladder and bile ducts: ultrasound. Special course. RSNA, syllabus. Oak Brook, IL: RSNA Publications, 1991:273.
104. Jeffrey RB, Laing FC, Wong W, et al. Gangrenous cholecystitis: diagnosis by ultrasound. Radiology 1983; 148:219.
105. Kane RA. Ultrasonographic diagnosis of gangrenous cholecytitis and empyema of the gallbladder. Radiology 1980; 134:191.
106. Teefey SA, Baron RL, Radke HM, et al. Gangrenous cholecystitis: new observations on sonography. J Ultrasound Med 1991; 10:603.
107. Teefey SA, Baron RL, Bigler SA. Sonography of the gallbladder: the significance of striated (layered) thickening of the gallbladder wall. AJR Am J Roentgenol 1991; 156:945.
108. Simeone JF, Brink JA, Mueller PR, et al. The sonographic diagnosis of acute gangrenous cholecystitis: importance of the Murphy sign. AJR Am J Roentgenol 1989; 152:289.
109. Madrazo BL, Francis I, Hricak H, et al. Sonographic findings in perforation of the gallbladder. AJR Am J Roentgenol 1982; 139:491.
110. Forsberg L, Anderson R, Hederstrom E, et al. Ultrasonography and gallbladder perforation in acute cholecystitis. Acta Radiol 1988; 29:203.
111. Bergman AB, Neiman HL, Kraut B. Ultrasonographic evaluation of pericholecystic abscesses. AJR Am J Roentgenol 1979; 132:201.
112. Chau WK, Wong KB, Chan SC, et al. Ultrasonic hole sign: a reliable sign of perforation of the gallbladder. JCU J Clin Ultrasound 1992; 20:294.
113. Soiva M, Aro K, Pamilo M, et al. Ultrasonography in carcinoma of the gallbladder. Acta Radiol 1987; 28:711.
114. Teefey SA, Wechter DG. Sonographic evaluation of pericholecystic abscess with intrahepatic extension. J Ultrasound Med 1987; 6:659.
115. Nyberg DA, Laing FC. Ultrasonographic findings in peptic ulcer disease and pancreatitis that simulate primary gallbladder disease. J Ultrasound Med 1983; 2:303.
116. Madrazo BL, Hricak H, Sandler MA, et al. Sonographic findings in complicated peptic ulcer. Radiology 1981; 140:457.
117. Chinn DH, Miller El, Piper N. Hemorrhagic cholecystitis sonographic appearance and clinical presentation. J Ultrasound Med 1987; 6:313.
118. Jenkins M, Golding RH, Cooperberg PL. Sonography and computed tomography of hemorrhagic cholecystitis. AJR Am J Roentgenol 1983; 140:1197.
119. Hunter ND, Macintosh PK. Acute emphysematous cholecystitis: an ultrasonic diagnosis. AJR Am J Roentgenol 1980; 134:592.
120. Parulekar SG. Sonographic findings in acute emphysematous cholecystitis. Radiology 1982; 145:117.
121. Bloom RA, Libson E, Lebensart PD, et al. The ultrasound spectrum of emphysematous cholecystitis. JCU J Clin Ultrasound 1989; 17:251.
122. Nemcek AA Jr, Gore RM, Vogelzang RL, et al. The effervescent gallbladder: a sonographic sign of emphysematous cholecystitis. AJR Am J Roentgenol 1988; 150:575.
123. White M, Simeone JF, Mueller PR. Imaging of cholecystocolic fistulas. J Ultrasound Med 1983; 2:181.
124. Pedersen PR, Petersen KK, Topp SW. Value of ultrasonography in the diagnosis of gallstone ileus. Radiology 1988; 28:479.
125. Lassandro F, Gagliardi N, Scuderi M, et al. Gallstone ileus analysis of radiological findings in 27 patients. Eur J Radiol 2004; 50:23.
126. Shuman WP, Rogers JV, Rudd TG, et al. Low sensitivity of sonography and cholescintigraphy in acalculous cholecystitis. AJR Am J Roentgenol 1984; 142:531.
127. Raduns K, McGahan JP, Beal S. Cholecystokinin sonography: lack of unity in diagnosis of acute calculous cholecystitis. Radiology 1990; 175:463.
128. Mirvis SE, Vainright JR, Nelson AW, et al. The diagnosis of acute acalculous cholecystitis: a comparison of sonography, scintigraphy, and computed tomography. AJR Am J Roentgenol 1986; 147:1171.
129. Cornwell EE III, Rodriquez A, Mirvis SE, et al. Acute acalculous cholecystitis in critially injured patients. Preoperative diagnostic imaging. Ann Surg 1989; 210:52.
130. Johnson LB. The importance of early diagnosis of acute acalculous cholecystitis. Surg Gynecol Obstet 1987; 164:197.
131. Barie PS, Eachempati SR. Acute acalculous cholecystitis. Curr Gastroenterol Rep 2003; 5:302.
132. Jeffrey RB Jr, Sommer FG. Follow-up sonography in suspected acalculous cholecystitis: preliminary clinical experience. J Ultrasound Med 1993; 12:183.
133. Puc MM, Tran HS, Wry PW, et al. Ultrasound is not a useful screening tool for acute acalculous cholecystitis in critically ill trauma patients. Am Surg 2002; 68:65.
134. Blankenberg R, Wirth R, Jeffrey RB Jr, et al. Computed tomography as an adjunct to ultrasound in the diagnosis of acute acalculous cholecystitis. Gastrointest Radiol 1991; 16:149.
135. Hanada K, Nakata H, Nakayama T, et al. Radiologic findings in xanthogranulomatous cholecystitis. AJR Am J Roentgenol 1987; 148:727.
136. Bluth El, Katz MM, Merritt CRB, et al. Echographic findings in xanthogranulomatous cholecystitis. JCU J Clin Ultrasound 1979; 7:213.
137. Lichtman JB, Varma VA. Ultrasound demonstration of xanthogranulomatous cholecystitis. JCU J Clin Ultrasound 1987; 15:342.
138. Solanki RL, Arora HL, Gaur SK, et al. Xanthogranulomatous cholecystitis (XGC): a clinicopathological study of 21 cases. Indian J Pathol Microbiol 1989; 32:256.

139. Safadi RR, Abu-Yousef MM, Farah AS, et al. Preoperative sonographic diagnosis of gallbladder torsion: report of two cases. J Ultrasound Med 1993; 12:296.
140. Yeh HC, Weiss MF, Gerson CD. Torsion of the gallbladder: the ultrasonographic features. JCU J Clin Ultrasound 1989; 17:123.
141. Quinn SF, Fazzio F, Jones E. Torsion of the gallbladder: findings on CT and sonography and role of percutaneous cholecystostomy. AJR Am J Roentgenol 1987; 148:881.
142. Cameron EW, Beale TJ, Pearson RH. Case report: torsion of the gallbladder on ultrasound—differentiation from acalculous cholecystitis. Clin Radiol 1993; 47:285.
143. Zeman R. Cholelithiasis and cholecystitis. In: Gore RM, Levine MS, Laufer I, eds. Gastrointestinal Radiology. Philadelphia: WB Saunders, 1994:1655.
144. Frykberg ER, Duong TC, LaRosa JJ, et al. Chronic acalculous gallbladder disease: a clinical variant. South Med J 1988; 81:1353.
145. Raptopoulos V, Compton CC, Doherty P, et al. Chronic acalculous gallbladder disease: multiimaging evaluation with clinical-pathologic correlation. AJR Am J Roentgenol 1986; 147:721.
146. Lewandowski B, Winsberg F. Gallbladder wall thickness distortion by ascites. AJR Am J Roentgenol 1981; 137:519.
147. Shlaer WJ, Leopold GR, Scheible FW. Sonography of the thickened gallbladder wall: a nonspecific finding. AJR Am J Roentgenol 1981; 136:337.
148. Sanders RC. The significance of sonographic gallbladder wall thickening. JCU J Clin Ultrasound 1980; 8:143.
149. Ralls PW, Quinn MF, Juttner HU. Gallbladder wall thickening: patients without intrinsic gallbladder disease. AJR Am J Roentgenol 1981; 137:65.
150. Fiske CE, Laing FC, Brown TW. Ultrasonographic evidence of gallbladder wall thickening in association with hypoalbuminemia. Radiology 1980; 135:713.
151. Carroll BA. Gallbladder wall thickening secondary to focal lymphatic obstruction. J Ultrasound Med 1983; 2:89.
152. Cohan RH, Mahoney BS, Bowie JD, et al. Striated intramural gallbladder lucencies on ultrasound studies: predictors of acute cholecystitis. Radiology 1987; 164:31.
153. Sharma MP, Dasarathy S. Gallbladder abnormalities in acute viral hepatitis: a prospective ultrasound evaluation. J Clin Gastroenterol 1991; 13:697.
154. Maresca G, De Gaetano AM, Mirk P, et al. Sonographic patterns of the gallbladder in acute viral hepatitis. JCU J Clin Ultrasound 1984; 12:141.
155. Juttner H-U, Ralls PW, Quinn MF, et al. Thickening of the gallbladder wall in acute hepatitis: ultrasound demonstration. Radiology 1982; 142:465.
156. Romano AJ, VanSonnenberg E, Casola G, et al. Gallbladder and bile duct abnormalities in AIDS: sonographic findings in eight patients. AJR Am J Roentgenol 1988; 150:123.
157. Tsujimoto F, Miyamoto Y, Tada S. Differentiation of benign from malignant ascites by sonographic evaluation of gallbladder wall. Radiology 1985; 157:503.
158. Huang Y-S, Lee S-D, Wu J-C, et al. Utility of sonographic gallbladder wall patterns in differentiating malignant from cirrhotic ascites. JCU J Clin Ultrasound 1989; 17:187.
159. Marchal G, deVoorde V, Dooren MV, et al. Ultrasonic appearance of the filled and contracted normal gallbladder. JCU J Clin Ultrasound 1980; 8:439.
160. Marchal GJ, Holsbeeck MV, Tshiwabwa-Ntumba E. Dilatation of the cystic veins in portal hypertension: sonographic demonstration. Radiology 1985; 154:187.
161. Wachsberg RH. Evaluation of patients before laparroscopic cholecystectomy: imaging findings. AJR Am J Roentgenol 1995; 164:1419.
162. Ralls PW, Mayekawa DS, Lee KP, et al. Gallbladder wall varices: diagnosis with color flow doppler sonography. JCU J Clin Ultrasound 1988; 16:595.
163. West MS, Garra BS, Horri SC, et al. Gallbladder varies: imaging findings in patients with poral hypertension. Radiology 1991; 179:179.
164. Saigh J, Williams S, Cawley K, et al. Varices: a cause of focal gallbladder wall thickening. J Ultrasound Med 1985; 4:371.
165. Kane RA, Jacobs R, Katz J, et al. Porcelain gallbladder: ultrasound and computed tomography appearance. Radiology 1984; 152:137.
166. Shimizu M, Miura J, Tanaka T, et al. Porcelain gallbladder: relation between its type by ultrasound and incidence of cancer. J Clin Gastroenterol 1989; 11:471.
167. Lichtenstein J. Adenomatosis and cholesterolosis: the "hyperplastic cholecystoses." In: Gore RM, Levine MS, Laufer I, eds. Gastrointestinal Radiology. Philadelphia: WB Saunders, 1994:1705.
168. Kidney M, Goiney R, Cooperberg PL. Adenomyomatosis of the gallbladder: a pictorial exhibit. J Ultrasound Med 1986; 5:331.
169. Detweiler DG, Biddinger P, Staab EV, et al. The appearance of adenomyomatosis with the newer imaging modalities: a case with pathologic correlation. J Ultrasound Med 1982; 1:295.
170. Raghavendra BN, Subramanyam BR, Balthazer EJ, et al. Sonography of adenomyomatosis of the gallbladder: radiologic-pathologic correlation. Radiology 1983; 146:747.
171. Lafortune M, Gariepy G, Dumont A, et al. The V-shaped artifact of the gallbladder. AJR Am J Roentgenol 1986; 147:505.
172. Lichtenstein J. Adenomatosis and cholesterolosis: the "hyperplastic cholecystoses." In: Gore RM, Levine MS, Laufer I, eds. Gastrointestinal Radiology. Philadelphia: WB Saunders, 1994:1709.
173. Price RJ, Stewart ET, Foley WD, et al. Sonography of polypoid cholesterolosis. AJR Am J Roentgenol 1982; 139:1197.
174. Ruhe AH, Zachman JP, Mulder BD, et al. Cholesterol polyps of the gallbladder: ultrasound demonstration. JCU J Clin Ultrasound 1979; 7:386.
175. Shinchi K, Kono S, Honjo S, et al. Epidemiology of gallbladder polyps: an ultrasonographic study of male self-defense officials in Japan. Scand J Gastroenterol 1994; 29:7.
176. Farinon AM, Pacella A, Cetta F, et al. Adenomatous polyps of the gallbladder adenomas of the gallbladder. HPB Surg 1991; 3:251.
177. Koga A, Watanabe K, Fukuyama T, et al. Diagnosis and operative indications for polypoid lesions of the gallbladder. Arch Surg 1988; 123:26.
178. Ishikawa O, Ohhigashi H, Imaoka S, et al. The difference in malignancy between pedunculated and sessile polypoid lesions of the gallbladder. Am J Gastroenterol 1989; 84:1386.
179. Myers RP, Shaffer EA, Beck PL. Gallbladder polyps: epidemiology, natural history and management. Can J Gastroenterol 2002; 16:187.
180. Boulton RA, Adams DH. Gallbladder polyps: when to wait and when to act. Lancet 1997; 349:817. (Erratum in Lancet 1997; 349:1032).
181. Hallgrimsson P, Skaane P. Hypoechoic solitary inflammatory polyp of the gallbladder. JCU J Clin Ultrasound 1988; 16:603.
182. Ward E, Stephens D. Neoplasms. In: Gore RM, Levine MS, Laufer I, eds. Gastrointestinal Radiology. Philadelphia: WB Saunders, 1994:1717.
183. Lane J, Buck JL, Zeman RK. Primary carcinoma of the gallbladder: a pictorial essay. Radiographics 1989; 9:209.
184. Rooholamini SA, Tehrani NS, Razavi MK, et al. Imaging of gallbladder carcinoma. Radiographics 1994; 14:291.
185. Tsuchiya Y. Early carcinoma of the gallbladder: macroscopic features and US findings. Radiology 1991; 179:171.
186. Weiner SN, Koenigsberg M, Morehouse H, et al. Sonography and computed tomography in the diagnosis of carcinoma of the gallbladder. AJR Am J Roentgenol 1984; 142:735.
187. Kumar A, Aggarwal S, Berry M, et al. Ultrasonography of carcinoma of the gallbladder—an analysis of 80 cases. J Clin Ultrasound 1990; 18:715.
188. Oikarinen H, Paivansalo M, Lahde S, et al. Radiological findings in cases of gallbladder carcinoma. Eur J Radiol 1993; 17:179.
189. Hayakawa S, Goto H, Hirooka Y, et al. Colour Doppler-guided spectral analysis of gall-bladder wall flow. J Gastroenterol Hepatol 1998; 13:181.
190. Li D, Dong BW, Wu YL, et al. Image-directed and color Doppler studies of gallbladder tumors. JCU J Clin Ultrasound 1994; 22:551.
191. Cunningham CC, Zibari GB, Johnston LW. Primary carcinoma of the gall bladder: a review of our experience. J La State Med Soc 2002; 154:196.
192. Ferin P, Lerner RM. Contracted gallbladder: a finding in hepatic dysfunction. Radiology 1985; 154:769.

193. Bret PM, de Stempel JV, Atri M, et al. Intrahepatic bile duct and portal vein anatomy revisited. Radiology 1988; 169:405.
194. Lim JH, Ryu KN, Ko YT, et al. Anatomic relationship of intrahepatic bile ducts to portal veins. J Ultrasound Med 1990; 9:137.
195. Bressler El, Rubin JM, McCracken S, et al. Sonographic parallel channel sign: a reappraisal. Radiology 1987; 164:343.
196. Conrad MR, Landay MJ, Janes JO. Sonographic "parallel channel" sign of biliary tree enlargement in mild to moderate obstructive jaundice. AJR Am J Roentgenol 1978; 130:279.
197. Weill F, Eisencher A, Zeltner F. Ultrasonic study of the normal and dilated biliary tree: the "shotgun" sign. Radiology 1978; 127:221.
198. Ralls PW, Mayekawa, Lee KP, et al. The use of color Doppler sonography to distinguish dilated intrahepatic ducts from vascular structures. AJR Am J Roentgenol 1989; 152:291.
199. Laing FC, London LA, Filly RA. Ultrasonographic indentification of dilated intrahepatic bile ducts and their differentiation from portal vein structures. JCU J Clin Ultrasound 1978; 6:90.
200. Wing VW, Laing FC, Jeffrey RB. Sonographic differentiation of enlarged hepatic arteries from dilated intrahepatic bile ducts. AJR Am J Roentgenol 1985; 145:57.
201. Zeman RK, Lee C, Stahl RS, et al. Ultrasonography and hepatobiliary scintigraphy in the assessment of biliary-eneric anastomoses. Radiology 1982; 145:109.
202. Lewandowski BJ, Withers C, Winsberg F. The air-filled left hepatic duct: the saber sign as an aid to the radiographic diagnosis of pneumobilia. Radiology 1984; 153:329.
203. MacCarty RL. Noncalculous inflammatory disorders of the biliary tract. In: Gore RM, Levine MS, Laufer I, eds. Gastrointestinal Radiolology. Philadelphia: WB Saunders, 1994:1737.
204. Carroll BA, Oppenheimer DA. Sclerosing cholangitis: sonographic demonstration of bile duct wall thickening. AJR Am J Roentgenol 1982; 139:1016.
205. Dolmatch BL, Laing FC, Federle MP, et al. AIDS-related cholangitis: radiographic findings in nine patients. Radiology 1987; 163:313.
206. Da Silva F, Boudghene F, Lecomte I, et al. Sonography in AIDS-related cholangitis: prevalence and cause of an echogenic nodule in the distal end of the common duct. AJR Am J Roentgenol 1993; 160:1205.
207. Chung CJ, Sivit CJ, Rakusan TA, et al. Hepatobiliary abnormalities on sonography in children with HIV infection. J Ultrasound Med 1994; 13:205.
208. Teixidor HS, Godwin TA, Ramirez EA. Cryptosporidiosis of the biliary tract in AIDS. Radiology 1991; 180:51.
209. Lim JH, Ko YT, Lee DH, et al. Oriental cholangiohepatitis: sonographic findings in 48 cases. AJR Am J Roentgenol 1990; 155:511.
210. Ralls PW, Colletti PM, Quinn MF, et al. Sonography in recurrent oriental pyogenic cholangitis. AJR Am J Roentgenol 1981; 136:1010.
211. White LM, Wilson SR. Hepatic arterial calcification: a potential pitfall in the sonographic diagnosis of intrahepatic biliary calculi. J Ultrasound Med 1994; 13:141.
212. Benhamou JP. Congenital hepatic fibrosis and Caroli's syndrome. In: Schiff L, Schiff ER, eds. Diseases of the Liver. Vol. 1. Philadelphia: JB Lippincott, 1993:1204.
213. Mittelstaedt CA, Volberg FM, Fisher GJ, et al. Caroli's disease sonographic findings. AJR Am J Roentgenol 1980; 134:585.
214. Middleton WD. Ultrasound: The Requisites. St Louis, Mosby-Year Book, 1996:69.
215. Marchal GJ, Desmer VJ, Proesmans WC, et al. Caroli's disease: high-frequency ultrasound and pathologic findings. Radiology 1986; 158:507.
216. Choi BI, Yeon KM, Kim SH, et al. Caroli disease: central dot sign in CT. Radiology 1990; 174.
217. Lee, Cho KS, Auh YH, et al. Hepatic arterial color Doppler signals in Caroli's disease. Clin Imaging 1992; 16:234.
218. Toma P, Lucigrai G, Pelizza A. Sonographic patterns of Caroli's disease: report of 5 new cases. JCU J Clin Ultrasound 1991; 19:155.
219. Parulekar SG. Ultrasound evaluation of common bile duct size. Radiology 1979; 133:703.
220. Kurtz AB, Middleton WD. Bile ducts. In: Ultrasound: The Requisites. St Louis: Mosby-Year Book, 1996:55.
221. Cooperberg P. High-resolution real-time ultrasound in the evaluation of the normal and obstructed biliary tract. Radiology 1978; 129:477.
222. Niederau C, Muller J, Sonnenberg A, et al. Extrahepatic bile ducts in healthy subjects, in patients with cholelithiasis, and in postcholecystectomy patients: a prospective ultrasonic study. JCU J Clin Ultrasound 1983; 11:23.
223. Behan M, Kazam E. Sonography of the common bile duct: value of the right anterior oblique view. AJR Am J Roentgenol 1978; 130:701.
224. Wachsberg RH. Respiratory variation of extrahepatic bile duct diameter during ultrasonography. J Ultrasound Med 1994; 13:617.
225. Bowe JD. What is the upper limit of normal for the common bile duct on ultrasound: how much do you want it to be? Am J Gastroenterol 2000; 95:897.
226. Wu CC, Ho YH, Chen CY. Effect of aging on common bile duct diameter: a real-time ultrasonographic study. JCU J Clin Ultrasound 1984; 12:473.
227. Perret RS, Sloop GD, Borne JA. Common bile duct measurements in an elderly population. J Ultrasound Med 2000; 19:727.
228. Bruneton JN, Roux P, Fenart D, et al. Ultrasound evaluation of common bile duct size in normal adult patients and following cholecystectomy. A report of 750 cases. Eur J Radiol 1981; 1:171.
229. Bachar GN, Cohen M, Belenky A, et al. Effect of aging on the adult extrahepatic bile duct: a sonographic study. J Ultrasound Med 2003; 22:879.
230. Horrow MM, Horrow JC, Niakosari A, et al. Is age associated with size of adult extrahepatic bile duct: sonographic study. Radiology 2001; 221:411.
231. Carroll BA, Oppenheimer DA, Muller HH. High-frequency real-time ultrasound of the neonatal biliary system. Radiology 1982; 145:437.
232. Hernanz-Schulman M, Ambrosino MM, Freeman PC, et al. Common bile duct in children: sonographic dimensions. Radiology 1995; 195:193.
233. Graham MF, Cooperberg PL, Cohen MM, et al. The size of the normal common hepatic duct following cholecystectomy: an ultrasonographic study. Radiology 1980; 135:137.
234. Mueller PR, Ferrucci JT, Simeone JF, et al. Postcholecystectomy bile duct dilatation: myth or reality? AJR Am J Roentgenol 1981; 136:355.
235. Graham MF, Cooperberg PL, Cohen MM, et al. Ultrasonographic screening of the common hepatic duct in symptomatic patients after cholecystectomy. Radiology 1981; 138:137.
236. Bucceri AM, Brogna A, Ferrara R. Common bile duct caliber following cholecystectomy: a two-year sonographic survey. Abdom Imaging 1994; 19:251.
237. Escedy G, Mundi B, Farkas I, et al. Über den diagnostischen wert der sog., postcholecystektomischen gallengangserweiterung. Chirurg 1990; 61:387.
238. Feng B, Song Q. Does the common bile duct dilate after cholecystectomy? Sonographic evaluation in 234 patients. AJR Am J Roentgenol 1995; 165:859.
239. Hunt DR, Scott AJ. Changes in bile duct diameter after cholecystectomy: a 5-year prospective study. Gastroenterology 1989; 97:1485.
240. Laing F. The gallbladder and bile ducts. In: Rumack CM, Wilson SR, Charboneau JW, eds. Diagnostic Ultrasound. Vol. 1. St. Louis, MO: Mosby-Year Book, 1991:132.
241. Chang VH, Cunningham JJ, Fromkes JJ. Sonographic measurement of the extrahepatic bile duct before and after retrograde cholangiography. AJR Am J Roentgenol 1985; 144:753.
242. Sauerbrei EE, Cooperberg PL, Gordon P, et al. The discrepancy between radiographic and sonographic bileduct measurements. Radiology 1980; 137:751.
243. Davies RP, Downey PR, Moore WR, et al. Contrast cholangiography versus ultrasonographic measurement of the "extrahepatic" bile duct: a two-fold discrepancy revisited. J Ultrasound Med 1991; 10:653.
244. Berland LL, Lawson TL, Foley WD. Porta hepatis: sonographic discrimination of bile ducts from arteries with pulsed Doppler with new anatomic criteria. AJR Am J Roentgenol 1982; 138:833.
245. Jacobson JB, Brody PA. The transverse common duct. AJR Am J Roentgenol 1981; 136:91.

246. Gore RM, Ghahremani GG, Fernbach SK. Anomalies and anatomic variants. In: Gore RM, Levine MS, Laufer I, eds. Gastrointestinal radiology. Philadelphia: WB Saunders, 1994:1628.
247. Parulekar SG. Sonography of the distal cystic duct. J Ultrasound Med 1989; 8:367.
248. Laing FC, Jeffrey RB, Wing VW. Improved visualization of choledocholithiasis by sonography. AJR Am J Roentgenol 1984; 143:949.
249. Dong B, Chen M. Improved sonographic visualization of choledocholithiasis. JCU J Clin Ultrasound 1987; 15:185.
250. Ikeda S, Sera Y, Akagi M. Serial ultrasonic examination to differentiate biliary atresia from neonatal hepatitis: special reference to changes in size of the gallbladder. Eur J Pediatr 1989; 148:396.
251. Kirks DR, Coleman RE, Filston HC, et al. An imaging approach to persistent neonatal jaundice. AJR Am J Roentgenol 1984; 142:461.
252. Siegel MJ. Liver and biliary tract. In: Siegel MJ, ed. Pediatric Sonography. New York: Raven Press, 1991:115.
253. Majd M. 99mTc-IDA scintigraphy in the evaluation of neonatal jaundice. Radiographics 1983; 3:88.
254. Weinberger E, Blumhagen JD, Odell JM. Gallbladder contraction in biliary atresia. AJR Am J Roentgenol 1987; 149:401.
255. Han BK, Babcock DS, Gelfand MH. Choledochal cyst with bile duct dilatation: sonography and 99mTc-IDA cholescintigraphy. AJR Am J Roentgenol 1981; 136:1075.
256. Kimura K, Ohto T, Ono T, et al. Congenital cystic dilatation of the common bile duct: relationship to anomalous pancreatico-biliary ductal union. AJR Am J Roentgenol 1977; 128:571.
257. Savader SJ, Benenati JF, Venbrux AC, et al. Choledochal cysts: classification and cholangiographic appearance. AJR Am J Roentgenol 1991; 156:327.
258. Aggarwal S, Kumar A, Roy S, et al. Massive dilatation of the common bile duct resembling a choledochal cyst. Trop Gastroenterol 2001; 22:219.
259. Laing FC, Jeffrey RB Jr, Wing VW. Biliary dilatation: defining the level and cause by real-time ultrasound. Radiology 1986; 160:39.
260. Koenigsberg M, Weiner SN, Walzer A. The accuracy of sonography in the differential diagnosis of obstructive jaundice: a comparison with cholangiography. Radiology 1979; 133:157.
261. Haubek A, Pedersen JH, Burcharth F, et al. Dynamic sonography in the evaluation of jaundice. AJR Am J Roentgenol 1981; 136:1071.
262. Malini S, Sabel J. Ultrasonography in obstructive jaundice. Radiology 1977; 123:429.
263. Honickman SP, Mueller PR, Wittenberg J, et al. Ultrasound in obstructive jaundice: prospective evaluation of site and cause. Radiology 1983; 147:511.
264. Baron RL, Stanley RJ, Lee JKT, et al. A prospective comparison of the evaluation of biliary obstruction using computed tomography and ultrasonography. Radiology 1982; 145:91.
265. Gibson RN, Yeung E, Thompson J, et al. Bile duct obstruction: radiologic evaluation of level, cause and tumor resectability. Radiology 1986; 160:43.
266. Weinstein BJ, Weinstein DP. Biliary tract dilatation in the nonjaundiced patient. AJR Am J Roentgenol 1980; 134:899.
267. Zeman R, Taylor KJW, Burrell MI, et al. Ultrasound demonstration of anicteric dilatation of the biliary tree. Radiology 1980; 134:689.
268. Shawker TH, Jones BL, Girton ME. Distal common bile duct obstruction: an experimental study in monkeys. JCU J Clin Ultrasound 1981; 9:77.
269. Zeman RK, Taylor KJW, Rosenfield AT, et al. Acute experimental biliary obstruction in the dog: sonographic findings and clinical implications. AJR Am J Roentgenol 1981; 136:965.
270. Raptopoulos V, Smith EH, Cummings T, et al. Bile-duct dilatation after laparotomy: a potential effect of intestinal hypomotility. AJR Am J Roentgenol 1986; 147:729.
271. Muhletaler CA, Gerlock AJ Jr, Fleischer AC, et al. Diagnosis of obstructive jaundice with nondilated bile ducts. AJR Am J Roentgenol 1980; 134:1149.
272. Burrell MI, Zeman RK, Simeone JF, et al. The biliary tract: imaging for the 1990s. AJR Am J Roentgenol 1991; 157:223.
273. Mueller PR, Ferrucci JT, Simeone JF, et al. Observations of the distensibility of the common bile duct. Radiology 1982; 142:467.
274. Scheske GA, Cooperberg PL, Cohen MM, et al. Dynamic changes in the caliber of the major bile ducts, related to obstruction. Radiology 1980; 135:215.
275. Glazer GM, Filly RA, Laing FC. Rapid change in caliber of the nonobstructed common duct. Radiology 1981; 140:161.
276. Simeone JF, Butch RJ, Mueller PR, et al. The bile ducts after a fatty meal: further sonographic observations. Radiology 1985; 154:763.
277. Willson SA, Gosnik BB, vanSonnenberg E. Unchanged size of a dilated common bile duct after fatty meal: results and significance. Radiology 1986; 160:29.
278. Willson SA. The fatty meal in biliary tree diagnosis. In: Raymond HW, Zwiebel WJ, eds. Semin Ultrasound CT MR 1987; 8:114.
279. Darweesh RM, Dodds WJ, Hogan WJ. Fatty meal sonography for evaluating patients with suspected partial common duct obstruction. AJR Am J Roentgenol 1988; 151:63.
280. Quinn RJ, Meredith C, Slade L. The effect of the Valsalva maneuver on the diameter of the common hepatic duct in extrahepatic biliary obstruction. J Ultrasound Med 1992; 11:143.
281. Laing FC, Jeffrey RB. The pseudo-dilated common bile duct: ultrasonographic appearance created by the gallbladder neck. Radiology 1980; 135:405.
282. Laffey PA, Brandon JC, Teplick SK, et al. Ultrasound of hemobilia: a clinical and experimental study. JCU J Clin Ultrasound 1988; 16:167.
283. Laing FC. Ultrasound diagnosis of choledocholithiasis. Semin Ultrasound CT MR 1987; 8:103.
284. Hai S, Tanaka H, Kubo S, et al. Choledocholithiasis caused by migration of a surgical clip into the biliary tract following laparoscopic cholecystectomy. Surg Endosc 2003; 17:2028.
285. Kaji M, Asano N, Tamura H, et al. Common bile duct stone caused by a fish bone: report of a case. Surg Today 2004; 34:268.
286. Gross BH, Harter LP, Gore RM, et al. Ultrasonic evaluation of common duct stones: prospective comparison with endoscopic retrograde cholangiopancreatography. Radiology 1983; 146:471.
287. Cronan J. Ultrasound diagnosis of choledocholithiasis: a reappraisal. Radiology 1986; 161:133.
288. Hunt DR. Common bile duct stones in non-dilated bile ducts? An ultrasound study. Australas Radiol 1996; 40:221.
289. Parulekar SG, McNamara M. Ultrasonography of choledocholithiasis. J Ultrasound Med 1983; 2:395.
290. Mueller PR, Cronan JJ, Simeone JF, et al. Choledocholithiasis: ultrasonographic caveats. J Ultrasound Med 1983; 2:13.
291. Majeed AW, Ross B, Johnson AG, et al. Common duct diameter as an independent predictor of choledocholithiasis: is it useful? Clin Radiol 1999; 54:170.
292. Gore RM. Endoscopic retrograde cholangiopancreatography. In: Gore RM, Levine MS, Laufer I, eds. Gastrointestinal Radiology. Philadelphia: WB Saunders, 1994:1596.
293. Jackson VP, Lappas JC. Sonography of the Mirizzi syndrome. J Ultrasound Med 1984; 3:281.
294. Becker CD, Hassler H, Terrier F. Preoperative diagnosis of the Mirizzi syndrome: limitations of sonography and computed tomography. AJR Am J Roentgenol 1984; 143:591.
295. Koehler RE, Melson GL, Lee JKT, et al. Common hepatic duct obstruction by cystic duct stone: mirizzi syndrome. AJR Am J Roentgenol 1979; 132:1007.
296. Barton P, Maier A, Steininger R, et al. Biliary sludge after liver transplantation. 1. Imaging findings and efficacy of various imaging procedures. AJR Am J Roentgenol 1995; 164:859.
297. Pezzilli R, Billi P, Barakat B, et al. Ultrasonographic evaluation of the common bile duct in biliary acute pancreatitis patients: comparison with endoscopic retrograde cholangiopancreatography. J Ultrasound Med 1999; 18:391.
298. Biggi E, Derchi L, Cicio GR, et al. Sonographic findings of hydatid cyst of the liver ruptured into the biliary duct. JCU J Clin Ultrasound 1979; 7:381.
299. Subramanyam BR, Balthazar EJ, Naidich DP. Ruptured hydatid cyst with biliary obstruction: diagnosis by sonography and computed tomography. Gastrointest Radiol 1983; 8:341.
300. Lang EV, Pinckney LE. Spontaneous resolution of bileplug syndrome. AJR Am J Roentgenol 1991; 156:1225.
301. Pfieffer W, Robinson L, Balsara V. Sonographic features of bile plug syndrome. J Ultrasound Med 1986; 5:161.

302. Schulman A, Roman T, Dalrymple R, et al. Sonography of biliary worms (ascariasis). JCU J Clin Ultrasound 1982; 10:77.
303. Cerri GG, Leite GJ, Simoes JB, et al. Ultrasonographic evaluation of ascariasis in the biliary tract. Radiology 1983; 146:753.
304. Schulman A, Loxton AJ, Heydenrych JJ, et al. Sonographic diagnosis of biliary ascariasis. AJR Am J Roentgenol 1982; 139:485.
305. Fawzy RK, Salem AE, Osman MM. Ultrasonographic findings in the gallbladder in human fascioliasis. J Egypt Soc Parasitol 1992; 22:827.
306. Mairiang E, Elkins DB, Mairiang P, et al. Relationship between intensity of *Opisthorchis viverrini* infection and hepatobiliary disease detected by ultrasonography. J Gastroenterol Hepatol 1992; 7:17.
307. Khuroo MS, Zargar SA, Mahajan R, et al. Sonographic appearance in biliary ascariasis. Gastroenterology 1987; 93:267.
308. Khuroo MS, Zargar SA, Yattoo GN, et al. Sonographic findings in gallbladder ascariasis. JCU J Clin Ultrasound 1992; 20:587.
309. Aslam M, Dore SP, Verbanck JJ, et al. Ultrasonographic diagnosis of hepatobiliary ascariasis. J Ultrasound Med 1993; 12:573.
310. Lim JH. Radiologic findings of clonorchiasis. AJR Am J Roentgenol 1990; 155:1000.
311. Lim JH, Ko YT, Lee DH. Clonorchiasis: sonographic findings in 59 proved cases. AJR Am J Roentgenol 1989; 152:761.
312. Berger J, Lindsell DRM. Case report: thickening of the walls of non-dilated bile ducts. Clin Radiol 1997; 52:474.
313. Middleton WD, Surratt RS. Thickened bile duct wall simulating ductal dilatation on sonography. AJR Am J Roentgenol 1992; 159:331.
314. Denys A, Hélénon O, Lafortune M, et al. Thickening of the wall of the bile duct due to intramural collaterals in three patients with portal vein thrombosis. AJR Am J Roentgenol 1998; 171:455–456.
315. Chow L, Jeffrey RB Jr. Intramural varices of the bile duct: an unusual pattern of cavernous transformation of the portal vein. AJR Am J Roentgenol 1999; 173:1255.
316. Dumortier J, Vaillant E, Boillot O, et al. Diagnosis and treatment of biliary obstruction caused by portal cavernoma. Endoscopy 2003; 35:446.
317. Ward EM, Stephens DH. Neoplasms. In: Gore RM, Levine MS, Laufer I, eds. Gastrointestinal Radiology. Philadelphia: WB Saunders, 1994:1718.
318. Nesbit GM, Johnson CD, James EM, et al. Cholangiocarcinoma: diagnosis and evaluation of resectability by CT and sonography as procedures complementary to cholangiograpy. AJR Am J Roentgenol 1988; 151:933.
319. Choi BI, Lee JH, Han MC, et al. Hilar cholangiocarcinoma: comparative study with sonography and CT. Radiology 1989; 172:689.
320. Meyer DG, Weinstein BJ. Klatskin tumors of the bile ducts: sonographic appearance. Radiology 1983; 148:803.
321. Takayasu K, Muramatsu Y, Shima Y, et al. Hepatic lobar atrophy following obstruction of the ipsilateral portal vein from hilar cholangiocarcinoma. Radiology 1986; 160:389.
322. Neumaier CE, Bertolotto M, Perrone R, et al. Staging of hilar cholangiocarcinoma with ultrasound. JCU J Clin Ultrasound 1995; 23:173.
323. Subramanyam BR, Raghavendra BN, Balthazar EJ, et al. Ultrasonic features of cholangiocarcinoma. J Ultrasound Med 1984; 3:405.
324. Levine E, Maklad NF, Wright CH, et al. Computed tomographic and ultrasonic appearances of primary carcinoma of the common bile duct. Gastrointest Radiol 1979; 4:147.
325. Donaldson JS. Gallbladder and biliary tract. In. Gore RM, Levine MS, Laufer I, eds. Gastrointestinal Radiolology. Philadelphia: WB Saunders, 1994:2425.
326. Williams AJ, Sheward S. Ultrasound appearance of biliary rhabdomyosarcoma. JCU J Clin Ultrasound 1986; 14:63.
327. Haller JO. Sonography of the biliary tract in infants and children. AJR Am J Roentgenol 1991; 157:1051.
328. Robledo R, Prieto ML, Perez M, et al. Carcinoma of the hepaticopancreatic ampullar region: role of US. Radiology 1988; 166:409.
329. Tio TL, Tytgat GNJ, Cikot RJ, et al. Ampullopancreatic carcinoma: preoperative TNM classification with endosonography. Radiology 1990; 175:455.
330. vanSonnenberg E, Ferrucci JT. Bile duct obstruction in hepatocellular carcinoma (hepatoma)—clinical and cholangiographic characteristics: report of 6 cases and review of the literature. Radiology 1979; 130:7.
331. Maffessanti MM, Bazzochi M, Melato M. Sonographic diagnosis of intraductal hepatoma. JCU J Clin Ultrasound 1982; 10:397.
332. Kirk JM, Skipper D, Joseph AE, et al. Intraluminal bile duct hepatocellular carcinoma. Clin Radiol 1994; 49:886.
333. Park CM, Cha IH, Chung KB, et al. Hepatocellular carcinoma in extrahepatic bile ducts. Acta Radiol 1991; 32:34.
334. Ward EM, Stephens DH. Neoplasms. In: Gore RM, Levine MS, Laufer I, eds. Gastrointestinal Radiology. Philadelphia: WB Saunders, 1994:1725.
335. Zegal HG, Kurtz AB, Perlmutter GS, et al. Ultrasonic characteristics of bilomas. JCU J Clin Ultrasound 1981; 9:21.
336. Esensten M, Ralls PW, Colletti P, et al. Posttraumatic intrahepatic biloma: sonographic diagnosis. AJR Am J Roentgenol 1983; 140:303.
337. Ghahremani GG. Postsurgical and traumatic lesions of the biliary tract. In: Gore RM, Levine MS, Laufer I, eds. Gastrointestinal Radiology. Philadelphia: WB Saunders, 1994:1762.
338. Weissman HS, Chun KJ, Frank M, et al. Demonstration of traumatic bile leakage with cholescintigraphy and ultrasonography. AJR Am J Roentgenol 1979; 133:843.
339. Mueller PR, Ferrucci JT, Simeone JF, et al. Detection and drainage of bilomas: special considerations. AJR Am J Roentgenol 1983; 140:715.
340. Teefey SA, Soper NJ, Middleton WD, et al. Imaging of the common bile duct during laparoscopic cholecystectomy: sonography versus videofluoroscopic cholangiography. AJR Am J Roentgenol 1995; 165:847.
341. Palazzo L, Girollet PP, Salmeron M, et al. Value of endoscopic ultrasonography in the diagnosis of common bile duct stones: comparison with surgical exploration and ERCP. Gastrointest Endosc 1995; 42:225.
342. Rao AV, Champine JG, Forte T. 3-D sonographic evaluation of common bile duct morphology: correlation with traditional 2-D measurement [abstr]. AJR Am J Roentgenol 2001; 176:51.

Peripheral Vascular System

Sandra J. Allison, Daniel A. Merton, Laurence Needleman, and Joseph F. Polak

18

BASIC ANATOMY

Venous Anatomy of the Lower Extremities

The lower extremity venous system is composed of deep and superficial veins (Table 1 and Figs. 1 and 2).

From the foot, three sets of deep veins serve as the main conduits: anterior tibial, posterior tibial, and peroneal veins. Typically, these veins are duplicated and accompany, by definition, the arteries of the same names. The anterior tibial veins drain the dorsum of the foot and the muscles within the anterior compartment of the calf. They are easily visualized sonographically because they lie anterior to the interosseous membrane and between the tibia and fibula. They drain the anterior compartment of the calf and are rarely the site of isolated thrombi. The posterior tibial veins originate from the plantar (superficial and deep) veins of the foot. They run cephalad from the medial malleolus just deep to the soleus muscle medially. They become more difficult to visualize in the upper quarter of the calf, where they lie deep to the medial head of the gastrocnemius muscle. The peroneal veins lie behind and medial to the fibula. They are difficult to visualize sonographically in their entirety because they lie deep to the flexor hallucis longus as well as to the soleus muscle in the lower two-thirds of the calf. In the upper calf, the peroneal veins lie deep to the bulk of the soleus and gastrocnemius muscles as they parallel the path of the posterior tibial veins. The posterior tibial veins join the peroneal veins to form the popliteal vein.

Deep muscular veins of the calf include the soleal and gastrocnemius veins. The soleal veins drain the soleus muscle and can join either the posterior tibial or peroneal veins. The gastrocnemius veins are paired and drain into the popliteal veins; they accompany an artery. Less well defined and valveless arcades (sinusoidal veins) also drain into the posterior tibial and peroneal veins. Although some soleal and gastrocnemius veins can be readily visualized, most of the deep-lying sinusoidal veins may be difficult to image.

The popliteal vein originates from the confluence of the anterior tibial, posterior tibial, and peroneal veins. The popliteal vein lies deep to the two heads of the gastrocnemius muscle and then deep to the semimembranosus muscle. Duplicated popliteal veins occur in approximately 30% to 35% of the population. The popliteal vein becomes the femoral vein when it transits through the hiatus in the tendinous portion of the adductor magnus muscle, at approximately the lower third of the thigh. The femoral vein then lies deep in the adductor (Hunter's) canal, a space deep to the sartorius muscle, bounded by the vastus medialis and adductor longus muscles. The femoral vein may be duplicated in 20% to 30% of cases. The region of the adductor canal, close to the adductor hiatus, is a difficult region to evaluate with sonography because of the relative thickness of the soft tissues overlying the artery and vein. The deep femoral vein (profunda femoris vein) drains the deep muscles of the proximal two-thirds of the thigh. It joins the femoral vein approximately 8 cm to 10 cm below the

TABLE 1 ■ Normal Venous Flow Dynamics of the Lower Extremity

Pattern	Association
Phasic variation of venous flow, decreasing with inspiration	Normal, from increased intra-abdominal pressure during inspiration
Augmentation of venous flow following external squeeze of calf or voluntary dorsiflexion of foot	Emptying of blood from calf veins causing increased velocity of blood flow
Low-velocity signals in (superficial) saphenous veins	Low volume of blood flow from skin to saphenous veins; blood flow is also from superficial to deep veins through perforating veins
Decreased venous blood flow during Valsalva maneuver or deep inspiration	Increased intra-abdominal pressure decreasing venous return (blood flow)
Transient reversal of blood flow during Valsalva maneuver	Reversal of blood flow accounting for amount of blood necessary to force closure of venous valves
Dampened cyclic variation in blood flow as sampling is done more distally in leg veins	Attenuation of effects of respiration on column of blood

inguinal ligament to become the common femoral vein. A venous connection between the popliteal vein and the deep femoral vein is seen sonographically in 30% to 40% of limbs. This can serve as an accessory pathway for venous drainage when thrombosis is limited to a segment of the femoral vein.

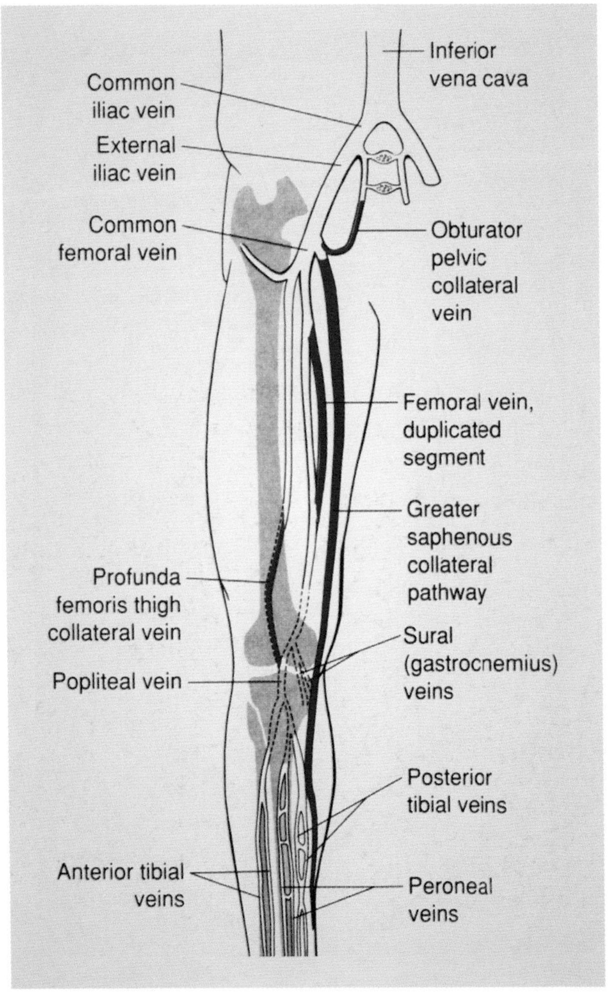

FIGURE 1 ■ Diagram of the major veins of the leg. Potential collateral pathways are shown in purple.

The great and small saphenous veins are bounded by muscular fascia below and saphenous fascia above. The small saphenous vein drains the subcutaneous tissues from the medial malleolus and then stays posteriorly as it rises to the saphenopopliteal junction, although this connection is variable (1). The great saphenous vein lies medially as it drains the medial calf and then ascends the thigh to join the common femoral vein. The superficial veins can be easily visualized sonographically in most patients. Perforating veins connect the deep and superficial veins at multiple levels in the calf. There are fewer perforators in the thigh. These veins drain blood from the skin to the deep veins.

Above the inguinal ligament, the external iliac vein ascends along the pelvic brim to join the internal iliac vein. The common iliac vein on the right then joins the left iliac vein to become the inferior vena cava at the superior aspect of the pelvis. The left common iliac vein courses under the right common iliac artery. This anatomic relationship causes a mild compression on the vein and is thought to account for stasis and a slightly greater preponderance of left-sided deep venous thrombosis (DVT).

Arterial Anatomy of the Lower Extremities

The common iliac arteries are the two major terminal branches of the distal abdominal aorta. The right common iliac artery is slightly longer than the left iliac artery. They typically bifurcate into the internal and external iliac arteries slightly cephalad to the iliac vein bifurcations. The internal iliac artery supplies the walls and viscera of the pelvis and is shorter than the external iliac artery. The external iliac artery passes obliquely downward and laterally along the inner margin of the pelvic side wall to exit the pelvis anterior to the pubic bone and beneath Poupart's ligament. The external iliac veins lies posterior to the arteries. After passing under Poupart's ligament, the external iliac artery enters the thigh to become the common femoral artery.

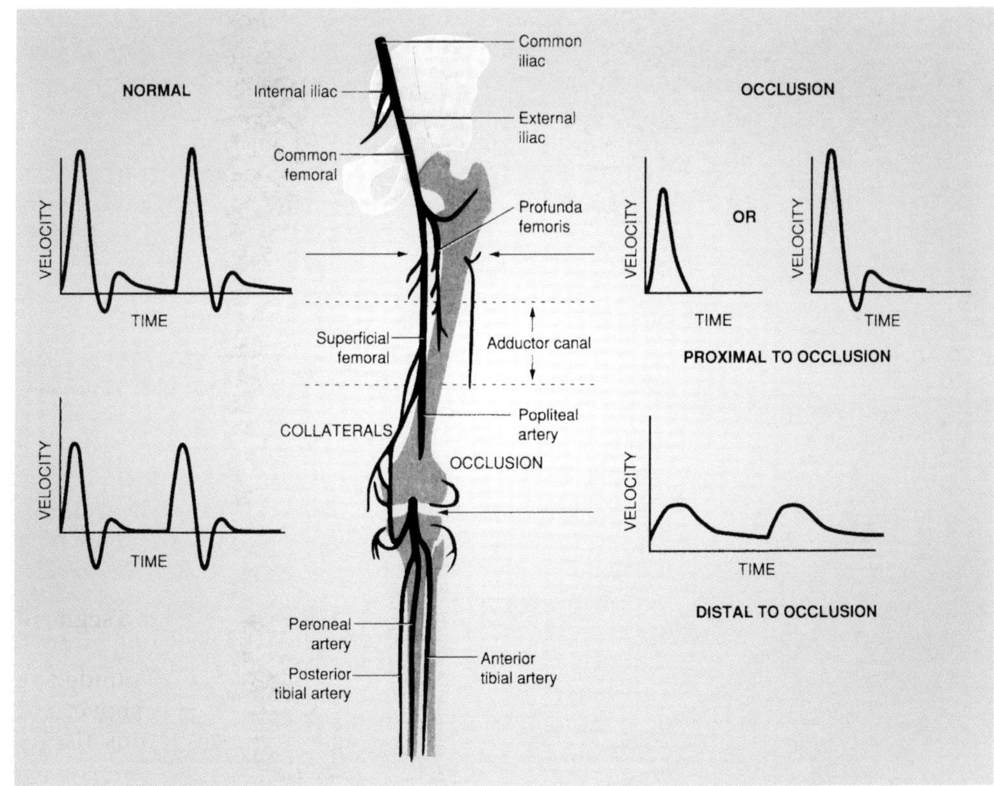

FIGURE 2 ■ Diagram of the major arteries of the leg. Normal Doppler waveforms are shown on the *left*. The waveforms shown on the *right* are "typical" of those seen with an occlusion of the popliteal artery.

The common femoral artery (CFA) is very superficial and immediately lateral to the femoral vein. There are several small branches arising from the CFA including the superficial epigastric and superficial circumflex arteries. These small vessels in the groin can be injured during vascular interventional procedures. The CFA bifurcates into the deep femoral artery (profunda femoris artery) and the superficial femoral artery approximately 2 cm to 4 cm above the common femoral vein bifurcation. The superficial femoral artery (SFA) typically lies anterior to the vein and serves mainly as a conduit for blood to the popliteal artery. The SFA courses from its superficial location at the proximal thigh downward along the anteriomedial aspect of the leg gradually getting deeper to enter Hunter's canal above the knee. The deep femoral artery supplies muscles and tissues in the proximal two thirds of the thigh while the SFA supplies muscles and tissues in the distal third of the thigh.

The SFA becomes the popliteal artery at the opening of the adductor magnus muscle. The popliteal artery is anterior to the popliteal vein and courses downward behind the knee joint through the popliteal space where it is not covered by muscle. Several small arteries arise from the popliteal artery before it branches into the anterior and posterior tibial arteries at the upper calf.

The anterior tibial artery passes through the interosseous membrane and descends along the anterior surface of the membrane to reach the tibia near the ankle joint where it becomes the dorsalis pedis artery (DPA). One branch then continues to join the lateral plantar artery of the posterior tibial artery as the plantar arch. Integrity of the plantar arch is typically evaluated when lower extremity arterial bypass surgery is planned.

The posterior tibial artery (PTA) is relatively large in diameter and courses approximately 2 cm to 3 cm before giving rise to the peroneal artery. In some patients there is a short common tibioperoneal trunk from which the posterior tibial and peroneal arteries branch. The PTA descends along the inner side of the leg posterior to the tibia, and terminates in the medial and lateral (internal and external) plantar arteries at the heel. The peroneal artery descends along the inner aspect of the fibula.

Venous Anatomy of the Upper Extremities

The deep and the superficial veins of the arm drain into the axillary vein (Figs. 3 and 4).

At the level of the wrist, the deep veins draining the palm of the hand form the radial and ulnar veins. These are duplicated and they ascend the forearm to the level of the elbow. The interosseous branches ascend along the interosseous membrane between the ulna and the radius. They also join the radial and ulnar veins to form the brachial veins just below the elbow. The brachial veins ascend the arm to form the axillary vein.

The superficial veins originate from a superficial dorsal arch of the hand. The cephalic vein takes a lateral course and joins the axillary vein just medial to the shoulder. The basilic vein courses medially and joins with the brachial veins in the upper arm, thereby becoming the axillary vein. The basilic and cephalic systems can communicate with each other at the elbow.

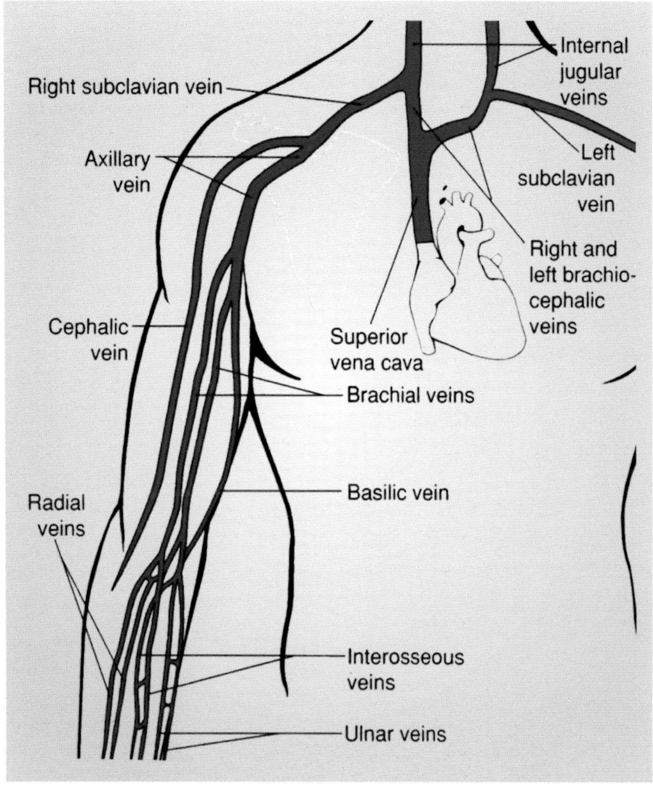

FIGURE 3 ■ Diagram of the major veins of the arm.

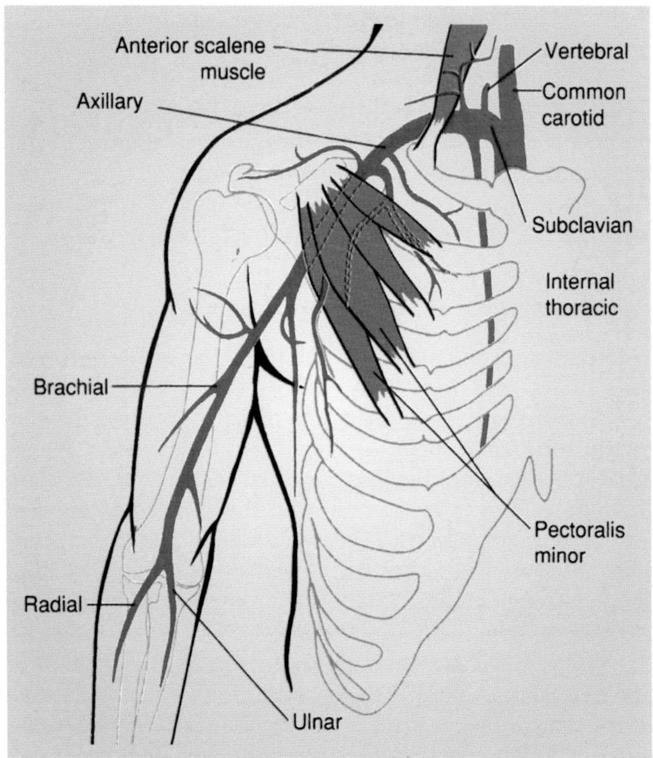

FIGURE 4 ■ Diagram of the major arteries of the arm. Sites of extrinsic compression include the level of the first rib at the scalene muscle and the level of the pectoralis muscle.

The axillary vein extends between the outer border of the teres major muscle and the outer margin of the first rib. Sonographic access to the axillary veins requires placement of the transducer in the axilla, with the patient's arm raised. The subclavian vein runs from the first rib to its confluence with the internal jugular vein. Access of the subclavian vein depends on whether the peripheral portion or central portion of the vein is studied. The peripheral (lateral) portion of the subclavian vein is imaged from a window inferior to the clavicle. Compressibility of the vein can be evaluated to the level of the clavicle. The central (medial) portion of the subclavian vein is best evaluated sonographically using an acoustic window superior to the clavicle.

The internal jugular vein drains the head and joins the subclavian vein to form the brachiocephalic veins. The left brachiocephalic vein crosses beneath the sternum to reach the right brachiocephalic vein. Both these veins combine to form the superior vena cava (SVC). The peripheral portions of the brachiocephalic veins can be insonated from a supraclavicular approach, although the central portions and SVC are less commonly evaluated. The longer course of the left brachiocephalic vein is thought to account for the higher incidence of left-sided venous thrombosis. When performing sonography of this region, probe compression maneuvers cannot be performed on the central subclavian and brachiocephalic veins but these vessels can be evaluated using gray scale sonography, color flow imaging, and spectral Doppler analysis.

Arterial Anatomy of the Upper Extremities

The brachiocephalic (innominate) artery originates from the aortic arch, gives rise to the right common carotid artery, and becomes the right subclavian artery. The left subclavian artery has a separate origin from the aorta. The branches arising from the subclavian arteries include the vertebral arteries, the costoclavicular trunk and the internal mammary arteries. The subclavian veins lie close behind the clavicles inferior and anterior to the arteries. The subclavian arteries become the axillary arteries after crossing the first ribs on the left and right sides.

The axillary artery courses from the first rib to the lower border of the tendon of the teres major muscle. The vessel is deeper at its origin where it is covered by the pectoralis muscle and more superficial in the upper extremity where it continues as the brachial artery. The brachial artery courses parallel to the brachial vein downward along the inner aspect of the arm to a point a few centimeters below the elbow joint before terminating in the radial and ulnar arteries. The radial artery, while appearing to be a continuation of the brachial artery, is typically smaller than the ulnar artery. It courses along the radial side of the forearm to the wrist. The ulnar artery courses along the ulnar side of the forearm.

The arterial supply of blood to the hand and digits is ensured by the superficial palmar arch. The superficial palmar arch is typically a continuation of the ulnar artery that anastomoses with the radial artery in the proximal palm. In the vast majority of patients, the ulnar artery is dominant so that radial arterial lines or radial harvest for coronary artery bypass grafting is possible. The deep palmar arch provides an additional pathway for collateral flow between branches of the ulnar and radial arteries. Arterial flow to the thumb is primarily via the two dorsalis pollicis arteries (branches from the radial artery) while the remaining digital arteries arise from the palmar arch.

PERIPHERAL VENOUS SONOGRAPHY

Normal Gray Scale Appearance

The peripheral vein is normally larger than its accompanying artery. The vein shape is often oval and its size will vary with respiration. The vein lumen is usually echo-free (anechoic) and the wall is thin and smooth. Because of the low pressure within, the lumen can be obliterated when a small amount of extrinsic transducer pressure is applied. Valves, if present, may be associated with slight dilatation in the vein lumen. They appear as delicate linear structures that move freely in the lumen. Blood is usually echo-free but in some patients echoes can be seen within the vein. Blood echogenicity may also be observed if the blood is slowly moving or if evaluated with high frequency probes.

Blood Flow Patterns in the Lower Extremities

Typically, spectral Doppler analysis is performed from long axis images of the vein. The deep system veins of the legs have low velocity blood flow on which is superimposed a cyclic variation resulting from respiration (Table 1 and Fig. 5). During inspiration, flow decreases because of the increase in intra-abdominal pressure. During expiration, venous return and blood flow increase. This cyclic pattern ("phasic respiratory variation") is easily appreciated in the common femoral and proximal femoral veins but is less apparent at the popliteal vein and posterior

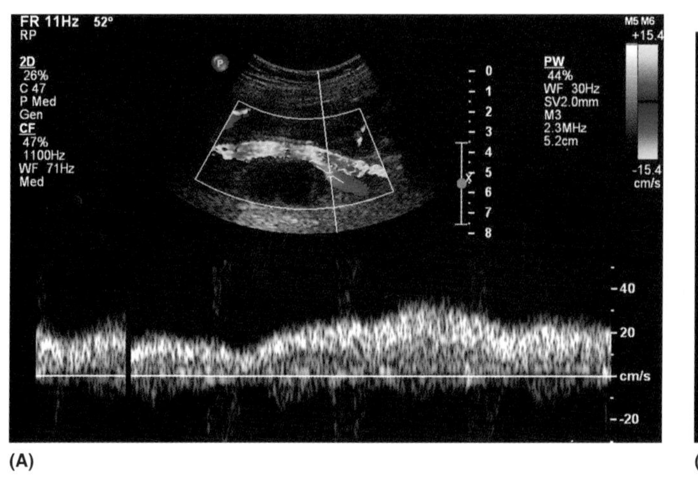

(A)

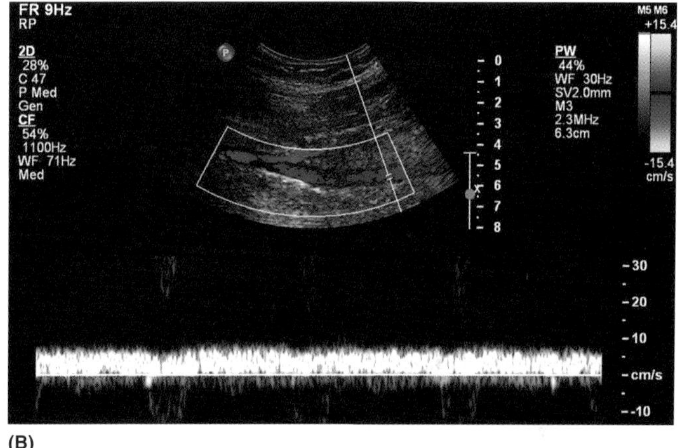

(B)

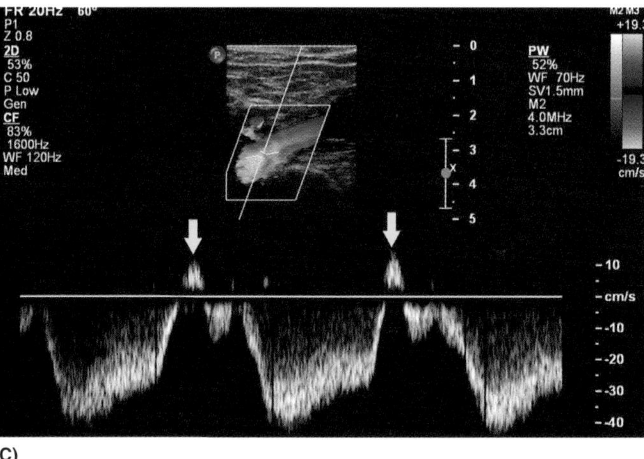

(C)

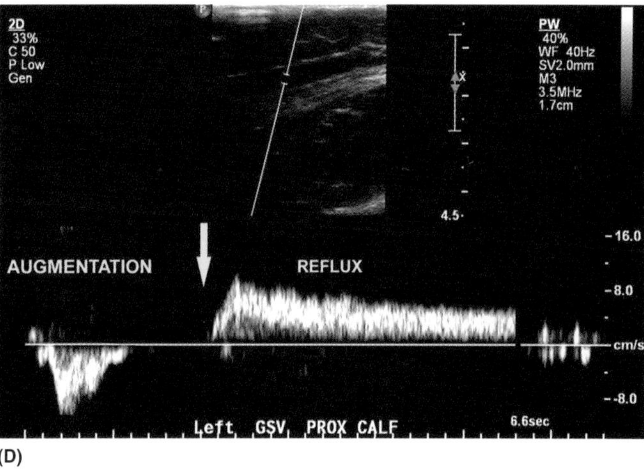

(D)

FIGURE 5 A–D ■ Normal and abnormal venous Doppler waveforms. Spectral Doppler analysis from the left femoral vein **(A)** demonstrates normal respiratory phasicity, while the waveform from the right femoral vein **(B)** is asymmetric with loss of phasicity due to central obstruction from a nodal mass compressing the iliac vein. In a different patient with right heart failure **(C)**, there is abnormally pulsatile flow with transient flow reversal (*arrows*) in the femoral vein. (**D**) Spectral Doppler analysis of flow in the greater saphenous vein (GSV) demonstrates normal flow (below the baseline) during distal augmentation and reflux (above the baseline) after rapid release (*arrow*) of distal limb compression.

TABLE 2 ■ Normal Venous Flow Dynamics of the Upper Extremity

Pattern	Association
Pulsatile cyclic variations in blood flow in jugular, subclavian, and brachiocephalic veins	Transmission of cardiac A and V waves through patent venous channels
Poor augmentation of blood flow on squeezing arm	Small volume of blood stored in forearm veins
Emptying of vein and apposition of walls of subclavian vein during rapid inspiration or "sniff"	Increased venous return caused by negative intrathoracic pressure
Absent to near absent pulsatile variation in blood flow velocity in peripheral veins	Low blood volumes in arm veins

tibial veins. It may not be perceived in the peroneal or anterior tibial veins.

Blood flow velocity in the veins can be increased by emptying the calf veins by externally compressing or squeezing the calf or by having patients dorsiflex or plantarflex their feet. Prompt augmentation of flow signals (flow accentuation) indicates a patent venous return and the likely absence of significant obstruction to venous flow.

Blood Flow Patterns in the Upper Extremities

The jugular, mid and central subclavian, and brachiocephalic veins normally show pronounced pulsatility because of transmission of the cardiac A and V waves in addition to respiratory phasicity. The pulsatility is typically attenuated or even lost at the peripheral subclavian and axillary veins (Table 2 and Fig. 6). Respiratory phasicity is still present although it may be less striking than in the lower extremity veins. A short inspiration or sniff by the patient may cause a normal central vein to collapse, which can substitute for probe compression if the vein compresses completely.

Venous Blood Flow Abnormalities

Doppler flow signals can be absent from a vein if the segment is occluded. Respiratory phasicity is blunted (a "continuous" signal) or, in upper veins, pulsatility is blunted or absent if the patient has a proximal obstruction

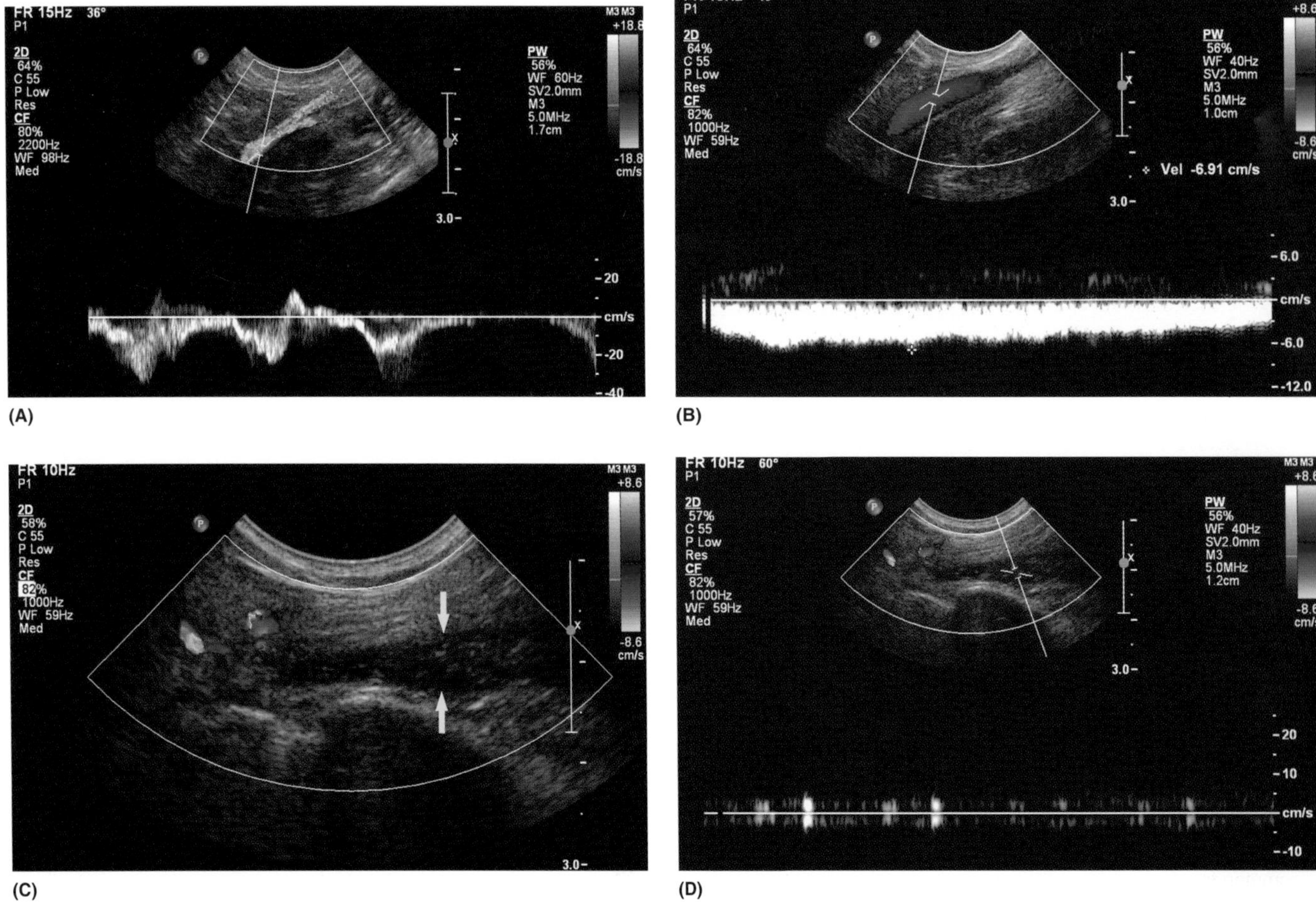

FIGURE 6 A–D ■ Findings of central obstruction. In this patient with left arm swelling a spectral Doppler waveform from the normal right axillary vein **(A)** demonstrates normal pulsatility and phasicity, while the waveform from the left axillary vein **(B)** lacks the normal pulsatility and phasicity. Longitudinal color Doppler **(C)** of the left subclavian vein (*arrows*) reveals a near complete absence of flow and echogenic material filling the vessel lumen compatible with thrombosis. Spectral Doppler analysis **(D)** detects a low amplitude, low velocity flow signal.

(Figs. 5 and 6). Comparison to the contralateral side may be helpful in subtle cases. Prior thrombosis with collateral flow may also create a blunted flow signal. Overly prominent pulsations can be due to right-sided heart failure and may be a manifestation of tricuspid valve regurgitation (Fig. 5).

Venous stenosis elevates flow velocities through the region of luminal narrowing. Stenosis can be seen in the upper extremities but is rare to observe in the lower extremity veins. Obstructive venous stenosis may produce blunt flow peripheral to it.

Venous reflux is typically diagnosed after rapid release of distal limb compression (Fig. 5D). Reflux through an incompetent valve may be observed during Valsalva or proximal limb compression. The reflux examination should not be performed with the patient in the supine position because it may yield false-positive results. Since the values must be given time to close, the duration of flow reversal (reflux) must exceed 0.5 sec to be considered siginificant (2).

Venous Thrombosis

Venous thromboembolic disease is a common clinical entity that affects many medical and surgical patients in both the hospital and outpatient setting. It can lead to postthrombotic syndrome and venous insufficiency. If untreated, venous thrombi can detach and embolize to the pulmonary circulation in up to 50% of patients (3,4). Because 80% of emboli to lungs arise from leg thrombi, lower extremity venous ultrasound examinations play an important role in screening for venous thrombosis. A variety of anatomical factors can contribute to the development of lower extremity DVT (Table 3).

With a sensitivity of 86–89% and specificity of 94–99% for symptomatic above-knee DVT, and 73–95% sensitivity for symptomatic calf DVT, sonography has established itself as the diagnostic mainstay replacing venography as the study of choice (5–11). Its value for asymptomatic screening is more limited. Calf and popliteal thromboses are more common than iliofemoral thrombosis, particularly in orthopedic and other post-surgical patients. Symptoms of calf and popliteal DVT include pain and swelling in the calf which tend to increase with ambulation and are relieved with rest (12). Warmth, redness and tenderness may accompany these symptoms.

TABLE 3 ■ Relation Between Deep Venous Thrombosis (DVT) and Lower Extremity Anatomy

Anatomic fact	Association with DVT
High density of venous valves in tibioperoneal veins	Increased sites for thrombus formation
	Greater likelihood of thrombus formation in calf than in thigh
Large muscular vein sinuses (soleus muscle)	Sites of stasis inducive for DVT formation
Duplication of popliteal vein (prevalence: 30–40%) and femoral vein (prevalence: 20–30%)	Increased number of valves and sites for early thrombus formation
Proximity of deep femoral vein to femur	Propensity for femoral vein thrombosis in hip fracture
Absence of valves in common femoral vein	Low incidence of isolated common femoral vein
Great saphenous vein junction at common femoral vein	Extension of superficial thrombosis into femoral vein
Crossing of left iliac vein deep to right iliac artery	Compression of vein associated with greater prevalence of left-sided DVT than right-sided DVT

Patients with iliofemoral DVT, on the other hand, present with pain in the buttock or groin region which may extend into the medial thigh. Proximal leg swelling may be present. A group of patients who may develop iliofemoral thrombus are peripartum patients, over 90% of the time affecting the left leg possibly resulting from the longer length as well as compression of left common iliac vein by right iliac artery. DVT associated with pelvic masses, antiphospholipid antibody syndrome, or recent pelvic surgery is also associated with this distribution (13–15).

Asymptomatic DVT is surprisingly common. As many as 50–80% of patients presenting for screening venography after major surgical orthopedic procedures have DVT, some even with the use of effective prophylaxis. The lack of symptoms is due to the small size of thrombi which often do not cause occlusion. Most postoperative thrombi are calf DVT and most resolve spontaneously without complication (16–18).

Upper extremity thrombosis has been increasing due to the proliferation of central venous catheters. In multiple studies, 28–61% of patients with upper extremity DVT had some form of indwelling catheter (19–22). Patients with malignancy are particularly prone to upper extremity DVT both due to alterations in coagulation factors, compression of veins by tumor, radiation-related narrowing and use of indwelling catheters (23). Published reports indicate that 12–36% of patients with upper extremity clot get pulmonary emboli (24–26). Other sequelae of DVT includes postthrombotic syndrome, loss of vascular access, SVC syndrome and septic thrombophlebitis. Upper extremity DVT may be asymptomatic due to the presence of a large collateral network.

Duplex Doppler sonography examinations have been shown in multiple studies to be accurate in the diagnosis of upper extremity DVT with a sensitivity range of 78–100% and specificity range of 82–100% (19,27,28). Thus, duplex Doppler sonography has replaced venography as the primary screening examination for DVT (29).

Lower Extremity Scanning Technique

Evaluation of the lower extremity venous system is performed with the patient supine, preferably with mild elevation of the head of the bed to promote venous pooling in the legs. The leg is externally rotated and flexed at the knee. Compression is performed in the transverse (short) axis because in the long axis, the transducer may slide off the vein and result in a false negative examination. The transducer is placed transversely in the groin and just enough pressure is applied to completely coapt the vein walls. This maneuver is repeated every 1 cm to 2 cm along the course of the common femoral, femoral, and popliteal veins to the level of the calf veins. Particular attention should be paid to the saphenofemoral function and the confluence of the femoral and deep femoral veins. Compression of the segment of the femoral vein in the adductor canal is sometimes difficult due to its deep location and relative thickness of overlying soft tissues. Inability to compress may lead to false positive results (30). Compression in this area can be aided by placing the free hand underneath the thigh and trapping the vein between that hand and the transducer. The popliteal vein is usually imaged in the decubitus or prone position.

The paired peroneal and posterior tibial veins can be imaged together as they share a parallel course along the posterior tibialis muscle, with the peroneal veins anterolateral to the posterior tibial veins. They can be imaged from either a posteromedial or posterior approach with the patient either sitting or supine. It is sometimes possible to identify both pairs from a posteromedial approach in long axis. The paired anterior tibial veins course lateral to the tibia on the interosseous membrane and are imaged from an anterolateral approach. Because isolated thrombosis of the anterior tibial veins is uncommon, some suggest that their examination is not necessary unless the patient is symptomatic (31).

Color Doppler imaging and pulsed Doppler with spectral analysis provide different information. Pulsed Doppler is used to exclude or diagnose obstruction while color Doppler demonstrates the presence or lack of intraluminal filling defects. Pulsed Doppler should be a part of all venous examinations. Color Doppler imaging is used in all upper extremity exams, in some lower extremity protocols, as well as in cases when there are technical difficulties or diagnostic uncertainties.

Augmentation of calf flow is performed by compressing the calf caudal to the level of imaging manually or by having the patient dorsiflex and plantarflex the foot. Increased venous flow (detected with CDI or spectral Doppler analysis) suggests an absence of occlusive thrombus between the site of compression and insonation. Augmentation to increase venous flow may also help to locate venous segments in otherwise technically limited examinations. This maneuver is optional as it is often uncomfortable for the patient and has not been shown to provide additional information to an already negative examination. Instead, when there are equivocal findings, augmentation may aid in establishing a diagnosis (32). The gastrocnemius and soleal veins are well known sites of early thrombus formation and should be included in a complete examination of the leg.

Upper Extremity Scanning Technique

Evaluation of the upper extremity venous system uses the same principles as the lower extremities albeit with more dependence on color Doppler and spectral Doppler analysis. The patient is imaged in a supine position with their arm abducted approximately 60 degrees from their body. The subclavian and brachiocephalic veins cannot be compressed and diagnosis in this area uses a combination of gray scale, color Doppler, and spectral Doppler findings. A small footprint transducer using a supraclavicular and suprasternal approach can be used for examinations of the central subclavian and brachiocephlic veins. Compression of the internal jugular, axillary, brachial, cephalic, and basilic veins is performed in short axis. Long axis color Doppler and spectral Doppler analysis are used for all of the central veins including the axillary, internal jugular, subclavian, and (optionally) the brachiocephalic veins. Care must be taken to avoid oversaturation of the color flow signals which may obscure small intraluminal partially obstructing thrombi (33). Doppler is also useful for detection of areas with stenosis which may be related to prior catheterization, thrombosis, or radiation and can serve as a predisposing risk factor for thrombosis. Gray scale evaluation of the veins can also be helpful but intraluminal echoes in the vein may be real or artifactual from reverberation, slow flow, or beam width artifact.

Additional interrogation of the contralateral veins should be performed as waveform asymmetry may indicate more central obstruction that is not visualized directly. In cases in which a diagnosis of central obstruction is considered on the basis of dampening of spectral waveform, comparison should be made with the contralateral side to confirm that the pattern is present only on the symptomatic side. (Fig. 6) (34).

Diagnostic Criteria for Acute Deep Venous Thrombosis

Inability to completely obliterate the vein lumen with manual probe compression is the principal criterion for the diagnosis of DVT (11,12,35,36). This maneuver proves that a space-occupying lesion (clot) is present in the vein. Other findings are less sensitive and specific.

Acute thrombus presents as heterogeneous echoes within the vein lumen and it frequently distends the vein diameter. Acute DVT may be poorly echogenic; therefore, echogenicity is not a useful or reliable way to determine the age of the thrombus (Fig. 7) (37). When symptomatic, thrombus tends to fill most of the vein lumen. The proximal edge may not be attached to the wall, instead being surrounded by anechoic blood flow or color flow signals (Fig. 8). This likely represents the most recently formed portion of the thrombus and may be seen sonographically as mobile or free floating within the lumen. When an acute (and especially a mobile) clot is detected, care must be taken not to dislodge the thrombus by excessive manipulation. Rarely probe compression maneuvers can result in dislodgement of thrombus and pulmonary embolism (38).

Color Doppler imaging may demonstrate a filling defect within the thrombus involved segment (Fig. 9) (10,39). Spectral Doppler analysis will not detect flow from an occluded vessel or from within a thrombus. If incompletely obstructed, spectral Doppler will demonstrate spectral signals from the patent portion. If there is obstruction, there is a loss of phasicity distally (40). Loss

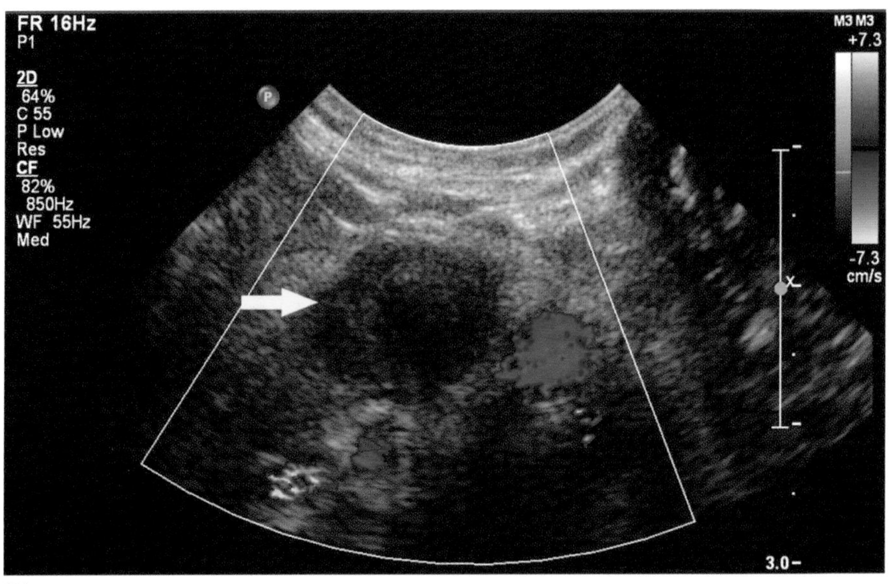

(A)

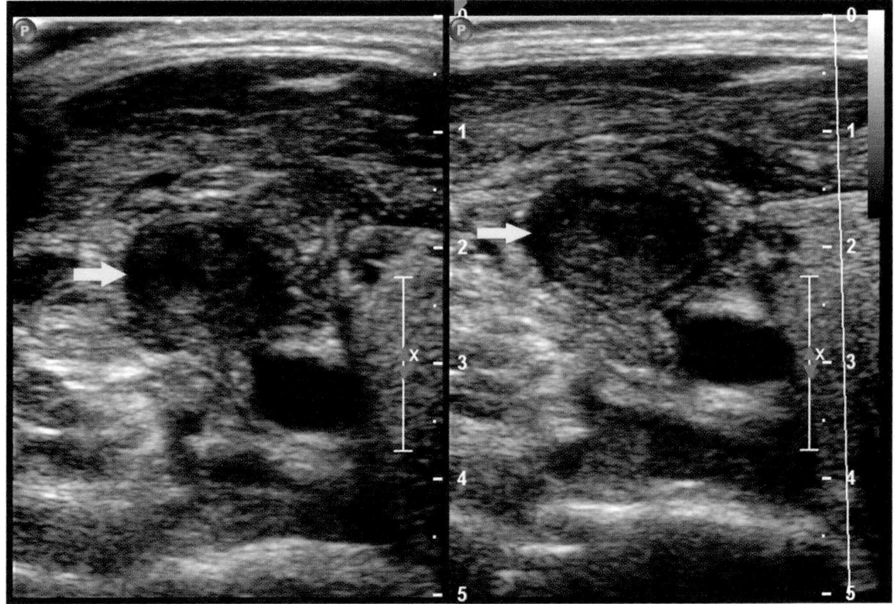

(B)

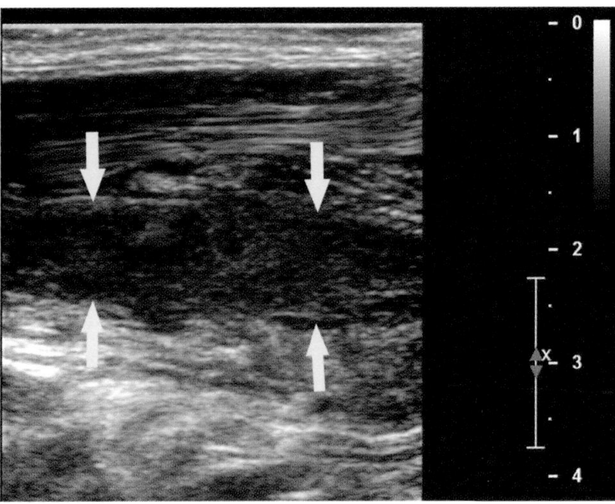

(C)

FIGURE 7 A–C ■ Acute deep venous thrombosis of the upper extremity. Color Doppler imaging of the axillary vein **(A)** demonstrates hypoechoic material (*arrow*) representing obstructive thrombus within the distended lumen and no detectable flow. The adjacent axillary artery is patent. Transverse images of the right internal jugular vein. **(B)** obtained without (*left*) and with (*right*) compression. Heterogeneous echogenic material fills the lumen of the vein and the inability to fully coapt the vein walls confirms the presence of thrombus. Longitudinal view **(C)** of the right internal jugular vein (*arrows*) shows distension of the vein by the heterogeneous clot, typical of acute thrombosis.

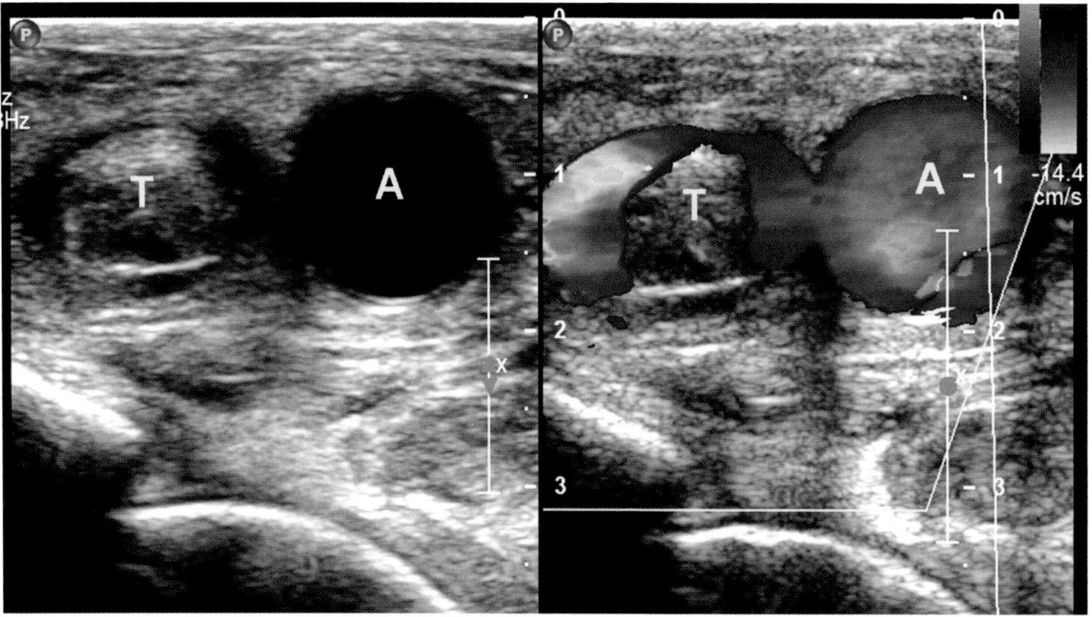

(A)

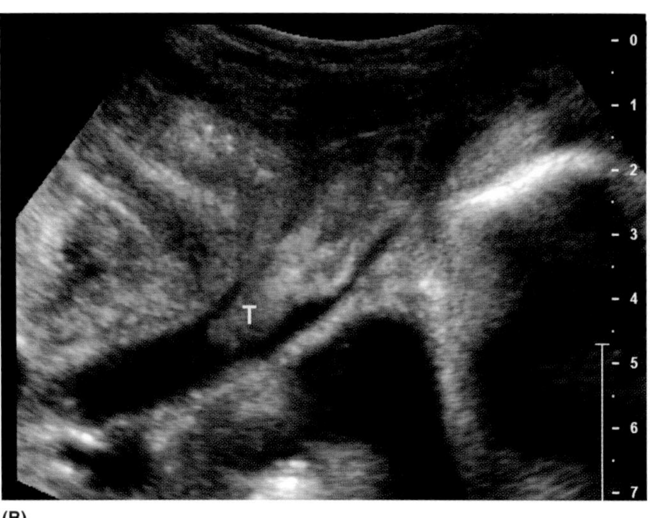

(B)

FIGURE 8 A AND B ■ Other findings in acute DVT. **(A)** In this transverse view of the left common femoral vein, gray scale imaging (*left*) demonstrates an echogenic thombus (T) that appears to fill the vein lumen. However, color flow imaging (*right*) reveals blood flow around the thrombus. A, common femoral artery. **(B)** A longitudinal view of the proximal end of the thrombus shows the thrombus in the middle of the vessel lumen; it was mobile on real time imaging. This represents the most recently formed portion of the thrombus and is said to "float freely" within the lumen.

of phasicity in the absence of thrombus implies a non-visualized central obstruction. This is the rationale for performing bilateral common femoral vein spectral Doppler to indirectly detect disease in the iliac veins or inferior vena cava. With proximal obstruction, it is impossible to determine whether the obstruction is intrinsic to the vein (DVT) or extrinsic as a result of compression of the more proximal vein. The level of the abnormality must be imaged directly to make a specific diagnosis (41).

The same diagnostic criteria for acute DVT in the lower extremity veins are applied to the upper extremity veins. Pulsed Doppler with spectral analysis can document the presence of a total occlusion, but it lacks diagnostic accuracy for detecting partly obstructing thrombus (42). Nonpulsatile flow or reduced phasicity detected with spectral Doppler analysis suggests the presence of central venous obstruction, stenosis, or extrinsic compression by mass (Fig. 6). Evaluation for bilateral symmetry is highly recommended in all cases. Care must be taken not to confuse flow detected in a patent collateral vessel with a normal vessel and miss the thrombosed vein.

Indwelling catheters themselves should not affect blood flow in the venous channels (43). However, pericatheter thrombi or fibrin sleeves may develop (Fig. 10) (44).

Chronic Changes after Acute Thrombosis

As a thrombus ages and reendothelializes, it retracts and recanalizes (Table 4). Sonographically it becomes more irregular, stiff, and echogenic (Fig. 11). As a thrombus ages it may also resolve completely. Residual changes such as wall thickening, scarring, synechiae, or calcification are common. The vein may appear narrowed or of normal caliber. Wall thickening can prevent compression,

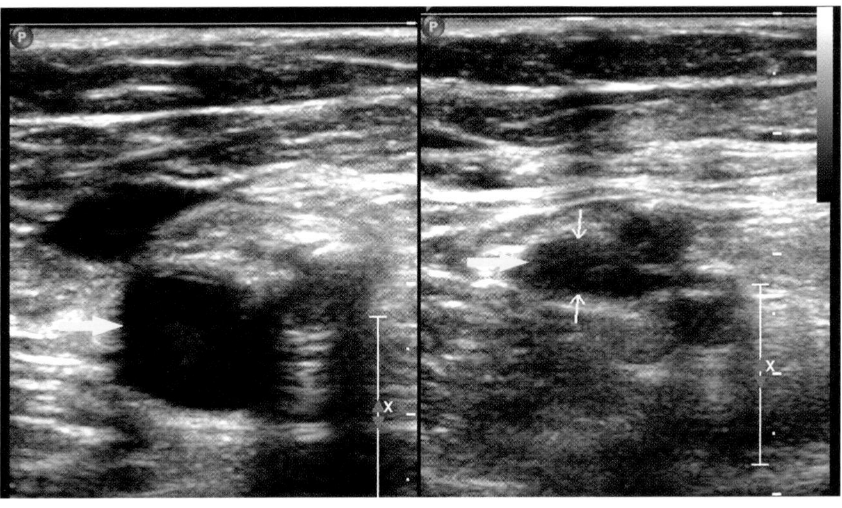

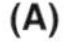
(A)

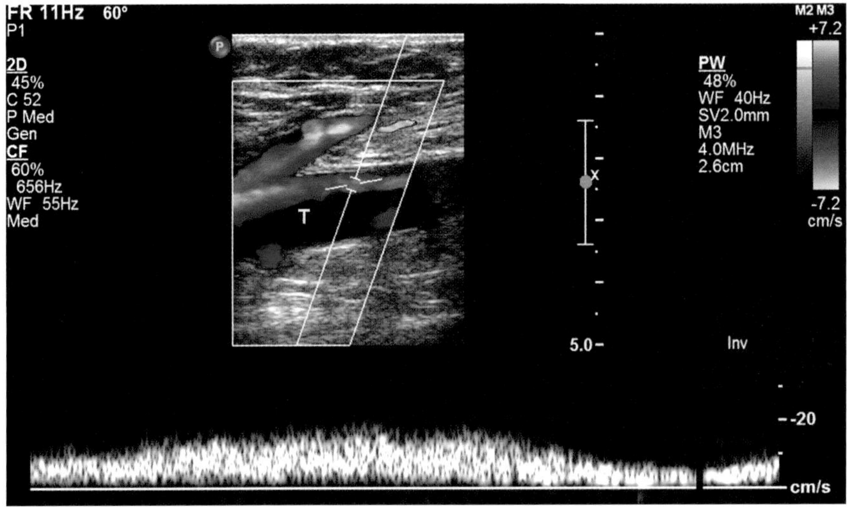

(B)

FIGURE 9 A AND B ■ Nonobstructive acute venous thrombosis. Transverse images **(A)** of the left common femoral vein (*arrows*) without (*left*) and with (*right*) compression demonstrates hypoechoic DVT with incomplete compressibility of the vein at that level. The acute DVT can be deformed (flattened) with probe compression. Color and pulsed Doppler of the same vein in long axis **(B)** demonstrate the presence of normal phasic flow around the hypoechoic venous thrombus.

which can mimic non-occlusive thrombus (Fig. 11). This needs to be recognized to avoid unnecessary anticoagulation. Color Doppler imaging can aid in demonstrating a circumferentially thickened wall or demonstrate flow signals in an irregular eccentric lumen. Respiratory phasicity (detected with spectral Doppler analysis) may normalize after an acute thrombus or may remain decreased or absent (Fig. 9). Valves may be damaged resulting in venous insufficiency. In some cases the thrombosed vein remains permanently occluded and collateral vessels

TABLE 4 ■ Characteristics of Acute Deep Venous Thrombosis (DVT) and Chronic Changes (Scarring)

Acute obstructive DVT	Acute nonobstructive DVT	Chronic scarring
Distended vein	Normal diameter vein	Normal to small diameter vein
Noncompressible but deformable, possibly spongy	Noncompressible, likely spongy	Noncompressible and stiff
Smooth	Smooth	Irregular
Obstruction to blood flow	Nonobstructive	Incomplete or complete obstruction possible
Central location with blood flow surrounding it, free floating possible	Eccentric or central location with blood flow surrounding it, free floating possible	Eccentric location with scar against wall and blood flow in central portion of vein lumen, diffuse wall thickening possible
Possible collateral channels	No collateral channels	Collateral channels likely

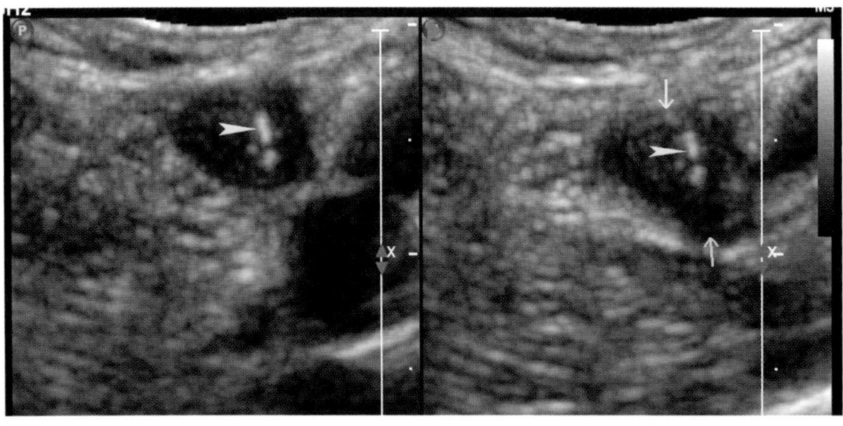

(A)

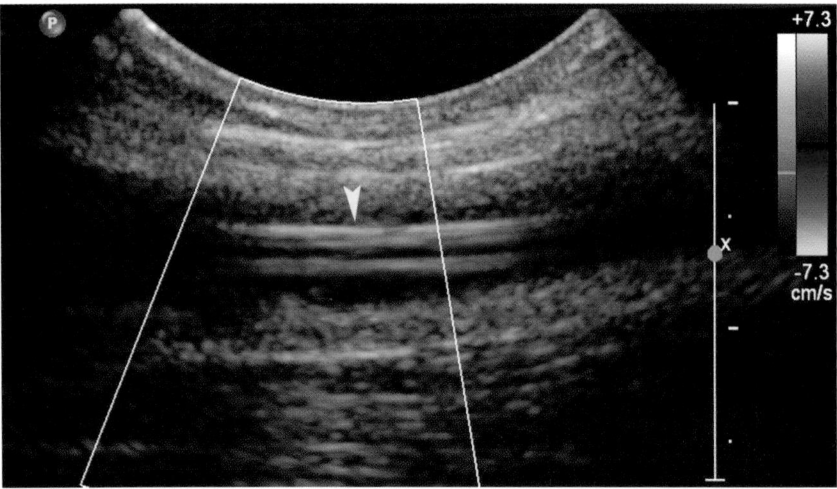

(B)

FIGURE 10 A AND B ■ Indwelling venous catheter. Transverse images of the basilic vein **(A)** demonstrate a central echogenic indwelling catheter (*arrowheads*). Echogenic material surrounds the catheter. The image on the right was obtained during compression and demonstrates no change confirming the presence of pericatheter thrombus. A longitudinal color Doppler image of the same basilic vein **(B)** demonstrates the indwelling catheter (*arrowhead*) but no flow around the catheter consistent with venous occlusion.

may be found in the vicinity (Fig. 12) (45). The only manifestation of prior thrombosis may be an inability to locate a vein in its expected anatomic location because it is occluded and fibrosed. A patent vein without an accompanying artery should raise suspicion that the main vein is thrombosed and a collateral vessel is being imaged.

Pitfalls of Venous Sonography

Internal echoes in the presence of a compressible vein can be seen in the setting of slow flow or Rouleaux formation (Fig. 13). In areas that cannot be compressed this can be sufficiently echogenic to mimic the appearance of clot (46). If the flow is slow enough it may not be detected with color flow imaging. If the echoes are due to slow but otherwise normal flow, or due to Rouleaux, optimized spectral Doppler analysis will typically detect it. Distal compression or other maneuvers that augment venous flow can be helpful to exclude thrombosis. Echogenic blood with no flow detected with Doppler ultrasound is more worrisome.

Vascular duplication may pose a problem if thrombus within one vessel of a duplicated segment is missed and compression of the normal segment is misinterpreted as a negative examination. Close attention to the size of the "normal" vessel and attention to a previous (baseline) study is useful (47).

Recurrent thrombosis or acute thrombosis superimposed on chronic scarring is a difficult diagnostic dilemma (Fig. 14). It is important to recognize that 50% of patients with acute DVT have abnormalities on ultrasound imaging at least 6 months after the initial event (48–50). In addition, pain and swelling is a symptom of both acute thrombosis and post-thrombotic syndrome. A new site of acute thrombus remote from the original thrombus is the most reliable finding. Some authors have used an increase of ≥2 mm in the size of a non-compressible segment as criterion for recurrent DVT but these measurements are subject to error (50). Acute thrombosis may not distend veins in the setting of scarred walls; this may also decrease the usefulness of this sign. In the patient with symptoms and a history of prior DVT, a careful search for acute changes such as dilatation, free floating thrombus, and deformable smooth filling defects should be sought even if other signs of scarring are present. The presence of collateral vessels does not rule out acute clot superimposed on chronic disease as collateral formation has been described to occur in early thrombosis.

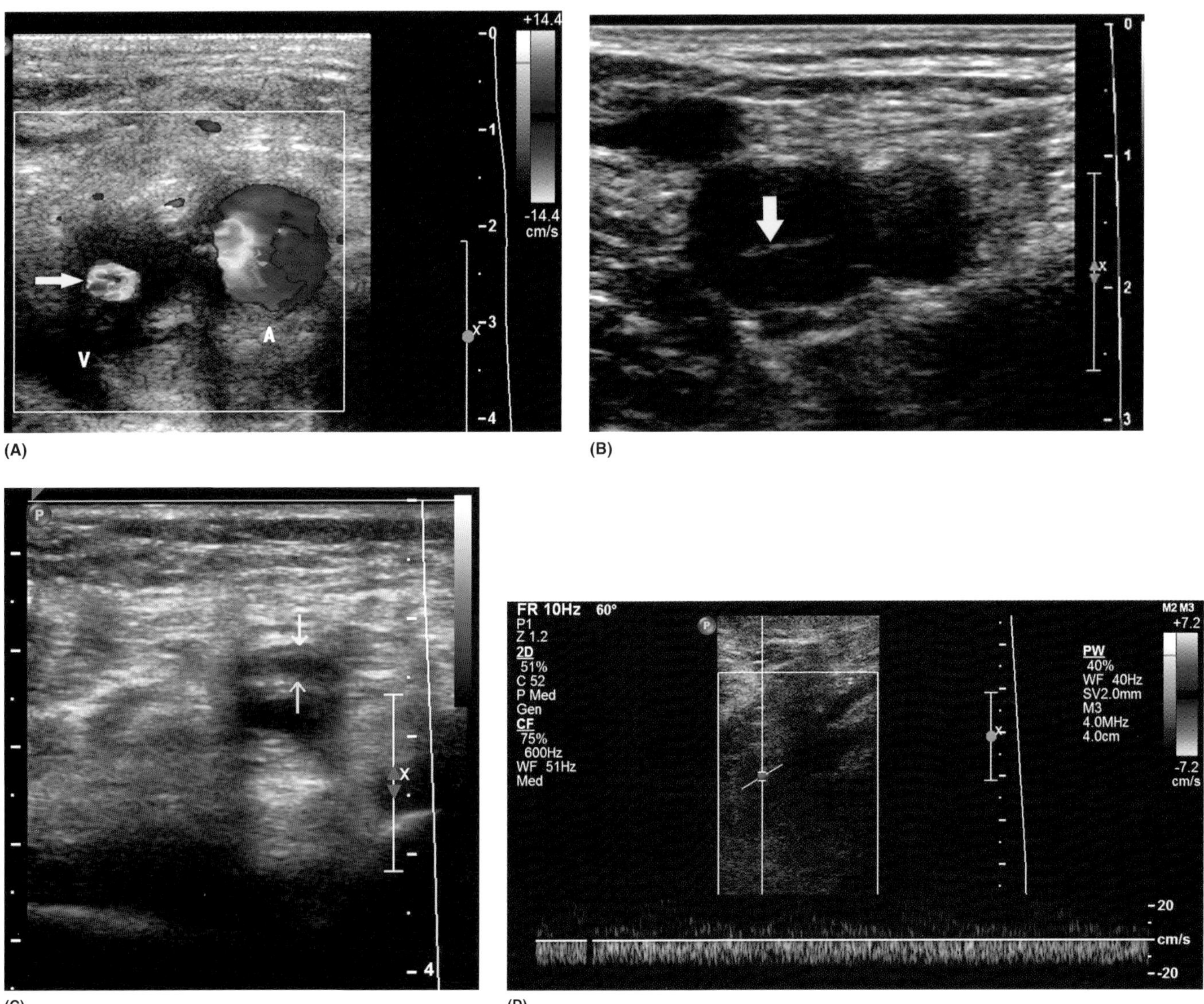

FIGURE 11 A–D ■ Venous scarring. **(A)** A transverse color Doppler image demonstrates flow in the center of the left external iliac vein (*arrow*) with circumferential scarring on the vessel wall. As the thrombus lyses, recanalization will occur resulting in thickened walls and a patent central lumen. V, external iliac vein; A, external iliac artery. **(B)** Post-thrombotic venous scarring can lead to synechiae formation. This transverse view of a patient's left common femoral vein demonstrates a linear echogenic structure (*arrow*) within the lumen representing a synechia. As the DVT attached to the wall lyses, it evolves into a fibrous band (synechia or web-like changes). **(C)** Cross-sectional image obtained during probe compression of a different patient's left popliteal vein shows eccentric wall thickening (*arrows*), limiting compressibility of the vein. **(D)** A spectral Doppler waveform of flow in this popliteal vein demonstrates loss of phasicity, which is not a result of central obstruction but in this case is related to diffuse narrowing and scarring of the vein from prior DVT.

Should Bilateral Examinations Be Performed? Should the Asymptomatic Leg Be Imaged?

Every patient, even those with a single symptomatic leg, should get bilateral spectral Doppler evaluations of the common femoral veins. Isolated unilateral clot in the asymptomatic extremity of a patient with contralateral symptoms is present in 1% of patients and does not warrant routine evaluation of that leg except in patients with particular risk factors such as malignancy, joint surgery, or hypercoagulable state (51–54). In patients where clot was found in the asymptomatic leg, greater than 75% of patients already had clot in the symptomatic leg (48,55).

Should Ultrasound Imaging Be Performed if Both Legs Are Symptomatic?

In the absence of risk factors, only 1 of 37 patients with bilateral symptoms and no risk factors have DVT, with the majority of the patients suffering from cardiac disease or peripheral vascular disease as the cause of swelling (55–57). On the other hand, patients with risk factors will have bilateral disease. In one series, 77% of patients with bilateral swollen legs and DVT had malignancy, trauma, or orthopedic surgery (57). Ten percent to 23% of cancer patients with bilateral lower extremity swelling present with DVT (53,58). Loud and Klippenstein divided patients

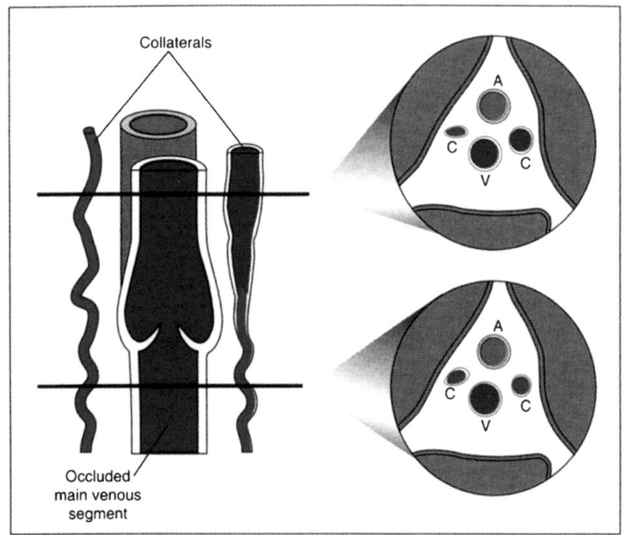

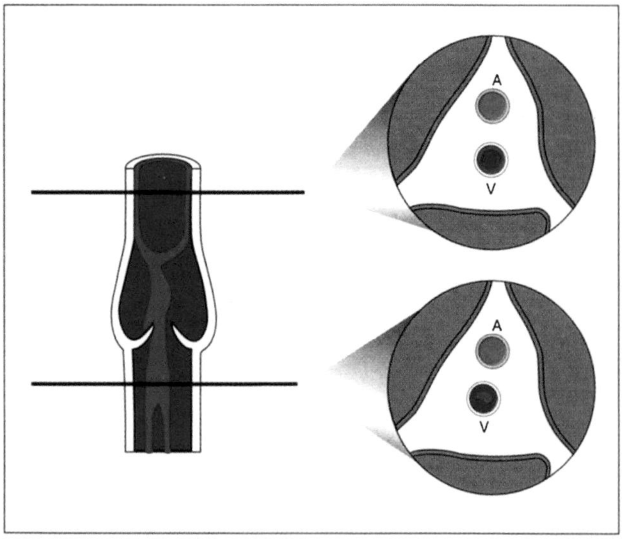

FIGURE 12 A AND B ■ Diagram showing the appearance of chronic as compared with acute deep venous thrombosis. **(A)** shows that collateral branches have developed around an obstructed venous segment. An acute thrombus is seen in one of these branches. **(B)** A cross-sectional image through the vein shows diffuse wall thickening (*purple*), affecting the circumference of the vein wall with blood flow (*blue*) in the center. An acute thrombus (*purple*) is shown to occupy the center of the vein lumen at a slightly higher level. Blood flow (*blue*) surrounds the thrombus.

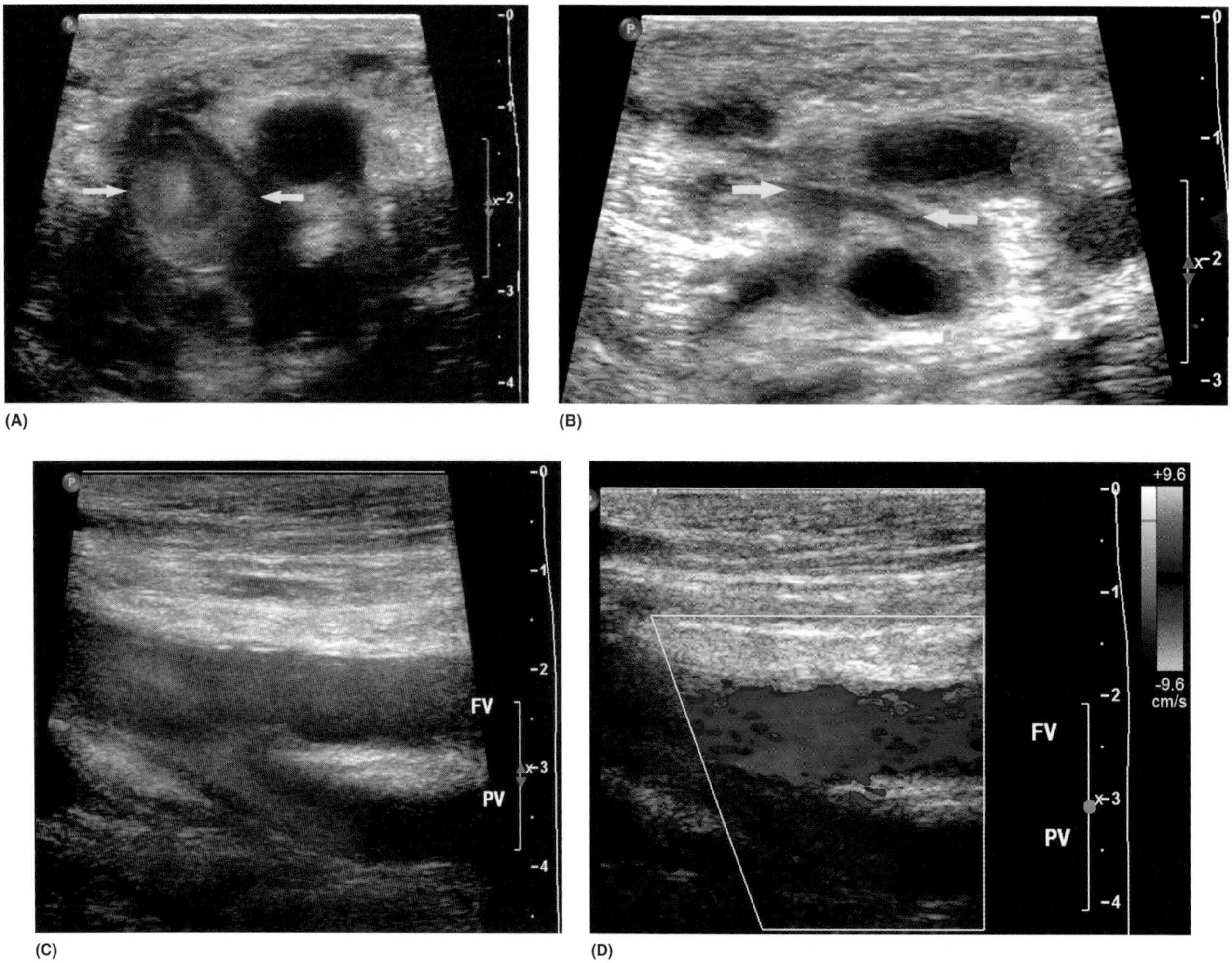

FIGURE 13 A–D ■ Potential pitfalls in venous sonography. This transverse view **(A)** of the left common femoral vein (*arrows*) and artery demonstrates echogenicity in the vein lumen suggesting the presence of thrombus. However, when probe compression is applied **(B)** the vein walls (*between arrows*) completely coapt excluding thrombosis in this vessel segment. A longitudinal gray scale image **(C)** of the common femoral (FV) and profunda femoral (PF) veins in the same patient again demonstrates echogenicity within the vein lumen but color Doppler imaging **(D)** reveals flow. (Flow in the PF vein is not detected as a result of signal attenuation.) The echogenicity within the veins in this case was related to extremely slow flow within the veins and Rouleau formation (i.e., stacking of the red blood cells). Real-time imaging was useful to make this distinction.

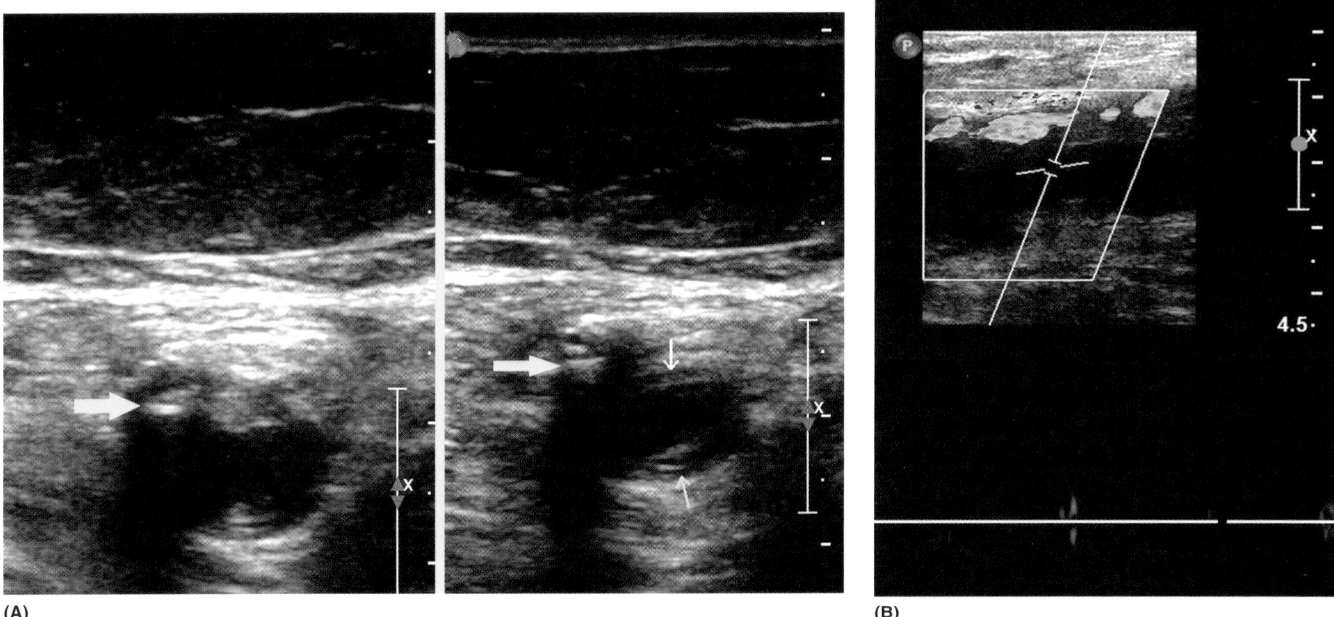

FIGURE 14 A AND B ■ Recurrent DVT. Transverse images **(A)** of the common femoral vein without (*left*) and with (*right*) probe compression reveals that the vein does not completely compress due to anechoic acute thrombosis. Irregular echogenic thickening of the vein wall indicates scarring formation from prior thrombosis. Note calcified shadowing atherosclerotic plaque (*yellow arrows*) in the adjacent common femoral artery. Pulsed Doppler with spectral analysis **(B)** confirms occlusion of the distended vein by acute anechoic thrombus.

with bilateral swelling into two groups: symmetric and asymmetric symptoms, noting that the latter had an increased incidence of DVT (59).

Therefore, it makes sense that a bilateral examination should be performed in patients with significant underlying risk for DVT. In the absence of risk factors, an attempt to exclude heart disease or other etiology causing bilateral edema should be made before performing the ultrasound examination.

Clinical and Imaging Strategies

The relative roles of clinical assessment, venous ultrasound, and the D-dimer blood test are ongoing. A variety of strategies have been proposed. A clinical practice guideline for primary care patients jointly issued by the American Academy of Family Physicians and the American College of Physicians recommends clinical prediction rules be applied prior to subsequent testing (5). In selected patients with low pretest probability and a negative high-sensitivity D-dimer, no further imaging is necessary. For those with intermediate or high risk, an ultrasound examination is warranted. These D-dimer test and the prediction rules apply best in younger patients without comorbidities. Additionally, D-dimer also has limitations for those with a history of venous thromboembolism (VTE) or with a long duration of symptoms. After a negative ultrasound study, some patients may require a repeat ultrasound examination or venogram (5).

Another proposed strategy is the complete venous ultrasound examination from the thigh to the calf including the major calf veins. Different studies apply different protocols, specifically in the number of positions used and the use of color flow imaging. A study by Cornuz et al. demonstrated that in patients without risk factors for DVT, a negative venous study can help exclude the presence of clinically important DVT if the examination includes color Doppler and gray scale evaluations of calf veins (60). In their study, no clinically important cases of DVT were present at a 3-month follow-up. Elias et al. and Subramaniam et al. demonstrated that it is safe to withhold anticoagulation after negative complete lower extremity duplex ultrasound examinations (61,62). Another advantage of a complete evaluation of the leg veins is that it increases the likelihood of detecting other causes of the patient's symptoms (Fig. 15) (61,63). Some have criticized this approach because it has the potential to lead to over treatment of some patients with self limited calf vein thrombosis (64,65).

After a negative ultrasound scan which does not evaluate the calf, a second test 5 to 7 days after the first sufficiently rules out DVT (66). This approach focuses on the more important larger veins at a cost of repeated testing. The follow-up ultrasound study has only a 2% yield.

Another approach investigated for patients with suspected first-time DVT is to follow a negative limited ultrasound examination with a D-dimer blood test (67). These two negative tests combined are effective to exclude VTE for this group. Patients with a positive D-dimer exam or moderate to high clinical scores are candidates for repeat ultrasound imaging studies.

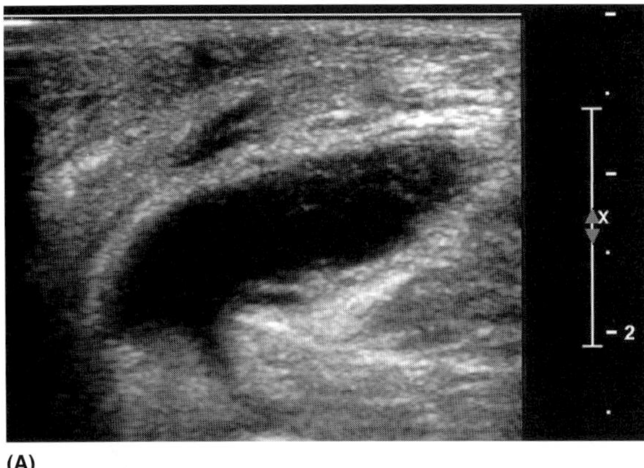

(A)

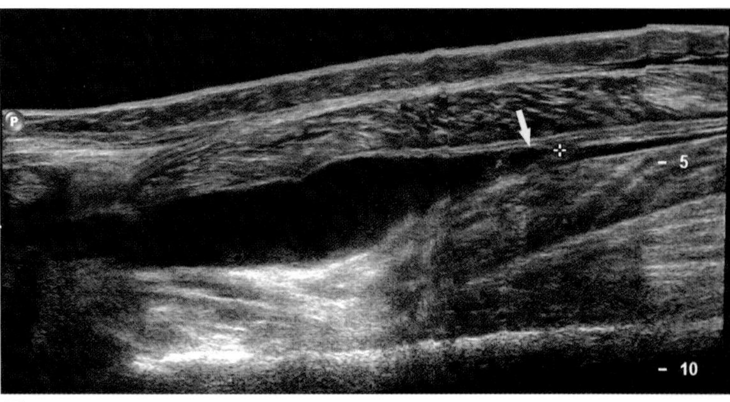

(B)

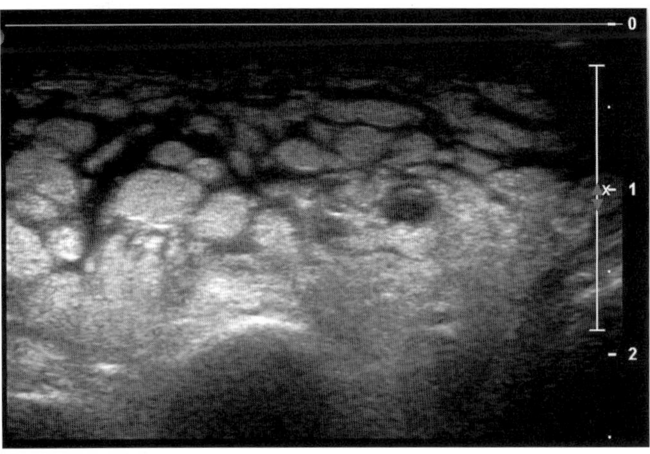

(C)

FIGURE 15 A–C ■ Nonvascular pathology encountered during venous sonography. This is a transverse view of cystic lesion **(A)** is located in the popliteal fossa. The mass is located in the space between the medial head of the gastrocnemius muscle and the semimembranous tendon. The cystic mass represents the bursa distended with fluid and is diagnostic of a Baker's cyst (synonyms include synovial cyst or popliteal cyst), a common incidental finding in patients presenting with calf pain. In a different patient an extended field of view display **(B)** demonstrates a pointed configuration (*arrow*) of the inferior margin of a large (~14 cm long) Baker cyst with fluid tracking along the fascia. This appearance implies that the cyst has recently ruptured. Patients with Baker cysts can present with acute calf pain that can mimic symptoms of deep venous thrombosis. In a patient with lymphedema **(C)** interdigitating linear hypoechoic or anechoic regions are seen in the subcutaneous tissues of the lower extremity.

In symptomatic patients found to have DVT, isolated calf vein thrombosis is detected in approximately 15% of patients although comprehensive ultrasound assessment does detect a higher number proportion, up to 45% (65,68). Isolated calf DVT is rarely associated with pulmonary embolism but 20% of patients subsequently propagate or develop femoropopliteal DVT (69–71).

There are several studies that report the safety of a thigh sonogram (72,73). Gottlieb et al. demonstrated that scanning the calf focally if there are calf symptoms, or eliminating it in the 43% of those without calf symptoms, did not have an adverse outcome compared to a complete calf ultrasound study (72). These findings may have been affected by a low rate of calf DVT in their population.

There is an increasing trend to treat symptomatic isolated calf thrombosis due to its potential to propagate and cause post thrombotic syndrome (74,75). The current practice recommendations established by the American College of Radiology and American Institute of Ultrasound in Medicine indicate that at the very minimum, the calf should be included in the examination of patients with calf symptoms (76,77).

The decision of how best to incorporate a complete sonography study for all, D-dimer, or serial sonography exams is ultimately dictated by many factors including a history of previous DVT, location and duration of symptoms, comorbidities, and clinical risk.

Follow-up Sonography Studies

A reported 22–38% of patients treated for DVT with heparin demonstrate some clot propagation. Therefore, this finding does not indicate a complication or failure of therapy (78). Repeat ultrasound exams during the initial period of treatment is not generally recommended but they are appropriate at the end of anti-coagulation therapy and may serve as a new baseline if the patient develops subsequent symptoms. If a patient has calf DVT and is not treated, follow-up sonography studies should be performed. A repeat scan every week for 2 weeks is recommended to confirm that there is no propagation of DVT into more central veins (75).

Chronic Venous Disease

Doppler sonography is extremely useful for the evaluation of venous insufficiency and may become the new standard (79). Time to recanalization after an episode of acute DVT is related to the likelihood of venous insufficiency (20). The likelihood of ulceration also appears linked to the magnitude of the reflux detected by sonography (80,81).

Duplex ultrasound is used to manage chronic venous disease (2). The aim of the study is both physiologic (to document the site and source of venous reflux) and anatomic (to map the size of the superficial veins as well as the perforating and communicating veins of interest). The study concentrates on the size and extent of reflux in the great and small sapheous veins. It documents the status of other veins that may show reflux including perforating veins. Evaluation also includes assessment of the deep system to document obstruction, scarring, incompetence. Rarely is hypoplasia, aplasia, or acute thrombosis detected as well. Duplex ultrasound is widely used to plan venous ablation but can also evaluate other patients with this common condition.

ARTERIAL SONOGRAPHY EVALUATIONS

Blood Flow Patterns in the Lower Extremity Arteries

Blood flow in the leg arteries has a typical multiphasic pattern (Fig. 2). There is a larger antegrade forward phase followed by a smaller, shorter second phase of flow reversal in diastole. In many patients a third smaller antegrade wave is noted, yielding a triphasic wave form. Some patients may show a biphasic waveform while still others may demonstrate more than three flow phases.

Late diastolic antegrade flow is decreased by vasoconstriction in response to cold or is increased after vasodilatation resulting from exercise. Doppler waveforms are not the same shape as either pressure or flow waveforms. Peak systolic velocity decreases from an average of 120 cm/sec in the iliac and common femoral arteries to, at the level of the popliteal, an average of 70 cm/sec (Table 5) (82).

Blood Flow Patterns in the Upper Extremity Arteries

The upper extremity arteries have a pattern of blood flow similar to that seen in the leg arteries. The peak systolic velocity varies from 100 cm/sec to 120 cm/sec in the proximal subclavian artery and decreases to approximately 80 cm/sec to 90 cm/sec in the axillary artery.

Arterial Stenosis and Occlusion

Arterial stenosis may occur in one or multiple vessels. Diameter narrowing of 50% or more is considered a hemodynamically significant stenosis (Figs. 16 and 17). This degree of stenosis generally produces a pressure drop across the stenosis and decreased flow in the vessel (Table 6).

Occlusions can occur in a portion of the artery or through its length. If focal, blood flow is often reconstituted by collaterals (Fig. 18). Absent CDI and pulsed Doppler spectral signals confirm occlusion of an arterial segment (Fig. 18). The Doppler gain needs to be set sufficiently high and the velocity scale [pulse repetition frequency

TABLE 5 ■ Normal Peak Systolic Velocities of Blood Flow in the Lower Extremities

Artery	Peak systolic velocity ± SD (cm/sec)
External iliac	119.3 ± 21.7
Common femoral	114.1 ± 24.9
Superficial femoral (proximal)	90.8 ± 13.6
Superficial femoral (distal)	93.6 ± 14.1
Popliteal	68.8 ± 13.5

Source: From Ref. 82.

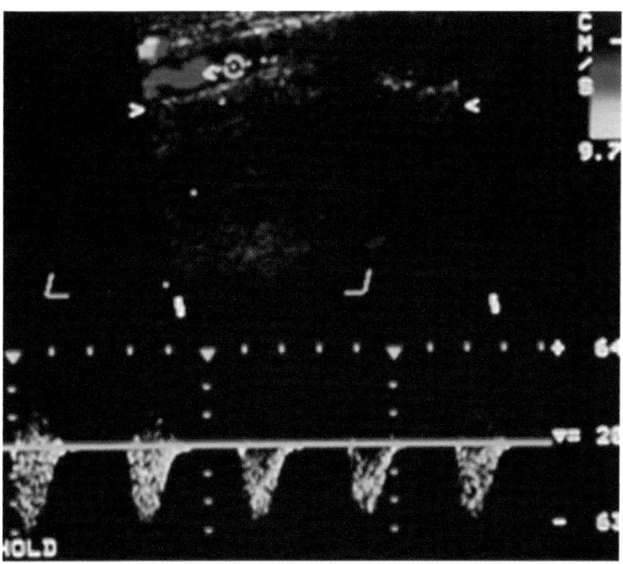

FIGURE 16 ■ Doppler analysis proximal to an arterial stenosis or occlusion. Color Doppler-guided spectral Doppler analysis demonstrates a monophasic staccato waveform proximal to an atherosclerotic arterial occlusion (not shown). When a monophasic staccato waveform is detected the examination should be focused distally to identify the site of stenosis/occlusion.

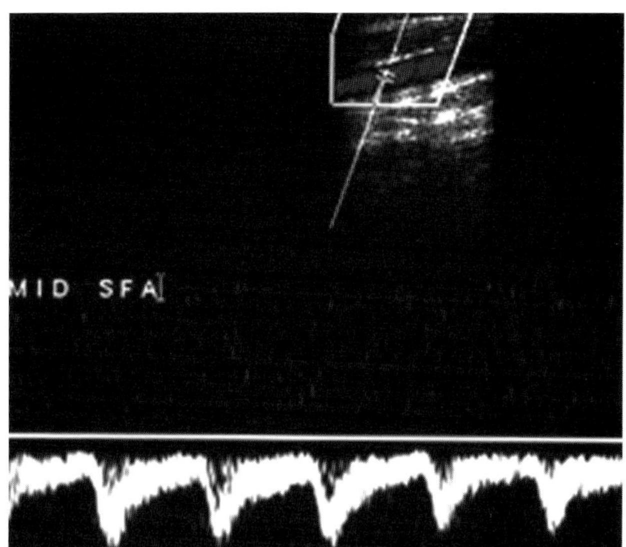

FIGURE 17 ■ Spectral Doppler analysis distal to a stenosis or occlusion. This monophasic continuous spectral Doppler waveform was obtained distal to a hemodynamically significant stenosis. A similar waveform can be detected distal to an occlusion when collaterals have developed. When a monophasic continuous waveform is detected the examination should be focused proximally to identify the site of stenosis/occlusion.

TABLE 6 ■ Arterial Stenosis and Occlusions: Arterial Flow Patterns and Correlates

Observed flow pattern	Correlate
Multiphasic signal	Normal resting signals with early systolic reversal indicating compliant distal arterial bed and sufficient runoff
Jet of focally elevated velocity associated with narrowing; peak systolic velocity ratio greater than 2	Stenosis greater than 50% diameter stenosis
Jet of focally elevated systolic and antegrade diastolic flow	Hemodynamically significant stenosis
Spectral broadening; excessive low velocity flow near baseline; simultaneous forward and reverse flow; ill-defined edge of spectral envelope	Post-stenotic disturbed flow or turbuence
Monophasic staccato waveform	Arterial occlusion *distal* to sampling site. May be seen in hemodynamically significant stenoses less commonly
Monophasic continuous waveform with antegrade systolic *and* diastolic flow remote from focal stenosis. This can be called tardus–parvus if initial upstroke is slowed. If remote from stenosis, velocity tends to be low or normal	Significant stenosis or occlusion *proximal* to site of sample. Pressure drop through the stenosis creates most of the waveform change
Continuous signal with elevated velocity and little difference between systole and diastole	Arteriovenous fistula
Forward systolic and extended reversed flow during diastole (to-and-fro)	Neck of pseudoaneurysm; artery with profound venous obstruction (e.g., renal transplant venous occlusion)

(PRF)] set sufficiently low to detect signals of low strength. The selected settings should permit the visualization of flow signals in adjacent veins and artery segments above and below the occluded segment.

With stenoses of less than 50%, spectral Doppler waveforms demonstrate no or modest velocity increases and may show some spectral broadening. On CDI narrowing of the lumen, a change of color related to the velocity change or aliasing is demonstrated. A distinct color jet at the site of maximal narrowing emerges and extends up to 2–4 cm distal to the stenosis. The highest peak systolic velocity in the stenosis is the "jet." A stenosis of 50% diameter reduction is associated with a doubling of the peak systolic velocity. A stenosis with a 75% diameter reduction is associated with an increase of 370% in the peak systolic velocity (83,84). A stenosis of 75% is associated with an increase of 370% (84). Spectral broadening and turbulence occurs distal to the stenosis.

Further distal from a high-grade lesion or an occlusion in a proximal arterial segment, the downstream peak systolic velocity in the distal segment decreases (parvus), whereas the time to reach this peak systolic

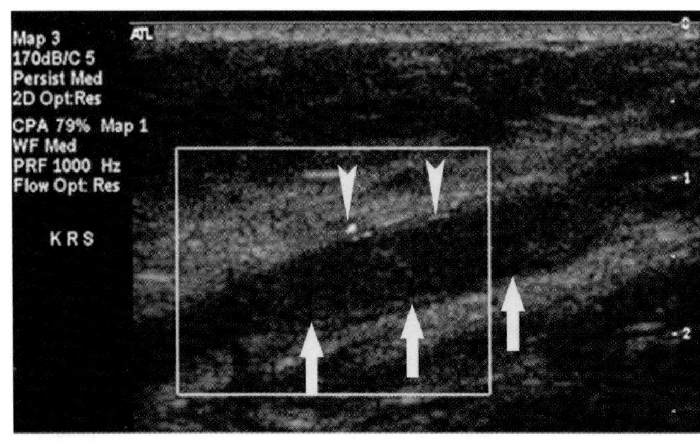

(A)

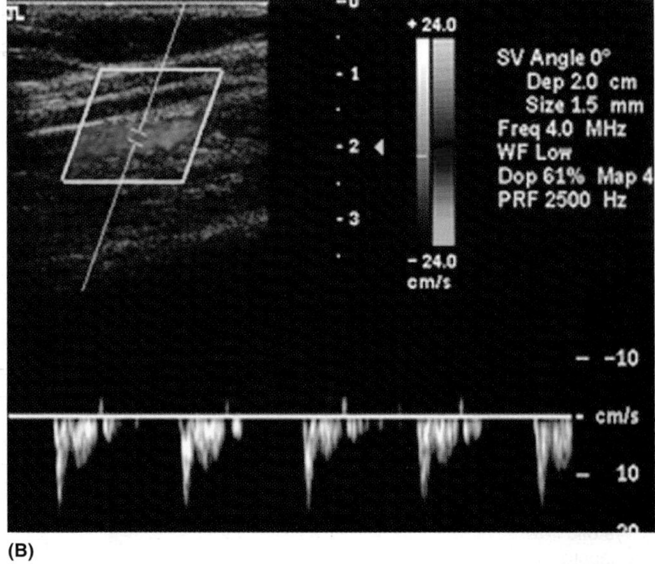

(B)

FIGURE 18 A AND B ■ Acute brachial artery occlusion resulting from trauma. This power Doppler image **(A)** demonstrates no flow in the vessel lumen which is filled with heterogenous clot (*arrows*). Flow in vasa vasorum is demonstrated (*arrowheads*). The spectral waveform obtained proximal to the region of occlusion **(B)** demonstrates a pulsatile waveform with no end diastolic flow. The oscillations are related to the high resistance of flow in the arm.

velocity is delayed (tardus) (85). These distal waveforms also affect diastole which becomes antegrade—the monophasic continous pattern. The jet within a stenosis may also demonstrate antegrade systolic and diastolic flow but the peak systolic velocity is high. In the continous signal downstream from the jet, the peak velocity is normal or low. The monophasic continous pattern is useful for identifying a significant stenosis but is not useful for distinguishing stenosis from occlusion (86). Proximal to occlusion, a short systolic antegrade waveform followed by no flow may be detected (Fig. 16). This monophasic staccato waveform may be less commonly found proximal to stenoses.

PERIPHERAL ARTERIAL DISEASE

Duplex sonography is a useful method for detecting the presence of peripheral arterial disease (87–89). It can help to determine if the lesion is suitable for angioplasty or stenting and can be used to select the site and suitability for surgical bypass (87,90,91). Doppler sonography with CDI is the most useful noninvasive approach for monitoring the occurrence of postoperative vein graft stenosis. Duplex sonography may be helpful to monitor stents (87, 92–94).

Native Disease

A velocity ratio or a fixed velocity threshold can be used to estimate the severity of peripheral arterial stenoses (Table 7). Since various peripheral arteries have different normal velocities, the velocity threshold varies by vessel. In the femoral arteries, a peak systolic velocity cut-off point of 200 cm/sec is typcailly utilized (normal peak systolic velocity is 110 cm/sec). For the popliteal artery a selected cut-off point of 150 cm/sec suffices because the average peak systolic velocities, in this vessel is 70 cm/sec.

The ratio of the peak systolic velocities is a more useful measurement (Fig. 19). It compensates for the level of the arterial segment under study and for variations in cardiac output (83). Measurement of the jet (i.e., the highest peak systolic velocity at the site of stenosis), commonly demonstrated as a region of aliasing on color Doppler, is typically made with color Doppler-guided spectral Doppler analysis (90). This velocity measurement is then divided by the peak systolic velocity at a point proximal to this lesion (normally 4 cm) to calculate the peak systolic velocity ratio. A ratio of 2 (i.e., a doubling of the peak systolic velocity) represents a hemodynamically significant stenosis with a greater than 50% diameter lumen narrowing. Some authors, however, have reported different ratios (87). Immediately distal to a stenosis the flow becomes disordered and turbulent. This is characterized by spectral broadening, filling in of the spectral window, and loss of a well-defined spectral envelope, often with simultaneous forward and reverse flow. Further distal from a high-grade lesion or an occlusion in a proximal arterial segment the downstream peak systolic velocity in the distal segment, decreases (parvus), whereas the time to reach this peak-systolic velocity is delayed (tardus) (95). High-grade proximal lesions also result in a loss of the normal triphasic Doppler waveform, replacing it with a monophasic continuous pattern. Identifying antegrade diastolic flow is useful for identifying a significant stenosis but are not useful for distinguishing stenosis from occlusion (96).

The sensitivity and specificity for the detection of arterial lesions, above 50% stenosis and of occlusions, are approximately 80% to 90% (83,84,86,90,97). A meta-analysis demonstrated a sensitivity of 93% with a specificity of 95% for color-guided duplex Doppler exams (Fig. 20) (87).

A common pitfall is inadvertent sampling of a collateral branch that is parallel to an occluded vessel segment (Fig. 18) (90,98). This is more likely to occur in the region of the adductor canal and leads to a false-positive ultrasound diagnosis of a high-grade stenosis, whereas the arterial segment is in fact occluded. Other findings of arterial stenoses and occlusions are listed in Table 7.

Doppler velocity estimates also often overestimate the severity of focal lesions when compared with arteriography (87). Color flow imaging has principally been used to evaluate the femoral and popliteal arteries. The runoff arteries of the calf can also be evaluated, although

TABLE 7 ■ Arterial Stenoses and Occlusions: Findings and Correlates

Finding	Correlate
Absence of color Doppler or pulsed Doppler signals	Absence of flow
Echogenic material in artery	Thrombosis associated with occlusion; thrombus typically extends between two largest collaterals
Large collateral branches seen during color flow imaging	Indicates high likelihood of more distal occlusion
Persistent antegrade flow during systole and diastole—monophasic continuous waveform	Significant stenosis or occlusion proximal to site of sampling
Systolic flow without reverse component—monophasic staccato waveform	Significant stenosis or occlusion distal to site of sampling
False low-amplitude systolic signals in occluded segment	Signals due to motion of thrombus in occluded segment
False flow signals detected at level of occlusion	Inadvertent sampling of collateral branch near occluded segment
Failure to detect signals in patent arterial segment	Poor sensitivity of Doppler (generally due to depth or poor sensitivity or inappropriate settings); calcification; subtotal occlusion

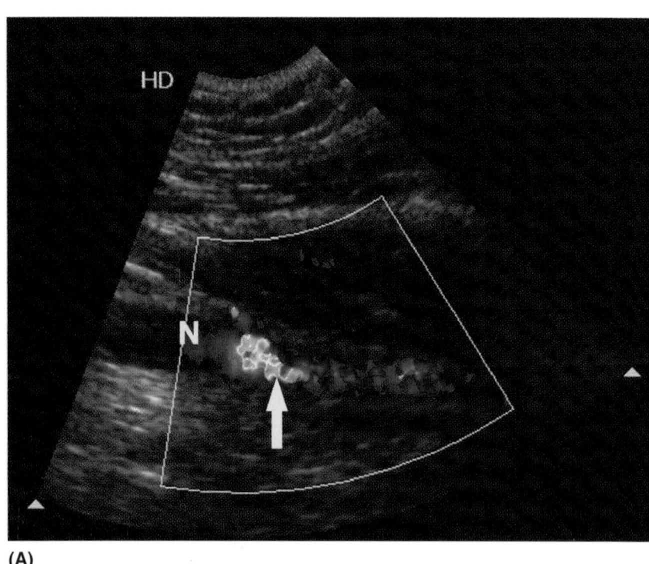

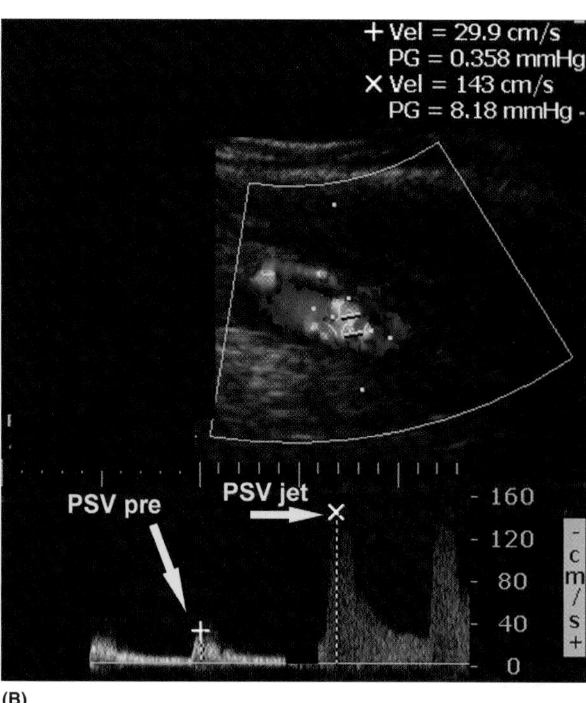

(A) (B)

FIGURE 19 A AND B ■ Calculation of the peak systolic velocity ratio in a native artery. Color Doppler imaging **(A)** demonstrates an area of aliasing at the site of stenosis (*arrow*). N, non-aliased CDI from the pre-stenotic region. Spectral Doppler analysis **(B)** demonstrates a velocity at the site of stenosis of 143 cm/sec (PSV jet) while the velocity proximal to the stenosis (PSV pre) is 30 cm/sec resulting in a PSV ratio of 4.8, indicating a hemodynamically significant stenosis.

this study is time consuming (40). A comprehensive measurement of arterial stenoses in the calf may be possible in nondiabetic patients. For diabetics, however the high prevalence of multiple lesions in the tibioperoneal arteries makes this task more difficult. The iliac arteries are also amenable to color flow or duplex Doppler evaluations. Sonographic examination of the pelvic arteries can be improved when patients have had bowel preparation to minimize bowel gas (99). If multiple lesions are present, the most proximal lesion may be interpreted, but the second and other distal lesions are less easily detected, approximating 60–65% (87).

Color flow imaging and duplex sonography have been used for the triage of patients with suspected arterial disease and to establish, with a specificity of 93%, those patients who may benefit from angioplasty (87,88). This concept has been expanded to the triage of patients among conservative therapy, angioplasty, or surgery, further reducing the need for diagnostic arteriography in 22% to 62% of cases (89). In skilled hands, duplex Doppler sonography can be used to select the most appropriate vessel for infrapopliteal bypass grafts (87).

Diagnostic criteria for the presence of focal stenosis in the arm arteries are similar to those in the leg arteries. More central lesions at the origin of the subclavian artery can be missed and care must be taken to evaluate the vessel for the presence of aneurysms or stenoses associated with thoracic outlet syndrome. Demonstration of the parvus–tardus waveforms while patients move their arms in various positions can be used to diagnose thoracic outlet syndrome.

Synthetic Vascular Bypass Grafts

Synthetic vascular bypass grafts are easily evaluated by sonography but surveillance of synthetic grafts are not recommended as it may not influence long-term outcome (87). In the early postoperative period, gas within the wall of the synthetic material impairs imaging of the graft lumen. Sonography is also useful for evaluating masses adjacent to the bypass graft, such as hematomas or pseudoaneurysm formation (100). Sonography can confirm graft occlusions and detect graft stenoses. Stenoses are more likely to occur at the anastomotic sites and are likely due to fibro-intimal hyperplasia (101). This type of stenosis typically manifests within the first 2 years after surgery. Imaging of older grafts often shows a more diffuse deposition of thrombus and fibro-intimal reaction within the graft.

Autologous Vein Grafts

Sonography is routinely used to map veins and assess their adequacy for use in a variety of surgical procedures including arterial bypass grafts and arteriovenous fistulas and grafts. Color flow imaging and duplex Doppler sonography are now the preferred examinations for postoperative graft surveillance (Fig. 21). Duplex sonography is recommended for routine surveillance after venous conduits at 3, 6, and 12 months and then yearly (87). The diagnostic sensitivity and specificity are much higher than those of serial monitoring with ankle-brachial indices or segmental pressures (90,102). Case-control studies looking at the natural history of bypass grafts with early lesions have shown that lesions above 70% diameter narrowing are

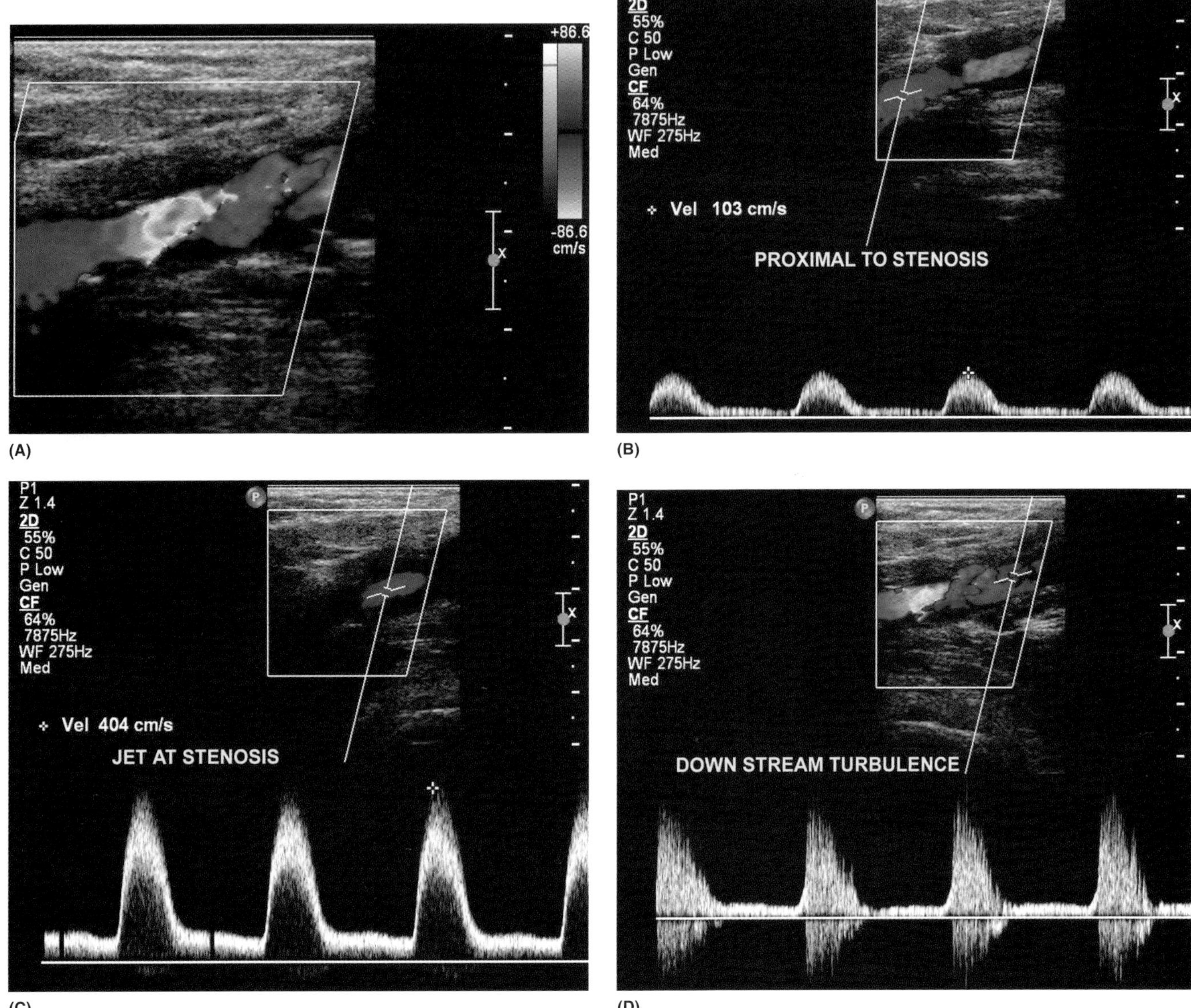

FIGURE 20 A–D ■ Common femoral artery (CFA) stenosis. Color Doppler imaging (**A**) of the CFA demonstrates color aliasing indicating the presence of a stenosis in this vessel segment. Spectral Doppler analysis proximal to the region of color aliasing (**B**) provides a velocity of 103 cm/sec, while the velocity at the narrowed segment (**C**) is 404 cm/sec yielding an elevated peak systolic velocity ratio of 3.9. Spectral Doppler analysis also confirms down stream turbulence (**D**) which completes the findings of a hemodynamically significant stenosis.

almost always associated with total occlusion of the bypass graft within 3 to 6 months after detection (91). A stenosis in the range of 50–70% has a 30% likelihood of occluding within 3 to 6 months and probably warrants more careful monitoring. Once lesions reach hemodynamic significance, they should be repaired since doing so improves graft patency rates to above 80% (103).

Vein bypass grafts may be in situ (the valves must be removed) or reversed. The diameter of the vein graft conduit at the proximal and distal arterial anastomosis can be markedly different. With a reversed bypass graft, the proximal portion of the graft has a small diameter, whereas the distal segment is large. In situ bypass graft diameters more closely match artery diameter at the proximal and distal anastomoses. Flow velocities within the bypass graft should approximate those detected within the native arterial tree. In general, however, early diastolic reversal can be short and barely perceptible (104). The principal utility of sonography for the postoperative monitoring of vein bypass grafts is to detect stenosis and to confirm possible occlusion (Fig. 22) (105).

For the first month after surgery, early bypass graft failures are due mainly to technical defects (106,107). These defects include clamp injuries, poor anastomoses, and communicating arteriovenous fistulas that develop after surgery. After this critical month, fibro-intimal hyperplasia

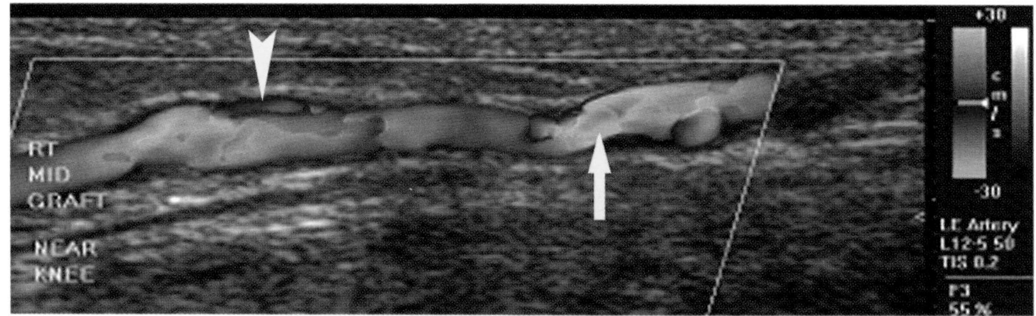

FIGURE 21 ■ Color Doppler of a fem-pop venous bypass graft. An area of color aliasing (*arrow*) identifies an area of elevated velocity associated with a stenosis in the graft from fibro-intimal hyperplasia. In this case the functional lumen is over-written by color Doppler signals—a potential pitfall in estimating functional lumen size. An additional minor flow disturbance (*arrowhead*) is demonstrated that is associated with a slightly dilated area of the vein where a valve had been resected.

mainly produces stenoses, often at the site of lysed valves or at anastomoses. Stenotic lesions cause a focal area of increased flow velocity (108,109). As the lesion progresses, the velocity at the stenosis increases. With high-grade lesions the mean velocity elsewhere in the bypass graft drops because volume flow decreases. The average peak systolic velocity (the average of 3 to 4 samples through the graft avoiding areas of turbulence and stenosis) is another criterion for a graft at risk. Average velocities below 45 cm/sec in a normal-diameter bypass graft suggest a low

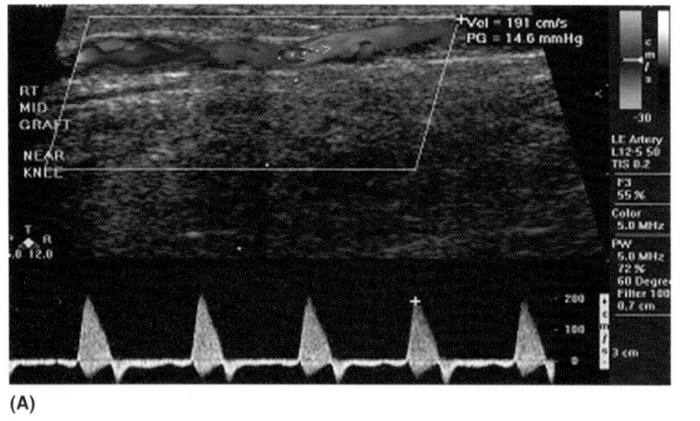

(A)

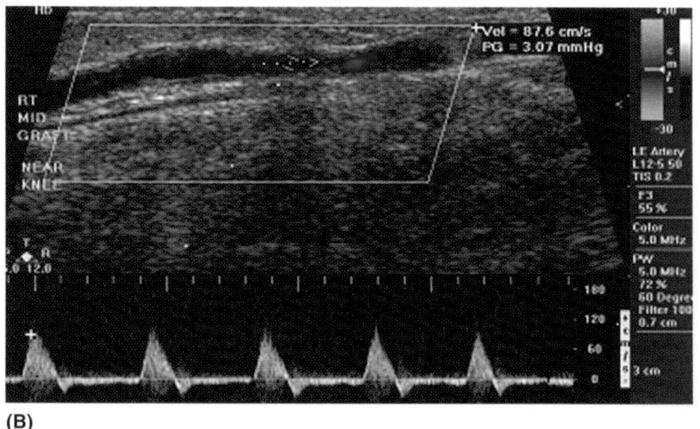

(B)

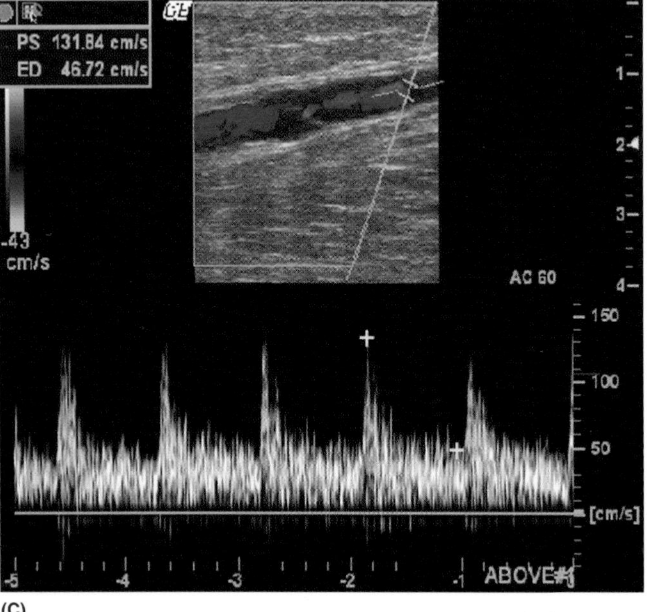

(C)

FIGURE 22 A–C ■ Bypass graft stenosis. The velocity at the site of stenosis is 191 cm/sec **(A)** while the velocity proximal to the stenosis **(B)** is 88 cm/sec resulting in a PSV ratio of 2.2 indicating a hemodynamically significant stenosis. Note: The color flow image shown in **(A)** was obtained in systole and the color display in **(B)** was obtained in diastole, which accounts for the paucity of color. (**C**) False-positive elevated velocity from an arterio-venous fistula in an in-situ vein bypass graft. Spectral Doppler analysis demonstrates an increase in blood flow velocity with turbulence (irregular contour of Doppler spectrum) producing a "picket fence" appearance. This abnormality can be mistaken for a focal stenosis. The cause of the fistula was a venous branch that was not ligated at the time of surgery (not shown).

volume flow, which can result from a variety of causes (102). This last stage precedes complete failure and thrombosis of the bypass graft (90,92). This criterion should not be used for large veins (greater than 6 mm in diameter) or grafts bypassed into a small distal vessel. Management of graft surveillance has been proposed based on a combination of detection of stenosis, average graft velocity, and ankle brachial indices (110). Atherosclerotic lesions can also lead to graft difficulties, typically as a late complication. New lesions proximal to the graft or in the run-off vessels may compromise the graft. Over time, plaque may also develop in the vascular bypass.

Percutaneous Angioplasty and Atherectomy

Vascular sonography can be used in triage of patients either to vascular surgery or to a percutaneous intervention (88,89). In general, short, focal lesions, occlusions, or high-grade stenoses are treated by percutaneous angioplasty because long-term results show that angioplasty offers reasonable patency rates (111,112). The ankle-brachial index and segmental pressures cannot distinguish between long segmental occlusions and short focal stenoses. Doppler sonography offers high sensitivity and specificity for the detection of stenotic lesions and can be used for screening as well as for triage of patients (87–89,97).

Doppler sonography can also be used to monitor the success of the vascular intervention. Persistent doubling of the peak systolic velocity is associated with significant focal lesions. These warrant more careful monitoring because they may indicate recurrence of the lesion. An early post-angioplasty flow abnormality may predict long-term patency (or lack thereof) better than a postprocedure arteriogram (113). This observation has not been confirmed (114). Sequential color flow imaging or duplex sonographic examinations can, however, predict long-term successes (115).

Aneurysms

An aneurysm is a focal dilatation of an artery having at least a 50% increase compared to the expected normal diameter (116). It may be determined by a 50% increase in diameter compared with an adjacent segment of the vessel. Gray scale sonography remains the standard for evaluating peripheral aneurysms since it can determine the outer dimensions of the arterial wall, the length of the affected segment, and the presence of intraluminal thrombus (117).

Dissections, Arteriovenous Fistulas, and Pseudoaneurysms

Vascular dissections are readily identified by the appearance of a free flap seen on gray scale sonography (118). Transverse imaging is useful in confirming the presence of this lesion. Doppler velocity measurements can confirm whether both channels are patent and can identify the true lumen of the dissection (119).

The common femoral artery and vein are common access sites for a variety of catheter-based interventional procedures including diagnostic angiography and cardiac angioplasty. Other vessels that may be used for vascular access include the radial artery and vein, subclavian vessels, and dialysis grafts. Furthermore, peripheral vascular injuries can result from other causes including needle sticks and blunt or penetrating trauma.

Potential complications of vascular catheterization procedures include ecchymosis, arteriovenous fistulas, pseudoaneurysms (PSAs) and dissections (120,121).

Arteriovenous fistulas (AVFs) can result when there is puncture of an artery and vein with a direct communication between the two injured vessels (Fig. 23). A significant pressure gradient will result in a focal area of significantly increased velocity at the site of the AVF with flow directed from the artery to the vein (122,123). Color Doppler imaging of AVFs will often demonstrate a bruit artifact and/or a thrill may be palpable. Spectral Doppler analysis of the effected artery above the AVF will demonstrate a mono-phasic continuous waveform with elevated systolic and diastolic velocities (Fig. 22). Flow in the injured artery distal to the AVF will generally have normal pulsatility. Spectral Doppler analysis of the effected vein central to the AVF will demonstrate "arterialized flow" with pulsations during systole and a lack of respiratory phasicity. Although ultrasound-guided compression repair (described below) has been used to treat iatrogenic AVFs, the success of the technique is not as high as when the technique is used to treat PSAs (124).

Pseudoaneurysms occur when an arterial puncture site does not adequately close which allows blood to escape into the perivascular tissues and form a focal collection. (Fig. 23) The presence of pain or swelling in the groin after vascular access is the most common presentation of a PSA. Swelling from a large PSA (with or without ecchymosis) may result in compression of nerves and vessels with associated neuropathy, venous thrombosis, or claudication. PSAs, which differ from true aneurysms as they lack an endothelial lining, are more common in patients receiving antithrombotic and antiplatelet therapy (125). If the PSA is not causing severe pain, serial observation is generally considered appropriate with the hope that the PSA will thrombose. However, if the patient is in pain or the PSA is enlarging over time, treatment is indicated (123).

The sensitivity of duplex sonography for the detection of PSA is 94% with a specificity of 97% (124). PSAs typically appear on gray scale imaging as a hypoechoic mass (hematoma) in the region of a previous percutaneous vascular access (126–128). PSAs can also result from leakage of blood around surgical anastomoses and around grafts (129). A communicating tract (neck) of varying length and diameter will allow blood to flow from the injured artery into the PA during systole and blood will drain out the same channel throughout diastole, resulting in a characteristic to-and-fro waveform on spectral Doppler analysis (Fig. 23). Color flow imaging will demonstrate blood flow from the injured vessel through the communicating neck and into the PA and a swirling flow pattern within the mass. Swirling flow within PSAs can also be detected with high resolution gray scale sonography. PSAs can be unilocular or multilocular with communicating

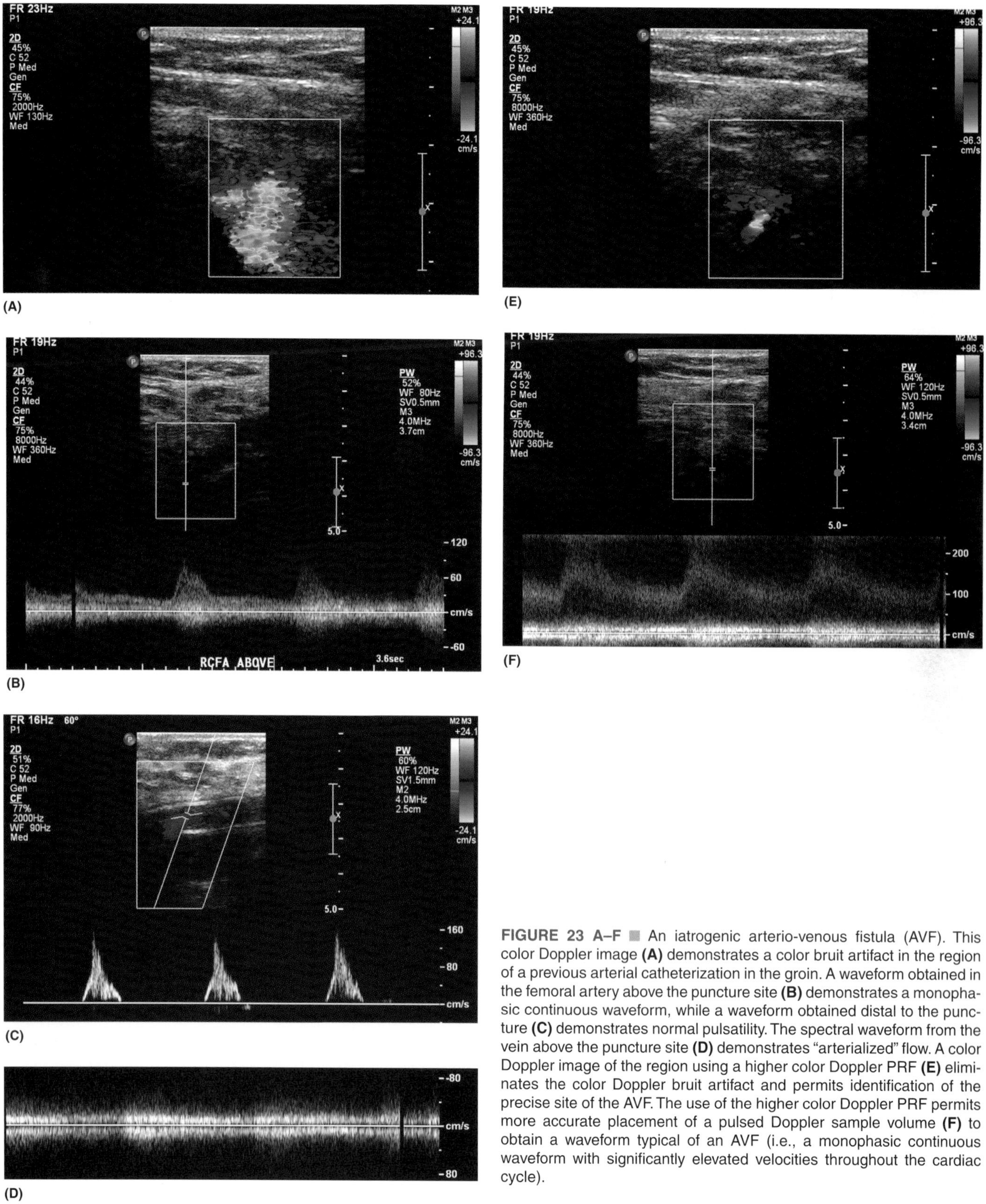

(A)

(E)

(B)

(F)

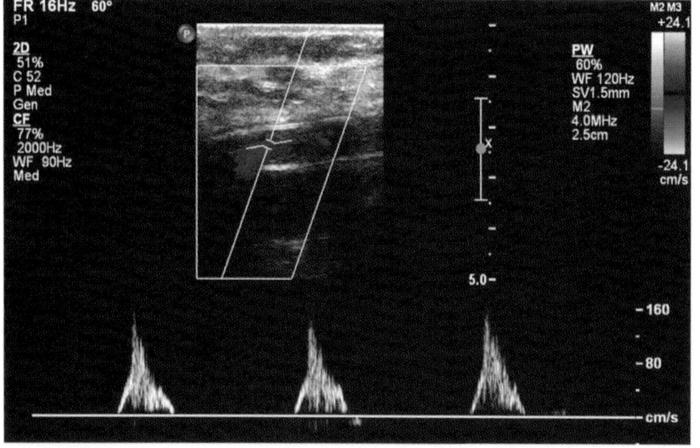

(C)

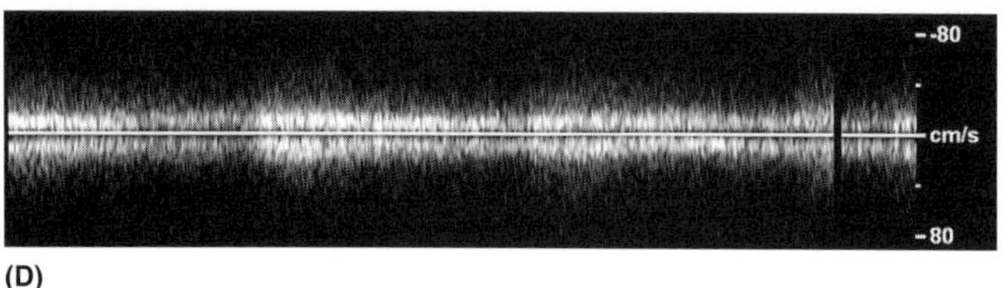

(D)

FIGURE 23 A–F ■ An iatrogenic arterio-venous fistula (AVF). This color Doppler image **(A)** demonstrates a color bruit artifact in the region of a previous arterial catheterization in the groin. A waveform obtained in the femoral artery above the puncture site **(B)** demonstrates a monophasic continuous waveform, while a waveform obtained distal to the puncture **(C)** demonstrates normal pulsatility. The spectral waveform from the vein above the puncture site **(D)** demonstrates "arterialized" flow. A color Doppler image of the region using a higher color Doppler PRF **(E)** eliminates the color Doppler bruit artifact and permits identification of the precise site of the AVF. The use of the higher color Doppler PRF permits more accurate placement of a pulsed Doppler sample volume **(F)** to obtain a waveform typical of an AVF (i.e., a monophasic continuous waveform with significantly elevated velocities throughout the cardiac cycle).

tracts between each loculation. PSAs may contain varying degrees of thrombus around their inner walls. Over time, PSAs can spontaneously thrombose, persist, or rupture (130). The risk of rupture increases in cases of PSAs larger than 3 cm in diameter, when symptoms are severe, and/or when the PSA is enlarging over time (123). Sonography has also been used to confirm the high rate of spontaneous thrombosis of pseudoaneurysms (131,132).

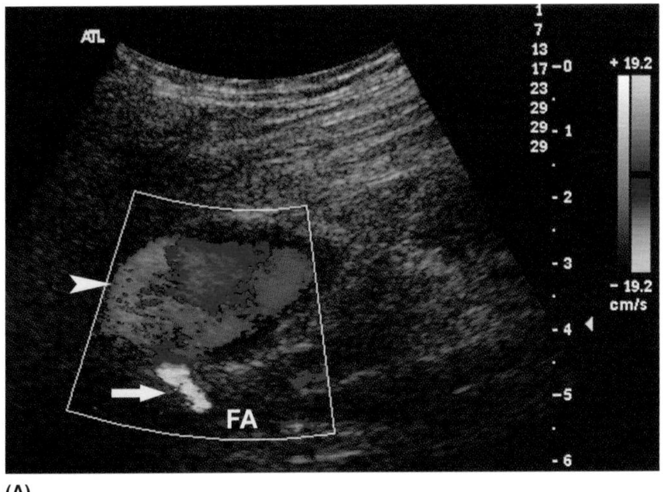

(A)

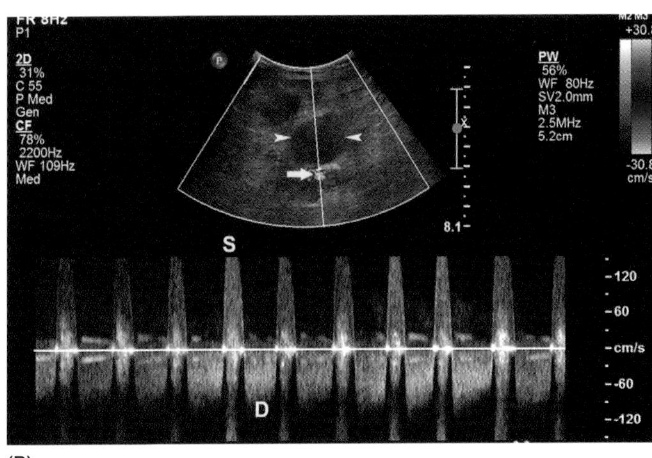

(B)

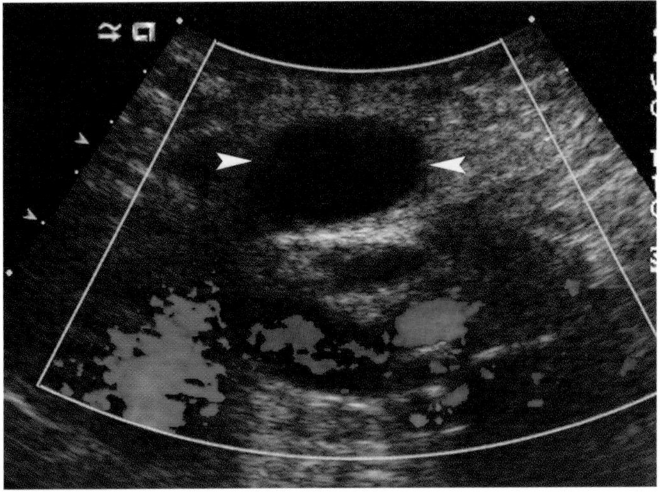

(C)

FIGURE 24 A–C ■ Pseudoaneurysm (PSA) pre- and post-thrombin injection. Color Doppler imaging (**A**) demonstrates a "ying/yang" blood flow pattern in the PSA (*arrowhead*) and the neck (*arrow*) connecting it to the femoral artery (FA). Pulsed Doppler with spectral analysis of flow through the neck (**B**) demonstrates flow into the PSA (*arrowheads*) in systole (S) and holo-diastolic flow reversal (to-and-fro sign). After thrombin injection (**C**) CDI demonstrated no residual flow in the PSA (*arrowheads*) or neck but flow in the more deeply situated native vessels.

In the early 1990s ultrasound-guided compression repair (UGCR) was described as an alternative to conventional surgery (128,133). Since that time additional treatment methods have been developed including ultrasound-guided thrombin injection and the use of specialized devices (133).

The goal of UGCR of PSAs is to use ultrasound imaging to first localize the communicating tract and then to compress the neck with the ultrasound probe in order to occlude flow into the PSA (128). Care must be taken not to occlude flow in the femoral artery; thus, distal pulses should be monitored manually. The use of UGCR has been reported for iatrogenic injuries in vessels other than the femoral artery (134–137).

The use of ultrasound-guided thrombin injections (UGTI) has become the preferred treatment method for iatrogenic PSAs (Fig. 24) (138–140). Thrombin allergy and coexistent AVFs are contraindications to UGTI. After identification of the PSA, using sterile technique, a gray scale ultrasound imaging is used to guide a 22–25 gauge needle into the PSA. Aliquots of 50 to 300 units of commercially available thrombin are injected into the PSA until no flow is visualized with color Doppler imaging. The procedure is concluded when there is no flow detected in the PSA. Thrombin should never be injected directly into the tract because this increases the likelihood of thrombosis of the native vessel (6). With UGTI a clot is created within the PSA within seconds of injection. This method offers significant advantages over UGCR, which can take significantly longer. The reported success of UGTI is typically greater than 90% (141–144). The technique has also been used to treat injuries of other vessels (145). Although this is an off-label use of thrombin, the technique has gained wide-spread clinical utilization (125).

REFERENCES

1. Cavezzi A, Labropoulost N, Partscht H, et al. Duplex ultrasound investigation of the veins in chronic venous disease of the lower limbs: UIP consensus document – Part II: Anatomy. Rev Port Cir Cardiotorac Vasc. 2007 April–June; 14(2):99–108.
2. Coleridge-Smith P, Labropoulos N, Partsch H, et al. Duplex ultrasound investigation of the veins in chronic venous disease of the lower limbs – UIP Consensus Document Part I: Basic principles. Rev Port Cir Cardiotorac Vasc. 2007 January–March; 14(1): 53–61.

3. Partsch H, Oburger K, Mostbeck A, et al. Frequency of pulmonary embolism in ambulant patients with pelvic vein thrombosis: a prospective study J Vasc Surg 1992; 16:715–722.
4. Sevitt S. Venous thrombosis and pulmonary embolism. Their prevention by oral anticoagulants. Am J Med 1962; 33:703–716.
5. Qaseem A, Snow V, Barry P, Hornbake ER, et al. Current diagnosis of venous thromboembolism in primary care: A clinical practice guideline from the American Academy of Family Physicians and the American College of Physicians. Ann Intern Med, March 20, 2007; 146(6):454–458.
6. Murphy TP, Cronan JJ. Evolution of deep venous thrombosis: a prospective evaluation with US. Radiol 1990; 177:543–548.
7. Heijboer H, Buller HP, Lensing AW et al. A comparison of real time compression ultrasonography with impedance plethysmography for the diagnosis of deep vein thrombosis in symptomatic outpatients N Engl J Med 1993; 329:1365–1369.
8. 12. Yucel EK, Fisher JS, Egglin TK, et al. Isolated calf venous thrombosis: diagnosis with compression US. Radiology 1991; 179:443–446.
9. White RH, McGahan JP, Daschbach MM, et al. Diagnosis of deep-vein thrombosis using duplex ultrasound. Ann Intern Med 1989; 111:297–304.
10. Rose SC, Zwiebel WJ, Nelson BD, et al. Symptomatic lower extremity deep venous thrombosis: accuracy, limitations, and role of color duplex flow imaging in diagnosis. Radiology 1990; 175:639–644.
11. Lensing AW, Prandoni P, Brandjes D, et al. Detection of deep vein thrombosis by real-time B mode ultrasonography. N Engl J Med 1989; 320:342–345.
12. Cogo A, Lensing AW, Prandoni P, et al. Distribution of venous thrombosis in patients with symptomatic deep vein thrombosis: implications for simplifying the diagnostic process with compression ultrasound. Arch Intern Med 1993; 153; 2777–2780.
13. Ginsberg JS, Brill-EdwardsP, Burrows RF, et al. Venous thrombosis during pregnancy: leg and trimester of presentation. Thromb Haemost. 1992; 67:519–520.
14. Brockman, SK, Vasko JS. Phlegmasia cerulea dolens. Surg Gynecol Obstet. 1965; 121:1347–1356.
15. Lockshin MD. Antiphospholipid antibody syndrome. Rheum Dis Clin North Am 1994; 20:45–59.
16. Girard P, Sanchez O, Leroyer C, et al. Deep venous thrombosis in patients with acute pulmonary embolism: prevalence, risk factors and clinical significance. Chest 2005; 128:1593–1600.
17. Robinson KS, Anderson DR, Gross M, et al. Ultrasonographic screening before hospital discharge for deep venous thrombosis after arthroplasty: the post-arthroplasty screening study. Ann Intern Med 1997; 127:439–445.
18. Clagett GP, Anderson FA Jr, Heit J, et al. Prevention of venous thromboembolism. Chest 1995; 108(suppl 4):312S–334S.
19. Luciani A, Clement O, Halimi P, et al. Catheter-related upper extremity deep venous thrombosis in cancer patients: a prospective study based on Doppler US. Radiology 2001; 220:655–660.
20. Mustafa S, Stein PD, Patel KC, et al. Upper extremity deep venous thrombosis. Chest 2003; 123:1953–1956.
21. Gaitini D, Beck-Razi N, Haim N, et al. Prevalence of upper extremity deep venous thrombosis diagnosed by color Doppler duplex sonography in cancer patients with central venous catheters. J Ultrasound Med 2006; 25:1297–1303.
22. Giess CS, Thaler H, Bach AM, et al. Clinical experience with upper extremity venous sonography in a high-risk cancer population. J Ultrasound Med 2002; 21:1365–1370.
23. Letai A, Kuter DJ. Cancer, coagulation and anticoagulation. Oncologist 1999; 4:443–449.
24. Horattas MC, Trupiano J, Hopkins S, et al. Changing concepts in long-term central venous access: catheter selection and cost savings. Am J Infect Control. 2001; 29:32–40.
25. Prandoni P, Polistena P, Bernardi E, et al. Upper extremity deep vein thrombosis. Risk factors diagnosis, and complications. Arch Intern Med 1997; 157:57–62.
26. Hingorani A, Ascher E, Hanson J et al. Upper extremity versus lower extremity deep venous thrombosis. Am J Surg 1997; 174:214–217.
27. Koksoy C, Kuzu A, Kutlay J, et al. The diagnostic value of colour Doppler ultrasound in central venous catheter related thrombosis. Clin Radiol 1995; 50:687–689.
28. Joffee HV, Goldhaber SZ. Upper extremity deep vein thrombosis. Circulation 2002; 106:1874–1880.
29. Falk RL, Smith DF. Thrombosis of upper extremity thoracic inlet veins: Diagnosis with duplex Doppler sonography. AJR 1987; 149:677–682.
30. Wright DJ, Shepard AD, McPharlin M, et al. Pitfalls in lower extremity venous duplex scanning. J Vasc Surg 1990; 11:675–679.
31. Kazmers A, Groehn H, Meeker-Ferguson C. Is interrogation of the anterior tibial veins necessary during venous duplex? J Vasc Tech 2001; 25:7–9.
32. Lockhart ME, Sheldon HI, Robbin ML. Augmentation in lower extremity sonography for the detection of deep venous thrombosis. AJR 2005; 184(2):419–422.
33. Machi J, Sigel B, Roberts AB, et al. Oversaturation of color may obscure small intralminal partial occlusions in color Dopper imaging. J Ultrasound Med 1994; 13:735–741.
34. Patel MC, Berman LH, Moss HA, et al. Subclavian and internal jugular veins at Doppler US: abnormal cardiac pulsatility and respiratory phasicity as a predictor of complete central occlusion. Radiology 1999; 211:579–583.
35. Cronan JJ, Dorfman GS, Scola FH, et al. Deep venous thrombosis: US assessment using vein compression. Radiology 1987; 162:191–194.
36. White RH, McGahan JP, Daschbach MM, et al. Diagnosis of deep-vein thrombosis using duplex ultrasound. Ann Intern Med 1989; 111:297–304.
37. Cronan JJ, Leen V. Recurrent deep venous thrombosis: Limitations of US. Radiology 1989; 170:739–742.
38. Schroder WB, Bealer JF. Venous Duplex ultrasonography causing acute pulmonary embolism: a brief report. J Vasc Surg 1992; 15: 1082–1083.
39. Foley WD, Middleton WD, Lawson TL et al. Color Doppler ultrasound imaging of lower extremity venous disease. AJR 1989; 152:371–376.
40. Bach AM, Hann LE. When the common femoral vein is revealed as flattened on spectral Doppler sonography: is it a reliable sign for diagnosis of proximal venous obstruction? AJR 1997; 168:733–736.
41. Lin EP, Bhatt S, Rubens D, et l. The importance of monophasic Doppler waveforms in the common femoral vein: a retrospective study. J Ultrasound Med 2007; 26:885–891.
42. Grassi CJ, Polak JF. Axillary and subclavian venous thrombosis: follow-up evaluation with color Doppler flow US and venography. Radiology 1990; 175:651–654.
43. Cronan JJ, Leen V. Recurrent deep venous thrombosis: Limitations of US. Radiology 1989; 170:739–742.
44. Haire WD, Lynch TG, Lieberman RP, et al. Utility of duplex ultrasound in the diagnosis of asymptomatic catheter-induced subclavian vein thrombosis. J Ultrasound Med 1991; 10:493–496.
45. Murphy TP, Cronan JJ. Evolution of deep venous thrombosis: a prospective evaluation with US. Radiology 1990; 177:543–548.
46. Machi J, Sigel B, Beitler SC, et al. Relation of in vivo blood flow to ultrasound echogenicity. J Clin Ultrasound 1983; 11:3–10.
47. Quinn KL, Vandeman FN. Thrombosis of a duplicated superficial femoral vein. Potential error in compression ultrasound diagnosis of lower extremity deep venous thrombosis. J Ultrasound Med 1990; 9:235–238.
48. Cronin JJ. Venous thromboembolic disease: the role of ultrasound. Radiol 1993; 186:619–630.
49. Prandoni P, Lensing AW, Bernardi E, et al. The diagnostic value of compression ultrasonography in patients with suspected recurrent deep vein thrombosis. Thromb Haemost 2002; 88:402–406.
50. Prandoni P, Lensing AW, Cattelan AM, et al. Outcome of abnormal compression ultrasonography after acute DVT and its implications for diagnosis of recurrent DVT. Thromb Haemost 1991; 66:1175.
51. Miller N, Obrand D, Tousignant L, Gascon I, Rossignol M. Venous duplex scanning for unilateral symptoms: when do we need a contralateral evaluation? Eur. J. Vasc. Endovasc. Surg. 1998; 15: 18–23.
52. Cronan JJ. Deep venous thrombosis: one leg or both legs? Radiology 1996; 200:323–324.
53. Naidich JB, Torre JR, Pellerito JS, et al. Suspected deep venous thrombosis: Is US of both legs necessary? Radiology 1996; 200: 429–431.

54. Beecham RP, Dorfman GS, Cronan JJ et al. Is bilateral lower extremity compression sonography useful and cost-effective in the evaluation of suspected pulmonary embolism? AJR 1993; 161:1289–1292.
55. Sheiman RG, McArdle CR. Bilateral lower extremity US in the patient with unilateral symptoms of deep venous thrombosis: assessment of need. Radiology 1995; 194:171–173.
56. Sheiman RG, Weintraub JL, McArdle CR. Bilateral lower extremity US in the patient with bilateral symptoms of deep venous thromboss: assessment of need. Radiology 1995; 196:379–381.
57. Anderson FA, Wheeler HB. Physcian practices the management of venous thromboembolism: a community wide survey. J Vasc Surg 1992; 15:707–714.
58. Gless CS, Bach AM, Hann LE. Lower extremity venous sonography in the high risk cancer population: one leg or two? AJR 2001; 176:1049–1062.
59. Loud PA, Klippenstein DL. Lower extremity deep venous thromboss in cancer patients: correlation of presenting symptoms with venous sonographic findings. J Ultrasound Med 1998; 17: 693–698.
60. Cornuz J, Pearson SD, Polak JF. Deep venous thrombosis: complete lower extremity venous US evaluation in patients without known risk factors – outcome study. Radiology 1998; 211:637–641.
61. Elias A, Mallard L, Elias M, et al. A single complete ultrasound investigation of the veous network for the diagnostic managemet of patients with a clinically suspected first empisode of deep venous thrombosis of the lower limbs. Thromb Haemost 2003; 89:221–227.
62. Subramaniam RM, Heath R, Chou T, et al. Deep venous thrombosis: withholding anticoagulation therapy after negative complete lower limb US findings. Radiology 2005; 237:348–352.
63. Quinlan DJ, Alikhan R, Gishen P, et al. Variations in Lower Limb Venous Anatomy: Implications for US diagnosis of Deep Vein Thrombosis. Radiology 2003; 228:443–448.
64. Bounameaux H, Righini M, Perrier A. Diagnosing deep vein thrombosis: the case for compression ultrasonography limited to the proximal veins. J Thromb Haemost 2004; 2:2260–1.
65. El Kheir D, Büller H. One-time comprehensive ultrasonography to diagnose deep venous thrombosis: is that the solution? [Editorial] Ann Intern Med. 2004; 140:1052–3.
66. Birdwell BG, Raskob GE, Whitsett TL, et al. The clinical validity of normal compression ultrasonography in outpatients suspected of having deep venous thrombosis. Ann Intern Med 1998 128:1–7.
67. Kearon C, Ginsberg JS, Douketis J, Crowther MA, Turpie AG, Bates SM, et al. A randomized trial of diagnostic strategies after normal proximal vein ultrasonography for suspected deep venous thrombosis: D-dimer testing compared with repeated ultrasonography. Ann Intern Med. 2005; 142:490–6.
68. Bradley MJ, Spencer PA, Alexander L, et al. Colour flow mapping in the diagnosis of calf vein thrombosis. Clin Radiol 1993; 47:399–402.
69. Meibers DJ, Baldridge ED, Ruoff BA, et al. The significance of calf muscle thrombosis. J Vasc Surg 1988; 12:143–149.
70. Moser KM, LeMoine JR. Is embolic risk conditioned by location of deep venous thrombosis? Ann Intern Med 1981; 94:439–444.
71. Philbrick JT, Becker DM. Calf deep venous thrombosis: a wolf in sheeps clothing? Arch Intern Med 1998; 148:2131–2138.
72. Gottlieb RH, Voci SL, Syed L, et al. Randomized prospective study comparing routine versus selective use of sonography of the complete calf in patients with suspected deep venous thrombosis. AJR 2003; 180:241–245.
73. Vaccaro JP, Cronan JJ, Dorfman GS. Outcome analysis of patients with normal compression US examnations. Radiology 1990; 10:443–446.
74. Hyers TM, Agnelli G, Hull RD et al. Antithrombotic therapy for venous thromboembolic disease. Chest 2001; 119(suppl 1):176S–193S.
75. The Seventh ACCP Conference on Antithrombotic and Thrombolytic Therapy: Evidence-Based Guidelines. Hirsh J, Guyatt G, Albers GW, Schünemann HJ. Chest 126:172S–173S.
76. ACR Practice Guideline for the performance of peripheral venous ultrasound examination. 2006 Revision.
77. AIUM Practice Guideline for the performance of a peripheral venous ultrasound examination. 2006.
78. Krupsk WC, Bass A, Dilley RB et al. Propagation of deep venous thrombosis identified by duplex ultrasonography. J Vasc Surg 1990; 12:467–475.
79. Araki CT, Back TL, Padberg FTJ, et al. Refinements in the ultrasonic detection of popliteal vein reflux. J Vasc Surg 1993; 18:742.
80. Meissner MH, Manzo RA, Bergelin RO, et al. Deep venous insufficiency: the relationship between lysis and subsequent reflux. J Vasc Surg 1993; 18:596.
81. Weingarten MS, Branas CC, Czeredarczuk M, et al. Distribution and quantification of venous reflux in lower extremity chronic venous stasis disease with duplex scanning. J Vasc Surg 1993; 18:753.
82. Jager KA, Ricketts HJ, Strandness DE. Duplex scanning for the evaluation of lower limb arterial disease. In: Bernstein EF, editor. Noninvasive Diagnostic Techniques in Vascular Disease. St. Louis: CV Mosby Co; 1985.
83. Kohler TR, Nance DR, Cramer MM, et al. Duplex scanning for diagnosis of aortoiliac and femoropopliteal disease: a prospective study. Circulation 1987; 76:1074.
84. Ranke C, Creutzig A, Alexander K. Duplex scanning of the peripheral arteries: correlation of the peak velocity ratio with angiographic diameter reduction. Ultrasound Med Biol 1992; 18:433.
85. Kotval PS. Doppler waveform parvus and tardus: a sign of proximal flow obstruction. J Ultrasound Med 1989; 8:435.
86. Hutchison K, Karpinski E. Stability of flow patterns in the in vivo post-stenotic velocity field. Ultrasound Med Biol 1988; 14:269.
87. Hirsch AT, Haskal ZJ, Hertzer NR, et al. ACC/AHAGuidelines for the Management of Patients with Peripheral Arterial Disease (Lower Extremity, Renal, Mesenteric, and Abdominal Aortic): A Collaborative Report from the American Association for Vascular Surgery/Society for Vascular Surgery, Society for Cardiovascular Angiography and Interventions, Society of Interventional Radiology, Society for Vascular Medicine and Biology, and the American College of Cardiology/American Heart Association Task Force on Practice Guidelines (Writing Committee to Develop Guidelines for the Management of Patients With Peripheral Arterial Disease). J Am Coll Cardiol 2006; 47:1239–1312.
88. Cossman DV, Ellison JE, Wagner WH, et al. Comparison of contrast arteriography to arterial mapping with color-flow duplex imaging in the lower extremities. J Vasc Surg 1989; 10:522.
89. Polak JF, Karmel MI, Meyerovitz MF. Accuracy of color Doppler flow mapping for evaluation of the severity of femoropopliteal arterial disease: a prospective study. J Vasc Interv Radiol 1991; 2:471.
90. Edwards JM, Goldwell DM, Goldman ML, et al. The role of duplex scanning in the selection of patients for transluminal angioplasty. J Vasc Surg 1991; 13:69.
91. Elsman BH, Legemate DA, van der Heijden FH, et al. Impact of ultrasonographic duplex scanning on therapeutic decision making in lower limb arterial disease. Br J Surg 1995; 82:630.
92. Mills JL, Harris EJ, Taylor LM Jr, et al. The importance of routine surveillance of distal bypass grafts with duplex scanning: a study of 379 reversed vein grafts. J Vasc Surg 1990; 12:379.
93. Idu MM, Blankestein JD, de Gier P, et al. Impact of a color-flow duplex surveillance program on infrainguinal vein graft patency: a five-year experience. J Vasc Surg 1993; 17:42.
94. Mills JL, Bandyk DF, Gathan V, et al. The origin of infrainguinal vein graft stenosis: a prospective study based on duplex surveillance. J Vasc Surg 1995; 21:16.
95. Kotval PS. Doppler waveform parvus and tardus: a sign of proximal flow obstruction. J Ultrasound Med 1989; 8:435.
96. Hutchison K, Karpinski E. Stability of flow patterns in the in vivo post-stenotic velocity field. Ultrasound Med Biol 1988; 14:269.
97. Whelan FF, Barry MH, Moir JD. Color flow Doppler ultrasonography: comparison with peripheral arteriography for the investigation of peripheral arterial disease. J Clin Ultrasound 1992; 20:369.
98. Sacks D, Robinson ML, Marinelli DL, et al. Peripheral arterial Doppler ultrasonography: diagnostic criteria. J Ultrasound Med 1992; 11:95.
99. Moneta GL, Yeager RA, Lee RW, et al. Noninvasive localization of arterial occlusive disease: a comparison of segmental pressures and arterial duplex mapping. J Vasc Surg 1993; 17:578.

100. Polak JF, Donaldson MC, Whittemore AD, et al. Pulsatile masses surrounding vascular prostheses: real-time US color flow imaging. Radiology 1989; 170:363.
101. Sanchez LA, Suggs WD, Veith FJ, et al. Is surveillance to detect failing polytetrafluoroethylene bypasses worthwhile: twelve-year experience with 91 grafts. J Vasc Surg 1993; 18:981.
102. Berkowitz HD, Greenstein SM. Improved patency in reversed femoral-infrapopliteal autogenous vein grafts by early detection and treatment of the failing graft. J Vasc Surg 1987; 5:755.
103. Cohen JR, Mannick JA, Couch NP, et al. Recognition and management of impending vein-graft failure: importance for long-term patency. Arch Surg 1986; 121:758.
104. Bandyk DF, Seabrook GR, Moldenhauer P, et al. Hemodynamics of vein graft stenosis. J Vasc Surg 1988; 8:688.
105. Bandyk DF, Schmitt DD, Seabrook GR, et al. Monitoring functional patency of in situ saphenous vein bypasses: the impact of a surveillance protocol and elective revision. J Vasc Surg 1989; 9:286.
106. Whittemore AD, Clowes AW, Couch NP, et al. Secondary femoropopliteal reconstruction. Ann Surg 1981; 193:35.
107. Bandyk DF, Jorgensen RA, Towne JB. Intraoperative assessment of in situ saphenous vein arterial bypass grafts using pulsed Doppler spectral analysis. Arch Surg 1986; 121:292.
108. Grigg MJ, Nicolaides AN, Wolfe JH. Detection and grading of femorodistal vein grafts stenoses: duplex velocity measurements compared with angiography. J Vasc Surg 1988; 8:661.
109. Polak JF, Donaldson MC, Dobkin GR, et al. Early detection of saphenous vein arterial bypass graft stenosis by color-assisted duplex sonography: a prospective study. AJR Am J Roentgenol 1990; 154:857.
110. Bandyk DF. Ultrasound assessment during and after peripheral intervention. In: Introduction to vascular ultrasonography. 5th Edition. Zwiebel WJ, Pellerito JS eds. Philadelphia, PA. Elsiver / Saunders. 2005. 357–379.
111. Hunink. MGM, Magruder CD, Meyerovitz MF, et al. Risks and benefits of femoropopliteal percutaneous balloon angioplasty. J Vasc Surg 1993; 17:183.
112. Hunink M, Wong J, Donaldson M, et al. Revascularization for femoropopliteal disease: a decision and cost-effectiveness analysis. JAMA 1995; 274:165.
113. Mewissen MW, Kinney EV, Bandyk DF, et al. The role of duplex scanning versus angiography in predicting outcome after balloon angioplasty in the femoropopliteal artery. J Vasc Surg 1992; 15:860.
114. Sacks D, Robinson ML, Summers TA, et al. The value of duplex sonography after peripheral artery angioplasty in predicting subacute stenosis. AJR 1994; 162:179.
115. Vroegindeweij D, Tielbeek A, Buth J, et al. Recanalization of femoropopliteal occlusive lesions: a comparison of long-term clinical, color duplex US, and arteriographic follow-up. J Vasc Interv Radiol 1995; 6:331.
116. Johnston KW, Rutherford RB, Tilson MD, Shah DM, Hollier L, Stanley JC. Suggested standards for reporting on arterial aneurysms. Subcommittee on Reporting Standards for Arterial Aneurysms, Ad Hoc Committee on Reporting Standards, Society for Vascular Surgery and North American Chapter, International Society for Cardiovascular Surgery. J Vasc Surg 1991; 13(3):452–8.
117. MacGowan SW, Saif MF, O'Neil G, et al. Ultrasound examination in the diagnosis of popliteal artery aneurysms. Br J Surg 1985; 72:528.
118. Bluth El, Shyn PB, Sullivan MA, et al. Doppler color flow imaging of carotid artery dissection. J Ultrasound Med 1989; 8:149.
119. Kotval PS, Babu SC, Fakhry J, et al. Role of the intimal flap in arterial dissection: sonographic demonstration. AJR Am J Roentgenol 1988; 150:1181.
120. Liu JB, Merton DA, Mitchell DG, Needleman L, Kurtz AB, Goldberg BB: Color Doppler imaging of the iliofemoral region. Radiographics. 1990 10:403–412.
121. Mitchell DG, Merton DA, Liu JB, Goldberg BB: Superficial masses with color flow Doppler imaging. J Clinical Ultrasound. 1991 19:555–560.
122. Helvie MA, Rubin J. Evaluation of traumatic groin arteriovenous fistulas with duplex Doppler sonography. J Ultrasound Med 1989; 8:21.
123. Roubidoux MA, Hertzberg BS, Carroll BA, et al. Color flow and image-directed Doppler ultrasound evaluation of iatrogenic arteriovenous fistulas in the groin. J Clin Ultrasound 1990; 18:463.
124. Fellmeth BD, Roberts AC, Bookstein JJ, Freischlag JA, Forsythe JR, Buckner NK, Hye RJ. Postangiographic femoral artery injuries: nonsurgical repair with US-guided compression. Radiology. 1991; 178:671–675.
125. Webber GW, Jang J, Gustavson S, Olin JW. Contemporary Management of Postcatheterization Pseudoaneurysms Circulation 2007; 115; 2666–2674.
126. Coughlin BF, Paushter DM. Peripheral pseudoaneurysms: evaluation with duplex US. Radiology 1988; 168:339.
127. Helvie MA, Rubin JM, Silver TM, et al. The distinction between femoral artery pseudoaneurysms and other causes of groin masses: value of duplex Doppler sonography. AJR Am J Roentgenol 1988; 150:1177.
128. Fellmeth BD, Baron SB, Brown PR, et al. Repair of postcatheterization femoral pseudoaneurysms by color flow ultrasound guided compression. Am Heart J 1992; 123:547.
129. Polak JF, Donaldson MC, Whittemore AD, et al. Pulsatile masses surrounding vascular prostheses: real-time US color flow imaging. Radiology 1989; 170:363.
130. McCann RL, Schwartz LB, Pieper KS. Vascular complications of cardiac catheterization. J Vasc Surg 1991; 14:375.
131. Kresowik TF, Khoury MD, Miller BV, et al. A prospective study of the incidence and natural history of femoral vascular complications after percutaneous transluminal coronary angioplasty. J Vasc Surg 1991; 13:328.
132. DiPrete DA, Cronan JJ. Compression ultrasonography: treatment for acute femoral artery pseudoaneurysms in selected cases. J Ultrasound Med 1992; 11:489.
133. Feld R, Patton GM, Carabsi RA, et al. Treatment of iatrogenic femoral artery injuries with ultrasound-guided compression. J Vasc Surg 1992; 16:832–840.
134. Rooker KT, Morgan CA, Haseman MK, Hofer GA, Fellmeth BD. Color flow-guided repair of axillary artery pseudoaneurysm. J. Ultrasound Med. 1992; 11:625–626.
135. Henney SE, Bhattacharya V, Sarker BA. Iatrogenic pseudoaneurysm resulting in transection of the radial artery. J Ultrasound Med. 2004; 23:1091–1093.
136. Salour M, Dattilo JB, Mingloski PM, Brewer WH. Femoral vein pseudoaneurysm: uncommon complication of femoral vein puncture. J Ultrasound Med. 1998; 17:577–579.
137. Zehnder T, Mahler CF, Do D. Successful ultrasonographically guided compression repair of a dialysis fistula pseudoaneurysm. J Ultrasound Med 2000; 19:329–331.
138. La Perna L, Olin JW, Goines D, Childs MB, Ouriel K. Ultrasound-guided thrombin injection for the treatment of postcatheterization pseudoaneurysms. Circulation. 2000; 102:2391–2395.
139. Taylor BS, Rhee RY, Muluk S, et al. Thrombin injection versus compression of femoral artery pseudoaneurysms. J Vasc Surg. 1999; 30:1052–1059.
140. Weinmann EE, Chayen D, Kobzantzev ZV, Zaretsky M, Bass A. Treatment of postcatheterisation false aneurysms: ultrasound-guided compression vs ultrasound-guided thrombin injection. Eur J Vasc Endovasc Surg. 2002; 23:68–72.
141. Grewe PH, Mugge A, Germing A, Harrer E, Baberg H, Hanefeld C, Deneke T. Occlusion of pseudoaneurysms using human or bovine thrombin using contrast-enhanced ultrasound guidance. Am J Cardiol. 2004; 93:1540–1542.
142. Khoury M, Rebecca A, Greene K, et al. Duplex scanning-guided thrombin injection for the treatment of iatrogenic pseudoaneurysms. J Vasc Surg. 2002; 35:517–521.
143. Krueger K, Zaehringer M, Strohe D, et al. Postcatheterization pseudoaneurysm: results of US-guided percutaneous thrombin injection in 240 patients. Radiology. 2005; 236:1104–1110.
144. Kruger K, Zahringer M, Sohngen FD, et al. Femoral pseudoaneurysms: management with percutaneous thrombin injections–success rates and effects on systemic coagulation. Radiology. 2003; 226:452–458.
145. Ghersin E, Karram T, Gaitini D, et al: Percutaneous ultrasonographically guided thrombin injection of iatrogenic pseudoaneurysms in unusual sites. J Ultrasound Med 2003; 22:809–816.

Carotid ● Mark E. Lockhart and Lincoln L. Berland

19

INTRODUCTION

Carotid sonography is most commonly performed to grade the severity of carotid and vertebral artery (VA) atherosclerotic disease, employing flow characteristics and velocity criteria. The goal of carotid evaluation is determining which patients will benefit from intervention, usually carotid endarterectomy (CEA) or stenting. A detailed understanding of the anatomy, sonographic techniques, diagnostic criteria, and potential pitfalls is essential for optimal evaluation. In this chapter, we address the key issues in carotid ultrasound, including efforts to standardize the diagnostic criteria and highlight areas requiring further study. We incorporate the findings of the consensus conference on carotid ultrasound, sponsored by the Society of Radiologists in Ultrasound (SRU) in 2002 (1).

NORMAL ANATOMY

The extracranial arteries supplying the brain include (*i*) the common carotid artery (CCA), (*ii*) the internal carotid artery (ICA), (*iii*) the external carotid artery (ECA), and (*iv*) the VA. These arteries arise from the aortic arch or one of its branches. Typically, the brachiocephalic artery, the first major aortic arch branch, divides into the right common carotid and the right subclavian arteries. Occasionally, the right CCA is the first branch and an aberrant right subclavian artery arises beyond the left subclavian artery origin. The second major artery arising from the aortic arch is the left CCA, which is usually separate from the third major branch, the left subclavian artery. The right VA originates from the right subclavian artery and the left vertebral from the left subclavian artery. Rarely, the left VA originates directly from the aortic arch, between the left carotid and the left subclavian origin.

Both CCAs ascend posterolateral to the thyroid, deep and medial to the internal jugular vein and sternocleidomastoid muscles. Each CCA bifurcates at the level of the upper margin of the thyroid cartilage into the ECA and the ICA. In short necks, the bifurcation may lie higher. The ICA lies more posterior in the neck without branching. The ECA is anteromedial to the ICA with several branches.

The VAs are lateral to the vertebrae and join at the base of the skull to form the basilar artery, which supplies the posterior brain circulation. They provide collateral circulation through the circle of Willis in the setting of significant carotid occlusion. They also provide collateral flow to the arm in stenosis of the subclavian artery origin.

EXAMINATION TECHNIQUE

Patient Positioning

Optimal sonographic technique first depends on a proper imaging setting and patient positioning, ideally in a sonographic suite. Properly reduced lighting and freedom from distractions decrease exam difficulty. Carotid artery examinations are performed with the patient recumbent or supine, the neck slightly extended, the ipsilateral shoulder lowered as if the patient is reaching toward the feet, and the head turned away from the side being examined. Hyperextension of the neck facilitates examination of obese patients and is accomplished by placing a pillow under the shoulders, allowing the head to rest on the table. The sonographer sits at the patient's side or head.

The SRU consensus conference recommends that all carotid ultrasounds be performed by a registered vascular sonographer using standards of an accreditation organization such as the American College of Radiology (ACR) or the American Institute of Ultrasound in Medicine (AIUM). A standard carotid ultrasound includes (*i*) gray-scale examination, (*ii*) color Doppler evaluation, and (*iii*) spectral Doppler analysis (1). All three techniques contribute to the evaluation of disease and must be used in concert for diagnosis. In discrepancies between Doppler and gray-scale image information, finding the source of disagreement is critical. In a patient with large plaques but normal velocities, the gray-scale images may allow correct detection of a long-segment stenosis. Color Doppler often helps explain apparent discrepancies between image and spectral Doppler information (2).

Gray-Scale Examination

The sonographic evaluation employs a linear high-frequency transducer; we often begin with a 5 to 7.5MHz probe. Transducers employ a continuous range of frequencies, and we select the highest frequency range allowing good penetration. We initially obtain transverse images of the CCA at the base of the neck and progress cranially, obtaining representative images to the angle of the mandible, with special attention to the carotid bulb and proximal ICA. Inferior angulation of the transducer in the supraclavicular area demonstrates the origin of the right CCA. The left CCA origin is deeper and more elusive. In the mid neck, the common carotid mildly dilates (the carotid bulb) and then bifurcates into the ICA and ECA. We obtain longitudinal gray-scale images of the CCA from its origin through the bifurcation. The bifurcation is imaged from two transducer positions, optimizing visualization of the origins of the ICA and the ECA relative to the carotid bulb. The location and severity of any plaques, which may be eccentric, or any visible narrowing should be noted. Careful selection of the proper plane avoids overestimating or underestimating the disease. Some studies demonstrate the association of plaque ulceration (Fig. 1) or heterogeneity with higher risk of rupture and thrombosis (3,4). Therefore, plaque heterogeneity by ultrasound should be reported because increased risk of stroke renders vulnerable plaques surgical lesions in appropriate settings, even if the stenosis is less than 50% by Doppler criteria (2).

Color and Power Doppler Evaluation

Color Doppler provides useful information beyond the presence or absence of flow. Longitudinal color survey of the extracranial carotid and vertebral arterial system can identify regions of turbulent, high velocity flow for subsequent spectral Doppler analysis. Within areas of very high-flow velocity, the color representation will "wrap" to the opposite end of the spectrum, a phenomenon known as aliasing (Fig. 2). Using this signal as a guide, the sonographer uses spectral Doppler to quantitate the peak flow velocity. Avoiding error requires proper color Doppler settings of scale and filter. A large scale may lack

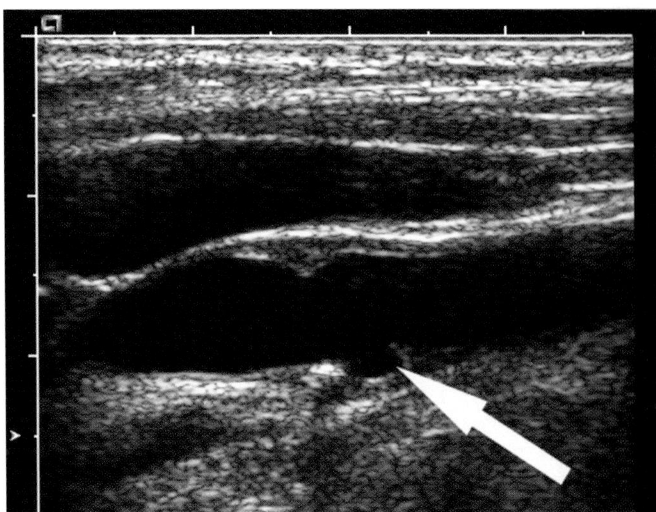

FIGURE 1 ■ Plaque ulceration. This carotid bulb demonstrates an irregular plaque with an apparent ulceration (*arrow*). However, depending on its age, the ulcer may have re-epithelialized, decreasing the risk of thromboembolism.

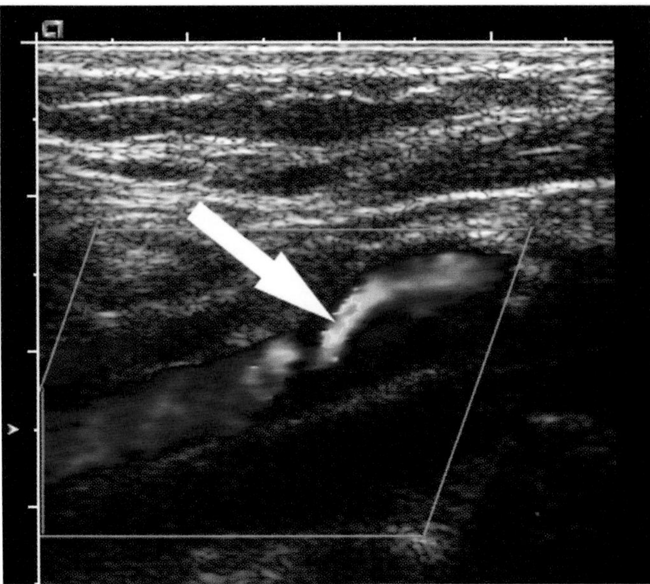

FIGURE 2 ■ Internal carotid artery (ICA) stenosis with aliasing. The blue color throughout the common and internal carotid arteries indicates antegrade flow. However, a focus of high-velocity flow with orange-yellow color is seen at a stenosis (*arrow*) at the origin of the ICA. This does not indicate reversed flow but rather represents color Doppler aliasing or color "wrap-around." This sign can be used to determine the best location to interrogate the artery with spectral Doppler. The Doppler angle cursor should be oriented parallel to the flow jet rather than to the vessel walls.

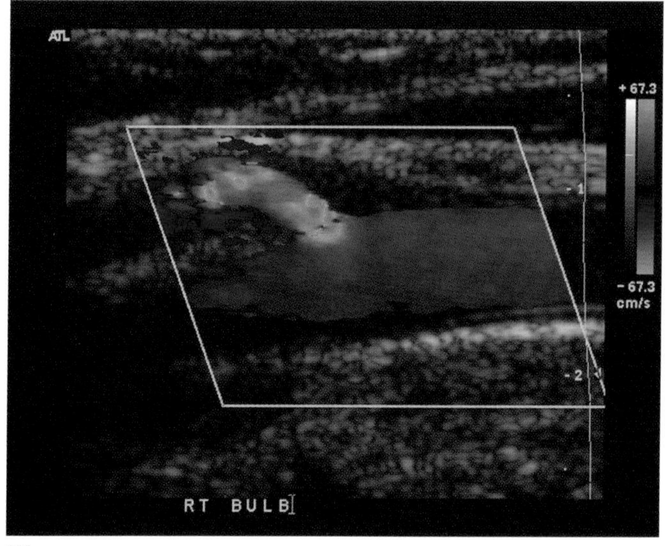

(A)

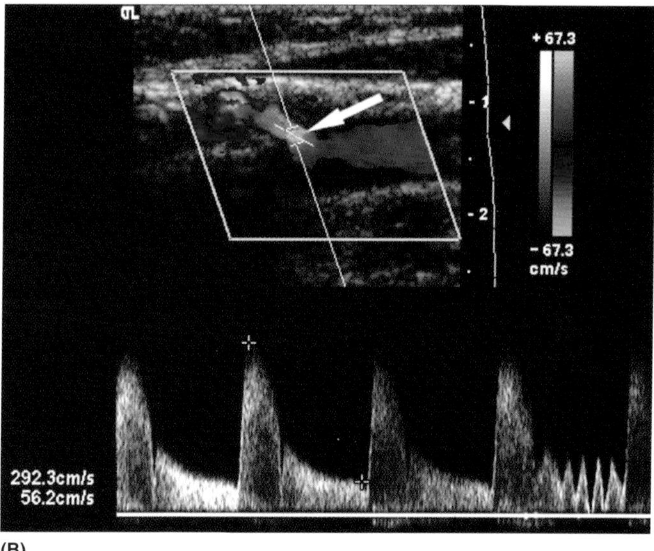

(B)

FIGURE 3 A AND B ■ External carotid artery (ECA) stenosis. (**A**) Color Doppler image of the common carotid artery (CCA) demonstrates a small focus of color aliasing at the origin of the ECA. However, the color image suggests that the origin is widely patent. (**B**) Spectral Doppler of the ECA origin (*arrow*) reveals an elevated velocity of 2.9 m/sec, indicating a stenosis that was obscured by color "bleeding" or overwriting the stenotic plaque.

sensitivity for increased flow detection, while a small scale may create excessive aliasing and noise. Newer machines have greatly improved color optimization, and some platforms automatically adjust the color settings. Power Doppler is the most sensitive technique for detecting blood flow, although it does not depict the direction. Both color and power Doppler can be useful for detecting hypoechoic or anechoic plaque, demonstrated as a focal signal void. However, color "bleeding" into tissue adjacent to flow may also obscure such plaques (Fig. 3A and B). Color or power Doppler may also be helpful in detecting flow in tortuous vessels. For detecting small channels of slow flow in areas of near occlusion, power Doppler may still be more sensitive than color Doppler (5). However, advances in color Doppler have reduced this difference.

Spectral Doppler Analysis

Spectral Doppler should be used to interrogate any region of aliasing detected by color Doppler and to characterize flow in standardized parts of the carotid system. We obtain flow velocities and waveforms from the proximal, mid, and distal CCA; the proximal, mid, and distal ICA; the proximal ECA, and the proximal VA (Fig. 4A and B). A Doppler gate must nearly fill the lumen of the artery (Fig. 5). The scale and gain should show strong flow signals that use most of the scale to display the waveform, a process nearly automated by newer machines. The Doppler angle cursor should be parallel to the flow, not parallel to the vessel wall, allowing definition of the angle between the transducer line of sight and the direction of blood flow. This Doppler angle allows conversion of frequencies to flow velocities.

On spectral Doppler, we achieve the greatest frequency shift when flow parallels the transducer line of sight (Doppler angle = 0), maximizing the cosine. Because this angle is rarely achievable in carotid Doppler, the SRU consensus panel recommends an angle less than 60° for spectral analysis (1). Velocity values are standardized based on this angle of interrogation, and velocity measurement error is substantially increased for angles of insonation greater than 60°. One study suggests we should thus use a consistent angle near 60° for follow-up ultrasound exams of patients with moderate disease (6).

Spectral Doppler helps differentiate the ECA from the ICA, because the ECA's anteromedial location may be difficult to confirm if the examiner cannot visualize the ECA's branches. Because the temporal artery is a branch of the ECA, repetitive tapping of its supra-auricular segment sends pulsations to the ECA, allowing differentiation from the ICA (Fig. 6) (7). Although transmitted pulsations have been described in the ICA from this maneuver, their amplitude is usually much smaller than within the ECA (7,8).

VA Evaluation

VA evaluation is integral to the carotid system examination. In a patient with symptoms of dizziness or altered mental status, vertebrobasilar insufficiency is one possible cause. Spectral Doppler determines patency and direction of flow in the VAs. We place the transducer lateral to the carotid in a longitudinal orientation and angle it laterally using color Doppler to locate the VA. Color Doppler is performed along the visualized length of the artery to detect aliasing or turbulence. A spectral Doppler waveform of the extracranial VA is obtained near the base of the

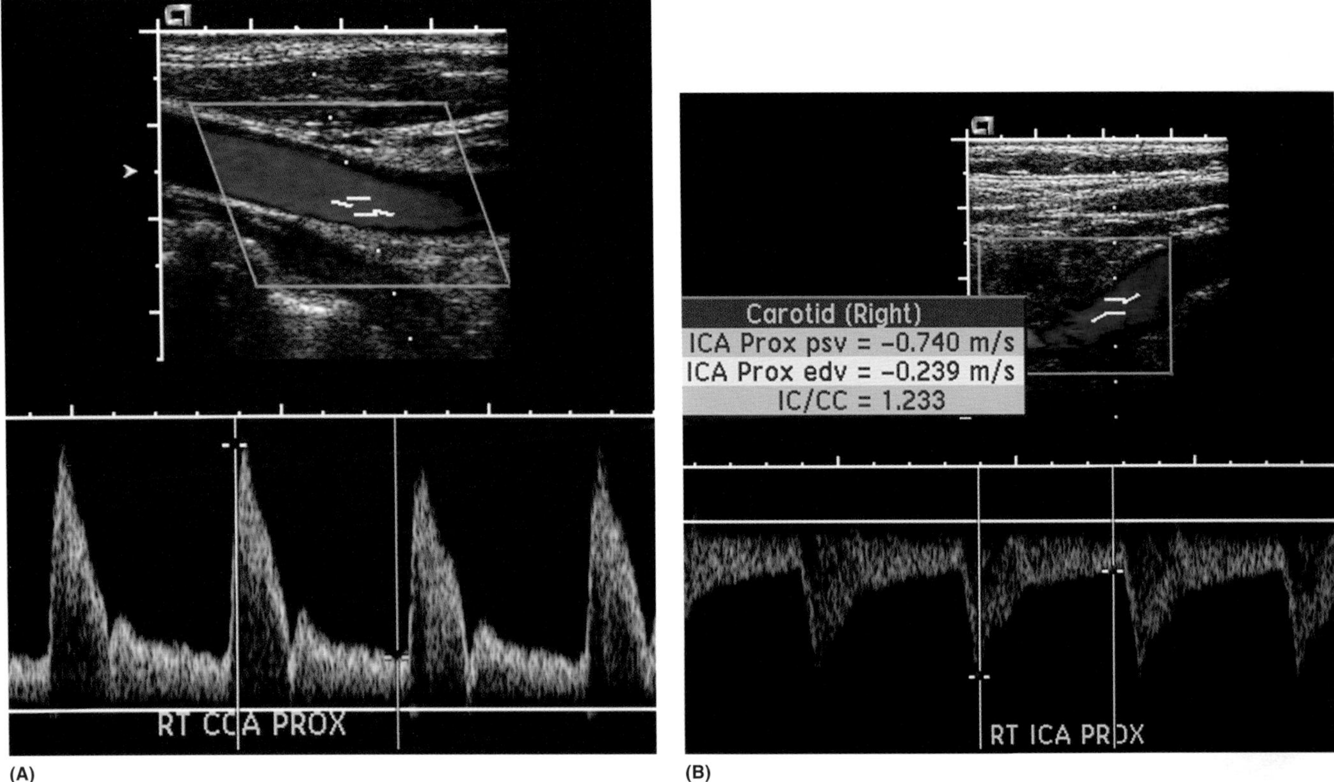

FIGURE 4 A AND B ■ (**A**) Normal Common carotid artery (CCA) Doppler. The spectral tracing demonstrates a sharp envelope and normal peak and end-diastolic velocity. The resistivity index is 0.80. This degree of spectral broadening is normal. (**B**) Normal Internal carotid artery (ICA) Doppler. This is a different patient, in whom the tracing is also normal. The resistivity index is lower at 0.68 (the relative diastolic flow is higher).

neck and at any point of suspected stenosis suggested by color Doppler aliasing.

DIAGNOSTIC ISSUES IN CAROTID ULTRASOUND

Indications

In patients with substantial risk, symptoms, or signs of cerebral atherosclerotic disease, carotid ultrasound triages patients to medical management or surgery. The Asymptomatic Carotid Atherosclerosis Study (ACAS) showed improved morbidity and mortality with CEA in asymptomatic patients with stenoses greater than 60% (9). The North American Symptomatic Carotid Endarterectomy Trial (NASCET) study showed clinical benefit from surgery in symptomatic patients with carotid stenoses greater than 70% (10). Accepted indications for carotid sonography are (*i*) unexplained stroke or transient ischemic attack (TIA), (*ii*) cervical bruit, (*iii*) to follow the progression of known atherosclerotic disease, (*iv*) to follow the results of prior carotid surgery or intervention, and (*v*) to evaluate carotid stent flow. Because carotid ultrasound also evaluates the VAs, additional indications include (*vi*) evaluation for subclavian steal syndrome, and (*vii*) workup of suspected vertebrobasilar insufficiency. Performing carotid ultrasound before some major (particularly cardiovascular) surgical procedures is common but is not universally accepted.

Intraoperative sonography of the carotid arteries differs from the standard evaluation. The most common indication is documentation of flow after a difficult CEA or concern for dissection during surgery. We perform limited gray-scale, color Doppler, and spectral Doppler unilaterally; the surgeon may desire only documentation of arterial patency or the presence of intimal flaps or dissection. In some cases, visualization of a carotid patch may exclude any intravascular debris or flap.

Diagnostic Criteria—Carotid

More than a decade after the results of large randomized trials showed benefits for surgical therapy in carotid atherosclerotic disease, a large number of ultrasound trials demonstrate variable success in predicting which patients benefit from surgery. The NASCET (10,11), a benchmark study on the use of CEA in North America, invoked stopping rules in 1991, with a mean of 18 months followup for the severe group arm of the trial. The risk of ipsilateral hemisphere stroke at two years was 26% in the medical group and only 9% in the surgical group. For major or fatal stroke in the same hemisphere, 13.1% occurred in the medical group and only 2.5% in the surgical group. The best clinical benefit came at the 70% threshold, as published in the NASCET report (10,11). This standard is now widely accepted. Percent stenosis in this trial was defined as minimum proximal ICA diameter

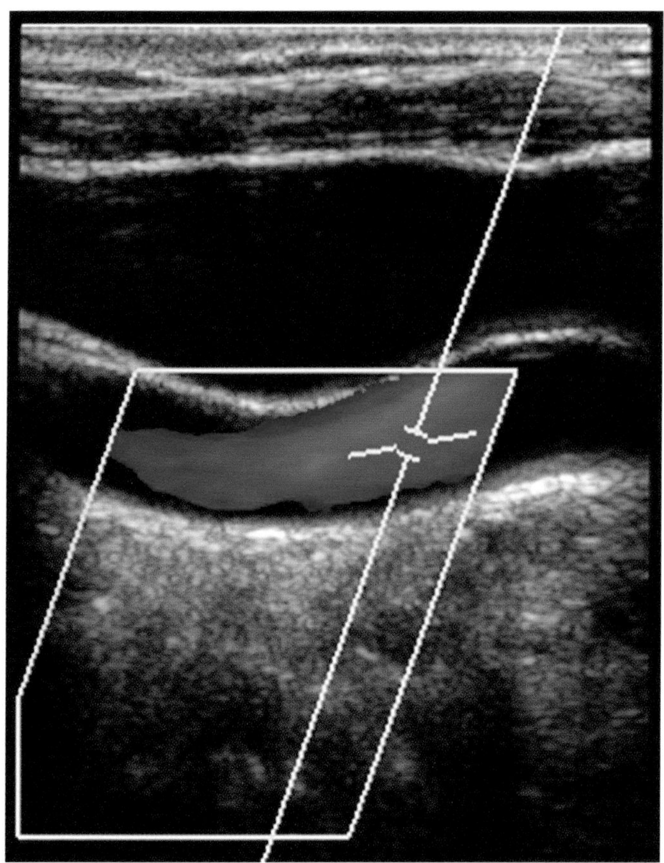

FIGURE 5 ■ Doppler gate placement. This color Doppler image of the common carotid artery demonstrates the proper placement of the cursor within the center of the vessel with the cursor angled parallel to the vessel walls.

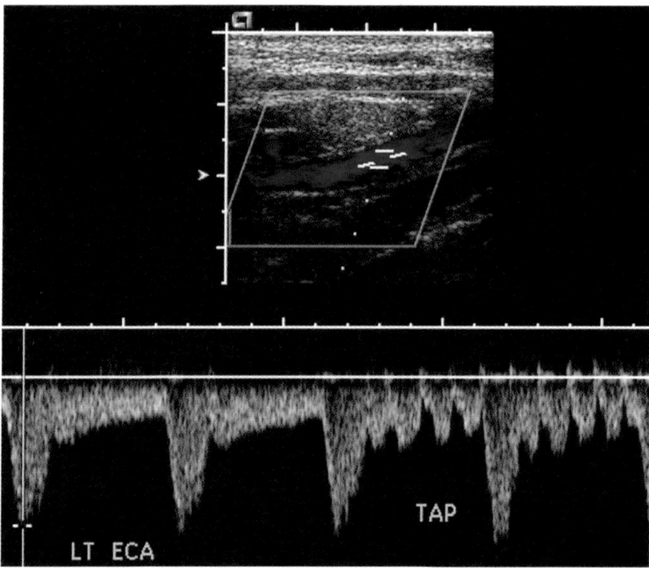

FIGURE 6 ■ Temporal tap. At the time of the third pulse, the supra-auricular temporal artery was tapped, demonstrating a sawtooth pattern on the spectral Doppler tracing, indicating that this is in direct continuity with the temporal artery and confirming its identity as the external carotid artery.

divided by nontapering ICA beyond the narrowing, which is now the standard measure of stenosis severity (11).

The European Carotid Surgery Trial (ECST) found similar beneficial results for surgery in symptomatic patients with ICA stenoses greater than 70% (12). The ACAS reports that even asymptomatic patients with greater than 60% stenosis benefit from endarterectomy, finding a 5.8% absolute decreased incidence of stroke within two years (9). These investigators also found a 55% relative benefit of surgery over medical therapy. The benefit may be greater in males since there is significantly higher rate of poor outcomes in males with high-grade stenoses than in females with similar stenoses (13).

The sonographic criteria for diagnosing stenosis vary among authors and include peak systolic velocity (PSV), minimum or end-diastolic velocity, spectral broadening, resistive index, ratios between the peak velocities of ICA and the peak velocities of CCA, ratios between the minimum diastolic velocities of ICA and the minimum diastolic velocities of CCA, ratios between right and left ICAs, and flow direction in the VAs. Given the remarkable diversity of opinion regarding these criteria, there is a remarkable unanimity regarding this test's high accuracy. Most studies indicate 90% to 95% accuracy rates for Doppler ultrasound (14,15), regardless of the criteria chosen.

In 2002, the SRU convened a consensus conference on carotid ultrasound to help standardize the criteria and predictive success of the varied classifications. This conference included leaders from vascular surgery, neurology, radiology, and others who use sonography for carotid evaluation (1). Many prior studies of carotid ultrasound (16–22) have applied variable thresholds for stenosis and threshold velocity values, while still finding high levels of specificity, sensitivity, and accuracy. However, these studies have also demonstrated that at breakpoints of stenosis, such as 50% to 60% and 70% to 80%, the curves that plot stenosis versus PSV and end-diastolic velocity (EDV) show abrupt changes (17,20). These breakpoints thus represent substantial physiologic thresholds of hemodynamically significant stenosis and explain the high levels of accuracy, despite differing criteria. However, at lower degrees of stenosis where such breakpoints do not exist, determining precise degrees of stenosis is not reproducible, accounting for some of the discrepancy in velocity values.

Prior to the development of the consensus criteria, Neale et al. (18) indicated that a PSV of 270 cm/sec was 96% sensitive and 86% specific for 70% stenosis. An EDV of 110 cm/sec was 91% sensitive and 93% specific. With both criteria applied simultaneously, sensitivity was 96%, specificity was 91%, and accuracy was 93%. Moneta et al. (23), using 260 cm/sec PSV and 70 cm/sec EDV for 60% stenosis, had an accuracy of 90%. Values of 290 cm/sec PSV and an EDV of 80 cm/sec achieved a 95% positive predictive value for 60% stenoses. Similar results were obtained with a PSV of 260 cm/sec and a PSV ICA/CCA ratio of 3.2 to 3.5. These authors also noted that prior studies list criteria for 70% as a PSV of 325 cm/sec and a PSV ICA/CCA ratio of 4.

TABLE 1 ■ Spectral Doppler Parameters from SRU Consensus Criteria for Classification of Carotid Stenosis

Percentage of stenosis	PSV (cm/sec)		EDV (cm/sec)	PSV ICA/CCA ratio
Normal	<125	and	<40	<2.0
0–50	<125	and	<40	<2.0
50–69	125–230	and	40–100	2.0–4.0
70–near occlusion	>230	and	>100	>4.0
Near occlusion	Variable		Variable	Variable
Occlusion	No flow		No flow	–

Abbreviations: PSV, peak systolic velocity; EDV, end-diastolic velocity; ICA, internal carotid artery; CCA, common carotid artery; SRU, Society of Radiologists in Ultrasound.

Source: From Ref. 1.

To satisfy the need to detect stenoses at the 60% and 70% levels based on the NASCET, ECST, and ACAS reports and to account for the success of investigators using various threshold criteria, the SRU consensus panel created six broad categories and criteria (Table 1) (1). They also recommended using three primary criteria for diagnosing ICA stenosis—PSV, EDV, and PSV ICA/CCA ratio (Figs. 7 and 8) (1). PSV is the most widely used and evaluated, and EDV adds information in high-grade stenoses. The PSV ratio, calculated as the PSV of the proximal ICA divided by the PSV of the distal CCA, may help to confirm a stenosis (1). It may also serve as the primary means of diagnosis in tandem carotid stenosis.

Although these criteria lack independent validation in large patient populations, they reflect a combination of criteria gleaned from several of the reports referenced herein. This scheme optimizes sensitivity and recognizes the uncertainty reflected in inconsistencies in the literature. The panel also acknowledged the inability of carotid sonography to finely categorize mild-to-moderate degrees of stenosis (1). The recommendations should be guidelines for institutions without internally validated criteria and are not intended to replace criteria at programs that have their own validated data. These criteria address grading of ICA stenosis, primarily for single lesions in the proximal ICA. Several potential pitfalls limit their applicability for certain individuals and will be discussed in detail near the end of this chapter.

Diagnostic Criteria—Vertebral

Sonographic evaluation of the VAs has not received as much attention as carotid ultrasound, likely because no consensus exists on optimal therapy for VA stenosis (24) and because the origins of the VAs often cannot be seen. Nevertheless, VA disease may be detected incidentally, and clinicians may request sonograms to evaluate symptoms originating from VA disease or subclavian artery disease that can affect VA waveforms. Therefore, the sonographer should obtain vertebral spectral waveforms in every patient and the interpreting physician should be alert to the manifestations of vertebral disease.

Little data in the literature addresses grading of VA stenoses. Segments showing spectral broadening or color Doppler aliasing should be interrogated further. Using angle correction and signal optimization similar to carotid evaluation, a PSV should be measured at the point of stenosis.

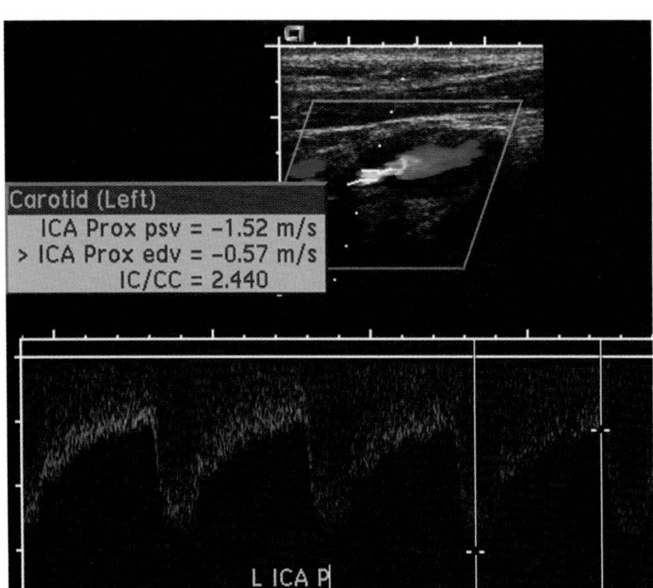

FIGURE 7 ■ Patient with 50% to 69% internal carotid artery stenosis. The peak systolic velocity exceeds the threshold of 1.25 m/sec. Also, there is mild spectral broadening with spectral energy filling within the envelope to the baseline.

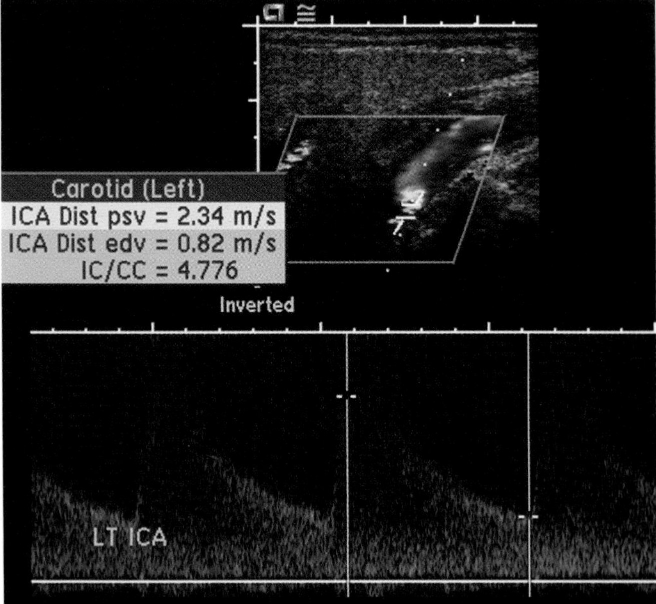

FIGURE 8 ■ Proximal internal carotid artery (ICA) stenosis of greater than 70%. The peak systolic velocity exceeds the threshold of 2.3 m/sec. The spectrum has greater intensity signal at lower energies and the signal from the envelope is weaker and more ill defined.

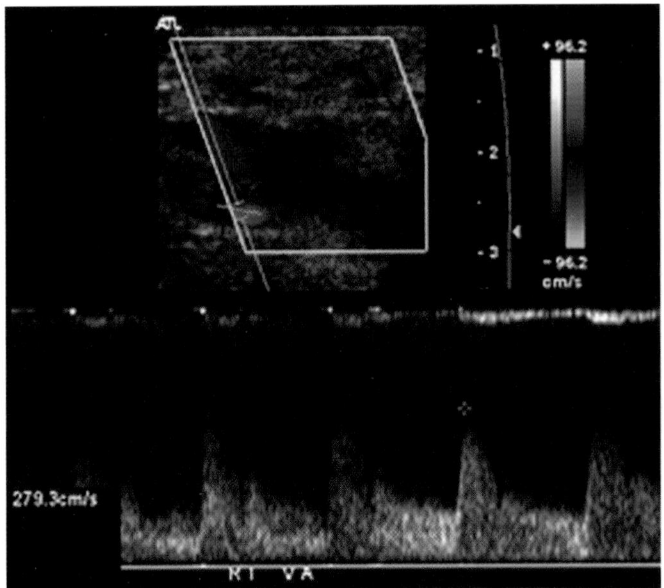

FIGURE 9 ■ Vertebral stenosis. Although the stenosis is not visualized within the vertebral artery, the peak systolic velocity exceeds 2.7 m/sec. Spectral broadening to various degrees is normal in a vertebral artery and cannot be used alone to demonstrate stenosis.

The normal VA waveform has rapid systolic acceleration (upstroke) and antegrade diastolic flow. Normal PSV of the VA is less than 60 cm/sec (25). A PSV above 100 cm/sec correlates with stenosis at the VA origin (Fig. 9) (26), although this value has not been widely reproduced and is not part of the consensus criteria. Poststenotic spectral broadening and other secondary changes may exist cranial to the origin, but velocity criteria have not been developed for stenoses in these areas. Elevated PSV with a PSV ratio above 1.5 relative to the artery immediately caudal to the level of stenosis warrants further evaluation (27). Elevated velocities may occur in nonstenotic VAs secondary to compensatory flow in the setting of contralateral VA occlusion or hypoplasia.

Comparison with Magnetic Resonance Angiography, CT Angiography, and Conventional Angiography

Because of its accuracy, low cost, absence of risk, and nearly universal availability, ultrasound is the initial test of choice for suspected carotid disease. Magnetic resonance angiography (MRA) has gained increased acceptance in recent years, but its high costs, contraindications such as pacemakers, concerns such as claustrophobia, and the need for intravenous injection have constrained its use. Computed tomography angiography (CTA) has also become increasingly popular because of improved resolution and speed, but the need for intravenous contrast and ionizing radiation limits its use. Ultrasound, MRA, and CTA are usually compared to conventional angiography as the reference standard. Ultrasound may underestimate the severity of disease and is more operator dependent. Magnetic resonance imaging (MRI) may overestimate disease and is degraded by motion artifacts, limiting its use in uncooperative or impaired patients. For MRA, a combination of contrast-enhanced MRA and three-dimensional (3D) time-of-flight imaging is highly sensitive and specific (28). Multiplanar reformatted CTA is very sensitive for carotid stenosis, as compared to rotational angiography, although it may slightly underestimate the degree of stenosis (29).

Unfortunately, an assumption that has not been widely challenged is that angiography is the appropriate reference standard. It was the first effective test for carotid stenosis, was widely studied, and generates easily understandable and reproducible images. However, angiography has not been directly compared to these alternative tests for stroke predictive value, but it has maintained its role as the designated standard because of its early success.

Additionally, the now commonplace digital subtraction angiography may not correlate best with conventional angiography, with at least one study (30), indicating that ultrasound correlates better with direct angiography than digital angiography. Angiography may also underestimate the severity of a stenosis (31,32). The two-dimensional (2D) images may be inaccurate for measuring eccentric plaques even using three projections (33), and ultrasound, MRA, and CTA may better visualize the entire cross section of the vessels. Also, these methods directly depict the plaque and lumen, whereas angiography demonstrates only the residual lumen.

Furthermore, because of the 2D limitations of angiography, the standard criterion became percent diameter stenosis. However, the percentage area stenosis is more relevant to flow limitation and depends on plaque shape (34). For example, a discrete semicircular plaque, viewed in profile, creating a 50% diameter stenosis may cause an approximately 50% area stenosis, whereas a circumferential plaque creating the same 50% diameter stenosis causes a 75% area stenosis.

To satisfy the historical standard of angiography, ultrasound empirically converts physiologic parameters of flow to percentage diameter stenosis. PSV is a valuable parameter to calculate stenosis because fluid flowing in a closed tube must increase its speed of flow through a narrowed area to maintain the same volumetric flow rate. Flow is the product of velocity and cross-sectional area, and velocity elevations correlate well with angiographic narrowing despite flow-rate variations. Velocity values are preferred to visual area calculation because ultrasound is unable to reliably identify the actual residual lumen size secondary to plaque irregularity, spatial resolution limitations, and calcification in plaques commonly causing shadowing.

As noted earlier, conclusions of prior research regarding risk of stroke are based entirely on the empirical association of increased risk with stenoses exceeding 60% to 70%. Despite elucidating much of the pathophysiology of embolic stroke, we remain without satisfactory means of identifying the source of emboli in individual patients (35). We have yet to determine whether ultrasound, angiography, or another test will prove superior for predicting the risk of stroke.

In recent years, ultrasound's high specificity has firmly entrenched it as the preliminary test for carotid disease. A negative study reduces the need for carotid angiography, with its approximately 1% morbidity and mortality in carotid stenosis (36). The role of MRA and CTA as diagnostic adjuncts is evolving, and in departments without good sonographic studies, they may be the primary diagnostic modalities. Angiographers have the unique advantage that they can treat a detected lesion, mainly by stenting. Angiography and MRA have the advantage of depicting extensive areas of the intracranial cerebral circulation, allowing direct display of atherosclerotic lesions beyond the areas visualized by ultrasound. Many laboratories employ these tests in sequence, first identifying the risk of substantial stenosis with ultrasound, MRA, or CTA, then confirming severity and defining the pattern with angiography.

Plaque Characterization

The value of sonographically characterizing plaques remains controversial. Much research has recently examined measuring the intima-medial thickness (IMT) as an early predictor of atherosclerotic disease prior to the appearance of discrete plaques (Fig. 10). To improve the consistency of technical and diagnostic criteria, a recent consensus conference was convened (37). Increased IMT is associated with early vascular disease and is common in older populations. The clinical utility of increased IMT has not been determined, but it is an independent predictor of stroke (38).

Pathologic studies have shown that internal plaque hemorrhage increases risk for forming superficial clots in plaques that subsequently embolize (39–42). Some authors contend that identifying high-risk plaques by their heterogeneous sonographic characteristics and low-level echoes with hypoechoic or anechoic areas is highly reliable (Fig. 11). Some studies show direct correlation of cerebrovascular risk with the presence of hypoechoic or anechoic content (43). Patients with echolucent plaques have significantly higher rate of stroke after carotid stenting (44). One difficulty is a paucity of evidence regarding interobserver variability for identifying plaque heterogeneity. Although computerized gray-scale median quantification of plaque echolucency has been used, visual evaluation correlates well and may be used in general practice (45).

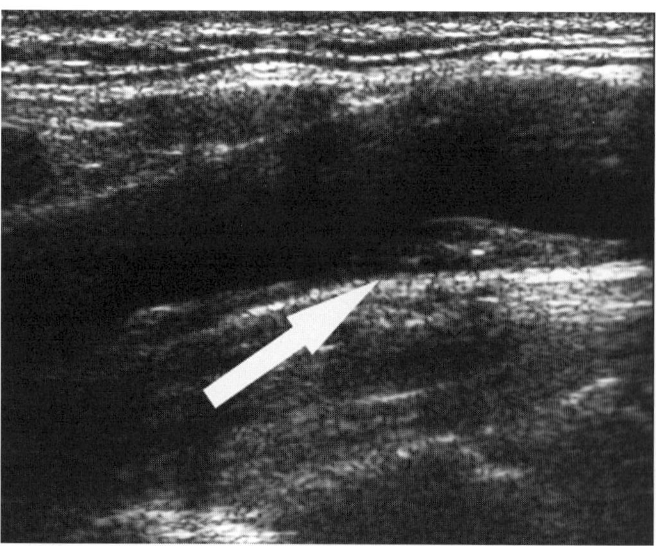

FIGURE 11 ■ Plaque heterogeneity. The plaque surface is difficult to discern (*arrow*). Also, areas of decreased echogenicity are present, indicating possible internal plaque hemorrhage and an increased risk of rupture and embolization.

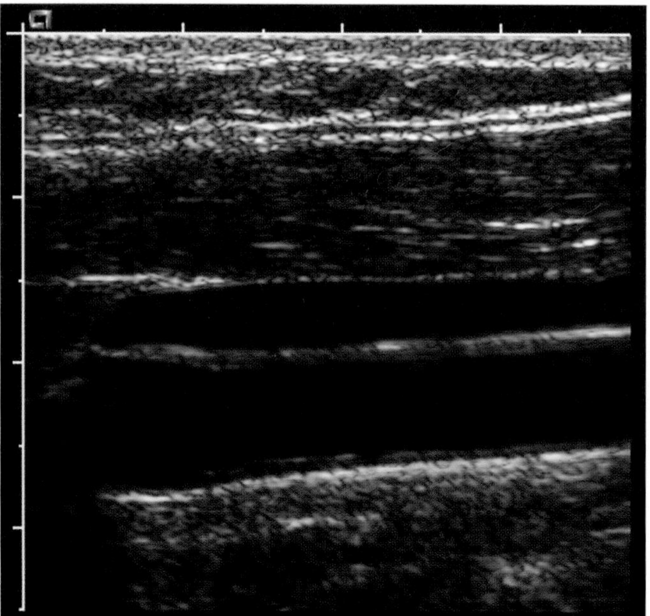

FIGURE 10 ■ Intimal thickening. This view of a common carotid artery to the bifurcation demonstrates diffuse intimal thickening with a mildly irregular intimal surface.

Markedly hypoechoic plaques are associated with increased risk of ulceration and cerebrovascular events (46,47). For each level of stenosis severity, angiographically irregular plaques have an increased risk of symptoms and stroke compared with smooth plaques (3,4). Hypoechoic plaques have a higher fatty composition than echogenic fibrous plaques (48) and may blend on real-time gray-scale imaging with the anechoic vascular lumen. Color Doppler may detect such high-risk plaques by demonstrating flow voids. More echogenicity indicates increased fibrosis with a lower risk of complications, and calcifications within plaques do not worsen the prognosis. MRI detection of a lipid core within plaques is also a poor prognostic indicator with an increased 68% risk versus 31% in lipid poor plaques (49).

Surgery Based upon Sonography Alone

Many surgeons will forego angiography before endarterectomy when noninvasive imaging is conclusive. Some will operate based solely upon sonographic findings or using data from ultrasound and MRA. In these institutions, quality assurance is essential for providing the surgeon with the necessary information.

Alternative Interventions for Carotid Atherosclerosis

Endovascular carotid angioplasty and stenting is an increasingly used alternative to CEA for cerebrovascular disease. Now that CEA, at least for severe stenosis of more than 70%, has been validated, interest has risen in developing randomized clinical trials comparing it to nonsurgical interventions. In a Cochrane Systematic Review of 1269 patients in five randomized clinical trials, there was no difference between CEA and carotid stenting in terms of death or stroke at 30-day safety monitoring or one-year followup (50). Although a carotid stent may develop in-stent stenosis, this is rare (3.6% of stents) and responds well to endovascular therapy (51). The risk is higher in women and diabetics (52). Based on systematic data, endarterectomy and stenting appear equally efficacious, with less nerve injury in the stenting group. A distal balloon protection system may further reduce the risk of embolic events during stenting (53). The Stenting and Angioplasty with Protection in Patients at High Risk for Endarterectomy (SAPPHIRE) study has suggested carotid stenting with distal protection may reduce adverse events relative to CEA (54). However, one source has shown that as many as 36% of patients cannot receive a carotid stent, usually due to excessive carotid tortuosity (55).

Risk and Cost of Diagnostic Workup and Treatment

Although the NASCET, ACAS, and ECST studies have demonstrated the value of endarterectomy for symptomatic patients with greater than 70% stenosis and asymptomatic patients with greater than 60% stenosis, several aspects of the workup and treatment remain unresolved. Ultrasound is generally the first imaging study performed for suspected carotid stenosis because it is inexpensive and noninvasive. The role of MRA and CTA varies among institutions, as their cost is several times that of ultrasound. Still, MRA and CTA are useful in preventing unnecessary angiograms in cases of equivocal ultrasound. In a cost-effectiveness analysis of the evaluation of patients with prior TIA or minor stroke using modeling from a societal perspective, ultrasound alone was the most cost-effective tool. Although MRA increased the diagnostic sensitivity and specificity, the costs per additional quality-adjusted-life-year were well beyond what is generally considered within reason for a widespread health strategy (56). For high-risk surgical patients, CEA appears more cost-effective than carotid stenting, although the efficacy is similar (57).

As screening for carotid disease has increased, guidelines for selecting patients require standardization to ensure cost-effectiveness. Other screening initiatives, such as whole body screening computed tomography (CT), have met with limited success or were implemented without scientific validation or economic analysis (58). While the ACAS study showed that asymptomatic patients with greater than 60% stenosis benefit from therapy, Lovelace et al. demonstrated that patients with less than 60% stenosis but PSV above 175 cm/sec have a significantly increased rate of progression into the above 60% category. Therefore, these patients require close monitoring on a semiannual basis regardless of symptoms (59).

Potential of Microbubble Contrast Agents for Carotid Evaluation

Although not yet approved in the USA for noncardiac indications, microbubble ultrasound contrast agents are widely used in Europe, Asia, and Canada, and have shown excellent safety profiles. These contrast agents use tiny stabilized bubbles to increase the reflection of sound waves, increasing the signal from perfused vessels and tissues. Many ultrasound vendors have developed specific packages to detect the sonographic reflections of microbubbles. As a result, studies have shown improved visualization of carotid stenosis after intravenous injection of microbubble contrast (60). However, until Food and Drug Administration (FDA) approval occurs for noncardiac indications, use in the United States remains mainly limited to research.

PITFALLS AND ARTIFACTS

The potential pitfalls and artifacts in carotid sonography are separated into four categories: (*i*) anatomic pitfalls, (*ii*) physiologic pitfalls, (*iii*) technical errors, and (*iv*) artifacts.

Anatomic Pitfalls

Distinguishing the ICA from the ECA

The ICA may be difficult to correctly differentiate from the ECA. Distinguishing features are listed in Table 2. In about 95% of patients, the ICA is posterior and lateral to the ECA; but it can ascend posterolateral or lateral. One reliable distinguishing feature of the ECA is branching vessels; the ICA has no branches in the neck. A temporal tap maneuver also helps to confirm the identity of the ECA. Rapid tapping of the supra-auricular area of the temporal artery transmits pulsations (a sawtooth pattern) on spectral Doppler as noted in the Examination Technique section above (Fig. 6) (7). This waveform may occasionally be seen in the ICA with the tap maneuver but is usually dampened.

Tortuous Carotids

The carotid arteries are commonly tortuous and elongated in chronically hypertensive and elderly patients

TABLE 2 ■ Distinguishing Features of the Normal Internal and External Carotid Arteries

Feature	ICA	ECA
Neck branches	No	Yes
Temporal tap	No	Transmitted pulsations
Orientation	Posteriorly, toward spine	Anteriorly, toward face
Doppler waveform	Low-resistance flow	High-resistance flow

Abbreviations: ICA, internal carotid artery; ECA, external carotid artery.

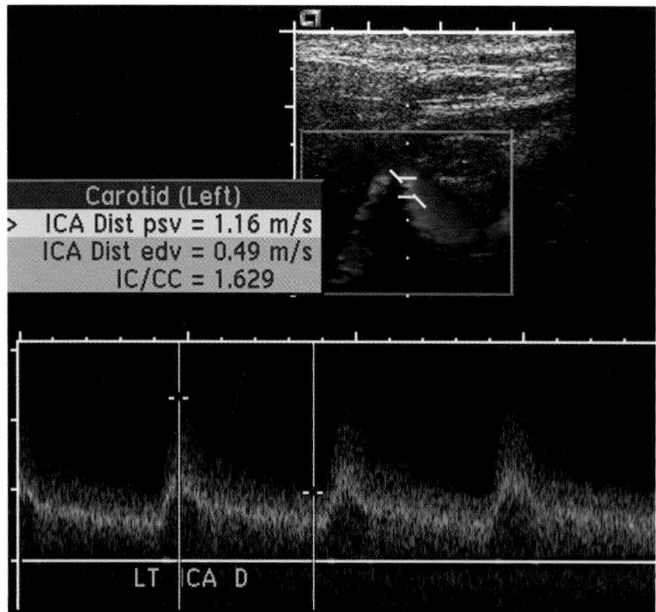

FIGURE 12 ■ Tortuous internal carotid artery (ICA). This ICA is markedly tortuous. This may be a cause of spectral broadening, even without stenosis. The spectral tracing demonstrates a more ill-defined envelope and distribution of spectral energy to the mid range of the spectrum. Color Doppler aliasing is present at the arc of tortuosity.

and may be difficult to interrogate with Doppler (Fig. 12). Artifactually high velocities may follow misapplication of the angle correction cursor and approach at a nonstandard insonation angle. Signs such as abnormal waveform characteristics may provide some warning, but reporting the level of certainty is advisable, especially when velocity values are in borderline ranges.

High Bifurcation

In some patients, particularly those with relatively short necks, the high positions of the carotid bifurcations and proximal ICAs may obscure them. Visualization of the ICA may be limited by the mandibular angle. This situation is one of the uncommon causes of a nondiagnostic study. MRA or CTA may better evaluate these patients.

Postoperative Changes

Patients after CEA are commonly followed with carotid ultrasounds. Although recurrent stenosis in the treated carotid is rare, progressive disease is more common in the contralateral carotid within approximately two years (61). These patients should receive yearly surveillance unless clinical considerations necessitate more frequent followup. In patients with at least 50% contralateral ICA stenosis, follow-up studies should be performed as often as 6 to 12 months (62). Over a longer period of time, re-stenosis of the ipsilateral carotid may occur.

The SRU consensus criteria have not been validated in patients with previous CEA or stenting. Thus, categorizing specific degrees of stenosis may not be accurate in these settings. Velocity of flow in patients with prior carotid surgery or other interventions varies. Spectral broadening often persists after CEA without residual or recurrent disease (2,63–65) and is often striking in vein patch graft carotid surgery (2). Spectral analysis may demonstrate discordantly high or low velocities in the area of the vein patch graft, suggesting markedly disturbed flow even when color Doppler shows a widely patent graft. Incorrect assumptions of the true Doppler angle in these areas of disturbed flow can result in erroneous velocity determinations. Relatively normal flow in the CCA proximal to and in the ICA distal to the graft suggests no occlusion or severe stenosis. In these patients, MRA is a good alternative unless a metallic stent has been placed, since the metal will create artifact obscuring the proximal ICA lumen. In the immediate postoperative setting, gas in the tissues surrounding the carotid may impair sonographic visualization. This gas usually resolves within one to two days.

Physiologic Pitfalls

High-Resistance Flow in the ICA or CCA

Distal ICA occlusions or high-grade stenoses often cause a high-resistance flow pattern with little or no diastolic flow, represented by a high resistive index in the CCA or proximal ICA. This may be associated with low-velocity systolic "thump" waveforms in the proximal ICA. Because the high-resistance pattern is similar to the normal flow pattern in the ECA, the appearance may be termed "externalization" of ICA flow (Fig. 13). Absence of diastolic flow in the CCA should suggest occlusion or severe stenosis of the ICA. When present in the proximal ICA, externalization may signify one of several conditions, as shown in Table 3. Most of the conditions listed here have associated clinical signs or historical information, which should be specifically elicited. Also, because of the common occurrence

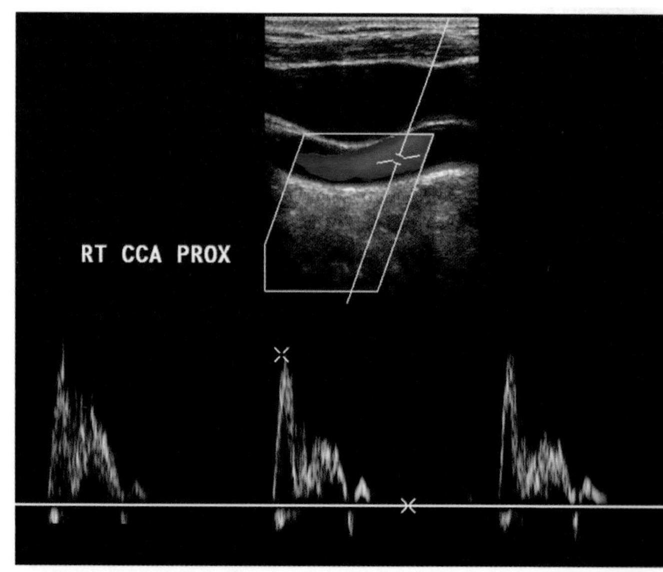

FIGURE 13 ■ High-resistance common carotid artery (CCA) spectral tracing shows minimal reversal of flow in early diastole with no persistent diastolic flow, indicating a resistivity index of greater than 1.0. This pattern can be found in patients with occlusion of the internal carotid artery.

TABLE 3 ■ Causes and Features of High-Resistance Flow in the ICA

Cause or feature	Symmetry	Velocities
Low cardiac output	Yes	Low in all normal vessels[a]
Aortic valvular insufficiency	Yes	Normal to high peak[b]
Distal ICA stenosis	No	Low peak
Distal small vessel disease	Possible	Normal or low peak
Increased intracranial pressure	Yes	Normal or low peak

[a]Confirm by studying other systems such as the femoral arteries.
[b]Aortic insufficiency may also be accompanied by reversed flow component in early diastole.
Abbreviation: ICA, internal carotid artery.

of multiple sites of vascular disease, combinations of these conditions should be considered.

Abnormally Low-Resistance Flow in the ICA or CCA

Severe stenosis or near occlusion proximal to the area of insonation may cause dampened flow in the CCA or ICA, recognized by low-amplitude waveforms with rounded peaks and little difference between the peak systolic and the end-diastolic flow velocities (low resistive index) (Fig. 14A). The stenosis may be at the origin of either CCA or within the brachiocephalic artery if the right CCA is affected. Slightly lesser degrees of stenosis cause elevated diastolic flow with elevated systolic peaks. In either case, when the vessel is sampled near the stenosis, spectral broadening is prominent. Uncommonly, carotid-cavernous sinus fistulae, usually due to trauma, cause a high-PSV with high diastolic flow.

Low-Resistance Flow in the ECA

While ICA stenosis may suppress diastolic velocity within the CCA and proximal ICA, it may also elevate diastolic velocity in the ECA. Occlusion of the ICA produces collateral circulation to the carotid siphon through the ECA and ophthalmic arteries secondary to complex intracranial–extracranial anastomoses, second only to the circle of Willis in degree of collateral. This decreased resistive index, thus, may represent recruitment of the ECA to the low-resistance cerebral circulation, termed "internalization" of ECA flow (Fig. 15).

With ICA occlusion and ECA collateral flow to the internal circulation, the ICA may not be visible, and the primary collateralized trunk of the ECA can be dilated with an ICA-like waveform. In such cases, the ECA may be mistaken for the ICA, and the first ECA branch may be mistaken for the main ECA. Thus, one may miss complete

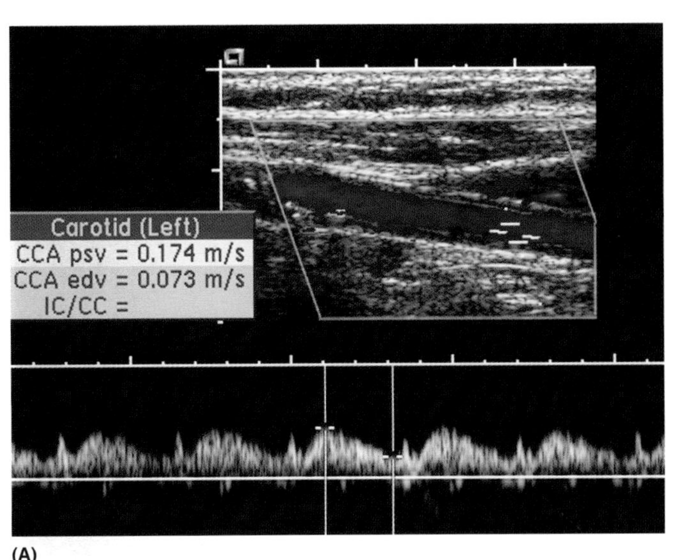

(A)

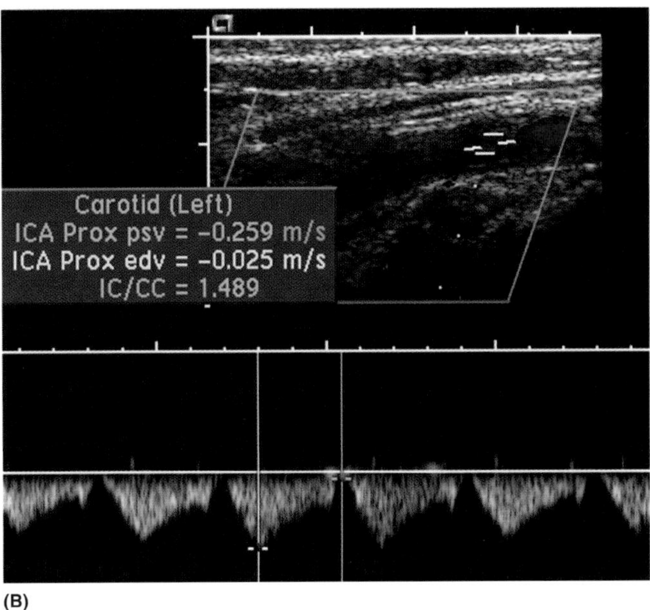

(B)

FIGURE 14 A AND B ■ Severe internal carotid artery (ICA) stenosis. (**A**) Markedly abnormal spectral Doppler signals in the common carotid artery (CCA) are secondary to a high-grade proximal CCA stenosis. (**B**) The ICA in this same patient demonstrates a delayed systolic upstroke, also reflecting the more proximal stenosis. However, if velocity criteria alone had been used to diagnose stenosis, this condition would not have been detected.

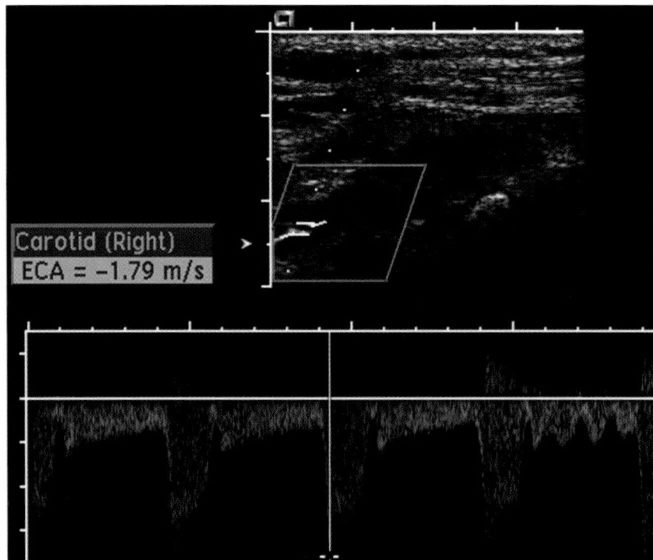

FIGURE 15 ■ Internalization of external carotid artery (ECA). Flow within the ECA has unusually strong diastolic flow but is confirmed as the ECA by the temporal tap maneuver as seen on the fourth diastolic segment. This is termed "internalization" of ECA flow and reflects collateralization in a patient with a flow-limiting internal carotid artery lesion.

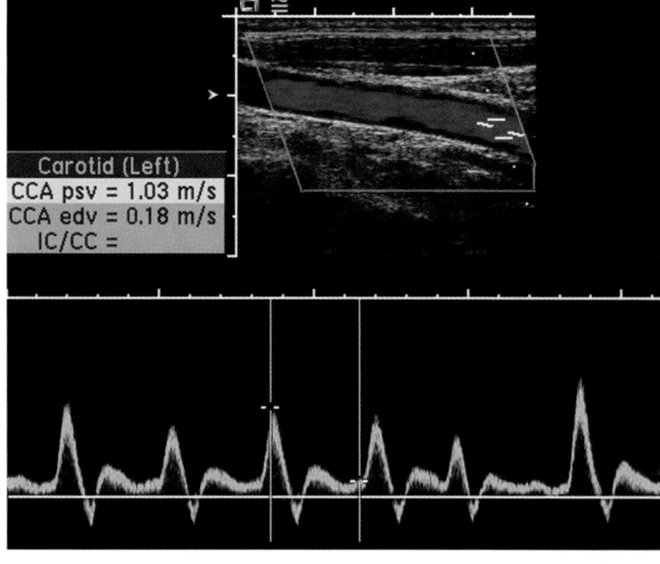

FIGURE 16 ■ Aortic regurgitation. Flow within the common carotid artery in this patient has an early diastolic flow reversal. This may be seen in aortic valvular regurgitation. This patient also has an irregular heart rate from atrial fibrillation. The peak systolic pulse following a long pause, as seen near the end of this tracing, is artifactually elevated and should not be used for measuring for stenosis.

or near-complete ICA occlusion. The temporal tap maneuver usually resolves this question.

Low-Velocity ICA Flow

Generalized low-amplitude, low-velocity ICA flow occurs in several situations. If flow through a stenosed artery is critically restricted, flow velocity begins to decline before complete occlusion (Fig. 14B). This waveform features a distorted signal with spectral broadening, but resembling low-resistance flow.

A severe brachiocephalic or proximal CCA stenosis may reduce flow and produce spuriously decreased velocity measurements (66,67). In these patients, there is often a downstream delay in the systolic upstroke associated with low velocities. Tandem stenoses proximal and distal to the point of interrogation may cause low velocity and distorted flow signals. Cardiac disease may also create a low-flow, low-velocity state. These possibilities are summarized in Table 4.

Effects of Cardiac Disease

Cardiovascular pathophysiology, such as cardiac arrhythmias, aortic valvular lesions, and severe cardiomyopathies, can produce abnormal carotid artery flow waveforms and alter carotid velocity measurements. These situations limit Doppler flow velocity analysis for quantifying stenosis. Hypertension may result in higher-velocity measurements than in normotensive patients with comparable carotid artery narrowing. Conversely, hypotension or poor cardiac output can decrease both systolic and diastolic velocities. Bradycardia may result in increased systolic velocities due to increased stroke volume (68,69).

Cardiac Arrhythmia ■ An irregular heart rate may cause velocities that are variable from beat to beat. After a prolonged diastole, the subsequent PSV often abnormally increases. In diagnosing stenosis, the peak velocity from a beat immediately after a normal-length beat of about one second, provides the best value (Fig. 16). With

TABLE 4 ■ Causes and Features of Low-Velocity Flow in the ICA

Cause or feature	Symmetry	Resistive index[a]	Peak
Low cardiac output	Yes	Low	Sharp
Aortic valvular stenosis	Yes	Low	Rounded
Proximal ICA stenosis	No	Low	Rounded
Tandem, other proximal lesions	No	Low	Rounded
Distal small vessel disease	Possible	Normal, high	Sharp
Increased intracranial pressure	Yes	High	Sharp

[a]Resistive index = (PSV − EDV)/PSV.

Abbreviations: ICA, internal carotid artery; PSV, peak systolic velocity; EDV, end-diastolic velocity.

tachycardia or bradycardia, peak-flow velocities may be unpredictably altered. These circumstances reduce the certainty of results, and one must cautiously grade the severity of stenoses using Doppler criteria, reporting these concerns.

Intermittent Reversal of Flow in the Carotid Arteries ■ CCA occlusion can cause bidirectional flow in the ICA in a patient with a patent ICA and ECA. Collateral flow through the circle of Willis and ECA create a peculiar to-and-fro circle of flow into and out of the ICA and ECA with reversed ECA flow supplying blood to the brain (70). Alternatively, aortic valvular incompetence can lead to intermittent backflow during diastole, while the systolic flow remains antegrade (Fig. 16).

Symmetric High-Velocity Flow without Apparent Vascular Cause ■ At times, flow velocities appear elevated without apparent substantial carotid atherosclerotic disease. The differential diagnosis is outlined in Table 5.

Contralateral ICA Stenosis

Recommended diagnostic criteria for grading of carotid stenosis may not be valid if there is severe disease of the contralateral CCA or ICA, because high-grade stenosis may significantly alter contralateral flow (71–73), through collateral shunting and increased velocity, particularly in areas of stenosis. Once patients have undergone CEA or stenting, the elevated velocities in the contralateral ICA decrease (74–76). In one series, stenosis severity category by ultrasound decreased after a contralateral endarterectomy in about half the patients (76). Similarly, an ipsilateral high-grade intracranial artery stenosis may reduce anticipated peak velocity at a proximal ICA stenosis. Therefore, it is important to extend the Doppler interrogation of the ICA as far cephalad as possible (16).

Carotid Artery Occlusion vs. Residual Trickle of Flow

In internal carotid occlusion, distinguishing complete and near-complete occlusion requires additional efforts. This is a critical distinction because a high-grade stenosis is a candidate for surgical endarterectomy or carotid stent placement, whereas complete occlusion is not. Duplex ultrasound may not detect all cases of minimal residual flow (77–81). Conversely, angiography may rarely fail to detect minimal residual flow suggested by Doppler ultrasound.

As a stenosis approaches occlusion, the high-velocity blood flow reduces to a trickle. Early pulsed Doppler systems were unable to detect these low-amplitude, low-flow velocities. The introduction of color Doppler and advances in the sensitivity of flow detection has largely ameliorated this problem (82–84). Power Doppler is currently the most sensitive sonographic technique for detecting minimal flow (5), although its high sensitivity may lead to falsely identifying flow. However, a trickle of flow may go undetected if there is suboptimal visualization (81). Further imaging by MRA, CTA, or angiography may be necessary to avoid denying a patient the potential benefit of treatment when minimal residual flow exists. Small systolic "blips" do not indicate patency (Fig. 17), because the thrombus or plaque within the ICA can conduct transmitted pulsations, creating this signal.

TABLE 5 ■ Differential Diagnosis of Symmetric High-Velocity Flow without Carotid Vascular Disease

- Hypertension
- Systemic arteriovenous fistula
- Intracardiac shunt
- Hyperpyrexia
- Other causes of increased cardiac output

Partly or Completely Reversed VA Flow

Subclavian steal syndrome is caused by a proximal subclavian artery stenosis or occlusion (67), in which the subclavian artery "steals" blood flow from the basilar circulation through retrograde VA flow. This process can produce symptoms of vertebrobasilar insufficiency, most pronounced during arm exercise and in certain head positions. Subclavian steal is suggested when Doppler spectral tracings or color Doppler ultrasound images demonstrate reversed or partially reversed high-resistance VA flow.

The presence or severity of a subclavian steal can be studied with provocative maneuvers. If a blood pressure cuff is inflated above arterial pressure on the arm with the abnormal VA flow, the flow should partly or completely revert to normal, because flow to the stealing arm is obstructed. On releasing the cuff, there is usually a rapid reperfusion of the briefly ischemic arm,

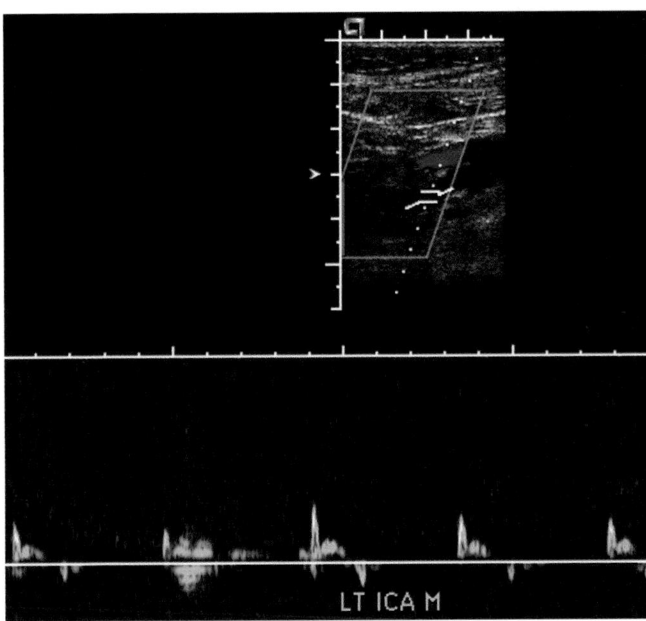

FIGURE 17 ■ Internal carotid artery (ICA) occlusion. The Doppler signal in this occluded ICA probably does not represent residual flow but rather motion of the thrombus from transmitted pulsations from the common carotid artery.

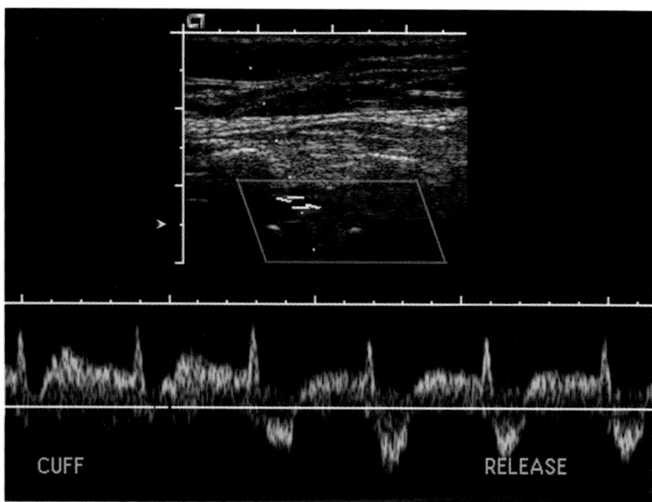

FIGURE 18 ■ Vertebral artery reversal. The first three pulses in this vertebral artery were performed after application of an inflated blood pressure cuff, limiting the ability of the subclavian artery to siphon blood from the vertebral artery. Following release of the cuff, there is a stronger reversed component of flow as the now ischemic arm vasodilates and draws more blood from the vertebral artery.

leading to an accentuated reversal of flow before returning to the baseline appearance (Fig. 18). Conversely, exercising the arm often accentuates vertebral retrograde flow.

Incomplete subclavian steals may not demonstrate this reversed VA flow without provocative maneuvers. A partial subclavian steal may also appear on Doppler with retrograde flow in systole and antegrade flow in diastole (85). Kliewer et al. categorized the severity of partial reversal of VA flow using a four-point scale. Even minor deceleration of flow during systole without reversal was still associated with an increased prevalence of subclavian stenosis, with the prevalence of stenosis increasing with worsened decelerations of systolic flow (86). To avoid mistaking flow reversal in a subclavian steal as normal pulsatile vertebral venous flow, spectral Doppler analysis may identify the arterial nature of the signal in a single visualized vessel.

Other Unusual Distorted Carotid and Vertebral Waveforms

In VA occlusion near its origin, flow is shunted to the thyrocervical and costocervical axes, with compensatory enlargement of the opposite VA. Collateral circulation arising from occlusion of large branches of the aortic arch travels through the intercostal and internal mammary arteries to the subclavian and then through the branches of the thyrocervical and costocervical axes to the vertebral and carotid arteries. Other uncommon situations include proximal innominate artery occlusion, carotid dissection, and cavernous sinus fistulas. When odd waveforms present in situations defying accurate diagnosis of lesion localization, MRA, CTA, or angiography can assess locations of disease other than the carotid arteries.

Technical Errors

ECA

In the carotid ultrasound evaluation, only the origin of the ECA is evaluated because plaque in the ECA is rarely clinically significant. There are no standardized criteria for quantification of stenosis at the ECA origin. However, stenosis of the ECA, as suggested by high-PSV and turbulent flow, may cause a cervical bruit in the absence of ICA stenosis (Fig. 3A and B).

Gray-Scale Errors in Estimating Stenosis

Gray-scale measurements should not be used to calculate the severity of stenosis because they correlate poorly with angiography and were not used in NASCET or ACAS studies. However, they may clarify or corroborate Doppler results (Fig. 19) in situations such as severe plaques with normal velocity criteria.

Assigning Doppler Angle

Inaccurate Doppler angle correction is probably the most common error in carotid sonography. Angles greater than 60° can artifactually elevate calculated flow velocity. Angling the Doppler cursor parallel to the vessel walls rather than to the direction of the flow jet caused by the stenosis, which is often oblique to the wall in high-grade stenoses (Fig. 2), leads to underestimated peak velocities. Since the original endarterectomy studies oriented the Doppler angle parallel to the artery wall, this concept is controversial.

Artifacts

Color "Bleed"

Color Doppler may overestimate residual lumen diameter, because the color may "bleed" into the gray-scale image

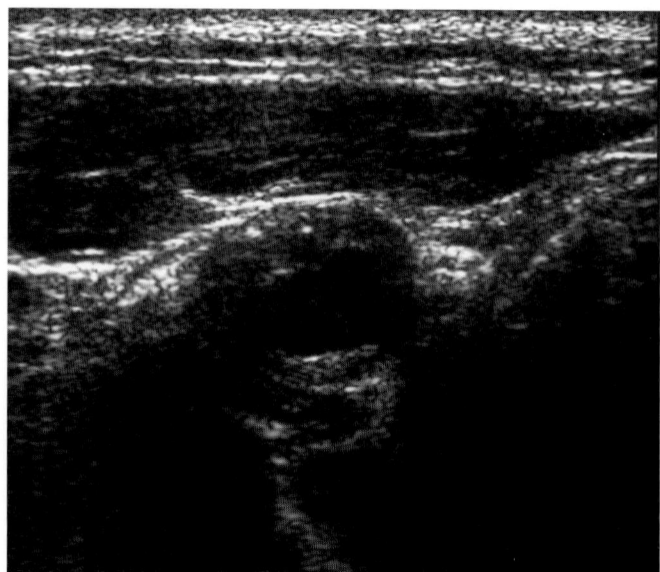

FIGURE 19 ■ This transverse image of the carotid bulb demonstrates severe asymmetric thickening of the wall. Such images do not reliably estimate stenosis but can be used to corroborate a stenosis calculated from velocity criteria.

and obscure small plaques, a problem less pronounced in newer units. Doppler adjustments can minimize this effect of color bleed (16) but may not eliminate it because of limitations in color spatial resolution and other technical variations based on color frequency, variations in equipment, and technical settings.

The use of a non-Doppler technique, B-flow, can show the flow of blood without any color bleed, and its use may increase color Doppler accuracy in visualizing stenoses (87,88). This technique demonstrates blood flow without the color Doppler format and does not suffer from color bleed. However, B-flow is not available in all ultrasound machines.

Calcification Shadowing

Factors contributing to poor visualization of a high-grade stenosis include irregular plaque or plaque-containing calcification, which may shadow and obscure the vessel lumen (Fig. 20A and B). It is surprisingly uncommon for this to lead to a nondiagnostic examination if a qualified operator examines the vessel carefully. Secondary criteria, such as high-resistance flow in the vessel proximal to the calcification or turbulence distal to the calcification with a dampened low-amplitude flow pattern, suggest a possible stenosis (66). For cases with severe carotid calcification-limiting evaluation, MRA or CTA may prove diagnostic.

Soft Plaque

Noncalcified carotid plaque may have acoustic properties similar to those of blood and may be almost invisible on gray-scale images. In some cases, the vessel may be anechoic or hypoechoic and yet be totally occluded (89,90). Color Doppler and power Doppler can readily distinguish between these hypoechoic lesions and flowing blood (82).

Spurious Flow Voids

When the angle of insonation approaches 90°, areas of flow within the vessel may not generate any Doppler signal. Spurious flow voids in color Doppler images may erroneously suggest plaque or may overestimate plaque severity and luminal narrowing, a problem in very tortuous vessels. These flow voids can also occur with inappropriate Doppler power and gain settings (16). Analysis of the color Doppler region using sonographic steering with linear phased arrays and maintaining a Doppler angle less than 60° can prevent this problem.

Spectral Broadening without Stenosis

Spectral broadening in the carotid artery does not always correlate with vessel narrowing. The magnitude of spectral broadening is affected by the Doppler sampling site, the flow velocity, and the size of the sample volume (91–94) and may occur at points of vessel curvature (Fig. 12). In small vessels with greater friction effects at their walls, spectral broadening may occur because of more slowly moving blood near the wall than at the center.

Disturbed Flow

Unusual flow patterns occur in both normal and diseased vessels. Kinks, dives, curves, and arterial branching may produce flow disturbances in normal vessels. Examples include the physiologic flow separation (locally reversed flow) that may occur near the wall of the carotid bulb (Fig. 21) (82,95–97).

Aliasing on Spectral Doppler

Another potential source of error in Doppler analysis is aliasing on spectral Doppler, caused by an inability to detect the true peak velocities because of an overly slow Doppler sampling rate [pulse repetition frequency (PRF)]. Aliasing allows identification of potential stenoses on color Doppler, but it may create a confusing

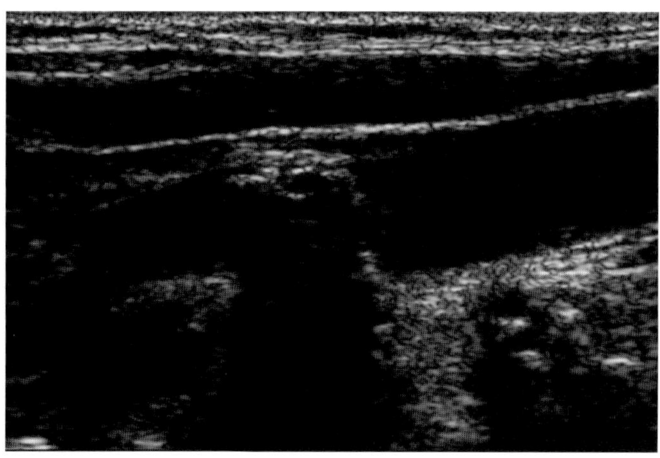

(A)

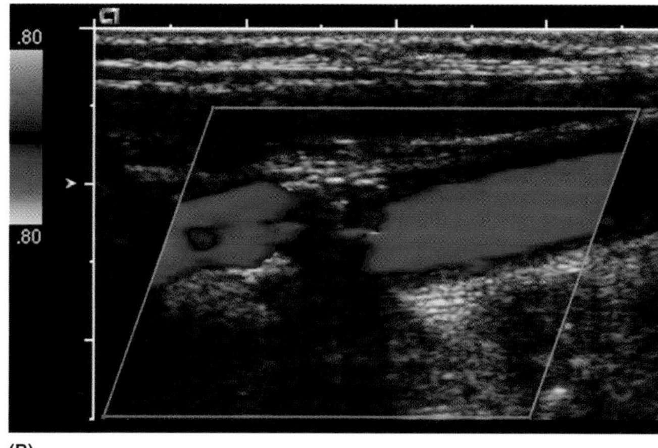

(B)

FIGURE 20 A AND B ■ Calcified carotid plaque. (**A**) The origin of this internal carotid artery contained a calcified plaque that prevented sonographic penetration. (**B**) The Doppler evaluation also demonstrates this shadow. Often, a jet of high velocity flow can be seen distal to the obscured area or the area can be examined by changing the orientation of the transducer to the vessel. However, occasionally, the plaque may limit the examination of this area.

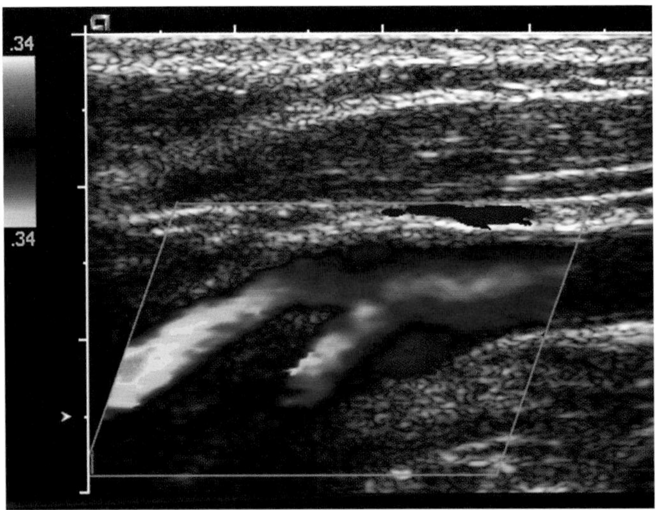

FIGURE 21 ■ Flow separation in carotid bulb. In this patient, red color flow represents small foci of reversed flow at the carotid bulb. This is a normal variant.

waveform on spectral Doppler analysis, where the highest velocities are truncated and wrap around, appearing below the baseline. This effect may lead an inexperienced examiner to underestimate the peak velocity. Aliasing can be reduced or eliminated by increasing the Doppler angle, thereby decreasing the detected Doppler shift, or by decreasing the insonating sound-beam frequency. Increasing the PRF increases the detectable frequency shift. However, the PRF increase is limited by the depth of the vessel and by the center frequency of the transducer.

Variations in Velocity Measurements Based on Equipment

Although most ultrasound machines are calibrated to accurately measure velocity, accuracy varies among manufacturers and in different machines or transducers produced by the same vendor. The degree of deviation is not well established because of the variety of products and their rapid change. However, a 14% to 18% mean

TABLE 6 ■ Sonographic Findings of Carotid Stenosis

Normal carotid ultrasound
- No intimal–medial thickening or plaque
- Flow separation in carotid bulb
- Normal waveforms
- Cross-sectional measurements are reliable

1% to 50% carotid stenosis
- Intimal–medial thickening (>1.2 mm) and mild plaque
- Possible spectral broadening
- Possible loss of flow separation
- Cross-sectional measurements remain reliable

50% to 69% carotid stenosis
- Moderate plaque
- Spectral broadening
- Cross-sectional measurements are not reliable

70% to 99% carotid stenosis
- Severe plaque
- More severe spectral broadening
- Represents hemodynamically significant (flow-restricting) disease

Near occlusion
- Severe plaque
- Longitudinal pulsation (cephalocaudad movement, rather than solely normal transverse pulsation)
- Small systolic spikes possibly caused by transmitted pulsations
- Possible increased resistance in CCA (externalization)
- Possible decreased resistance in ECA (internalization of ECA from collateral flow)
- Spectral broadening with distorted waveform, including rounded peaks, loss of sharp envelope, and accentuation of spectral energy in lower ranges
- Values of calculated parameters that exceed those listed in tables

Carotid occlusion
- No visible or Doppler-detectable flow
- Possible visible thrombus in ICA
- Longitudinal pulsation
- Small systolic spikes possibly caused by transmitted pulsations
- CCA externalization and ECA internalization

Abbreviations: ICA, internal carotid artery; CCA, common carotid artery; ECA, external carotid artery.

error for detecting a 60% stenosis (98) may be seen. Some have suggested that each laboratory create local criteria for stenosis based on angiographic correlation at their own institution. This is probably impractical and unnecessary, given the variety of criteria that have been validated.

Pitfalls in Grading Carotid Stenosis

Despite a relatively large body of literature on carotid ultrasound, velocity criteria have been validated in a narrow patient population. Therefore, the SRU consensus threshold criteria should be applied cautiously in several less common situations. Patients with tandem stenoses, prior surgery, and CCA stenosis are a few examples. In patients with findings that do not suggest a single proximal stenosis in a noninstrumented ICA and cases with inconsistent or confusing data or confounding factors, such as cardiac disease, we propose using secondary criteria (Table 6).

Pitfalls in Grading VA Stenosis

Diagnostic criteria are not well validated for the vertebral system. Furthermore, aplasia or hypoplasia of the VA is more common than in the carotid system. In the carotid, absence of flow in the expected location of the artery usually arises from atherosclerotic disease. In the VA, absence of flow may indicate occlusion. However, other etiologies such as a hypoplastic VA may also have only a small amount of high-resistance flow.

High-velocity flow in a nonstenotic VA may be caused by compensatory flow from occlusion of a carotid artery or the contralateral VA. Turbulent flow may be simulated by spectral broadening due to tortuosity of the artery near its origin. Unlike the carotid arteries, high-resistance flow is not a specific sign in the VA (99). Although high-resistance flow may suggest distal or intracranial stenosis, there may be normal diastolic flow if the stenosis is above the level of the posterior inferior cerebellar artery (100).

CONCLUSIONS

In summary, there have been significant advances in carotid ultrasound during the last two decades. As other imaging modalities have arisen, ultrasound has remained the first-line modality for imaging carotid disease. The examination continues to require excellent technical ability of the sonographer coupled with close attention to detail and thorough understanding of carotid physiology and potential pitfalls by the interpreting physician.

ACKNOWLEDGMENTS

We would like to thank Trish Thurman for her invaluable assistance in administrative support and Sanjiv Bajaj for his editorial assistance.

REFERENCES

1. Grant EG, Benson CB, Moneta GL, et al. Carotid artery stenosis: grayscale and Doppler ultrasound diagnosis—Society of Radiologists in Ultrasound Consensus Conference. Ultrasound Q 2003; 19(4):190–198.
2. Carroll BA. Carotid sonography. Radiology 1991; 178(2):303–313.
3. Fisher M, Paganini-Hill A, Martin A, et al. Carotid plaque pathology: thrombosis, ulceration, and stroke pathogenesis. Stroke 2005; 36(2):253–257.
4. Rothwell PM, Gibson R, Warlow CP. Interrelation between plaque surface morphology and degree of stenosis on carotid angiograms and the risk of ischemic stroke in patients with symptomatic carotid stenosis. On behalf of the European Carotid Surgery Trialists' Collaborative Group. Stroke 2000; 31(3):615–621.
5. AbuRahma AF, Jarrett K, Hayes DJ. Clinical implications of power Doppler three-dimensional ultrasonography. Vascular 2004; 12(5):293–300.
6. Logason K, Bärlin T, Jonsson ML, et al. The importance of Doppler angle of insonation on differentiation between 50–69% and 70–99% carotid artery stenosis. Eur J Vasc Endovasc Surg 2001; 21:311–313.
7. Budorick NE, Rojratanakiat W, O'Boyle MK, et al. Digital tapping of the superficial temporal artery: significance in carotid duplex sonography. J Ultrasound Med 1996; 15(6):459–464.
8. Kliewer MA, Freed KS, Hertzberg BS, et al. Temporal artery tap: usefulness and limitations in carotid sonography. Radiology 1996; 201(2):481–484.
9. National Institute of Neurological Disorders and Stroke. Clinical advisory. Bethesda, National Institute of Health. September 28 1994.
10. North American Symptomatic Carotid Endarterectomy Trial (NASCET) Steering Committee. North American Symptomatic Carotid Endarterectomy Trial: methods, patient characteristics, and progress. Stroke 1991; 22:711–720.
11. North American Symptomatic Carotid Endarterectomy Trial Collaborators. Beneficial effect of carotid endarterectomy in symptomatic patients with high grade carotid stenosis. N Engl J Med 1991; 325(7):445–453.
12. Charles W. MRC European Carotid Surgery Trial: interim results for symptomatic patients with severe (70–99%) or with mild (0–29%) carotid stenosis. Lancet 1991; 337(8752):1235–1243.
13. Dick P, Sherif C, Sabeti S, et al. Gender differences in outcome of conservatively treated patients with asymptomatic high grade carotid stenosis. Stroke 2005; 36(6):1178–1183.
14. Zwiebel WJ. Duplex sonography of the cerebral arteries: efficacy, limitations, and indications. AJR Am J Roentgenol 1992; 158(1):29–36.
15. Sabeti S, Schillinger M, Mlekusch W, et al. Quantification of internal carotid artery stenosis with duplex US: comparative analysis of different flow velocity criteria. Radiology 2004; 232(2):431–439.
16. Zwiebel WJ. Color-duplex features of normal and abnormal carotid arteries. In: Zwiebel W, ed. Introduction to Vascular Ultrasonography. Vol. 3. 3rd ed. Philadelphia: WB Saunders Company, 1992:105–121.
17. Strandness DE Jr. Extracranial arterial disease. In: Duplex Scanning in Vascular Disorders. New York: Raven Press Ltd., 1990:92–120.
18. Neale ML, Chambers JL, Kelly AT, et al. Reappraisal of duplex criteria to assess significant carotid stenosis with special reference to reports from the North American Symptomatic Carotid Endarterectomy Trial and the European Carotid Surgery Trial. J Vasc Surg 1994; 20(4): 642–649.
19. Carroll BA. Duplex sonography in patients with hemispheric symptoms. J Ultrasound Med 1989; 8(1):535–540.
20. Bluth EI, Stavros AT, Marich KW, et al. Carotid duplex sonography: a multicenter recommendation for standardized imaging and Doppler criteria. Radiographics 1988; 8(3):487–506.
21. Withers CE, Gosink BB, Keightley AM, et al. Duplex carotid sonography. Peak systolic velocity in quantifying internal carotid artery stenosis. J Ultrasound Med 1990; 9(6):345–349.
22. Branas CC, Weingarten MS, Czeredarczuk M, et al. Examination of carotid arteries with quantitative color Doppler flow imaging. J Ultrasound Med 1994; 13(2):121–127.
23. Moneta GL, Edwards JM, Papanicolaou G, et al. Screening for asymptomatic internal carotid artery stenosis: duplex criteria for discriminating 60% to 99% stenosis. J Vasc Surg 1995; 21(6):989–994.

24. Coward LJ, Featherstone RL, Brown MM. Percutaneous transluminal angioplasty and stenting for vertebral artery stenosis. Cochrane Database Syst Rev 2005; (2):CD000516.
25. Bendick PJ, Jackson VP. Evaluation of the vertebral arteries with duplex sonography. J Vasc Surg 1986; 3(3):523–530.
26. Sidhu PS. Ultrasound of the carotid and vertebral arteries. Br Med Bull 2000; 56(2):346–366.
27. Ackerstaff RG, Grosveld WJ, Eikelboom BC, et al. Ultrasonic duplex scanning of the prevertebral segment of the vertebral artery in patients with cerebral atherosclerosis. Eur J Vasc Surg 1988; 2(6):387–393.
28. Fellner C, Lang W, Janka R, et al. Magnetic resonance angiography of the carotid arteries using three different techniques: accuracy compared with intraarterial x-ray angiography and endarterectomy specimens. J Magn Reson Imaging 2005; 21(4): 424–431.
29. Berg M, Zhang Z, Ikonen A, et al. Multi-detector row CT angiography in the assessment of carotid artery disease in symptomatic patients: comparison with rotational angiography and digital subtraction angiography. Am J Neuroradiol 2005; 26(5):1022–1034.
30. Fontenelle LJ, Simper SC, Hanson TL. Carotid duplex scan versus angiography in evaluation of carotid artery disease. Am Surg 1994; 60(11):864–868.
31. Elgersma O, Buijs PC, Wüst AF, et al. Maximum internal carotid arterial stenosis: assessment with rotational angiography versus conventional intraarterial digital subtraction angiography. Radiology 1999; 213(3):777–783.
32. Porsche C, Walker L, Mendelow D, et al. Evaluation of cross-sectional luminal morphology in carotid atherosclerotic disease by use of spiral CT angiography. Stroke 2001; 32:2511–2515.
33. Schulte-Altedorneburg G, Droste DW, Kollar J, et al. Measuring carotid artery stenosis. Comparison of postmortem arteriograms with the planimetric gold standard. J Neurol 2005; 252(5):575–582.
34. Stavros AT, Harshfield D. Renal Doppler, renal artery stenosis, and renovascular hypertension: direct and indirect duplex sonographic abnormalities in patients with renal artery stenosis. Ultrasound Q 1994; 4:217–263.
35. Polak JF, O'Leary DH, Kronmal RA, et al. Sonographic evaluation of carotid artery atherosclerosis in the elderly: relationship of disease severity to stroke and transient ischemic attack. Radiology 1993; 188(2):363–370.
36. Asymptomatic Carotid Atherosclerosis Study. Endarterectomy for asymptomatic carotid artery stenosis. Executive Committee for the Asymptomatic Carotid Atherosclerosis Study. J Am Med Assoc 1995; 273(18):1421–1428.
37. Touboul PJ, Hennerici MG, Meairs S, et al. Mannheim intima-media thickness consensus. Cerebrovasc Dis 2004; 18(4): 346–349.
38. Rosvall M, Janzon L, Berglund G, et al. Incidence of stroke is related to carotid IMT even in the absence of plaque. Atherosclerosis 2005; 179(2):325–331.
39. Bluth EI, McVay LV III, Merritt CR, et al. The identification of ulcerative plaque with high resolution duplex carotid scanning. J Ultrasound Med 1988; 7(2):73–76.
40. Maiuri F, Gallicchio B, Iaconetta G, et al. Intraplaque hemorrhage of the carotid arteries: diagnosis by duplex scanning. J Neurosurg Sci 1994; 38(2):87–92.
41. Bluth EI, Kay D, Merritt CR, et al. Sonographic characterization of carotid plaque: detection of hemorrhage. AJR Am J Roentgenol 1986; 146(5):1061–1065.
42. Weinberger J, Marks SJ, Gaul JJ, et al. Atherosclerotic plaque at the carotid artery bifurcation. Correlation of ultrasonographic imaging with morphology. J Ultrasound Med 1987; 6(7):363–366.
43. Polak JF, Shemanski L, O'Leary DH, et al. Hypoechoic plaque at US of the carotid artery: an independent risk factor for incident stroke in adults aged 65 years or older. Radiology 1998; 208:649–654.
44. Biasi GM, Froio A, Diethrich EB, et al. Carotid plaque echolucency increases the risk of stroke in carotid stenting: the Imaging in Carotid Angioplasty and Risk of Stroke (ICAROS) study. Circulation 2004; 110(6):756–762.
45. Mayor I, Momjian S, Lalive P, et al. Carotid plaque: comparison between visual and grey-scale median analysis. Ultrasound Med Biol 2003; 29(7):961–966.
46. Gronholdt ML, Nordestgaard BG, Schroeder TV, et al. Ultrasonic echolucent carotid plaques predict future strokes. Circulation 2001; 104(1):68–73.
47. Mathiesen EB, Bonaa KH, Joakimsen O. Echolucent plaques are associated with high risk of ischemic cerebrovascular events in carotid stenosis: the tromso study. Circulation 2001; 103(17):2171–2175.
48. Gronholdt ML, Wiebe BM, Laursen H, et al. Lipid-rich carotid artery plaques appear echolucent on ultrasound B-mode images and may be associated with intraplaque haemorrhage. Eur J Vasc Endovasc Surg 1997; 14(6):439–445.
49. Ouhlous M, Flach HZ, de Weert TT, et al. Carotid plaque composition and cerebral infarction: MR imaging study. Am J Neuroradiol 2005; 26(5):1044–1049.
50. Coward LJ, Featherstone RL, Brown MM. Safety and efficacy of endovascular treatment of carotid artery stenosis compared with carotid endarterectomy: a Cochrane systematic review of the randomized evidence. Stroke 2005; 36(4):905–911.
51. Setacci C, de Donato G, Setacci F, et al. In-stent restenosis after carotid angioplasty and stenting: a challenge for the vascular surgeon. Eur J Vasc Endovasc Surg 2005; 29(6):601–607.
52. Reina-Gutierrez T, Serrano-Hernando FJ, Sanchez-Hervas L, et al. Recurrent carotid artery stenosis following endarterectomy: natural history and risk factors. Eur J Vasc Endovasc Surg 2005; 29(4):334–341.
53. Vitek JJ, Al-Mubarak N, Iyer SS, et al. Carotid artery stent placement with distal balloon protection: technical considerations. Am J Neuroradiol 2005; 26(4):854–861.
54. Yadav JS, Wholey MH, Kuntz RE, et al. Protected carotid-artery stenting versus endarterectomy in high-risk patients. N Engl J Med 2004; 351(15):1493–1501.
55. Chong PL, Salhiyyah K, Dodd PD. The role of carotid endarterectomy in the endovascular era. Eur J Vasc Endovasc Surg 2005; 29(6):597–600.
56. Buskens E, Nederkoorn PJ, Buijs-Van Der Woude T, et al. Imaging of carotid arteries in symptomatic patients: cost-effectiveness of diagnostic strategies. Radiology 2004; 233(1):101–112.
57. Arrebola-Lopez M, Hernandez-Osma E, Gomez-Moya B, et al. Carotid stenosis in high risk patients. The SAPPHIRE study versus a decision analysis. Which is the best therapeutic option? Rev Neurol 2005; 40(8):449–452.
58. Beinfeld MT, Wittenberg E, Gazelle GS. Cost-effectiveness of whole-body CT screening. Radiology 2005; 234(2):415–422.
59. Lovelace TD, Moneta GL, Abou-Zamzam AM Jr, et al. Optimizing duplex follow-up in patients with an asymptomatic internal carotid artery stenosis of less than 60%. J Vasc Surg 2001; 33(1):56–61.
60. Kono Y, Pinnell SP, Sirlin CB, et al. Carotid arteries: contrast-enhanced US angiography—preliminary clinical experience. Radiology 2004; 230(2):561–568.
61. Pross C, Shortsleeve CM, Baker JD, et al. Carotid endarterectomy with normal findings from a completion study: is there need for early duplex scan? J Vasc Surg 2001; 33(5):963–967.
62. AbuRahma AF, Cook CC, Metz MJ, et al. Natural history of carotid artery stenosis contralateral to endarterectomy: results from two randomized prospective trials. J Vasc Surg 2003; 38(6):1154–1161.
63. Cook JM, Thompson BW, Barnes RW. Is routine duplex examination after carotid endarterectomy justified? J Vasc Surg 1990; 12(3):334–340.
64. Glover JL, Bendick PJ, Dilley RS, et al. Restenosis following carotid endarterectomy. Evaluation by duplex ultrasonography. Arch Surg 1985; 120(6):678–684.
65. Russell D, Bakke SJ, Wiberg J, et al. Patency and flow velocity profiles in the internal carotid artery assessed by digital subtraction angiography and Doppler studies three months following endarterectomy. J Neurol Neurosurg Psychiatry 1986; 49(2):183–186.
66. Robinson ML. Duplex sonography of the carotid arteries. Semin Roentgenol 1992; 27(1):17–27.
67. Erickson SJ, Mewissen MW, Foley WD, et al. Color Doppler evaluation of arterial stenoses and occlusions involving the neck and thoracic inlet. Radiographics 1989; 9(3):389–406.
68. Jacobs NM, Grant EG, Schellinger D, et al. Duplex carotid sonography: criteria for stenosis, accuracy, and pitfalls. Radiology 1985; 154(2):385–391.

69. Zwiebel WJ, Crummy AB. Sources of error in Doppler diagnosis of carotid occlusive disease. AJR Am J Roentgenol 1981; 137(1):1–12.
70. Belkin M, Mackey WC, Pessin MS, et al. Common carotid artery occlusion with patent internal and external carotid arteries: diagnosis and surgical management. J Vasc Surg 1993; 17(6):1019–1027.
71. Beckett WW Jr, Davis PC, Hoffman JC Jr. Duplex Doppler sonography of the carotid artery: false-positive results in an artery contralateral to an artery with marked stenosis. Am J Neuroradiol 1990; 11(5):1049–1053.
72. Hayes AC, Johnston KW, Baker WH, et al. The effect of contralateral disease on carotid Doppler frequency. Surgery 1988; 103(1):19–23.
73. Fujitani RM, Mills JL, Wang LM, et al. The effect of unilateral internal carotid arterial occlusion upon contralateral duplex study: criteria for accurate interpretation. J Vasc Surg 1992; 16(3):459–467.
74. Abou-Zamzam AM Jr, Moneta GL, Edwards JM, et al. Is a single preoperative duplex scan sufficient for planning bilateral carotid endarterectomy. J Vasc Surg 2000; 31(2):282–288.
75. Sachar R, Yadav JS, Roffi M, et al. Severe bilateral carotid stenosis. The impact of ipsilateral stenting on Doppler-defined contralateral stenosis. J Am Coll Cardiol 2004; 43(8):1358–1362.
76. Busuttil SJ, Franklin DP, Youkey JR, et al. Carotid duplex overestimation of stenosis due to severe contralateral disease. Am J Surg 1996; 172(2):144–147.
77. Bodily KC, Phillips DJ, Thiele BL, et al. Noninvasive detection of internal carotid artery occlusion. Angiology 1981; 32(8):517–521.
78. Bornstein NM, Beloev ZG, Norris JW. The limitations of diagnosis of carotid occlusion by Doppler ultrasound. Ann Surg 1988; 207(3):315–317.
79. Bridges SL. Clinical correlates of Doppler/ultrasound errors in the detection of internal carotid artery occlusion. Stroke 1989; 20(5):612–615.
80. Lubezky N, Fajer S, Barmeir E, et al. Duplex scanning and CT angiography in the diagnosis of carotid artery occlusion: a prospective study. Eur J Vasc Endovasc Surg 1998; 16(2):133–136.
81. AbuRahma AF, Pollack JA, Robinson PA, et al. The reliability of color duplex ultrasound in diagnosing total carotid artery occlusion. Am J Surg 1997; 174(2):185–187.
82. Middleton WD, Foley WD, Lawson TL. Color-flow Doppler imaging of carotid artery abnormalities. AJR Am J Roentgenol 1988; 150(2):419–425.
83. Erickson SJ, Mewissen MW, Foley WD, et al. Stenosis of the internal carotid artery: assessment using color Doppler imaging compared with angiography. AJR Am J Roentgenol 1989; 152(6):1299–1305.
84. Berman SS, Devine JJ, Erdoes LS, et al. Distinguishing carotid artery pseudo-occlusion with color-flow Doppler. Stoke 1995; 26(3):434–438.
85. Kotval PS, Babu SC, Shah PM. Doppler diagnosis of partial vertebral/subclavian steals convertible to full steals with physiologic maneuvers. J Ultrasound Med 1990; 9(4):207–213.
86. Kliewer MA, Hertzberg BS, Kim DH, et al. Vertebral artery Doppler waveform changes indicating subclavian steal physiology. AJR Am J Roentgenol 2000; 174(3):815–819.
87. Tola M, Yurdakul M, Cumhur T. Combined use of color duplex ultrasonography and B-flow imaging for evaluation of patients with carotid artery stenosis. Am J Neuroradiol 2004; 25(10):1856–1860.
88. Yurdakul M, Tola M, Cumhur T. B-flow imaging of internal carotid artery stenosis: comparison with power Doppler imaging and digital subtraction angiography. J Clin Ultrasound 2004; 32(5): 243–248.
89. Carroll BA. Carotid sonography: pitfalls and color flow. Appl Radiol 1988; 6:15.
90. O'Leary DH, Polak JF. High-resolution carotid sonography: past, present, and future. AJR Am J Roentgenol 1989; 153(4):699–704.
91. Douville Y, Johnston KW, Kassam M. Determination of the hemodynamic factors which influence the carotid Doppler spectral broadening. Ultrasound Med Biol 1985; 11(3):417–423.
92. Campbell JD, Hutchison KJ, Karpinski E. Variation of Doppler ultrasound spectral width in the post-stenotic velocity field. Ultrasound Med Biol 1989; 15(7):611–619.
93. van Merode T, Hick P, Hoeks AP, et al. Limitations of Doppler spectral broadening in the early detection of carotid artery disease due to the size of the sample volume. Ultrasound Med Biol 1983; 9(6):581–586.
94. Knox RA, Phillips DJ, Breslau PJ, et al. Empirical findings relating sample volume size to diagnostic accuracy in pulsed Doppler cerebrovascular studies. J Clin Ultrasound 1982; 10(5):227–232.
95. Zierler RE, Phillips DJ, Beach KW, et al. Noninvasive assessment of normal carotid bifurcation hemodynamics with color-flow ultrasound imaging. Ultrasound Med Biol 1987; 13(8):471–476.
96. Ku DN, Giddens DP, Phillips DJ, et al. Hemodynamics of the normal human carotid bifurcation: in vitro and in vivo studies. Ultrasound Med Biol 1985; 11(1):13–26.
97. Phillips DJ, Greene FM Jr, Langlois Y, et al. Flow velocity patterns in the carotid bifurcations of young, presumed normal subjects. Ultrasound Med Biol 1983; 9(1):39–49.
98. Fillinger MF, Baker RJ Jr, Zwolak RM, et al. Carotid duplex criteria for a 60% or greater angiographic stenosis: variation according to equipment. J Vasc Surg 1996; 24(5):856–864.
99. Nicolau C, Gilabert R, Chamorro A, et al. Doppler sonography of the intertransverse segment of the vertebral artery. J Ultrasound Med 2000; 19:47–53.
100. Saito K, Kimura K, Nagatsuka K, et al. Vertebral artery occlusion in duplex color-coded ultrasonography. Stroke 2004; 35:1068–1072.

Diagnostic Criteria for Transcranial Doppler Ultrasound

Annabelle Lao, Vijay K. Sharma, Mira L. Katz, and Andrei V. Alexandrov

20

INTRODUCTION

Transcranial Doppler (TCD) is an ultrasound test that evaluates the intracranial arterial system (1). Accuracy of the TCD examination is based on proper technique, intracranial arterial identification criteria, clinical diagnostic criteria, and experience. It is critical to understand that TCD measures the velocity of the blood and does not measure cerebral blood flow. Increases in the velocity of the blood in intracranial arteries may be due but not limited to an increased volume flow without a lumen diameter change, a decrease in lumen diameter (stenosis) without a change in volume flow, or a combination of an increase in volume flow and a decrease in lumen diameter.

The TCD examination is performed using a low-frequency (1–2 MHz), focused, pulsed Doppler transducer with the received ultrasound signal displayed as a uni- or bidirectional spectral waveform. The conventional signal display shows blood flow toward the transducer above the zero baseline and blood flow away from the transducer below the baseline. Spectral Doppler waveforms are displayed in real time and pertinent quantifications [i.e., mean velocity, pulsatility index (PI)] are calculated and automatically updated with each display sweep. The TCD examination may be performed at the patients' bedside if necessary and may also be used to provide continuous monitoring if required for the evaluation of patients. When performing TCD examinations, the most reliable and reproducible results are obtained by using proper instruments and instrument control settings, careful patient positioning, proper utilization of examination sites, and accurate vessel identification (2). The TCD examination has been evaluated and validated in several different clinical applications (3).

Every institution that performs TCD examinations should have a written protocol that includes a description of the clinical indications, correct patient positioning, proper instrument and instrument control settings, appropriate transducer selection and placement, measurement depths and samples to be recorded, diagnostic velocity criteria (depth of the sample volume, presence and direction of blood flow, and Doppler spectral waveform characteristics), and documentation of examination limitations. Accreditation of institutions that perform TCD examination, such as that offered by the Intersocietal Commission for the Accreditation of Vascular Laboratories, requires documentation and consistent application of a standardized protocol (4). The official final report of a TCD examination should contain, at minimum (*i*) the date of the examination, (*ii*) the clinical indication, (*iii*) a description of the examination that was performed, (*iv*) the reasons for a technically limited evaluation, (*v*) a description of the data obtained, (*vi*) the interpretation of the ultrasound data, (*vii*) a comparison with results from previous examinations where available, (*viii*) the clinical implications of the study, and (*ix*) the typed name and signature of the medical staff.

The diagnostic criteria presented in this chapter represent a summary of previously published criteria for TCD examinations and those internally generated by the STAT Neurosonology Service at the Barrow Neurological

Institute (5). These criteria may be used as a guide to establish a TCD vascular ultrasound department; however, each institution needs to validate the TCD examinations performed at their institution with an appropriate reference standard. This chapter will describe the normal values associated with a TCD examination and the diagnostic criteria being used for the (*i*) diagnosis of intracranial vascular disease (stenosis and occlusion), (*ii*) monitoring vasospasm and hyperemia, (*iii*) assessment of intracranial collateral pathways, (*iv*) detection of cerebral emboli, (*v*) increased intracranial pressure (ICP), (*vi*) monitoring cerebral circulatory arrest, (*vii*) documentation of a subclavian steal, and (*viii*) detection of right-to-left shunts.

NORMAL VALUES

Intracranial arterial velocities recorded during TCD examinations often reveal some variation. This is due to underlying anatomic, physiologic, and technical variables that may affect the intracranial arterial velocities. These variables include but are not limited to anatomy of the circle of Willis, quality of the TCD ultrasound window, age of the patient, patient's hematocrit, velocity modulation with the patient's breathing patterns, autoregulatory responses, cardiac output, chronic hypertension, brain activity, side-to-side differences because of the transducer's angle of insonation, and operator variability. Therefore, each person must be considered individually because of the variety of factors that may affect the intracranial arterial hemodynamics. Absolute velocity values have less significance than the Doppler spectral waveform configuration, the symmetry of the intracranial findings, and the comparative velocity findings between the intracranial vessels in each individual.

Proper identification of the intracranial arteries is based on the (*i*) depth of the sample volume, (*ii*) angle of the transducer, (*iii*) direction of blood flow relative to the transducer, (*iv*) spatial relationship of one Doppler signal to another, and (*v*) traceability of an artery in a set depth range. Previous studies have established normal ranges for the TCD examination in adults (6–8). Mean blood flow velocities are usually reported for TCD examinations since this parameter is less affected by changes of central cardiovascular factors such as cardiac output and peripheral resistance.

In each individual, the side-to-side velocity asymmetry should be minimal. The velocity difference between sides should be less than 30% for normal vessels and undisturbed anatomy of the circle of Willis. This difference may be attributable to the difference in the angle of insonation and/or associated with normal variations in patients' breathing patterns. Asymmetries in the posterior cerebral and intracranial vertebral arteries are difficult to interpret due to dominance, hypoplasia, and/or the tortuous course of these arteries. These intracranial arteries may have side-to-side velocity differences greater than 30%. Similarly, segments of the same intracranial artery may also have velocity differences. For example, the M2 segment of the middle cerebral artery (MCA) may have velocities significantly less than the M1 segment because of the artery's smaller lumen and the tortuosity of the M2 branches. Additional observations of the intracranial arterial velocities are that the mean velocities usually follow a hierarchical pattern: MCA ≥ anterior cerebral artery (ACA) ≥ internal carotid artery (ICA) siphon ≥ posterior cerebral artery (PCA) ≥ basilar artery (BA) ≥ vertebral artery (VA). The velocities may be equal between these arterial segments or sometimes they may be slightly increased by 5 to 10 cm/sec (i.e., ACA > MCA or BA > ICA) usually due to the angle of insonation or an anatomic variation.

Individuals free of hypertension while breathing room air have a positive end-diastolic velocity (EDV) of approximately 25% to 50% of the peak systolic velocity (PSV). The pulsatility index (PI) considers the resistance that is encountered with each cardiac cycle and is calculated as PI = PSV–EDV/mean velocity (9). Normally, the PI from the intracranial arteries ranges from 0.5 to 1.1. During a TCD examination, the ophthalmic artery (OA) is the only high-resistance (PI ≥ 1.2) Doppler signal that should be recorded because it supplies the orbital structures including muscles and it anastomoses with branches of the external carotid artery (ECA). The PI, however, may be increased in an individual due to aging, chronic hypertension, increased cardiac output, and during hyperventilation. The resistance to blood flow may also be expressed using the resistance index (RI) described by Pourcellot and this index is calculated as RI = PSV–EDV/PSV (10). The PI, however, is the parameter more widely reported for TCD examinations.

Based on this information, the STAT Neurosonology Laboratory at the Barrow Neurological Institute has adopted the diagnostic criteria listed in Table 1 for a complete normal TCD examination in an adult (5). These criteria are based on the presence of adequate TCD (transtemporal, transorbital, suboccipital, and submandibular) windows and assuming a 0° angle of insonation. A typical TCD waveform from an intracranial artery is displayed in Figure 1.

DIAGNOSIS OF INTRACRANIAL VASCULAR DISEASE

Stenosis

Intracranial arterial stenoses cause characteristic alterations in the Doppler spectral waveform that include focal increases in velocity, local turbulence, and a poststenotic drop in velocity (11–22). These changes associated with a stenosis occur assuming that volume flow is maintained. Stenoses may also produce low-frequency enhancement around the baseline (bruit), band-shaped enhancements symmetrical and parallel to the baseline (musical murmur), compensatory blood flow velocity increase in branching vessels, and microembolic signals (MES) found in distal arterial segments.

The higher the focal velocity increase recorded during a TCD examination, the greater the confidence that a significant intracranial stenosis has been identified. It is important not to overestimate the degree of stenosis from the TCD information because mild and moderate intracranial

TABLE 1 ■ Intracranial Arterial Identification Criteria

Window	Artery	Depth (mm)	Direction[a]	Mean flow velocity[b] (cm/sec)
Transtemporal	MCA	30–65	Toward	62 + 12
	ACA	62–75	Away	50 + 11
	Terminal ICA	55–70	Toward	39 + 9
	PCA	55–65	Toward	39 + 10
Transorbital	ICA siphon	58–75	Bi, toward, away	47 + 14
	OA	40–62	Toward	21 + 5
Suboccipital	BA	>80	Away	41 + 10
	VA	45–80	Away	38 + 10
Submandibular	ICA	35–75	Away	37 + 9

[a]Relative to the TCD transducer.

[b]Assuming zero degree of insonation.

Abbreviations: ACA, anterior cerebral artery; BA, basilar artery; Bi, bidirectional; ICA, internal carotid artery; MCA, middle cerebral artery; OA, ophthalmic artery; PCA, posterior cerebral artery; VA, vertebral artery; TCD, transcranial doppler.

arterial disease is difficult to demonstrate with angiography. An intracranial stenosis should be suspected when the normal hierarchy (MCA ≥ ACA ≥ ICA ≥ PCA ≥ BA ≥ VA) of intracranial arterial velocities is disrupted (Table 2). TCD can reliably detect significant stenoses (≥50% diameter reduction) located in the M1 segment of the MCA, the ICA siphon, the terminal vertebral arteries, the proximal BA, and P1 segment of the PCA. The sensitivity of TCD to identify an intracranial stenosis in the anterior circulation ranges from 85% to 90%, the specificity ranges from 90% to 95%, the positive predictive value is 85%, and the negative predictive value is 98%. Identification of a stenosis in the posterior circulation is not as accurate. The sensitivity to measure intracranial arterial velocities without aliasing is limited in patients with deep (>65 mm) stenoses due to the limitations of the TCD instrument (7,8,23). If this occurs, the EDV can be measured and used to approximate the mean velocity. If the EDV exceeds 80 cm/sec, the mean velocity likely exceeds 100 cm/sec. Stenoses of M2 (MCA), A2 (ACA), and P2 (PCA) segments are usually difficult to identify because of suboptimal angle of insonation or anatomic variation. Additionally, intracranial collaterals and hyperemia may mimic stenotic flow. Although not described in this chapter, TCD is also used in the pediatric population. TCD has been instrumental in the evaluation of children with sickle-cell disease by the prevention of the first stroke (24).

Middle Cerebral Artery

A focal stenosis greater than 50% diameter reduction will usually be detected by TCD because it usually causes at least a "doubling" of the velocity compared to the normal segment. Absolute velocity criteria for the diagnosis of an intracranial arterial stenosis are not reliable, due to the many velocity alterations caused by nonvascular variables (i.e., age, hematocrit). Additionally, the status of the cerebral tissue perfused can also have considerable impact on intracranial arterial velocity profiles. A mean velocity of ≥80 cm/sec or is the threshold causing

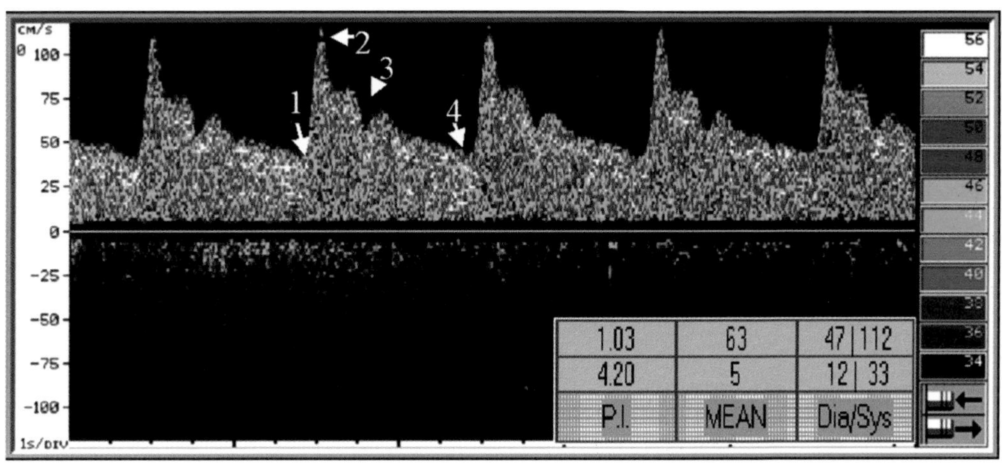

FIGURE 1 ■ A TCD waveform from a normal intracranial artery. The arrows point to (*1*) beginning systole, (*2*) peak systole, (*3*) diacrotic notch, and (*4*) end diastole.

TABLE 2 ■ TCD Mean Velocity Thresholds for an Intracranial Arterial Stenosis

Artery	Depth (mm)	Mean velocity (cm/sec)[a]	Velocities for WASID ≥50% stenosis[a]
M1-M2 MCA	30–65	≥80	≥100 cm/sec
			1: ≥2 prestenotic to stenotic velocity ratio
A1 ACA	60–75	≥80	N/A
ICA siphon	60–65	≥70	≥90 cm/sec
			1: ≥2 prestenotic to stenotic velocity ratio
PCA	60–72	≥50	N/A
BA	80–100+	≥60	≥80 cm/sec
			1: ≥2 prestenotic to stenotic velocity ratio
VA	40–80	≥50	≥80 cm/sec
			1: ≥2 prestenotic to stenotic velocity ratio

[a]Assuming zero degree of insonation.
Abbreviations: ACA, anterior cerebral artery; BA, basilar artery; ICA, internal carotid artery; MCA, middle cerebral artery; N/A, not applicable; PCA, posterior cerebral artery; VA, vertebral artery; WASID, warfarin–aspirin symptomatic intracranial disease.

concern while ≥100 cm/sec is more predictive of a ≥50% stenosis. Other diagnostic criteria reported for MCA stenosis have included an increase in PSV (≥140 cm/sec) and/or interhemispheric mean velocity difference (≥30 cm/sec) in adults free of abnormal circulatory conditions (7). A stenosis of the proximal M2-distal M1 segment of the MCA is present if the focal velocity increase is located at a depth of 40 to 50 mm and a stenosis of the proximal M1 segment of the MCA is usually found at depths of 55 to 65 mm from the transtemporal approach. Chimowitz et al. in the warfarin-aspirin symptomatic intracranial disease (WASID) study adopted diagnostic criteria for a stenosis that used a mean velocity of ≥100 cm/sec to indicate a ≥50% diameter reduction of the M1 segment of the MCA (25). To improve the predictive value of the 100 cm/sec mean velocity threshold, calculate a ratio using the highest velocity recorded in the stenosis and the velocity from the homologous or a proximal MCA segment (nonstenotic). A ≥50% stenosis is usually associated with a ratio of ≥2 and a stenosis of ≥70% diameter reduction of the MCA will usually produce a ratio of ≥3 (Fig. 2) (16).

If an individual's intracranial arterial velocities are affected by anemia, congestive heart failure and other circulatory conditions, then a focal mean velocity difference of ≥30% between adjacent or homologous arterial segments should be used as the diagnostic criteria. The velocity should usually double with a significant, i.e., ≥50% diameter reduction stenosis. Adults with anemia or hyperthyroidism often have MCA mean velocities in the range of 60 to 110 cm/sec.

If intracranial velocities are increased throughout the length of the M1 segment of the MCA, the differential diagnosis includes MCA stenosis, terminal ICA or ICA siphon stenosis, hyperemia or compensatory blood flow increase in the presence of contralateral ICA stenosis, ACA occlusion, or incorrect vessel identification.

An MCA subtotal stenosis or near occlusion may actually produce a decrease in velocity. The characteristic TCD waveform from the MCA is "blunted" with slow or delayed systolic acceleration, slow systolic flow deceleration, decreased velocities, and the mean velocity is usually less than the velocity recorded from the ACA or other intracranial arteries (26,27). Decreased or minimal flow

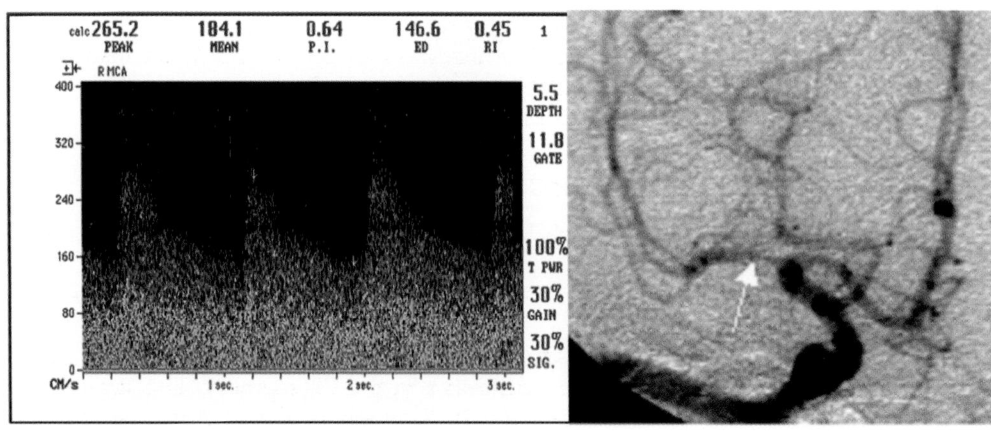

FIGURE 2 ■ A TCD waveform from the MCA. The mean velocity is >180 cm/sec, indicating a stenosis. The arrow on the corresponding angiogram points to the MCA stenosis. MCA, middle cerebral artery.

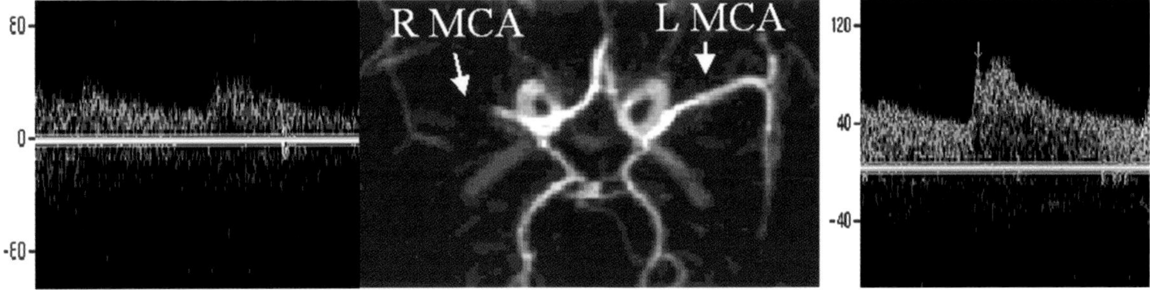

FIGURE 3 ■ Acute near occlusion of the M1 segment of the right MCA. At a depth of 55 mm, the right MCA TCD waveform is "blunted" compared to the MCA waveform from the left side. The MRA shows a flow signal void (*arrow*) on the right side due to slow and diminished blood flow in the mid-M1 MCA segment with some flow reconstitution in the distal branches. MCA, middle cerebral artery; R, right; L, left.

velocities with slow systolic acceleration can be found due to a tight elongated MCA stenosis or thrombus causing near occlusion or a proximal ICA obstruction (28,29). The "blunted" waveform is common in patients with acute ischemic stroke, particularly in those presenting with a hyperdense MCA sign on noncontrast computed tomography (CT) scan or a flow gap on magnetic resonance angiography (MRA) (Fig. 3). A false-positive diagnosis of MCA subtotal stenosis may occur because of vessel misidentification and/or because of a suboptimal angle of insonation or too shallow an ultrasound insonation. To confirm the presence of a flow-limiting lesion, branching vessels should also be evaluated. This is because an MCA (M1-M2) subtotal stenosis is usually accompanied by flow diversion to the ACA and/or compensatory flow increase in the PCA, indicating transcortical collateralization of flow (26,27).

Anterior Cerebral Artery

Diagnostic criteria for an ACA stenosis includes a mean velocity ≥80 cm/sec, a focal significant increase in ACA velocity (ACA > MCA), a ≥30% difference between the proximal and distal ACA segments, and/or a ≥30% velocity difference compared to the contralateral ACA (8,26). Collateralization via the anterior communicating artery (ACoA) can be excluded by normal ACA flow direction and the absence of stenotic signals at midline (depth of 75 mm). Usually, a stenosis of the A1 segment of the ACA is detected at a depth of 60 to 75 mm. Additional findings may include turbulence and a flow diversion into the MCA and/or compensatory flow increase in the contralateral ACA. The differential diagnosis includes cross-filling via the anterior cerebral arteries due to proximal contralateral carotid artery disease.

Decreased or minimal flow velocities in the A1 segment of the ACA may indicate a suboptimal angle of insonation from the ipsilateral transtemporal window, an atretic or tortuous A1 segment, or a near occlusion of the A1 segment of the ACA. Since the A2 segment of the ACA cannot be assessed directly by TCD, its obstruction can be suspected only if a high resistance flow is found in the distal dominant A1 segment (70–75 mm) of the ACA. Common interpretation errors associated with the diagnosis of an ACA stenosis include the incorrect identification of the artery (terminal ICA vs. ACA), and velocity underestimation (suboptimal angle of insonation, poor window, and weak signals).

Terminal ICA and ICA Siphon

A stenosis of the terminal ICA and ICA siphon may be difficult to identify because these arterial segments are usually not evaluated in their entirety during a TCD examination. Additionally, the TCD examination via the transorbital window may identify blood flow toward, away, or bidirectional from the ultrasound transducer at depths from 58 to 65 mm in adults depending on the segment (parasellar, supraclinoid, or genu) insonated. Deeper insonation via the transorbital window is possible but vessel identification is less reliable since a velocity signal from the ACA may be detected. From the transtemporal approach, the terminal ICA is usually located at a depth of 55 to 70 mm. An ICA siphon or terminal ICA stenosis produces a focal significant increase in mean velocity (ICA > MCA), an ICA mean velocity ≥70 cm/sec, and/or a ≥30% difference between arterial segments (30).

The differential diagnosis includes moderate proximal ICA stenosis and/or compensatory velocity increase from a contralateral ICA stenosis. Additional findings in the presence of an ICA stenosis may include turbulence, blunted ipsilateral MCA (poststenotic flow), increase in OA velocity, and/or reversal of blood flow direction with low pulsatility. The ICA siphon velocity may decrease due to siphon near occlusion (a blunted siphon signal) or distal obstruction (i.e., MCA occlusion or increased intracranial cerebral pressure). Interpretation errors include vessel misidentification (MCA vs. ICA), an insonation depth of >65 mm, and blood flow collateralization misinterpreted as an arterial stenosis.

Posterior Cerebral Artery

A stenosis in the PCA produces a focal increase in mean velocity of ≥50 cm/sec (PCA > ACA or ICA) (31). From the transtemporal window, the PCA velocity signal is located at a depth of 55 to 65 mm with blood flow toward the transducer in the P1 segment and blood flow away from the transducer in the P2 segment. The top-of-the-basilar and the P1 segment of the PCA can usually be located at midline (65–75 mm) in most adults. Additional findings may include turbulence and a compensatory flow increase in the MCA. The differential diagnosis includes collateral blood flow via the posterior communicating artery (PCoA) and siphon stenosis. By using transcranial color Doppler imaging, it may be possible to differentiate PCA stenosis from collateralization by using the color Doppler and velocity information (32). Common sources of error include unreliable vessel identification, presence of an arterial occlusion, and top-of-the-basilar stenosis.

Basilar Artery

The presence of a BA stenosis include a focal increase in velocity BA ≥ 60 cm/sec, BA > MCA or ACA or ICA, and/or ≥30% difference between arterial segment (33–36). The reported depth range for the BA has varied in previous studies (34,35). The variation in BA depth may be due to the size of the individual's neck and the technical skills of the operator (35). In adults, the proximal BA is located at ≥75 mm, the mid-BA segment is located at 90 mm, and the distal BA is located at depths ≥100 mm (5,35). The differential diagnosis includes terminal VA stenosis if elevated velocities are found proximally. If elevated velocities are found throughout BA and the vertebral arteries have increased velocity, the differential diagnosis includes compensatory flow increase.

BA subtotal stenosis or near occlusion produces a decrease (≤30% difference between arterial segments and/or BA < VA) in velocity, resulting in a blunted waveform (37). The differential diagnosis includes a fusiform BA with or without thrombus since an enlarged vessel diameter may be responsible for the decrease in velocity. If EDV is absent, the differential diagnosis includes BA occlusion. Additional findings may include signs of turbulence and disturbed signals distal to the stenosis, compensatory flow increase in VAs and posterior inferior cerebellar arteries (PICAs) indicating cerebellar collateralization, collateral supply via PCoAs to PCAs, and reversed distal BA.

Common sources of error include a tortuous basilar ("not identified" is "not diagnostic of occlusion"), an elongated BA obstruction, and distal BA lesions that were not insonated because of technical limitation. Application of power Doppler, ultrasound contrast, and color Doppler imaging may help detection of the distal basilar segment, tortuosity, and distal branches (38,39). Also, collateral flow from the posterior to the anterior circulation in the presence of carotid lesions may increase velocity changes associated with mild stenosis and/or tortuosity. In the case of blood flow collateralization, the dominant VA velocities are also increased (40).

Vertebral Artery

Intracranial VA stenosis includes a significant focal increase in velocity (VA ≥ 50 cm/sec, VA > BA) (5,33,40). A terminal VA stenosis may also cause a high resistant (PI ≥ 1.2) velocity signal in one of the vertebral arteries and/or a blunted decreased velocity signal (37). The terminal VA is usually located at depths of 45 to 80 mm depending on the size of the individual's neck (40).

Additional findings may include signs of turbulence or disturbed flow signal distal to the stenosis, a compensatory flow increase in the contralateral VA or its branches (cerebellar collaterals), low BA velocities (hemodynamically significant lesion and hypoplastic contralateral VA) and low-resistance blood flow distal to stenoses (compensatory vasodilation). The differential diagnosis includes proximal BA or contralateral terminal VA stenoses and a compensatory flow increase in the presence of a contralateral VA occlusion or carotid stenosis (7).

Common sources of interpretation error include a compensatory flow increase due to hypoplastic contralateral VA, low velocities in both VAs due to suboptimal angle of insonation, extracranial VA stenosis or occlusion with well-developed muscular collaterals, elongated VA stenosis/hypoplasia, and incorrect vessel identification (i.e., PICA).

Occlusion

The diagnosis of acute intracranial arterial occlusion with TCD is more complex and yields more information about intracranial thrombus than described in previously published criteria (11,13,30,41–45). The operator must be experienced and the best results are usually obtained for the M1 segment of the MCA, the terminal ICA and ICA siphon, and the BA. The lack of a Doppler signal from an intracranial artery cannot be interpreted as an arterial occlusion. If the Doppler signal is not identified, it may be due to an inadequate ultrasound window, poor technique including the angle of insonation, anatomic variability, or congenital aplasia or severe hypoplasia. To diagnose an arterial occlusion, there must be a good TCD; other patent arteries should be identified through the same TCD window, and/or a contrast agent should be used. In addition to the absence of a TCD signal at the site of an occlusion or velocity asymmetry between the homologous segments on TCD in acute ischemic stroke (13,30,41–45), a variety of flow signals around a thrombus may be detected (46). To determine the presence of an acute arterial occlusion, it is important to depart from a simplistic concept of asymmetry in blood flow velocities between affected and nonaffected sides. An acute lesion may represent a complete occlusion, subtotal stenosis, or partial, yet hemodynamically significant blood flow obstruction. Instead of relying on velocity measurements, the TCD operator should focus on the shape of the velocity waveforms and signs of blood flow diversion or collateralization. This approach leads to a greater yield of abnormal TCD findings that are highly predictive of the presence of a thrombus on corresponding angiography (26,46).

To achieve better sensitivity to slow and weak blood flow, a single-gate TCD instrument should be set at maximum power and a large (12–15 mm) sample volume should be used during the examination. When using a power M-mode TCD instrument, the sample volume should be small (3 mm) and the depth range set at the depth of the presumed arterial occlusion. In approximately 75% of cases with acute intracranial occlusion, some residual flow signals can be detected from presumed clot location (46,47). Waveform shape discloses

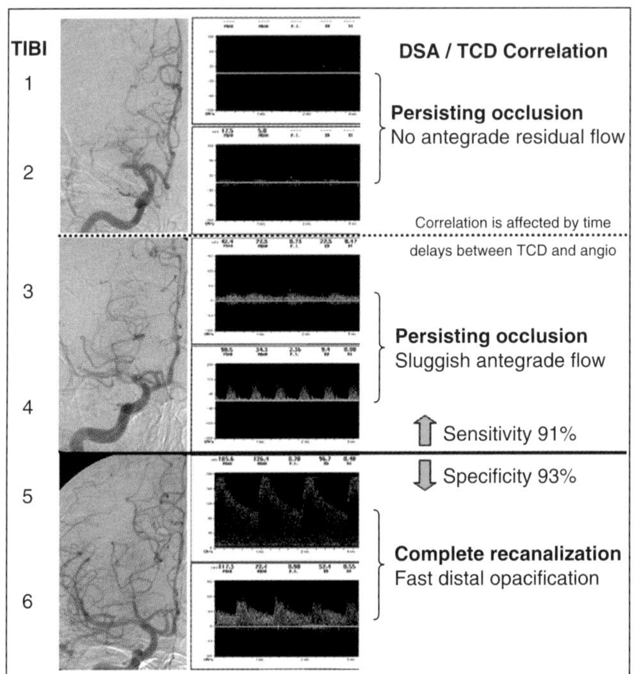

FIGURE 4 ■ Thrombolysis in brain ischemia residual flow grading system.

important information about clot location, hemodynamic significance of the obstruction, and resistance in the distal vasculature than an absolute velocity difference by itself. Moreover, if the MCA on the affected side has mean velocity <30% than nonaffected side and it also has delayed systolic acceleration, these findings suggest a proximal ICA obstruction and not necessarily an MCA lesion (29). Further waveform analysis of the distal MCA and PCA is required to establish the presence of an additional lesion in the MCA. Doppler waveform analysis also allows determination of the patency of small perforating arteries in the proximal MCA stem (48). This finding is often helpful in explaining distribution of the neurological deficits in the acute stroke patient. The thrombolysis in brain infarction (TIBI) flow grading system was developed to predict the success of intracranial clot lysis and short-term improvement after ischemic stroke (Fig. 4) (46).

Both acute and chronic intracranial occlusions can present with TIBI flow grades of ≤3 and accurate differentiation may not be possible. An acute occlusion is more likely to be found with recent stroke symptoms or fluctuating neurological deficits and signs of flow diversion and elevated velocities in the branching vessels. A chronic

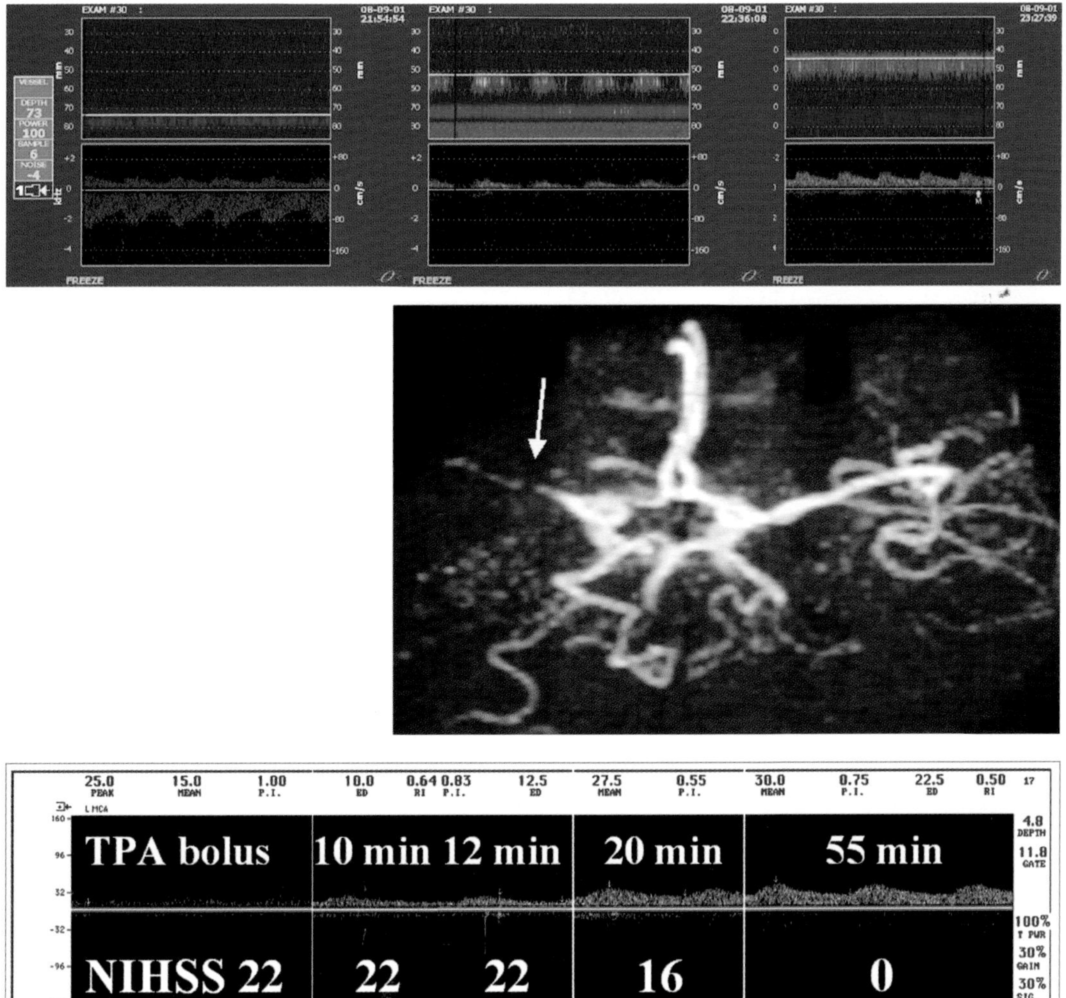

FIGURE 5 ■ Appearance of an acute proximal M1 middle cerebral artery occlusion and recanalization.

occlusion is often associated with well-developed major collateral channels and lower velocities.

Based on the previous studies (11,13,41–45) and correlations with invasive angiography, detailed criteria have been described for intracranial occlusions on TCD (29,37). For the diagnosis of the MCA occlusion, the abnormal waveforms have to be found between 40 and 65 mm via the transtemporal approach (Fig. 5). Secondary findings are (*i*) flow diversion/compensatory velocity increase in the ipsilateral ACA and/or PCA; (*ii*) no blood flow signals from the ACA and ICA with PCA flow–identified possible "T"-type terminal ICA occlusion (Fig. 6); (*iii*) diastolic blood flow and overall velocity decrease from the terminal ICA to the distal MCA; and (*iv*) Zanette asymmetry index of 21% for MCA, 27% for ACA and 28% for PCA (43).

These findings help to localize MCA occlusion, i.e., M2 segment, distal M1 segment, proximal M1 segment with or without residual flow to perforators, or extending from the terminal ICA. If findings are uncertain or multiple lesions are suspected, these findings need to be confirmed by insonation across the midline from the contralateral temporal window if technically possible and when time permits.

With the intracranial, or terminal ICA occlusion (C1–C2 segments), the abnormal waveforms are found at depths of 62 to 70 mm via the transorbital approach. For example, with ICA occlusion above the origin of the OA, a high resistance or dampened ICA siphon signal can be found from the transorbital approach. The hallmark of an isolated distal ICA occlusion is the presence of patent MCA signals (normal or blunted) throughout M1-proximal M2 segments and the presence of collateralization of flow, indicating a hemodynamically significant lesion in the ICA.

With a proximal ICA occlusion, the most common findings include a blunted MCA signal and reversed blood flow direction in the OA (Fig. 7) or the absence of Doppler signals from the OA and ICA siphon from the transorbital approach. The TCD examination by itself cannot differentiate complete extracranial ICA occlusion from hemodynamically significant proximal high-grade stenosis and carotid duplex imaging should be used to answer this question. TCD can help to determine an extension of the proximal ICA occlusion into the supraclinoid siphon or terminal ICA, tandem MCA and ICA lesions, and the presence of collateral blood flow channels. Secondary findings for any ICA occlusion site include (*i*) collateral flow in the PCoA and/or cross-filling via the ACoA; (*ii*) contralateral ICA compensatory velocity increase; and (*iii*) possible frequent microemboli in the ipsilateral terminal ICA or MCA.

With an occlusion in the BA, the abnormal waveforms are found at depths of ≥80 mm from the suboccipital approach (Fig. 8). Usually, the proximal BA is located at a depth of 80 mm, the mid-BA at 90 mm, and distal BA depths of 100 mm. Secondary findings may include (*i*) a flow velocity increase in one or both of the VAs or PICAs,

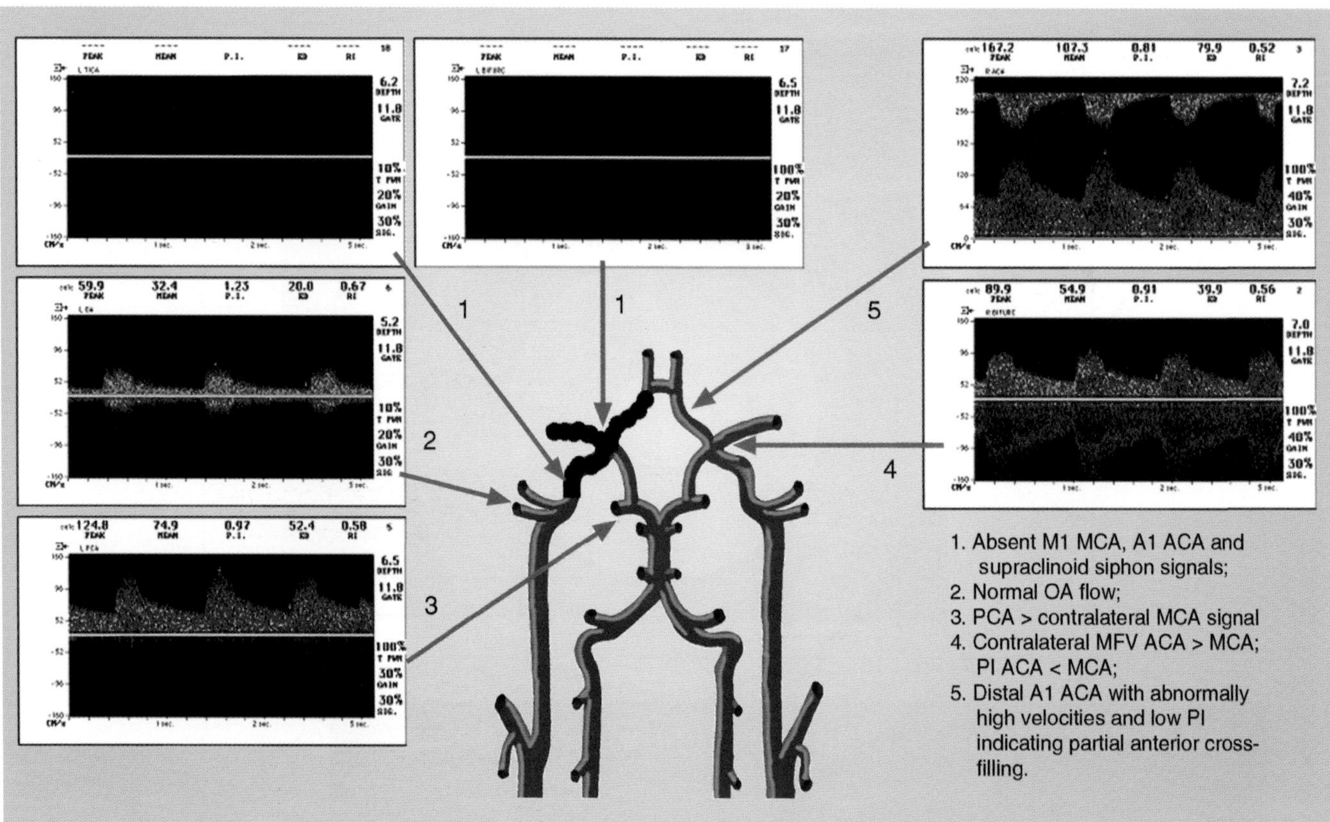

FIGURE 6 ■ Carotid "T"-type occlusion documented by TCD. MCA, middle cerebral artery; ACA, anterior cerebral artery; OA, ophthalmic artery; PCA, posterior cerebral artery; MFV, mean blood flow velocity; PI, pulsatility index. *Source*: From Ref. 37.

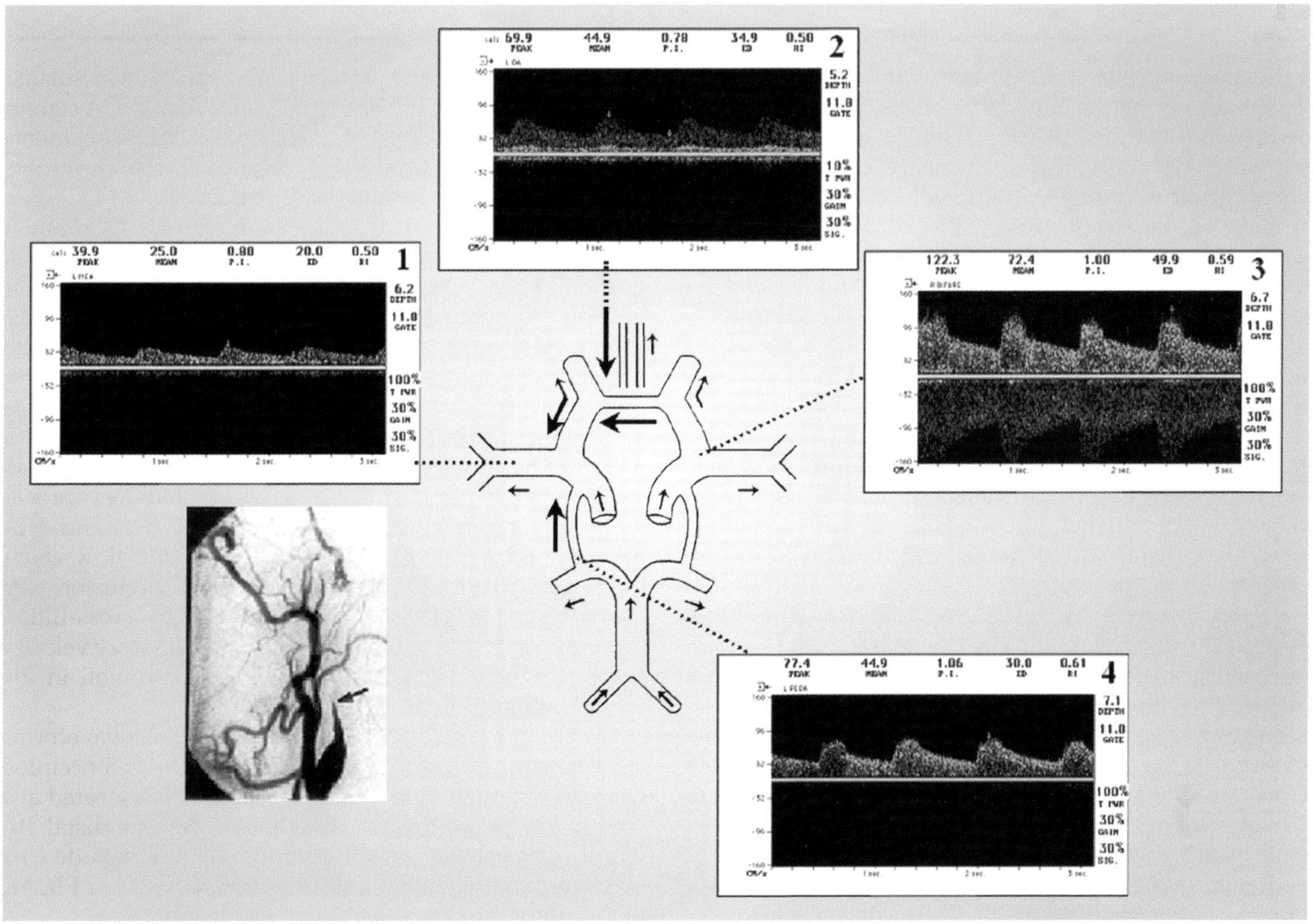

FIGURE 7 ■ Proximal ICA occlusion. The most common site of a proximal ICA occlusion is its extracranial portion particularly at the level of the carotid bulb (DSA image). If TCD is performed without angiographic correlation, the location of a hemodynamically significant ICA obstruction may only be reported as proximal to the ophthalmic artery origin. Correlation with carotid duplex imaging is necessary to determine the presence of an occlusion or a hemodynamically significant stenosis in the proximal extracranial ICA. 1—Blunted signal in the MCA ipsilateral to ICA occlusion; 2—Reversed blood flow direction and low resistant signal from the ophthalmic artery (inverted image); 3—Contralateral ACA > MCA indicating collateral blood flow via anterior cross-filling. MCA, middle cerebral artery; ICA, internal carotid artery; DSA, digital subtraction angiography; ACA, anterior cerebral artery.

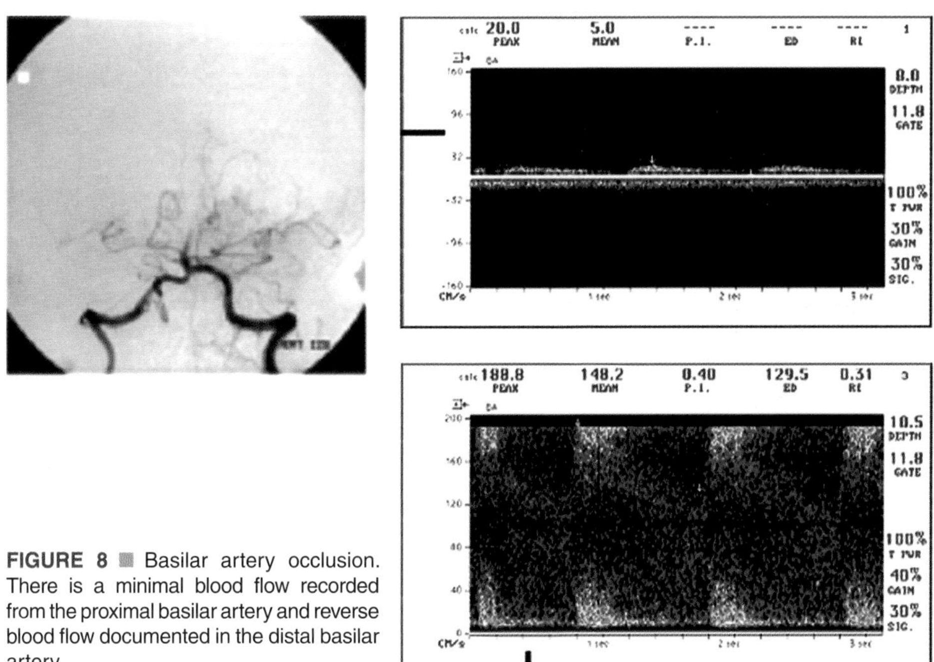

FIGURE 8 ■ Basilar artery occlusion. There is a minimal blood flow recorded from the proximal basilar artery and reverse blood flow documented in the distal basilar artery.

indicating cerebellar collateral flow; (*ii*) a high-resistance flow signal in one or both VAs, indicating proximal BA occlusion; (*iii*) a high-resistance flow signal at the origin of the BA, indicating distal BA occlusion; (*iv*) retrograde (low resistance, stenotic) blood flow toward the transducer at the top of the BA (proximal BA occlusion collateralized via PCoAs); (*v*) functional PCoAs with flow directed away from the transducer via the temporal window; and (*vi*) low distal BA velocities with top-of-the-BA occlusion.

The TCD diagnosis of the distal basilar occlusion or subtotal stenosis without obvious PCoA or cross-cerebellar blood flow is particularly challenging (49,50). CT-angiography or three-dimensional contrast-enhanced TCD or color Doppler imaging with power mode may be techniques of choice if a distal BA occlusion is suspected (37,49,50). Special attention must be paid when only relatively low distal BA velocities are found without any other abnormal findings.

The diagnosis of the VA occlusion is difficult to establish using TCD alone since an extracranial segmental occlusion may be present (51). The most accurate diagnosis with TCD can be made for a terminal VA occlusion (52); however, the sensitivity of abnormal blood flow signals is approximately 60% (37,51,53). Normal intracranial TCD examination cannot completely rule out VA occlusion particularly with a proximal location of a segmental and collateralized VA occlusion or hypoplasia (53). Figure 9 shows a typical finding with asonic terminal VA occlusion. Secondary findings may include normal blood flow signals directed toward the transducer on the side of occlusion indicating collateralization of blood flow from the contralateral side and filling of the PICAs.

MONITORING VASOSPASM AND HYPEREMIA

Vasospasm

Arterial vasospasm is a complication of subarachnoid hemorrhage (SAH), which becomes symptomatic in more than 25% of patients, leading to a delayed ischemic neurologic deficit (DIND) (54). DIND usually occurs when vasospasm results in a severe (≤1 mm) intracranial arterial narrowing producing blood flow depletion with extremely high velocities (55). Vasospasm may affect proximal segments and distal branches of intracranial arteries with the most common locations being the MCA, terminal ICA, ACA, and BA (56). Vasospasm may coexist with hydrocephalus, edema, and cerebral infarction. The differential diagnosis with TCD should always consider the hyperdynamic state that we will refer to as hyperemia. Hyperemia may be induced by spontaneous cardiovascular responses to SAH or induced by the hypertension-hemodilution-hypervolemia (HHH) therapy (57). Although inadequate, the term "hyperemia" is used to describe velocity changes on TCD. The blood flow velocity measured by TCD is not a direct measurement of cerebral blood flow volume (58). However, focal or global velocity changes can help to differentiate between spasm and hyperemia. Both conditions may coexist since most SAH patients with spasm routinely receive components of HHH therapy.

Although quantitative criteria have been studied extensively, grading vasospasm severity is difficult, and the interpretation of TCD findings should be individualized to the patient. Daily TCDs may detect considerable blood flow velocity and pulsatility changes that should be related to the patient's clinical condition, medications, blood pressure, time after day 0, and ICP findings.

Proximal vasospasm in any intracranial artery results in a focal (or diffuse along one or two branching segments) elevation of mean velocities without parallel velocity increase in the feeding extracranial arteries (intracranial/extracranial artery ratio ≥3). Distal vasospasm in any intracranial artery may produce a focal pulsatile flow, indicating increased resistance (PI ≥ 1.2) distal to the site of insonation. This PI increase has to be differentiated with effects of hyperventilation or increased cardiac output. No increase in mean velocity may be found if vasospasm is located distal to the site of insonation (59). Additional findings may include daily changes

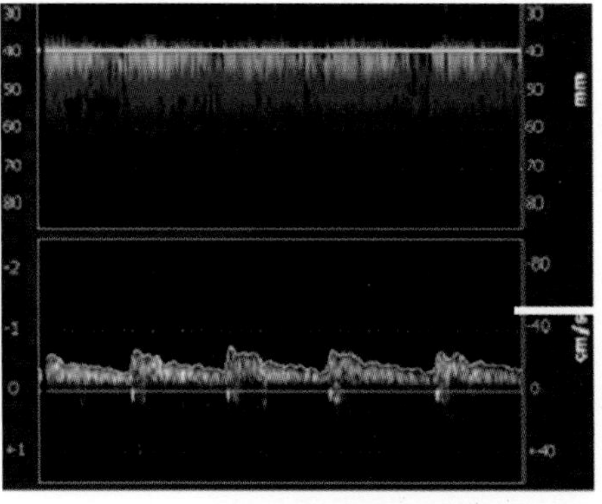
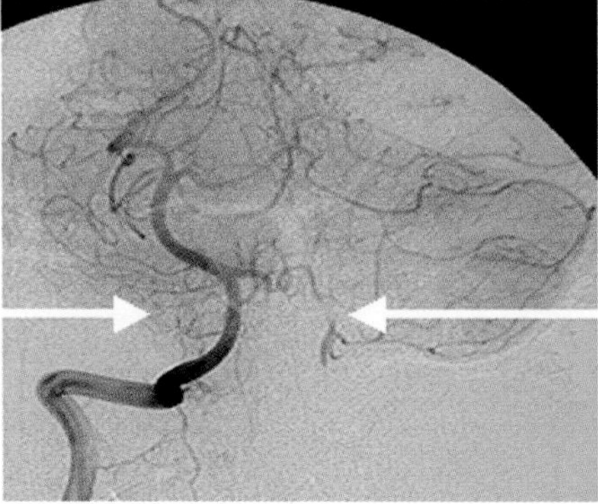
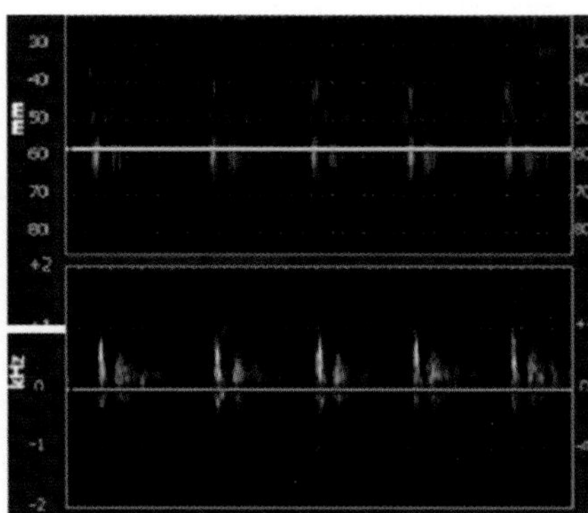

FIGURE 9 ■ Terminal vertebral artery occlusion. DSA image shows retrograde filling of the left terminal vertebral artery and posterior inferior cerebellar arteries from a right vertebral artery injection. TCD shows a high resistant minimal blood flow signal in the reversed part of the left terminal vertebral artery just distal to its occluded segment at the atlas loop. DSA, digital subtraction angiography.

TABLE 3 ■ TCD Criteria for Proximal Middle Cerebral Artery Vasospasm

Mean velocity (cm/sec)	MCA/ICA mean velocity ratio	Interpretation
<120	≤3	Hyperemia
>80	3–4	Hyperemia + possible mild spasm
≥120	3–4	Mild spasm + hyperemia
≥120	4–5	Moderate spasm + hyperemia
>120	5–6	Moderate spasm
≥180	6	Moderate-to-severe spasm
≥200	≥6	Severe spasm
>200	4–6	Moderate spasm + hyperemia
>200	3–4	Hyperemia + mild (often residual) spasm
>200	<3	Hyperemia

Abbreviations: ICA, internal carotid artery; MCA, middle cerebral artery; TCD, transcranial Doppler.

TABLE 4 ■ Predictors of Adverse Outcomes in Patients with Subarachnoid Hemorrhage

Parameter	TCD findings
Velocity	Early appearance of MCA mean velocity ≥180 cm/sec
	Rapid (>20% or >65 + cm/sec) increase in mean velocity daily during critical days 3–7
Ratio	MCA/ICA ratio ≥6
Pulsatility	Abrupt appearance of high-resistance PI ≥ 1.2 due to increased ICP (hydrocephalus)
	Appearance of PI ≥ 1.2 due to distal spasm

Abbreviations: MCA, middle cerebral artery; ICA, internal carotid artery; ICP, increased cerebral pressure; PI, pulsatility index; TCD, transcranial Doppler.

in velocities, ratios, and PIs during the first two weeks but are particularly pronounced during the critical days 3 to 7 after the onset of SAH.

Middle Cerebral Artery

The MCA findings on TCD were most rigorously validated and correlated with the diameter of the residual lumen on digital subtraction angiography (DSA) (Table 3) (55,60–63). According to Lindegaard, the MCA mean velocity of 200 cm/sec or more predicts residual lumen of 1 mm or less (55). The differential diagnosis includes hyperemia, combination of vasospasm and hyperemia in the same vessel, residual vasospasm and hyperemia. Unlike focal atherosclerotic lesions, vasospasm may affect longer segments of the terminal ICA and MCA. Vasospasm may be unequally distributed along the MCA stem and branches. However, the presence of hyperdynamic cardiovascular state and HHH-therapy may promote high velocities even in the presence of severe spasm affecting multiple segments. TCD findings that may be used to predict adverse outcomes in patients are summarized in Table 4 (54).

Other Intracranial Arteries

Grading vasospasm severity in other intracranial arteries is difficult (54,55). It has been suggested to report vasospasm in these arteries as possible, probable, and definite (Table 5) (54). The key indicator of a significant vasospasm is a focal, asymmetrical, and disproportionate velocity increase that may occur in an artery distant from the aneurysm site or blood clot collection on CT. The differential diagnosis includes hyperemia and its combination with vasospasm in these arteries.

An ongoing individual correlation of digital subtraction angiography with same day TCD findings may improve the accuracy of TCD to detect vasospasm onset. A focal increase in flow velocities that is disproportionate to therapy indicates the development of vasospasm. For example, an MCA mean velocity increase by 50 + cm/sec may indicate 20% diameter reduction of the vessel, and since velocity is inversely proportionate to the vessel radius, a 30% diameter reduction usually doubles the velocity on TCD (64). Therefore, TCD may be more sensitive to intracranial artery diameter changes than angiography, particularly at the early phases of spasm development. Since TCD is a screening tool, the velocity criteria should be adjusted to a higher sensitivity to detect any degree of vasospasm in order to institute HHH therapy. At the same time, higher specificity threshold should be used for severe vasospasm to minimize the number of false-negative angiograms, particularly if TCD is used to select patients for angioplasty.

Vasospasm that affects the BA stem, the PCAs, or ACAs may cause compensatory velocity increase in the MCAs with low Lindegaard ratios (MCA/distal extracranial ICA). Therefore, a complete daily TCD examination may reveal more significant hemodynamic changes that can be used to identify patients with spasm in arteries other than MCA.

Hyperemia

Hyperemia is suspected with elevated velocities in the intracranial and feeding extracranial vessels. Hyperemic changes on TCD are common in patients with SAH receiving HHH therapy. The use of the Lindegaard ratio (62) and new flow and area indexes (64) may help to minimize false-positive TCD results and better predict the diameter of the residual lumen on angiography.

Otherwise, hyperperfusion syndrome may develop after carotid endarterectomy or angioplasty due to limited or impaired capacity of the brain to regulate restored blood flow volume (65–68). Patients frequently experience headache and seizures. TCD often shows ≥30% increase in MCA mean velocity ipsilateral to the reconstructed

TABLE 5 ■ Mean Velocity Criteria for Grading Vasospasm in Intracranial Arteries[a]

Artery	Possible vasospasm[b] (cm/sec)	Probable vasospasm[b] (cm/sec)	Definite vasospasm[b] (cm/sec)
ICA	>80	>110	>130
ACA	>90	>110	>120
PCA	>60	>80	>90
BA	>70	>90	>100
VA	>60	>80	>90

[a]Optimized criteria were modified from the review by Sloan (47).

[b]After hyperemia has been ruled out by the focal velocity increase and by the intracranial artery/extracranial ICA ratio ≥3 except for posterior circulation vessels.

Abbreviations: ACA, anterior cerebral artery; BA, basilar artery; ICA, internal carotid artery; PCA, posterior cerebral artery; VA, vertebral artery.

carotid artery and low pulsatility waveforms compared to the contralateral side, indicating decreased capacity of the distal vasculature to regulate the reestablished blood flow volume. The PI may decrease >20% compared to the contralateral side. These changes are often found immediately after cross-clamp release during a carotid endarterectomy. The diagnosis of hyperperfusion is when the MCA mean velocity is 1.5 times the pre–cross-clamp values and persists at that level without corrective measures (69).

ASSESSMENT OF INTRACRANIAL COLLATERAL PATHWAYS

TCD can detect the following collateral pathways (70–74):

1. The ACoA providing a channel from hemisphere to hemisphere
2. The PCoA providing blood flow between the posterior and the anterior circulations
3. The OA providing a channel from the extracranial ECA to the intracranial ICA through the orbit

The intracranial collateral channels are dormant under normal circulatory conditions. A collateral channel is active when a pressure gradient develops between the two anastomosing arterial systems. Increased velocity is detected during a TCD examination and the blood flow direction depends on the direction of collateralization. When present, collateral flow patterns rarely imply anatomic variants but most often the presence of a flow-limiting lesion proximal to the recipient arterial system.

The direction of blood flow in the collateral channel indicates which arterial system is the donor (the source) and which is the recipient (the blood flow destination). TCD provides information on functioning collateral channels and direction of the collateral blood flow. An expanded battery of TCD parameters may be used to refine the evaluation of the severity of ICA lesions, particularly when multiple lesions are found or the applicability of other tests is limited due to the presence of the distal ICA lesions (75,76).

Anterior Communicating Artery

The most commonly found collateral pattern in response to significant extracranial carotid disease is via the ACoA. Collateral blood flow through ACoA cannot be reliably distinguished from the neighboring ACAs because of its small length and diameter. The ultrasound characteristics of this collateral pathway include (*i*) an increase in the velocity from the contralateral (donor) A1 segment of the ACA resulting in ACA > MCA; (*ii*) a turbulent Doppler signal with increased velocity at midline; and (*iii*) a normal or low mean velocity in the ipsilateral A1 segment of the ACA (with or without ACA blood flow reversal) (Fig. 10).

The differential diagnosis includes distal A1 ACA stenosis and compensatory flow increase if one A1 segment is atretic. Identification of the reversed A1 segment depends on the skill of the operator. The following are four typical observations made by TCD:

1. Only increased donor ACA velocities are documented: the differential diagnosis includes A1 ACA stenosis and atresia of the contralateral A1 segment. The donor A1 segment supplies both A2 segments (may be present in normal individuals due to anatomic variations of the circle of Willis as well as in patients with ICA- or MCA-obstructive lesions).
2. An increased donor ACA velocity is found with stenotic flow at midline: the differential diagnosis includes distal A1 stenosis, ICA siphon stenosis, and cross-filling via ACoA.
3. An increased donor ACA mean velocity is documented with a reversed blood flow direction in the contralateral A1; this indicates probable proximal ICA stenosis.
4. An increased donor ACA mean velocity is documented with stenotic-like blood flow at midline and a reversed blood flow direction in the contralateral A1 ACA; there is a definite proximal ICA stenosis or occlusion.

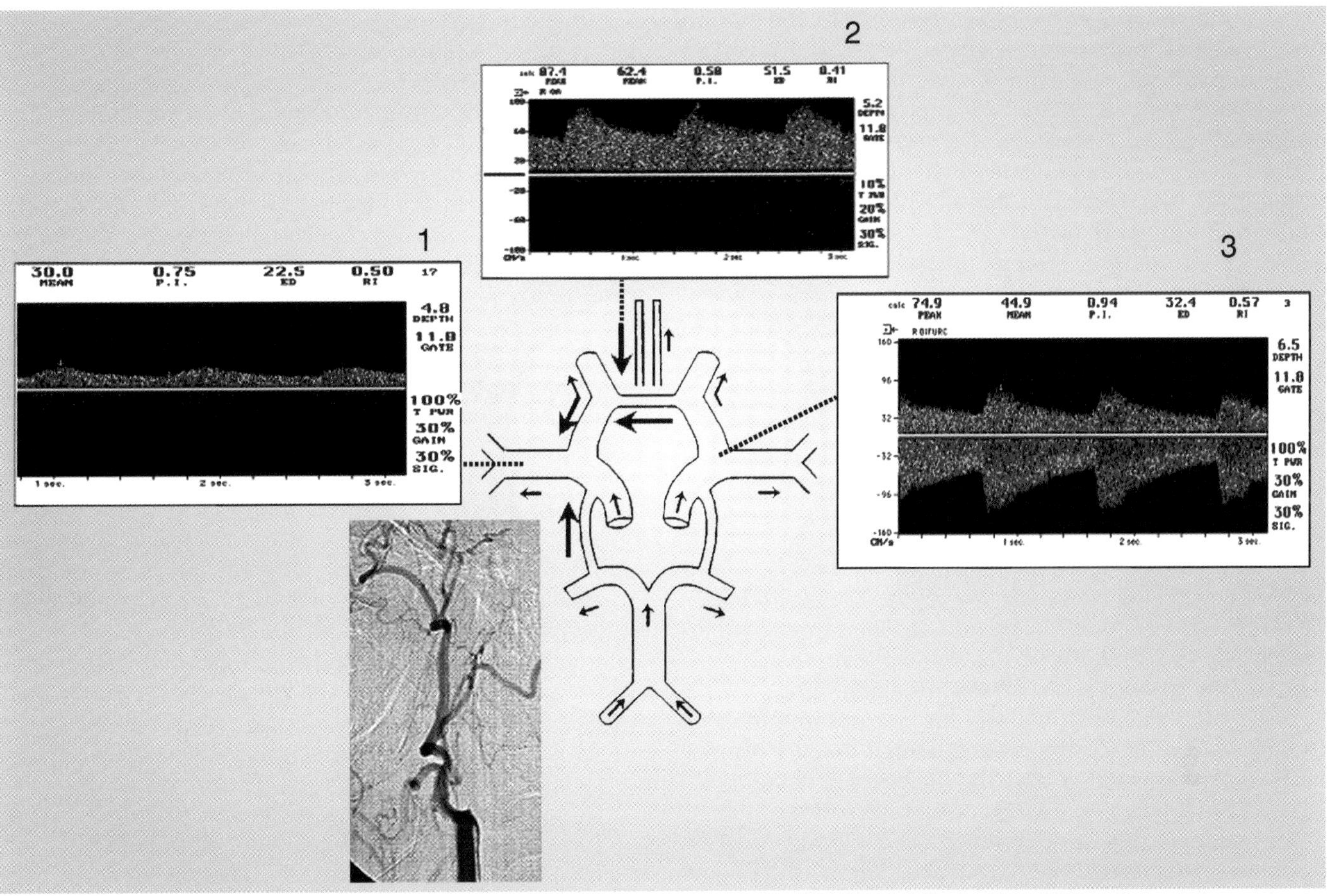

FIGURE 10 ■ Collateral blood flow pathways documented in an individual with an extracranial ICA occlusion 1. Recipient MCA Doppler signal has a delayed systolic acceleration and is "blunted." 2. Collateral blood flow via the OA (*arrow*). The Doppler signal has a low pulsatility index and blood flow direction is away from the probe (inverted image). 3. Anterior Cross-filling via the ACoA. There is increased velocity in the contralateral anterior cerebral artery (>MCA) of the donor side. 4. Collateral blood flow via PCoA. The mean velocity is usually greater than the velocity in the recipient artery where the delayed systolic flow acceleration is also visualized. ICA, internal carotid artery; MCA, middle cerebral artery; OA, ophthalmic artery; ACoA, anterior communicating artery; PCoA, posterior communicating artery.

Posterior Communicating Artery

Collateral perfusion from the posterior to the anterior circulation or from the anterior circulation to the posterior circulation via increased velocity through the PCoA can be detected by TCD. The PCoA usually lies in a favorable angle of insonation from the transtemporal window. When functioning, it may be detected as a flow signal consistently present at varying depths from 60 to 75 mm via the transtemporal approach (Fig. 10). Under normal conditions, this area usually has no detectable blood flow when the transducer is angled posteriorly from the ICA bifurcation to locate the PCA. The direction of blood flow in the PCoA corresponds to collateralization: anterior to posterior collateral blood flow is directed away from the transducer, whereas the posterior to anterior collateral blood flow is directed toward the transducer. Vessel identification is difficult since the PCoA and the PCA are prone to anatomic variations. The velocity range is similar to or higher than those detected in the M1 MCA and ICA bifurcation (anterior to posterior collateral flow), or BA (posterior to anterior collateral flow). A possible stenotic-like blood flow signal may be found at 60 to 75 mm with similar transducer angulation. The differential diagnosis includes a terminal ICA or PCA stenoses.

Ophthalmic Artery

An abnormal OA signal includes low pulsatility flow directed primarily away from the transducer via the transorbital window at 50 to 62 mm depth (Fig. 10). Check arterial identification since an ICA siphon flow signal may be insonated in the presence of low-velocity OA signals. Additional findings may include no substantial difference in mean velocities detected in the OA and siphon and high velocities in the ICA siphon, suggesting a high-grade proximal ICA and/or siphon stenosis; and no Doppler signals at depths of ≥60 mm, suggesting an ICA occlusion.

If the reversed OA is the only abnormal finding, this indicates possible ICA occlusion or severe stenosis proximal to the OA origin and inadequate intracranial collaterals. Occasionally, this may be the only sign of an ICA dissection or occlusion. Do not overestimate bidirectional Doppler signals found at depths of 30 to 55 mm in the orbit. True reversed blood flow in the OA should demonstrate low resistance with no velocity elevation in the siphon since collateral flow enters a larger vessel. If a reversed OA is found with a delayed systolic flow acceleration in the ipsilateral MCA, there is a probable proximal ICA occlusion or severe stenosis. If a reversed OA is found with at least one other collateral channel (anterior cross-filling or PCoA), there is a definite proximal ICA occlusion or high-grade stenosis.

Common sources of error include shallow or deep OA insonation, ICA dissection with considerable residual flow, terminal ICA occlusion distal to the OA origin, and retrograde filling of the ICA siphon with normal OA direction. Furthermore, a normal OA direction does not rule out proximal ICA stenosis.

DETECTION OF CEREBRAL EMBOLI

Ultrasound can detect embolism in real time (77), and TCD can detect this process in the cerebral vessels (78–80). TCD is used to monitor carotid and cardiac surgery, angioplasty/stenting and stroke patients with presumed cardiac or arterial sources for brain embolization.

The MES detected by TCD are asymptomatic since the size of the particles producing them is usually comparable to or even smaller than the diameter of brain capillaries (81). However, the MES cumulative count is related to the incidence of neuropsychological deficits after cardiopulmonary bypass (79,82,83), stroke after carotid endarterectomy (70,80,84–86), and the significance of MES as a risk factor for ischemic stroke is emerging.

It is important to know how to detect and identify MES. Occasionally, a TCD operator may be the only witness to cerebral microembolization during a routine examination and this finding may suggest a vascular origin of the neurological event and point to the potential sources of embolism (heart chambers and septum, aortic arch, arterial stenosis or dissection) (87–94).

Strict standards should be followed when an interpreter documents and reports microemboli on TCD (95). The gold standard for MES identification still remains the on-line interpretation of real-time, video- or digitally taped flow signals (95–97). The spectral recording should be obtained with minimal gain at a fixed angle of insonation with a small (<10 mm) sample volume. The probe should be maintained with a fixation device during at least 0.5 to 1 hour monitoring. The use of a two-channel simultaneous registration and a prolonged monitoring period may improve the yield of the procedure. Multigated or multiranged registration at different insonation depths may improve differentiation of embolic signals from artifacts.

According to the International Cerebral Hemodynamics Society definition (98), MES have the following characteristics (Fig. 11): (*i*) random occurrence during the cardiac cycle, (*ii*) brief duration (usually <0.1 sec), (*iii*) high intensity (>3 dB over background), (*iv*) primarily unidirectional signals (if fast Fourier transformation is used), and (*v*) an audible component (chirp, pop). The International Consensus Group on Microembolus Detection states that for the quality control of studies that report microemboli, the documentation should include the following parameters: ultrasound device, transducer frequency, type and size, insonated artery, insonation depth, algorithms for signal intensity measurement, scale settings, detection threshold, axial length of sample volume, fast Fourier transform (FFT) size (number of points used), FFT length (time), FFT overlap, transmitted ultrasound frequency, high-pass filter settings, and the recording time (95). There is an agreement that no current system of automated embolus detection has the required sensitivity and specificity for clinical use. Therefore, the interpreting physician has to review every stored signal, listen to the sound characteristics, determine the difference between the signal and background (dB), and attempt to determine the source of microemboli.

Recently, MES originating at the MCA stenosis that were associated with changes in stenotic flow velocity were described (99), as well as detected clusters of slow-moving MES with dissolving MCA thrombi in patients with crescendo transient ischemic attacks (TIAs) (100).

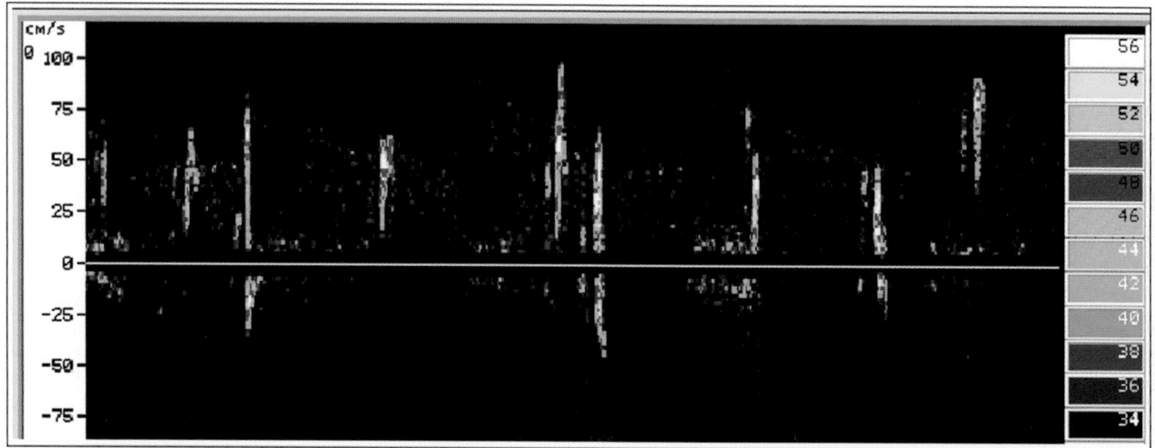

FIGURE 11 ■ Microembolic signals. A single-gated TCD recording from the MCA shows multiple high-intensity transient and primarily unidirectional signals after intravenous injection of agitated saline in a patient with a right-to-left cardiac shunt. TCD, transcranial Doppler; MCA, middle cerebral artery.

These findings indicate larger size of emboli that can change blood flow velocity and cerebral perfusion.

INCREASED ICP

A normal, low-resistance intracranial waveform is detected by TCD since the brain is a low-resistance vascular system with low ICP values. When ICP increases up to the diastolic pressure of the resistance vessels, EDV decreases and flow deceleration occurs more rapidly. Changes on TCD are noted with ICP values of 20 mmHg or higher (101–111). The following changes can be observed on TCD with increasing ICP: (*i*) EDV decreases, (*ii*) PI increases (PI ≥ 1.2 for previously normotensive young individuals), (*iii*) RI increases, (*iv*) trans-systolic time shortens, and (*v*) peak and mean velocities decrease.

When ICP becomes greater than diastolic blood pressure but less than systolic pressure, the result is either a triphasic waveform as seen in the peripheral arteries or a sharply peaked systolic signal and an absent end-diastolic component. Further increase in ICP may lead to cerebral circulatory arrest (Fig. 12).

Increased ICP may result in high-resistance waveforms: PI ≥ 1.2, decreased or absent EDV, and triphasic or reverberating flow. The following algorithm is used that may help to differentiate among the mechanisms of increased resistance to flow:

If the PI ≥ 1.2 and positive end-diastolic flow are present in: (*i*) all arteries then suspect hyperventilation, increased cardiac output, hypertension, increased ICP, (*ii*) unilaterally: then suspect compartmental ICP increase, stenoses distal to the site of insonation, (*iii*) one artery: then suspect distal obstruction (spasm, stenosis, edema).

If the PI ≥ 2.0 and end-diastolic flow is absent (*i*) in all arteries: then arterial occlusion, extremely high ICP, and possible arrest of cerebral circulation is suspected, (*ii*) unilaterally: then compartmental ICP increase and occlusion distal to insonation site is suspected, (*iii*) in one artery: then distal obstruction (occlusion, severe spasm, and edema) is suspected.

MONITORING CEREBRAL CIRCULATORY ARREST

Progressive elevation of ICP due to brain edema or mass effect produces stepwise compression of small and large intracranial arteries, eventually leading to cerebral circulatory arrest. A prolonged absence of brain perfusion can be detected using oscillating (reverberating) flow pattern (Fig. 12), systolic spike, or absent flow signals (23,112–123), and this process will lead to brain death (124). TCD is a reliable tool to confirm cerebral circulatory arrest with accuracy parameters close to 100% at experienced centers (23,112–123).

Based on previous published studies, reviews, and criteria (23,112–123) and our clinical experience, we developed the following algorithm if cerebral circulatory arrest is suspected: (*i*) document arterial blood pressure at the time of TCD examination, (*ii*) if there is presence of positive MCA or BA end-diastolic flow then there is no cerebral circulatory arrest, (*iii*) if there is absent end-diastolic flow then there is uncertain cerebral circulatory arrest (too early or too late), (*iv*) if there is reversed minimal end-diastolic flow then there is possible cerebral circulatory arrest (continue monitoring), and (*v*) if there is reverberating flow then there is probable cerebral circulatory arrest (confirm in both MCA's at 50–60 mm and BA at 80–90 mm, then monitor arrest for 30 minutes).

TCD "cannot" be used to diagnose brain death since this is a clinical diagnosis (124). TCD can be used to confirm cerebral circulatory arrest in adults and children "except" in infants less than six months (23,112–123). TCD can be used to monitor progressive flow changes toward cerebral circulatory arrest. Once a reverberating signal is found, it should be monitored for at least 30 minutes in both MCAs and BA to avoid false-positive findings. Also, avoid insonation of bifurcations, i.e., MCA/ACA, since bidirectional reverberating signals may overlap, creating an illusion of positive EDV.

SA-transient cerebral circulatory arrest can occur in patients with SAH and head trauma due to A-waves of ICP. TCD can also be used to determine the appropriate

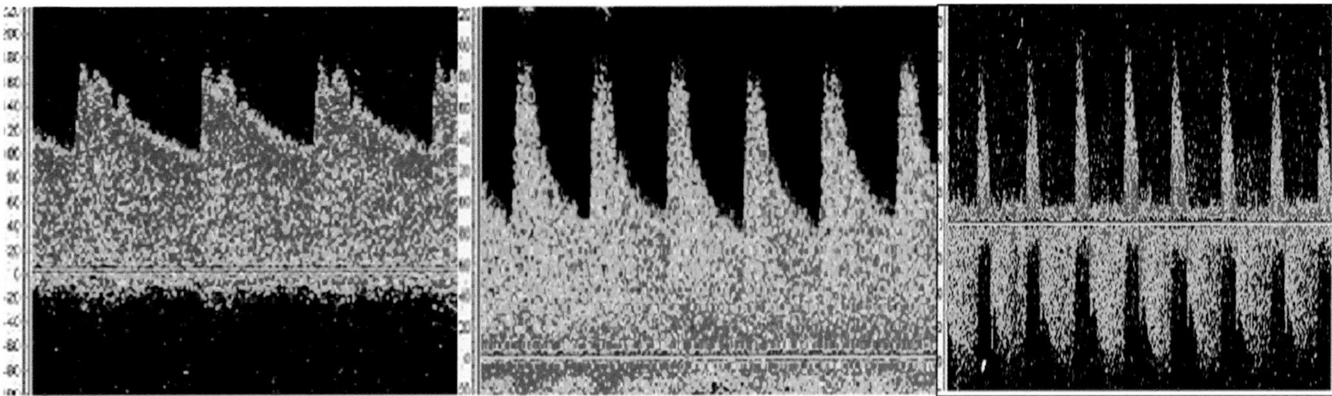

FIGURE 12 ■ Increased ICP and cerebral circulatory arrest. TCD waveforms in a patient with progressively increasing ICP following subarachnoid hemorrhage. Reverberating flow pattern is documented in this patient. ICP, intracranial cerebral pressure.

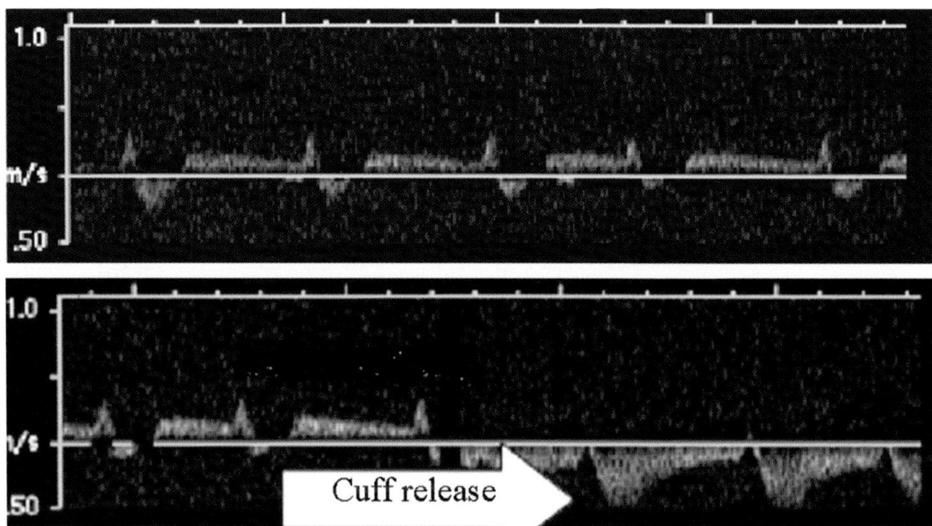

FIGURE 13 ■ Bidirectional blood flow signal documented in the vertebral artery. After the blood pressure cuff is quickly released from the arm, changes in the Doppler signal direction and velocity are documented.

time for other confirmatory tests (i.e., to minimize studies with residual cerebral blood flow) and to discuss the consequent issues with the patient's family.

DOCUMENTATION OF SUBCLAVIAN STEAL

Subclavian steal is a hemodynamic condition of reversed flow in one VA to compensate for a proximal stenosis or occlusion of the left subclavian, the innominate, or the right subclavian arteries proximal to the origin of the VA (125). A stenosis at this location may cause the pressure in the upper extremity to be lower than normal. Thus, blood flow is diverted or "stolen" from the brain to feed the arm. Subclavian steal is usually an incidental finding since it rarely produces neurological symptoms. If the patient is asymptomatic, it is considered the "subclavian steal phenomenon" and it usually indicates widespread atherosclerosis of the aortic branches. If symptoms of vertebrobasilar ischemia are present, it is considered the "subclavian steal syndrome"(125).

Subclavian steal is well studied with ultrasound (Fig. 13) (126–146). When a subclavian steal is suspected, a standard TCD examination should be performed with special attention focused on blood flow direction and velocities in the vertebral and basilar arteries. If a steal is present at rest, the main findings usually include a difference in blood pressure between arms of ≥20 mmHg and reversed blood flow direction in the vertebral and/or BA. Often, reversed blood flow direction is only found in the VA, suggesting a possible vertebral to vertebral steal. Right-to-left subclavian steal is found in 85% of cases due to the anatomic differences in the origin of these arteries.

If the blood pressure difference between arms is 10 to 20 mmHg and in the absence of blood flow reversal at rest, or if alternating blood flow direction is observed, the involved upper extremity should be stressed (hyperemia test) to reduce outflow resistance, thereby revealing the hemodynamics of a potentially latent steal. A blood pressure cuff is applied to the arm ipsilateral to the arterial stenosis/occlusion. The blood pressure cuff is above systolic pressure (>20 mmHg above systolic) and maintained about 1 to 1.5 minute (maximum three minutes, if tolerated by patient). The cuff should be rapidly deflated (quickly released from the arm) and changes in blood flow direction and velocity recorded. This procedure may be repeated with monitoring of the contralateral VA and the BA. A 5- to 10-minute rest period is necessary for the return of baseline arterial hemodynamics between evaluations.

TABLE 6 ■ International Concensus Criteria: Right-to-Left Shunt

Diagnosis	Microbubbles
Negative	0
Positive	1–10
	>10 and no curtain[a]
	Curtain

[a]Curtain is a shower of microbubbles, where a single bubble cannot be identified.

TABLE 7 ■ Spencer Logarithmic Scale

Shunt grade	Embolic signals
0	0
1	1–10
2	11–30
3	31–100
4	101–300
5	>300

Note: Shunt grades have to be provided for injections at rest and with Valsalva.

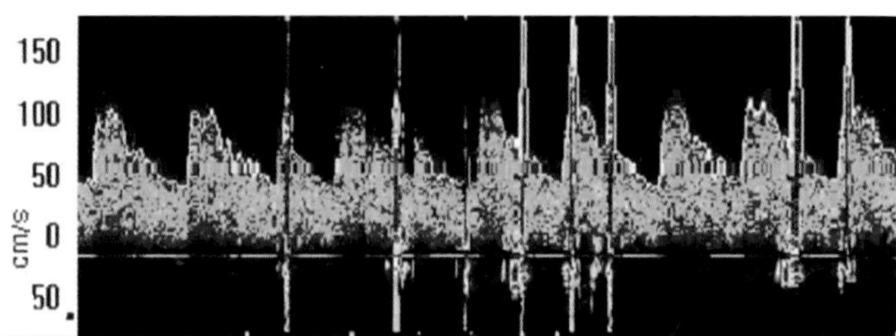

FIGURE 14 ■ Microbubbles (1–10) were documented in the middle cerebral artery after injection of agitated saline in a patient with a right-to-left shunt.

DETECTION OF RIGHT-TO-LEFT SHUNTS

Research studies have proposed TCD as an alternative noninvasive technique for the detection of right-to-left shunts that commonly occur with a patent foramen ovale (PFO) (147–153). A PFO is estimated to be present in 25% of the population and may be present in up to 40% of individuals who have suffered a stroke. TCD is less invasive compared to the gold standard, transesophageal echocardiography (TEE). Investigators have reported a wide range for TCD's sensitivity (63–100%) and its specificity has been reported to be 100% (147–153). One report suggests superior accuracy of power motion (M-mode) TCD compared to the single-gate TCD, with comparable diagnostic capabilities of the power motion TCD and TEE determined during cardiac catheterization (154).

The TCD examination for right-to-left shunt, also called the "bubble" test, is done with TCD insonation of the MCA (50–55 mm) via the transtemporal approach. A mixture of 9 mL of saline + 1 mL of air is prepared with a three-way stopcock by exchange of saline/air mixture between the syringes and injected as a bolus. The suspension is rapidly injected into the antecubital vein and is monitored at rest and with Valsalva maneuver. The diagnostic criteria for right-to-left shunt are listed in Tables 6 and 7 and an example is shown in Figure 14.

CONCLUSION

Interpretation of the TCD results should include consideration of the (*i*) patient's neurologic signs and symptoms, (*ii*) various physiological factors (i.e., age, hematocrit) that can influence intracranial arterial hemodynamics, and (*iii*) results of the extracranial carotid/vertebral studies. When these factors are taken into account, the results of the TCD examination provide useful clinical information for patient management. Currently, TCD is one of the recommended neuroimaging technologies for developing a comprehensive stroke center (155).

REFERENCES

1. Aaslid R. Transcranial Doppler Sonography. New York: Wien Springer Verlag, 1986.
2. Katz ML, Alexandrov AV. A Practical Guide To Transcranial Doppler Examinations. Littleton, CO: Summer Publishing, 2003.
3. Babikian VL, Feldmann E, Wechsler LR, et al. Transcranial Doppler ultrasonography: year 2000 update. J Neuroimaging 2000; 10:101–115.
4. Intersocietal Commission for the Accreditation of Vascular Laboratories (ICAVL). http://www.icavl.org/icavl/index.htm. Retrieved March 2006.
5. Alexandrov AV, Tegeler CH. Diagnostic criteria for transcranial Doppler sonography: a model for quality assurance and laboratory accreditation. Vascular Ultrasound Today 1999; 4:1–24.
6. Hennerici M, Rautenberg W, Schwartz A. Transcranial Doppler ultrasound for the assessment of intracranial arterial flow velocity—Part I. Examination technique and normal values. Surg Neurol 1987; 27:439–448.
7. Otis SM, Ringelstein EB. The transcranial Doppler examination: principles and applications of transcranial Doppler sonography. In: Tegeler CH, Babikian VL, Gomez CR, eds. Neurosonology. St Louis: Mosby, 1996:140–155.
8. Babikian V, Sloan MA, Tegeler CH, et al. Transcranial Doppler validation pilot study. J Neuroimaging 1993; 3:242–249.
9. Gosling RG, King DH. Arterial assessment by Doppler-shift ultrasound. Proc Roy Soc Med 1974; 67:447–449.
10. Pourcellot L. Applications cliniques de l'examen Doppler transcutane. Les colloques de l'Institute national de la Sante et de la Recherche medicale. INSERM 1974; 213–240.
11. Lindegaard KF, Bakke SJ, Aaslid R, Nornes H. Doppler diagnosis of intracranial artery occlusive disorders. J Neurol Neurosurg Psychiatry 1986; 49:510–518.
12. de Bray JM, Joseph PA, Jeanvoine H, Maugin D, Dauzat M, Plassard F. Transcranial Doppler evaluation of middle cerebral artery stenosis. J Ultrasound Med 1988; 7(11):611–616.
13. Ley-Pozo J, Ringelstein EB. Noninvasive detection of occlusive disease of the carotid siphon and middle cerebral artery. Ann Neurol 1990; 28:640–647.
14. Schwarze JJ, Babikian V, DeWitt LD, et al. Longitudinal monitoring of intracranial arterial stenoses with transcranial Doppler ultrasonography. J Neuroimaging 1994; 4:182–187.
15. Rother J, Schwartz A, Rautenberg W, Hennerici M. Middle cerebral artery stenoses: assessment by magnetic resonance angiography and transcranial Doppler ultrasound. Cerebrovasc Dis 1994; 4: 273–279.
16. Alexandrov AV, Bladin CF, Norris JW. Intracranial blood flow velocities in acute ischemic stroke. Stroke 1994; 25:1378–1383.
17. Wong KS, Li H, Lam WW, Chan YL, Kay R. Progression of middle cerebral artery occlusive disease and its relationship with further vascular events after stroke. Stroke 2002; 33(2):532–536.
18. Segura T, Serena J, Castellanos M, Teruel J, Vilar C, Davalos A. Embolism in acute middle cerebral artery stenosis. Neurology 2001; 56(4):497–501.
19. Arenillas JF, Molina CA, Montaner J, Abilleira S, Gonzalez-Sanchez MA, Alvarez-Sabin J. Progression and clinical recurrence of symptomatic middle cerebral artery stenosis: a long-term follow-up transcranial Doppler ultrasound study. Stroke 2001; 32(12): 2898–2904.
20. Felberg RA, Christou I, Demchuk AM, Malkoff M, Alexandrov AV. Screening for intracranial stenosis with transcranial Doppler: the accuracy of mean flow velocity thresholds. J Neuroimaging 2002; 12(1):9–14.
21. Mattle H, Grolimund P, Huber P, Sturzenegger M, Zurbrugg HR. Transcranial Doppler sonographic findings in middle cerebral artery disease. Arch Neurol 1988; 45(3):289–295.
22. Brass LM, Duterte DL, Mohr JP. Anterior cerebral artery velocity changes in disease of the middle cerebral artery stem. Stroke 1989; 20(12):1737–1740.
23. Hennerici M, Neuerburg-Heusler D. Vascular Diagnosis With Ultrasound: Clinical References with Case Studies. Stuttgart: Thieme, 1998:96.
24. Adams RJ. TCD in sickle cell disease: an important and useful test. Pediatr Radiol 2005; 35:229–234.
25. Chimowitz MI, Kokkinos J, Strong J, et al. The Warfarin-Aspirin Symptomatic Intracranial Disease Study. Neurology 1995; 45(8):1488–1493.

26. Alexandrov AV, Demchuk AM, Wein TH, Grotta JC. Yield of transcranial Doppler in acute cerebral ischemia. Stroke 1999; 30:1604–1609.
27. Alexandrov AV, Demchuk AM, Felberg RA, Grotta JC, Krieger DW. Intracranial clot dissolution is associated with embolic signals on transcranial Doppler. J Neuroimaging 2000; 10(1):27–32.
28. Lindegaard K, Bakke S, Grolimund P, Aaslid R, Huber P, Nornes H. Assessment of intracranial hemodynamics in carotid artery disease by transcranial Doppler ultrasound. J Neurosurg 1985; 63(6): 890–898.
29. Schneider P, Rossman M, Bernstein E, Torem S, Ringelstein E, Otis S. Effect of internal carotid artery occlusion on intracranial hemodynamics: transcranial Doppler evaluation and clinical correlation. Stroke 1988; 19:589–593.
30. Razumovsky AY, Gillard JH, Byran RN, Hanley DF, Oppenheimer SM. TCD, MRA and MRI in acute cerebral ischemia. Acta Neurol Scand 1999; 99:65–76.
31. Steinke W, Mangold J, Schwartz A, Hennerici M. Mechanisms of infarction in the superficial posterior cerebral artery territory. J Neurol 1997; 244(9):571–578.
32. Kimura K, Minematsu K, Yasaka M, Wada K, Yamaguchi T. Evaluation of posterior cerebral artery flow velocity by transcranial color-coded real-time sonography. Ultrasound Med Biol 2000; 26(2):195–199.
33. de Bray JM, Missoum A, Dubas F, Emile J, Lhoste P. Detection of vertebrobasilar intracranial stenoses: transcranial Doppler Sonography versus angiography. J Ultrasound Med1997; 16(3):213–218.
34. Ringelstein EB. Ultrasonic diagnosis of the vertebrobasilar system. II. Transnuchal diagnosis of intracranial vertebrobasilar stenoses using a novel pulsed Doppler system. Ultraschall Med 1985; 6(2):60–67. German.
35. Budingen HJ, Staudacher T. Identification of the basilar artery with transcranial Doppler sonography. Ultraschall Med 1987; 8(2): 95–101. German.
36. Volc D, Possnigg G, Grisold W, Neuhold A. Transcranial Doppler sonography of the vertebro-basilar system. Acta Neurochir (Wien) 1988; 90(3–4):136–138.
37. Demchuk AM, Christou I, Wein TH, et al. Accuracy and criteria for localizing arterial occlusion with transcranial doppler. J Neuroimaging 2000; 10:1–12.
38. Droste DW, Nabavi DG, Kemeny V, et al. Echocontrast enhanced transcranial colour-coded duplex offers improved visualization of the vertebrobasilar system. Acta Neurol Scand 1998; 98(3):193–199.
39. Postert T, Federlein J, Przuntek H, Büttner T. Power-based versus conventional transcranial color-coded duplex sonography in the assessment of the vertebrobasilar-posterior system. J Stroke Cerebrovasc Dis 1997; 6:398–404.
40. Baumgartner RW, Mattle HP, Schroth G. Assessment of ≥50% and <50% intracranial stenoses by transcranial color-coded duplex sonography. Stroke 1999; 30(1):87–92.
41. Grolimund P, Seiler RW, Aaslid R, Huber P, Zurbruegg H. Evaluation of cerebrovascular disease by combined extracranial and transcranial Doppler sonography. Experience in 1,039 patients. Stroke 1987; 18:1018–1024.
42. Halsey J. Prognosis of acute hemiplegia estimated by transcranial Doppler sonography. Stroke 1988; 19:648–649.
43. Zanette EM, Fieschi C, Bozzao L, et al. Comparison of cerebral angiography and transcranial Doppler sonography in acute stroke. Stroke 1989; 20:899–903.
44. Kaps M, Damian MS, Teschendorf U, Dorndorf W. Transcranial Doppler ultrasound findings in the middle cerebral artery occlusion. Stroke 1990; 21:532–537.
45. Carmelingo M, Casto L, Censori B, Ferraro B, Gazzaniga GC, Mamoli A. Transcranial Doppler in acute ischemic stroke of the middle cerebral artery territories. Acta Neurol Scand 1993; 88:108–111.
46. Demchuk AM, Burgin WS, Christou I, et al. Thrombolysis in brain ischemia (TIBI) transcranial Doppler flow grades predict clinical severity, early recovery, and mortality in patients treated with tissue plasminogen activator. Stroke 2001; 32:89–93.
47. Burgin WS, Malkoff M, Felberg RA, et al. Transcranial Doppler ultrasound criteria for recanalization after thrombolysis for middle cerebral artery stroke. Stroke 2000; 31:1128–1132.
48. El-Mitwalli A, Saad M, Christou I, Malkoff M, Alexandrov AV. Clinical and sonographic patterns of tandem ICA/MCA occlusion in TPA treated patients. Stroke 2002; 33:99–102.
49. Brandt T, Knauth M, Wildermuth S, et al. CT angiography and Doppler sonography for emergency assessment in acute basilar artery ischemia. Stroke 1999; 30(3):606–612.
50. Klotzsch C, Bozzato A, Lammers G, Mull M, Noth J. Contrast-enhanced three-dimensional transcranial color-coded sonography of intracranial stenoses. AJNR Am J Neuroradiol 2002; 23(2):208–212.
51. Delcker A, Diener HC. Various ultrasound methods for studying the vertebral artery—a comparative evaluation. Ultraschall Med 1992; 13(5):213–220. German.
52. Niederkorn K, Myers LG, Nunn CL, Ball MR, McKinney WM. Three-dimensional transcranial Doppler blood flow mapping in patients with cerebrovascular disorders. Stroke 1988; 19(11): 1335–1344.
53. Toole JF. Cerebrovascular Disorders. 5th ed. Philadelphia: Lippincott Williams & Wilkins, 1999.
54. Sloan MA. Transcranial Doppler monitoring of vasospasm after subarachnoid hemorrhage. In: Tegeler CH, Babikian VL, Gomez CR, eds. Neurosonology. St Louis: Mosby, 1996:156–171.
55. Lindegaard KF, Nornes H, Bakke SJ, Sorteberg W, Nakstad P. Cerebral vasospasm after subarachnoid haemorrhage investigated by means of transcranial Doppler ultrasound. Acta Neurochir (Wien) 1988; 42 suppl:P81–P84.
56. Newell DW, Grady MS, Eskridge JM, Winn HR. Distribution of angiographic vasospasm after subarachnoid hemorrhage: implications for diagnosis by transcranial Doppler ultrasonography. Neurosurgery 1990; 27:574–577.
57. Awad IA, Carter LP, Spetzler RF, Medina M, Williams FC. Clinical vasospasm after subarachnoid hemorrhage: response to hypervolemic hemodilution and arterial hypertension. Stroke 1987; 18:365–372.
58. Kontos HA. Validity of cerebral arterial blood flow calculations from velocity measurements. Stroke 1989; 20:1–3.
59. Mizuno M, Nakajima S, Sampei T, et al. Serial transcranial Doppler flow velocity and cerebral blood flow measurements for evaluation of cerebral vasospasm after subarachnoid hemorrhage. Neurol Med Chir (Tokyo) 1994; 34(3):164–171.
60. Sloan MA, Haley EC Jr, Kassell NF, et al. Sensitivity and specificity of transcranial Doppler ultrasonography in the diagnosis of vasospasm following subarachnoid hemorrhage. Neurology 1989; 39(11): 1514–1518.
61. Newell DW, Winn HR. Transcranial Doppler in cerebral vasospasm. Neurosurg Clin N Am 1990; 1(2):319–328.
62. Lindegaard KF. The role of transcranial Doppler in the management of patients with subarachnoid haemorrhage: a review. Acta Neurochir Suppl 1999; 72:59–71.
63. Lysakowski C, Walder B, Costanza MC, Tramer MR. Transcranial Doppler versus angiography in patients with vasospasm due to a ruptured cerebral aneurysm: a systematic review. Stroke 2001; 32(10):2292–2298.
64. Piepgras A, Hagen T, Schmiadek P. Reliable prediction of grade of angiographic vasospasm by transcranial Doppler sonography [abstr]. Stroke 1994; 25:260.
65. Reigel MM, Hollier LH, Sundt TM Jr, Piepgras DG, Sharbrough FW, Cherry KJ. Cerebral hyperperfusion syndrome: a cause of neurologic dysfunction after carotid endarterectomy. J Vasc Surg 1987; 5(4):628–634.
66. Powers AD, Smith RR. Hyperperfusion syndrome after carotid endarterectomy: a transcranial Doppler evaluation. Neurosurgery 1990; 26(1):56–59.
67. Schoser BG, Heesen C, Eckert B, Thie A. Cerebral hyperperfusion injury after percutaneous transluminal angioplasty of extracranial arteries. J Neurol 1997; 244(2):101–104.
68. Dalman JE, Beenakkers IC, Moll FL, Leusink JA, Ackerstaff RG. Transcranial Doppler monitoring during carotid endarterectomy helps to identify patients at risk of postoperative hyperperfusion. Eur J Vasc Endovasc Surg 1999; 18(3):222–227.
69. Spencer MP. Transcranial Doppler monitoring and causes of stroke from carotid endarterectomy. Stroke 1997; 28(4):685–691.

70. Padayachee TS, Kirkham FJ, Lewis RR, Gillard J, Hutchinson MC, Gosling RG. Transcranial measurement of blood velocities in the basal cerebral arteries using pulsed Doppler ultrasound: a method of assessing the Circle of Willis. Ultrasound Med Biol 1986; 12(1):5–14.
71. Bass A, Krupski WC, Dilley RB, Bernstein EF, Otis SM. Comparison of transcranial and cervical continuous-wave Doppler in the evaluation of intracranial collateral circulation. Stroke 1990; 21(11):1584–1588.
72. Byrd S, Wolfe J, Nicolaides A, et al. Vascular surgical society of Great Britain and Ireland: transcranial doppler ultrasonography as a predictor of haemodynamically significant carotid stenosis. Br J Surg 1999; 86(5):692–693.
73. Schneider PA, Rossman ME, Bernstein EF, Ringelstein EB, Otis SM. Noninvasive assessment of cerebral collateral blood supply through the ophthalmic artery. Stroke 1991; 22(1):31–36.
74. Rutgers DR, Klijn CJ, Kappelle LJ, van Huffelen AC, van der Grond J. A longitudinal study of collateral flow patterns in the circle of Willis and the ophthalmic artery in patients with a symptomatic internal carotid artery occlusion. Stroke 2000; 31(8):1913–1920.
75. Wilterdink JL, Feldmann E, Furie KL, Bragoni M, Benavides JG. Transcranial Doppler ultrasound battery reliably identifies severe internal carotid artery stenosis. Stroke 1997; 28:133–136.
76. Christou I, Felberg RA, Demchuk AM, et al. Accuracy parameters of a broad diagnostic battery for bedside transcranial Doppler to detect flow changes with internal carotid artery stenosis or occlusion. J Neuroimaging 2001; 11:236–242.
77. Spencer MP, Campbell SD, Sealey JL, Henry FC, Lindbergh J. Experiments on decompression bubbles in the circulation using ultrasonic and electromagnetic flowmeters. J Occup Med 1969; 11(5):238–244.
78. Padayachee TS, Gosling RG, Bishop CC, Burnand K, Browse NL. Transcranial measurement of blood velocities in the basal cerebral arteries using pulsed Doppler ultrasound: a method of assessing the circle of Willis. Ultrasound Med Biol 1986; 12(1):5–14.
79. Deverall PB, Padayachee TS, Parsons S, Theobold R, Battistessa SA. Ultrasound detection of micro-emboli in the middle cerebral artery during cardiopulmonary bypass surgery. Eur J Cardiothorac Surg 1988; 2(4):256–260.
80. Spencer MP, Thomas GI, Nicholls SC, Sauvage LR. Detection of middle cerebral artery emboli during carotid endarterectomy using transcranial Doppler ultrasonography. Stroke 1990; 21(3): 415–423.
81. Brucher R, Russel D. Background and principles. In: Tegeler CH, Babikian VL, Gomez CR, eds. Neurosonology. St. Loius: Mosby, 1996:231–234.
82. Clark RE, Brillman J, Davis DA, Lovell MR, Price TR, Magovern GJ. Microemboli during coronary artery bypass grafting. Genesis and effect on outcome. J Thorac Cardiovasc Surg 1995; 109(2): 249–257.
83. Diegeler A, Hirsch R, Schneider F, et al. Neuromonitoring and neurocognitive outcome in off-pump versus conventional coronary bypass operation. Ann Thorac Surg 2000; 69(4):1162–1166.
84. Jansen C, Moll FL, Vermeulen FE, van Haelst JM, Ackerstaff RG. Continuous transcranial Doppler ultrasonography and electroencephalography during carotid endarterectomy: a multimodal monitoring system to detect intraoperative ischemia. Ann Vasc Surg 1993; 7(1):95–101.
85. Ackerstaff RG, Jansen C, Moll FL, Vermeulen FE, Hamerlijnck RP, Mauser HW. The significance of microemboli detection by means of transcranial Doppler ultrasonography monitoring in carotid endarterectomy. J Vasc Surg 1995; 21(6):963–969.
86. Ackerstaff RG, Moons KG, van de Vlasakker CJ, et al. Association of intraoperative transcranial doppler monitoring variables with stroke from carotid endarterectomy. Stroke 2000; 31(8):1817–1823.
87. Georgiadis D, Grosset DG, Kelman A, Faichney A, Lees KR. Prevalence and characteristics of intracranial microemboli signals in patients with different types of prosthetic cardiac valves. Stroke 1994; 25(3):587–592.
88. Tong DC, Bolger A, Albers GW. Incidence of transcranial Doppler-detected cerebral microemboli in patients referred for echocardiography. Stroke 1994; 25(11):2138–2141.
89. Tong DC, Albers GW. Transcranial Doppler-detected microemboli in patients with acute stroke. Stroke 1995; 26(9):1588–1592.
90. Nabavi DG, Georgiadis D, Mumme T, et al. Clinical relevance of intracranial microembolic signals in patients with left ventricular assist devices. A prospective study. Stroke 1996; 27(5):891–896.
91. Sliwka U, Lingnau A, Stohlmann WD, et al. Prevalence and time course of microembolic signals in patients with acute stroke. A prospective study. Stroke 1997; 28(2):358–363.
92. Koennecke HC, Mast H, Trocio SS Jr, Sacco RL, Thompson JL, Mohr JP. Microemboli in patients with vertebrobasilar ischemia: association with vertebrobasilar and cardiac lesions. Stroke 1997; 28(3):593–596.
93. Nadareishvili ZG, Choudary Z, Joyner C, Brodie D, Norris JW. Cerebral microembolism in acute myocardial infarction. Stroke 1999; 30(12):2679–2682.
94. Rundek T, Di Tullio MR, Sciacca RR, et al. Association between large aortic arch atheromas and high-intensity transient signals in elderly stroke patients. Stroke 1999; 30(12):2683–2686.
95. Ringelstein EB, Droste DW, Babikian VL, et al. Consensus on microembolus detection by TCD. International Consensus Group on Microembolus Detection. Stroke 1998; 29:725–729.
96. Cullinane M, Reid G, Dittrich R, et al. Evaluation of new online automated embolic signal detection algorithm, including comparison with panel of international experts. Stroke 2000; 31(6): 1335–1341.
97. Markus HS. Transcranial Doppler ultrasound. Br Med Bull 2000; 56(2):378–388.
98. The International Cerebral Hemodynamics Society Consensus Statement. Stroke 1995; 26:1123.
99. Gao S, Wong KS. Characteristics of mircoembolic signals detected near their origins in middle cerebral artery stenosis. J Neuroimaging 2003; 13(2):124–132.
100. Segura T, Serena J, Molins A, Davalos A. Clusters of microembolic signals: a new form of cerebral microembolism presentation in a patient with middle cerebral artery stenosis. Stroke 1998; 29:722–724.
101. Nornes H, Angelsen B, Lindegaard KF. Precerebral arterial blood flow pattern in intracranial hypertension with cerebral blood flow arrest. Acta Neurochir 1977; 38:187–194.
102. Harders A. Neurosurgical Applications of Transcranial Doppler Sonography. Wien: Springer-Verlag, 1986:45.
103. Fischer AQ, Livingstone JN. Transcranial Doppler and real-time cranial sonography in neonatal hydrocephalus. J Child Neurol 1989; 4(1):64–69.
104. Homburg AM, Jakobsen M, Enevoldsen E. Transcranial Doppler recordings in raised intracranial pressure. Acta Neurol Scand 1993; 87(6):488–493.
105. Hanlo PW, Peters RJ, Gooskens RH, et al. Monitoring intracranial dynamics by transcranial Doppler—a new Doppler index: trans systolic time. Ultrasound Med Biol 1995; 21(5):613–621.
106. Mayer SA, Thomas CE, Diamond BE. Asymmetry of intracranial hemodynamics as an indicator of mass effect in acute intracerebral hemorrhage. A transcranial Doppler study. Stroke 1996; 27(10):1788–1792.
107. Lewis S, Wong M, Myburgh J, Reilly P. Determining cerebral perfusion pressure thresholds in severe head trauma. Acta Neurochir Suppl 1998; 71:174–176.
108. Richards HK, Czosnyka M, Whitehouse H, Pickard JD. Increase in transcranial Doppler pulsatility index does not indicate the lower limit of cerebral autoregulation. Acta Neurochir Suppl 1998; 71:229–232.
109. Treib J, Becker SC, Grauer M, Haass A. Transcranial doppler monitoring of intracranial pressure therapy with mannitol, sorbitol and glycerol in patients with acute stroke. Eur Neurol 1998; 40(4):212–219.
110. Czosnyka M, Smielewski P, Piechnik S, et al. Hemodynamic characterization of intracranial pressure plateau waves in head-injury patients. J Neurosurg 1999; 91(1):11–19.
111. Rainov NG, Weise JB, Burkert W. Transcranial Doppler sonography in adult hydrocephalic patients. Neurosurg Rev 2000; 23(1): 34–38.
112. Grolimund P, Seiler RW, Mattle H. Possibilities and limits of transcranial Doppler sonography. Ultraschall Med 1987; 8(2):87–94. German.

113. Klingelhofer J, Conrad B, Benecke R, Sander D. Intracranial flow patterns at increasing intracranial pressure. Klin Wochenschr 1987; 65(12):542–545.
114. Kirkham FJ, Levin SD, Padayachee TS, Kyme MC, Neville BG, Gosling RG. Transcranial pulsed Doppler ultrasound findings in brain stem death. J Neurol Neurosurg Psychiatry 1987; 50(11):1504–1513.
115. Ropper AH, Kehne SM, Wechsler L. Transcranial Doppler in brain death. Neurology 1987; 37(11):1733–1735.
116. Hassler W, Steinmetz H, Gawlowski J. Transcranial Doppler ultrasonography in raised intracranial pressure and in intracranial circulatory arrest. J Neurosurg 1988; 68(5):745–751.
117. Bode H, Sauer M, Pringsheim W. Diagnosis of brain death by transcranial Doppler sonography. Arch Dis Child 1988; 63(12): 1474–1478.
118. Newell DW, Grady MS, Sirotta P, Winn HR. Evaluation of brain death using transcranial Doppler. Neurosurgery 1989; 24(4): 509–513.
119. Petty GW, Mohr JP, Pedley TA, et al. The role of transcranial Doppler in confirming brain death: sensitivity, specificity, and suggestions for performance and interpretation. Neurology 1990; 40(2):300–303.
120. van der Naalt J, Baker AJ. Influence of the intra-aortic balloon pump on the transcranial Doppler flow pattern in a brain-dead patient. Stroke 1996; 27(1):140–142.
121. Ducrocq X, Hassler W, Moritake K, et al. Consensus opinion on diagnosis of cerebral circulatory arrest using Doppler-sonography: Task Force Group on cerebral death of the Neurosonology Research Group of the World Federation of Neurology. J Neurol Sci 1998; 159:145–150.
122. Ducrocq X, Braun M, Debouverie M, Junges C, Hummer M, Vespignani H. Brain death and transcranial Doppler: experience in 130 cases of brain dead patients. J Neurol Sci 1998; 160(1): 41–46.
123. Hadani M, Bruk B, Ram Z, Knoller N, Spiegelmann R, Segal E. Application of transcranial doppler ultrasonography for the diagnosis of brain death. Intensive Care Med 1999; 25(8):822–828.
124. Wijdicks EF. The diagnosis of brain death. N Engl J Med 2001; 344(16):1215–1221.
125. Voigt K, Kendel K, Sauer M. Subclavian steal syndrome. Bloodless diagnosis of the syndrome using ultrasonic pulse echo and vertebral artery compression. Fortschr Neurol Psychiatr Grenzgeb 1970; 38(1):20–33. German.
126. Grossman BL, Brisman R, Wood EH. Ultrasound and the subclavian steal syndrome. Radiology 1970; 94(1):1–6.
127. Reutern GM, Budingen HJ, Freund HJ. The diagnosis of obstructions of the vertebral and subclavian arteries by means of directional Doppler sonography. Arch Psychiatr Nervenkr 1976; 222(2–3): 209–222. German.
128. von Reutern GM, Budingen HJ. Doppler sonographic study of the vertebral artery in subclavian steal syndrome. Dtsch Med Wochenschr 1977; 102(4):140–141. German.
129. Yoneda S, Nukada T, Tada K, Imaizumi M, Takano T. Subclavian steal in Takayasu's arteritis. A hemodynamic study by means of ultrasonic Doppler flowmetry. Stroke 1977; 8(2):264–268.
130. Pourcelot L, Ribadeau-Dumas JL, Fagret D, Planiol T. Contribution of the Doppler examination to the diagnosis of subclavian steal syndrome. Rev Neurol (Paris) 1977; 133(5):309–323. French.
131. Walker DW, Acker JD, Cole CA. Subclavian steal syndrome detected with duplex pulsed Doppler sonography. AJNR Am J Neuroradiol 1982; 3(6):615–618.
132. Ringelstein EB, Zeumer H. Delayed reversal of vertebral artery blood flow following percutaneous transluminal angioplasty for subclavian steal syndrome. Neuroradiology 1984; 26(3): 189–198.
133. Ackerstaff RG, Hoeneveld H, Slowikowski JM, Moll FL, Eikelboom BC, Ludwig JW. Ultrasonic duplex scanning in atherosclerotic disease of the innominate, subclavian and vertebral arteries. A comparative study with angiography. Ultrasound Med Biol 1984; 10(4):409–418.
134. Pokrovskii AV, Volynskii IuD, Kuntsevich GI, Buianovskii VL, Berdikian SIa. Ultrasonic angiography in the diagnosis of lesions of the brachiocephalic branches of the aorta. Kardiologiia 1985; 25(10):82–86. Russian.
135. Kuperberg EB, Grozovskii IuL, Agadzhanova LP. Functional test of reactive hyperemia in the diagnosis of the vertebro-subclavian steal syndrome using ultrasonic dopplerography. Zh Nevropatol Psikhiatr Im S S Korsakova 1986; 86(1):28–34. Russian.
136. Bornstein NM, Norris JW. Subclavian steal: a harmless haemodynamic phenomenon? Lancet 1986; 2(8502):303–305.
137. Ackermann H, Diener HC, Dichgans J. Stenosis and occlusion of the subclavian artery: ultrasonographic and clinical findings. J Neurol 1987; 234(6):396–400.
138. Ackermann H, Diener HC, Seboldt H, Huth C. Ultrasonographic follow-up of subclavian stenosis and occlusion: natural history and surgical treatment. Stroke 1988; 19(4):431–435.
139. Klingelhofer J, Conrad B, Benecke R, Frank B. Transcranial Doppler ultrasonography of carotid-basilar collateral circulation in subclavian steal. Stroke 1988; 19(8):1036–1042.
140. Bornstein NM, Krajewski A, Norris JW. Basilar artery blood flow in subclavian steal. Can J Neurol Sci 1988; 15(4):417–419.
141. Lunev DK, Pokrovskii AV, Nikitin IuM, Lunes AM. Cerebrovascular disorders in various types of the subclavian steal syndrome. Zh Nevropatol Psikhiatr Im S S Korsakova 1991; 91(1):10–14. Russian.
142. Nicholls SC, Koutlas TC, Strandness DE. Clinical significance of retrograde flow in the vertebral artery. Ann Vasc Surg 1991; 5(4):331–336.
143. de Bray JM, Zenglein JP, Laroche JP, et al. Effect of subclavian syndrome on the basilar artery. Acta Neurol Scand 1994; 90(3):174–178.
144. Rossum AC, Steel SR, Hartshorne MF. Evaluation of coronary subclavian steal syndrome using sestamibi imaging and duplex scanning with observed vertebral subclavian steal. Clin Cardiol 2000; 23(3):226–229.
145. Mukhtar OM, Miller AP, Nanda NC, et al. Transesophageal echocardiographic identification of left subclavian artery stenosis with steal phenomenon. Echocardiography 2000; 17(2):197–200.
146. AbuRahma AF, Robinson PA, Jennings TG. Carotid-subclavian bypass grafting with polytetrafluoroethylene grafts for symptomatic subclavian artery stenosis or occlusion: a 20-year experience. J Vasc Surg 2000; 32(3):411–418.
147. Teague SM, Sharma MK. Detection of paradoxical cerebral echo contrast embolization by transcranial Doppler ultrasound. Stroke 1991; 22:740–745.
148. Nemec JJ, Marwick TH, Lorig RJ, et al. Comparison of transcranial Doppler ultrasound and transesophageal contrast echocardiography in the detection of interatrial right-to-left shunts. Am J Cardiol 1991; 68:1498–1502.
149. Karnik R, Stolberger C, Valentin A, Winkler WB, Slany J. Detection of patent foramen ovale by transcranial contrast Doppler ultrasound. Am J Cardiol 1992; 69:560–562.
150. Di Tullio M, Sacco RL, Venketasubramanian N, Sherman D, Mohr JP, Homma S. Comparison of diagnostic techniques for the detection of a patent foramen ovale in stroke patients. Stroke 1993; 24:1020–1024.
151. Job FP, Ringelstein EB, Grafen Y, et al. Comparison of transcranial contrast Doppler sonography and transesophageal contrast echocardiography for the detection of patent foramen ovale in young stroke patients. Am J Cardiol 1994; 74:381–384.
152. Jauss M, Kaps M, Keberle M, Haberbosch W, Dorndorf W. A comparison of transesophageal echocardiography and transcranial Doppler sonography with contrast medium for detection of patent foramen ovale. Stroke 1994; 25:1265–1267.
153. Anzola GP, Renaldini E, Magoni M, Costa A, Cobelli M, Guindani M. Validation of transcranial Doppler sonography in the assessment of patent foramen ovale. Cerebrovasc Dis 1995; 5:194–198.
154. Spencer M, Moehring M, Jesurum J, Gray W, Olsen J, Reisman M. Power M mode transcranial Doppler for diagnosis of patent foramen ovale and assessing transcatheter closure. J Neuroimaging 2004; 14:342–349.
155. Alberts MJ, Latchaw RE, Selman WR, et al; for the Brain Attack Coalition. Recommendations for comprehensive stroke centers: a consensus statement from the Brain Attack Coalition. Stroke 2005; 36:1597–1618.

Pediatric Brain • 21

Henrietta Kotlus Rosenberg, Vijay Viswanathan, and John Amodio

INTRODUCTION

The advent of high-resolution real-time ultrasonography in the 1980s revolutionized the imaging approach to the infant brain. This noninvasive, nonionizing imaging modality with portable and repeatable capabilities is not only cost effective but is also readily available and reliable for the evaluation and followup of a wide gamut of intracranial abnormalities in infants (1–9). This chapter reviews the technique for performing cranial ultrasonography, the normal ultrasonographic brain anatomy, and the many applications of this operator-dependent modality.

TECHNIQUE AND ANATOMY

Routine ultrasonography of the brain is performed through the anterior fontanelle, which remains patent in full-term infants until about 9 to 18 months of age (1). This sonic window to the brain may remain open for much longer periods of time in premature infants and in those with increased intracranial pressure. Scanning can also be accomplished through the posterior fontanelle in the coronal, sagittal, and oblique planes (10). In addition, axial images can be obtained through the squamosal suture, anterolateral or posterolateral fontanelles, or other bone windows in patients with closed fontanelles, who have craniotomy or Burr hole defects. The choice of transducer is related to the size of the cranial vault and the anterior fontanelle or other sonic window. To maximize resolution and allow for maximum depth penetration, the following guidelines are suggested: 9–4 MHz broadband curvilinear transducer for larger, older babies; 8–5 MHz small footprint phased array broad bandwidth transducer for newborn babies; and 12–5, 17–5, and 15 MHz (small footprint "hockey stick") linear broad bandwidth transducers for superficial scalp lesions and for assessing the internal content of a meningocele or encephalocele. All the transducers provide duplex/color Doppler imaging. A step-off pad may be necessary for evaluation of superficial structures.

To obtain images that encompass as much of the intracranial contents as possible, it is necessary to scan the brain in a sequential fashion from anterior to posterior in the coronal plane and then from the midline to the far lateral aspects of the cerebral hemispheres in the sagittal plane (Fig. 1). The ventricular system and cerebrospinal fluid (CSF) spaces are used as references for the identification of the cross-sectional anatomy. The convexities of the brain must be imaged as completely as possible with a high-frequency probe and by angling the beam as necessary.

The parasagittal view of the brain includes frontal horns and bodies of the lateral ventricles as well as the caudothalamic groove, a thin, echogenic band that lies between the slightly more echogenic caudate nucleus anteriorly and the thalamus posteriorly (Fig. 2A) (11). In the premature infant, the highly vascular germinal matrix is found inferolateral to the ependyma lining the floor of the lateral ventricle, anterior and superior to the caudothalamic groove. The examination of the lateral ventricles also includes images of the bodies and temporal and occipital horns. The

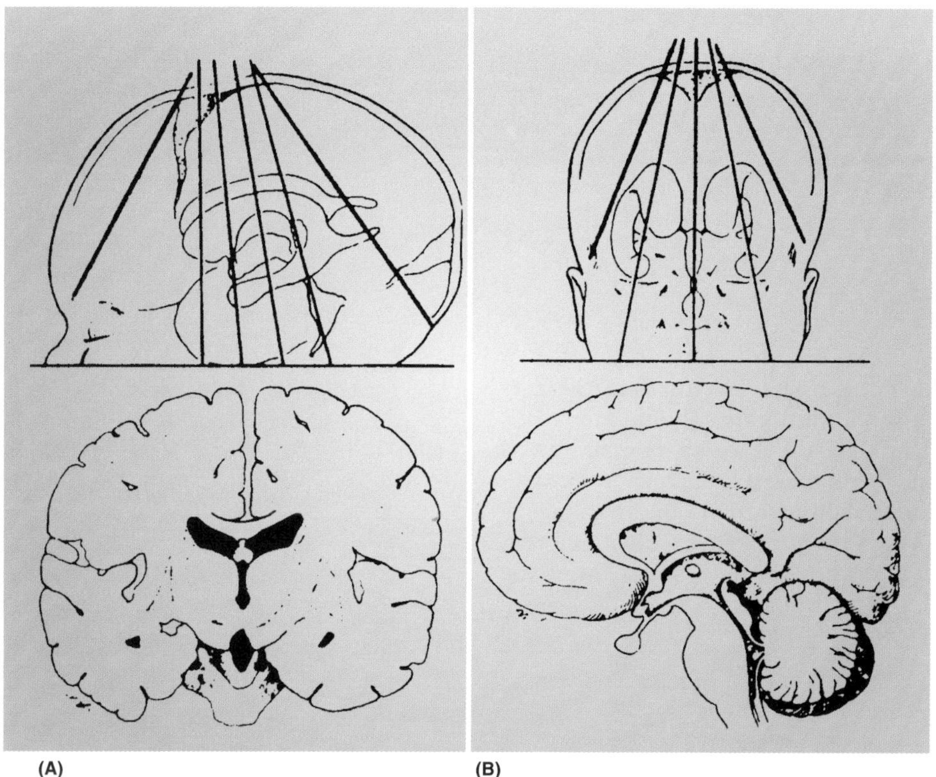

FIGURE 1 A AND B ■ Planes of ultrasonographic sections. (**A**) Coronal section. The brain is scanned sequentially from anterior to posterior. (**B**) Sagittal section. The brain is scanned in the midline (shown here) and parasagittal planes. *Source*: From Ref. 3.

choroid plexus of the lateral ventricle is seen within the atrium of the ventricle. The glomus of the choroid plexus is prominent and smooth, with the anterior-most portion tapering toward the caudothalamic groove as it courses inferiorly into the third ventricle and with the inferior-most portion tapering toward the temporal horn (12). The frontal horn of the lateral ventricle is more medially positioned than the posterior horn; therefore, to visualize the entire ventricle optimally, the anterior aspect of the transducer must be angled medially while the posterior aspect is angled posteriorly. The lateral ventricles are frequently asymmetric, and the occipital horns may

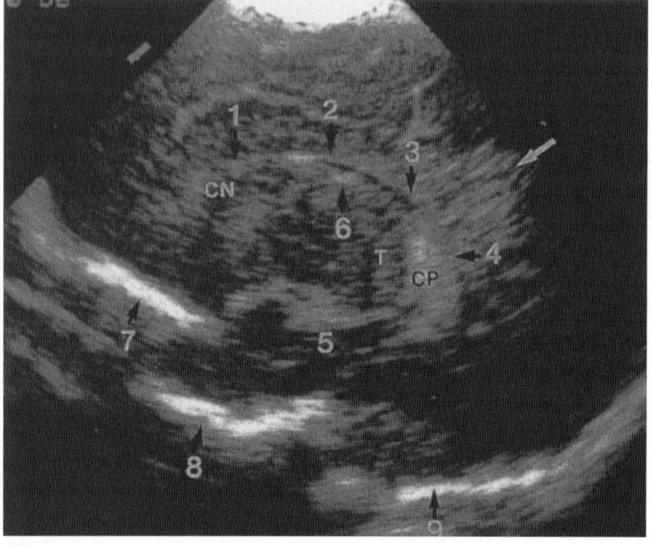

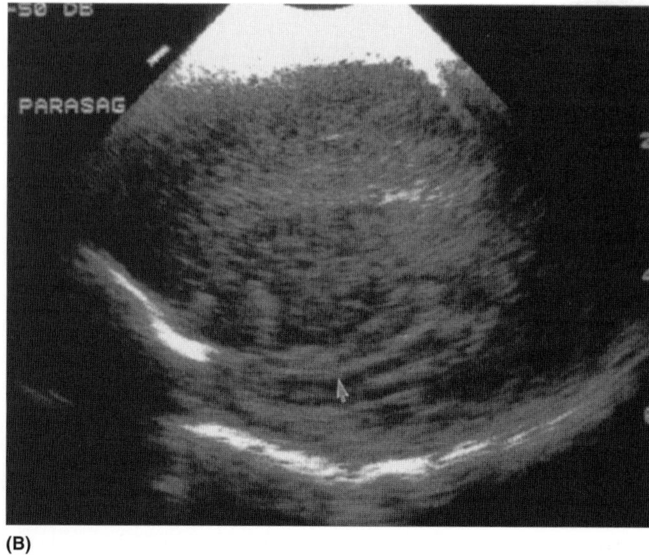

FIGURE 2 A–F ■ Sagittal scans of the brain. (**A**) Parasagittal views of the brain through the lateral ventricle. 1, frontal horn of lateral ventricle; 2, body; 3, atrium; 4, occipital horn; 5, temporal horn; 6, caudothalamic groove; 7, anterior cranial fossa; 8, middle cranial fossa; 9, posterior cranial fossa; CN, caudate nucleus; CP, choroid plexus; *white arrow*, periventricular blush; T, thalamus. (**B**) Far lateral parasagittal view of the brain. (*Continued*)

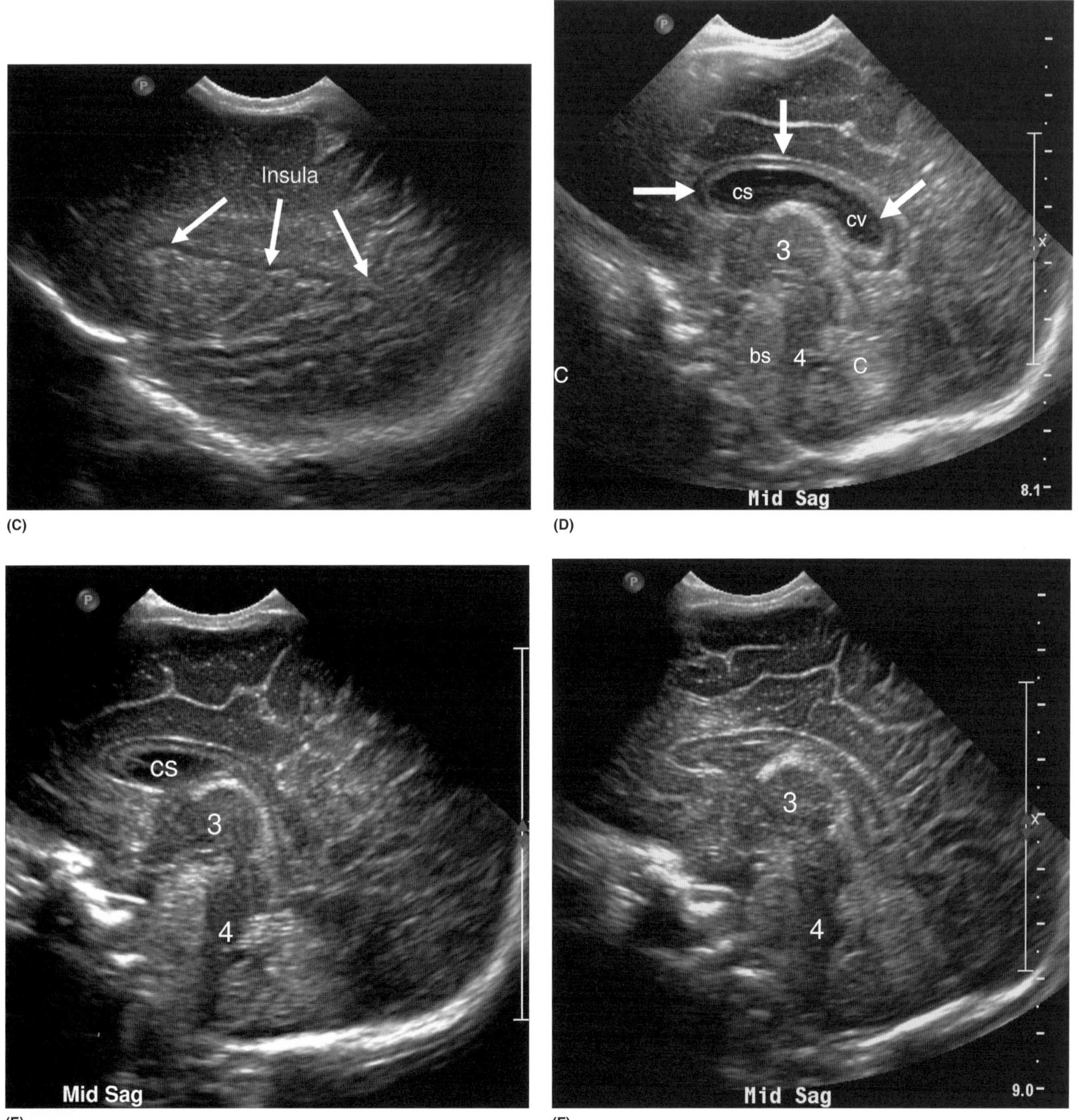

FIGURE 2 A–F ■ (*Continued*) (**C**) Farther lateral parasagittal view demonstrating the insula. Midline scan of the brain in two full-term infants (**D, E**) and in a premature infant (**F**). cs, cavum septum pellucidum; cv, cavum vergae; 3, third ventricle; 4, fourth ventricle; cm, cisterna magna.

be wider than the frontal horns. The ventricles become progressively smaller with increasing fetal age, so that by term, the frontal horns may appear almost slit-like, measuring less than 2 to 3 mm in depth. The amount of CSF seen in the lateral ventricles ranges from none seen behind the glomus of the choroid plexus to an obvious C-shaped collection filling the entire ventricle. The lateral ventricles are surrounded by frontal, parietal, occipital, and temporal lobes of the cerebral hemispheres. Posterior to the occipital horns, there is a periventricular blush of increased echogenicity. The echogenicity should not be greater than that of the choroid plexus and should not be coarse but should be rather like the lines created by an artist's brush stroke (13). It is hypothesized that this echogenic halo is related to the white-matter fibers and vascular plexus that extend from the cortex of the cerebral hemispheres to the subependymal layer of the ventricle. Parasagittal views show the brain parenchyma in the periventricular regions, the Sylvian fissure, and the insula (Fig. 2B and C). The midline sagittal images of the brain (Fig. 2C and D) are obtained by keeping the transducer parallel to the anteroposterior diameter of the cranial vault. The cavum septum pellucidum is seen as a fluid-filled structure lying between the frontal horns of the lateral ventricles. This fetal structure begins to close just before term and is often completely closed by the second postnatal month. The posterior extension of this structure, the cavum vergae, generally begins to close from posterior to anterior during the sixth gestational month and when present is imaged more posteriorly between the bodies of the lateral ventricles. The size of the cavae is quite variable. Occasionally, bright linear echogenicities representing septal veins are seen within these areas (14,15).

Above these midline fluid-filled structures is the corpus callosum, a thin, crescentic-shaped, hypoechoic structure, of which the genu, body, and splenium should be demonstrated (16). It is bound by the echogenic pericallosal sulcus, which contains the pericallosal arteries. Cephalad and superior to the sulcus of the corpus callosum is the cingulate gyrus, which appears as a broad, curvilinear hypoechoic band. This is separated from the more superficial gyri by a thin hyperechoic line, the cingulate sulcus. The presence, number, and configuration of the gyri are proportional to the gestational age of the infant (Fig. 3) (17). Generally, the sulci are not seen ultrasonographically until about 26 weeks' gestation. They increase in number and become more serpiginous in their configuration as the infant reaches term. With real-time imaging, the vascular pulsations of the branches of the anterior cerebral arteries can be seen within the cerebral sulci. The third and fourth ventricles are seen on the midline sagittal scans of the brain as hypoechoic structures because of their narrow width and the inability of the ultrasound beam to obtain a section that does not record reflections from the adjacent brain tissue. The bright area of echogenicity in the roof of the third ventricle is due to the presence of choroid plexus as it courses posteriorly to the suprapineal recess. The massa intermedia, a soft-tissue structure within the third ventricle, is generally only seen when the third ventricle is dilated. The quadrigeminal plate cistern is located posterior to the third

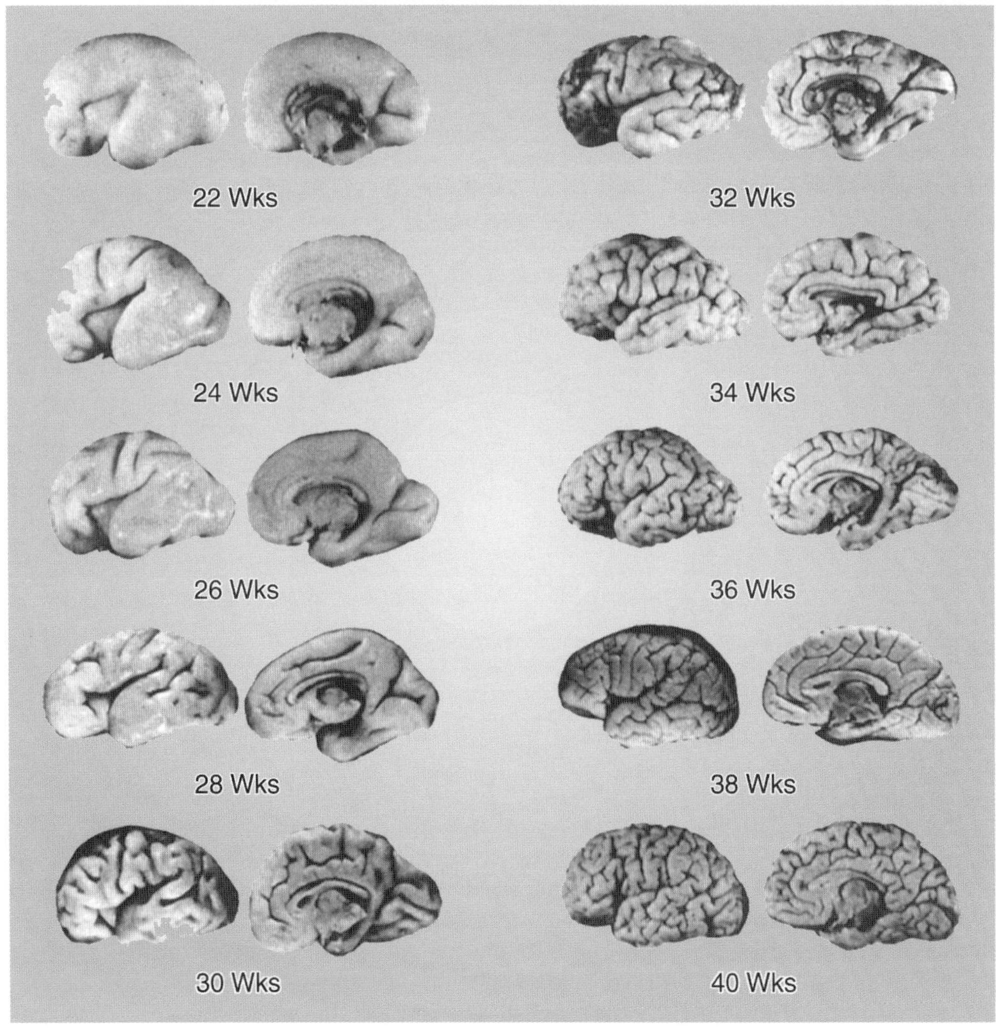

FIGURE 3 ■ Development of normal gyral markings in the neonatal brain as correlated to gestational age. *Source*: From Ref. 17.

ventricle and appears as a dense band. Below this cistern is the brightly echogenic cerebellar vermis, which is indented anteriorly by the triangular fourth ventricle. The anechoic cisterna magna is located inferior to the cerebellum and communicates with the fourth ventricle (18). The height of this cistern in the midsagittal plane should be 4.5 + 1.29 mm. The variably sized, anechoic torcular Herophili is a triangular or elongated structure located inferior to the occipital lobes, posterior to the cerebellum, just inside the cranial vault (19). The choroid plexus in the roof of the fourth ventricle cannot be seen ultrasonographically. The moderately echoic brain stem lies anterior to the fourth ventricle and posterior to the clivus.

Coronal plane imaging begins anteriorly and sweeps posteriorly (20,21). A far anterior view of the frontal hemispheres should include the anterior-most tips of the frontal horns of the lateral ventricles, the interhemispheric fissure, and the orbits (Fig. 4A). A second image (Fig. 4B) is obtained at the level of the frontal horns or bodies of the lateral ventricles, anterior to the foramina of Monroe. The anterior horns of the lateral ventricles are anechoic, crescentic, paramedian, fluid-filled spaces. The corpus callosum forms the roof of this portion of the lateral ventricles, the cavum septi pellucidi the medial walls, and the heads of the caudate nuclei the lateral borders. The lateral walls of the anterior portions of the lateral ventricles are normally concave. The brightly echogenic pericallosal sulcus separates the superior aspect of the corpus callosum from the hypoechoic cingulate gyrus. The putamen and globus pallidus are lateral and inferior to the caudate nucleus. The portions of the cerebral hemispheres imaged at this level include the hypoechoic frontal and temporal lobes. With real-time imaging, the pulsations of the branches of the anterior cerebral arteries may be observed in the interhemispheric fissure and those of the middle cerebral arteries in the sylvian fissures. The next scan (Fig. 4C) is obtained slightly posteriorly at the level of the foramen of Monroe, where the lateral and third ventricles communicate. The normal-sized third ventricle is more often not visualized on this view because of its small size. When visualized, it appears as a vertically oriented midline anechoic structure beneath the bodies of the lateral ventricles. The vascular pulsations from the anterior cerebral arterial branches and those from the middle cerebral artery may also be seen on this view. In addition, the relatively echogenic brain stem (pons and medulla) is seen on this image. The thalami are separated by the third ventricle. Echogenic material representing choroid plexus is seen in the roof of the third ventricle and in the groove between the thalamus and the lateral ventricle. The next image (Fig. 4D) is obtained at the level of the quadrigeminal plate cistern and the cerebellum. On this view, the cerebellar vermis appears as a midline pie-shaped area of bright echogenicity occupying the lower third of the brain with the anechoic cisterna magna posteriorly and inferiorly. The bodies of the lateral ventricles, bordered by the caudate nuclei and thalami, are seen superiorly and the temporal horns inferiorly. At this level, the pulsations of the middle cerebral and pericallosal arteries can be seen. The echogenic glomi of the choroid plexus are seen at the posterior aspects of the lateral ventricles at the level of the trigone (Fig. 4E). As the lateral ventricles diverge in this view, they are separated by the splenium of the corpus callosum. On this scan, the previously described periventricular blush is seen lateral to the posterior horns of the lateral ventricles. Inferiorly, the posterior-most part of the cerebellum is seen. The final image (Fig. 4F) is the most posterior view of the brain parenchyma in the coronal projection. This view is important for evaluation of the parenchyma because it includes the more superficial sulci and gyri of the occipital lobes, with the echogenic areas cephalad to the atria of the lateral ventricles representing white matter.

The size of the normal choroid plexus may be asymmetric depending on the position of the infant's head, with the choroid plexus on the nondependent side appearing more prominent because the choroid plexus is adherent to the roof plate in only one small area and is thus buoyed up by the CSF (Fig. 5) (22). Neuroepithelial cysts of the choroid plexus up to 7 mm in size may be visualized during routine ultrasonography. These are usually asymptomatic and clinically insignificant and have been shown to persist unchanged for 13 months. Most patients were found to have no associated ultrasonographic, neurologic, or chromosomal abnormalities, and no ultrasound followup is required (23).

The extra-axial fluid space can be most easily examined ultrasonographically in the midline. The extracerebral spaces, which can be prominent in premature infants, are best evaluated with a high-frequency linear transducer, usually with 12 to 15 MHz range. This technique allows demonstration of the extra-axial spaces, cerebral convexities as well as the extra-axial vessels, when color Doppler sonography is employed. Normally, the sinocortical width is 0.4 to 3.3 mm, the craniocortical width is 0.3 to 6.3 mm, and the interhemispheric width is 0.5 to 8.2 mm (Fig. 6) (24). The extra-axial fluid spaces located more laterally, anteriorly, or posteriorly can be examined, at least in part, by angling the transducer accordingly. Further discussion of this technique is found below.

Alternate Sonographic Imaging Techniques

When abnormalities are encountered that cannot be completely imaged with this protocol, additional views should be obtained using whatever approach can best elucidate the problem. This may include oblique views through the anterior fontanelle (e.g., to demonstrate a shunt tube), views through the posterior fontanelle (e.g., posterior fossa lesions not well delineated through the anterior fontanelle), or axial views (e.g., to delineate the course of a shunt tube, to better demonstrate an extra-axial fluid collection, or to image the brain stem, cerebral peduncles, middle cerebral and posterior cerebral arteries, and anterior communicating artery of the circle of Willis).

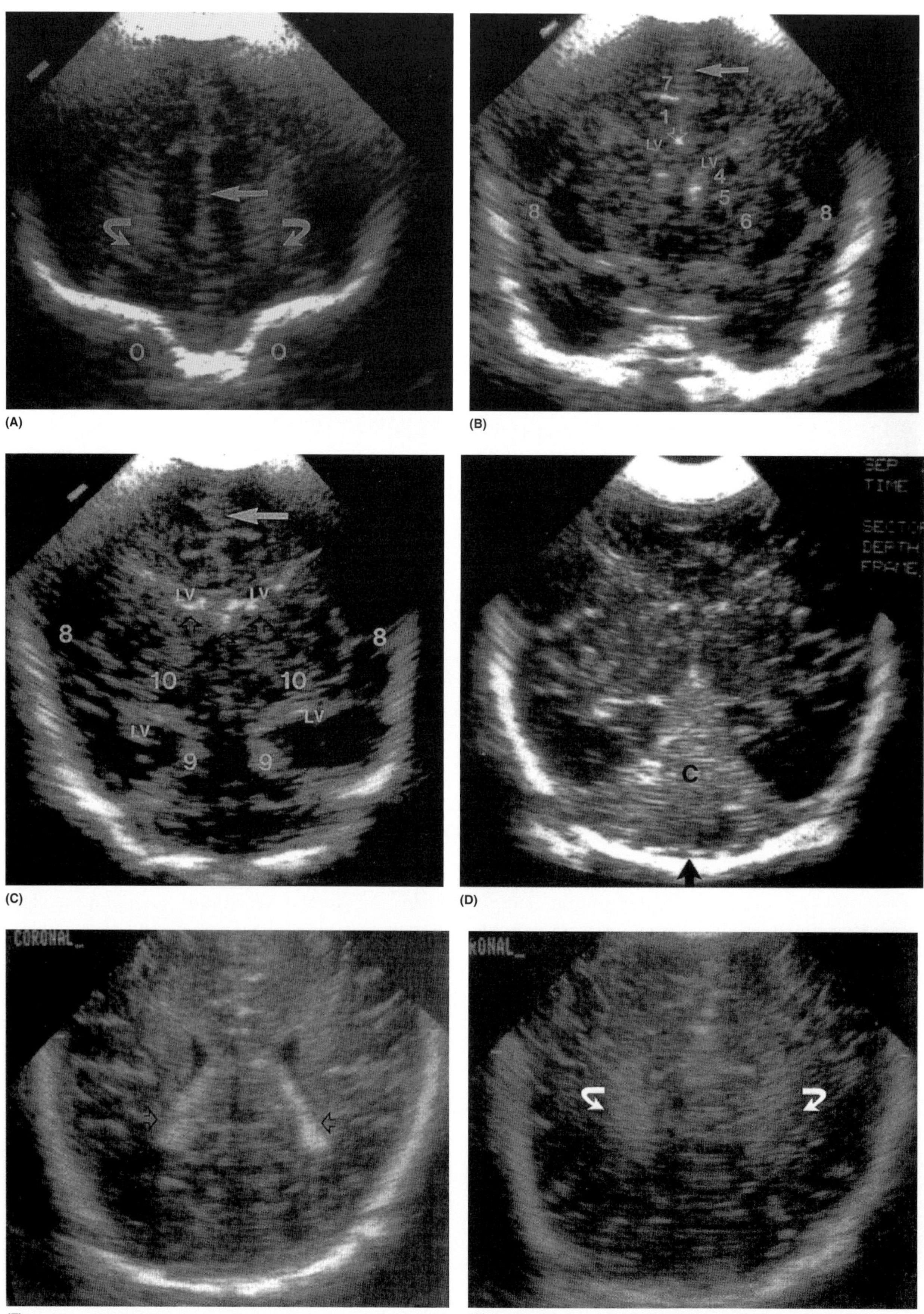

FIGURE 4 A–F ■ Coronal sonograms of the brain, anterior to posterior. 1, cingulate gyrus; 4, head of caudate nucleus; 5, anterior limb of internal capsule; 6, putamen; 7, cingulate sulcus; 8, sylvian fissure; 9, hippocampal gyrus; 10, thalamus; 11, brain stem. *Large white arrow*, interhemispheric fissure; *large black arrow*, cisterna magna; *curved arrows*, periventricular blush; *open white arrows*, corpus callosum; *small black arrow*, cavum septum pellucidum; *open black arrows*, choroid plexus; LV, lateral ventricles; O, orbits; C, cerebellum.

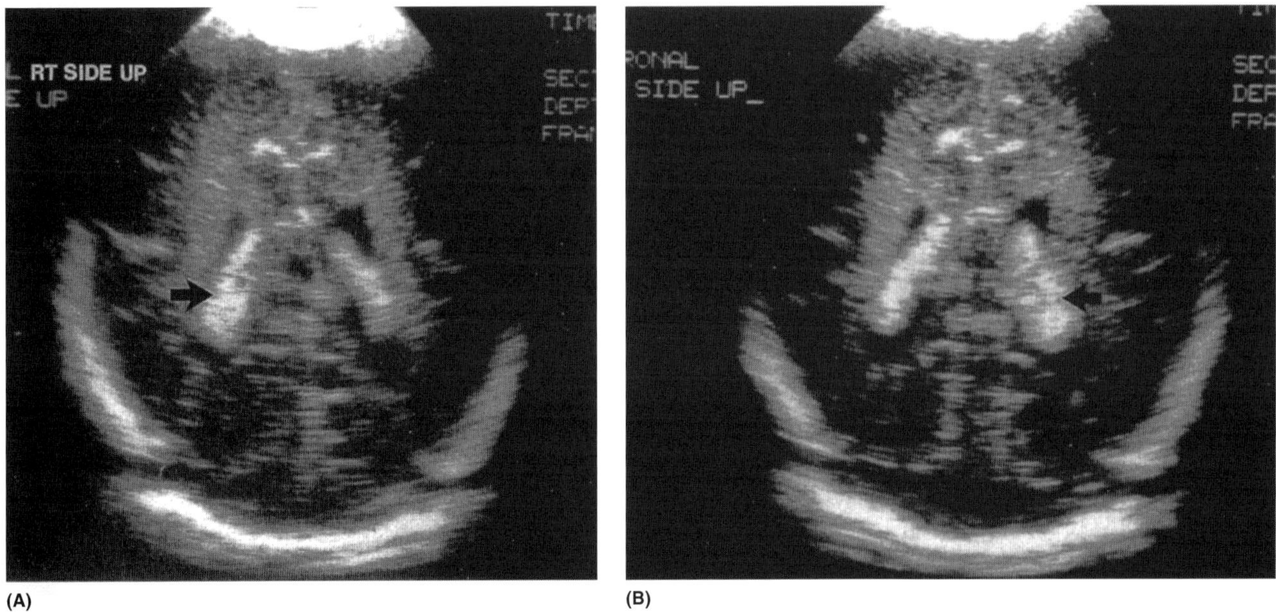

(A) (B)

FIGURE 5 A AND B ■ Choroid plexus in nondependent ventricle. Coronal scans performed in the right (**A**) and left (**B**) lateral decubitus positions. The choroid plexus appears larger in the nondependent ventricle (*black arrows*).

Posterior fontanelle imaging is recommended for examining posterior fossa abnormalities. In addition, it has been shown that posterior fontanelle sonography provides greater accuracy in detecting intraventricular hemorrhage (IVH) compared with anterior fontanelle imaging alone. This is especially true when the ventricles are not dilated (25). Using the posterior fontanelle as a sonographic window, differences in echogenicity between clot and choroid can be demonstrated. It also depicts clot in the occipital and temporal horns to a better advantage than anterior fontanelle imaging.

Another useful acoustical window, for examining the contents of the posterior fossa and brainstem, is the mastoid fontanelle. The transducer is positioned

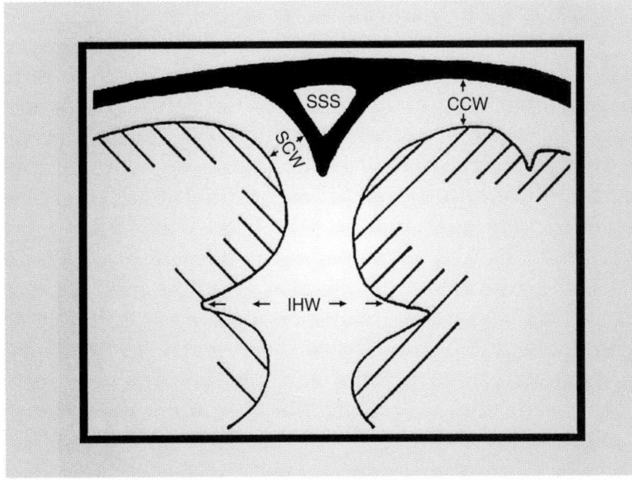

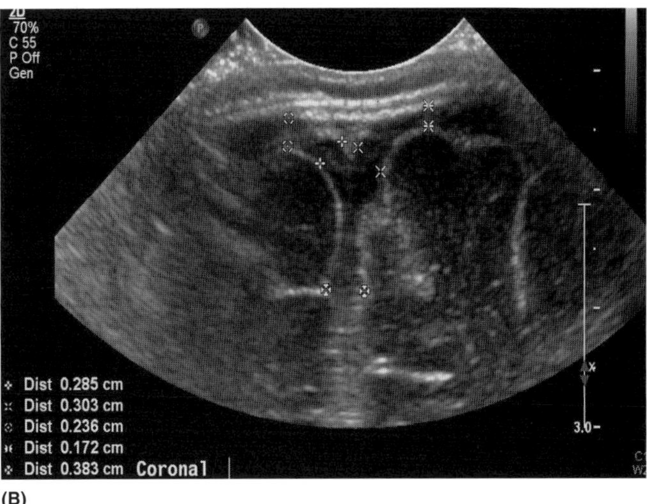

(A) (B)

FIGURE 6 A AND B ■ Anatomic landmarks and sonographic variables of the subarachnoid space in the coronal plane. (**A**) The SCW is defined as the shortest distance between the lateral wall of the triangular superior sagittal sinus and the surface of the adjacent cerebral cortex. The CCW is defined as the shortest vertical distance between the calvarium and the surface of the cerebral cortex. The IHW is defined as the widest horizontal distance and is not the same as the oblique distance between the sulci of the interhemispheric fissure. (**B**) Coronal US measurements of extra-axial fluid spaces. SCW, sinocortical width; CCW, craniocortical width; IHW, interhemispheric width; SSS, superior sagittal sinus. *Source*: From Ref. 24.

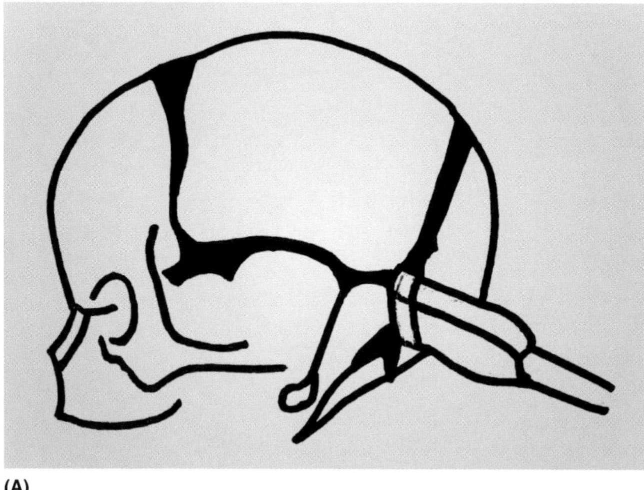

(A)

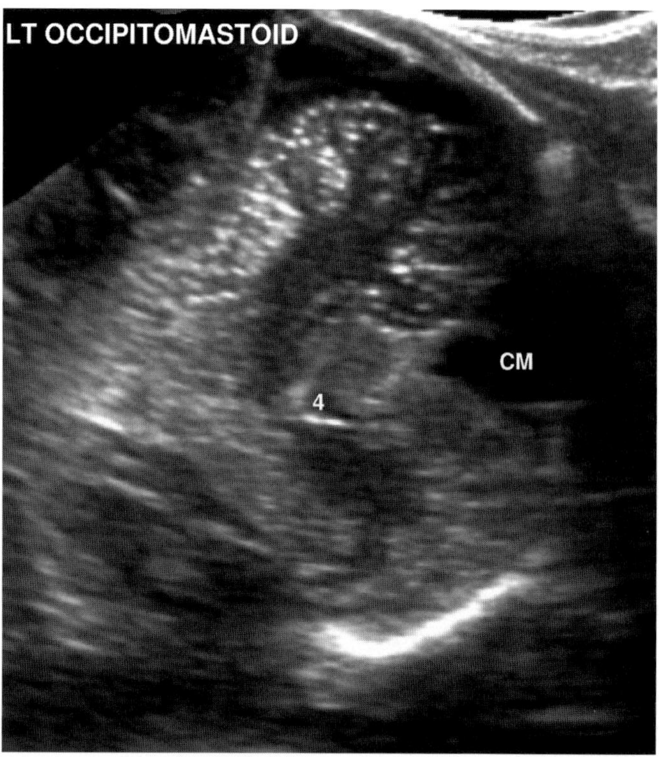

(B)

FIGURE 7 A AND B ■ (**A**) Drawing illustrates the neonatal skull (*lateral view*) with the major sutures as well as posterior and anterior fontanelles. An US transducer is positioned over the mastoid fontanelle. (**B**) Mastoid fontanelle imaging. US image of both lobes of the cerebellum and the cisterna magna (CM). 4, fourth ventricle.

approximately 1 cm posterior to the ear and 1 cm above the tragus. High-frequency transducers are more helpful in delineating brain pathology, using the mastoid fontanelle, than the traditional probes, especially with respect to delineating structures within the posterior fossa (Fig. 7).

Imaging through the mastoid fontanelle can be especially useful in detecting hemorrhage involving the brain stem, cerebellum, and subarachnoid cisterns. Mastoid fontanelle imaging also facilitates detection of clot within the fourth ventricle and cisterna magna. Small malformations of the posterior fossa, aqueductal stenosis, and holoprosencephaly are well demonstrated with this technique (26).

There has been some interest in three-dimensional ultrasound (3DUS) of the infant brain, although most 3DUS work is currently performed in obstetrics. 3DUS is based on data acquisition from two-dimensional ultrasound (2DUS) image data, which allows for 3D reconstructions of a volume of tissue. The technique is essentially simple, in which a 2DUS sweep in any plane can be performed, which is then reconstructed in 3D. The 3D images can be portrayed as a volume of tissue or reconstructed in orthogonal imaging planes. This technique is limited by quality of the original data acquisition as well as lack of patient motion. Furthermore, gain and depth correction cannot be performed during the acquisition. 3DUS of the infant brain may be helpful in delineating complex anatomical abnormalities, hydrocephalus, and cerebral hemorrhage (27).

Normal Variants and Artifacts

There are several normal variants and sonographic artifacts of the brain anatomy that one may encounter when performing cranial sonography. There is often asymmetry in size of the lateral ventricles with the left more often larger than the right (28–30) and often most pronounced in the most posterior portion of the occipital horn. The larger lateral ventricle is often associated with a larger ipsilateral choroid plexus.

Another normal variant that may be observed is coarctation of the lateral ventricles. This normal variant consists of a focal approximation of the ventricular walls at any point medial to their external angle. Coarctation of the lateral ventricles may be unilateral or bilateral and may have the appearance of a germinal matrix cyst or periventricular leukomalacia (PVL) (31). Coarctation may be distinguished by the fact that the false cystic image is seen at the external angle, whereas germinal matrix cysts and cystic PVL are below and above the external angle, respectively (30).

There are three normal variants that may be seen regarding the choroid plexus. The choroid at the level of the ventricular atrium may have a cleft appearance or a lobular appearance that may raise the concern for choroidal hemorrhage. This is known as a split choroid. Recognizing this variation is helpful in avoiding misdiagnosis. In addition, color Doppler imaging will show vascularity of the area in question, whereas choroidal hemorrhage is avascular. The second choroidal variant is the truncated choroid plexus, in which there is flattening of the rounded lower portion of the plexus. This variant may have the appearance of a solid-fluid level. Posterior fontanelle imaging can be helpful in this instance in demonstrating the absence of blood within the ventricle. The third choroidal variant to be aware of is the choroid cyst. A choroid cyst may be single or multiple and can vary in size. These cysts have been known to resolve on subsequent scans. Large cysts (>1 cm) have been found in association with chromosomal abnormalities, such as trisomy 18.

It is well known that the bilateral peritrigonal hyperechogenicity or "blush" is the result of anisotropic effect of scanning (13). The ultrasound beam through the anterior fontanelle strikes nerve fibers and blood vessels of the peritrigonal region in a perpendicular fashion producing this effect. It is typically found in preterm and in some full-term infants. Scanning through the posterior fontanelle will essentially eradicate this effect because the beam is more parallel to the nerve fibers. This fact should be kept in mind in differentiating this normal variant from PVL. In questionable cases, follow-up scanning may be required.

Scanning through the posterior fontanelle may produce an echogenic focus within the thalamus on parasagittal views, known as the thalamic pseudolesion. This artifact is the result of anisotropic scanning and is eliminated by scanning through the anterior fontanelle. Thus, the examiner should be aware of this artifact to prevent misinterpretation of a thalamic, an ischemic, or a hemorrhagic lesion.

When scanning through the mastoid fontanelle, the examiner may encounter an apparent wide communication between the fourth ventricle and the cisterna magna, simulating vermian agenesis. This artifact is the result of transducer angulation and the fact that the vermis in some newborns tilts slightly forward from the usual position. Pseudo absence of the inferior vermis may be eliminated by readjusting the angle or tilt of the transducer.

In infants who are under 34 gestational weeks, the occipital lobe may appear as a hypoechoic "mass" on parasagittal images. This artifact is the result of poor gyral development that contrasts with the well-developed hyperechoic tentorium and parieto-occipital fissure (30).

The calcar avis, which is a mound of white matter that protrudes into the medial aspect of the lateral ventricle, may simulate IVH on images taken through the posterior fontanelle. The calcar avis will be properly identified by tilting the transducer slightly more laterally, thus identifying its continuity with the brain and its echogenic fissures (30).

A cyst of the velum interpositum (CVI) is occasionally encountered. The velum interpositum, the choroid plexus of the third ventricle, forms the roof of the third ventricle, extending from above the pineal body anteriorly to the foramen of Monro posteriorly. During intrauterine or postnatal life, it becomes visible only when a cyst develops in this location. When the potential space between the layers of the tela choroidea, an extension of the quadrigeminal plate cistern, is filled with fluid, the term cavum velum interpositum is applied (32). A CVI is an incidental finding, is not associated with other abnormalities, and is consistent with a favorable postnatal outcome (32). Other entities that may resemble a CVI include vein of Galen malformation, enlarged third ventricle, interhemispheric cyst in association with agenesis of the corpus callosum, and arachnoid cyst. Color Doppler sonography will distinguish a vein of Galen malformation from CVI. Stability in size of a CVI and presence of the corpus callosum are helpful findings in distinguishing CVI from other cysts.

INTRACRANIAL HEMORRHAGE

Intracranial hemorrhage (ICH) is a leading cause of serious morbidity and mortality in neonates, especially premature infants. High-resolution ultrasonography is as sensitive and accurate as computed tomography (CT) in the detection of ICH, particularly hemorrhages occurring in the subependymal and intraventricular regions (33–35). Additionally, ultrasound is a powerful predictor of long-term outcome and cerebral palsy in low-birthweight neonates (36). The portable capability of ultrasonography allows for performance of the examination in the neonatal intensive care nursery without moving the infant or the vital life support equipment.

Neonatal ICH occurs most often in the developing, immature brain and is most common in premature infants younger than 32 weeks' gestational age or with a birthweight under 1500 g. The incidence of ICH in these tiny premature infants has been reported to be as high as 70%, if assisted ventilation is required (37). In the premature infant, ICH usually occurs within the first three days of life, with 36% of cases occurring on day 1, 32% on day 2, and 18% on day 3 (38). Most major hemorrhages (IVH with ventricular dilation or parenchymal hemorrhage) occur on day 1. By the sixth day, 91% of all cases of ICH have occurred (38).

Many risk factors have been identified as contributory factors in the development of ICH. The most common, as already mentioned, are prematurity (less than 32 weeks' gestation) and low birthweight (less than 1500 g). Extremely small premature infants weighing 500 to 700 g have a higher incidence of IVH than infants weighing 701 to 1500 g. The incidence of IVH was reported by Perlman et al. (39) to be 65% in these extremely small infants, compared with 25% in larger premature infants. These investigators also found that the IVH was more severe, occurred earlier, and was associated more often with a fatal outcome in the extremely small premature infants. Late and lethal hemorrhages were more likely to occur in these smaller infants. Other reported risk factors for ICH include sex (males 2:1), multiple gestations, trauma at delivery, prolonged labor, hyperosmolarity, hypocoagulation, pneumothorax, patent ductus arteriosus, and factors associated with increased or decreased cerebral blood flow (40).

The underlying etiologic factor in the pathophysiology of ICH is hypoxia (41,42). Hypoxia predisposes to the loss of autoregulation of the cerebral circulation and causes significant changes in systemic blood pressure. Loss of autoregulation allows fluctuations in blood pressure to be directly transmitted to the cerebral circulation. The cerebral vessels in the premature infant, particularly in the germinal matrix, are fragile and susceptible to hemorrhage. Hypertension, hypercapnia, acidosis, and vasoactive substances (e.g., prostaglandins) contribute to intracerebral vasodilation and subsequent hemorrhage (43).

ICH in the premature neonate has been divided into four grades. The most widely accepted classification is modified from that of Papile et al. (44): grade I, subependymal germinal matrix hemorrhage (GMH); grade II, GMH and IVH without ventricular dilation; grade III, GMH and IVH with ventricular dilation; grade IV, intraparenchymal hemorrhage (IPH) with IVH (45).

Based on an outcome study of 133 infants reported on in 1984 at the American Institute of Ultrasound in Medicine meeting, we further subdivided the infants with grade III IVH into grades IIIA, IIIB, and IIIC, which, respectively, indicate mild, moderate, and severe degrees of IVH and ventricular dilation (with or without subependymal hemorrhage). We employ this classification routinely because it allows for identification of infants in whom structural changes may be expected to resolve or progress and infants who may require intervention in the form of ventricular reservoirs, shunts, or lumbar punctures. Most infants with initial grade I and II IVH had normal follow-up cranial sonograms; most of the infants with grade IIIA IVH appeared normal on followup or remained the same; and those with grades IIIB and IIIC required treatment (Table 1).

The germinal matrix, a zone of neuronal and glial-cell production and proliferation, is a highly cellular, richly vascular, and metabolically active area in the developing brain. The germinal matrix lies beneath the ependyma of the lateral ventricles. The most prominent portion of the germinal matrix is the ganglionic eminence, which lies between the head of caudate nucleus and the thalamus just anterior to the caudothalamic notch. The germinal matrix usually involutes by 34 weeks' gestation (46–48). It is susceptible to hypoxic changes in the brain and is, thus, the usual initial site of ICH in the premature infant. GMH appears as a uniformly echogenic mass inferolateral to the frontal horns,

TABLE 1 ■ Classification of Intracranial Hemorrhage in Neonates

Grade	Description
I	GMH
II	IVH, normal-sized ventricles, ± GMH
III	A. Mild IVH, mild ventricular dilation, ± GMH
	B. Moderate IVH, moderate ventricular dilation, ± GMH
	C. Severe IVH, severe ventricular dilation, ± GMH
IV	IVH, IPH, ventricular dilation, ± GMH

Abbreviations: GMH, germinal matrix hemorrhage; IVH, intraventricular hemorrhage; IPH, intraparenchymal hemorrhage.

at a level just posterior to the foramen of Monroe (Fig. 8A and B). GMH may be unilateral or bilateral. Larger hemorrhages may cause focal compression of the inferolateral margin of the ventricle. It is important not to confuse hemorrhage in this location with a nonhemorrhagic entity referred to as the "hyperechoic caudate." The hyperechoic caudate nucleus (HCN) can mimic GMH but is thought to be either a normal finding or perhaps a result of ischemia. HCN tends to appear bilateral, symmetric, and tear-drop shaped as opposed to the typical unilateral, asymmetric hyperechogenicity of GMH (49). Even when GMH is bilateral, it typically appears as a region of asymmetric hyperechogenicity and a round shape. In addition, GMH occurs during the first week of life and either progresses or resolves. As the hemorrhage resolves, the focal echogenic lesion decreases in size and echogenicity. The hemorrhagic lesion frequently undergoes central liquefaction, resulting in a well-defined subependymal cyst (Fig. 8C) (48). In contrast, HCN tends to remain stable and occasionally develops small cysts, as seen in ischemia (Fig. 9) (49).

IVH may result from intraventricular extension of GMH and may be unilateral or bilateral. Blood within the ventricles appears as bright echoes within the ventricular lumen. If the ventricles are not dilated (i.e., grade II IVH), the clot may be difficult to identify. The presence of bright echoes within the frontal or occipital horn or a blood–CSF level may be the only sign of a grade II bleed (Fig. 10) (37). It can be difficult to separate intraventricular clot from the normal choroid plexus. The choroid plexus should be a symmetric structure with a smooth, tapered configuration that does not extend into the occipital horn or into the frontal horn anterior to the foramen of Monroe. Clot may become adherent to the choroid plexus, giving it a lumpy, bulbous configuration. In grade III IVH with ventricular dilation, the clot is easily detected. With severe hemorrhage, the entire ventricle is filled with blood, forming a cast of the ventricle (Fig. 11A and B) (37).

As the hemorrhage resolves in both grades II and III IVH, the intraventricular clot gradually decreases in size and echogenicity owing to internal liquefaction. The interior of the clot becomes more hypoechoic, surrounded by a densely echogenic clot margin. The clot gradually retracts away from the ventricular walls (Fig. 11C). Fragmentation of the clot may occur, resulting in small fragments that move freely within the ventricle. Resorption of clot continues until there is complete clearing. A residual intraventricular septation may persist. About seven days after the hemorrhagic event, the ependymal lining of the ventricle often becomes brightly echogenic and thicker. These changes usually disappear in about six weeks. Histologic studies in patients with echogenic ependymal walls have shown disruptions in the ependyma, with proliferation and extension of subependymal glial cells onto the ventricular surface (50).

Ventricular enlargement in grade III IVH initially is due to distention by hemorrhage. As the blood resorbs, ventriculomegaly may resolve spontaneously, persist, or progress. Posthemorrhagic hydrocephalus may result

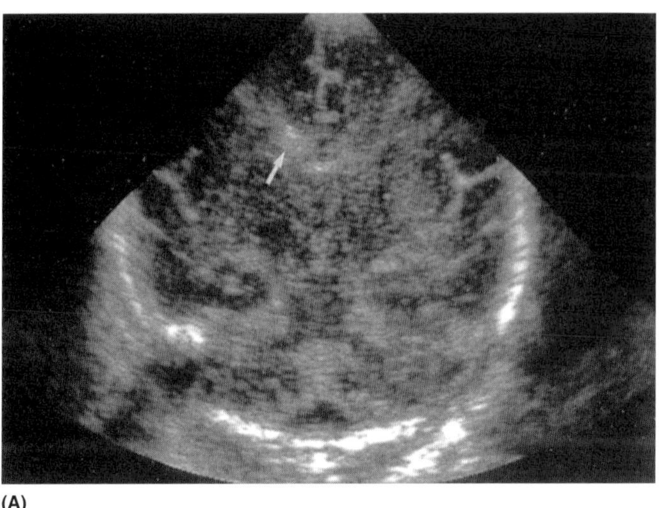
(A)

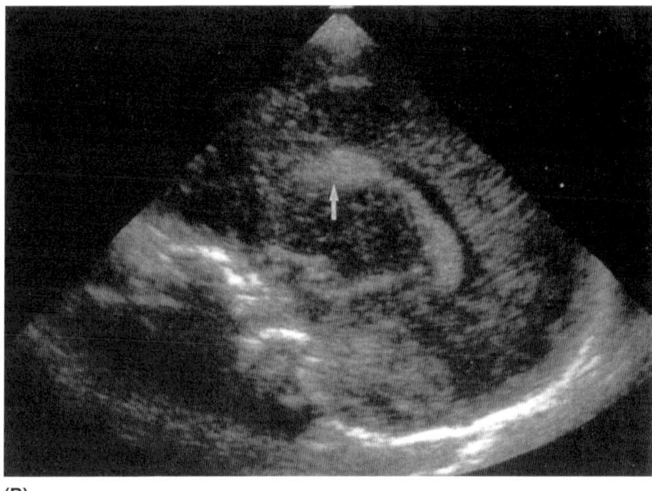
(B)

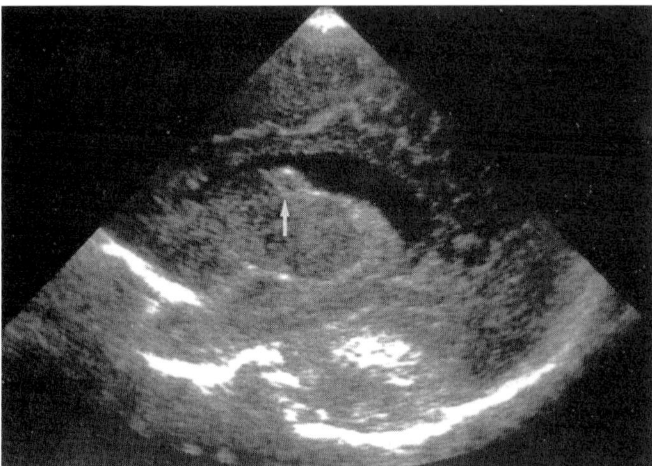
(C)

FIGURE 8 A–C ■ Grade I germinal matrix hemorrhage. Coronal (**A**) and sagittal (**B**) scans show an echogenic mass (*arrows*) in the caudothalamic notch representing a germinal matrix hemorrhage. (**C**) Follow-up sagittal scan shows a subependymal cyst (*arrow*) at the site of the previous germinal matrix hemorrhage. *Source*: From Ref. 45.

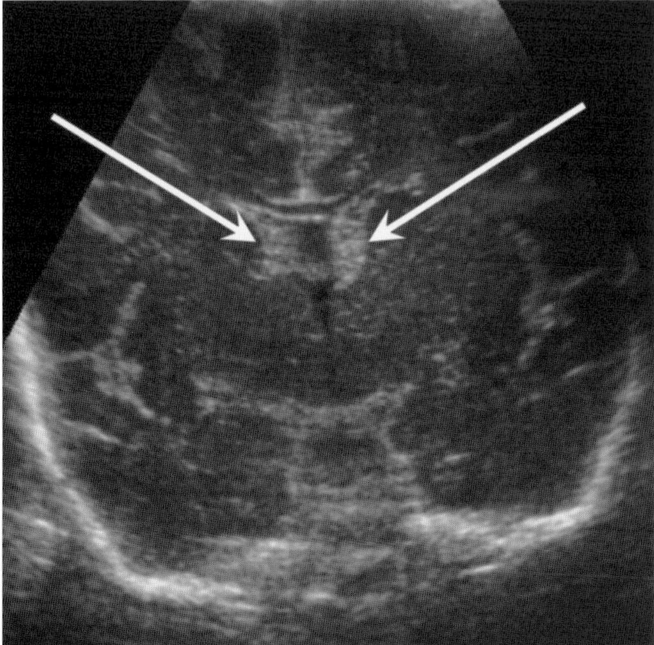

FIGURE 9 ■ Hyperechoic caudate nucleus (HCN). Coronal sonographic image shows HCN bilaterally (*both arrows*).

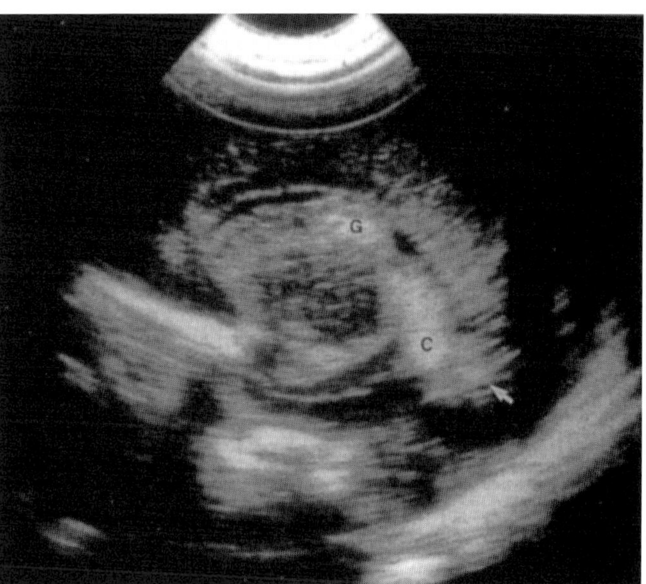

FIGURE 10 ■ Grade II intraventricular hemorrhage. Sagittal image shows a germinal matrix hemorrhage (G) and an intraventricular hemorrhage within the occipital horn (*arrow*). Note that the lateral ventricle is not dilated. c, choroid plexus. *Source*: From Ref. 45.

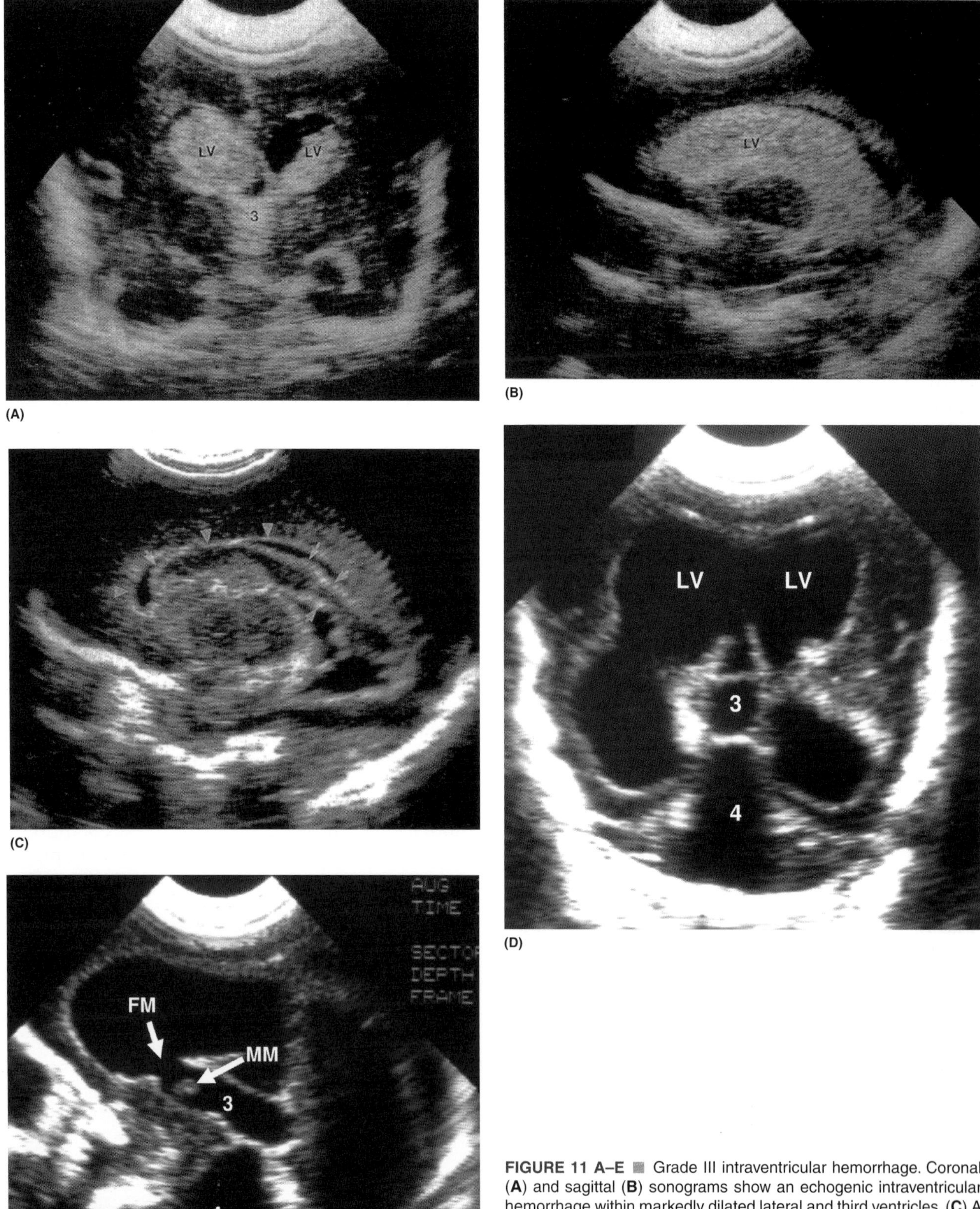

(A) (B) (C) (D) (E)

FIGURE 11 A–E ■ Grade III intraventricular hemorrhage. Coronal (**A**) and sagittal (**B**) sonograms show an echogenic intraventricular hemorrhage within markedly dilated lateral and third ventricles. (**C**) A 3 week follow-up sagittal sonogram in another patient with grade III hemorrhage shows retraction of the intraventricular clot (*arrows*) and echogenic thickened ependymal lining (*arrowheads*). Two months later, the baby developed panhydrocephalus. (**D**) Coronal and (**E**) mid sagittal views of the brain. LV, lateral ventricle; 3, third ventricle; 4, fourth ventricle; FM, foramen of Monroe; MM, massa intermedia.

from obstruction of the ventricular system by clot, septations, or debris (usually at the aqueduct) (51,52). A communicating form of hydrocephalus may develop secondary to arachnoiditis, in which CSF is not resorbed by the arachnoid granulations. An inflammatory ependymitis secondary to the IVH may also result in persistent ventriculomegaly (40). Infants with hydrocephalus may not present with the classical signs of hydrocephalus, i.e., macrocephaly, suture diastasis, and clinical findings of increased intracranial pressure, such as apnea, bradycardia, and mental status changes until days to weeks after the onset of ventriculomegaly (42,51). Initially, the trigones and occipital horns of the lateral ventricles dilate before the frontal horns. The lateral ventricles usually dilate more than the third or fourth ventricles. Ventricular dilatation usually improves commencing within approximately four weeks from the onset of ventriculomegaly, the degree of improvement directly proportional to the severity of ICH (51). Periodic lumbar puncture, a temporary ventricular reservoir, or a ventricular shunt may be required to control the hydrocephalus.

IPH is the most severe grade of ICH in the premature infant. Originally, it was believed that IPH was the result of direct extension of IVH into the adjacent brain parenchyma. More recent work indicates that IPH in most premature infants represents hemorrhage into areas that are already damaged by PVL, which is a form of hemorrhagic periventricular infarction (53,54) (hypoxic–ischemic encephalopathy). Parenchymal hemorrhage is associated with IVH in 80% of cases and usually occurs on the side of the cerebral hemisphere with the more severe IVH. The initial parenchymal bleed is brightly echogenic and often causes a mass effect. A frontoparietal distribution is most common. As the hemorrhage resolves, the central portion of the clot becomes less echogenic, central liquefaction occurs, and a peripheral echogenic rim persists. As the clot retracts, a porencephalic cyst forms at the site of the original infarcted hemorrhagic parenchyma. The mature porencephalic cyst usually communicates with the ipsilateral ventricle, which is dilated (Fig. 12) (55).

The morbidity and mortality associated with ICH increase with the severity and extent of the hemorrhage. Infants with grades I and II hemorrhage have the same risk for major neurologic damage (12–18%) as premature infants without hemorrhage (40). There is a marked increased incidence of major neurologic handicaps in grades III and IV IVH. These include developmental delay, mental retardation, and motor disabilities. A contralateral hemiparesis can result from an IPH (40).

ICH in the term infant is much less common than in the premature infant. Both GMH and IVH have been reported in term infants. Remnants of the germinal matrix are present at term in the periventricular tissue. Scattered islands of matrix cells may persist in the ventricular wall at term. GMH in the term infant can be clinically asymptomatic. Hayden et al. (56) reported that term infants with GMH were usually small for gestational age, vaginally delivered, and black. IVH in the full-term neonate is thought to arise primarily from the choroid plexus; there is no associated GMH. Etiologic factors associated with ICH in the term infant include asphyxia, birth trauma, apnea, seizures, and coagulation defects (38).

Other, much less common sites of ICH in the neonate are subarachnoid hemorrhage (SAH) and intracerebellar hemorrhage (CBH). Ultrasound is less accurate than CT in the detection of these two types of hemorrhage. SAH may occur secondary to IVH, with flow of bloody CSF through the fourth ventricular outlet foramina of Magendie and Luschka. Isolated SAH is more common in full-term neonates secondary to asphyxia, trauma, or disseminated intravascular coagulation (40). The ultrasonographic findings in SAH are increased echogenicity and widening of the horizontal portion of the sylvian fissure on coronal images (Fig. 13) (57). Widening of the sylvian fissure alone without increased echogenicity can be seen in cases of increased subarachnoid fluid associated with many conditions. The ultrasound findings of SAH are subtle and often only detectable with large amounts of blood. Therefore, CT is the preferred imaging modality in cases of suspected SAH.

Posterior fossa CBH is an uncommon event in both premature and full-term infants. The recent use of the mastoid fontanelle, the thinnest region of the temporal bone at the junction of the squamosal, lambdoidal, and occipital sutures, has significantly improved the diagnosis of this condition (58). Alternatively, using a very similar acoustic window, the posterolateral fontanelle, which is present at the junction of the temporal, parietal, and occipital bones, has also been helpful (59). The exact pathogenesis of CBH is unknown but is likely multifactorial. In preterm infants, this condition has been found to be associated with a number of prenatal, intrapartum, and early postnatal risk factors (58). In premature infants, CBH is usually associated with GMH and IVH. More recently, assisted methods of conception have been implicated in GMH and possibly CBH (60,61). Germinal matrix tissue has been identified in the subependymal tissues of the roof of the fourth ventricle up to 30 weeks' gestation (20). Therefore, this germinal matrix extension can be a source of hemorrhage. Intrapartum risk factors for CBH include abnormalities in fetal heart tracings, need for emergent cesarean section, low Apgar scores at one and five minutes, and fetal distress. Emergent cesarean section was found to be a significant independent risk factor for CBH. Early postnatal risk factors identified in the first five days of life include hemodynamic compromise, PDA, and acidosis (58). Cerebellar hemorrhage has also been implicated in infants undergoing extracorporeal membrane oxygenation (ECMO) (62). In the term neonate, CBH has been associated with traumatic delivery and coagulation defects. The use of mask ventilation has been reported as an etiologic factor in posterior fossa hemorrhage in low-birthweight

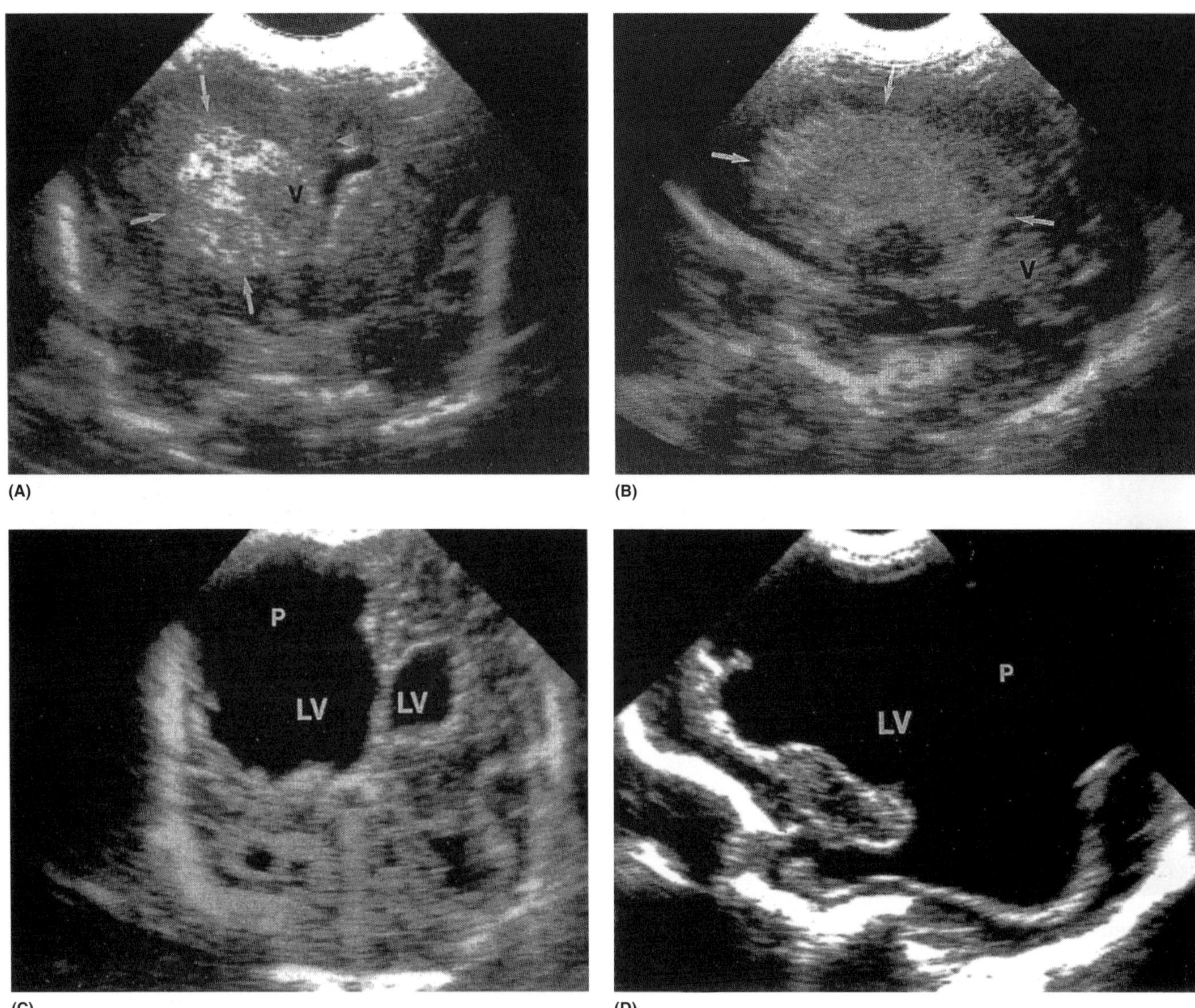

FIGURE 12 A–D ■ Intraparenchymal hemorrhage. Coronal (**A**) and right parasagittal (**B**) sonograms show a large intraparenchymal hemorrhage extending from the frontal to the posterior parietal lobes (*arrows*). The right lateral ventricle (V) is completely filled with blood. Note the mass effect with shift of the interhemispheric fissure to the left on the coronal scan. Eight-week follow-up coronal (**C**) and right parasagittal (**D**) scans show liquefaction of the right intraparenchymal hemorrhagic infarction with a developing porencephalic cyst. LV, lateral ventricle; P, porencephalic cyst.

and term infants (40,63). The prognosis is poor and frequently fatal in neonates with cerebellar hemorrhage. On ultrasound, the hemorrhage presents as an echodense area within the cerebellum below the tentorium (Fig. 14). The fourth ventricle is usually not visualized owing to compression or filling with clot. On sagittal midline scans, there is loss of the normal anatomic differentiation of the brain stem structures. The coronal images are usually the most definitive (20).

Subdural and epidural hemorrhages usually occur in term infants secondary to trauma. These peripheral fluid collections are difficult to detect on ultrasonography owing to the initial transducer artifact. Use of a stand-off pad, a high-frequency 7.5 or 10 MHz transducer, or axial scans through the temporal bone, however, may elucidate a collection with ultrasonography. The ultrasonographic findings of a subdural or epidural collection include visualization of the cortical gyral surface away from the cranial vault, widening of the interhemispheric fissure, a linear or elliptical fluid collection between the brain and the skull, and mass effect with displacement and distortion of the ventricles and midline structures (Fig. 15) (21). CT and magnetic resonance imaging (MRI) are the preferred imaging modalities for the evaluation of extra-axial hemorrhage and fluid collections.

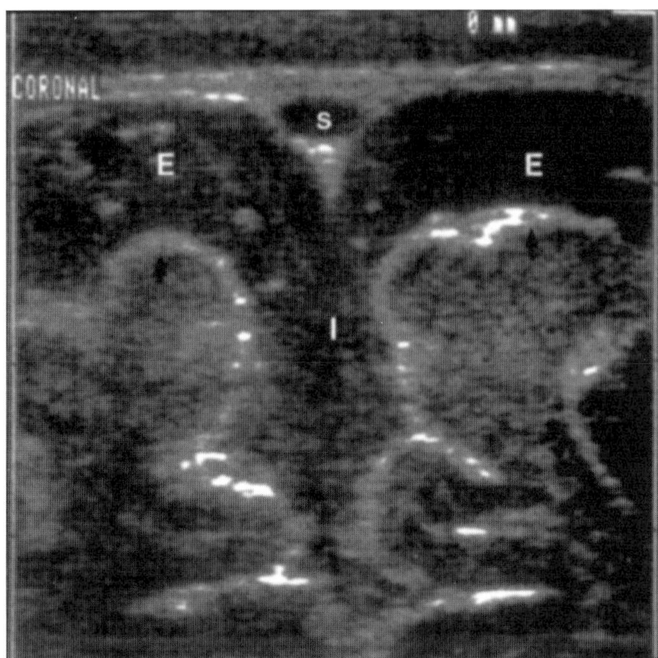

FIGURE 13 ■ Subarachnoid hemorrhage. Coronal sonogram of the extra-axial fluid space demonstrates widening of the extra-axial space and interhemispheric fissure, with internal echoes and increased echogenicity of the cortical surface (*arrows*). E, extra-axial space s, sagittal sinus; I, interhemispheric fissure.

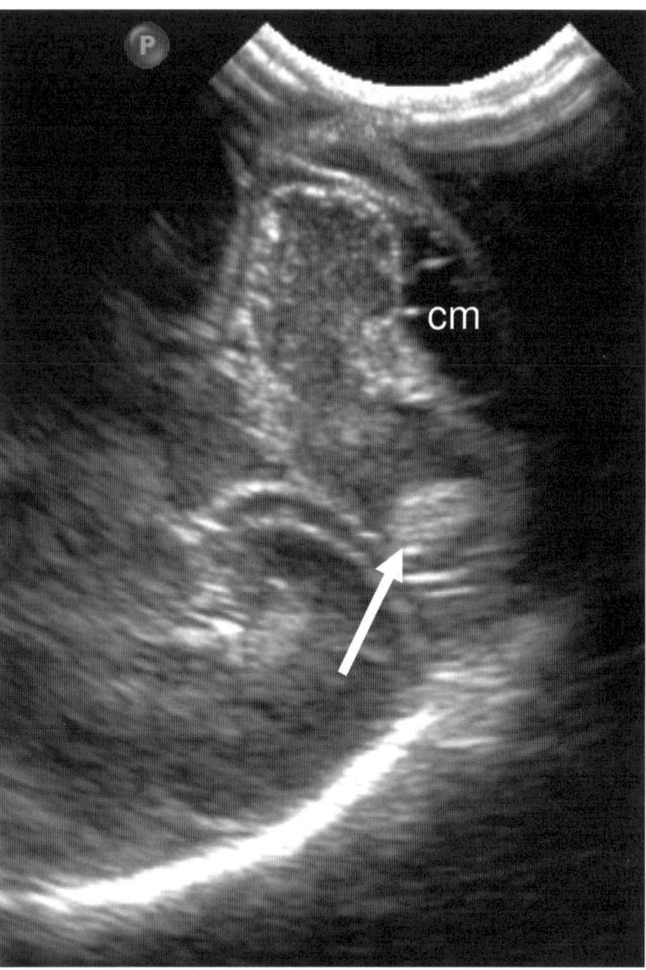

FIGURE 14 ■ Posterior fossa hemorrhage. Mastoid view shows a discrete, hyperechoic area within the cerebellum (*arrow*).

HYPOXIC–ISCHEMIC ENCEPHALOPATHY

Major neurologic and developmental deficits in infants and young children are the result of perinatal hypoxic–ischemic injury to the brain (Table 2). In the preterm infant, GMH–IVH is the most common manifestation of hypoxic brain injury. If there is a significant ischemic component to the insult, however, then infarction may result. PVL and periventricular hemorrhagic infarction (PVHI) are the primary manifestations of hypoxic–ischemic encephalopathy in the premature infant (64).

PVL is coagulation necrosis of the deep white matter. This white-matter infarction usually occurs at two common sites: at the external angle of the frontal horns near the foramen of Monroe and at the level of the optic radiations adjacent to the trigone. The distribution of these lesions is related to the vascular supply. The periventricular white matter in the premature infant is a watershed area between ventriculopedal and ventriculofugal arterial blood supplies (53,65,66). As a result, this junctional zone of end arteries lacks a collateral circulation and is vulnerable to ischemic changes. The prominence of these arterial end zones in the periventricular white matter is inversely related to gestational age (53). A second factor in the pathogenesis of PVL is the lack of cerebral autoregulation in the preterm brain. This results in a direct linear relation between systolic blood pressure and cerebral blood flow. There is also a limited capacity for

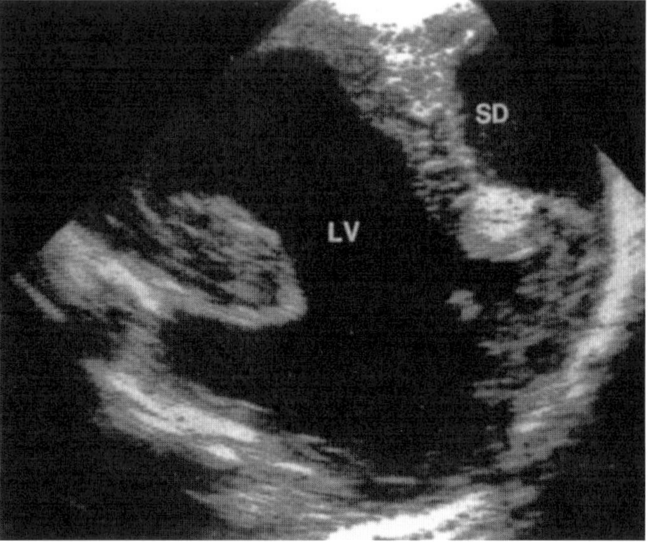

FIGURE 15 ■ Subdural hematoma. Left parasagittal sonogram demonstrates an extra-axial subdural hematoma in a patient with an Arnold–Chiari malformation type II. Rapid decompression of the ventricular system occurred after placement of a ventriculoperitoneal shunt in this premature infant. The lateral ventricle is severely dilated. SD, subdural hematoma; LV, lateral ventricle.

TABLE 2 ■ Hypoxic–Ischemic Encephalopathy

Manifestation	Risk factors	Ultrasound findings
Periventricular leukomalacia	Prematurity	Normal initially or coarse, increased echogenicity in periventricular white matter
		Evolves to multiple tiny cysts (2–3 wk)
		Cysts may collapse (1–3 mo)
		Larger cysts persist, resolve, or form porencephalic cysts
		White-matter gliotic scars
		Ventricles may enlarge
Periventricular hemorrhagic infarction	Prematurity	Asymmetric echogenicity radiating from external angle of lateral ventricle
		May evolve into porencephalic cyst
		80% associated with intraventricular hemorrhage
Perinatal asphyxia and cerebral edema	Full term	Focal or diffuse, hazy, increased cerebral echogenicity Slit-like ventricles
		Obliteration of extra-axial spaces and interhemispheric fissure
		Obliteration of sulci
Cerebral cortical infarction	Prematurity	Absence of gyral definition
	Asphyxia	Loss of vascular pulsations
	Congenital heart disease	Cystic spaces during resolution
	Polycythemia	
	Trauma	
	Meningitis	
	Thromboembolism	

vasodilation in the immature brain. This pressure-passive cerebral circulation renders the infant vulnerable to decreases in cerebral perfusion and leads to periventricular white-matter ischemia secondary to systemic hypotension (53). Third, the glial cells in the periventricular white matter are particularly vulnerable to injury because they are actively differentiating into astrocytes and oligodendroglia (53).

The earliest ultrasonographic abnormality in PVL consists of bilateral, coarse, globular, or broad bands of echodensity in the periventricular white matter (13). This finding usually develops within the first 10 days of life (67). The echodensities may be distributed diffusely in the periventricular white matter or localized along the external angles of the frontal horns and adjacent to the trigone of the lateral ventricles as well as within the

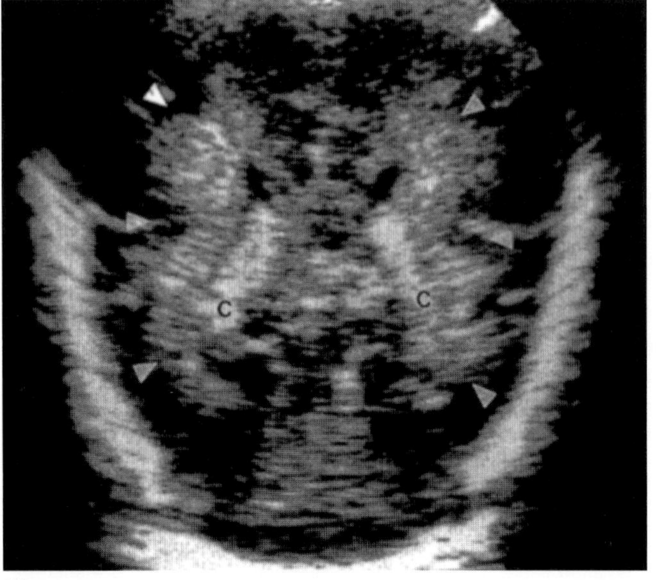

(A)

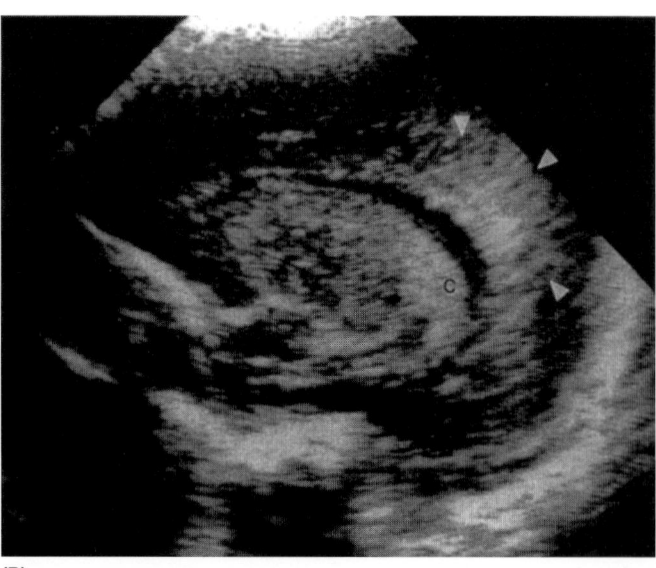

(B)

FIGURE 16 A–F ■ Periventricular leukomalacia. Coronal (**A**) and sagittal (**B**) scans show bilateral, symmetric bands of echogenicity in the white matter adjacent to the frontal horns and trigones (*arrowheads*). (*Continued*)

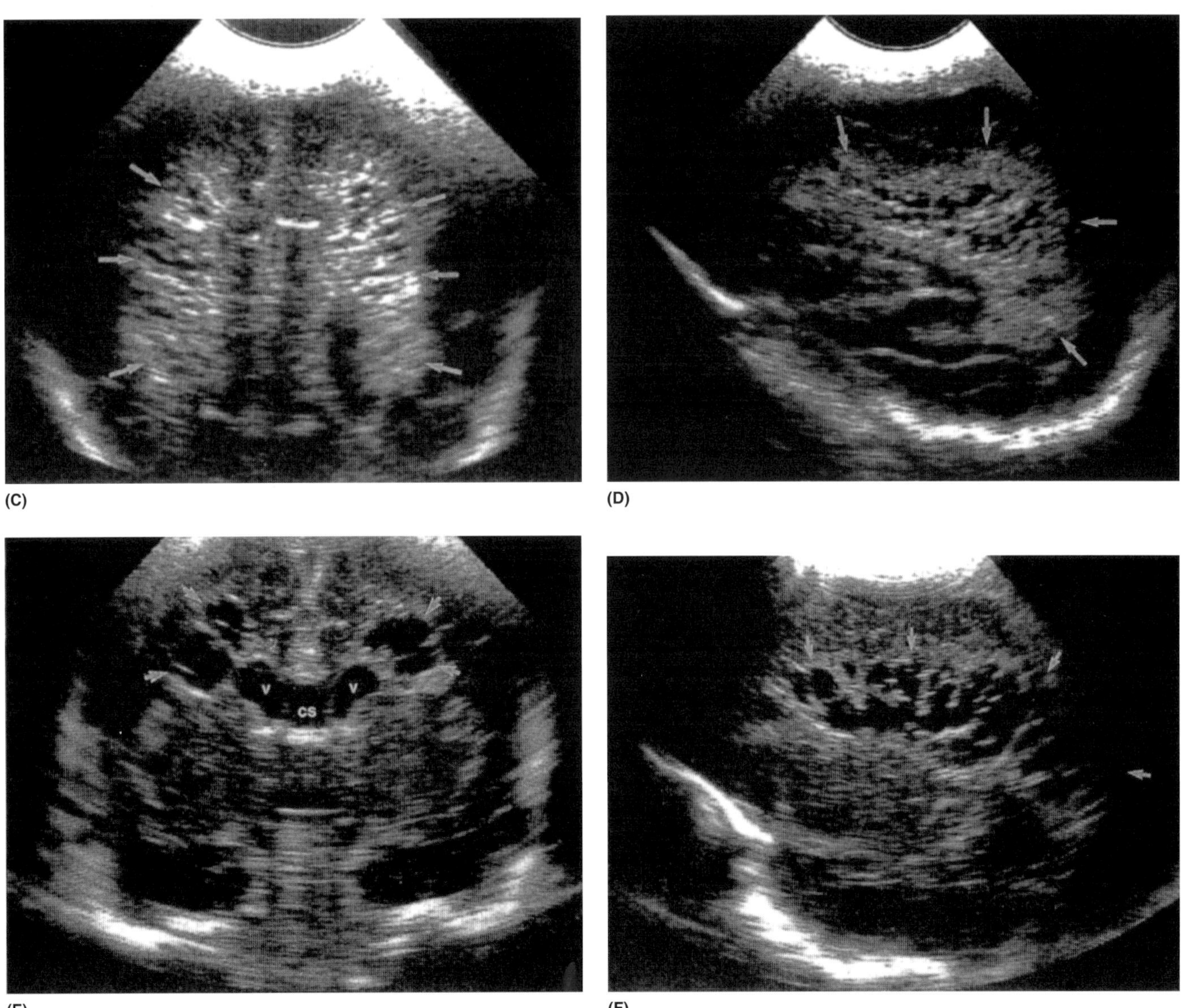

FIGURE 16 A–F ■ (*Continued*) Three weeks later, follow-up coronal (**C**) and sagittal (**D**) scans show multiple, tiny bilateral cysts in the periventricular deep white matter (*arrows*). Another 4 weeks later, coronal (**E**) and sagittal (**F**) scans show larger confluent cysts (*arrows*) in the periventricular white matter. The lateral ventricles are dilated owing to atrophy. A cavum septum pellucidum (cs) is seen. c, choroid plexus; V, lateral ventricle; cs, cavum septum pellucidum

corpus callosum (Fig. 16A and B) (68). PVL is almost always bilateral and symmetric. Secondary petechial hemorrhages can occur within areas of PVL; this is more common the more premature the infant (53). The bright periventricular echoes may represent hemorrhagic PVL; ultrasonography cannot differentiate between hemorrhagic and nonhemorrhagic forms. Increased periventricular echogenicity is not specific for PVL. This ultrasonographic finding is seen in other types of parenchymal injuries, including white-matter gliosis, he morrhage, and cortical infarction that extends into the deep white matter (69).

In the evolution of PVL, multiple small cysts develop at the sites of periventricular echodensity (Fig. 16C and D). Cyst formation usually occurs two to three weeks after the appearance of the echodensities. The cysts represent areas of necrosis and cavitation. Frequently, the small cavities collapse and disappear on ultrasound after one to four months, presumably due to resorption of fluid by the surrounding brain tissue (65,70,71). White-matter gliotic scars develop, resulting in decreased cerebral myelin and enlarged ventricles, especially in the region of the trigone and occipital horns. The larger cysts may either resolve or persist and form porencephalic cysts (Fig. 16E and F) (72). On CT, PVL initially appears as periventricular lucency, unless secondary hemorrhage has occurred. This periventricular hypodensity may be difficult to detect because of the normally low attenuation of the neonatal brain due to its high water content and unmyelinated fibers. During the later stage o f cyst formation, CT occasionally shows solitary or multiple focal low-density cysts in the periventricular white matter. CT is less sensitive than ultrasonography in the detection of these periventricular cysts, however, which is probably a result of volume averaging (67,73).

PVL occurs in about 25% to 40% of low-birthweight preterm neonates. Only 28% of lesions are detected in vivo with cranial ultrasonography (53). Although ultrasonography is more accurate than CT in the detection of periventricular cystic leukomalacia, neither modality is sensitive when compared with neuropathologic series (73,74). Although sonography is invaluable for this use, MRI has proven to be a useful diagnostic adjunct (75,76). The early detection of PVL is crucial because PVL is associated with major neurodevelopmental handicaps, in particular cerebral palsy. Spastic diplegia, in which the lower extremities are more affected than the upper extremities, is the most common clinical sequela of PVL. It is the result of necrosis involving the descending fibers from the motor cortex, which normally run in the periventricular frontal white matter. With more extensive lesions of PVL, spastic quadriparesis may develop. Severe visual impairment with cortical blindness may result from lesions involving the optic radiations adjacent to the trigone (77–79). Intellectual deficits are less common but can occur if extensive PVL involves the fibers associated with the visual, auditory, and somatesthetic functions necessary for learning (53). Recent evidence seems to indicate that the incidence of PVL can largely be reduced if impaired cerebral blood flow can be prevented (53).

Of note, congenital periventricular pseudocysts are diagnosed in approximately 1% of premature newborns undergoing sonography within the first 24 hours of life and may be confused with PVL (80). These pseudocysts are located in the caudothalamic groove or in the caudate nucleus, lateral to the wall of the frontal horn of the lateral ventricle. The pathogenesis of these lesions appears unclear, although hypoxia, hemorrhage, or infections have been postulated as possible etiologies. These pseudocysts are differentiated from the cysts of PVL by their different prognosis. Pseudocysts develop in the remnants of the germinal matrix where there are no axons, whereas PVL cysts develop in the unmyelinated white matter especially affecting the corona radiate and centrum semiovale. Because of this difference, pseudocysts are associated with a good prognosis, whereas neonates with PVL are prone to develop cerebral palsy and visual disturbances (80).

IPH is a serious sequela of hypoxic–ischemic injury to the brain of the preterm neonate. In most cases, IPH is associated with GMH and IVH. As a result, it was originally thought that IPH was a direct extension of hemorrhage from the subependymal germinal matrix or the ventricle (i.e., grade IV IVH). More recent studies have shown that IPH can occur in the absence of IVH, IPH can occur at a site distant from IVH, and IPH can develop 2 to 10 days after the initial IVH (54,81). These observations, in conjunction with neuropathologic data, indicate that these intraparenchymal lesions represent areas of hemorrhagic infarction. Volpe (53) uses the term periventricular hemorrhagic infarction (PVHI) to describe this lesion.

PVHI is an area of hemorrhagic necrosis in the periventricular white matter. It is usually a large, asymmetric lesion, and it coexists with large IVH in 80% of cases. The incidence is highest in very small premature infants. PVHI is most commonly located dorsal and lateral to the external angle of the lateral ventricle; half of lesions are more extensive and extend from the frontal to the parieto-occipital white matter (53,81).

On cranial ultrasound, PVHI is a unilateral or bilateral, asymmetric, globular or triangular fan-shaped echodensity, radiating from the external angle of the lateral ventricle. It can be localized or extensive in the periventricular white matter. Ultrasound may underestimate the extent of the infarction if the entire infarct is not hemorrhagic. Characteristically, these echodensities evolve into cystic cavities. These cysts are usually single and large, unlike those in PVL, which are small, multiple, and bilaterally symmetric. The cysts secondary to PVHI rarely disappear and usually progress to porencephaly (53).

PVHI is a venous infarction involving the terminal vein in the subependymal region, which drains the medullary veins in the periventricular white matter. The pathogenesis of PVHI is probably related to GMH–IVH. Eighty percent of parenchymal lesions are associated with large IVHs, usually on the side of the larger amount of intraventricular blood. In addition, PVHI usually develops and progresses after the occurrence of IVH, with peak occurrence on the fourth postnatal day. These data suggest that the GMH–IVH complex causes obstruction of the terminal vein with resultant hemorrhagic venous infarction. Other contributing etiologic mechanisms include the impairment of periventricular blood flow secondary to increased intraventricular pressure and the release of vasoactive compounds from the intraventricular blood.

Clinically, premature infants with PVHI have a poor prognosis. Spastic hemiparesis or asymmetric quadriparesis develops in 86% of survivors. Characteristically, the lower extremities are equally affected as the upper extremities. The overall mortality rate is 59%. Major intellectual deficits develop in 64%. The prognosis parallels the severity of the periventricular echodensity (81). Recent evidence suggests that by preventing germinal matrix–IVH, it may be possible to reduce the incidence of PVHI (53).

The ultrasonographic and CT manifestations of hypoxic–ischemic encephalopathy in the full-term neonate differ from those in the preterm infant. This difference in the pattern of brain injury is related to changes in the distribution of cerebral blood flow. In the premature infant, the watershed area is in the periventricular region. Toward the end of gestation, the watershed area begins moving more peripherally toward the cortex, beginning at 36 weeks' gestation. By 44 weeks, this watershed zone between the end fields of the anterior, middle, and posterior cerebral arteries has moved completely peripherally and involves the cortical and the subcortical white matter, sparing the periventricular area (82,83).

Perinatal asphyxia in the term infant can cause tiny slit-like ventricles, obliteration of the extra-axial fluid spaces, and hazy increased parenchymal echogenicity with decreased or no visualization of the sulci or the interhemispheric fissure (84,85). The abnormal parenchymal echogenicity may be diffuse or focal. During the first weeks of life, there is obliteration of the ventricles, sulci, and interhemispheric fissure, with diffuse homogenous increase in cerebral echogenicity (Fig. 17A and B). Babcock et al. (84) postulated that these findings are due to cerebral edema. The follow-up scans in these patients show signs of atrophy, with dilation of the ventricles and an increase in extra-axial fluid in the sulci and interhemispheric fissure. More severe anoxic insult can result in multicystic encephalomalacia (Fig. 17C) (86).

Focal areas of increased parenchymal echogenicity have also been described in the asphyxiated term infant. These can occur in the subcortical or periventricular white matter and in the thalamus and basal ganglia (85,87,88). The increase in echogenicity may be heterogeneous or homogenous. In reported series with pathologic correlation, these echodensities corresponded to areas of necrosis, although ultrasonography often underestimated the

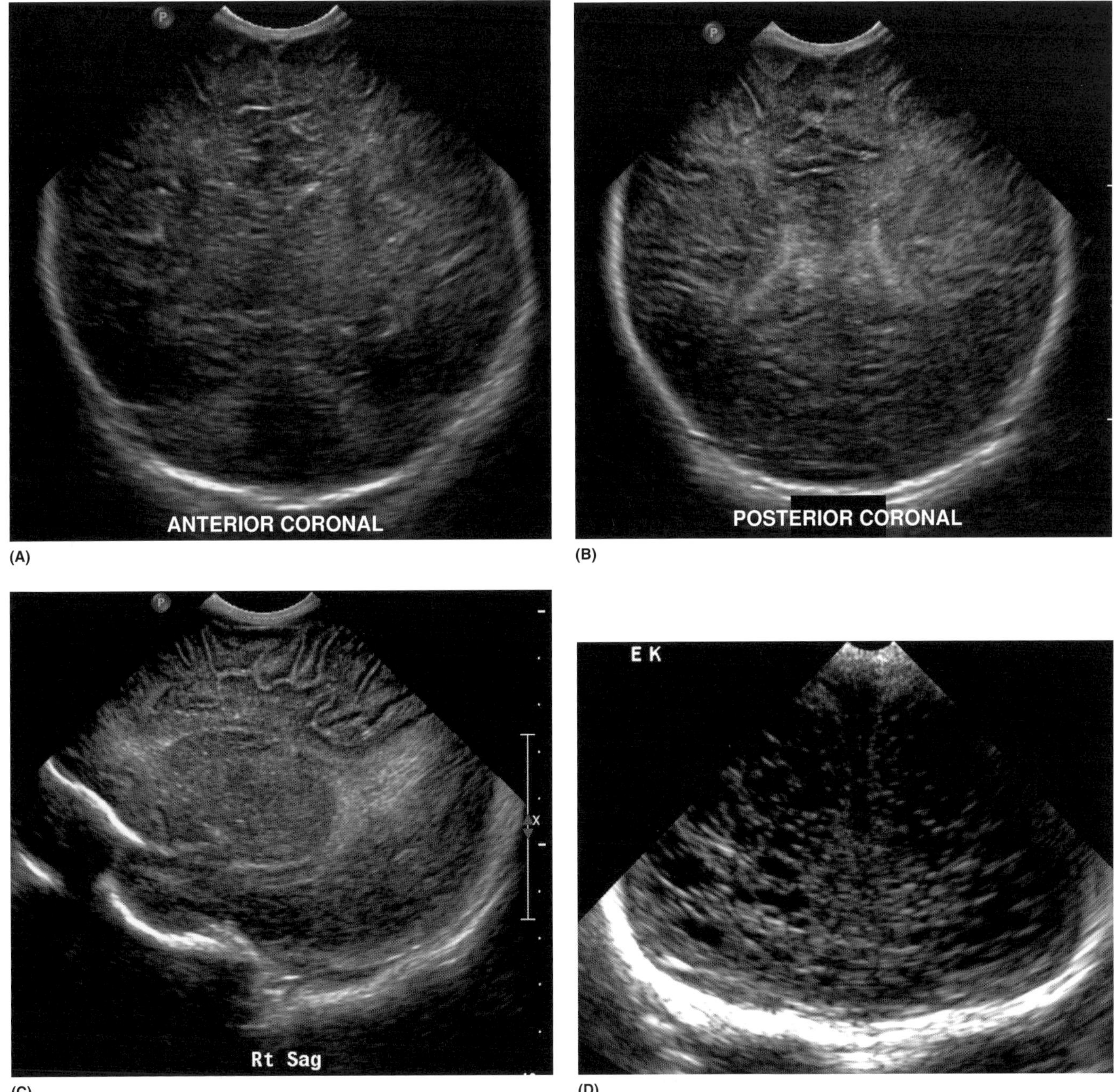

FIGURE 17 A–D ■ Cerebral edema in a full-term infant. Anterior coronal (**A**), posterior coronal (**B**), and sagittal (**C**) sonograms show markedly compressed ventricles, sulci, and interhemispheric fissure with diffuse hazy homogeneously increased cerebral echogenicity. (**D**) Sonogram of another infant shows diffuse heterogeneous cystic encephalomalacia. *Source*: From Ref. 45.

extent of disease. Subcortical cystic leukomalacia is another manifestation of hypoxic–ischemic encephalopathy in the term infant.

Cerebral cortical infarction is uncommon in neonates and young infants. Predisposing factors include prematurity, asphyxia, congenital heart disease, polycythemia and hyperviscosity, trauma, meningitis, and thromboembolism. The middle cerebral artery distribution is most commonly involved. In the acute stage, the characteristic ultrasound findings of cortical infarction are absence of gyral definition, absence of vascular pulsations, altered parenchymal echogenicity, and territorial distribution. If there is a significant amount of edema, usually with multiple infarcts, there may be midline shift and ventricular compression (89,90). The intensity of echogenicity does not reflect the presence or absence of secondary hemorrhage (Fig. 18). During the stage of resolution, there is gradual return of pulsations and the development of cystic spaces. With single vessel involvement, the return of pulsations usually begins peripherally and extends centrally; with multiple vessel infarctions, it begins at the base and extends toward the convexities (89). Although localized cerebral infarction can occur in the premature infant, it is uncommon. In four reported cases in premature infants, none had seizures, whereas in full-term infants, seizures and hemiplegia are common after stroke (91).

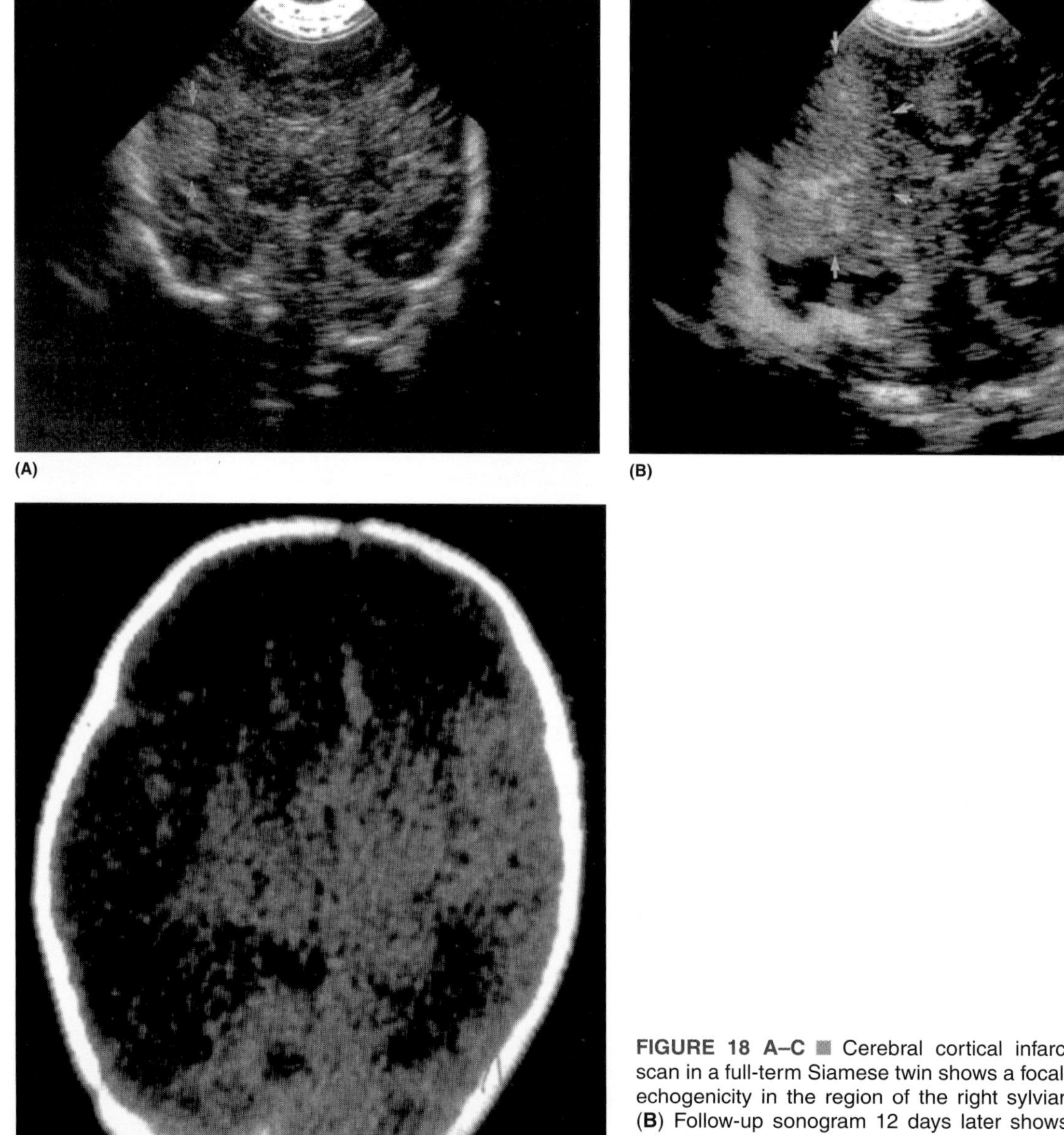

FIGURE 18 A–C ■ Cerebral cortical infarction. (**A**) Coronal scan in a full-term Siamese twin shows a focal area of increased echogenicity in the region of the right sylvian fissure (*arrows*). (**B**) Follow-up sonogram 12 days later shows progression and extension of the abnormal echogenicity within the right cerebral hemisphere (*arrows*). (**C**) CT scan performed at the time of the second sonogram shows extensive low-density nonhemorrhagic infarction involving the right hemisphere and left frontal lobe. *Source*: From Ref. 45.

CONGENITAL ANOMALIES

In 1971, DeMyer (92) classified congenital anomalies of the brain into three categories, according to the developmental stages involved: those resulting from errors in cytogenesis (development of molecules into cells), those resulting from errors in histogenesis (development of cells into tissues), and those resulting from errors in organogenesis (development of tissues into organs). Because the anomalies resulting from disturbances in histogenesis (Table 3) and organogenesis (Table 4) result in macroscopic anatomic changes, these congenital anomalies of the brain can be identified with ultrasonography (93,94).

Congenital anomalies of the brain can result from genetic or environmental factors. Most occur between the fourth and sixth weeks of embryonic life, a time when the embryologic development of the brain is particularly complex (92). Hydrocephalus is the most common congenital anomaly in neonates who survive to infancy. The presence of hydrocephalus is important to identify since only 38% of these patients go on to develop normal cognitive function (95). Indications for a sonographic examination include an enlarged head, prominent separation of the cranial sutures, a full fontanelle, or signs of neurologic abnormality.

Hydrocephalus is manifested as an increased volume of fluid within the ventricular system and can be characterized as either obstructive or nonobstructive. Although nonobstructive hydrocephalus can be seen due to (*i*) increased production of CSF as in choroid plexus papilloma, (*ii*) loss of brain tissue as in cortical atrophy, or (*iii*) merging of periventricular cysts, obstruction is the form of hydrocephalus most commonly seen in congenital anomalies. Obstructive hydrocephalus can be classified as noncommunicating, in which the point of obstruction occurs within the ventricular system and communicating, in which the obstruction occurs beyond the ventricular system, i.e., the arachnoid granulations. The most common causes of congenital hydrocephalus are aqueductal stenosis (Fig. 19), myelomeningocele in association with Arnold–Chiari malformation, communicating hydrocephalus, and Dandy–Walker malformation, conditions that will be described later in this section (95).

TABLE 4 ■ Disorders of Organogenesis

Disorders of closure
Cranioschisis
Meningocele
Encephalocele
Anencephaly
Lipomas of corpus callosum
Agenesis of corpus callosum
Teratoma
Arnold–Chiari malformation
Dandy–Walker syndrome
Disorders of diverticulation
Septo-optic dysplasia
Lobar holoprosencephaly
Alobar holoprosencephaly
Aventricular cerebrum
Disorders of sulcation and migration
Lissencephaly
Polymicrogyria
Schizencephaly
Heterotopias
Disorders of size
Microcephaly
Macrocephaly
Hydrocephalus with aqueductal stenosis
Megalencephaly
Destructive lesions
Hydranencephaly
Porencephaly
Hypoxia
Toxicosis
Inflammatory diseases
Rubella
Cytomegalic inclusion disease
Toxoplasmosis
Herpes simplex virus

TABLE 3 ■ Disorders of Histogenesis

Disorder	Pattern of inheritance	Ultrasound findings
Tuberous sclerosis	Autosomal dominant (70% new mutations)	Hamartomas in cerebrum, cerebellum, medulla, and spinal cord
		Mainly subependymal
		Commonly calcify
Neurofibromatosis	Type I autosomal dominant	Not usually seen until after closure of fontanelle
		Optic nerve gliomas may be seen with orbital ultrasound
Encephalotrigeminal angiomatosis (Sturge–Weber syndrome)	–	Findings rarely seen before two years of age and are therefore not seen on ultrasound
Neoplasia	–	See Table 13
Vascular lesions	–	Variable

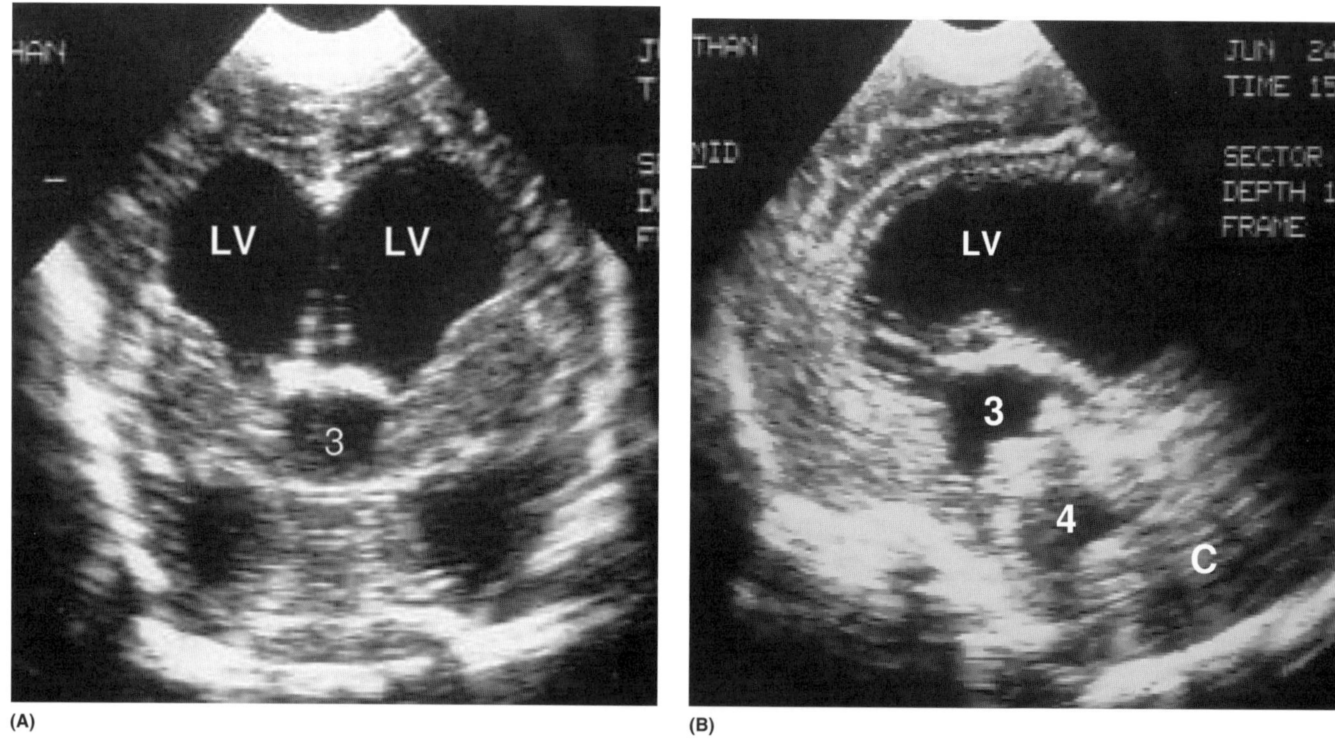

FIGURE 19 A AND B ■ Aqueductal stenosis acquired after severe grade III intraventricular hemorrhage. Coronal (**A**) and sagittal (**B**) cranial sonograms show moderately severe dilation of the lateral and third ventricles. LV, lateral ventricle; 3, third ventricle; 4, fourth ventricle; C, cerebellum; m, massa intermedia.

It is important to note the difference between the above conditions that result in hydrocephalus from an entity termed "benign hydrocephalus of infancy." This condition is also referred to as benign external hydrocephalus and is characterized by increasing head circumference that is out of proportion to body weight and length (96). The cause of this condition is presumably immature arachnoid villi that cannot absorb CSF as quickly as the choroid plexus produces it. Thus, CSF accumulates within the ventricles as well as within the cerebral convexities, typically in the frontal, subarachnoid region (Fig. 20) (97). Recent literature suggests that this

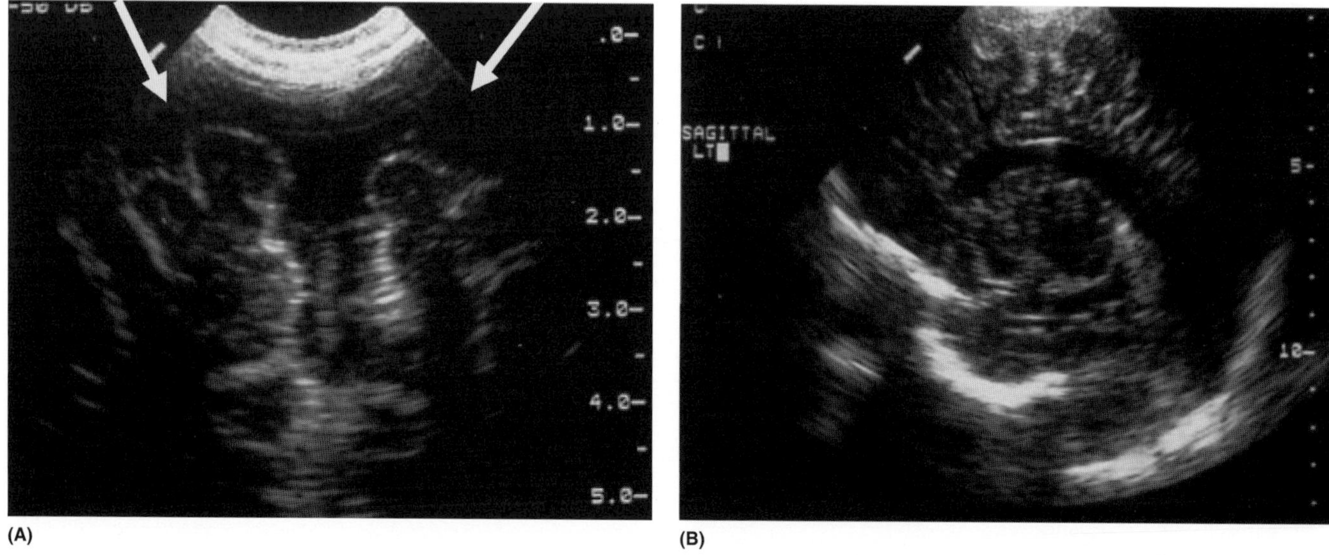

FIGURE 20 A AND B ■ Benign external hydrocephalus. (**A**) Coronal sonogram identifies enlarged extra-axial collections (*arrows*). (**B**) Parasagittal section shows prominence of the frontal horn and body of the lateral ventricle.

condition may be less benign than originally thought. Statistically larger intracranial volumes of adult patients with normal pressure hydrocephalus compared with age- and sex-matched control subjects suggest that this process begins in infancy, perhaps as external hydrocephalus (96). A similar condition may occur in the first year of life in normal babies in which there is prominence of the extra-axial fluid spores anterior to the frontal lobes with a normal size interhemispheric fissure, sometimes referred to as subdural effusions of infancy. These collections usually resolve by the second year of life (95). This topic is further discussed in the section entitled Vascular Abnormalities under Color Doppler Ultrasound of Extra-axial Fluid Collections to follow later in this chapter.

Other congenital anomalies include the disorders of closure, which result in anomalies such as cranioschisis (meningocele, encephalocele, and anencephaly), agenesis of the corpus callosum, teratoma, lipoma of the corpus callosum, Arnold–Chiari malformation, and Dandy–Walker syndrome.

Calvarial or cranial defects, also known as "cranium bifidum," are often associated with congenital malformations of the brain, meninges, or both (Fig. 21) (98,99). These defects most often present as a midline occipital mass and less often in the cranial base or in the frontoethmoidal region. When the cranial defect is small, only the meninges may herniate, resulting in a cranial meningocele or cranium bifidum with meningocele. On the other hand, when the defect is large, the meninges and part of the brain herniate, forming an encephalomeningocele (Fig. 22). When the brain tissue herniates along with a portion of the ventricle and meninges, a meningohydroencephalocele develops.

The corpus callosum is the largest of the medial interhemispheric commissures whose fibers interconnect the cerebral hemispheres, allowing them to share learning and memory (100,101). The corpus callosum forms during the third and fourth fetal months as a bud from the lamina terminalis and grows upward and backward as the primitive cerebral hemispheres grow laterally and then posteriorly. Primary complete agenesis occurs before the 12th gestational week as a result of an early vascular or inflammatory lesion of the commissural plate (102–104). Secondary dysgenesis may occur later in

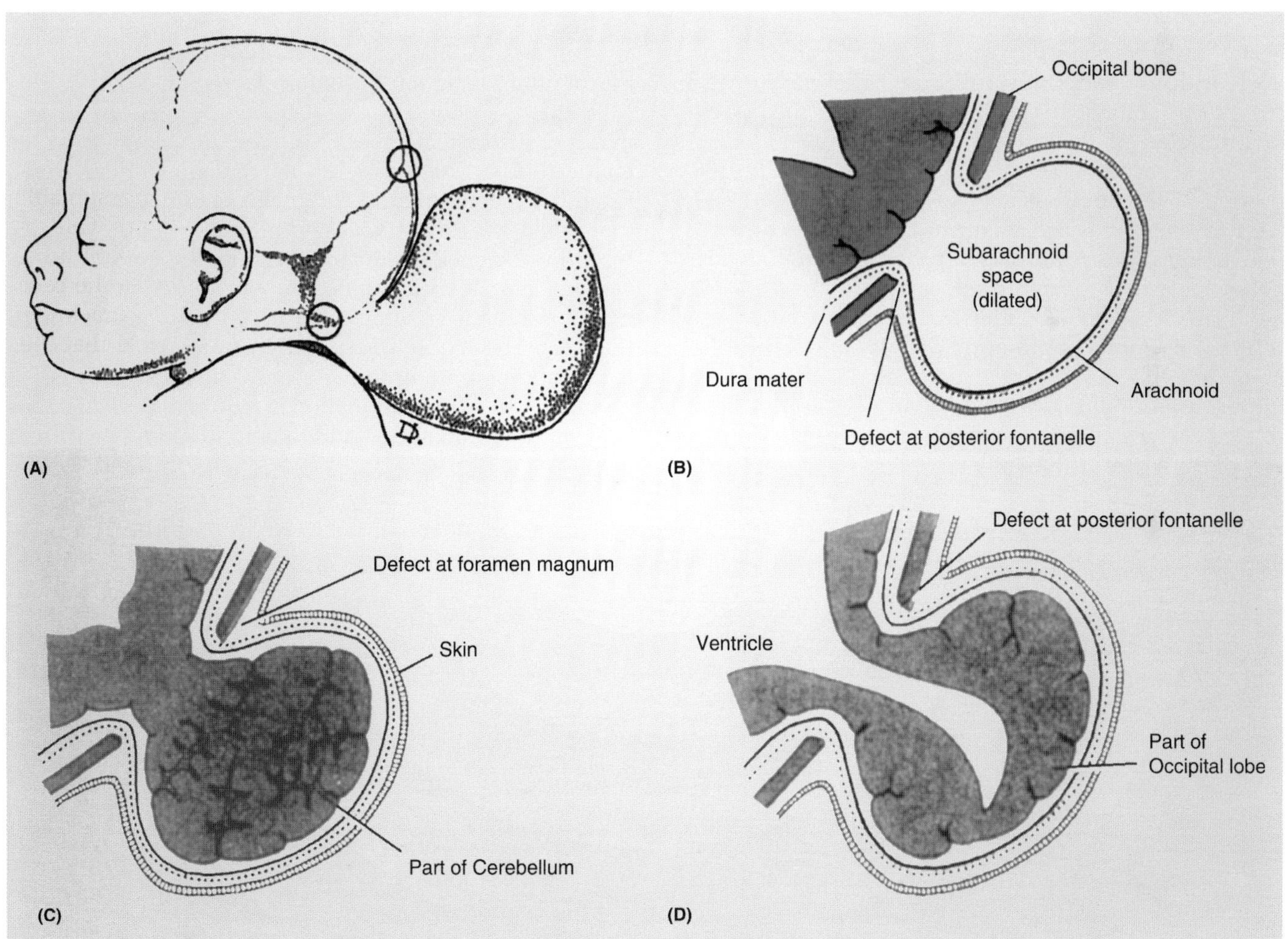

FIGURE 21 A–D ■ Schematic drawing showing cranium bifidum with various types of herniation. (**A**) Neonatal head with a large occipital protrusion. (**B**) Meningocele (meninges). (**C**) Meningoencephalocele (brain and meninges). (**D**) Meningohydroencephalocele (brain, meninges, and a portion of lateral ventricle). *Source*: From Ref. 98.

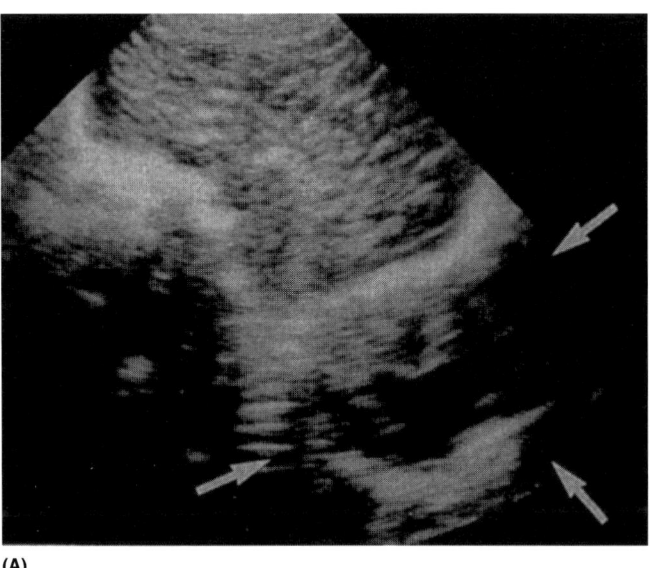

(A)

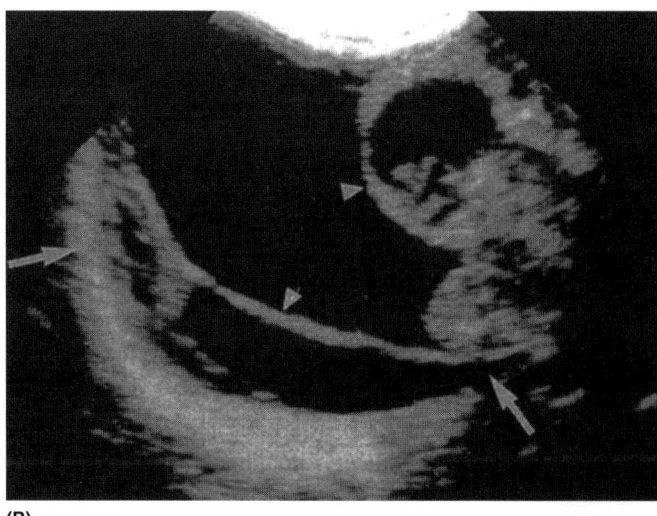

(B)

FIGURE 22 A AND B ■ Occipital encephalocele. (**A**) Midline sagittal scan of the brain showing a low-lying cerebellum herniated into a large occipital encephalocele (*arrows*). (**B**) Transverse image of encephalocele (*arrows*) posterior to portion containing herniated cerebellum, showing that the sac contains a large amount of fluid and multiple septations (*arrowheads*).

gestational life as partial or total destruction of a previously well-formed corpus callosum, secondary to a vascular or inflammatory process. Because of the direction of formation of the corpus callosum from anterior to posterior, partial agenesis usually affects the posterior portion of this midline structure. Associated anomalies seen with agenesis of the corpus callosum include midline lipomas, encephaloceles, arachnoid cysts, polymicrogyria, polymacrogyria, microcephaly, Dandy–Walker malformation, Arnold–Chiari malformation, holoprosencephaly, cyclopia, septo-optic dysplasia, porencephaly, aqueductal stenosis, and hydrocephalus. The psychomotor abnormalities noted clinically are generally related to the associated anomalies rather than the agenesis of the corpus callosum (Table 5).

Intracranial lipomas are generally seen at or near the midsagittal plane, most often in the region of the corpus callosum, occasionally associated with agenesis of this midline structure (105–107). Other, less common sites include the pericallosal region, the cerebellopontine angle, the tuber cinereum, and the quadrigeminal plate (108). Many patients do not have symptoms, and the lipoma is recognized coincidentally as a brightly hyperechoic mass arising from the corpus callosum, often extending into the interhemispheric fissures and laterally into adjacent sulci (Fig. 23). The highly dense, fatty elements and possible calcifications within the mass may cause acoustic shadowing. CT or MRI examination is required to identify the fatty nature of the lesion and to help differentiate it from hemorrhage.

TABLE 5 ■ Agenesis of Corpus Callosum

Malformation	Gestational age	Causes	Associated anomalies
Primary agenesis	12th gestational week	Vascular or inflammatory lesion of commissural plate	Lipoma
			Encephalocele
			Arachnoid cyst
			Migrational abnormality
Secondary dysgenesis	Later	Destruction of previously formed corpus callosum	Microcephaly Dandy–Walker syndrome
		Usually posterior	Arnold–Chiari malformation
			Holoprosencephaly
			Cyclopia
			Septo-optic dysplasia
			Porencephaly
			Aqueductal stenosis

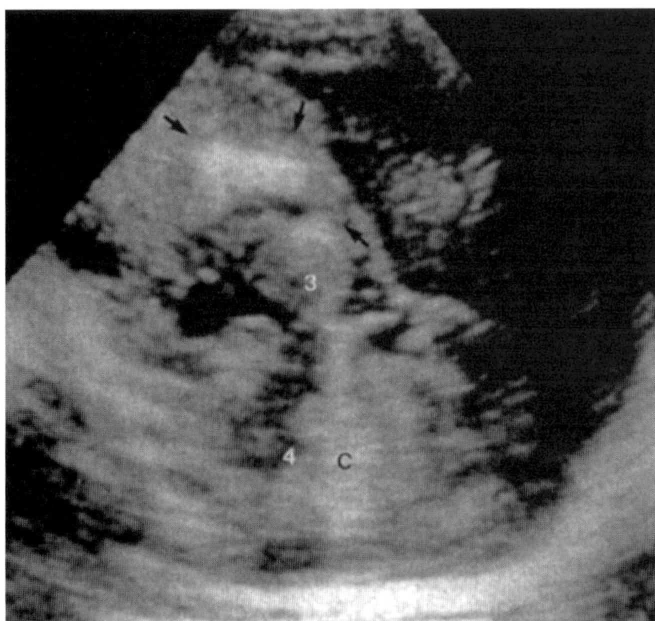

FIGURE 23 ■ Lipoma of the corpus callosum. Sagittal midline sonogram shows a bright hyperechoic mass (*arrows*) in the region of the absent corpus callosum. 3, third ventricle; 4, fourth ventricle; C, cerebellum. *Source*: Courtesy of Jeanette Pleasure, MD, Division of Neonatology, Hospital of the University of Pennsylvania, Philadelphia, PA, U.S.A.

The ultrasonographic findings of agenesis of corpus callosum include complete absence of the sonolucent band of fibers in the expected location of corpus callosum, when there is complete agenesis (Fig. 24) (102–104).

TABLE 6 ■ Agenesis of Corpus Callosum: Ultrasound Features

- Absence of sonolucent band in location of corpus callosum
- Widely separated frontal horns and bodies of lateral ventricles (double-horned appearance)
- Colpocephaly
- Concave medial borders of lateral ventricles
- Dilation and posterosuperior displacement of third ventricles
- Radial arrangement of medial cerebral sulci

With partial agenesis of the corpus callosum, there is absence of the posterior or middle and posterior aspects of the sonolucent band in the region of body and splenium of corpus callosum (Fig. 25). The frontal horns and bodies of lateral ventricles are widely separated, and the frontal horns are narrow, unless hydrocephalus is present. The lateral peaks of frontal horns and bodies of lateral ventricles are sharply angled, creating a double-horned appearance on coronal scans. The occipital horns are relatively dilated (colpocephaly). The medial borders of the lateral ventricles are concave, owing to protrusion of the Probst bundles–cingulate gyrus complex, and the foramina of Monroe are elongated. There is dilation and posterosuperior displacement of the third ventricle, resulting in interposition of the third ventricle between the lateral ventricles. The medial cerebral sulci have a radial arrangement around the roof of the third ventricle, resulting in echogenic serpiginous-like striations radiating superoposteriorly from the dorsal and posterior aspect of the third ventricle (Table 6).

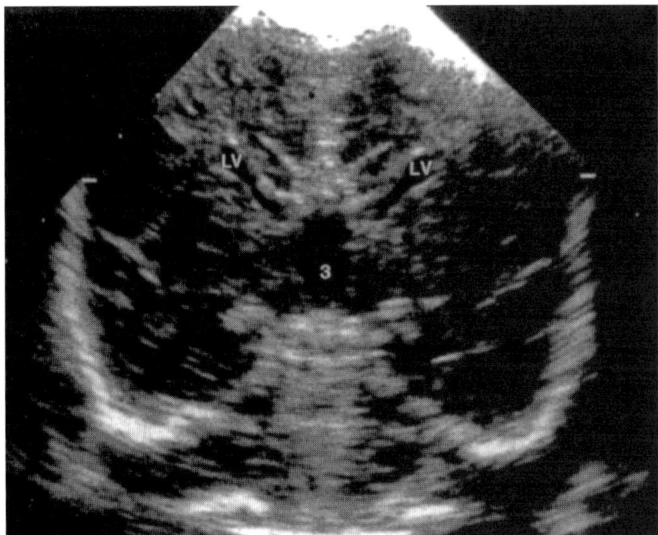

(A)

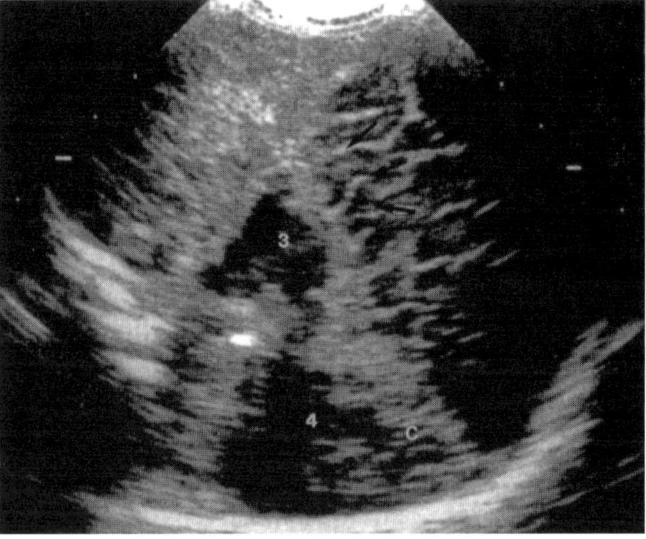

(B)

FIGURE 24 A AND B ■ Agenesis of the corpus callosum. (**A**) Coronal image of brain shows widely separated, slightly enlarged, sharply angled bodies of the lateral ventricles, creating a double-horned appearance. The medial borders of the lateral ventricles are concave, owing to protrusion of Probst bundles-cingulate gyrus complex. The dilated third ventricle is superiorly displaced. (**B**) Midsagittal scan showing superior and posterior displacement of dilated third ventricle with no evidence of corpus callosum superior to third ventricle. Note radial arrangement of medial cerebral sulci (*arrows*), which appear as serpiginous-like striations radiating from dorsal and superior aspects of the third ventricle. LV, lateral ventricle; 3, third ventricle; 4, fourth ventricle; C, cerebellum. *Source*: From Ref. 9.

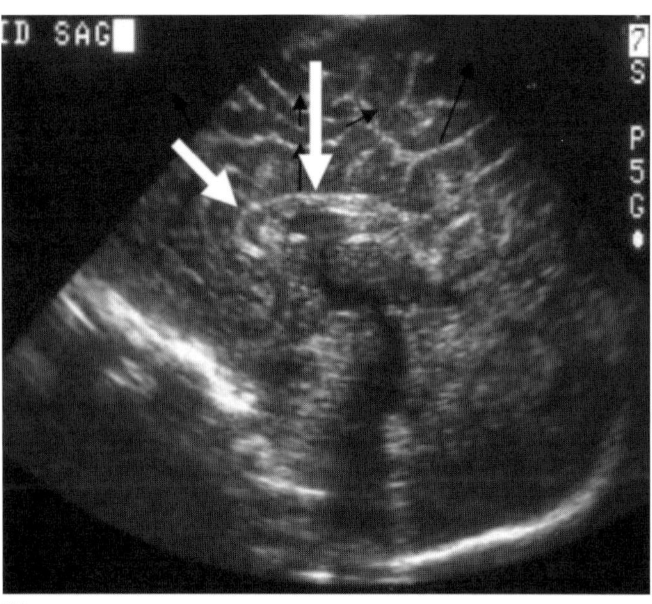

(A)

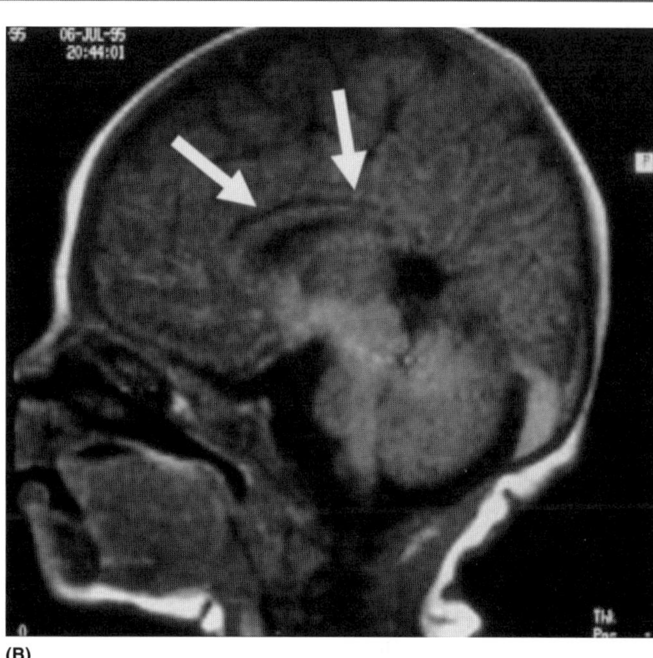

(B)

FIGURE 25 A AND B ■ Partial agenesis of the corpus callosum. Midsagittal ultrasound (**A**) and midsagittal T1-weighted MRI (**B**) show that the only remaining parts of the corpus callosum include the genu and the body. Notable is the absence of the splenium of the corpus callosum.

Dandy–Walker syndrome is characterized by cystic dilation of the fourth ventricle, hypoplastic cerebellar hemispheres, and absent or rudimentary vermis (Fig. 26) (109–112). Other associated cerebral malformations may be present, such as encephalocele, agenesis of the corpus callosum, holoprosencephaly, gyral anomalies, heterotopias, cleft palate, and polydactylism and syndactylism (Table 7). The lateral and third ventricles are dilated to variable degrees. Care must be taken to differentiate this condition from a mega cisterna magna (anatomic variant without clinical significance) and a trapped fourth ventricle (isolated fourth ventricle due to occlusion of the aqueduct of Sylvius and the foramina of Magendie and Luschka, most often due to previous subarachnoid cyst, which may invaginate between the two cerebellar hemispheres, causing nonvisualization of the fourth ventricle). With Dandy–Walker cyst, a large posterior fossa cyst, continuous with the fourth ventricle, is seen on ultrasound. The lateral and

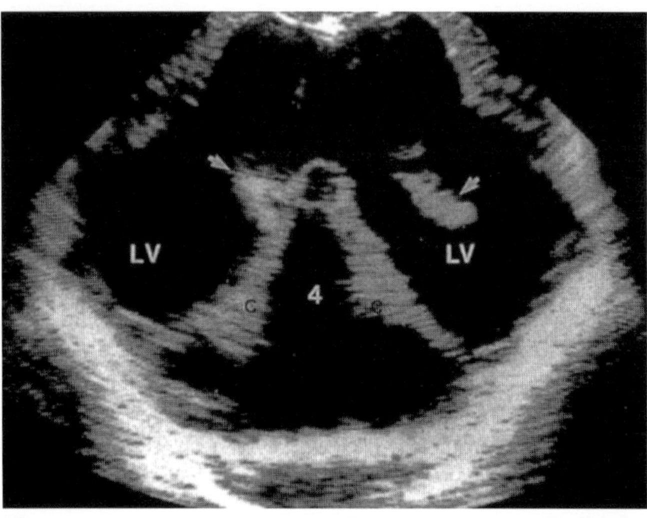

(A)

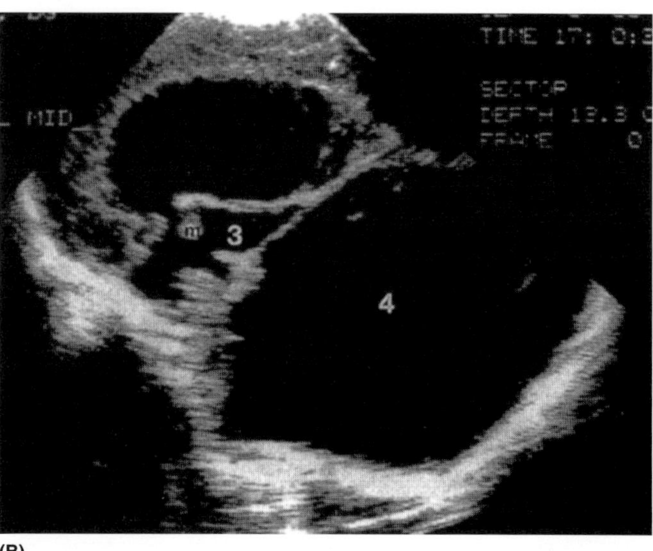

(B)

FIGURE 26 A AND B ■ Dandy–Walker cyst. Coronal (**A**) and sagittal (**B**) sonograms demonstrating massive lateral ventricular dilation, massive cystic dilation of the fourth ventricle, and rudimentary cerebellum. *Arrows*, choroid plexus. LV, lateral ventricle; 4, fourth ventricle; m, massa intermedia; C, cerebellum; 3, third ventricle. *Source*: From Ref. 9.

TABLE 7 ■ Dandy–Walker Cysts

Ultrasound features:
- Cystic dilation of the fourth ventricle
- Hypoplastic cerebellar hemispheres
- Absent or rudimentary vermis
- Large posterior fossa continuous with the fourth ventricle
- Variable degrees of hydrocephalus

Associated anomalies:
- Encephalocele
- Agenesis of the corpus callosum
- Holoprosencephaly
- Gyral anomalies
- Heterotopias
- Cleft palate
- Polysyndactylism

third ventricles are variably dilated with divergence of the occipital horns due to the large cyst and the associated elevation of the tentorium. The hypoplastic cerebellar hemispheres are shown to be displaced anteriorly.

In the late nineteenth century, the Arnold–Chiari malformations were described (Table 8) (113). Type I consists of inferior displacement of the tonsils and cerebellum without displacement of the fourth ventricle or the medulla. This is often accompanied by syringomyelia and skeletal malformations, including achondroplasia, platybasia, or the Klippel–Feil anomaly. The Arnold–Chiari malformation type II is the most common type seen in neonates and infants (Table 9) (114,115). This is a complex congenital brain malformation that includes a relatively small posterior fossa, elongation of the pons and fourth ventricle, and downward displacement of the medulla, fourth ventricle, and cerebellum into the cervical spinal canal, causing obliteration of the cisterna magna (Fig. 27). These infants usually present as newborns with obvious spina bifida and meningomyelocele. Most often, there is a variable degree of hydrocephalus with worsening after closure of the back defect. The lateral ventricles are frequently asymmetric with a colpocephalic configuration, owing to the relatively more dilated occipital horns and atria. Pointing of the frontal horns is often seen. The septum pellucidum may be partially or completely absent.

TABLE 8 ■ Arnold–Chiari Malformations

Type	Description
I	Inferior displacement of cerebellar tonsils without displacement of fourth ventricle or medulla
	Syringomyelia and skeletal dysplasias are additional features
II	Most common type (Table 9)
	Associated with spina bifida and myelomeningocele
III	Occipital or high cervical encephalocele
IV	Hypoplastic cerebellum without inferior displacement

TABLE 9 ■ Ultrasound Features of Arnold–Chiari Malformation Type II

- Pointing of the frontal horns
- Partial or complete absence of septum pellucidum
- Small posterior fossa
- Elongation of pons and fourth ventricle
- Downward displacement of medulla, fourth ventricle, and cerebellum into cervical spinal canal
- Obliteration of cisterna magna
- Hydrocephalus (often worse after closure of back defect)
- Colpocephaly
- Dilation of third ventricle with prominent massa intermedia

The third ventricle is usually dilated (owing to relative aqueductal stenosis), and the massa intermedia is markedly enlarged. The maximal thinning of the cerebral mantle involves the occipital regions. Occasionally, a prominent anterior commissure, herniation of the third ventricle into the suprasellar cistern, and an enlarged suprapineal recess are seen. With Arnold–Chiari malformation type III, there is an occipital encephalocele or high cervical encephalocele; with type IV, the cerebellum is hypoplastic without inferior displacement (113).

The disorders of diverticulation (Table 10) include septo-optic dysplasia, lobar and alobar holoprosencephaly, and aventricular cerebrum (109). Septo-optic dysplasia was first described by Morsier in 1956 (Fig. 28). It is a rare congenital malformation of anterior midline structures, occurring as early as two weeks' gestational age during the time when mesodermal induction of overlying ectoderm forms the neural plate (116,117). This entity includes agenesis of the septum pellucidum; dilation of the lateral ventricles, with flattening of the roofs of the frontal horns; hypoplasia of the optic chiasm, nerves, and infundibulum; and a primitive optic ventricle. It may include hypopituitarism if it extends into the hypothalamus. The chiasmatic and suprasellar cisterns are dilated owing to dysgenesis of the hypothalamus. In addition, diverticular expansion of the optic recess of the anterior third ventricle and cortical atrophy and dilated sulci may be seen. Most affected patients are first-born girls of healthy mothers, who develop seizures and hypotonia during the first few days of life. One or both optic discs are hypoplastic, optic nerves are small, and half of the infants have diabetes insipidus.

Holoprosencephaly results from a disorder of the diverticulation of the fetal brain, in which there is a defect in the midline cleavage of the prosencephalon, causing failure of formation of separate cerebral hemispheres and resulting in a holosphere cerebrum (118,119). The degree of separation of the holosphere determines the varying degrees of the disorder. The most severe form of holoprosencephaly is the alobar type in which there is no division of the cerebral tissue into hemispheres, a large horseshoe-shaped single ventricular cavity, and fused thalami (Fig. 29). A thin, pancake-like primitive cerebrum is situated anteriorly. Associated facial anomalies may

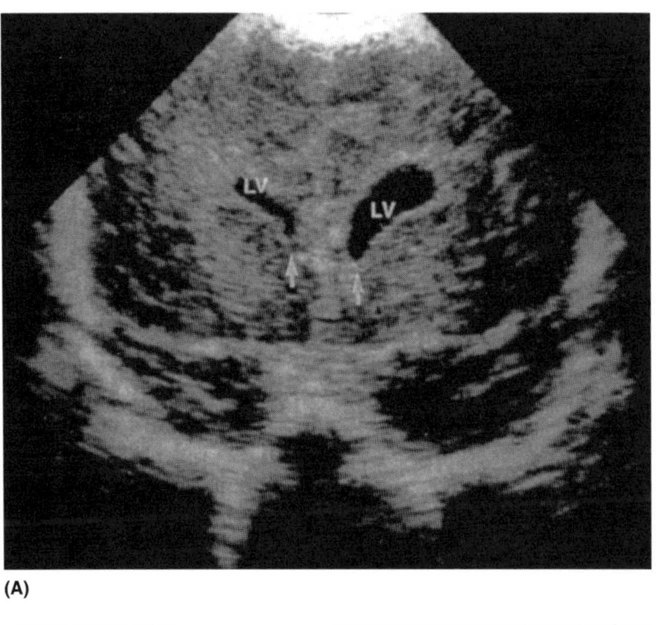

(A)

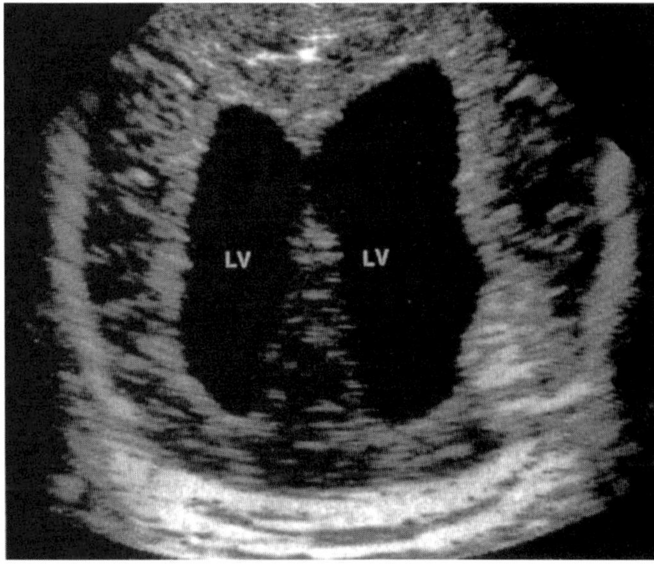

(B)

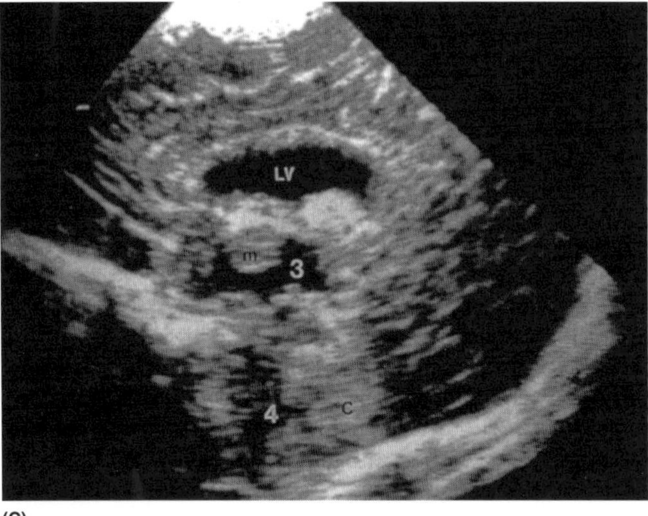

(C)

FIGURE 27 A–C ■ Arnold–Chiari malformation type II. (**A**) Anterior coronal sonogram of brain showing asymmetric dilation of the lateral ventricles with pointing of the frontal horns (*arrows*). (**B**) Posterior coronal scan demonstrating more severe enlargement of the occipital horns of the asymmetrically dilated lateral ventricles (colpocephaly). The posterior fossa is small. (**C**) Midline sagittal view demonstrating enlarged third ventricle, prominent massa intermedia, normal-sized fourth ventricle, and low-lying cerebellum with obliteration of the cisterna magna. LV, lateral ventricle; 4, fourth ventricle; m, massa intermedia; C, cerebellum; 3, third ventricle.

include cyclopia, ethmocephalus, cebocephaly, median cleft lip, and philtrum–premaxilla anlage. Although the cause is unknown, there is some association with some chromosomal aberrations [trisomy 13 (most commonly) and the 18p and 13q karyotypes], maternal diabetes mellitus, toxoplasmosis, amino acid abnormalities, endocrine dysgenesis, and intrauterine rubella. Semilobar holoprosencephaly is associated with normal formation of the dura and interhemispheric fissure. However, this condition is associated with partially separated thalami, a rudimentary third ventricle, and sometimes presence of the splenium of the corpus callosum (Fig. 30). With lobar and semilobar holoprosencephaly, there is partial separation of the cerebral hemispheres, but the frontal horns are always fused, and the sagittal falx cerebri is only partially developed.

The disorders of sulcation and migration include lissencephaly, polymicrogyria, schizencephaly, and heterotopias (Table 11) (120). During the third and sixth months of human fetal development, the neuroblasts formed in the subependymal germinal matrix migrate through the periventricular tissue to the forming cerebral cortex. At the same time as this radial migration, a second tangential migration occurs through the cortex. If there is disturbance in the neuronal migration, the cortical mantle develops abnormally. If it becomes too thick, then lissencephaly, pachygyria, or macrogyria may result, with a moderate reduction in the number of sulci of the cerebrum, sometimes with enlargement of the brain substance and gyri (121–123). If the cortical mantle becomes too flat, then polymicrogyria results, with numerous small convolutions (96). When the cortical mantle is too folded, heterotopias result (120).

Lissencephaly (agyria and pachygyria), or "smooth brain," is a rare malformation consisting of failure of development of the cerebral sulci and gyri, with increased depth of the gray matter underlying the smooth part of the brain (Fig. 31) (121–124). The subarachnoid space is

TABLE 10 ■ Disorders of Diverticulation

Malformation	Ultrasound findings
Septo-optic dysplasia	Agenesis of septum pellucidum
	Dilation of lateral ventricles with flattened roofs
	Hypoplastic optic chiasm, nerves, and infundibulum
	Dilation of chiasmatic and suprasellar cisterns
	Expansion of optic recess of third ventricles
Holoprosencephaly:	
Alobar	No division of the cerebral hemispheres
	Large, horseshoe-shaped single ventricular cavity
	Thin, anteriorly placed cerebrum
	Fused thalami
Semilobar	Normal formation of dural, interhemispheric fissure and falx
	Partially separated thalami
	Rudimentary third ventricle
	Splenium of corpus callosum may be present
Lobar	Hypoplastic frontal horns of lateral ventricles
	Interhemispheric fissure missing rostrally
	Fusion of frontal lobes
	Body and splenium of corpus callosum present
	Hypoplastic anterior aspect of falx
Aventricular cerebrum	Ventricles not seen

widened, and in severe cases, the only visible indentations externally over the brain are the sylvian fissures, which have shorter and more oblique courses, with the groove appearing wide and linear rather than the usual T- or Y-shaped configuration of the fissure. There is also a lack of opercularization of the insula, with the ascent of the middle cerebral artery assuming a straight line, resulting in lack of visualization of the pulsations of the middle cerebral arteries in the sylvian grooves. The ventricles are mildly to moderately dilated. Normal interdigitation of gray and white matter is not seen, and there is a relative increase in echogenicity in the periventricular region.

Heterotopia, or heterotopic gray matter, is a developmental brain anomaly resulting from migratory arrest of primitive neuroblasts in the developing fetal

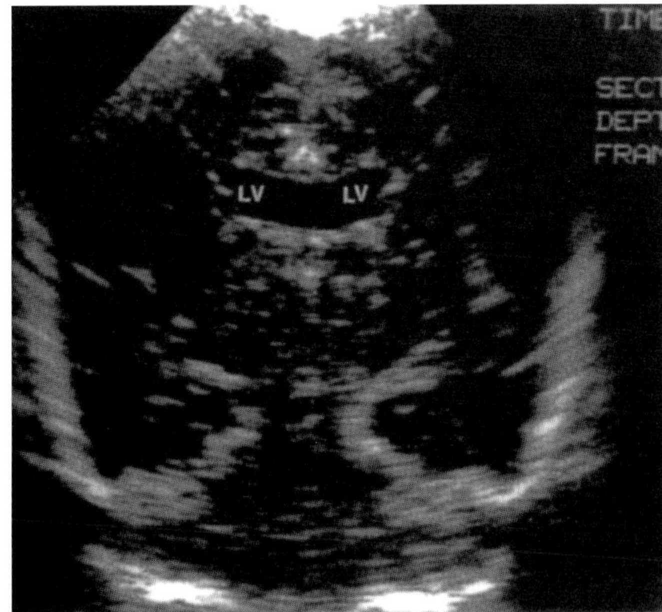

FIGURE 28 ■ Septo-optic dysplasia. Coronal scan of neonatal brain showing flat roofs of moderately dilated lateral ventricles (LV) and absence of the septum pellucidum.

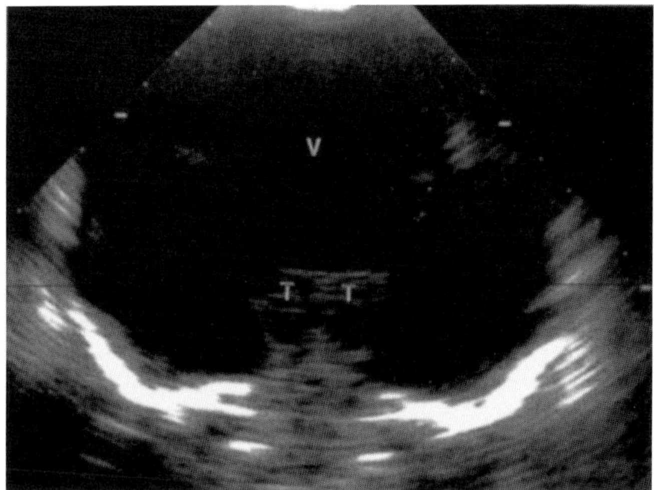

FIGURE 29 ■ Alobar holoprosencephaly. Coronal sonogram of an infant with midline facial deformities showing fusion of the thalami (T) and lateral ventricles with a single horseshoe-shaped ventricle (V). The cerebral hemispheres are markedly compressed and barely visible.

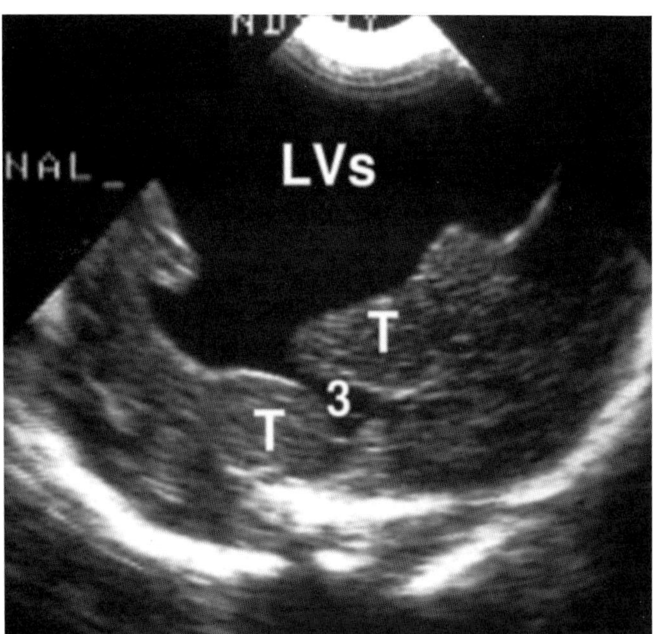

FIGURE 30 ■ Semilobar holoprosencephaly. The thalami (T) are partially separated, the third ventricle (3) is rudimentary, and the lateral ventricles (LVs) are dilated and fused. This condition is associated with normal formation of the dura and interhemispheric fissure (especially posteriorly). The splenium of the corpus callosum may also be present in this condition.

cerebrum (120). They are subependymal in location and involve the frontal horns, bodies, and occipital horns more commonly than the temporal horns (Fig. 32). Other congenital malformations may be associated. Heterotopic brain tissue protrudes into the ventricular cavity and has the same echogenicity as normal gray matter.

Schizencephaly is another rare congenital malformation of the brain, in which there are clefts in the brain that are usually bilateral and nearly symmetric (125). The clefts, which are lined by cortical gray matter, extend from the ventricle to the brain surface, often lying along an axis of normal future fissure development, particularly the sylvian fissure (Fig. 33). The lips of the cleft may be opposed ("closed lip") or gaping ("open lip"). There may be associated ventricular dilation, heterotopias, and polymicrogyria. The malformation may be related to a vascular abnormality (126).

The disorders of size include microcephaly and macrocephaly, the latter of which can be familial or associated with neurofibromatosis (126). Various forms of hydrocephalus may be the underlying cause of macrocephaly.

The congenital anomalies of the brain due to destructive lesions include hydranencephaly, porencephaly, hypoxia, toxicosis, and inflammatory disease such as rubella, cytomegalic inclusion disease, toxoplasmosis, and herpes simplex virus (Table 12) (113).

TABLE 11 ■ Disorders of Sulcation and Migration

Malformation	Causes	Ultrasound findings
Lissencephaly ("smooth" brain, agyria, pachygyria)	Failure of development of sulci and gyri	Increased depth of gray matter
		Widened subarachnoid space
		Minimal or no visible indentations except sylvian fissure
		Sylvian fissures shorter and more oblique
		Lack of opercularization of insula
		Lack of ascent of MCA
		Absent pulsation of MCA in sylvian groove
		Mild-to-moderate ventricular dilation
		Increased periventricular echogenicity
		No normal gray–white interdigitation
Polymicrogyria	–	Flat cortical mantle
		Numerous small convolutions
Schizencephaly	May be related to failure of formation of germinal matrix or failure of migration of primitive neuroblasts	Clefts in brain, often bilateral
		Clefts lined by gray matter
		Often along axis of normal fissure development
		May be associated with ventricular dilation, heterotopia, polymicrogyria
Heterotopic gray matter	Migratory arrest of primitive neuroblasts	Cortical mantle top folded
		Subependymal, protrudes into lateral ventricle
		Frontal horns and bodies affected more than temporal horns
		Isoechoic with gray matter

Abbreviation: MCA, middle cerebral artery.

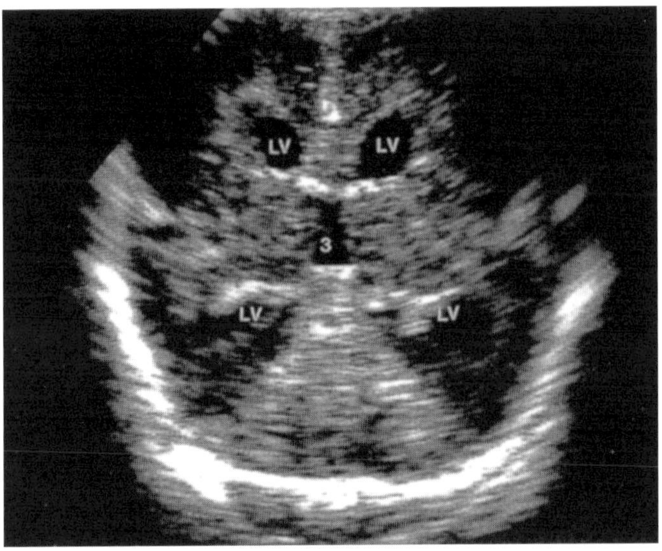

(A)

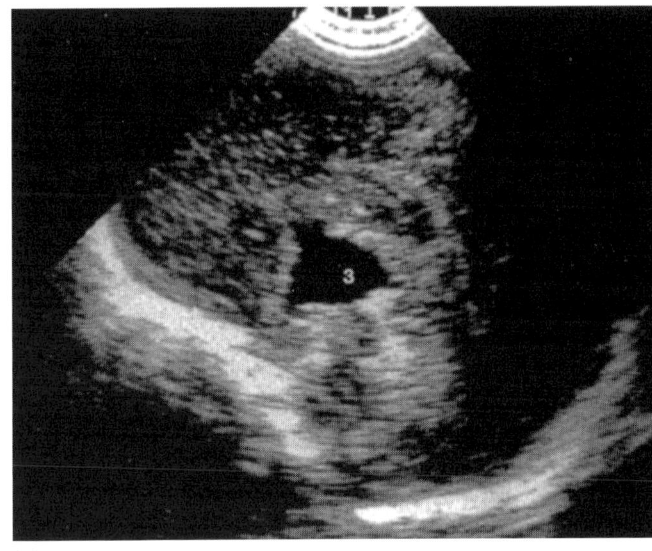

(B)

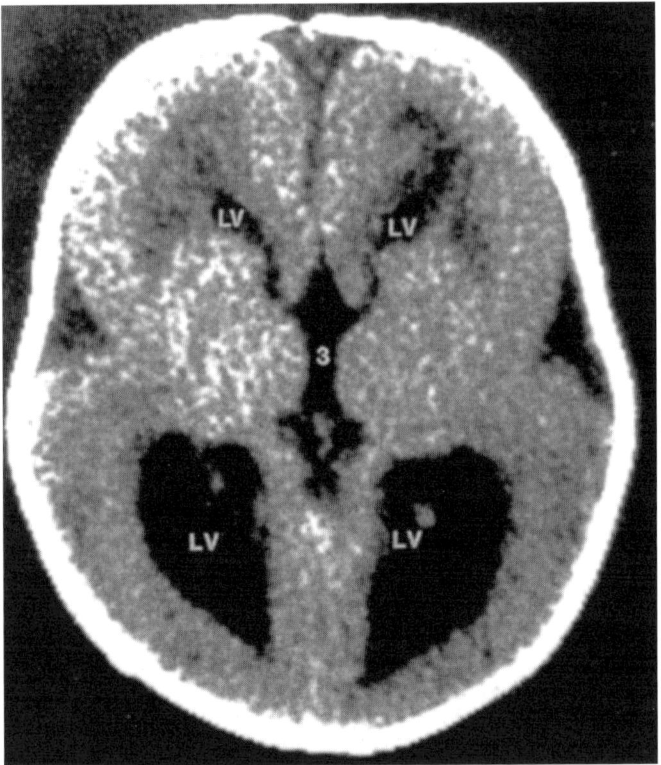

(C)

FIGURE 31 A–C ■ Lissencephaly. Four-month-old infant with markedly retarded development. Note the absence of convolutional markings and moderate dilation of the lateral and the third ventricles. The normal interdigitation of gray and white matter is also absent. (**A**) Coronal view. (**B**) Sagittal view. (**C**) CT scan. LV, lateral ventricle; 3, third ventricle.

Hydranencephaly is a congenital disorder in which the cerebral hemispheres are replaced by thin sacs of CSF (127,128). The cranial vault, meninges, and falx are intact. It is thought to be due to cerebral infarction resulting from in utero occlusion of the carotid arteries. Suggested etiologies include ionizing radiation, trauma, and infectious causes including toxoplasmosis and herpes virus.

Porencephaly is an area of cavitation within the cerebral hemisphere due to a hypoxic–ischemic insult, periventricular hemorrhage, infection, trauma, or surgery, resulting in injury to and encystment of necrotic brain tissue (55,129–131). These cysts, which may be multiple, are not lined by ependyma, even though they may communicate with the ventricular system. At times, septation within the ventricles resulting from previous ventriculitis leads to compartmentalization of the ventricles due to bands and adhesions that create isolated areas of hydrocephalus.

The disorders of histogenesis include tuberous sclerosis, neurofibromatosis, Sturge–Weber syndrome (encephalotrigeminal angiomatosis), neoplasia, and vascular lesions (Table 3) (132–140).

The phakomatoses are neuroectodermal dysplasias in which there is a tendency to develop tumors in the skin, viscera, and central nervous system. Tuberous sclerosis is a hereditary disorder characterized by epilepsy,

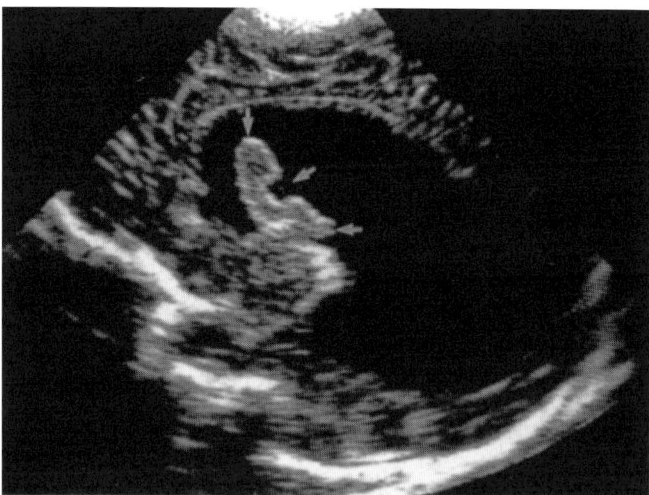

FIGURE 32 ■ Heterotopic brain tissue. Unusually shaped isoechoic area of brain tissue (*arrows*) arising from the subependymal region of the dilated lateral ventricle in this infant with Arnold–Chiari malformation type II.

mental retardation, and adenoma sebaceum. Although it is inherited as an autosomal-dominant trait, about 70% of cases are apparently due to spontaneous mutation (132,133). There is abnormal proliferation of cells (usually astrocytes) within the brain. Hamartomatous foci are primarily seen in the cerebrum, but the cerebellum, medulla, and spinal cord may also be affected. The nodules are mainly located in the subependyma in the floor of the lateral ventricle and, in fact, may occlude the interconnecting foramina and cause hydrocephalus. They may also be found in the brain parenchyma in cortical and subcortical locations. These nodules are frequently calcified and most often benign, but low-grade astrocytomas have also been seen.

Neurofibromatosis type I (von Recklinghausen disease) is a hereditary hamartomatous disorder that involves the neuroectoderm, mesoderm, and endoderm. It is probably of neural crest origin and has the potential to appear in any organ system of the body (130,131). Neurofibromatosis type I occurs in a hereditary form transmitted by autosomal dominance in half of cases and sporadically in the other half. It appears to be transmitted on the long arm of chromosome 17. Complications of this condition include neurofibromas; cutaneous pigmentary changes (many café-au-lait spots); skeletal abnormalities (bone dysplasias and pseudoarthrosis of a long bone); a predilection for certain tumors, particularly within the central nervous system (optic pathway gliomas and cerebellar, brain stem, and cerebral astrocytomas); and vascular and endocrine abnormalities. With the exception of macrocranium, however, the intracranial complications are not generally seen until long after the anterior fontanelle closes and therefore cannot be diagnosed with ultrasonography. Associated optic nerve gliomas can be identified with orbital ultrasound, but intracranial extension cannot be shown.

Intracranial tumors are uncommon in children younger than two years of age, with 35% seen during the

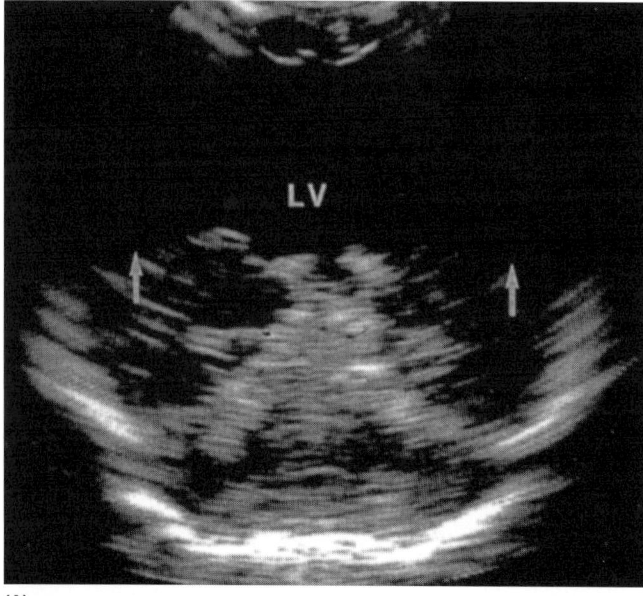

(A)

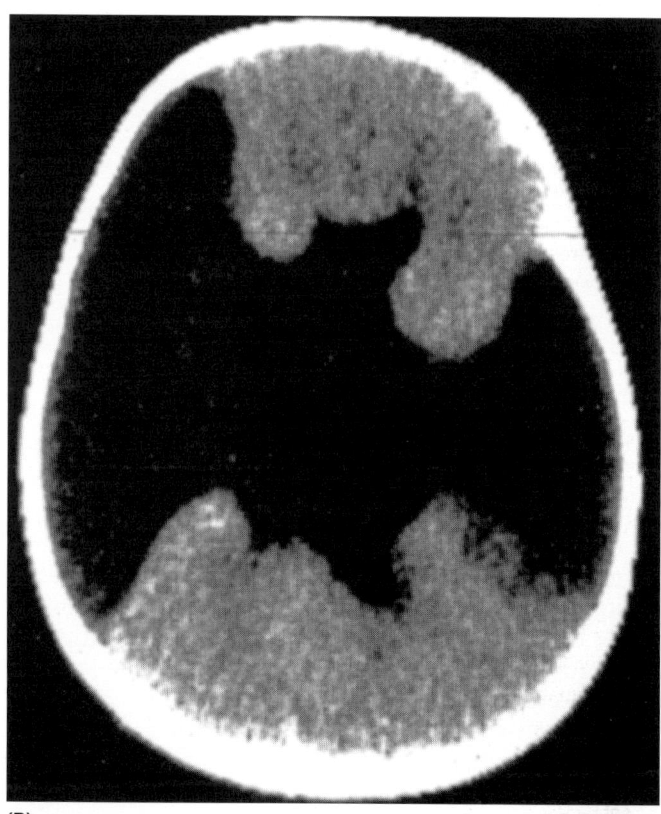

(B)

FIGURE 33 A AND B ■ Schizencephaly. (**A**) Large fluid-filled clefts (*arrows*) in the region of the sylvian fissures communicate with the massively dilated, fused lateral ventricles (LV) on this coronal sonogram. (**B**) Correlative CT scan.

TABLE 12 ■ Destructive Lesions

Abnormality	Causes	Ultrasound findings
Hydranencephaly	Cerebral infarction secondary to in utero occlusion of carotid arteries	Cerebral hemispheres replaced by thin sacs of cerebrospinal fluid
		Cranial vault, meninges, and falx are intact
Porencephaly	Hypoxic–ischemic insult	Encystment of necrotic brain tissue
	Periventricular hemorrhage	
	Infection	Cysts may communicate with ventricle
		No ependymal lining
Hypoxia		See Table 2
Toxicosis		
Inflammatory diseases	Rubella	See Table 16
	Cytomegalovirus	
	Toxoplasmosis	
	Herpes simplex virus	

first year of life and only 2% in the neonatal period (Table 13) (137–148). Supratentorial tumors are more common in younger infants than infratentorial neoplasms, unlike the distribution observed in older children. The neurologic criteria that can be used in young infants are limited, and therefore the signs of a brain tumor may not be easy to detect unless there is obvious macrocranium, tumor erosion through the calvarium, or clinical evidence of increased intracranial pressure. The origin of brain tumor in the neonate is neuroectodermal, and teratoma is the most frequent type (50%) in younger infants, followed by glioma, astrocytoma, lipoma of the corpus callosum, primitive neuroectodermal tumor, choroid plexus papilloma, ependymoma, and ganglioglioma.

TABLE 13 ■ Intracranial Neoplasms

Infratentorial

- Brain stem glioma
- Cerebellar astrocytoma
- PNET
- Ependymoma
- Choroid plexus tumors
- Metastatic disease

Supratentorial

- Optic pathway glioma
- Hypothalamic glioma
- Craniopharyngioma
- Germinoma
- Adenoma
- Teratoma
- Epidermoid
- Hamartoma
- Histiocytoma
- Metastasis

Abbreviation: PNET, primitive neuroectodermal tumor.

No specific ultrasonographic findings can allow for differentiation of the various cell types, but the size and location of the masses can give clues that can limit the differential diagnosis. Intracranial teratomas are notoriously large echogenic lesions containing cystic spaces and superimposed bright echogenic areas with acoustic shadowing due to calcifications (137,138). These uniformly fatal tumors are primarily located in the pineal region, followed by the suprasellar and posterior fossae. They may be so extensive that they obstruct or erode into the ventricular system or through the cranial vault. Lesions in the brain stem are more likely to be due to gliomas and are generally hyperechoic compared with the cerebral hemispheres, as are most brain tumors (Fig. 34) (149–151). Therefore, it may be difficult to recognize a tumor on ultrasound in the normally hyperechoic cerebellum. Regardless of the type of tumor, in the setting of fetal brain neoplasm, sonography can be valuable in identifying the presence of hydrocephalus, since it can be a decisive factor in the choice of treatment and time of delivery (152).

Intracranial arachnoid cysts account for 1% of space-occupying lesions in children (145,153) and are the most common congenital cystic abnormality of the brain. They are fluid-filled cavities caused by abnormal leptomeningeal formation with splitting of the arachnoid (primary arachnoid cyst) or by entrapment of CSF by arachnoid adhesions (secondary arachnoid cyst; Fig. 35). They may also result from infection and trauma. These cysts lie between two membranes contiguous at the cyst margin with normal arachnoid matter, and they may or may not communicate with the subarachnoid space. They may be supratentorial or infratentorial. They are most often located in the sylvian fissure or temporal region. Less frequently, they are found in the suprasellar region, posterior

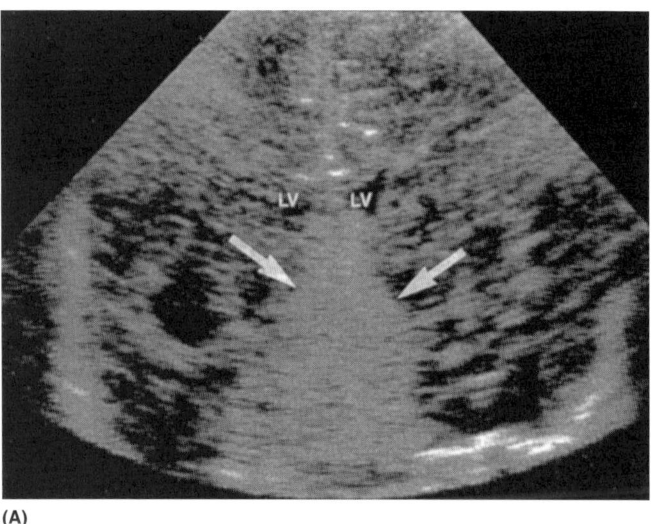

(A)

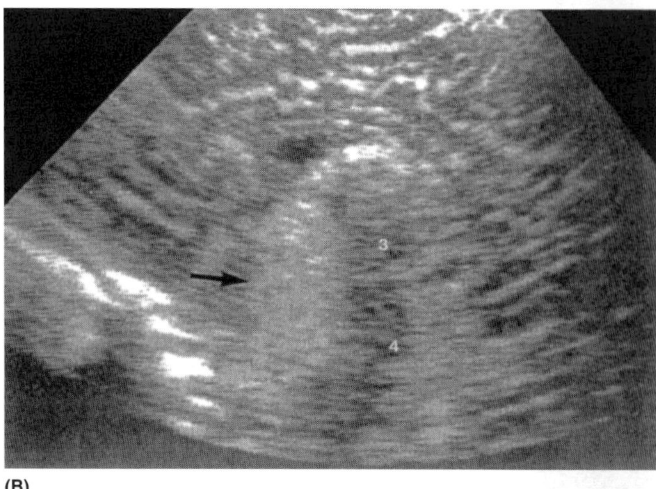

(B)

FIGURE 34 A AND B ■ Brain stem glioma. (**A**) Coronal section of the brain in a 4-month-old boy with diencephalic syndrome. A brightly echogenic mass is seen in the region of the brain stem (*arrows*). The lateral ventricles are of normal size. (**B**) A midline sagittal section in the same patient shows the echogenic mass (*arrow*) arising from the brain stem with posterior displacement of the third and fourth ventricles. LV, lateral ventricle; 4, fourth ventricle; 3, third ventricle.

fossa, and collicular (quadrigeminal) region (Fig. 36). They are most often recognized because of a mass effect and resultant hydrocephalus.

VASCULAR ABNORMALITIES

With the advent of duplex and color Doppler ultrasound (154–162), the demonstration of arteriovenous malformations of the brain has been remarkably simplified. The large, more centrally located malformations, such as vein of Galen aneurysms, are easily differentiated from other cystic-appearing lesions. The former appear as an anechoic cystic mass separate from and posterior to the third ventricle, generally with a tubular structure that fans out to the torcular Herophili (Fig. 37) (Table 14). The feeding arteries and draining veins, as well as associated ventricular dilation, can be seen on duplex and color Doppler ultrasound. Brain atrophy may be apparent, with calcifications in the brain parenchyma as a result of shunting of

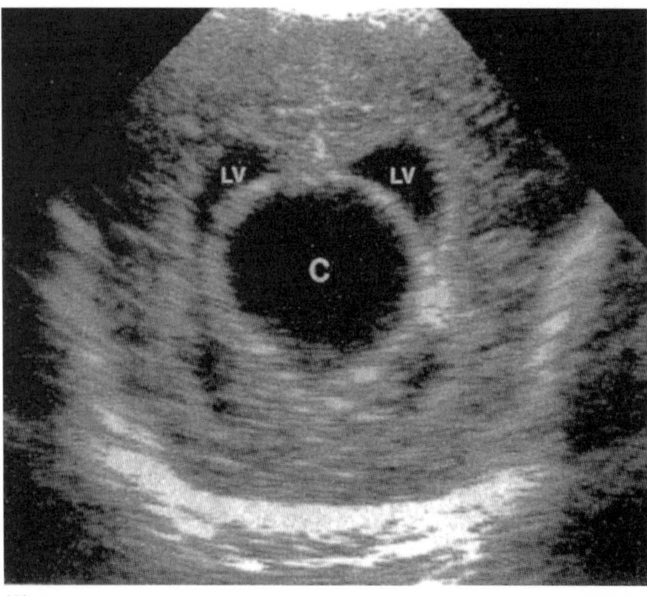

(A)

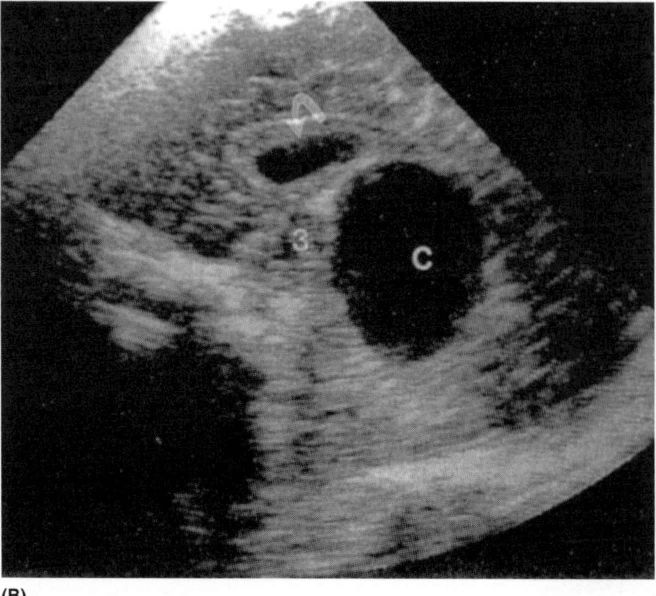

(B)

FIGURE 35 A AND B ■ Arachnoid cyst. (**A**) A large midline cyst obstructs the lateral ventricles on this coronal scan in an infant with an enlarged head circumference. (**B**) Sagittal section demonstrates that the cyst is located posterior to the third ventricle. The curved arrow shows the cavum septum pellucidum. LV, lateral ventricle; C, cyst; 3, third ventricle.

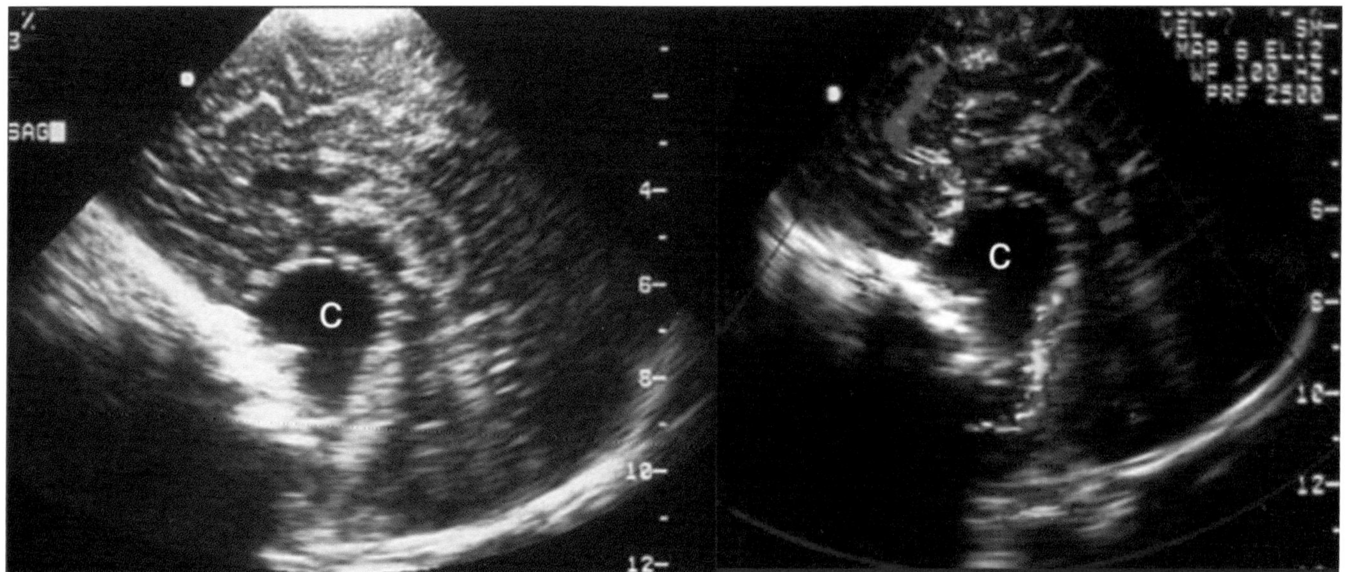

FIGURE 36 ■ Arachnoid cyst. Sagittal scan shows a cystic mass (C) in the suprasellar recess. Doppler flow shows no vascularity, excluding other diagnoses such as a vein of Galen aneurysm.

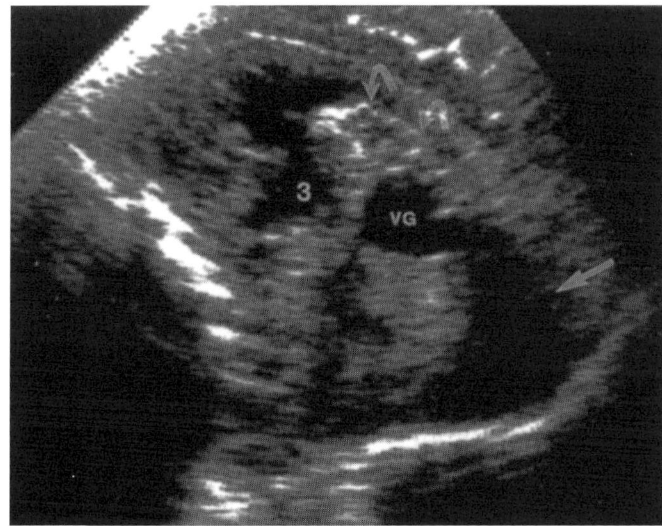

(A)

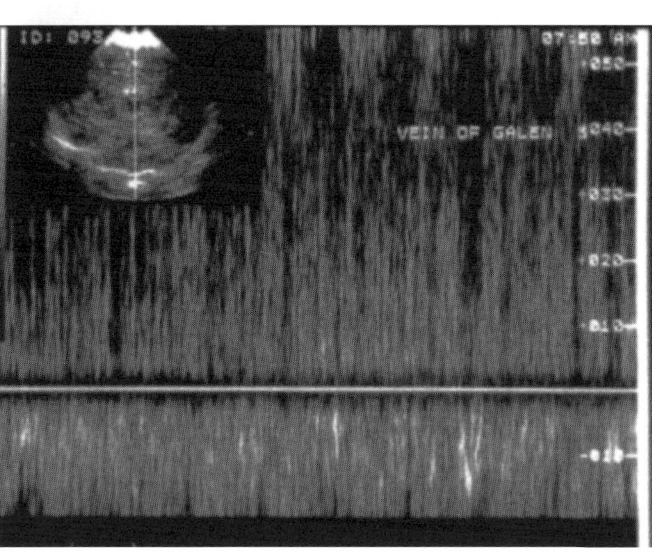

(C)

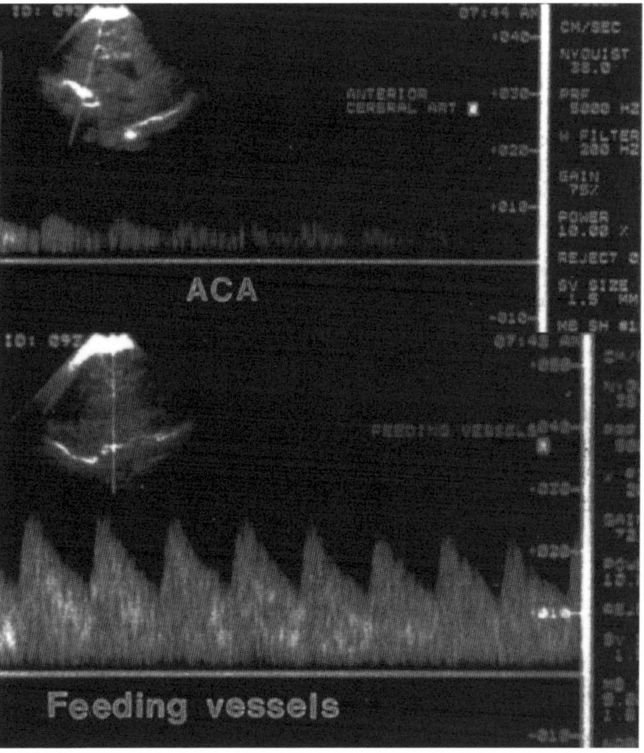

(B)

FIGURE 37 A–C ■ Vein of Galen aneurysm in a newborn with seizures and an intracranial bruit. (**A**) Midsagittal section of brain demonstrating cystic area (VG) posterior to third ventricle that fanned out to the enlarged torcular Herophili (*straight arrow*). Curved arrows indicate echogenic feeding arteries, which were vigorously pulsating during real-time scanning. (**B**) Sagittal scans show normal arterial flow in the anterior cerebral artery on the left and tremendously high systolic peaks and diastolic valleys in the region of the feeding arteries. (**C**) Coronal image demonstrating loud, turbulent flow in the aneurysm. 3, third ventricle; ACA, anterior cerebral artery. *Source*: From Ref. 9.

TABLE 14 ■ Vein of Galen Malformation: Ultrasound Findings

- Anechoic, cystic mass posterior to the third ventricle fans out to torcular Herophili
- Feeding arteries and draining veins may be seen with duplex or color Doppler
- Ventricular dilation
- Brain atrophy with calcifications

blood from the cerebral cortex ("vascular steal") during fetal life. The smaller, more peripheral vascular lesions may be difficult to identify, even with Doppler. Arteriovenous malformations may be recognized clinically because of seizures, congestive heart failure, cardiomegaly, intracranial bruit, or signs of hydrocephalus. They may be difficult to identify, however, if overlying ICH obscures the underlying congenital anomaly.

Duplex and color Doppler techniques can be used to evaluate cerebral blood flow and velocity, using either transfontanellar or transcranial approach (163–172). Color-flow mapping allows for more rapid and precise identification of the vessels requiring more quantitative duplex insonation (173,174).

Studies of healthy term infants show that all the intracranial arterial signals are diphasic, with forward flow continuing during diastole (154). The velocities increase with gestational age because the intracranial arteries serve a low-resistance vascular bed in the brain of the full-term infant (163,164). Because there is no laminar plug flow in the small arteries of the infant brain, the spectral pattern is that of turbulence and spectral broadening, creating a Doppler tracing with the sonic window completely filled in. In gestationally mature infants, antegrade flow is seen during both systole and diastole. Forward flow, however, may be absent during diastole in infants younger than 30 weeks' gestation.

Using conventional duplex Doppler, the flow velocities are highest in the basilar artery, internal carotid arteries, and anterior cerebral arteries (163–165). The resistive index (RI) of the intracranial vessels (peak systolic velocity minus end diastolic velocity divided by the peak systolic velocity) decreases with increasing gestational age, as the cerebrovascular resistance decreases. The average RI in a full-term infant is 75 ± 10 SD (163). The RI may be elevated due to intracranial or extracranial abnormalities that influence cerebral blood flow. When the intracerebral resistance is elevated due to intracranial processes such as ICH, hydrocephalus, brain edema due to hypoxic–ischemic disease or cerebritis, increased extra-axial fluid collections, and PVL, the RI is accordingly affected (163,166–168).

With the presence of a hypoxic–ischemic episode, loss of vascular autoregulation as the result of asphyxia leads to an increase in diastolic flow and a low RI. A low RI (less than 60) without corresponding gray-scale abnormalities can be used to predict a significant hypoxic–ischemic injury (175). RIs will increase with a loss of forward diastolic flow as cerebral edema increase. Premature infants with GMHs have been found to have a greater mean velocity and lower RIs in the lenticulostriate vessels. Thus, transcranial Doppler may be useful in predicting which neonates are at risk for IVH and periventricular leukomalacia (175).

Transcranial Doppler may also be useful in the assessment of hydrocephalus. Ventriculomegaly in association with increased intracranial pressure causes a decrease in diastolic flow and an increase in RI. It is imperative that a baseline exam be performed so that serial measurements can be compared to the initial study. A shunt may be indicated in an infant with increasing RI and ventriculomegaly in the appropriate clinical setting (176).

Extracranial processes may cause decreased cerebral perfusion and thus elevate the RI, such as in the presence of cardiac failure, hypotension, and patent ductus arteriosus (169–172).

Color Doppler Ultrasound of Extra-Axial Fluid Collections

Prominence of the extra-axial spaces is common in infancy and is thought to be the result of immature arachnoid villi and impaired CSF resorption (177). Affected infants usually present with macrocrania or rapid head growth. Extra-axial fluid collections can also be assessed by color Doppler ultrasound. Although it has generally been accepted that the presence of extra-axial veins traversing the collections usually indicates that they are subarachnoid in position, this is not necessarily the case. It has been reported that subdural veins may also traverse a subdural collection. This is important to be aware of when evaluating infants with external hydrocephalus in which prominent extra-axial subarachnoid spaces are encountered. In this condition, known as benign hydrocephalus of infancy, the extra-axial subarachnoid collections may put tension on subdural veins, resulting in a subdural hematoma (178). Clues that a subdural is present are the relative decrease in number of traversing veins, compression of these veins beneath a dural membrane, and complex appearing extra-axial fluid (178).

Duplex and color Doppler ultrasound are particularly useful in the evaluation of the brains of infants requiring treatment with ECMO. In this technique, cannulas are placed into the right common carotid artery and jugular vein, allowing for shunting of deoxygenated blood from the right atrium to an external membrane for oxygenation, then returning to the aorta through the carotid artery (173,174,179–185). As a result of ligating the carotid artery (179–185), the right cerebral hemisphere is perfused using collateral flow from the basilar artery and contralateral common carotid artery through the circle of Willis. However, patients may demonstrate right-sided brain abnormalities after receiving ECMO. These include neuromotor abnormalities, abnormal electroencephalography (EEG) findings, infarction, and brain atrophy (186) as well as large parenchymal hemorrhages, cerebellar hemorrhage, and diffuse cerebral edema (182). Color Doppler plays an important role in these patients by providing a noninvasive means of evaluating the presence and direction of collateral pathways and the presence of flow within the cerebral hemispheres (185). Doppler may play a role in evaluating neonates exposed to cocaine in utero. These infants may demonstrate increased flow velocities in the anterior cerebral artery related to vasospasm, without corresponding real-time abnormalities (171,187).

Duplex Doppler may also play a role in the diagnosis of brain death by demonstrating absence of flow or reduction of flow velocities and retrograde flow during early diastole when the larger intracerebral vessels are interrogated (188–192). Reversed diastolic flow alone is not conclusive evidence of brain death, as evidenced by two patients who recovered despite diastolic reversal. One patient was a one-month-old boy with status epilepticus and increased intracranial pressure, whose diastolic reversal disappeared after medical therapy. The other was a six-month-old girl with a choroid plexus papilloma, who had reversal of diastolic flow during an abrupt clinical deterioration; her diastolic reversal cleared after emergent surgical removal of the tumor. Completely absent blood flow intracranially is an indicator of brain death. However, brain death may be present despite intracranial blood flow (193). Clinical evaluation is essential in such patients (192).

INTRACRANIAL INFECTION

High-resolution real-time ultrasonography of the brain is highly valuable in the evaluation of intracranial infections in infants (Table 15). Neonatal and infantile meningitis is a serious illness often associated with permanent neurologic damage despite early antibiotic therapy. About 25% of newborns with bacterial sepsis develop meningoencephalitis (194). In the neonate, group B streptococcus and *Escherichia coli* are the most common causative organisms. After the neonatal period, *Haemophilus influenzae, Streptococcus pneumoniae, and Neisseria meningitides* are the more common causes of bacterial meningitis. The organisms enter the central nervous system through the choroid plexus of the lateral ventricles, and thus ventriculitis is a common complication. Perinatal intracranial infections may also be secondary to viral or protozoan agents. These infections may be acquired in utero, during birth, or in the first few weeks of life. The most common viral and protozoan organisms to infect the neonate are cytomegalovirus (CMV), *Toxoplasma gondii*, rubella, and herpes simplex virus type 2 (194). In utero, infection by one of these organisms can cause teratogenic (developmental) effects on the central nervous system as well as destructive lesions (Table 16).

The ultrasonographic features of perinatal meningitis are not specific for a particular infecting organism. The spectrum of ultrasound findings is related to the inflammation, edema, and vasculitis common to all cerebral infections. Abnormalities that can be detected with ultrasonography include echogenic sulci, extra-axial fluid collections, hydrocephalus, ventriculitis, abnormal parenchymal echogenicity, abscess, encephalomalacia, and calcifications (194–197).

In meningitis, there is an increase in echogenicity of the cortical sulci and widening of the sulcal echoes.

TABLE 15 ■ Complicated Bacterial Intracranial Infection: Spectrum of Ultrasound Findings

Infection	Common causes	Ultrasound findings
Meningitis	Neonatal	Normal cranial sonogram
	Escherichia coli	Echogenic sulci
	Group B streptococcus	Extra-axial fluid collections
	Infant	Focal or diffuse increased parenchymal echogenicity
	Haemophilus influenzae	Hydrocephalus
	Streptococcus pneumoniae	
	Neisseria meningitides	
Ventriculitis	(Same organisms as above)	Ventricles initially may be slit-like
		Dilated ventricles
		Thickened, irregular, hyperechoic ependyma
		Irregular, hyperechoic choroid plexus
		Intraventricular septations
Cerebritis	(Same organisms as above)	Abnormal parenchymal echogenicity
		May be focal, diffuse, or patchy
		Increased gyral echogenicity
		Decreased vascular pulsations
Abscess	*Proteus mirabilis*	Well-circumscribed lesion
	Citrobacter diversus	Hypoechoic center, fluid–debris level
		Thick, echogenic wall
		May compress ventricle or cause midline shift

TABLE 16 ■ Congenital Infections

Pathogen	Ultrasound findings
Cytomegalovirus	Gyral abnormalities: agyria, poly-microgyria, focal microgyria
	Calcification (usually periventricular)
	Hypoplastic cerebellum
Toxoplasmosis	Calcification (periventricular and cortical)
	Microcephaly
	Hydrocephalus
	Atrophy
	Porencephaly
Herpes simplex virus	Diffuse cerebral edema
	Diffuse cerebral atrophy
	Multicystic encephalomalacia
	Punctate or gyriform calcification
	Cerebellar involvement
Rubella	Areas of ischemic necrosis
	Scattered calcifications (basal ganglia, white matter, and periventricular)
	Ventriculomegaly
	Microcephaly

These two findings are attributed to the accumulation of an inflammatory exudate within the sulci and fissures. This exudate can also accumulate in the subarachnoid space and result in the development of extra-axial fluid collections. These fluid collections are usually small to moderate in size. They can be detected with ultrasonography using either a stand-off pad or a 7.5 MHz transducer with magnification. These extra-axial collections cause widening of the interhemispheric fissure and displacement of the brain away from the cranial vault such that the cortical gyri are well visualized over the convexity of the brain. Both the echogenic sulci and the extra-axial fluid collections are transient findings seen in the acute stage of illness and are not associated with significant neurologic sequelae (194–197). Subdural effusions (sterile) also occur occasionally. Subdural effusions occur in 20% to 50% of cases of infants with meningitis who are less than one year of age (198) and are thought to be the result of leakage of fluid and protein into the subdural space. These effusions are most frequently found over the frontal and parietal convexities as well as within the interhemispheric fissure. Sterile collections are commonly anechoic, whereas infected fluid may have low-level echoes (199). These low-level echoes are thought to represent increase protein content and fibrinous strands. It should be emphasized that sterile and infected subdural collections cannot be differentiated on the basis of ultrasound. Aspiration and analysis of the subdural fluid is required in such cases. Subdural empyemas are uncommonly seen and are usually associated with complicated cases of bacterial meningitis that are not responding appropriately to antibiotic treatment (Fig. 38).

Ventricular enlargement can occur early or late in the course of the illness. In the acute stage, the ventricles may be slit-like and associated with a diffuse increase in parenchymal echogenicity. This finding is thought to be secondary to diffuse brain edema and inflammation (195). The ventricular system, however, can also be mildly to moderately dilated acutely. This dilation is thought to be the result of a communicating hydrocephalus in which arachnoiditis interferes with CSF resorption (194–197). The development of ventriculitis, which occurs in 65% to 90% of neonates with bacterial meningitis, increases morbidity and mortality. The lateral and third ventricles become dilated, and the ependymal lining becomes thickened, hyperechoic, and irregular. Low-level echoes develop within the ventricular lumen secondary to inflammatory cells and debris (Fig. 39). The choroid plexus becomes irregular and hyperechoic. Intraventricular septations or bands may develop owing to glial proliferation (200,201). These septations can compartmentalize and obstruct portions of the ventricular system, resulting in an obstructive hydrocephalus. Ultrasonography has been found to be superior to CT in the detection of these intraventricular echoes and septations (202,203). An unsuspected trapped or compartmentalized ventricle can be a source of continued infection or reinfection after otherwise adequate intravenous or intraventricular antibiotic treatment.

Abnormal parenchymal echogenicity is associated with meningoencephalitis. The increase in cerebral parenchymal echogenicity may be focal or diffuse and unilateral

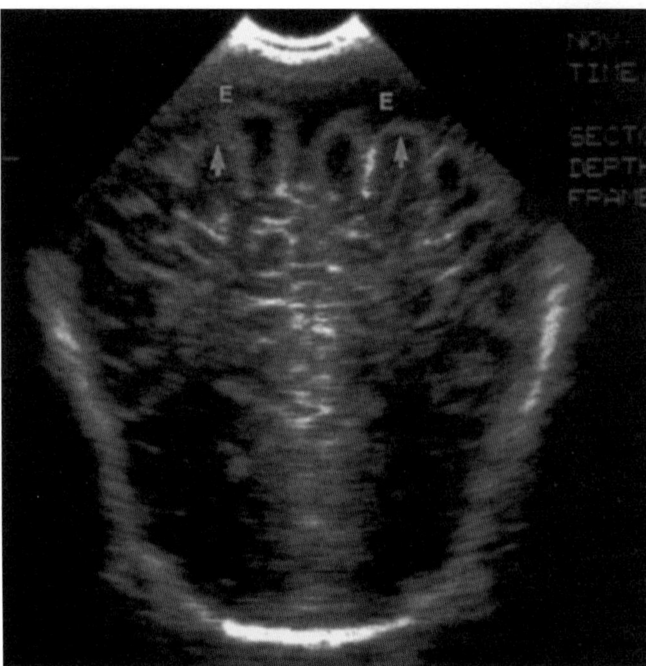

FIGURE 38 ■ *Haemophilus influenzae* empyema. Four-week-old infant with cerebrospinal fluid positive for *H. influenzae* and increased head circumference. Note the wide extra-axial fluid space and bright convolutional markings (*arrows*) consistent with empyema. E, extra-axial fluid space.

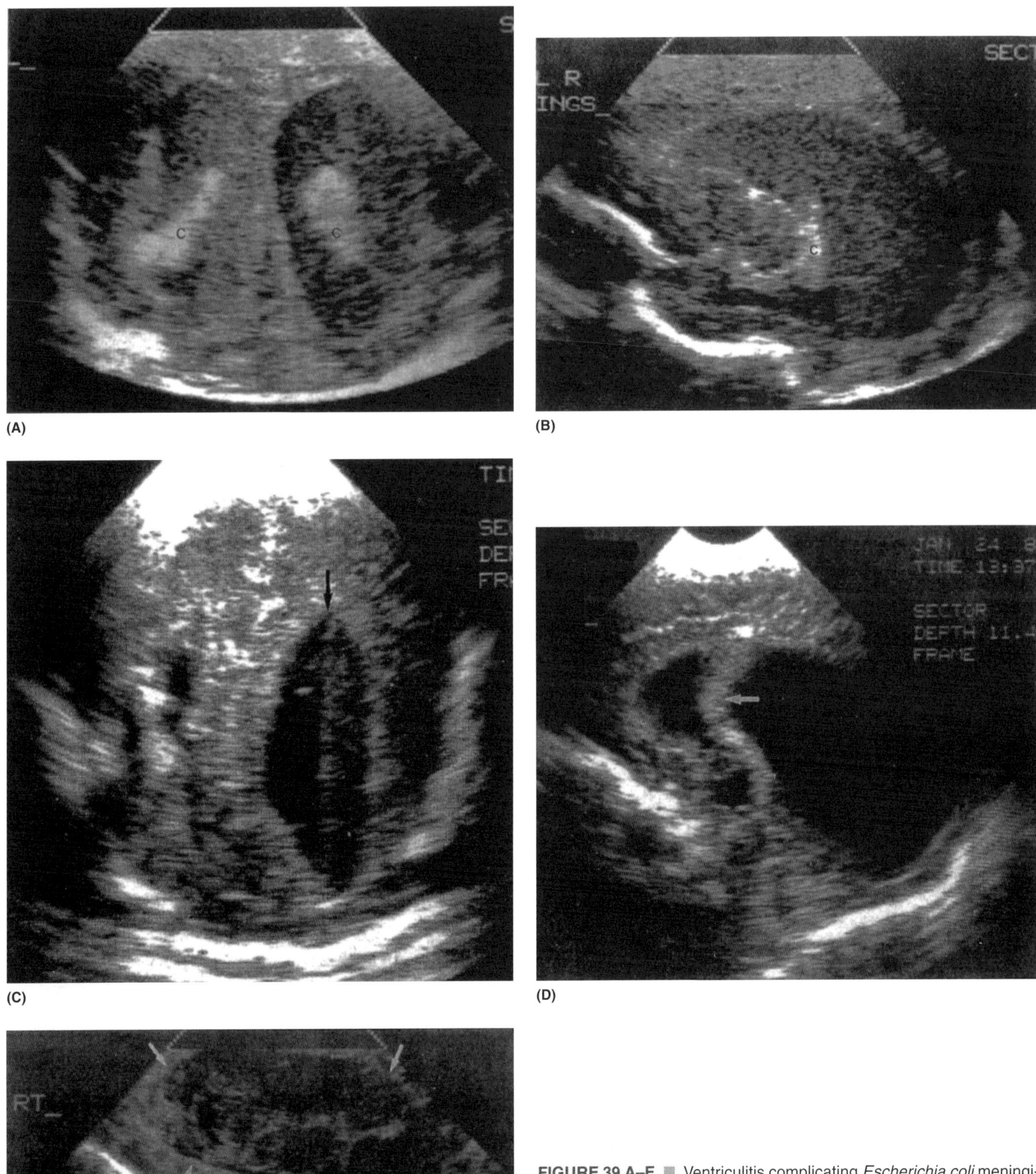

FIGURE 39 A–E ■ Ventriculitis complicating *Escherichia coli* meningitis in a one-week-old infant with spina bifida and Arnold–Chiari malformation type II. Posterior coronal (**A**) and left parasagittal (**B**) sonograms show severe ventricular dilation and moderately echogenic cerebrospinal fluid due to purulent material. (**C**) Note the fluid–debris level (*arrow*) in the left lateral ventricle with the cranial vault in the left lateral decubitus position. (**D**) Eleven days later, the left lateral ventricle is dilated, and a well-defined thick septation (*arrow*) is seen in the anterior horn. (**E**) Two-week followup in another patient with spina bifida, *E. coli* sepsis, and right ventriculoperitoneal shunt failure demonstrates coalesced dense material within the dilated ventricles. Arrows outline the massively dilated right ventricle. c, choroid plexus. *Source*: From Ref. 196.

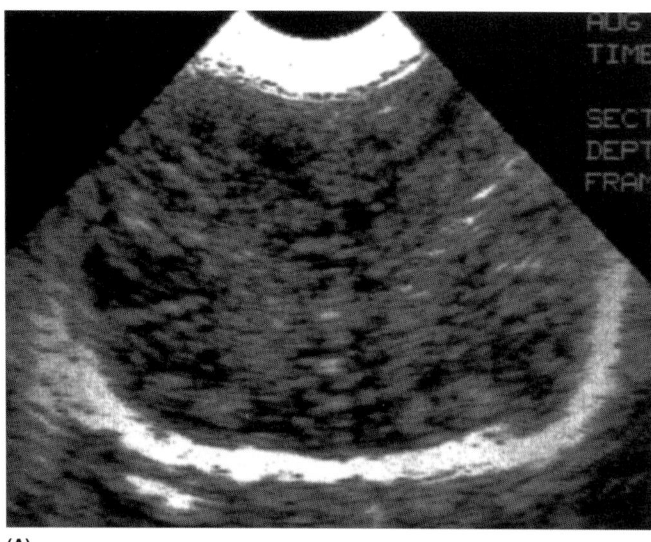

(A)

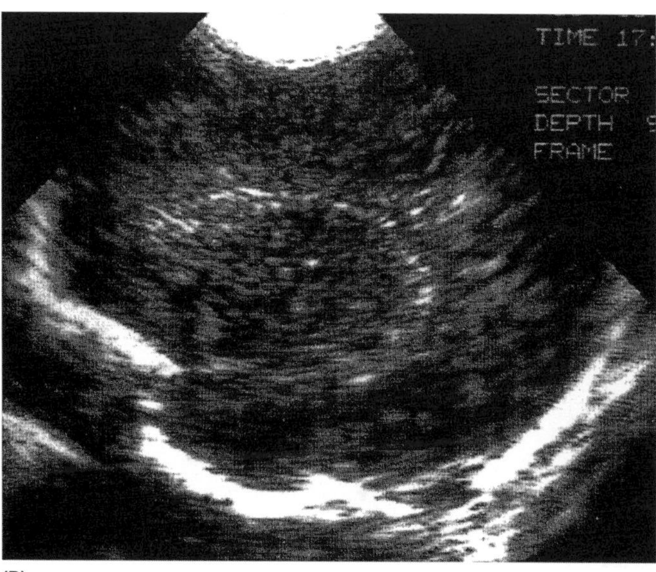

(B)

FIGURE 40 A AND B ■ *Haemophilus influenzae* meningitis with cerebritis. Seventeen-day-old girl with sepsis and *H. influenza*-positive blood and cerebrospinal fluid cultures. Coronal (**A**) and sagittal (**B**) sonograms of brain show diffuse, hazy increased echogenicity with marked compression of the ventricles and obliteration of the interhemispheric fissure and sulcal markings, consistent with brain edema. *Source*: From Ref. 196.

or bilateral (Fig. 40). Focal abnormalities are usually multiple, patchy areas of hyperechogenicity. The increase in echogenicity is thought to be secondary to edema, cerebritis, or infarction. Increased gyral echogenicity represents infarction of cortical gray matter and corresponds to gyral enhancement on CT (204).

Meningitis may lead to vasculitis and venous thrombosis, most commonly involving the cortical veins and dural sinuses (204), which in turn may result in infarction. The sonographic appearance of an intravascular thrombus is an area of increased echogenicity on gray-scale imaging and absent flow on color Doppler imaging. Venous occlusion results in infarction in 30% of patients. Doppler imaging in the region of infarction may reveal absent flow, although luxury perfusion to the infarcted area may result in increased flow in the periphery of the region.

The meninges may be thickened in cases of meningoencephalitis and such thickening can be seen sonographically. Meninges are considered to be thickened when the sonographic measurements are greater than 1.3 mm on the surface of a gyrus or 2 mm within a sulcus (205). However, the absence of meningeal thickening does not exclude meningitis. Brain edema and rapid toxic shock are thought to be responsible for visual absence of meningeal thickening. It should also be noted that clinical outcome of bacterial meningitis cannot be predicted by the absence or presence of meningeal thickening as the only sonographic abnormality (205).

Abscess formation is an uncommon complication of meningoencephalitis in healthy newborns. It usually develops in cases of virulent gram-negative infections, such as *Proteus mirabilis* or *Citrobacter diversus* (194,195). Newborns with IgA deficiency have also been reported to develop brain abscesses (206,207). Serratia marcescens may also be a cause of cerebral abscess in newborns in the neonatal intensive care unit (208). An abscess usually develops within a previously abnormal echogenic

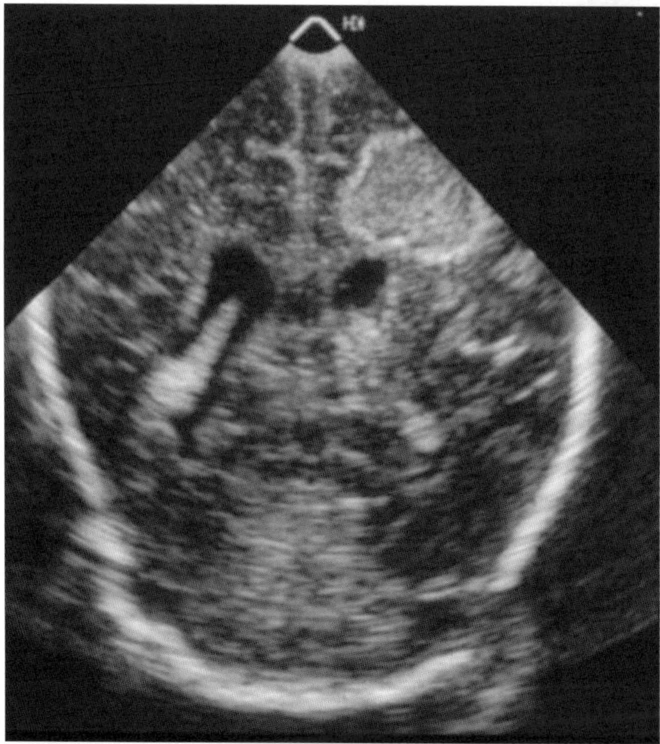

FIGURE 41 ■ Abscess complicating infection by *Serratia arborescens*. Coronal section of the brain shows a large hypoechoic collection with a hyperechoic rim within the left parietal cortex.

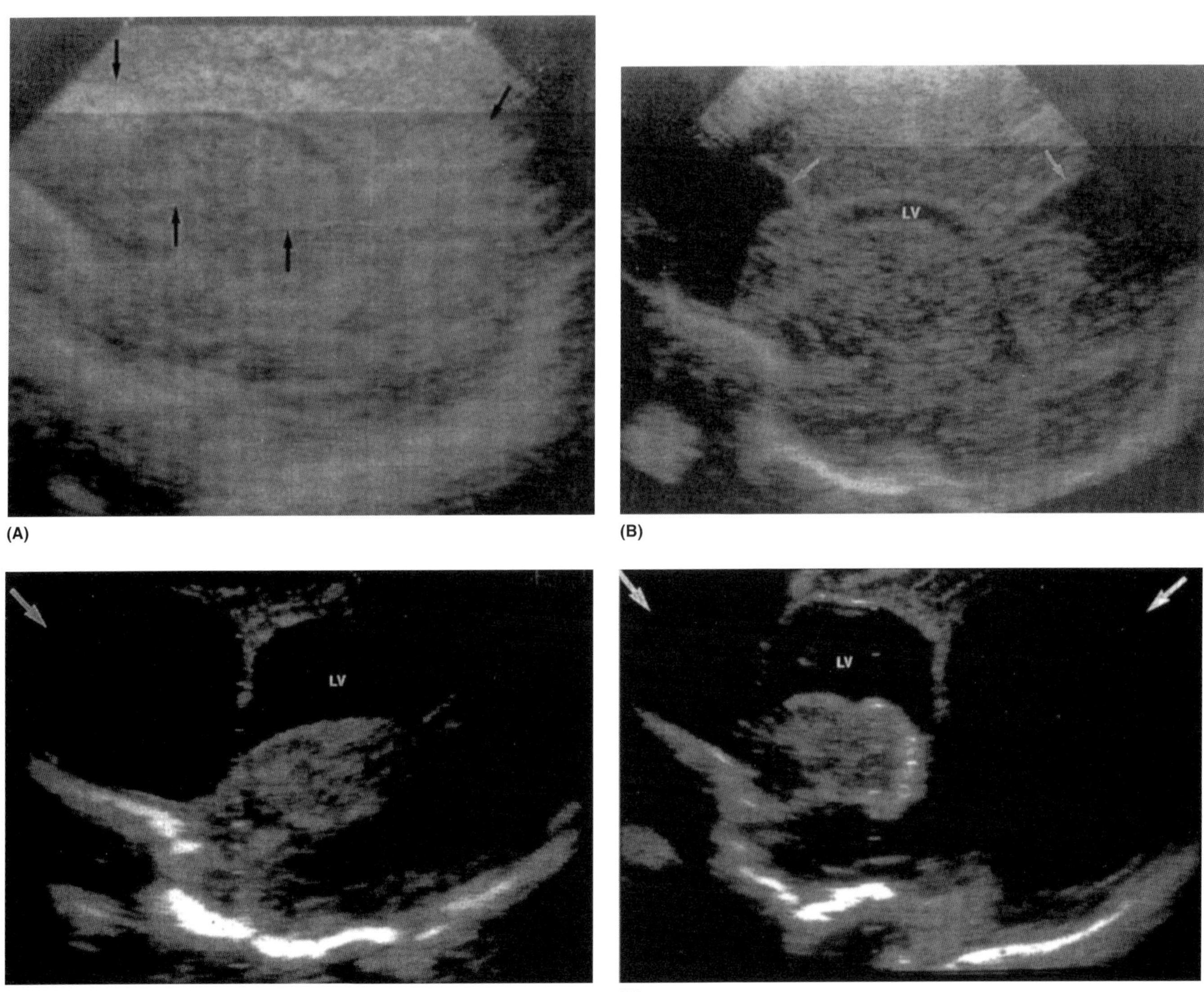

FIGURE 42 A–D ■ *Citrobacter diversus* meningitis with porencephaly. Nine-day-old full-term boy with *C. diversus* meningitis complicated by brain atrophy and encephalomalacia with porencephalic cysts. (**A**) Left parasagittal scan of the brain shows focal areas (*arrows*) of bright echogenicity in the frontal, parieto-occipital, basal ganglia, and thalamic areas with overall diffuse, hazy, increased echogenicity and diminution of the sulcal definition. (**B**) A few weeks later, focal anechoic areas replace the previously hyperechoic densities in the frontal and parieto-occipital regions. The left lateral ventricle is mildly dilated. (**C** and **D**) At 50 days of age, the anechoic areas (*arrows*) in the frontal and parieto-occipital areas have massively enlarged and are consistent with communicating porencephalic cysts. LV, lateral ventricle. *Source*: From Ref. 209.

area of parenchyma that was a focus of cerebritis or infarction (194–197). On ultrasonography, an abscess appears as a well-circumscribed lesion with a thick echogenic wall and a relatively hypoechoic center, which may contain a fluid–debris level (Fig. 41). Associated mass effect may compress the ipsilateral ventricle or displace the midline.

Multicystic encephalomalacia can be the end-stage result of meningoencephalitis. Anechoic areas of cystic degeneration develop in previously abnormal echogenic parenchyma. It is the result of vasculitis and hypoxia leading to cerebral necrosis (Fig. 42).

Dystrophic calcification (Table 17) is most common in infections from CMV, toxoplasmosis, and herpes simplex virus. The calcifications may or may not cause acoustic shadowing. A periventricular distribution of calcification is common in CMV infection and to a lesser extent in herpes simplex virus type 2 (Fig. 43). CMV may rarely cause schizencephaly as well, as seen in Figure 44 in a patient with Dandy–Walker malformation. Toxoplasmosis may cause calcified granulomas in the meninges, brain parenchyma, ependyma, and the eye. Herpes simplex virus type 2 has been reported to produce veil-like calcifications over atrophic hemispheres (194). In tuberculous meningitis, calcifications tend to develop near the basal cisterns. Calcifications in the gyri and convolutions of the cerebral cortex have been reported rarely in purulent meningitis (194).

TABLE 17 ■ Dystrophic Calcification

Cause	Most common location
Cytomegalovirus	Periventricular
Herpes simplex virus type 2	May be periventricular Veil-like calcifications over atrophic hemispheres
Toxoplasmosis	Calcified granulomas of the meninges, parenchyma, ependyma, and eye
Tuberculosis	Calcification near basal cisterns

Ultrasonography can also be used to demonstrate noncalcific inflammation and mineralization in infants with vasculitis related to congenital infection (such as CMV, rubella, or syphilis), chromosomal abnormality (trisomy 13 syndrome), idiopathic, hypoxia/ischemia, fetal alcohol and drug exposure, twin–twin transfusion, diabetic fetopathy, cardiac disease, rotavirus (210), neonatal lupus, neonatal hypoglycemia, prematurity, encephalitis, or head injury (211,212). With mineralizing vasculopathy, also known as lenticulostriate vasculopathy or hyalinization of the lenticulostriate vessels, abnormally brightly echogenic vasculature is seen in the branching vessels of the lenticulostriate arteries supplying the basal ganglia and thalami (Fig. 45). Pathologically, the walls of these vessels are thickened because of deposition of amorphous basophilic material. Because these linear densities are not calcific, CT examination does not confirm the ultrasound findings. Interestingly, there has been long-term neuropsychiatric followup in children who, as infants, had sonographic evidence of lenticulostriate vasculopathy on an idiopathic basis. It has been determined that such individuals have a significant increase in development of neuropsychiatric disorders by seven to nine years of age (213).

INTRAOPERATIVE ULTRASOUND

Ultrasound plays an important role in the neurosurgical operating room by providing guidance during placement of ventricular and cyst shunt tubes, needle biopsy of solid or complex masses, aspiration of cysts, and

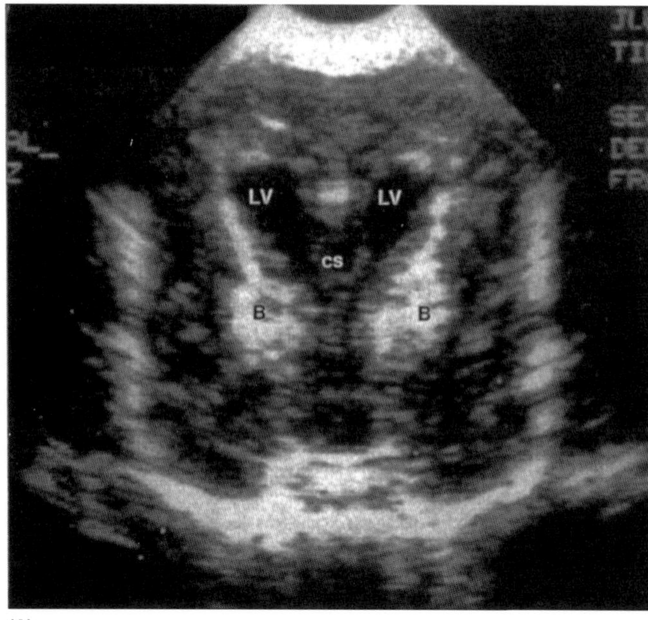

(A)

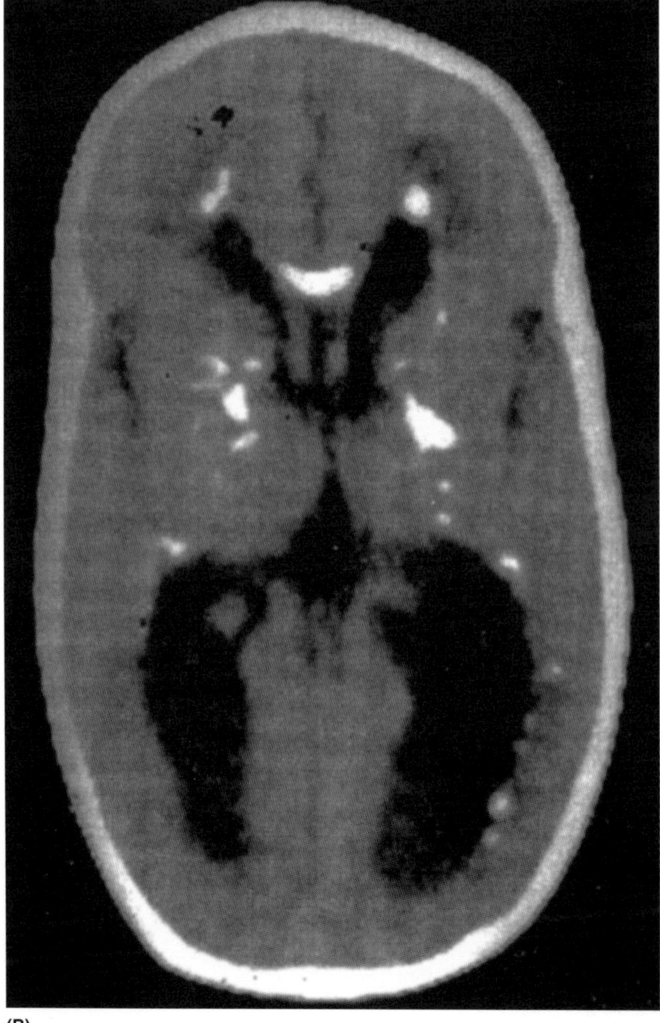

(B)

FIGURE 43 A AND B ■ Cytomegalovirus infection. Two-and-one-half-month-old Indian girl with cytomegalovirus infection and hypotonia. (A) Coronal, relatively anterior ultrasonographic section through the bodies of the lateral ventricles and cavum septum pellucidum shows moderately dilated lateral ventricles and strikingly bright echogenicity in the periventricular regions and the basal ganglia as well as scattered in several areas throughout the brain parenchyma. (B) Axial CT scan confirms the ventricular dilation and calcification in the periventricular regions and basal ganglia. LV, lateral ventricle; cs, cavum septum pellucidum; B, basal ganglia. *Source*: From Ref. 196.

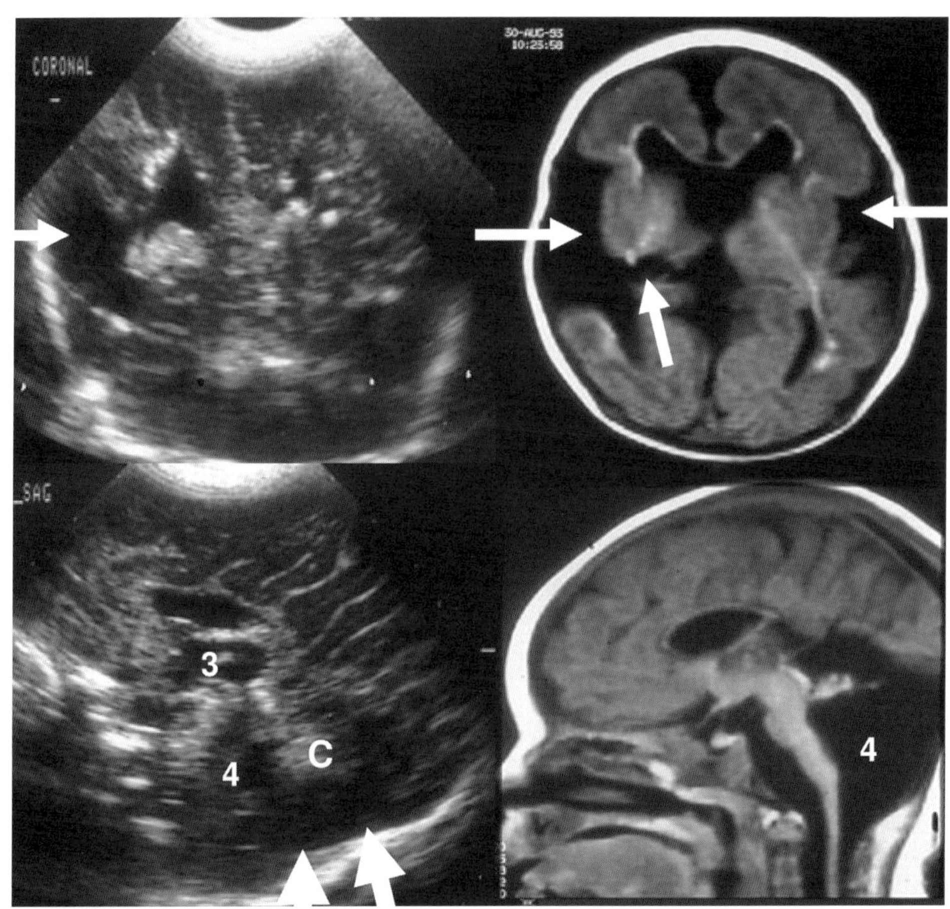

FIGURE 44 ■ Open lip schizencephalv as a sequelae of cytomegalovirus infection in a patient with Dandy–Walker malformation. Coronal sonogram and accompanying axial T1MR image show a wide cleft in the region of the right sylvian fissure, which communicates with the dilated right lateral ventricle and the third ventricle. Midsagittal sonogram and accompanying sagittal T1MR image shows a cystic fourth ventricle and a hypoplastic cerebellum, consistent with Dandy–Walker syndrome. 4, fourth ventricle; C, cerebellum; 3, third ventricle.

localization of intracranial neoplasms and arteriovenous malformations before resection. Ultrasound also is important in the assessment of residual disease before closure (214–221).

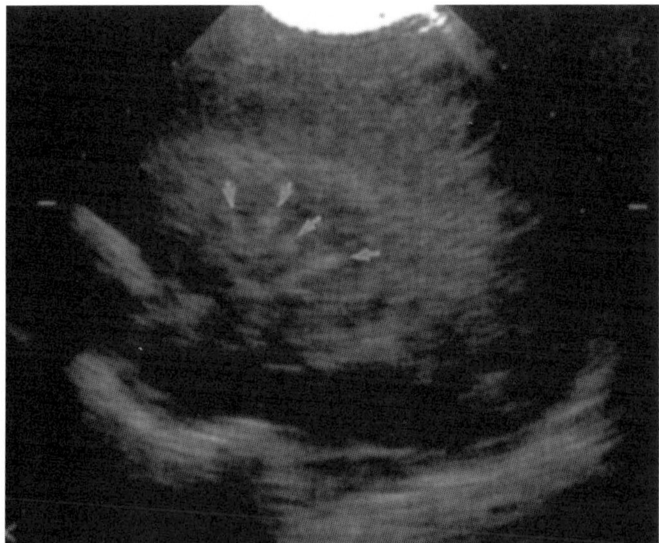

FIGURE 45 ■ Mineralizing vasculopathy. Human immunodeficiency virus-positive newborn with serologic findings of cytomegalovirus and syphilis. Parasagittal ultrasound reveals bright linear echogenicity corresponding to the branches of the lenticulostriate arteries (*arrows*). *Source*: From Ref. 196.

The technique used for intraoperative ultrasound of the brain depends on whether or not sterile conditions must be maintained (215–219). During shunt tube placement, scanning is done through the anterior fontanelle or a Burr hole outside the surgical field, and sterile technique is not necessary. The shunt catheter can be observed as it is passed into the lateral ventricle and then advanced anteriorly into the frontal horn, anterior to the foramen of Monroe. The catheter can be repositioned if it is noted that it is improperly positioned in the temporal horn or in the region of the choroid plexus. Ultrasound guidance during shunt placement is especially helpful when the ventricular system is minimally dilated because it establishes whether or not the shunt has been properly positioned within the ventricular system. The position of the shunt tube should be assessed in both coronal and sagittal planes. If there is any question as to the appropriateness of the position, sterile saline may be injected through the shunt catheter, with the contained microbubbles acting as a contrast agent (219). The same holds true for the placement of shunt catheters into intracranial cysts. Intraoperative ultrasonography allows for immediate observation of complications from a procedure, such as hemorrhage from the brain tissue or the choroid plexus. Both short-term and long-term complications have been reduced when ultrasound guidance is used during shunt tube placement.

Not all shunt, aspiration, and needle biopsy procedures can be accomplished by scanning through the anterior fontanelle or a previous Burr hole, and therefore, when ultrasonography is performed in a sterile operative field through a craniotomy defect or a Burr hole, strict sterile technique must be used at all times (216). The size of the "window" must be carefully planned with thorough knowledge of the size of the transducer. At times, a second window or Burr hole may be necessary to observe a procedure being carried out through a small craniotomy defect or another Burr hole, particularly when a needle guidance system cannot be applied directly over the acoustic window created. First, the ultrasound equipment and transducer must be washed antiseptically. Then, a sterile acoustical gel is placed into a sterile sheath, which is carefully draped over the transducer and the cable wire to ensure that the outside of these parts of the system remain sterile. All gas bubbles must be eliminated from within the gel to avoid image degradation. Sterile saline is then used as a coupling agent at the operative site between the sheathed transducer and the dural or brain surface. The choice of transducer frequency depends on the depth of the lesion. Generally, a 5 MHz phased array transducer with a small footprint or a mechanical sector scan head is sufficient for the deeper masses, whereas a 7.5 or 10 MHz transducer is used for the more superficial lesions. Multifrequency probes are particularly advantageous because once the transducer is sheathed, the frequency may be changed with ease. Generally, the area of suspicion is scanned before opening the dura. The brain is then scanned in multiple planes, with an attempt to achieve appropriate orientation in reference to the falx, interhemispheric fissure, tentorium, and ventricular system. It is important to obtain images that demonstrate the anatomy in coronal and sagittal planes, even when the point of contact with the dural or the brain surface may create a feeling of disorientation, owing to the obliquity of the image.

Once the dura is removed in patients with underlying masses, it is not uncommon for the brain surface to appear normal or to have normal consistency when gently palpated by the neurosurgeon. It is in these cases that intraoperative ultrasonography plays an indispensable role in noninvasively identifying the underlying abnormality, thus avoiding unnecessary brain dissection, cortical incisions, and incorrect "blind" biopsies (Fig. 46). The depth from the brain surface can be measured as well as the size of the lesion and the related and surrounding vasculature. Ultrasonography can help differentiate intraventricular from extraventricular lesions, and duplex and color Doppler imaging can outline vascular structures that must be avoided or that are the area of interest (e.g., arteriovenous malformation). Using high-frequency probes, the mass can be distinguished from surrounding hyperechoic vasogenic edema; however, this distinction may be difficult because of the hyperechoic nature of the underlying tumor. In addition, when an abnormality is known to be adjacent to vital areas, such as the motor strip, ultrasonography can help to outline other paths through which a biopsy needle may course more safely.

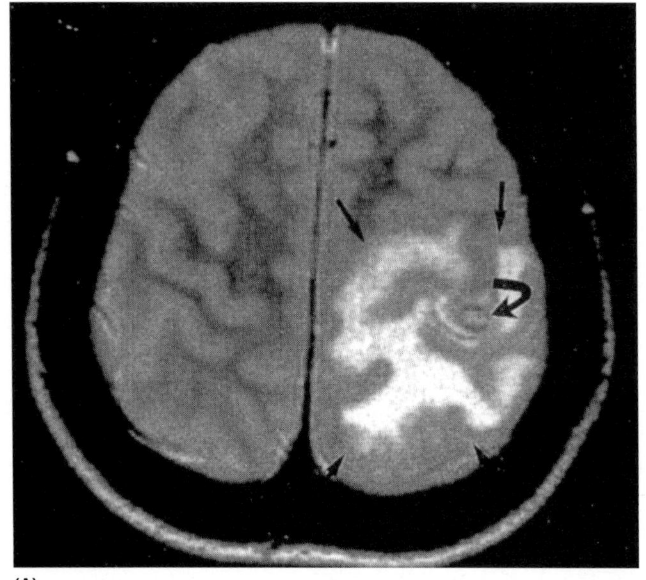

(A)

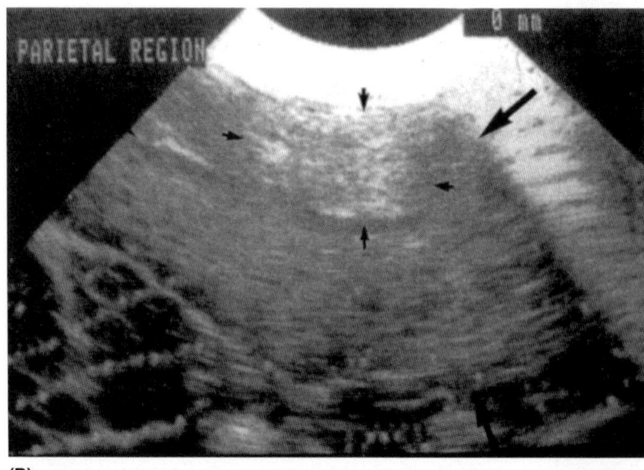

(B)

FIGURE 46 A AND B ■ Intraoperative ultrasound. This 15-year-old Cambodian girl presented with right-sided weakness and headaches. Outside CT showed a left temporal parietal lesion. (**A**) TR 5000/TE 50 MRI showed a small hyperintense mass (*curved arrow*) in the posterior left parietal lobe associated with a hypointense rim and extensive edema (*straight arrows*) involving the central and the subcortical white matter. (**B**) Intraoperative ultrasound revealed an oval-shaped area of inhomogeneously increased echogenicity (*large arrows*) beneath the brain surface in the left parietal region, thought to be due to edema. More superficially, a more echogenic, fairly well-defined area (*small arrows*) was identified and removed. At pathology, this proved to be an abscess secondary to fish fluke *Metagonimus yokogawai* infection. *Source*: From Ref. 196.

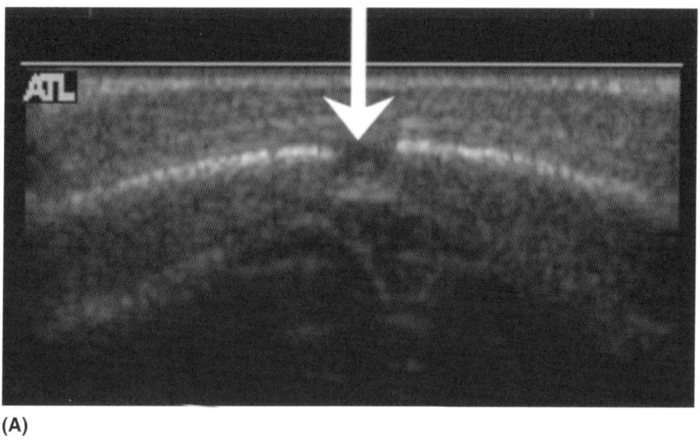

(A)

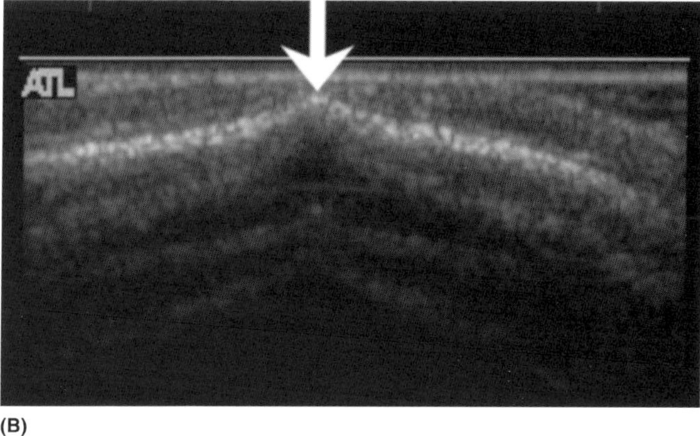

(B)

FIGURE 47 A AND B ■ (**A**) Coronal view of a normally open sagittal suture (*arrow*). (**B**) Axial view of the coronal suture shows premature closure in an infant with craniosynostosis.

The ultrasound beam is kept as perpendicular as possible to the orientation of the needle to ensure maximum visualization of the needle and its tip.

Although used for guidance, 2D intraoperative ultrasound imaging can vary in image quality (222,223). Recently, the incorporation of neuronavigational software programs with 3D ultrasound imaging has made this technique quite helpful to navigate down to a lesion with a high degree of precision. Intraoperative MRI has several drawbacks, which include high investment and running costs, limited working space, and special surgical equipment. 3D ultrasound with neuronavigational software appears to be quite promising as an alternative to intraoperative MRI (224).

SUTURE EVALUATION WITH ULTRASOUND

The major sutures of the skull can be visualized using ultrasound. Although skull radiographs are the first line of imaging for sutural patency, they have a 15% rate of false-positive or false-negative diagnoses when compared to surgical and pathologic findings (177). High-resolution sonography is an alternative method in evaluating suture patency. A normal suture on sonography appears as a hypoechoic band extending through both tables of the skull where the suture is expected anatomically (Fig. 47). Craniosynostosis is indicated if the hypoechoic zone does not cross the inner and the outer

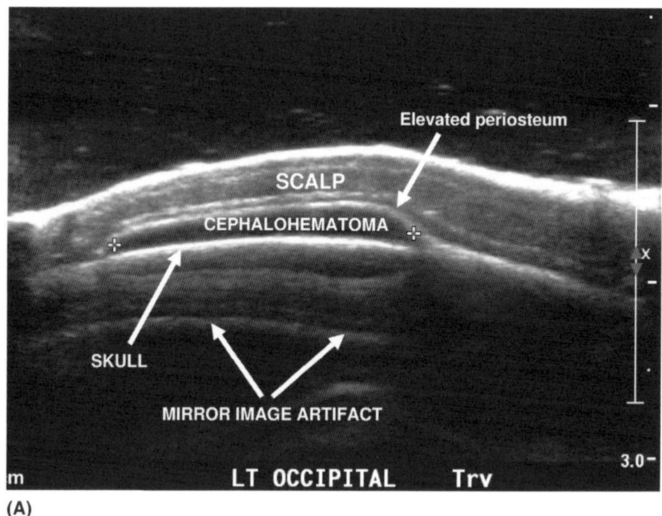

(A)

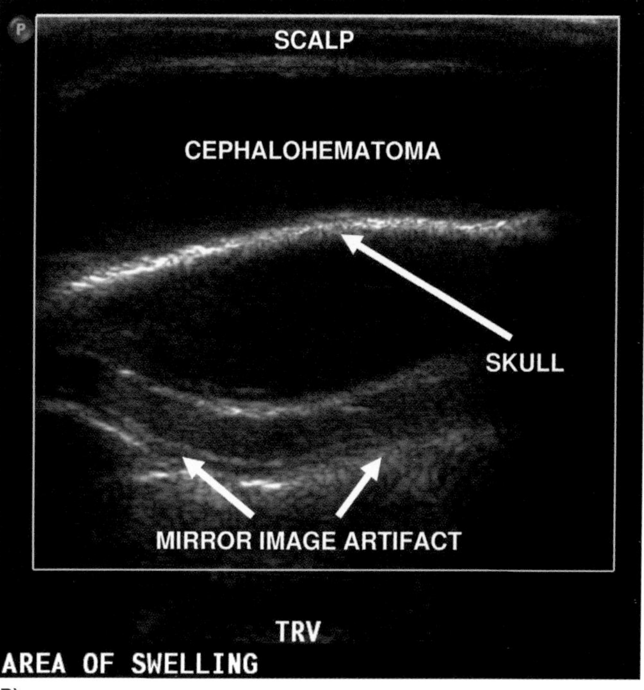

(B)

FIGURE 48 A AND B ■ (**A**) Small and (**B**) large cephalohematoma. Coronal sonogram shows a subperiosteal, elliptical hypoechoic collection, compatible with cephalohematoma.

tables or does not run the whole course of the suture. Thus, sonography is an alternative imaging method for suture evaluation, taking advantage of the lack of radiation, relative ease, and low cost compared to CT. Plagiocephaly can also be distinguished from sutural closure using ultrasound (225).

Cephalohematoma

The most common calvarial injury in the newborn period is a cephalohematoma. Cephalohematomas are secondary to birth trauma. They present as a soft-tissue abnormality most frequently in the parietal region followed by the occipital region. A cephalohematoma is a subperiosteal hemorrhage and therefore bound by the sutures, as opposed to caput succedaneum and subgaleal bleeds, which are superficial and not bound by the sutures. The diagnosis of cephalohematoma is usually made clinically, but ultrasound may be useful in questionable cases. On sonography, cephalohematoma appears as an elliptical hypoechoic collection that can have areas of increased echogenicity representing blood in different states (Fig. 48). This collection does not cross the suture, which can readily be seen with sonography.

CONCLUSION

Ultrasound is an indispensable, cost-effective, noninvasive, nonionizing, portable imaging technique that requires neither intravenous contrast material nor sedation, and is ideal for serial imaging. It can be used for the diagnosis and followup of many diseases that affect the infant brain.

REFERENCES

1. Allan WC, Roveto CA, Sawyer LR, et al. Sector scan ultrasound imaging through the anterior fontanelle. Am J Dis Child 1980; 134:1028.
2. Grant EG, Schellinger D, Borts FT, et al. Real-time sonography of the neonatal and infant head. AJR Am J Roentgenol 1981; 136:265.
3. Slovis TL, Kuhns LR. Real-time sonography of the brain through the anterior fontanelle. AJR Am J Roentgenol 1981; 136:277.
4. Skelly AC, Appareti KE, Johnson ML. Real-time evaluation of normal intracranial anatomy in the premature infant. Med Ultrasound 1981; 5:11.
5. Edwards MK, Brown DL, Muller J, et al. Cribside neurosonography: real-time sonography for intracranial investigation of the neonate. AJR Am J Roentgenol 1981; 136:271.
6. Babcock DS, Han BK. The accuracy of high resolution, real-time ultrasonography of the head in infancy. Radiology 1981; 139:665.
7. Shuman WP, Rogers JV, Mack LA, et al. Real-time sonographic sector scanning of the neonatal cranium: technique and normal anatomy. AJR Am J Roentgenol 1981; 137:821.
8. Mack LA, Alvord EC Jr. Neonatal cranial ultrasound: normal appearances. Semin Ultrasound 1982; 3:216.
9. Kirby CL, Rosenberg HK. The infant brain. In: Goldberg BB, Pettersson H, eds. The NICER Yearbook 1996: Ultrasonography. Oslo, Norway: The NICER Institute, 1996:483.
10. Grant EG, Schellinger D, Richardson JD. Real-time ultrasonography of the posterior fossa. J Ultrasound Med 1983; 2:73.
11. Naidich TP, Yousefzadeh DK, Gusnard DA, et al. Sonography of the internal capsule and basal ganglia in infants. II. Localization of pathologic processes in the sagittal section through the caudothalamic groove. Radiology 1986; 161:615.
12. Fiske CE, Filly RA, Callen PW. The normal choroid plexus: ultrasonographic appearance of the neonatal head. Radiology 1981; 141:467.
13. DiPietro MA, Brody BA, Teele RL. Peritrigonal echogenic "blush" on cranial sonography: pathologic correlates. AJR Am J Roentgenol 1986; 146:1067.
14. Lemire RJ, Loeser JD, Leexh RW, et al. Normal and Abnormal Development of the Human Nervous System. New York: Harper & Row, 1975:264.
15. Babcock DS, Han BK. Cranial Ultrasonography in Infants. Baltimore: Williams & Wilkins, 1981.
16. Atlas SW, Shkolnik A, Naidich TP. Sonographic recognition of agenesis of the corpus callosum. AJNR Am J Neuroradiol 1985; 6:369.
17. Dolan CL, Dorovini ZIS. Gestational development of the brain. Arch Pathol Lab Med 1977; 101:192–195.
18. Goodwin L, Quisling RG. The neonatal cisterna magna: ultrasonic evaluation. Radiology 1983; 149:691.
19. Segal SR, Rosenberg HK. Sonographic appearance of the torcular Herophili. AJR Am J Roentgenol 1986; 146:109.
20. Naidich TP, Gusnard DA, Yousefzadeh DK. Sonography of the internal capsule and basal ganglia in infants. I. Coronal sections. AJNR Am J Neuroradiol 1985; 6:909.
21. Naidich TP, Yousefzadeh DK, Gusnard DA. Sonography of the normal neonatal head. Supratentorial structures: state-of-the-art imaging. Neuroradiology 1986; 28:408.
22. Sivo JJ. Postural changes in the sonographic appearance of the neonatal choroid plexus: an aid in differentiating choroid from IVH. Med Ultrasound 1984; 8:50.
23. Riebel T, Nasir R, Weber K. Choroid plexus cysts: a normal finding on ultrasound. Pediatr Radiol 1992; 22:410.
24. Libicher M, Troger J. Ultrasound measurement of the subarachnoid space in infants: normal values. Radiology 1992; 184:749.
25. Correa F, Enriquez G, Rossello J, et al. An acoustic window into the neonatal brain. Am J Neuroradiol 2004; 25:1274–1282.
26. Di Salvo D. A new view of the neonatal brain: clinical utility of supplemental neurologic US imaging windows. Radiographics 2001; 21:943–955.
27. Riccabona M. Pediatric three—dimensional ultrasound: basics and potential clinical value. J Clin Imaging 2005; 29:1.
28. Horbar JD, Leahy KA, Lucey JF. Ultrasound identification of lateral ventricular asymmetry in the human neonate. J Clin Ultrasound 1983; 11:67–69.
29. Shen EY, Huang FY. Sonographic finding of ventricular asymmetry in the neonatal brain. Arch Dis Child 1989; 64:730–732.
30. Enriquez G, Correa F, Lucaya J, et al. Potential pitfalls in cranial sonography. Pediatr Radiol 2003; 33:110.
31. Rosenfeld D, Schonfeld S, Underberg-Davis S. Coarctation of the lateral ventricles: an alternative explanation for subependymal pseudocysts. Pediatr Radiol 1997; 27:895–897.
32. Eisenberg V, Zalel Y, Chen H, et al. Prenatal diagnosis of cavum velum interpositum cysts: significance and outcome. Prenat Diagn 2003; 23:779–783.
33. Grant EG, Borts FT, Schellinger D, et al. Realtime ultrasonography of neonatal intraventricular hemorrhage and comparison with computed tomography. Radiology 1981; 139:687.
34. London DA, Carroll BA, Enzmann DR. Sonography of ventricular size and germinal matrix hemorrhage in premature infants. AJR Am J Roentgenol 1980; 135:559.
35. Mack LA, Wright K, Hirsch JH, et al. Intracranial hemorrhage in premature infants: accuracy of sonographic evaluation. AJR Am J Roentgenol 1981; 137:245.
36. Pinto-Martin JA, Riolo S, Cnaan A, et al. Cranial ultrasound prediction of disabling and non-disabling cerebral palsy at age two in a low birth weight population. Pediatrics 1995; 95:249.
37. Bowerman RA, Donn SM, Silver TM, et al. Natural history of neonatal periventricular/intraventricular hemorrhage and its

complications: sonographic observations. AJR Am J Roentgenol 1984; 143:1041.
38. Rumack CM, Manco-Johnson ML, Manco-Johnson MJ, et al. Timing and course of neonatal intracranial hemorrhage using realtime ultrasound. Radiology 1985; 154:101.
39. Perlman JM, Volpe JJ. Intraventricular hemorrhage in extremely small premature infants. Am J Dis Child 1986; 140:1122.
40. Rumack CM, Johnson ML. Perinatal and Infant Brain Imaging. Chicago: Year Book, 1984:117.
41. Fleischer AC, Hutchison AA, Allen JH, et al. The role of sonography and the radiologist-ultrasonologist in the detection and follow-up of intracranial hemorrhage in the preterm neonate. Radiology 1981; 139:733.
42. Allan WC. Intraventricular hemorrhage. J Child Neurol 1989; 4:S12.
43. van de Bor M, van Bel F, Lineman R, et al. Perinatal factors and periventricular-intraventricular hemorrhage in preterm infants. Am J Dis Child 1986; 140:1125.
44. Papile L, Burstein J, Burstein R, et al. Incidence and evolution of subependymal and intraventricular hemorrhage. J Pediatr 1978; 92:529.
45. Sherman NH, Rosenberg HK. Ultrasound essential for imaging neonatal brains. Diagn Imaging 1994; 16:108.
46. Sauerbrei EE, Digney M, Harrison PB, et al. Ultrasonic evaluation of neonatal intracranial hemorrhage and its complications. Radiology 1981; 139:677.
47. Bowie JD, Kirks DR, Rosenberg ER, et al. Caudothalamic groove: value in identification of germinal matrix hemorrhage by sonography in preterm neonates. AJR Am J Roentgenol 1983; 141:1317.
48. Shackelford GD, Fulling KH, Glasier CM. Cysts of the subependymal germinal matrix: sonographic demonstration with pathologic correlation. Radiology 1983; 149:117.
49. Schlesinger AE, Shackelford GD, Adcock LM. Hyperechoic caudate nuclei: a potential mimic of germinal matrix hemorrhage. Pediatr Radiol 1998; 28:297–302.
50. Gaisie G, Roberts MS, Boulden TW, et al. The echogenic ependymal wall in intraventricular hemorrhage: sonographic-pathologic correlation. Pediatr Radiol 1990; 20:297.
51. Hill A. Ventricular dilatation following intraventricular hemorrhage in the premature infant. Can J Neurol Sci 1983; 10:81–85.
52. Hill A, Shackelford GD, Volpe JJ. A potential mechanism of pathogenesis for early posthemorrhagic hydrocephalus in the premature newborn. Pediatrics 1984; 73:19–21.
53. Volpe JJ. Current concepts of brain injury in the premature infant. AJR Am J Roentgenol 1989; 153:243.
54. Schellinger D, Grant EG, Manz HJ, et al. Intraparenchymal hemorrhage in preterm neonates: a broadening spectrum. AJR Am J Roentgenol 1988; 150:1109.
55. Grant EG, Kerner M, Schellinger D, et al. Evolution of porencephalic cysts from intraparenchymal hemorrhage in neonates: sonographic evidence. AJR Am J Roentgenol 1982; 138:467.
56. Hayden CK, Shattuck KE, Richardson CJ, et al. Subependymal germinal matrix hemorrhage in full-term neonates. Pediatrics 1985; 75:714.
57. Ennis MG, Kaude JV, Williams JL. Sonographic diagnosis of subarachnoid hemorrhage in premature newborn infants: a retrospective study with histopathologic and CT correlation. J Ultrasound Med 1985; 4:183.
58. Limperopoulos C, Benson CB, Bassan H, Disalvo DN, Kinnamon DD, Moore M, Ringer SA, Volpe JJ, du Plessis AJ. Cerebellar hemorrhage in the preterm infant: ultrasonographic findings and risk factors. Pediatrics 2005; 116(3):717–724.
59. Merrill JD, Piecuch RE, Fell SC, Barkovich J, Goldstein RB. A new pattern of cerebellar hemorrhages in preterm infants. Pediatrics 1998; 102(6):E62.
60. Stromberg B, Dahlquist G, Ericson A, Finnstrom O, Koster M, Stjernqvist K. Neurological sequelae in children born after in-vitro fertilization: a population-based study. Lancet 2002; 359: 461–465.
61. Linder N, Haskin O, Levit O, et al. Risk factors for intraventricular hemorrhage in very low birth weight premature infants: a retrospective case-control study. Pediatrics 2003; 111(5). Available at: www.pediatrics.org/cgi/content/full/111/5/e590
62. Bulas DI, Taylor GA, Fitz CR, Revenis ME, Glass P, Ingram JD. Posterior fossa intracranial hemorrhage in infants treated with extracorporeal membrane oxygenation: sonographic findings. Am J Roentgenol 1991; 156:571–575.
63. Peterson CM, Smith WL, Franken EA. Neonatal intracerebellar hemorrhage: detection by realtime ultrasound. Radiology 1984; 150:391.
64. Hay TC, Rumack CM, Horgan JG. Cranial sonography: intracranial hemorrhage, periventricular leukomalacia, and asphyxia. Clin Diagn Ultrasound 1989; 24:25.
65. Bowerman RA, Donn SM, DiPietro MA, et al. Periventricular leukomalacia in the pre-term newborn infant: sonographic and clinical features. Radiology 1984; 151:383.
66. Rushton DI, Preston PR, Durbin GM. Structure and evolution of echodense lesions in the neonatal brain: a combined ultrasound and autopsy study. Arch Dis Child 1985; 60:798.
67. Schellinger D, Grant EG, Richardson JD. Cystic periventricular leukomalacia: sonographic and CT findings. AJNR Am J Neuroradiol 1984; 5:439.
68. Coley BD, Hogan MJ. Cystic periventricular leukomalacia of the corpus callosum. Pediatr Radiol 1997; 27:583–585.
69. Carson SC, Hertzberg BS, Bowie JD, et al. Value of sonography in the diagnosis of intracranial hemorrhage and periventricular leukomalacia: a postmortem study of 35 cases. AJNR Am J Neuroradiol 1990; 11:677.
70. Dubowitz LMS, Bydder GM, Mushin J. Developmental sequence of periventricular leukomalacia. Arch Dis Child 1985; 60: 349–355.
71. Trounce JQ, Levene MI. Diagnosis and outcome of subcortical cystic leukomalacia. Arch Dis Child 1985; 60:1041–1044.
72. Bejar R, Coen RW, Merritt TA, et al. Focal necrosis of the white matter (PVL): sonographic pathologic and EEG features. AJNR Am J Neuroradiol 1986; 7:1073.
73. Chow PP, Horgan JG, Taylor KSW. Neonatal periventricular leukomalacia: realtime sonographic diagnosis with CT correlation. AJR Am J Roentgenol 1985; 145:155.
74. Baarsma R, Laurini RN, Baerts W, et al. Reliability of sonography in non-hemorrhagic periventricular leukomalacia. Pediatr Radiol 1987; 17:189.
75. De Vries LS, Dubowitz LMS, Pennock JM, Bydder GM. Extensive cystic leucomalacia: correlation of cranial ultrasound, magnetic resonance imaging and clinical findings in sequential studies Clin Radiol 1989; 40:158–166.
76. Baker LL, Stevenson DK, Enzmann DR. End-stage periventricular leukomalacia: MR evaluation. Radiology 1988; 168:809–815.
77. Fawer CL, Diebold P, Calame A. Periventricular leukomalacia and neurodevelopmental outcome in preterm infant. Arch Dis Child 1987; 62:30.
78. Monset-Couchard M, de Bethmann O, Radvanyl-Bouvet MF, et al. Neurodevelopmental outcome in cystic periventricular leukomalacia. Neuropediatrics 1988; 19:124.
79. Bennett FC, Silver G, Leung E, et al. Periventricular echodensities detected by cranial ultrasonography: usefulness in predicting neurodevelopmental outcome in low-birth-weight, preterm infants. Pediatrics 1990; 85:400.
80. Malinger G, Lev D, Sira LB, Kidron D, Tamarkin M, Lerman-Sagie T. Congenital periventricular pseudocysts:prenatal sonographic appearance and clinical implications. Ultrasound Obstet Gynecol 2002; 20:447–451.
81. Guzzetta F, Shackelford GD, Volpe S, et al. Periventricular intraparenchymal echodensities in the premature newborn: critical determinant of neurologic outcome. Pediatrics 1986; 78:995.
82. Hill A, Volpe JJ. Pathogenesis and management of hypoxic-ischemic encephalopathy in the term newborn. Neurol Clin 1985; 3:31.
83. Huang CC, Ho MY, Shen EY. Sonographic changes in a parasagittal cerebral lesion in an asphyxiated newborn. J Clin Ultrasound 1987; 15:68.
84. Babcock DS, Ball W. Postasphyxial encephalopathy in full-term infants: ultrasound diagnosis. Radiology 1983; 148:417.
85. Siegel MJ, Shackelford GD, Perlman JM, et al. Hypoxic ischemic encephalopathy in term infants: diagnosis and prognosis evaluated by ultrasound. Radiology 1984; 152:395.

86. Slovis TL, Shankaran S, Bedard MP, et al. Intracranial hemorrhage in the hypoxic-ischemic infant: ultrasound demonstration of unusual complications. Radiology 1984; 151:163.
87. Hertzberg BS, Pasto ME, Needleman L, et al. Postasphyxial encephalopathy in term infants: sonographic demonstration of increased echogenicity of the thalamus and basal ganglia. J Ultrasound Med 1987; 6:197.
88. Shen EY, Huang CC, Chyou SC, et al. Sonographic finding of the bright thalamus. Arch Dis Child 1986; 61:1096.
89. Hernanz-Schulman M, Cohen W, Genieser NB. Sonography of cerebral infarction in infancy. AJR Am J Roentgenol 1988; 150:897.
90. Hill A, Martin DJ, Daneman A, et al. Focal ischemic cerebral injury in the newborn: diagnosis by US and correlation with computed tomographic scan. Pediatrics 1983; 71:790.
91. DeVries LS, Regev R, Connell JA, et al. Localized cerebral infarction in the premature infant: an ultrasound diagnosis correlated with computed tomography and MRI. Pediatrics 1988; 81:36.
92. DeMyer W. Classification of cerebral malformations. Birth Defects 1971; 7:78.
93. Babcock DS. Cranial sonography: congenital anomalies. In: Babcock DS, ed. Clinics in Diagnostic Ultrasound: Neonatal and Pediatric Ultrasonography. New York: Churchill Livingstone, 1989:1.
94. Babcock DS. Sonography of congenital malformations of the brain. Neuroradiology 1986; 28:428.
95. Benson JE, Bishop MR, Cohen HL. Intracranial neonatal neurosonography: an update. Ultrasound Q 2002; 18(2):89–114.
96. Bradley WG, Safar FG, Hurtado C, Ord J, Alksne JF. Increased intracranial volume: a clue to the etiology of idiopathic normal-pressure hydrocephalus? Am J Neuroradiol 2004; 25: 1479–1484.
97. Suara RO, Trouth AJ, Collins M. Benign subarachnoid space enlargement of infancy. J Natl Med Assoc 2001; 93(2):70–73.
98. Moore KL. The nervous system. In: Before We Are Born. 3rd ed. Philadelphia: WB Saunders, 1989.
99. Moore KL. The nervous system. In: Moore KL, ed. The Developing Human: Clinically Oriented Embryology. 4th ed. Philadelphia: WB Saunders, 1988:364.
100. Bull J. The corpus callosum. Clin Radiol 1967; 18:2.
101. Babcock DS. The normal, absent and abnormal corpus callosum: sonographic findings. Radiology 1984; 151:449.
102. Hernanz-Schulman M, Dohan FC, Jones T, et al. Sonographic appearance of callosal agenesis: correlation with radiologic and pathologic findings. AJNR Am J Neuroradiol 1985; 6:361.
103. Gebarski SS, Gebarski KS, Bowerman RA, et al. Agenesis of the corpus callosum: sonographic features. Radiology 1984; 151:443.
104. Baarsma R, Martijn A, Okken A. The missing pericallosal artery on sonography: a sign of agenesis of the corpus callosum in the neonatal brain? Neuroradiology 1987; 29:47.
105. Boechat MI, Kangarloo H, Diament MJ, et al. Lipoma of the corpus callosum: sonographic appearance. J Clin Ultrasound 1983; 11:447.
106. Christensen RA, Pinckney LE, Higgins S, et al. Sonographic diagnosis of lipoma of the corpus callosum. J Ultrasound Med 1987; 6:449.
107. Imaizumi SO, Pleasure JR, Zubrow AB. Lesion mistaken for hemorrhage in a premature infant: lipoma of corpus callosum. Pediatr Neurol 1988; 4:313.
108. Ickowitz V, Eurin D, Rypens F, Sonigo P, Simon I, David P, Brunelle F, Avni FE. Prenatal diagnosis and postnatal follow-up of pericallosal lipoma: report of seven new cases. Am J Neuroradiol 2001; 22:767–772.
109. Funk KC, Siegel MJ. Sonography of congenital midline brain malformations. Radiographics 1988; 8:11.
110. Suzuki Y, Mimaki T, Tagawa T, et al. Dandy-Walker cyst associated with occipital meningocele. Pediatr Neurol 1989; 5:191.
111. Serlo W, Kirkinen P, Heikkinen E, et al. Ante- and postnatal evaluation of the Dandy-Walker syndrome. Childs Nerv Syst 1985; 1:148.
112. Tritrakarn A, Khanjanasthiti P, Bhoopat W. Ultrasound diagnosis of Dandy-Walker cyst. J Med Assoc Thai 1989; 72:52.
113. Urich H. Malformations of the nervous system, perinatal damage and related conditions in early life. In: Blackwood W, Corsellis JAN, eds. Greenfield's Neuropathology. 3rd ed. London: Edward Arnold, 1976:361.
114. Naidich TP, McLone DG, Felling KH. The Chairi II malformation. IV. The hindbrain deformity. Neuroradiology 1983; 25:179.
115. Babcock DS, Han BK. Cranial sonographic findings in meningomyelocele. AJNR Am J Neuroradiol 1980; 1:493.
116. Kuban KCK, Teele RL, Wallman J. Septo-optic-dysplasia-schizencephaly: radiographic and clinical features. Pediatr Radiol 1989; 19:145.
117. Nowell M. Ultrasound evaluation of septo-optic dysplasia in the newborn. Neuroradiology 1986; 28:491.
118. McGahan JP, Nyberg DA, Mack LA. Sonography of facial features of alobar and semilobar holoprosencephaly. AJR Am J Roentgenol 1990; 154:143.
119. Britton CA. Semilobar holoprosencephaly with associated Arnold-Chiari variant. J Clin Ultrasound 1989; 17:374.
120. Smith AS, Blaser SI. Magnetic resonance imaging of disturbances in neuronal migration: illustration of an embryologic process. Radiographics 1989; 9:509.
121. Ramirez RE. Sonographic recognition of lissencephaly (agyria). AJNR Am J Neuroradiol 1984; 5:830.
122. Motte J, Gomes H, Morville P, et al. Sonographic diagnosis of lissencephaly. Pediatr Radiol 1987; 17:362.
123. Babcock DS. Sonographic demonstration of lissencephaly (agyria). J Ultrasound Med 1983; 2:465.
124. Trounce JQ, Fagan DG, Young ID, et al. Disorders of neuronal migration: sonographic features. Dev Med Child Neurol 1986; 28:467.
125. DiPietro MA, Brody BA, Kuban K, et al. Schizencephaly: rare cerebral malformation demonstrated by sonography. AJNR Am J Neuroradiol 1984; 5:196.
126. Babcock DS, Han BK, Dine MS. Sonographic findings in infants with macrocrania. AJR Am J Roentgenol 1988; 150:1359.
127. Crome L. Hydrencephaly. Dev Med Child Neurol 1972; 14:224.
128. Sylvester PE. Hydranencephaly (hydrencephaly). Arch Dis Child 1958; 33:235.
129. Mack LA, Rumack CM, Johnson ML. Ultrasound evaluation of cystic intracranial lesions in the neonate. Radiology 1980; 137:451.
130. Suarez JC, Sfaello ZM, Albarenque M, et al. Porencephalic congenital cysts with hydrocephalus. Childs Brain 1984; 11:77.
131. Hansen NB, Kopechek J, Miller RR, et al. Prognostic significance of cystic intracranial lesions in neonates. Dev Behav Pediatr 1989; 10:129.
132. Christopher C, Bartholome J, Blum D, et al. Neonatal tuberous sclerosis: US, CT, and MR diagnosis of brain and cardiac lesions. Pediatr Radiol 1989; 19:446.
133. Legge M, Sauerbrei E, MacDonald A. Intracranial tuberous sclerosis in infancy. Radiology 1984; 153:667.
134. Holt JF. Neurofibromatosis in children. AJR Am J Roentgenol 1978; 130:615.
135. Kuhns LR. Macrocranium and macrocephaly in neurofibromatosis. Skeletal Radiol 1978; 1:25.
136. Sturge WA. Case of rare vaso-motor disturbance in the leg. Trans Clin Soc Lond 1879; 12:156.
137. Takaku A, Kodama N, Ohara H, et al. Brain tumor in newborn babies. Childs Brain 1978; 4:365.
138. Odell JM, Allen JK, Badura RJ, et al. Massive congenital intracranial teratoma: a report of two cases. Pediatr Pathol 1987; 7:333.
139. Han BK, Babcock DS, Oestreich AE. Sonography of brain tumors in infants. AJR Am J Roentgenol 1984; 143:31.
140. Buetow PC, Smirniotopoulos JG, Done S. Congenital brain tumors: a review of 45 cases. AJNR Am J Neuroradiol 1990; 11:793.
141. Chuang S, Harwood-Nash D. Tumors and cysts. Neuroradiology 1986; 28:463.
142. Roosen N, Deckert M, Nicola N, et al. Congenital anaplastic astrocytoma with favorable prognosis: case report. J Neurosurg 1988; 69:604.
143. Hanquinet S, Christophe C, Rummens E, et al. Ultrasound, computed tomography and magnetic resonance of a neonatal ganglioglioma of the brain. Pediatr Radiol 1986; 16:501.
144. Osborn RA, McGahan JP, Dublin AB. Sonographic appearance of congenital malignant astrocytoma. AJNR Am J Neuroradiol 1984; 5:814.

145. Madrazo BL, Sanders WP, Mehta B, et al. Computed tomographic and sonographic characterizations of central nervous system masses. Henry Ford Hosp Med J 1985; 33:69.
146. Higer H-P, Dittrich M, Just M, et al. Long-term follow-up of children with magnetic resonance imaging and ultrasound after treatment of brain tumors. Neurosurg Rev 1987; 10:141.
147. Chow PP, Horgan JG, Burns PN, et al. Choroid plexus papilloma: detection by real-time and Doppler sonography. AJNR Am J Neuroradiol 1986; 7:168.
148. Cappe IP, Lam AH. Ultrasound in the diagnosis of choroid plexus papilloma. J Clin Ultrasound 1985; 13:121.
149. Hatfield MK, Rubin JM, Gebarski SS, et al. Intraoperative sonography in low-grade gliomas. J Ultrasound Med 1989; 8:131.
150. Morof DF, Levine D, Stringer KF, Grable I, Folkerth R. Congenital glioblastoma multiforme prenatal diagnosis on the basis of sonography and magnetic resonance imaging. J Ultrasound Med 2001; 20:1369–1375.
151. Lee D, Kim Y, Yoo S, Cho B, Chi JG, Kim IO, Wang K. Congenital glioblastoma diagnosed by fetal sonography. Childs Nerv Syst 1999; 15:197–201.
152. Cavalheiro S, Moron AF, Hisaba W, Dastoli P, Silva NS. Fetal brain tumors. Childs Nerv Syst 2003; 19:529–536.
153. Locatelli D, Bonfanti N, Sfogliarini R, et al. Arachnoid cysts: diagnosis and treatment. Childs Nerv Syst 1987; 3:121.
154. Grant EG, White EM, Schellinger D, et al. Cranial duplex sonography of the infant. Radiology 1987; 163:177.
155. Mitchell DG, Merton D, Needleman L, et al. Neonatal brain: color Doppler imaging. I. Technique and vascular anatomy. Radiology 1988; 167:303.
156. Mitchell DG, Merton D, Desai H, et al. Neonatal brain: color Doppler imaging. II. Altered flow patterns from extracorporeal membrane oxygenation. Radiology 1988; 167:307.
157. Cubberley DA, Jaffe RB, Nixon GW. Sonographic demonstration of galenic arteriovenous malformations in the neonate. AJNR Am J Neuroradiol 1982; 3:435.
158. Langer R, Kaufmann HJ. Arteriovenous malformation of the great cerebral vein (of Galen) in a newborn: diagnosis by ultrasound and digital subtraction angiography. Eur J Pediatr 1987; 146:87.
159. Sivakoff M, Nouri S. Diagnosis of vein of Galen arteriovenous malformation by two-dimensional ultrasound and pulsed Doppler method. Pediatrics 1982; 69:84.
160. Soto G, Daneman A, Hellman J. Doppler evaluation of cerebral arteries in a Galenic vein malformation. J Ultrasound Med 1985; 4:673.
161. Nicholson AA, Hourihan MD, Hayward C. Arteriovenous malformations involving the vein of Galen. Arch Dis Child 1989; 64:1653.
162. O'Donnabhain D, Duff DF. Aneurysms of the vein of Galen. Arch Dis Child 1989; 64:1612.
163. Seibert JJ, McCowan TC, Chadduck WM, et al. Duplex pulsed Doppler US versus intracranial pressure in the neonate: clinical and experimental studies. Radiology 1989; 171:155.
164. Horgan JG, Tumack CM, Hay T, et al. Absolute intracranial blood-flow velocities evaluated by duplex Doppler sonography in asymptomatic preterm and term neonates. AJR Am J Roentgenol 1989; 152:1059.
165. Raju TNK, Zikos E. Regional cerebral blood velocity in infants: a real-time transcranial and fontanellar pulsed Doppler study. J Ultrasound Med 1987; 6:497.
166. Bada HS, Miller JE, Menke JA, et al. Intraventricular pressure and cerebral arterial pulsatile flow measurements in neonatal intraventricular hemorrhage. J Pediatr 1982; 100:291.
167. Bode H, Eden A. Transcranial Doppler sonography in children. J Child Neurol 1989; 4:S68–S76.
168. Hill A, Volpe JJ. Decrease in pulsatile flow in the anterior cerebral arteries in infantile hydrocephalus. Pediatrics 1982; 69:4.
169. Cowan F, Thoresen M. The effects of intermittent positive pressure ventilation on cerebral arterial and venous blood velocities in the newborn infant. Acta Paediatr Scand 1987; 76:239.
170. van Bel F, den Ouden L, van de Bor M, et al. Cerebral blood-flow velocity during the first week of life of preterm infants and neurodevelopment at two years. Dev Med Child Neurol 1989; 31:320.
171. van de Bor M, Walther FJ, Sims ME. Increased cerebral blood flow velocity in infants of mothers who abuse cocaine. Pediatrics 1990; 85:733.
172. Bode H, Harders A. Transient stenoses and occlusions of main cerebral arteries in children: diagnosis and control of therapy by transcranial Doppler sonography. Eur J Pediatr 1989; 148:406.
173. Mitchell DG, Merton DA, Mirsky PJ, et al. Circle of Willis in newborns: color Doppler imaging of 53 healthy full-term infants. Radiology 1989; 172:201.
174. Tatsuno M, Kubota T, Okuyama K, et al. Intracranial vessels with color Doppler echoencephalography in infants. Brain Dev 1989; 11:125.
175. Blackenberg FG, Loh N-N, Norbash AM, et al. Impaired cerebrovascular autoregulation after hypoxic-ischemic injury in extremely low birth weight neonates: detection with power and pulsed wave Doppler US. Radiology 1997; 25:425–428.
176. Lowe L, Bulas D. Transcranial Doppler imaging in children: sickle cell screening and beyond. Pediatr Radiol 2005; 35:54–65.
177. Siegel MA. Pediatric Sonography. 3rd ed. Philadelphia, PA: Lippincott Williams and Wilkins.
178. Amodio J, Spektor V, Pramanik B, et al. Spontaneous development of bilateral subdural hematomas in an infant with benign infantile hydrocephalus: color Doppler assessment of vessels traversing extra-axial spaces. Pediatr Radiol 2005; 35: 1113–1117.
179. Raju TNK, Kim SY, Meller JL, et al. Circle of Willis blood velocity and flow direction after common carotid artery ligation for neonatal extracorporeal membrane oxygenation. Pediatrics 1989; 83:343.
180. Mitchell DG, Merton DA, Graziani LJ, et al. Right carotid artery ligation in neonates: classification of collateral flow with color Doppler imaging. Radiology 1990; 175:117.
181. Taylor GA, Glass P, Fitz CR, et al. Neurologic status in infants treated with extracorporeal membrane oxygenation: correlation of imaging findings with developmental outcome. Radiology 1987; 165:679.
182. Taylor GA, Fitz CR, Miller MK, et al. Intracranial abnormalities in infants treated with extracorporeal membrane oxygenation: imaging with US and CT. Radiology 1987; 165:675.
183. Luisiri A, Graviss R, Weber T, et al. Neurosonographic changes in newborns treated with extracorporeal membrane oxygenation. J Ultrasound Med 1988; 7:429.
184. Babcock DS, Han BK, Weiss RG, et al. Brain abnormalities in infants on extracorporeal membrane oxygenation: sonographic and CT findings. AJR Am J Roentgenol 1989; 153:571.
185. Graziani LJ, Streletz LJ, Mitchell DG, et al. Electroencephalographic, neuroradiologic, and neurodevelopmental studies in infants with subclavian steal during ECMO. Pediatr Neurol 1994; 10:97.
186. Schumacher R, Barks J, Johnston M, et al. Right sided brain lesions in infants following extracorporeal membrane oxygenation. Pediatrics 1988; 82:155–161.
187. King TA, Perlman JM, Laptook AR, et al. Neurologic manifestations of in utero cocaine exposure in nearterm and term infants. Pediatrics 1995; 96:259.
188. Newell DW, Grady MS, Sirotta P, et al. Evaluation of brain death using transcranial Doppler. Neurosurgery 1989; 24:509.
189. Petty GW, Mohr JP, Pedley TA, et al. The role of transcranial Doppler in confirming brain death: sensitivity, specificity and suggestions for performance and interpretation. Neurology 1990; 40:300.
190. Bode H, Sauer M, Pringsheim W. Diagnosis of brain death by transcranial Doppler sonography. Arch Dis Child 1988; 63:1474.
191. Powers AD, Graeber MC, Smith RR. Transcranial Doppler ultrasonography in the determination of brain death. Neurosurgery 1989; 24:884.
192. Chiu NC, Shen EY, Lee BS. Reversal of diastolic cerebral blood flow in infants without brain death. Pediatr Neurol 1994; 11:337.
193. Lupetin AR, Davis DA, Beckman I, et al. Transcranial Doppler sonography. Part 2. Evaluation of intracranial and extracranial abnormalities and procedural monitoring. Radiographics 1995; 15:179–191.
194. Frank JL. Sonography of intracranial infection in infants and children. Neuroradiology 1986; 28:440.

195. Rosenberg HK, Levine RS, Stoltz K, et al. Bacterial meningitis in infants: sonographic features. AJNR Am J Neuroradiol 1983; 4:822.
196. Rosenberg HK, Kessler A. Sonography of neonatal intracranial infection. In: Sanders RC, Hill MC, eds. Ultrasound Quarterly. Vol. 11. No 2. New York: Raven Press, 1993:125.
197. Han BK, Babcock DS, McAdams L. Bacterial meningitis in infants: sonographic findings. Radiology 1985; 154:645.
198. Egelhoff JC. Infections of the central nervous system. In: Ball WS Jr, ed. Pediatric Neuroradiology. Philadelphia: Lippincott-Raven, 1997:273–318.
199. Chen C-Y, Chou T-Y, Zimmerman RA, et al. Pericerebral fluid collection: differentiation of enlarged subarachnoid spaces from subdural collections with color Doppler US. Radiology 1996; 201:389–392.
200. Grant EG, White EM, Schellinger D, et al. Low level echogenicity in intraventricular hemorrhage versus ventriculitis. Radiology 1987; 165:471.
201. Carey BM, Arthur RJ, Houlsby WT. Ventriculitis in congenital rubella: ultrasound demonstration. Pediatr Radiol 1987; 17:415.
202. Vachon L, Mikity V. Computed tomography and ultrasound in purulent ventriculitis. J Ultrasound Med 1987; 6:269.
203. Hill A, Shackelford GD, Volpe JJ. Ventriculitis with neonatal bacterial meningitis: identification by realtime ultrasound. J Pediatr 1981; 99:133.
204. Babcock DS, Han BK. Sonographic recognition of gyral infarction in meningitis. AJR Am J Roentgenol 1985; 144:833.
205. Jequier S, Jequier J. Sonographic nomogram of the leptomeninges (pial-glial plate) and its usefulness for evaluating bacterial meningitis in infants. AJNR Am J Neuroradiol 1999; 20:1359–1364.
206. Rozmanic V, Ahel V, Dessardo S, et al. Sonographic detection of multiple brain abscesses in a newborn with IgA deficiency. J Clin Ultrasound 2001; 29:479–481.
207. Ruebenacker C, Heary R, Baredes S. Type A immunoglobulin deficiency presenting as a mixed polymicrobial brain abscess: case report. Neurosurgery 1999; 44:411.
208. Messerschmidt A, Prayer D, Olischar M. Brain abscess after Serratia marcescens infection on a neonatal intensive care unit: differences on serial imaging. Neuroradiology 2004; 46:148–152.
209. Levine RS, Rosenberg HK, Zimmerman R, et al. Complications of Citrobacter meningitis in infants: assessment by realtime cranial sonography correlated with CT. AJNR Am J Neuroradiol 1983; 4:668.
210. Coley B, Rusin J, Boue D. Importance of hypoxic/ischemic conditions in the development of cerebral lenticulostriate vasculopathy. Pediatr Radiol 2000; 30:846–855.
211. Teele RL, Hernanz-Schulman M, Sotrel A. Echogenic vasculature in the basal ganglia of neonates: a sonographic sign of vasculopathy. Radiology 1988; 169:423.
212. Wang HS, Kuo MF, Chang TC. Sonographic lenticulostriate vasculopathy in infants: some associations on a hypothesis. AJNR Am J Neuroradiol 1995; 16:97.
213. Wang H, Kuo M. Sonographic lenticulostriate vasculopathy in infancy with tic and other neuropsychiatric disorders developed after 7 to 9 years of follow up. Brain Dev 2003; 25:S43–S47.
214. Quencer RM, Montalvo BM. Intraoperative cranial sonography. Neuroradiology 1986; 28:528.
215. Knake JE, Bowerman RA, Silver TM, et al. Neurosurgical applications of intraoperative ultrasound. Radiol Clin North Am 1985; 23:73.
216. Quencer RM, Montalvo BM. Time requirements for intraoperative neurosonography. AJR Am J Roentgenol 1986; 146:815.
217. Shkolnik A, McLone DG. Intraoperative realtime ultrasonic guidance of intracranial shunt tube placement in infants. Radiology 1982; 144:573.
218. Madrazo BL. Intraoperative sonography: localizing brain lesions. Diagn Imaging 1986; 106.
219. Gooding GAW, Boggan JE, Weinstein PR. Characterization of intracranial neoplasms by CT and intraoperative sonography. AJNR Am J Neuroradiol 1984; 5:517.
220. Pery M, Borovich B, Kaftori JK, et al. Intraoperative ultrasonography in cystic brain lesions. Isr J Med Sci 1988; 24:405.
221. Rubin JM, Hatfield MK, Chandler WF, et al. Intracerebral arteriovenous malformations: intraoperative color Doppler flow imaging. Radiology 1989; 170:219.
222. Koivukangas J, Louhisalmi Y, Alakuijala J, et al. Ultrasound-controlled neuronavigator-guided brain surgery. J Neurosurgery 1993; 79:36–42.
223. Woyd M, Krone A, Becker G, et al. Correlation of intra-operative ultrasound with histopathologic findings after tumor resection in supratentorial gliomas: a method to improve gross total tumour resection. Acta Neurochir 1996; 138:1391–1398.
224. Unsgaard G, Ommedal S, Muller T, et al. Neuronavigation by intraoperative three-dimensional ultrasound: initial experience during brain tumor resection. Neurosurgery 2002; 50:804–812.
225. Sobeleski D, Mussari B, McCloskey D, et al. High resolution sonography of the abnormal cranial suture. Pediatr Radiol 1998; 28:79–82.

Pediatric Neck • *Henrietta Kotlus Rosenberg and Ada Kessler*

22

INTRODUCTION

Despite the development of higher technological imaging modalities, duplex/color Doppler [ultrasound (US)] remains the modality of choice in children for the evaluation of soft-tissue abnormalities of the neck (1,2). Information may be quickly and easily obtained regarding the size, shape, borders, location (relationship to adjacent neck structures and extension into the mediastinum), internal consistency, and vascularity of the area or mass in question and whether or not there is displacement and/or encasement of the major neck vessels (3–6). The efficacy of US for both diagnosis and followup of soft-tissue abnormalities of the neck is emphasized, in order to reduce radiation exposure, risk of iodinated contrast, need for preparation and sedation, and cost. If the US field of view (FOV) is insufficient for visualization of an entire mass or if malignancy is suspected, then computed tomography (CT) and/or magnetic resonance imaging (MRI) are generally indicated (7). Correlating the sonographic characteristics with the clinical information helps narrow the differential diagnosis so that appropriate therapeutic decisions can be made. When indicated, interventional procedures can be performed under US guidance.

SCANNING TECHNIQUE

The pediatric neck is generally scanned in the supine position with the neck held in hyperextension. A sponge, pad, or roll of material such as a towel is centered under the shoulders to optimize examination of the soft tissues and vasculature of the neck from the mandible to the thoracic inlet. A high-frequency (17–5 or 12–5 MHz) broad bandwidth duplex/color Doppler linear transducer is preferred to maximize the FOV in the near surface and to enhance the fine detail. It may be necessary to use a curvilinear transducer and/or extended FOV technology for very large lesions. At times, a gel standoff pad may be applied to visualize the structures just below the skin surface. A 15–7 MHz miniature "hockey stick" shaped linear duplex/color Doppler transducer is very useful for evaluation of the neck in very small infants. In addition, it may be helpful at times to allow the patient to suck on a pacifier or a lollipop, or to drink, not only for purposes of relaxing the patient to gain better cooperation but also to observe swallowing, which can help to assess anatomical detail and pathologic findings involving the tongue and the esophagus. When drinking, the patient should be turned to the side to reduce the chance of tracheal aspiration. Images are obtained in transverse, sagittal, and, if necessary, oblique positions. When there is a question of extension of a neck mass into the mediastinum, a small footprint probe may be placed on the suprasternal notch or over the parasternal intercostal spaces to visualize the relationship of the mass to the anterior superior mediastinal structures including thymus and major vasculature.

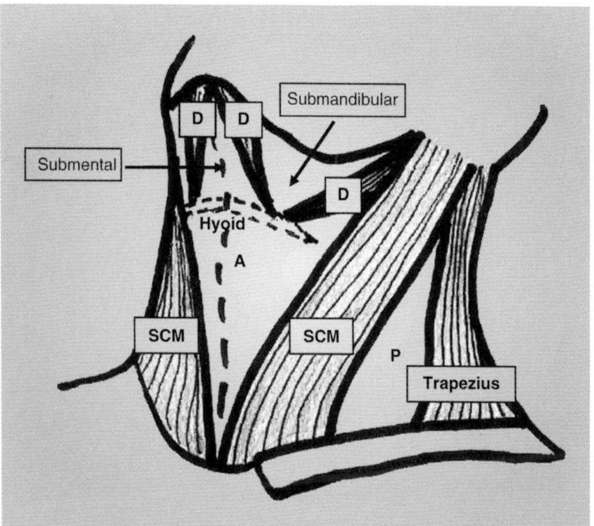

FIGURE 1 ■ Triangles of the neck. The sternocleidomastoid (SCM) muscle divides the neck into anterior (A) and posterior (P) triangles. The hyoid bone divides the anterior triangle into a suprahyoid and an infrahyoid component. D, digastric muscle.

NORMAL GROSS ANATOMY

The neck comprises the distance between the mylohyoid muscle superiorly and the first rib inferiorly. The mylohyoid muscle forms the boundary between the floor of the mouth and the neck. By dividing the neck into triangular components, one can understand and locate the various structures in specific parts of the neck. The sternocleidomastoid (SCM) muscle separates the posterior triangle from the anterior triangle of the neck (Fig. 1). The superior attachment of this large muscle is the mastoid process, which is located immediately posterior to the external ear (auricle). The SCM then courses anteriorly and inferiorly to its attachment on the clavicle and the sternum (8,9). The anterior triangles meet in the midline with the body of the mandible superiorly, the midline of the neck medially, and the SCM muscles posteriorly. The anterior triangle of the neck can be further subdivided into submental and submandibular triangles. The submental triangle is inferior to the anterior belly of the digastric muscle and superior to the hyoid bone and the midline of the neck with the floor formed by the mylohyoid muscle. The triangle is most noted for the presence of several submental lymph nodes that drain the floor of the oral cavity, tip of the tongue, and lower lip. The submandibular (digastric) triangle is located between the posterior and the anterior bellies of the digastric muscle and the inferior border of the mandible with its floor formed by the mylohyoid, hyoglossus, and middle constrictor muscles. The posterior triangle is bordered by the SCM muscle anteriorly, the trapezius muscle posteriorly, the deep cervical fascia superiorly, and the clavicle inferiorly.

The lymph nodes in the neck are divided into two groups: superficial (e.g., parotid, submandibular, facial, and occipital) and deep (sublingual, retropharyngeal, and anterior cervical between the two carotid sheaths, and lateral cervical) (10,11). The superficial group of nodes courses along the external jugular vein from the base of the skull to its junction with the brachiocephalic vessels. The nodes of the internal jugular chain are the largest in the upper neck and follow the course of the internal jugular veins. These nodes drain the major structures of the head and neck, including nasopharynx, oropharynx, tonsils, hypopharynx, and larynx. It is not unusual to find small lymph nodes (usually 5 mm or less in diameter) in the neck of asymptomatic children (Fig. 2) (2). These nodes appear as flattened or oval hypoechoic structures with an echogenic linear hilum in which color Doppler imaging demonstrates blood flow (12). Normal and reactive lymph nodes are generally found in submandibular, parotid, upper cervical, and posterior triangle regions and appear hypoechoic and oval, with the exception of

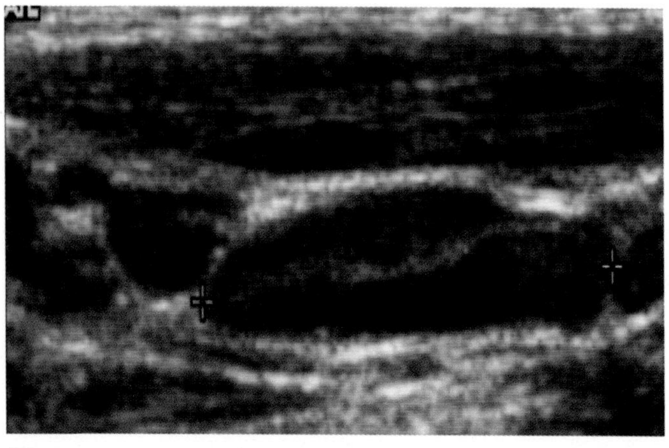

(A)

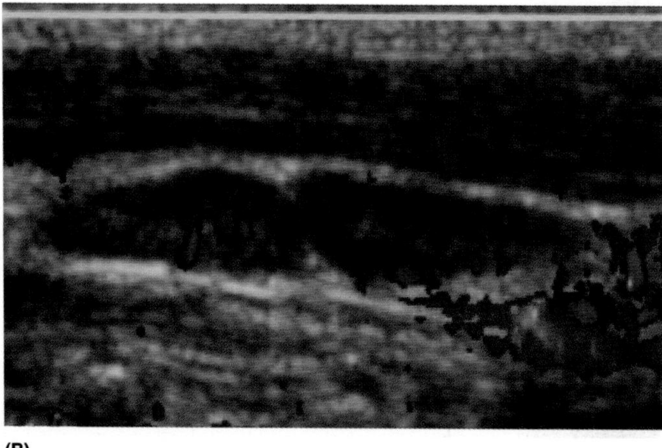

(B)

FIGURE 2 A AND B ■ Normal cervical lymph nodes. Normal lymph nodes are flat or oval in configuration, usually measure <5 mm in maximum diameter, and appear hypoechoic with an echogenic linear hilum (**A**) in which color Doppler imaging demonstrates blood flow (**B**).

the submandibular and parotid nodes, which are usually round. Both normal and reactive cervical nodes generally have an echogenic hilus and are likely to be hypoechoic compared with the adjacent muscles and oval [short-axis-to-long-axis ratio (S/L) < 0.5] except for submandibular and parotid nodes, which are usually round (S/L ≥ 0.5) (11). Gray-scale US is useful to evaluate number, location, size, configuration, borders, matting, adjacent soft-tissue edema, and internal architecture of cervical lymph nodes (e.g., reticulation, calcification, and vascularity). Sonographic features that help to differentiate abnormal nodes include shape (round), absent hilus, intranodal necrosis, reticulation, calcification, matting, soft-tissue edema, and peripheral vascularity (13). On color and power Doppler, normal cervical nodes predominantly show hilar vascularity. On spectral Doppler, normal and reactive nodes generally show low vascular resistance [resistance index (RI) and pulsatility index (PI)]. Increased blood-flow velocity is often seen in reactive lymph nodes due to vasodilatation in the presence of inflammation (11).

INFLAMMATORY DISEASE

The majority of pediatric neck masses are due to acute lymphadenitis secondary to a viral (adenovirus, rhinovirus, and enterovirus) or bacterial (*Staphylococcus aureus* most often, group A β-hemolytic Streptococcus less often) etiology, should resolve with appropriate medical treatment, and do not require imaging. These infections are likely due to tonsillar and pharyngeal infections, upper respiratory tract infections, and recent dental work. The child usually presents with enlarged painful cervical masses, most often due to inflamed submandibular and deep cervical (jugular chain) nodes. However, if the child appears toxic or has symptoms that increase despite administration of antibiotic therapy, imaging is frequently performed to assess the extent of the inflammatory process, to differentiate nonsuppurative adenopathy from abscess and to demonstrate the presence of complications such as jugular vein compression, venous thrombosis, and narrowing of the internal carotid artery (14,15). With more advanced pharyngeal infection, peritonsillar and retropharyngeal space infection may ensue and the clinical findings may include stridor, drooling, and unusual neck posturing due to airway obstruction, mediastinal extension, and jugular venous thrombosis (16).

US, along with clinical correlation, often provides sufficient information to determine that the symptomatology is indicative of an inflammatory process. Sonographically, cervical adenitis appears as homogeneous, hypoechoic, round-to-oval-shaped masses, typically larger than 5 mm in diameter, with an echogenic hilum that demonstrates central vascularity traced from the hilum (Fig. 3) (17,18). It is not unusual for the nodes to be matted together and appear as a single conglomerate mass (19). The major complication of cervical adenitis is abscess formation, which generally appears sonographically as a hypoechoic or anechoic mass with variable wall thickness with absence of the central hilar stripe (20,21). During the early suppurative phase of inflammation, the abscess may appear homogeneous and hypoechoic (Figs. 4 and 5). As the process progresses, the lesion becomes heterogeneous and may be multilocular, containing debris, septations, or air (bright echogenic foci with dirty shadowing) (Fig. 6). The demonstration of gas bubbles in the soft tissues of the neck is quite helpful in the early recognition of the anaerobic nature of an infection (22). With frank pus, the internal content may be quite echogenic and the wall may be irregular. Color Doppler imaging shows flow around the periphery of the lesion and none within the central cavity. US may also be used to guide aspiration biopsy (23–25).

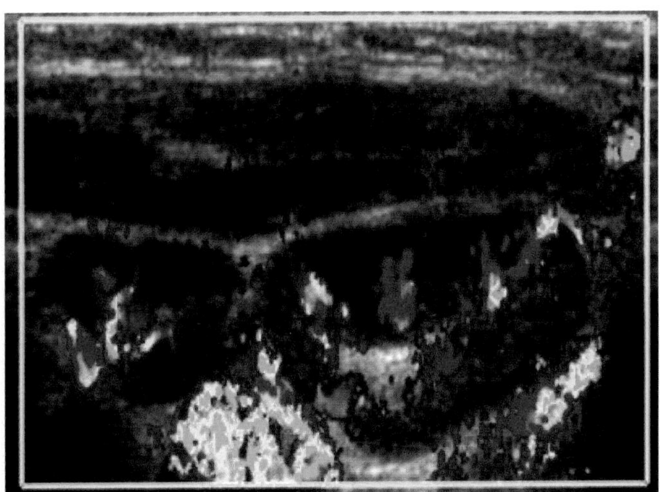

FIGURE 3 ■ Cervical adenitis. The nodes are typically >5 mm in diameter with preservation of the echogenic hilum in the presence of increased vascularity. At times, multiple nodes are matted and appear as a single conglomerate mass.

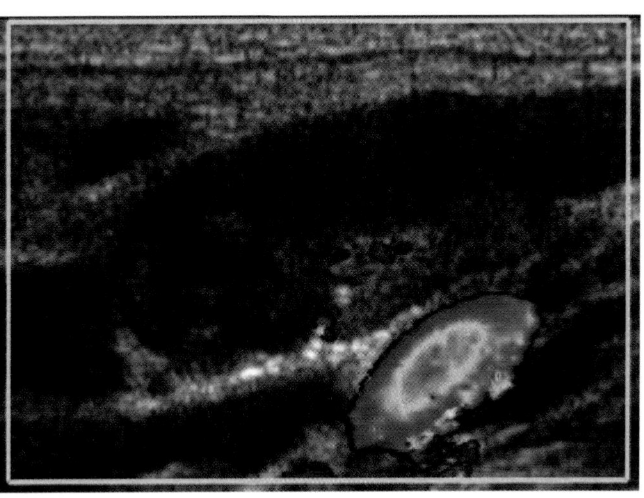

FIGURE 4 ■ Cervical adenitis with suppuration. Note the nodal enlargement with heterogeneous echotexture, reduced hilar stripe, and decreased color Doppler flow.

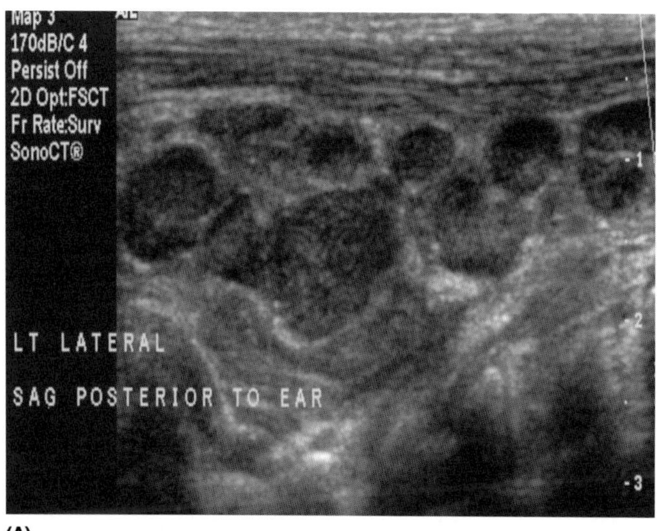

(A)

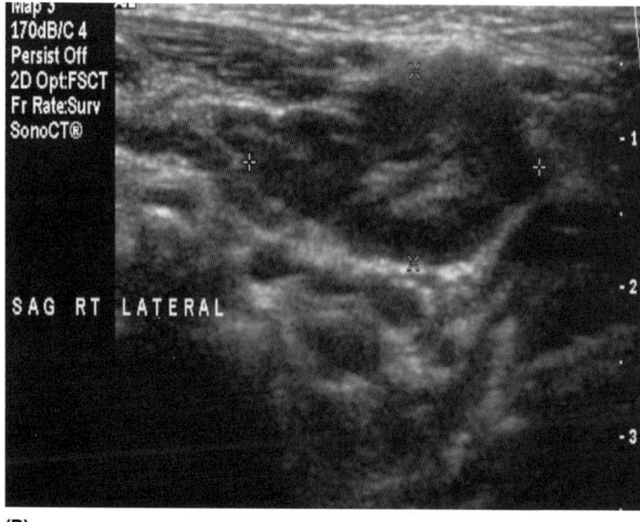

(B)

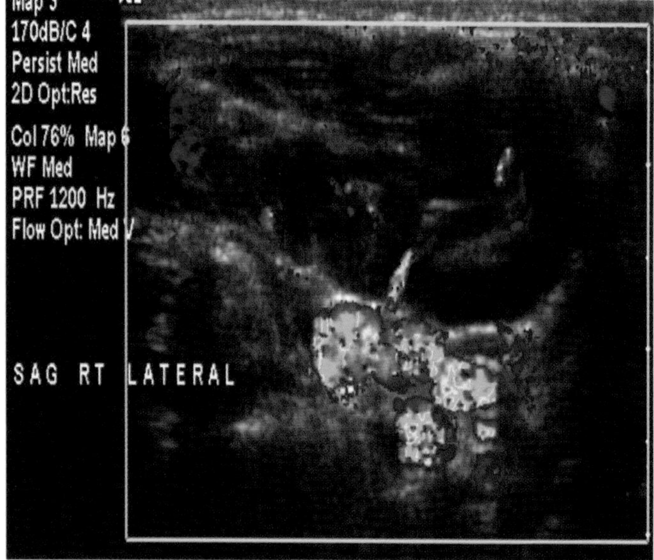

(C)

FIGURE 5 A–C ■ Conglomeration of inflamed nodes bilaterally with suppuration on right side. Multiple variable size lymph nodes are noted on the left side (**A**) with heterogeneity throughout, along with reduced central hilar stripes. On the right side, there is a conglomeration of enlarged heterogeneous lymph nodes with loss of the central stripe (**B**) and decreased color flow (**C**).

Other less common etiologies for cervical nodal infection include tuberculosis, fungus, cat-scratch disease, mononucleosis, acquired immunodeficiency syndrome (AIDS), sinus histiocytosis with massive lymphadenopathy, and sarcoidosis.

Patients with mycobacterial disease may present with firm, nontender, and often matted, enlarged cervical lymph nodes. The US patterns of nodal involvement may represent the different stages of the disease with enlargement being a nonspecific effect of early inflammatory disease. Later on, caseation, necrosis, and suppuration may occur, which result in an US appearance of an inhomogeneous hypoechoic mass with irregular borders, a variable degree of posterior acoustic enhancement, and occasionally containing calcifications. As the disease progresses, the nodal masses often conglomerate, abscess may form, and the process may spread into the adjacent soft-tissue structures (26). Different stages of the disease may be noted simultaneously within a given patient. On the other hand, nontuberculous mycobacterial nodal disease has similar findings in the nodes but lacks the surrounding cellulitis and myositis (27–29). Cat-scratch disease is not uncommon in children and should be considered as a cause of cervical adenopathy without significant associated cellulitis in any child with a history of exposure to cats (14). Mononucleosis should also be considered in a child without evidence of cellulitis, who presents with significant cervical adenopathy and associated enlargement of the adenoids and tonsils. In patients with AIDS, cervical nodal enlargement may present in combination with nasopharyngeal lymphoid hyperplasia and parotid lesions (30,31). Nodal enlargement in AIDS has been correlated with decreasing CD4 lymphocyte counts. The possibility of non-Hodgkin's lymphoma should be considered in the presence of enlarging nodes in these patients.

Pyriform sinus fistula is a congenital branchial pouch abnormality that is often overlooked as a cause of recurrent left-sided neck infection or acute suppurative thyroiditis in the pediatric patient (32,33). Pyriform sinus

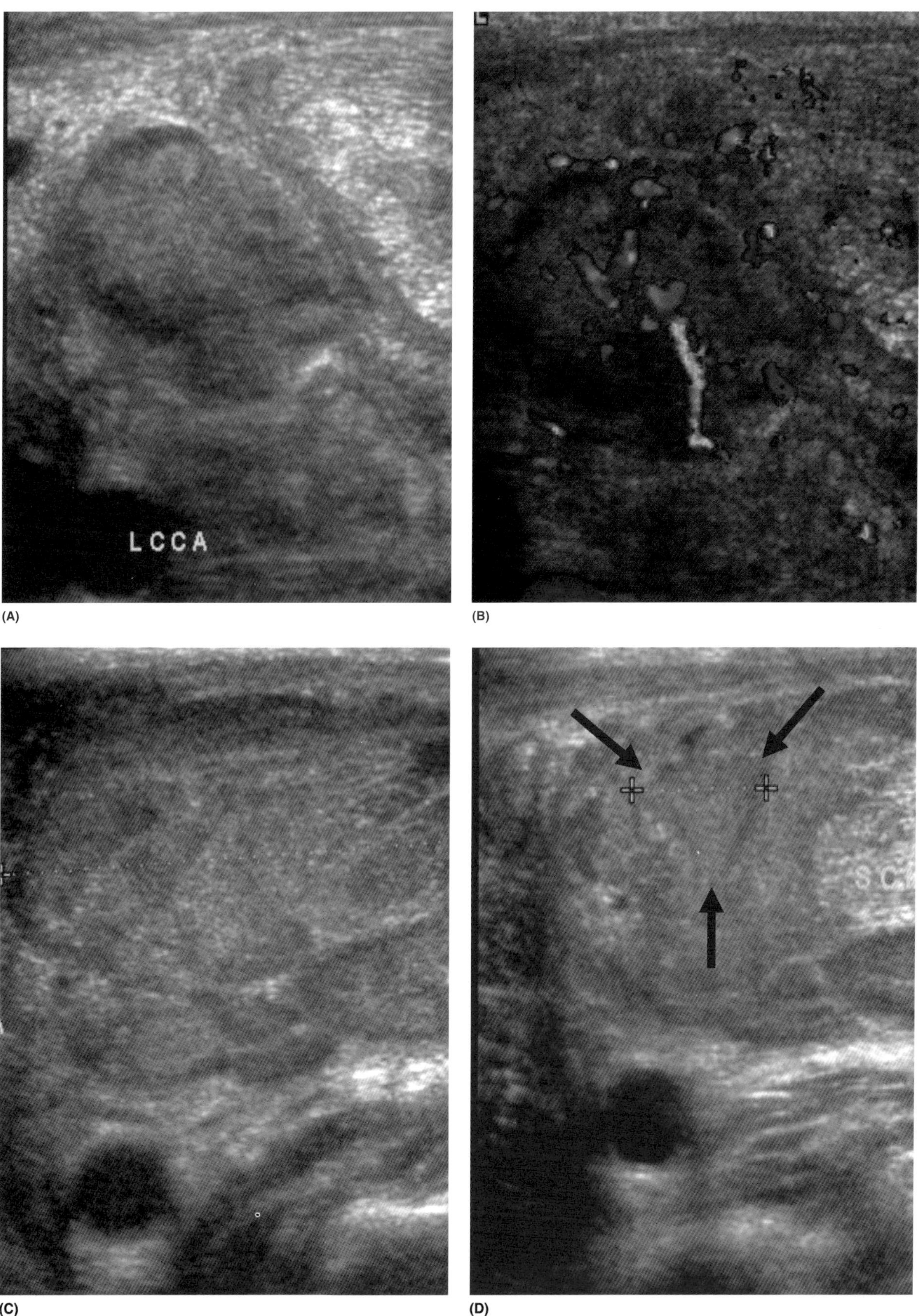

FIGURE 6 A–E ■ Inflammatory mass with abscess formation. This 14-year-old male with HIV presented to the emergency room with a fixed painful 5 cm mass on left side of his neck, which shows loss of the normal nodal architecture (**A**) and reduced color Doppler flow. (**B**) Four days later, the mass was unchanged in size and more painful, and the patient developed spiking fevers developed despite antibiotics. The echotexture appears more heterogeneous. (**C**) and a central area of internal liquefaction containing mobile isoechoic fluid was noted during real-time observation (**D**). (*Continued*)

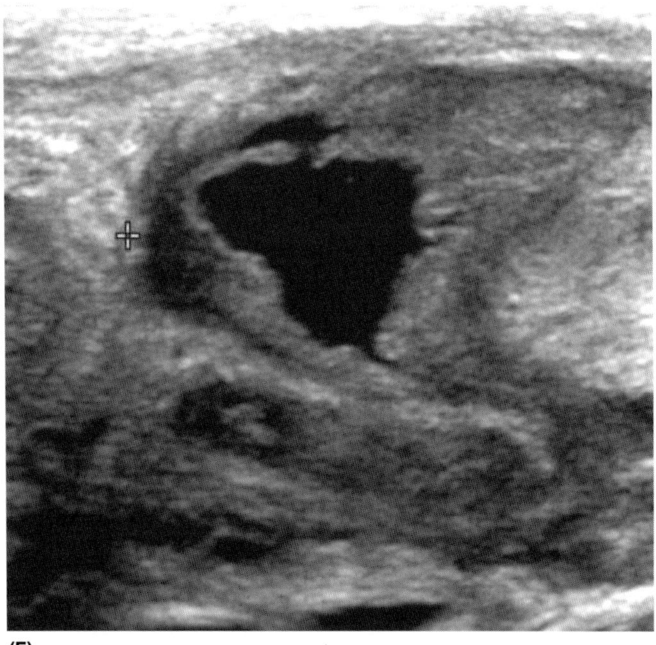

(E)

FIGURE 6 A–E ■ (*Continued*) Four days later, the central area demonstrated irregular thick walls and internal liquefaction, consistent with formation of an abscess (**E**).

fistulae usually originate from the tip of the left pyriform sinus and are thought to be remnants of either the third or the fourth pharyngeal pouches. The fistula courses anteroinferiorly and ends blindly in the parenchyma of the thyroid gland or in the perithyroid soft tissue. Infection usually follows an upper respiratory tract infection due to accumulation of contaminated secretions in the pharynx and the fistulous tract. Depending on the course of the tract, suppurative thyroiditis or neck abscesses may occur. Gas pockets may be noted in the neck due to gas-forming bacilli, external cutaneous drainage, or from the pyriform sinus via the fistula. Barium esophagography helps to confirm the presence of the pyriform sinus fistula and delineates its extent prior to surgical treatment.

CERVICAL MASSES

The majority of cervical masses in infants and children are benign, either on a congenital (fibromatosis colli, thyroglossal duct cyst, branchial cleft cyst, cystic hygroma, thymic ectopia, thymic cyst, hemangioma, teratoma, ranulas, lymphatic malformations, bronchogenic cyst, and gastrointestinal duplication cyst) or on an inflammatory basis (lymphadenopathy or abscess lesions). Less commonly, lymphoma, neuroblastoma, and rhabdomyosarcoma are seen. Of all childhood neoplasms, 5% occur in the head and neck. Metastatic disease may occur in the neck from thyroid, pulmonary, genitourinary, and gastrointestinal origin (3,7,34–38). A differential diagnosis may be derived based on the location of the mass (midline or lateral), clinical history (congenital or acquired and presence or absence of fever and tenderness), and imaging characteristics (cystic vs. solid) (34,38).

The specificity of gray-scale US for the diagnosis of cervical soft-tissue masses is approximately 40%. Color Doppler US serves to increase observer confidence but does not significantly increase specificity. If the full extent of a lesion can be established sonographically, there is no need for further imaging, but if the lesion is too large to be completely imaged within the FOV available or malignancy is suspected, computed radiography (CT) or MRI are required prior to surgical removal (7,39). Scintigraphy is reserved for evaluation of midline masses that are thought to be most likely due to ectopic thyroid in order to determine preoperatively if the "mass" is the patient's only functioning thyroid tissue (39–41).

Fibromatosis Colli

Fibromatosis colli or SCM tumor of infancy occurs in neonates (42–47). This benign lesion of the SCM is at times confused clinically with neoplasm. The neonates who present with the condition are usually between two and four weeks of age, and they manifest a unilateral anterior neck mass that is right sided in 75% of cases. The head is generally tilted toward the affected side of the neck (torticollis) and there is an associated ipsilateral SCM soft-tissue mass. There is frequently a history of breech or difficult delivery (requiring forceps). The etiology of the "mass" is not clear but it may result from intramuscular hemorrhage or fibrosis, which leads to shortening of the SCM, which in turn causes torticollis, all of which may be due to abnormal fetal positioning. The entire length of the muscle may be involved, but the lower two-thirds of the muscle are most affected. Sonographically, the muscle mass is often elliptical in shape and slightly hyperechoic as compared with the SCM with which it blends (Fig. 7). The echotexture of the "mass" may be homogeneous or heterogeneous. There may be a rim of decreased echoes thought to represent compressed normal adjacent SCM. The ratio of fibrosis to normal muscle can be used to guide therapy. This condition usually regresses over four to eight months of life with conservative management in the form of physical therapy (48). Surgical transaction is reserved for babies with persistent facial hemihypoplasia (49).

Thyroglossal Duct Cyst

Thyroglossal duct cyst (TDC) is the most common congenital neck mass, accounting for 70% of congenital neck anomalies, and it is the second most common benign neck mass, after infectious lymphadenopathy (34,35,50–52). TDC forms anywhere along the course of the thyroglossal duct, from the foramen cecum of the tongue to the pyramidal lobe of the thyroid gland, due to incomplete involution of the embryonic duct (53). Enlargement of the thyroglossal duct occurs secondary to the accumulation of secretions produced by the epithelial lining. Approximately 50% of the patients present before 20 years of age during the first decade of life, with no

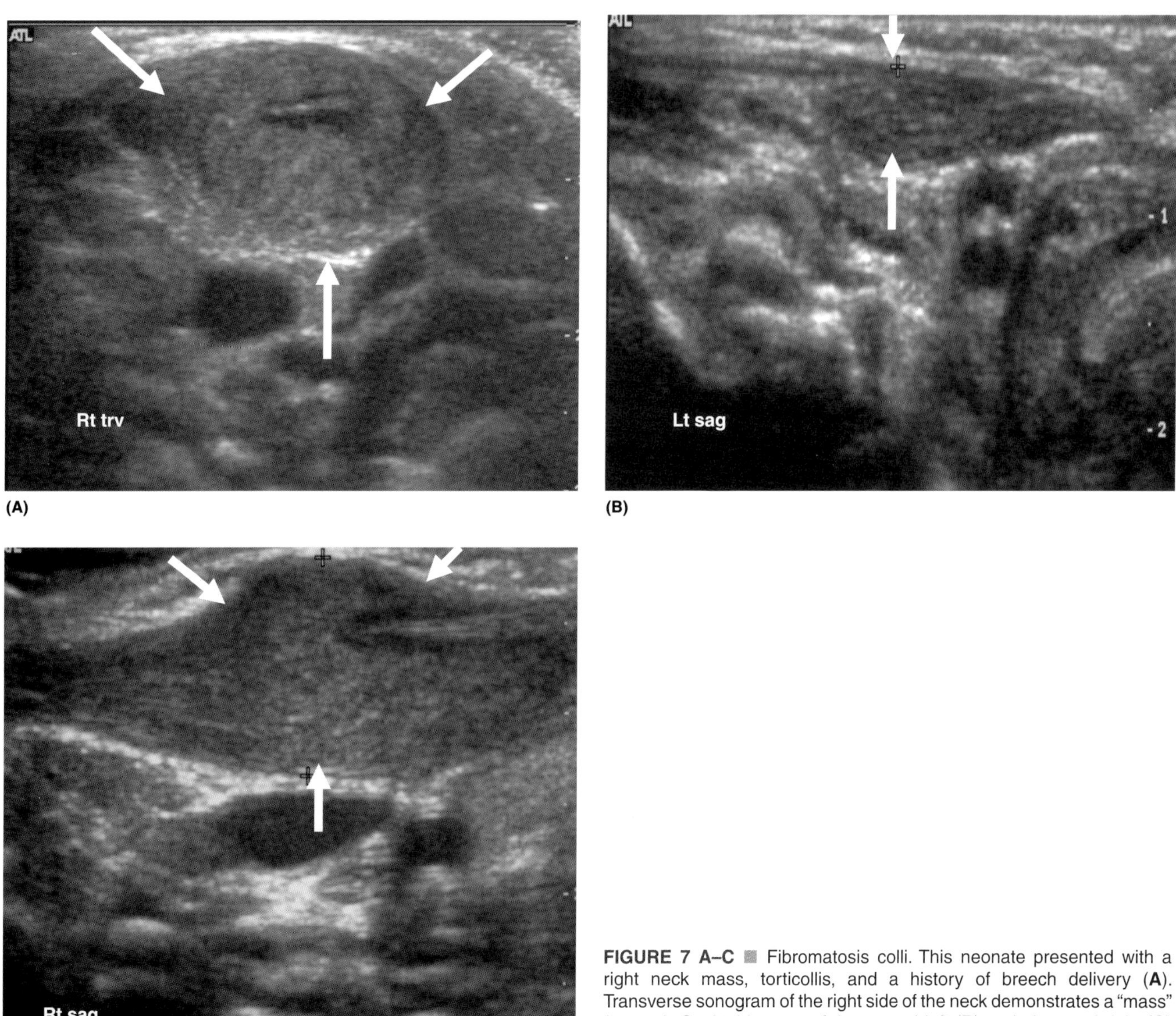

FIGURE 7 A–C ■ Fibromatosis colli. This neonate presented with a right neck mass, torticollis, and a history of breech delivery (**A**). Transverse sonogram of the right side of the neck demonstrates a "mass" (*arrows*). Sagittal images of the normal left (**B**) and abnormal right (**C**) sternocleidomastoid muscles confirm that there is swelling of the belly of the right SCM muscle with no evidence of a discrete mass.

gender predilection. There is a typical history of a fluctuating or gradually enlarging painless soft or semifirm mass in the midline of the neck (75% of cases) or slightly off midline (25% of cases), but always within 2 cm of the midline. For unknown reasons, most cysts located in a paramedian location are on the left side. Approximately 75% are located either at or below the level of the hyoid bone, 20% above the hyoid bone, and 15% at the level of the hyoid bone (54). Those located below the hyoid bone may have both midline and off-midline components. Rarely will a thyroglossal duct cyst present as a mass in the floor of the mouth (55). The mass moves cephalad with swallowing or tongue extension, which is a reflection of the origin of the duct at the foramen cecum. The size of the cyst ranges from 0.5 to 6 cm in diameter, with most between 1.5 and 3 cm.

Sonographically, thyroglossal duct cyst appears as a cyst-like, well-marginated, thin-walled, anechoic or hypoechoic mass with posterior acoustic enhancement, either in the midline of the anterior neck at the level of the hyoid bone or within the strap muscles just off the midline (Fig. 8). Demonstration of an associated connecting duct is helpful in confirming the diagnosis (56). When the cyst contains highly proteinaceous material (secreted by the wall), blood, or purulent material, the internal content may appear quite coarse and hyperechoic and a fluid/debris level may be present (Fig. 9) (57). The real-time observation of shimmering within the mass aids in the differentiation of dense mucus and solid mass. When the cyst becomes infected, the walls may become thick and internal septa may be identified. The cyst wall is generally avascular in the absence of infection. On the other hand,

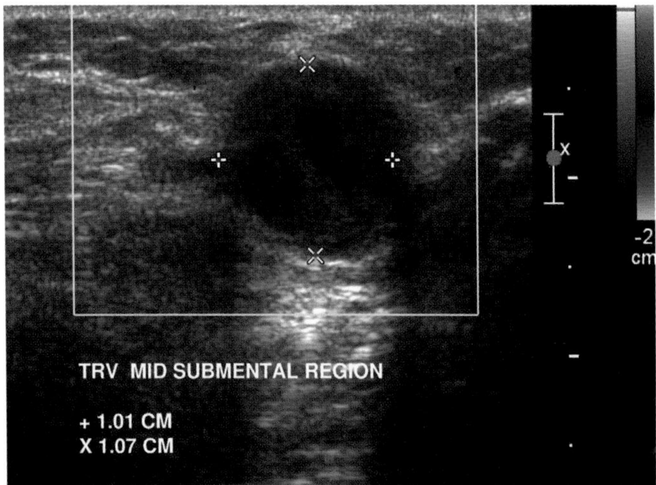

FIGURE 8 ■ Thyroglossal duct cyst. This 2-month-old presented with recurrent soft tissue swelling in the midline of the submental region. US demonstrates a round, 1.0 cm diameter heterogenous cystic structure which contains mobile internal echoes and no evidence of internal vascularity.

color Doppler flow may be demonstrated within the cyst wall and the surrounding tissues in the presence of infection. Because of the potential risk for infection and malignant degeneration, surgical excision is performed (Sistrunk procedure), which includes excision of the cyst, the entire remnant tract, and a central portion of the hyoid bone (58,59). About 1% of thyroglossal duct abnormalities are associated with thyroid carcinoma arising from ectopic rests of thyroid tissue within the duct and not from the duct itself. Most (80%) of the malignancies arising within a thyroglossal duct cyst are of the papillary type (Fig. 10). Nodal spread is much less common in these neoplasms, occurring within the duct, which, in primary carcinomas, arise within the thyroid gland itself (60).

In addition to thyroglossal duct cyst, the differential diagnosis of a midline mass includes ectopic thyroid tissue, dermoid, and adenopathy. Gray-scale demonstration confirming the presence of a normal thyroid and color Doppler demonstration of the typical appearance of a hilum of a lymph node are most helpful for differentiation (61).

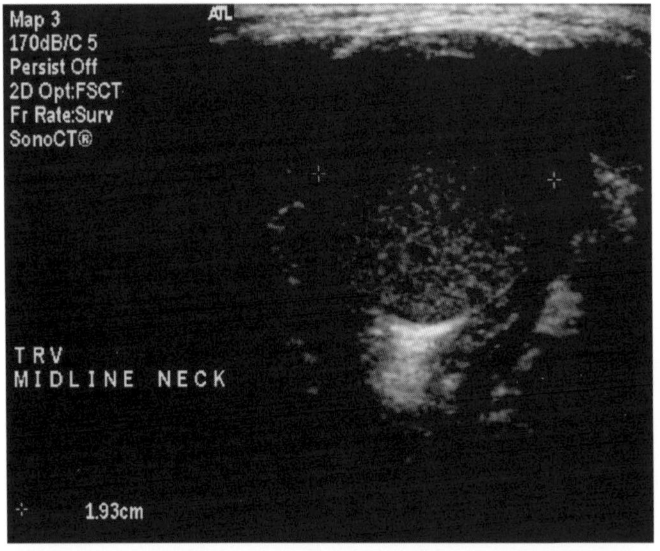

(A)

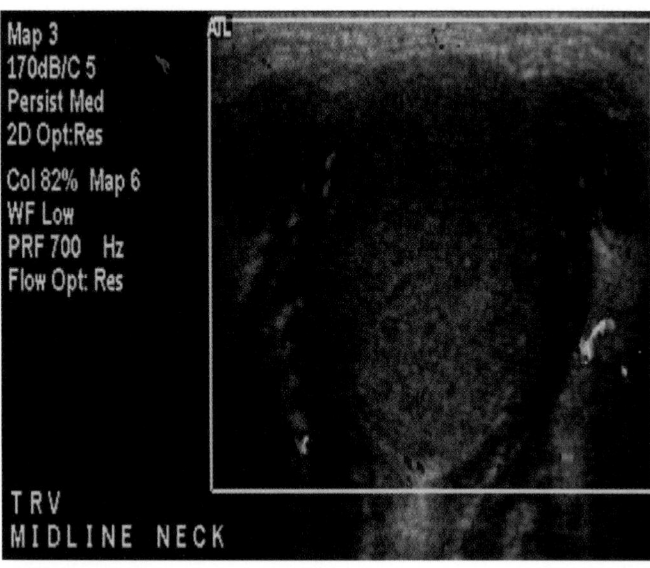

(B)

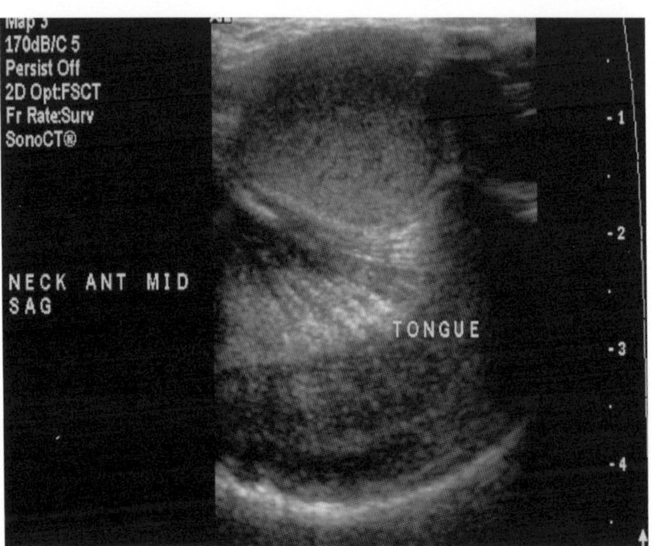

(C)

FIGURE 9 A–C ■ Infected thyroglossal duct cyst. This four-year-old female had a history of an intermittent painful swelling in the submandibular region. A tender round hypoechoic mass is demonstrated (**A**), (**B**) in the upper mid anterior neck in the transverse plane. The mass is separate from the thyroid gland (not shown), contains a fluid/debris level, and is devoid of color Doppler flow except in the wall (**B**). With swallowing, the image obtained in the sagittal projection (**C**) clearly showed that the mass is contiguous with and attached to the tongue.

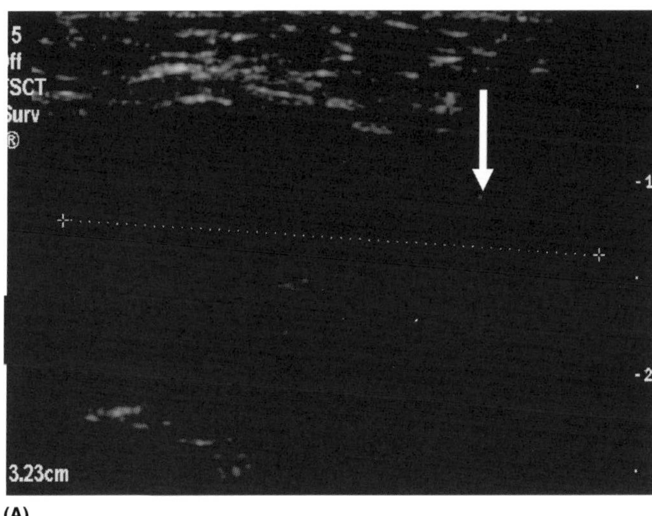

(A)

FIGURE 10 A AND B ■ Papillary carcinoma in thyroglossal duct cyst. The patient presented with a mass arising from the internal wall of the left side of the cyst (**A**) with evidence of tiny bright punctuate echodensities within the solid component (*arrow*).

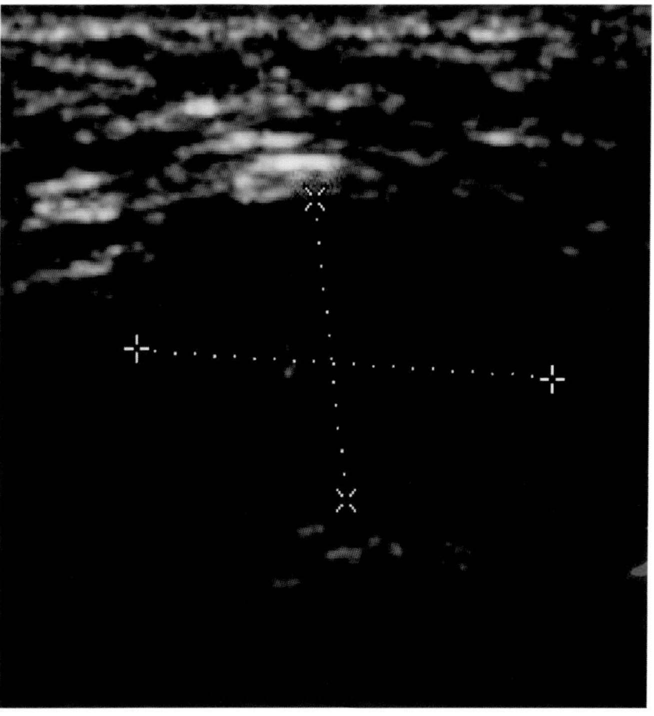

(B)

Branchial Cleft Cyst

Branchial apparatus structures develop between the fourth and sixth weeks of gestation and consist of six pairs of mesodermal branchial arches separated by five paired endodermal pharyngeal pouches internally and five paired ectodermal branchial clefts externally. Branchial apparatus anomalies take the form of branchial cleft cysts, sinus tracts, or fistulae, with branchial apparatus cysts the most common branchial apparatus anomaly that requires imaging. These anomalies develop when there is failure of obliteration of the cervical sinus of His or the first or second branchial clefts or pouches, with 90% of the branchial abnormalities arising from the second branchial cleft, 8% from the first branchial cleft, and 2% from the third branchial cleft (62–66). While a branchial sinus opens externally to the skin and a fistula communicates externally with the skin and internally with the pharynx, a cyst has no internal or external openings. Almost all (95%) branchial cleft cysts arise from the second branchial cleft (67). The branchial cleft cyst typically presents in later childhood or adolescence, in contrast to fistulas or sinuses, which most often present during the first decade of life. The clinical presentation is generally one of a painless, fluctuant, smooth lateral neck mass, or if it becomes infected, a painful tender mass. A history of a recurrent inflammatory mass at the same location in the anterolateral aspect of the neck suggests an infected branchial cleft cyst. The cysts are usually found in the anterior triangle of the neck anterior to the SCM, posterior to the submandibular gland, and lateral to the thyroid gland and to the carotid sheath, with most of them located near the angle of the mandible in the submandibular space. Because of the anatomic relationship of the second branchial apparatus and the cervical sinus, a branchial cleft cyst can occur anywhere along a line from the oropharyngeal tonsillar fossa to the supraclavicular region of the neck (68). At times, cysts may protrude between the internal and the external carotid arteries. Larger cysts may extend posteriorly under the SCM muscle and displace the carotid sheath structures posteromedially, or they may be found in the parapharyngeal spaces or within the substance of the parotid gland.

Sonographically, the sec;ond branchial cleft cyst appears as a well-defined, round or oval mass anterior to the SCM, lateral to the thyroid gland, and anterolateral to the carotid artery and jugular vein (Fig. 11) (69). A noninfected cyst has a thin, uniform wall surrounding hypoechoic fluid. An infected cyst is more likely to demonstrate irregularity and thickening of the walls and increased echogenicity of the contained fluid. At times, the internal debris may be due to cholesterol crystals (Fig. 12).

LYMPHATIC MALFORMATION

Lymphatic malformations are vascular malformations composed of primitive embryonic lymph sacs of varying sizes. Cystic hygroma is the most common form of lymphangioma and constitutes approximately 5% of all benign tumors of infancy and childhood (70). They typically occur in areas within loose areolar tissue, such as the neck and axilla, with 75% of these malformations occurring in the neck, particularly in the posterior triangle, and a lesser number in the oral cavity (39). These lesions may extend into the adjacent soft tissues, invade the muscle, surround vascular structures, and grow into the mediastinum (approximately 2–10%). They are

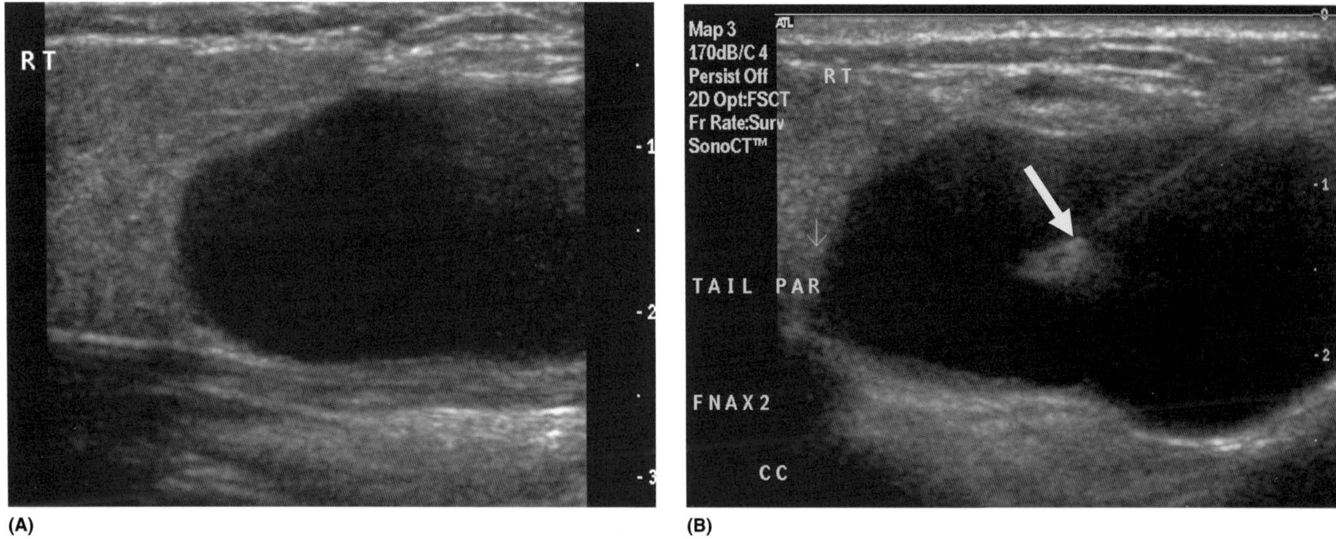

FIGURE 11 A AND B ■ Branchial cleft cyst. This older teenager presented with a nontender swelling in the submandibular region. A purely anechoic cyst (**A**) with thin smooth walls is demonstrated. The cyst was easily aspirated (**B**). *Arrow*, needle.

thought to develop when there is incomplete or lack of drainage of the lymphatic system into the superior vena cava (71). Other hypotheses include abnormal budding of the lymphatic structures or sequestrations of primitive embryonic lymph sacs early in embryogenesis. Capillary and cavernous lymphangiomas are most frequent in areas with fibrous tissue or muscle, such as the skin, retroperitoneum (kidneys), and abdomen (colon, spleen, and liver). They may also occur in skeletal structures and within the scrotum. They probably enlarge either because of inadequate drainage of the central lymphatic channels into the internal jugular veins or because of excessive secretion from the lining cells. In general, lymphatic malformations may be categorized according to their size as lymphangioma simplex, cavernous lymphangioma, and cystic hygroma with the latter being the largest one and

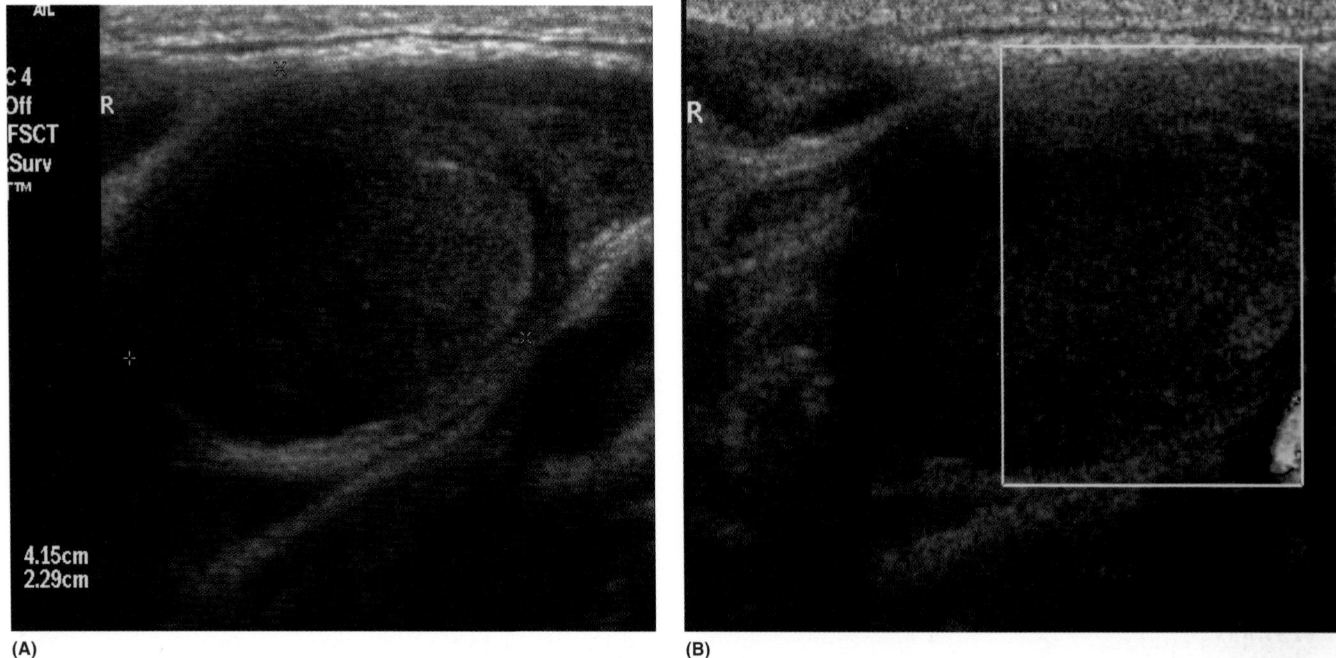

FIGURE 12 A AND B ■ Infected branchial cleft cyst. This teenage female presented with a painful swelling in her submandibular region. Gray-scale (**A**) and color Doppler (**B**) imaging demonstrate an avascular hypoechoic solid-appearing mass with no internal blood flow. Close observation during real-time imaging showed that the mass was filled with mobile echogenic material. Very thick purulent material was aspirated by fine-needle aspiration.

the most common type. The lesions consist of large, dilated cystic lymphatic spaces (72). It is currently believed that cystic hygromas and the other three types of lymphangioma (cavernous lymphangioma, capillary or simple lymphangioma, and vasculolymphatic malformations) are manifestations of the same disease process. The nature of the stroma surrounding the malformation helps to differentiate between the four types. The lesion is most likely to be a cystic hygroma when loose connective tissue surrounds the lymphatic anomaly, whereas a firmer surrounding texture is more likely seen in the other types of lymphangioma (73). Cystic hygromas are composed of multiple, dilated cystic spaces separated by minimal thin intervening stroma. The cysts vary in diameter from a few millimeters to more than 10 cm and most contain chylous fluid. If the mass is very large, it may extend across the midline. They typically increase in size as the child grows, and they may show rapid increase in size in association with upper respiratory infection (viral, with large amounts of lymphatic fluid produced from the lymphoid follicles in the cyst wall) or intralesional hemorrhage (spontaneous or secondary to trauma) (74). Most occur in children with normal karyotype, but there is an increased incidence in genetic syndromes such as Noonan's syndrome, Turner's syndrome, and trisomy 21.

Cystic hygromas typically present as painless soft or semifirm masses in the posterior triangle of the neck. The very large mass may fill one side of the neck and if there is mediastinal extension, esophageal and/or airway compression may result. Other reported clinical manifestations include facial nerve paralysis, dysphagia, or other feeding problems (75). Chylothorax and chylopericardium may occur as complications of mediastinal involvement.

Sonographically, cystic hygroma is typically a well-defined multilocular cystic mass with thin walls and contains hypo- or anechoic fluid (Fig. 13). Less commonly, cystic hygromas are unilocular (74). The mass usually contains septa of variable thickness. Solid echogenic components may arise from the septa or cyst wall. Phleboliths (small punctate calcifications) may be observed within the lesion. In the presence of infection or hemorrhage within the mass, the internal contents may be heterogeneously echogenic with possible septations. Infiltration into adjacent soft tissues is common with larger lesions. With color Doppler, the mass is predominantly avascular, although color signal may be observed within the soft-tissue components.

The preferred treatment of lymphatic malformations is surgical excision, but complete excision may be difficult when the lesions are microcystic and infiltrative. The treatment for macrocystic lesions may include percutaneous sclerotherapy (including alcohol solution), cyclophosphamide, bleomycin, doxycycline, and OK-432 (76–79). OK-432 is proven to be an effective treatment modality for macrocystic-type lymphangiomas in the head and neck region as it has no complications, and surgical excision in case of failure is not compromised by fibrosis as it can be in other types of sclerotherapy (79).

Cervical Thymic Cysts

During embryonic life, the thymus descends from the third branchial pouch into the mediastinum and maintains a connection via the thymopharyngeal duct, which generally involutes during embryonic life (Fig. 14). Cervical thymic cysts arise from vestiges of the thymopharyngeal duct or from areas of cystic degeneration of the thymus gland and may be found anywhere along the path of the thymopharyngeal duct, immediately adjacent to the carotid sheath from the angle of the mandible to the

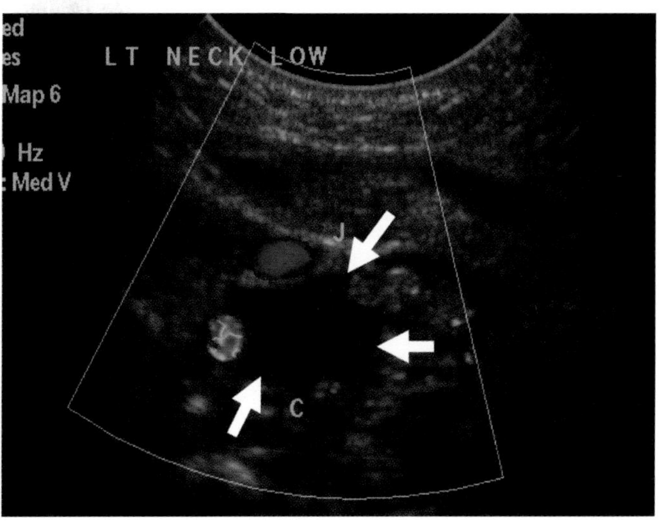

(A)

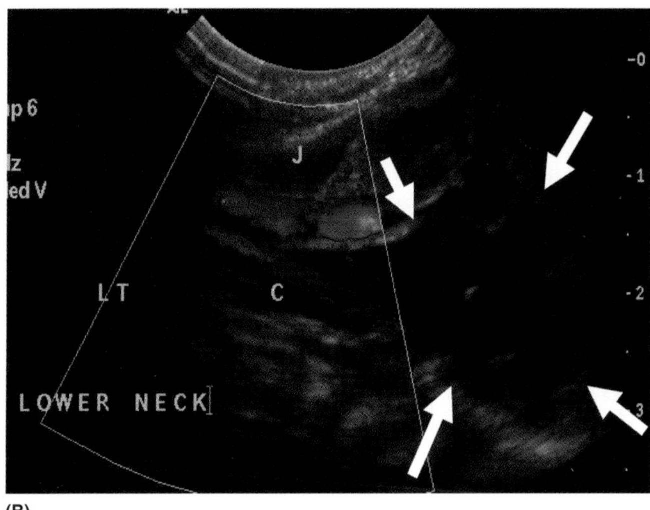

(B)

FIGURE 13 A–E ■ Cystic hygroma extending into the mediastinum. Gray-scale/color Doppler imaging in transverse (**A**) and sagittal (**B**) planes shows complex space-occupying lesion composed of multiple fluid collections invaginated between and displacing the carotid artery and the jugular vein. (*Continued*)

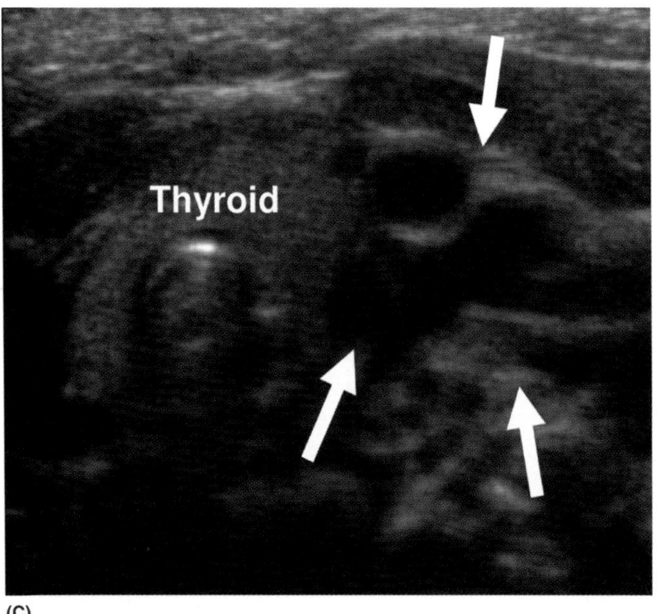

(C)

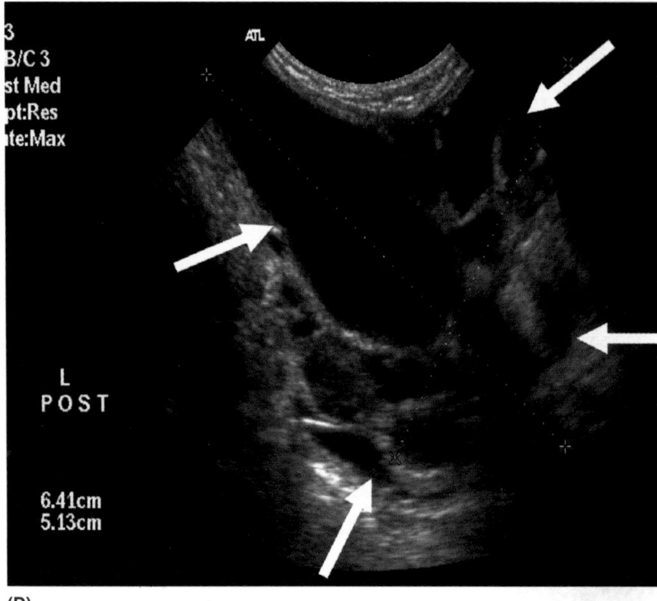

(D)

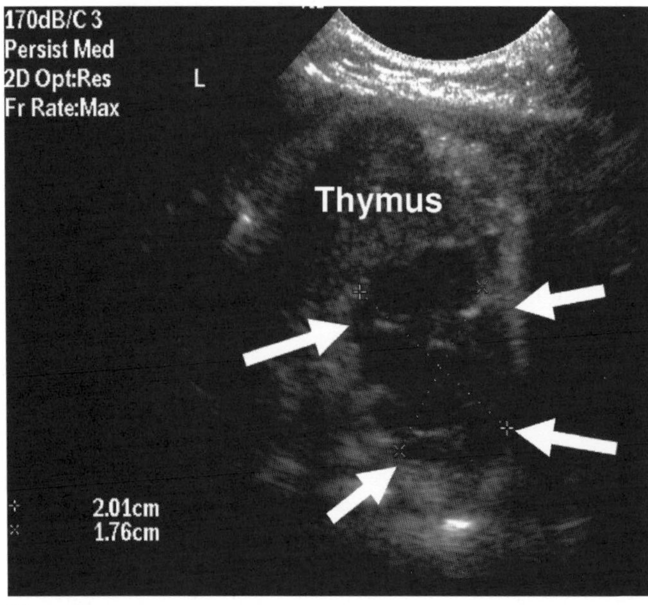

(E)

FIGURE 13 A–E ■ (*Continued*) In (**C**), the lesion extends lateral to the left lobe of the thyroid, displacing this structure anterosuperiorly with the bulkiest portion extending posterolaterally (**D**) and the most inferior extent posterolateral to the normal appearing thymus (**E**). *Arrows*, lesion in all images.

thoracic inlet (80,81). They may splay the carotid artery and jugular vein, especially when they involve the suprahyoid neck. Up to 50% of cervical thymic cysts will be continuous with the mediastinal thymus (82). The lesions have been observed by some authors to be more commonly located on the left side (81). Their shape is quite variable with a spectrum ranging from a 1 cm round cyst to a 26 cm long persistent thymopharyngeal duct cyst that extends into the mediastinum (83). Thymic cysts present as slowly growing, painless, and nontender masses in the lateral aspect of the lower third of the neck, either anterior or deep in the SCM muscle (81,84). Cervical thymic cysts are very uncommon lesions, with approximately 75% diagnosed during the first decade of life and the remainder in the second and third decades. Most of the lesions are asymptomatic and are discovered incidentally (75,82,85). However, they may less commonly present with dysphagia, stridor, or hoarseness, and with respiratory distress in the newborn (85–88). They may suddenly enlarge during a Valsalva maneuver (due to elevation of the thymus of vascular engorgement from increased intrathoracic pressure) or may enlarge secondary to hemorrhage or viral infection (85).

Sonographically, the thymic cyst is a well-marginated, hypoechoic mass that is generally unilocular but may be multilocular. The mass extends downward, parallel to the SCM muscle, and may extend into the mediastinum (83,86). When the cyst contains blood or protein, the echogenicity within the contained fluid increases. Most often, the masses are found anterior to the SCM muscle, although they can extend posterior to it. Sonography lends itself extremely well to demonstrating

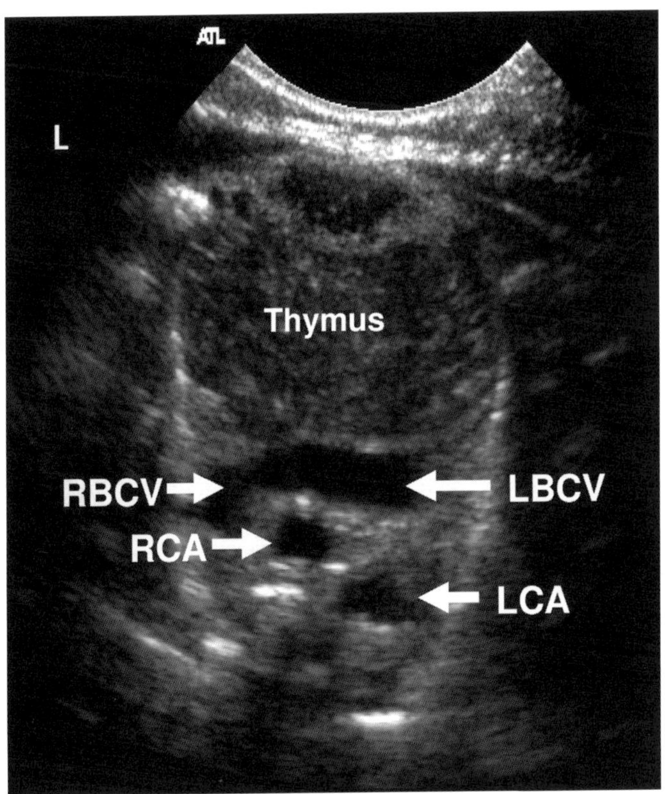

(A)

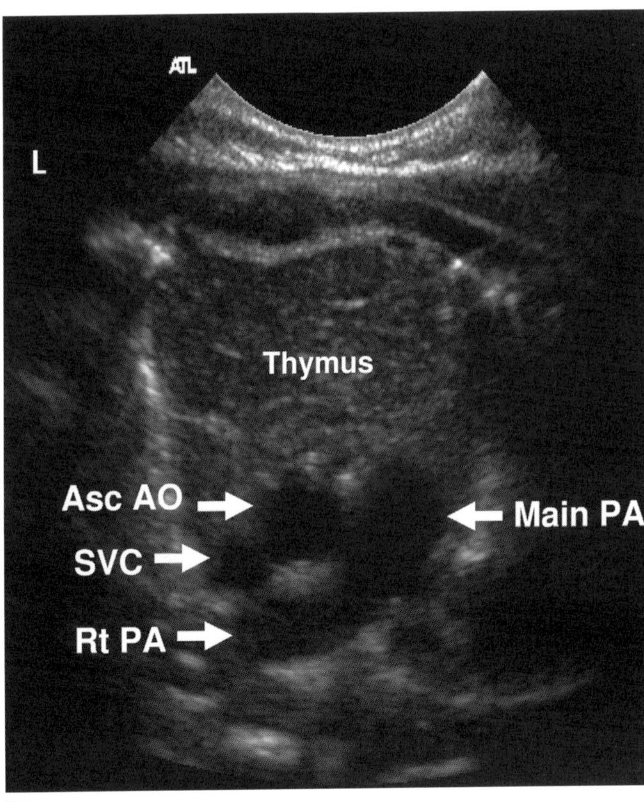

(B)

FIGURE 14 A AND B ■ Normal thymus. Transverse images of the thymus at the level of the brachiocephalic veins (**A**) and at the level of the great vessels (**B**) demonstrate the typical echopattern of normal thymic tissue: multiple linear echoes and discrete echogenic foci throughout that represent connective-tissue septa and blood vessels within the septa. RBCV, right brachiocephalic vein; RCA, right carotid artery; LBCV, left brachiocephalic vein; LCA, left carotid artery; Asc Ao, ascending aorta; SVC, superior vena cava; Rt PA, right pulmonary artery; main PA, main pulmonary artery.

the continuity of the cyst with the mediastinal thymus by using a suprasternal notch and intercostal scanning approach.

Cervical Thymus

The aberrant cervical thymus is an uncommon entity that is most often seen in infants and young children (89–91). If the descent of the thymus is arrested during embryonic life, the thymus may be located in the neck and present as a lateral or midline soft neck mass above the level of the left brachiocephalic vein. The echotexture of the mass is that of normal thymus and can be shown to be in anatomic continuity with the normally positioned thymus in the superior anterior mediastinum (Fig. 15). In order to confirm that the mass is in fact cervical thymus, one must demonstrate the typical echopattern of normal thymic tissue, which includes multiple linear echoes and discrete echogenic foci throughout, which represent connective-tissue septa and blood vessels within the septa (92).

This condition does not require therapy or surgery unless it causes symptoms or problems, as one would not choose to remove the thymus that plays an important role in the development of the immune system (93).

Hemangiomas and Hemangiolymphangiomas

Hemangiomas and hemangiolymphangiomas are usually found in younger patients, localized to the skin or involving the deeper soft tissues of the neck. They are benign masses composed of vascular channels lined by endothelial cells. The two major histologic types include capillary hemangiomas (capillary-sized vascular spaces with few, if any, recognizable erythrocytes) and cavernous hemangiomas (contain larger, dilated, erythrocyte-filled vascular spaces). At times, both types may be contained within the same lesion (94).

Hemangiomas result from endothelial proliferation with hyperplasia of these cells that grow rapidly. They typically present as soft, fluctuant masses or as diffuse infiltrative skin lesions in children less than six months of age. They gradually increase in size over the next two years and spontaneously involute over the next five to seven years. The overlying skin may have a bluish discoloration and the lesion is usually compressible. Bruits may be heard over the lesions and other similar lesions may be noted elsewhere in the body. At times, the children with very large hemangiomas develop the Kasabach–Merritt syndrome (thrombocytopenic coagulopathy),

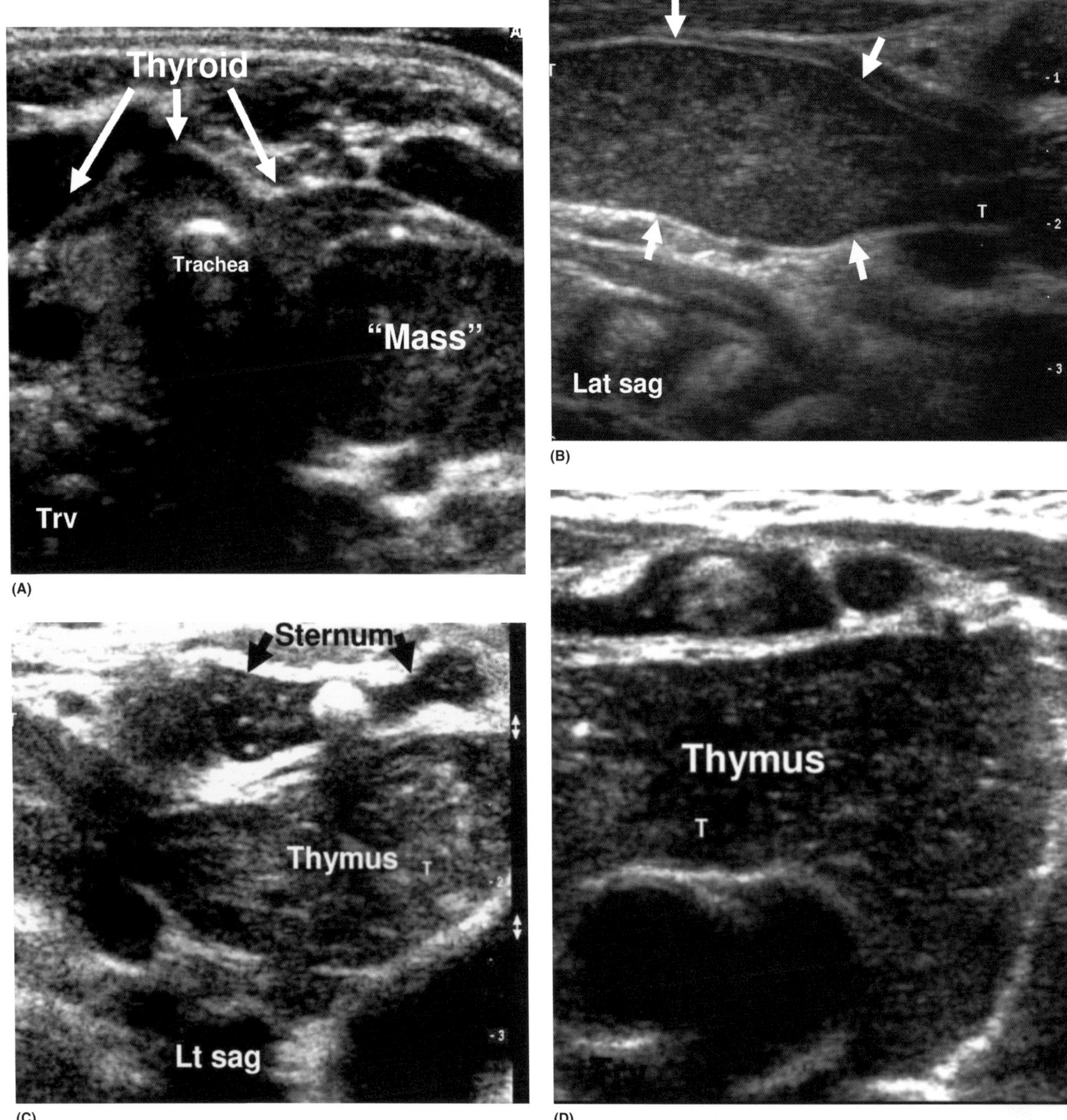

FIGURE 15 A–D ■ Ectopic thymus. Asymptomatic left-sided neck mass was noted coincidentally. Transverse sonogram at the level of the thymus (**A**) shows a solid "mass," which on sagittal view (**B**) is noted in the upper mediastinum. The mass passes posterior to the sternum (**C**) and is in continuity with the normal-appearing thymus in the anterior superior mediastinum (**D**).

which has a poor prognosis with a 30% to 40% mortality rate (95,96).

During the stage of involution, they demonstrate decrease in size and evidence of fatty infiltration. In the infant, treatment consists of watchful waiting. In the infant with airway compromise or associated significant loss of skin integrity, steroids, interferon, and rarely, surgery are employed. In the older child who presents with a similarly appearing mass without a history of hemangioma in infancy, the question of sarcoma rather than hemangioma must be raised. Sonographically, hemangiomas are hypoechoic masses. The smaller masses are usually homogeneous and the larger masses tend to be heterogeneous due to the presence of a multitude of interfaces, proteinaceous material, or areas of thrombosis and fibrosis.

Hemangiomas are usually well defined, although larger lesions may infiltrate adjacent soft tissues. At times, they contain small punctate echodensities, representing phleboliths. Color/pulsed Doppler imaging is extremely helpful in documenting the hypervascular nature of the lesion and the feeding arteries (94). Unlike hemangiomas, vascular malformations are composed of morphologically normal vascular tissue, which can include arterial, capillary, venous, lymphatic, or a combination of the four tissue types. These do not regress spontaneously but tend to grow proportionately with the child. Both hemangiomas and vascular malformations demonstrate a highly vascular lesion with the internal vessels clustered in close contiguity (95,96). Hemangiomas typically demonstrate a high diastolic flow and low resistive index. The Doppler findings are variable in vascular malformations and dependent on the predominant vascular tissue type present. Venous malformations are congenital anomalies that generally do not present until adolescence and may invade adjacent muscle and bone. These may result in disfigurement and are characterized by stasis. Thrombus and phleboliths may be present within the variable-size large-venous channels. Venous malformations are typically compressible with little flow and low vessel density characteristic.

Conservative management of hemangiomas is usual, as these lesions usually regress spontaneously. If vital airway structures are compromised, corticosteroids, interferon, laser, embolization, and surgical excision are potential therapies. On the other hand, therapy for symptomatic vascular malformations is necessary, as these lesions do not regress spontaneously. Treatment can include embolization, surgical resection, and laser ablation (97–100).

Duplex/color Doppler imaging is very useful not only to demonstrate the vascular nature of a mass and the depth, but also to demonstrate other reasons for the neck mass that may in fact be jugular phlebectasia (jugular vein enlarges during Valsalva maneuver) or an ectatic carotid artery (Figs. 16 and 17) (31,101).

Teratomas, Dermoid Cysts, and Epidermoid Cysts

The neck is the second most common location for teratomas after the sacrum (102). Those located in the neck have less malignant potential than those found in the sacrum. Teratoma is a developmental lesion arising from pluripotential embryonal cells and contains elements from all three germ layers (ectoderm, endoderm, and mesoderm). These lesions have both solid and cystic components

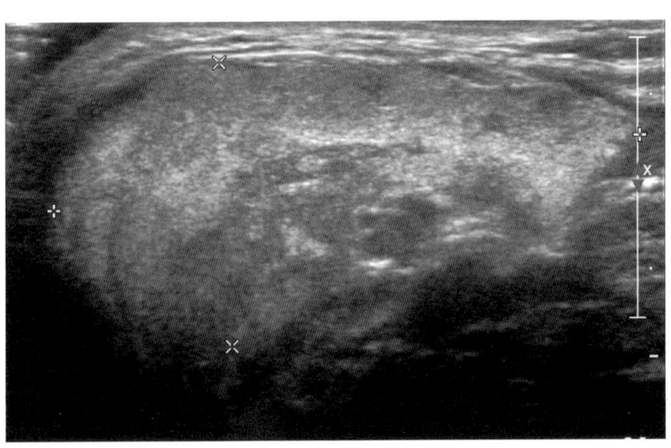
(A)

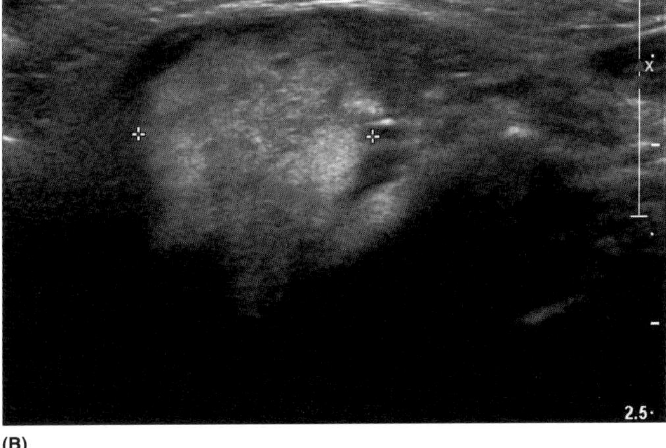

(B)

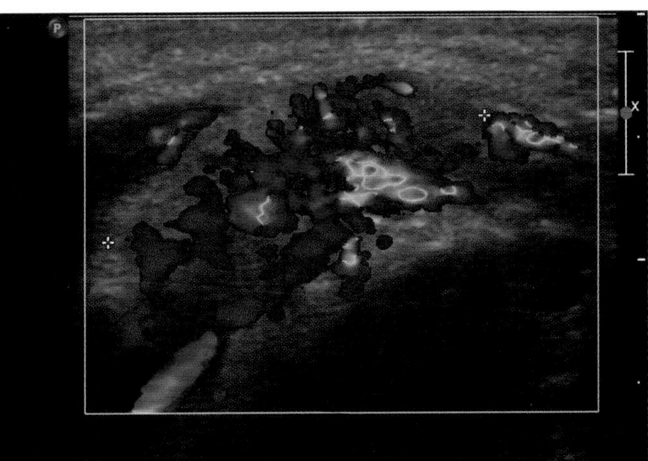
(C)

FIGURE 16 A–C ■ Hemangioma. Thirteen-month-old infant with right neck mass posterior to sternocleidomastoid muscle. Sagittal (**A**) and transverse (**B**) grayscale US images demonstrate a fairly well defined subcutaneous mass which is clearly hypervascular with color Doppler imaging (**C**).

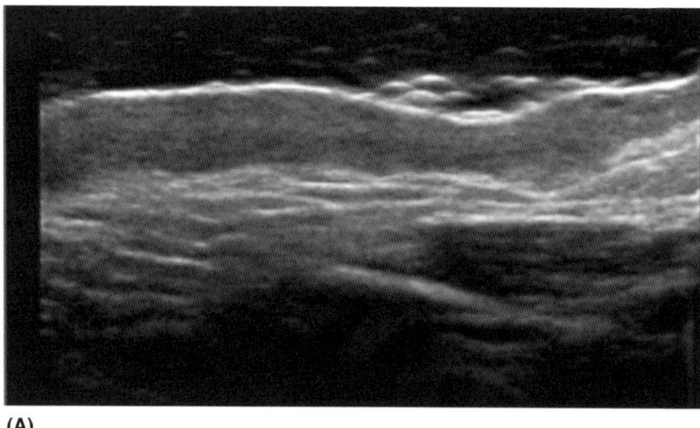
(A)

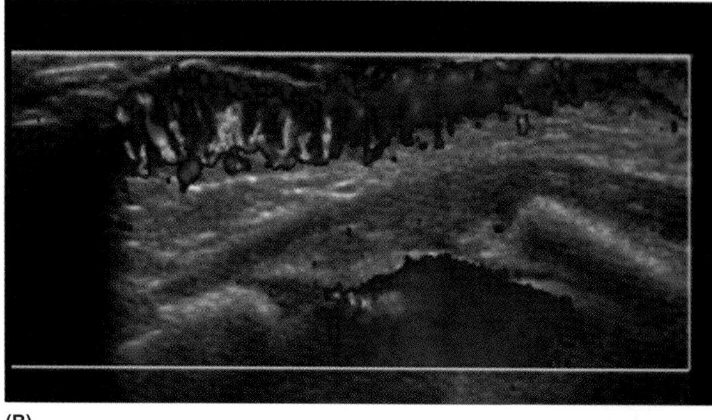
(B)

FIGURE 17 A AND B ■ Hemangioma. Two-month-old with reddish colored, firm left shoulder/neck mass. US requested to determine the depth of the lesion for treatment planning. Grayscale (**A**) and color Doppler (**B**) imaging demonstrated the well-defined nature of this cutaneous mass. Note the extreme hypervascularity.

as well as elements of fat and calcifications. In the rare situation when a teratoma is purely cystic, it may mimic a branchial cleft cyst or thyroglossal duct cyst.

When they are very large and bulky, the children may have stridor, dyspnea, or dysphagia and it is therefore extremely important to rapidly establish the extent of the mass so that complete resection can be accomplished, as there is high morbidity and mortality associated with recurrence (103).

Dermoid cysts are developmental lesions arising from pluripotential embryonal cells and contain elements from two germ layers (ectoderm and mesoderm) (104). Dermoid cysts may contain squamous epithelium and skin appendages such as hair follicles, sweat glands, and sebaceous glands. Epidermoid cysts contain only squamous epithelium. These lesions are very rare and when they do occur, they are due to entrapment of ectodermal elements underneath the skin present in the submental region above the hyoid bone or off midline, adjacent to or within a thyroid lobe (105). These lesions are generally hypoechoic to subcutaneous fat and demonstrate well-defined walls. They often contain echogenic areas reflecting the presence of fat, calcification, or soft tissue.

Carotid Body Tumors

Carotid body tumors are located high in the neck in the notch of the carotid bifurcation. They are generally solid, slightly heterogeneous masses that range in size from 1.2 to 5.0 cm (Fig. 18) (106). They and other glomus-type tumors are fed by the external carotid artery and are highly vascular with a high diastolic flow pattern in the external carotid artery.

Neoplasms

Lymphoma is the third most common malignant tumor in children and accounts for approximately 50% of head and neck malignances in children (107). Rhabdomyosarcoma accounts for approximately 10% to 15% of cervical malignancies with other tumors including neuroblastoma, other sarcomas (neurofibrosarcoma, fibrosarcoma), and Langerhans' histiocytosis (108,109). Rarely, squamous-cell carcinoma occurs in the head and neck in children. Castleman's disease and Rosai–Dorfman syndrome may be confused with malignant neck masses (110).

Lymphoma

Approximately 60% of cervical involvement with lymphoma is due to Hodgkin's disease and 40% due to non-Hodgkin's lymphoma. There are no imaging characteristics to differentiate between these types. The small, noncleaved histologic subtype of non-Hodgkin's lymphoma is the most common type in the pediatric neck while the nodular sclerosing form is the most common histologic subtype of Hodgkin's disease in children. The children with non-Hodgkin's disease are typically younger than 10 years of age and those with Hodgkin's are more likely to be in the second decade of life. They present with painless, enlarged cervical adenopathy most likely in the upper neck, either in a unilateral or in a bilateral distribution. The appearance of the mass(es) may simulate cervical adenitis, making tissue sampling mandatory for differentiation. Lymphomatous nodes are frequently larger and more extensive than inflammatory adenopathy (107).

In Hodgkin's lymphoma and non-Hodgkin's lymphoma, lymph nodes tend to be round, hypoechoic, without an echogenic hilum and tend to show intranodal reticulation (Fig. 19). The nodes may be discretely enlarged or appear as a conglomerate soft-tissue mass (107–111). With pulsed Doppler, there is moderate flow (20–50 cm/sec) and high RI and PI values. With color Doppler imaging, both hilar and peripheral flow may be seen (112,113).

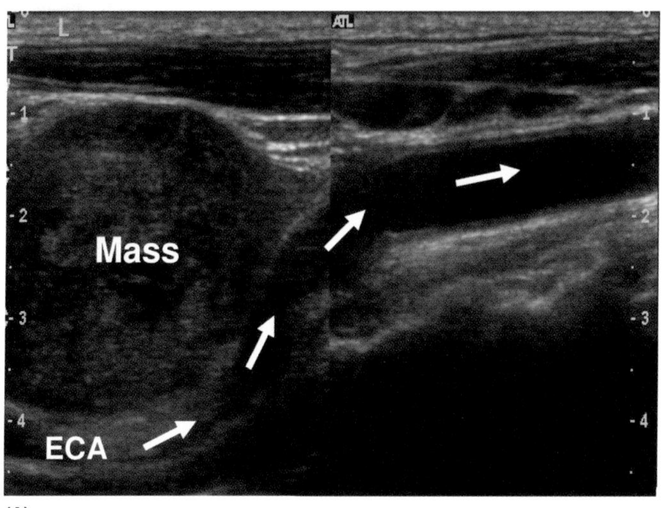

(A)

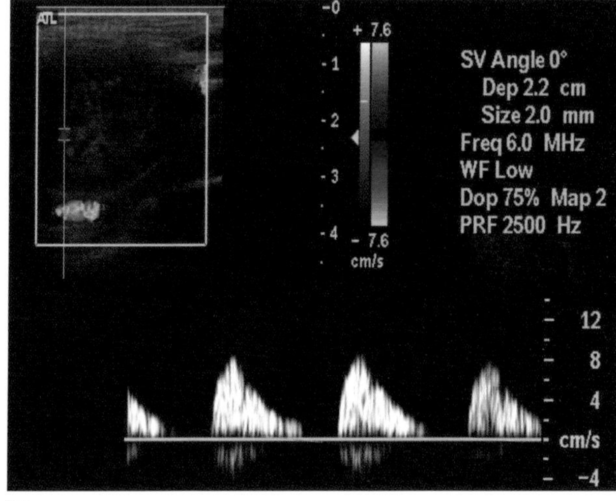

(B)

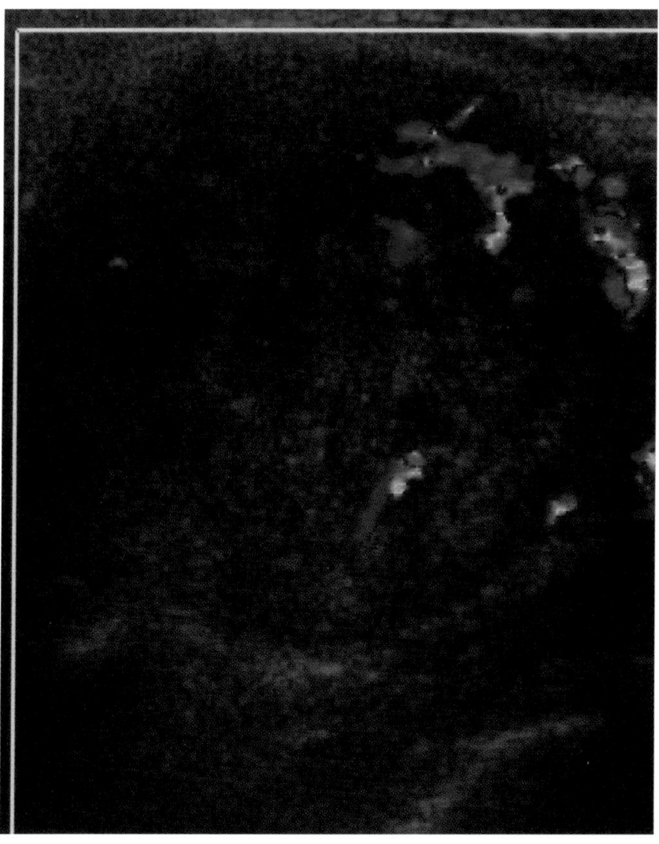

(C)

FIGURE 18 A–C ■ Carotid body tumor. A solid lesion is demonstrated in the neck at the level of the bifurcation of the common carotid bifurcation, which compresses and deviates the external carotid artery branch posteriorly (**A**). The lesion is hypervascular by color and pulsed Doppler (**B**) and (**C**).

Neurogenic Tumors

Neuroblastomas (Fig. 20) and neurofibromas constitute the most common neurogenic tumors found in the neck region of children, with ganglioneuromas and schwannomas (Fig. 21) occurring less often (114,115). Neuroblastoma is the most common malignant tumor in children less than one year of age, with most lesions arising from the adrenal gland or the retroperitoneum. Less than 10% of neuroblastomas arise in the neck and are most often due to metastatic disease. The children typically present with a painless, firm, lateral neck mass, although at times, the tumor may cause airway obstruction, dysphagia, hoarseness, Horner's syndrome (ptosis, miosis, and anhidrosis), paralysis of the lower cranial nerves, and opsoclonus, myoclonus, and cerebellar ataxia.

Sonographically, neurogenic tumors are elliptical or round, hypoechoic solid masses posterior to the carotid sheath vessels in a paraspinal location, with or without intraspinal extension and with or without calcifications.

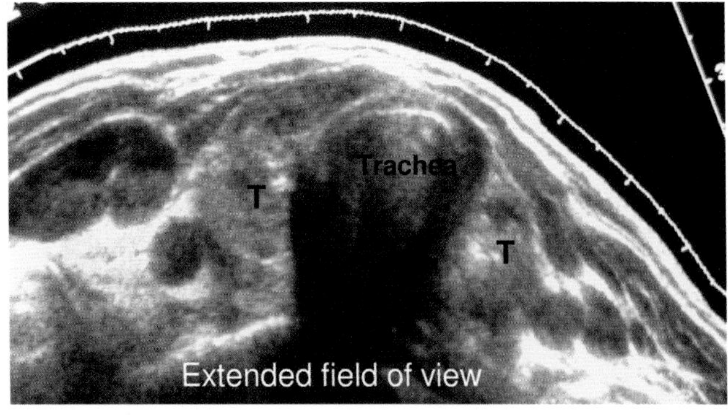

(A)

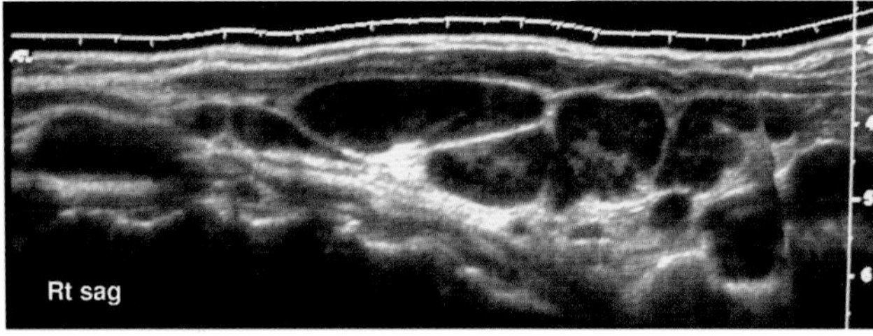

(B)

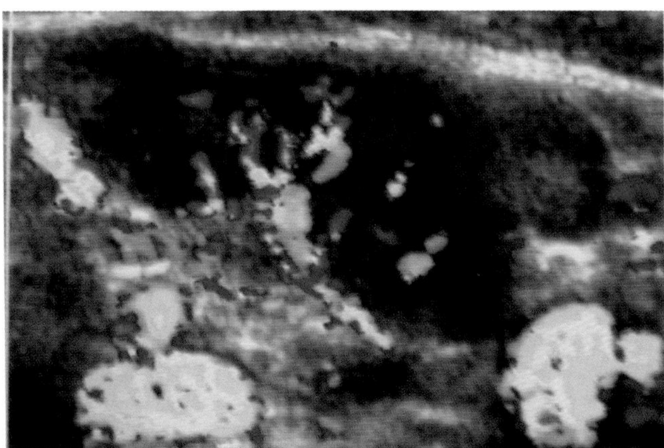

(C)

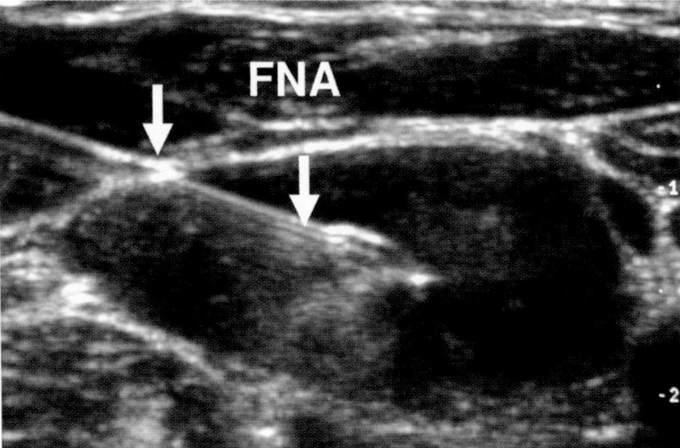

(D)

FIGURE 19 A–D ■ Lymphoma. Transverse (**A**) scan at the level of the thyroid gland shows multiple enlarged lymph nodes bilaterally with distortion of the internal architecture of the nodes. The extended field of view (**B**) demonstrates the extent of the nodes on the left side of the neck. Color Doppler imaging (**C**) shows hypervascularity of the irregular-appearing vessels within the nodes. Fine-needle aspiration performed under US guidance (**D**) proved the presence of lymphoma.

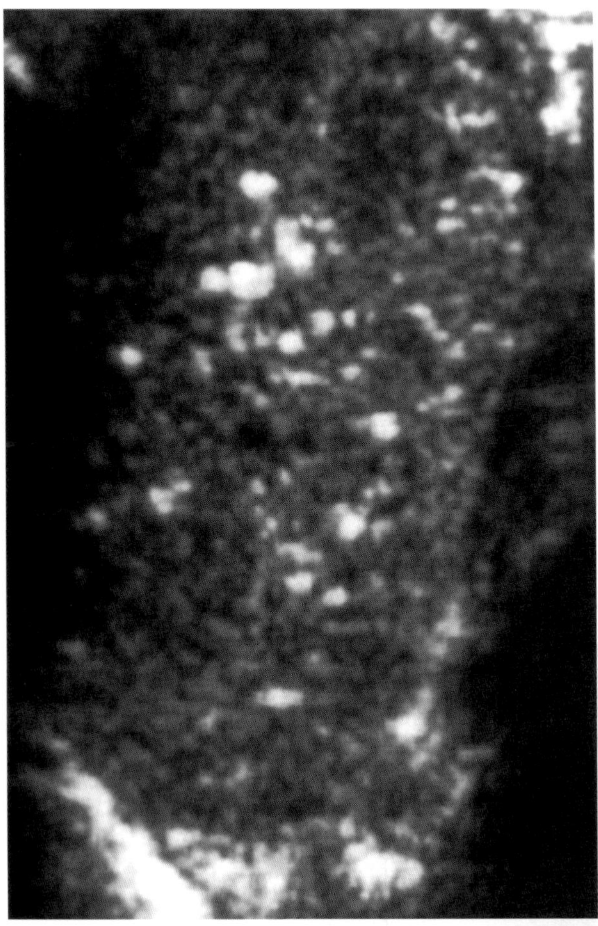

FIGURE 20 ■ Neuroblastoma. One-year-old with difficulty breathing presented with a solid neck mass that extended into the retropharyngeal space. Fine calcifications are noted throughout the mass. *Source*: From Ref. 4.

Fifty percent of the tumors contain calcifications and the tumors often infiltrate the surrounding soft tissues, contain irregular margins, encase regional blood vessels, and extend into the spinal canal. MRI is indicated to establish the entire extent of the tumor including intraspinal extension. Rarely, cystic neuroblastoma may occur and be confused with cystic hygroma or teratoma.

Rhabdomyosarcoma

Rhabdomyosarcoma is the most common soft-tissue sarcoma of childhood with approximately 35% to 40% of all rhabdomyosarcomas occurring in the head and neck in children, with the embryonal form being the most common histologic subtype in the head and neck (109,116). The children are generally less than 10 years of age and present with an enlarging painless mass. Rhabdomyosarcoma is an aggressive, infiltrating malignancy that grows rapidly, tends to invade adjacent structures, and metastasizes to regional lymph nodes, lung, bone, bone marrow, brain, and liver. Other sarcomas (malignant fibrous histiocytoma, fibrosarcoma,

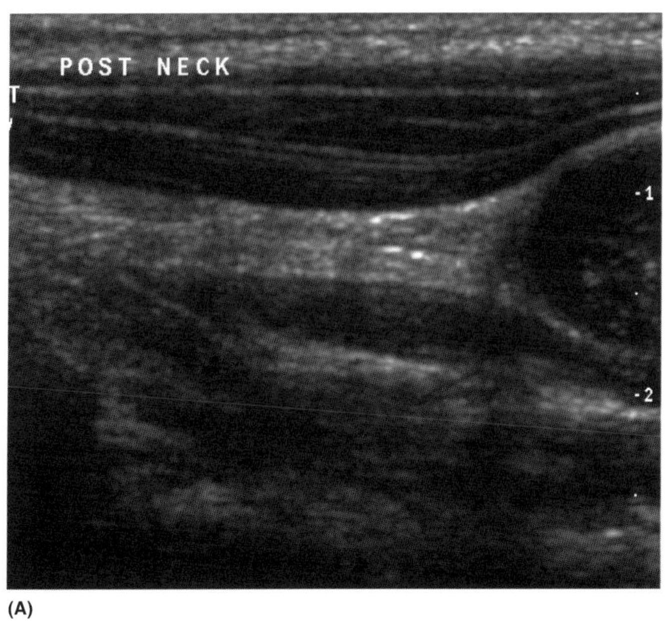

(A)

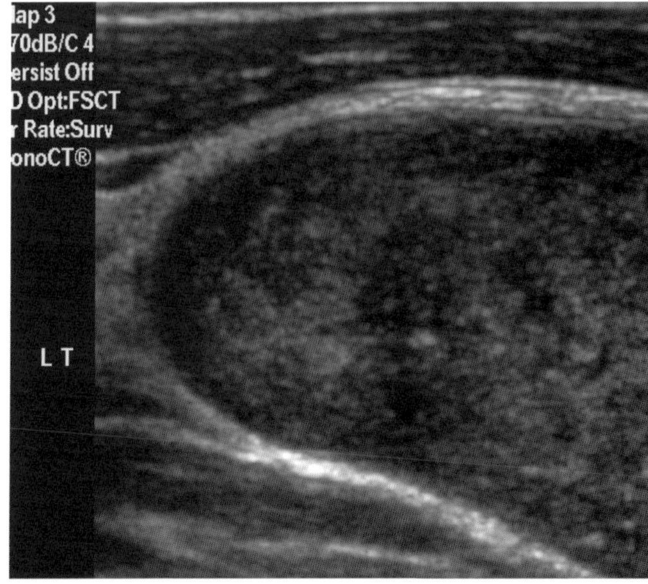

(B)

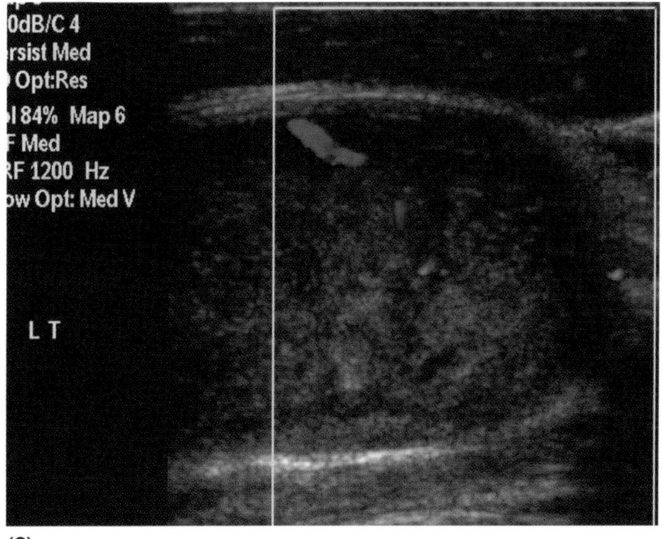

(C)

FIGURE 21 A–C ■ Schwannoma. Sagittal sonograms of this solid mass show that the mass arises from a nerve (**A**), is solid (**B**), and is mildly vascular (**C**).

myosarcoma, neurofibrosarcoma, and angiosarcoma) occur more rarely (117).

Sonographically, rhabdomyosarcoma resembles neuroblastoma as regards echotexture and vascular encasement. The arterial velocity is markedly increased, however, with the arterial flow velocity greater than 1 m/sec on spectral Doppler. MRI is indicated for determination of extent of disease (117).

PAROTID GLAND

There are three major groups of salivary glands: the parotid glands, the submandibular glands, and the sublingual glands (118). The parotid gland is the largest of the salivary glands and is bound anteriorly by the ramus of the mandible and the masseter muscle and posteriorly by the mastoid process and the SCM muscle. The normal gland is hyperechoic compared with the adjacent masseter muscle, reflecting the presence of fatty glandular tissue (Fig. 22). The gland is often homogeneous, but it may appear heterogeneous when it contains multiple lymph nodes (119). The gland has an elliptical shape on coronal images and appears round or oval in shape on transverse scans. The submandibular gland is bordered superiorly by the mylohyoid muscle and laterally by the body of the mandible while the sublingual glands lie in the floor of the mouth deep in the mylohyoid muscle and superficial to the hypoglossus muscle.

Salivary gland neoplasms are rare in childhood, accounting for 8% of all pediatric head and neck tumors. The ratio of benign to malignant salivary gland neoplasms varies from 50% to 70% with most (80–95%) tumors occurring in the parotid gland (120,121). During infancy and early childhood, the most common salivary gland neoplasms are due to vascular lesions such as

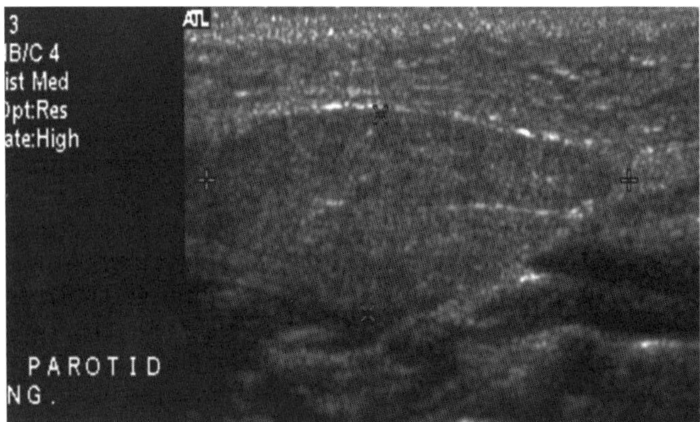

FIGURE 22 ■ Normal parotid gland. The normal parotid gland is elliptical shaped in the sagittal plane), is generally hyperechoic in comparison with the masseter muscle, and is homogeneous, except when the gland contains lymph nodes.

hemangiomas, hemangioendotheliomas, or lymphangiomas. These lesions usually present as nontender masses. Bluish discoloration of the skin may be noted with underlying hemangiomatous lesions (Fig. 23). Malignant neoplasms are usually (60%) due to mucoepidermoid and acinar cell carcinomas, the former most common in childhood (107,121). Less often, undifferentiated cancer, adenocarcinoma, malignant mixed tumor, adenoid cystic cancer, squamous-cell cancer, embryoma, and sialoblastoma are seen. The children usually present with a painless, enlarging lump in the salivary gland. There are no clinical features that differentiate with certainty between benign and malignant lesions. Features suggesting malignancy would include history of rapid growth, fixation to the skin or deep tissues, cervical lymphadenopathy, and/or presence of facial nerve weakness or paralysis. The best opportunity for cure lies in complete surgical removal of the neoplasm at the time of initial treatment.

Most salivary gland enlargements are due to either acute or chronic inflammatory process, either unilateral or bilateral (122). Acute salivary gland inflammation is usually due to viral or bacterial etiology. It is usually unilateral, although it can be bilateral. Conditions such as tuberculosis, mycobacterial infections, toxoplasmosis, sarcoidosis, and AIDS may cause salivary gland inflammation, enlargement, and dysfunction of the gland associated with enlarged lymph nodes into and outside the parotid gland. The US findings include heterogeneity of the gland due to multiple hypoechoic nodules, which are thought to be due to intraparotid nodes or abscesses (Figs. 24 and 25). Inflammation of either the Stenson or the Wharton duct due to an obstruction near the orifice of the duct can lead to sialodochitis with calculi noted within the ductal structures. Calculi may also be seen within the parenchyma of the gland. Associated cervical adenopathy may be present as well. Color Doppler imaging demonstrates increased vascularity within the gland (119,123). With human immunodeficiency virus, which is often a bilateral process, parotid enlargement is seen with a heterogeneous echo pattern due to multiple hypoechoic or anechoic areas separated by thickened septa that show no acoustic enhancement, reflecting the presence of lymphoid infiltration and lymphoepithelial cysts within the substance of the gland (124). Chronic or recurrent inflammation of the parotid glands or their associated ducts is generally manifested by intermittent unilateral or bilateral swelling of the parotid glands, neck pain, fever, and malaise. It may be due to recurrent bacterial infections, autoimmune disease, prior irradiation, granulomatous disease, or cystic fibrosis (119,125). Sonographically, the

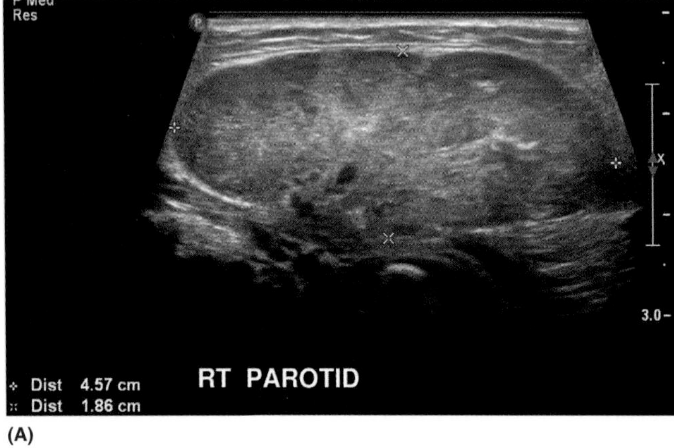

(A)

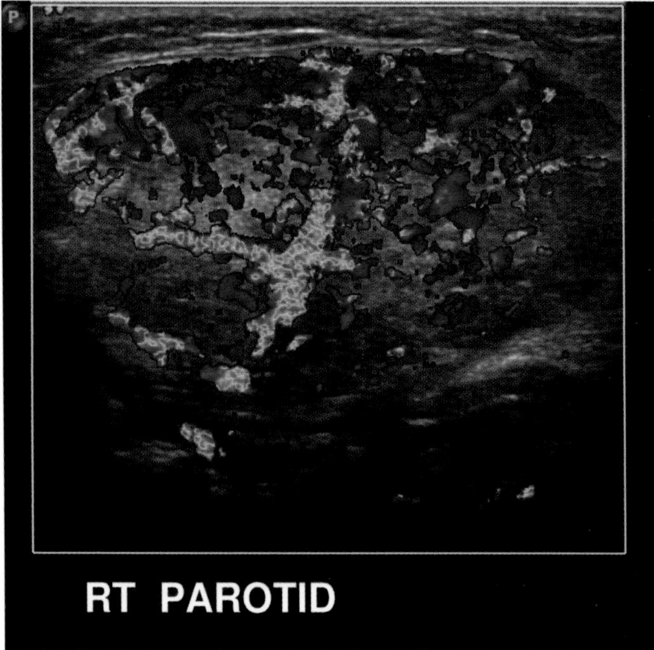

(B)

FIGURE 23 A AND B ■ Parotid hemangioma. This 3-month-old baby presented with a 2 week history of a right neck mass. Sonography revealed a 4.6 × 1.9 × 3.6 cm heterogenous solid mass (A) that totally replaced the right parotid gland and demonstrates marked hypervascularity.

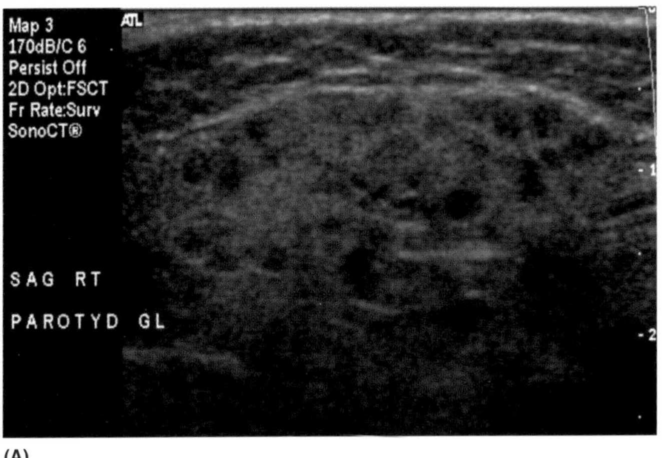

(A)

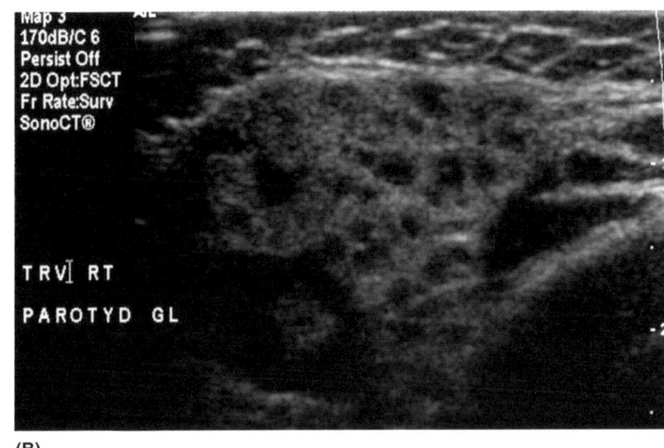

(B)

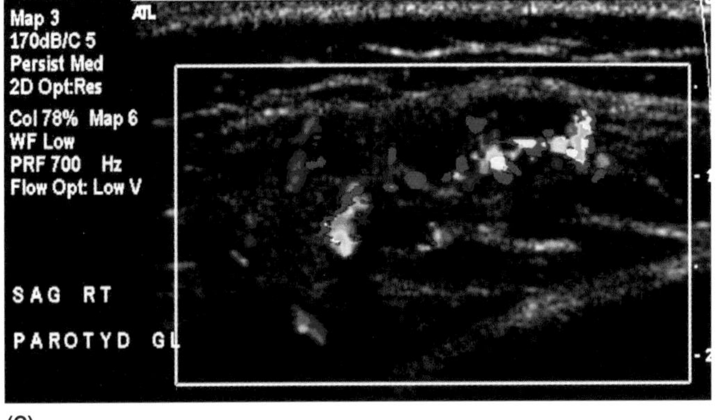

(C)

FIGURE 24 A–C ■ Parotitis. This 10-year-old girl presented with swelling on one side of her neck. The parotid gland is enlarged and there are multiple, small, hypoechoic areas seen throughout the gland on both sagittal (**A**) and transverse (**B**) scans. Color Doppler imaging (**C**) shows the hypervascular nature of the gland.

chronically inflamed gland appears heterogeneous due to small punctate echogenic densities due to parenchymal calcifications, mucus within areas of ductal ectasia or the walls of ectatic ducts, and multiple hypoechoic areas (measuring 2–4 mm in diameter) that are thought to be due to sialectasis of the peripheral ducts and surrounding lymphocytic infiltration (125–127).

THYROID AND PARATHYROID GLANDS

Normal Anatomy and Congenital Abnormalities

The thyroid gland develops from a thickening of the primitive pharyngeal floor, the thyroid primordium, which is first recognizable in the human embryo approximately one month after conception. The developing thyroid tissue then migrates caudally, traveling through the base of the tongue and the floor of the mouth and is finally positioned anterior to the larynx and the strap muscles in the inferior part of the neck. The gland maintains its connection with the base of the tongue via the thyroglossal duct. Once the gland reaches its final destination in the lower neck, the duct atrophies and virtually disappears, with the exception of a remnant in the tongue, the foramen cecum (128).

The thyroid gland consists of paired right and left lobes on either side of the trachea in the lower anterior neck (Fig. 26). The lobes are joined at the midline by a thin bridge of thyroid tissue, the isthmus, which is draped over the anterior aspect of the trachea at the junction of the middle and lower thirds of the gland. Occasionally, an extra lobe, the pyramidal lobe, extends superiorly from the isthmus in the midline. The lobes of the gland are bordered posterolaterally by the common carotid artery and the internal jugular vein and medially by the trachea on the right and the esophagus on the left. In the upper neck, the internal jugular veins lie lateral and posterior to the common carotid artery, whereas in the lower neck, they lie anterior and lateral to the carotid artery. The SCM muscle and strap muscles (sternohyoid, sternothyroid, thyrohyoid, and omohyoid) are anterolateral to each lobe and the longus colli muscles are posterolateral to each lobe. A fibrous capsule covers the gland and fixes it to the deep pretracheal fascia, causing it to move upward with swallowing. The size of the thyroid varies with age, body surface, and weight. In infants and young children, the lateral lobe measures 1 to 1.5 cm in transverse diameter, 2 to 3 cm vertically, and 0.2 to 1.2 cm in anteroposterior diameter. In adolescents and adults, the lateral lobes measure 2 to 4 cm in transverse diameter, 5 to 8 cm vertically, and 1 to 2.5 cm in anteroposterior diameter. The right lobe is usually larger than the left (129). The gland generally appears homogeneous sonographically and relatively hyperechoic in comparison with the adjacent neck muscles. At times, tiny (3 mm) diameter anechoic areas without acoustic enhancement are seen, which are thought to be due to colloid follicles (5,130).

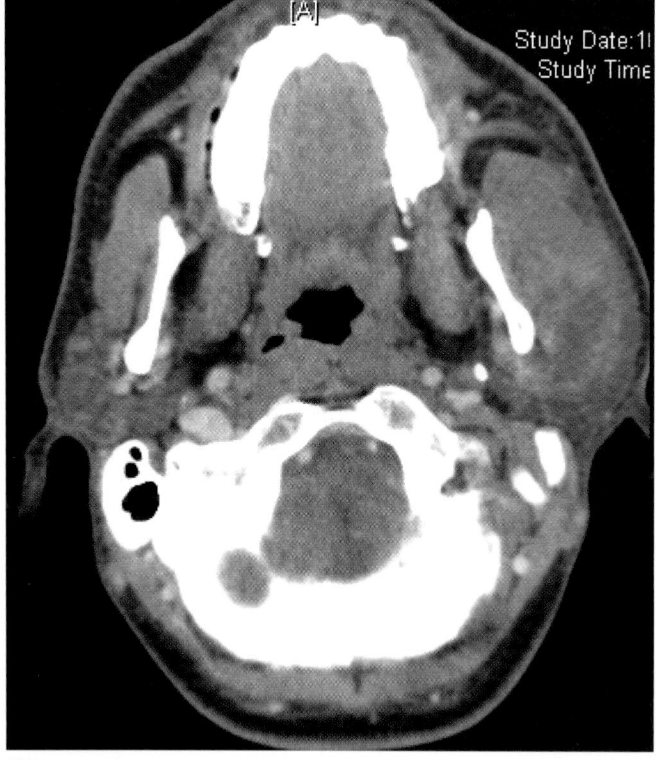

(A)

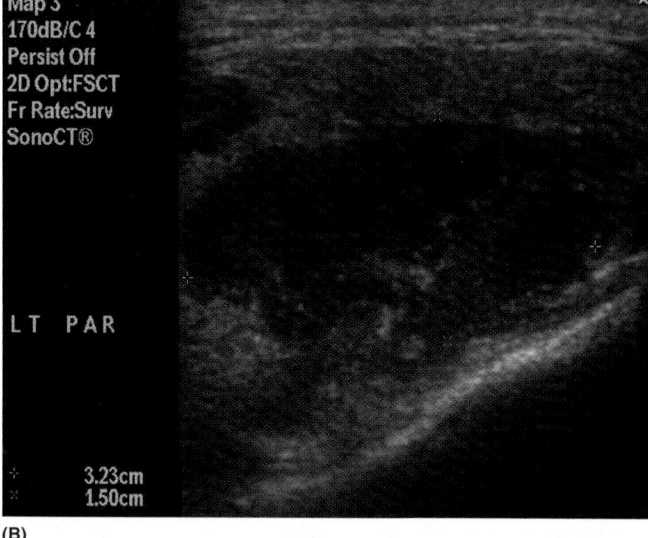

(B)

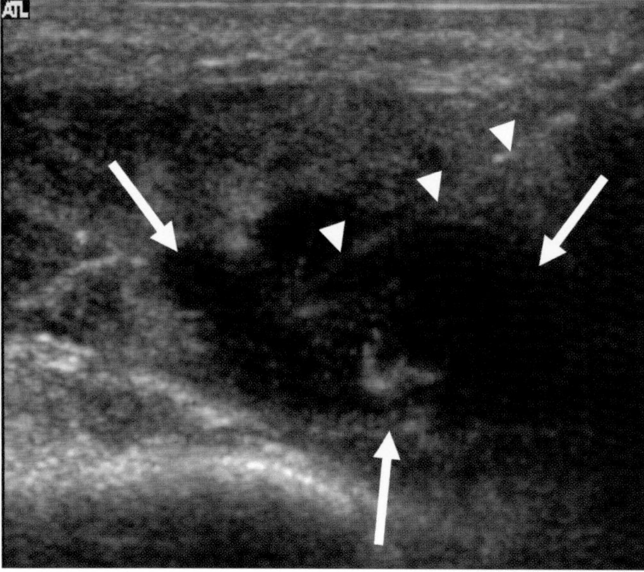
(C)

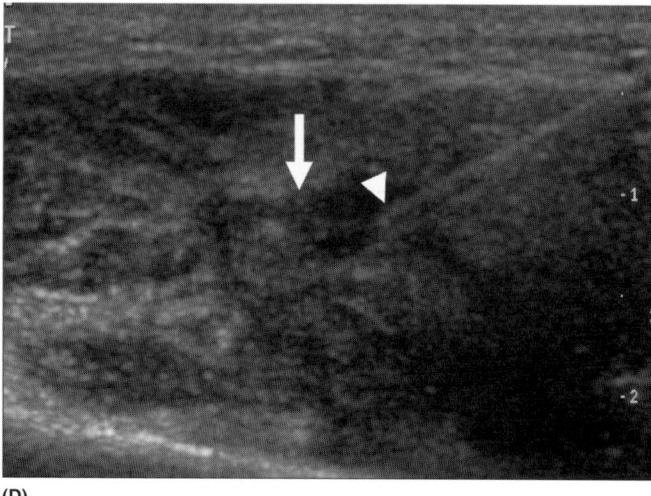
(D)

FIGURE 25 A–D ■ Parotid abscess. The child presented with swelling of the left cheek and high fever. Sagittal scan (**A**) demonstrates heterogeneity of the parotid gland with a large focal area of low-level echoes. Axial contrast-enhanced CT scan (**B**) confirms the presence of an abscess. Fine-needle aspiration under US guidance (**C**) resulted in the aspiration of 5 cc of pus. The cavity was completely empty following aspiration. (**D**) *Arrow*, abscess cavity; *arrowheads*, aspiration needle.

The normal color Doppler examination of the thyroid shows small vessels coursing throughout the thyroid parenchyma. The parathyroid glands are not usually identified but occasionally are seen as hypoechoic masses along the posteromedial aspects of the thyroid lobes.

Congenital hypothyroidism is due to a genetic enzymatic deficiency or a developmental defect in thyroid morphogenesis or dysgenesis. Dysgenesis of the thyroid gland is the most common cause accounting for at least 90% of the cases and is may be due to aplasia, hypoplasia, or ectopia. If any or all of the primordial thyroid tissue fails to descend, ectopic thyroid tissue remains in that arrested position, anywhere along the tract of the thyroglossal duct. Descent beyond the normal distance results in a mediastinal thyroid component. In 90% of cases, complete failure of descent from the foramen cecum may result in a lingual thyroid (41). In most cases, the lingual thyroid is the only functioning thyroid tissue (40). Ectopic thyroid tissue has been described in more distal locations such as the chest (heart, trachea, and thymus), abdomen (liver, gallbladder, and pancreas), axilla, and pelvis (vagina) (131,132). Hypothyroidism in patients

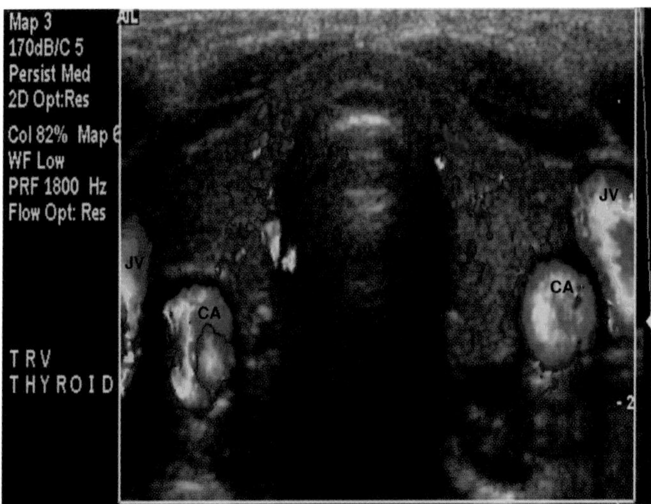

FIGURE 26 ■ Normal thyroid. The thyroid gland consists of paired right and left lobes on either side of the trachea in the lower anterior neck. The lobes are joined at the midline by a thin bridge of thyroid tissue, the isthmus, which is draped over the anterior aspect of the trachea at the junction of middle and lower thirds of the gland. CA, carotid artery; JV, jugular vein.

with an ectopic thyroid may not be detected at birth due to residual functional activity of the gland and presents later with clinical symptoms of hypothyroidism or a lingual or upper neck mass. When thyroid remnants are supernumerary to the normal thyroid gland in the neck, they may be mistaken for lymph nodes of the anterior triangle or metastases. As described earlier in this chapter, persistence of portions of the thyroglossal duct may result in a thyroglossal duct cyst (53).

Agenesis of the thyroid is uncommon and causes cretinism, leading to retardation of both physical and intellectual growth. Congenital hypothyroidism may also be caused by a genetic enzymatic deficiency, most commonly due to absence of peroxidase with failure of oxidation of iodide to iodine, resulting in trapping of iodide but no organification. In this condition, the thyroid is normally positioned and demonstrates normal echotexture. The thyroid-stimulating hormone (TSH) is elevated, which leads to enlargement, particularly of the pyramidal lobe of the thyroid (131). Rare causes of hypothyroidism in neonates include end-organ unresponsiveness to thyroid hormones and maternal medications for the treatment of hyperthyroidism.

Thyroid Nodules

Thyroid nodules are rare in children and most often benign (Fig. 27). The adenoma is the most common cause of a thyroid nodule in children and is thought to result from cycles of hyperplasia and involution of thyroid lobules. This lesion is also known as nodular adenomatous goiter, adenomatous goiter, and adenomatous nodule. Most adenomas are hypoechoic relative to the normal thyroid gland, although some are hyperechoic and a few isoechoic (133,134). About 60% of cases demonstrate a hypoechoic halo or rim around the lesion, which measures 1 to 2 mm in depth and may represent pericapsular inflammatory infiltrate, compressed thyroid parenchyma, or the fibrous capsule. They may contain shadowing calcifications and hypoechoic or anechoic areas due to internal hemorrhage and necrosis. Colloid follicles may be visualized as small cystic areas and may contain echogenic inspissated colloid. The sonographic appearance of a nodule being completely hypoechoic or anechoic is most often associated with benign lesions. Color Doppler imaging usually demonstrates a vascular rim or border and at times, prominent central vascularity. Simple or hemorrhagic cysts within the thyroid gland are usually due to cystic degeneration of a follicular adenoma and may appear sonographically as simple cysts or hyperechoic or complex masses with internal septations, debris, and fluid–fluid levels.

Malignant Thyroid Nodules

Carcinoma of the thyroid gland is very rare in the pediatric age range, constituting 1% to 1.5% of all malignancies before the age of 15 years (135). Sixty-six percent occur in girls between 7 and 12 years of age. The typical presentation is a palpable thyroid nodule, cervical adenopathy, or both. Large tumors may cause hoarseness from pressure

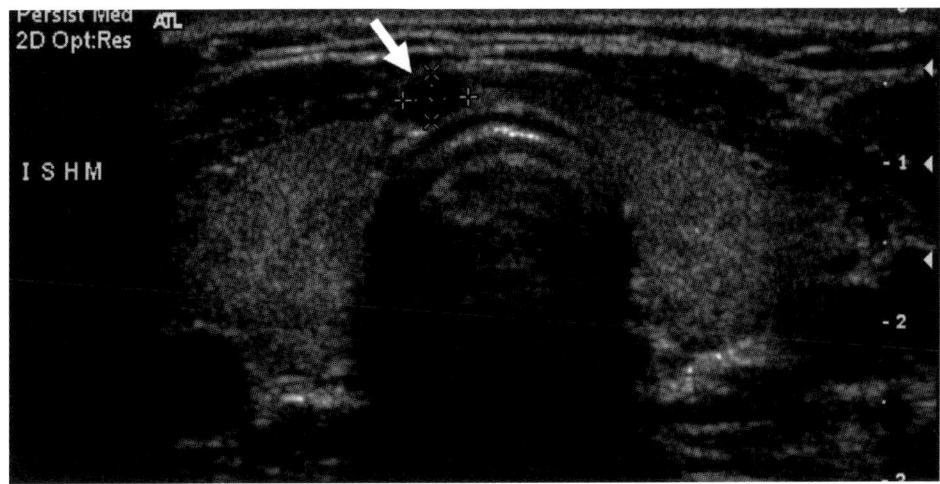

FIGURE 27 ■ Colloid nodule. Transverse sonogram of the thyroid demonstrates a small hypoechoic nodule in the isthmus of the gland (*arrow*).

on the recurrent laryngeal nerve or airway obstruction. Thyroid neoplasms are either follicular derived [papillary, follicular and Hurthle (oncocytic) variants of papillary or follicular cell lesions] or C-cell derived (medullary carcinoma) (136). The diagnosis of these tumors can usually be made at the histologic level, with immunohistochemical stains necessary in some circumstances. The most common (70–90%) subtype of thyroid cancer in childhood is papillary carcinoma (Fig. 28). This tumor spreads by direct invasion or nodal metastases. About 10% to 20% of thyroid malignancies are follicular, which may spread hematogenously to lung, bone, or cervical nodes. Thyroid malignancies in children may also present with mixed papillary and follicular histology. Hurthle-cell carcinoma is a less common histology of the thyroid cancer occurring in less than in 1.5% to 10%. About 1% to 10% is medullary and may spread to lymph nodes and bone. This tumor is familial (inherited as an autosomal-dominant trait) and is commonly multicentric and bilateral. It is also associated with multiple endocrine neoplasia (MEN) type II syndromes. Medullary carcinoma arises from parafollicular or C-cells, may secrete calcitonin, and may be multicentric and bilateral. MEN IIA is defined by medullary thyroid carcinoma (MTC), pheochromocytoma (about 50%), and hyperparathyroidism caused by parathyroid gland hyperplasia (about 20%). MEN IIB is defined by medullary thyroid tumor, pheochromocytoma, and mucosal neuromas (137). Less common thyroid tumors include tall-cell and cribriform-morular variants of papillary carcinoma, hyalinizing trabecular tumor, mucoepidermoid and sclerosing mucoepidermoid carcinoma with eosinophilia, poorly differentiated (insular) carcinoma, and undifferentiated (anaplastic) carcinoma and sarcoma. Less differentiated malignancies carry a very poor prognosis (138).

Thyroid cancer in children tends to present at a later stage than in adults, usually with cervical lymphadenopathy and pulmonary or osseous metastases; however, in spite of more advanced presentation, the prognosis is more favorable (139).

Sonographically, most thyroid cancers are hypoechoic relative to the normal thyroid parenchyma. The borders of the tumor may be irregular and ill defined or smooth and well delineated. A sonolucent rim or halo may completely or partially surround the lesion. Punctate echogenic foci are detectable in medullary carcinoma. US-guided biopsy is an important tool in diagnosis.

There is an increased incidence of benign and malignant tumors present in thyroid, parathyroid, and salivary glands after radiation. Up to 30% of patients develop thyroid nodules and up to 9% develop carcinoma, which are frequently multicentric and bilateral.

Lymphoma may involve the thyroid gland and sonographically presents as solitary or multiple hypoechoic nodules, which may totally replace the gland (140).

Diffuse Thyroid Disease

Diffuse thyroid enlargement is generally due to inflammatory or infectious conditions such as acute suppurative

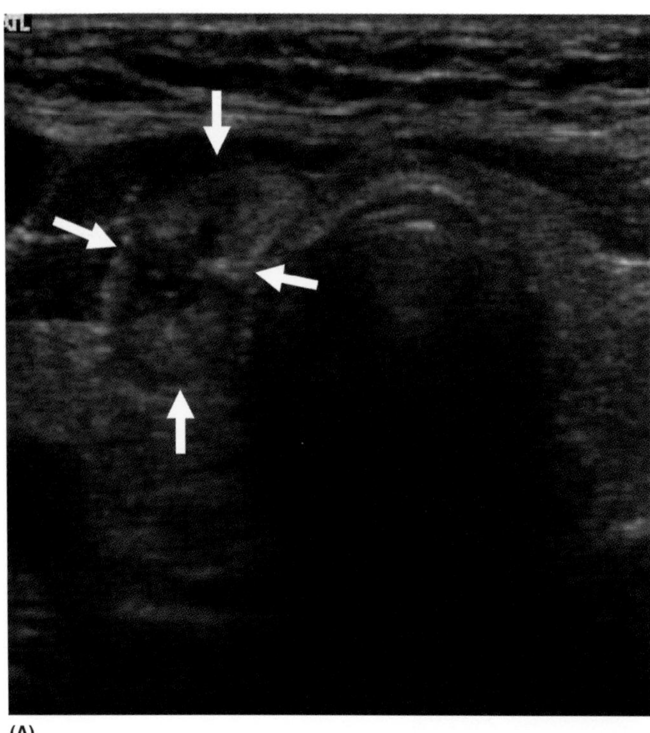

(A)

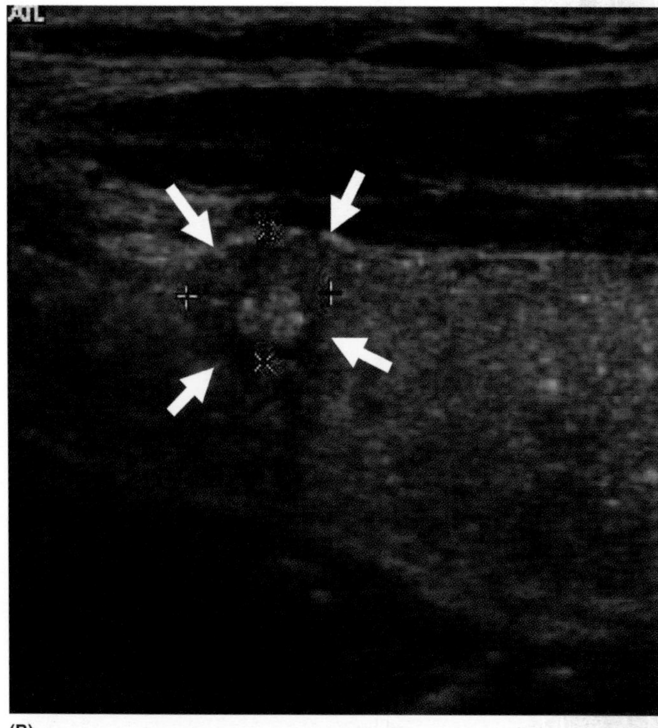

(B)

FIGURE 28 A AND B ■ Papillary carcinoma. There is a heterogeneous solid mass with a hypoechoic halo seen on the transverse sonogram (**A**) at the junctions of the right side of the isthmus and the right lobe of the gland. On the sagittal image (**B**), tiny nonshadowing calcifications are noted with the mass.

and subacute (de Quervain's) thyroiditis, autoimmune processes [chronic lymphocytic (Hashimoto's) thyroiditis and Graves' disease] and colloid goiter. Acute suppurative thyroiditis is usually caused by a bacterial infection with Staphylococcal, Streptococcal, and other skin flora organisms, which may develop into an abscess. Rarely, a fistula with a pyriform sinus may be a cause (32). Sonographic findings include single or multiple hypoechoic or complex masses.

Subacute or de Quervain's thyroiditis is a self-limited transient disease that is caused by a viral infection and may initially present with mild thyrotoxicosis followed by mild hypothyroidism (141). Sonographically, the thyroid may appear lobulated with decreased echogenicity especially in the periphery of the gland.

Graves' disease is an autoimmune disease caused by circulating immunoglobulins with the ability to stimulate the TSH receptors, resulting in a markedly hyperstimulated gland and thyrotoxicosis (5,135). The typical sonographic appearance includes glandular enlargement with lobulated borders and a coarse heterogeneous echotexture. Duplex/color Doppler US evaluation is quite helpful in demonstrating the typical "thyroid inferno" sign of Graves' disease with marked parenchymal hypervascularity along with high systolic and diastolic flow velocities, ranging between 50 and 120 cm/sec. Arteriovenous shunting and enlarged vessels around the periphery of the gland may be noted as well (Fig. 29) (142).

Hashimoto's or chronic lymphocytic thyroiditis is an autoimmune disease in which there is significant lymphocytic infiltration with follicular atrophy and fibrosis (135). There is familial association as well as association with Turner's syndrome, Klinefelter's syndrome, Down's syndrome, other autoimmune and connective tissue diseases, and other endocrine disorders. Sonographically the gland is enlarged with coarse heterogeneous echogenicity (Fig. 30) (143). Associated lymphadenopathy is common.

Multinodular goiter, also known as adenomatous goiter, colloid goiter, nodular hyperplasia, or adenomatous hyperplasia, may be idiopathic due to congenital defects of thyroid hormone synthesis or iodide organification due to dietary iodine insufficiencies and ingestion of excess iodine or thyrotropic medications. The

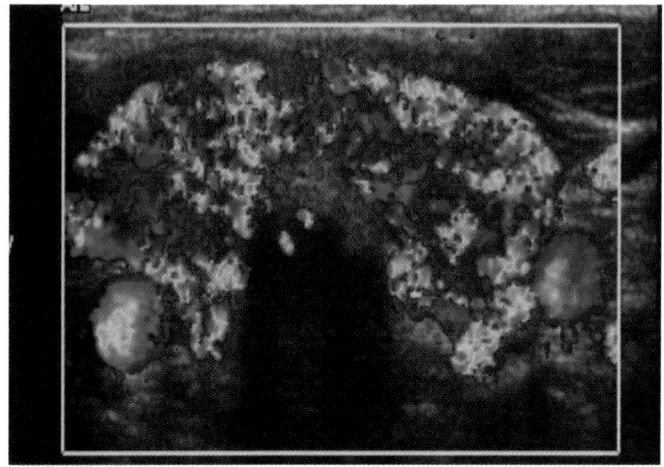

(A)

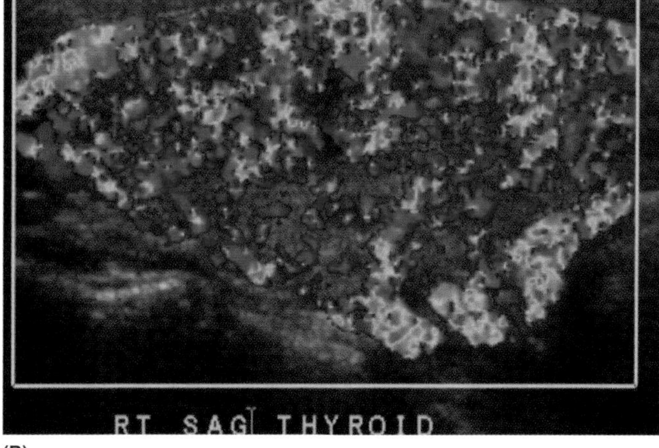

(B)

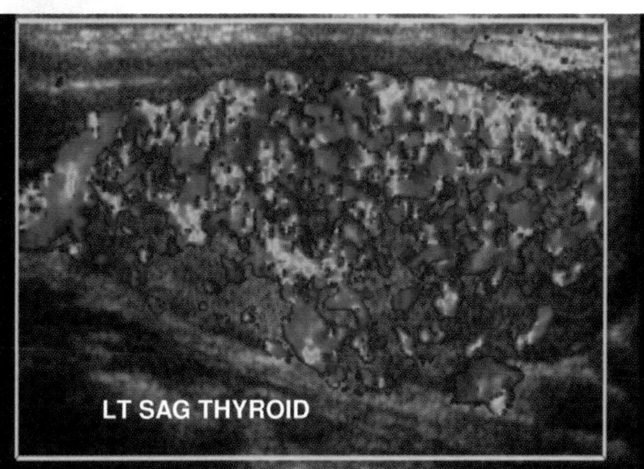

(C)

FIGURE 29 A–C ■ Graves' disease. The thyroid gland in this patient with thyrotoxicosis is diffusely enlarged on both transverse (**A**) and both sagittal images (**B,C**) and demonstrates intense hypervascularity ("inferno sign").

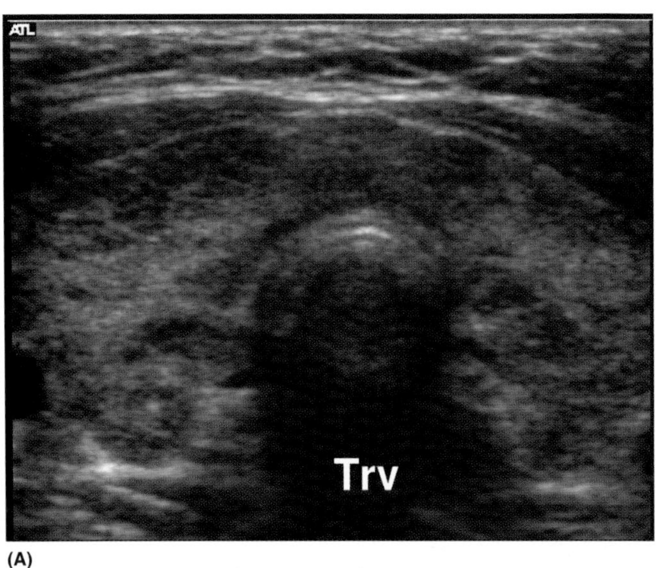

(A)

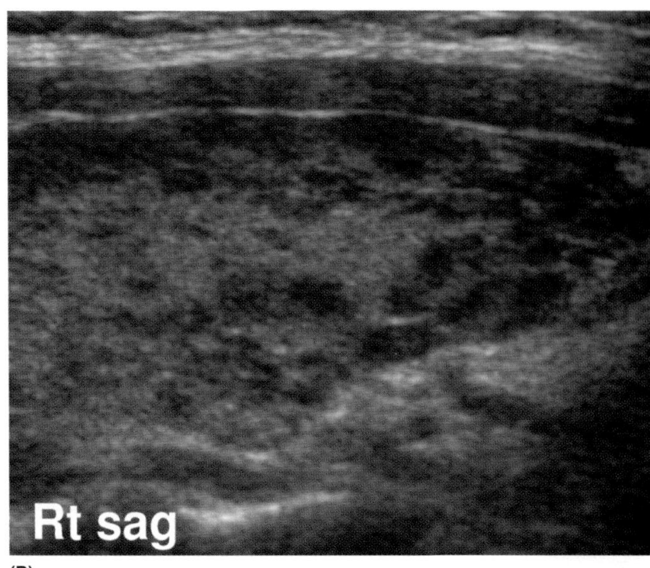

(B)

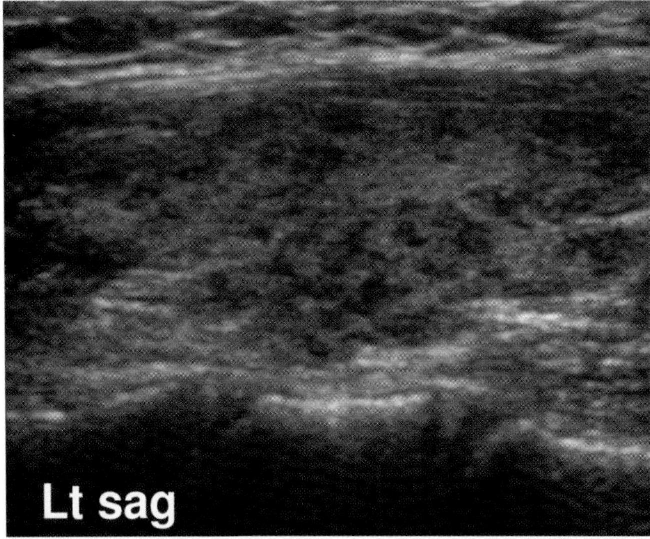

(C)

FIGURE 30 A–C ■ Hasimoto's thyroiditis. Teenager with anterior neck swelling and evidence of autoimmune thyroiditis. The gland is generally enlarged and contains multiple, small, hypoechoic round/oval lesions, some of which are confluent in both lobes as well as in the isthmus. (**A**) Transverse sonogram. (**B**) Right sagittal scan. (**C**) Left sagittal scan.

gland appears enlarged sonographically with heterogeneous echogenicity and multiple hyperechoic areas (Fig. 31) (144).

Parathyroid Glands and Hyperparathyroidism

Excess parathormone production results in hyperparathyroidism. Primary hyperparathyroidism is caused by a simple parathyroid adenoma in about 89% of cases, by multiglandular hyperplasia in about 20% of cases, and by carcinoma or a parathyroid cyst in less than 1% (145,146). Since the treatment for hyperparathyroidism is surgical exploration and subtotal parathyroidectomy, preoperative imaging, such as US and Tc-99m-Sestamibi with Tc-pertechnetate or I-123 subtraction is helpful in establishing the location of the parathyroids and the echotexture (147). Scintigraphic and MRI studies are particularly valuable for detection of lesions in an ectopic location. The suspicious nodules may be biopsied under US guidance (148). In patients who may not be surgical candidates, percutaneous ethanol ablation may be useful.

The use of intraoperative radiation probes has also been found very useful for localization, especially in a previously operated neck (149).

Most patients have four parathyroid glands, two superior and two inferior. The superior glands tend to be located more posterior and the inferior more anterior, and they are fed by the superior and inferior thyroidal artery, respectively (150). Most parathyroid adenomas or hyperplastic lesions are anechoic and rounded if less than 1 cm and more oval and lobulated if larger than 1 cm, without the through transmission typical of a cyst (Fig. 32). Parathyroid cysts are infrequently visualized and arise from third and fourth pharyngeal pouches or from cystic degeneration of parathyroid glands, most commonly of the inferior. A hyperechoic appearance is rare and may represent a lipoadenoma. Calcifications in the parathyroid adenomas are infrequent.

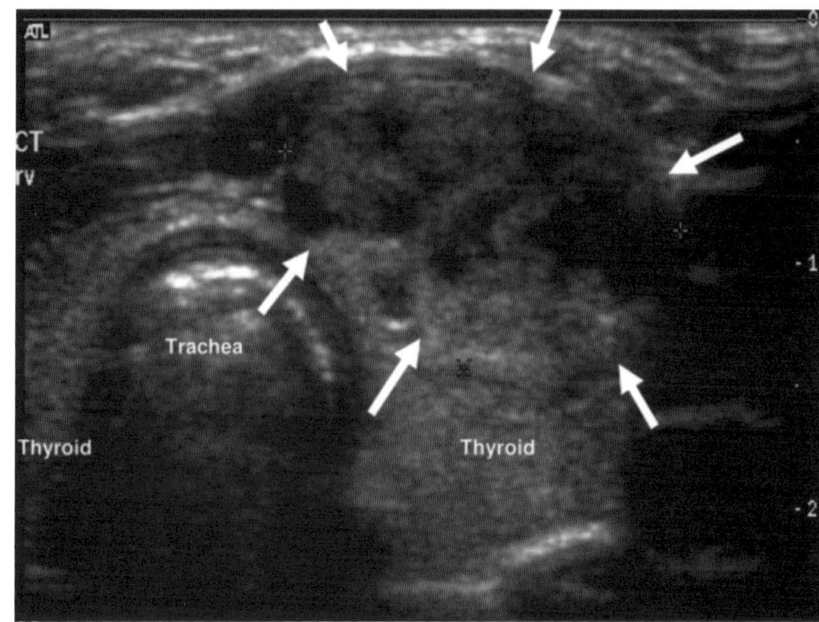

FIGURE 31 ■ Colloid goiter. A complex lesion (*arrow*) is demonstrated in the left lobe of the thyroid gland in this nine-year-old.

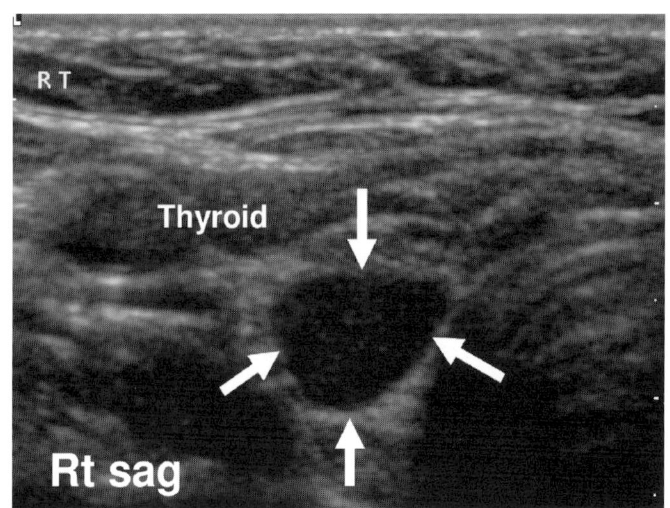

(A)

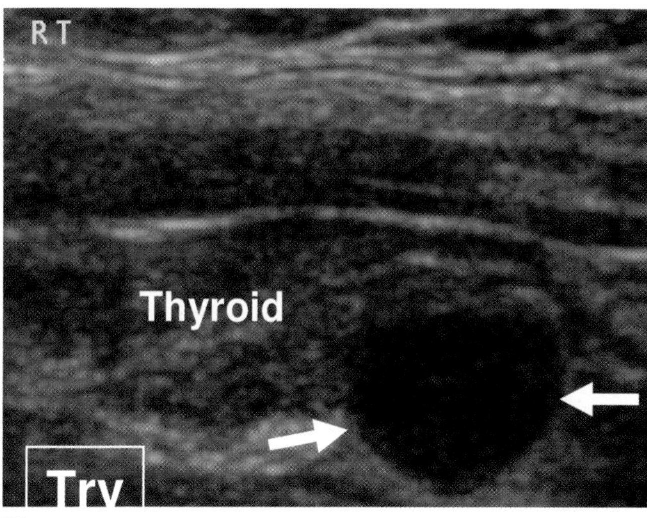

(B)

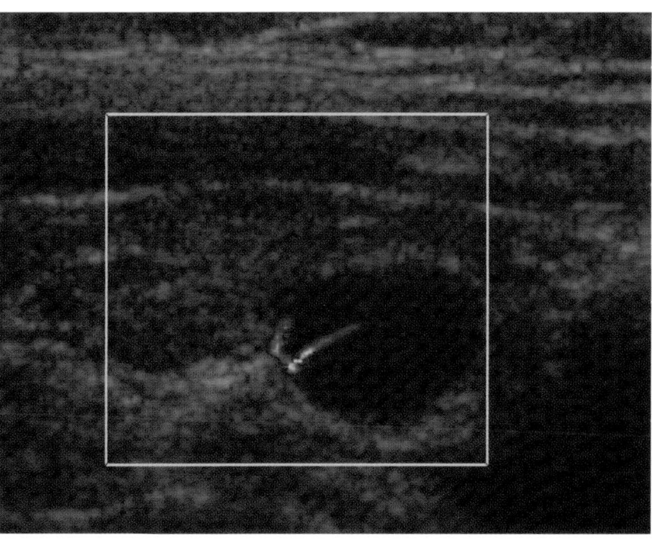

(C)

FIGURE 32 A–C ■ Parathyroid adenoma. There is an oval-shaped hypoechoic solid mass caudal and posterior to the lower pole of the right lobe of the thyroid on the sagittal (**A**) and the transverse (**B**) sonograms with evidence of a blood vessel entering the center of the adenoma (**C**).

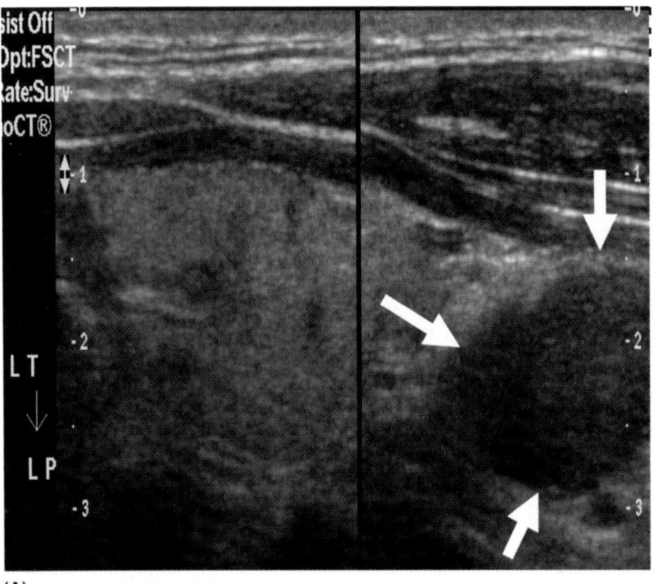

(A)

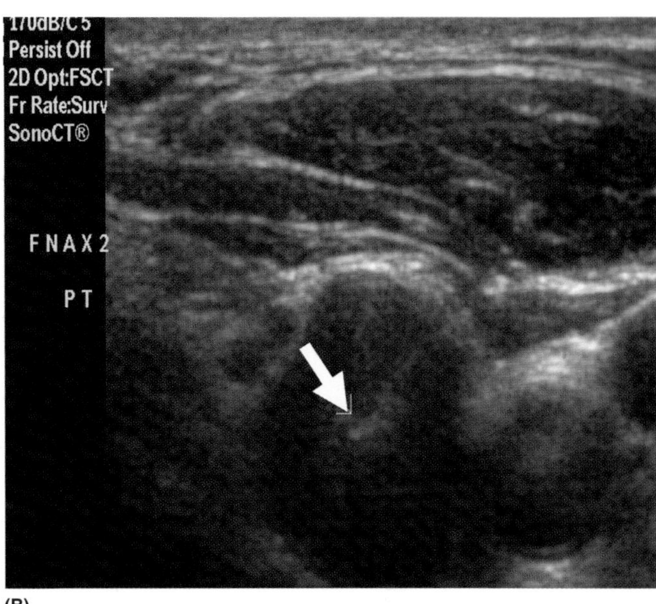

(B)

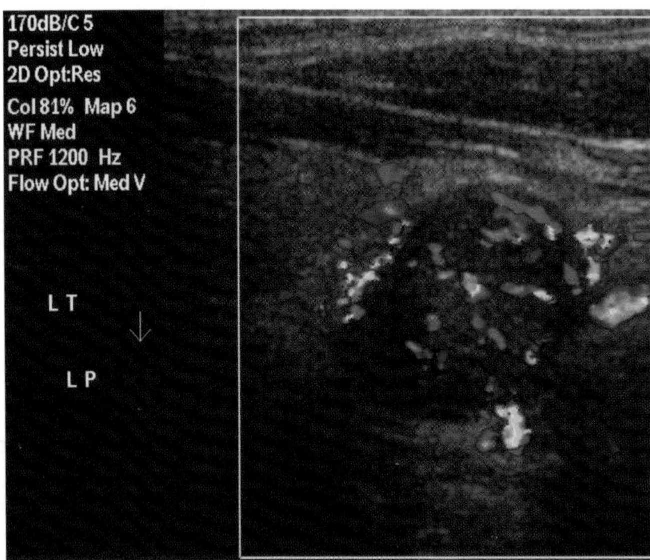

(C)

FIGURE 33 A–C ■ Metastasis of papillary thyroid carcinoma to paratracheal lymph node mimicking parathyroid. There is a solid hypoechoic round solid mass (**A**) adjacent to the thyroid gland, which contains a calcification (*arrow*) (**B**) and multiple chaotic vessels (**C**).

Parathyroid abnormalities are also associated with MEN syndromes types I and IIA. MEN I affects the parathyroid glands, the pancreatic islets (causing gastrinoma, insulinoma, glucagonoma, vasoactive intestinal peptide tumor, or pancreatic polypeptide-producing tumor), and the anterior pituitary (causing prolactinoma, somatotropinoma, corticotropinoma, or nonfunctioning tumors) (151). Associated tumors include lipomas, angiofibromas, or those located in the adrenal gland cortex. MEN IIA is defined by MTC, pheochromocytoma (about 50%), and hyperparathyroidism caused by parathyroid gland hyperplasia (about 20%).

Parathyroid cysts and malignancies are much less common causes of hyperthyroidism, representing less than 5% of the cases. Supernumerary parathyroid glands are frequently ectopic in location. Ectopic parathyroids are located in the thymus (17%), within the thyroid gland (10%), within the carotid sheath and in the retroesophageal space (3.6%). A lymph node may mimic a parathyroid adenoma and care should be taken to confirm the usual US characteristics of a lymph node, which may include the presence of a hilum with a vascular pedicle and a hyperechoic center. Parathyroid and thyroid cysts are indistinguishable by US and may, on occasion, mimic a parathyroid adenoma (150). At times, a papillary carcinoma of the thyroid may spread to a paratracheal lymph node and mimic a parathyroid gland (Fig. 33).

CONCLUSION

Duplex/color Doppler US remains the modality of choice for the evaluation of soft tissue abnormalities of the pediatric neck. If the US field of view is insufficient for complete visualization of a mass, or if malignancy is suspected, then CT or MRI is generally indicated.

ACKNOWLEDGMENT

The authors acknowledge the assistance of Dr. Steve B. Losik, Mt. Sinai Medical Center, New York, New York.

REFERENCES

1. Siegel MJ. Face and neck. In: Siegel MJ, ed. Pediatric Sonography. 3rd ed. Philadelphia: Lippincott Williams & Wilkins, 2002: 123–166.
2. Solbiati L, Cioffi V, Ballarati E. Ultrasonography of the neck. Radiol Clin North Am 1992; 30:941–954.
3. Sherman NH, Rosenberg HK, Heyman S, et al. Ultrasound evaluation of neck masses in children. Ultrasound J Med 1985; 4: 127–134.
4. Greenberg SB, Seibert JJ, Seibert RW. Pediatric head and neck masses. In: Rumack CM, Wilson SR, Charboneau JW, et al., eds. Diagnostic Ultrasound. Vol. 2. 3rd ed. St. Louis: Elsevier Mosby, 2005:1755–1791.
5. Hopkins CR, Reading CC. Thyroid, parathyroid, and other glands. In: McGahan JP, Goldberg BB, eds. Diagnostic Ultrasound: A Logical Approach. Philadelphia: Lippincott-Raven, 1998: 1087–1114.
6. Oates CP, Wilson AW, Ward-Booth RP, et al. Combined use of Doppler and conventional ultrasound for the diagnosis of vascular and other lesions in the head and neck. Int J Oral Maxillofac Surg 1990; 19:235–239.
7. Meuwly J, Lepori D, Theumann N, et al. Multimodality imaging evaluation of the pediatric neck: techniques and spectrum of findings. Radiographics 2005; 25:931–948.
8. Bielamowicz SA, Storper IS, Jabour BA, et al. Spaces and triangles of the head and neck. Head Neck 1994; 16:383–388.
9. Smoker WRK. Normal anatomy of the neck. In: Som PM, Curtin HD, eds. Head and Neck Imaging. 3rd ed. St. Louis: Mosby, 1995:711–737.
10. Som PM. Lymph nodes. In: Som PM, Durtin HD, eds. Head and Neck Imaging. 3rd ed. St. Louis: Mosby-Year Book, 1996:772–793.
11. Ahuja AT, Ying M. Sonographic evaluation of cervical lymph nodes. AJR Am J Roentgenol 2005; 184:1691–1699.
12. Marchal, Oyen R, Verschakelen J, et al. Sonographic appearance of normal nodes. J Ultrasound Med 1985; 4:417–419.
13. Ahuja AT, Ying M. Sonographic evaluation of cervical lymph nodes. AJR Am J Roentgenol 2004; 184:1691–1699.
14. Bodenstein L, Altman RP. Cervical lymphadenitis in infants and children. Semin Pediatr Surg 1994; 3:134–141.
15. Hudgins PA, Dorey JH, Jacobs IN. Internal carotid artery narrowing in children with retropharyngeal lymphadenitis and abscess. AJNR Am J Neuroradiol 1998; 19:1841–1843.
16. Glasier CM, Stark JE, Jacobs RF, et al. CT and ultrasound imaging of retropharyngeal abscesses in children. AJNR Am J Neuroradiol 1992; 13:1191–1195.
17. Hajek PC, Salomonowitz E, Turk R, et al. Lymph nodes of the neck: evaluation with US. Radiology 1986; 158:739–742.
18. Na GD, Kun HK, Byun HS, et al. Differential diagnosis of cervical lymphadenopathy: usefulness of color Doppler sonography. AJR Am J Roentgenol 1997; 168:1311–1316.
19. van den Brekel MWM, Castelijns JA, Snow GB. Imaging of cervical lymphadenopathy. Neuroimag Clin North Am 1996; 6:417–434.
20. Quraishi MS, OHalpin DR, Blayney AW. Ultrasonography in the evaluation of neck abscesses in children. Clin Otolaryngol 1997; 22:30–33.
21. Kusumi RK. Infections. In: Cummings CW, Fredrickson JM, Harker LA, et al., eds. Otolaryngology: Head and Neck Surgery. 2nd ed. St. Louis: CV Mosby, 1993:1566–1577.
22. Tovi F, Barki Y, Hertzanu Y. Imaging case study of the month—ultrasound detection of anaerobic neck infection. Ann Otol Rhinol Laryngol 1993; 102(2):157–159.
23. Yusa H, Yoshida H, Ueno E, et al. Ultrasound-guided surgical drainage of face and neck abscesses. Int J Oral Maxillofac Surg 2002; 31:327–329.
24. Yeow K, Chun-Ta L, Shen-Po H. US-guided needle aspiration and catheter drainage as an alternative to open surgical drainage for uniloculated neck abscesses. J Vasc Interv Radiol 2001; 12:589–594.
25. Baatenburg de Jong RJ, Rongen RJ, Lameris JS, et al. Ultrasound-guided percutaneous drainage of deep neck abscesses. Clin Otolaryngol Allied Sci 1990; 15(2):159–166.
26. Baatenburg de Jong, Rongen RJ, Lameris JS. Ultrasound in the diagnosis of cervical tuberculous adenitis. Auris Nasus Larynx 1998; 25(1):67–72.
27. Nadel DM, Bilianiuk L, Handler SC. Imaging of granulomatous neck masses in children. Int J Pediatr Otorhinoloaryngol 1996; 37:151–162.
28. Hazra R, Robson CD, Perez-Atay de AR, et al. Lymphadenitis due to nontuberculous mycobacteria in children: presentation and response to therapy. Clin Infect Dis 1999; 28:123–129.
29. Robson CD, Hazra R, Barnes PD, et al. Nontuberculous mycobacterial infection of the head and neck in immunocompetent children: CT and MR findings. AJNR Am J Neuroradiol 1999; 20:1829–1835.
30. Soberman N, Leonidas JC, Berdon WE, et al. Parotid enlargement in children seropositive for human immunodeficiency virus: imaging findings. AJR Am J Roentgenol 1991; 157:553–556.
31. Sander S, Elicevik M, Unal M, et al. Jugular phlebectasia in children: is it rare or ignored? J Pediatr Surg 1999; 34:1829–1832.
32. Gan Y, Lam SL. Imaging findings in acute neck infection due to pyriform sinus fistula. Ann Acad Med Singapore 2004; 33:636–640.
33. Lucaya J, Berdon WE, Enriquez G. Congenital pyriform sinus fistula: a cause of acute left-sided suppurative thyroiditis and neck abscess in children. Pediatr Radiol 1990; 21:27–29.
34. Kan JH. Congenital pediatric neck masses. Appl Radiol 2001; 30(7):31–37.
35. Koch BL. The child with a neck mass. Appl Radiol 2005; 34(8):8–22.
36. Cunningham MJ. The management of congenital neck masses. Am J Otolaryngol 1992; 13:78–92.
37. McQuirt WF. Differential diagnosis of neck masses. In: Cummings CW, Frederickson JM, Harker LA, et al. Otolaryngology: Head and Neck Surgery. 3rd ed. St. Louis: Mosby, 1998:1686–1699.
38. Telander RL, Filston HC. Review of head and neck lesions in infancy and childhood. Surg Clin North Am 1992; 72:1429–1447.
39. Koeller KK, Alamo L, Adair FA, et al. From the archives of the AFIP–Congenital cystic masses of the neck: radiologic-pathologic correlation. Radiographics 1999; 19:121–146.
40. Noyek AM, Friedberg J. Thyroglossal duct and ectopic thyroid disorders. Otolaryngol Clin North Am 1981; 14:187–201.
41. Yousem DM, Scheff AM. Thyroid and parathyroid. In: Som PM, Curtin HD, eds. Head and Neck Imaging. 3rd ed. St. Louis: Mosby-Year Book, 1996:952–975.
42. Brown RL, Azizkhan RG. Pediatric head and neck lesions. Pediatr Clin North Am 1998; 45:889–905.
43. Youkilis RA, Koch B, Myer CMI. Ultrasonographic imaging of sternocleidomastoid tumor of infancy. Ann Otol Rhinol Laryngol 1995; 104:323–325.
44. Chan YL, Cheng JC, Metreweli C. Ultrasonography of congenital muscular torticollis. Pediatr Radiology 1992; 22:356–360.
45. Yamaguchi M, Matsuo S. Ultrasonic evaluation of pediatric superficial masses. J Clin Ultrasound 1987; 15:107–113.
46. Hsu TC, Wang, CL, Wong MK, et al. Correlation of clinical and ultrasonographic features in congenital muscular torticollis. Arch Phys Med Rehabil 1999; 80:637–641.
47. Cheng JC, Metreweli C, Chen TM, et al. Correlation of ultrasonographic imaging of congenital muscular torticollis with clinical assessment in infants. Ultrasound Med Biol 2000; 26:1237–1241.
48. Lin JN, Chou ML. Ultrasonographic study of the sternocleidomastoid muscle in the management of congenital muscular torticollis. J Pediatr Surg 1997; 32:1648–1651.

49. Cheng JC, Tang SP. Outcome of surgical treatment of congenital muscular torticollis. Clin Orthop 1999; 362:190–200.
50. Thomas JR. Thyroglossal-duct cysts. Ear Nose Throat J 1979; 58:510–514.
51. Pounds LA. Neck masses of congenital origin. Pediatr Clin North Am 1981; 28:841–844.
52. Allard R. The thyroglossal duct cyst. Head Neck Surg 1982; 5:134–146.
53. Sadler TW. Langman's Medical Embryology. 6th ed. Baltimore: Williams & Wilkins, 1990:297–327.
54. Weissman JL. Nodal masses of the neck. In: Som PM, Curtin HD, eds. Head and Neck Imaging. 3rd ed. St. Louis: Mosby-Year Book, 1996:794–822.
55. McDonald D. Thyroglossal duct cyst in the mouth floor: an unusual location. Otolaryngol Head Neck Surg 1994; 119:580–583.
56. McDonald D. Thyroglossal cysts and fistulae. Int J Oral Surg 1974; 3:342–346.
57. Wadsworth D, Siegel M. Thyroglossal duct cysts: variability of sonographic findings. AJR Am J Roentgenol 1994; 163:1475–1477.
58. Ghaneim A, Atkins P. The management of thyroglossal duct cysts. Int J Clin Pract 1997; 51:512–513.
59. Deane S, Telander R. Surgery for thyroglossal duct and branchial cleft anomalies. Am J Surg 1978; 136:348–353.
60. Hays LL, Marlowe JF Jr. Papillary adenocarcinoma arising in a thyroglossal duct cyst. Laryngoscope 1968; 78:2189–2203.
61. Lim-Dunham J, Feinstein K, Yousefzadeh D, et al. Sonographic demonstration of a normal thyroid gland excludes ectopic thyroid in patients with thyroglossal duct cyst. AJR Am J Roentgenol 1995; 164:1489–1491.
62. Benson MT, Dalen K, Mancuso AA, et al. Congenital anomalies of the branchial apparatus: embryology and pathologic anatomy. Radiographics 1992; 12:943–960.
63. Karmody CS. Developmental anomalies of the neck. In: Bluestone CD, Stool SE, Kenna MA, eds. Pediatric Otolaryngology. 3rd ed. Philadelphia: WB Saunders, 1996:1557–1583.
64. Maran ADG, Buchanan DR. Branchial cysts, sinuses and fistulae. Clin Otolaryngol 1978; 3:77–92.
65. Olsen KD, Maragos NE, Weiland LH. First branchial cleft anomalies. Laryngoscope 1980; 90:423–436.
66. Mukherji SK, Fatterpekar G, Castillo M, et al. Imaging of congenital anomalies of the branchial apparatus. Neuroimaging Clin N Am 2000; 10:75–93, vii.
67. Donegan JO. Congenital neck masses. In: Cummings CW, Fredrickson JM, Harker LA, et al., eds. Otolaryngology: Head and Neck Surgery. 2nd ed. St. Louis: Mosby, 1994:1555–1565.
68. Harnsberger H, Mancuso A, Muraki A, et al. Branchial cleft anomalies and their mimics: computed tomographic evaluation. Radiology 1984; 152:739–748.
69. Reynolds JH, Wolinski AP. Sonographic appearance of branchial cyst. Clin Radiol 1993; 48:109–110.
70. Parker G, Harnsberger H, Smoker W. The anterior and posterior cervical spaces. Semin US CT MR 1991; 12:257–273.
71. Zadvinskis DP, Benson MT, Kerr HH, et al. Congenital malformations of the cervico-thoracic lymphatic system: embryology and pathogenesis. Radiographics 1992; 12:1175–1189.
72. Gallagher PG, Mahoney MJ, Gosche JR. Cystic hygroma in the fetus and newborn. Semin Perinatol 1999; 23:341–356.
73. Emory P, Bailey C, Evans J. Cystic hygroma of the head and neck. J laryngol Otol 1984; 98:613–619.
74. Sheath S, Nussbaum A, Hutchins G, et al. Cystic hygromas in children: sonographic-pathologic correlation. Radiology 1987; 162:821–824.
75. Faerber E, Swartz J. Imaging of neck masses in infants and children. Crit Rev Diag Imaging 1991; 31:283–314.
76. Dubois J, Garel L, Abela A, et al. Lymphangiomas in children: percutaneous sclerotherapy with an alcoholic solution of zein. Radiology 1997; 204:651–654.
77. Turner C, Gross S. Treatment of recurrent suprahyoid cervicofacial lymphangioma with intravenous cyclophosphamide. Am J Pediatr Hematol Oncol 1994; 16:325–328.
78. Molitch HI, Unger EC, Witte CL, et al. Percutaneous sclerotherapy of lymphangiomas. Radiology 1995; 194:343–347.
79. Sichel J, Udassin R, Gozal D. OK-432 therapy for cervical lymphangioma. Laryngoscope 2004; 114:1805–1809.
80. Zarbo R, McClatchey K, Areen R, et al. Thymopharyngeal duct cyst: a form of cervical thymus. Ann Otol Rhinol Laryngol 1983; 92:284–289.
81. Ellis H. Cervical thymic cysts. Br J Surg 1967; 54:17–20.
82. Guba AM, Adam AE, Jaques DA, et al. Cervical presentation of thymic cysts. Am J Surg 1978; 136:430–436.
83. Boyd J, Templer J, Harvey A, et al. Persistent thymopharyngeal duct cyst. Otolaryngol Head Neck Surg 1993; 109:135–139.
84. Fahmy S. Cervical thymic cysts: their pathogenesis and relationship to branchial cysts. J Laryngol Otol 1974; 86:47–60.
85. Wagner C, Vanocur C, Weintraub W, et al. Respiratory complications in cervical thymic cysts. J Pediatr Surg 1988; 23:657–660.
86. Rosevear W, Singer M. Symptomatic cervical thymic cyst in a neonate. Otolaryngol Head Neck Surg 1981; 89:738–741.
87. Jones J, Hession B. Cervical thymic cysts. Ear Nose Throat J 1996; 75:678–680.
88. Miller M, DeVito M. Cervical thymic cyst. Otolaryngol Head Neck Surg 1995; 112:586–588.
89. Han BK, Yoon H, Suh Y. Thymic ultrasound II. Diagnosis of aberrant cervical thymus. Pediatr Radiol 2001; 31:480–487.
90. Millman B, Pransky S, Castillo J, et al. Cervical thymic anomalies. 1999; 47:29–39. J Pediatr Otorhinol 1999; 47(1):29–39.
91. Loney DA, Bauman NM. Ectopic cervical thymic masses in infants. A case report and review of the literature. Int J Pediatr Otorhinol 1998; 43:77–84.
92. Han BK, Suh Y, Yoon H. Thymic ultrasound I. Intrathymic anatomy in infants. Pediatr Radiol 2001; 31:474–479.
93. Cacciaguerra S, Rizzo L, Tranchina MG, et al. Ultrasound features of ectopic cervical thymus in a child. Pediatr Surg Int 1998; 13:597–599.
94. Fordham LA, Chung CJ, Donnelly LF. Imaging of congenital vascular and lymphatic anomalies of the head and neck. Neuroimag Clin N Am 2000; 10:117–136.
95. Mulliken JB, Glowacki J. Hemangiomas and vascular malformations in infants and children: a classification based on endothelial characteristics. Plast Reconstr Surg 1982; 69:412–422.
96. Burrows PE, Mulliken JB, Fellows KE, et al. Childhood hemangiomas and vascular malformation: angiographic differentiation. AJR Am J Roentgenol 1983; 141:483–488.
97. Clymer MA, Furtune DS, Reinisch L, et al. Interstitial Nd: YAG photocoagulation for vascular malformations and hemangiomas in childhood. Pediatr Radiol 1999; 29:879–893.
98. Dubois J, Garel L. Imaging and therapeutic approach of hemangiomas and vascular malformations in the pediatric age group. Pediatr Radiol 1999; 29:879–893.
99. Greinwald JH, Burke DK, Bonthius DJ, et al. An update on the treatment of hemangiomas in children with interferon alfa-2a. Arch Otolaryngol Head Neck Surg 1999; 125(1):21–27.
100. Armstrong DC, ter Brugg K. Selected interventional procedures for pediatric head and neck vascular lesions. Neuroimag Clin N Am 2000; 10:271–292.
101. Kwok KL, Lam HS, Ng DKK. Unilateral right-sided internal jugular phlebectasis in asthmatic children. J Paediatr Child Health 2000; 36:517–519.
102. Carr MM, Thorner P, Phillips JH. Congenital teratomas of the head and neck. J Otolaryngol 1997; 26:246–252.
103. April MM, Ward RF, Garelick JM. Diagnosis, management, and follow-up of congenital head and neck teratomas. Laryngoscope 1997; 108:1398–1401.
104. Smitniotopoulos JG, Chiechi MV. Teratomas, dermoids and epidermoids of the head and neck. Radiographics 1995; 15: 1437–1455.
105. Vittore CP, Goldber KN, McClatchey KD. Cystic mass at the suprasternal notch of a newborn: congenital suprasternal dermoid cysts. Pediatr Radiol 1998; 28:984–986.
106. Derchi LE, Serafini G, Rabbia C. Carotid body tumors: US evaluation. Radiology 1992; 182:457–459.
107. Cunningham MJ, McGuirt WF Jr, Myers EN. Malignant tumors of the head and neck. In: Bluesone, CD Stool SE, Kenna MA, eds.

Pediatric Otolaryngology. 3rd ed. Philadelphia: WB Saunders, 1996:1557–1583.

108. Rosenfeld RM. Cervical adenopathy. In: Bluestone CD, Stool SE, Kenna MA, eds. Pediatric Otolaryngology. 3rd ed. Philadelphia: WB Saunders, 1996:1557–1583.
109. Latack JT, Hutchinson RJ, Heyn RM. Imaging of rhabdomyosarcomas of the head and neck. AJNR Am J Neuroradiol 1987; 8:353–359.
110. Ying M, Ahuja A. Sonography of neck lymph nodes. I. Normal lymph nodes. Clin Radiol 2003; 58:351–358.
111. Ahuja A, Ying M, Sonography of neck lymph nodes. II. Abnormal lymph nodes. Clin Radiol 2003; 58:359–366.
112. Ying M, Ahuja AT, Yuen HY. Grey-scale and power Doppler sonography of unusual cervical lymphadenopathy. Ultrasound Med Biol 2004; 30:449–454.
113. Steinkamp H-J, Mueffelmann M, Bock JC, et al. Differential diagnosis of lymph node lesions: a semiquantitative approach with colour Doppler ultrasound. Br J Radiol 1998; 71:828–833.
114. Abrahmson SJ, Berdon WE, Ruzal-Shapiro C. Cervical neuroblastoma in eleven infants: a tumor with favorable prognosis. Clinical and radiologic findings. Pediatr Radiol 1993; 23:253–359.
115. Smith MC, Smith RJ, Bailey CM. Primary cervical neuroblastoma in infants. J Laryngol Otl 1985; 99:209–214.
116. Wiener ES. Head and neck rhabdomyosarcoma. Semin Pediatr Surg 1994; 3:203–206.
117. Lewis GJS, Leithiser RE Jr, Glasier CM, et al. Ultrasonography of pediatric neck masses. Ultrasound Q 1989; 7:315–355.
118. McGahan JP, Water JP, Bernstein L. Evaluation of the parotid gland. Radiology 1984; 152:453–458.
119. Garcia CJ, Flores PA, Arce JD, et al. Ultrasonography in the study of salivary gland lesions in children. Pediatr Radiol 1998; 28: 418–425.
120. Bianchi A, Cudmore RE. Salivary gland tumors in children. Pediatr Surg 1978; 13:519–521.
121. Shikhani AH, Johns ME. Tumors of the major salivary glands in children. Head Neck Surg 1988; 10(4):257–263.
122. Martinoli C, Derchi LE, Solbiati L, et al. Color Doppler sonography of salivary glands. AJR Am J Roentgenol 1994; 163:933–941.
123. Grunebaum M, Ziv N, Mankuta DJ. Submaxillary sialadenitis with a calculus in infancy diagnosed by ultrasonography. Pediatr Radiol 1985; 15:191–192.
124. Goddart D, Francois A, Ninane J, et al. Parotid gland abnormality found in children seropositive for the human immunodeficiency virus (HIV). Pediatr Radiol 1990; 20:354–357.
125. Nozaki H, Harasawa A, Hara A, et al. Ultrasonographic features of recurrent parotitis in childhood. Pediatr Radiol 1994; 24: 98–100.
126. Rubaltelli L, Sponga T, Candiani F, et al. Infantile recurrent sialectatic parotitis: the role of sonography and sialography in diagnosis and follow-up. Br J Radiol 1987; 60:1211–1214.
127. Seibert RW, Seibert JJ. High resolution ultrasonography of the parotid gland in children. Part II. Pediatr Radiol 1988; 19:13–18.
128. Burgos R, Murphy T, Ruess L. Thyroid disease beyond the thyroid: multisystemic radiologic manifestations of developmental, benign, and malignant thyroid disorders. Radiologist 2002; 9(3):155–163.
129. Williams RH, ed. Textbook of Endocrinology, Philadelphia: WB Saunders, 1981:117–427.
130. James EM, Charboneau JW. High-frequency (10 MHz) thyroid ultrasonography. Semin Ultrasound CT MR 1989; 143:1369–1372.
131. Kuffner HA, McCook BM, Swaminatha R, et al. Controversial ectopic thyroid: a case report of thyroid tissue in the axilla and benign total thyroidectomy. Thyroid 2005; 15(9):1095–1097.
132. MacCormick J, Carpenter B. Pediatric intratracheal ectopic thyroid tissue: case study and review of the literature. J Otolaryngol 2005; 34(5):365–369.
133. Wienke JR, Chong WK, Fielding JR, et al. Sonographic features of benign thyroid nodules: interobserver reliability and overlap with malignancy. J Ultrasound Med 2003; 22:1027–1031.
134. Desjardins JG, Khan AH, Montupet P, et al. Management of thyroid nodules in children: a 20-year experience. J Pediatr Surg 1987; 22:736–739.
135. Skinner MA. Thyroid and parathyroid. In: Oldham KT, Colombani PM, Folgia RP, eds. Surgery of Infants and Children. Philadelphia: Lippincott-Raven, 1997:857–868.
136. Muir A, Telander RL. Papillary carcinoma of the thyroid in children. Semin Pediatr Surg 1994; 3:182–187.
137. Skinner MA, DeBeneditti MK, Moley JF, et al. Medullary thyroid carcinoma in children with multiple endocrine neoplasia types 2 and 2B. J Pediatr Surg 1996; 31(1):177–181.
138. Hunt JL. Unusual thyroid tumors: a review of pathologic and molecular diagnosis. Expert Rev Mol Diag 2005; 5(5):725–734.
139. Chaukar DA, Rangarajan V, Nair N, et al. Pediatric thyroid cancer. J Surg Oncol 2005; 92(2):130–133.
140. Fiorillo A, Migliorati R, Fiore M, et al. Non-Hodgkin's lymphoma in childhood presenting as thyroid enlargement. Clin Pediatr 1987; 26:152–154.
141. Birchall IWJ, Chow CC, Metreweli C. Ultrasound appearances of de Quervain's thyroiditis. Clin Radiol 1990; 41:57–59.
142. Ralls PW, Mayakawa DS, Lee KP, et al. Color-flow Doppler sonography in Graves disease: "thyroid inferno." AJR Am J Roentgenol 1988; 150:781–784.
143. Hayashi N, Tamaki N, Konishi J, et al. Sonography of Hashimoto's thyroiditis. J Clin Ultrasound 1986; 14:123–126.
144. Garcia CJ, Daneman A, Thorner P, et al. Sonography of multinodular thyroid gland in children and adolescents. Am J Dis Child 1992; 146:811–816.
145. DeLellis R. The endocrine system. In: Cotran RS, Kumar V, Robbins SL, eds. Robbins Pathologic Basis of Disease. 4th ed. Philadelphia: WB Saunders, 1989:1214.
146. Stratakis CA, Chrousos GP. Endocrine tumors. In: Pizzo PA, Poplack DG, eds. Principles and Practices of Pediatric Oncology. 3rd ed. Philadelphia: Lippincott-Raven, 1997:947–976.
147. Burke GJ, Wei JP, Binet EF. Parathyroid scintigraphy with iodine-123 and 99 mTc-sestamibi: imaging findings. AJR Am J Roentgenol 1993; 161:1265.
148. Kang YS, Rosen K, Clark OH, et al. Localization of abnormal parathyroid glands of the mediastinum with MR imaging. Radiology 1993; 189:137.
149. Shimotake T, Tsuda T, Aoi S, Fumino S, Iwai N. Iodine 123 metaiodobenzylguanidine radio-guided navigation surgery for recurrent medullary thyroid carcinoma in a girl with multiple endocrine neoplasia type 2B. J Pediatr Surg 2005; 40(10):1643–1646.
150. Gooding GAW. Parathyroid ultrasound: the why and wherefore. Radiologist 2005; 7(1).
151. Randel SB, Gooding GAW, Clark OH, et al. Parathyroid variants: US evaluation. Radiology 1987; 165:191–194.

Pediatric Spine

Rebecca Stein-Wexler and Eugenio O. Gerscovich

23

INTRODUCTION

Spinal dysraphism is the second most common congenital abnormality after cardiac malformations. Ultrasound (US) provides an excellent means for imaging the spine in infants up to three to six months of age (1), when the predominantly cartilaginous dorsal elements provide a window that allows evaluation of the spinal cord, conus medullaris, filum terminale, nerve roots, and cauda equina. As ossification progresses, the role of US becomes more limited, yielding to the "gold standard" magnetic resonance imaging (MRI) some time between 6 and 12 months, depending on the rapidity with which ossification progresses. However, even after that time, US can be useful in evaluating the postoperative child or the child with spinal dysraphism, due to the absence of posterior bony elements (2).

US has the advantages of being inexpensive and noninvasive, with no ionizing radiation or need for sedation. Furthermore, although image quality is usually better if the infant is transported to the US suite, portable examination is possible, and this can be essential in the unstable infant. US also allows real-time evaluation of the movement of the spinal cord and cauda equina, which provides important information in assessing for tethered cord. However, even in a technically adequate study of the complete spine, US can miss subtle findings such as dorsal dermal sinus, small lipomas, and thickened filum terminale (3–6). Fortunately, US will usually discern the often-associated tethered cord, triggering additional workup. MRI is generally needed to clarify abnormalities discovered on US and then delineates additional problems (7) such as dorsal dermal sinus.

CLASSIFICATION OF DEFECTS

Spinal dysraphism can be divided into three general categories (8). With "occult dysraphism" (spina bifida occulta), dysraphism is present but there is no associated mass. There is tremendous variety in severity of lesions that fall into this category, including tethered cord, tight filum terminale, spinal lipoma, diastematomyelia, hydromyelia, anterior sacral or lateral thoracic meningocele, caudal regression syndrome, and dorsal dermal sinus. The second category consists of a "dorsal mass covered with skin" ("spina bifida cystica"). Lipomyelomeningocele, myelocystocele, and posterior meningocele constitute these anomalies. Dysraphism associated with a "dorsal mass that is not covered with skin" constitutes the third category ("spina bifida aperta"), consisting of myelomeningocele and myelocele. US is contraindicated in their evaluation, as there is no protective skin covering these lesions. However, US may be performed to evaluate for associated defects. Table 1 presents a summary of these defects. Isolated bony "spina bifida occulta" refers simply to incomplete fusion of the dorsal neural arch, usually at L5 or S1. If limited to one level, this is of no clinical significance, but if it occurs at two or more levels, there may be associated abnormalities.

TABLE 1 ■ Classification of Forms of Spinal Dysraphism

Spinal dysraphism without a back mass (spina bifida occulta)

Simple

- Tethered cord, including tight filum terminale
- Intradural lipoma
- Lipoma of the filum terminale
- Hydromyelia and syringomyelia
- Dorsal dermal sinus

Complex

- Diastematomyelia
- Caudal regression syndrome

Spinal dysraphism with a skin-covered back mass (spina bifida cystica)

- Lipomyelomeningocele and lipomyelocele
- Terminal myelocystocele
- Posterior meningocele
- Anterior sacral meningocele
- Lateral meningocele

Spinal dysraphism with a non–skin-covered back mass (spina bifida aperta)

- Myelocele
- Myelomeningocele

EMBRYOLOGY

The fetal nervous system forms between weeks 3 and 8.5 of gestation. The spinal cord, which forms from the ectoderm, undergoes neurulation, canalization, and retrogressive differentiation. With neurulation, the neural plate infolds and the two sides approach each other dorsally at the midline. The tube initially closes at the midpoint and then progresses to close first cranially and then, at about four weeks, caudally. Meanwhile, overlying ectoderm separates from the underlying neural tube, and mesenchyme around the neural tube forms muscle, bone, and meninges. Many dysraphic defects occur at this time—the dorsal dermal sinus probably resulting from incomplete separation of ectoderm, neuroectoderm, and mesenchyme; the myelomeningocele/lipomyelomeningocele resulting from more extensively disordered separation. Canalization then takes place, beginning at about 30 days. At this time, the distal end of the neural tube elongates to form a caudal cell mass, and simultaneously ependyma lines the central portion of the neural tube. Abnormal formation of the caudal cell mass probably accounts for tethered cord, intradural lipoma, and sacrococcygeal teratoma. The final major event is retrogressive differentiation, when the size of both the central lumen and the caudal cell mass decrease, and the recognizable structures of the spinal cord, filum terminale, conus medullaris, and central canal form.

Fusion of the bony portion of posterior elements is complete by one year of age, but since this fusion progresses from caudal to cranial, the thecal sac can be obscured by fused dorsal elements in the lumbar region as early as three months (9).

INDICATIONS FOR ULTRASOUND

Ultrasonographic screening is indicated in two general groups of infants: those with cutaneous markers that place them at risk for dysraphism and those with syndromes that are associated with an increased incidence of dysraphism, including vertebral defects, cardiac anomalies, anal atresia, tracheoesophageal fistula, renal anomalies, and limb dysplasia associations. In general, associated symptoms such as bowel and bladder dysfunction and gait disorders become apparent when ultrasonographic evaluation is no longer an option.

Only specific cutaneous stigmata serve as markers for spinal dysraphism. The simple dimple, that is, one that is less than 5 mm in diameter, less than 2.5 cm from the anus, and unaccompanied by additional cutaneous stigmata, is not associated with increased risk for spinal dysraphism (6). Spinal US is therefore not necessary, although it can be comforting to parents. In contrast, if the dimple is more than 2.5 cm from the anus and larger than 5 mm, it is considered atypical and at risk. If associated with a capillary hemangioma, cutis aplasia, or upraised hairy patch or skin tag, occult dysraphism may be present in between 39% and 67% of patients (6). A palpable dorsal soft-tissue mass can be evaluated with US, although MRI will usually prove necessary as well. US may be employed to evaluate the spinal axis distant from an open defect that lacks skin covering, but scanning directly over such a lesion is absolutely contraindicated.

The spine can also be evaluated if birth trauma is suspected or after a possibly traumatic lumbar puncture. In older children with spinal dysraphism, US can be helpful to evaluate for postoperative problems.

TECHNIQUE

Spinal US is usually performed with the infant prone and the torso draped over a small, rolled-up towel to facilitate opening of the dorsal elements and improve the acoustic window. Occasionally, the infant may lie in the lateral decubitus position. The neck should be flexed when the craniocervical junction is evaluated. If a meningocele is suspected, the infant may be positioned upright to facilitate its filling with cerebrospinal fluid (CSF). A linear-array high-frequency transducer is employed in the majority of spinal ultrasound; rarely, a curved-array transducer is useful in older dysraphic patients (7–12 MHz). Occasionally, a standoff pad is helpful for evaluating a dorsal sinus tract, but copious gel often provides better visualization, as the standoff pad may compress structures and slide around.

The spine is imaged in sagittal and axial planes. Although it is common to evaluate only the lower thoracic, lumbar, and upper sacral spine, lesions may be missed unless the entire spine is examined (4). If the patient is older than three months, US may be unsuccessful, but visualization can sometimes be improved by paramedian scanning. Three-dimensional US is promising (10). A recent study

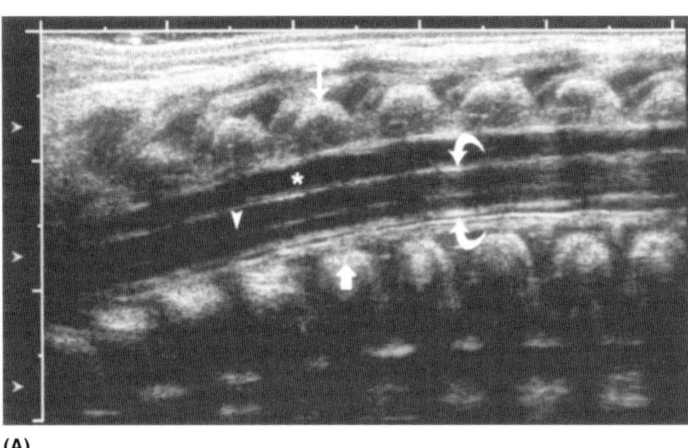
(A)

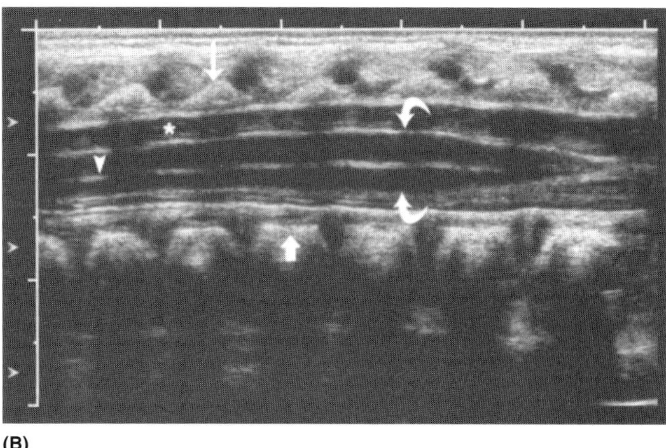
(B)

FIGURE 1 A AND B ■ Longitudinal US of the thoracic (**A**) and upper lumbar (**B**) spine and spinal cord demonstrate ossified portions of spinous processes (*thin arrows*), vertebral bodies (*thick arrows*), spinal cord (*curved arrows*), cerebrospinal fluid (*asterisks*), and central echogenic complex (*arrowhead*). Note that the cerebrospinal fluid in (**B**) appears more echogenic than in (**A**) due to the presence of more numerous nerve roots in this area.

correlating US with MRI found that 92% of ultrasound errors resulted from the following: acoustic shadowing from either ossified posterior elements or cutaneous stigmata and incomplete evaluation of the spine, i.e., not evaluating the upper thoracic spine or lower sacrum (4).

NORMAL ANATOMY

The spinal cord is normally widest in the cervical and the lumbar spine, where large exiting nerve roots are present. It is relatively narrow in the thoracic spine and widens distally to form the conus medullaris, which then tapers to a conical end (Fig. 1). The spinal cord is predominantly hypoechoic, but there is a "central echo complex" that is echogenic. Although this was originally thought to represent the central canal, histologic evaluation has found that this echogenicity results from the interface of the border between the myelinated ventral white commissure and the central portion of the anterior median fissure (11). Occasionally, a "ventriculus terminalis," or "fifth ventricle," is present, a small, ependyma-lined cavity limited to the conus (12) or proximal filum (Fig. 2) (13). The cavity is anechoic and sharply demarcated; unlike a syrinx, it does not extend

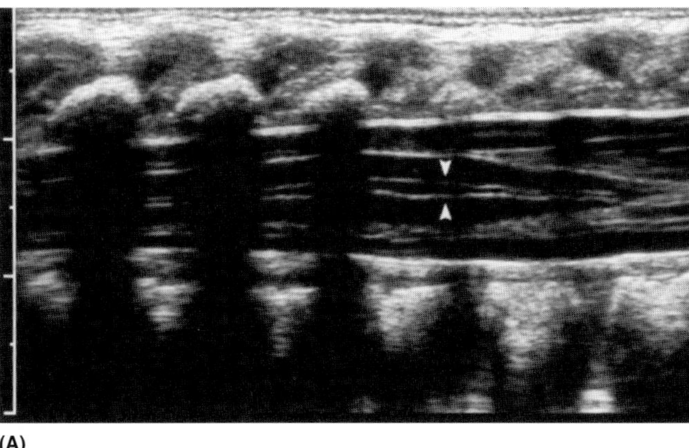
(A)

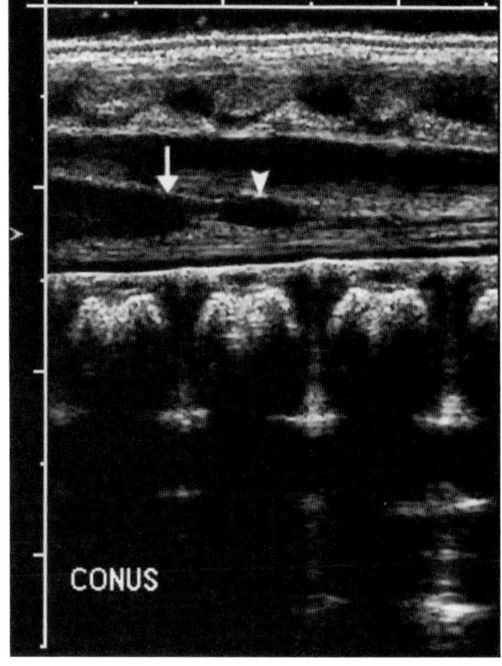

(B)

FIGURE 2 A AND B ■ Longitudinal US of lower thoracic and lumbar spine demonstrates ventriculus terminalis. (**A**) Demonstrates slight widening of the central canal (*arrowheads*) in the conus medullaris. (**B**) Demonstrates ventriculus terminalis (*arrowhead*) in the proximal filum. Note tip of conus (*arrow*).

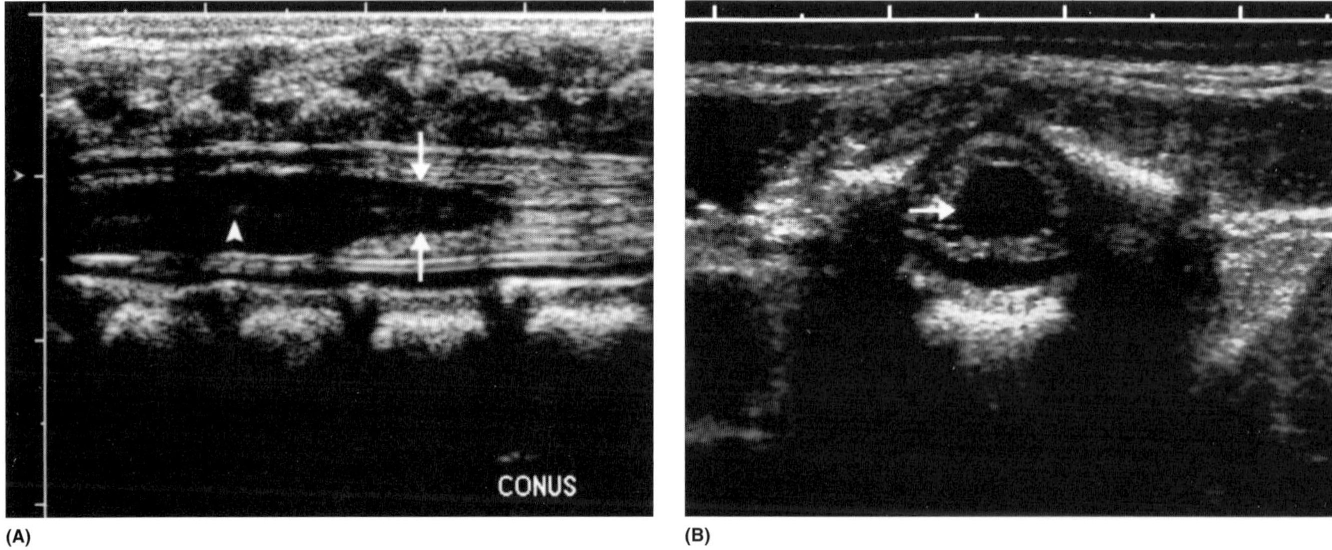

(A) (B)

FIGURE 3 A AND B ■ Longitudinal US demonstrates conus medullaris. In (**A**), the central echogenic area (*arrowhead*) and tapering conus (*arrows*) are readily appreciated. Also, observe the surrounding fibers of the cauda equina. In (**B**), the conus medullaris (*arrow*) is seen in transverse view.

superiorly (14). Thought to result from altered retrogressive differentiation, the ventriculus terminalis can be considered a remnant of normal embryologic development (13).

For the first few months, the conus may lie as low as upper L3, but it should subsequently terminate above L2/3 (3). The spinal cord should be positioned either ventrally or centrally within the thecal sac; a dorsal position may indicate tethering.

The filum terminale consists of a thin strand of glial-ependymal tissue that extends from the tip of the conus medullaris to the coccyx, piercing the dura at about S2, which is the normal distal extent of the thecal sac. The filum terminale should measure less than 2 mm in diameter.

Echogenic, paired dorsal and ventral nerve roots can be observed exiting the spinal cord, angled progressively more caudad as the more distal portion of the spinal canal is imaged. After the termination of the cord in the conus medullaris (Fig. 3), the multiple echogenic nerve roots constitute the cauda equina. Occasionally it is difficult to differentiate the normal cord-like, echogenic filum terminale from the surrounding cauda equina (Fig. 4). Echogenic dentate ligaments pass laterally from the cord. The arachnoid space is normally filled with anechoic CSF, and this is then surrounded by echogenic arachnoid-dura mater.

Vertebral level can be determined in various ways (Fig. 5). In the normal infant, L5/S1 constitutes the transition from the straight lumbar spine to the lordotic sacrum, so S1 is the first vertebra with dorsal tilt. Alternatively, one can count cephalad from S5, which should be the last ossified vertebra in the neonatal period, the coccyx being

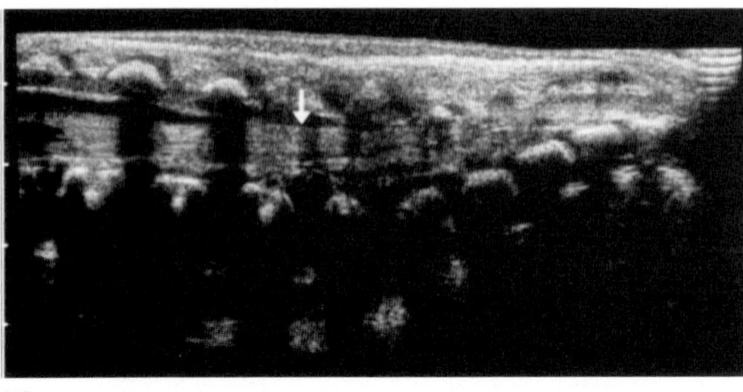

(A)

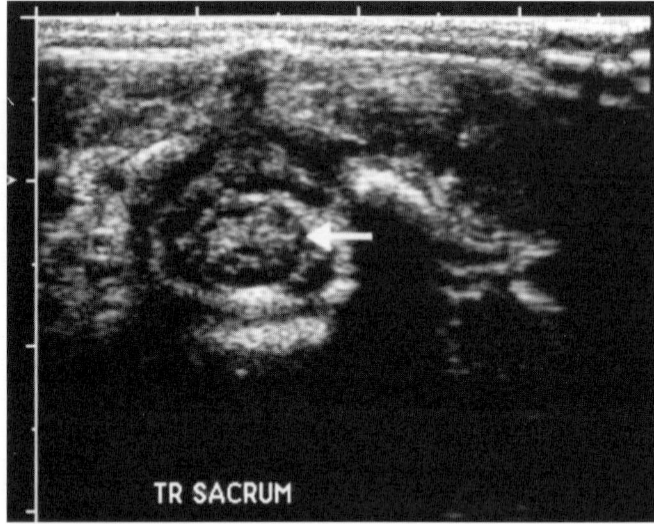

(B)

FIGURE 4 A AND B ■ The multiple echogenic nerve roots of the cauda equina (*arrow*) cannot be readily differentiated from the filum terminale on these longitudinal (**A**) and transverse (**B**) US views.

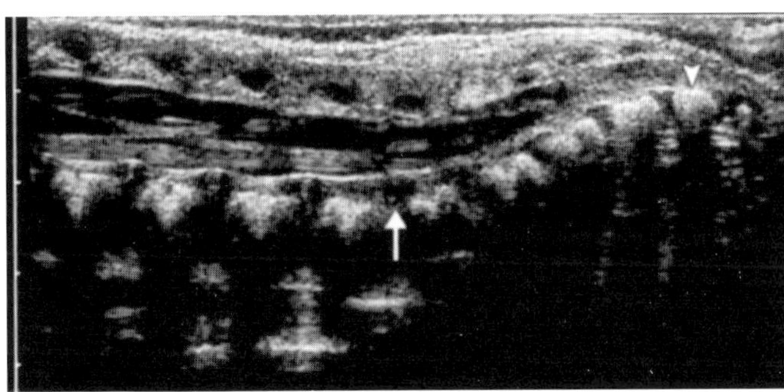

FIGURE 5 ■ A longitudinal US of the lower thoracic spine, lumbar spine, and sacrum demonstrates possible means for determining vertebral level. S5 (*arrowhead*) is the last fully ossified vertebra. The lumbosacral junction (*arrow*) is just above S1, the first vertebra with a dorsal tilt.

cartilaginous or at most partially ossified at this time. Another approach is counting cephalad from S2, which should be the most distal extent of the thecal sac. If there is inconsistency between these levels, and if the cord is borderline tethered, one can tape a radio-opaque marker to the skin and correlate with radiography. Configuration of vertebral bodies and dorsal elements should be assessed, as splayed dorsal elements may be present with dysraphism, and segmentation abnormalities may also coexist.

In addition to anatomic assessment, it is important to observe spinal cord and nerve root motion in real time. The normal cord and nerve roots demonstrate dorsoventral oscillations at the pulse rate as well as movement with respiration (5). When tethering is present, movement may be decreased.

CONGENITAL ANOMALIES

Spinal Dysraphism without Mass

Occult Spinal Dysraphism: Simple

Tethered Cord, Including Tight Filum Terminale Syndrome ■ The spinal cord is tethered, resulting in a low position of the conus medullaris in 50% of patients (8), below L3 in a neonate and below L2/3 in older patients (Fig. 6). The conus is positioned relatively dorsally within the thecal sac, and tethering may result in decreased pulsatility of the cord. Symptoms result from vascular insufficiency due to stretching of the cord. The filum terminale is thickened to more than 2 mm by fibrous or lipomatous tissue, a result of overgrowth of the fat cells that normally occur in the pia and the arachnoid (8), overgrown ectodermal rests (8), or incomplete involution of the distal cord during embryogenesis (15). If there is a lipoma of the filum terminale, it will usually appear echogenic, but if the filum is merely thickened this may not be appreciated on US (4). Tight filum terminale syndrome may occur in the absence of tethering of the cord, in which case the filum is thickened but the conus is at the normal level. Symptoms include bladder dysfunction and orthopedic deformities (15). A small percentage of patients with tethered cord have associated diastematomyelia, hydromyelia, or Chiari I, necessitating evaluation of the remainder of the neuroaxis; a dorsal dermal sinus may be associated as well.

Intradural Lipoma ■ The intradural lipoma is relatively uncommon, constituting only 4% of spinal lipomas, whereas lipomyelocele/lipomyelomeningocele and fibrolipoma of the filum terminale are more common at 84% and 12%, respectively (16). The intradural lipoma consists of a collection of lipomatous tissue that adheres to but does not invade the surface of the spinal cord. The lipoma also adheres to the adjacent dura, resulting in tethering of the cord. If located at the conus, the cord is low lying as well. The intradural lipoma is an isolated lesion, occurring in the absence of myelocele or myelomeningocele.

On sonography, the fatty mass appears highly echogenic, possibly compressing the adjacent cord. Tethering may be demonstrated. Multilevel spina bifida may be associated, and the spinal canal may demonstrate focal enlargement at the level of the lipoma.

Lipoma of Filum Terminale ■ If isolated, this echogenic lesion is typically of no clinical significance, being found on autopsy in 4% to 6% of patients with otherwise normal

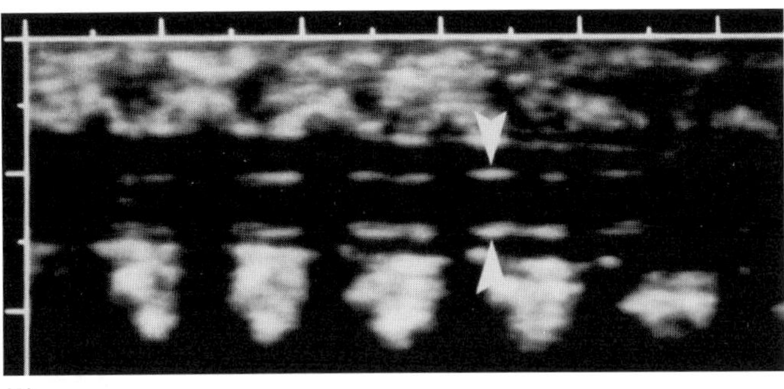

(A)

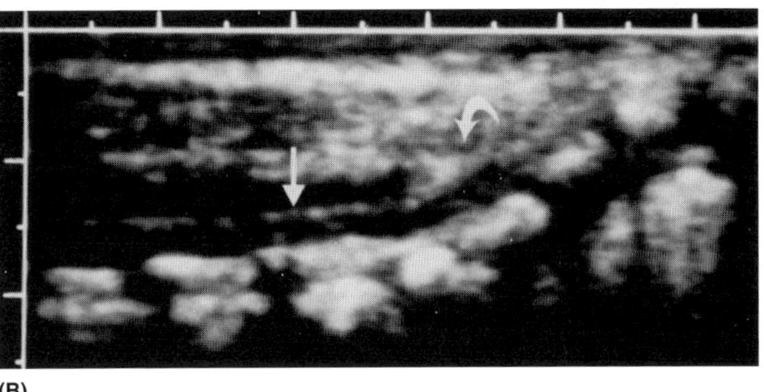

(B)

FIGURE 6 A AND B ■ Longitudinal US of tethered cord with thick filum (**A**) demonstrates the taut cord at the lumbar level (*arrowheads*), and (**B**) demonstrates the thick, stretched filum (*arrow*) as well as the site of dorsal tethering at the lumbosacral area (*curved arrow*). *Source*: Courtesy of Sandra Wootton-Gorges, M.D., University of California Medical Center, Davis, CA.

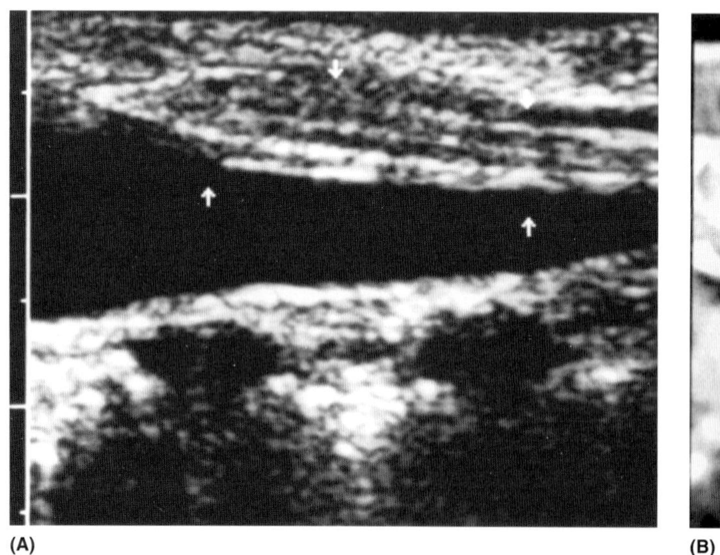
(A)

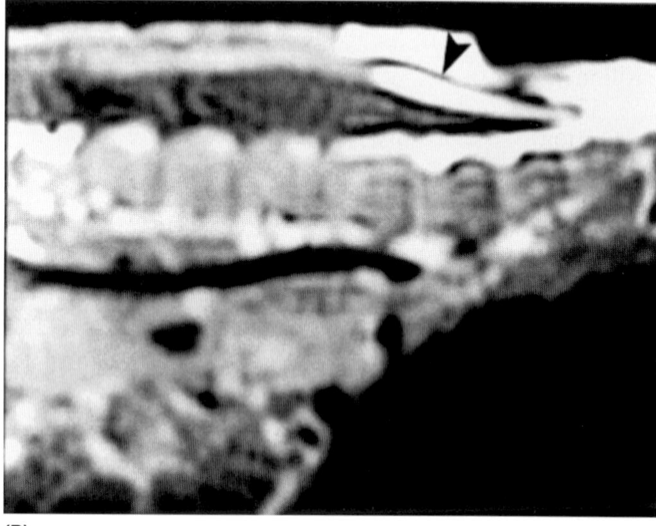
(B)

FIGURE 7 A AND B ■ Lipoma of filum terminale. Sagittal US (**A**) demonstrates a thick fatty filum (*arrows*). In the corresponding sagittal T1-weighted MRI (**B**), the fatty filum (*arrowhead*) appears markedly hyperintense. *Source*: From Ref. 2; courtesy of American Institute of Ultrasound in Medicine.

fila (15). It may also accompany a tethered cord, however (Fig. 7).

Hydromyelia and Syringomyelia ■ Disturbance of CSF flow or dysraphic malformation results in the abnormal accumulation of CSF, either within the paracentral cavities (syringomyelia) or within the central canal (hydromyelia). Imaging does not differentiate between these two entities, demonstrating a central fluid collection within the cord in both (Fig. 8). These malformations can be asymptomatic or present with scoliosis or sensorimotor disturbances. It is important to search for an associated Chiari I or II malformation, diastematomyelia, and myelomeningocele.

Dorsal Dermal Sinus ■ This is an epithelium-lined tract that extends from the skin to the arachnoid, cauda equina, or spinal cord and results from localized failure of superficial ectoderm to separate from neural ectoderm. Occurring most often in the lumbosacral area, it is recognized by a small ostium, often accompanied by a hemangioma, hairy nevus, or localized hyperpigmentation (6). Although it is often sonographically occult (4), when recognized, it appears as a hypoechoic linear structure in

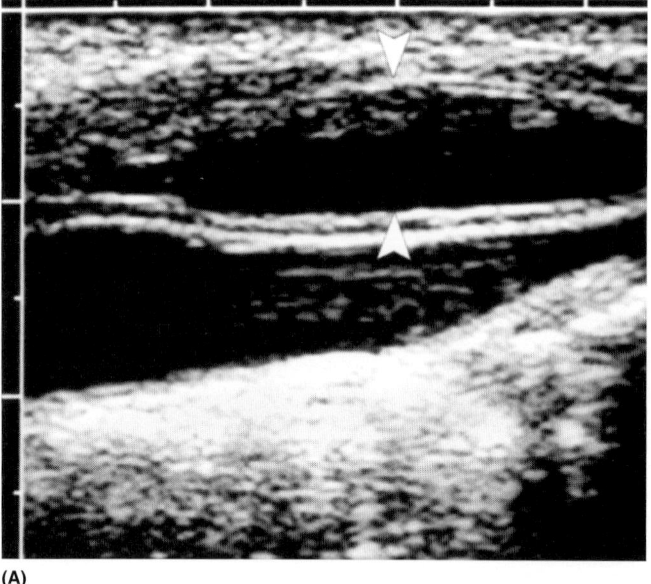
(A)

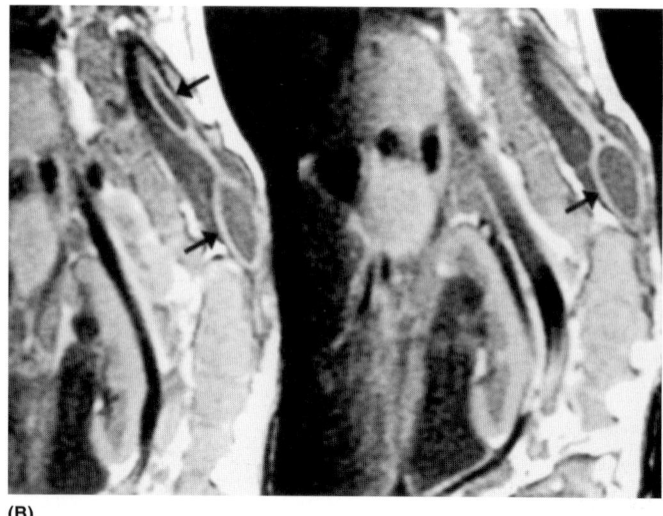
(B)

FIGURE 8 A AND B ■ Hydromyelia. The longitudinal US (**A**) demonstrates a dilated, fluid-filled central cord (*arrowheads*). The accompanying T1-weighted longitudinal MRI of the spine (**B**) demonstrates the thin, stretched cord with dilated center (*arrows*). *Source*: From Ref. 2; courtesy of American Institute of Ultrasound in Medicine.

the subcutaneous soft tissues, whereas in the thecal sac it appears echogenic with respect to the CSF. It is usually midline but can be paramedian. Of dorsal dermal sinuses, 11% (12) to 50% terminate in an intraspinal dermoid or epidermoid cyst, usually with resultant tethering of the spinal cord (8); there may also be dermal or epidermal cysts along the more superficial portion of the tract, although these can be difficult to visualize on US (16). The cutaneous opening results in spinal infection in almost two-thirds of cases (16), often recurrent.

The dorsal dermal sinus must be differentiated from the pilonidal sinus, which may terminate blindly or in a simple cyst. No tract connects this to neural structures, and there are no associated intraspinal anomalies or increased risk of spinal infection (although localized infection can occur). The tract of the pilonidal sinus extends straight or caudally, whereas dorsal dermal sinus tracts extend cranially (12). Terminating at or below the coccyx (17), the pilonidal sinus may be recognized at physical examination by apparent deepening of the tract as the skin is pulled cephalad, implying caudal deep attachment (16).

Occult Spinal Dysraphism: Complex

Diastematomyelia ■ An osseous or fibrous sagittal ridge results in often-asymmetric splitting of the spinal cord, usually limited to one or two vertebral levels and often associated with localized bony abnormalities such as focally increased interpediculate distance, laminar fusion, and spina bifida (16). Most often encountered in females, it usually occurs near the thoracolumbar junction. A patch of silky hair or other cutaneous stigmata occur in 50% to 75% of patients (15).

Diastematomyelia is recognized ultrasonographically by the presence of localized duplication of the spinal cord, both hemicords readily recognized in cross section (Fig. 9), unless they are obscured by an ossified septum. Occasionally, an artifact results in apparent duplication of a cord that is indeed normal; it is important to scan off midline to clarify this issue (18). Approximately 75% of patients also have tethering of the cord, and a syrinx is present in 50% (15). Thickened filum terminale is also common, as are clubfoot, scoliosis, and spina bifida.

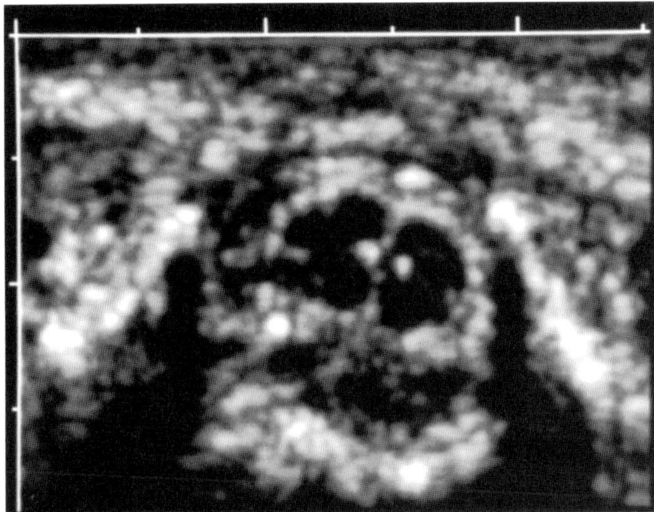

FIGURE 9 ■ Transverse US of lower thoracic spine demonstrates duplicated hemicords of diastematomyelia. *Source*: Courtesy of Sandra Wootton-Gorges, M.D., University of California Medical Center, Davis, CA.

Caudal Regression Syndrome ■ This constitutes a spectrum of abnormalities involving the trunk and the lower extremities and can present with relatively mild partial agenesis of the sacrococcygeal spine or severe spinal deformity with fusion of the lower extremities (sirenomelia). Often accompanied with genitourinary abnormalities such as renal agenesis, hydronephrosis, and Mullerian duct anomalies, as well as imperforate anus, it is associated with maternal diabetes. The etiology is abnormal retrogression of the caudal mesoderm.

There are two groups of spinal cord malformations that occur with caudal regression. The first type consists of blunt-ended, spade-shaped high conus medullaris, terminating above L1 (Fig. 10). There may also be a dilated central canal or a distal cyst, and sacral abnormalities are severe. The second type consists of a tethered cord (Fig. 11), with a thick, elongated filum and possibly an intraspinal lipoma. Patients in group 2 have more serious neurological abnormalities.

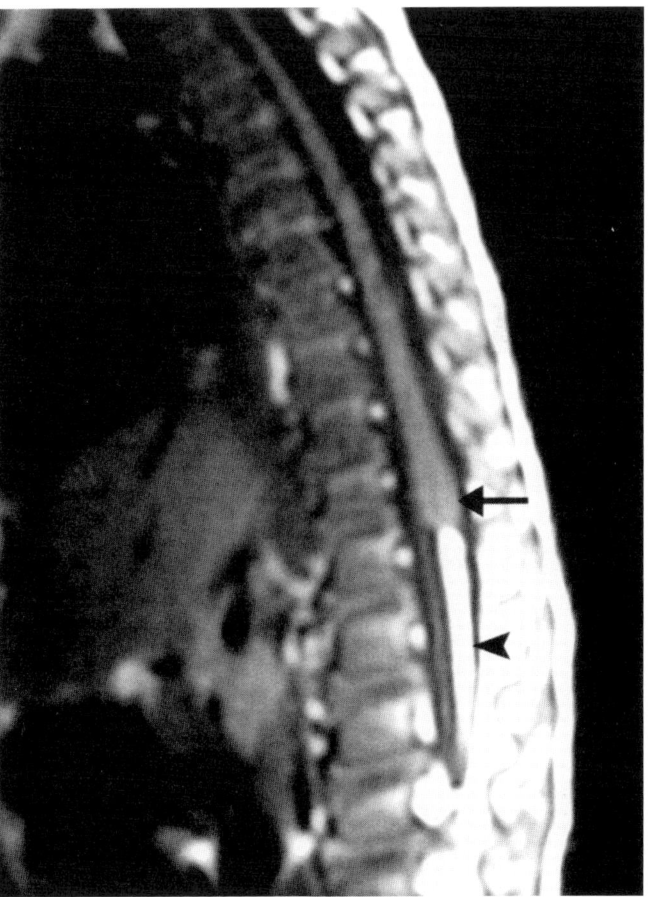

FIGURE 10 ■ Caudal regression, Type I. This sagittal T1-weighted MRI demonstrates a high, blunt conus (*arrow*) and thick lipoma of the filum terminale (*arrowhead*). Distal vertebral segments are disordered and incomplete.

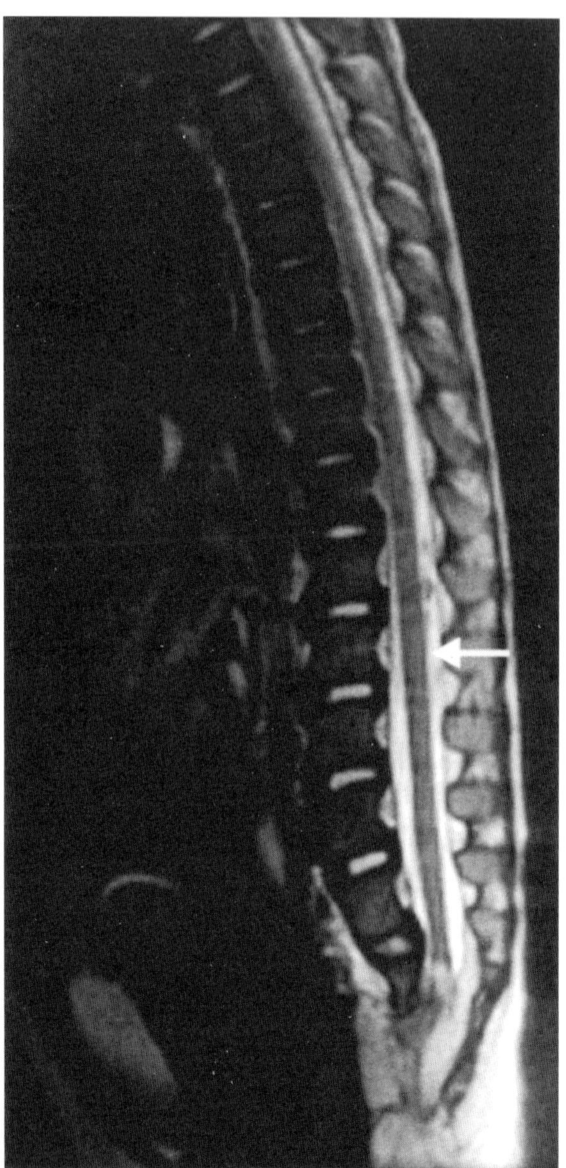

FIGURE 11 ■ Caudal regression, Type II. This sagittal T2-weighted MRI demonstrates an elongated, tethered cord (*arrow*) and disordered, incomplete distal vertebrae.

Spinal Dysraphism with a Skin-Covered Mass

Lipomyelomeningocele and Lipomyelocele

The lipomyelomeningocele/lipomyelocele constitutes a lipoma that extends from the intraspinal region, through a dysraphic defect, to the deep subcutaneous tissue of the back. The spinal cord inserts into the fatty tissue, resulting in tethering, and there is an accompanying meningomyelocele or myelocele. Cutaneous stigmata, such as dermal sinus, hemangioma, and nevus may be present. The term "lipomyelomeningocele" is employed if the distal spinal cord herniates posteriorly with the subarachnoid space, whereas "lipomyelocele" indicates that the meninges do not bulge posteriorly (Fig. 12). The lipomyelomeningocele is the most common occult dysraphic lesion (17).

The lipomatous portion appears highly echogenic and can be shown to be continuous from subcutaneous fat to the spinal canal (normal subcutaneous fat is hypoechoic) (16). The spinal cord can be observed to herniate into the meningeal sac if a lipomyelomeningocele is present, or it may be displaced anteriorly by the fatty mass if a lipomyelocele is present (16).

Terminal Myelocystocele

The terminal myelocystocele is rare, consisting of a dilated central canal in the distal portion of a bifid, tethered cord that terminates as a meningocele that protrudes through a posterior spina bifida defect. The terminal cyst in the spinal cord communicates with neither the subarachnoid space of the spinal canal nor that of the meningocele, although the latter spaces are in continuity. The defect is covered with skin and presents as a lumbosacral mass, often accompanied with anorectal and genitourinary anomalies. Alterations in CSF circulation result in distal hydromyelia and disruption of dorsal mesenchyme.

US demonstrates a large amount of fluid surrounding a bifid cord as well as hydromyelia. There is characteristic flaring of the central canal as it enlarges into the cystic mass, allowing differentiation from myelomeningocele (15). Nerve roots exit the cord ventrally.

Posterior Meningocele

A posterior meningocele consists of a CSF-filled sac lined with dura and arachnoid that herniate through a dysraphic defect, usually limited to one or two vertebrae (8). A skin-covered mass results, usually lumbar or sacral in location, though occasionally in the cervical or thoracic spine. The sac contains no neural tissue, but the cord may be tethered to its neck (12). US demonstrates an anechoic mass continuous with the anechoic CSF of the thecal sac (Fig. 13).

Anterior Sacral Meningocele and Lateral Meningocele

Much less common than the posterior meningocele, these are associated with mesenchymal disorders such as neurofibromatosis I, Marfan syndrome, and Ehlers–Danlos syndrome. These meningoceles consist of dura that protrudes laterally through an intervertebral foramen or anteriorly through a bony defect in the sacrum or the coccyx. Single or multiple, lateral meningoceles are most common in the thoracic and the lumbar spine and are associated with expansion of the associated intervertebral foramen or spinal canal. They are located in paraspinal, intrathoracic, or retroperitoneal areas and may be asymptomatic or result in scoliosis. US demonstrates a cystic mass displacing the spinal cord. Anterior meningoceles may be asymptomatic, or patients may present with bowel or bladder dysfunction. On ultrasound interrogation, there is an anechoic mass, anterior to the sacrum.

Spinal Dysraphism with a Non–Skin-Covered Mass

Myelocele and Myelomeningocele

Localized failure of neural folds to fuse dorsally results in an open spinal cord that causes deranged development of mesenchyme and ectoderm. The neural placode and leptomeninges are attached to an open skin defect, and,

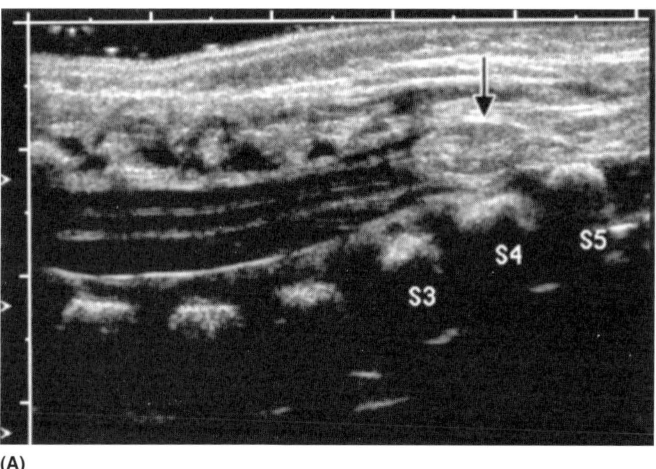

(A)

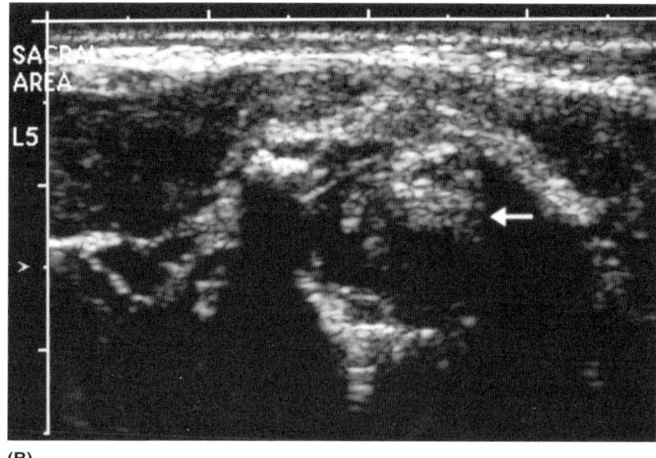

(B)

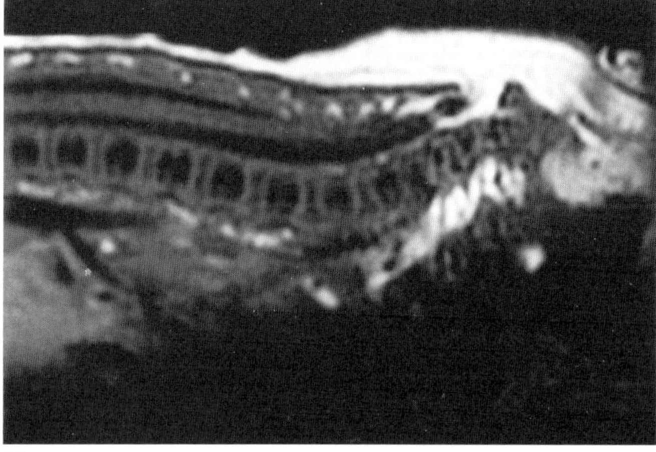

(C)

FIGURE 12 A–C ■ Lipomyelocele. (**A**) Sagittal US image of the lumbosacral spine shows a tethered cord terminating distally in echogenic fat (*arrow*) that is continuous with subcutaneous fatty tissue. (**B**) Transverse US image demonstrates the dorsal lipoma displacing the distal cord anteriorly. (**C**) Longitudinal T1-weighted MRI of the distal spine portrays the distal lipoma as well as a defect in the dorsal elements.

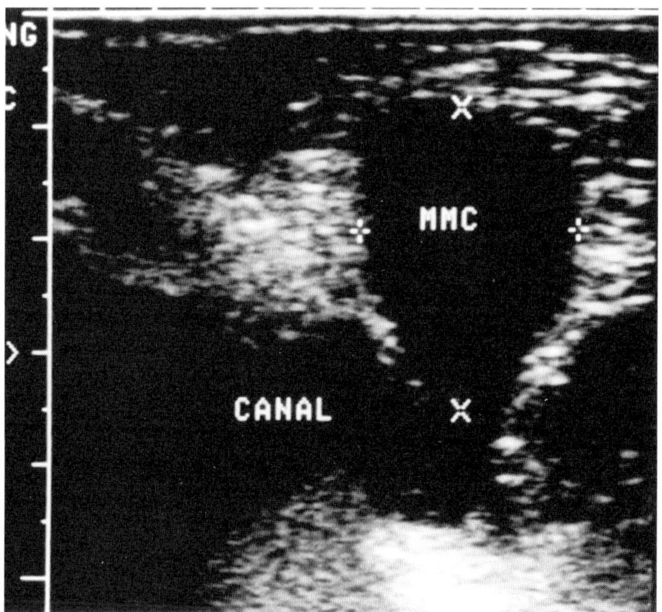

FIGURE 13 ■ Posterior meningocele. Longitudinal US of lumbosacral spine in a newborn demonstrates an anechoic, fluid-filled sac that protrudes dorsally into the soft tissues of the back. *Source*: From Ref. 19; courtesy of Anderson Publishing Ltd.

because mesenchyme cannot migrate posteriorly, dorsal elements are everted. The myelocele lies flush with the skin of the patient's back, whereas the myelomeningocele protrudes dorsally, secondary to expansion of ventral subarachnoid space (16). Most common in the thoracolumbar spine (44%), these defects also occur in the lumbar spine (22%), thoracolumbar spine (32%), and thoracic spine (2%) (20). Infants exhibit asymmetric loss of motor function in the lower extremities or other neural deficits. Later in life, loss of bladder or bowel function may become apparent.

Preoperative imaging of the defect is not recommended due to the dual risks of infection and injury. However, the high frequency of accompanying abnormalities, such as Chiari II malformation, tethered cord, syrinx, diastematomyelia, and arachnoid cyst mandates thorough evaluation of the remainder of the neural axis, and this can be accomplished ultrasonographically. Chiari II malformation, which occurs in 99% of patients, is recognized by downward herniation of the cerebellar tonsils and kinking of the cervical cord. Tethering occurs in all patients with a lumbosacral defect and in 70% to 90% of all cases; imaging findings have been discussed earlier. Hydro- or syringomyelia is found in 40% to 80% and occurs cephalad

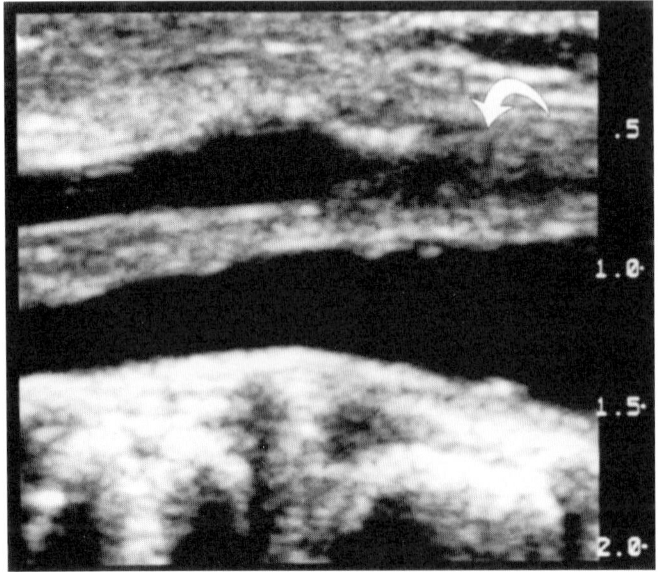

(A)

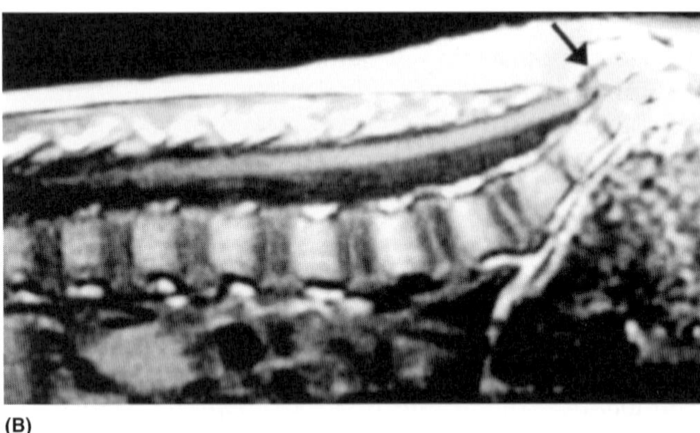

(B)

FIGURE 14 A AND B ■ Re-tethering after surgery for myelomeningocele. (**A**) Longitudinal US demonstrates dorsal scar tissue (*curved arrow*), with adjacent tethered cord. (**B**) In the accompanying longitudinal T1-weighted MRI, tethering is apparent (*arrow*). *Source*: From Ref. 2; courtesy of American Institute of Ultrasound in Medicine.

to the defect. Diastematomyelia accompanies 20% to 40% of cases, whereas arachnoid cysts are found in only 2% (20). Lipomas are found in up to 74% of patients (16).

US may be possible in postoperative evaluation of the repaired defect, as the splayed dorsal vertebral elements often provide an adequate acoustic window, although scarring may prohibit ultrasonographic interrogation (2). Postoperative development of scoliosis—or worsening or recurrence of symptoms—may signify re-tethering of the cord, secondary to postoperative scarring or changes in the dura (Fig. 14). US demonstrates posterior positioning of a taut cord with decreased pulsations. Note that the actual position of the conus is not useful, as de-tethering does not correct the position of the already-low cord. Increase in size of dermoids, epidermoids, or lipomas (Fig. 15) may also be observed postoperatively as an area of decreased or mixed echogenicity positioned between the cord and the closure (16); worsening hydrosyringomyelia may also be identified.

ACQUIRED ABNORMALITIES OF THE SPINAL CORD

Birth Injury: Intraspinal Hematoma and Cord Injury

Forceps delivery and breech presentation are associated with these entities. Affected infants may present with peripartal asphyxia, hypotonia, abnormal deep tendon reflexes,

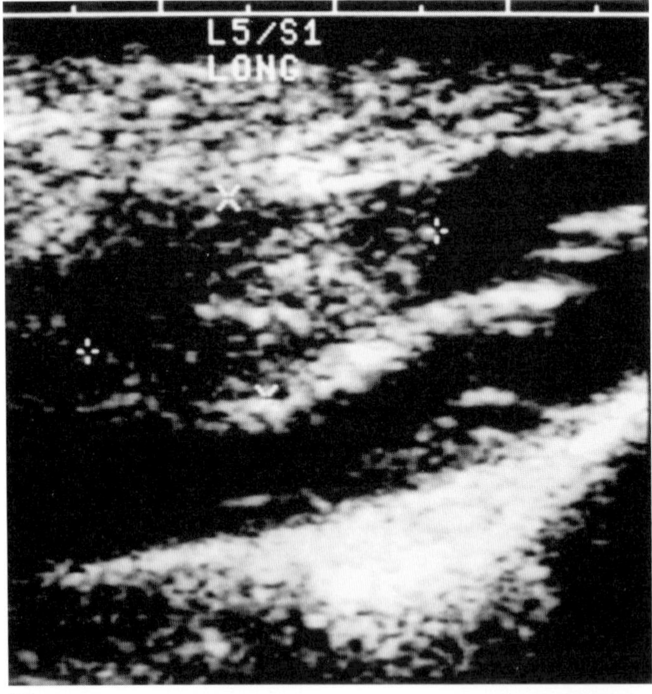

(A)

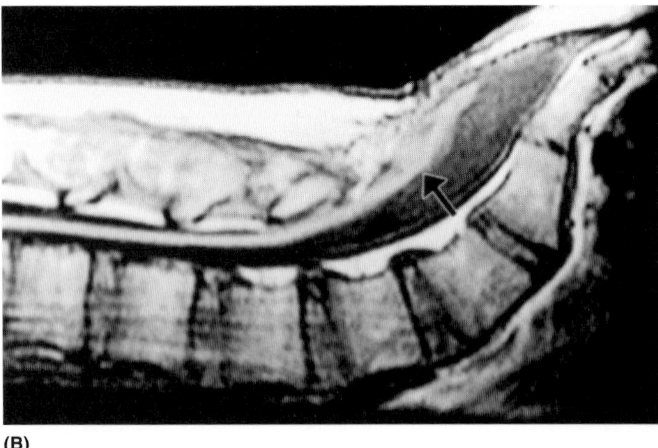

(B)

FIGURE 15 A AND B ■ (**A**) Longitudinal US of sacral spine after myelomeningocele repair. There is an intraspinal mass with adherent cord (US markers). (**B**) The accompanying T1-weighted MRI demonstrates a low cord adjacent to an epidermoid tumor (*arrow*). *Source*: From Ref. 2; courtesy of American Institute of Ultrasound in Medicine.

or paradoxical respiration. There can be (*i*) epidural hemorrhage due to meningeal damage, (*ii*) nerve root laceration or avulsion, and (*iii*) laceration, distortion, or transaction of the cord (21). US may demonstrate extra-axial hemorrhage with cord compression, increased echogenicity of the cord (resulting from edema or hemorrhage), and cord transection. Follow-up US may demonstrate decrease in size of the fluid collections as well as pathologic thinning of the spinal cord (22).

Lumbar Puncture

If lumbar puncture results in dural or leptomeningeal laceration and resultant leak of CSF, subdural or epidural fluid collections may develop, surrounding the neural structures with resultant compression of nerve roots or cauda equina. US demonstrates a fluid collection that tapers cephalad as well as mass effect on crowding and thinning of nerve roots (23).

REFERENCES

1. Kangarloo H et al. High-resolution spinal sonography in infants. AJR Am J Roentgenol 1984; 142(6):1243–1247.
2. Gerscovich EO et al. Spinal sonography and magnetic resonance imaging in patients with repaired myelomeningocele: comparison of modalities. J Ultrasound Med 1999; 18(9):655–664.
3. DiPietro MA. The conus medullaris: normal US findings throughout childhood. Radiology 1993; 188(1):149–153.
4. Hughes JA et al. Evaluation of spinal ultrasound in spinal dysraphism. Clin Radiol 2003; 58(3):227–233.
5. DiPietro MA, Venes JL. Real-time sonography of the pediatric spinal cord: horizons and limits. Concepts Pediatr Neurosurg 1988; 8:120–132.
6. Kriss VM, Desai NS. Occult spinal dysraphism in neonates: assessment of high-risk cutaneous stigmata on sonography. AJR Am J Roentgenol 1998; 171(6):1687–1692.
7. Rohrschneider WK et al. Diagnostic value of spinal US: comparative study with MR imaging in pediatric patients. Radiology 1996; 200(2):383–388.
8. Byrd SE, Darling CF, McLone DG. Developmental disorders of the pediatric spine. Radiol Clin North Am 1991; 29(4):711–752.
9. Kriss VM, Kriss TC, Babcock DS. The ventriculus terminalis of the spinal cord in the neonate: a normal variant on sonography. AJR Am J Roentgenol 1995; 165(6):1491–1493.
10. Hughes JA et al. Three-dimensional sonographic evaluation of the infant spine: preliminary findings. J Clin Ultrasound 2003; 31(1):9–20.
11. Nelson MD Jr, Sedler JA, Gilles FH. Spinal cord central echo complex: histoanatomic correlation. Radiology 1989; 170(2):479–481.
12. Rossi A et al. Imaging in spine and spinal cord malformations. Eur J Radiol 2004; 50(2):177–200.
13. Unsinn KM et al. Sonography of the ventriculus terminalis in newborns. AJNR Am J Neuroradiol 1996; 17(5):1003–1004.
14. Sigal R et al. Ventriculus terminalis of the conus medullaris: MR imaging in four patients with congenital dilatation. AJNR Am J Neuroradiol 1991; 12(4):733–737.
15. Dick EA, de Bruyn R. Ultrasound of the spinal cord in children: its role. Eur Radiol 2003; 13(3):552–562. Epub 2002.
16. Naidich TP, Radkowski MA, Britton J. Real-time sonographic display of caudal spinal anomalies. Neuroradiology 1986; 28(5–6): 512–527.
17. Korsvik HE. Ultrasound assessment of congenital spinal anomalies presenting in infancy. Semin Ultrasound CT MR 1994; 15(4):264–274.
18. Austin MJ et al. Sonographic duplication artifact of the spinal cord in infants and children. J Ultrasound Med 2004; 23(6):799–803.
19. Gerscovich EO, McGahan JP. Ultrasound of the spinal canal in the young child. Appl Radiol 2001; 30:21–26.
20. Unsinn KM et al. US of the spinal cord in newborns: spectrum of normal findings, variants, congenital anomalies, and acquired diseases. Radiographics 2000; 20(4):923–938.
21. Towbin A. Latent spinal cord and brain stem injury in newborn infants. Dev Med Child Neurol 1969; 11(1):54–68.
22. Babyn PS et al. Sonographic evaluation of spinal cord birth trauma with pathologic correlation. AJR Am J Roentgenol 1988; 151(4):763–766.
23. Kiechl-Kohlendorfer U et al. Cerebrospinal fluid leakage after lumbar puncture in neonates: incidence and sonographic appearance. AJR Am J Roentgenol 2003; 181(1):231–234.

Pediatric Chest ● *Marilyn J. Siegel*

24

INTRODUCTION

Chest radiography remains the initial imaging study to evaluate diseases of the pediatric chest. Computed tomography (CT) and magnetic resonance imaging (MRI) have become the studies of choice to further assess an abnormality when chest radiography is equivocal or nonconfirmatory. In selected clinical instances, ultrasonography also can be useful as a secondary test to further evaluate abnormalities of the chest detected on conventional radiographic studies (1–5). Ultrasonography is particularly helpful in evaluating pleural effusions, peripheral lung opacities, mediastinal widening, diaphragmatic abnormalities, and chest-wall lesions.

This chapter reviews the technique of chest sonography, the diagnostic applications of sonography in a wide variety of disease processes of the chest in children, and the characteristic sonographic features of the common pleural, pulmonary, mediastinal, chest-wall, and vascular lesions in childhood.

TECHNIQUE

Imaging Approaches

Conventional chest radiography should be performed in all patients before the sonographic examination to define the area of interest for insonation. Ultrasonography is performed with the patient in supine, prone, or decubitus position, depending on the location of the lesion. Images are obtained in transverse and longitudinal planes, supplemented by oblique planes when needed to enhance lesion conspicuity.

Useful acoustic windows are shown in Figure 1. Supraclavicular and suprasternal approaches are helpful in examining lung apices, anterior mediastinum, and great vessels. Transsternal and parasternal approaches also facilitate evaluation of the anterior mediastinum, particularly in infants who have large thymus glands and an unossified sternum, which allow transmission of the ultrasound beam. Intercostal scanning allows imaging of the pleural space and peripheral lung parenchyma. Using liver and spleen as acoustic windows can facilitate evaluation of the deep sulcal spaces (inferior thoracic cavity). The subxiphoid and subdiaphragmatic approaches are used to image juxtaphrenic lesions, while the posterior paraspinal approach is used to evaluate paravertebral lesions.

Transducers

The choice of transducer varies with the size of the patients and the area being examined. Higher-frequency (7.5 or 10.0 MHz) transducers usually suffice for the evaluation of the chest in infants and young children, whereas lower-frequency transducers (5.0 MHz) are required in older children and adolescents. Curved or linear-array transducers are useful to insonate via transsternal and parasternal approaches. Sector or vector transducers are preferred for insonation above the suprasternal notch, between the ribs, and below the diaphragm and subxiphoid spaces. Color Doppler sonography is valuable for examining the mediastinal vascular anatomy and the relationship of mediastinal vessels to intrathoracic

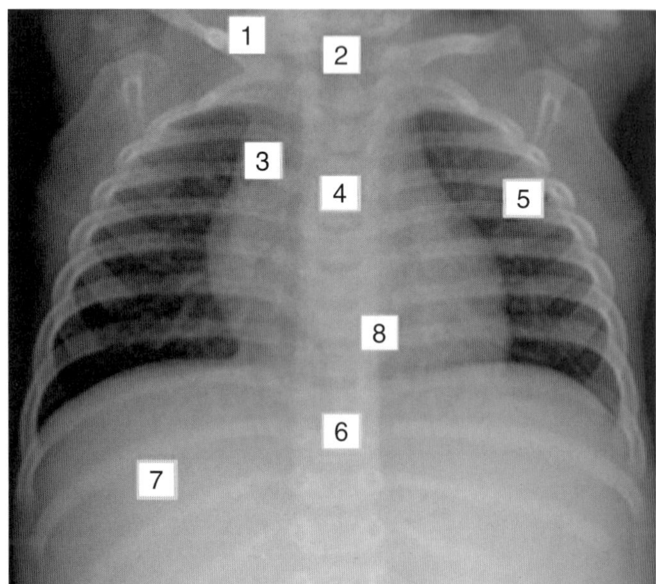

FIGURE 1 ■ Acoustic windows for thoracic sonography. (1) Supraclavicular; (2) suprasternal; (3) parasternal; (4) transsternal; (5) intercostal; (6) subxiphoid; (7) subdiaphragmatic; and (8) posterior paraspinal. *Source*: Courtesy of Brian D. Coley, M.D., Columbus, OH.

lesions and it may be helpful in characterizing a lesion by demonstrating the internal vascularity and flow pattern. It also is helpful in identifying anomalous vessels such as those that occur in pulmonary sequestration.

NORMAL ANATOMY

Thymus

The thymus is relatively large compared with the rest of the thorax in neonates and infants and is easily evaluated by sonography. Because it abuts the chest wall and the sternum anteriorly, it can be readily seen using suprasternal, transsternal, or parasternal approaches (1). It usually extends from the horizontal portion of the left brachiocephalic vein cephalad to the origin of the great vessels caudally and has a quadrilateral shape and smooth margins. On sonography, it is hypoechoic to the thyroid gland and nearly isoechoic to the liver. The normal thymus is mildly heterogeneous and has regular linear and punctate echogenicities scattered throughout the parenchyma (Fig. 2) (5–7). Even when large, it drapes around adjacent mediastinal structures without displacing or deforming them. It is hypovascular or nearly avascular on color Doppler sonography (5,6).

Occasionally, the thymus extends either cranially above the brachiocephalic vessels and may bulge into the neck or it may extend into the posterior thorax. The sonographic findings that allow confident recognition of the ectopically positioned thymus are its direct continuity with the thymic tissue in the anterior mediastinum, an echopattern similar to that of normal thymic tissue, and the lack of compression of adjacent vessels (Fig. 3) (5,8,9).

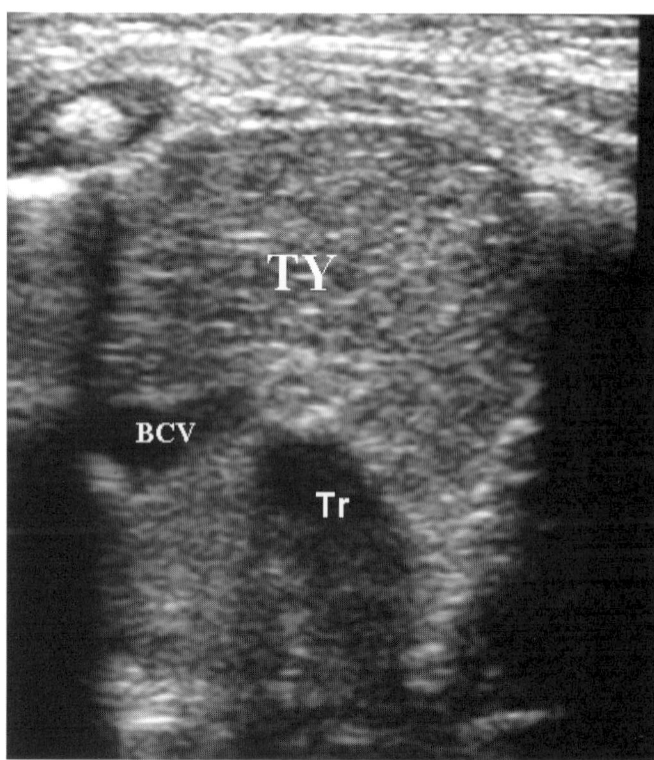

FIGURE 2 ■ Normal thymus. Transverse sonogram shows a mildly heterogeneous thymus (TY) with characteristic linear and punctate echodensities. BCV, brachiocephalic vein; Tr, trachea.

The acoustic limitations imposed by the small size of the thymus, aerated lung in the anterior mediastinum, and the ossified sternum limit the usefulness of sonography in imaging the thymus in older children and adolescents. In

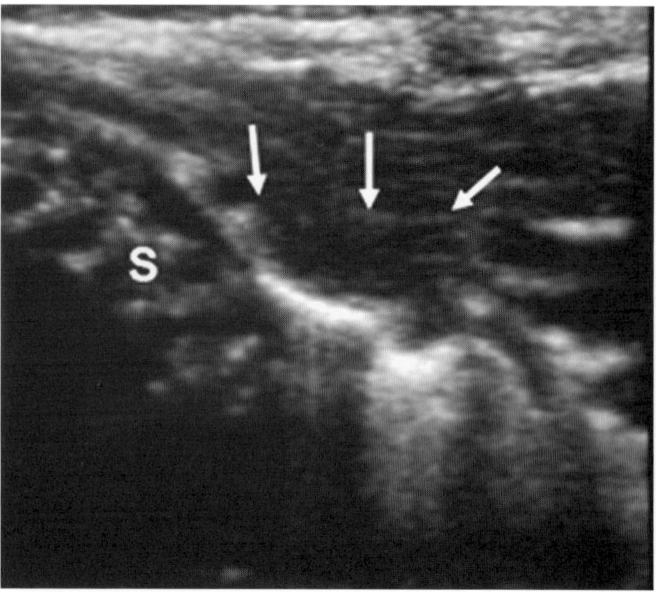

FIGURE 3 ■ Superior extension into the neck. Longitudinal scan to the left of midline shows normally echogenic thymus (*arrows*) anterior to the cervical spine (S).

this age group, CT and MRI are the preferred imaging modalities for evaluating thymic pathology.

Pleura and Lung

The normal pleural surface produces a hyperechoic line beneath the chest wall and ribs. The acoustic interface of the chest wall with normal aerated lung produces multiple strong posterior reverberations and mirror image artifacts (Fig. 4). With respiration, aerated lung can be noted to move along the parietal pleural surface (termed the "gliding sign").

Great Vessels

The deeper vascular structures, such as the thoracic aorta and superior vena cava, can be evaluated sonographically in neonates and young infants, but they become more difficult to recognize in older children. However, in this population, sonography remains a useful tool to evaluate abnormalities of the subclavian and brachiocephalic vessels.

Normal vessels have thin, smooth echogenic walls and anechoic lumina. Because they lack valves, the central veins show the effects of respiratory and cardiac activity. They increase in size during inspiration and decrease in size during expiration. The Doppler flow pattern is characterized by a biphasic flow profile with systolic and diastolic peaks and even reversal of flow with atrial systole (Fig. 5) (10,11).

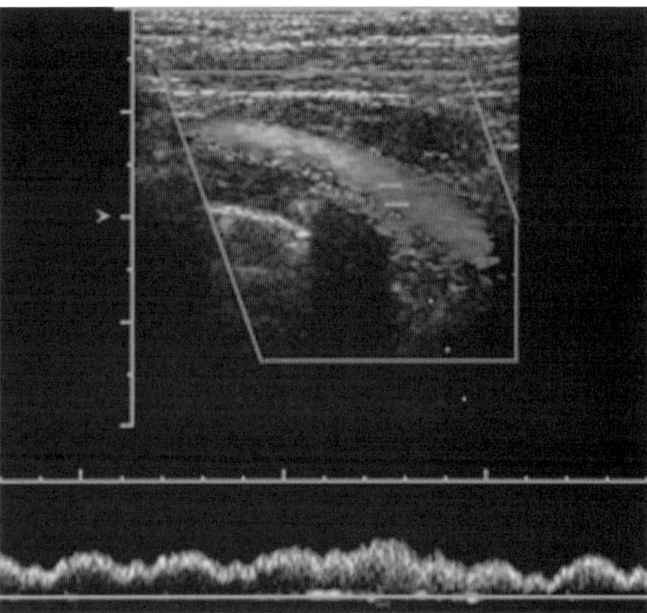

FIGURE 5 ■ Normal mediastinal veins. Transverse scan through a suprasternal approach shows a patent left subclavian vein (*cursor*) with normal pulsatility, reflecting transmitted cardiac pulsations.

Diaphragm

The diaphragm is the musculotendinous structure that separates thoracic and abdominal cavities and it is also the primary muscle of respiration. The right hemidiaphragm is easy to image using the right lobe of the liver as an acoustic window. The left hemidiaphragm is best visualized using the spleen, the left lobe of the liver, or the fluid-filled stomach as acoustic windows. The diaphragm appears as a relatively smooth, slightly undulating echogenic band (Fig. 6). The crural parts are seen as relatively hypoechoic, linear structures near the midline.

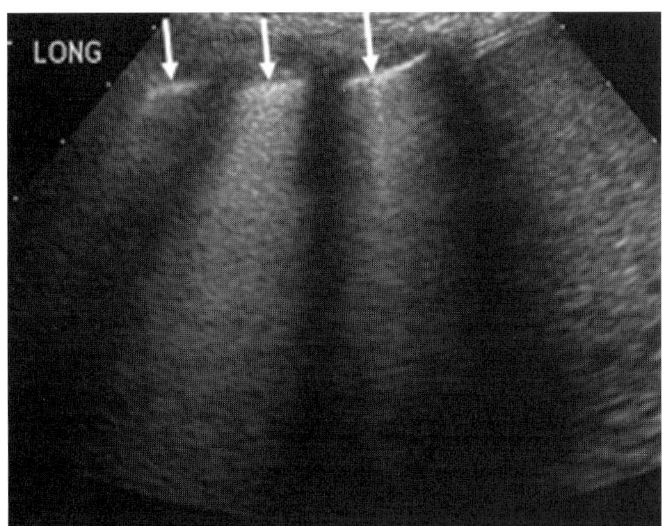

FIGURE 4 ■ Normal lung. Longitudinal image of the lateral chest using a linear transducer shows the echogenic pleura (*arrows*) and the subadjacent highly echogenic air-filled lung. The ribs are recognized because they cast acoustic shadows.

Diaphragmatic motion is assessed on scans obtained during inspiration and expiration (12,13). The transverse plane allows simultaneous identification of both hemidiaphragms. Measurements for normal diaphragmatic excursion on longitudinal scans have been established in the neonate (14). The excursion of the middle and posterior thirds of the diaphragm is greater than that of the anterior third. In the longitudinal plane, the mean excursion (and

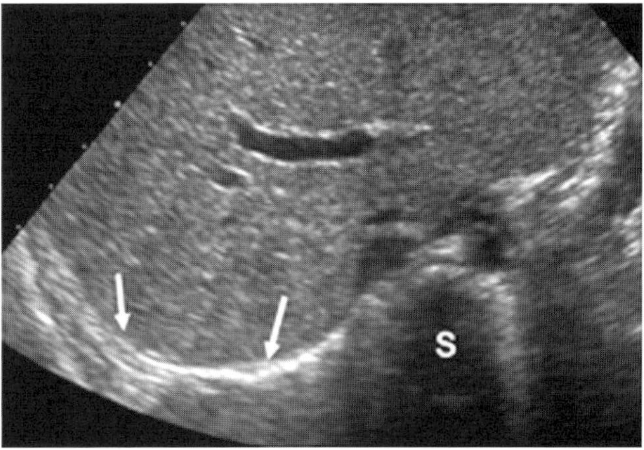

FIGURE 6 ■ Normal diaphragm. Transverse subxiphoid scan demonstrates the echogenic diaphragm (*arrows*). S, spine.

standard deviation) for anterior, middle, and posterior thirds of the diaphragm are 2.6 ± 0.1, 3.6 ± 0.2, and 4.5 ± 0.2 mm, respectively.

INDICATIONS

The indications for sonography of the chest include (*i*) differentiation of pleural from parenchymal disease in a child with an opaque hemithorax on chest radiography and guidance for intervention; (*ii*) characterization of focal parenchymal masses seen on chest radiography; (*iii*) evaluation of an abnormal mediastinal contour (which often is an unusual-shaped thymus); (*iv*) assessment of vascular abnormalities; (*v*) evaluation of diaphragmatic motion and peridiaphragmatic masses; and (*vi*) characterization of palpable chest-wall lesions.

PLEURAL DISEASES

Pleural Effusions

Pleural fluid collections are ideal for imaging with sonography because they transmit acoustic sound. Conventional chest radiography usually suffices for the evaluation of pleural effusion and parenchymal lung disease, but if the diagnosis is equivocal, sonography can enable differentiation of pleural effusion from infiltrate and it also can help guide percutaneous drainage.

Sonography is superior to CT in demonstrating septations within the fluid collections. Recognition of the presence of septations or a multiloculated fluid collection is important because it means that fibrinolytic therapy may be required to attain adequate catheter drainage (15).

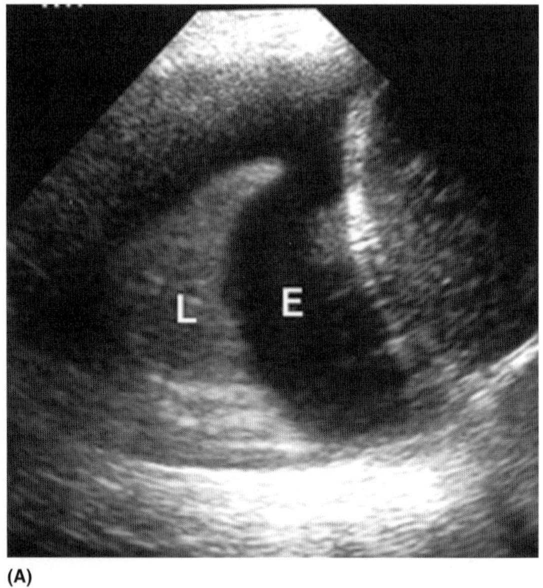

(A)

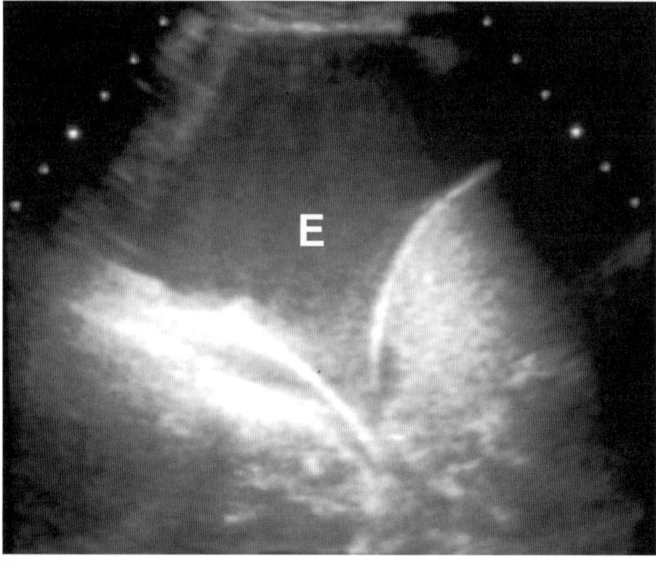

(B)

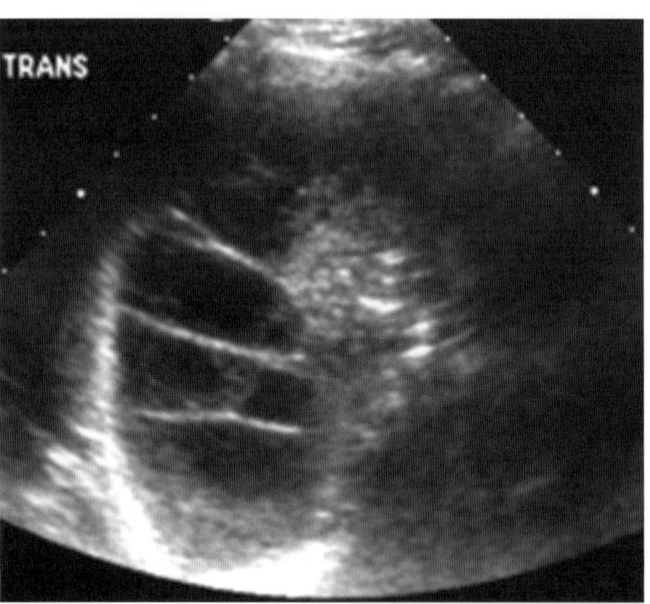

(C)

FIGURE 7 A–C ■ Pleural effusions. (**A**) Simple effusion. Longitudinal sonogram in a one-year-old girl demonstrates a large anechoic pleural effusion (E) and atelectatic lung (L). Aspiration revealed serous fluid. (**B**) Empyema. Longitudinal sonogram in another patient shows a pleural effusion (E) with diffuse low-level echoes. Aspiration yielded purulent material. (**C**) Intercostal transverse scan in a 10-year-old girl demonstrates multiple loculations in the pleural space. These were not mobile with changes in respiration. Aspiration yielded purulent fluid.

There are four major types of pleural fluid collections: serous (transudate), purulent (exudate), hemorrhagic, and chylous. Serous effusions are usually of parapneumonic origin, but they also occur with a number of other conditions, including acute glomerulonephritis, nephrotic syndrome, congestive heart failure, cirrhosis, subphrenic abscess, and pancreatitis. Purulent collections (i.e., empyemas) are virtually always a complication of bacterial infection. Hemorrhagic fluid usually follows blunt or penetrating chest trauma. Chylous effusion can be a complication of thoracic or cardiac surgery or it can be idiopathic.

The sonographic appearance of pleural fluid ranges from completely anechoic (usually representing serous or chylous effusions) to hypoechoic collections with mobile or floating particles (hemorrhagic, purulent, or chylous effusions) to septated collections (usually purulent collections) (Fig. 7) (16). On color Doppler imaging, the mobile debris scatters the sound and produces color Doppler signal within the fluid (termed the "fluid color sign") (17,18).

Sonographic features that are useful in identifying fluid that is amenable to aspiration include changes in the shape of the fluid with changes in patient respiration or patient position and the demonstration of mobile echogenic particles or bands. The demonstration of the "fluid color sign" is also a useful finding for identifying free-flowing fluid. The gliding sign is preserved. These findings generally indicate a relatively low viscosity fluid collection.

Purulent fluid collections contain fibrous strands, which initially are thin and mobile. With these findings, the fluid can usually be aspirated. As purulent fluid collections organize, the strands or septa thicken and increase in number, resulting in multiple loculations or a honeycomb appearance. The fluid no longer changes configuration with changes in respiration or patient position and the gliding sign is lost. The parietal and visceral pleura may be thickened and the interface between the pleura and the adjacent lung parenchyma is often indistinct. These findings generally imply a high viscosity collection or pleural thickening and indicate that thoracentesis will be difficult.

Empyema may progress to a fibrothorax, which appears as an echogenic pleural mass, with or without small loculated fluid collections, encasing the lung (Fig. 8). In this situation, thoracentesis is usually not successful, and thoracotomy with pleural debridement may be required (3).

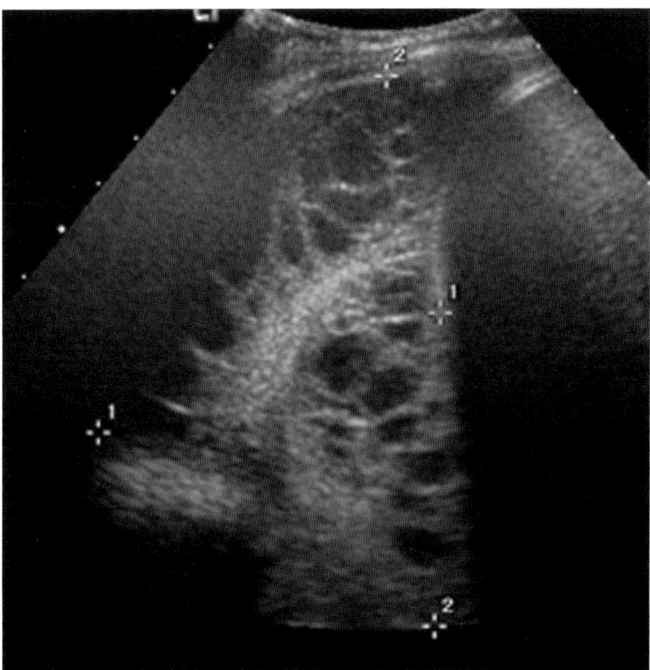

FIGURE 8 ■ Fibrothorax. Transverse sonogram in a three-year-old boy shows thickened visceral and parietal pleura (*calipers*). Small anechoic fluid collections are noted in the pleural space.

Pleural Masses

Pleural masses in children are more often the result of metastatic disease or leukemia rather than primary neoplasm. Sonographic findings of pleural metastases include echogenic pleural nodules and pleural effusion, which is often hemorrhagic and contains echogenic debris.

Pneumothorax

Sonography does not have a role in the diagnosis of pneumothorax, but knowledge of the sonographic findings is important because a pneumothorax may be detected incidentally during an examination performed for another clinical indication. In pneumothorax, the gliding motion of the lung is absent and the normal reverberations at the pleural–lung interface are replaced by a homogeneous posterior acoustic shadow (19–21). Mobile air-fluid levels and loss of the normal gliding have been described in hydropneumothorax (22).

PULMONARY PARENCHYMA

Consolidation and Atelectasis

When the normally aerated lung becomes consolidated or atelectatic, it allows transmission of the ultrasound beam (23). The airless lung has an echogenicity and echotexture similar to that of liver and spleen. This echogenic area of lung usually contains multiple bright punctate and branching linear structures, corresponding to air trapped within the bronchi. This appearance is termed a "sonographic air bronchogram" (Fig. 9A) (23,24). Occasionally, the bronchi are filled with fluid or mucoid material. In these instances, sonography demonstrates anechoic or hypoechoic branching structures, termed a "sonographic fluid bronchogram" (Fig. 9B).

In consolidation, the lung volume is normal or increased and the bronchi maintain their normal branching pattern. In atelectasis, the overall lung volume is diminished and as a result, the bronchi are closer together. However, in practice, the distinction between consolidation and atelectasis is often difficult on sonography and is better appreciated on chest radiography or CT. In consolidated and atelectatic

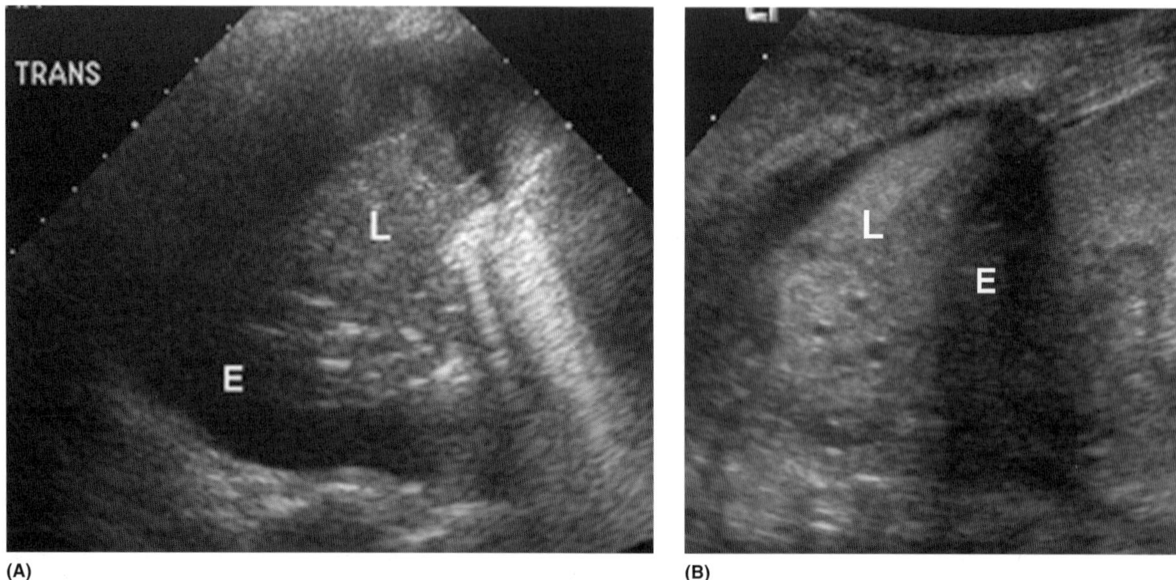

FIGURE 9 A AND B ■ Consolidated lung. Nine-year-old boy with pneumonia. (**A**) Air-bronchograms. Transverse scan through the right lung base shows consolidated lung (L) with echogenic linear branching structures, which represent air bronchograms. (**B**) Fluid-filled bronchi. Longitudinal image slightly more medially through the right lung base demonstrates echogenic consolidated lung (L) containing branching anechoic tubular structures, which represent bronchi filled with fluid or mucus. E, pleural effusion.

lung, color Doppler imaging shows branching pulmonary vessels (18). Normal pulmonary vessels are not seen in aerated lung by sonography and their identification is another finding of consolidation or atelectasis.

Lung abscess refers to an area of tissue suppuration surrounded by a well-formed capsule. In children, lung abscesses develop either as a primary lesion or secondarily in an area of abnormal lung, such as a sequestration, lung cyst, or pneumatocele. In patients with peripheral pleural opacity, sonography can be useful to diagnose lung abscess and can also characterize associated fluid and consolidation. The sonographic appearance of a pulmonary abscess is that of a spherical or ovoid hypoechoic mass with thick, irregular walls. Air-fluid levels may be observed within the cavity, particularly if the patient is scanned in an erect or semierect position. When the abscess abuts the pleural surface, the hyperechoic pleural line is lost and the gliding motion of the underlying lung is no longer seen (25). Sonography can also be used to guide percutaneous needle aspiration for therapeutic management.

Congenital Parenchymal Masses

Congenital lung lesions are usually cystic adenomatoid malformations and pulmonary sequestrations. Most are diagnosed on prenatal sonography or MRI or on postnatal chest radiographs obtained for evaluation of respiratory distress or for persistent or chronic recurrent pneumonia. (1,3,5,26). In some instances, the lesion is an incidental finding on radiographs obtained for other clinical indications. In neonates and infants, sonography can clarify the diagnosis when other imaging studies are equivocal. In older patients, CT and MRI are the preferred imaging studies to diagnose these congenital lung lesions.

Cystic adenomatoid malformation is a mass of disorganized pulmonary tissue that has a normal communication with the bronchial tree and normal vascular supply and drainage. There are three histologic types: Type I (accounting for 50% of cases) contains large cysts greater than 2 cm in diameter; Type II (40% of cases) contains multiple small cysts less than 2 cm in diameter; and Type III (10% of cases) appears solid on visual inspection but contains microscopic cysts (27). The sonographic appearance mirrors the histologic findings, demonstrating variable sized cysts and echogenic parenchyma (Fig. 10).

Bronchopulmonary sequestration is a mass of nonfunctioning pulmonary tissue that has no normal connection with the tracheobronchial tree and is supplied by an anomalous systemic artery arising from the aorta. When the sequestered lung is confined within the normal visceral pleura and has venous drainage to the pulmonary veins, it is termed "intralobar or acquired." The sequestered lung is termed "extralobar or congenital" when it has its own pleura and venous drainage to systemic veins. Extralobar sequestration can be associated with pleural effusions, hydrops and polyhydramnios, cystic adenomatoid malformation, usually Type II, and Bochdalek hernia (28). The sonographic appearance of sequestration can be similar to that of cystic adenomatoid malformation and ranges from a homogeneous solid-appearing mass to a complex echogenic mass with cysts (Fig. 11) (29–31). These two lesions can also coexist (Fig. 12).

When a complex or homogeneous mass is found, particularly in the lung bases, color Doppler imaging may be helpful to differentiate between cystic adenomatoid malformation and pulmonary sequestration. The pathognomonic finding diagnostic of sequestration is the anomalous

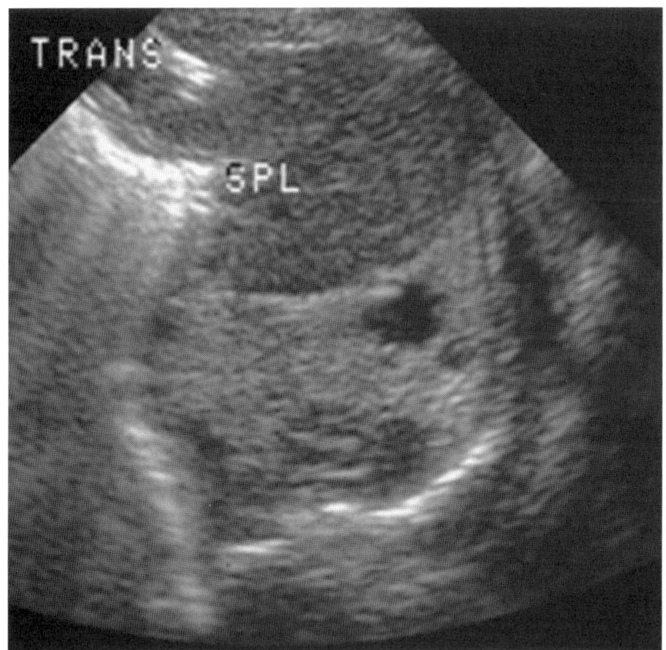

FIGURE 10 ■ Congenital cystic adenomatous malformation. Neonate with a mass in the left lower thorax. Transverse scan demonstrates a complex mass containing small cysts and echogenic soft-tissue components. The mass is adjacent to the spleen (SPL).

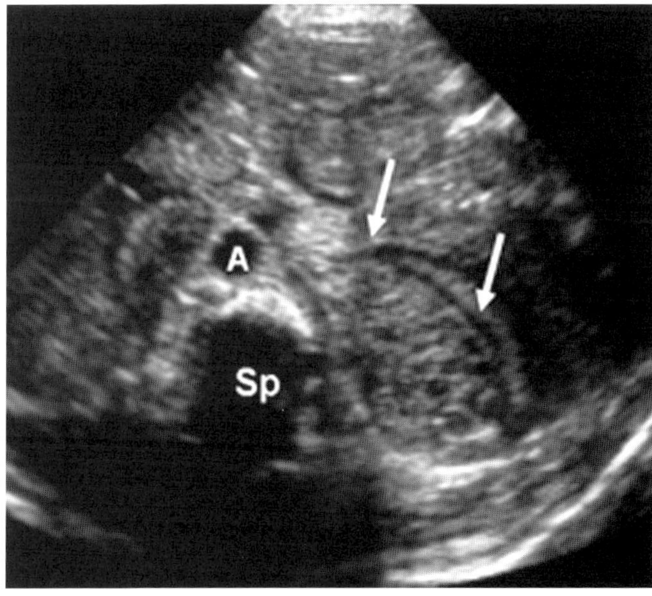

FIGURE 12 ■ Extralobar sequestration with cystic adenomatoid malformation. Transverse sonogram shows an echogenic mass with cystic components (*arrows*) that were shown to be elements of cystic adenomatoid malformation at pathologic sectioning. Sp, spine; A, aorta. *Source*: From Ref. 5.

systemic arterial supply arising from the aorta and supplying the mass (Fig. 11) (18,29–32). Differentiation between cystic changes in a sequestration and an associated cystic adenomatoid malformation cannot be done by sonography and will require tissue sampling.

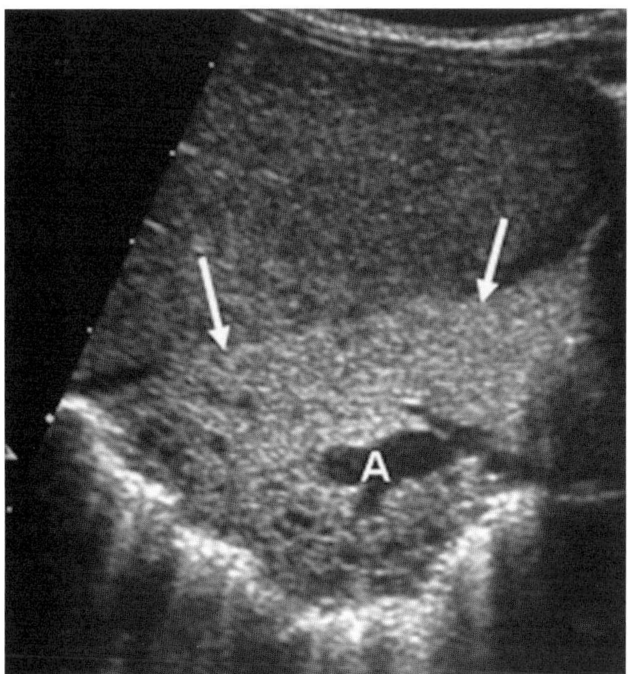

FIGURE 11 ■ Intralobar sequestration. Neonate with a right lower lobe opacity and right-sided aortic arch on chest radiography. Transverse sonogram shows an echogenic mass (*arrows*) in the right lung base. The feeding artery (A) supplying the mass arises from the right-sided aorta.

Tumors

Most parenchymal tumors in children represent metastases. Primary malignant tumors of the lung are rare. The most common malignant tumor is the pulmonary blastoma. Other lesions include rhabdomyosarcoma, leiomyosarcoma, hemangiopericytoma, and bronchogenic carcinoma. Pulmonary blastomas are usually found peripherally in the lung and they are often large at presentation. Sonography can confirm the presence of a peripheral mass in a patient with a pleural effusion or an opacified hemithorax on chest radiographs. Pulmonary masses appear sonographically echogenic.

MEDIASTINUM

In neonates and young infants, thymic masses, foregut cysts, and neurogenic tumors comprise the majority of mediastinal masses. Sonography is not commonly used in the evaluation of the mediastinum, but it can be helpful in neonates and young infants with mediastinal widening on chest radiography to differentiate a normal thymus from a mediastinal mass and it can help characterize middle and posterior mediastinal masses. In children below one year of age, the thymus is relatively large compared with other structures and the sternal centers are not yet ossified. As a result, the thymus can be used as an acoustic window to evaluate the mediastinum. In older infants and children, the most common mediastinal masses are those due to lymphoma, lymphadenopathy, and neurogenic tumors. In this population, acoustic windows are limited, making CT or MRI the imaging procedures of choice to further evaluate mediastinal widening on chest radiography. The use of sonography in assessment of mediastinal masses in neonates and infants will be emphasized in the following discussion.

An abnormally shaped or enlarged thymus can mimic a mediastinal mass or upper lobe consolidation or atelectasis on conventional radiography. In these cases, the characteristic sonographic findings of normal thymic tissue can confidently exclude pathology and obviate further imaging evaluation.

Causes of thymic masses in neonates and young infants are lymphangioma (also termed "cystic hygroma"), thymic cysts, and teratomas. Lymphangiomas are congenital malformations of the lymphatic channels (33). Pathologically, they contain dilated lymphatic spaces that are separated by connective tissue. Most affected children present in the first year of life with cervical masses posterior to the sternocleidomastoid muscle. Approximately 10% of these tumors extend into the anterior mediastinum. The classic sonographic findings are thin-walled anechoic cysts with intervening echogenic septa (Fig. 13). Increased echogenicity or fluid-debris levels may be noted if there is superimposed hemorrhage or infection. Color Doppler imaging shows a predominantly avascular mass with scattered flow in the soft-tissue components. An associated finding is aneurysmal dilatation of the jugular vein (34).

Thymic cysts arise from remnants of the thymopharyngeal duct or from degeneration of the thymus subsequent to mediastinal trauma or surgery. Typically, they are unilocular masses with thin walls and anechoic contents. Multiple thymic cysts, associated with diffuse thymic enlargement, have been reported in human immunodeficiency virus (HIV) infection (35,36).

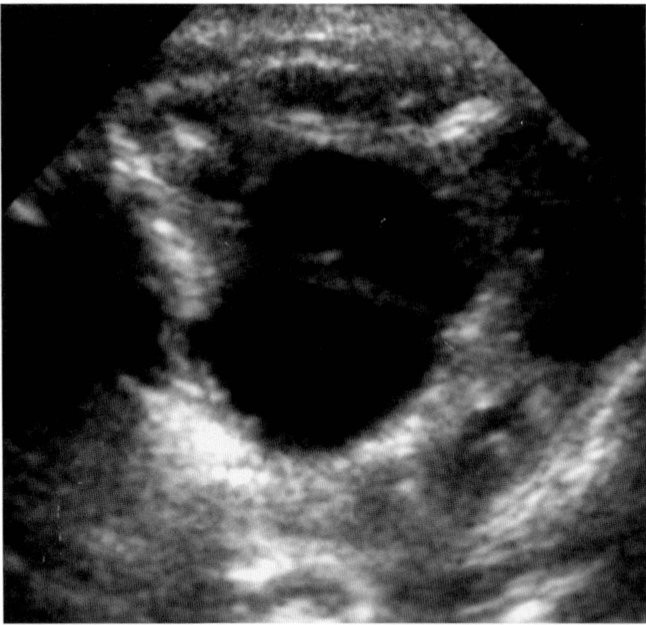

FIGURE 13 ■ Mediastinal cystic hygroma. Transverse sonogram of the superior hemithorax shows a large cystic mass with a thin septation that is characteristic of cystic hygroma (also referred to as lymphangioma). *Source*: From Ref. 5.

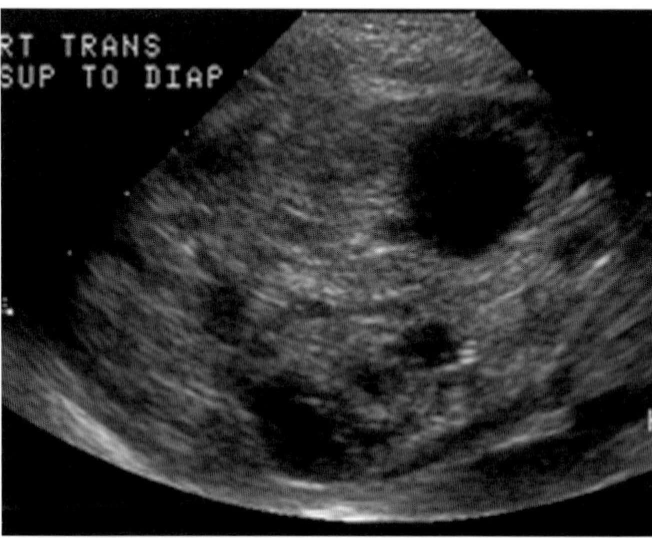

FIGURE 14 ■ Mediastinal teratoma. Transverse sonogram in a neonate demonstrates a complex mass with cystic and solid components. *Source*: Courtesy of Brian Coley, M.D., Columbus, OH.

Teratomas are also found in the anterior mediastinum and most arise within the thymus. Sonographically, they have well-circumscribed walls and contain an admixture of tissues, including sebum or serous fluid, which appear hypoechoic and hair, calcifications, bone, or fat that appear hyperechoic (Fig. 14) (1,2,5,37). They are typically hypovascular or avascular on color flow Doppler imaging.

Middle mediastinal masses include foregut cysts (bronchogenic and enteric) and pericardial cysts. Bronchogenic cysts are usually located in the right paratracheal and subcarinal regions, whereas enteric cysts are more common in the inferior mediastinum, close to or within the esophageal wall. On sonography, both lesions appear as thin-walled hypoechoic lesions with increased through transmission (Fig. 15). The internal echogenicity increases if the contents of the cyst contain mucoid or proteinaceous material, debris, or air. Uncomplicated cysts are avascular. Flow may be noted in the wall if the cyst is infected. Pericardial cysts are most common in the right cardiophrenic angle, but they can be found adjacent to any part of the pericardium. The sonographic findings are similar to those of the foregut cysts.

Posterior mediastinal masses are usually of neurogenic origin, and the most common neurogenic tumor in neonates and infants are neuroblastoma and ganglioneuroblastoma. These lesions are best visualized using a posterior thoracic or subxiphoid approach. Neural tumors appear as fusiform paraspinal masses. They are iso- or hyperechoic relative to thymus or chest-wall muscle and they may contain cystic areas, representing necrosis or degeneration, and echogenic areas, due to calcification (Fig. 16). Sonography can also demonstrate intraspinal extension through the neural foramen and neoplastic invasion of the chest wall, although CT and MRI are the preferred studies for assessing extramediastinal extension.

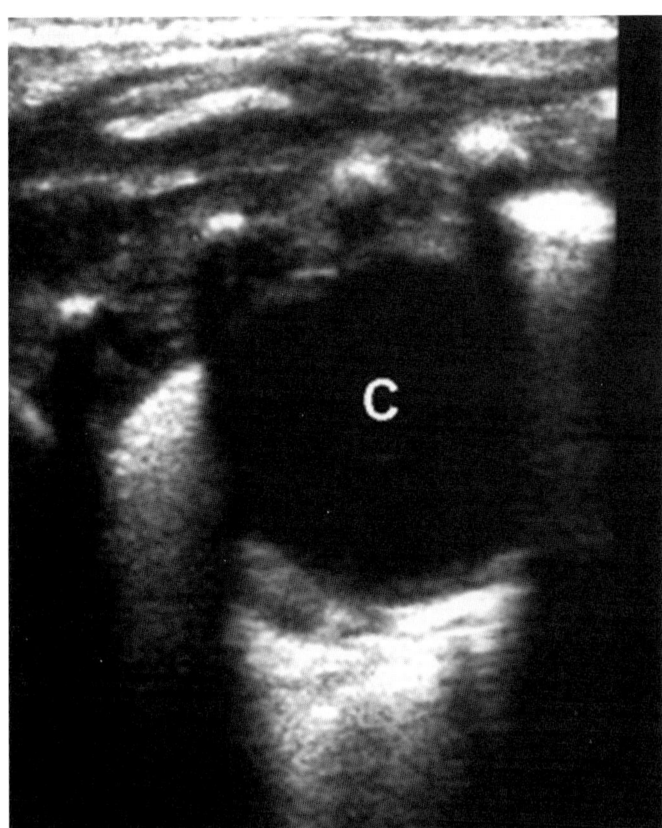

FIGURE 15 ■ Bronchogenic cyst. Chest radiography in a newborn boy with mild dyspnea showed a right mediastinal mass. Longitudinal sonogram shows a fluid-filled cyst (C) just beneath the ribs. The sonographic appearances of duplication and bronchogenic cysts are similar and histologic examination is required for a specific diagnosis.

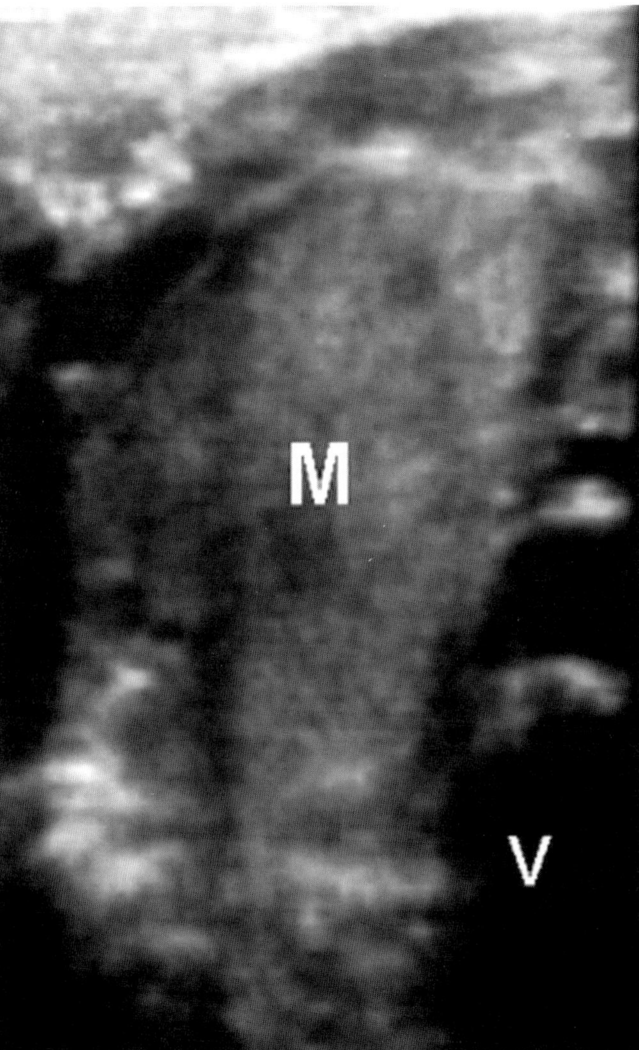

FIGURE 16 ■ Neuroblastoma. One-year-old girl with a right apical mass on chest radiography. Transverse scan through the upper chest shows an echogenic mass (M) adjacent to a vertebral body (V).

THORACIC GREAT VESSELS

Venous Thrombosis

The most common indication for sonography of the intrathoracic vessels is suspected venous thrombosis. Acute thrombosis is most often the sequela of an indwelling vascular catheter and appears as echogenic material expanding the vessel lumen (Fig. 17) (38). With chronic occlusion, the echogenicity of the thrombus decreases, so that the clot appears hypoechoic or anechoic, and collateral vessels form. Doppler findings of thrombosis include absence of flow and loss of the normal biphasic waveform.

Arterial Stenosis and Aneurysms

Arterial stenosis and aneurysm formation can occur in association with vascular disorders, such as Kawasaki disease, or as a complication of vascular access procedures. In aneurysms, gray-scale sonography can detect the vessel dilatation and Doppler sonography can confirm the presence of arterial flow in the enlarged segment and in some cases even show turbulent flow. Stenosis is recognizable by its narrowed vascular lumen and elevated peak systolic flow and delayed systolic upstroke. If the stenosis is severe, there may be elevated flow in diastole.

DIAPHRAGMATIC LESIONS

The common indications for sonography of the diaphragm are evaluation of a suspected diaphragmatic hernia or eventration, delineation of juxtadiaphragmatic masses, and evaluation of diaphragmatic motion.

Diaphragmatic Hernias

Diaphragmatic hernias in the pediatric population are usually congenital in origin and diagnosed in utero. The most common hernia is the Bochdalek hernia, which is typically located on the left and is easily diagnosed on chest radiography, which characteristically shows air-filled loops of stomach or bowel in the thorax. Sometimes, however, the diagnosis is not obvious, especially if the hernia contains solid viscera or fluid-filled bowel loops. In these instances, sonography becomes a valuable diagnostic tool to show the discontinuity of the diaphragm and the herniated intra-abdominal contents (Fig. 18) (1,4,5,39).

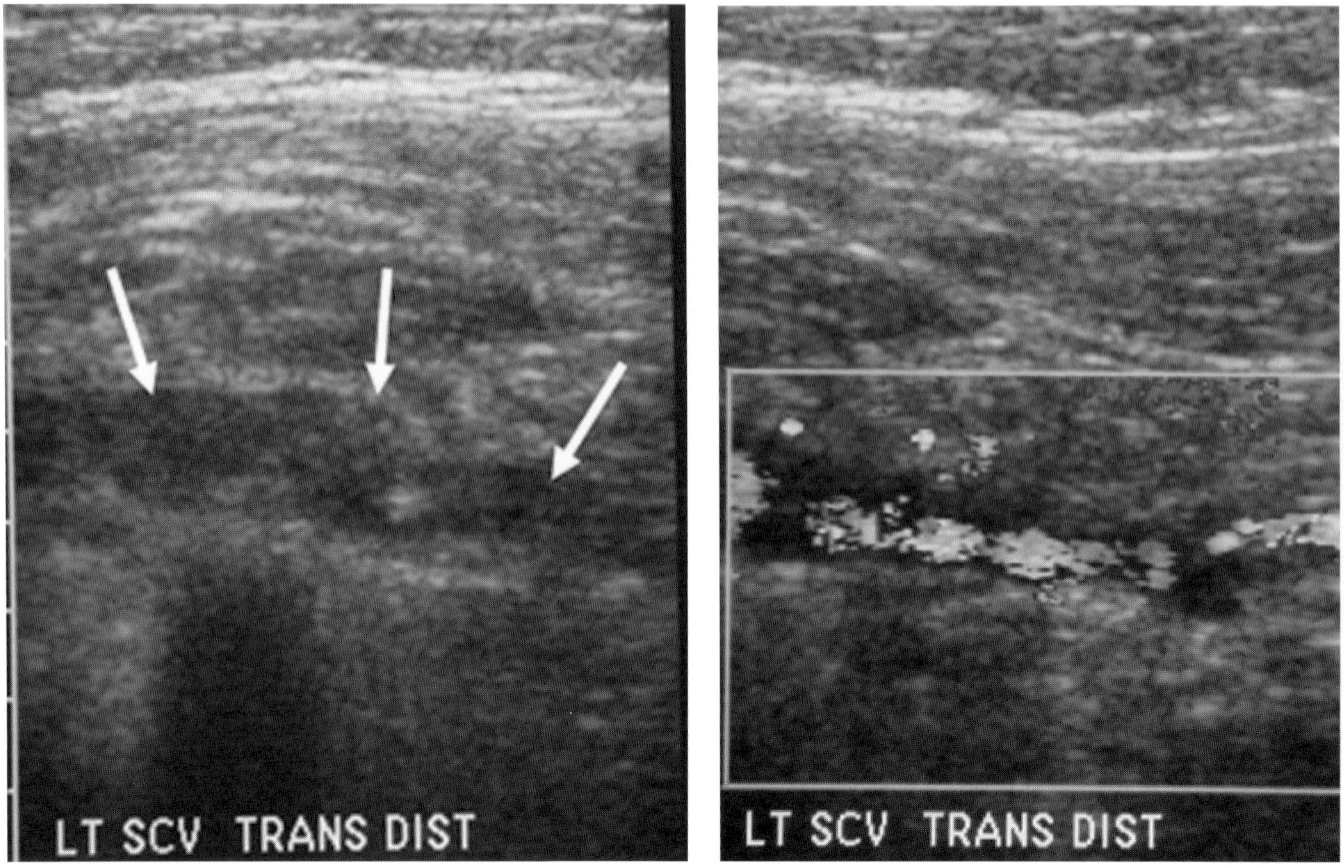

(A) (B)

FIGURE 17 A AND B ■ Brachiocephalic vein thrombosis. (**A**) Transverse sonogram in a child with a swollen upper extremity and a previous indwelling catheter in the left brachiocephalic vein. Echogenic thrombus (*arrows*) is present in the distal left subclavian vein (*arrow*). (**B**) Color Doppler imaging shows nonocclusive thrombus.

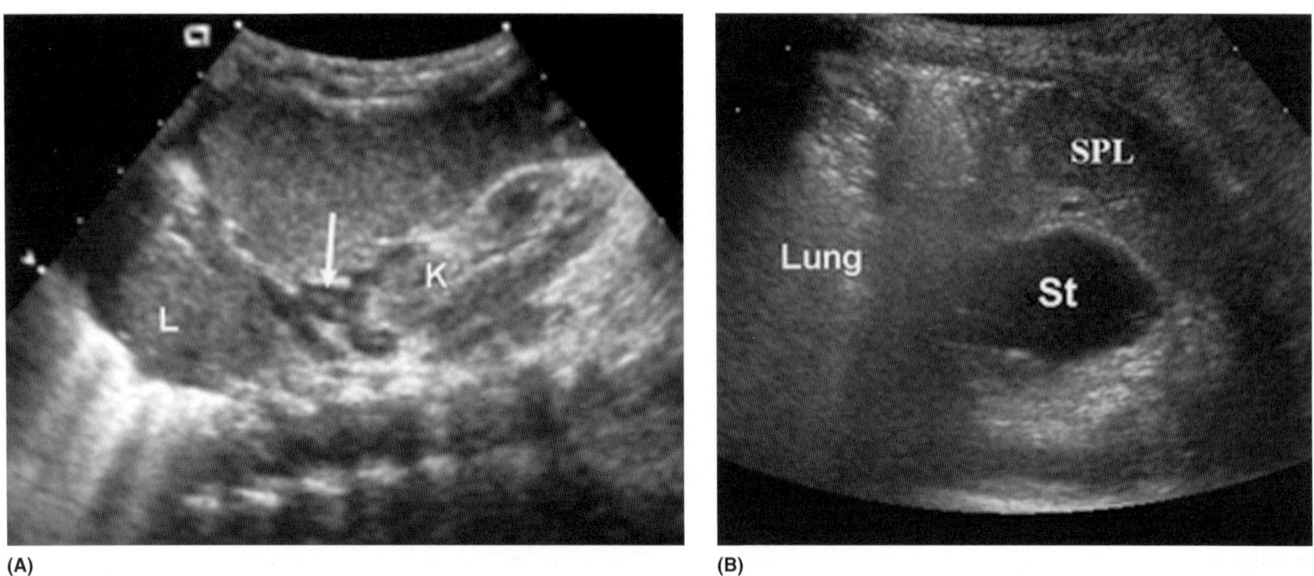

(A) (B)

FIGURE 18 A AND B ■ Bochdalek hernia. (**A**) Neonate with a mass in the right lower hemithorax on chest radiography. Transverse sonogram shows liver (L), right adrenal gland (*arrow*), and kidney (K) in the right lower chest. (**B**) Transverse sonogram in another newborn with an opacified left hemithorax shows fluid-filled stomach (St) and spleen (SPL) in the lower chest. In both cases, the diaphragm was nearly completely absent.

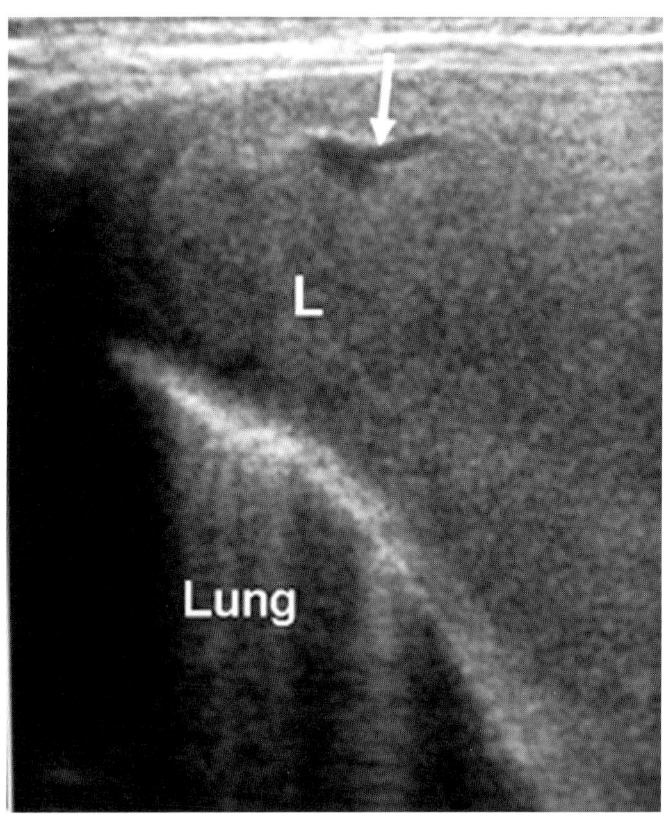

FIGURE 19 ■ Morgagni hernia in a four-month-old boy. Chest radiograph demonstrated a right cardiophrenic mass. Longitudinal scan demonstrates liver (L) anterior to the lung. *Arrows*, hepatic vein.

Another less common congenital hernia is the Morgagni hernia. It is typically located on the right and usually contains liver and omentum and occasionally transverse colon, which are demonstrated easily by sonography (Fig. 19).

Eventration

Eventration of the diaphragm results from a congenital weakness or thinness of the central tendon or muscle. It is more often left sided than right sided and the defect occurs in the anteromedial portion of the diaphragm (Fig. 20). Most eventrations are clinically insignificant and detected incidentally on chest radiographs. Sonographic findings of eventration are a focally thinned but intact diaphragm that protrudes into the ipsilateral hemithorax.

Paralysis

Diaphragmatic paralysis and paresis usually result from phrenic nerve injury following surgery or trauma. The sonographic hallmark of paralysis is absent or paradoxical diaphragmatic excursion during inspiration and expiration. Transverse imaging allows comparison of both hemidiaphragms and is particularly helpful for evaluating unilateral paralysis (Fig. 21). In patients with diaphragmatic paralysis, the degree of excursion is similar in the anterior, middle, and posterior portions of the diaphragm, in contrast to the normal situation where the excursion of the middle and posterior thirds is greater than that of the anterior third.

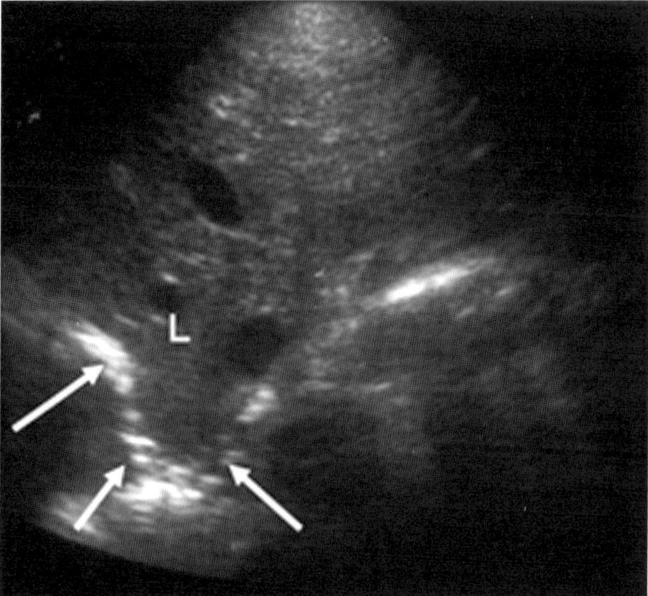

FIGURE 20 ■ Eventration. Transverse scan of the right hemidiaphragm demonstrates a focal herniation of an intact diaphragm (*arrows*) into the chest. Liver (L) is noted in the eventrated area. *Source*: From Ref. 5.

Juxtadiaphragmatic Masses

Juxtadiaphragmatic masses are uncommon and include lipomas, hemangiomas, and rhabdomyosarcomas (40). The role of sonography is to identify the abnormality and characterize its echotexture. Further imaging is usually required with CT or MRI.

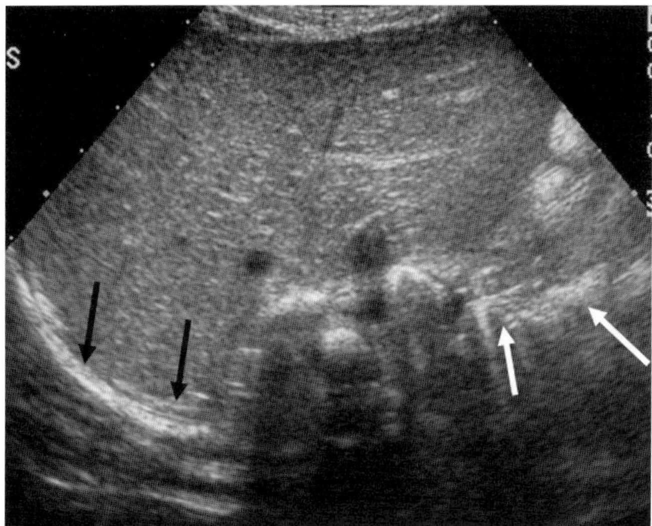

FIGURE 21 ■ Diaphragmatic paralysis. Four-month-old boy with a history of repair of congenital heart disease. Transverse sonogram during expiration. The left hemidiaphragm (*white arrows*) moves anteriorly, which is normal. The right hemidiaphragm (*black arrows*) showed no motion.

CHEST-WALL LESIONS

Soft-Tissue Masses

Sonography with Doppler interrogation can provide information about the cystic, solid, or vascular nature of a chest-wall mass. Cystic and vascular masses are more likely to be benign than are solid masses. Most benign masses are soft and nontender on palpation.

Benign Masses

The common benign masses include hemangiomas, lymphangiomas, lipomas, hematomas, and abscesses (1,5,41). Hemangiomas typically are well-circumscribed masses, usually located in the subcutaneous tissues. On gray-scale imaging, hemangiomas have variable echogenicity, depending on the size of the vascular channels and the amount of thrombus and fatty stroma (Fig. 22). On Doppler sonography, hemangiomas show high color Doppler signal and high Doppler frequency shifts (42,43).

Lymphangiomas (cystic hygroma) have variable sized cysts with interspersed echogenic septa (Fig. 23). The cyst fluid is usually anechoic, but it may be hyperechoic if there has been hemorrhage or infection. The septa show some flow on Doppler imaging. Lymphangiomas can occur anywhere in the chest but are most common in the axilla.

Lipomas are usually located in the subcutaneous tissues. Typically, they are well circumscribed and echogenic because of their fat content. Color Doppler shows minimal or absent flow.

Hematomas usually are the result of trauma, but they can occur spontaneously or be associated with bleeding diatheses. The acute hematoma has ill-defined margins and a hyperechoic matrix due to the presence of fibrin. The chronic hematoma is usually a well-circumscribed hypoechoic mass. At this stage, it may not be readily differentiated from a cyst. Abscesses appear as hypoechoic masses with scattered internal debris and thick hypervascular walls. Associated osteomyelitis of a rib manifests as disruption or irregular thickening of the cortex.

Malignant Neoplasms

Malignant chest-wall masses include rhabdomyosarcoma, fibrosarcoma, and Ewing family of tumors. These lesions have variable internal echogenicity, ranging from hypoechoic to highly echogenic, and variable margins, which may be well defined or infiltrative. Color Doppler

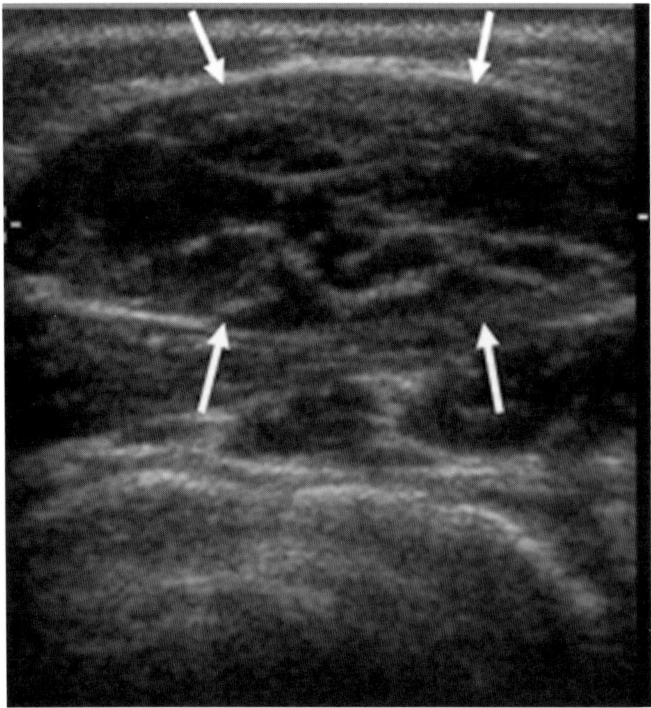

(A)

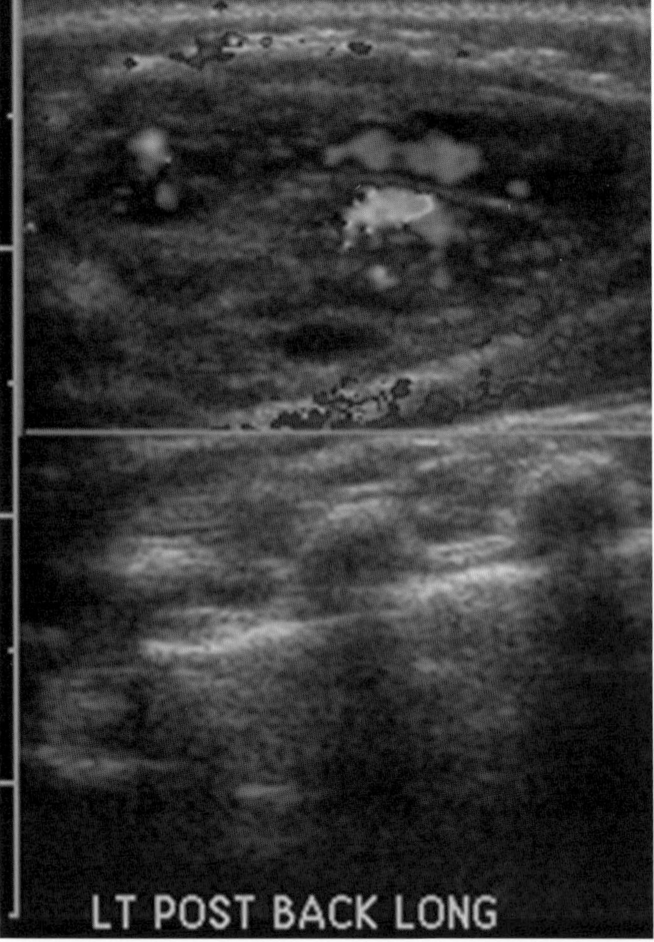

(B)

FIGURE 22 A AND B ■ Hemangioma. Eleven-month-old girl with a palpable soft-tissue mass over the anterior lateral chest wall. (**A**) Transverse sonogram shows an echogenic mass (*arrows*) in the subcutaneous tissues. The areas of higher echogenicity represent fatty stroma, while the hypoechoic channels are vessels. (**B**) Color Doppler scan shows multiple vascular channels coursing through the lesion.

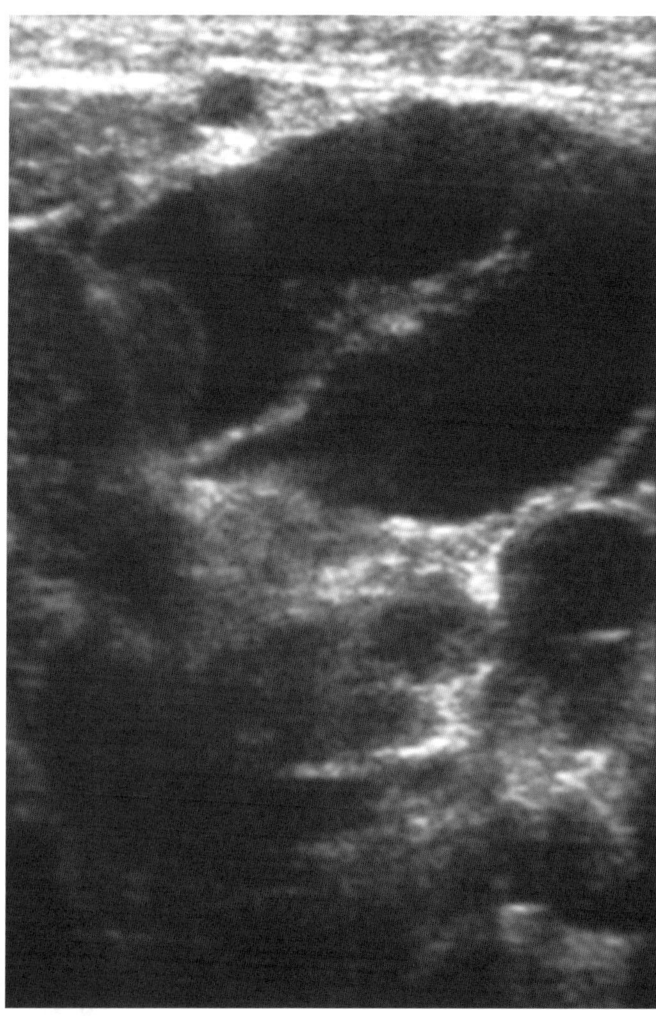

FIGURE 23 ■ Soft-tissue lymphangioma. Transverse scan over the chest wall shows a poorly defined complex mass with cystic and solid components. The multilocular appearance is characteristic of lymphangioma.

flow is usually increased. Associated findings include chest wall and rib destruction. Similar to other imaging studies, sonography cannot provide a specific histologic diagnosis, and some benign lesions, such as acute hematomas and abscesses, may show aggressive sonographic findings. Tissue sampling, which can be guided by sonography, is usually required for diagnosis.

Osseous Lesions

Cartilaginous or rib abnormalities, such as asymmetric cartilaginous costochondral junctions, anomalous rib ends, osteochondromas, and healing rib fractures can present as firm chest-wall masses. These are readily confirmed by sonography when chest radiographs are equivocal. Cartilaginous abnormalities are typically hypoechoic masses (Fig. 24). Rib fractures show disruption of the cortical surface and there may be adjacent hematoma or callous formation depending on the age of the injury (44).

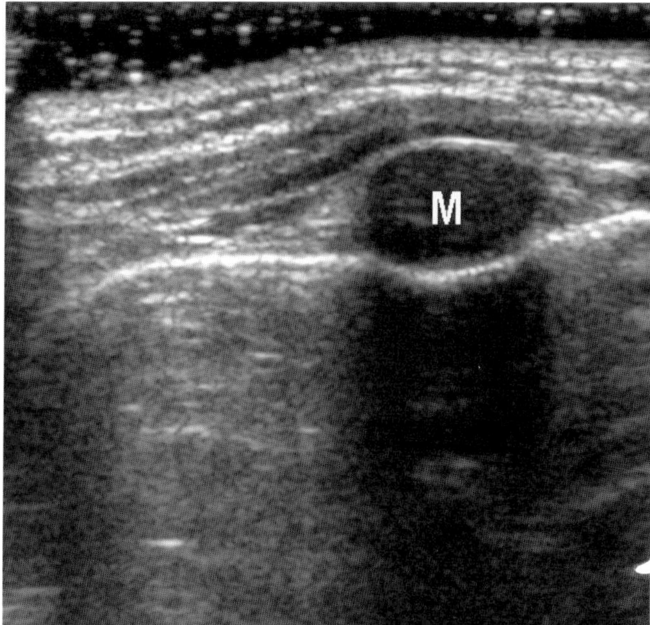

FIGURE 24 ■ Prominent costochondral junction. A six-year-old boy with a firm palpable anterior chest-wall mass (M). Longitudinal sonogram shows a hypoechoic mass at the end of a rib, representing prominent cartilage.

REFERENCES

1. Coley BD. Pediatric chest ultrasound. Radiol Clin North Am 2005; 43:405–418.
2. Ben-Ami TE, O'Donovan JC, Yousefzadeh DK. Sonography of the chest in children. Radiol Clin North Am 1993; 31:517–531.
3. Kim H, Kim WS, Kim MJ, Jung JY, Suh JH. Ultrasound in the diagnosis of pediatric chest diseases. Radiographics 2000; 20:653–671.
4. Koh D, Burke S, Davies N, et al. Transthoracic US of the chest: clinical uses and applications. Radiographics 2002; 22:1e.
5. Siegel MJ. Chest. In: Siegel MJ, ed. Pediatric Sonography. Philadelphia: Lippincott Williams-Wilkins, 2002:167–211.
6. Adam EJ, Ignotus PI. Sonography of the thymus in healthy children: frequency of visualization, size, and appearance. AJR Am J Roentgenol 1993; 161:153–155.
7. Han BK, Babcock DS, Oestreich AE. The normal thymus in infancy: sonographic characteristics. Radiology 1989; 170:471–474.
8. Han B, Yoon H, Suh Y. Thymic ultrasound: diagnosis of aberrant cervical thymus. Pediatr Radiol 2001; 31:480–487.
9. Koumanidou C, Vakaki M, Theophanopoulou M, et al. Aberrant thymus in infants: sonographic evaluation. Pediatr Radiol 1998; 28:987–989.
10. Hammerli M, Meyer RA. Doppler evaluation of central venous lines in the superior vena cava. J Pediatr 1993; 122:S104–S108.
11. Nazarian G, Foshager M. Color Doppler sonography of the thoracic inlet veins. Radiographics 1995; 15:1257–1371.
12. Gersovich E, Cronan M, McGahan J, et al. Ultrasonographic evaluation of diaphragmatic motion. J Ultrasound Med 2001; 20:597–604.
13. Houston JG, Fleet M, Cowan MD, McMillan NC. Comparison of ultrasound with fluoroscopy in the assessment of suspected hemidiaphragmatic movement abnormality. Clin Radiol 1995; 50:95–98.
14. Laing IA, Teel RL, Stark AR. Diaphragmatic movement in newborn infants. J Pediatr 1988; 112:638–643.
15. Wells R, Havens P. Intrapleural fibrinolysis for parapneumonic effusion and empyema in children. Radiology 2003; 228:370–378.
16. Chen K, Liaw Y, Wang H, et al. Sonographic septations: a useful prognostic indicator of acute thoracic empyema. J Ultrasound Med 2000; 19:837–843.

17. Wu RG, Yang PC, Kuo SH, Luh KT. "Fluid color" sign: a useful indicator for discrimination between pleural thickening and pleural effusion. J Ultrasound Med 1995; 14:767–769.
18. Yang P. Applications of colour Doppler ultrasound in the diagnosis of chest diseases. Respirology 1997; 2:231–238.
19. Dulchavsky S, Schwarz R, Kirkpatrick A, et al. Prospective evaluation of thoracic ultrasound in the detection of pneumothorax. J Trauma 2001; 50:201–205.
20. Rowan K, Kirkpatrick A, Liu D, et al. Traumatic pneumothorax detection with thoracic US: correlation with chest radiography and CT—initial experience. Radiology 2002; 225:210–214.
21. Targhetta R, Bourgeois M, Chavagneux R, et al. Diagnosis of pneumothorax by ultrasound immediately after ultrasonically guided aspiration biopsy. Chest 1992; 101:855–856.
22. Targhetta R, Bourgeois M, Chavagneux R, et al. Ultrasonographic approach to diagnosing hydropneumothorax. Chest 1992; 101:931–934.
23. Targhetta R, Chavagneux R, Bourgeois JM, Dauzat M, Balmes P, Pourcelot L. Sonographic approach to diagnosing pulmonary consolidation. J Ultrasound Med 1992; 11:667–672.
24. Mathias G. Thorax sonography—part II: peripheral pulmonary consolidation. Ultrasound Med Biol 1997; 23:1131–1153.
25. Yang PC, Luh KT, Lee YC, et al. Lung abscesses: US examination and US-guided transthoracic aspiration. Radiology 1991; 180: 171–175.
26. Dhingsa R, Coakley F, Albanese C, et al. Prenatal sonography and MR imaging of pulmonary sequestration. AJR Am J Roentgenol 2003; 180:433–437.
27. Rosado-de-Christenson ML, Stocker JT. Congenital cystic adenomatoid malformation. Radiographics 1991; 11:865–886.
28. Rosado-de-Christenson ML, Frazier AA, Stocker JT, Templeton PA. Extralobar sequestration: radiologic-pathologic correlation, Radiographics 1993; 13:425–441.
29. Benya EC, Bulas DI, Selby DM, Rosenbaum KN. Cystic sonographic appearance of extralobar pulmonary sequestration. Pediatr Radiol 1993; 23:605–607.
30. Ceola AF, Angtuaco TL. US case of the day: extralobar pulmonary sequestration. Radiographics 1999; 19:817–819.
31. Schlesinger AE, DiPietro MA, Statter MB, Lally KP. Utility of sonography in the diagnosis of bronchopulmonary sequestration. J Pediatr Surg 1994; 29:52–55.
32. Smart LM, Hendry GMA. Imaging of neonatal pulmonary sequestration including Doppler ultrasound. Br J Radiol 1991; 64:324–329.
33. Zadvinskis DP, Benson MT, Kerr HH, et al. Congenital malformations of the cervico-thoracic lymphatic system: embryology and pathogenesis. Radiographics 1992; 12:1175–1189.
34. Gorenstein A, Katz S, Rein A, Schiller M. Giant cystic hygroma associated with venous aneurysm. J Pediatr Surg 1992; 27:1504–1506.
35. Kontny H, Sleasman J, Kingma D, et al. Multilocular thymic cysts in children with human immunodeficiency virus infection: clinical and pathologic aspects. J Pediatr 1997; 131:264–270.
36. Leonidas JC, Berdon WE, Valderrama E, et al. Human immunodeficiency virus infection and multilocular thymic cysts. Radiology 1996; 198:377–379.
37. Wu T, Wang H, Chang Y, et al. Mature mediastinal teratoma: sonographic and imaging patterns and pathologic correlation. J Ultrasound Med 2002; 21:759–765.
38. Babcock DS. Sonographic evaluation of suspected pediatric vascular diseases. Pediatr Radiol 1991; 21:486–489.
39. Yeh HC, Halton KP, Gray CE. Anatomic variations and abnormalities in the diaphragm seen with US. Radiographics 1990; 10:1019–1030.
40. Gupta AAK, Mitra DK, Berry M. Primary embryonal rhabdomyosarcoma of the diaphragm in a child: case report. Pediatr Radiol 1999; 29:823–825.
41. Donnelly L, Frush D. Abnormalities of the chest wall in pediatric patients. AJR Am J Roentgenol 1999; 173:1595–1601.
42. Dubois J, Patriquin HB, Garel L, et al. Soft-tissue hemangiomas in infants and children: diagnosis using Doppler sonography. AJR Am J Roentgenol 1998; 171:247–252.
43. Dubois J, Garel, David M, et al. Vascular soft-tissue tumors in infancy: distinguishing features on Doppler sonography. AJR Am J Roentgenol 2002; 178:1541–1545.
44. Mathias G. Thorax sonography. Part 1: chest wall and pleura. Ultrasound Med Biol 1997; 23:1131–1139.

Pediatric Liver, Spleen, and Pancreas

Sandra L. Wootton-Gorges

25

INTRODUCTION

Ultrasonographic examination of the pediatric abdominal solid organs is performed with the patient supine, using a linear or curved array transducer, usually 5 to 7.5 MHz (1). The patient should be fasting for three or four (infants) to six to eight (older children) hours prior to the examination. Scanning in the oblique or decubitus position may be helpful if bowel gas obscures the organ being examined. In addition, giving water may also improve the acoustic window.

The liver is examined in both transverse and sagittal planes. For the normal hepatic anatomy as well as normal hepatic vascular waveform patterns, please refer to Chapter 26. The normal hepatic parenchyma is homogeneous, finely granular, and slightly lower in echogenicity than the spleen (2). Longitudinal normal dimensions of the liver, based upon patient age and height, are given in Table 1 (3). Although the portal and hepatic arterial waveforms are similar in children and adults, only about 40% of children have the adult hepatic venous triphasic pattern. Instead, children (especially infants) may demonstrate a monophasic hepatic venous waveform (4).

The normal gallbladder varies in size based upon age. In infants, it measures from 1.3 to 3.4 cm in length (5); in 2 to 16 year olds, it measures 2.9 to 8 cm in length. The gallbladder wall should be less than 3 mm thick in the fasting state (6). The cystic duct is not usually seen in children. The common duct, seen anterior to the portal vein and hepatic artery, should not exceed 1 mm in neonates, 2 mm in infants younger than 1 year, and 4 mm in children 1 to 10 years of age (5).

The normal spleen is a curved, wedge-shaped organ. Its normal longitudinal dimension, based upon age and height, is given in Table 2 (3). It is slightly more echogenic than the liver or the renal cortex.

The pancreas is a nonencapsulated, multilobular gland in the anterior pararenal space. Its echotexture is similar to the liver. The pancreatic duct should be less than 2 mm in diameter (7). The normal pancreatic size based on age is shown in Table 3 (8,9).

LIVER

Hepatic Neoplasms

A liver mass in a child is most commonly due to metastases, usually Wilms' tumor, neuroblastoma (Fig. 1), or lymphoma. Primary liver tumors account for 15% of abdominal neoplasms and about 1% of all neoplasms in children, and about two-thirds of these primary hepatic tumors are malignant.

Hepatoblastoma

Hepatoblastoma is the most common primary pediatric hepatic tumor (10). It usually occurs in patients less than three to five years of age, and is more common in boys. Most children present with an asymptomatic abdominal mass or abdominal distension. Anorexia, weight loss, and pain

TABLE 1 ■ Longitudinal Dimensions of Right Lobe of Liver vs. Height and Age

Subjects		Longitudinal dimensions (mm) of right lobe of the liver			
		Percentile		Suggested limits of normal	
Body height (cm)	Age range (mo)	5th	95th	Lowermost	Uppermost
48–64	1–3	48	82	40	90
54–73	4–6	53	86	45	95
65–78	7–9	70	90	60	100
71–92	12–30	68	98	65	105
85–109	36–59	63	105	65	115
100–130	60–83	77	124	70	125
110–131	84–107	90	123	75	130
124–149	108–131	83	128	75	135
137–153	132–155	95	136	85	140
143–168	156–179	94	136	85	140
152–175	180–200	104	139	95	145

Source: From Ref. 3.

may be present. α-fetoprotein levels are elevated in 90% of cases. Hepatoblastoma has been associated with Beckwith–Wiedemann syndrome, hemihypertrophy, fetal alcohol syndrome, biliary atresia, maternal ingestion of oral contraceptives and gonadotropin, familial polyposis, and Gardner syndrome (11).

Sonography correctly predicts the extent of hepatoblastoma in three-quarters of cases (12). The tumor appears as a well-defined, hyperechoic, septated, complex intrahepatic mass with a lobulated outline (Figs. 2 and 3) (12–14). Foci of hypoechogenicity may be cysts, necrosis, hemorrhage, or extramedullary hematopoiesis. Calcification is seen by sonography in up to half of cases. Invasion of one or more branches of the portal vein or hepatic veins is an important sonographic feature of malignancy (15). High-velocity flow in the hepatic artery has been associated with neovascularity in hepatoblastoma. Ascites is associated with metastases.

Hepatocellular Carcinoma

Children with hepatocellular carcinoma (HCC) are older than children with hepatoblastoma and usually present with an abdominal mass or an enlarging abdomen. The peak age for HCC is 12 to 15 years. Presenting symptoms may also include pain, constitutional symptoms, and jaundice. Laboratory evaluation may demonstrate elevated transaminase, alkaline phosphatase, α-fetoprotein and bilirubin. HCC in childhood has been associated with

TABLE 2 ■ Longitudinal Dimensions of Spleen vs. Height and Age

Subjects		Longitudinal dimensions (mm) of right lobe of the liver			
		Percentile		Suggested limits of normal	
Body height (cm)	Age range (mo)	5th	95th	Lowermost	Uppermost
48–64	1–3	40	65	30	70
54–73	4–6	47	67	40	75
65–78	7–9	53	74	45	80
71–92	12–30	55	82	50	85
85–109	36–59	61	88	55	95
100–130	60–83	70	100	60	105
110–131	84–107	69	100	65	105
124–149	108–131	70	100	65	110
137–153	132–155	81	108	75	115
143–168	156–179	85	118	80	120
152–175	180–200	88	115	85	120

Source: From Ref. 3.

TABLE 3 ■ Normal Anteroposterior Dimension of the Pancreas

Age	Anteroposterior diameter (cm)		
	Head	Body	Tail
<1 mo	0.6–1.4	6.4–0.8	0.6–1.4
1–6 yr	1.0–1.9	0.4–1.2	0.8–2.2
7–12 yr	1.2–2.0	0.6–1.0	1.3–1.6
13–18 yr	1.8–2.2	0.7–1.2	1.3–1.8

Source: From Refs. 8, 9.

hepatitis B exposure, hereditary tyrosinemia, biliary cirrhosis, methotrexate therapy, type I glycogen storage disease, α1-antitrypsin deficiency, cystinosis, Wilson's disease, giant-cell hepatitis, androgenic anabolic steroid therapy, neurofibromatosis, ataxia–telangiectasia, and familial polyposis. The fibrolamellar type of HCC is more commonly seen in children than in adults; it carries a better patient prognosis than the more typical HCC.

Sonography defines the presence, site, and extent of the tumor. The tumor involves both lobes in half of cases, is multicentric in one-third, but also may have isolated right-lobe or left-lobe involvement (Fig. 4) (16). Diffuse hepatic involvement should be suspected if the sonogram reveals a diffusely inhomogeneous echogenicity, sometimes with distortion of the vascular anatomy (17). Focal masses are predominantly hyperechoic (14,17) although necrosis and hemorrhage are hypoechoic. HCC is often hypervascular (18). The preoperative evaluation must accurately define local extent and distant spread of the tumor. Exact hepatic segmental involvement must be determined. Local spread may occur into the nodes in the porta hepatis. Distant metastases occur most frequently in the lungs and less frequently in the skeleton and brain.

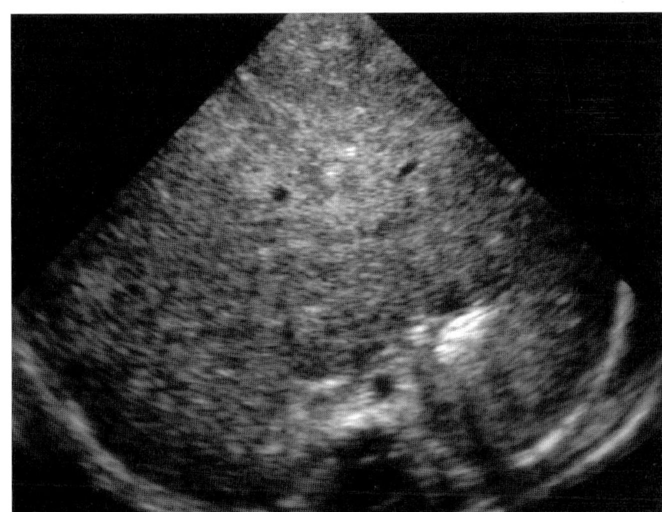

FIGURE 1 ■ Six-week-old girl with 4S neuroblastoma. Transverse ultrasound image shows diffuse infiltration of the liver with liver enlargement and inhomogeneous echogenicity.

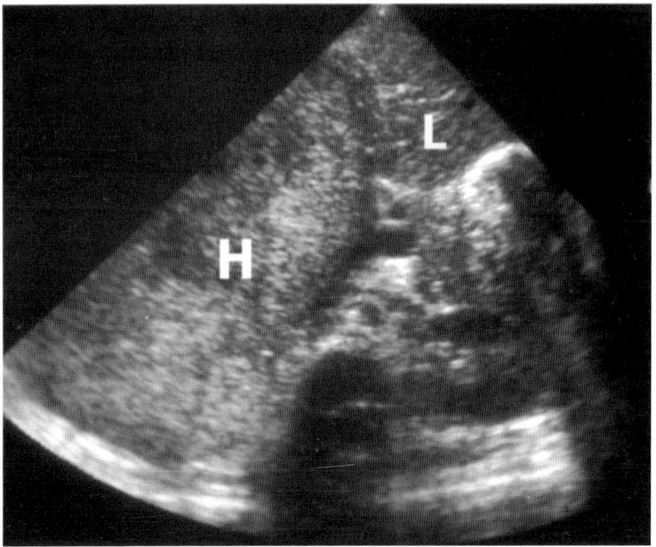

FIGURE 2 ■ Hepatoma. Transverse ultrasound image of a three-year-old girl with hepatoblastoma (H) involving the right lobe and medial segment of the left lobe of the liver. The lateral segment (L) of the left lobe is spared.

Hemangioendothelioma

Benign liver tumors account for approximately one-third of all primary neoplasms of the liver in children. Infantile hemangioma, also known as capillary hemangioma and infantile hemangioendothelioma, accounts for one-half to three-fourths (19) of these benign tumors. The disease is more common in girls. Eighty-five percent of patients present before six months of age (20). Presenting symptoms

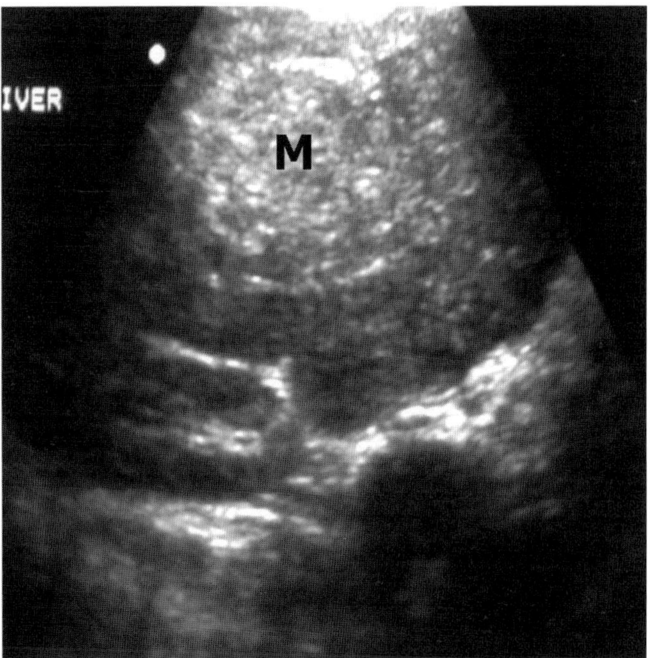

FIGURE 3 ■ Hepatoblastoma. Transverse ultrasound image of a three year old with hepatoblastoma demonstrating a hyperechoic mass (M) in the right lobe of the liver.

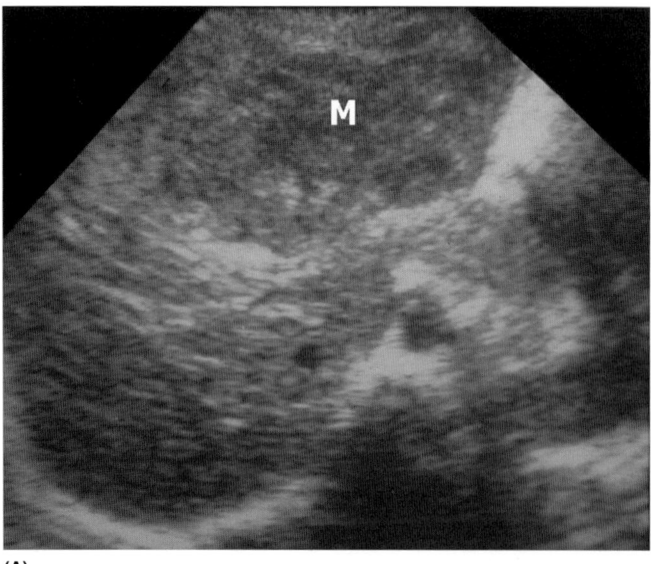

(A)

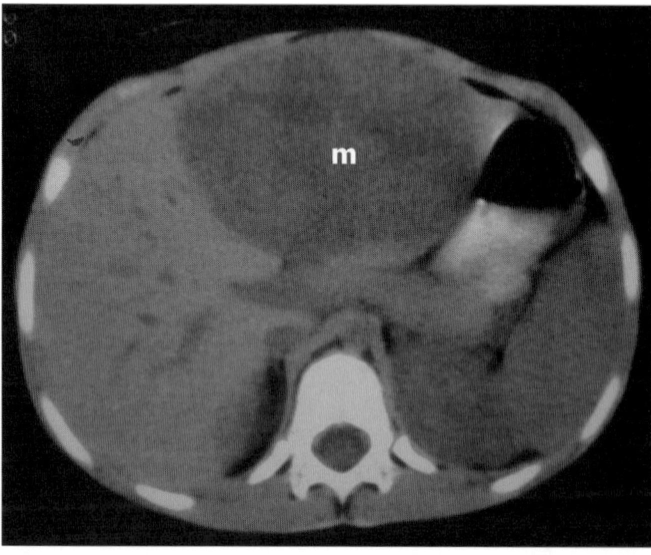

(B)

FIGURE 4 A AND B ■ Hepatocellular carcinoma. (**A**) Transverse image of a teenager with hepatocellular carcinoma demonstrating an ill-defined left-lobe liver mass (M). (**B**) The noncontrast CT correlates well with the ultrasound findings, showing the hypodense left lobe mass (m).

vary from none to florid congestive heart failure (19). About three-quarters have an abdominal mass or hepatic enlargement. Cutaneous hemangiomas are present in half (21). Other presenting symptoms include jaundice or platelet consumption coagulopathy (Kasabach–Merritt syndrome). Liver function studies are typically normal, but α-fetoprotein levels are elevated in about half.

Sonography will localize the tumor to the liver. The tumor is predominantly discrete, solid and may be single or multifocal (Fig. 5) (22), large or small (23), and hypoechoic or hyperechoic. Echogenic stroma and septa may be seen within it. Dilatation of the proximal aorta with abrupt decrease below the celiac axis, enlargement of the celiac artery and hepatic artery, and dilatation of the hepatic veins are important signs of shunting in this vascular tumor (20,24). Differentiation of hemangioendothelioma from hepatoblastoma may be difficult in the very young neonate (25,26). The natural history of infantile hemangioma is one of growth for six months to one year and then involution.

Mesenchymal Hamartoma

Mesenchymal hamartoma (Fig. 6) is the second most common benign liver mass in children with about three-quarters diagnosed within the first two years of life. It is a benign developmental malformation consisting of cysts, bile ducts, hepatocytes, mesenchyme, and branches of the portal vein. These cases usually come to medical attention because of an abdominal mass or respiratory distress. Eighty percent arise in the right lobe of the liver, and one-fifth are pedunculated. Mesenchymal hamartoma characteristically is a well-defined multiseptate cystic mass (27) but may be solid (28). It is avascular centrally. The cysts may be variable in size and are divided by septae of variable thickness (29). Debris may be present within the cysts. Round hyperechoic parietal nodules within the cystic spaces may be seen (30). Solid portions are hyperechoic. Increased portal venous flow may be documented by Doppler evaluation (31).

Parenchymal Disease

Hepatitis usually results from viral infection, including hepatitis A, B, and C-E, cytomegalovirus, Epstein–Barr, HIV, and others (1). Toxins, drugs, and autoimmune diseases are noninfectious causes. In most cases of acute hepatitis, the liver appears ultrasonographically normal (32), but in severe cases, hepatomegaly, parenchymal hypoechogenicity, periportal hyperechogenicity (Fig. 7), thickening of gallbladder wall, and periportal nodes may be seen.

Cat scratch disease (Fig. 8), caused by the gram-negative *Bartonella henselae*, usually results in regional adenopathy (33). Involved nodes are enlarged, hypoechoic, and highly vascularized. The liver and spleen are involved in at least one-third (33) of patients, even in the absence of abdominal complaints. Round, well-defined hypoechoic lesions of different sizes up to 2 cm may be seen acutely (34). Subsequently, the lesions may calcify (35). The differential diagnosis of the lesions includes malignant processes such as lymphoma or metastases, granulomatous disease, and other infectious processes. The diagnosis may be confirmed with serologic testing in the setting of a cat or kitten bite or scratch.

Cirrhosis of the liver in children may result from many causes, including chronic hepatitis, biliary atresia, cystic fibrosis, metabolic disease, hemochromatosis, prolonged total parenteral nutrition, venous outflow obstruction (Budd–Chiari syndrome), and drugs (1). On ultrasonography, one sees a small liver with coarsened increased hepatic echotexture, enlargement of the caudate lobe, and nodularity of the liver.

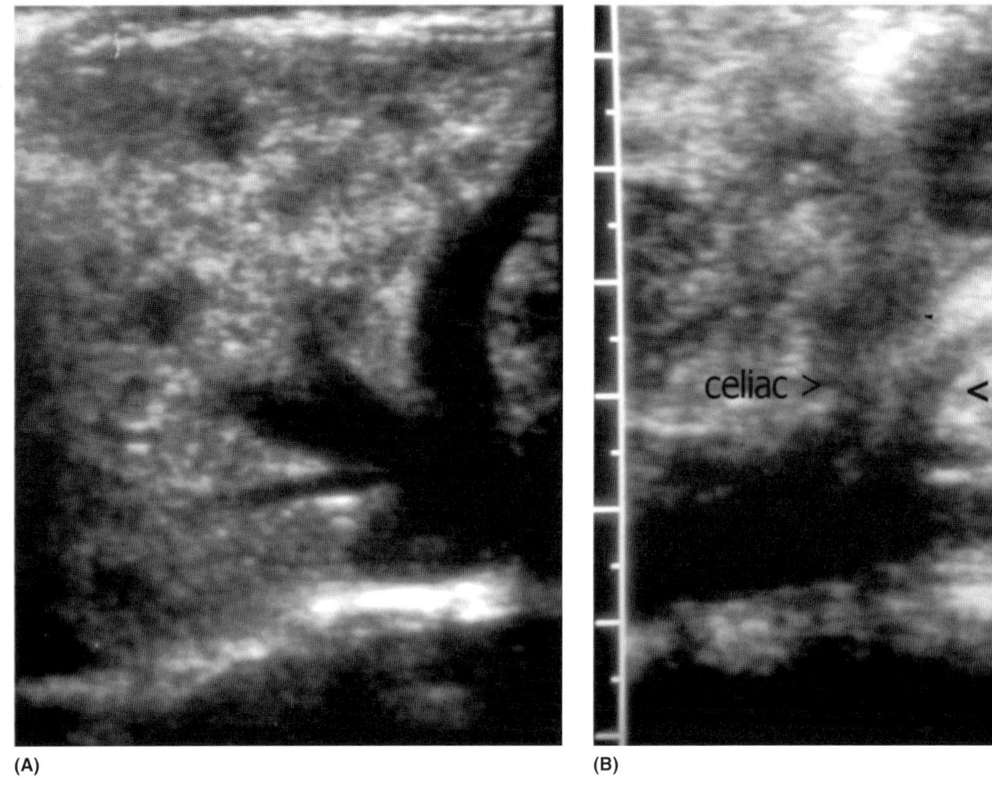

(A) (B)

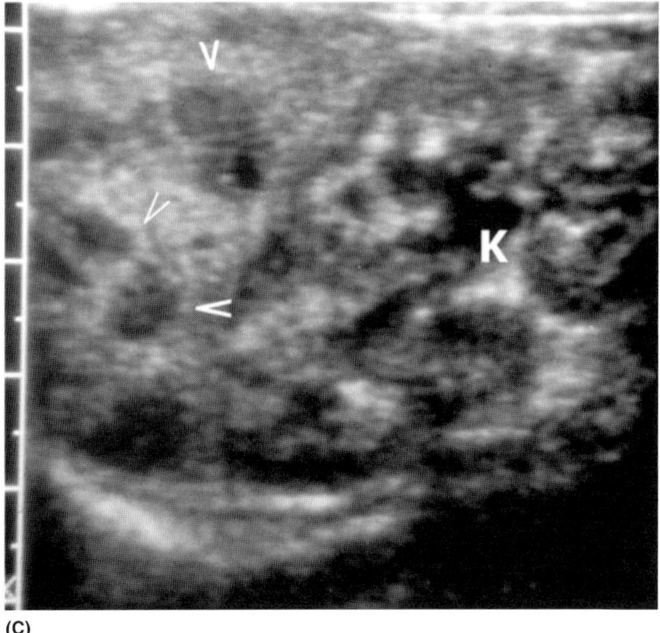

(C)

FIGURE 5 A–C ■ One-month-old infant with multiple hepatic hemangiomas and congestive heart failure. (**A**) Transverse ultrasound image shows multiple hypoechoic tumors within the liver as well as enlargement of the hepatic vein-s from shunting. (**B**) Longitudinal image shows abrupt tapering of the aorta (due to shunting into the liver) after the celiac and superior mesenteric artery (SMA) takeoff. (**C**) Longitudinal image of the liver and kidney (K) show more hypoechoic liver lesions (*arrowheads*) as well as nephrocalcinosis resulting from furosemide therapy for the congestive heart failure.

Cavernous Transformation of the Portal Vein

Cavernous deformity of the portal vein is an uncommon cause of portal hypertension (36). In children, it may be idiopathic or may result from collateral development after portal vein thrombosis (resulting from omphalitis, umbilical vein catheterization, pancreatitis, etc.) (37). This diagnosis may be suggested by absence of a normal portal vein with replacement by anechoic tubular, irregular spaces that exhibit color Doppler flow (Fig. 9). Prominent hepatic arterial inflow may also be seen (38). Splenomegaly (Fig. 9c) and abdominal collateral venous varices are commonly observed. Other findings of portal hypertension, including ascites, thickening of the lesser omentum, and signs of cirrhosis may also be seen.

Hepatic Trauma

Injuries are the most common cause of death in children. Abdominal trauma in children usually results from blunt

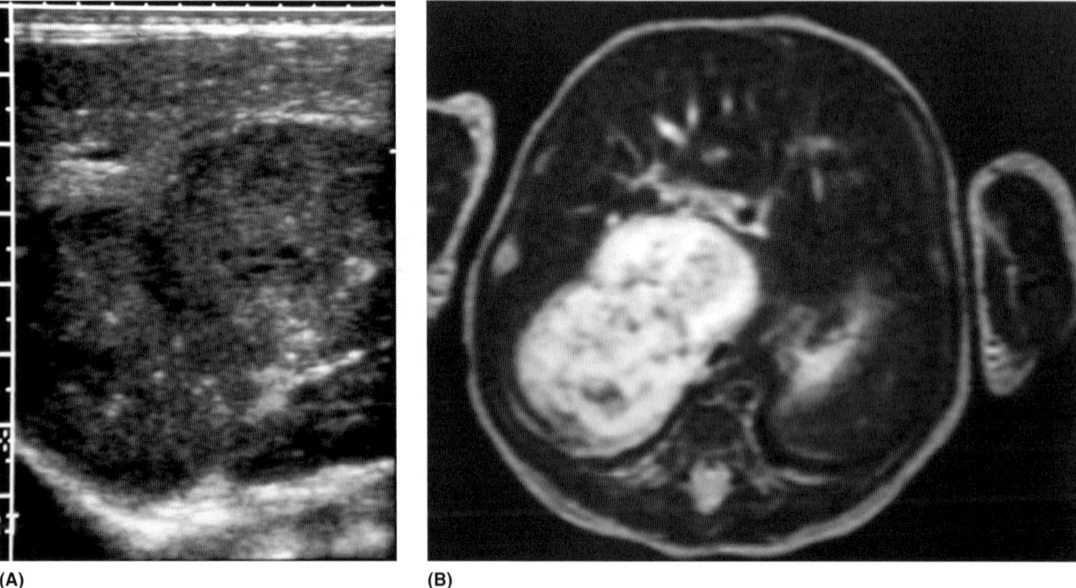

(A) (B)

FIGURE 6 A AND B ■ Mesenchymal hamartoma. (**A**) Transverse image of the liver in a young boy with mesenchymal hamartoma. The bilobed tumor is hypoechoic and has central areas of linear hyperechogenicity. (**B**) T2-weighted MRI defines the high-signal mass in the posterior aspect of the right lobe of the liver.

force such as motor vehicle accidents, falls, blows to the abdomen, and child abuse (39). Although ultrasonography is readily available, it cannot match the accuracy of computed tomography (CT) in detecting and depicting pediatric abdominal injuries (40,41). The focused abdominal sonogram for trauma scan (42) that evaluates for free fluid as a sign of solid organ injury also has not been shown to be useful in children (43).

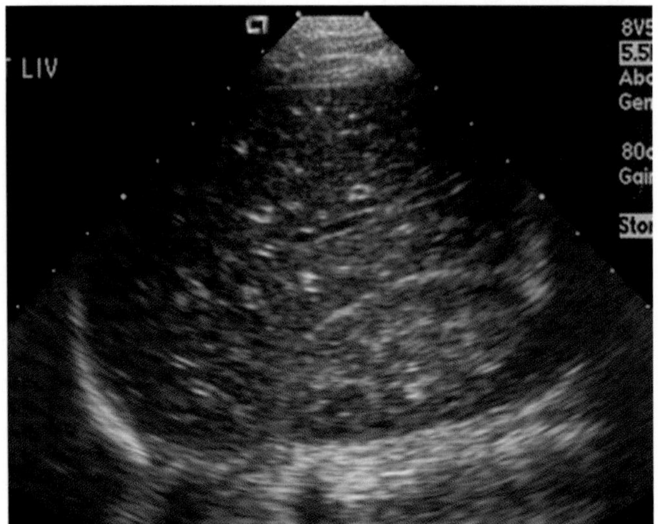

FIGURE 7 ■ Longitudinal ultrasound image of a four-year-old boy with viral hepatitis. Periportal increased echogenicity gives a "starry sky" appearance.

GALLBLADDER AND BILIARY TREE

Cholelithiasis and cholecystitis have become more common in the pediatric population (44) in recent years. In many patients, a cause such as hemolytic disease, major surgery, parenteral nutrition, pregnancy, prior ileal resection, cystic fibrosis, and metabolic liver disease may be found (45). One study found the majority of gallstones in children were black pigment or calcium carbonate (46); this is different than the cholesterol stones that are most common in adults. Gallstones, as in adults, are mobile, usually shadowing, echogenic foci found in the dependent portion of the gallbladder (Fig. 10). Rarely, the stone(s) may be adherent to the mucosa or may float within the bile. The sonographic signs of acute cholecystitis are also similar to those found in adults, including a thickened hyperechoic gallbladder wall (>3 mm), pericholecystic fluid, and gallstones or sludge. Other causes of gallbladder wall thickening include hepatitis, hypoproteinemia, ascites, Henoch–Schonlein purpura (47), hemangioma, or gallbladder contraction (48). Pericholecystic abscess, and gallbladder empyema and perforation are very rare in children (48). Acalculous cholecystitis is associated with recent surgery, sepsis, burns, and prolonged bile stasis.

Hydrops of the gallbladder is defined as dilatation of the gallbladder with thinning of its wall. The gallbladder is usually filled with stagnant bile. The biliary tree is not dilated. Causes may include sepsis, Kawasaki syndrome, hyperalimentation, narcotics, starvation, vomiting, and electrolyte imbalance. It may predispose the patient to acalculous cholecystitis (49).

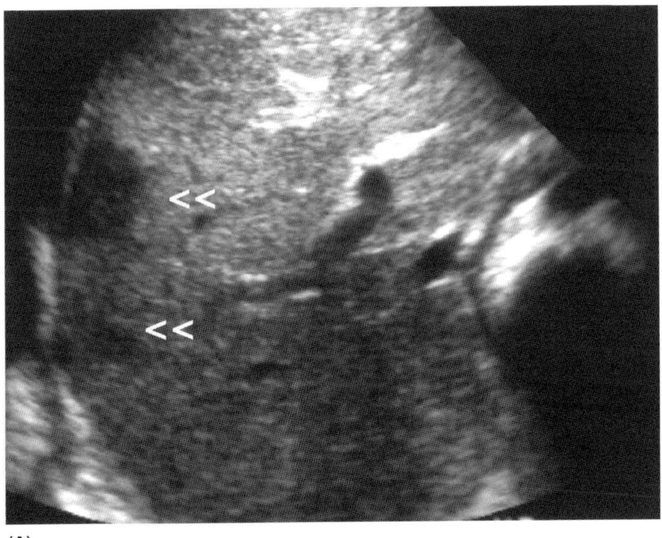

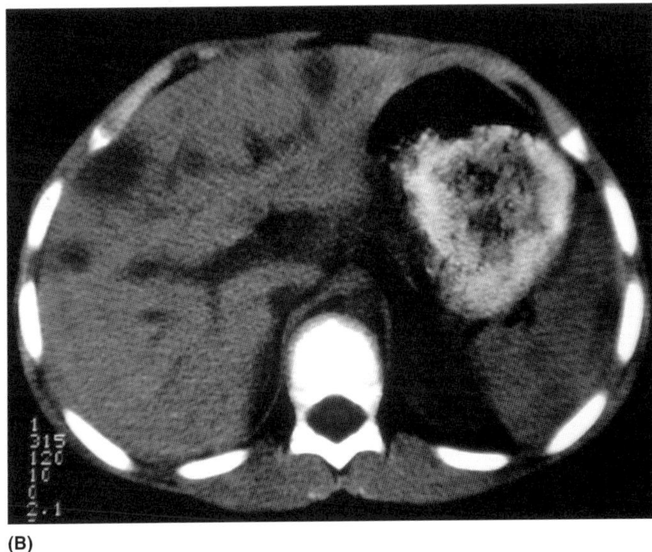

(A) (B)

FIGURE 8 A AND B ■ Cat scratch disease. (**A**) Transverse ultrasound shows hypoechoic lesions (*arrowheads*) within the liver. (**B**) Noncontrast CT scan defines multiple hypodense lesions of varying size.

Jaundice in the newborn may result from direct (conjugated) or indirect (unconjugated) hyperbilirubinemia. Anatomical abnormalities usually result in prolonged (greater than 14–21 days) direct hyperbilirubinemia. The list of causes of neonatal cholestasis is long (Table 4), but the most common differential possibilities in the newborn referred for imaging include neonatal hepatitis and extrahepatic biliary atresia. Ultrasonography and Technetium-99m-iminodiacetic acid (Tc-99m-IDA) imaging are the two major tools in differentiating these entities. Magnetic resonance cholangiography may also be useful (51). Liver biopsy, though, may be the single most informative test (50).

In neonatal hepatitis (Fig. 11), the liver is normal to large in size and has hepatic parenchyma, which is normal to hyperechoic and coarse. The biliary tree, including the gallbladder, appears normal (52). Differential difficulty (with biliary atresia) results from cases of severe hepatitis, where decrease in bile production causes the gallbladder to appear small. If a gallbladder is seen, it is useful to feed the infant and assess for gallbladder contraction and emptying (53), which implies a patent extrahepatic biliary tract. However, very rare cases of biliary atresia may also initially demonstrate gallbladder emptying with feeding (54). Tc-99m-IDA imaging will show

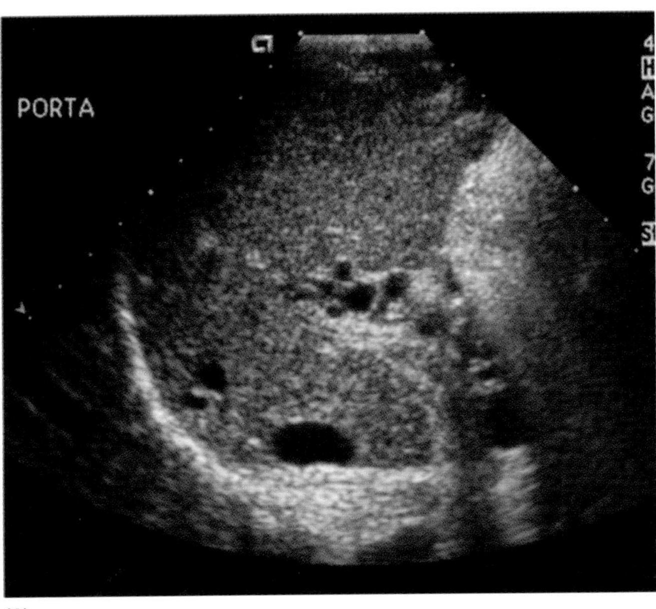

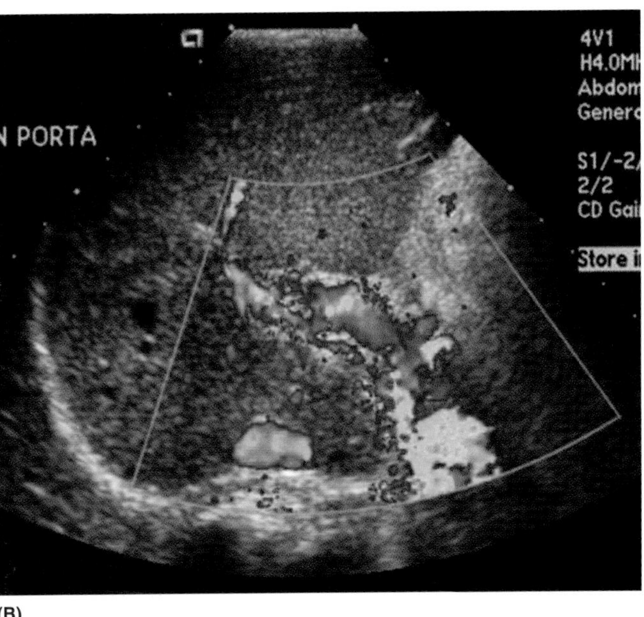

(A) (B)

FIGURE 9 A–C ■ Eight-year-old boy with cavernous transformation of the portal vein. (**A**) Transverse ultrasound image of the porta shows multiple tubular structures and no normal portal vein. (**B**) Color Doppler image demonstrates these are collateral blood vessels. (*Continued*)

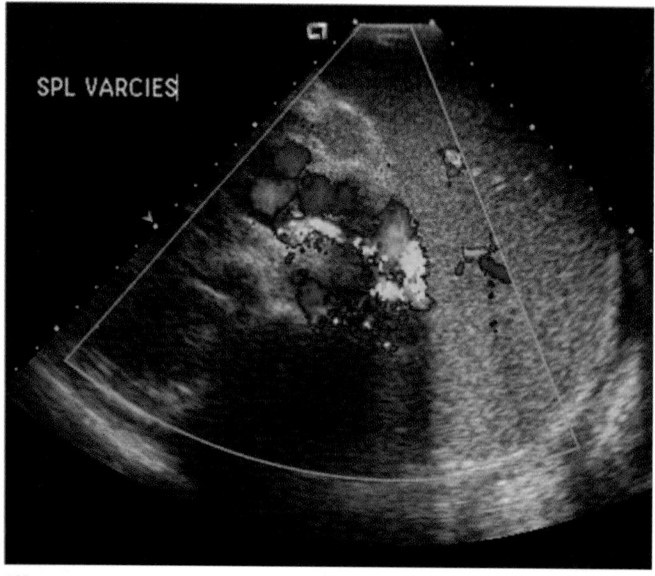

(C)

FIGURE 9 A–C ■ (*Continued*) (**C**) Transverse image of the spleen shows splenic varices and splenomegaly.

TABLE 4 ■ Causes of Neonatal Cholestasis

Biliary tree anomalies:
Biliary atresia
Choledochal cyst
Biliary tree obstruction
■ Gallstones
■ Inspissated bile syndrome
Infection:
Sepsis
Hepatic infection
TORCH, viral
Metabolic and inherited disorders such as:
α-1 antitrypsin deficiency
Alagille syndrome
Cystic fibrosis
Gaucher disease
Zellweger syndrome
Other causes:
Hypopituitarism, hypothyroidism, and hypoadrenalism
Chromosomal disorders
Toxic exposure
Vascular abnormalities

Source: From Ref. 50.

delayed uptake by the liver but eventual excretion of the radiopharmaceutical into the small bowel.

Extrahepatic biliary atresia is more common in boys and is a progressive, obliterative process of the bile ducts, which begins at birth or antenatally. The liver may be normal or enlarged, and its echotexture may be normal or hyperechoic. The intrahepatic ducts are not dilated, and the gallbladder is small [<1.5 cm in length (55)] or undetectable. A triangular or tubular echogenic cord (Fig. 12) of fibrous tissue seen in the porta hepatis is relatively specific in the diagnosis of biliary atresia (56–58) and has been termed the "triangular cord sign." Biliary cysts (Fig. 13) are also associated with biliary atresia (59). It is important to evaluate the spleen in patients with biliary atresia, as about 10% have polysplenia. The diagnosis of biliary atresia is confirmed with Tc-99m-IDA imaging,

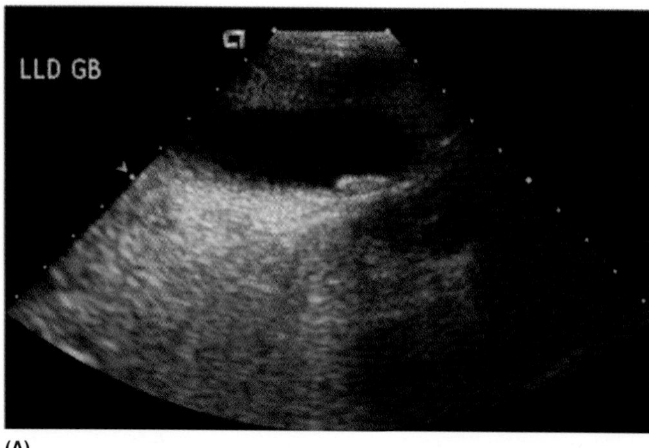

(A)

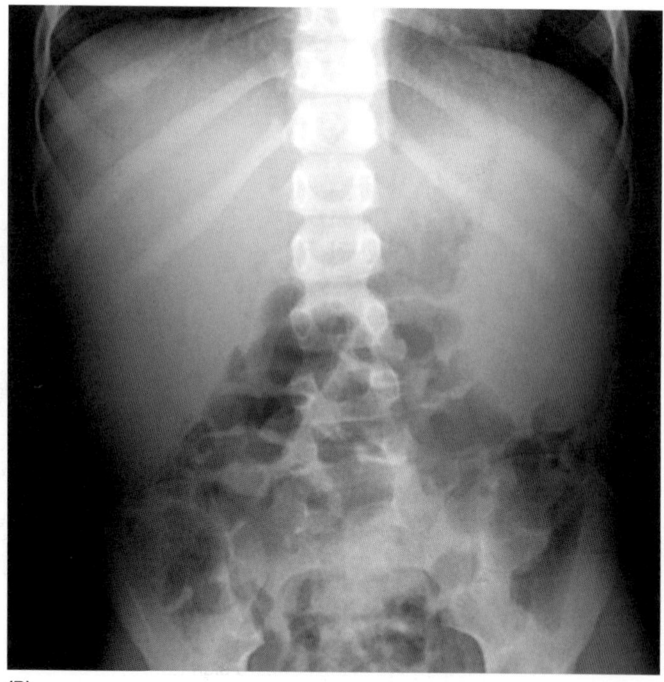

(B)

FIGURE 10 A AND B ■ Spherocytosis. (**A**) Longitudinal image of the gallbladder in an eight-year-old boy with spherocytosis shows a shadowing gallstone in the fundus of the gallbladder. (**B**) Plain film image of the upper abdomen in this same boy demonstrates splenomegaly.

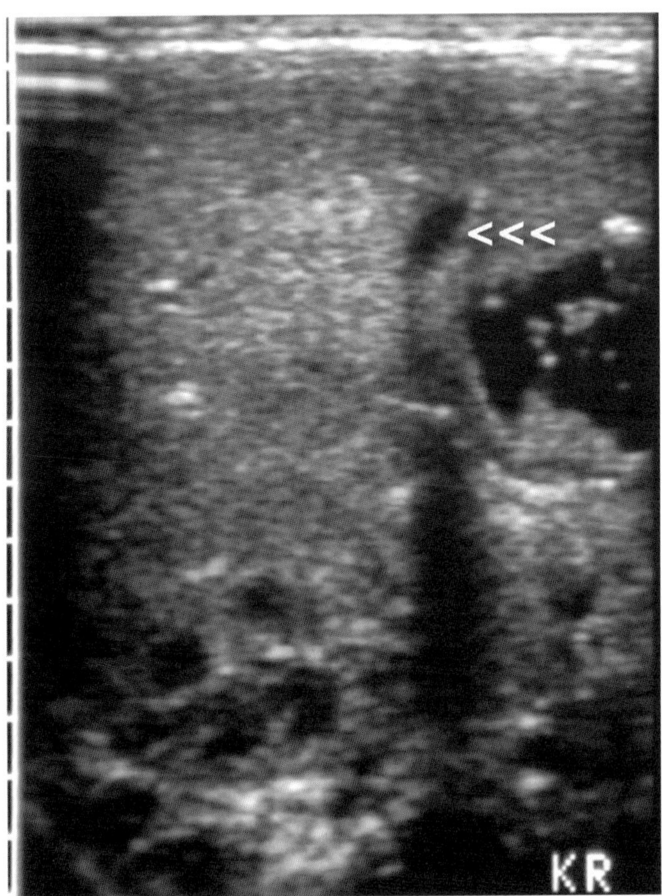

FIGURE 11 ■ Newborn with neonatal hepatitis. Transverse ultrasound image shows a small gallbladder is present (*arrowheads*).

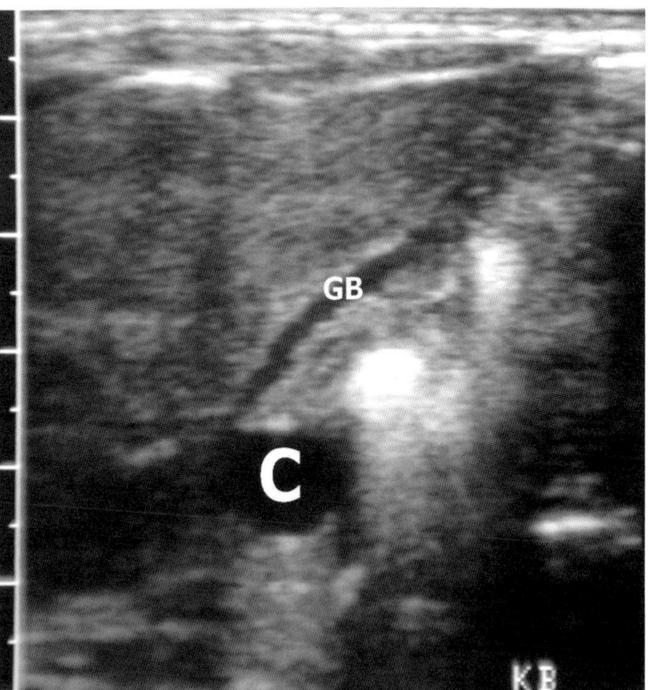

FIGURE 13 ■ Newborn with proven biliary atresia. Longitudinal images show a small gallbladder (GB) and a biliary cyst (C) just anterior to the portal vein.

where hepatic uptake is normal, but no radiopharmaceutical is excreted into the small bowel. It is important to make the diagnosis of biliary atresia promptly, as the best results from Kasai portoenterostomy are obtained if the patient is operated on before 60 days old (52).

Patients with Alagille syndrome, or arteriohepatic dysplasia, may have biliary hypoplasia and present with a similar clinical picture to biliary atresia (52). Additional clinical findings to suggest the diagnosis include butterfly vertebrae, pulmonic stenosis, congenital heart disease, and abnormal facies.

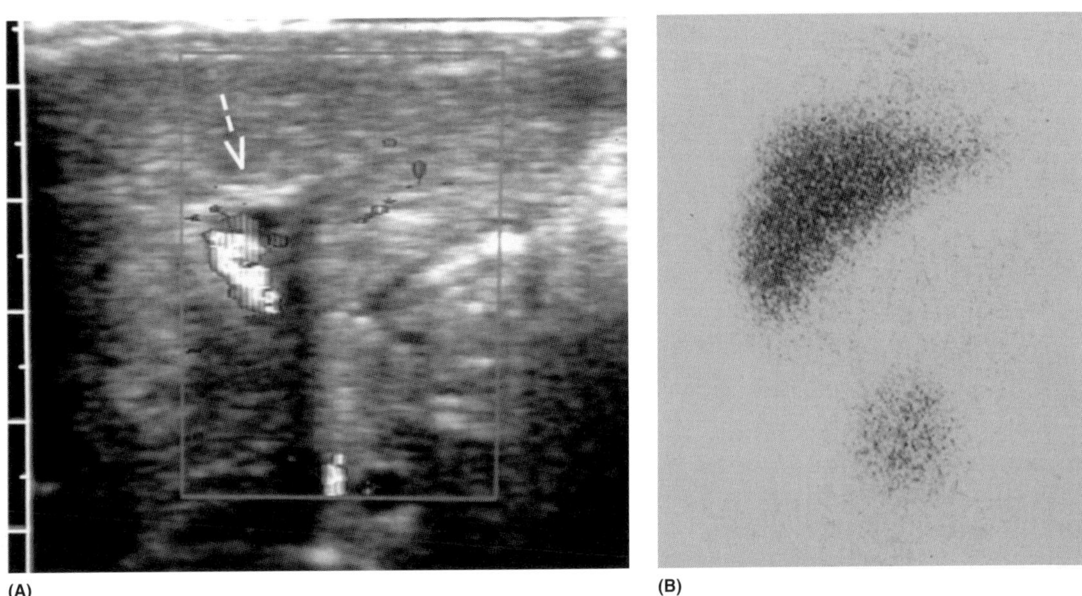

FIGURE 12 A AND B ■ Newborn with biliary atresia. (**A**) Black and white image of a color Doppler exam showing the triangular cord sign (*arrow*) just anterior to the portal vein. No gallbladder was found. (**B**) Biliary scan demonstrating no excretion into the bowel.

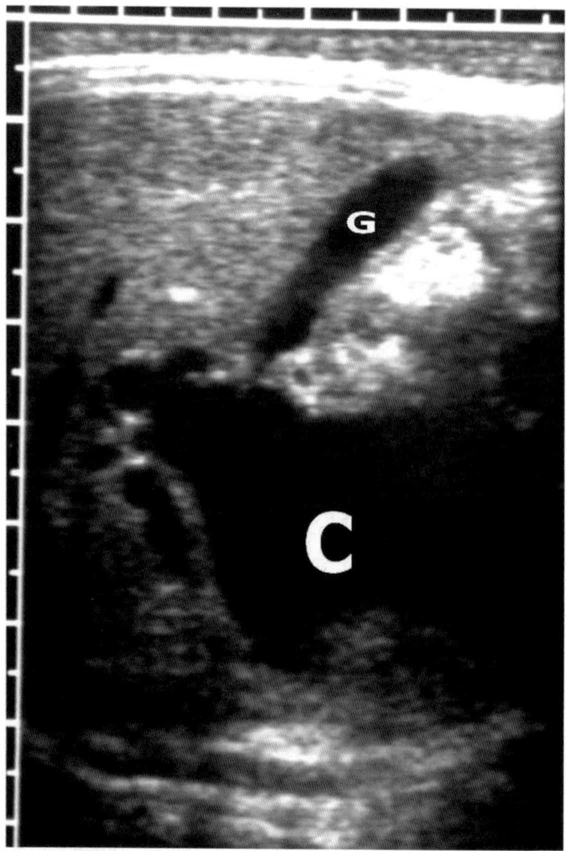

FIGURE 14 ■ Transverse ultrasound image of a four-year-old girl with a type IA choledochal cyst. Intrahepatic dilated ducts are seen to extend into the cystic mass (C) located posterior to the gallbladder. The gallbladder (G) neck opens into the dilated common duct.

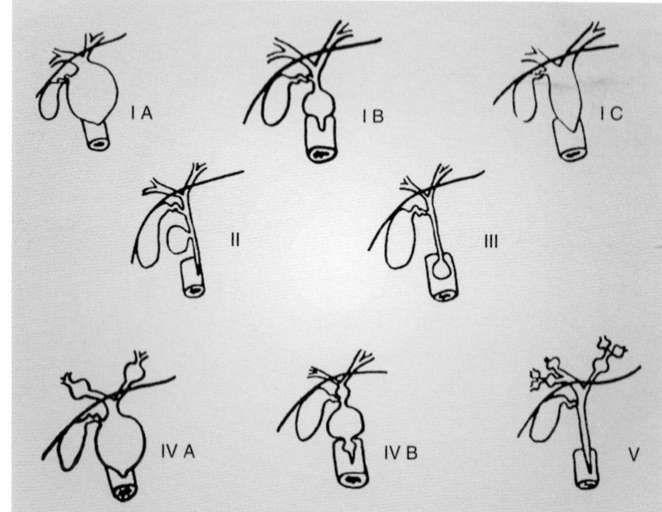

FIGURE 15 ■ Types of choledochal cysts using the system of Todani et al. Type IA—marked cystic dilatation all or part of the extrahepatic biliary tree. The gallbladder arises from the cyst. Type IB—focal dilatation of the common bile duct (usually distal), with a normal duct between the cyst and the cystic duct. Type IC—fusiform dilatation of the common bile duct along with cylindrical dilatation of the common hepatic duct and common bile duct. The gallbladder arises from the dilated common bile duct. Type II—choledochal diverticulum. Type III—choledochocele. Type IVA—cystic dilatation of the intrahepatic and extrahepatic biliary tree. Type IV B—multiple segmental dilatation of the common bile duct. Type V—dilatation of intrahepatic bile ducts (Caroli disease). *Source*: From Ref. 61.

Choledochal cysts (Fig. 14) are a relatively rare congenital abnormality of the biliary tree and probably result in abnormal connection between the pancreatic duct and the common bile duct (60), allowing chronic reflux of pancreatic enzymes into the common bile duct and ductal irritation and dilatation. Choledochal cysts are more common in girls and are most frequently diagnosed in children less than 10 years of age. The classic triad of pain, jaundice, and a right upper quadrant mass is seen in the minority of patients.

Choledochal cysts may be classified into four types (61), as shown in Figure 15. Type I accounts for 80% to 90% of cases (52). On ultrasonography, a cystic mass, separate from the gallbladder but communicating with the biliary tree, is seen. The intrahepatic ducts may or may not be dilated. Complications may include chole(docho)lithiasis, pancreatitis, infection, malignancy, and cirrhosis (52).

Spontaneous perforation of the common bile duct is rare, but it is the second most common cause of jaundice amenable to surgical treatment in infants (62). The pathogenesis is not known, but distal obstruction (stenosis, stone), weakness of the bile duct wall, and trauma have been proposed. The typical history is a normal infant who develops jaundice, ascites, and abdominal distension. Ultrasonographic findings in this diagnosis include a cystic collection in the porta (pseudocholedochal cyst), a nondilated biliary tree, and ascites (Fig. 16) (62).

Rhabdomyosarcoma of the biliary tract (Fig. 17) is a rare tumor in children. The median age at presentation is three years, and the tumor is slightly more common in boys. Patients usually present with jaundice and abdominal distension. Ultrasound imaging will demonstrate intrahepatic biliary ductal dilatation and an intraductal mass (63). Cystic areas may be seen in larger tumors and may represent areas of necrosis. If the tumor is large and grows into the liver, it may be difficult to distinguish from other primary liver masses. The most common site of metastatic spread is the liver.

SPLEEN

Situs anomalies are a relatively rare continuum of cardiac, vascular, and visceral anomalies. Situs ambiguous, or heterotaxy, refers to indeterminate visceral malposition and dysmorphism (64). Several genes as well as teratogenic exposures (especially maternal diabetes) have been implicated in its development (65). Although these anomalies occur along a continuum, these patients tend to be divided into those in whom right-sided structures predominate and those in whom left-sided structures predominate (66). Sonographic evaluation of the abdomen must include (*i*) position of venous drainage relative to midline, (*ii*) position of the aorta, (*iii*) position of the stomach, (*iv*)

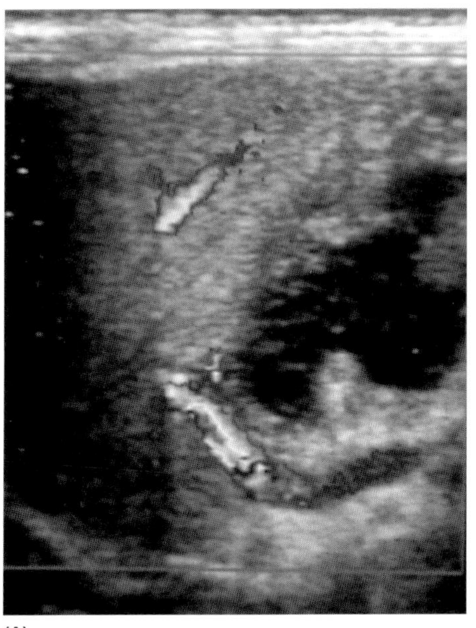
(A)

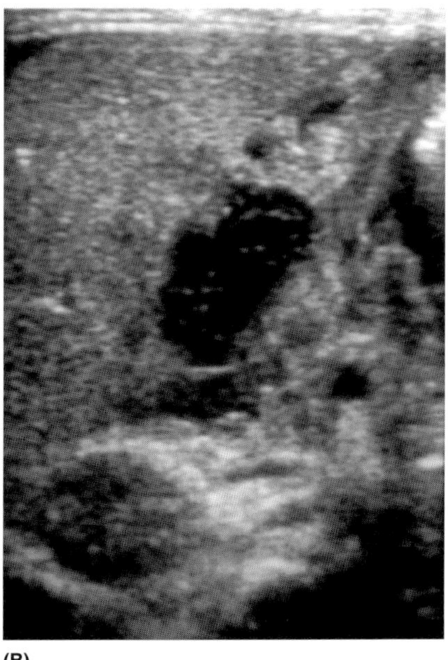
(B)

FIGURE 16 A–E ■ Two-month-old with spontaneous perforation of the biliary tree. He presented with jaundice and a right upper quadrant mass. (**A**) Longitudinal black and white ultrasound image of a color Doppler exam shows an irregular cystic mass with internal echoes in the porta that displaces the portal vein posteriorly. (**B**) Transverse image demonstrating this same mass. (**C**) CT further defines this irregular fluid-density mass (P) as well as ascites (*arrowheads*). (**D**) Three hour delayed image from a Tc-99m-IDA exam shows biliary ascites. (**E**) Intrahepatic gallbladder cholangiogram shows leakage of contrast after spontaneous perforation of the biliary tree.

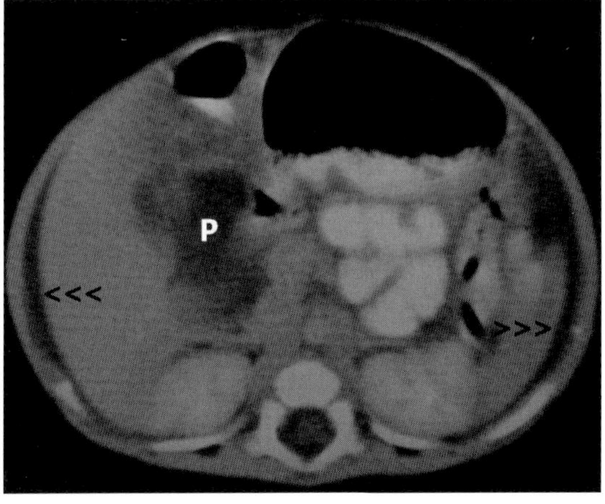

(C)

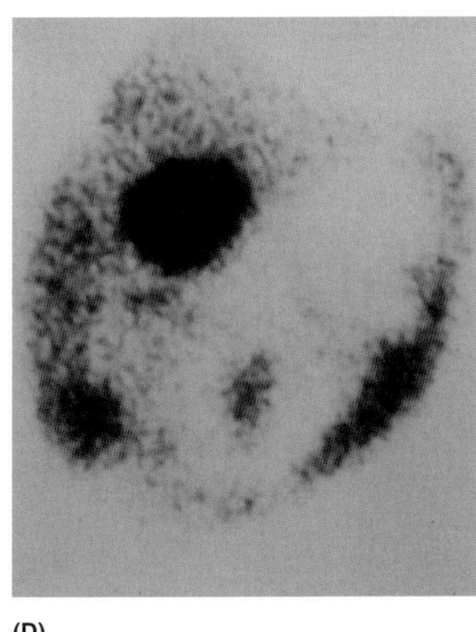
(D)

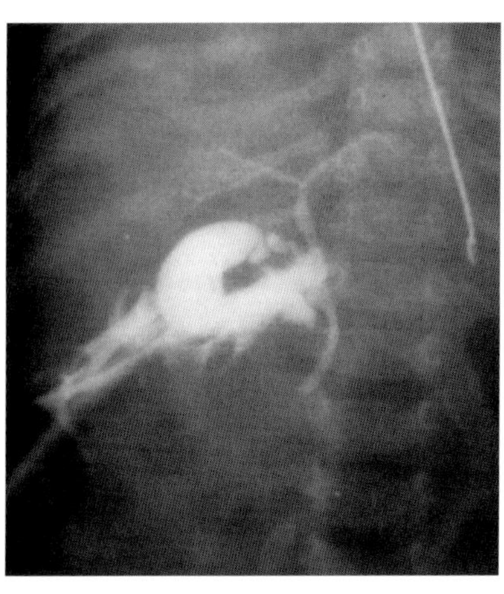
(E)

presence of small bowel malrotation, (*v*) position of the liver and gallbladder, and (*iv*) presence, position, and appearance of splenic tissue.

With right-sided isomerism, or Ivemark syndrome, abdominal findings include a transverse liver and a midline (often small) stomach and small bowel malrotation. The aorta and inferior vena cava may appear on the same side of the spine. Splenic tissue is absent or rudimentary, increasing the risk for sepsis. Subdiaphragmatic total anomalous pulmonary venous connections may be noted (66). The adrenal glands may be horseshoe in appearance (67). These patients also have complex congenital heart disease and bilateral trilobed lungs.

With left-sided isomerism, abdominal findings include a transverse liver (Fig. 18), an indeterminate stomach, and multiple, retrogastric splenuli (Fig. 18c). Other findings include interruption of the inferior vena cava with azygos continuation, preduodenal portal vein, biliary atresia (Fig. 18d) (68), and small bowel malrotation. The lungs are bilobed bilaterally, and congenital heart disease is less severe than with right-sided isomerism.

Wandering spleen and splenic torsion are rare in children (69). This lesion usually results from congenital maldevelopment of the dorsal mesogastrium (70), resulting in incomplete fixation by the lienorenal and gastrosplenic ligaments. Most commonly, the child will present with a mass and pain; many will have an acute abdomen requiring emergent surgical treatment (71). Ultrasound imaging will show low position of the spleen and splenomegaly (from vascular congestion). The splenic parenchyma will appear granular, and hypoechoic echotexture (72) and Doppler interrogation will show absence of parenchymal flow if torsion and infarction have occurred (73). A whorled appearance of the splenic hilum may result from the twisted splenic pedicle intermixed with fat (74).

Splenomegaly (Table 5) in children may result from chronic liver disease with portal hypertension, infiltrative disease, metabolic disorders, hematological disease, infection, and splenic masses (75). Splenic tumors other than leukemia and lymphoma are very rare. Splenic cysts (Fig. 19) may be congenital or secondary from trauma,

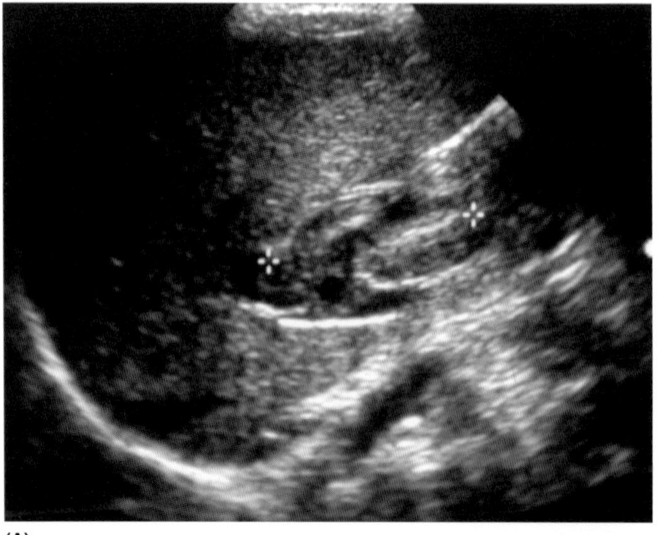

(A)

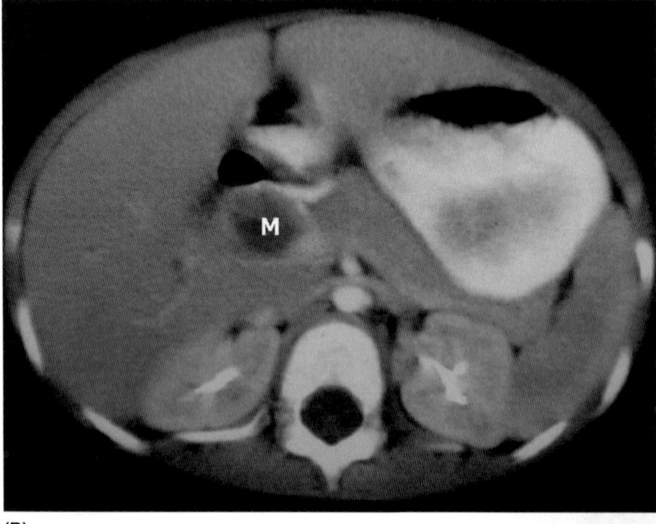

(B)

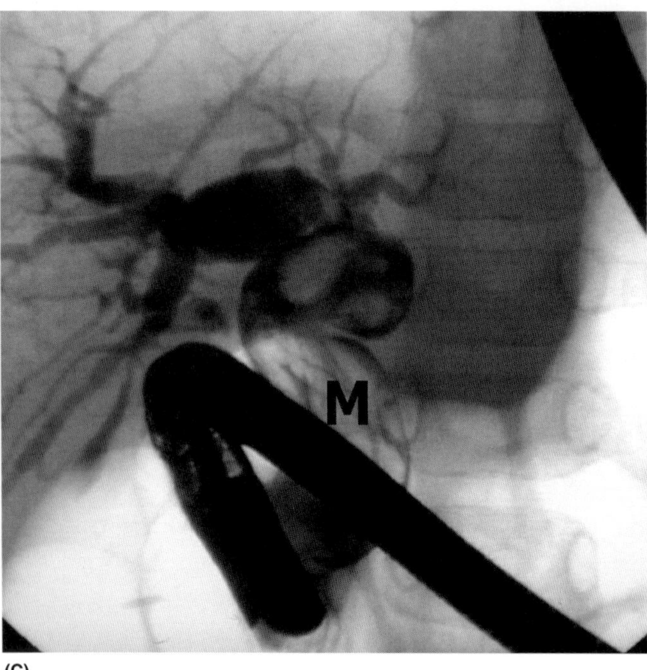

(C)

FIGURE 17 A–C ■ Biliary rhabdomyosarcoma. (**A**) Longitudinal image of the porta in a four year old with jaundice and biliary rhabdomyosarcoma showing an inhomogeneous mass (*cursors*). (**B**) CT in this same patient defines a low-density mass (M) extending into the common bile duct in the head of the pancreas. (**C**) Endoscopic retrograde cholangiopancreatography outlines a lobular mass (M) in the common bile duct.

infarction, or hydatid disease. Congenital cysts are lined by epithelium (76) and are usually solitary. Their margin may be echogenic and they are surrounded by normal splenic tissue. A sonolucent mass with septations or internal debris should suggest abscess or hematoma.

As discussed in the liver section above, ultrasonography has not proven to be useful compared with CT in the detection of solid organ injury in children. However, it can be helpful in following splenic injury (77) and in documenting splenic healing. The more severe the injury, the longer it takes to heal.

PERITONEAL CAVITY

Mesenteric cysts (Fig. 20) are benign, cystic lymphangiomas that contain chyle or serous material. They are thought to be developmental abnormalities of the lymphatic system rather than true tumors (78). Patients usually present with abdominal distension and may have pain, anorexia, vomiting, or fever (79,80). These lesions appear as well-defined, thin-walled cystic or multicystic masses, often with internal fine septations. They are most common in the ileal mesentery, and displace adjacent structures to the periphery of the abdomen. When very large, lymphangiomas may be difficult to distinguish from severe ascites. Differentiating features suggesting ascites rather than lymphangioma include separation of bowel loops, fluid collecting in the perihepatic spaces and cul-de-sac, and lack of septations (81).

Cerebrospinal fluid (CSF) pseudocyst (Fig. 21) is a complication resulting from ventriculoperitoneal shunting. Children can present with abdominal pain, distension, or

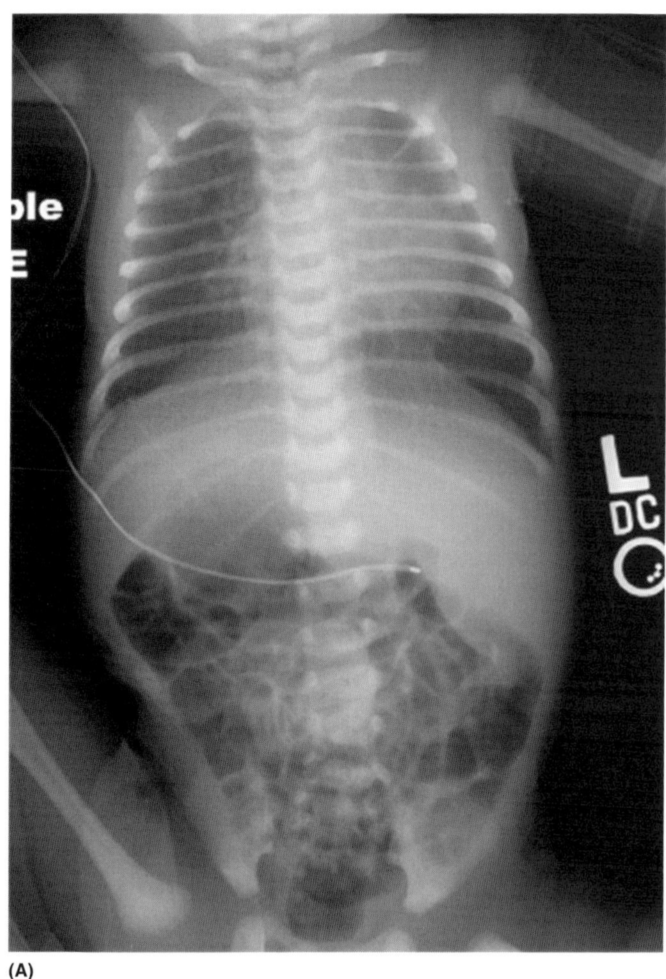

(A)

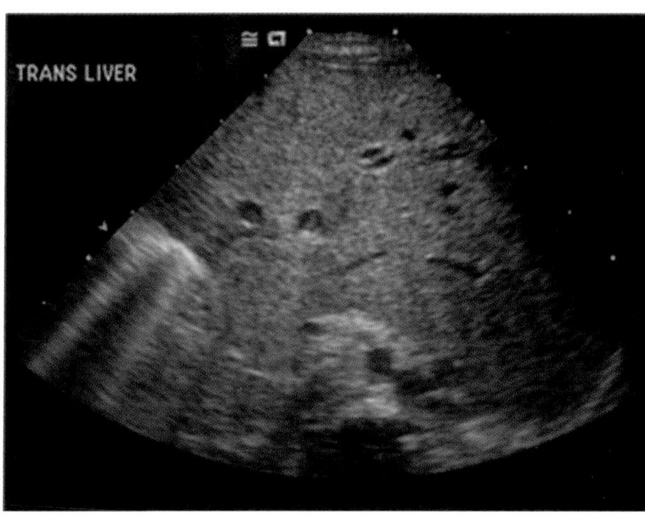

(B)

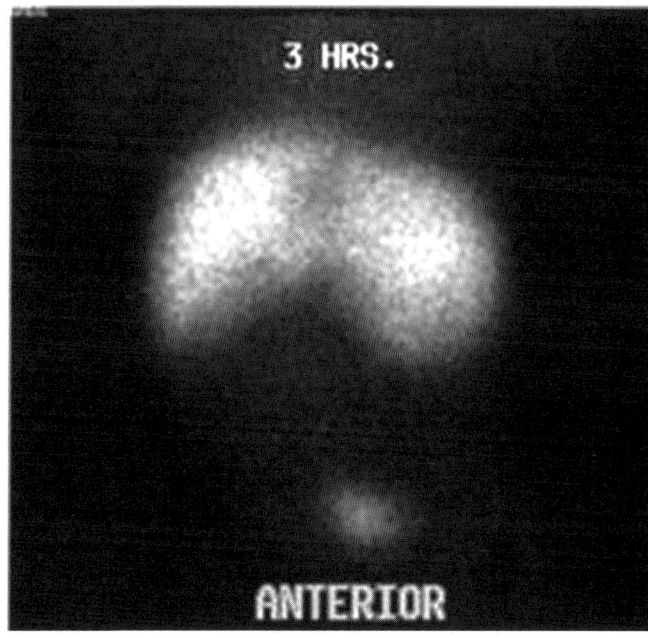

(D)

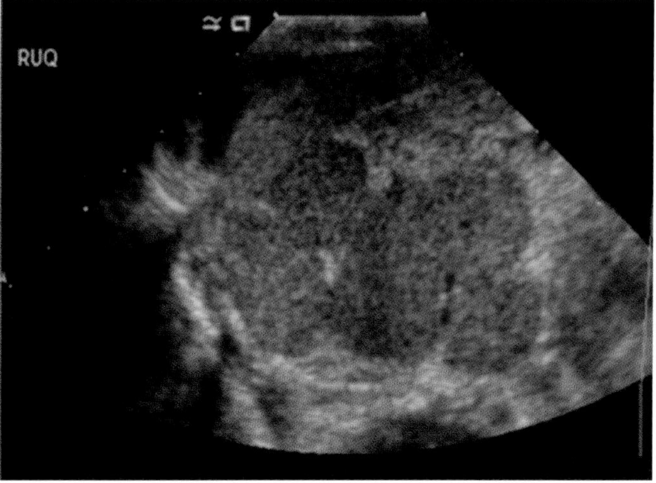

(C)

FIGURE 18 A–D ■ Newborn with left-sided isomerism. (**A**) Babygram shows a left-sided cardiac apex, a transverse liver and a right-sided stomach. (**B**) Transverse ultrasound of a left-sided liver crossing the midline. (**C**) Transverse image showing multiple splenules in the right upper quadrant in the retrogastric region. (**D**) Biliary scintigraphy demonstrates no biliary excretion in this patient with biliary atresia.

mass. Larger pseudocysts tend to be sterile, whereas smaller pseudocysts are more often infected. Ultrasound shows a well-defined cystic mass with the shunt catheter tip identified within the collection. A noninfected shunt pseudocyst appears homogeneous, whereas an infected collection will demonstrate septations, a fluid-fluid level, or internal debris (82).

PANCREAS

Pancreas divisum, in which there is absent or incomplete fusion between dorsal and ventral ducts of the pancreas, is the most common anatomic variant of the pancreas. With this anomaly, the majority of the pancreatic gland drains via the minor papilla, and only the head and uncinate

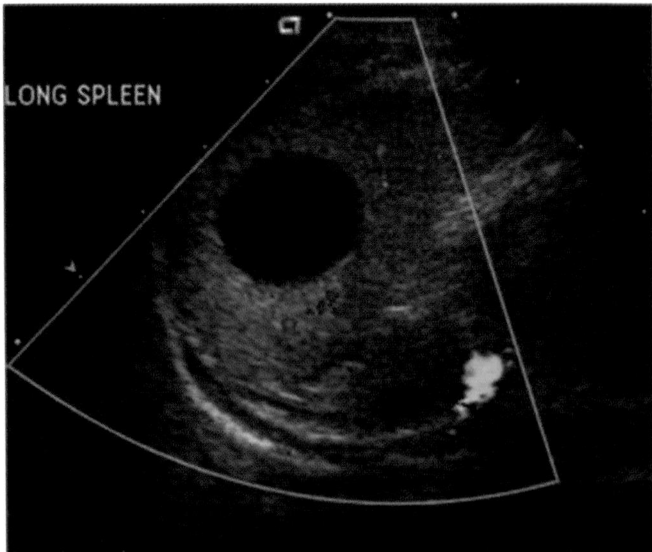

FIGURE 19 ■ Splenic cyst. Longitudinal image of the spleen in a four month old shows a well-defined congenital splenic cyst.

TABLE 5 ■ Causes of Splenomegaly

Diffuse
Portal hypertension
Infiltrative disease
■ Leukemia, lymphoma
■ Langerhans-cell histiocytosis
Hematological
■ Sickle-cell anemia
■ Hemolytic anemia
Metabolic disorders
■ Gaucher disease
Collagen vascular disease
Infection
Focal
Splenic cyst
Infection
■ Cat scratch
■ Abscess
■ Fungal
Vascular malformation
Hematoma

process drain via the major papilla. This diagnosis is not usually made by sonography; the imaging modality of choice is magnetic resonance cholangiopancreatography or endoscopic retrograde cholangiopancreatography.

Annular pancreas develops from a bifid ventral pancreatic bud or abnormal adherence of the ventral pancreatic duct to the duodenum before rotation (8,9). It results in pancreatic tissue encasing the duodenum and is associated with duodenal stenosis or atresia. On ultrasound, a ring of pancreatic tissue surrounding a dilated proximal duodenum may be seen (83).

Congenital pancreatic cysts, caused by maldevelopment of the pancreatic ducts, are usually single and located in the body or tail of the pancreas (84). Multiple cysts may be seen with autosomal-dominant polycystic kidney disease or von Hippel Lindau syndrome.

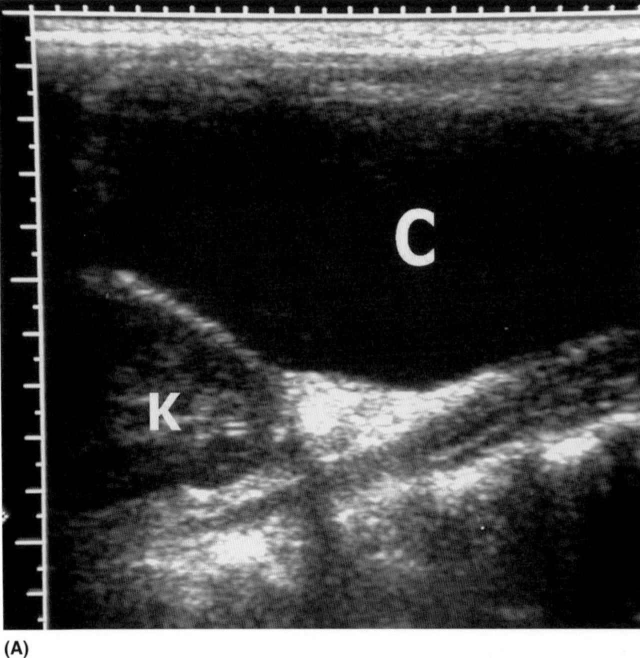

(A)

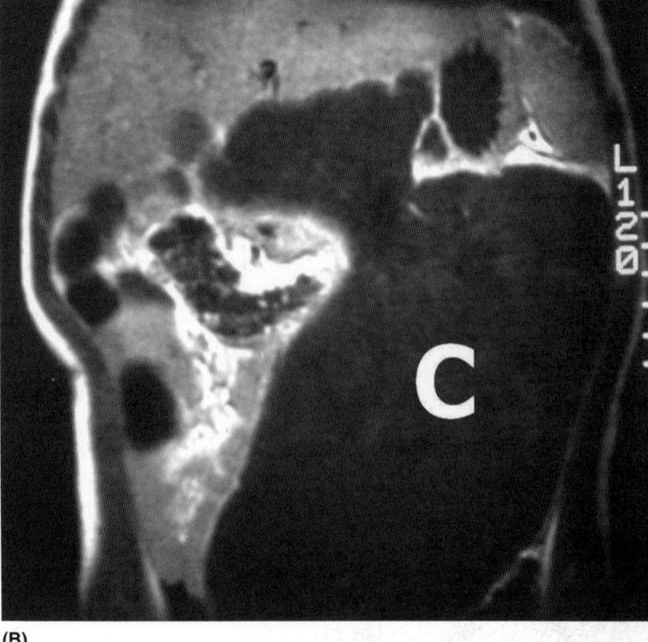

(B)

FIGURE 20 A AND B ■ Mesenteric cyst. (**A**) Longitudinal ultrasound image shows a large, thin-walled cystic mass (C) filling the abdomen. The kidney (K) is seen posterior to the mass. (**B**) Coronal post-gadolinium MRI further defines this large mesenteric cyst (C).

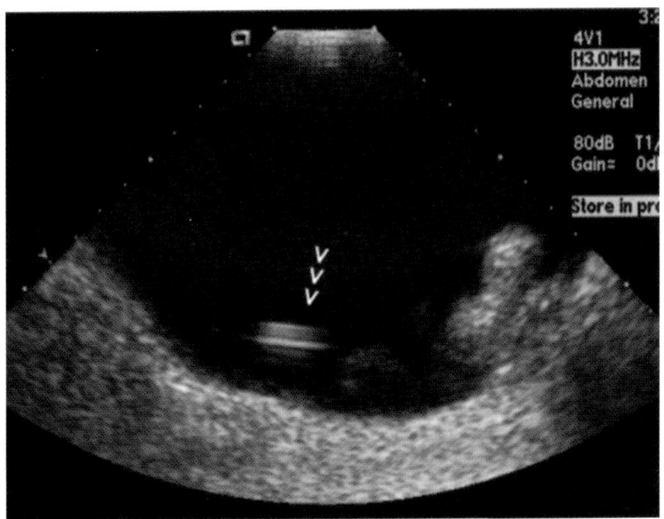

FIGURE 21 ■ Fourteen year old with shunt pseudocyst. The catheter (*arrowheads*) is identified within the cystic fluid collection.

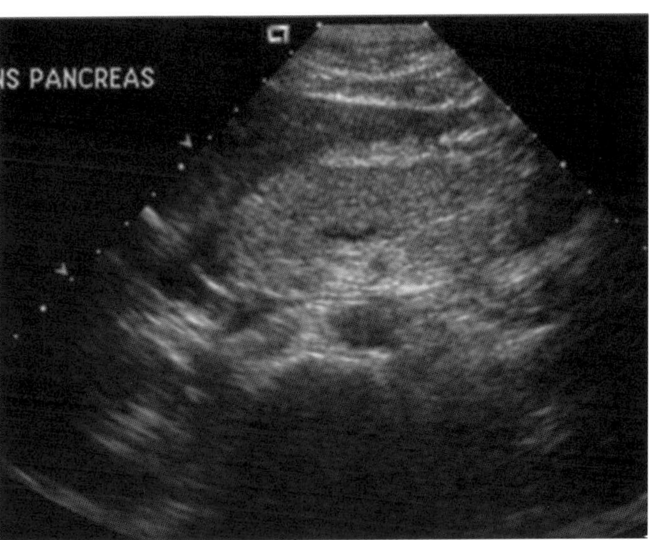

FIGURE 23 ■ Fourteen-year-old girl with acute pancreatitis. Transverse ultrasound shows an enlarged, somewhat echogenic pancreas and mild prominence of the pancreatic duct.

Patients with cystic fibrosis have abnormal chloride transport across the membrane of epithelial cells that express the cystic fibrosis transmembrane conductance regulator (85). Within the pancreas, this leads to accumulation of thick intraluminal secretions, ductal ectasia, acinar tissue atrophy, fibrosis, and exocrine or endocrine pancreatic insufficiency. The result is fibrofatty replacement of the pancreas (Fig. 22), enlargement due to lipomatous pseudohypertrophy, diffuse fibrosis or atrophy of the pancreas, and/or cystic transformation (8,86). Sonographic findings, seen in virtually every patient with cystic fibrosis, include an increase in pancreatic echogenicity (8), a decrease in the pancreatic size, and a loss of the fine normal echo pattern of the gland. Calcifications may be seen (87).

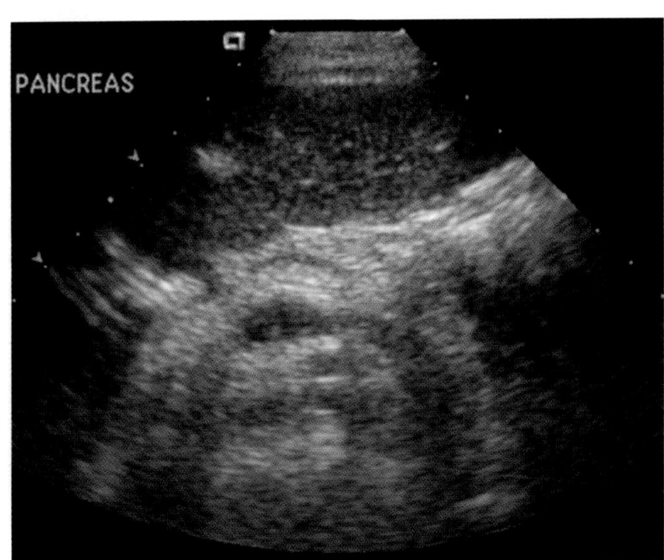

FIGURE 22 ■ Transverse ultrasound image of the pancreas in a 16 year old with cystic fibrosis. The pancreas is replaced with fibrofatty tissue and is small and echogenic.

Pancreatic cystosis is seen as multiple, thin-walled cysts with interspersed pancreatic tissue. However, the appearance of the pancreas does not correlate well with pancreatic function (85).

The most common cause of acute pancreatitis in children is trauma (8). Other causes include infection (viral), vasculitis, sepsis, hemolytic uremic syndrome, drugs (L-asparaginase, steroids, etc.), hyperlipidemia, hypercalcemia, gallstone pancreatitis, and embryologic anomalies of pancreatic drainage (9). Sonographic findings (Fig. 23) include focal or diffuse pancreatic enlargement, increased (9) or decreased (8) pancreatic echogenicity, poorly defined pancreatic borders, peripancreatic fluid, and pancreatic ductal dilatation. Complications may include pseudocyst formation (most common), abscess, hemorrhage, necrosis, and thrombosis of the splenic or portal vein.

Hereditary pancreatitis, cystic fibrosis, hyperparathyroidism, malnutrition, and Shwachman–Diamond syndrome are causes of chronic pancreatitis in the pediatric population (8,9). With chronic pancreatitis, the gland is small, irregular, and has increased echogenicity and calcifications. Ductal dilatation may also be seen.

Pancreatic tumors are rare in children. Metastatic disease is more frequent than primary neoplasm, with Burkitt lymphoma seen most frequently. This may appear as solitary or multiple hypoechoic masses, or diffuse glandular infiltration (8). Other metastatic tumors may include sarcomas or neuroblastoma. Primary tumors include exocrine, endocrine, and cystic tumors (7).

Exocrine tumors include adenocarcinoma (Fig. 24) and pancreatoblastoma (88). Pancreatoblastoma is most often seen between the ages of one and eight years. This tumor is more common in males and in Asians. A congenital cystic form is associated with Beckwith–Wiedemann syndrome. It is slowly growing and typically

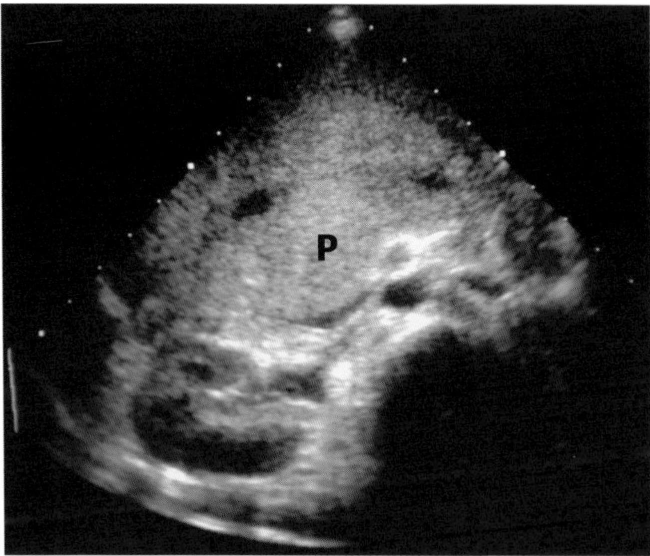

FIGURE 24 ■ Five-year-old boy with pancreatic adenocarcinoma. Transverse image through the pancreas (P) shows an infiltrative mass enlarging the pancreas.

quite large at diagnosis, with symptoms usually relating to mass effect. Obstructive jaundice may be seen. Serum α-fetoprotein, adrenocorticotropic hormone and lactate dehydrogenase may be elevated. Pancreatoblastoma is seen as a well defined and at least partially circumscribed, lobulated mass with a mixed echotexture. Defining the pancreas as the organ of origin may be difficult, as large tumors may extend into the duodenum and porta hepatis. The liver is the most frequent site of metastases, but metastases may also be seen in the omentum or peritoneum.

Endocrine tumors arise from the islet cells and may be functional or nonfunctional (9). Functioning tumors may produce insulin, gastrin, vasoactive intestinal polypeptide, or glucagon. They are associated with multiple endocrine neoplasia type I and von Hippel Lindau disease. The tumors may be small and difficult to detect; they are usually hypoechoic and well-defined small masses.

The most common cystic tumor is the solid-cystic papillary tumor. It is seen more frequently in females and in Asians and those of African decent (89). This tumor is found in the head of the pancreas in half of cases and is usually well defined. It contains areas of hemorrhage or cystic degeneration (90). Calcification may be seen in about a third of patients. This tumor may invade adjacent structures or may show metastatic spread to the liver or lymph nodes. Other rare cystic pancreatic tumors in children include serous or mucinous cystadenoma, cystadenocarcinoma, teratoma, or hamartoma (9).

REFERENCES

1. Siegel MJ. Liver. Pediatric sonography. 3rd ed. Philadelphia, PA: Siegel, Lippincott Williams and Wilkins, 2002.
2. Teele RL, Share JC. Ultrasonography of the biliary tree in infants and children. Appl Radiol 1992; 21:15–29.
3. Konus OL, Ozdemir A, Akkaya A, Erbas G, Celik H, Isik S. Normal liver, spleen and kidney dimensions in neonates, infants and children: evaluation with sonography. AJR Am J Roentgenol 1998; 171:1693–1698.
4. Jequier S, Jequier JC, Gong J, et al. Doppler waveform of hepatic veins in healthy children. AJR AM J Roentgenol 2000; 175:85–90.
5. Siegel MJ. Gallbladder and biliary tract. Pediatric Sonography. 3rd ed. Philadelphia, PA: Siegel, Lippincott Williams and Wilkins, 2002.
6. McGahan JP, Phillips HE, Cox KL. Sonography of the normal pediatric gallbladder and biliary tree. Radiology 1982; 144:873–875.
7. Siegel MJ. Adrenal glands, pancreas, and other retroperitoneal structures. Pediatric Sonography. 3rd ed. Philadelphia, PA: Siegel, Lippincott Williams and Wilkins, 2002.
8. Berrocal T, Prieto C, Pastor I, Gutierrez J, Al-Assir I. Sonography of pancreatic disease in infants and children. Radiographics 1995; 15:301–313.
9. Nijs E, Callahan MJ, Taylor GA. Disorders of the pediatric pancreas: imaging features. Pediatr Radiol 2005; 35:358–373.

Hepatic Neoplasms

10. Helmberger TK, Ros PR, Mergo PJ, Tomczak R, Feiser MF. Pediatric liver neoplasms: a radiologic-pathologic correlation. Eur Radiol 1999; 9:1339–1347.
11. Stoupis C, Ros PR. Imaging findings in hepatoblastoma associated with Gardner's syndrome. AJR AM J Roentgenol 1993; 161:593–594.
12. deCampo M, deCampo JF. Ultrasound of primary hepatic tumours in childhood. Pediatr Radiol 1988; 19:19–24.
13. Dachman AH, Pakter RL, Ros PR, et al. Hepatoblastoma: radiologic-pathologic correlation in 50 cases. Radiology 1987; 164:15–19.
14. Miller JH, Greenspan BS. Integrated imaging of hepatic tumors in childhood. Radiology 1985; 154:83–90.
15. Graif M, Manor A, Itzchak Y. Sonographic differentiation of extra and intrahepatic masses. AJR Am J Roentgenol 1983; 141:553–556.
16. Exelby PR, Filler RM, Grosfeld JL. Liver tumors in children in the particular reference to hepatoblastoma and hepatocellular carcinoma: American Academy of Pediatrics Surgical Section Survey 1974. J Pediatr Surg 1975; 10:329–337.
17. Taylor KJW, Ramos I, Morse SS, et al. Focal liver masses: differential diagnosis with pulsed Doppler US. Radiology 1987; 164:643–647.
18. Sato M, Ishida H, Konno K, et al. Liver tumors in children and young patients: sonographic and color Doppler findings. Abdom Imaging 2000; 25(6):596–601.
19. Luks FI, Yazbeck S, Brandt ML, et al. Benign liver tumors in children: a 25-year experience. J Pediatr Surg 1991; 11:1326–1330.
20. Dachman AH, Lichtenstein JE, Friedman AC, et al. Infantile hemangioendothelioma of the liver: a radiographic-pathologic-clinical correlation. AJR Am J Roentgenol 1983; 140:1091–1096.
21. Lucaya J, Enriquez G, Amat L, et al. Computed tomography of infantile hepatic hemangioendothelioma. AJR Am J Roentgenol 1985; 144:821–826.
22. Chen CC, Kong MS, Yang CP, Hung IJ. Hepatic hemangioendothelioma in children: analysis of thirteen cases. Acta Paediatr Tw 2003; 44:8–13.
23. Klein MA, Slovis TL, Chang CH, et al. Sonographic and Doppler features of infantile hepatic hemangiomas with pathologic correlation. J Ultrasound Med 1990; 9:619–624.
24. Burrows PE, Dubois J, Kassarjian A. Pediatric hepatic vascular anomalies. Pediatr Radiol 2001; 31:533–545.
25. Ingram JD, Yerushalmi B, Connell J, Karrer FM, Tyson RW, Sokol RJ. Hepatoblastoma in a neonate: a hypervascular presentation mimicking hemangioendothelioma. Pediatr Radiol 2000; 30:794–797.
26. von Schweinitz D, Gluer S, Midenberger H. Liver tumors in neonates and very young infants: diagnostic pitfalls and therapeutic problems. Eur J Pediatr Surg 1995; 5:72–76.
27. Stanley P, Hall TR, Woolley MM, Diament MJ, Gilsanz V, Miller JH. Mesenchymal hamartomas of the liver in childhood: sonographic and CT findings. AJR Am J Roentgenol 1986; 147:1035–1039.
28. Stringer MD, Alizai NK. Mesenchymal hamartoma of the liver: a systematic review. J Pediatr Surg 2005; 40:1681–1690.

29. Ros PR, Goodman ZD, Ishak KG, et al. Mesenchymal hamartoma of the liver: radiologic-pathologic correlation. Radiology 1986; 158:619–624.
30. Koumanidou C, Vakaki M, Papadaki M, Pitsoulakis G, Savvidou D, Kakavakis K. New sonographic appearance of hepatic mesenchymal hamartomas in childhood. J Clin Ultrasound 1999; 27:164–167.
31. von Schweinitz D. Neonatal liver tumours. Semin Neonat 2003; 8:403–410.

Parenchymal Disease

32. Giorgio A, Amoroso P, Fico P, et al. Ultrasound evaluation of uncomplicated and complicated acute viral hepatitis. J Clin Ultrasound 1986; 14:675–679.
33. Garcia CJ, Varela C, Abarca K, Ferres M, Prado P, Vial PA. Regional lymphadenopathy in cat-scratch disease: ultrasonographic findings. Pediatr Radiol 2000; 30:640–645.
34. Danon O, Duval-Arnould M, Osman Z, et al. Hepatic and splenic involvement in cat-scratch disease: imaging features. Abdom Imaging 2000; 25:182–183.
35. Talenti E, Cesaro S, Scapinello A, et al. Disseminated hepatic and splenic calcifications following cat-scratch disease. Pediatr Radiol 1994; 24:342–343.
36. Barakat M. Doppler sonographic findings in children with idiopathic portal vein cavernous deformity and variceal hemorrhage. J Ultrasound Med 2002; 21:825–830.
37. Philips RL. Cavernous transformation of the portal vein. Australas Radiol 1988; 32:239–241.
38. Galleto C, Velasco M, Marcuello P, Tejedor D, DeCampo L, Friera A. Congenital and acquired anomalies of the portal venous system. Radiographics 2002; 22:141–159.

Hepatic Trauma

39. Division of Injury Control—Center for Environmental Health and Injury Control—Centers for Disease Control. Childhood injuries in the United States. Am J Dis Child 1990; 144:527–646.
40. Benya EC, Lim-Dunham JE, Landrum O, Statter M. Abdominal sonography in examination of children with blunt abdominal trauma. AJR Am J Roentgenol 2000; 174:1613–1616.
41. Taylor GA, Kaufman RA. Emergency department sonography in the initial evaluation of blunt abdominal injury in children. Pediatr Radiol 1993; 23:161–163.
42. McGahan JP, Richards J, Gillen M. The focused abdominal sonography for trauma scan: pearls and pitfalls. J Ultrasound Med 2002; 21:789–800.
43. Mutabagani KH, Coley BD, Zumberge N, et al. Preliminary experience with focused abdominal sonography for trauma (FAST) in children: is it useful? J Pediatr Surg 1999; 34:48–52.

Biliary Tree

44. Kumar R, Nguyen K, Shun A. Gallstones and common bile duct calculi in infancy and childhood. Aust NZ J Surg 2000; 70:188–191.
45. Reif S, Sloven DG, Lebenthal E. Gallstones in children. Characterization by age, etiology and outcome. Am J Dis Child 1991; 145:105–108.
46. Stringer MD, Taylor DR, Soloway RD. Gallstone composition: are children different? J Pediatr 2003; 142:435–440.
47. Pery M, Alon U, Latcher JH, et al. The value of ultrasound in Schoenlein-Henoch purpura. Eur J Pediatr 1990; 150:92–94.
48. Haller JO. Sonography of the biliary tract in infants and children. AJR Am J Roentgenol 1991; 157:1051–1058.
49. Slater H, Goldfarb IW. Acute septic cholecystitis in patients with burn injuries. J Burn Care Rehabil 1989; 10:445–447.
50. McKiernan PJ. Neonatal cholestasis. Sem Neonatol 2002; 7:153–165.
51. Norton KI, Glass RB, Kogan D, Lee JS, Emre S, Shneider BL. MR cholangiography in the evaluation of neonatal cholestasis: initial results. Radiology 2002; 222:687–691.
52. Gubernick JA, Rosenberg HK, Ilaslan H, Kessler A. US approach to jaundice in infants and children. Radiographics 2000; 20:173–195.
53. Ikeda S, Sera Y, Akagi M. Serial ultrasonic examination to differentiate biliary atresia from neonatal hepatitis—special reference to change in size of the gallbladder. Eur J Pediatr 1989; 148:396–400.
54. Ikeda S, Sera Y, Ohshiro H, Uchino S, Akizuki M, Kondo Y. Gallbladder contraction in biliary atresia: a pitfall of ultrasound diagnosis. Pediatr Radiol 1998; 28:451–453.
55. Kendrick APT, Phua KB, Subramaniam R, Goh ASW, Ooi BC, Tan CE. Making the diagnosis of biliary atresia using the triangular cord sign and gallbladder length. Pediatr Radiol 2000; 30:69–73.
56. Choi SI, Park WH, Lee HU, Woo Sk. Triangular cord: a sonographic finding applicable in the diagnosis of biliary atresia. J Pediatr Surg 1996; 31:363–366.
57. Kanegawa K, Akasaka Y, Kitamura E, et al. Sonographic diagnosis of biliary atresia in pediatric patients using the "triangular cord" sign versus gallbladder length and contraction. AJR Am J Roentgenol 2003; 181:1387–1390.
58. Kim MJ, Park YN, Han SJ, et al. Biliary atresia in neonates and infants: triangular area of high signal intensity in the porta hepatis at T2-weighted MR cholangiography with US and histopathologic correlation. Radiology 2000; 215:395–401.
59. Betz BW, Bisset GS III, Johnson ND, Daugherty CC, Balistreri WF. MR imaging of biliary cysts in children with biliary atresia: clinical associations and pathologic correlation. Am J Roentgenol 1994; 160:167–171.
60. Babbitt DP, Starshak RJ, Clemett AR. Choledochal cyst: a concept of etiology. AJR Am J Roentgenol 1973; 119:57–62.
61. Kim OH, Chung HJ, Choi BG. Imaging of the choledochal cyst. Radiographics 1995; 15:69–88.
62. Haller JO, Condon VR, Berdon WE, et al. Spontaneous perforation of the common bile duct in children. Radiology 1989; 172: 621–624.
63. Roebuck DJ, Yang WT, Lam WW, Stanley P. Hepatobiliary Rhabdomyosarcoma in children: diagnostic radiology. Pediatr Radiol 1998; 28:101–108.

Spleen

64. Applegate KE, Goske MJ, Pierce G, Murphy D. Situs revisited: imaging of the heterotaxy syndrome. Radiographics 1999; 19:837–852.
65. Belmont JW, Mohapatra B, Towbin JA, Ware SM. Molecular genetics of heterotaxy syndromes. Curr Opin Cardiol 2004; 19:216–220.
66. Hernanz-Schulman M, Ambrosino MM, Genieser NB, et al. Current evaluation of the patient with abnormal viseroatrial situs. AJR Am J Roentgenol 1990; 154:797–802.
67. Strouse PJ, Haller JO, Berdon WE, et al. Horseshoe adrenal gland in association with asplenia: presentation of six new cases and review of the literature. Pediatr Radiol 2002; 32:778–782.
68. Abramson SJ, Berdon WE, Altman RP, Amodio JB, Levy J. Biliary atresia and noncardiac polysplenic syndrome: US and surgical considerations. Radiology 1987; 163:377–379.
69. Desai DC, Hebra A, Davidoff AM, Schnaufer L. Wandering spleen: a challenging diagnosis. South Med J 1997; 90:439–443.
70. Buehner M, Baker MS. The wandering spleen. Surg Gynecol Obstet 1992; 175:373–387.
71. Allen KB, Andrews G. Pediatric wandering spleen—the case for splenopexy: review of 35 reported cases in the literature. J Pediatr Surg 1989; 24:432–435.
72. Bakir B, Poyanli A, Yekeler E, Acunas G. Acute torsion of a wandering spleen: imaging findings. Abdom Imaging 2004; 29: 707–709.
73. Karmazyn B, Steiberg R, Gayer G, Grozovski S, Freud E, Kornreich L. Wandering spleen—the challenge of ultrasound diagnosis: report of 7 cases. J Clin Ultrasound 2005; 33:433–438.
74. Swischuk LE, Williams JB, John SD. Torsion of wandering spleen: the whorled appearance of the splenic pedicle on CT. Pediatr Radiol 1993; 23:476–477.
75. Buonomo C, Taylor GA, Share JC, Kirks DR. In: Kirks DR, Griscom NT, ed. Gastrointestinal Tract. Practical Pediatric Imaging. 3rd ed. Philadelphia: Lippincott-Raven, 1998.
76. Daneman A, Martin DJ. Congenital epithelial splenic cysts in children. Emphasis on sonographic appearances and some unusual features. Pediatr Radiol 1982; 12:119–125.
77. Emery KH, Babcock DS, Borgman AS, Garcia VF. Splenic injury diagnosed with CT: US follow-up and healing rate in children and adolescents. Radiology 1999; 212:515–518.

Peritoneal Cavity

78. Khong PL, Cheung SC, Leong LL, Ooi CG. Ultrasonography of intra-abdominal cystic lesions in the newborn. Clin Radiol 2003; 58:449–454.
79. Bliss DP Jr, Coffin CM, Bower RJ, Stockmann PT, Ternberg JL. Mesenteric cysts in children. Surgery 1994; 115:571–577.
80. Chung MA, Brandt ML, St-Vil D, Yazbeck S. Mesenteric cysts in children. J Pediatr Surg 1991; 26:1306–1308.
81. Lugo-Olivieri CH, Taylor GA. CT differentiation of large abdominal lymphangioma from ascites. Pediatr Radiol 1993; 23:129–130.
82. Pathi R, Sage M, Slavotinek J, Hanieh A. Abdominal cerebrospinal fluid pseudocyst. Australas Radiol 2004; 48:61–63.

Pancreas

83. Orr LA, Powell RW, Melhem RE. Sonographic demonstration of annular pancreas in the newborn. J Ultrasound Med 1992; 11:373–375.
84. Auringer ST, Ulmer JL, Sumner TE, Turner CS. Congenital cyst of the pancreas. J Pediatr Surg 1993; 28:1570–1571.
85. Berrocal T, Pajares MP, Zubillaga AF. Pancreatic cystosis in children and young adults with cystic fibrosis: sonographic, CT and MRI findings. AJR Am J Roentgenol 2005; 184:1305–1309.
86. Agrons GA, Corse WR, Markowitz RI, Suarez ES, Perry DR. Gastrointestinal manifestations of cystic fibrosis: radiologic-pathologic correlation. Radiographics 1996; 16:871–893.
87. Iannaccone G, Antonelli M. Calcification of the pancreas in cystic fibrosis. Pediatr Radiol 1980; 9:85–90.
88. Montemarano H, Lonergan GJ, Bulas DI, Selby DM. Pancreatoblastoma: imaging findings in 10 patients and review of the literature. Radiology 2000; 214:476–482.
89. Friedman AC, Lichtenstein JE, Fishman EK, et al. Solid and papillary epithelial neoplasm of the pancreas. Radiology 1985; 154: 333–337.
90. Buetow PC, Buck JL, Pantongrag-Brown L, Beck KG, Ros PR, Adair CF. Solid and papillary epithelial neoplasm of the pancreas: imaging-pathologic correlation on 56 cases. Radiology 1996; 199:707–711.

Pediatric Bowel

Sandra L. Wootton-Gorges

26

INTRODUCTION

Transabdominal sonography of the pediatric gastrointestinal (GI) tract is an important tool in the diagnosis of many pediatric GI diseases. It can be particularly useful in the vomiting infant, and in the pediatric acute abdomen (1). This chapter will discuss the pediatric GI processes in which ultrasonography currently plays a major diagnostic role.

TECHNIQUE

Sonography of the pediatric GI tract is best achieved using an at least 5 MHz or higher linear-array probe. Graded compression may be useful in displacing overlying gas and may improve resolution by bringing the bowel closer to the transducer. It also allows the examiner to assess the flexibility of the bowel, with normal loops easily displaced and compressed by the pressure of the overlying transducer. Color Doppler evaluation may be helpful.

NORMAL ANATOMY

The bowel wall has five layers, including an innermost hyperechoic superficial mucosa, an inner hypoechoic layer of deeper superficial mucosa, a middle hyperechoic submucosa, an outer hypoechoic muscularis propria, and an outer hyperechoic serosa (Fig. 1) (2). Often with transabdominal examination, the inner three layers blend and appear as a single hyperechoic layer. The thickness of the fluid-distended bowel (measured from the inner aspect of the superficial mucosa to the outer aspect of the muscular layer) should not exceed 3 mm (3). The small bowel wall, when collapsed, may measure 5 to 7 mm in thickness.

Normal bowel shows little color Doppler signal (3). Hypervascularity may suggest an inflammatory process.

MALROTATION

Intestinal malrotation is a major diagnostic challenge in infants and children. Initially the midgut is a straight tube. During the fourth through the 10th gestational week, the bowel herniates into the yolk sac and then returns to the fetal abdomen while performing three 90° counterclockwise turns. This results in the normal duodenal sweep with the duodenal–jejunal junction in the left upper quadrant and fixed to the retroperitoneum as well as the normal position of the cecum in the right lower quadrant. The mesentery of the small bowel thus reaches from the left upper quadrant to the right lower quadrant. If this normal rotation does not occur, the small bowel mesenteric pedicle is short, and the bowel may twist on this vascular pedicle, resulting in midgut volvulus. Midgut volvulus is a true surgical emergency, as vascular compromise of the bowel will result in ischemia and infarction.

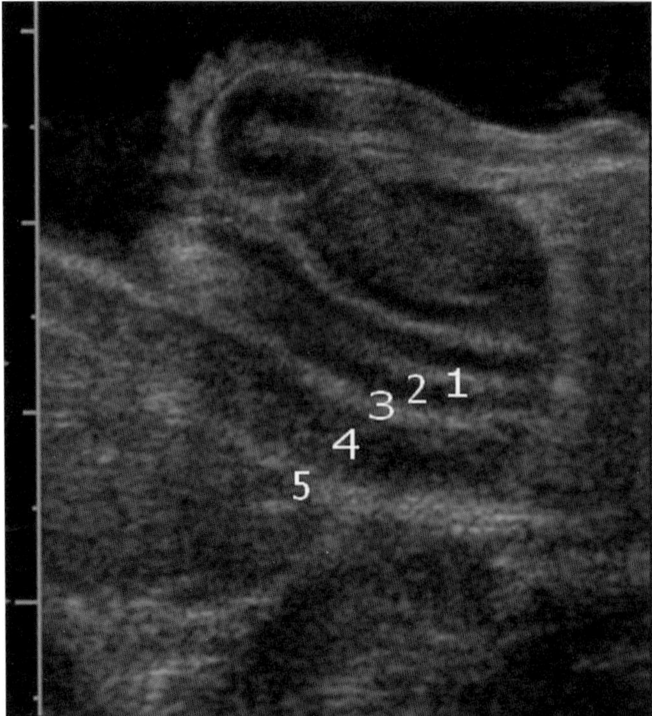

FIGURE 1 ■ Bowel layers. Infant with pyloric stenosis and a posteriorly placed pylorus behind the stomach antrum. All five layers of the bowel wall are seen: 1—(echogenic) superficial mucosa, 2—(hypoechoic) deeper superficial mucosa, 3—(echogenic) submucosa, 4—(hypoechoic) muscularis propria, and 5—(echogenic) serosa.

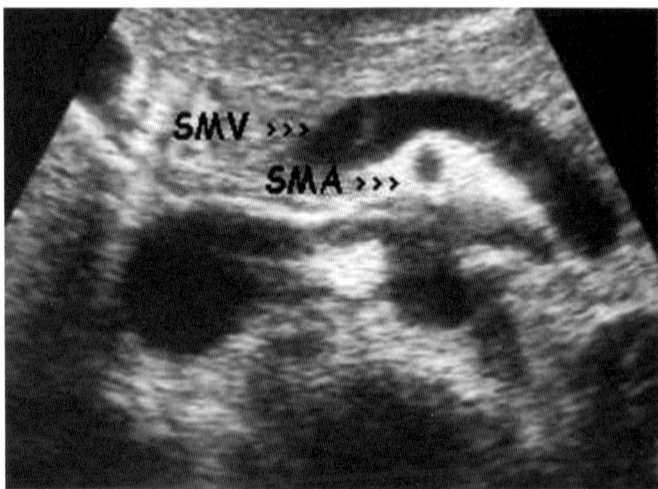

FIGURE 2 ■ Normal SMA/SMV axial ultrasound image of the normal SMV and SMA orientation with the SMV to the right of the SMA. SMA, superior mesenteric artery; SMV, superior mesenteric vein.

Most cases of midgut volvulus occur during the neonatal period (1,4), and the usual history is an infant with acute onset of bilious emesis and abdominal distension. Malrotation and midgut volvulus are typically evaluated using contrast radiography. Ultrasonography of the relative positions of the most cranial aspects of the superior mesenteric artery (SMA) and superior mesenteric vein (SMV) may be useful in more atypical cases. The SMV normally lies to the right of the SMA on axial images (Fig. 2) (5,6). If the SMV is to the left of the left lateral margin of the SMA (Fig. 3), then there is a high chance of malrotation, and further evaluation is warranted (7,8). If the SMV is directly ventral to the SMA, about one-quarter will have malrotation (6,7). However, the literature clearly and repeatedly reports that a normal orientation of the SMV and SMA does *not* exclude the diagnosis of malrotation (6,8,9). Findings suggestive of midgut volvulus include a clockwise whirlpool sign (10–12), best seen with color Doppler, due to the mesentery wrapping around the SMA, duodenal dilatation with distal tapering (13), fixed midline

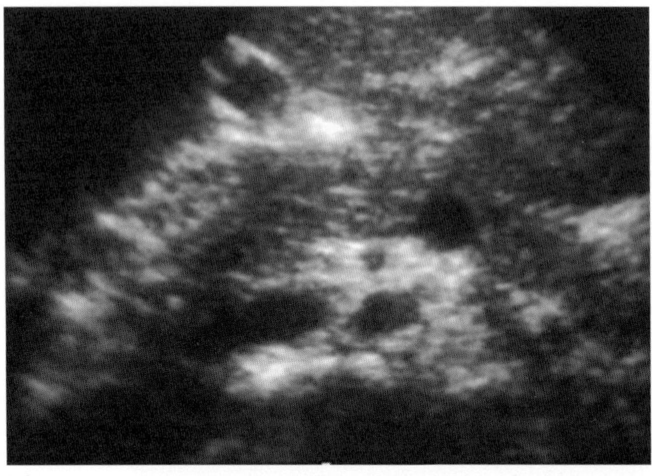

(A)

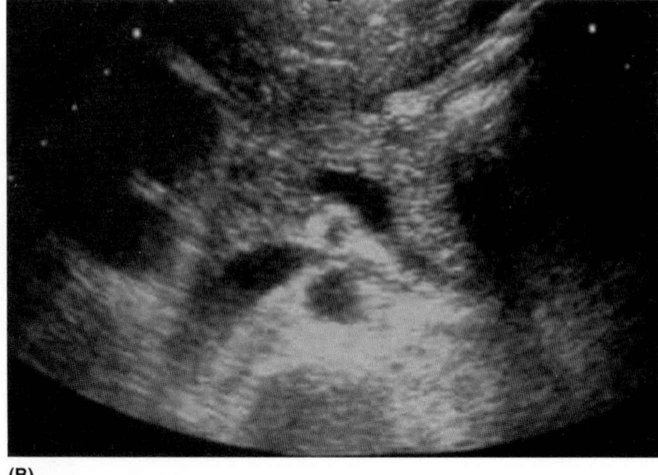

(B)

FIGURE 3 A AND B ■ Malrotation. (A) Axial ultrasound image of an inverted superior mesenteric vein (SMV) and superior mesenteric artery (SMA) orientation in an infant with malrotation. (B) Axial ultrasound image showing the SMV directly ventral to the SMA in another infant with malrotation.

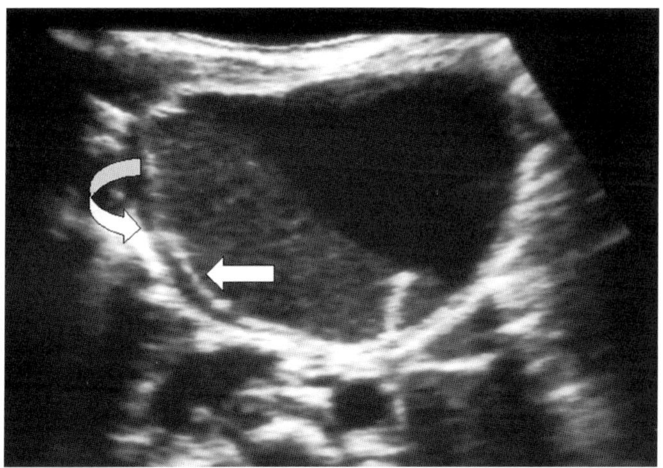

FIGURE 4 ■ Duplication cyst. Ultrasound of an ileal duplication cyst projecting into the right upper quadrant in a newborn. Note the hyperechoic inner (*arrow*) and hypoechoic outer (*curved arrow*) layers. The debris within it is old hemorrhage.

bowel, dilatation of the distal SMV, and a solitary hyperdynamic pulsating SMA (14).

DUPLICATION CYSTS

Enteric duplication cysts (Fig. 4) are most commonly found in the ileal region but may occur anywhere along the GI tract (15). These lesions are located in or adjacent to the bowel wall. They typically are hypoechoic and round or tubular, and they have a distinctive hyperechoic inner mucosal layer and a hypoechoic outer smooth muscular layer (16). Debris within the cystic lesion may be from hemorrhage, infection, or inspissated material (17). Duplication cysts may be small or large and may or may not communicate with the adjacent lumen. These lesions may result in intestinal obstruction, small bowel volvulus, or act as a lead point for intussusception, though some are asymptomatic. If the duplication contains

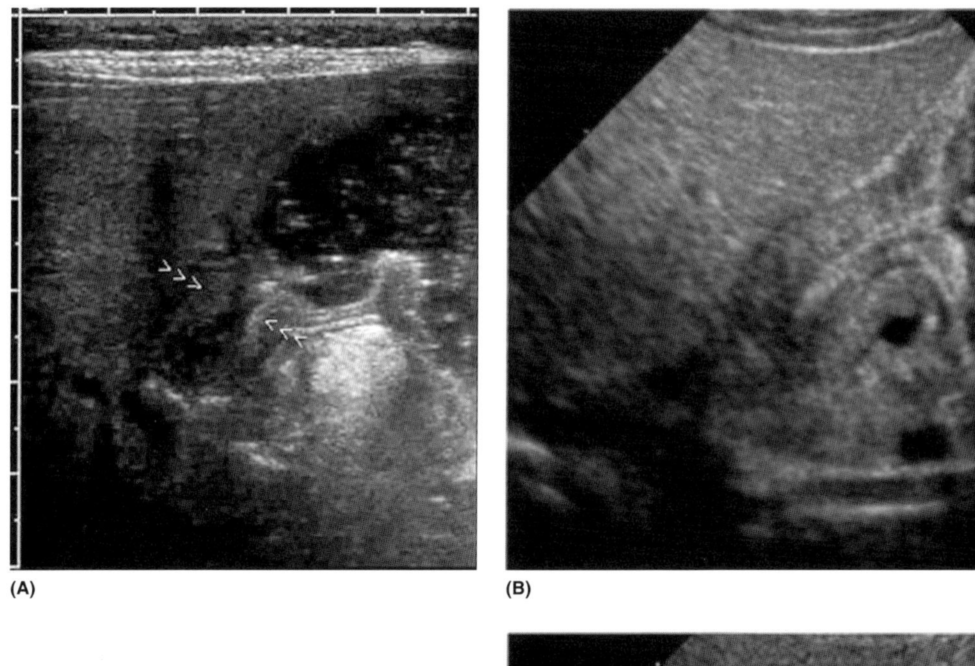

(A) (B)

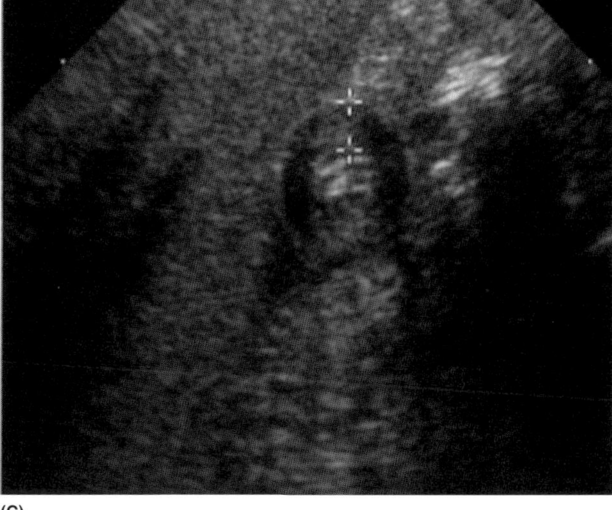

(C)

FIGURE 5 A–C ■ Normal pylorus. (**A**) Ultrasonographic image of the normal pylorus. The open pyloric channel is seen between the arrowheads, with fluid passing through it. (**B**) Longitudinal ultrasonographic image of pyloric stenosis, demonstrating the typical "cervix" sign of the thickened, elongated pylorus. (**C**) Transverse ultrasound image of the pylorus demonstrating the thickened pyloric muscle (*cursors*).

ectopic, gastric, or pancreatic mucosa and communicates with the bowel lumen, bleeding may occur.

HYPERTROPHIC PYLORIC STENOSIS

Hypertrophic pyloric stenosis (HPS) results from idiopathic thickening of the circular muscle layer of the pylorus, resulting in gastric outlet obstruction (18). Classically, HPS is clinically suggested by projectile, nonbilious vomiting in a previously healthy (usually male) infant. Symptoms may occur as early as birth or as late as several months of age, but typically, the infants are about six weeks old. Persistent symptoms may lead to dehydration, weight loss, and electrolyte imbalance. If the clinician can palpate an olive-like mass at the pylorus, the diagnosis is confirmed and no further imaging is required. In the present day, though, palpation of an olive is unusual.

Since its first use in 1977 by Teele and Smith (19), ultrasonography has become the imaging modality of choice for the diagnosis of clinically suspected pyloric stenosis. Using a high-resolution (5–10 MHz) linear transducer placed obliquely over the right upper quadrant, adjacent to the gallbladder, the pylorus can be defined with an echogenic mucosa, a hypoechoic muscularis mucosa, echogenic submucosa, and a hypoechoic muscular layer (Fig. 5). Many authors have studied the value of measuring pyloric canal muscle thickness, canal length, canal width, and canal volume in this diagnosis. The normal antropyloric canal increases in length, width, and muscle thickness with increasing gestational age (20,21). At 26 to 28 gestational weeks, the mean pyloric muscle thickness is 1.05 ± 0.09 mm and the length is 8.28 ± 1.19 mm, and at term, the mean muscle thickness is 1.76 ± 0.24 mm and the length 11.56 ± 1.15 mm (20). Normal infants show regular peristaltic waves leading to fluid passage through the open pyloric channel. In contrast, infants with HPS show a thickened, elongated pyloric channel (Fig. 1) that does not allow passage of gastric contents. In fact, there may be gastric hyperperistalsis and retrograde peristalsis. The mucosa appears redundant and thickened, and color Doppler demonstrates hypervascularity of the muscle (22). Investigators report a variety of upper normal limits for pyloric dimensions, but good "ballpark" values include a pyloric length of 15 mm, a pyloric diameter of 11 mm, and a single-wall muscle thickness of 3 mm (23). With these values, the accuracy for the diagnosis approaches 100%. However, there is some overlap of the measurements between normal infants and those with HPS (24).

There are several pitfalls in the diagnosis of HPS (25). Tangential angled cross-sectional images may result in pseudothickening of the muscle. Nonuniform echogenicity of the hypertrophied pyloric muscle may be caused by the anisotropic effect related to the orientation of the ultrasound beam with respect to the circular muscle fibers of the pylorus (26). Overdistension of the stomach may cause the pylorus to be posteriorly directed, which makes it more difficult to evaluate. HPS must also be differentiated from other entities. Pylorospasm (Fig. 6) is probably the

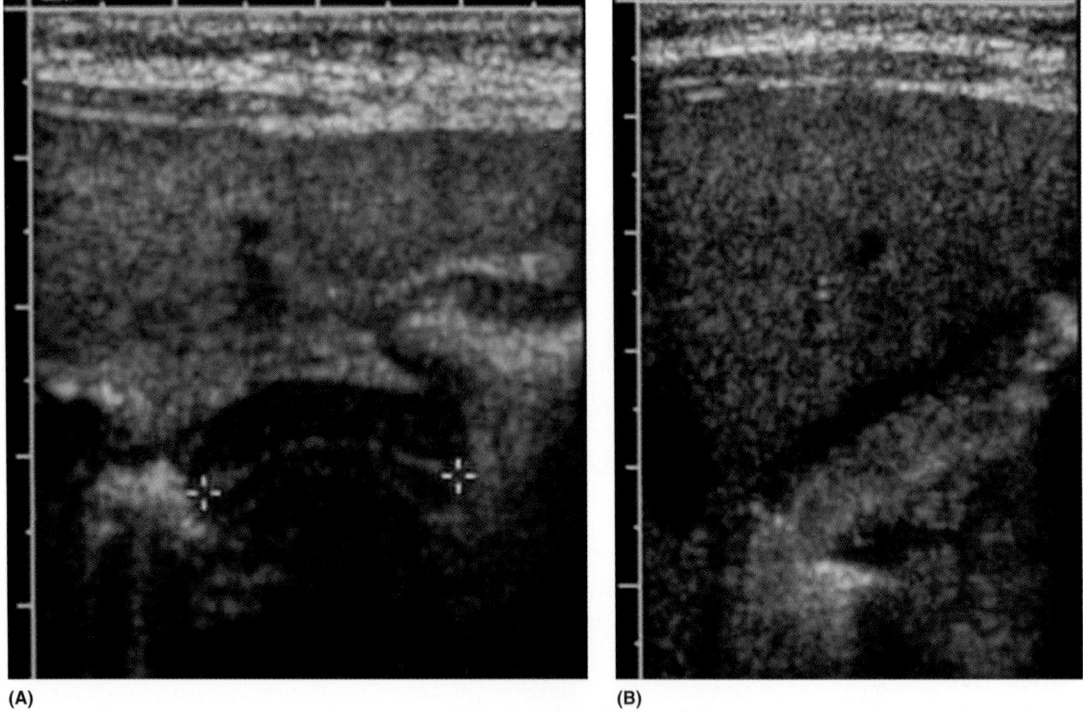

FIGURE 6 A AND B ■ Pylorospasm. (**A**) Ultrasonographic image of pylorospasm, mimicking pyloric stenosis. However, a minute later, the pylous is seen to open (**B**) and appears normal.

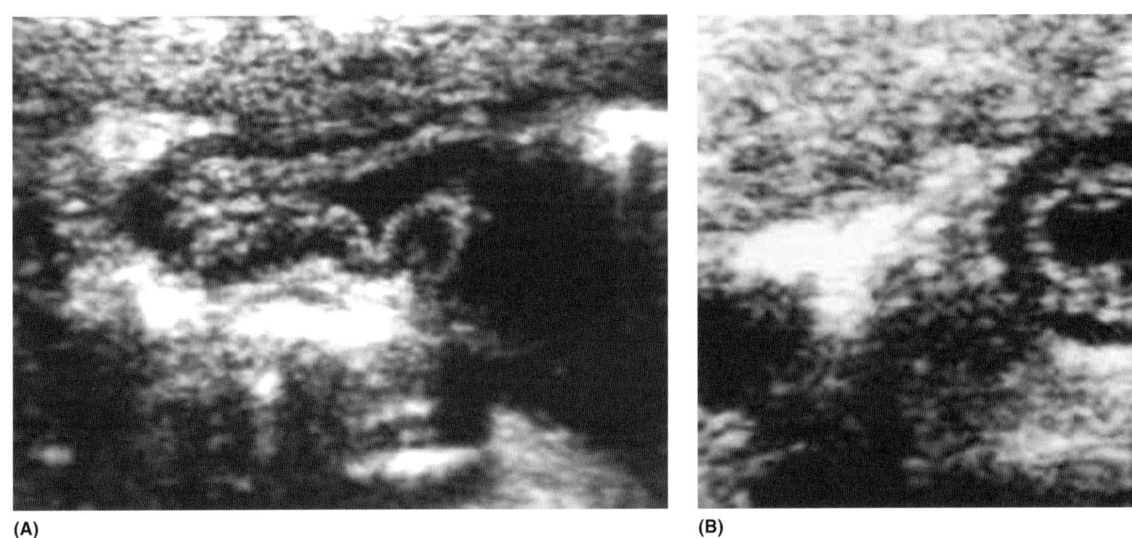

FIGURE 7 ■ Gastritis. Ultrasonographic image of gastritis. The mucosa appears thickened but the muscle is not.

most frequently encountered differential diagnosis. In these cases, the configuration of the pylorus initially resembles that of HPS, but over time, the muscle becomes less prominent and gastric fluid traverses the pyloric channel (27). Gastritis will cause mucosal thickening without thickening of the muscle (Fig. 7). Prostaglandin infusion, used to maintain patency of the ductus arteriosus in infants with cyanotic heart disease, may result in antral mucosal hyperplasia that causes gastric outlet obstruction (28,29). In these cases, the pylorus often appears elongated, but the muscle does not appear thickened.

INTUSSUSCEPTION

"Idiopathic" intussusception is one of the most common causes of acute abdominal pain in the child between three months and two years of age. Hypertrophy of the lymphoid tissue in terminal ileal Peyer patches allows the ileum to be drawn through the ileocecal valve into the colon, resulting in an ileocolic intussusception. Intussusception resulting from a pathological lead point [such as Meckel diverticulum, duplication cyst, polyp, or tumor (lymphoma)] is more common in infants under 30 days of age, in children older than five years, and in cases restricted to the small intestine (30).

The clinical diagnosis may be difficult to make. Less than one-half of infants present with the classic clinical triad of colicky abdominal pain, currant-jelly stools, and a palpable abdominal mass. Many children have nonspecific symptoms including vomiting and lethargy. Failure to diagnose intussusception may result in bowel ischemia, perforation, and peritonitis (31).

Many studies have documented the usefulness and sensitivity (30) of ultrasonography in the diagnosis of intussusception, with an accuracy reported at 100% (32) and a negative predictive value of 100% (33). The intussusception appears as a 3 to 5 cm mass along the course of the colon, most often in the subhepatic region (30). When viewed in an axial plane with respect to the intussusception, multiple concentric rings or a target (Fig. 8) or "crescent in doughnut" (34) appearance results from the intussusceptum and its mesentery being dragged into the intussuscipiens. On longitudinal images, the intussusception resembles a sandwich (Fig. 9) (32) or "hayfork" sign (35). Trapped peritoneal fluid within an intussusception suggests ischemia and irreducibility (36). Blood flow documented within the intussusception by color Doppler suggests reducibility (37), while lack of blood flow by color Doppler correlates with a lower rate of reduction (38) and potential bowel necrosis (37). If a pathologic lead point is the cause of an intussusception, it can be detected

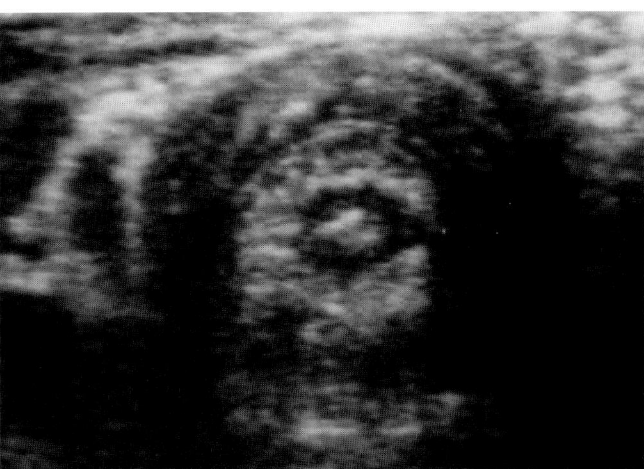

FIGURE 8 ■ Intussusception. Axial image of an idiopathic intussusception demonstrating the target sign. Concentric rings of hyperechoic mucosa and hypoechoic muscular layer are seen. Mesenteric fat is hyperechoic.

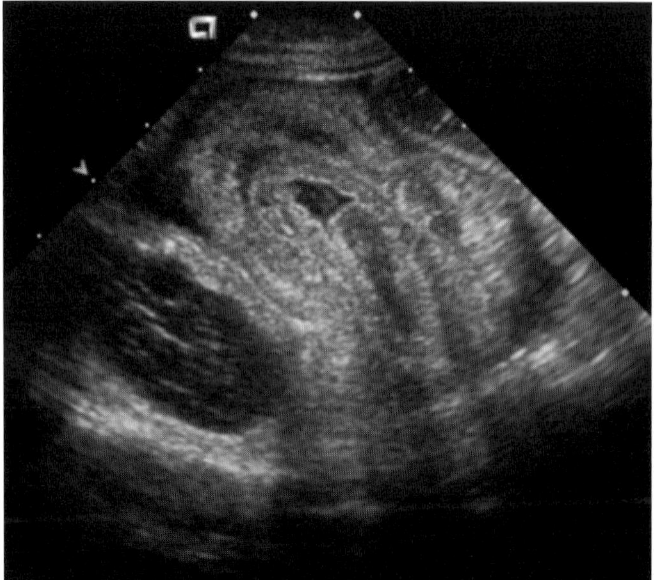

FIGURE 9 ■ Intussusception. Longitudinal image demonstrating the "sandwich sign" of intussusception.

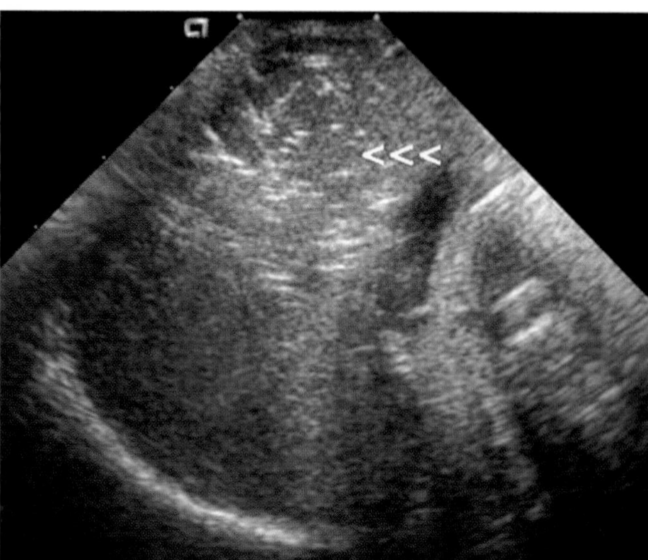

FIGURE 10 ■ Portal venous gas. Portal venous gas seen in the periphery of this infant's right lobe of the liver (*arrowheads*).

by sonography in about two-thirds of cases (39). The main imaging differential for intussusception is another cause of bowel wall thickening, such as inflammation, edema, hematoma, or volvulus (31). Other intra-abdominal pathology may also be detected by sonography (32) when no intussusception is found.

The high accuracy of ultrasonography in the diagnosis or exclusion of intussusception has made it the primary imaging modality in many centers. In some centers in the Far East, ultrasound-guided saline (40) or pneumatic (41) reduction has been performed, but this is not widely used in the United States.

NECROTIZING ENTEROCOLITIS

Necrotizing enterocolitis (NEC) is an inflammatory bowel disease of predominantly preterm infants (42). Its exact etiology is unknown, but its pathology resembles ischemic necrosis. Inflammation begins in the mucosa and spreads through the bowel wall. It may be patchy or diffuse, with the distal ileum and proximal colon most frequently involved. Symptoms include abdominal distension, feeding intolerance, bloody stool, diarrhea, lethargy, apnea, and temperature and blood pressure instability.

Abdominal radiography has been the standard method for evaluation for NEC. However, ultrasonography has been shown to be useful in this diagnosis. Sonographic findings in NEC include thick-walled, fluid-filled bowel with diminished peristalsis (43). Pneumatosis intestinalis and portal venous gas (Fig. 10) may also be detected (44). Color Doppler is particularly useful, with absent perfusion as well as bowel wall thinning (<1 mm), suggesting bowel necrosis (45). Normal or increased color Doppler signal may be seen in less severe disease.

CROHN'S DISEASE

Crohn's disease is a chronic inflammatory bowel disease that results from altered immunoregulatory action of the intestine. It is common in the pediatric (especially adolescent) population as well as in adults. Clinical symptoms may include crampy abdominal pain, diarrhea, weight loss, and fever. Extraintestinal manifestations may include arthritis, hepatitis, skin rashes, and uveitis or episcleritis.

Crohn's disease is characterized by asymmetric, focal, transmural bowel inflammation. The terminal ileum is most commonly involved, but any part of the intestinal tract can be affected. While the initial diagnosis is usually made by endoscopy and contrast-enhanced radiography, sonography has proved useful in evaluation of ongoing disease (46–48). Actively involved bowel will be thickened and hyperemic (Fig. 11) (47,48) and may show decreased compressibility as well as lack of normal wall stratification. Increased SMA flow volume (46,49) and decreased SMA resistive index (SMA RI) (48) also correlate with disease activity. Successful treatment may result in normalization of these imaging parameters (47).

APPENDICITIS

Acute appendicitis is one of the most common causes of abdominal pain in children. Although most children present with typical clinical features, about one-third will have atypical findings (50), making clinical diagnosis more difficult. The technique of graded compression sonography, first described in the adult population by Puylaert in 1986 (51), has proven very effective in the pediatric population as well, with a sensitivity of 80% to

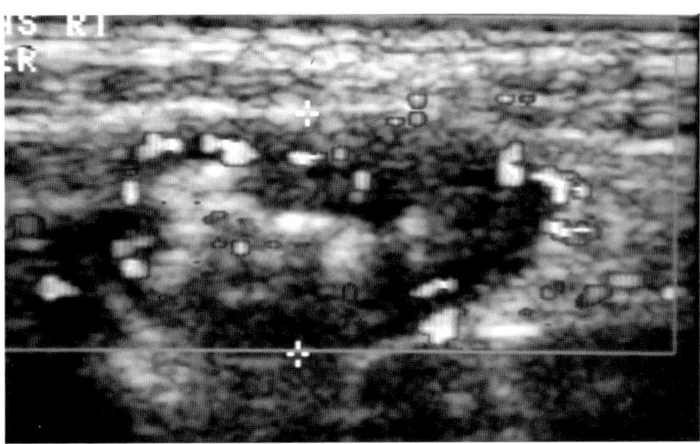

FIGURE 11 ■ Crohn's disease. Axial black-and-white image of color Doppler ultrasound showing thickened, hyperemic ileum in this 12-year-old with Crohn's disease.

100%, a specificity of 90% to 97%, and an overall accuracy of 90% to 97% (52,53).

As with adults, an abnormal appendix appears as a noncompressible, tubular structure at least 6 mm in diameter (Fig. 12) (54). Other associated findings may include an appendicolith (55), loss of the echogenic submucosal layer, a fluid-filled appendiceal lumen, increased pericecal echogenicity, or a loculated fluid collection suggesting periappendiceal abscess (Fig. 13). Free fluid does not correlate with the presence or absence of appendicitis (54). The best predictors of perforation include loss of the echogenic submucosal layer of the appendix and the presence of a loculated periappendiceal fluid collection (56). Demonstration of hyperemia of the appendiceal wall or of a right lower quadrant mass or fluid collection by color Doppler (53,57–59) may be a useful adjunctive finding to the diagnosis as well.

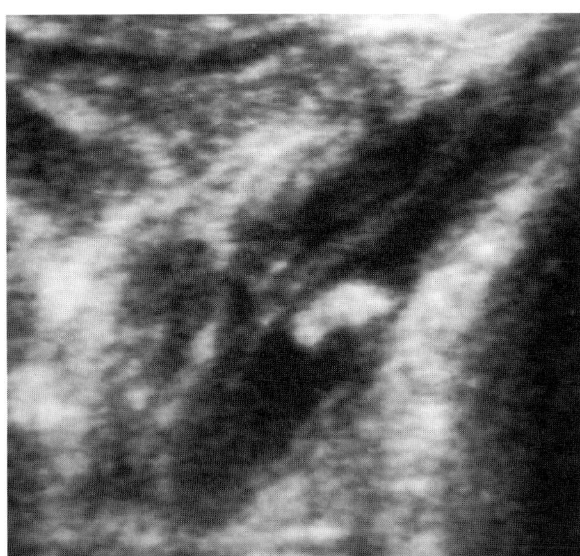

FIGURE 12 ■ Appendicitis. Longitudinal image demonstrating a fluid-filled noncompressible appendix containing an appendicolith in this child with right lower quadrant pain.

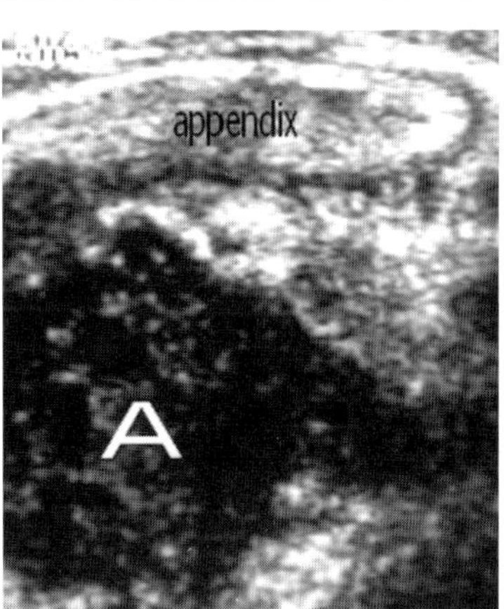

FIGURE 13 ■ Appendicitis. Longitudinal image demonstrating a noncompressible appendix (*arrow*) anterior to an appendiceal abscess (*arrowhead*) in this eight-year-old girl.

REFERENCES

Introduction

1. Hayden CK Jr. Ultrasonography of the gastrointestinal tract in infants and children. Abdom Imaging 1996; 21:9–20.

Technique

2. Deignan RW, Malone DE, McGrath FP. High-resolution ultrasound in assessment of the gastrointestinal tract. Crit Rev Diagn Imaging 1994; 35:257–311.
3. Sivit CJ, Siegel MJ. Gastrointestinal tract. Pediatric Sonography. 3rd ed. Philadelphia: Lippincott Williams and Wilkins, 2002.

Malrotation

4. Jamieson D, Stringer DA. Small Bowel. Pediatric Gastrointestinal Imaging and Intervention. 2nd ed. Hamilton, ON: Stringer and Babyn, 2000.
5. Zerin JM, DiPietro MA. Mesenteric vascular anatomy at CT: normal and abnormal appearances. Radiology 1991; 179:739–742.
6. Dufour D, Delaet MH, Dassonville M, et al. Midgut malrotation, the reliability of sonographic diagnosis. Pediatr Radiol 1992; 22:21–23.
7. Weinberger E, Winters WD, Liddell RM, et al. Sonographic diagnosis of intestinal malrotation in infants: importance of the relative positions of the superior mesenteric vein and artery. AJR Am J Roentgenol 1992; 159:825–828.
8. Zerin JM, DiPietro MA. Superior mesenteric vascular anatomy at US in patients with surgically proved malrotation of the midgut. Radiology 1992; 183:693–694.
9. Ashley LM, Allen S, Teele RL. A normal sonogram does not exclude malrotation. Pediatr Radiol 2001; 31:354–356.
10. Pracros JP, Sann L, Genin G, et al. Ultrasound diagnosis of midgut volvulus: the "whirlpool" sign. Pediatr Radiol 1992; 22:18–20.
11. Shimanuki Y, Aihara T, Takano H, et al. Clockwise whirlpool sign at color Doppler US: an objective and definite sign of midgut volvulus. Radiology 1996; 199:261–264.
12. Yeh WC, Wang HP, Chen C, et al. Preoperative sonographic diagnosis of midgut malrotation with volvulus in adults: the "whirlpool" sign. J Clin Ultrasound 1999; 27:279–283.
13. Chao HC, Kong MS, Chen JY, et al. Sonographic features related to volvulus in neonatal intestinal malrotation. J Ultrasound Med 2000; 19:371–376.
14. Smet MH, Marchal G, Ceulemans R, Eggermont E. The solitary hyperdynamic pulsating superior mesenteric artery: an additional dynamic sonographic feature of midgut volvulus. Pediatr Radiol 1991; 21:156–157.

Duplication Cysts

15. Berrocal T, Lamas M, Gutierrez J, et al. Congenital anomalies of the small intestine, colon and rectum. Radiographics 1999; 19:1219–1236.
16. Barr LL, Hayden CK, Stansberry SD, Swischuk LE. Enterid duplication cysts in children: are their ultrasonographic wall characteristics diagnostic? Pediatr Radiol 1990; 20:326–328.
17. Kangarloo H, Sample WF, Hansen G, et al. Ultrasonic evaluation of abdominal gastrointestinal tract duplication in children. Radiology 1979; 131:191–194.

Hypertrophic Pyloric Stenosis

18. Hernanz-Schulman M. Infantile hypertrophic pyloric stenosis. Radiology 2003; 227:319–331.
19. Teele RL, Smith EH. Ultrasound in the diagnosis of idiopathic hypertrophic pyloric stenosis. N Engl J Med 1977; 296:1149–1150.
20. Argyropoulou MI, Hadjigeorgi CG, Kiortsis DN. Antro-pyloirc canal values from early prematurity to full-term gestational age: an ultrasound study. Pediatr Radiol 1998; 28:933–936.
21. Hallam D, Hansen B, Bodker B, et al. Pyloric size in normal infants and in infants suspected of having hypertrophic pyloric stenosis. Acta Radiol 1995; 36:261–264.
22. Hernanz-Schulman M, Zhu Y, Stein SM, et al. Hypertrophic pyloric stenosis in infants: US evaluation of vascularity of the pyloric canal. Radiology 2003; 229:389–393.
23. Rohrschneider WK, Mittnacht H, Darge K, et al. Pyloric muscle in asymptomatic infants: sonographic evaluation and discrimination from idiopathic hypertrophic pyloric stenosis. Pediatr Radiol 1998; 28:429–434.
24. Blumhagen JD, Maclin L, Drauter D, et al. Sonographic diagnosis of hypertrophic pyloric stenosis. AJR Am J Roentgenol 1988; 150: 1367–1370.
25. Swischuk LE, Hayden CK, Stansberry SD. Sonographic pitfalls in imaging of the antropyloric region in infants. Radiographics 1989; 9:437–447.
26. Spevak MR, Ahmadijian JM, Kleinman PK, et al. Sonography of the hypertrophic pyloric stenosis: frequency and cause of nonuniform echogenicity of the thickened pyloric muscle. AJR Am J Roentgenol 1992; 158:129–132.
27. Cohen HL, Zinn HL, Haller JO, et al. Ultrasonography of pylorospasm: findings may simulate hypertrophic pyloric stenosis. J Ultrasound Med 1998; 17:705–711.
28. Mercado-Deane MG, Burton EM, Brawley AV, et al. Prostaglandin-induced foveolar hyperplasia simulatin pyloric stenosis in an infant with cyanotic heart disease. Pediatr Radiol 1994; 24:45–46.
29. Babyn P, Peled N, Manson D, et al. Radiologic features of gastric outlet obstruction in infants after long-term prostaglandin administration. Pediatr Radiol 1995; 25:41–43.

Intussusception

30. del-Pozo G, Albillos JC, Tejedor D, et al. Intussusception in children: current concepts in diagnosis and enema reduction. Radiographics 1999; 19:299–319.
31. Daneman A, Navarro O. Intussusception. Part 1: a review of diagnostic approaches. Pediatr Radiol 2003; 33:79–85.
32. Pracos JP, Tran-Minh Va, Morin DE, et al. Acute intestinal intussusception in children: contribution of ultrasonography (145 cases). Ann Radiol 1987; 30:525–530.
33. Verschelden P, Filiatrault D, Garel L, et al. Intussusception in children: reliability of US in diagnosis—a prospective study. Radiology 1992; 184:741–744.
34. del-Pozo G, Albillos JC, Tejedor D. Intussusception: US findings with pathologic correlation—the crescent-in-doughnut sign. Radiology 1996; 199:688–692.
35. Alessi V, Salerno G. The "hay-fork" sign in the ultrasonographic diagnosis of intussusception. Gastrointest Radiol 1985; 10:177–179.
36. del-Ppozo G, Gonzalez-Spinola J, Gomez-Anson B, et al. Intussusception: trapped peritoneal fluid detected with US—relationship to reducibility and ischemia. Radiology 1996; 201:379–386.
37. Lim HK, Bae SH, Lee KH, et al. Assessment of reducibility of ileocolic intussusception in children: usefulness of color Doppler sonography. Radiology 1994; 191:781–785.
38. Kong MS, Wong HF, Lin SL, et al. Factors related to detection of blood flow by color Doppler ultrasonography in intussusception. J Ultrasound Med 1997; 16:141–144.
39. Navarro O, Dugougeat F, Kornecki A, et al. The impact of imaging in the management of intussusception owing to pathologic lead points in children. Pediatr Radiol 2000; 30:594–603.
40. Woo SK, Kim JS, Suh SJ, et al. Childhood intussusception: US-guided hydrostatic reduction. Radiology 1992; 182:77–80.
41. Yoon CH, Kim HJ, Goo HW. Intussusception in children: US-guided pneumatic reduction—initial experience. Radiology 2001; 218:85–88.

Necrotizing Enterocolitis

42. Buonomo C. The radiology of Necrotizing enterocolitis. Rad Clin North Am 1999; 37:1187–1198.
43. Patel U, Leonidas JC, Furie D. Sonographic detection of Necrotizing enterocolitis in infancy. J Ultrasound Med 1990; 9:673–675.
44. Robberecht EA, Afschrift M, De Bel CE, et al. Sonographic demonstration of portal venous gas in necrotizing enterocolitis. Eur J Pediatr 1988; 147:192–194.
45. Faingold R, Daneman A, Tomlinson G, et al. Necrotizing enterocolitis: assessment of bowel viability with color Doppler US. Radiology 2005; 235:587–594.

Crohn's Disease

46. van Oostayen JA, Wasser MNJM, van Hogenzand RA, et al. Activity of Crohn's disease assessed by measurement of superior mesenteric artery flow with Doppler US. Radiology 1994; 193:551–554.
47. Ruess L, Nussbaum Blask AR, Bulas DI, et al. Inflammatory bowel disease in children and young adults: correlation of sonographic and clinical parameters during treatment. AJR Am J Roentgenol 2000; 175:79–84.
48. Yekeler E, Danalioglu A, Movasseghi B, et al. Crohn's disease activity evaluated by Doppler ultrasonography of the superior mesenteric artery and the affected small-bowel segments. J Ultrasound Med 2005; 24:59–65.
49. van Oostayen JA, Wasser MNJM, van Hogenzand RA, et al. Doppler sonography evaluation of superior mesenteric artery flow to assess Crohn's disease activity: correlation with clinical evaluation, Crohn's disease activity index, and alpha1-antitrypsin clearance in feces. AJR Am J Roentgenol 1997; 168:429–433.

Appendicitis

50. Siegel MJ. Acute appendicitis in childhood: the role of US. Radiology 1992; 185:341–342.
51. Puylaert JBCM. Acute appendicitis: US evaluation using graded compression. Radiology 1986; 158:355–360.
52. Sivit CJ, Newman DK, Boenning DA, et al. Appendicitis: usefulness of US in diagnosis in a pediatric population. Radiology 1992; 185:549–552.
53. Quillin SP, Siegel MJ. Appendicitis: efficacy of color Doppler sonography. Radiology 1994; 191:557–560.
54. Sivit CJ. Diagnosis of acute appendicitis in children: spectrum of sonographic findings. AJR Am J Roentgenol 1993; 161:147–152.
55. Kao SCS, Smith WL, Abu-Yousef, et al. Acute appendicitis in children: sonographic findings. AJR Am J Roentgenol 1989; 153:375–379.
56. Quillin SP, Siegel MJ, Coffin CM. Acute appendicitis in children: value of sonography in detecting perforation. AJR Am J Roentgenol 1992; 159:1265–1268.
57. Quillin SP, Siegel MJ. Appendicitis in children: color Doppler sonography. Radiology 1992; 184:745–747.
58. Quillin SP, Siegel MJ. Color Doppler US of children with acute lower abdominal pain. Radiographics 1993; 13:1281–1293.
59. Quillin SP, Siegel MJ. Diagnosis of appendiceal abscess in children with acute appendicitis: value of color Doppler sonography. AJR

Ultrasonography of the Pediatric Kidney and Adrenal Gland

Sandra L. Wootton-Gorges

27

INTRODUCTION

Ultrasonography plays an important role in the evaluation of the pediatric kidney. Sector or curved-array probes can be used to examine the kidney for abnormalities including structural anomalies, hydronephrosis, and mass. Doppler imaging is useful in evaluation of vascular diseases. In both gray-scale and Doppler imaging, the liver and spleen are used as acoustic windows. The patient may be examined in the supine or decubitus position; prone positioning may be useful as well.

NORMAL DEVELOPMENT

The kidneys form from the metanephros, which begins to develop during the fifth gestational week (1). The metanephros includes the ureteric bud, which gives rise to the ureter, renal pelvis, calyces and renal tubules, and a metanephric mass of mesoderm that gives rise to the renal parenchyma. Initially, the kidneys are located in the pelvis, but they migrate cranially with differential growth of the body. During this migration, the kidneys are supplied by arteries at successively higher levels, with concomitant involution of the more inferior arteries. Initially, the hila of the kidneys face ventrally, but during ascent turn 90° to become medially placed.

The kidneys increase in size through infancy and childhood. Many studies have been performed comparing the kidney size to weight, height, age, and body surface area (2–9). Tables 1 and 2 provide normative data for renal length in children (6).

The normal infant kidney (Fig. 1) looks sonographically different from the kidney of an older child or adult. Because the infant renal cortex has increased cellularity (10), the renal cortex of the infant kidney is usually equal or slightly more echogenic than the liver or spleen (11). The more premature the infant, the more likely that the renal cortex will be hyperechoic (12). The renal cortex becomes less echogenic than the liver or spleen by about 12 months of age. The renal pyramids in the infant kidney are markedly hypoechoic and prominent, again likely due to their relatively larger size (3). This relative medullary hypoechogenicity diminishes over the first 12 months of life. Lastly, the renal sinus is not as echogenic in infants, as there is less fat present (11).

Doppler flow indices are higher in young children than in adults (13,14) and decrease with increasing age. This results from maturation of renal function, including age-dependent decrease in active plasma rennin levels (15,16). Debate exists as to the exact age at which adult values should be attained, with study results varying from 4 to 10 years of age (17,18). Table 3 gives normal resistive index values for healthy infants and children (19). It should be noted that in infants the Doppler flow parameters are significantly higher in the central renal arteries than in the intraparenchymal arteries (20).

TABLE 1 ■ Longitudinal Dimensions of Right Kidney vs. Height and Age

Subjects		Longitudinal dimensions (mm) of right kidney			
		Percentile		Suggested limits of normal	
Body height (cm)	Age range (mo)	5th	95th	Lowermost	Uppermost
48–64	1–3	58	–	35	65
54–73	4–6	50	64	40	70
65–78	7–9	52	66	70	–
71–92	12–30	55	65	50	75
85–109	36–59	59	75	55	80
100–130	60–83	65	83	60	85
110–131	84–107	70	91	65	95
124–149	108–131	69	89	65	100
137–153	132–155	82	100	70	105
143–168	156–179	85	102	75	110
152–175	180–200	83	102	75	110

Source: From Ref. 6.

The cortex of the adrenal gland develops from mesoderm, while the medulla develops from neuroectoderm. The cortex first appears adjacent to the root of the dorsal mesentery during the sixth week of gestation. During the seventh week, cells from the adjacent sympathetic ganglia migrate to and are gradually encapsulated by the cortex, forming the adrenal gland.

The adrenal gland has a Y or V shape on longitudinal images (Fig. 2) and a linear, V or Y configuration on transverse images (21). In newborns, the gland has convex margins and is large in relation to the body size. It has a hypoechoic cortex a hyperechoic medulla (22). By six months of age, the corticomedullary differentiation is lost, and the gland appears smaller and diffusely hyperechoic. After one year of age, the adrenal gland attains an adult appearance and is diffusely hypoechoic.

CONGENITAL ANOMALIES

A number of developmental anomalies of the kidneys may occur. If the ureteric bud fails to develop, renal agenesis will occur. Sonographic findings include absence of the kidney, elongation and flattening of the ipsilateral adrenal gland (Fig. 3), and an absent ipsilateral renal artery. Ipsilateral genital anomalies are common.

Renal ectopia results from abnormal ascent of the kidneys during early gestation. The ectopic kidney may be located anywhere from the pelvis to the posterior thorax. The ectopic kidney may remain on its normal side (simple ectopia) or may cross to the opposite side (crossed ectopia). A crossed ectopic kidney (Fig. 4) is usually fused to the orthotopic kidney and is typically smaller and malrotated (11). The ureter of the crossed ectopic kidney

TABLE 2 ■ Longitudinal Dimensions of Left Kidney vs. Height and Age

Subjects		Longitudinal dimensions (mm) of right kidney			
		Percentile		Suggested limits of normal	
Body height (cm)	Age range (mo)	5th	95th	Lowermost	Uppermost
48–64	1–3	42	59	35	65
54–73	4–6	47	64	40	70
65–78	7–9	54	68	45	75
71–92	12–30	57	72	50	80
85–109	36–59	61	76	55	85
100–130	60–83	70	87	60	95
110–131	84–107	73	93	65	100
124–149	108–131	75	97	65	105
137–153	132–155	77	102	70	110
143–168	156–179	84	110	75	115
152–175	180–200	90	110	80	120

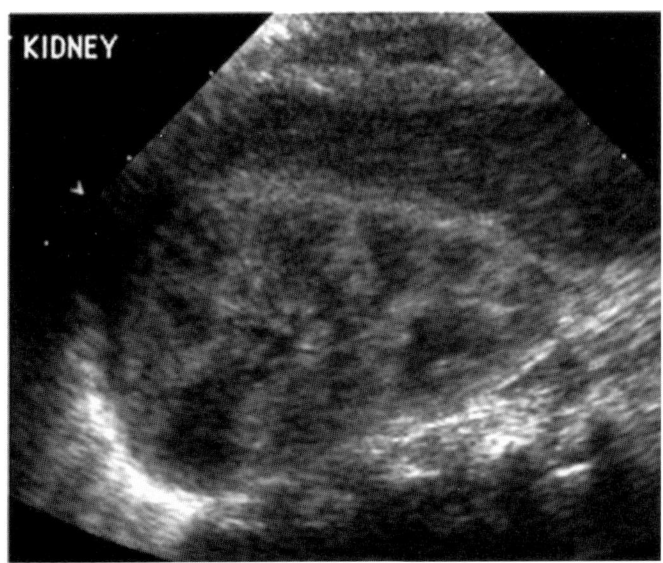

FIGURE 1 ■ Normal newborn kidney. Longitudinal ultrasound of the right kidney. The normal newborn kidney cortex is hyperechoic when compared with an older child or an adult kidney. The medullary pyramids are prominent and hypoechoic.

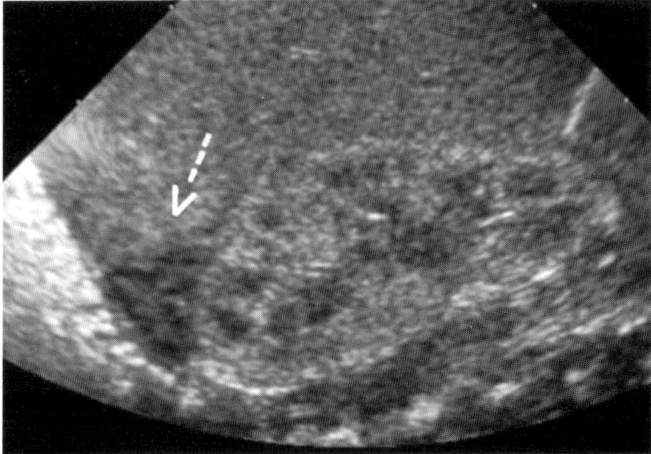

FIGURE 2 ■ Normal newborn adrenal. Longitudinal ultrasound of the right adrenal gland. The normal newborn adrenal gland is prominent (*arrow*), with a Y or V configuration. It has a hyperechoic medulla and a hypoechoic cortex.

crosses back across the midline to insert into its normal position at the trigone of the bladder.

Horseshoe kidney (Fig. 5) is the most common fusion anomaly (23). The two kidneys lie parallel to the spine, caudal to their normal position, and are joined, usually inferiorly, by an isthmus of tissue. The renal pelves are oriented anteriorly (24). Hydronephrosis, renal dysplasia, and stone formation may also be seen.

Duplication of the renal collecting system is a common anomaly of the urinary tract (23,25). Complete duplication (Fig. 6) occurs when two ipsilateral ureteric buds form. Sonographically, the duplex kidney (Fig. 7) will be longer than normal and will have a split renal sinus. Pelviectasis of the lower pole moiety may result from reflux, while pelviectasis and hydroureter of the upper pole moiety may result from obstruction. The upper pole moiety ureter inserts inferomedial to the normal position at the trigone (Weigert–Meyer rule) and may be associated with an ectopic ureterocele (Fig. 8). The ectopic ureter may insert into the bladder or bladder neck, but in girls, it may also insert into the urethra, vagina, uterus, or rectum. In boys, the ectopic ureter may insert into the posterior urethra, ejaculatory ducts, seminal vesicles, vas deferens, or rectum.

Multicystic dysplastic kidney (MCDK) (Fig. 9) results from pyeloinfundibular atresia in early gestation. Ultrasound will demonstrate multiple noncommunicating cysts of various sizes in the affected renal fossa, and the renal parenchyma is absent or dysplastic. The largest cyst is nonmedial in location, and the renal sinus is not seen (26). Renal scintigraphy can help to confirm the diagnosis of MCDK by demonstrating absence of function. Contralateral abnormalities such as vesicoureteral reflux or ureteropelvic junction obstruction may be seen in up to

TABLE 3 ■ Renal Resistive Indices in Children

Synopsis of mean renal RI data vs. age		
Age (yr)	**Mean RI ± SD**	**Range of RIs**
0.0–0.4	0.71 ± 0.06	0.58–0.85
0.5–0.9	0.64 ± 0.04	0.58–0.69
1.0–3.9	0.64 ± 0.05	0.54–0.72
4.0–6.9	0.62 ± 0.05	0.53–0.70
≥7.0	0.59 ± 0.04	0.52–0.66
Adult	0.58 ± 0.05	–

Abbreviations: RI, resistive index; SD, standard deviation.
Source: From Ref. 18.

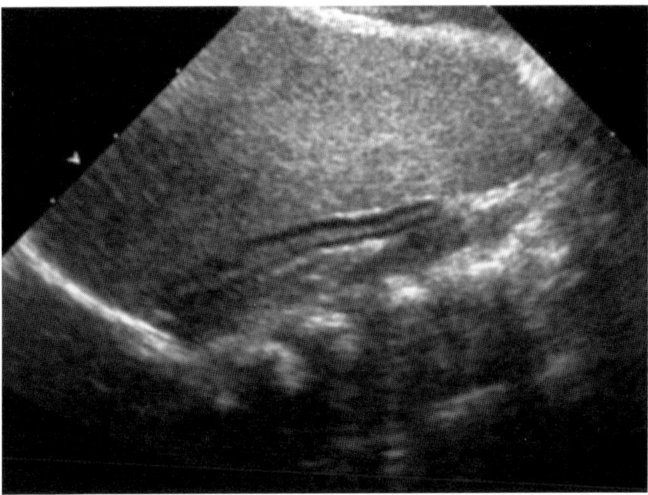

FIGURE 3 ■ Right renal agenesis. Longitudinal ultrasound of the right renal fossa. No right kidney is present in this newborn. The right adrenal gland is flattened and prominent.

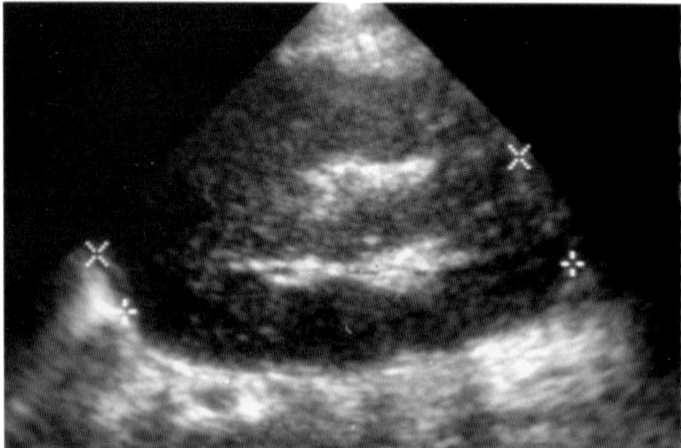

FIGURE 4 ■ Crossed renal ectopia. Longitudinal ultrasound of crossed fused ectopia. The kidneys lie adjacent to each other and are fused medially.

40% of patients (27). The MCDK cysts usually involute spontaneously (28,29); this may be confirmed with serial sonography. It is rare to see long-term complications of hypertension or tumor development (30).

HYDRONEPHROSIS

Dilatation of the renal collecting system can result from obstruction, vesicoureteral reflux, infection, or increased urine production. Hydronephrosis in children may be graded as follows (Fig. 10) (31): grade 0—no hydronephrosis, grade 1—renal pelvis only is visualized, grade 2—renal pelvis and a few calyces are visualized, grade 3—renal pelvis and all calyces are seen, and grade 4—parenchymal thinning is seen in addition to the renal pelvis and all calyces being visualized.

Prenatal sonography has had a major effect upon the diagnosis of hydronephrosis in children (32). The incidence of neonatal hydronephrosis and asymptomatic hydronephrosis has increased, allowing for intervention before symptoms and renal damage occur. Immediate postpartum dehydration and decreased glomerular filtration rate may result in underestimation of hydronephrosis diagnosed in utero. Thus, sonographic reevaluation of antenatal hydronephrosis should not be performed until

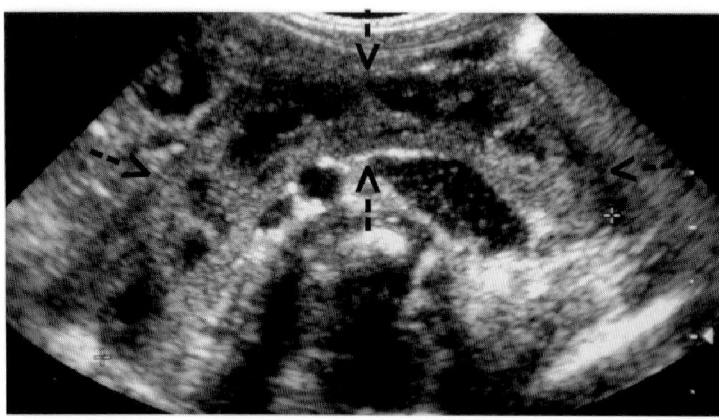

FIGURE 5 ■ Horseshoe kidney. Transverse ultrasound of a horseshoe kidney, showing the isthmus crossing the spine (*arrows*). Renal parenchyma is seen extending both to the right and to the left.

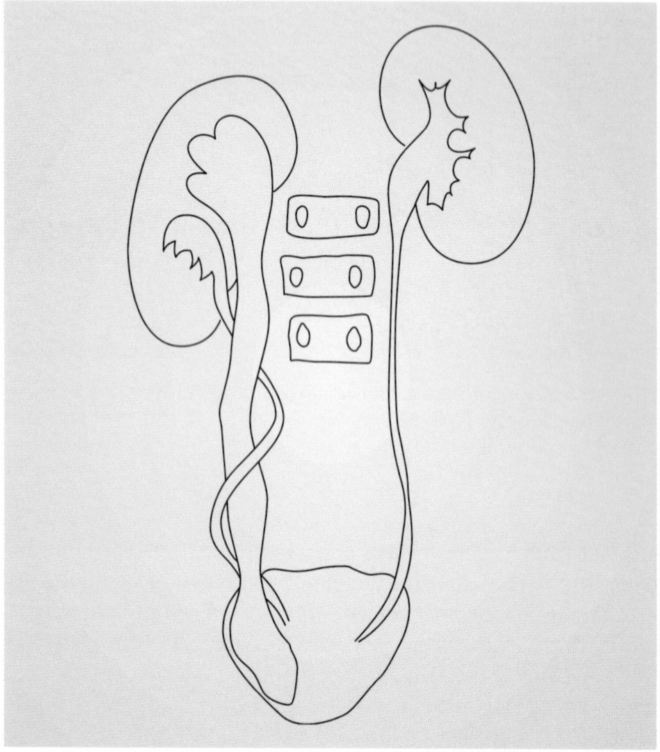

FIGURE 6 ■ Diagram of a duplex collecting system. The upper pole moiety ureter inserts inferomedial to the normal position at the trigone of the bladder. It tends to be associated with an ectopic ureterocele, and the upper pole may be obstructed. The lower pole moiety ureter inserts normally into the trigone and tends to reflux.

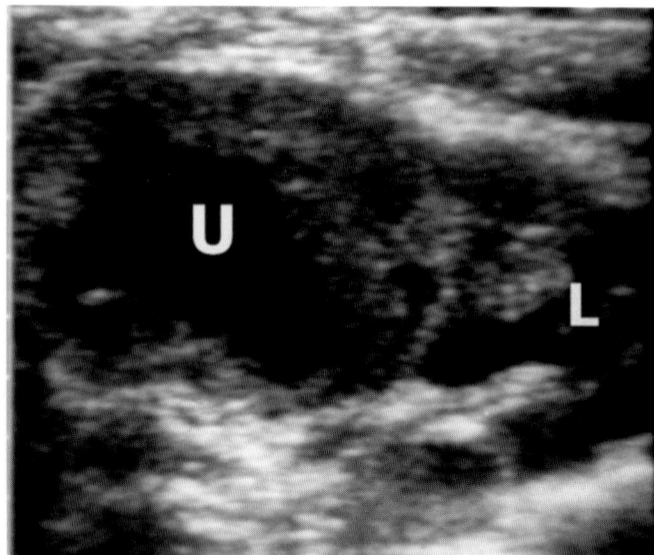

FIGURE 7 ■ Duplex collecting system. Longitudinal ultrasound of a duplex kidney in a one-year-old boy. The upper pole moiety (U) is dilated due to obstruction, while the lower pole moiety (L) is dilated due to reflux.

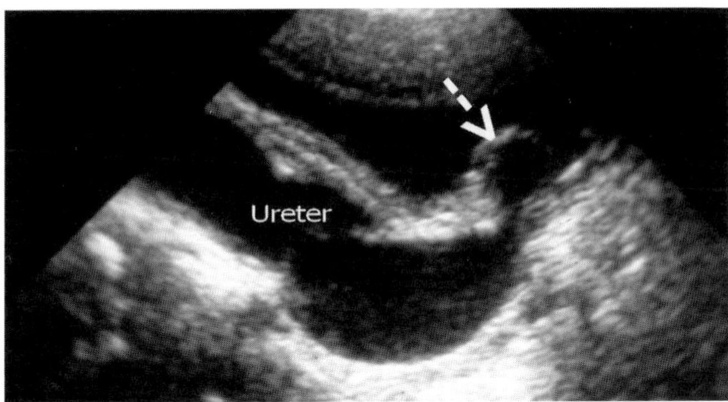

FIGURE 8 ■ Ureterocele. Longitudinal ultrasound of the pelvis defining a dilated upper pole moiety ureter terminating in an ectopic ureterocele (*arrow*).

at least four to seven days after birth and, in fact, may be best obtained at several weeks of age (33,34).

The most common cause of unilateral hydronephrosis in children is ureteropelvic junction obstruction (Fig. 11) (32,35), caused by an aberrant renal artery, idiopathic stenosis, or aperistaltic ureteral segment. Ultrasound demonstrates dilatation of the renal pelvis and calyces of the affected kidney but no ureteral dilatation. Other causes of hydronephrosis include posterior urethral valves, vesicoureteral reflux, ectopic ureterocele, and ureterovesical junction obstruction. In these cases, the ureter is also dilated and tortuous.

The triad of urinary tract anomalies, cryptorchidism, and hypoplastic or absent abdominal wall musculature characterizes Eagle–Barrett or prune-belly syndrome (36). Other anomalies include clubfoot, hip dysplasia, congenital heart disease, imperforate anus, and intestinal malrotation. The most common sonographic appearance is a large bladder, with tortuous, dilated, hypoperistaltic ureters, and varying degrees of hydronephrosis.

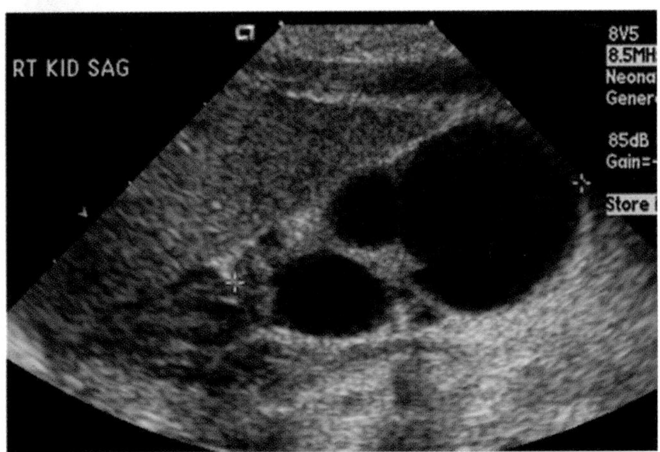

FIGURE 9 ■ Multicystic dysplastic kidney. Longitudinal ultrasound of the right renal fossa in a newborn. Multiple, noncommunicating cysts of various sizes are seen in this baby with a right multicystic dysplastic kidney.

URINARY TRACT INFECTION

Bacterial infection of the urinary tract is an important cause of morbidity in children. Radiographic evaluation is used in these patients to (*i*) detect structural or functional abnormalities such as hydronephrosis and (*ii*) detect effects of infection, such as scarring (37). The long-term goal in the evaluation and treatment of childhood urinary tract infection (UTI) is the prevention of renal damage (glomerulosclerosis, tubular atrophy, and vascular changes) leading to hypertension and renal insufficiency (38,39). Renal scarring occurs in 5% to 20% of children after a febrile UTI. Although vesicoureteral reflux is an important risk factor developing renal scarring after UTI, postinfectious renal scarring may also occur in the absence of reflux (40).

Ultrasonography has been widely used in the initial workup of children with UTI. It can readily identify structural abnormalities and hydronephrosis as well as the anatomy of the bladder (41). Ultrasound findings of acute pyelonephritis include renal swelling, loss of corticomedullary differentiation, altered renal echogenicity, or focal mass (lobar nephronia, Fig. 12). However, these findings are observed in only 11% to 69% of affected children (39,42). Power Doppler sonography increases the detection rate for acute pyelonephritis to about 77% (43). Renal ultrasonography is insensitive to the accurate detection of vesicoureteral reflux (44) and thus does not obviate the need for voiding cystourethrography (VCUG) or nuclear cystography. It is less sensitive than DMSA renal scintigraphy in the detection of renal scars (45), seen as cortical thinning/defects most common at the renal poles (Fig. 13). Renal growth retardation may also be a sign of vesicoureteral reflux (46).

Despite its limitations, ultrasonography remains an important mainstay in the evaluation of children with UTI. The American Academy of Pediatrics practice parameters recommends ultrasonography of the kidneys in infants and children up to two years of age with the first febrile UTI (47), and the Swedish guidelines also recommend ultrasonography in children older than two years with their first UTI (48). Others disagree (44,49), stating that ultrasound alone had little impact on the patients' management.

Echo-enhanced cystosonography (50–52) using ultrasonographic contrast agents such as galactose suspension (and others) has been reported to be comparable to VCUG in the detection of vesicoureteral reflux. It may be useful in follow-up examinations for reflux, or for screening (53), but has not been widely used in the United States.

Ultrasonography is frequently utilized in the postoperative evaluation of children treated for vesicoureteral reflux. Typical findings after ureteral reimplantation include thickening of the posterior bladder wall, pseudodiverticular sacculations, bladder asymmetry, and transitory hydroureteronephrosis (54). Abnormal findings include persistent hydroureteronephrosis, urinoma, hematomas, bladder lithiasis, and diverticula. After submucosal injection of tissue-augmenting substances (55)

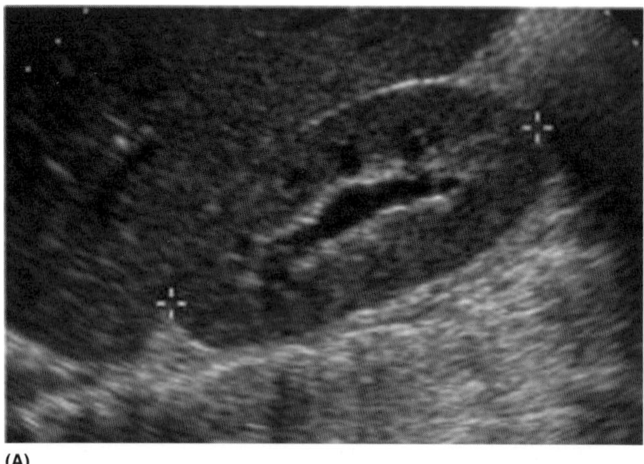

(A)

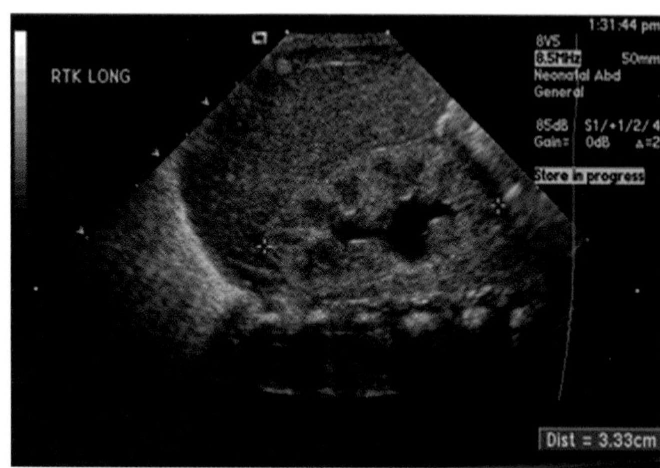

(B)

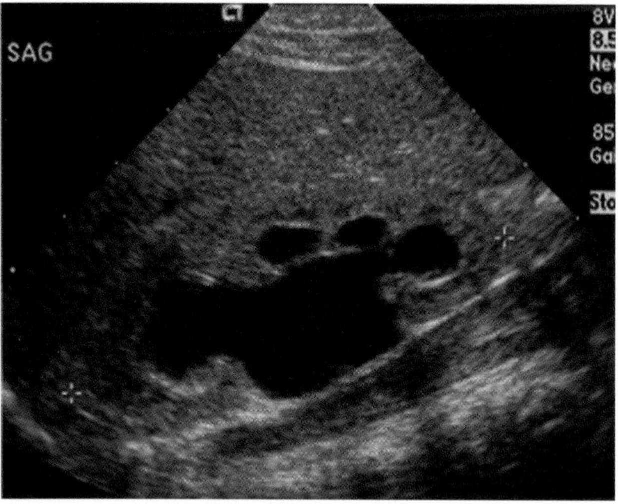

(C)

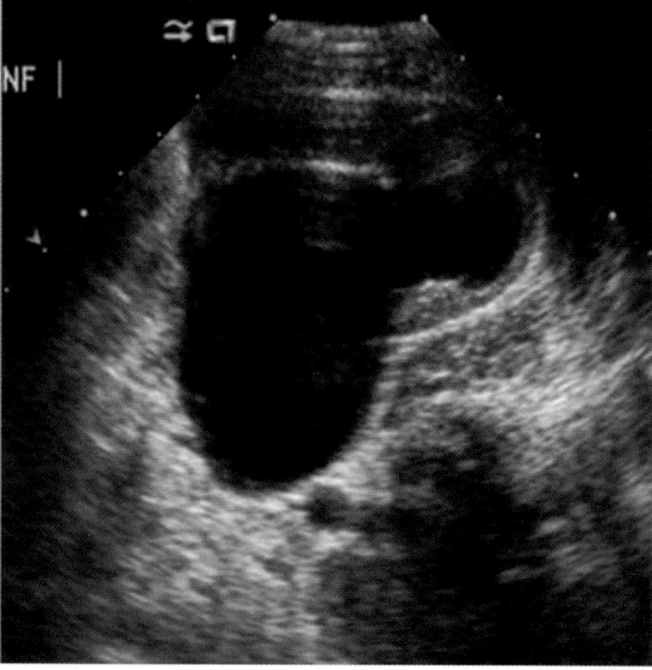

(D)

FIGURE 10 A–D ■ Hydronephrosis. (**A**) Longitudinal image of grade 1 hydronephrosis, seen as mild dilatation of the renal pelvis. (**B**) Longitudinal ultrasound of grade 2 hydronephrosis, seen as dilatation of the renal pelvis and a few calyces. (**C**) Longitudinal ultrasound of grade 3 hydronephrosis, seen as moderate dilatation of the renal pelvis and all of the calyces. (**D**) Transverse ultrasound of grade 4 hydronephrosis, with marked pelvis and calyceal dilatation as well as parenchymal thinning.

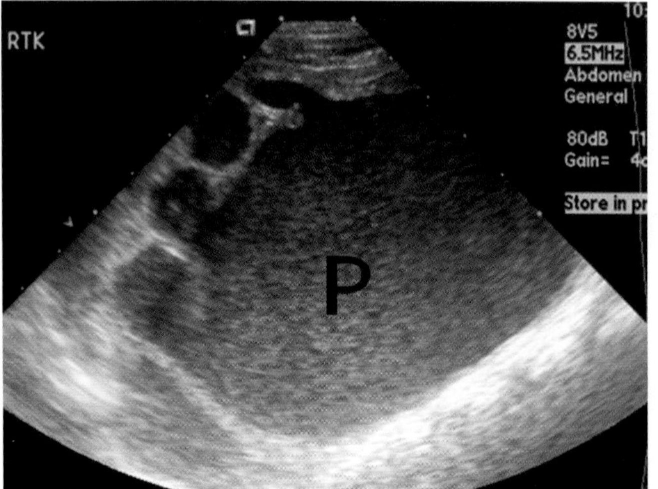

FIGURE 11 ■ Uteropelvic junction obstruction.

such as polytetrafluoroethylene, collagen, polydimethylsiloxane or chondrocytes, a subureteric mound of the injected material should be seen (Fig. 14). Depending on its chemical character, it may be hyperechoic (54) or isoechoic with the bladder base. Absence of the subureteric mound or multilobed mounds is associated with persistent reflux (56). Other abnormal findings may include persistent hydroureteronephrosis, granuloma formation, or ectopic intracavitary particles.

RENAL CYSTIC DISEASE

There are many different cystic diseases of the kidney that present in children. Simple renal cysts, a common finding in adults, are seen in fewer than 1% of children (57). They are typically single, and below 1 cm in size.

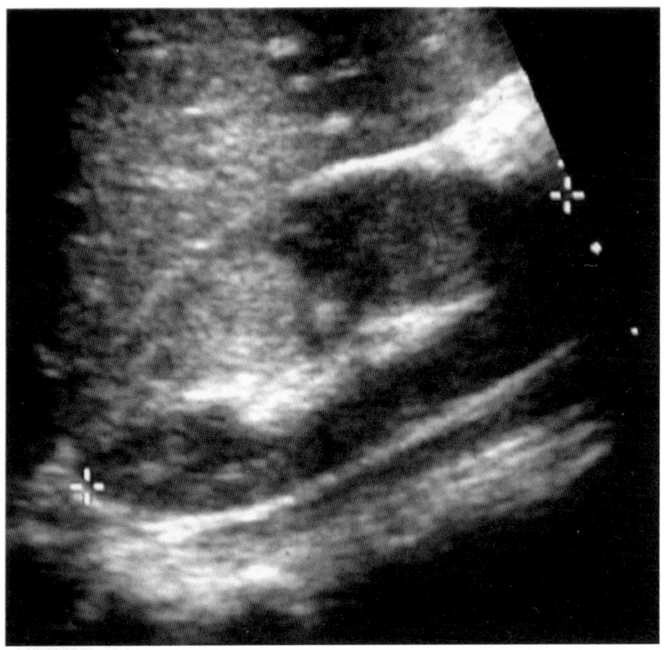

FIGURE 12 ■ Lobar nephronia. Longitudinal ultrasound of a hyperechoic mass-like wedge-shaped area (*cursors*) in the right upper pole in this girl with pyelonephritis.

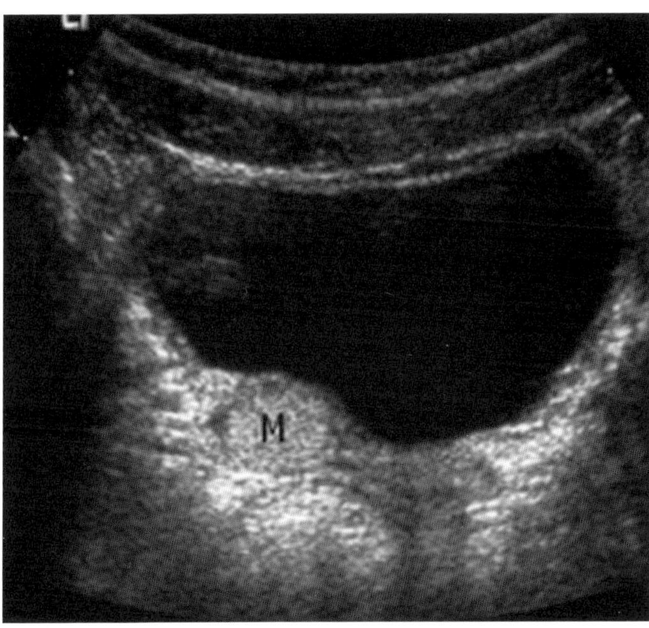

FIGURE 14 ■ Subureteric mound. Transverse ultrasound of the bladder in a patient after a subtrigonal injection procedure. A right subureteric mound (M) is noted. *Source*: Courtesy of Harriet Paltiel, M.D.

Autosomal-recessive polycystic kidney disease (Fig. 15) is the most common heritable cystic renal disease presenting in infancy and childhood (58). It is a disease of renal collecting tubular malformation and ectasia. There is associated congenital hepatic fibrosis with abnormal bile duct formation. There is considerable variability in presentation of this disease, but there tends to be an inverse relationship: children with severe renal disease tend to have milder hepatic disease and vice versa. Severe renal disease, with diminished urine output, results in prenatal oligohydramnios, Potter facies, and pulmonary hypoplasia. The kidneys are symmetrically and smoothly enlarged as a result of the dilated collecting ducts. The radial orientation of the ducts with respect to the ultrasound beam results in increased echogenicity. Corticomedullary differentiation is poor, and macrocysts may also be present. These macrocysts tend to be smaller than in autosomal-dominant polycystic disease and are often medullary in position (59). Renal calcifications may be seen and correlate with the degree of renal failure (60).

Although autosomal-dominant polycystic kidney disease (ADPKD) is considered a disease of adults, it is a

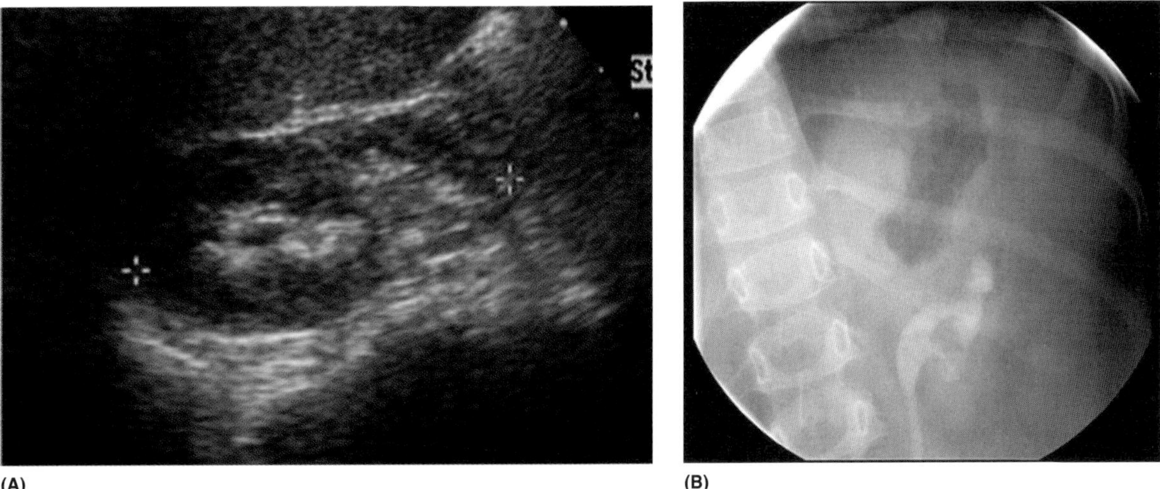

(A) (B)

FIGURE 13 A AND B ■ Renal scarring. (**A**) Longitudinal image of a five year old with left lower pole renal scarring. The lower pole parenchyma is thinned when compared with the upper pole. (**B**) Voiding cystourethrogram defines grade III left lower pole vesicoureteral reflux.

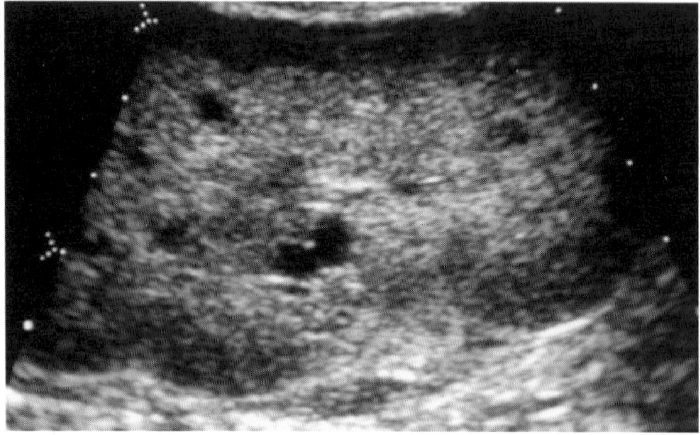

FIGURE 15 ■ Autosomal-recessive polycystic renal disease. Longitudinal ultrasound image of an infant with autosomal-recessive polycystic kidney disease shows the kidney to be echogenic and markedly enlarged for age. Several small hypoechoic cysts are also seen.

heritable disorder that begins in childhood. Sonographic findings of ADPKD in childhood include increased renal size (61), increased corticomedullary differentiation (59), and renal cysts. Sixty percent of children who carry the *PKD-1* gene have cysts detected by five years of age, and 80% have cysts by 18 years of age (61). Progression of disease manifests as an increase in cyst number and an increase in renal size.

Renal cysts in a child with seizures and developmental retardation should raise the consideration of tuberous sclerosis (TS) (Fig. 16). These cysts are relatively common in children with TS, are usually small, multiple and bilateral, and have a distinct lining of hyperplastic cells (62). They are distinct from the angiomyolipomas also commonly seen in TS (Fig. 17). Other syndromes and disorders associated with renal cysts include von Hippel-Lindau and Zellweger syndrome (63).

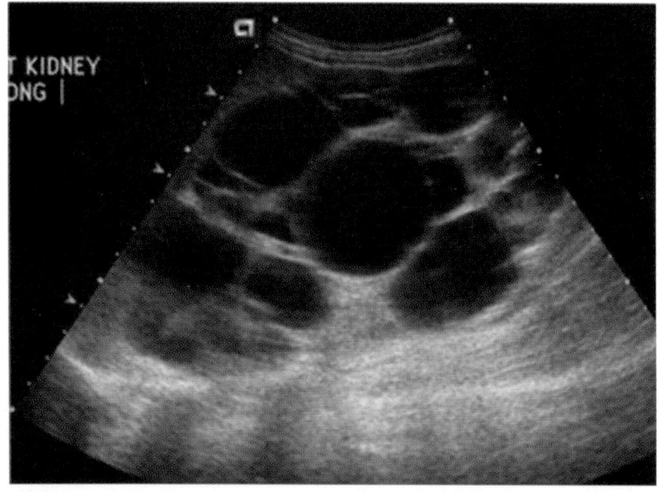

(A)

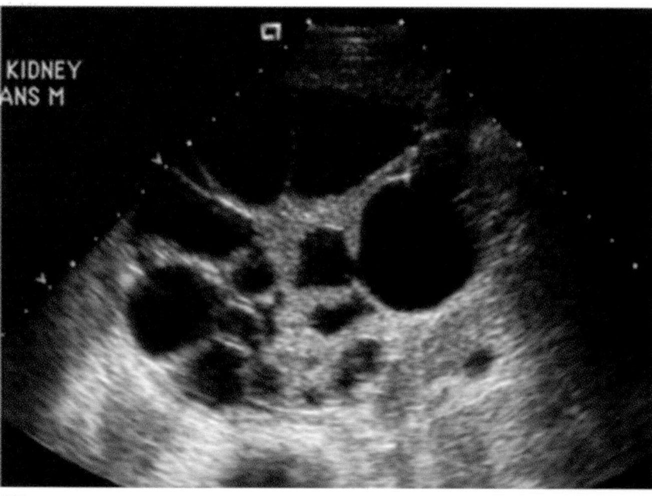

(B)

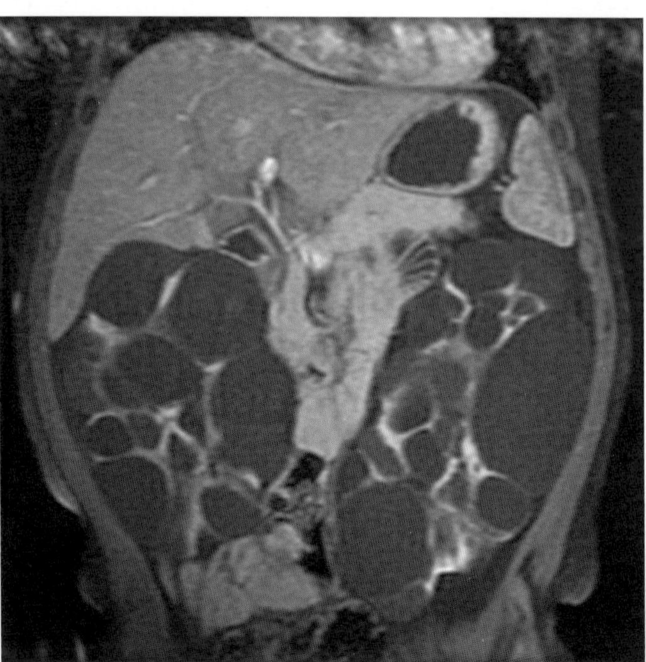

(C)

FIGURE 16 A–C ■ Tuberous sclerosis. Longitudinal (**A**) and transverse (**B**) ultrasound images of the right kidney in a young boy with tuberous sclerosis. (**C**) Coronal postgadolinium MRI further defines the bilateral renal cysts in this child.

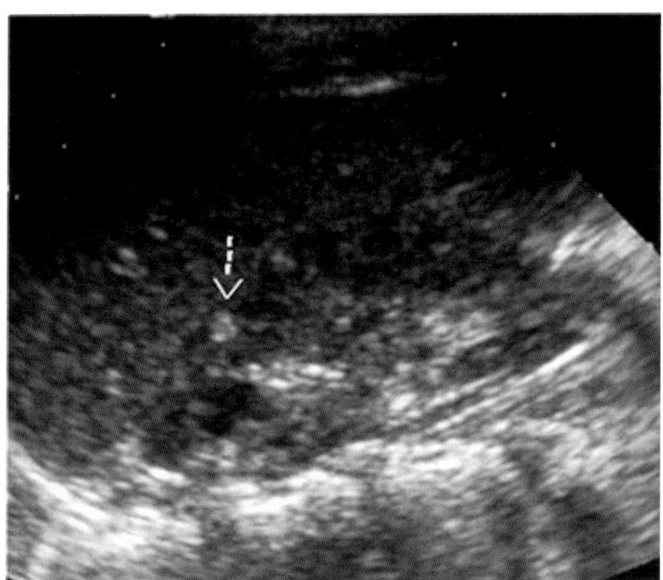

FIGURE 17 ■ Angiomyolipomas. Longitudinal ultrasound showing multiple tiny hyperechoic foci in this patient with tuberous sclerosis and multiple renal angiolipomas. One is marked with an arrow.

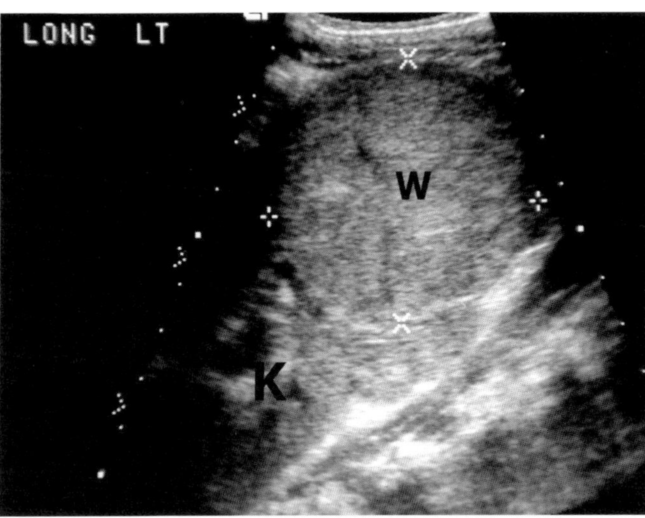

FIGURE 18 ■ Wilms' tumor. Longitudinal ultrasound showing a hyperechoic renal mass (W) in this child with left Wilms' tumor. The normal upper pole is marked (K). An enlarged node is seen medial to the tumor.

RENAL NEOPLASMS

Wilms' tumor (nephroblastoma) is both the most common renal tumor and the most common intra-abdominal tumor of childhood (64). The disease is seen equally in boys and girls, and most patients present between one and five years of age; Wilms' tumor is unusual in the first year of life.

An asymptomatic unilateral abdominal mass is the most common presentation of Wilms' tumor. Other symptoms may include hypertension, malaise, abdominal pain, and hematuria. A new left varicocele in a boy should raise suspicion for a left-sided Wilms' tumor with invasion of the left renal vein. Congenital anomalies associated with Wilms' tumor may include sporadic aniridia, hemihypertrophy, Beckwith–Wiedemann syndrome, Sotos syndrome, Perlmann syndrome, malformations of the genitourinary system (cryptorchidism, hypospadias, gonadal dysgenesis, and horseshoe kidney), Drash syndrome, and neurofibromatosis. Both the diffuse and the multifocal forms of nephroblastomatosis, or persistence of metanephric blastema, are associated with Wilms' tumor (65).

Ultrasonography will demonstrate Wilms' tumor as an intrarenal (usually) hyperechoic mass when compared with normal renal or hepatic parenchyma (Fig. 18) (66). Areas of necrosis and cysts (Fig. 19), if present, are hypoechoic. The renal vein and inferior vena cava must be carefully evaluated, including the use of color Doppler, to assess for vascular extension of tumor. The renal vein is involved in 15% of patients, the inferior vena cava in up to 10%, and the tumor extends into the right atrium in less than 1% (67). Sonography has been reported as more sensitive than computed tomography (CT) in evaluating vascular tumor extension. The involved vessels are focally enlarged and filled with echogenic tumor (Fig. 20) (68). Fixation of the tumor thrombus to the vascular wall suggests invasion. It may be helpful to scan the patient in the upright position to distend the inferior vena cava. Adenopathy may be reactive or may result from tumor infiltration. The liver is evaluated for the presence of metastases.

The opposite kidney must also be examined, as 5% of tumors are bilateral, with two-thirds of these being synchronous and one-third, metachronous. Rests of nephroblastomatosis (Fig. 21) (a precursor to Wilms' tumor) are typically nodular and hypoechoic (69), though occasionally they are isoechoic, hyperechoic, cystic, or diffuse in appearance.

Staging of Wilms' tumor is surgical. Stage I Wilms' tumors are limited to the kidney and are completely resected (70). In stage II, tumor extends into the perirenal

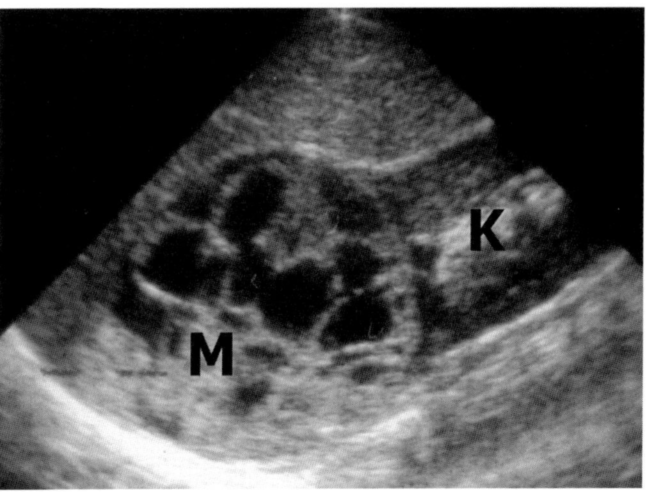

FIGURE 19 ■ Cystic Wilms' tumor. A complex, partially cystic mass (M) is seen in the upper pole of the kidney in this child with Wilms' tumor. The normal renal parenchyma (K) is also seen on the longitudinal image.

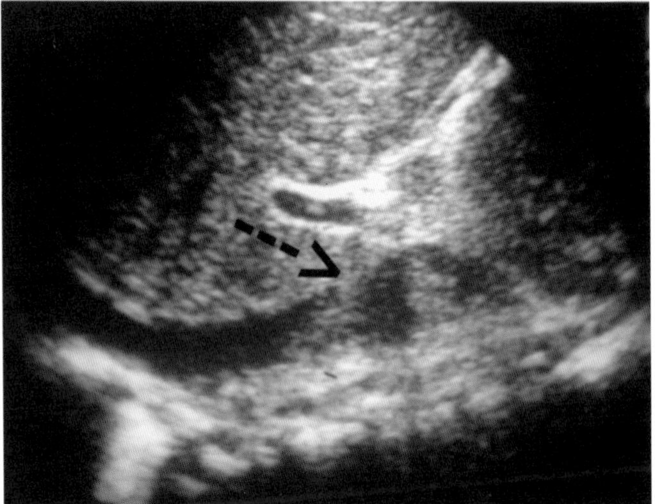

FIGURE 20 ■ Longitudinal image showing Wilms' tumor growing into the inferior vena cava (*arrow*).

soft tissues, periaortic lymph nodes, or veins, but resection is complete. In stage III, residual tumor is present after resection. In stage IV, hematogenous metastases are present. Distant metastases occur most often to the lungs, less frequently to the liver, and rarely to the bones or brain. In stage V, both kidneys are involved, either at the time of diagnosis or subsequently.

Followup of patients treated for Wilms' tumor includes periodic evaluation of the tumor bed for local recurrence. A new soft-tissue mass in the renal fossa suggests recurrence. The opposite kidney is carefully evaluated for the development of a metachronous tumor, especially if the removed kidney contained nephroblastomatosis. Another complication is susceptibility of the remaining kidney to hyperfiltration injury, suggested by increasing parenchymal echogenicity over time (71). Second malignant neoplasms may also develop, with leukemia and lymphoma being the most common (72).

The kidneys are the most frequent extranodal site of metastases from lymphoma (73). The most common pattern observed is bilateral nephromegaly with increased cortical echogenicity (74) resulting from diffuse infiltration of the parenchyma (Fig. 22). A second pattern seen is focal hypoechoic masses (Fig. 23) (75). Obstructive uropathy may result from pelvic or retroperitoneal masses or uric acid stones (76).

Multilocular cystic nephroma is a rare pediatric renal tumor. There is debate as to whether this tumor is hamartomatous or if it results from maldevelopment of the ureteral bud. Two-thirds occur in children below two years of age, and there is a male predominance in this age group.

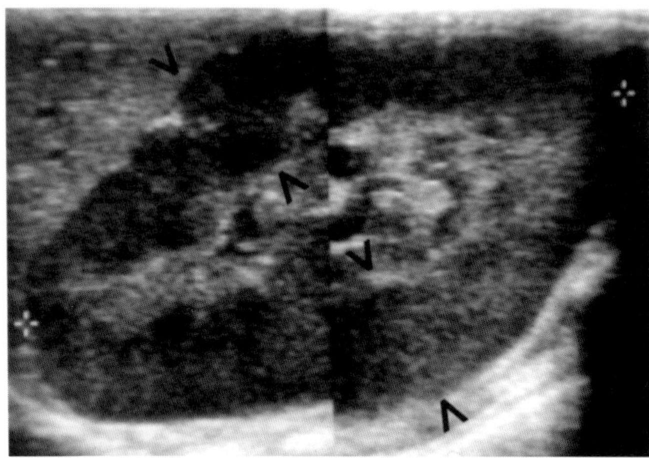

FIGURE 21 ■ Nephroblastomatosis. Longitudinal split-frame image showing diffuse, relatively hypoechoic nephroblastomatosis (*arrowheads*) completely encasing the kidney of this two year old. The kidney is markedly enlarged for age.

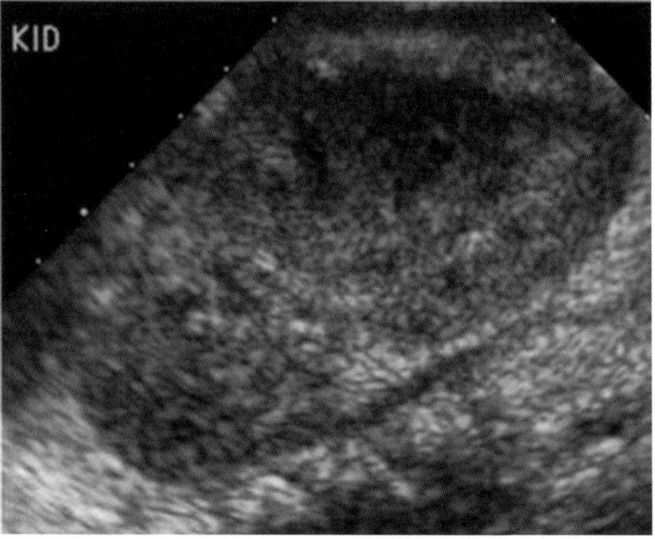

(A)

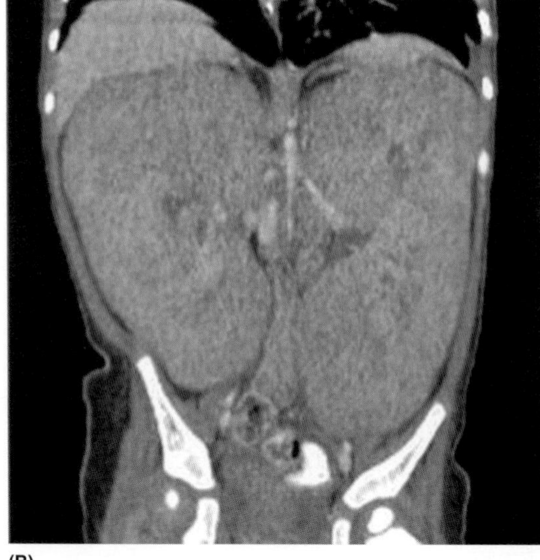

(B)

FIGURE 22 A AND B ■ Leukemia of the kidneys. (**A**) Longitudinal image of the right kidney in this one-year-old patient with leukemia/lymphoma. The kidney is markedly enlarged and is hyperechoic. (**B**) Corresponding coronal postcontrast CT reconstruction shows massive bilateral nephromegaly.

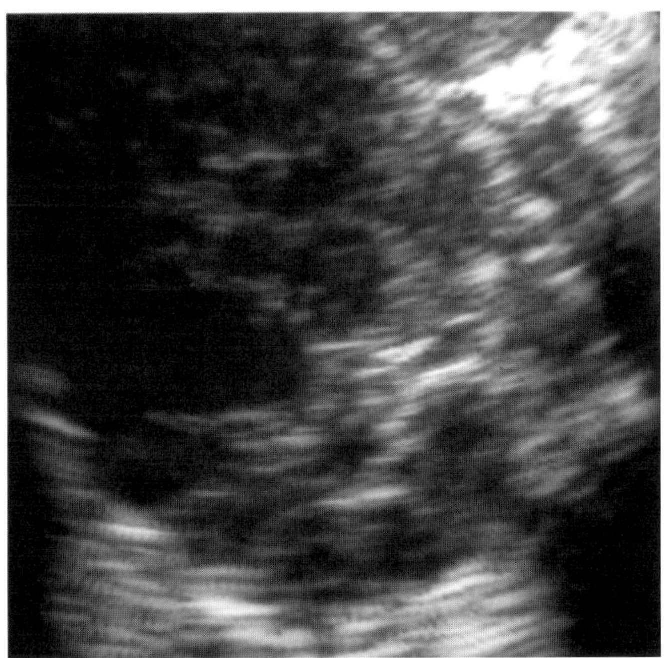

FIGURE 23 ■ Renal lymphoma. Transverse ultrasound image showing multiple hypoechoic foci in this patient with lymphomatous involvement of the kidney.

Most present with a painless abdominal mass, but hypertension, hematuria, and flank pain may be seen. Ultrasonography demonstrates a well-defined, multiseptated mass with noncommunicating cysts and septa of varying thickness (Fig. 24). Calcification is uncommon. Herniation of the cysts into the renal pelvis can cause hydronephrosis (77).

Congenital mesoblastic nephroma (fetal renal hamartoma) is the most common renal tumor in neonates and is histologically distinct from Wilms' tumor. Affected infants usually have a nontender abdominal mass; additional signs and symptoms may include hematuria, hypertension, anemia, and hypercalcemia. Associated abnormalities may include polyhydramnios, gastrointestinal tract malformations, neuroblastoma, and genitourinary tract anomalies. Sonography will demonstrate a well-defined hypoechoic mass. The presence of concentric echogenic and hypoechoic rings is a helpful diagnostic feature (78). A more complex pattern results from hemorrhage, cyst formation, and necrosis (Fig. 25).

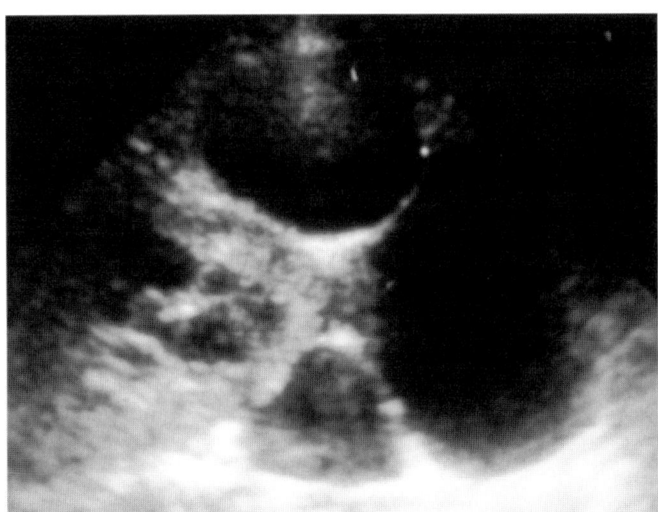

FIGURE 24 ■ Multilocular cystic nephroma. Transverse image showing multiple cysts in this patient with proven multilocular cystic nephroma. The tumor replaced and was exophytic from the lower pole of the kidney.

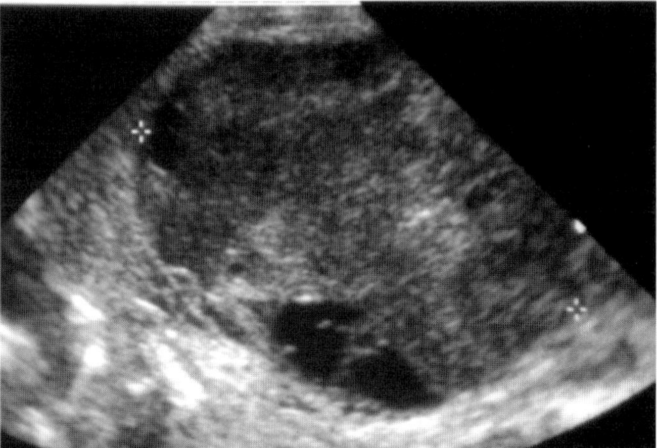

FIGURE 25 ■ Congenital mesoblastic nephroma. Longitudinal image showing a massive, inhomogeneous tumor (*cursors*) in this newborn with congenital mesoblastic nephroma.

MEDICAL RENAL DISEASE

Increased renal parenchymal echogenicity usually indicates parenchymal disease. Common medical diseases that may cause increased parenchymal echogenicity in children include nephrotic syndrome, glomerulonephritis, glycogen storage disease, hemolytic uremic syndrome, pyelonephritis, sickle-cell anemia, renal dysplasia, chronic renal failure, and acquired immunodeficiency syndrome (73).

Hemolytic-uremic syndrome (Fig. 26) occurs in children typically below five years of age. These children present with thrombocytopenia, renal failure, anemia, and hypertension. Endothelial damage from an antigen–antibody reaction to a bacterial toxin results in vasculitis, with microthrombi and platelet consumption. The kidneys may be mildly enlarged and are hyperechoic due to glomerular swelling, platelet aggregates, and fibrin thrombi (79). During the oliguric or anuric phase of the disease, intrarenal arterial flow may be absent or diastolic flow may be diminished, absent, or reversed (80).

Hyperechoic renal medullary pyramids may result from a number of causes in the pediatric population (Fig. 27). Most cases of nephrocalcinosis have hypercalciuria. If hypercalcemia is also present, likely etiologies include drugs (furosemide) (81), steroids, vitamin D, Bartter syndrome, Williams syndrome, or hyperparathyroidism (82). Patients with hypercalciuria and normal blood calcium levels may have renal tubular acidosis, medullary sponge kidney, or primary hypercalciuria. If urine calcium

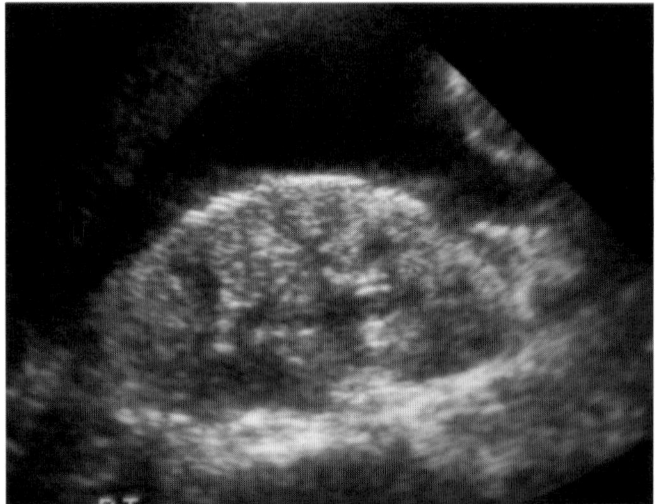

FIGURE 26 ■ Hemolytic-uremic syndrome. Longitudinal ultrasound of a three year old with hemolytic-uremic syndrome. The kidney is hyperechoic, and there is ascites.

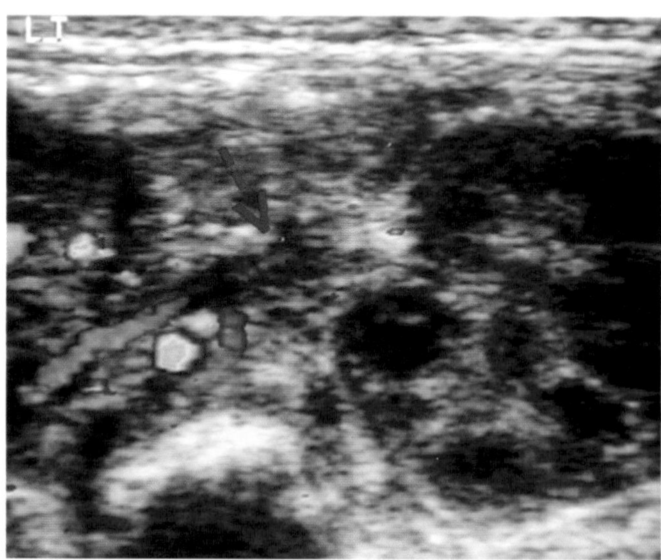

FIGURE 28 ■ Newborn with renal vein thrombosis. Transverse color Doppler image shows no flow in the proximal main renal vein (*arrow*).

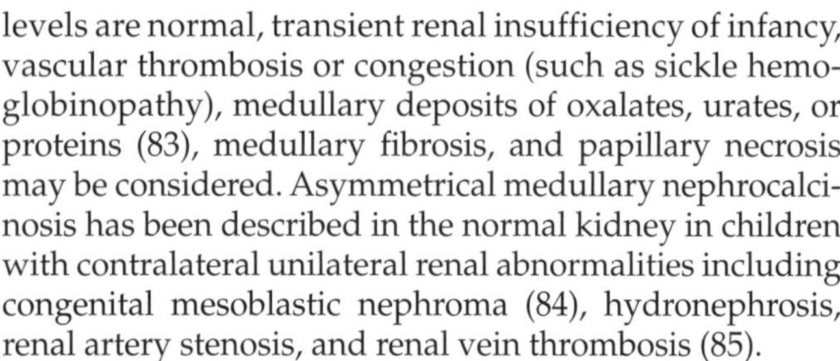

levels are normal, transient renal insufficiency of infancy, vascular thrombosis or congestion (such as sickle hemoglobinopathy), medullary deposits of oxalates, urates, or proteins (83), medullary fibrosis, and papillary necrosis may be considered. Asymmetrical medullary nephrocalcinosis has been described in the normal kidney in children with contralateral unilateral renal abnormalities including congenital mesoblastic nephroma (84), hydronephrosis, renal artery stenosis, and renal vein thrombosis (85).

RENAL VEIN THROMBOSIS

Renal vein thrombosis is the most common vascular condition in the newborn kidney. Risk factors include dehydration, sepsis, birth asphyxia, maternal diabetes, polycythemia, or indwelling umbilical venous catheters (86). There is an association with adrenal hemorrhage as well (87).

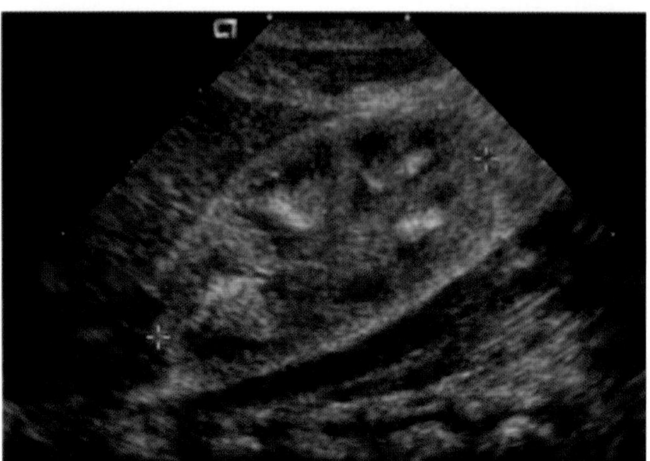

FIGURE 27 ■ Nephrocalcinosis. Longitudinal ultrasound of an infant with nephrocalcinosis related to diuretic therapy.

The ultrasonographic appearance of the affected kidney depends on both the extent and the stage of the thrombus. Initially, the kidney swells and becomes echogenic with prominent hypoechoic medullary pyramids. Echogenic intramedullary streaks (88) result from interlobular and interlobar thrombus (86). The thrombus within the renal vein may be echolucent or echogenic. After the first week, the kidney appears heterogeneous and loses its corticomedullary differentiation. The echogenic intramedullary streaks disappear. There may be echolucency at the apex of or surrounding the renal pyramids (89). The clot will retract and may calcify. The kidney may recover completely or may atrophy.

Duplex and color Doppler may be useful (90). Initially, renal venous flow will be absent (Fig. 28). Renal arterial diastolic flow may be decreased and the resistive index elevated. Over time, renal venous flow may be documented as the clot retracts and collaterals develop.

ABDOMINAL NEUROBLASTOMA

Neuroblastoma arises from primitive neuroblasts of the embryonic neural crest, adrenal medulla, and sympathetic ganglia. It is the most common extracranial solid tumor of childhood (91) and the most common malignant tumor in infancy. Abdominal neuroblastoma accounts for about half of all cases of neuroblastoma. The median age at diagnosis is two years, and the tumor is unusual in children more than 10 years of age.

Neuroblastoma is usually clinically silent until it invades or compresses adjacent structures, metastasizes, or causes a paraneoplastic syndrome [myoclonic encephalopathy ("dancing eyes, dancing feet") or watery diarrhea, hypokalemia, and achlorhydria]. Half to two-thirds of children have tumor beyond the primary site at presentation. Neuroblastoma has been reported with increased frequency in patients with neurofibromatosis, Beckwith–Wiedemann syndrome, nesidioblastosis, fetal hydantoin syndrome, and total aganglionosis of the colon.

Nearly half of children with abdominal neuroblastoma have an abdominal mass at presentation. Metastases to the liver can cause hepatomegaly. Almost all children with neuroblastoma have increased 24-hour urinary levels of catecholamine metabolites (92). A rise or fall in these metabolites after therapy parallels growth or regression of the tumor, respectively.

Abdominal sonography reveals the tumor to be an inhomogeneous, echogenic, poorly defined, extrarenal mass (Fig. 29) (93). If adrenal in origin, the mass displaces the kidney inferiorly. Hypoechoic regions may be due to hemorrhage, necrosis, or cyst formation. Areas of calcification are hyperechoic. A characteristic well-defined echogenic lobule (94) has been related to aggregates of tumor cells surrounded by collagen. Aggressive tumors can invade the kidney and thus may lead to an erroneous diagnosis of an exophytic Wilms' tumor. Features that suggest neuroblastoma with renal invasion (95), rather than Wilms' tumor, include displacement of the kidney by a predominant suprarenal mass, growth across the midline, multifocal calcification within the mass, and displacement of the great vessels.

The primary tumor or retroperitoneal adenopathy may encase the great vessels, celiac axis, or superior mesenteric vessels, splaying and displacing them anteriorly (Fig. 30). Hepatic metastases may be identified as discrete, hypoechoic masses or diffuse, ill-defined hyperechogenicity (Fig. 31) (91). The extent of metastatic disease to the liver may be inadequately assessed by ultrasonography, especially in younger children with diffuse hepatic infiltration (93). Prior to ossification of the posterior elements, intraspinal extension can be imaged by sonography.

The international neuroblastoma staging system (96,97) utilizes radiologic findings, lymph node involvement, bone marrow involvement, and surgical resectability in determining the tumor stage. Stage 1 tumors are confined to the area of origin, are completely grossly resected, and have no nodal involvement. Stage 2A tumors are localized but incompletely resected and have negative nodes. Stage 2B tumors are unilateral and may be completely or incompletely resected. There are positive ipsilateral but negative contralateral nodes. Stage 3 tumors include those crossing midline, unilateral tumor with contralateral positive nodes, or midline tumor with bilateral nodal involvement. Stage 4 includes disseminated tumor. Stage 4S disease includes a localized primary tumor (stage 1, 2A, or 2B) with dissemination limited to the skin, liver, or bone marrow (<10% tumor cells) in infants below one year of age.

Treatment of neuroblastoma may include surgical resection, chemotherapy, and radiation therapy. Age, stage, and location of the primary tumor are the major prognostic factors, with the single most important factor being age at diagnosis (98). Children with tumors in the abdomen have a poorer prognosis than those with extra-abdominal tumors.

Appropriate imaging of children during and after the completion of treatment for neuroblastoma depends on the initial site, stage, and extent of tumor. With response to chemotherapy, the tumor usually decreases in size and increases in calcification.

Recent work (99–101) describes a connection between neuroblastoma treated in young infants and subsequent development of renal-cell carcinoma. These renal-cell carcinomas (Fig. 32) develop as early as two years and up to 30 years after the neuroblastoma diagnosis and do not appear associated with prior radiation or chemotherapy. Other second malignant neoplasms seen in patients treated for neuroblastoma include bone and soft-tissue sarcomas, leukemia, and lymphoma (102).

Other adrenal masses, including adrenocortical tumor (ACT, adenoma/carcinoma) and pheochromocytoma, are

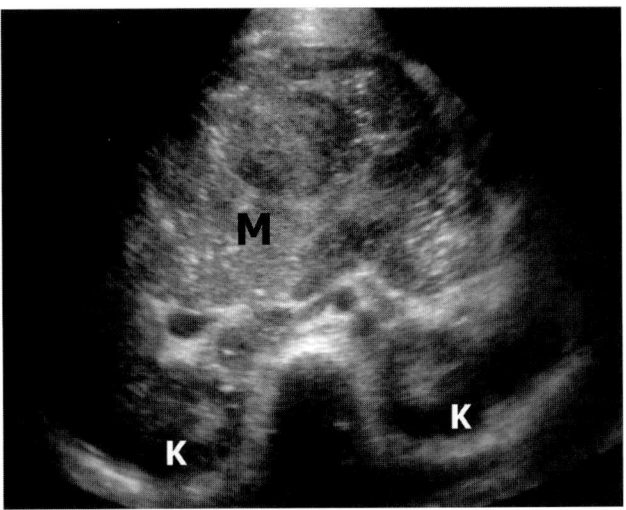

(A)

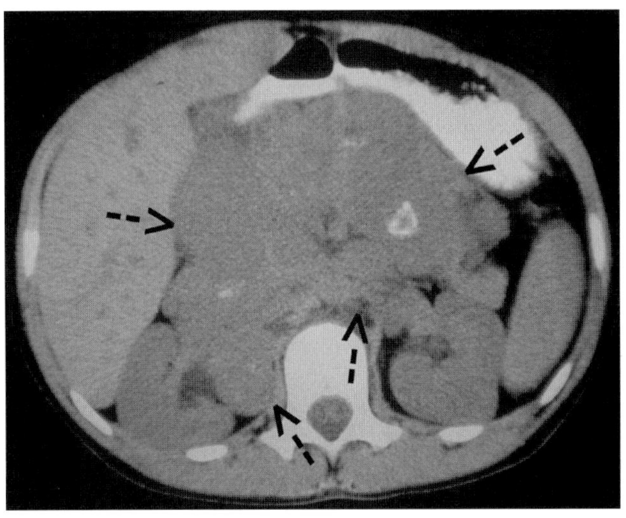

(B)

FIGURE 29 A AND B ■ Transverse image of a young girl with neuroblastoma. **(A)** The tumor (M) crosses the midline and is inhomogeneous in its echotexture. **(B)** This same tumor (*arrows*) is seen on noncontrast CT to contain areas of calcification. K, kidney.

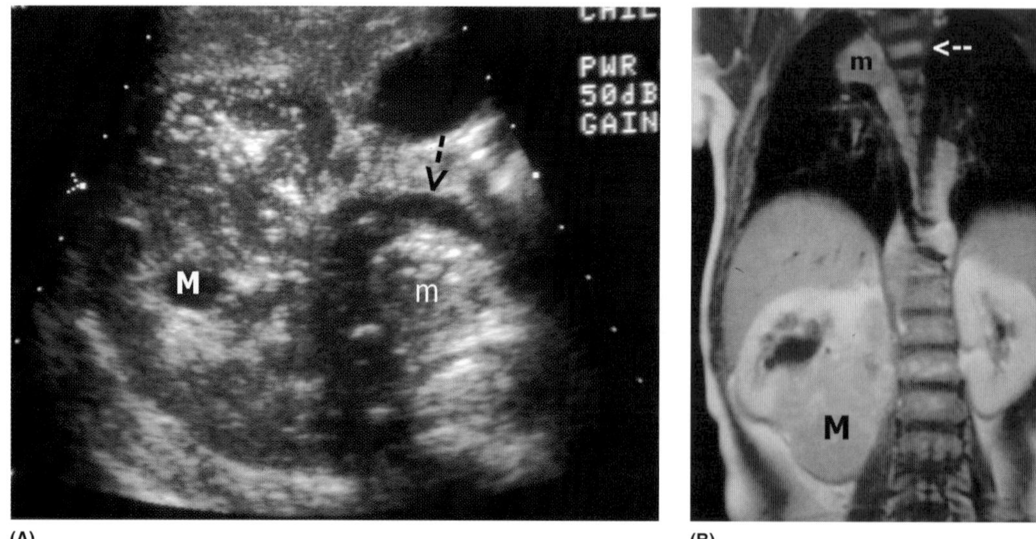

(A) (B)

FIGURE 30 A AND B ■ Neuroblastoma. (**A**) Transverse ultrasound image of a two-year-old boy with neuroblastoma. The tumor (M) is primarily in the right abdomen but extends (m) posteriorly to uplift the inferior vena cava. (**B**) A coronal postgadolinium MRI shows the tumor displacing the right kidney upward and laterally. The mass extends along both sides of the spine, to the right suprahilar region, where it inferiorly displaces the azygos vein. Increased signal is seen on a thoracic vertebra (*arrow*), indicating bony metastases.

rare in children (93). ACT is usually seen in children less than five years of age and are more common in girls. It is associated with Li–Fraumeni syndrome (103), Beckwith–Wiedemann syndrome, and hemihypertrophy. The presenting manifestations depend upon the type of adrenocortical hormone secreted and may include virilizing, feminizing, Cushing, and Conn syndromes. These tumors are typically large (>6 cm) at presentation (104) and are well defined. They may contain calcifications as well as central necrosis or hemorrhage (103). They may be locally aggressive and may invade the inferior vena cava (IVC) (105). Metastatic spread occurs to the liver, lungs, or regional lymph nodes.

Pheochromocytoma (Fig. 33) is a tumor of neural crest origin. Children typically present with sustained hypertension (98). This tumor is located in the adrenal gland in about three-quarters of cases and may be multiple (93). They are associated with neurofibromatosis, von Hippel-Lindau disease, Sturge–Weber syndrome, and multiple endocrine neoplasia.

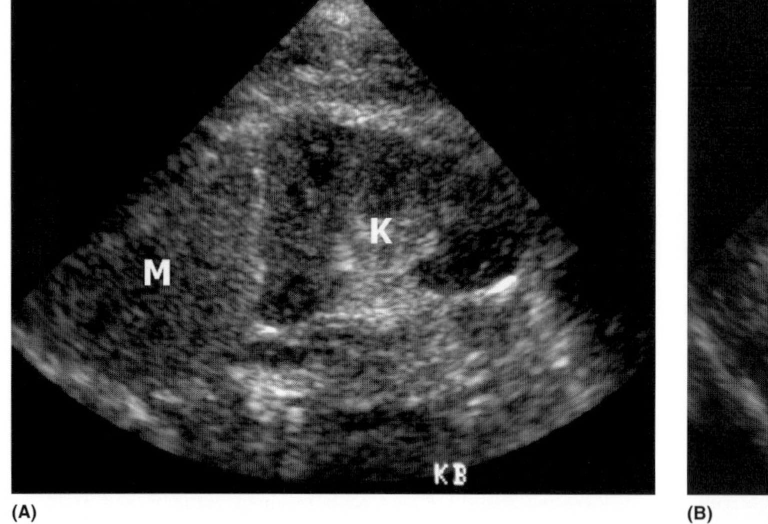

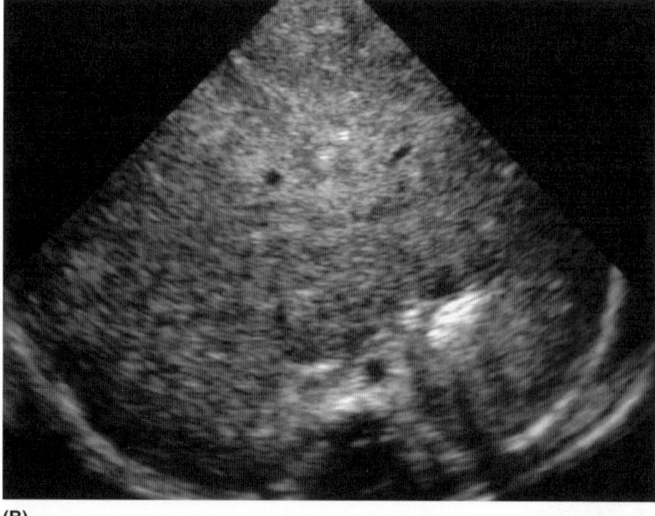

(A) (B)

FIGURE 31 A AND B ■ Neuroblastoma. (**A**) Longitudinal ultrasound of the left renal fossa showing a mass in the suprarenal region (M), distorting the upper aspect of the kidney in this six week old. (**B**) On this transverse image, the liver is seen to be coarse in echotexture, enlarged, and echogenic due to diffuse metastatic involvement in this infant with Stage 4S neuroblastoma. K, kidney.

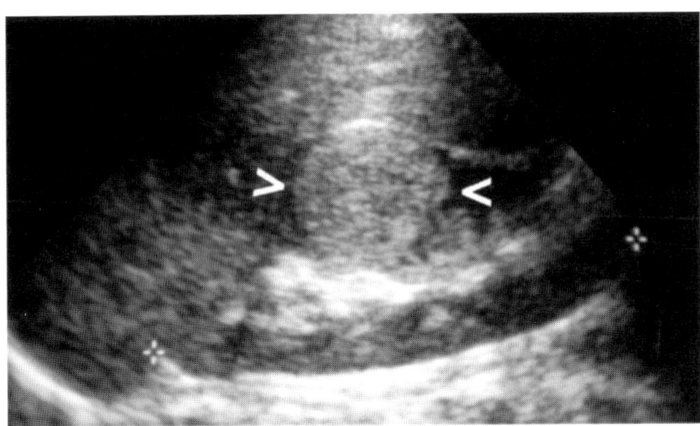

FIGURE 32 ■ Renal cell carcinoma. Longitudinal image of the kidney showing a well-defined hyperechoic mass (*arrowheads*), proven to be renal cell carcinoma, in this patient who had had neuroblastoma as a child.

ADRENAL HEMORRHAGE

Spontaneous neonatal adrenal hemorrhage is most common in term, large-for-gestational-age infants. Other risk factors (106) include infants of diabetic mothers and those with sepsis, hypoxia, and coagulopathy. Adrenal hemorrhage may be incidentally discovered (107), or the patient may have a flank mass, anemia, or jaundice (108). Rarely, massive intraperitoneal bleeding may occur. Acute scrotal swelling may rarely be seen with adrenal hemorrhage (109). The hemorrhage may occur prenatally but is most common around birth. It may be unilateral or bilateral and is more common on the right. The hemorrhage will replace the normal adrenal gland. Acutely, it will appear as a solid hyperechoic mass (108). As the clot liquefies, the hemorrhage will become cystic and hypoechoic (Fig. 34). Over a few weeks, the cyst involutes (110). It may calcify along its periphery (106,107). Lack of evolution and resolution of a suspected hemorrhage should raise the concern for coexisting neuroblastoma (106).

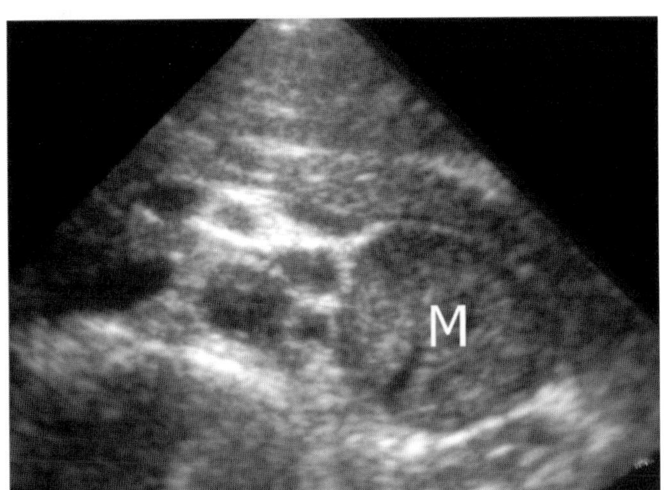

FIGURE 33 ■ Pheochromocytoma. Transverse ultrasound image showing a left suprarenal well-defined mass (M) proven to be pheochromocytoma.

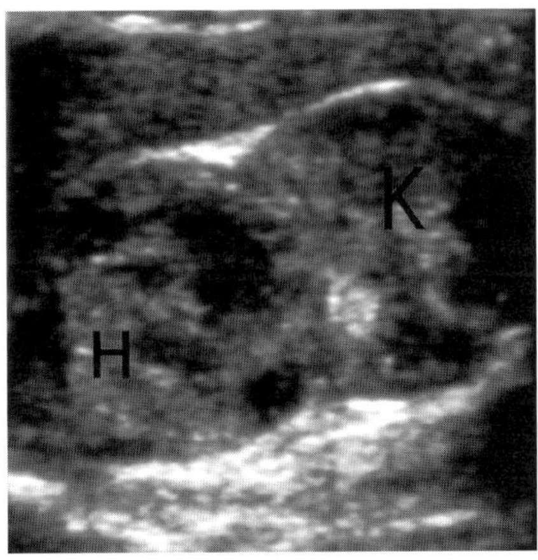

(A)

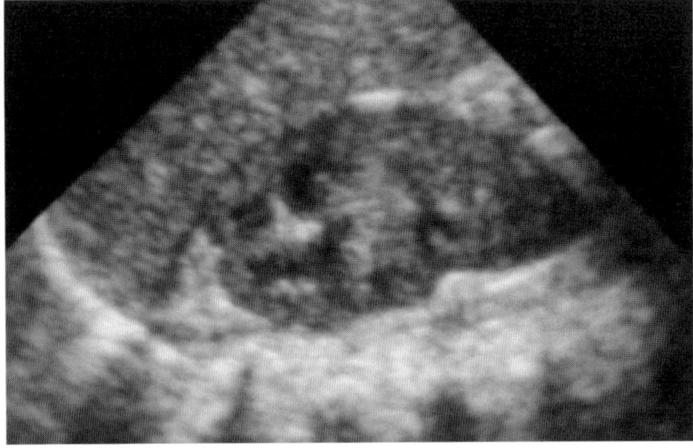

(B)

FIGURE 34 A AND B ■ Adrenal hemorrhage. (**A**) Longitudinal image of the right kidney (K) in a newborn showing a suprarenal heterogeneous mass (H) distorting the kidney. This proved to be an adrenal hemorrhage. (**B**) Follow-up longitudinal image several months later shows resolution of the hemorrhage and calcification of the adrenal gland.

REFERENCES

Normal Development

1. Moore KL. The urogenital system. The Developing Human. 2nd ed. Philadelphia: W. B. Saunders, 1977:220–228.
2. Safak AA, Simsek E, Bahcebasi T. Sonographic assessment of the normal limits and percentile curves of liver, spleen and kidney dimensions in healthy school-aged children. J Ultrasound Med 2005; 24:1359–1364.
3. Han BK, Babcock DS. Sonographic measurements and appearance of normal kidneys in children. AJR Am J Roentgenol 1985; 145:611–616.
4. Dremsek PA, Kritschner H, Bohm G, Hochberger O. Kidney dimensions in ultrasound compared to somatometric parameters in normal children. Pediatr Radiol 1987; 17:285–290.
5. Rosenbaum DM, Korngold E, Teele RL. Sonographic assessment of renal length in normal children. AJR Am J Roentgenol 1984; 142:467–469.
6. Konus OL, Ozdemir A, Akkaya A, Erbas G, Celik H, Isik S. Normal liver, spleen and kidney dimensions in neonates, infants and children: evaluation with sonography. AJR Am J Roentgenol 1998; 171:1693–1698.
7. Chu LW, Lu MY, Tsau YK. Sonographic measurements of renal size in normal children and children with compensatory renal hypertrophy. Acta Paediatr Taiwan 1999; 40:18–21.

8. Zerin JM, Meyer RD. Sonographic assessment of renal length in the first year of life: the problem of "spurious nephromegaly." Pediatr Radiol 2000; 30:52–57.
9. Loftus WK, Gent RJ, LeQuesne GW, Metreweli C. Renal length in Chinese children: sonographic measurement and comparison with western data. J Clin Ultrasound 1998; 26:349–352.
10. Vade A, Lau P, Smick J, et al. Sonographic renal parameters as related to age. Pediatr Radiol 1987; 17:212–215.
11. Siegel MJ. Urinary tract. Pediatric Sonography. 3rd ed. Philadelphia, PA: Siegel, Lippincott Williams and Wilkins, 2002.
12. Cramer B, Jequier S, de Chadarevian JP. Factors associated with renal parenchymal echogenicity in the newborn. J Ultrasound Med 1986; 5:633–638.
13. Kuzmic AC, Brkljacic B, Ivankovic D, Galesic K. Doppler sonographic renal resistance index in healthy children. Pediatr Radiol 2000; 10:1644–1648.
14. Andriani G, Persico A, Tursini S, Ballone E, Dirotti D, Lelli Chiesa P. The renal-resistive index from the last 3 months of pregnancy to 6 months old. BJU Int 2001; 87:562–564.
15. Arant BS Jr. Postnatal development of renal function during the first year of life. Pediatr Nephrol 1987; 1:308–313.
16. Fiselier T, Derkx F, Monnens L, Van Munster P, Peer P, Schalencamp M. The basal levels of active and inactive plasma rennin concentration in infancy and childhood. Clin Sci 1984; 67:383–387.
17. Vade A, Subbaiah P, Kalbhen CL, Ryva JC. Renal resistive indices in children. J Ultrasound Med 1993; 12:383–387.
18. Bude RO, DiPietro MA, PlattJR, Rubin JM, Miesowica S, Lundquist C. Age dependency of the renal resistive index in healthy children. Radiology 1992; 184:469–473.
19. Yildirim H, Gungor S, Cihangiroglu MM, Aygun AD. Doppler studies in normal kidneys of preterm and term neonates: changes in relation to gestational age and birth weight. J Ultrasound Med 2005; 24:623–627.
20. Stavel M, Zibolen M, Kolarovszka H, Murgas D. Comparison of Doppler parameters of central versus intraparenchymal renal arteries in physiologically normal newborns. Pediatr Radiol 2004; 34:552–555.
21. Yeh HC. Adrenal gland and nonrenal retroperitoneum. Urol Radiol 1987; 9:127–140.
22. Kangarloo H, Diament MJ, Gold RH, et al. Sonography of adrenal glands in neonates and children: changes in appearance with age. J Clin Ultrasound 1986; 14:43–47.

Congenital Anomalies

23. Decter RM. Renal duplication and fusion anomalies. Pediatr Clin North Am 1997; 44:1323–1341.
24. Teele RL, Share JC. Renal screening. In: Teele, Share, eds. Ultrasonography of Infants and Children. Philadelphia, PA: W. B. Saunders Co., 1991.
25. Fernbach SK, Feinstein KA, Spencer K, Lindstrom CA. Ureteral duplication and its complications. Radiographics 1997; 17: 109–127.
26. Stuck KJ, Koff SA, Silver TM. Ultrasonic features of multicystic dysplastic kidney: expanded diagnostic criteria. Radiology 1982; 143:217–221.
27. Karmazyn B, Zerin JM. Lower urinary tract abnormalities in children with multicystic dysplastic kidney. Radiology 1997; 203:223–226.
28. Strife JL, Souza AS, Kirks DR, Strife CF, Gelfand MJ, Wacksman J. Multicystic dysplastic kidney in children: US follow-up. Radiology 1993; 186:785–788.
29. Avni EF, Thoua Y, Lalmand B, Didier F, Droulle P, Schulman CC. Multicystic dysplastic kidney: natural history from in utero diagnosis and postnatal follow-up. J Urol 1987; 138:1420–1424.
30. Rottenberg GT, Gordon I, De Bruyn R. The natural history of the multicystic dysplastic kidney in children. Br J Radiol 1997; 70:347–350.

Hydronephrosis

31. Fernbach SK, Maizels M, Conway JJ. Ultrasound grading of hydronephrosis: introduction to the system used by the society for fetal urology. Pediatr Radiol 1993; 23:478–480.
32. Brown T, Mandell J, Lebowitz RL. Neonatal hydronephrosis in the era of sonography. AJR Am J Roentgenol 1987; 148:959–963.
33. Clautice-Engle T, Anderson NG, Allan RB, Abbott GD. Diagnosis of obstructive hydronephrosis in infants: comparison sonograms performed 6 days and 6 weeks after birth. AJR Am J Roentgenol 1995; 164:963–967.
34. Laing FC, Burke VD, Wing VW, Jeffrey RB, Hashimoto B. Postpartum evaluation of fetal hydronephrosis: optimal timing for follow-up sonography. Radiology 1984; 152:423–424.
35. Mahaffey SM, Ryckman FC, Martin LW. Clinical aspects of abdominal masses in children. Semin Roentgenol 1988; 23:161–174.
36. Taybi H, Lachman RS. Prune-Belly syndrome. Radiology of Syndromes, Metabolic Disorders and Skeletal Dysplasias. 4th ed. St. Louis: Mosby, 1996:405–406.

Urinary Tract Infection

37. Lebowitz RL, Mandell J. Urinary tract infection in children: putting radiology in its place. Radiology 1987; 165:1–9.
38. Dillon MJ, Goonasekera CDA. Reflux nephropathy. J Am Soc Nephrol 1998; 9:2377–2383.
39. Slovis TL. Is there a single most appropriate imaging workup of a child with an acute febrile urinary tract infection? Pediatr Radiol 1995; 25:S46–S49.
40. Jakobsson B, Jacobson SH, Hjalmas K. Vesico-ureteric reflux and other risk factors for renal damage: identification of high- and low-risk children. Acta Paediatr Suppl 1999; 431:31–39.
41. Hayden CK, Swischuk LE, Fawcett HD, Rytting JE, McCord G. Urinary tract infections in childhood: a current imaging approach. Radiographics 1986; 6:1023–1037.
42. Sty JR, Wells RG, Starshak RJ, Schroeder BA. Imaging in acute renal infection in children. AJR Am J Roentgenol 1987; 148:471–477.
43. Dacher JN, Pfister C, Monroc M, Eurin D, La Dosseur P. Power Doppler sonographic pattern of acute pyelonephritis in children: comparison with CT. AJR Am J Roentgenol 1996; 166:1451–1455.
44. Zamir G, Sakran W, Horowitz Y, Koren A, Miron D. Urinary tract infection: is there a need for routine renal ultrasonography? Arch Dis Child 2004; 89:466–468.
45. Stokland E, Hellstrom M, Jakobsson B, Sixt R. Imaging of renal scarring. Acta Paediatr Suppl 1999; 431:13–21.
46. Ginalski JM, Michaud A, Genton N. Renal growth retardation in children: sign suggestive of vesicoureteral reflux? AJR Am J Roentgenol 1985; 145:617–619.
47. Committee on quality improvement: subcommittee on urinary tract infection. Practice parameter: the diagnosis, treatment and evaluation of the initial urinary tract infection in febrile infants and young children. Pediatrics 1999; 103:843–852. Errata. Pediatrics 1999; 103:1052 and Pediatrics 1999; 104:118.
48. Jodal U, Lindberg U. Guidelines for management of children with urinary tract infection and vesico-ureteric reflux. Recommendations from a Swedish start-of-the-art conference. Acta Paediatr Suppl 1999; 431:97–99.
49. Alon US. Should renal ultrasonography be done routinely in children with first urinary tract infection? Clin Pediatr 1999; 38:21–25.
50. Berrocal T, Gaya F, Arjonilla A, Lonergan GJ. Vesicoureteral reflux: diagnosis and grading with echo-enhanced cystosonography versus voiding cystourethrography. Radiology 2001; 221:359–365.
51. Bosio M. Cystosonography with echocontrast: a new imaging modality to detect vesicoureteric reflux in children. Pediatr Radiol 1998; 28:250–255.
52. Piaggio G, degk'Innocenti ML, Toma P, Calevo MG, Perfumo F. Cystosonography and voiding cystourethrography in the diagnosis of vesicoureteral reflux. Pediatr Nephrol 2003; 18:18–22.
53. Riccabona M. Cystography in infants and children: a critical appraisal of the many forms with special regard to voiding cystourethrography. Eur Radiol 2002; 12:2910–2918.
54. Rypens F, Avni EF, Bank WO, Schulman CC, Struyven J. The ureterovesical junction in children: sonographic findings after surgical or endoscopic treatment. AJR Am J Roentgenol 1992; 158:837–843.
55. Chertin B, Puri P. Endoscopic management of vesicoureteral reflux: does it stand the test of time? Eur Urol 2002; 42:598–606.
56. Paltiel HJ, Diamond DA, Zurakowski D, Drubach LA, Atala A. Endoscopic treatment of vesicoureteral reflux with autologous chondrocytes postoperative sonographic features. Radiology 2004; 232:390–397.

Renal Cystic Disease

57. McHugh K, Stringer DA, Hebert D, Babiak CA. Simple renal cysts in children: diagnosis and follow-up with US. Radiology 1991; 178:383–385.
58. Lonergan GJ, Rice RR, Suarez ES. Autosomal recessive polycystic kidney disease: radiologic-pathologic correlation. Radiographics 2000; 20:837–855.
59. Avni FE, Guissard G, Hall M, et al. Hereditary polycystic kidney diseases in children: changing sonographic patterns through childhood. Pediatr Radiol 2002; 32:169–174.
60. Lucaya J, Enriquez G, Nieto J, et al. Renal calcifications in patients with autosomal recessive polycystic kidney disease: prevalence and cause. AJR Am J Roentgenol 1993; 160:359–362.
61. Fick-Brosnahan, Tran ZV, Johnson AM, et al. Progression of autosomal-dominant polycystic kidney disease in children. Kidney Int 2001; 59: 1654–1662.
62. Bernstein J. Renal cystic disease in the tuberous sclerosis complex. Pediatr Nephrol 1993; 7:490–495.
63. Luisiri A, Sotelo-Avila C, Silberstein MJ, et al. Sonography of the Aellweger syndrome. J Ultrasound Med 1988; 7:169–173.

Neoplasms

64. Donaldson JS, Shkolnik A. Pediatric renal masses. Semin Roentgenol 1988; 23:194–204.
65. Montgomery P, Kuhn JP, Berger PE, et al. Multifocal nephroblastomatosis: clinical significance and imaging. Pediatr Radiol 1984; 14:392–395.
66. Jaffe MH, White SJ, Silver TM, et al. Wilms' tumor: ultrasonic features, pathologic correlation, and diagnostic pitfalls. Radiology 1981; 140:147–152.
67. Weese DL, Applebaum H, Taber P. Mapping intravascular extension of Wilms' tumor with magnetic resonance imaging. J Pediatr Surg 1991; 26:64–67.
68. Slovis TL, Philippart AI, Cushing B, et al. Evaluation of the inferior vena cava by sonography and venography in children with renal and hepatic tumors. Radiology 1981; 140:767–772.
69. White KS, Kirks DR, Bove KE. Imaging of nephroblastomatosis: an overview. Radiology 1992; 182:1–5.
70. Cohen MD, Bugaieski EM, Haliloglu M, Faught P, Siddiqui A. Visual presentation of the staging of pediatric solid tumors. Radiographics 1996; 16:523–545.
71. Teele RL, Share JC. Ultrasonography of Infants and Children. Philadelphia: W. B. Saunders, 1991:252–255, 269–271.
72. Breslow NE, Takashima JR, Whitton JA, Moksness J, D'Angio GJ, Green DM. Second malignant neoplasms following treatment for Wilms' tumor: a report from the National Wilms' Tumor Study Group. J Clin Oncol 1995; 13(8):1851–1859.
73. Kraus RA, Gaisie G, Young LW. Increased renal parenchymal echogenicity: causes in pediatric patients. Radiographics 1990; 10:1009–1081.
74. Strauss S, Libson E, Schwartz E, et al. Renal sonography in American Burkitt lymphoma. AJR Am J Roentgenol 1986; 146:549–552.
75. Charboneau JW, James EM, Reading CC. Sonography case of the day: case 3: Burkitt lymphoma with diffuse renal involvement. AJR Am J Roentgenol 1984; 142:1075–1079.
76. Alford DA, Coccia PF, L'Heureux. Roentgenographic features of American Burkitt's lymphoma. Radiology 1977; 124:763–770.
77. Agrons GA, Wagner BJ, Davidson AJ, Suarez GS. Multilocular cystic renal tumors in children: radiologic-pathologic correlation. Radiographics 1995; 15:653–669.
78. Chan HSL, Cheng MY, Mancer K, et al. Congenital mesoblastic nephroma: a clinicoradiologic study of 17 cases representing the pathologic spectrum of the disease. J Pediatr 1987; 111:64–70.

Medical Renal Disease

79. Choyke PL, Grant EG, Hoffer FA, Tina L, Dorec S. Cortical echogenicity in the hemolytic uremic syndrome: clinical correlation. J Ultrasound Med 1988; 7:439–442.
80. Patriquin HB, O'Regan S, Robitaille P, Paltiel H. Hemolytic-uremic syndrome: intrarenal arterial Doppler patterns as a useful guide to therapy. Radiology 1989; 172:625–628.
81. Pearse DM, Kaude JV, Williams JL, Bush D, Wright PG. Sonographic diagnosis of furosemide-induced Nephrocalcinosis in newborn infants. J Ultrasound Med 1984; 3:553–556.
82. Shultz PK, Strife JL, Strife CF, McDaniel JD. Hyperechoic renal medullary pyramids in infants and children. Radiology 1991; 181:163–167.
83. Jequier S, Kaplan BS. Echogenic renal pyramids in children. J Clin Ultrasound 1991; 19:85–92.
84. Ozturk A, Haliloglu M, Akpinar E, Tekgul S. Cellular congenital mesoblastic nephroma with Contralateral medullary Nephrocalcinosis. Br J Radiol 2004; 77:436–437.
85. Navarro O, Daneman A, Kooh SW. Asymmetric medullary nephrocalcinosis in two children. Pediatr Radiol 1998; 28:687–690.

Renal Vein Thrombosis

86. Hibbert J, Howlett DC, Greenwood KL, MacDonald LM, Saunders AJS. The ultrasound appearances of neonatal renal vein thrombosis. Br J Radiol 1997; 70:1191–1194.
87. Orazi C, Fariello G, Malena S, et al. Renal vein thrombosis and adrenal hemorrhage in the newborn: ultrasound evaluation of 4 cases. J Clin Ultrasound 1993; 21:163–169.
88. Lin GJ, Yang PH, Wang ML. Neonatal renal venous thrombosis—a case report describing serial sonographic changes. Pediatr Neprol 1994; 8:589–591.
89. Wright NB, Blanch G, Walkinshaw S, Pilling DW. Antenatal and neonatal renal vein thrombosis: new ultrasonic features with high frequency transducers. Pediatr Radiol 1996; 26:686–689.
90. Laplante S, Patriquin HB, Robitaille P. Renal vein thrombosis in children; evidence of early flow recovery with Doppler US. Radiology 1993; 189:37–42.

Neuroblastoma

91. Bousvaros A, Kirks DR, Grossman H. Imaging of neuroblastoma: an overview. Pediatr Radiol 1986; 16:89–106.
92. Hayes FA, Smith EI. Neuroblastoma. In: Pizzo PA, Poplack DG, eds. Principles and Practice of Pediatric Oncology. Philadelphia: JB Lippincott, 1989:607–622.
93. Abramson SJ. Adrenal neoplasms in children. Radiol Clin North Am 1997; 35(6):1415–1453.
94. Amundson GM, Trevenen CL, Mueller DL, et al. Neuroblastoma: a specific sonographic tissue pattern. AJR Am J Roentgenol 1987; 148:943–945.
95. Peretz GS, Lam AH. Distinguishing neuroblastoma from Wilms' tumor by computed tomography. J Comput Assist Tomogr 1985; 9:889–893.
96. Brodeur GM, Pritchard J, Berthold F, et al. Revisions of the international criteria for neuroblastoma diagnosis, staging, and response to treatment. J Clin Oncol 1993; 11:1466.
97. Brodeur GM, Seeger RC, Barrett A, et al. International criteria for diagnosis, staging, and response to treatment in patients with neuroblastoma. J Clin Oncol 1988; 6:1874–1881.
98. Daneman A. Adrenal neoplasms in children. Semin Roentgenol 1988; 23:205–215.
99. Donnelly LF, Rencken IO, Shardell K, et al. Renal cell carcinoma after therapy for neuroblastoma. AJR Am J Roentgenol 1996; 167:915–917.
100. Medeiros LJ, Palmedo G, Krigman HR, Kovacs G, Beckwith JB. Oncocytoid renal cell carcinoma after neuroblastoma: a report of four cases of a distinct clinicopathologic entity. Am J Surg Path 1999; 23(7):772–780.
101. Fleitz JL, Wootton-Gorges SL, Wyatt-Ashmead J, et al. Renal cell carcinoma following treatment of advanced stage neuroblastoma in early childhood. Pediatr Radiol 2003; 33:540–545.
102. Meadows AT, Baum E, Fossati-Gellani F, et al. Second malignant neoplasms in children: an update from the late effects study group. J Clin Oncol 1985; 3:532–538.
103. Ribeiro RC, Michalkiewicz EL, Figueiredo BC, et al. Adrenocortical tumors in children. Braz J Med Bio Res 2000; 33:1225–1234.
104. Boothroyd A, Dicks-Mireau C, Malone M. Adrenal cortical tumors in children. Eur J Radiol 1994; 18:199–204.
105. Godine L, Berdon W, Brasch R, et al. Adrenocortical carcinoma with extension into inferior vena cava and right atrium: report of three cases in children. Pediatr Radiol 1990; 20:166–168.

Adrenal Hemorrhage

106. Westra SJ, Zaninovic AC, Hall TR, Kangarloo H, Boechat MI. Imaging of the adrenal gland in children. Radiographics 1994; 13:1323–1340.
107. Heij HA, Taets van Amerongen AHM, Ekkelkamp S, Vos A. Diagnosis and management of neonatal adrenal hemorrhage. Pediatr Radiol 1989; 19:391–394.
108. Wu CC. Sonographic spectrum of neonatal adrenal hemorrhage: report of a case simulating solid tumor. J Clin Ultrasound 1989; 17:45–49.
109. Yang WT, Ku KW, Metreweli C. Case report: neonatal adrenal hemorrhage presenting as an acute right scrotal swelling (hematoma)—value of ultrasound. Clin Radiol 1995; 50:127–129.
110. Nader EP, Barksdale EM Jr. Adrenal masses in the newborn. Sem Pediatr Surg 2000; 9:156–164.

The Pediatric Pelvis

Rebecca Stein-Wexler

28

INTRODUCTION

Transabdominal ultrasound constitutes the principal approach to the pediatric pelvis. The acoustic window provided by a full bladder greatly assists in evaluation of pelvic organs, but this can be difficult to achieve in the child who has not yet developed control of bladder function. However, the bladder can usually be adequately filled by orally administered fluid; rarely is placement of a urethral catheter for retrograde filling necessary. Water enema can help differentiate normal bowel from pathologic processes, though this too is rarely necessary. Coronal and axial images are obtained with the patient supine; oblique positioning often helps delineate the ovaries. Depending on patient size, a 5 to 10 MHz transducer is employed. Although transvaginal ultrasound can provide significant additional information (1), it has little application in pediatric radiology, being useful only in older girls who have had sexual intercourse or a speculum examination.

Transperineal ultrasound is helpful in evaluating disorders of the urethra, vagina, and bladder base. With the patient in a modified lithotomy position, evaluation is performed with a 5 MHz or higher transducer positioned over the perineum (2,3).

NORMAL DEVELOPMENT

Uterus

The newborn's uterus, stimulated by maternal estrogens, is relatively large, having a mean length of 3.4 cm (4). It usually has a spade-like or tubular configuration with the anteroposterior (AP) diameter of the cervix (mean 1.41 cm) being larger than that of the uterine body (mean 1.26 cm) (Fig. 1) (4). The endometrial cavity can be defined in 97% of patients (4), and endometrial fluid is seen in 23% of newborns (5).

As estrogen levels wane, the size of the uterine body and cervix decreases. The uterus assumes a more uniformly tube-like configuration as the AP diameter of uterine body and cervix become similar (Fig. 2) (4), although some patients retain the configuration of the relatively large cervix (6). Uterine length ranges from 2.5 to 4 cm, and AP thickness up to 1 cm, with the size remaining stable from three to six months until approximately seven years (6,7). Uterine volume then gradually begins to increase, and the uterine body becomes larger than the cervix (7–10). Finally, with onset of puberty, the uterus assumes an adult configuration, and cyclic changes in the endometrium become apparent (Chapter 36). Normal uterine measurements can be found in Table 1, but a practical upper value for prepubertal girls is 4.5 cm for length and 1 cm for thickness (11).

Doppler interrogation of the uterine artery can help determine whether onset of puberty is imminent, as the flow pattern changes from a narrow band of systolic flow in prepubertal girls to a systolic–diastolic flow wave at puberty (12), perhaps as the growing uterus undergoes angiogenesis. Simultaneously, with puberty the pulsatility index drops from a mean of

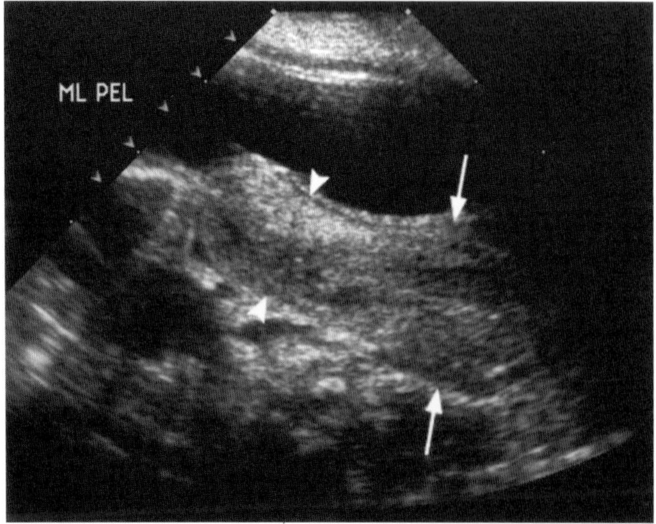

FIGURE 1 ■ Newborn uterus. On this sagittal midline US, the uterus is relatively large, and the cervix (*arrows*) is bigger than the fundus (*arrowheads*).

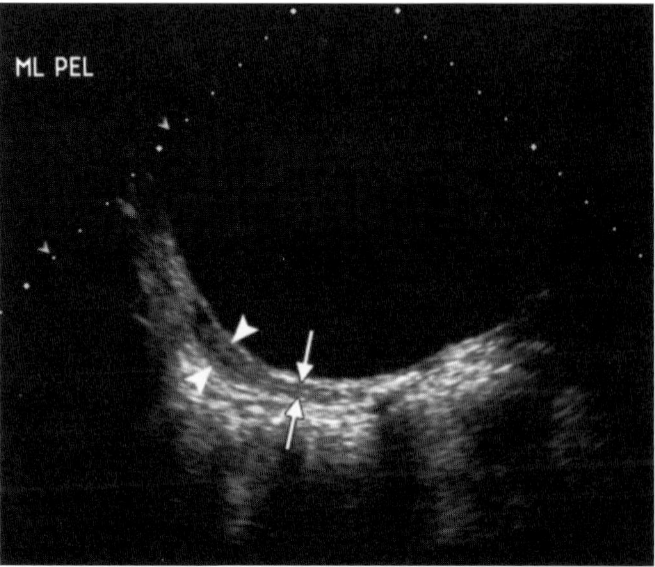

FIGURE 2 ■ Child uterus. This sagittal midline US of an eight-year-old girl reveals the typical tube-like configuration of the uterine cervix (*arrowheads*) and fundus (*arrows*) throughout most of childhood.

6.27 to a mean of 3.7; at the end of puberty, it is less than three (12). Assessment of pulsatility index can assist with evaluation of sexual precocity (13).

Ovaries

Ovarian position in neonates is quite variable. Although most often found along the superior margin of the posterior fold of the broad ligament, the ovaries can be located anywhere from the inferior margin of the kidney to the broad ligament, reflecting their normal pattern of descent (14). The ligaments that support the ovary are quite flexible, which allows ovarian position to change, depending on factors such as bladder fullness and ovarian size (15).

Ovarian volume is stable until approximately nine years, lagging two years behind uterine enlargement. Ovarian growth is then relatively rapid, reaching an average

TABLE 1 ■ Uterine Diameters and Volume[a]

		Uterine diameters (mm)				Uterine volume (cm^3)	
Age (yr)	No. of patients	TUL (mean ± SD)	COAP (mean ± SD)	CEAP (mean ± SD)	COAP/CEAP (mean ± SD)	By chronologic age (mean ± SD)	By bone age (mean ± SD)
2	7	33.1 ± 4.4	7.0 ± 3.4	8.3 ± 2.0	0.84 ± 0.29	1.98 ± 1.58	1.76 ± 0.72
3	8	32.4 ± 4.3	6.4 ± 1.3	7.6 ± 2.2	0.89 ± 0.29	1.63 ± 0.81	1.80 ± 0.74
4	15	32.9 ± 3.3	7.6 ± 1.8	8.6 ± 1.8	0.90 ± 0.22	2.10 ± 0.57	1.97 ± 0.74
5	7	33.1 ± 5.5	8.0 ± 2.8	8.4 ± 1.6	0.95 ± 0.28	2.36 ± 1.39	2.19 ± 1.16
6	9	33.2 ± 4.1	6.7 ± 2.9	7.5 ± 1.8	0.86 ± 0.18	1.80 ± 1.57	1.65 ± 0.93
7	9	32.3 ± 3.9	8.0 ± 2.2	7.7 ± 2.5	1.08 ± 0.26	2.32 ± 1.07	2.81 ± 1.44
8	11	35.8 ± 7.3	9.0 ± 2.8	8.4 ± 1.7	1.05 ± 0.20	3.12 ± 1.52	2.70 ± 1.43
9	11	37.1 ± 4.4	9.7 ± 3.0	8.8 ± 2.0	1.10 ± 0.24	3.70 ± 1.62	2.69 ± 1.83
10	13	40.3 ± 6.4	12.8 ± 5.3	10.7 ± 2.6	1.17 ± 0.31	6.54 ± 3.78	4.66 ± 3.03
11	13	42.2 ± 5.1	12.8 ± 3.1	10.7 ± 2.6	1.22 ± 0.26	6.66 ± 2.87	6.24 ± 3.07
12	6	54.3 ± 8.4	17.3 ± 5.3	14.3 ± 5.2	1.23 ± 0.16	16.18 ± 9.15	8.88 ± 3.65
13	5	53.8 ± 11.4	15.8 ± 4.5	15.0 ± 2.4	1.03 ± 0.15	13.18 ± 5.64	15.55 ± 5.98

[a]As determined by ultrasonography in 114 girls from age 2 to 13 years.

Abbreviations: TUL, total uterine length; COAP, anteroposterior diameter of the corpus; CEAP, anteroposterior diameter of the cervix.

Source: From Ref. 6.

TABLE 2 ■ Ovarian Volumes in Girls Aged 1 Day to 24 Months[a]

Age	No. of patients	No. of ovaries imaged	Ovarian volume (cm³) Mean (SD)	95% CI
1 day to 3 mo	34	34	1.06 (0.96)	0.03–3.56
4–12 mo	21	34	1.05 (0.67)	0.18–2.71
13–24 mo	22	30	0.67 (0.35)	0.15–1.68

[a]Volumes are based on measurements made on sonograms.
Source: From Ref. 17.

TABLE 4 ■ Ovarian Volume by Decade of Life

Decade	Mean volume (cm³)	Standard deviation	No. of ovaries	95% CI (cm³)[a]
1	1.7	1.4	19	0.2–4.9
2	7.8	4.4	83	1.7–18.5
3	10.2	6.2	308	2.6–23.1
4	9.5	5.4	358	2.6–20.7
5	9.0	5.8	206	2.1–20.9
6	6.2	3.6	57	1.6–14.2
7	6.0	3.8	44	1.0–15.0

[a]Calculated on the basis of cube root values, then transformed back to cubic centimeters.
Source: From Ref. 16.

volume of 4.2 mL (1 SD = 2.3 mL) just before menarche (6). Subsequent normal ovarian volume can be much greater [9.8 mL, 1 SD = 5.8 mL (16)]. Age-specific values can be found in Tables 2 to 4 but a practical upper limit of normal for the premenarchal ovary is 4.5 mL (11).

Small follicular cysts (Fig. 3), which are numerous throughout childhood, occur in response to pulsatile gonadotropin-releasing hormone. Microcysts (<9 mm) are described in as many as 84% of neonatal or infant ovaries (17) and 68% of ovaries in older girls (Fig. 4) (18), although other recent studies have found a much lower incidence in the older age group (19).

The incidence of larger cysts is somewhat controversial. With early ultrasound equipment, macrocysts were not identified in girls less than 12 years old (6), but modern equipment demonstrates cysts much more readily; overall the incidence of macrocysts (>9 mm) is 18% in newborns and infants up to 24 months old (17) and approximately 11% in girls between 2 and 12 years of age (18). Cysts larger than 2 cm are much more common in girls less than two years old (17,19), initially because of residual maternal placental chorionic gonadotropins and later due to transient neonatal production of gonadotropins (19). However, a recent study of 139 girls less than 14 years old found no cysts larger than 2 cm (9).

TABLE 3 ■ Ovarian Volume[a]

Age (yr)	No. of patients	Ovarian volume (cm³) By chronologic age (mean ± SD)	By bone age (mean ± SD)
2	5	0.75 ± 0.41	0.78 ± 0.38
3	6	0.66 ± 0.17	0.64 ± 0.18
4	14	0.82 ± 0.36	1.00 ± 0.45
5	4	0.86 ± 0.02	0.95 ± 0.52
6	9	1.19 ± 0.36	1.05 ± 0.65
7	8	1.26 ± 0.59	1.23 ± 0.47
8	10	1.05 ± 0.50	1.29 ± 0.33
9	11	1.98 ± 0.76	1.35 ± 0.71
10	12	2.22 ± 0.69	1.47 ± 0.56
11	12	2.52 ± 1.30	2.45 ± 0.86
12	6	3.80 ± 1.40	3.10 ± 1.29
13	4	4.18 ± 2.30	4.38 ± 2.74

[a]As determined by ultrasonography in 101 girls from age 2 to 13 years.
Source: From Ref. 6.

NEONATAL PELVIS

Ovarian Cysts

As discussed above, cysts are a common feature of the neonatal ovary. Neonatal ovarian cysts are almost always benign and represent follicular or corpus luteal cysts. As maternal hormonal stimulation and fetal pituitary follicle-stimulating hormone secretion decrease significantly after birth, many ovarian cysts, especially those smaller

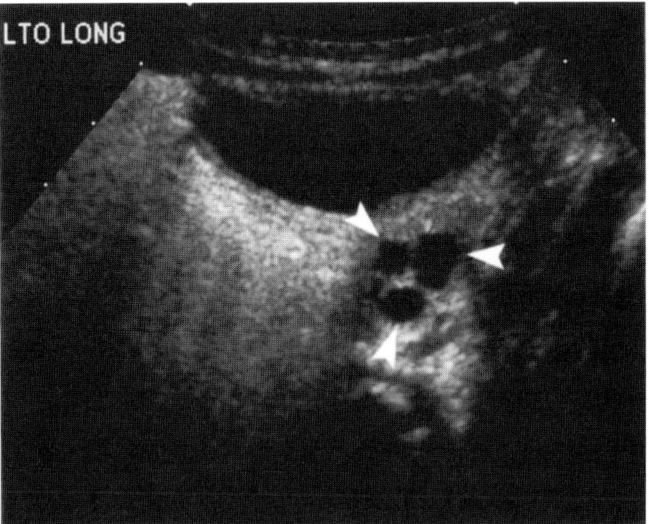

FIGURE 3 ■ Normal newborn ovary. Longitudinal US demonstrates three small follicular cysts within a normal ovary (*arrowheads*).

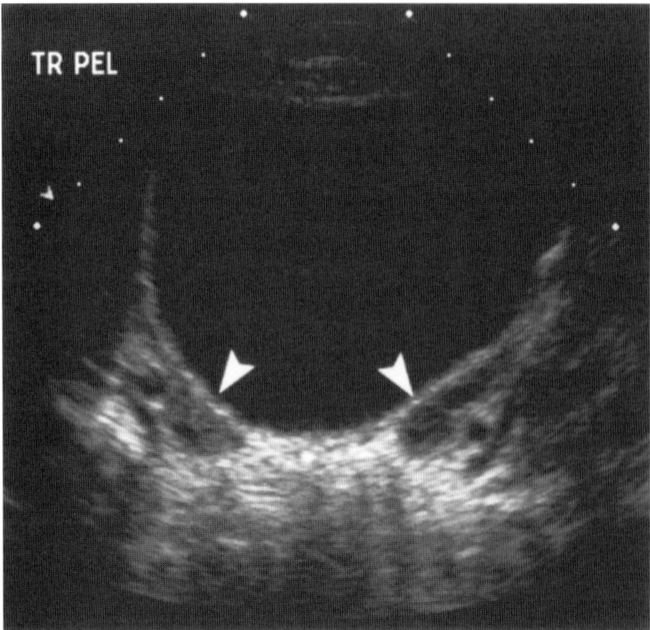

FIGURE 4 ■ Normal ovaries in childhood. This transverse US demonstrates both right and left ovaries (*arrowheads*) in a nine-year-old girl, with bilateral microcysts evident.

than 5 cm in diameter (20–22), spontaneously regress by about six months (20,23). Simple ovarian cysts in the neonate are anechoic and have an imperceptible wall (24). A simple ovarian cyst must be differentiated from a torsed cyst, hydrometrocolpos, meconium pseudocyst, urachal cyst, bowel obstruction, renal cyst, lymphangioma, and an anterior meningocele (Table 5). If the cyst is complex, neoplasm is also a consideration, although the likelihood of malignancy is extremely low [there being one case of ovarian malignancy in a child below two years old in the literature (25)].

TABLE 5 ■ Cystic Mass in Neonate

Differential diagnosis for cystic pelvic mass in the neonate	Properties
Simple ovarian cyst	Anechoic, thin-walled
Torsed ovarian cyst	Complex, fluid–fluid level
Hydrometrocolpos	Echogenic fluid common
	Identifiable thick-walled uterus
Urachal cyst	Cephalad to bladder
Meconium pseudocyst	Snowstorm calcifications, possible bowel obstruction
Bowel duplication	Adjacent to bowel
Bowel obstruction	Multiple dilated bowel loops
Renal cyst	Adjacent to kidney
Anterior meningocele	Anterior sacral defect
Cystic sacrococcygeal teratoma	Complex, cystic, or solid
	Close to coccyx
Bladder	Volume varies during examination

Neonatal Ovarian Torsion

The normal Fallopian tube and ovary are very mobile, and this predisposes these structures to torsion (26). Although torsion can occur postnatally, it is more common in utero (20). The newborn is usually asymptomatic (24), but presenting signs can include pain, vomiting, fever, abdominal distension, and leukocytosis (21). Differentiating between the torsed ovary and the simple ovarian cyst is important but can be problematic. Although there are exceptions, cysts greater than 5 cm are more prone to torsion, and it is therefore usually safe to observe smaller simple cysts with serial ultrasound (19,20,22,23). Aspiration for cysts greater than 4 or 5 cm can be helpful (25,27). Torsed ovaries in neonates are usually intra-abdominal rather than intrapelvic in location (28) and are of follicular origin (24).

However, if the cyst has complex characteristics (beyond a few thin septations), such as a fluid–fluid or fluid–debris level suggesting hemorrhage (28), or if it is filled with echogenic material that may represent retracting clot, torsion may have already occurred (Fig. 5) (20,24,26,29), although perinatal stress may also result in hemorrhage (21). Treatment is controversial. Percutaneous cyst puncture has proven helpful in several cases (20,23,30), but this does not allow fixation of the contralateral ovary, which is recommended by some (26). Many cases of neonatal ovarian torsion are treated surgically with oophorectomy or cystectomy (20), and laparoscopy has been successful (30). However, some recommend a conservative approach in asymptomatic infants, removing or draining only those cysts that are symptomatic (31) and allowing the others to involute and eventually calcify.

Uterine Obstruction

High levels of maternal estrogen stimulation can result in abundant mucus secretion from the fetus's endometrial and cervical glands (32,33). If there is obstruction to egress of this material, hydrocolpos (fluid-filled vagina) or hydrometrocolpos (fluid-filled uterus and vagina) develops. For patients exposed to lower levels of maternal estrogen, obstruction may manifest at menarche with hematocolpos or hematometrocolpos; later diagnosis is also more likely if the obstruction does not accompany obvious abnormalities such as urogenital sinus and cloaca. Should mucus enter the peritoneal cavity via the Fallopian tubes, hydrometros may give rise to peritonitis, similar to meconium peritonitis (34). Note that a small amount of vaginal fluid can be a normal finding in young girls due to reflux of urine from the bladder into the vagina during voiding in the supine position.

Hydrocolpos is more common than hydrometrocolpos. With hydrocolpos, the vagina appears as an elongated, thin-walled tubular structure posterior to the bladder, containing fluid of variable echogenicity (Fig. 6). The thick-walled uterus can usually be seen extending cephalad from the distended vagina, and occasionally fluid is also seen within the uterine cavity (hydrometrocolpos). The walls of

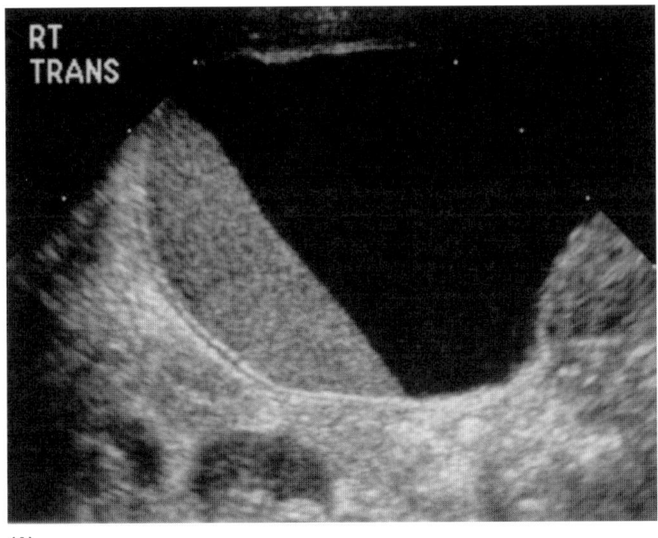

(A)

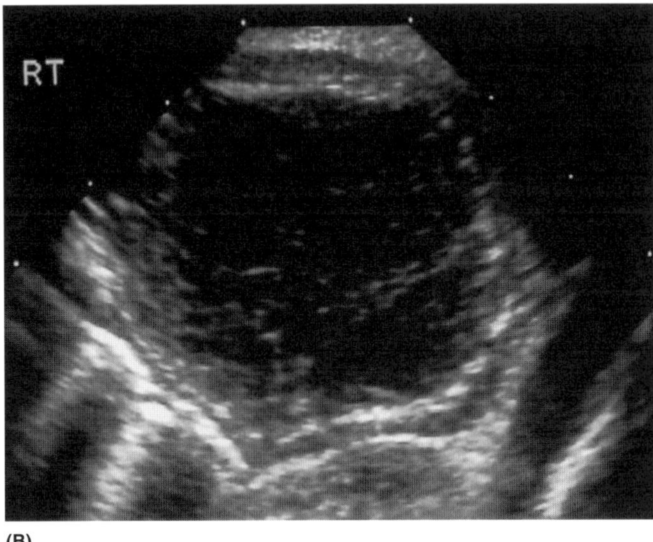

(B)

FIGURE 5 A AND B ■ Torsed ovarian cysts in neonates. (**A**) The fluid–debris level indicates that torsion has probably occurred. (**B**) This cyst is filled with echogenic thrombus, another finding that indicates torsion.

the uterus are much thicker than are those of the vagina, and in the neonate they are less plastic. Consequently, the uterus dilates much less than the vagina, and the fluid-filled vagina appears relatively large (35).

In neonates, vaginal obstruction is usually associated with urogenital sinus or cloaca, anomalies that occur most often with intersex states, especially with virilization due to elevated testosterone levels seen with congenital adrenal hyperplasia (35); these cases usually come to medical attention due to ambiguous genitalia. Uterine duplication may also be present. Although obstruction can also result from isolated imperforate hymen, vaginal septum, or vaginal atresia/stenosis (34,35), these cases are more likely to present in adolescence with amenorrhea or a pelvic mass. Differential considerations for a cystic midline mass or a midline mass with internal echoes or a debris–fluid level in the newborn include ovarian cyst, bowel duplication cyst, meconium pseudocyst, and rectovesical fistula. Hydro(metro)colpos can also be mistaken for the bladder if the bladder is collapsed.

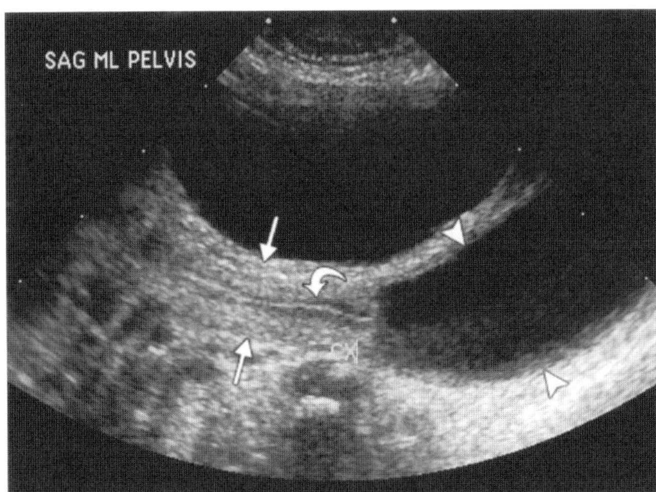

FIGURE 6 ■ Hydrocolpos in a small infant with congenital adrenal hyperplasia. The distended vagina (*arrowheads*) is filled with complex fluid, secondary to communication with a urogenital sinus. The uterus (*arrows*) is seen as echogenic soft tissue projecting cephalad; note the endometrial stripe (*curved arrow*).

Hydronephrosis and Renal Anomalies

Hydronephrosis and renal anomalies commonly accompany these disorders, and therefore both renal and adrenal ultrasounds are important adjuncts to pelvic ultrasound in the patient with hydrocolpos. Other anomalies such as esophageal, duodenal, or anal atresia, as well as congenital heart disease, may also accompany these abnormalities. Hydronephrosis may also occur simply secondary to mass effect on the distal ureters.

In the absence of urogenital sinus or cloaca, hemato(metro)colpos is more likely to present in adolescence, due to vaginal atresia, vaginal septum, or imperforate hymen. Imperforate hymen is a simple disorder, readily diagnosed by recognition of thin mucosa bulging into the introitus and easily remedied by an incision. Transperineal ultrasound demonstrates the lack of significant soft tissue separating the dilated vagina from perineal skin (3). Occurring as an isolated problem, imperforate hymen is not accompanied by renal or other genital anomalies.

The thickness of vaginal septum or extent of the atresia can also be quantified by transperineal ultrasound (3,36,37). Vaginal atresia and uterine anomalies can present as part of the Mayer–Rokitansky–Kuster–Hauser syndrome, thought to occur when a toxic substance or genetically induced event interferes with Müllerian, Wolffian, metanephros, and mesodermal interactions (38). These patients have a 50% chance of unilateral renal agenesis (38). If the atresia is high, the uterus may dilate in the absence of vaginal dilation.

Uterine and vaginal duplications occur when the septum between the two fused portions of the uterus and vagina fails to involute. This is discussed more fully in Chapter 36, when it becomes important to fertility. In childhood, duplicated genitalia are usually diagnosed when they are complicated by obstruction or ambiguous genitalia (39).

Intersex States

Ultrasound provides critical information in the workup of a patient with ambiguous genitalia, and in the neonate it must be performed promptly to facilitate early gender assignation. It is essential to determine whether a uterus and ovaries are present, and this is most easily done in the early neonatal period, when these structures are relatively large due to maternal hormonal stimulation. It is also very important to try to locate the gonads—whether they are pelvic, inguinal, or perineal (Fig. 7). Their echotexture must be assessed: Ovaries typically appear heterogeneous, possibly with identifiable small cysts (40), whereas testes appear uniformly homogeneous. An ovotestis may demonstrate both characteristics. When the gonads are located in the inguinal area, their superficial position makes their echotexture especially easy to assess (41).

Some understanding of the embryological development of the genitalia sheds light on the complex topic of intersex states. The Fallopian tubes, uterus, and upper vagina develop from the paired Müllerian ducts, which fuse to form the uterus and vagina and then undergo tubulation. In the male, Müllerian inhibitory substance diffuses from the adjacent testis, causing the ipsilateral Müllerian duct to involute. Stimulated by testosterone produced in the fetal testis, Wolffian structures (vas deferens, epididymis, and seminal vesicles) develop (42). In the absence of Müllerian inhibitory substance and testosterone, female genitalia develop. Table 6 summarizes the four intersex states.

The female pseudohermaphrodite is the most common intersex state and was also addressed in the section entitled Uterine Obstruction in the Neonate. This state occurs most often when increased levels of testosterone precursors accumulate in an XX fetus, due to deficiency of the enzyme 21-α hydroxylase (43), but increased maternal circulating androgen levels also give rise to this disorder. Masculinization of the external genitalia results in overgrowth of the genital tubercle and consequent clitoral enlargement, a variable degree of fusion of the labioscrotal folds, and persistence of the urogenital sinus, which consists of fusion of the distal vagina with what is often a masculinized urethra. Depending on when this insult occurs, the degree of masculinization of the external genitalia is more or less severe (43). Two ovaries and the uterus are present (42) and can usually be identified ultrasonographically (44). The adrenal glands can be but are not always enlarged from their normal thickness of 3 to 6 mm (for one limb) (43). They can also appear as redundant rope-like coils of hypertrophied cortical tissue (45). Adrenal cortical dysfunction results in a variable degree of salt wasting (46). Renal anomalies are common.

The other three intersex states are encountered much less frequently. Male pseudohermaphrodites have XY karyotype but androgen deficiency or end-organ insensitivity to normal androgen levels. These patients have normal testes, but they are cryptorchid, often located in the inguinal canal. Lacking either testosterone or the ability to react to it, the external genitalia appear feminized. Neither the uterus or ovaries are present (42). True hermaphrodites are quite rare and have both male and female gonadal tissue, consisting of one testis and one ovary, or, most often, two ovotestes. Their most common karyotype is a 46XY/46XX mosaic. Multiple scattered cysts in the ovotestes result in heterogeneous parenchyma (47). The gonads can be intra-abdominal, cryptorchid, or scrotal in location,

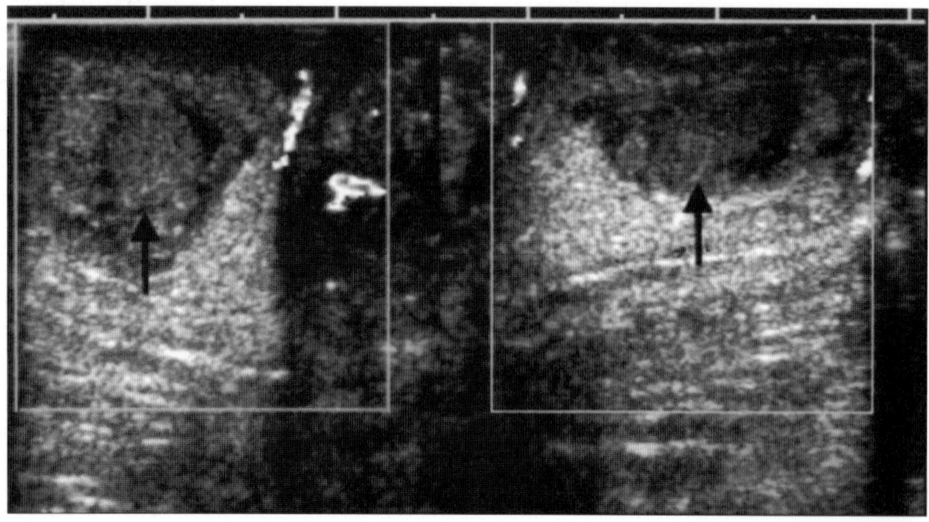

FIGURE 7 ■ Testes (*arrows*) and epididymi appear high in "labia" in a newborn male pseudohermaphrodite, with female-appearing external genitalia but no uterus or ovaries.

TABLE 6 ■ Intersex States

Condition	Mechanism	Manifestation	Ultrasound
Female pseudohermaphroditism	XX Elevated testosterone precursors Deficient 21-α hydroxylase Elevated maternal androgen	Masculinized external genitalia Fused labioscrotal folds Persistent urogenital sinus	Uterus 2 ovaries Possible enlarged adrenals Renal anomalies Possible hydrocolpos
Male pseudohermaphroditism	XY Androgen deficiency End-organ insensitivity to androgens	Feminized external genitalia	No uterus or ovaries Testes often cryptorchid
True hermaphrodite	Variable 46XY/XX mosaic most common	Male or female external genitalia Enlarged clitoris	Uterus: normal, bicornuate, hypoplastic Ovary and testis or 2 ovotestes in variable location
Mixed gonadal dysgenesis	XO/XY mosaic Deficient production of Müllerian inhibitory substance	Ambiguous external genitalia	Uterus 1 dysgenetic testis 1 streak ovary

and the uterus may be normal, bicornuate, or hypoplastic. Genital anatomy can resemble that of a normal male or appear female with slight clitoral enlargement. Mixed gonadal dysgenesis constitutes the fourth variety of intersex state, and these patients are usually mosaic 45XO/XY. They have deficient production of Müllerian inhibitory substance. Although a uterus is present, only one gonad, a dysgenetic testis, can be identified. The other consists of a "streak" ovary. External genitalia are usually ambiguous. These patients are at risk for gonadoblastoma, other germ-cell tumors, and Wilms tumor (42).

PELVIC ULTRASOUND POST INFANCY

Pelvic Masses

Most ovarian masses in young girls are cystic and benign, such as functional cysts, hemorrhagic cysts, and mature teratomas. Ovarian torsion can mimic an ovarian germ-cell tumor, but it is usually smaller and may show characteristic follicles. In older girls, the differential for cystic lesions is much broader and, in addition to functional and hemorrhagic cysts, mature teratomas, endometriomas, and tubo-ovarian abscesses, includes malignancy. Malignancy is more likely if the mass is solid (Table 7).

Ovarian Cysts

Even after the newborn period, ovarian cysts are common, accounting for more than 70% of ovarian masses (14). Cysts can be hemorrhagic or simple, follicular or corpus luteal cysts. The presence of a daughter cyst adjacent to a large cyst has a strong correlation with ovarian etiology (48); the daughter cyst is a follicular cyst. Normal follicular cysts are less than 3 cm in diameter. Functional but otherwise simple cysts are usually 4 to 10 cm and appear anechoic (Fig. 8). Surgical resection is recommended for symptomatic cysts; aspiration tends to be unsuccessful in older girls, as cysts may recur (25).

Hemorrhagic Cysts

These occur due to hemorrhage into either a corpus luteal or a follicular cyst. The appearance of hemorrhagic cysts

TABLE 7 ■ Pelvic Masses After Infancy

Cystic	Solid
Ovarian cyst	Torsed ovary (Possible peripheral cysts?)
Hemorrhagic cyst	Solid teratoma (greater risk for immaturity and malignancy)
Torsed ovarian cyst	Massive ovarian edema
Endometrioma	Tubo-ovarian abscess
Tubo-ovarian abscess	Germ-cell tumor Dysgerminoma Immature teratoma Endodermal sinus tumor Embryonal carcinoma Primary choriocarcinoma
Cystic teratoma	Sex cord/stromal tumors Juvenile granulosa-theca cell tumor Sertoli–Leydig cell tumor
Appendiceal abscess	Leukemia/lymphoma recurrence
Paraovarian cyst	
Epithelial cyst	

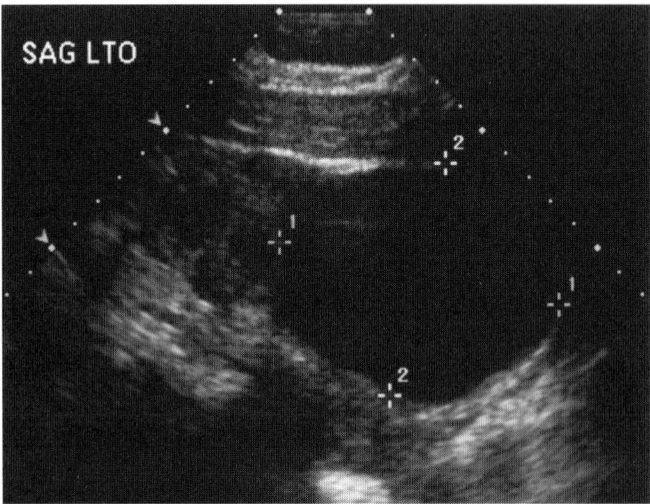

FIGURE 8 ■ Large simple ovarian cyst. This cyst, though large, demonstrates none of the complex characteristics that would suggest that hemorrhage, torsion, or tumor is present.

varies from anechoic to hypoechoic to moderately cystic; they can have thick walls and demonstrate septations (Fig. 9) (49). A hyperechoic mass within an anechoic ovarian mass suggests a hemorrhagic cyst, although this appearance can also be seen with teratomas, endometriomas, and abscesses (50). Almost all show enhanced through sound transmission, which allows differentiation from solid lesions. However, they can be difficult to differentiate from torsion, tubo-ovarian abscess, and cystic ovarian neoplasms. On followup, clot lysis should be apparent (49), and their size should decrease.

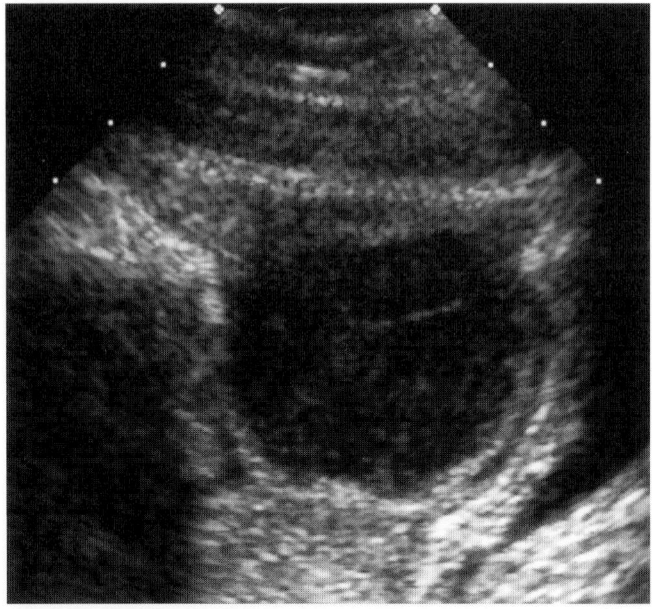

FIGURE 9 ■ Hemorrhagic cyst. The heterogeneous echotexture is typical of a hemorrhagic cyst.

Paraovarian Cysts

Located in the broad ligament and clearly separate from the ovary, these too may torse, necrose, or cause pain or mass effect if large (14).

Ovarian Torsion

Ovarian torsion occurs when the ovary, which is usually enlarged to greater than 5 cm in diameter, rotates on its axis, leading to arterial, venous, and lymphatic stasis, edema, and eventually hemorrhagic infarction (51). Like appendicitis, it presents with pain, but 50% of patients with torsion report similar previous episodes (49,52). Although chronic recurrent pain is considered typical, the average duration of symptoms in one study was approximately three days (53). Nausea and vomiting are also quite common, and approximately half of all patients demonstrate leukocytosis. Presentation thus mimics appendicitis, and, further confounding the situation, approximately 70% of torsions occur on the right (53).

The torsed ovary may be midline (51,53) or adnexal (28) in location. An adnexal location occurs more often in pubertal girls (28). The typical appearance of torsion in the pubertal girl is that of a solid mass with peripheral follicular cysts (28,54), whereas in young girls it is more likely cystic or solid with peripheral cysts (Fig. 10) (28). If cystic, it may be hypo- or hyperechoic but should demonstrate good through sound transmission (51). Peripheral follicular enlargement is attributed to transudation of fluid into follicles that results from ovarian congestion secondary to circulatory impairment (54). Torsed ovaries can demonstrate the "double wall" or "muscular rim" sign of hyperechogenic mucosa rimmed with hypoechoic muscularis that has been thought to be specific to hollow gastrointestinal tract structures (23,55). The presence of free fluid in the cul de sac is variable but may be seen in one-third of patients (51,56).

Doppler interrogation is generally not able to differentiate normal from torsed ovaries, as absence of flow is nonspecific (28,51,57,58) and normal arterial wave forms can be seen in ovaries that have undergone torsion (59). This is probably because the ovary is supplied with arterial flow both from the ovarian artery and from ovarian branches of the uterine artery that reach the ovary via the infundibular ligament (59). However, the presence of central venous flow in a torsed ovary suggests viability (60).

Ovarian Tumors

Ovarian tumors are rare in children, and most are benign. They constitute approximately 1.5% of malignancies in children (61). The probability of an ovarian mass being malignant increases with patient age. In girls less than eight years, approximately 3% of ovarian masses prove malignant, whereas approximately one-third are malignant in older girls (62). The most common benign masses include ovarian cysts (with or without torsion) and teratomas. Malignant masses are most often germ-cell tumors and occasionally epithelial tumors (62).

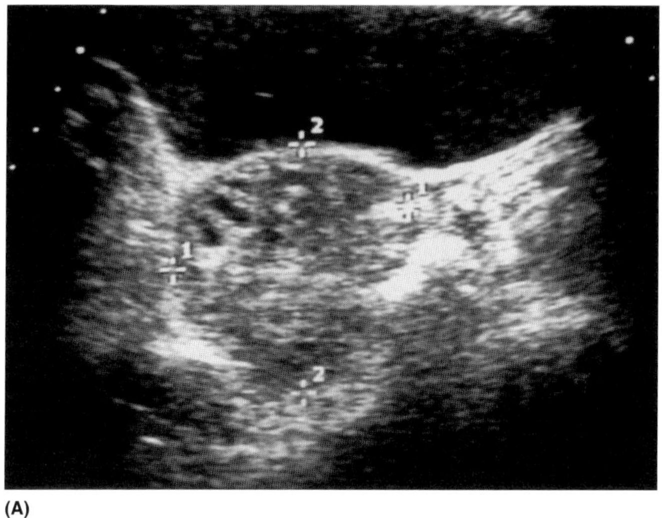
(A)

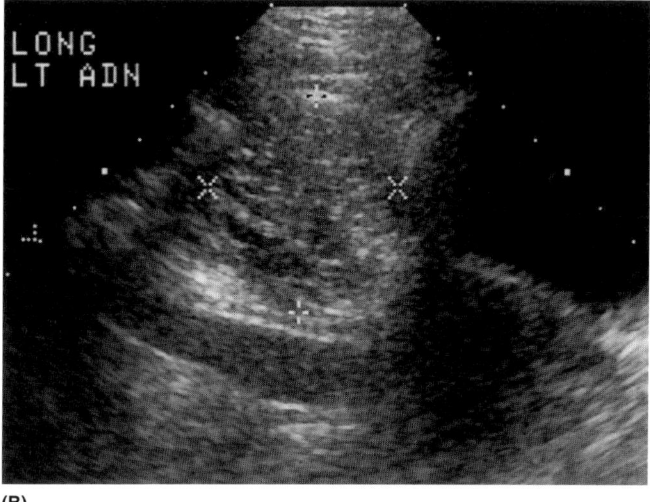

(B)

FIGURE 10 A AND B ■ Two examples of ovarian torsion demonstrate solid ovarian masses with small peripheral cystic structures.

Ovarian Teratomas

Approximately two-thirds of pediatric ovarian tumors are of germ-cell origin, usually mature teratomas (51). These congenital tumors are derived from pluripotent germ cells and consist of all three germ-cell layers (63). The vast majority is benign, or "mature." Ovarian teratomas average 10 cm at presentation and are bilateral in up to 10% of children (though as many as 25% of adults) (63). They usually present as an asymptomatic mass, but 33% can present with pain due to hemorrhage or torsion (51,64). They are usually diagnosed after puberty (58).

The typical appearance of a benign teratoma is that of a hypoechoic mass with a mural nodule that demonstrates posterior acoustic shadowing, but the appearance is variable (Fig. 11). Although their internal imaging characteristics vary, posterior shadowing is typical. Approximately 60% appear complex at ultrasound, the others appearing uniformly hypo- or hyperechoic (64). Pure sebum, which is liquid at body temperature, appears anechoic or hypoechoic and may layer above serous fluid, resulting in a fluid–fluid level. Hyperechoic lines and dots may be evident, attributed to hair (65). A dermoid plug (also known as a Rokitansky protuberance), which is a conglomerate mass of fatty/sebaceous material, hair, soft tissue, calcification, and teeth, appears echogenic, often occurring as a mural nodule and often (depending on the amount of hair present) demonstrating posterior shadowing (66). If the dermoid plug is very large and constitutes the entire teratoma, all that will be seen is an echogenic mass (66), but predominantly solid teratomas are also more likely to be malignant or "immature"(67). Predominantly solid teratomas often demonstrate peripheral hypoechogenicity, which constitutes fluid (68).

Ovarian teratomas that are diagnosed prior to puberty are less likely to demonstrate typical sonographic features, such as a mural nodule, acoustic shadowing, or a fluid–fluid level (64). Differential diagnosis includes hemorrhage into a pelvic mass (which should demonstrate enhanced through sound transmission), endometrioma, and perforated appendicitis with appendicolith. Teratomas can also simulate a distended urinary bladder or echogenic bowel (69).

Immature teratomas are composed of a wider variety of tissue elements, in varying states of differentiation, and, importantly, include embryonal elements that are often neurologic (67). Immature teratomas are most often found in the first decade. They demonstrate rapid growth and capsule penetration but, aside from a tendency to be more solid, appear similar to mature teratomas on ultrasound.

Malignant Ovarian Tumors

Ovarian malignancies are much more common in the second decade of life than in the first (62) but are still uncommon, accounting for 1% to 2% of childhood cancer (61). They present with abdominal pain, mass, premature vaginal bleeding, or precocious puberty. Those that occur in childhood are classified as germ cell (60–90%), stromal (10–12%), and epithelial (5–10%) in origin (70). They typically appear as a large mass with complex but predominantly solid sonographic characteristics.

Ultrasonographic differentiation of the various malignant ovarian tumors that occur during childhood is limited (62), and indeed ultrasonography is poor at characterizing lesions as malignant or benign (71). However, a solid ovarian mass in a child must be considered malignant until proven otherwise (61). Doppler differentiation of malignant and benign masses is controversial and discussed in Chapter 36 (72–74). Malignant ovarian masses tend to be larger than benign tumors [average diameter 20–26 cm (62), although tumor size does not correlate with outcome (75,76)]. Coarse calcifications can be seen in immature teratomas, more scattered than in their benign counterparts (75), whereas dysgerminomas may demonstrate finely stippled calcifications (51).

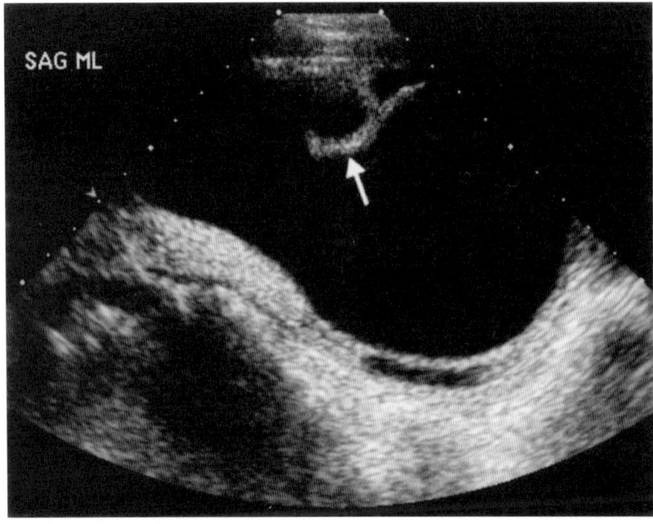

(A)

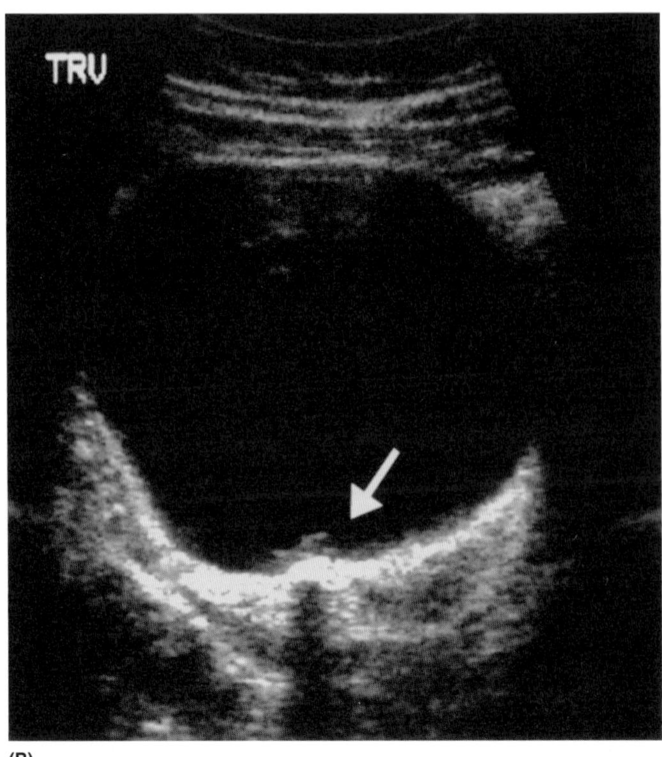

(B)

FIGURE 11 A AND B ■ Ovarian teratomas. Moderately thick septations are seen in (**A**) (*arrow*), whereas (**B**) demonstrates a shadowing echogenic mural nodule (*arrow*).

As a group, malignant germ-cell tumors are the most common malignant ovarian neoplasm. Subtypes include dysgerminoma, immature teratoma, endodermal sinus tumor, embryonal carcinoma, and primary choriocarcinoma, listed in decreasing order of frequency (70). Malignant germ-cell tumors present with mass, pain, and, occasionally, fever (75). In general, they appear solid or mixed solid and cystic; they may demonstrate irregular margins, papillary masses, and thick septae.

Dysgerminomas are usually solid and echogenic (Fig. 12) (67), though if large may show central necrosis (14). They can demonstrate a relatively specific finding of a homogeneous mass with irregular linear hypoechoic areas that demonstrate prominent flow, corresponding to fibrovascular septa (77). Immature teratomas are more commonly solid than their mature counterparts. The appearance of endodermal sinus tumor varies from that of an echogenic solid mass [reportedly most common (67)] to that of a complex mass with cystic areas. However, these cystic areas that represent either epithelial-lined cysts or coexisting mature teratomas (75) are better seen on computed tomography than on ultrasound (78). Malignant mixed germ-cell tumors have a variable appearance, depending on their constituents, but they are rarely purely cystic, and most are complex and predominantly solid (75).

Evaluation of serum α fetal protein (AFP), β human chorionic gonadotropin (BHCG), and α antitrypsin (AAT) can help suggest the diagnosis in the patient with a complex pelvic mass. Some ovarian malignancies, such as endodermal sinus tumor (78), are extremely aggressive, and abnormal laboratory values may trigger a rapid workup as the ultrasonographic appearance of these tumors can mimic benign disease such as tubo-ovarian abscess, appendiceal abscess, hemorrhagic cyst, or torsion. Approximately one-half to three-fourths of all germ-cell tumors generate elevated AFP or BHCG (62), and indeed most endodermal sinus tumors produce AFP (63,75,78) although they may have elevated AAT levels as well (67). Approximately 50% to 60% of immature teratomas also have elevated AFP levels. BHCG is elevated in dysgerminomas and choriocarcinomas.

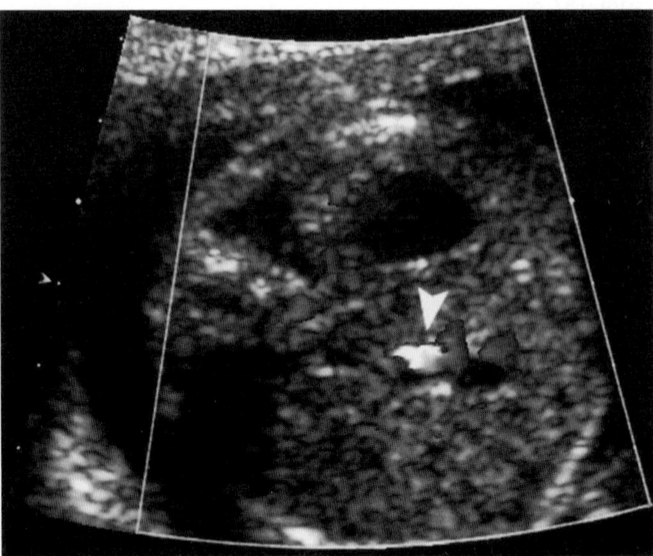

FIGURE 12 ■ Solid dysgerminoma. A solid, heterogeneous ovarian mass demonstrates flow (*arrowhead*).

Peritoneal spread occurs with both immature teratomas and with endodermal sinus tumors (75) and is particularly likely if a large amount of free fluid is present (78).

The sex cord/stromal tumors are unusual in girls and usually accompanied by androgen or estrogen production; diagnosis is often triggered by precocious puberty or virilization. Of these tumors, the estrogen-secreting juvenile granulosa-theca cell tumor is most common, occurring at the mean age of 13 years and resulting in 10% of cases of precocious puberty. This tumor is associated with both Ollier and Mafucci syndromes. Its typical appearance is that of an echogenic solid mass (67,79). Sertoli–Leydig cell tumors are virilizing tumors that occur rarely in girls; they constitute only 0.5% of ovarian neoplasms and have a variable appearance but are most often small, solid, and hypoechoic (79). Fibromas and steroid cell tumors are primarily limited to adults. Epithelial tumors, such as mucinous cystadenocarcinoma, papillary cystadenocarcinoma, papillary serous carcinoma, and endometrioid carcinoma, are very uncommon (51,62).

The ovary is also an important site of recurrence in leukemia and lymphoma (80); this manifests as a large, solid ovarian mass.

Massive Ovarian Edema

An exception to the rule that solid ovarian masses in children are malignant, this is a solid, virilizing, benign tumor-like condition that occurs in adolescents and is thought to result from partial or intermittent torsion and consequent venous and lymphatic obstruction (81,82) with subsequent fluid accumulation. The patient presents with acute pain, intermittent discomfort, or signs of virilization (82,83). Approximately 75% of cases occur in the right ovary, probably because this ovary is less tolerant of torsion as the ovarian vein pressure is higher because it drains directly into the inferior vena cava (81,84). The tumor can be solid, multicystic, or mixed, and the ovary ranges from 5 to 40 cm (mean diameter 11.5 cm) (83).

Vaginal Bleeding Prior to Puberty

Rhabdomyosarcoma is by far the most common primary vaginal or uterine tumor, usually occurring prior to the age of six years. It presents with vaginal hemorrhage or with a polypoid mass that prolapses through the introitus (85). Being intraluminal, it is of the subtype "botryoides," discussed more fully in the later section entitled Pelvic Rhabdomyosarcoma.

Vaginal foreign bodies can sometimes be recognized by virtue of an almost universal indentation that occurs in the posterior bladder wall (86). The foreign body itself is rarely evident, but it may demonstrate increased echogenicity and/or posterior shadowing. A foreign body accounts for 50% of vaginal bleeding without accompanying discharge and 18% of vaginal bleeding when discharge is also present (11).

Disorders of Puberty

Amenorrhea

Amenorrhea can occur due to anatomic outlet obstruction, physiologic hormonal immaturity or failure, inadequate nutrition or obesity, hypothyroidism, ovarian tumors, and psychological disturbance (Table 8) (14). Delayed menarche denotes absence of menses by age 16 or 5 years after onset of puberty; absence of secondary signs of sexual development may trigger an earlier workup.

Anatomic Outlet Obstruction

With uterine obstruction, hematocolpos or hematometrocolpos occur, secondary to accumulation of menstrual blood behind imperforate hymen, vaginal atresia, or vaginal septum (87). These disorders are discussed more fully in the section entitled Neonatal Pelvis, as they are often diagnosed at that time. However, if maternal estrogen levels were relatively low and little mucus accumulated in a fetus with normal external genitalia, they will manifest as amenorrhea or a pelvic mass in the pubescent girl (Fig. 13) (32). The appearance is similar to that in the neonate, with a distended cervix and possibly uterus containing material of variable echogenicity; fluid/debris levels are less common in this age group as there is usually no communication with the bladder or rectum via a urogenital sinus or cloaca (35). In this age group, the fluid usually appears as diffuse low-level echogenicity or predominantly anechoic (87).

Polycystic Ovary Syndrome (PCOS) or Stein–Leventhal Syndrome

This describes an association of obesity, oligomenorrhea, amenorrhea, hirsutism, and, classically, enlarged polycystic ovaries that results from a self-perpetuating cycle of endocrine imbalance that leads to infertility. Stein–Leventhal syndrome may manifest around puberty. Although the classic appearance is one of enlarged multicystic ovaries with multiple follicles in various stages of maturation (Fig. 14) (15), ovarian volume can be normal in 29% (88,89), and the classic appearance may be seen in only one-third of patients (90). This disorder is biologically quite variable, and therefore strict criteria cannot be applied in evaluation of the ovaries (91). Principal findings are unusually numerous follicular cysts (88,89) and increased echogenicity of ovarian stroma (91), but the latter finding is subjective and best assessed on transvaginal ultrasound, which is not performed in many teens; if both ovarian volumes are greater than 10 mL, PCOS has been found to be likely (92). However, this volume does overlap with the normal upper limit in a postmenarchal ovary (16).

Turner Syndrome

Gonadal dysgenesis is very common in patients with this disorder, and neither uterus nor ovaries may be demonstrable. When present, they are often small (Fig. 15) (93,94). Administration of exogenous steroids may result in uterine and ovarian development, which can be followed with serial ultrasonography.

TABLE 8 ■ Disorders of Puberty

Amenorrhea	Anatomic outlet obstruction	Hematocolpos Hematometrocolpos	
	Polycystic ovary syndrome	Normal ovaries in 29%	
	Turner syndrome	Small uterus and ovaries	
	Feminizing tumors	Granulosa-theca cell tumor	
	Masculinizing tumors	Arrhenoblastoma	
		Hilus-cell tumor	
		Adrenal-cell tumor	
	Physiologic hormonal imbalance		
	Inadequate nutrition		
	Obesity		
	Hypothyroidism		
	Psychological disturbance		
Precocious puberty	True (common)	Bilateral prematurely large ovaries	Premature activation of hypothalamic-pituitary-gonadal axis
	Pseudo (less common)	Ovarian cyst or mass	Functioning cyst or ovarian tumor causes pubertal changes

Tumors

The granulosa-theca cell tumors, which are feminizing, rarely cause amenorrhea. Masculinizing tumors such as arrhenoblastoma, hilus-cell, and adrenal-cell tumors are also very unusual causes of amenorrhea.

Precocious Puberty

This is defined as the expression of secondary sexual characteristics before the age of eight years. Premature thelarche refers to isolated premature breast development and usually occurs between ages one and four. Premature

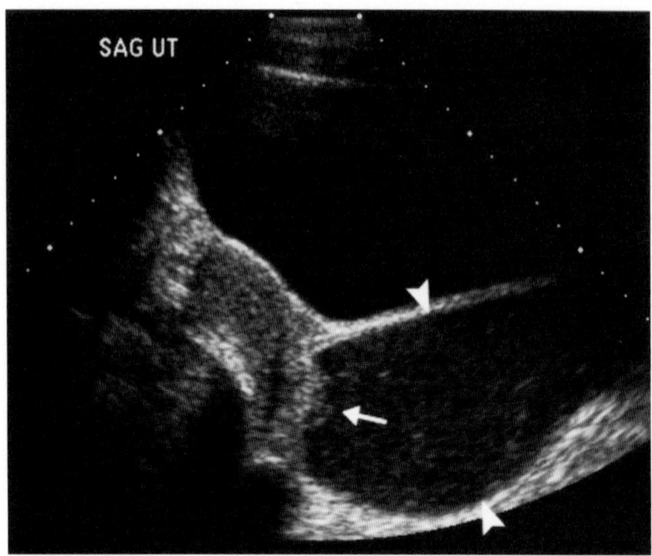

FIGURE 13 ■ Hematocolpos. Sagittal midline US demonstrating the vagina distended with echogenic hemorrhagic material; the cervix (*arrow*) protrudes into the vaginal lumen (*arrowheads*).

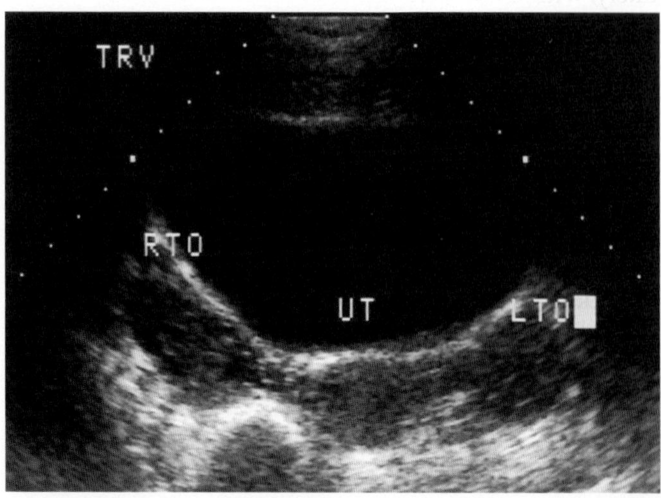

FIGURE 14 ■ Polycystic ovaries. Transverse US demonstrates uterus with bilateral ovaries, each appearing equal in size to the uterus and containing innumerable tiny cysts.

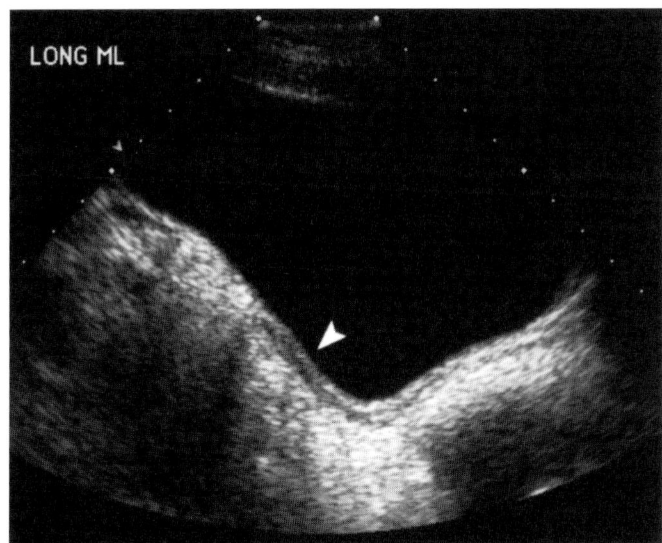

FIGURE 15 ■ Turner syndrome. This midline sagittal US in a 16-year-old girl with amenorrhea demonstrates a tiny uterus (*arrowhead*).

adrenarche denotes precocious appearance of axillary and pubic hair. Precocious puberty is divided into the much-more-common "true" versus unusual "pseudo" precocious puberty. This differentiation is based on whether there has been premature activation of the hypothalamic-pituitary-gonadal axis ("true") or whether a functioning cyst or tumor is causing pubertal changes, which occurs with pseudo precocious puberty. Ultrasound is important for assessing accelerated uterine growth, determining ovarian volumes, and diagnosing the functional cyst or tumor that very rarely causes premature maturation.

In true isosexual precocious puberty, the uterus and both ovaries are relatively large for age, in the range of more than 4.6 mL compared with normal of lesser than 1 mL (95,96); as in normal girls, microcysts (<9 mm) are common, but larger cysts are unusual (96).

If unilateral ovarian enlargement is present, usually due to a single macrocyst, pseudosexual precocity is more likely, with the development of secondary sexual characteristics resulting from the presence of a functioning ovarian cyst or tumor (96). An estrogen-secreting 1 to 6 cm follicular cyst is usually responsible and may resolve spontaneously, but occasionally these must be resected (97). Tumors are very unusual and are ovarian (granulosa-theca cell tumor, gonadoblastoma, and cystadenoma) or adrenal in origin (98). Precocious puberty is also associated with McCune–Albright syndrome. If the uterus and both ovaries are normal in size for age, the patient is considered to have "early puberty," which starts early but should progress slowly such that onset of menstruation occurs at a normal age (95).

BLADDER

Congenital bladder abnormalities include urachal anomalies, wherein part or all of the urachus persists, resulting in patent urachus or urachal cyst, sinus, or remnant.

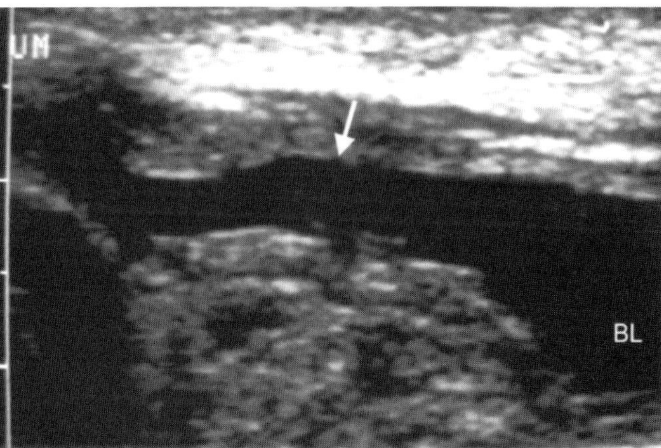

FIGURE 16 ■ Urachal remnant. A sagittal midline US obtained above the bladder demonstrates fluid within a tubular urachal remnant (*arrow*).

A hypoechoic or complex mass or tract may be apparent adjacent to the bladder dome (Fig. 16). Delayed risk of neoplasia necessitates excision.

Evaluation of the bladder is usually performed for hematuria, outlet obstruction, or urinary tract infection. The normal bladder wall thickness is up to 3 mm if full and up to 5 mm if the bladder is empty; measurements are best performed at the posteroinferior wall, lateral to the trigone (99). Diffuse thickening can be seen with muscular hypertrophy in cases of bladder outlet obstruction or neurogenic bladder; this, as well as more focal thickening, also occurs with various forms of cystitis and neoplasia.

Diffuse Bladder Wall Thickening

If this results from neurogenic bladder, diverticuli may be present, and calculi are not unusual. Assessment of postvoid residual is often clinically useful, and ureteral dilation may result from increased pressure due to large bladder volume or vesicoureteral reflux. Some centers evaluate for reflux with ultrasonography, but this practice is not widespread.

Posterior urethral valves also result in diffuse bladder wall thickening, and therefore, in the appropriate clinical setting, evaluation of the urethra should be attempted in male patients to help exclude the keyhole appearance of a dilated prostatic segment, though voiding cystourethrogram is considered definitive. Transperineal ultrasound may image the valve itself (2).

Various forms of cystitis, especially inflammatory, hemorrhagic, and that secondary to cytoxan toxicity, result in diffuse bladder wall thickening.

Focal Bladder Wall Thickening

More focal thickening can occur with inflammatory and hemorrhagic cystitis, but other entities should also be considered. Pseudotumoral cystitis is a self-limiting inflammatory process that encompasses a variety of disorders, most commonly eosinophilic cystitis and granulomatous cystitis (100). It is infectious or allergic in etiology.

It may consist of localized edema of the lamina propria and result in many round, cyst-like elevations of the mucosa that protrude into the lumen and resemble rhabdomyosarcoma. Alternatively, it can appear as a solid, broad-based intravesical mass with smooth or irregular outline or diffuse mucosal thickening (100). Like rhabdomyosarcoma, it most often involves the trigone (100,101), but unlike rhabdomyosarcoma it is confined to the mucosa whereas the underlying muscle layer appears normal (100).

Benign cystitis can also mimic bladder rhabdomyosarcoma, for although benign cystitis can appear diffuse with decreased bladder capacity, it also presents as focal or multifocal wall thickening. The less common bullous form consists of multiple small, rounded cystic areas. The mucosa is intact (102). Increasing bladder distension results in alteration in the contour of these hypoechoic masses, whereas rhabdomyosarcoma, being noncompliant, does not change. Two-week followup is also helpful to differentiate both benign cystitis and pseudotumoral cystitis from rhabdomyosarcoma, as the former entities should improve (Fig. 17) (102).

Hemangioma presents as a thickened bladder wall containing serpiginous anechoic spaces and is accompanied with cutaneous hemangiomas in one-fourth to one-third of patients (103). Neurofibromatosis is an unusual cause of massive thickening of the bladder wall (104). Transitional cell carcinoma is uncommon in children and when present is less aggressive than in adults (105).

Distal Ureteral Obstruction

Urinary tract infection is associated with ureteral dilatation resulting from reflux and ureteroceles that result in obstruction; the ureterocele appear as a thin-walled rounded structure protruding into the bladder lumen (Fig. 18). These may contain more complex fluid if obstructed. Simple ureteroceles insert in a normal position, whereas those that are ectopic insert more centrally in the bladder, in the urethra, or in the vagina. If an ureterocele is encountered, it is important to evaluate the upper urinary tracts to determine the presence of accompanying renal duplications and/or hydronephrosis (Chapter 26). After incision of a ureterocele, redundant collapsed tissue can appear mass-like (106).

Distal ureteral or bladder calculi can occasionally be recognized on pelvic ultrasound by the presence of an echogenic mass with distal acoustic shadowing.

Rhabdomyosarcoma

This is the most common tumor of the lower genitourinary tract in children, has a male preponderance, and usually occurs between the ages of three and six years (107), with a smaller peak in 15 to 19 year olds (108). It has been reported in neonates and is thus presumed to occur in utero (109). Rhabdomyosarcoma constitutes approximately 5% to 10% of malignant solid childhood tumors (110) and occurs often [in 15–30% of cases (109,111)] in the genitourinary tract, second in frequency to head and neck (111). Bladder and prostate rhabdomyosarcoma occur in males; pelvic rhabdomyosarcoma in females is usually vaginal or cervical but can be located in the bladder. This tumor arises from unsegmented, undifferentiated mesoderm (110). Although there are four subtypes, the vast majority of those occurring in the pelvis are embryonal (111). Within the subtype embryonal rhabdomyosarcoma, the botryoid group is common in the pelvis, where grape-like clusters of tumor arise in a submucosal intraluminal location. Metastases are present in

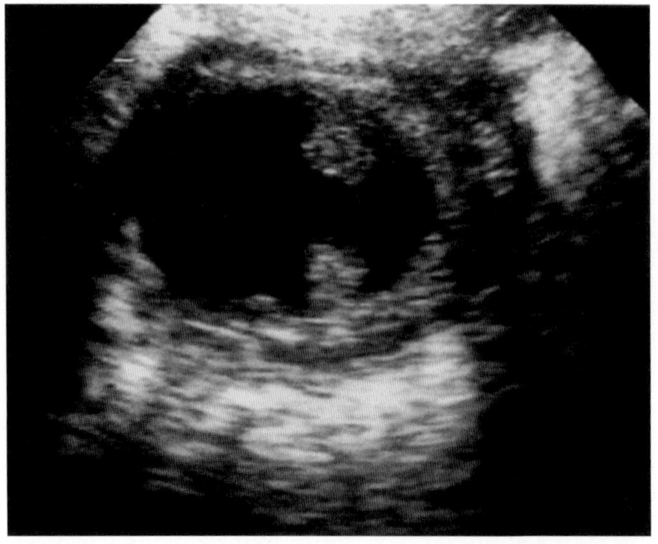

(A)

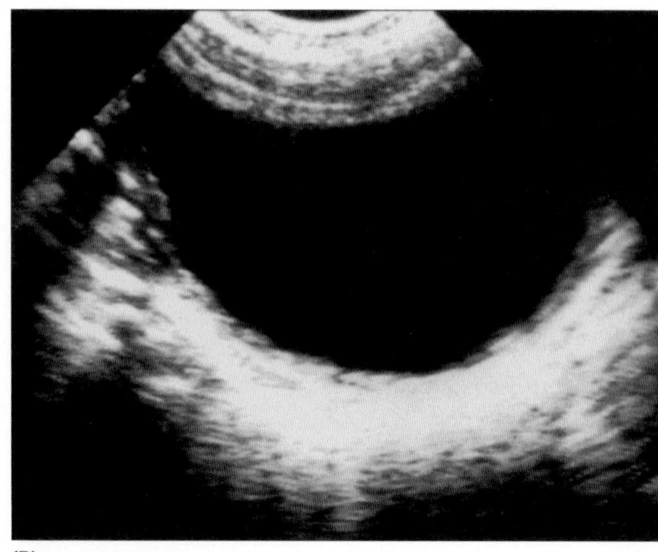

(B)

FIGURE 17 A AND B ■ Cystitis in this teenager initially manifested as multiple areas of focal bladder wall nodularity (**A**), but after two weeks of antibiotic therapy, the bladder wall became normal (**B**).

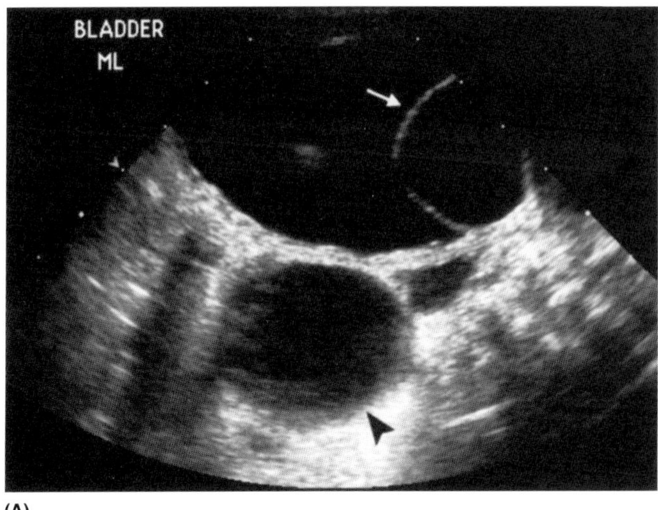

(A)

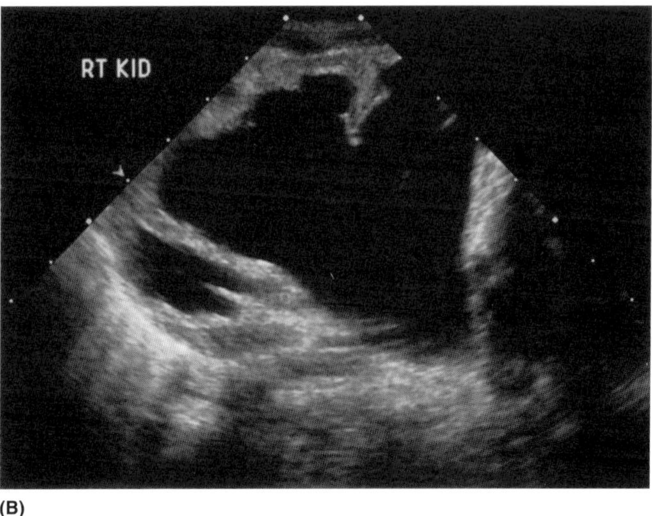

(B)

FIGURE 18 A AND B ■ (**A**) Both the thin-walled ureterocele (*arrow*) and portions of a tortuous, dilated distal ureter (*arrowhead*) are demonstrated. (**B**) A sagittal US of the corresponding kidney demonstrates a duplicated system with marked hydronephrosis of the lower pole.

10% to 20% of patients at the time of diagnosis, the most common sites being lungs, cortical bone, and lymph nodes; less frequent sites of involvement include bone marrow and liver (111).

Botryoid rhabdomyosarcoma in females occurs within the vagina in young girls, often presenting as a grape-like mass at the introitus, but the cervix is a more common location in adolescents (112). Differential considerations include prolapsed ureterocele, paraurethral cyst, and hydro(metro)colpos (85).

Bladder rhabdomyosarcoma arises in submucosa and infiltrates the bladder wall, protruding into the bladder lumen as a lobulated mass or masses (Fig. 19). Most originate in the trigone, and most prostatic rhabdomyosarcomas grow cephalad into the bladder, so it is often difficult to determine the organ of origin. Consequently, although prostatic rhabdomyosarcoma tends to disseminate more than that arising in the bladder, pelvic rhabdomyosarcoma in boys is often grouped as bladder/prostate (111). The exception to this is prostatic rhabdomyosarcoma that extends anteriorly into the space of Retzius, but this pattern of growth is highly unusual and more readily appreciated on magnetic resonance imaging (MRI) than on ultrasound (113). The treatment does differ, as bladder-sparing surgery

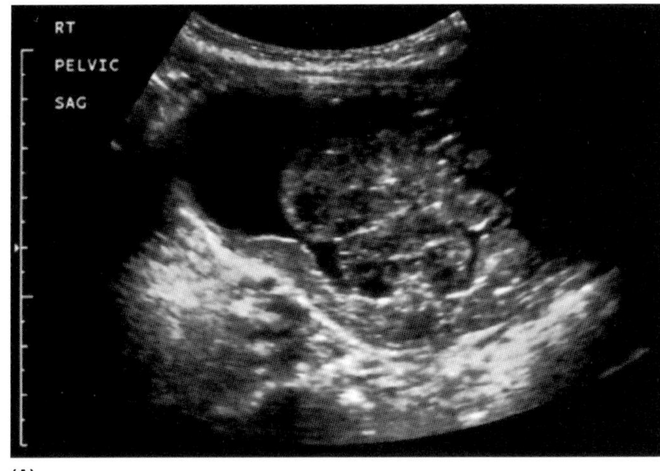

(A)

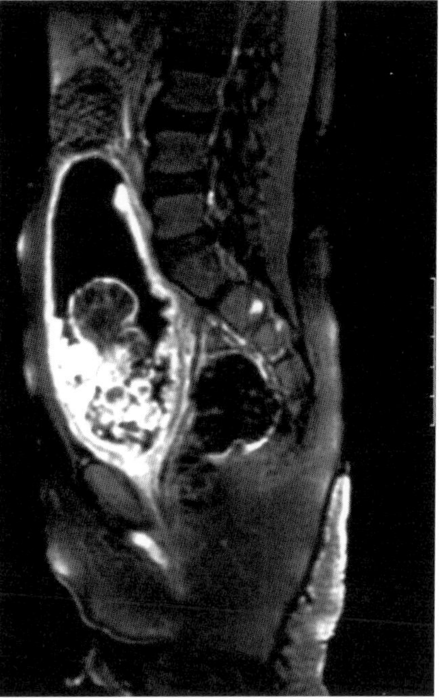

(B)

FIGURE 19 A AND B ■ Bladder rhabdomyosarcoma. Ultrasound (**A**) and sagittal T1 gadolinium-enhanced fat-suppressed MRI (**B**) demonstrate a multinodular soft-tissue mass extending upward from the bladder base, partially filling the bladder.

may be possible with this form of prostatic rhabdomyosarcoma. Bladder/prostate rhabdomyosarcoma presents with symptoms of bladder outlet obstruction; hematuria is unusual (111).

The ultrasonographic appearance of embryonal rhabdomyosarcoma is nonspecific and has been variably described as that of a hyper- or hypoechoic mass (111), which may be lobulated and can contain areas of necrosis and hemorrhage that appear anechoic (114). The botryoid form at the bladder base characteristically appears as a polypoid intraluminal mass resembling a bunch of grapes. MRI can assist in determining whether the tumor arose in the bladder or in the prostate.

The typical survival rate for treated nonmetastatic bladder/prostate rhabdomyosarcoma is now approximately 70%, and the prognosis for vaginal/cervical rhabdomyosarcoma is even better, with 80% 10-year survival (115).

SACROCOCCYGEAL TERATOMA

The differential diagnosis for a pelvic mass in an infant that does not arise from the bladder, prostate, uterus, cervix, or ovaries is broad. If in an anterior presacral location, diagnostic considerations include sacrococcygeal teratoma, neuroblastoma, anterior meningocele, duplication cyst, hemangioma/lymphangioma, and lipoma (116). Hemangiomas are usually accompanied with skin discoloration, and both hemangiomas and lipomas have a typical ultrasonographic appearance. Meningoceles and duplication cysts tend to be nonseptated. Sacrococcygeal

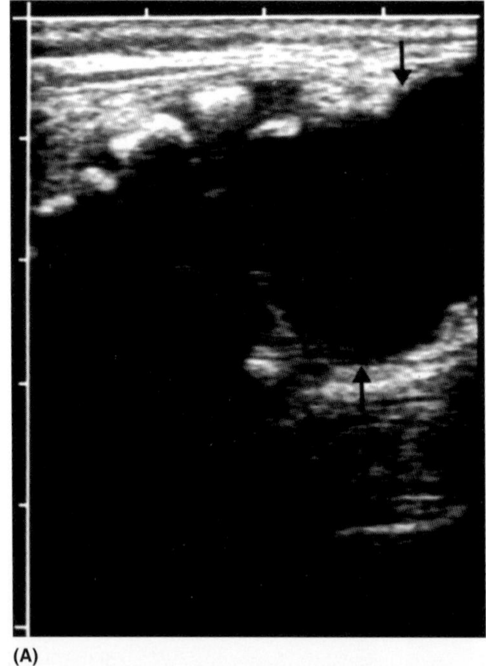
(A)

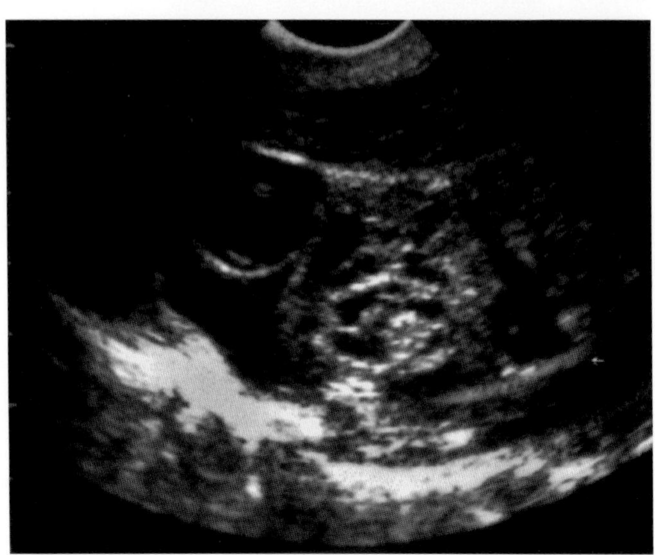
(B)

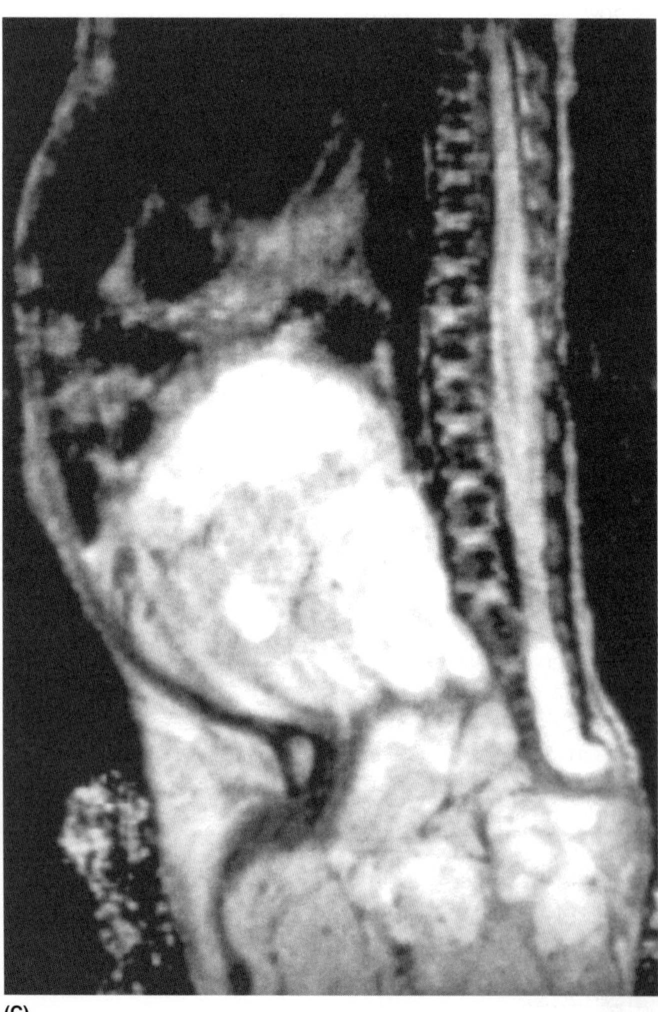
(C)

FIGURE 20 A–C ■ Sacrococcygeal teratoma. (**A**) is a sagittal paramidline dorsal US demonstrating a superficial cystic mass (*arrows*) that extends deep to the sacrum and coccyx. In a second case, a heterogeneous, more solid mass (**B**) has both internal and external components and demonstrates intraspinal extension as seen on the sagittal T2-weighted MRI (**C**).

teratoma and neuroblastoma are usually complex, although they too can be simply cystic; laboratory evaluation can help differentiate between these, as virtually all teratomas have elevated serum AFP levels (117) whereas urinary vanillylmandelic acid is elevated with neuroblastoma. Endodermal sinus tumors are related to sacrococcygeal teratomas but are much less common (see Chapter 26 for further discussion of neuroblastoma).

Sacrococcygeal teratomas arise from a totipotent primordial germ cell that has deviated from its normal migratory pathway from the yolk sac to the gonad during early embryogenesis (118). They are closely associated with the coccyx (Fig. 20), and, in order to prevent recurrence, treatment always involves resection of the coccyx. Immature teratomas contain primitive neuroectodermal tissue, tend to be larger (>10 cm), and are more likely to recur (118). Recurrences may be malignant.

If diagnosed prior to the age of two months, only 10% to 20% of sacrococcygeal teratomas are malignant, but, after that time, the likelihood of malignancy increases dramatically (117). They are four times more common in females than in males (119), but those in males are more likely to be malignant. These tumors have been categorized based on the percentage that is external versus internal (119). Those that are completely external (Type I) have a much lower incidence of malignancy than those that are entirely internal (Type IV) (Type II tumors are external and pelvic, whereas Type III are external, pelvic, and abdominal). Predominantly cystic sacrococcygeal teratomas are also more likely to be benign (119). Although sacrococcygeal tumors occur in infancy, entirely internal (or presacral) tumors tend to be diagnosed in older children (120) and, very rarely, adults (118). However, after infancy, they are essentially always malignant. MRI is useful for evaluating spinal involvement.

The most common appearance of sacrococcygeal teratoma is that of a large (up to 30 cm) (118), complex mass containing a roughly equal amount of cystic and solid areas. Cysts may be small or large, and there may be echogenic foci representing fat or bone. Alternatively, there may be a dominant cystic mass, with or without septations. Fluid–fluid levels are uncommon, and a completely solid mass is distinctly unusual but more likely to be malignant (118). As many as 18% of sacrococcygeal teratomas are accompanied with other congenital anomalies, many resulting from mass effect, such as imperforate anus, hydronephrosis, and dislocated hips; sacral agenesis and spinal dysraphism may also be associated (118).

REFERENCES

1. Bellah RD, Rosenberg HK. Transvaginal ultrasound in a children's hospital: is it worthwhile? Pediatr Radiol 1991; 21(8):570–574.
2. Cohen HL et al. Posterior urethral valve: transperineal US for imaging and diagnosis in male infants. Radiology 1994; 192(1): 261–264.
3. Teele RL, Share JC. Transperineal sonography in children. AJR Am J Roentgenol 1997; 168(5):1263–1267.
4. Nussbaum AR, Sanders RC, Jones MD. Neonatal uterine morphology as seen on real-time US. Radiology 1986; 160(3):641–643.
5. Ratani RS, Cohen HL, Fiore E. Pediatric gynecologic ultrasound. Ultrasound Q 2004; 20(3):127–139.
6. Orsini LF et al. Pelvic organs in premenarcheal girls: real-time ultrasonography. Radiology 1984; 153(1):113–116.
7. Haber HP, Mayer EI. Ultrasound evaluation of uterine and ovarian size from birth to puberty. Pediatr Radiol 1994; 24(1):11–13.
8. Salardi S et al. Pelvic ultrasonography in premenarcheal girls: relation to puberty and sex hormone concentrations. Arch Dis Child 1985; 60(2):120–125.
9. Herter LD et al. Ovarian and uterine sonography in healthy girls between 1 and 13 years old: correlation of findings with age and pubertal status. AJR Am J Roentgenol 2002; 178(6):1531–1536.
10. Ivarsson SA, Nilsson KO, Persson PH. Ultrasonography of the pelvic organs in prepubertal and postpubertal girls. Arch Dis Child 1983; 58(5):352–354.
11. Garel L et al. US of the pediatric female pelvis: a clinical perspective. Radiographics 2001; 21(6):1393–1407.
12. Ziereisen F et al. The role of Doppler evaluation of the uterine artery in girls around puberty. Pediatr Radiol 2001; 31(10): 712–719.
13. Battaglia C et al. Pelvic ultrasound and color Doppler findings in different isosexual precocities. Ultrasound Obstet Gynecol 2003; 22(3):277–283.
14. Haller JO et al. The normal and abnormal ovary in childhood and adolescence. Semin Ultrasound CT MR 1983; 4(3):206–225.
15. Hall DA. Sonographic appearance of the normal ovary, of polycystic ovary disease, and of functional ovarian cysts. Semin Ultrasound CT MR 1983; 4(3):149–165.
16. Cohen HL, Tice HM, Mandel FS. Ovarian volumes measured by US: bigger than we think. Radiology 1990; 177(1):189–192.
17. Cohen HL et al. Normal ovaries in neonates and infants: a sonographic study of 77 patients 1 day to 24 months old. AJR Am J Roentgenol 1993; 160(3):583–586.
18. Cohen HL et al. Ovarian cysts are common in premenarchal girls: a sonographic study of 101 children 2–12 years old. AJR Am J Roentgenol 1992; 159(1):89–91.
19. Millar DM et al. Prepubertal ovarian cyst formation: 5 years' experience. Obstet Gynecol 1993; 81(3):434–438.
20. Garel L et al. Antenatal diagnosis of ovarian cysts: natural history and therapeutic implications. Pediatr Radiol 1991; 21(3):182–184.
21. Muller-Leisse C et al. Ovarian cysts in the fetus and neonate–changes in sonographic pattern in the follow-up and their management. Pediatr Radiol 1992; 22(6):395–400.
22. Nussbaum AR et al. Spontaneous resolution of neonatal ovarian cysts. AJR Am J Roentgenol 1987; 148(1):175–176.
23. Schmahmann S, Haller JO. Neonatal ovarian cysts: pathogenesis, diagnosis and management. Pediatr Radiol 1997; 27(2):101–105.
24. Nussbaum AR et al. Neonatal ovarian cysts: sonographic-pathologic correlation. Radiology 1988; 168(3):817–821.
25. Strickland JL. Ovarian cysts in neonates, children and adolescents. Curr Opin Obstet Gynecol 2002; 14(5):459–465.
26. Mordehai J et al. Torsion of uterine adnexa in neonates and children: a report of 20 cases. J Pediatr Surg 1991; 26(10):1195–1199.
27. Luzzatto C et al. Neonatal ovarian cysts: management and follow-up. Pediatr Surg Int 2000; 16(1–2):56–59.
28. Stark JE, Siegel MJ. Ovarian torsion in prepubertal and pubertal girls: sonographic findings. AJR Am J Roentgenol 1994; 163(6): 1479–1482.
29. Bagolan P et al. Prenatal diagnosis and clinical outcome of ovarian cysts. J Pediatr Surg 1992; 27(7):879–881.
30. van der Zee DC et al. Laparoscopic approach to surgical management of ovarian cysts in the newborn. J Pediatr Surg 1995; 30(1):42–43.
31. Enriquez GDC, Toran N, Piqueras J, et al. Conservative versus surgical treatment for complex neonatal ovarian cysts: outcomes study. AJR Am J Roentgenol 2005; 185:501–508.
32. Burbige KA, Hensle TW. Uterus didelphys and vaginal duplication with unilateral obstruction presenting as a newborn abdominal mass. J Urol 1984; 132(6):1195–1198.
33. Mirk P, Pintus C, Speca S. Ultrasound diagnosis of hydrocolpos: prenatal findings and postnatal follow-up. J Clin Ultrasound 1994; 22(1):55–58.

34. Janus C, Godine L. Newborn with hydrometrocolpos and ambiguous genitalia: clinical significance. J Clin Ultrasound 1986; 14(9):739–741.
35. Blask AR, Sanders RC, Gearhart JP. Obstructed uterovaginal anomalies: demonstration with sonography. Part I. Neonates and infants. Radiology 1991; 179(1):79–83.
36. Graham D, Nelson MW. Combined perineal-abdominal sonography in the evaluation of vaginal atresia. J Clin Ultrasound 1986; 14(9):735–738.
37. Scanlan KA et al. Value of transperineal sonography in the assessment of vaginal atresia. AJR Am J Roentgenol 1990; 154(3):545–548.
38. Rosenberg HK et al. Mayer-Rokitansky-Kuster-Hauser syndrome: US aid to diagnosis. Radiology 1986; 161(3):815–819.
39. Brody JM, Koelliker SL, Frishman GN. Unicornuate uterus: imaging appearance, associated anomalies, and clinical implications. AJR Am J Roentgenol 1998; 171(5):1341–1347.
40. States LJ, Bellah RD. Imaging of the pediatric female pelvis. Semin Roentgenol 1996; 31(4):312–329.
41. Goske MJ, Emmens RW, Rabinowitz R. Inguinal ovaries in children demonstrated by high resolution real-time ultrasound. Radiology 1984; 151(3):635–636.
42. Wright NB et al. Imaging children with ambiguous genitalia and intersex states. Clin Radiol 1995; 50(12):823–829.
43. Bryan PJ et al. Ultrasound findings in the adreno-genital syndrome (congenital adrenal hyperplasia). J Ultrasound Med 1988; 7(12):675–679.
44. Kutteh WH, Santos-Ramos R, Ermel LD. Accuracy of ultrasonic detection of the uterus in normal newborn infants: implications for infants with ambiguous genitalia. Ultrasound Obstet Gynecol 1995; 5(2):109–113.
45. Hernanz-Schulman M, Brock JW III, Russell W. Sonographic findings in infants with congenital adrenal hyperplasia. Pediatr Radiol 2002; 32(2):130–137. Epub 2001 Nov 29.
46. Horowitz M, Glassberg KI. Ambiguous genitalia: diagnosis, evaluation, and treatment. Urol Radiol 1992; 14(4):306–318.
47. Eberenz W et al. True hermaphroditism: sonographic demonstration of ovotestes. Radiology 1991; 179(2):429–431.
48. Lee HJ et al. "Daughter cyst" sign: a sonographic finding of ovarian cyst in neonates, infants, and young children. AJR Am J Roentgenol 2000; 174(4):1013–1015.
49. Bass IS et al. The sonographic appearance of the hemorrhagic ovarian cyst in adolescents. J Ultrasound Med 1984; 3(11):509–513.
50. Baltarowich OH et al. The spectrum of sonographic findings in hemorrhagic ovarian cysts. AJR Am J Roentgenol 1987; 148(5): 901–905.
51. Surratt JT, Siegel MJ. Imaging of pediatric ovarian masses. Radiographics 1991; 11(4):533–548.
52. Cohen HL, Bober SE, Bow SN. Imaging the pediatric pelvis: the normal and abnormal genital tract and simulators of its diseases. Urol Radiol 1992; 14(4):273–283.
53. Helvie MA, Silver TM. Ovarian torsion: sonographic evaluation. J Clin Ultrasound 1989; 17(5):327–332.
54. Graif M, Itzchak Y. Sonographic evaluation of ovarian torsion in childhood and adolescence. AJR Am J Roentgenol 1988; 150(3):647–649.
55. Godfrey H, Abernethy L, Boothroyd A. Torsion of an ovarian cyst mimicking enteric duplication cyst on transabdominal ultrasound: two cases. Pediatr Radiol 1998; 28(3):171–173.
56. Meyer JS et al. Ovarian torsion: clinical and imaging presentation in children. J Pediatr Surg 1995; 30(10):1433–1436.
57. Quillin SP, Siegel MJ. Transabdominal color Doppler ultrasonography of the painful adolescent ovary. J Ultrasound Med 1994; 13(7):549–555.
58. Siegel MJ. Pediatric gynecologic sonography. Radiology 1991; 179(3):593–600.
59. Rosado WM Jr et al. Adnexal torsion: diagnosis by using Doppler sonography. AJR Am J Roentgenol 1992; 159(6):1251–1253.
60. Fleischer AC et al. Color Doppler sonography of adnexal torsion. J Ultrasound Med 1995; 14(7):523–528.
61. King DR. Ovarian cysts and tumors. In: Randolph JG, Welch KJ, Ravitch MM, et al. ed. Pediatric Surgery. 4th ed. Chicago, IL: Year Book Medical, 1986.
62. Brown MF et al. Ovarian masses in children: a review of 91 cases of malignant and benign masses. J Pediatr Surg 1993; 28(7):930–933.
63. Breen JL, Bonamo JF, Maxson WS. Genital tract tumors in children. Pediatr Clin North Am 1981; 28(2):355–367.
64. Sisler CL, Siegel MJ. Ovarian teratomas: a comparison of the sonographic appearance in prepubertal and postpubertal girls. AJR Am J Roentgenol 1990; 154(1):139–141.
65. Patel MD et al. Cystic teratomas of the ovary: diagnostic value of sonography. AJR Am J Roentgenol 1998; 171(4):1061–1065.
66. Sheth S et al. The variable sonographic appearances of ovarian teratomas: correlation with CT. AJR Am J Roentgenol 1988; 151(2):331–334.
67. Sutton CL et al. Ovarian masses revisited: radiologic and pathologic correlation. Radiographics 1992; 12(5):853–877.
68. Lee DK et al. Ovarian teratomas appearing as solid masses on ultrasonography. J Ultrasound Med 1999; 18(2):141–145.
69. Hertzberg BS, Kliewer MA. Sonography of benign cystic teratoma of the ovary: pitfalls in diagnosis. AJR Am J Roentgenol 1996; 167(5):1127–1133.
70. Siegel MJ. Pelvic tumors in childhood. Radiol Clin North Am 1997; 35(6):1455–1475.
71. Levine D et al. Sonography of ovarian masses: poor sensitivity of resistive index for identifying malignant lesions. AJR Am J Roentgenol 1994; 162(6):1355–1359.
72. Bromley B, Goodman H, Benacerraf BR. Comparison between sonographic morphology and Doppler waveform for the diagnosis of ovarian malignancy. Obstet Gynecol 1994; 83(3):434–437.
73. Jain KA. Prospective evaluation of adnexal masses with endovaginal gray-scale and duplex and color Doppler US: correlation with pathologic findings. Radiology 1994; 191(1):63–67.
74. Fleischer AC et al. Color Doppler sonography of benign and malignant ovarian masses. Radiographics 1992; 12(5):879–885.
75. Brammer HM III et al. From the archives of the AFIP. Malignant germ cell tumors of the ovary: radiologic-pathologic correlation. Radiographics 1990; 10(4):715–724.
76. Gribbon M, Ein SH, Mancer K. Pediatric malignant ovarian tumors: a 43-year review. J Pediatr Surg 1992; 27(4):480–484.
77. Kim SH, Kang SB. Ovarian dysgerminoma: color Doppler ultrasonographic findings and comparison with CT and MR imaging findings. J Ultrasound Med 1995; 14(11):843–848.
78. Levitin A et al. Endodermal sinus tumor of the ovary: imaging evaluation. AJR Am J Roentgenol 1996; 167(3):791–793.
79. Outwater EK et al. Sex cord-stromal and steroid cell tumors of the ovary. Radiographics 1998; 18(6):1523–1546.
80. Chu JY et al. Ovarian tumor as manifestation of relapse in acute lymphoblastic leukemia. Cancer 1981; 48(2):377–379.
81. Hall BP, Printz DA, Roth J. Massive ovarian edema: ultrasound and MR characteristics. J Comput Assist Tomogr 1993; 17(3):477–479.
82. Heiss KF, Zwiren GT, Winn K. Massive ovarian edema in the pediatric patient: a rare solid tumor. J Pediatr Surg 1994; 29(10): 1392–1394.
83. Hill LM, Pelekanos M, Kanbour A. Massive edema of an ovary previously fixed to the pelvic side wall. J Ultrasound Med 1993; 12(10):629–632.
84. Lee AR et al. Massive edema of the ovary: imaging findings. AJR Am J Roentgenol 1993; 161(2):343–344.
85. Nussbaum AR, Lebowitz RL. Interlabial masses in little girls: review and imaging recommendations. AJR Am J Roentgenol 1983; 141(1):65–71.
86. Caspi B et al. The role of sonography in the detection of vaginal foreign bodies in young girls: the bladder indentation sign. Pediatr Radiol 1995; 25(suppl 1):S60–S61.
87. Blask AR, Sanders RC, Rock JA. Obstructed uterovaginal anomalies: demonstration with sonography. Part II. Teenagers. Radiology 1991; 179(1):84–88.
88. Hann LE et al. Polycystic ovarian disease: sonographic spectrum. Radiology 1984; 150(2):531–534.
89. Yeh HC, Futterweit W, Thornton JC. Polycystic ovarian disease: US features in 104 patients. Radiology 1987; 163(1):111–116.
90. Orsini LF et al. Ultrasonic findings in polycystic ovarian disease. Fertil Steril 1985; 43(5):709–714.
91. Pache TD et al. How to discriminate between normal and polycystic ovaries: transvaginal US study. Radiology 1992; 183(2):421–423.

92. Herter LD, Magalhaes JA, Spritzer PM. Relevance of the determination of ovarian volume in adolescent girls with menstrual disorders. J Clin Ultrasound 1996; 24(5):243–248.
93. Haber HP, Ranke MB. Pelvic ultrasonography in Turner syndrome: standards for uterine and ovarian volume. J Ultrasound Med 1999; 18(4):271–276.
94. Massarano AA et al. Ovarian ultrasound appearances in Turner syndrome. J Pediatr 1989; 114(4 Pt 1):568–573.
95. Salardi S et al. Pelvic ultrasonography in girls with precocious puberty, congenital adrenal hyperplasia, obesity, or hirsutism. J Pediatr 1988; 112(6):880–887.
96. King LR, Siegel MJ, Solomon AL. Usefulness of ovarian volume and cysts in female isosexual precocious puberty. J Ultrasound Med 1993; 12(10):577–581.
97. Fakhry J et al. Sonography of autonomous follicular ovarian cysts in precocious pseudopuberty. J Ultrasound Med 1988; 7(11): 597–603.
98. Hedlund GL, Royal SA, Parker KL. Disorders of puberty: a practical imaging approach. Semin Ultrasound CT MR 1994; 15(1):49–77.
99. Jequier S, Rousseau O. Sonographic measurements of the normal bladder wall in children. AJR Am J Roentgenol 1987; 149(3): 563–566.
100. Friedman EP, de Bruyn R, Mather S. Pseudotumoral cystitis in children: a review of the ultrasound features in four cases. Br J Radiol 1993; 66(787):605–608.
101. Hoeffel JC et al. Pseudotumoral cystitis. Pediatr Radiol 1993; 23(7): 510–514.
102. Rosenberg HK et al. Benign cystitis in children mimicking rhabdomyosarcoma. J Ultrasound Med 1994; 13(12):921–932.
103. Pakter R, Nussbaum A, Fishman EK. Hemangioma of the bladder: sonographic and computerized tomography findings. J Urol 1988; 140(3):601–602.
104. Miller WB Jr, Boal DK, Teele R. Neurofibromatosis of the bladder: sonographic findings. J Clin Ultrasound 1983; 11(8):460–462.
105. Benson RC Jr, Tomera KM, Kelalis PP. Transitional cell carcinoma of the bladder in children and adolescents. J Urol 1983; 130(1): 54–55.
106. Fernbach SK, Feinstein KA. Abnormalities of the bladder in children: imaging findings. AJR Am J Roentgenol 1994; 162(5):1143–1150.
107. Poggiani C et al. Sonographic detection of rhabdomyosarcoma of the urinary bladder. Eur J Ultrasound 2001; 13(1):35–39.
108. Tannous WN et al. CT and ultrasound imaging of pelvic rhabdomyosarcoma in children. A review of 56 patients. Pediatr Radiol 1989; 19(8):530–534.
109. Onal B et al. Rhabdomyosarcoma of the prostate in a newborn: sonographic and CT findings. Eur J Radiol 1995; 21(2):106–108.
110. LaQuaglia M. Genitourinary rhabdomyosarcoma in children. Urol Clin North Am 1991; 18(3):575–580.
111. Agrons GA et al. From the archives of the AFIP. Genitourinary rhabdomyosarcoma in children: radiologic-pathologic correlation. Radiographics 1997; 17(4):919–937.
112. Brand E et al. Rhabdomyosarcoma of the uterine cervix. Sarcoma botryoides. Cancer 1987; 60(7):1552–1560.
113. Levin T et al. Three pediatric patients with extension of prostatic embryonal rhabdomyosarcoma anterior to the bladder into the space of Retzius. Pediatr Radiol 1992; 22(3):200–202.
114. McLeod AJ, Lewis E. Sonographic evaluation of pediatric rhabdomyosarcomas. J Ultrasound Med 1984; 3(2):69–73.
115. Maurer HM et al. The Intergroup Rhabdomyosarcoma Study-II. Cancer 1993; 71(5):1904–1922.
116. Kassarjian A, Davison BD, Blickman JG. Pediatric case of the day. Sacrococcygeal teratoma, type IV. AJR Am J Roentgenol 1999; 173(3):814, 817–818.
117. Kaste SC, Bridges JO, Marina NM. Sacrococcygeal yolk sac carcinoma: imaging findings during treatment. Pediatr Radiol 1996; 26(3):212–219.
118. Keslar PJ, Buck JL, Suarez ES. Germ cell tumors of the sacrococcygeal region: radiologic-pathologic correlation. Radiographics 1994; 14(3):607–620; quiz 621–622.
119. Altman RP, Randolph JG, Lilly JR. Sacrococcygeal teratoma: American Academy of Pediatrics Surgical Section Survey-1973. J Pediatr Surg 1974; 9(3):389–398.
120. Rescorla FJ et al. Long-term outcome for infants and children with sacrococcygeal teratoma: a report from the Childrens Cancer Group. J Pediatr Surg 1998; 33(2):171–176.

Pediatric Musculoskeletal Ultrasound

Rebecca Stein-Wexler

29

Ultrasonography lends itself readily to the evaluation of cartilaginous structures and can thus be employed to study a variety of disorders unique to the developing child. By far, the most common of these is developmental dysplasia of the hip (DDH). It can also define the presence or absence of hip effusions and evaluate the cartilaginous patella, popliteal cysts, foreign bodies, musculotendinous injuries, and soft-tissue infection.

DDH is a relatively common problem, occurring in 1% to 3% of infants (1–4); immature hips are found in as many as 13% of infants (5). Incidence varies with ethnicity, being more common among Navajo Indians (6) but almost nonexistent in African blacks (7). Untreated, it accounts for approximately 25% of osteoarthritis in adults (8).

PHYSICAL FINDINGS

Some cases can be diagnosed at clinical examination with manipulations that attempt to reduce a dislocated hip or dislocate a loose one (Table 1). These include, among others, the Ortolani maneuver and the Barlow maneuver. The Ortolani maneuver, developed by an Italian pediatrician in 1937, attempts to reduce a hip that is already dislocated. Holding the infant's leg with hip and knee flexed, the examiner attempts gentle abduction while lifting to slip the dislocated femoral head over the posterior labrum, returning it to the acetabulum. If the hip was dislocated, reducing it results in a "clunk." The Barlow maneuver, which was reported by an English orthopedic surgeon in 1962, attempts to dislocate a loose or unstable hip. The leg is held with the hip partially flexed and in adduction; the knee is then pushed superiorly, and the femoral head dislocates by sliding posteriorly over the acetabulum.

Additional physical findings that suggest DDH include asymmetric thigh folds, apparent decreased length of the affected thigh (due to telescoping secondary to dislocation), and decreased abduction (9). Some examiners have found an audible "click" to be significant (higher pitched than the aforementioned "clunk") (10,11), but this is controversial.

SCREENING

Although in the hands of skilled examiners physical examination can be reliable (12), studies have shown that DDH is often missed or overdiagnosed (12–16). Radiographs of the young infant provide limited diagnostic benefit, as the femoral heads are purely cartilaginous and thus radiolucent; furthermore, slight differences in patient positioning result in misleading findings. Over the past 25 years, the development of diagnostic hip ultrasound has provided an excellent method of diagnosing this important and relatively common disorder (17–22).

In some European countries, the hips of all newborn infants are screened ultrasonographically (23), but this may result in overtreatment of hips that would have normalized in the first month of life (10,20,24–27); a large randomized control study that followed patients for five years

TABLE 1 ■ Physical Diagnostic Maneuvers

Name	Maneuver	Significance
Ortolani	Gently abduct and lift flexed leg	Attempts to reduce a dislocated hip
Barlow	Gently adduct flexed leg while pushing posteriorly	Attempts to dislocate a loose or unstable hip
Push/pull	Gently push flexed leg posteriorly	Attempts to dislocate a loose or unstable hip

concluded that selective rather than universal screening is appropriate (28). In Great Britain and the United States, ultrasonographic screening is usually based on the combination of physical examination and incidence of risk factors, but this more-limited screening approach probably results in a few missed diagnoses that then present late (10,14,29–31).

ETIOLOGY

A combination of factors results in an increased risk for DDH (Table 2) (3,21). Girls are at significantly increased risk (three to five times more than boys), possibly due to increased sensitivity to estrogen/relaxin. Those with an affected family member (parent or sibling) are also at increased risk. Increased likelihood of DDH also results from fetal positioning that puts greater stress on the hips. For example, breech presentation, especially with knees extended, is associated with increased risk of DDH (32). Large infants (32), children of first pregnancies, and those complicated by oligohydramnios have increased risk for DDH, presumably because of restricted fetal motion resulting in reduced flexion and abduction at the hip (33). Additional risk factors, torticollis (34) and clubfoot, are probably associated with positioning issues as well. The left hip is four times more likely to be affected than is the right, probably because of fetal positioning, with the left side on the mother's spine, resulting in limited abduction on that side (33). Premature infants are less likely to be affected (35).

TABLE 2 ■ Clinical Indications for Ultrasound of Infant Hip

Abnormal findings on physical examination of the hip
- Positive Ortolani
- Positive Barlow
- Asymmetric hip crease
- Audible click or clunk

Family history of DDH
- Sibling
- Parent

Breech presentation at birth

Postural molding conditions
- Torticollis
- Foot deformity

Monitoring treatment of DDH

Abbreviation: DDH, developmental dysplasia of the hip.

It is now recognized that hip dislocation rarely occurs in utero, and hence this disorder is no longer labeled "congenital dislocation of the hip" but instead "DDH." Occasionally, an otherwise normal child will be born with a dislocated hip, in which case the dislocation is termed "atypical." When hip dislocation occurs prenatally as a result of an underlying neuromuscular disorder such as arthrogryposis or spina bifida, it is termed "teratologic" (36). In these infants, the acetabulum and femoral head are already severely deformed, and treatment options are more limited. Only 2% of cases of hip dislocation are teratologic (33).

However, the more typical case involves mild laxity of ligamentous structures, with resultant incongruity of the femoral head within the acetabulum. A close relationship between the femoral head and the acetabulum is required for normal development of both, and if mild laxity persists, then the acetabulum fails to form properly, allowing further increased mobility of the femoral head and greater acetabular dysplasia (33). If this situation progresses, complete dislocation can occur, nonreducible if the labrum becomes deformed and the acetabulum fills with fibrofatty pulvinar. With dislocation, there is also decreased mobility, resulting in soft-tissue contractures and further limiting potential reduction. However, if this process is addressed by three months, and the femoral head is positioned correctly within the acetabulum and not allowed to slip, the acetabulum will usually be able to form properly and eventually limit femoral head mobility. Earlier treatment results in a greater likelihood of a successful outcome.

TIMING OF ULTRASONOGRAPHIC EVALUATION

Numerous studies have addressed the question of ideal timing for evaluation of the hip, and although results conflict, some generalizations can be made (Table 3) (2,16,26,31,37–39). For the frankly abnormal hip—that is, one with a positive (or even equivocal) Ortolani or Barlow maneuver—the American Association of Pediatrics (AAP) practice guidelines recommend initial evaluation by an orthopedist, with subsequent ultrasonography, as needed, by two weeks (36). For more subtle physical findings (such as hip click, thigh asymmetry, limitation of abduction, or asymmetric creases), ultrasonography or orthopedic evaluation is recommended at approximately three to four weeks. However, if the sole findings are the history of breech presentation or a positive family history in a female, either ultrasound at six weeks or pelvic radiography at four months is recommended (36).

TABLE 3 ■ Recommendations for Timing of Ultrasound Evaluation

Indication	Timing for evaluation
Positive or equivocal Barlow or Ortolani	Orthopedic evaluation by 2 wks old Ultrasound as needed
Hip click Thigh asymmetry Limited abduction Asymmetric creases	Orthopedic evaluation or ultrasound at 3–4 wks
Breech presentation Positive family history	Ultrasound at 6 wks or radiograph at 4 mos

Source: From Ref. 36.

The reason for delaying evaluation is that many cases of mild instability result from neonatal capsular laxity (40) (probably secondary to circulating maternal hormones); such cases resolve promptly without treatment (2,16,31,41). An immature-appearing acetabulum can also normalize in this period. Furthermore, although there is some disagreement (3,42), orthopedic surgeons generally find satisfactory results from treatment of the mildly abnormal hip begun as late as three months after birth; some recommend initiating treatment even later (2).

The femoral head begins to ossify at between two and eight months in girls and slightly later in boys. Hip ultrasound is easily performed until shadowing from the ossifying femoral head nucleus limits visualization of the acetabulum, generally between six months and one year of age. However, some employ ultrasound to evaluate femoral head position in older children as well (43).

TREATMENT

In addition to the expense of overtreatment, intervention also results in an increased risk of avascular necrosis (AVN) of the femoral head (44). The hips must be fixed in flexion and abduction, but too much abduction can result in decreased blood flow to the femoral head and consequent AVN (44,45). The risk of AVN may also increase with application of greater force (44,45). However, the increased flexibility of young infants may partially protect them from this complication despite early treatment (3,42), although some have found that the incidence of AVN increases when treatment is begun at an early age (46). Promising studies suggest that power Doppler ultrasound (45) and gadolinium-enhanced magnetic resonance imaging (MRI) (47) may be able to assess femoral head perfusion and eventually assist the orthopedic surgeon in achieving maximal abduction while reducing the risk of AVN.

The Pavlik harness is usually employed in the United States and is a very effective form of treatment (48), but other abduction devices are common elsewhere. Ultrasound monitoring of treatment in the Pavlik harness is usually successful (48–50) and, if treatment is to be successful, should demonstrate improvement within three weeks (51). However, if more aggressive intervention becomes necessary, such as closed reduction or adductor tenotomy with abduction casting, ultrasound yields to limited computed tomography (CT) as the diagnostic method of choice. Investigators have attempted to monitor reduction ultrasonographically via a window created in the cast over the hip (52), but this may indeed result in a worse outcome (38,53), and limited CT is preferable.

HIP ANATOMY BY ULTRASOUND

Evaluation of femoral head position succeeds because the hyaline cartilage of the femoral head is relatively hypoechoic and thus allows through transmission of sound and visualization of the echogenic bony acetabulum (Fig. 1). The femoral head cartilage demonstrates alternating hypoechoic and echogenic columns, representing vascular channels alternating with columns of cartilage cells and mesenchymal stroma (55); this results in a specular appearance. The femoral head's articular surface is rimmed with anechoic articular cartilage, which is difficult to separate from a similar layer of anechoic cartilage that covers the acetabulum (55). However, rotation of the hip creates echogenic microbubbles within the joint, allowing definition of the femoral head from the acetabular cartilage (40). The cartilaginous labrum consists of hypoechoic hyaline cartilage, with a triangular echogenic tip of fibrocartilaginous cartilage. The femoral metaphysis adjacent to the growth plate appears echogenic.

Even before radiographically apparent ossification of the femoral head begins between two and eight months, the center of the femoral head nucleus alters ultrasonographically, demonstrating more focal multiple echogenic lines that represent vascular channels. This echogenic area gradually enlarges, eventually becoming evident on a radiograph (56). As the amount of shadowing posterior to the echogenic ossific nucleus increases, hip ultrasound becomes less successful, but radiographic assessment of exact femoral head position becomes possible. Thus, at some point between 6 and 12 months, hip ultrasound yields to the radiograph. It is helpful to note that ossification often lags in the dysplastic hip, which may extend the period of time when ultrasound is useful.

The acetabulum is composed of three echogenic bones: the ilium superiorly, the ischium posteroinferiorly, and the pubis anteroinferiorly. They are joined by the hypoechoic triradiate cartilage. By convention, the superior or anterior part of the hip is usually imaged to the left. The hypoechoic femoral head sits snugly within the acetabulum.

DEVELOPMENT OF HIP ULTRASOUND

Hip ultrasound was originally developed in the early 1980s (52,57–60). Two dominant approaches have emerged. Graf, working in Austria, employed A-mode sector scanning to create a static image of the acetabulum and femoral head in the coronal plane (61,62), focusing on the appearance of the acetabulum and measuring the angles both the ossified and the cartilaginous portions make with the horizontal margin of the ileum (61,62).

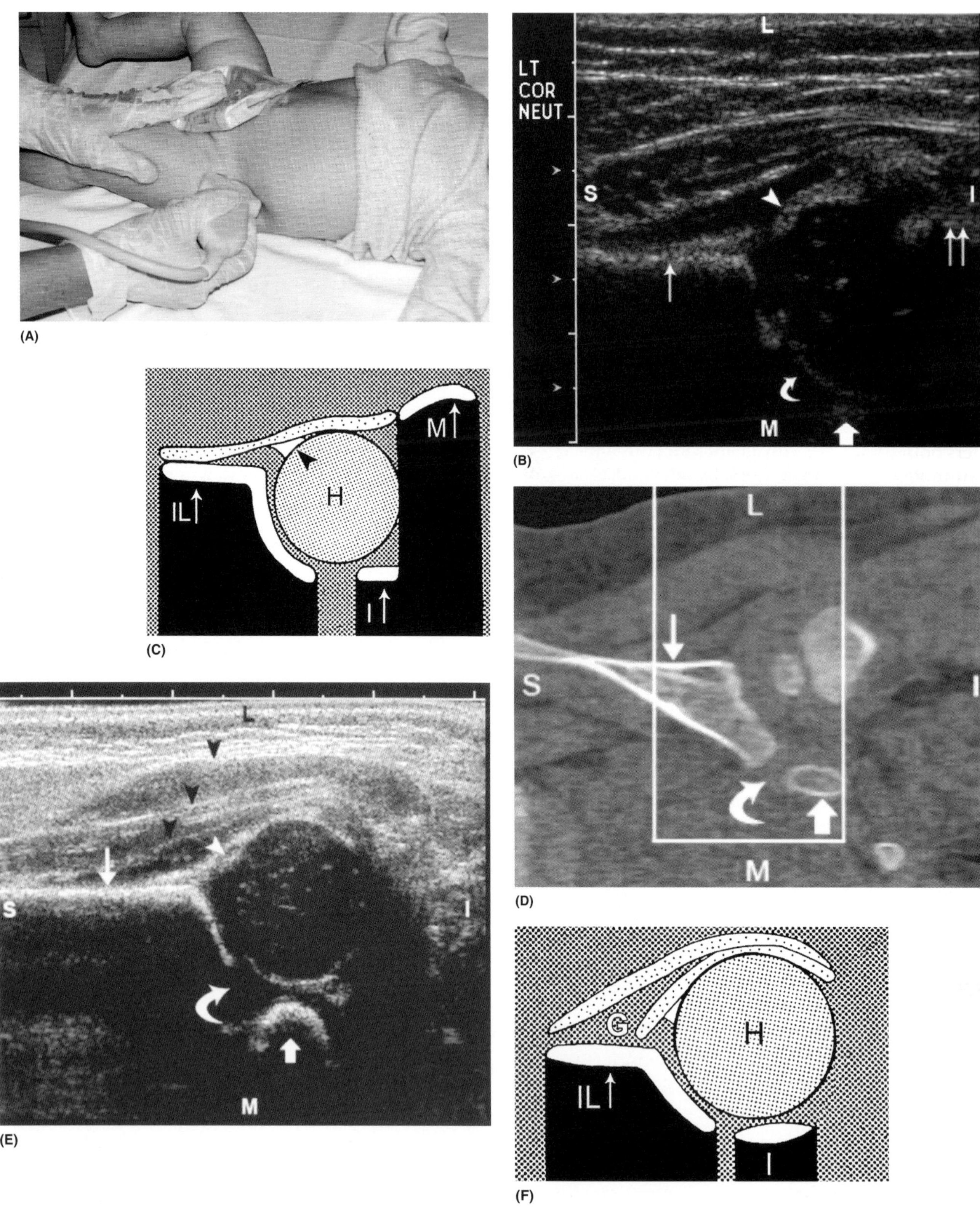

FIGURE 1 A–F ■ Normal coronal examination of the hip. (**A**) Note the slight tilt of the transducer as the infant is examined in coronal-neutral position. (**B**) Normal coronal-neutral hip US. Note the iliac bone (*straight arrow*), triradiate cartilage (*curved arrow*), ischium (*wide arrow*), echogenic fibrocartilaginous tip of labrum (*arrowhead*), and femoral metaphysis (*double arrow*). L, lateral; M, medial; S, superior; I, inferior. (**C**) Accompanying diagram demonstrates bony landmarks. Note fibrocartilaginous tip of the labrum (*arrowhead*). G, gluteal muscle; H, femoral head; I, ischium; IL, ileum; M, femoral metaphysis. (**D**) Corresponding image from coronal reconstruction of CT of a normal hip. The white box indicates the portion of the hip that is included in the ultrasound evaluation. Landmarks are similar to those indicated in (**B**). (**E**) Normal coronal-flexion hip ultrasound. Note the iliac bone (*straight white arrow*), triradiate cartilage (*curved white arrow*), ischium (*wide white arrow*), and echogenic fibrocartilaginous tip of labrum (*white arrowhead*). The black arrowheads point to the gluteus minimus, medius, and maximus muscles. Landmarks are similar to those in (**B**). (**F**) Accompanying diagram demonstrates bony landmarks similar to those in (**C**). *Source*: (**C,F**) from Ref. 54.

A short time later, Harcke, working in the United States, developed an approach based on dynamic B-mode scanning, which studied the motion of the femoral head within the acetabulum and characterized the acetabular contour without employing measurements (58). This assessment provided a closer parallel with the orthopedist's examination, for the ultrasonographer stressed and then reduced the hip in the manner of the Barlow and Ortolani maneuvers.

Some question the reliability and reproducibility of Graf's measurements, as the apparent angles vary depending on where the acetabulum is imaged (59,63,64). However, the Graf approach, with variations, is employed successfully in much of Europe (9,65). The Harcke approach is generally more accepted in the United States. However, Graf has also advocated an approach that considers both static acetabular angles and dynamic femoral head motion (66), and in 1993, Harcke and Graf agreed on a consolidation of their methods as the "dynamic standard minimum examination" (67). More recently, the American College of Radiology (ACR) and American Institute of Ultrasound in Medicine (AIUM) have developed guidelines for hip ultrasound that blend both approaches (Table 4) (68,69).

Other investigators have evaluated additional characteristics of the hip joint, with the percentage of femoral head being covered by the acetabulum being one of the more popular (43,59,70). Attempts have been made at three-dimensional imaging of the infant hip (71).

Graf and Harcke, as well as most other investigators discussed above, view the hip joint from a lateral or posterolateral approach—coronal for Graf, both coronal and transverse for Harcke. Others have evaluated the hip from an anterior or medial vantage point (39,52,60,72,73), which has some advantages if the patient is in a cast, but these approaches have not become widely accepted.

PERFORMING DYNAMIC HIP ULTRASOUND

There are two options available for patient positioning. The infant may be immobilized in a hammock-like device, in which case, they are held in the decubitus position. Alternatively, the infant may lie freely on the examining table and be positioned in supine and oblique decubitus positions as needed, the parents or an assistant helping to achieve immobility. Many examiners prefer the infant to be positioned perpendicular to the long axis of the examining table. The remainder of this discussion focuses on positioning when the hammock-like device is not used.

TABLE 4 ■ Essential Components of Dynamic Hip Ultrasound Recommended by AIUM and ACR

View	Assess
Coronal flexion or neutral	Acetabular contour
	Depth of femoral head
Transverse-flexion adduction	Instability
Transverse-flexion abduction	Reducibility

Abbreviations: ACR, American College of Radiology; AIUM, American Institute of Ultrasound in Medicine.

Source: From Refs. 68, 69.

Only the portion of diaper that covers the hip under evaluation is removed. To be an effective and reliable examination, the infant must be relaxed, possibly having just fed or being entertained and fed during the examination. The highest-frequency linear transducer that offers adequate penetration is employed, usually 5 to 7.5 MHz. To evaluate the left hip, the left leg is grasped in the examiner's left hand and the probe in their right. Evaluation of the right hip is performed with the probe in the left hand and the right leg grasped by the examiner's right hand. For ease of comparison, it is common to switch the orientation of the transducer so that the straight line of the ileum always appears horizontal on the left side of the image, whether examining the right hip or the left hip.

The minimum standard examination developed by the ACR and AIUM is discussed below. Additional optional maneuvers are presented later. It is essential that, although only one hip may be under suspicion, both must be interrogated. In addition, the hip must be evaluated in both the coronal and the transverse planes. Furthermore, in the coronal plane, the acetabular contour must be assessed, with angle measurement being optional (40). This is accomplished with the hip flexed and/or neutral. The hip must be stressed in a simulated Barlow maneuver, in the attempt to subluxate or dislocate an unstable hip. Finally, an Ortolani-like maneuver must be performed to determine reducibility of the unstable hip. The latter two maneuvers, stressing and then reducing the hip, are performed with the transducer oriented in the transverse plane and with the hip flexed; care must be taken to keep the femoral head and acetabulum in view during this maneuver, so that the same area is monitored in both abduction and adduction. Stressing the hip while in the coronal plane is optional.

Coronal View, Mid-Acetabular Plane

For the coronal views, the infant is positioned supine (Fig. 1). The acetabular configuration can be assessed with the hip either flexed or neutral, although the traditional angle measurements are usually obtained in neutral positioning. In either approach, the margin of the ileum above the acetabulum must appear as a straight line in order to be certain that the deepest portion of the acetabulum is being imaged. If the probe is too anterior, the iliac line inclines laterally; in this position, a normal hip can appear subluxated. If the probe is too posterior, the line appears concave, and a shallow acetabulum can appear normal. The proper position is achieved by rotating the superior edge of the transducer 15° to 20° posteriorly (68,69).

The normal femoral head appears as a hypoechoic round ball, lying against the concave, echogenic acetabulum, with a thin anechoic interface between the two, probably representing articular cartilage. As the femoral head is rotated within the acetabulum, the actual articular plane can be defined by the appearance of echoes (probably microbubbles) in the joint space. This appearance has been compared to an egg in a spoon, the egg corresponding to the femoral head, the cup of the spoon to the acetabulum, and the spoon's handle being the straight iliac line. The triradiate cartilage is recognized as a hypoechoic gap between the iliac portion of the acetabulum superiorly and the curved ischial portion inferiorly. The hypoechoic labrum with its echogenic tip is readily appreciated, extending the acetabular curve further over the femoral head. Layers of gluteus minimus, medius, and maximus demonstrate a striated muscle appearance, with echogenic bands separating the muscle planes.

At least half of the femoral head should be positioned within the bony acetabulum, below a theoretical line extending the straight margin of iliac bone across the acetabulum through the femoral head (70); another report suggests that even more (at least 55% for girls and 57% for boys) of the femoral head must be positioned below this line to be unequivocally normal (43), but a large number of hips fall in the indeterminate range (33–58% coverage) (59). If ossification of the femoral head has commenced, this more echogenic area should be central in the epiphysis, and the theoretical line should transect or be lateral to it. A subluxated femoral head is partially contained within the acetabulum (Fig. 2). If the femoral head is fully dislocated (Fig. 3), the deformed labrum and the fibrofatty pulvinar may become interposed between the femoral head and the acetabulum, resulting in the presence of echogenic material behind the femoral head. This can then prevent closed reduction of the femoral head, mandating surgical intervention. It is thus essential to note the configuration of the labrum and whether reduction is limited by abnormal acetabular contents.

The development of the acetabulum can be assessed in either coronal-neutral or coronal-flexed position. The normal acetabulum demonstrates a steep angle with the adjacent ileum. The immature acetabulum shows slight rounding of the corner but still has a steep angle, while the dysplastic acetabulum is shallow to varying degrees. The cartilaginous labrum may become deformed and echogenic with severe dysplasia (74).

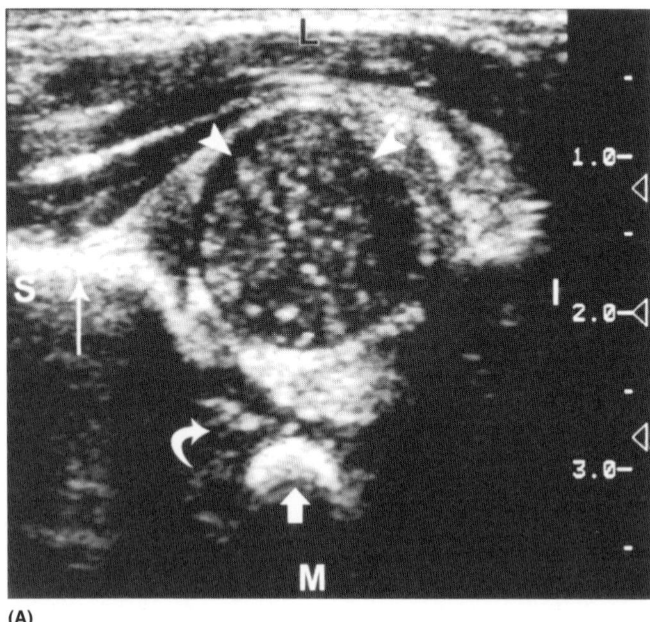

(A)

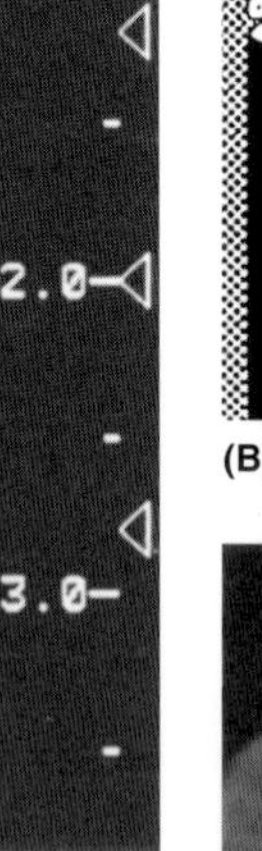

(B)

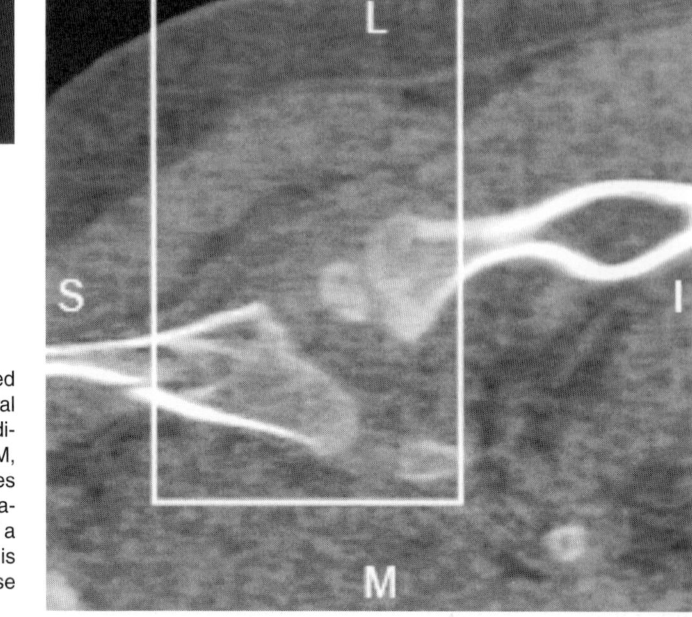

(C)

FIGURE 2 A–C ■ Subluxated hip (A) Coronal ultrasound of subluxated hip. Note that more than half of the femoral head (*arrowheads*) is lateral to the straight iliac line (*thin arrow*). The curved arrow indicates the triradiate cartilage, and the wide arrow points to the ischium. L, lateral; M, medial; S, superior; I, inferior. (B) Accompanying diagram demonstrates bony landmarks. H, femoral head; I, ischium; IL, ileum; M, femoral metaphysis. (C) Corresponding image from coronal reconstruction of CT of a subluxated hip. The white box indicates the portion of the hip that is included in the ultrasound evaluation. Landmarks are similar to those indicated in (A). *Source*: (B) from Ref. 54.

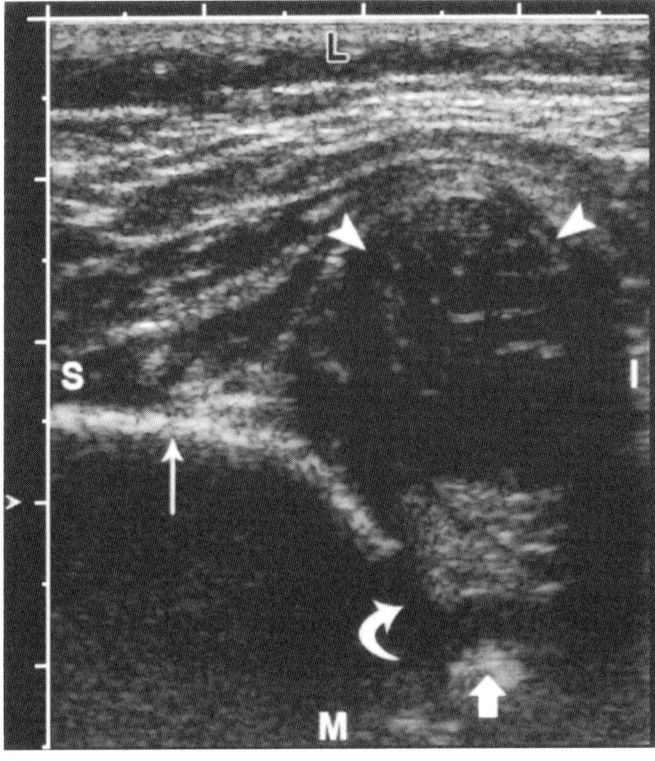

(A)

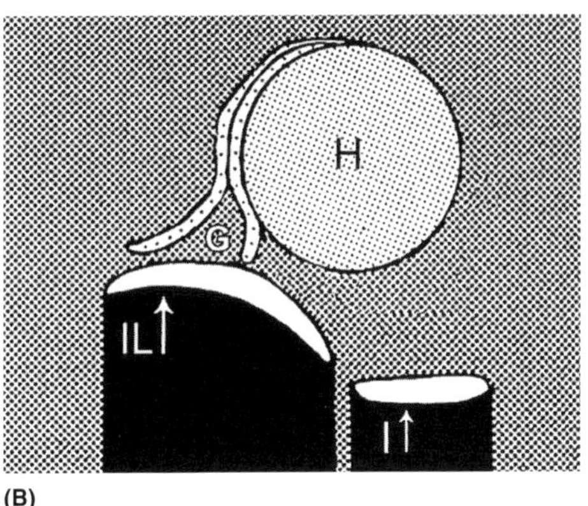

(B)

FIGURE 3 A AND B ■ Dislocated hip (**A**) Coronal ultrasound of a dislocated hip. The femoral head (*arrowheads*) is widely displaced lateral to the straight iliac line (*thin arrow*). Curved arrow indicates triradiate cartilage, and wide arrow points to the ischium. Note the echogenic pulvinar between ischium and femoral head as well as the shallow acetabulum. L, lateral; M, medial; S, superior; I, inferior. (**B**) Accompanying diagram demonstrates bony landmarks. G, gluteal muscle; H, femoral head; I, ischium; IL, ileum. *Source*: (**B**) From Ref. 54.

If the hip is in neutral position (which, in the infant, represents approximately 15–20° of hip flexion), the echogenic cortex of the proximal femur below the femoral head is seen distal to the acetabulum and femoral head. If the hip is flexed, the femoral cortex is out of the plane of view, unless the hip is dislocated posteriorly, in which case the femoral cortex blocks insonation of the acetabulum and landmarks are obscured. For this reason, many favor the neutral position for assessing the acetabulum and femoral head position in the coronal plane. Figure 1 delineates the anatomy of a normal hip viewed from coronal neutral versus coronal flexion.

Acetabular angle measurements are determined from a coronal image, usually with the hip neutral (Fig. 4). The angles are formed by the intersection of two different lines with the "baseline," which connects the bony acetabular convexity to the point where the joint capsule and perichondrium unite with the iliac bone. The "inclination line" connects the osseous convexity to the labrum, and the "acetabular roof line" connects the lower edge of the ilial bone to the osseous convexity (61). The α angle is formed by the angle between "baseline" and the "acetabular roof line"; it measures the convexity of the bony acetabulum; the greater the angle, the deeper, better formed is the bony acetabulum. An α angle of greater than 60° is normal, whereas 43° to 60° is likely normal in infants younger than three months of age (but merits followup and is suspicious in infants older than three months); less than 43° is abnormal (61,62). The β angle is formed by the "baseline" intersecting the "inclination line"; it can be thought of as measuring the form and size of the labrum. Normal is less than 55°, and equivocal (depending on age) is 55° to 77°; greater than 77° is clearly abnormal (Table 5) (61,62).

The acetabular cartilage is thicker in dysplastic hips [4.6 mm (1 SD. 71 mm)] than in normals [2.6 mm (1 SD. 37 mm)] (75), resulting in more separation of the femoral head from the acetabulum. This may be noted before acetabular dysplasia or hip instability is evident and may alone merit followup.

Transverse-Flexion View

For evaluation of the left hip, the patient is turned to a right posterior decubitus position, rotated approximately 30° off of the examining table (Fig. 5a). A rolled-up towel can be placed under the left torso, or a parent can assist in immobilization. Once again, the probe is grasped in the examiner's right hand, and the left holds the infant's leg, flexing both knee and hip. It is usually easiest to place the probe almost posteriorly over the ischium and then gradually sweep anteriorly until the acetabulum comes into view, with the final imaging position being posterolateral. If the transducer is placed too lateral (and insufficiently posterior), a normal hip can appear dislocated, yielding a false-positive examination.

From this approach, the acetabulum is composed of the pubic bone anteriorly and the ischium posteriorly (Fig. 5). The large curve of the ischium appears on the right side of the image, and the small portion of the visualized pubis appears inferior on the image. Once again, the triradiate cartilage can be seen as a hypoechoic gap separating the two echogenic curves of acetabular bone.

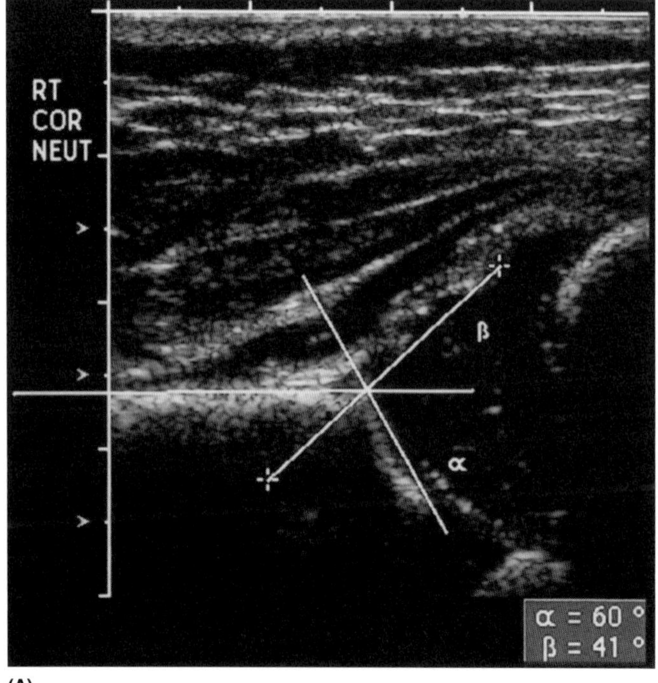

(A)

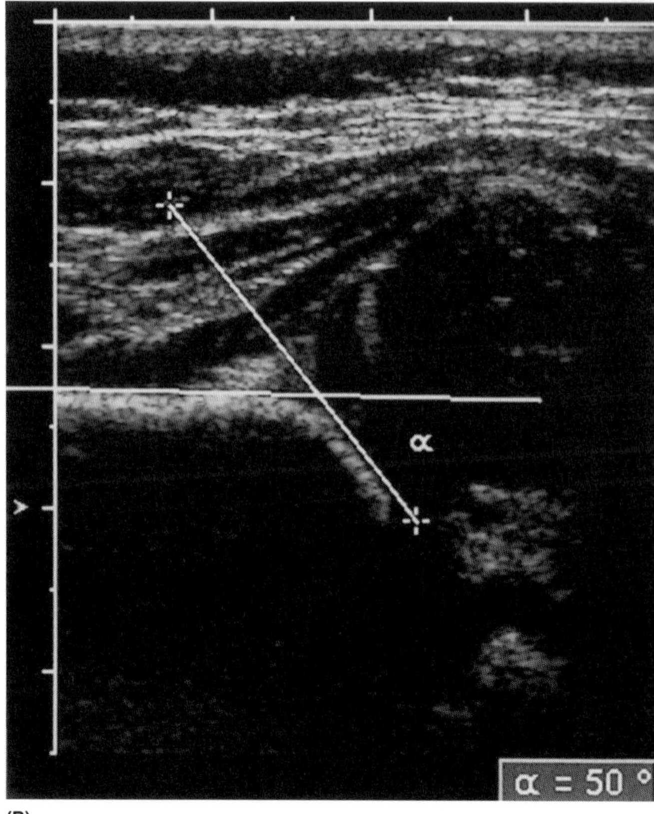

(B)

FIGURE 4 A AND B ■ (**A**) Coronal-neutral ultrasound image demonstrating a normal hip, with alpha and beta angles measured. (**B**) Coronal ultrasound view of a dysplastic acetabulum, with a shallow acetabulum and small alpha angle.

A third echogenic line, which should be relatively straight, consists of the echogenic metaphyseal plate adjacent to the growth plate of the femur. The hypoechoic femoral head nests within these structures, and the femoral shaft is not visible, being outside the plane of imaging. The posterior lip of the acetabulum can be seen at the superolateral portion of the screen; the femoral head should not overlie this structure.

Stability is evaluated by adducting the flexed thigh while at the same time gently pistoning the knee posteriorly in a Barlow-like maneuver. Held in this position, the femoral metaphyseal margin creates the left-hand line of a "V." An Ortolani-like maneuver is then performed, with abduction of the leg, and the metaphyseal line moves more medial in the acetabulum; this creates a "U" configuration.

With subluxation, the femoral head no longer nests deeply within the acetabulum but assumes a position displaced from the pubis, riding up against the posterolateral margin of ischium (Fig. 6). There is an increase in the thickness of moderately echogenic material between the femoral head and the pubis. With dislocation, the femoral head no longer rests within the confines of the acetabulum but perches on or is displaced posterolaterally from the ischial acetabular lip (Fig. 7). Dislocation may be so severe that normal acetabular landmarks cannot be defined in this plane. In the presence of either subluxation or dislocation, it is essential to check for reducibility by abducting the hip and attempting to reduce the femoral head into the acetabulum.

TABLE 5 ■ Acetabular Angle Measurements

Angle	Normal	Equivocal	Abnormal
α	>60	43–60	<43
β	<55	55–77	>77

Source: From Ref. 61.

Transverse Neutral

This optional approach, performed with the infant supine, evaluates femoral head position against the pubis anteriorly and the ischium posteriorly. The femoral head should demonstrate close contact with these bones (Fig. 8). A small amount of motion with pistoning maneuver can be normal in one-to-two-day-old neonates in this view, with posterior displacement of 4 to 6 mm being a normal response to the push maneuver (76). In older infants, the femoral head position should not change.

Posterior Lip, Coronal Flexion

Another optional imaging plane is performed with the infant supine and the hip flexed, the probe held as for coronal imaging but more posteriorly, over the posterior

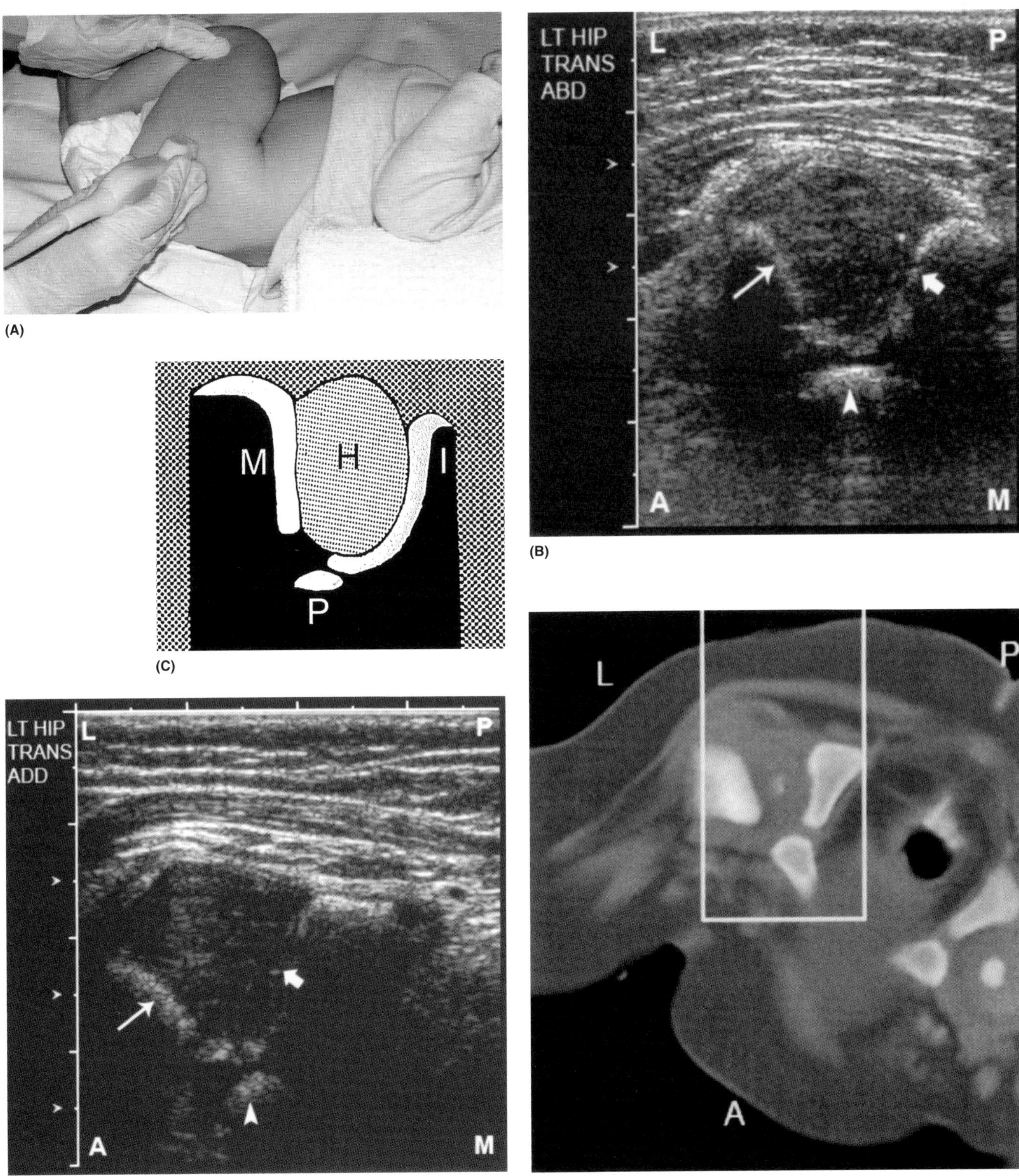

FIGURE 5 A–E ■ Transverse-flexion examination. (**A**) The infant is turned away from the transducer, and the transducer is positioned over the posterolateral hip. (**B**) Transverse-flexion ultrasound of a normal hip held in abduction, resulting in a "U" configuration. Recall that the transducer is posterolateral, not lateral. Note the pubis (*arrowhead*), ischium (*wide arrow*), and femoral metaphyseal plate (*thin arrow*) adjacent to hypoechoic femoral head. L, lateral; M, medial; A, anterior; P, posterior. (**C**) Accompanying diagram demonstrates bony landmarks. H, femoral head; I, ischium; M, femoral metaphysis; P, pubis. (**D**) Axial CT scan of normal hip positioned in flexion and abduction. The image is rotated to correspond to the accompanying ultrasound image. The white box indicates the portion of the hip that is included in the ultrasound evaluation. Landmarks same as in (**B**). (**E**) Normal transverse-flexion ultrasound with the hip held in adduction, resulting in a "V" configuration. Note that the femoral metaphyseal plate (*thin arrow*) is more angled than in abduction. The arrowhead denotes the pubis, and the wide arrow points to the ischium. *Source*: (**C**) from Ref. 54.

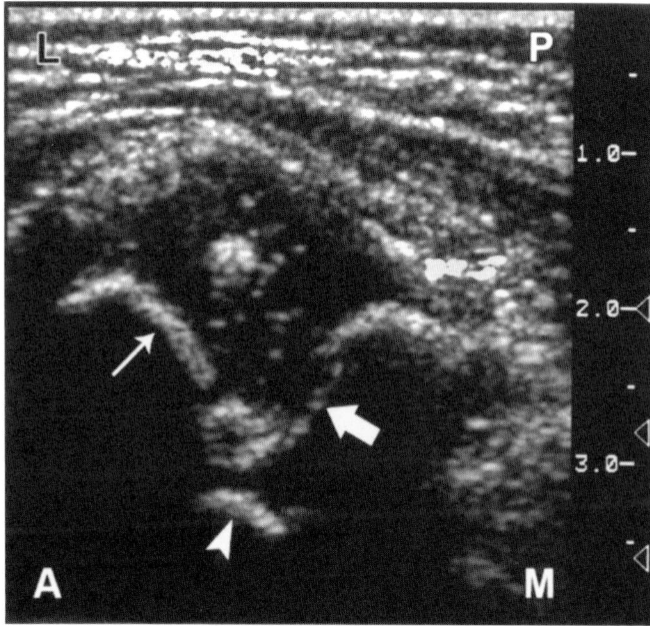

(A)

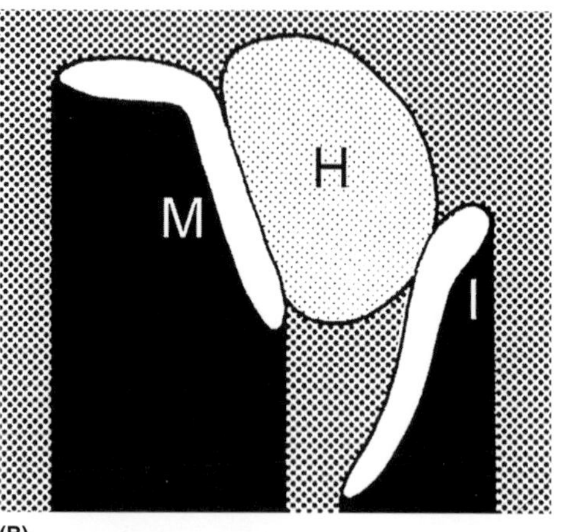

(B)

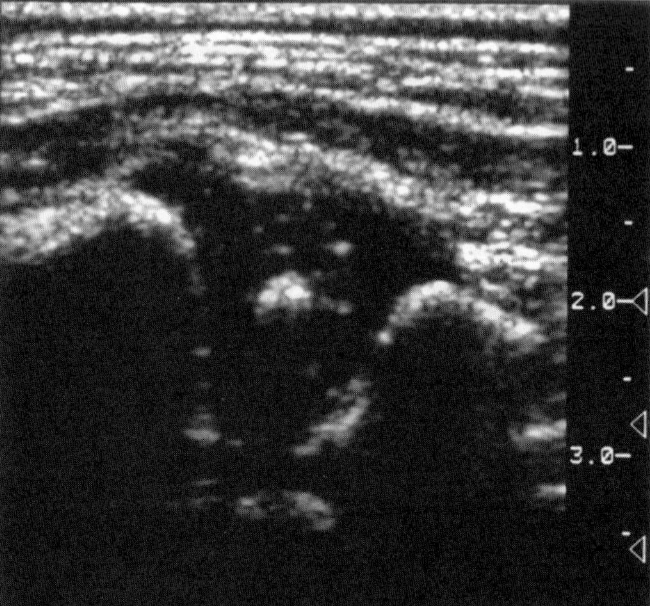

(C)

FIGURE 6 A–C ■ (**A**) Transverse-flexion adduction ultrasound of subluxated hip. Note the pubis (*arrowhead*), ischium (*wide arrow*), and femoral metaphyseal plate (*thin arrow*) adjacent to hypoechoic femoral head. The center of the femoral head has become echogenic as it begins to ossify. L, lateral; M, medial; A, anterior; P, posterior. (**B**) Accompanying diagram demonstrates bony landmarks. H, femoral head; I, ischium; M, femoral metaphysis. (**C**) Transverse-flexion abduction view of the same hip as in (**A**) shows that the femoral head reduces with abduction. Note that the femoral head is now seated deeply within the acetabulum. *Source*: (**B**) from Ref. 54.

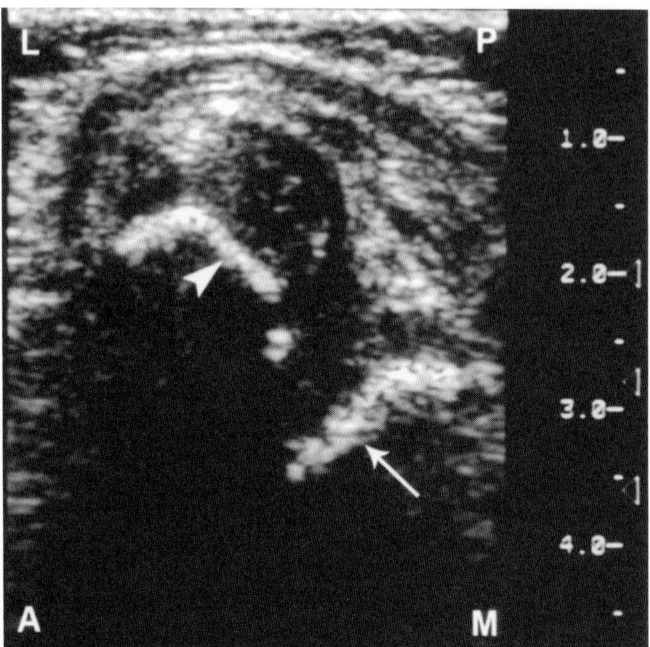

(A)

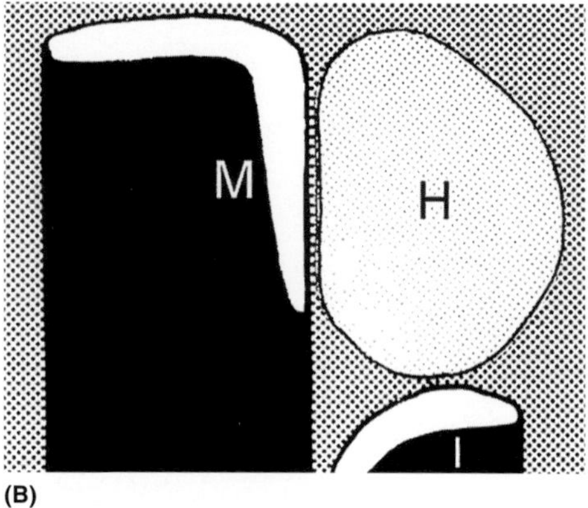

(B)

FIGURE 7 A–D ■ Transverse-flexion views of dislocated hip. (**A**) Transverse-flexion adduction ultrasound of dislocated hip. The pubis is no longer appreciable, due to a combination of increased distance from the transducer (now that the dislocated femoral head intervenes) and shadowing from the displaced metaphyseal plate (*arrowhead*). The ischium (*arrow*) is still evident. L, lateral; M, medial; A, anterior; P, posterior. (**B**) Accompanying diagram demonstrates bony landmarks. H, femoral head; I, ischium; M, femoral metaphysis. (*Continued*)

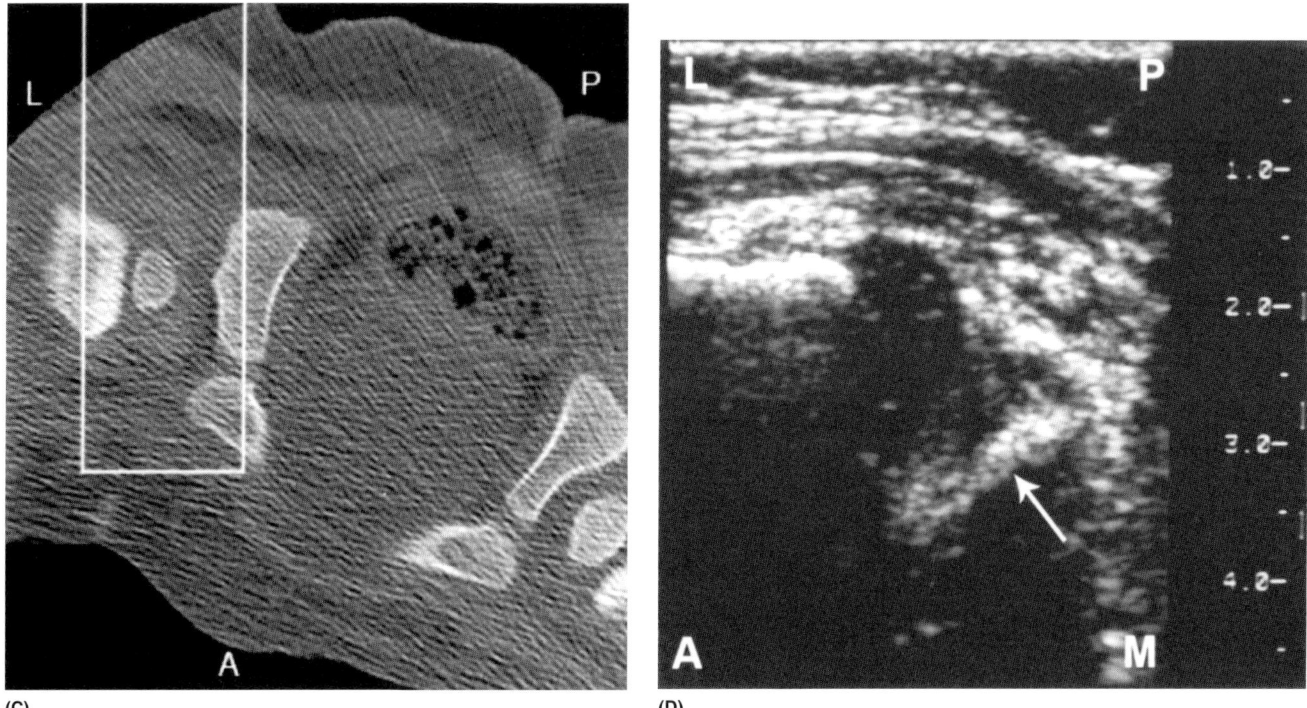

(C) (D)

FIGURE 7 A–D ■ (*Continued*) (**C**) Axial CT scan of dislocated hip held in flexion and abduction. The image is rotated to correspond to the accompanying ultrasound image. The white box indicates the portion of the image that is included in the ultrasound evaluation. (**D**) Transverse-flexion abduction view of minimally reducible hip. The arrow denotes the ischium. With abduction, the femoral head position corrects slightly. *Source*: (**B**) from Ref. 54.

portion of the acetabulum (Fig. 9). In this plane, the ilium and ischium are both horizontal, separated by the triradiate cartilage. In the normal hip, only the soft tissues of the hip musculature intervene between the hypoechoic triradiate cartilage and the transducer; the femoral head is not imaged. When hip instability is present, a small portion of the hypoechoic, round femoral head enters the plane of imaging, perhaps only when the joint is stressed by being pistoned posteriorly. If the triradiate cartilage is considered to be a mountain visible above the horizon formed by the horizontal ilium and ischium, the subluxating or dislocating femoral head can be considered to be the sunrise.

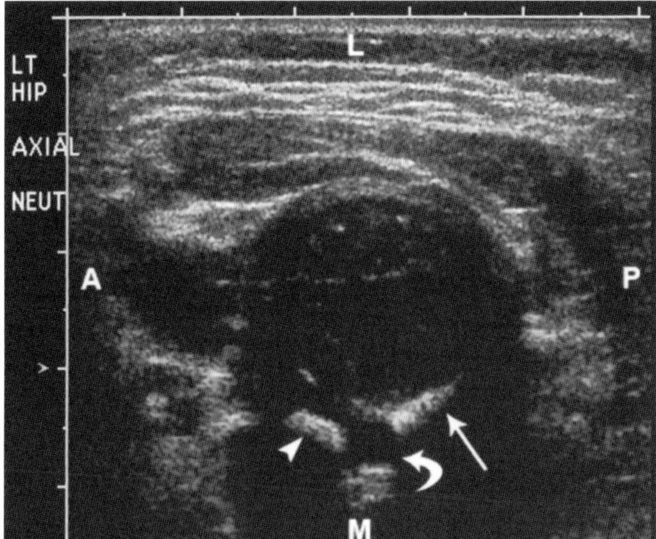

FIGURE 8 ■ Transverse-neutral view of normal hip. Note femoral head adjacent to pubis (*arrowhead*) and ischium (*arrow*). Curved arrow denotes triradiate cartilage. L, lateral; M, medial; A, anterior; P, posterior.

REPORTING HIP ULTRASOUND

The acetabulum is characterized as normal, immature, and mildly or severely dysplastic, depending on the degree of rounding of its edge and the steepness of the angle formed with the lateral margin of the ileum superior to the acetabulum. The cartilaginous component is characterized as normal, blunted, or displaced. If dysplastic, it may demonstrate increased echogenicity. Femoral head position is described in neutral, stressed, and attempted reduction positioning. The presence or absence of ossification of the femoral head should be noted. Asymmetry in degree of femoral head ossification merits mention but is not necessarily significant. The accompanying table summarizes the essential components of the hip ultrasound report, including discussion of optional views (Table 6).

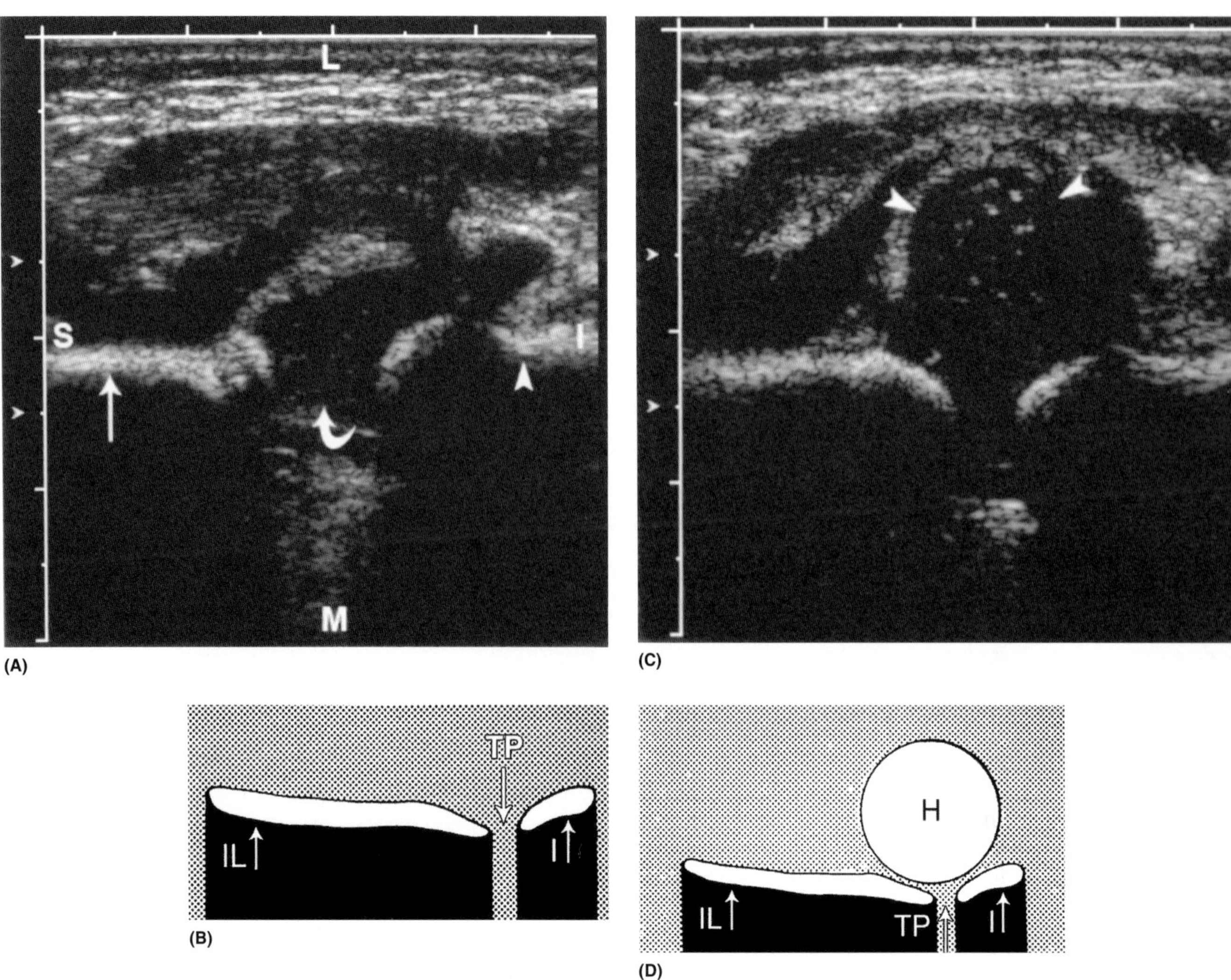

FIGURE 9 A–D ■ Coronal-flexion posterior lip views of normal and subluxatable hips. (**A**) Ultrasound of normal hip. Note the iliac bone (*straight arrow*) and ischium (*arrowhead*). The hypoechoic triradiate cartilage (*curved arrow*) can be regarded as a mountain rising out of a plain. (**B**) Accompanying diagram demonstrates bony landmarks. (**C**) Ultrasound of displaced hip. The speckled femoral head (*arrowheads*) is displaced into the image, visible as it overlaps the posterior plane of the acetabulum. It resembles a "sunrise" over the "mountain" of the triradiate cartilage. (**D**) Accompanying diagram demonstrates bony landmarks. L, lateral; M, medial; S, superior; I, inferior. (**B**) IL, ileum; I, ischium; TP, posterior lip of triradiate cartilage. *Source*: (**B,D**) from Ref. 54.

TABLE 6 ■ Ultrasound Views of the Hip

View	Appearance	Assess
Coronal neutral or Coronal flexion	Straight iliac line Curved acetabulum Posterior ischium	Acetabular contour Measurements (optional) Depth of femoral head below iliac line Shape of labrum
Coronal flexion	–	Femoral shaft may obscure acetabulum if hip dislocated
Transverse flexion Barlow: adduction Ortolani: abduction	Femoral metaphysis creates echogenic line on left Ischium creates echogenic line on right Pubis is relatively deep	"V": adduction. Determine if femoral head rises toward or perches on posterior acetabular margin (ischium) "U": abduction. Femoral head should seat tightly in acetabulum. Assess reducibility
Transverse neutral	Round femoral head nestles against ischium and pubis	Normal: femoral head close to acetabulum Abnormal: increased distance from ischium and pubis
Coronal flexion, posterior lip, with and without push/pull	Straight iliac line Curved "mountain" of triradiate cartilage	Femoral head should not be visible. If present ("sunrise"), indicates subluxation or dislocation

EXAMINING THE INFANT WHO IS UNDERGOING TREATMENT

During the initial phase of therapy for hip dysplasia, the infant wears a harness or other restraining device all the time (Fig. 10). The hip ultrasound exam is performed without removing the harness, and stress views are omitted, as they may be harmful to the stability of the femoral head. Only coronal-flexion and transverse-flexion views are obtained (40); mobility is assessed only within the confines of motion allowed by the harness. As the infant is gradually weaned from the harness, the examination can be performed out of the harness, but it is generally inadvisable to perform stress maneuvers until treatment nears completion and only when approved by the orthopedic surgeon. Ultrasound is performed at intervals of one to three weeks, depending on the severity of the instability.

EVALUATION OF HIP EFFUSIONS

The causes of hip pain in children are numerous, and the consequences of missing septic arthritis are profound; if an effusion can be excluded, a less aggressive therapeutic approach can be entertained. Ultrasound readily ascertains the presence of fluid within the hip joint (77–79), and this has important interventional and therapeutic implications.

A hip effusion can result from septic arthritis, osteomyelitis, Legg–Calve–Perthes disease, slipped capital femoral epiphysis, toxic synovitis, and other entities.

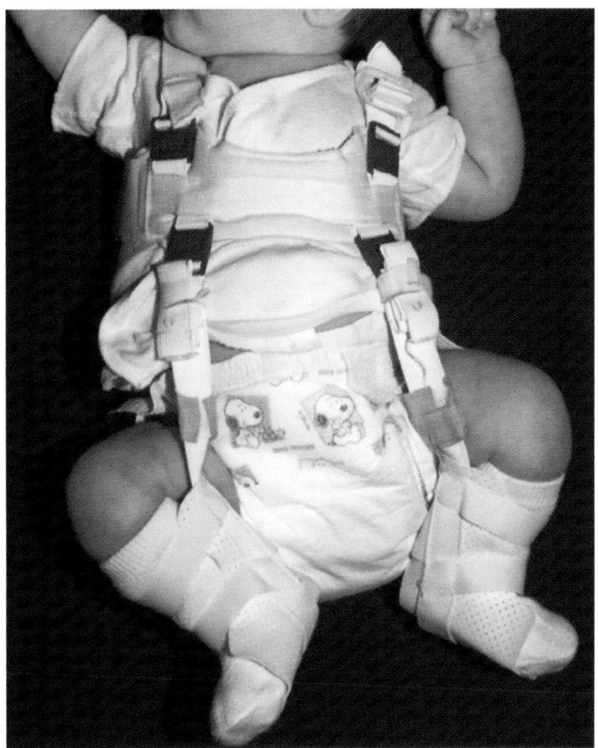

FIGURE 10 ■ Infant in Pavlik harness. The hips are symmetrically positioned in abduction and flexion.

Although early work found that the echo characteristics of the joint fluid and the thickness of the cartilage correlated with the etiology of hip pain (80), more recent work has found no such correlation (79,81). The principal use of ultrasonography in the evaluation of the painful hip is thus excluding or confirming the presence of a joint effusion, which if present must then be tapped to allow characterization of the fluid.

Technique

The child is positioned supine, with the legs extended and slightly externally rotated. A high-frequency 7 to 10MHz linear transducer is positioned longitudinally, parallel to the cortical margin of the femoral neck in the same oblique-sagittal plane as that of the femoral neck (Fig. 11a) (77). The femoral neck and femoral head are imaged, with particular attention paid to the soft tissues and possibly fluid anterior to the echogenic cortex of the femoral neck (Fig. 11). It is important to image both the symptomatic and the asymptomatic sides, as the width of the joint space must be compared.

Anatomy

Depending on the degree of ossification of the femoral head, it appears variably hypoechoic, echogenic, or centrally echogenic with peripheral, not-yet-ossified cartilage being hypoechoic. The cortex of the femoral neck appears gently curved and very echogenic, with posterior acoustic shadowing. The joint capsule appears as an echogenic band, and layers of gluteus minimus, medius, and maximus demonstrate striations of mixed echogenicity.

If there is no effusion, the fibrous capsule of the hip joint usually appears concave, resting adjacent to the cortex. There should be a gap of no more than 2mm between the cortex and the joint capsule, and there should be no more than a 2mm difference between the two sides (77,82).

Findings

If there is a discrepancy of greater than 2mm in the thickness of the joint fluid between the right and left hips, or if the hip capsule is convex rather than concave (Fig. 11c), an effusion is present. The quality of the fluid is not helpful in characterizing the pathologic process, as serous effusions can appear complex whereas purulent or hemorrhagic collections can appear simple (78,83). Absence of effusion does not exclude osteomyelitis, and further clinical and imaging evaluation may be necessary to diagnose or exclude this entity (78,83). The capsule does not thicken with transient synovitis (84). Doppler ultrasound is noncontributory, for flow is rarely elevated even when septic arthritis is present (85).

Although the articular cartilage of the femoral head may be thickened in Legg–Calve–Perthes disease, there is a significant overlap with normal hips (81). Atrophy of the quadriceps muscles may be apparent as well with this entity (81). It is recognized that a fragmented femoral head may be demonstrated when Legg–Calve–Perthes

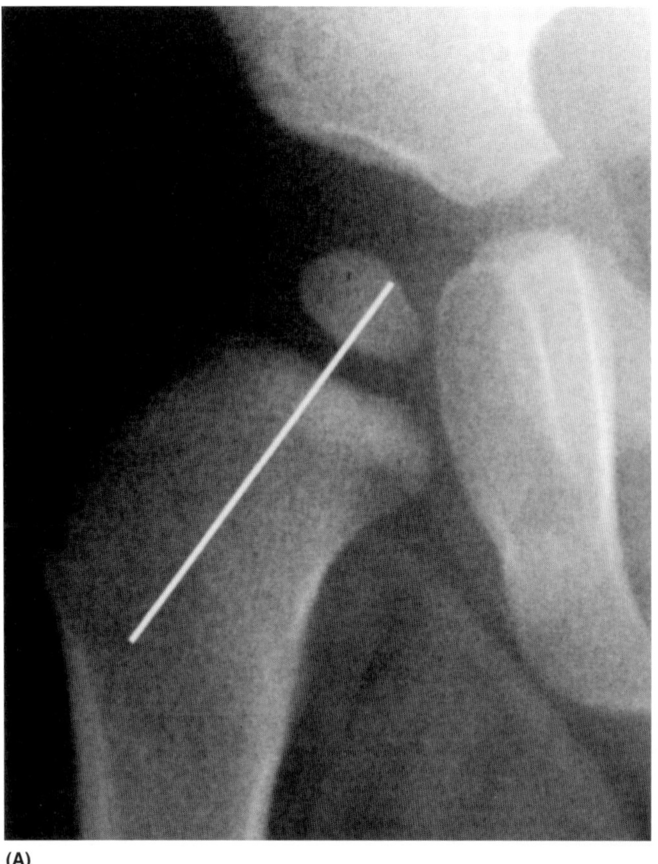

(A)

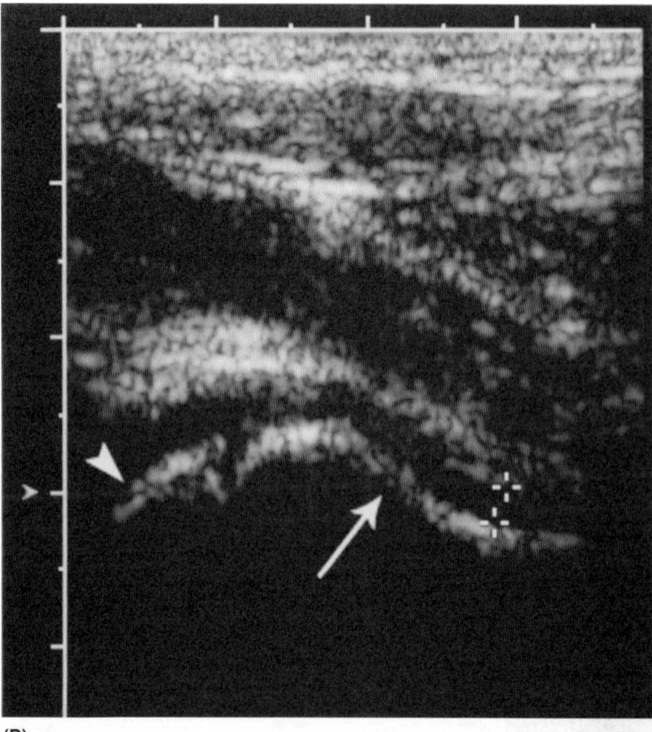

(B)

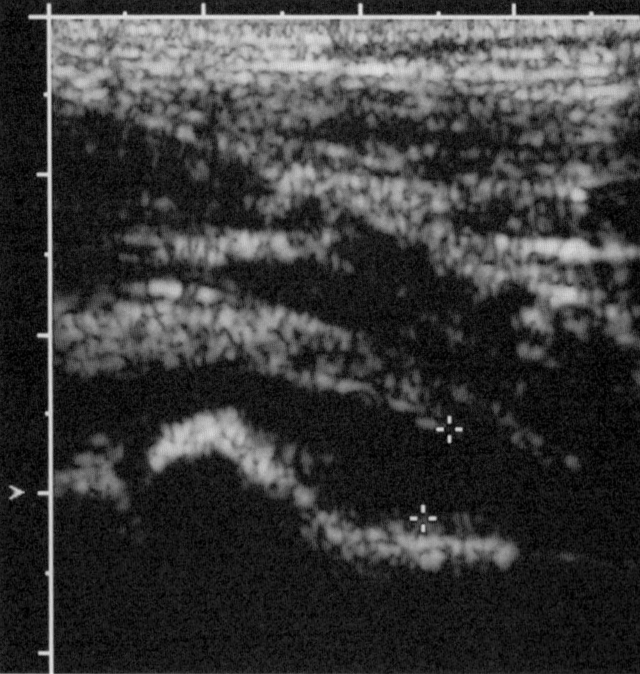

(C)

FIGURE 11 A–C ■ (**A**) Radiograph of a normal hip, demonstrating the correct oblique-sagittal placement of the ultrasound transducer (*white line*) for evaluation of effusion. (**B**) Normal oblique-sagittal ultrasound of the hip, demonstrating the rounded femoral head (*arrowhead*) and gently curved cortex of the femoral neck (*arrow*). The joint space is insignificant (ultrasound markers). (**C**) Oblique-sagittal ultrasound of hip with effusion. Note the large gap between femoral cortex and synovium (*ultrasound markers*) as well as the convex synovial contour.

disease is present, and a slipped capital femoral epiphysis may also be seen ultrasonographically.

INFECTIOUS PROCESSES

Ultrasound permits evaluation of fluid in additional joint spaces besides the hip, such as the wrist and shoulder (86); it can assist in localization for aspiration. It can also characterize inflammation of subcutaneous soft tissues and musculature, permitting definition of a phlegmon as a localized hypoechoic, ill-defined area, and then recognizing development of an abscess as a focal fluid collection (Fig. 12). Periosteal elevation and subperiosteal fluid can be demonstrated when osteomyelitis is present (87), but MRI is preferable (86).

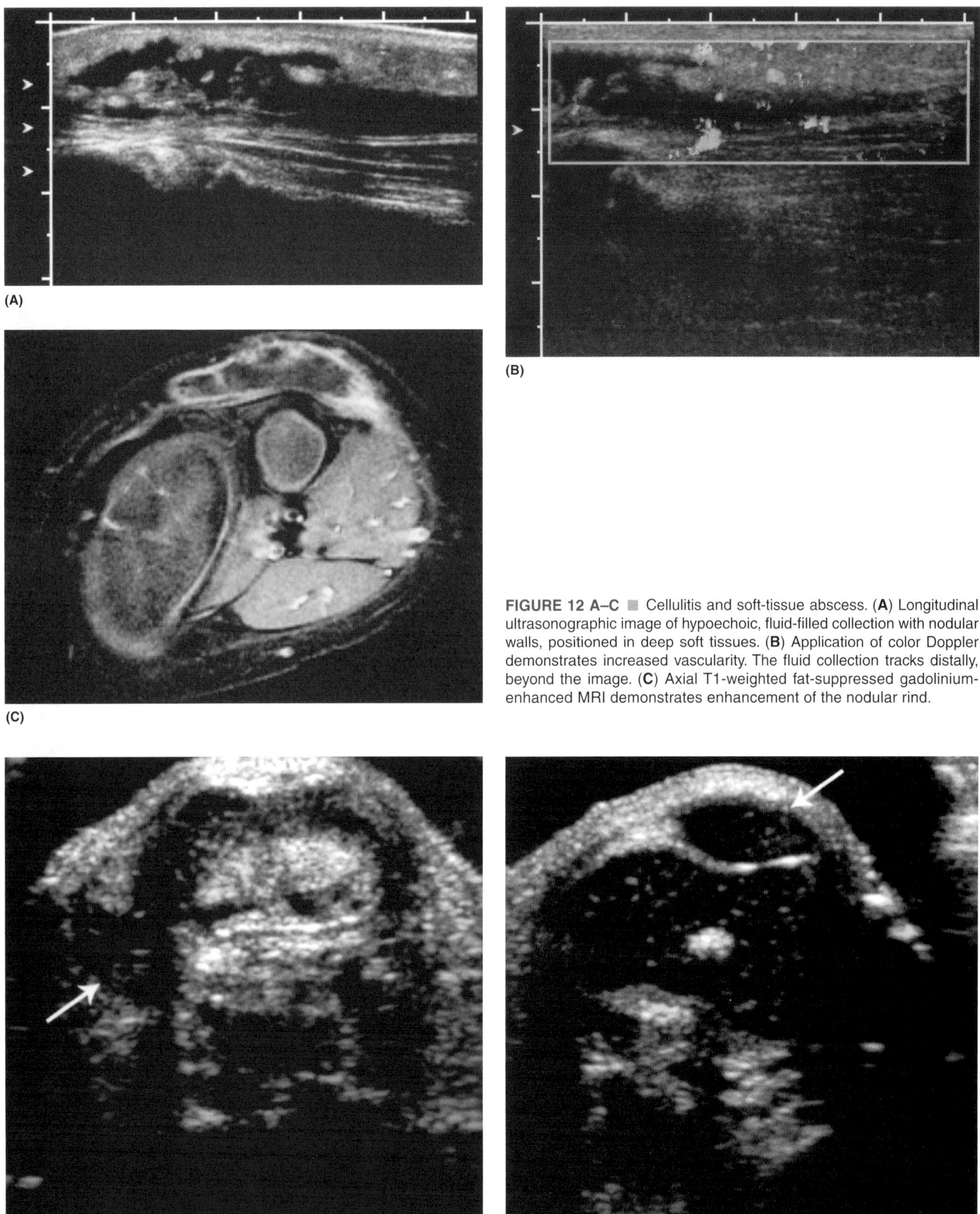

(A)

(B)

(C)

FIGURE 12 A–C ■ Cellulitis and soft-tissue abscess. (**A**) Longitudinal ultrasonographic image of hypoechoic, fluid-filled collection with nodular walls, positioned in deep soft tissues. (**B**) Application of color Doppler demonstrates increased vascularity. The fluid collection tracks distally, beyond the image. (**C**) Axial T1-weighted fat-suppressed gadolinium-enhanced MRI demonstrates enhancement of the nodular rind.

(A)

(B)

FIGURE 13 A AND B ■ Normal and dislocated cartilaginous patella in a three-month-old girl. (**A**) Transverse ultrasound of the knee at the level of the patella shows an empty femoral notch. The hypoechoic patella (*arrow*) is dislocated lateral to the posterolateral femoral condyle. (**B**) Transverse ultrasound of the contralateral knee demonstrates the patella (*arrow*) positioned normally between the medial and the lateral femoral condyles.

PATELLA

The nonossified patella is readily assessed by ultrasound. This is mainly important in evaluating patients with suspected congenital or developmental dislocation of the patella (88). The patella appears lentiform and hypoechoic, either positioned normally between the echogenic femoral condyles (Fig. 13a) or dislocated laterally or superiorly (Fig. 13b). Congenital patellar dislocation is associated with Trisomy 21, Larsen syndrome, arthrogryposis, nail-patella syndrome, and other syndromes (88). The extensor mechanism can also be evaluated during dynamic ultrasonographic interrogation (89).

REFERENCES

1. Tredwell SJ, Bell HM. Efficacy of neonatal hip examination. J Pediatr Orthop 1981; 1(1):61–65.
2. Burger BJ et al. Neonatal screening and staggered early treatment for congenital dislocation or dysplasia of the hip. Lancet 1990; 336(8730):1549–1553.
3. Dunn PM et al. Congenital dislocation of the hip: early and late diagnosis and management compared. Arch Dis Child 1985; 60(5):407–414.
4. Rosendahl K, Markestad T, Lie RT. Developmental dysplasia of the hip: prevalence based on ultrasound diagnosis. Pediatr Radiol 1996; 26(9):635–639.
5. Rosendahl K, Markestad T, Lie RT. Developmental dysplasia of the hip. A population-based comparison of ultrasound and clinical findings. Acta Paediatr 1996; 85(1):64–69.
6. Coleman SS. Congenital dysplasia of the hip in the navajo infant. Clin Orthop Relat Res 1968; 56:179–193.
7. Burke SW et al. Congenital dislocation of the hip in the American black. Clin Orthop Relat Res 1985; (192):120–123.
8. Lloyd-Roberts GC. Osteoarthritis of the hip; a study of the clinical pathology. J Bone Joint Surg Br 1955; 37-B(1):8–47.
9. Zieger M, Schulz RD. Ultrasonography of the infant hip. Part III: clinical application. Pediatr Radiol 1987; 17(3):226–232.
10. Boeree NR, Clarke NM. Ultrasound imaging and secondary screening for congenital dislocation of the hip. J Bone Joint Surg Br 1994; 76(4):525–533.
11. Jones DA, Powell N. Ultrasound and neonatal hip screening. A prospective study of "high risk" babies. J Bone Joint Surg Br 1990; 72(3):457–459.
12. Hadlow V. Neonatal screening for congenital dislocation of the hip. A prospective 21-year survey. J Bone Joint Surg Br 1988; 70(5): 740–743.
13. Berman L, Klenerman L. Ultrasound screening for hip abnormalities: preliminary findings in 1001 neonates. Br Med J (Clin Res Ed) 1986; 293(6549):719–722.
14. Jones D. Neonatal detection of developmental dysplasia of the hip (DDH). J Bone Joint Surg Br 1998; 80-B(6):943–945.
15. Bialik V et al. Developmental dysplasia of the hip: a new approach to incidence. Pediatrics 1999; 103(1):93–99.
16. Clarke NM, Clegg J, Al-Chalabi AN. Ultrasound screening of hips at risk for CDH. Failure to reduce the incidence of late cases. J Bone Joint Surg Br 1989; 71(1):9–12.
17. De Pellegrin M. Ultrasound screening for congenital dislocation of the hip. Results and correlations between clinical and ultrasound findings. Ital J Orthop Traumatol 1991; 17(4):547–553.
18. Clarke NM et al. Real-time ultrasound in the diagnosis of congenital dislocation and dysplasia of the hip. J Bone Joint Surg Br 1985; 67(3):406–412.
19. Toma P et al. Paediatric hip—ultrasound screening for developmental dysplasia of the hip: a review. Eur J Ultrasound 2001; 14(1):45–55.
20. Tonnis D, Storch K, Ulbrich H. Results of newborn screening for cdh with and without sonography and correlation of risk factors. J Pediatr Orthop 1990; 10(2):145–152.
21. Walter RS et al. Ultrasound screening of high-risk infants. A method to increase early detection of congenital dysplasia of the hip. Am J Dis Child 1992; 146(2):230–234.
22. Harcke HT. The role of ultrasound in diagnosis and management of developmental dysplasia of the hip. Pediatr Radiol 1995; 25(3):225–227.
23. Graf R, Tschauner C, Klapsch W. Progress in prevention of late developmental dislocation of the hip by sonographic newborn hip "screening": results of a comparative follow-up study. J Pediatr Orthop 1993; 2:115–121.
24. Castelein RM et al. Natural history of ultrasound hip abnormalities in clinically normal newborns. J Pediatr Orthop 1992; 12(4): 423–427.
25. Eastwood DM. Neonatal hip screening. Lancet 2003; 361(9357): 595–597.
26. Rosendahl K, Markestad T, Lie RT. Ultrasound screening for developmental dysplasia of the hip in the neonate: the effect on treatment rate and prevalence of late cases. Pediatrics 1994; 94(1):47–52.
27. Jones D et al. At the crossroads—neonatal detection of developmental dysplasia of the hip. J Bone Joint Surg Br 2000; 82(2):160–164.
28. Holen KJ et al. Universal or selective screening of the neonatal hip using ultrasound? a prospective, randomised trial of 15,529 newborn infants. J Bone Joint Surg Br 2002; 84(6):886–890.
29. Bache CE, Clegg J, Herron M. Risk factors for developmental dysplasia of the hip: ultrasonographic findings in the neonatal period. J Pediatr Orthop B 2002; 11(3):212–218.
30. Lewis K, Jones DA, Powell N. Ultrasound and neonatal hip screening: the five-year results of a prospective study in high-risk babies. J Pediatr Orthop 1999; 19(6):760–762.
31. Marks DS, Clegg J, Al-Chalabi AN. Routine ultrasound screening for neonatal hip instability. Can it abolish late-presenting congenital dislocation of the hip? J Bone Joint Surg Br 1994; 76(4):534–538.
32. Holen KJ et al. Ultrasonographic evaluation of breech presentation as a risk factor for hip dysplasia. Acta Paediatr 1996; 85(2): 225–229.
33. Murray KA, Crim JR. Radiographic imaging for treatment and follow-up of developmental dysplasia of the hip. Semin Ultrasound CT MR 2001; 22(4):306–340.
34. Walsh JJ, Morrissy RT. Torticollis and hip dislocation. J Pediatr Orthop 1998; 18(2):219–221.
35. Bick U, Muller-Leisse C, Troger J. Ultrasonography of the hip in preterm neonates. Pediatr Radiol 1990; 20(5):331–333.
36. Clinical Practice Guideline: early detection of developmental dysplasia of the hip. Committee on Quality Improvement, Subcommittee on Developmental Dysplasia of the Hip. American Academy of Pediatrics. Pediatrics 2000; 105(4 Pt 1):896–905.
37. Riboni G et al. Ultrasound screening for developmental dysplasia of the hip. Pediatr Radiol 2003; 33(7):475–481. Epub 2003.
38. Harcke HT. Screening newborns for developmental dysplasia of the hip: the role of sonography. AJR Am J Roentgenol 1994; 162(2): 395–397.
39. Andersson JE. Neonatal hip instability: results and experiences from ten years of screening with the anterior-dynamic ultrasound method. Acta Paediatr 2002; 91(8):926–929.
40. Harcke HT, Grissom LE. Performing dynamic sonography of the infant hip. AJR Am J Roentgenol 1990; 155(4):837–844.
41. Mackenzie IG. Congenital dislocation of the hip. The development of a regional service. J Bone Joint Surg Br 1972; 54(1):18–39.
42. Tredwell SJ, Davis LA. Prospective study of congenital dislocation of the hip. J Pediatr Orthop 1989; 9(4):386–390.
43. Terjesen T, Bredland T, and BergV. Ultrasound for hip assessment in the newborn. J Bone Joint Surg Br 1989; 71(5):767–773.
44. Iwasaki K. Treatment of congenital dislocation of the hip by the pavlik harness. Mechanism of reduction and usage. J Bone Joint Surg Am 1983; 65(6):760–767.
45. Bearcroft PW et al. Vascularity of the neonatal femoral head: in vivo demonstration with power doppler US. Radiology 1996; 200(1): 209–211.

46. Kalamchi A, Macewen GD. Avascular necrosis following treatment of congenital dislocation of the hip. J Bone Joint Surg Am 1980; 62(6):876–888.
47. Jaramillo D et al. Gadolinium-enhanced MR imaging demonstrates abduction-caused hip ischemia and its reversal in piglets. Pediatr Radiol 1995; 25(8):578–587.
48. Taylor GR, Clarke NM. Monitoring the treatment of developmental dysplasia of the hip with the pavlik harness. The role of ultrasound. J Bone Joint Surg Br 1997; 79(5):719–723.
49. Grissom LE et al. Ultrasound evaluation of hip position in the pavlik harness. J Ultrasound Med 1988; 7(1):1–6.
50. Hangen DH et al. The pavlik harness and developmental dysplasia of the hip: has ultrasound changed treatment patterns? J Pediatr Orthop 1995; 15(6):729–735.
51. Harding MG et al. Management of dislocated hips with pavlik harness treatment and ultrasound monitoring. J Pediatr Orthop 1997; 17(2):189–198.
52. Boal DK, Schwenkter EP. The infant hip: assessment with real-time US. Radiology 1985; 157(3):667–672.
53. Harcke HT, Kumar SJ. The role of ultrasound in the diagnosis and management of congenital dislocation and dysplasia of the hip. J Bone Joint Surg Am 1991; 73(4):622–628.
54. Harcke HT. Hip and Musculoskeletal US. In: Seibert JJ, ed. Syllabus: Current Concepts: A Categorical Course in Pediatric Radiology. Oak Brook: RSNA Publications, 1994.
55. Yousefzadeh DK, Ramilo JL. Normal hip in children: correlation of US with anatomic and cryomicrotome sections. Radiology 1987; 165(3):647–655.
56. Harcke HT et al. Ossification center of the infant hip: sonographic and radiographic correlation. AJR Am J Roentgenol 1986; 147(2): 317–321.
57. Graf R. The diagnosis of congenital hip-joint dislocation by the ultrasonic compound treatment. Arch Orthop Trauma Surg 1980; 97(2):117–133.
58. Harcke HT et al. Examination of the infant hip with real-time ultrasonography. J Ultrasound Med 1984; 3(3):131–137.
59. Morin C, Harcke HT, Macewen GD. The infant hip: real-time us assessment of acetabular development. Radiology 1985; 157(3): 673–677.
60. Novick G, Ghelman B, Schneider M. Sonography of the neonatal and infant hip. AJR Am J Roentgenol 1983; 141(4):639–645.
61. Graf R. Fundamentals of sonographic diagnosis of infant hip dysplasia. J Pediatr Orthop 1984; 4(6):735–740.
62. Graf R. Classification of hip joint dysplasia by means of sonography. Arch Orthop Trauma Surg 1984; 102(4):248–255.
63. Falliner A et al. Comparable ultrasound measurements of ten anatomical specimens of infant hip joints by the methods of Graf and Terjesen. Acta Radiol 2004; 45(2):227–235.
64. Rosendahl K et al. Reliability of ultrasound in the early diagnosis of developmental dysplasia of the hip. Pediatr Radiol 1995; 25(3):219–224.
65. Zieger M. Ultrasound of the infant hip. Part 2. Validity of the method. Pediatr Radiol 1986; 16(6):488–492.
66. Graf R. Hip sonography—how reliable? Sector scanning versus linear scanning? Dynamic versus static examination? Clin Orthop Relat Res 1992; (281):18–21.
67. Harcke HT, Grissom LE. Infant hip sonography: current concepts. Semin Ultrasound CT MR 1994; 15(4):256–263.
68. AIUM Practice Guideline for the performance of the ultrasound examination for detection of developmental dysplasia of the hip. J Ultrasound Med 2003; 22:1131–1136.
69. ACR Practice Guideline for the performance of the ultrasound examination for detection of developmental dysplasia of the hip. Practice Guidelines and Technical Standards. 2005, ed. A. C. O. Radiology. Reston, VA: ACR, 2005:753–757.
70. Holen KJ et al. Ultrasound screening for hip dysplasia in newborns. J Pediatr Orthop 1994; 14(5):667–673.
71. Gerscovich EO et al. Three-dimensional sonographic evaluation of developmental dysplasia of the hip: preliminary findings. Radiology 1994; 190(2):407–410.
72. Gomes H et al. Sonography of the neonatal hip: a dynamic approach. Ann Radiol (Paris) 1987; 30(7):503–510.
73. Andersson JE. Neonatal hip instability: normal values for physiological movement of the femoral head determined by an anterior-dynamic ultrasound method. J Pediatr Orthop 1995; 15(6):736–740.
74. Grissom LE, Harke HT. Developmental dysplasia of the pediatric hip with emphasis on sonographic evaluation. Semin Musculoskelet Radiol 1999; 5(4):359–369.
75. Soboleski DA, Babyn P. Sonographic diagnosis of developmental dysplasia of the hip: importance of increased thickness of acetabular cartilage. AJR Am J Roentgenol 1993; 161(4):839–842.
76. Keller MS et al. Normal instability of the hip in the neonate: US standards. Radiology 1988; 169(3):733–736.
77. Alexander JE et al. High-resolution hip ultrasound in the limping child. J Clin Ultrasound 1989; 17(1):19–24.
78. Marchal GJ et al. Transient synovitis of the hip in children: role of US. Radiology 1987; 162(3):825–828.
79. Miralles M et al. Sonography of the painful hip in children: 500 consecutive cases. AJR Am J Roentgenol 1989; 152(3): 579–582.
80. Dorr U, Zieger M, Hauke H. Ultrasonography of the painful hip. Prospective studies in 204 patients. Pediatr Radiol 1988; 19(1): 36–40.
81. Robben SG et al. US of the painful hip in childhood: diagnostic value of cartilage thickening and muscle atrophy in the detection of perthes disease. Radiology 1998; 208(1):35–42.
82. Adam R et al. Arthrosonography of the irritable hip in childhood: a review of 1 year's experience. Br J Radiol 1986; 59(699): 205–208.
83. Zawin JK et al. Joint effusion in children with an irritable hip: US diagnosis and aspiration. Radiology 1993; 187(2):459–463.
84. Robben SG et al. Anterior joint capsule of the normal hip and in children with transient synovitis: US study with anatomic and histologic correlation. Radiology 1999; 210(2):499–507.
85. Strouse PJ, Dipietro MA, Adler RS. Pediatric hip effusions: evaluation with power doppler sonography. Radiology 1998; 206(3):731–735.
86. Bureau NJ, Chhem RK, Cardinal E. Musculoskeletal infections: US manifestations. Radiographics 1999; 19(6):1585–1592.
87. Mah ET et al. Ultrasonic features of acute osteomyelitis in children. J Bone Joint Surg Br 1994; 76(6):969–974.
88. Koplewitz BZ, Babyn PS, Cole WG. Congenital dislocation of the patella. AJR Am J Roentgenol 2005; 184(5):1640–1646.
89. Miller TT et al. Sonography of patellar abnormalities in children. AJR Am J Roentgenol 1998; 171(3):739–742.

Skeletal and Superficial Soft Tissues

Viviane Khoury, Etienne Cardinal, and Rethy K. Chhem

30

Ultrasound (US) is an appealing technique for the evaluation of the musculoskeletal system. It has the advantages of being noninvasive and of relatively low cost, and it may be used for the initial investigation of a wide spectrum of musculoskeletal diseases. US also offers a unique opportunity to evaluate the soft tissues dynamically as muscles are contracted and joints mobilized, allowing the diagnosis of anomalies that may only be demonstrated during motion. Another interesting aspect of ultrasonography is that by probing a specific area with the transducer, the examiner can get information from the patient about the site of maximal pain, allowing establishment of an anatomic correlation. With the newer high-resolution transducers, smaller and more superficial structures can be studied. The diagnostic capabilities of US continue to increase and become more refined with the improved technology of transducers and more effective utilization of existing applications, such as Doppler imaging. Extended-field-of-view imaging has allowed for more easily interpretable images and more effective cross-specialty communication. Ultrasonography of the musculoskeletal system requires some training, but with careful evaluation and a systematic approach, its usefulness becomes apparent quickly.

NORMAL ANATOMY

Normal Skin and Subcutaneous Tissues

There are two basic types of ultrasonography with dermatological applications. One type is 20 MHz scanning, used in the imaging of borders of skin tumors and other focal skin lesions and in the assessment and measurement of skin thickness of inflammatory skin diseases such as scleroderma and psoriasis. This type of scanning has a well-established role in clinical dermatology (1). Detailed description of such applications is beyond the scope of this chapter.

The second type of ultrasonography in dermatology is 5 to 12 MHz scanning in the assessment of deeper or larger dermatological lesions. The most common dermatologic conditions that require US study include palpable mass, cellulitis, diffuse swelling of the extremities, and clinically suspected subcutaneous abscess (Table 1).

The normal skin is composed of epidermis, dermis, and subcutaneous fat. The epidermis is made up of a cellular layer with no blood vessels. The dermis consists of an extensive network of blood vessels distributed among hair follicles and sebaceous and sweat glands. The fatty subcutaneous tissue contains mainly fat associated with a variable amount of connective fibrous tissue. The US characteristics of normal skin are summarized in Table 2.

Normal Muscle

Normal skeletal muscle has a feathery or pennate aspect on longitudinal US scanning (Fig. 1A) (2,3). The individual muscle bundles are surrounded by fibroadipose septa (perimysium).

TABLE 1 ■ Role of US in Skin Disorders

- Detection of focal or diffuse lesion
- Compartmental localization of lesion (skin, subcutaneous fat)
- Characterization of lesion quality (solid or cystic, presence of calcification or gas)
- Assessment of tumor characteristics (borders, depth extension)
- Biopsy guidance
- Abscess drainage guidance

Abbreviation: US, ultrasound.

Muscle bundles of fibers are seen as hypoechoic zones and the septa are seen as hyperechoic lines separating the fibers. Surrounding the entire muscle is a fascia or aponeurosis, which is made up of thick connective tissue and is also hyperechoic relative to muscle.

On transverse scan (Fig. 1B), the echogenicity of muscle depends on the degree of contraction, while the septa and fascia appear bright, as seen on longitudinal scans. Contracted muscle is more echoic than relaxed muscle.

TABLE 2 ■ US Characteristics of Normal Skin Using a 7.5 to 10 MHz Transducer

- Epidermis and dermis: medium echogenicity
- Subcutaneous fat: hypoechoic layer with hyperechoic strands
- Skin appendages: not seen
- Nail: two parallel echoic lines

Abbreviation: US, ultrasound.

The general echogenicity of muscle is less than that of tendon, nerve, and subcutaneous tissue.

Normal Joint

Joint Space and Synovium

The diarthrodial joint is covered by synovium, which helps the lubrication of the joint. US demonstrates the joint capsule, articular recess, and intra-articular fat pad. The normal synovial membrane cannot be detected by US; however, the presence of an effusion is an indirect sign of a synovial disorder (Fig. 2). In synovitis, US often demonstrates accumulation of fluid in the joint space,

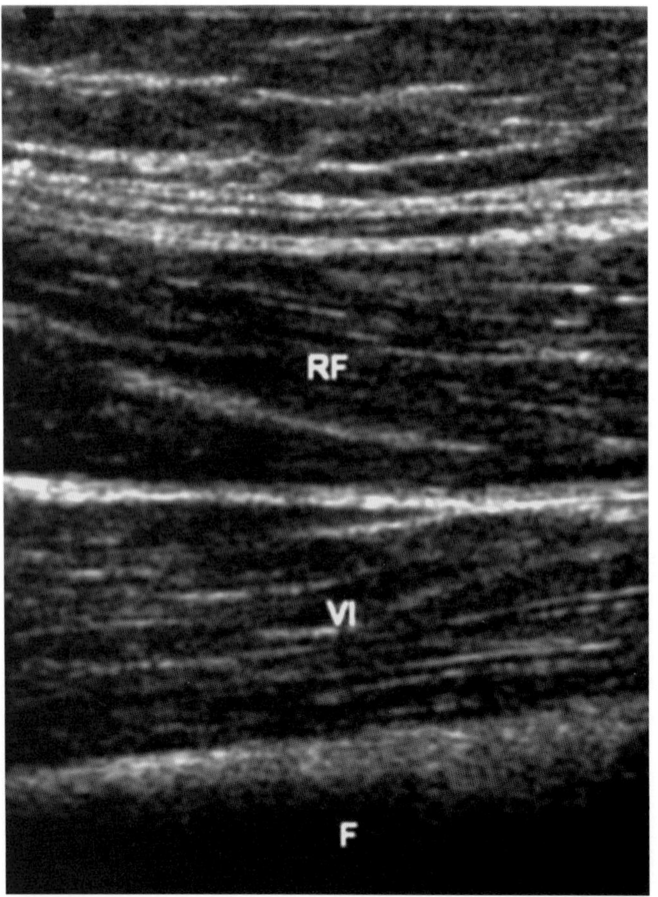

(A)

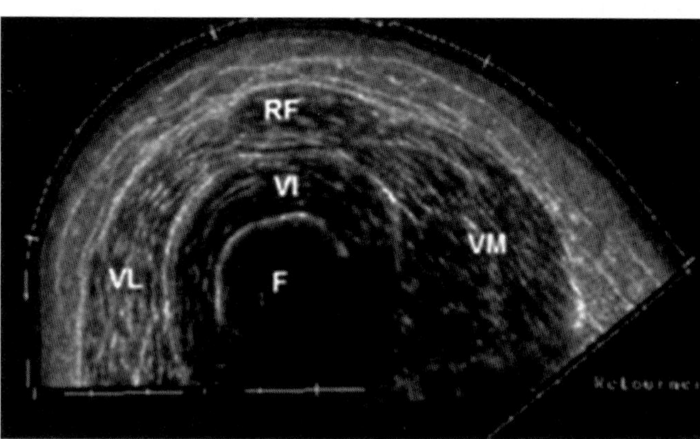

(B)

FIGURE 1 A AND B ■ Normal quadriceps muscle at the level of the midshaft of the femur. (**A**) Longitudinal sonogram of the anterior aspect of the thigh. The pennate pattern of the muscle is well demonstrated. (**B**) Panoramic transverse sonogram of the quadriceps group. RF, rectus femoris; VI, vastus intermedius; VM, vastus medialis; VL, vastus lateralis; F, femur.

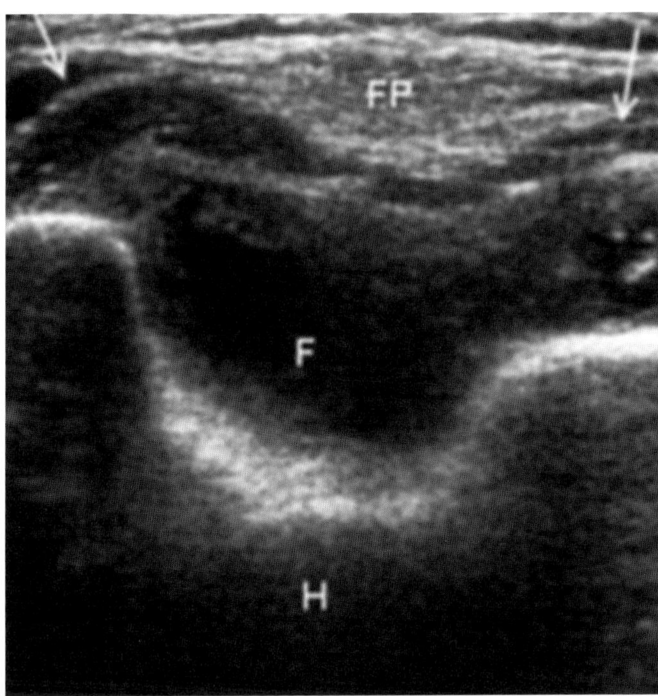

FIGURE 2 ■ Elbow joint effusion. Transverse sonogram along the olecranon fossa shows displacement of the posterior fat pad by the presence of intra-articular fluid. The distended joint capsule is shown (*arrows*). FP, fat pad; F, intra-articular fluid; H, distal humerus.

which can be associated with an abnormal hypertrophied synovium (4).

Bursa

Bursae are closed, connective, synovial sacs that normally contain a small amount of fluid. Their role is to facilitate gliding of one musculoskeletal structure on another. These structures include skin, tendon, ligament, and muscle gliding over bone. Three types of bursae have been described: superficial, deep, and adventitial.

On US, normal bursa appears as a small hypoechoic flat sac containing a small amount of normal fluid with a hyperechoic wall and peribursal fat (5).

The most commonly described bursae in radiology are the subacromial–subdeltoid (SASD) (2,5), olecranon (6), trochanteric (7), ischial (8), prepatellar, infrapatellar, and retrocalcaneal bursae (Fig. 3). Because of the multitude of these structures, the diagnosis of bursitis must be considered when fluid collection is demonstrated around a joint.

Among the myriad subcutaneous bursae, two are most commonly affected by inflammation: the olecranon bursa and the prepatellar bursa (Table 3).

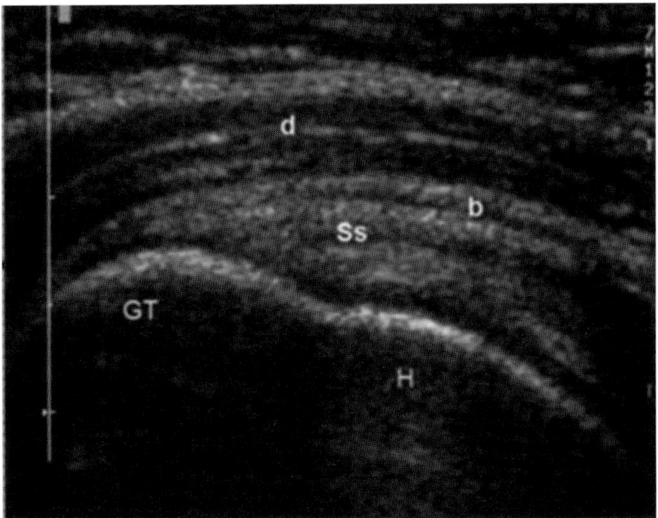

FIGURE 3 ■ Normal subacromial–subdeltoid bursa and supraspinatus tendon. Longitudinal sonogram along the course of the supraspinatus tendon. Insertion on the greater tuberosity is well demonstrated. The bursa appears as a thin hypoechoic line (*arrows*), delimited by two bright fat planes. The bursa lies deep to the deltoid muscle and superficial to the supraspinatus tendon. Ss, supraspinatus tendon; GT, greater tuberosity; H, humeral head; d, deltoid muscle; b, bursa.

TABLE 3 ■ Bursae Evaluated by US

Superficial
- Olecranon
- Trochanteric
- Prepatellar
- Ischial
- Pes anserine
- Achilles

Deep
- Subacromial–subdeltoid
- Iliopsoas
- Iliotibial band
- Infrapatellar
- Gastrocnemius–semimembranosus
- Retrocalcaneal

Abbreviation: US, ultrasound.

Ligament

Several ligaments have been imaged by US (Table 4) (5,9–13), which has proven useful for evaluating ligaments of both small and large joints. The evaluation of

TABLE 4 ■ Ligaments Evaluated by US

Shoulder: coracoacromial, transverse humeral

Elbow: ulnar collateral, medial collateral, annular

Wrist: scapholunate, (other intrinsic and extrinsic carpal ligaments, triangular fibrocartilage)

Hand: ulnar collateral of the thumb, collaterals of the metacarpophalangeal joints

Hip: iliofemoral

Knee: collateral, cruciate

Ankle: anterior and posterior talofibular, anterior and posterior tibiofibular, deltoid, calcaneofibular

Abbreviation: US, ultrasound.

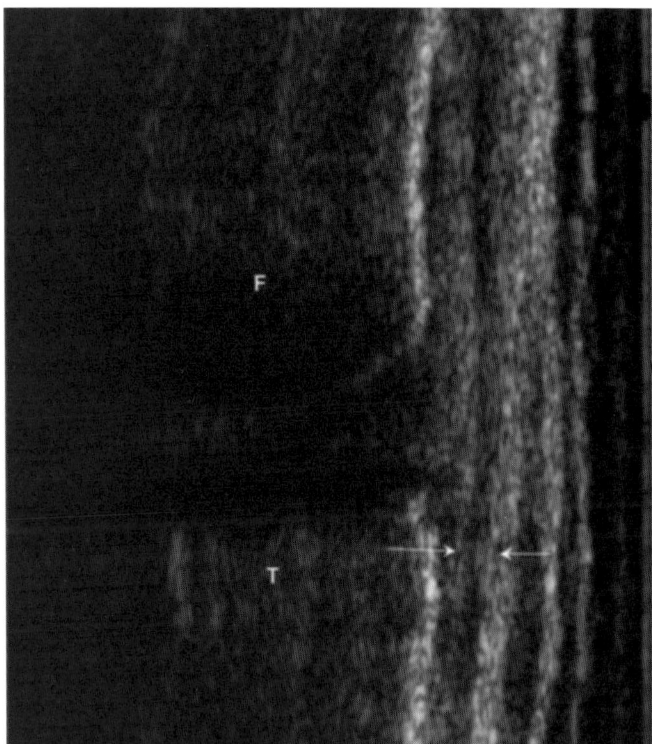

FIGURE 4 ■ Medial collateral ligament of the knee. Longitudinal sonogram of the medial aspect of the knee shows a hyperechoic linear structure representing the medial collateral ligament (*arrows*). This ligament is made up of two thick bundles, separated by a bursa or an areolar tissue. The deep component of the ligament is in close connection with the medial meniscus. F, femur; T, tibia.

some small ligaments, such as the intrinsic and extrinsic carpal ligaments, is particularly operator dependent and may be more challenging.

Depending on their orientation and that of the transducer, ligaments appear as cord-like or band-like structures that are usually hyperechoic (Figs. 4 and 5). This hyperechoic aspect is related to the histologic structure of a dense network of connective tissue.

Detection of normal ligament may be difficult in some patients in whom the ligament cannot be differentiated from surrounding hyperechoic fibroadipose tissue. Dynamic maneuvers to stretch the ligaments may improve their visualization.

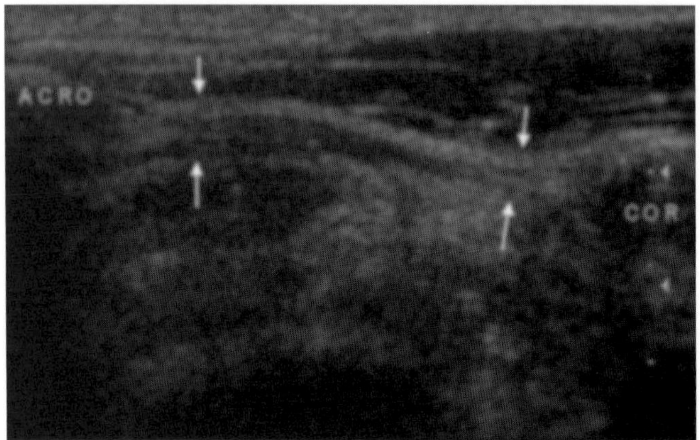

FIGURE 5 ■ Coracoacromial ligament of the shoulder. Oblique sonogram of superior aspect of the shoulder shows the normal fibrillar appearance of this ligament between the acromion (acro) and the coracoid process (cor).

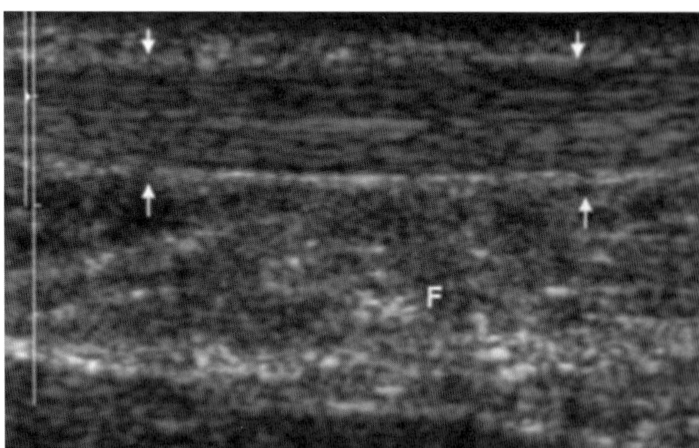

FIGURE 6 ■ Normal Achilles tendon. The tendon has a bright fibrillar pattern (*arrows*). The hypoechoic pre-Achillean fat is shown (F).

Tendon

Like ligaments, tendons consist of longitudinal collagen fibers and fibroblasts distributed in a thick and compact network. On longitudinal scan, a tendon appears as a band-like structure containing parallel hyperechoic lines (Figs. 3 and 6). This bright fibrillar structure is best visualized when the transducer is perfectly parallel—and the beam perpendicular—to the tendon. On transverse scan, tendons appear as bright oval-shaped structures (Fig. 7) surrounded by a thin hypoechoic halo when a synovial sheath is present. The enthesis, representing the bony insertion of the tendon, is also hypoechoic (14).

Some of tendons have synovial sheaths, but others do not (Table 5).

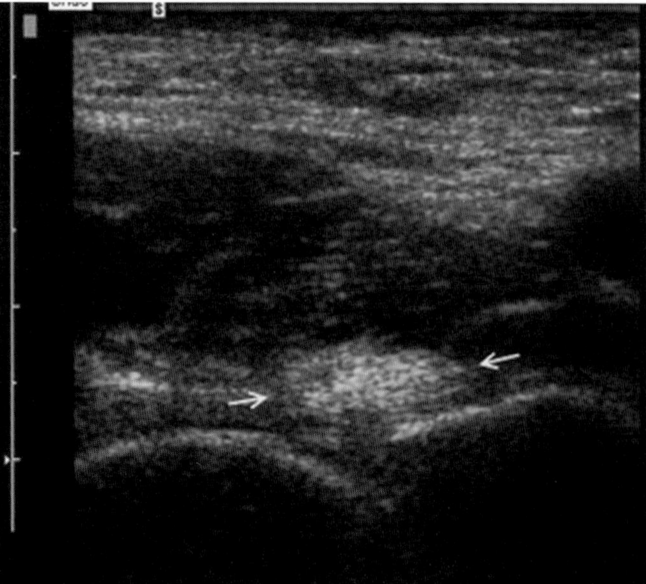

FIGURE 7 ■ Normal iliopsoas tendon. Transverse sonogram shows typical appearance of iliopsoas tendon, appearing as a bright oval-shaped structure (*arrows*).

TABLE 5 ■ Tendons with and without Synovial Sheaths

Tendons without sheaths

- *Shoulder*: rotator cuff
- *Elbow*: triceps, distal biceps, common extensor tendon, common flexor tendon
- *Hip*: iliopsoas
- *Knee*: quadriceps, biceps femoris, iliotibial band
- *Ankle*: Achilles

Tendons with sheaths

- *Shoulder*: long head of biceps
- *Wrist*: flexor, extensor
- *Ankle*: tibialis posterior, digitorum longus, hallucis longus, peroneus brevis and longus, tibialis posterior, extensor hallucis longus, extensor digitorum longus

Normal Bone

Although the primary purpose of US is not to study the bones, bony changes associated with soft-tissue or joint abnormalities can be detected and may help in the logical approach of the final diagnosis. Scanning of the bony surface may be challenging and difficult to interpret. Correlation with plain film is often necessary to prevent erroneous interpretation. One notable recent application is the use of US as a diagnostic tool for early inflammatory arthritis, as US is found to be more sensitive than radiography in the detection of erosions. As such, US is likely to have major implications for the practice of rheumatology (15).

The normal periosteum appears as a thin bright line running parallel to the cortex. The cortex is a hyperechoic smooth line without step or defect, and a posterior acoustic shadow is demonstrated (Fig. 8). No US transmission is seen beyond the cortical bone.

Normal Nerve

Peripheral nerves can be evaluated by US (Table 6) (16,17). A high-frequency linear transducer is used to evaluate superficial nerves such as the median nerve, while a deep-seated nerve such as the sciatic nerve is best imaged using a 5 MHz transducer. On longitudinal scan, nerves appear as parallel hypoechoic fascicles that are homogeneously distributed within hyperechoic connective tissue (Fig. 9).

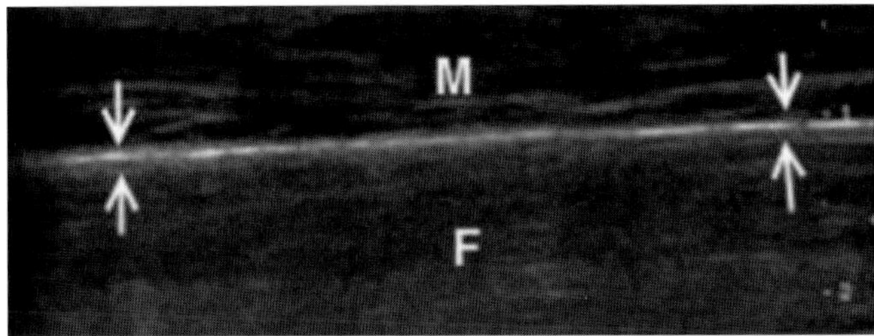

FIGURE 8 ■ Normal bone surface. Longitudinal sonogram of the proximal thigh. The bone surface of the femur appears as a smooth and regular echoic line (*arrows*). Posterior shadowing is best seen on transverse scan. The echostructure demonstrated beyond the cortex is related to artifacts. F, femur; M, muscle.

TABLE 6 ■ Large Nerves Studied by US

- Median
- Radial
- Ulnar
- Sciatic
- Tibial
- Popliteal
- Brachial plexus

Abbreviation: US, ultrasound.

Transverse scanning is the best plane to image the nerves, which appear as bright nodular structures (Fig. 10). Identification of nerves is based on these US characteristics and the specific anatomic landmarks. Nerves are discrete echoic structures, their echogenicity being between that of muscle and tendon. Their echogenicity is decreased in the elderly and in patients who have undergone previous regional surgery. In the wrist, the median nerve is easily discriminated from the surrounding flexor tendons, which are mobile during finger motion; the nerve is less mobile. On transverse scan, the median nerve is seen as an oval-shaped structure located in the carpal tunnel, deep to the flexor retinaculum.

The progressive refinement of broadband transducers with frequencies greater than 10 MHz and improved near-field resolution have enhanced the potential of sonography to evaluate not only larger nerves (median, radial, ulnar, sciatic, tibial, and popliteal) but their smaller branches as well (14,18,19).

ARTIFACTS

Two artifacts in musculoskeletal ultrasonography deserve mention: anisotropy and hypoechoic fat. The anisotropy of tendons and ligaments can mimic pathology (20).

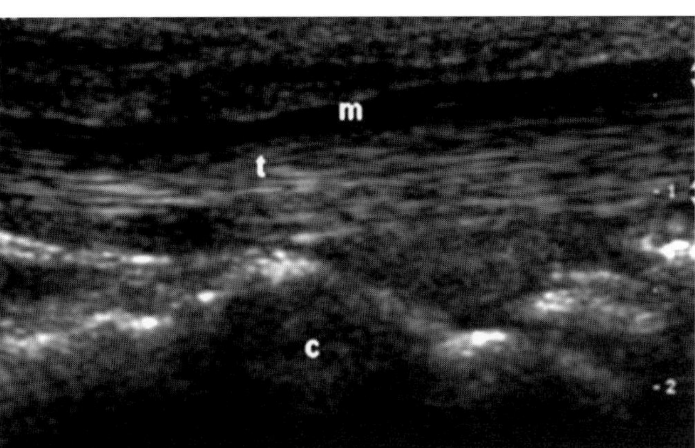

FIGURE 9 ■ Normal median nerve. Longitudinal scan along the palmar aspect of the carpal bones shows the median as a hyperechoic band lying underneath the skin, showing the characteristic homogeneously distributed parallel bright fibers of a normal nerve. c, carpal bones; m, median; t, flexor tendon.

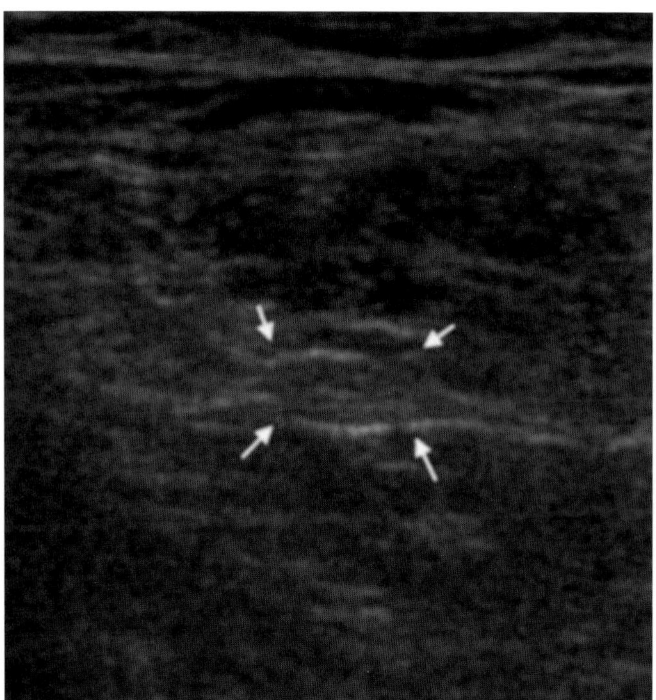

FIGURE 10 ■ Normal sciatic nerve. Transverse sonogram at the posterior aspect of the thigh shows the sciatic nerve as a well-defined structure with nodular internal echostructure.

Tendons and ligaments appear hyperechoic when imaged with the US beam perpendicular to its surface. If the beam is angled off a curved tendon, however, the tendon appears hypoechoic. This applies to both longitudinal and transverse sonograms. Anisotropy can be distinguished from edema or tendinopathy by simply correcting the transducer angle. On the other hand, anisotropy can be used to help identify tendons and ligaments when surrounded by hyperechoic fat. By modifying the beam angle, the appearance of the tendon varies between hyperechoic and hypoechoic, while the surrounding fat stays hyperechoic.

Alternatively, fat can be hypoechoic (21), mimicking fluid collection and joint effusion. This may be seen, for example, near the retrocalcaneal bursa and under the coracoacromial ligament.

TABLE 7 ■ Focal Skin Lesions

Cystic lesions of the epiderma
- Epidermal cyst
- Dermoid cyst
- Trichilemmal cyst
- Cutaneous ciliated cyst

Benign tumors of the epiderma
- Nevus
- Acanthoma
- Seborrheic keratosis

TABLE 8 ■ Vascular Palpable Pigmented Lesions Distinguished by Doppler

- Malignant melanoma
- Basal-cell papilloma
- Vascular lesions: angioma

ABNORMAL SKIN

Focal Skin Lesions

Focal skin lesions are numerous and include cysts, tumors, and inflammatory conditions (Table 7) (1,22–24). Ultrasonographic examination of focal skin lesions is performed to assess the size, shape, margin, echogenicity, and depth extension.

Despite its high sensitivity, the specificity of US examination of the skin is limited. The final diagnosis is based on correlation with clinical findings and histologic study.

Typical cystic lesions of the skin are easily confirmed by US study; however, these lesions may not appear totally anechoic, and posterior enhancement may be absent.

Most tumors of the skin are hypoechoic. US does not allow specific histologic diagnosis of skin tumors. Despite this limitation, the role of US is essential for the evaluation of the extension of the lesion, particularly in the deep soft tissue, which represents one of the most important prognostic criteria. In addition, US helps in planning the surgical procedure.

Doppler US has considerable potential as a screening tool to assist in the discrimination between pigmented skin lesions such as melanoma and other nonmelanocytic lesions such as basal-cell papilloma (23) as well as in their preoperative evaluation (Table 8) (24).

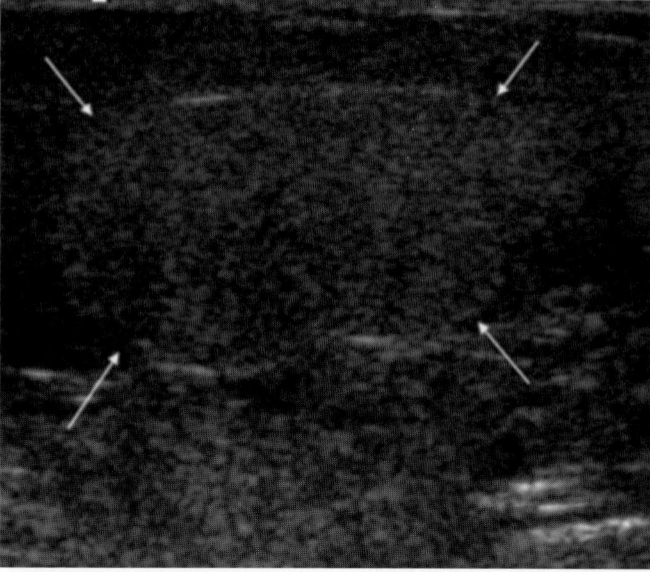

FIGURE 11 ■ Superficial lipoma. An oval-shaped mass (*arrows*) is seen in the subcutaneous soft tissue. The mass is well defined and compressible. This represents a typical lipoma.

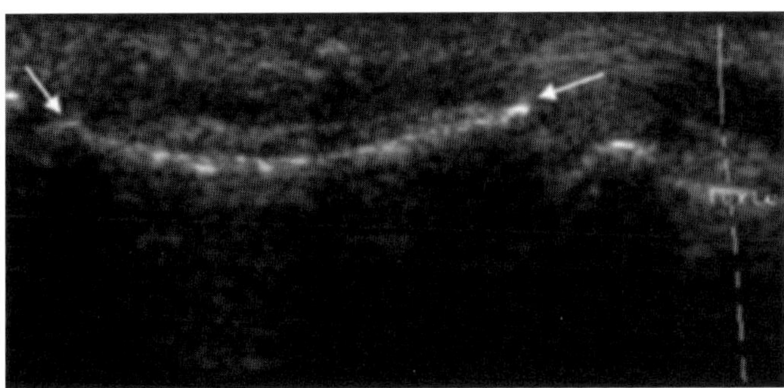

FIGURE 12 ■ Foreign body. Sonogram in sagittal plane of a finger shows a thorn (*arrows*) in the subcutaneous soft tissues. There is no posterior shadowing.

Subcutaneous Tissue Lesions

US plays a fundamental role in detecting subcutaneous masses, whether they are clinically palpated or not. Lipoma (Fig. 11) is one of the most common subcutaneous tumors. Classically, lipomas are described as being homogeneous and hyperechoic (25). Although in one study, sonography was stated to have a low accuracy in differentiation of soft-tissue lipomas from other masses (26), this has not been our experience. We find the sonographic features of lipomas—especially the feature of compressibility and low vascularity—to usually be quite characteristic.

Inflammatory masses may be seen in patients with systemic diseases such as rheumatoid arthritis, in gout, or in sarcoid and focal disorders such as foreign body inclusion (Fig. 12) (Table 9) (27). In diffuse soft-tissue infection, US may help in distinguishing primary disease from that associated with underlying abscess, such as subcutaneous abscess (Fig. 13), pyomyositis, or osteomyelitis. In addition, US plays a definite role in the guidance of percutaneous biopsy of solid lesions (28), the drainage of abscesses, and the aspiration of cystic lesions. US has also been used successfully for percutaneous removal of soft-tissue foreign bodies (29). In addition to cellulitis (Fig. 14),

TABLE 9 ■ Subcutaneous Tissue Lesions Evaluated by US

Tumor
■ Lipoma
■ Vascular malformation
■ Metastasis
■ Recurrence of soft-tissue sarcoma
Inflammation
■ Cellulitis
■ Abscess
Granuloma or inflammatory mass
■ Sarcoid
■ Foreign bodies
■ Rheumatoid nodule
■ Gout tophus
Trauma
■ Hematoma
■ Foreign body

Abbreviation: US, ultrasound.

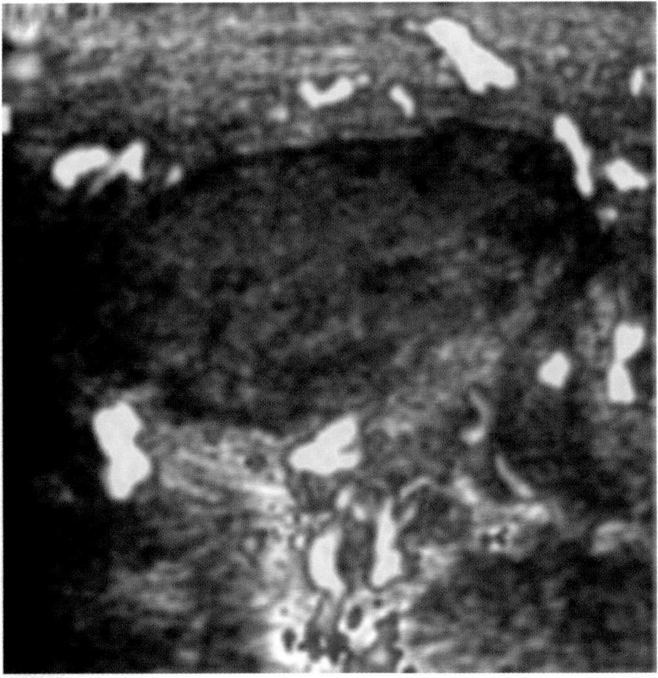

(A)

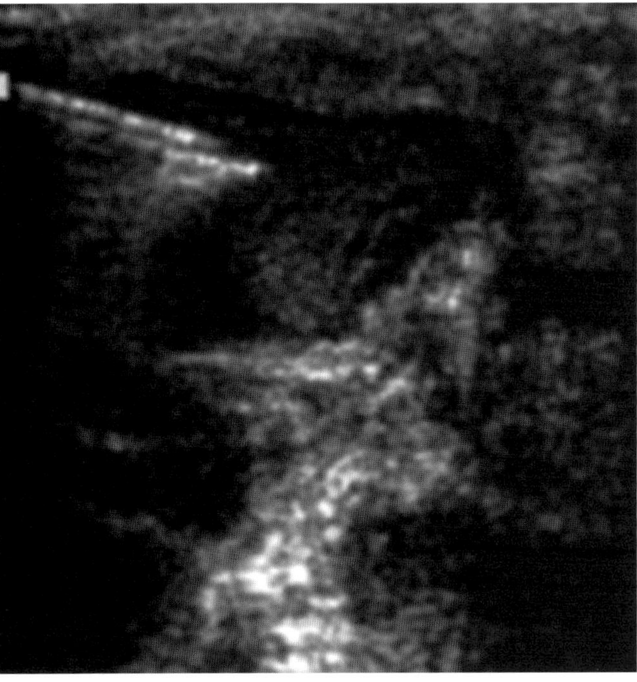

(B)

FIGURE 13 A AND B ■ (**A**) Abscess of the forearm. Transverse sonogram of the forearm shows an oval-shaped collection (*arrows*) in the subcutaneous soft tissue, with mass effect on the underlying muscle. Doppler interrogation demonstrates hypervascularity around the mass, in keeping with inflammatory mass. (**B**) Percutaneous drainage of abscess using ultrasound guidance.

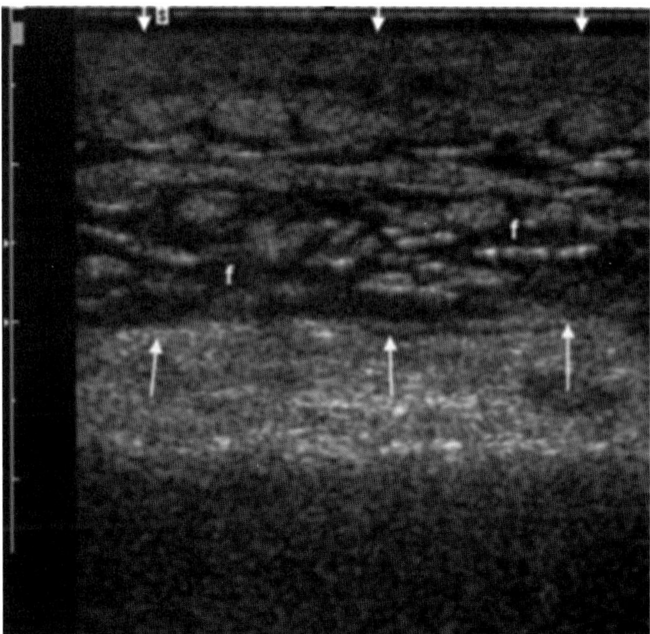

FIGURE 14 ■ Cellulitis. Transverse sonogram of the forearm shows a diffuse thickening of the subcutaneous soft tissue (*arrows*). Small areas of linear fluid collection are also seen. Other causes of subcutaneous edema may have a similar appearance. f, fluid collection.

the other causes of diffuse thickening of subcutaneous soft tissue include myxedema, lymphedema, and scleroderma. The extensive calcifications seen in scleroderma may prevent accurate assessment of soft-tissue thickening.

ABNORMAL MUSCLE

Edema of muscle fibers results in muscle enlargement. This phenomenon is nonspecific and is secondary to many types of muscle injuries. US demonstrates diffuse hypoechoic muscle bundles separated by hyperechoic fibroadipose septa. Edematous muscle may also be hyperechoic. Pain may be elicited by excessive compression of the transducer over the injured muscle.

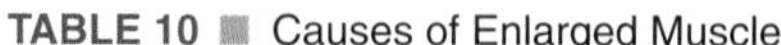

TABLE 10 ■ Causes of Enlarged Muscle

- Trauma (secondary to edema, hemorrhage, rupture)
- Abscess
- Tumor
- Rhabdomyolysis
- Myositis (trauma, infection, systemic disease)

Distortion of the muscular architecture with disappearance of the normal pennate characteristic is a feature of muscle infiltration by edema or hemorrhage.

Causes of muscle enlargement or distortion of muscle architecture are numerous and include muscle rupture, ischemia, infarction, infection (30), and rhabdomyolysis (Fig. 15) (31). Whatever the type of muscle injury, severe edema with secondary enlargement of the muscle belly in a nondistensible fascia may lead to compartment syndrome (Table 10).

Rhabdomyolysis is a muscular disorder that results from drug or alcohol abuse, infection, crush injuries, collagen disease, and extensive exercise (31). US may demonstrate a focal hypoechoic area in the muscle. This finding is not specific, however, and may also represent hematoma, abscess, or tumor necrosis.

Muscle injury may be classified as contusion, sprain, or tendon avulsion. Hematoma is a key sign of muscle injury. Contusion appears as altered echogenicity of the muscle. Muscle strains typically occur at the myotendinous junction and manifest as architectural disruption. Muscle rupture appears as a gap in the muscle belly or at the myotendinous junction (Fig. 16). In severe and complete muscle tear, the retracted muscle can be detected as a mass surrounded by hematoma (3).

Intramuscular masses can be easily detected by US. Characteristic features, such as echostructure, calcifications, size, margin, vascularity, and relation to the neurovascular bundle must be evaluated. The evaluation of these characteristics is much more important for the clinical management than speculating on the histologic diagnosis of these solid masses. The role of US in these cases is to differentiate solid from cystic masses, to assess the extension of the

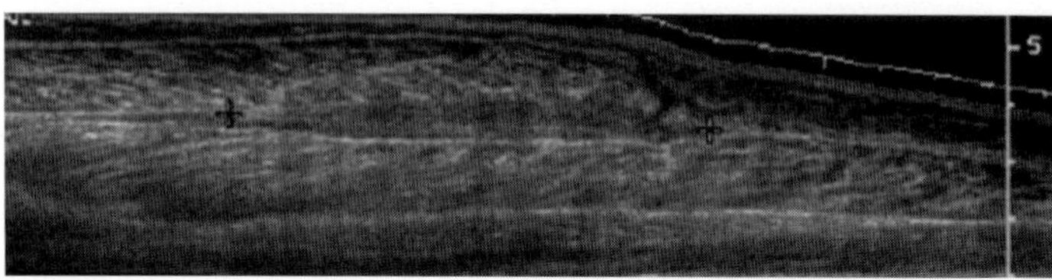

(A)

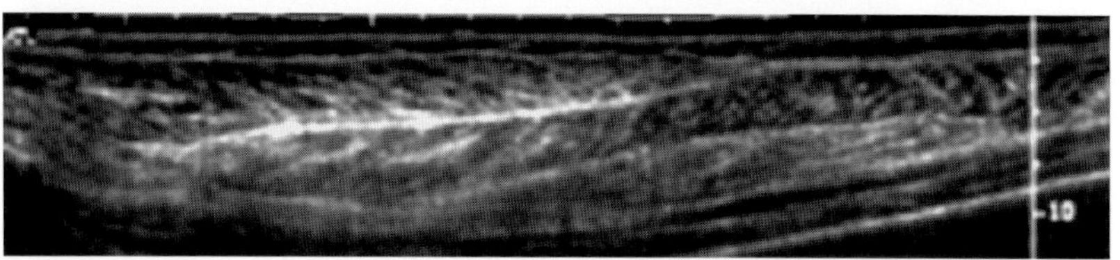

(B)

FIGURE 15 A AND B ■ Posttraumatic myositis. (**A**) Longitudinal sonogram of the anterior aspect of the thigh shows a hyperechoic semimembranosus muscle with loss of its normal pennate pattern indicating diffuse infiltration, in this case due to edema and inflammation. Differential diagnosis includes diffuse muscle infiltration by fat, malignancy, or hemorrhage. (**B**) Corresponding ^{99}Tc bone scan shows intense tracer uptake involving the same region of the hamstrings muscles.

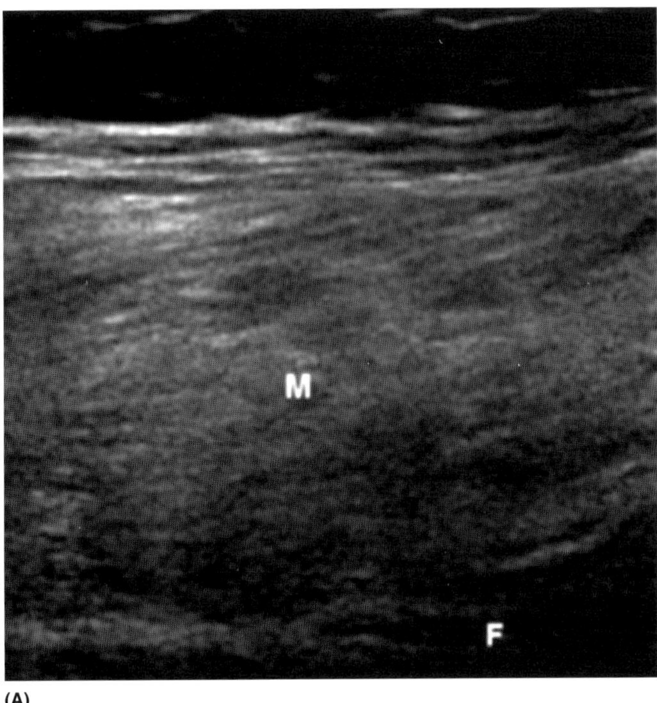

(A)

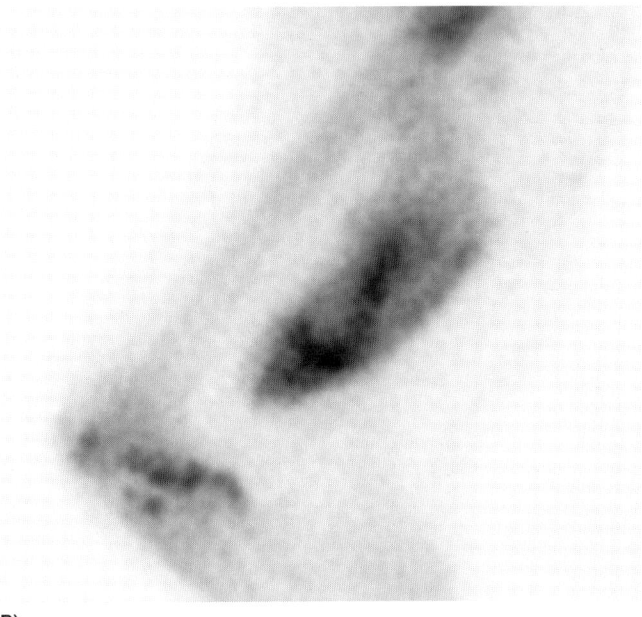

(B)

FIGURE 16 A AND B ■ (**A**) Chronic partial medial gastrocnemius muscle tear. Longitudinal panoramic sonogram of the posterior aspect of the lower leg demonstrates loss of the pennate pattern of muscle (M) and focal atrophy (*cursors*) at the myotendinous junction of the medial gastrocnemius. (**B**) Normal side for comparison. F, femur.

process, and to guide percutaneous biopsy. Causes of intramuscular solid masses are numerous and include benign and malignant neoplasms (Fig. 17) (2), pseudoneoplastic lesions such as heterotopic bone formation, granulomas, and scar tissue from old muscle tears (Table 11).

FIGURE 17 ■ Intramuscular mass. Transverse sonogram of the anterior aspect of the thigh shows a solid intramuscular mass. Differential diagnosis includes primary and secondary tumor, abscess, or hematoma with extensive blood clot. M, intramuscular mass.

Intramuscular or perimuscular fluid collection is a hypoechoic structure located in the muscle belly or at the margin of the muscle, limited by the fascia. It appears as a fusiform collection, and its size may be underestimated if there is excessive compression by the probe during the scanning process.

Intramuscular fluid collection may represent a hematoma, abscess, or necrotic tumor (Table 12). The roles of US are to confirm the cystic nature of the lesion and to guide a percutaneous needle aspiration to confirm the final diagnosis.

Interruption of the muscle fascia is a sign of traumatic muscle herniation. The protruded muscle through the fascia defect can be demonstrated with US (32). The edge of the muscle is hypoechoic, representing an artifact, most likely due to the angulation of the muscle fibers relative to the US beam. Dynamic scanning is important in confirming

TABLE 11 ■ Causes of Intramuscular Mass

- Abscess
- Tumor
- Benign: lipoma, vascular malformation
- Malignant: sarcoma, metastasis
- Pseudoneoplastic masses
- Myositis ossificans
- Granuloma
- Scar tissue (posttraumatic, postsurgical)

TABLE 12 ■ Causes of Intramuscular Fluid Collection

- Hematoma
- Abscess
- Tumor necrosis

the diagnosis because herniation may be demonstrated only during muscle contraction. Complete reduction of the herniated muscle can be obtained by excessive compression of the abnormal area by the transducer. It is also important to measure the size of the fascial defect.

ABNORMAL JOINT

Joint Cavity

Joint effusion is rarely located between the articular surfaces of two bones. It is usually accumulated in articular recesses (33). A thorough anatomic knowledge of these recesses is crucial for the search for joint effusion (Table 13).

Effusion

Injury to the synovial membrane leads to hyperemia, followed by hypersecretion and accumulation of fluid in the joint cavity. Joint effusion is one of the earliest signs of articular and periarticular disorders. Clinical diagnosis of joint effusion is not always easy. The presence of tendons, strong ligaments, or muscles around the joint often prevents dilation of articular recesses, making the clinical diagnosis inconclusive. In these cases, US plays a crucial role in confirming joint effusion associated or not with synovitis (Fig. 2).

Once the presence of effusion is confirmed, the next step is to establish a specific diagnosis. Unfortunately, the US patterns of joint effusion are nonspecific. Therefore, clinical correlation with US findings and the study of the synovial fluid obtained by fine-needle aspiration are imperative for the final diagnosis. In difficult cases, US may assist in the guidance of the arthrocentesis (33). The causes of joint effusion are numerous (Table 14).

TABLE 14 ■ Causes of Joint Effusion

- Trauma
- Inflammatory arthritis
- Infection
- Osteoarthritis
- Crystal-induced arthritis
- Synovial tumor or tumor-like lesions: pigmented villonodular synovitis, primary osteochondromatosis, lipoma arborescens

Intra-articular Mass

US may help in assessing intra-articular masses (2,5). The examination is easy when there is a joint effusion. The task becomes a real challenge when the intra-articular mass is not accompanied by effusion. Intra-articular masses can be solitary or multiple. They appear as a discrete mass and may be hypoechoic or hyperechoic, with a wide spectrum of echostructure. Acoustic shadowing may be present if there are associated calcifications. Loose bodies are confirmed if they move by mobilizing the patient's joint.

The causes of synovial masses are summarized in Table 15 (2,34). These synovial masses can be demonstrated by US.

TABLE 13 ■ US of Articular Recesses

Joint	Articular recess
Shoulder	Posterior
Elbow	Olecranon fossa
Wrist	Prestyloid
Hip	Anterior
Knee	Suprapatellar
Ankle	Anterior

Abbreviation: US, ultrasound.

TABLE 15 ■ Causes of Synovial Mass

- Infectious synovitis
- Inflammatory arthritis synovitis (rheumatoid, other)
- Amyloidosis
- Synovial osteochondromatosis
- Pigmented villonodular synovitis
- Lipoma
- Lipoma arborescens
- Synovial hemangioma
- Rare: intra-articular malignancy (e.g., synovial sarcoma)

Para-articular Mass

Para-articular masses are common clinical conditions. The clinician should assess whether the mass is solid or cystic because of different management approaches. For this purpose, US is the best and the most cost-effective option in the diagnosis. The most common cystic masses (Fig. 18) around the joint are synovial cyst, ganglion cyst (Figs. 19 and 20), bursitis, and neoplastic lesions (Table 16). Analysis of the content of the cyst is of little help in the final diagnosis. Anatomic landmarks contribute much more to the specific diagnosis (10,35).

Abnormal Tendon

The abnormal tendon may appear as a distortion of the internal architecture of the tendon, a change in diameter or position, a defect in the tendinous substance, an interruption of the tendon, or a calcific deposit in the tendon.

Abnormal Echostructure

When the normal echostructure of the tendon is diffusely altered, the most common cause is tendinopathy. This is usually manifested by attenuation or loss of the normal

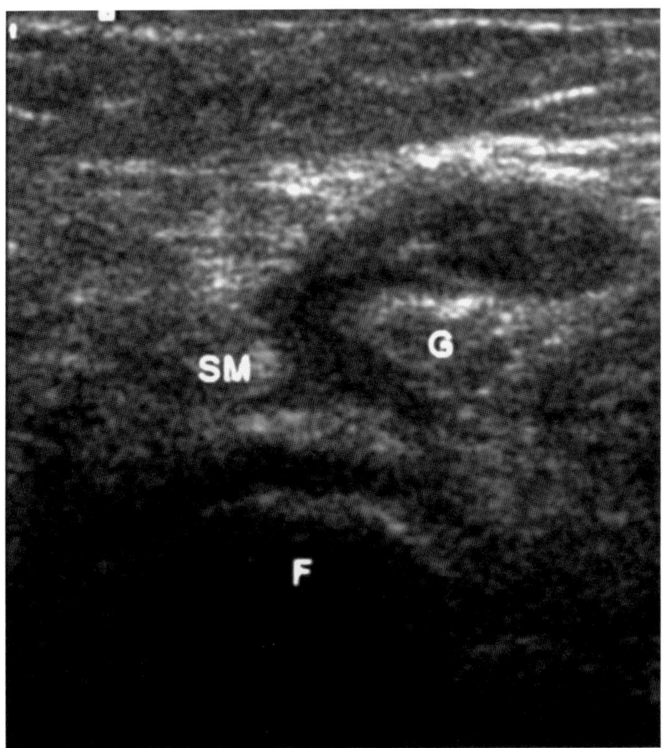

FIGURE 18 ■ Small Baker's cyst. Transverse sonogram of the posterior aspect of the distal femur shows typical appearance of a fluid-filled collection with a neck seen between medial gastrocnemius and semimembranosus tendon. Ultrasound may also help in the aspiration of large Baker's cysts. F, femur; G, gastrocnemius; SM, semimembranosus tendon.

fibrillar pattern of the tendon. A focal hypoechoic area in the tendon most commonly represents a partial tear (Fig. 21) or focal area of tendinopathy. Less commonly, it may be caused by a rheumatoid nodule, xanthoma (36), gouty tophus (37), or tumor. A bright spot in a tendon usually represents a calcification (calcium hydroxyapatite) (Fig. 22); posterior shadowing is not a constant associated finding. A longitudinal split is a sign of intrasubstance tear.

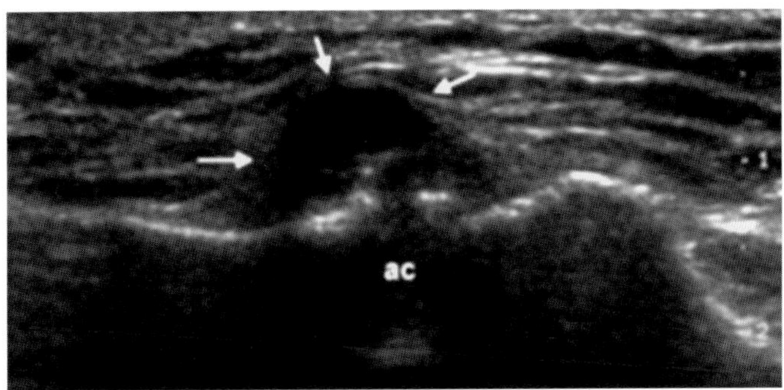

FIGURE 19 ■ Acromioclavicular joint (ac) cyst. Coronal sonogram shows a small cyst (*arrows*) associated with the ac joint, which shows mild degenerative changes. When palpable, these cysts may be mistaken clinically for tumor mass.

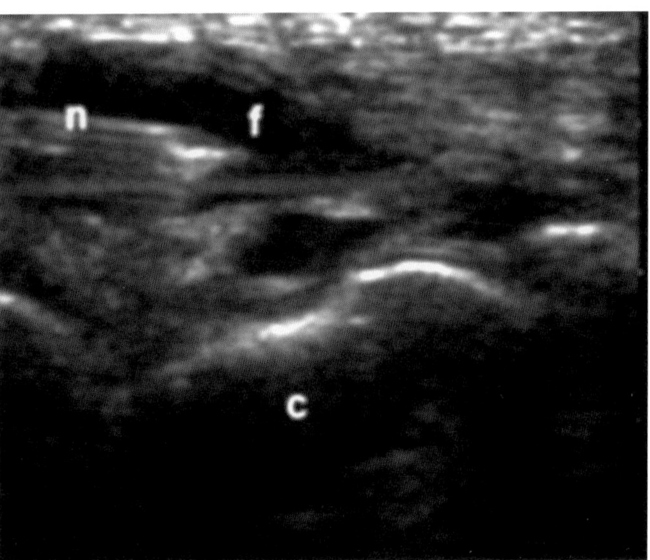

FIGURE 20 ■ Ultrasound-guided aspiration of dorsal ganglion cyst of the wrist. Sagittal sonogram of the dorsal aspect of the wrist shows a fluid-filled mass at the level of the radiocarpal joint. In this case, the cyst was aspirated percutaneously using ultrasound guidance. c, carpal bones; n, needle; f, fluid-filled mass.

Abnormal Size

The most common cause of enlargement of the tendon is chronic tendinopathy (Fig. 23) (2,5,14). The differential diagnosis includes acute tendinitis and granuloma seen in the healing phase of a tendon tear. Scar tissue seen in tendon repair may be another cause of diffuse thickening of the tendon. Chronic tendinopathy may less commonly manifest as tendon thinning rather than enlargement.

Abnormal Position and Nonvisualization

Nonvisualization of the tendon structure in the expected anatomic area is a sign of complete tear (Fig. 24) or tendon dislocation. This sign is commonly seen with tear of the rotator cuff or biceps tendon. Tendons most commonly dislocated are the long head of the biceps tendon (Fig. 25) and the peroneal tendons (38).

Tendon Interruption

Tendon interruption is a sign of full-thickness tendon tear (Fig. 26) (2,5,39). The gap may be filled with hematoma, blood clot, reactive tissue, or synovial fluid.

TABLE 16 ■ Cystic Lesions of the Knee

- Baker (popliteal) cyst
- Meniscal cyst
- Ganglion cyst
- Synovial cyst of proximal tibiofibular joint
- Bursitis: prepatellar, pes anserine, MCL, semimembranosus-MCL, iliotibial, and fibular collateral ligament-biceps femoris

Abbreviation: MCL, medial collateral ligament.

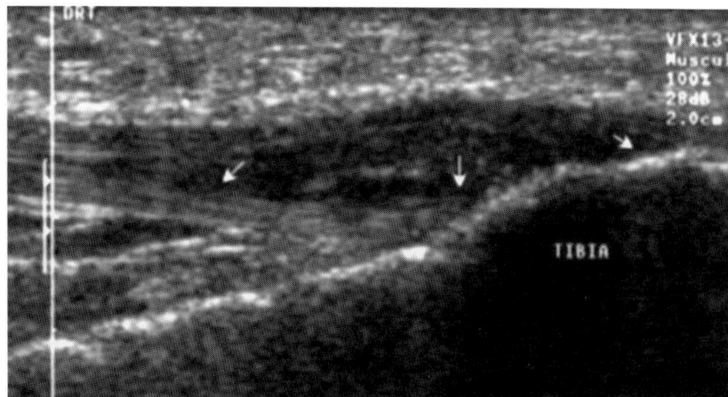

FIGURE 21 ■ Partial tear of the patellar tendon. Longitudinal sonogram of the patellar tendon shows a partial tear of the superficial aspect of the tendon at its insertion.

Abnormal Tendon Sheath

Because of its synovial-like structure, any injury to the tendon sheath may induce a diffuse thickening of that structure. In contrast to synovial thickening of the tendon sheath, effusion can be easily displaced by excessive compression of the tendon by the transducer. The most common cause of this feature is inflammation of the tendon and its sheath, called tenosynovitis (Fig. 27) (Table 17). Some sheaths (e.g., long head of the biceps, flexor hallucis longus, and iliopsoas) are or may be in direct communication with the joint space. The presence of fluid in the tendon sheath may therefore be an excellent indirect sign of joint effusion. Different types of masses have been reported to develop in the tendon sheath (Table 18) (34,40).

Abnormal Bursa

Bursal Effusion

Superficial bursal effusion is usually a primary bursal disorder, but deep bursal effusion is almost always a sign of an underlying joint disorder. Fluid accumulated in the joint is pumped into the bursa during joint motion.

Bursitis may be caused by trauma, systemic processes, or infection (Fig. 28). Systemic processes (41) that may affect bursa include rheumatoid arthritis, crystal-induced arthropathy, amyloidosis (42), and granulomatous disease (Table 19).

The only reliable sign of bursitis is its anatomic location around the joint. US demonstrates a fluid-filled collection with a well-defined margin, located next to the joint or close to the bony insertion of a tendon.

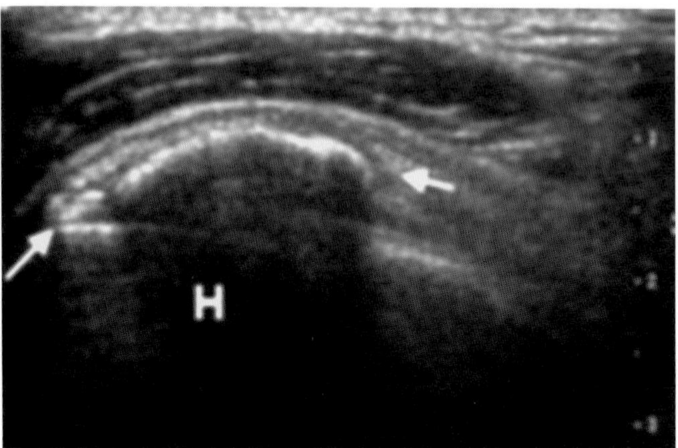

FIGURE 22 ■ Calcific deposit in supraspinatus tendon. Long axis sonogram of supraspinatus tendon shows intratendinous crescent-shaped calcification (*arrows*) with posterior shadowing. H, humeral head.

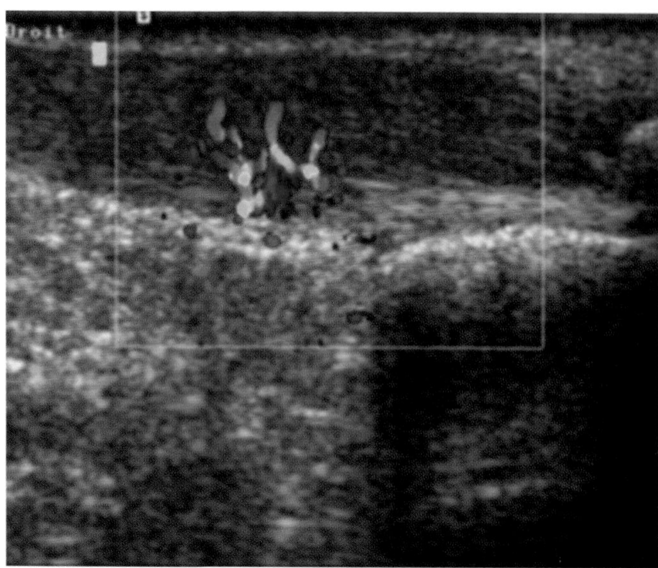

FIGURE 23 ■ Chronic Achilles tendinopathy. Longitudinal sonogram of the Achilles tendon shows a markedly swollen tendon that is hypoechoic. Note feature of hypervascularity as shown by color Doppler interrogation. No tendon defect is demonstrated.

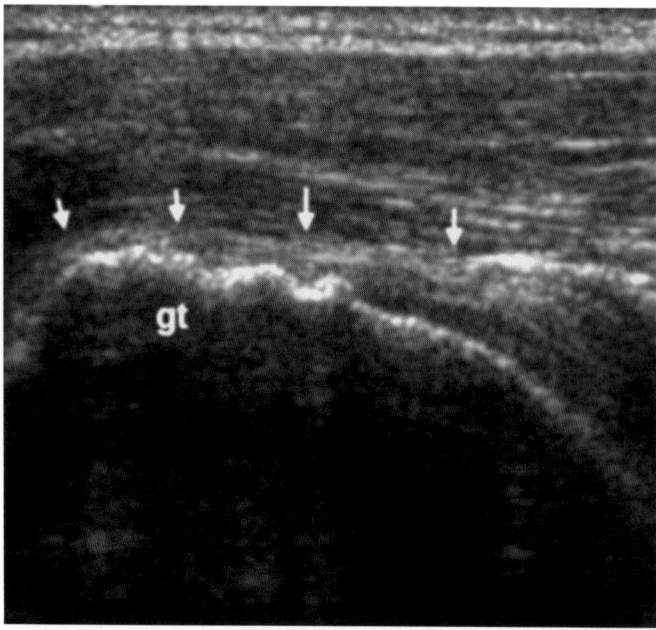

FIGURE 24 ■ Full-thickness tear of the supraspinatus tendon. Longitudinal sonogram along the supraspinatus tendon shows a torn and retracted tendon. The area is filled with fat of the peritendinous tissues. This is a characteristic sign of a full-thickness tear of the rotator cuff. The greater tuberosity (gt) is naked.

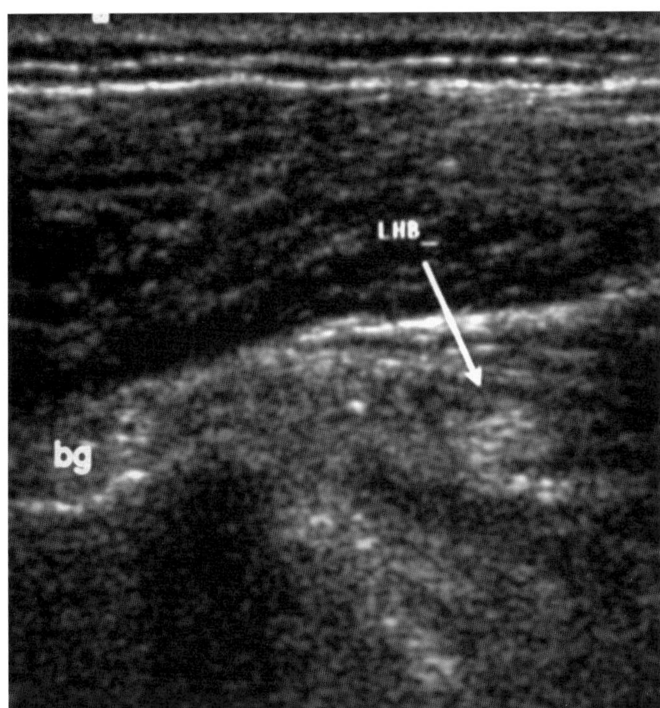

FIGURE 25 ■ Medial subluxation of the biceps tendon. Transverse sonogram of the anterior aspect of the shoulder demonstrates the long head of the biceps tendon (*arrow*) medially located relative to the bicipital groove. LHB, long head of the biceps; bg, bicipital groove.

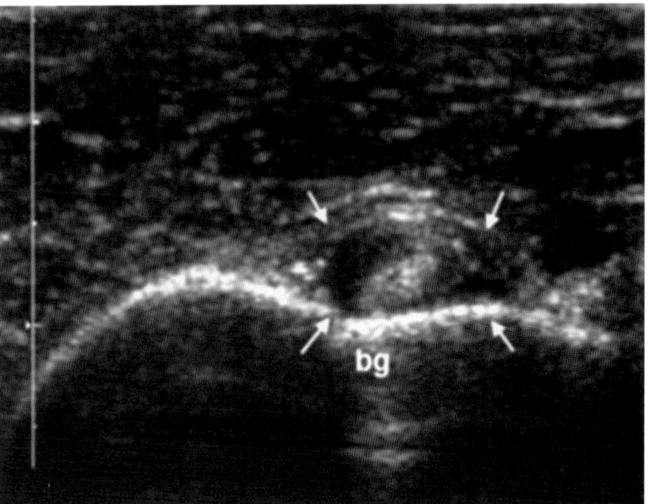

FIGURE 27 ■ Fluid in biceps tendon sheath. Transverse sonogram of the anterior aspect of the shoulder shows circumferential fluid in the biceps tendon sheath (*arrows*), in keeping with tenosynovitis of long head of biceps tendon. bg, bicipital groove.

The cause of bursitis cannot be determined on the basis of the US nature of the bursal effusion alone. The presence of synovial proliferation, however, is a sign of a more chronic process of effusion and is detectable by US (4).

Effusion of the SASD bursa deserves special mention because of the extensive and reliable use of US in the evaluation of the rotator cuff. Not all SASD bursal effusion is related to rotator cuff tendon tear despite its high association with this disorder (41). The other causes of SASD bursitis are the same as those mentioned earlier. Septic SASD bursitis is a rare but severe infection that needs surgical drainage. The main cause is steroid injection in the bursa. Fine-needle aspiration is the only means to confirm the sepsis.

Differentiating bursitis from periarticular cystic lesion depends on the type of joint involved. Around the knee, differential diagnosis of a hypoechoic lesion with posterior enhancement includes Baker cyst, meniscal cyst, ganglion cyst, hematoma, and neural tumor.

Iliopsoas bursitis should be distinguished from other groin masses (Table 20) (43).

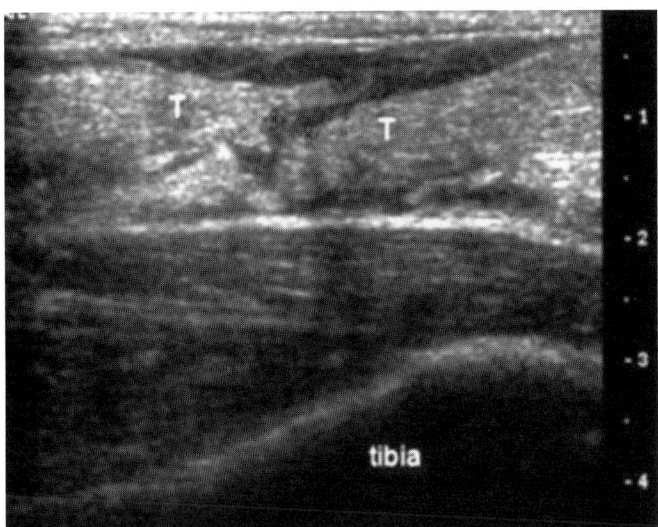

FIGURE 26 ■ Full-thickness tear of Achilles tendon. The two extremities (T) of the tendon are separated by a small gap of fluid (*cursors*). The tendon is hyperechoic and markedly thickened in keeping with chronic tendinopathy.

Thickening of the Bursal Wall

Bursal wall thickening is a sign of acute and severe bursitis or a chronic bursal process (Fig. 29). In the extreme case, chronic bursitis appears as a solid mass and may simulate other soft-tissue masses, including soft-tissue tumors, rheumatoid nodules, and gout tophi. US demonstrates a well-defined mass that appears echoic with or without fluid.

Intrabursal Mass

Possible masses in the bursal cavity include blood clot, loose bodies, inflammatory synovial pannus, osteochondromatosis, hemangioma, and pigmented villonodular synovitis (Table 21) (34,41).

TABLE 17 ■ Causes of Tenosynovitis

- Trauma
- Arthropathy (inflammatory, crystal-induced)
- Infection
- Foreign bodies

TABLE 18 ■ Synovial Masses in Tendon Sheath

- Synovial osteochondromatosis
- Pigmented villonodular synovitis
- Lipoma
- Giant-cell tumor of the tendon sheath
- Granulomatous disease
- Fibroma

Abnormal Ligament

All ligament injuries share the same common patterns. US features of acute complete ligament tear are disruption of the ligament with a variable gap size associated with edema, hematoma, or joint effusion. Acute partial tear appears as a thickened ligament associated with hypoechogenicity that represents edema or intrasubstance tear. Diffuse or focal hypertrophy of the ligament without discontinuity is a sign of chronic tear resulting from repetitive stress or from a healed remote ligament tear. Chronic ligament injuries can lead to focal or diffuse hyperechoic changes of the ligament. Ossification may be detected in and near the ligament. The most common ligaments evaluated by US are collateral ligament of the knee (10), ligaments of the ankle (11), and ulnar collateral ligament of the thumb (12) and elbow (13).

ABNORMAL BONE

Injuries to bone and soft-tissue lesions near bone can elicit periosteal reactions. Periosteal appositions are well known and readily described on conventional radiography. Single or multiple lamellar periosteal reactions appear as hyperechoic lines. The periosteum may be elevated by an underlying process such as hematoma, abscess (44), or tumor (Table 22) (45).

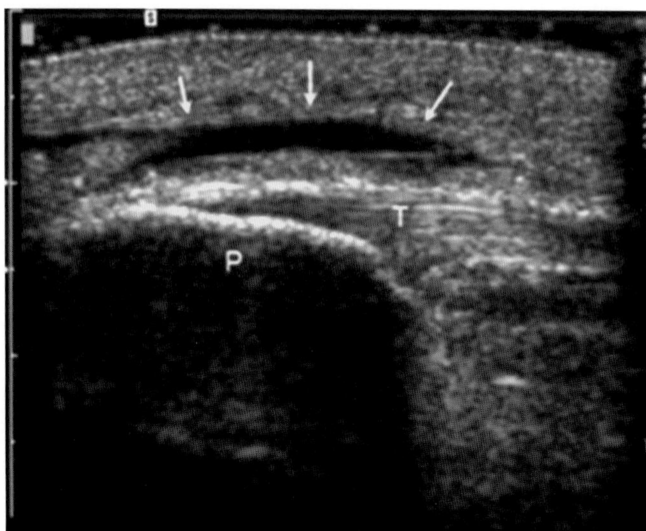

FIGURE 28 ■ Prepatellar bursitis. Longitudinal sonogram of the prepatellar region shows a small fluid collection (*arrows*) anterior to the patella and proximal aspect of the patellar tendon. P, patella; T, patellar tendon.

TABLE 19 ■ Causes of Bursitis

Superficial and deep
- Trauma
- Infection
- Inflammatory arthritis
- Crystal-induced arthropathy
- Metabolic disease (e.g., gout, amyloidosis)
- Granulomatous disease (e.g., sarcoidosis)
- Mass (Table 21)

Adventitial
- Hallux valgus
- Exostosis
- Amputation stump
- Clubfoot deformity

Spiculated periosteal reactions are bright echoic lines that run perpendicular to the axis of the cortex. These periosteal appositions are interrupted in aggressive lesions.

Some cortical bone abnormalities may be evaluated by US (46,47). These include cortical interruption, expansion, permeating destruction, and fracture.

Cortical interruption is seen as a discrete interruption in the regular echoic cortical line. This defect creates an acoustic window that allows study of the medullary cavity. Fine-needle aspiration may be performed through this window, guided by US. Permeating destruction of bone involves small, multiple defects in the cortex without a discrete interruption of the cortical line. The causes of cortical interruption include fracture, infection, and tumor.

Bone erosion may be detected while scanning a joint. Periarticular erosions are small notches seen in the marginal or paramarginal areas, articular surfaces of a joint, and epiphyseal or metaphyseal areas (48).

US has been described as an accurate tool for the detection of fracture in a particular context (Fig. 30). The diagnosis of a greater tuberosity fracture (49) is not uncommon while scanning the shoulder for rotator cuff pathology. Some of these fractures may be missed on the initial plain films.

The bone abnormalities found during assessment of the soft tissues of the extremities should be incorporated in the logical approach of the diagnosis. One or several of these findings may be present in association with soft-tissue abnormalities.

TABLE 20 ■ Causes of Mass in the Groin

- Iliopsoas bursitis
- Inguinal hernia
- Hematoma
- Adenopathy
- Tumor
- Lymphocele
- Aneurysm

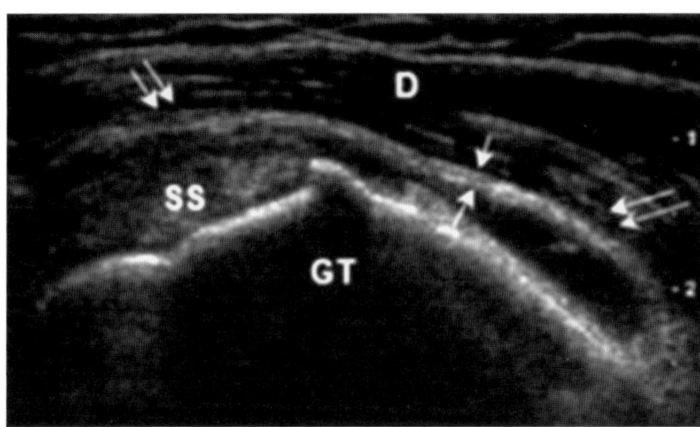

FIGURE 29 ■ Subacromial–subdeltoid (SASD) bursitis. Coronal sonogram shows distension on the SASD bursa (*double arrows*) situated around the greater tuberosity between deltoid muscle and rotator cuff. More laterally, bursa extends between deltoid muscle and humeral shaft. Note thickening of bursal wall in keeping with bursitis (*single arrows*). SS, supraspinatus; GT, greater tuberosity; D, deltoid muscle.

ABNORMAL NERVE

Neural Mass

Schwannoma, stump neuroma, and Morton's neuroma are the most common masses developed along the nerve course. Most neural masses are hypoechoic and thus cannot be differentiated from masses of other origin. More than its internal echostructure, the presence of a bright cord-like structure in continuity with the mass is a better sign of nerve sheath tumor or a stump neuroma (Fig. 31). A mass developed in the vicinity of a postamputation stump must be differentiated from adventitial bursitis.

TABLE 21 ■ Causes of Masses in Bursa

- Blood clot
- Loose bodies
- Chronic bursitis (trauma, rheumatoid arthritis, gout)
- Pigmented villonodular synovitis
- Lipoma arborescens

Morton neuroma is not a tumor but rather a lesion consisting of perineural fibrosis and local vascular proliferation involving the plantar digital nerves of the foot (Fig. 32) (50). This mass usually develops in the second or third intermetatarsal space. This must be differentiated from other masses of the region, such as ganglion cyst and intermetatarsal bursitis, gout tophus, rheumatoid nodule, or rarely giant-cell tumor of the tendon sheath.

Neoplastic nerve masses include benign tumors—schwannoma and neurofibroma—and malignant peripheral nerve-sheath tumor. The benign nerve tumors are usually fusiform in shape, oriented along the long axis of the nerve, with tapered ends that are in continuity with the nerve of origin. Although their sonographic appearance may be variable, benign peripheral nerve-sheath tumors are often hypoechoic with posterior acoustic enhancement, and so may simulate a ganglion cyst. The presence of intrinsic blood flow on color Doppler sonography and peripheral nerve continuity suggests the diagnosis of peripheral nerve-sheath tumor. Sonography cannot reliably distinguish neurofibromas from schwannomas (51). The "split fat" and the "target" sign, already described at magnetic resonance (MR) imaging, may also be seen with US (52). However, as with other imaging

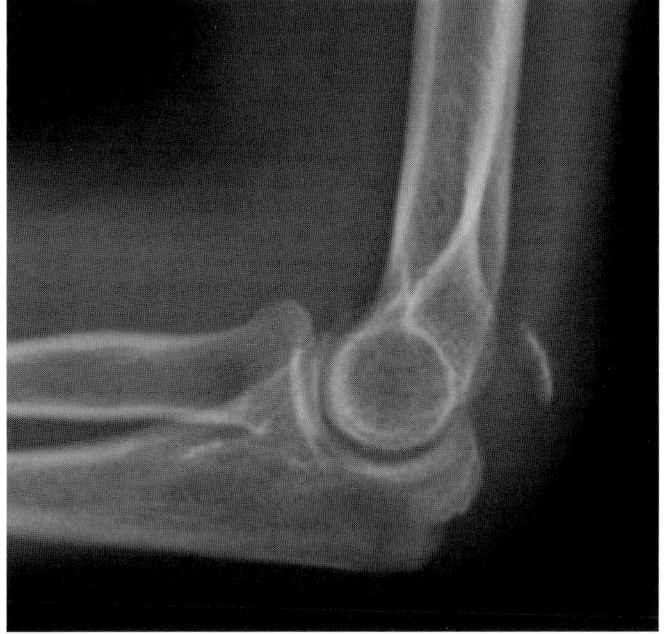

(A)

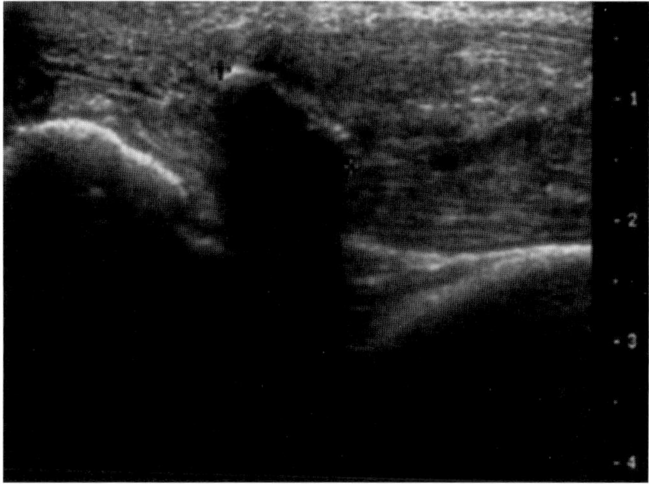

(B)

FIGURE 30 A AND B ■ Olecranon fracture. (**A**) Lateral radiograph of the elbow shows an avulsion fracture of the olecranon. (**B**) The bony fragment is well demonstrated by sonography (*cursors*).

TABLE 22 ■ Causes of Subperiosteal/Periosteous Fluid

- Infection (abscess, reactivation of chronic osteomyelitis)
- Hematoma
- Tumor

modalities, US cannot reliably differentiate between benign and malignant neurogenic masses.

Nerve Swelling

Fusiform nerve swelling has been described in patients with inflammatory changes caused by nerve compression as it courses through an osteofibrous tunnel. In association with this change in diameter, the echogenicity of the nerve is markedly decreased proximal to the site of compression. In the upper limb, this phenomenon is observed at the wrist where the median nerve is compressed in the carpal tunnel, the ulnar nerve at the cubital tunnel, and at the elbow where the ulnar nerve is compressed at the level of Guyon canal. Sonography of other nerve entrapment syndromes has also proven useful in clinical practice. In the upper limb, suprascapular neuropathy in the area of the spinoglenoid–supraspinous notch, the quadrilateral space syndrome (axillary neuropathy), radial neuropathy in the area of the spiral groove, the supinator syndrome (posterior interosseous neuropathy), the cubital tunnel syndrome (ulnar neuropathy), and the Kiloh–Nevin syndrome (anterior interosseous neuropathy) have all been shown (18).

In the lower limb, osteofibrous tunnels include the fibular neck for the common peroneal nerve, the tarsal tunnel for the posterior tibial nerve, and the intermetatarsal spaces for the interdigital nerves. US may also diagnose an associated cause of nerve entrapment, including tenosynovitis, ganglia, soft-tissue tumors, bone and joint abnormalities, and anomalous muscles (19).

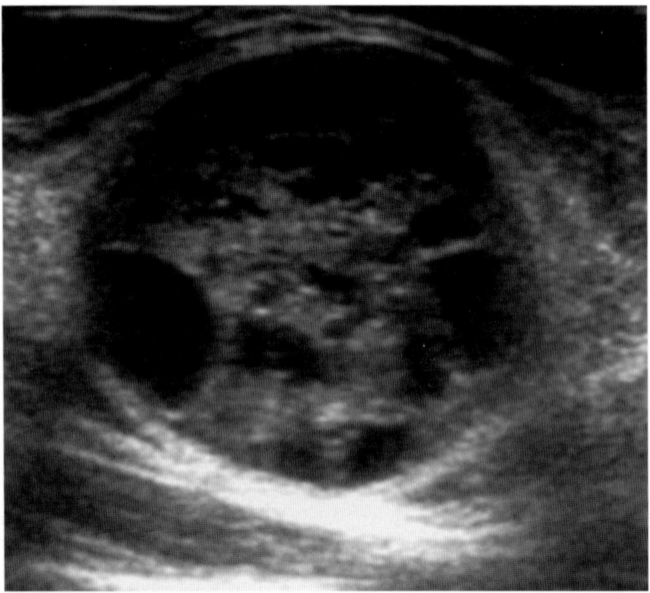

FIGURE 31 ■ Schwannoma. Longitudinal sonogram along the popliteal fossa in a patient with a solid mass. Ultrasound demonstrates a well-defined heterogenous mass containing small cystic areas. Visualizing a nerve entering and exiting the mass would be typical of nerve sheath tumor. Otherwise, the heterogenous appearance as shown here may not distinguishable from hematoma and from other solid soft-tissue masses, including malignancies.

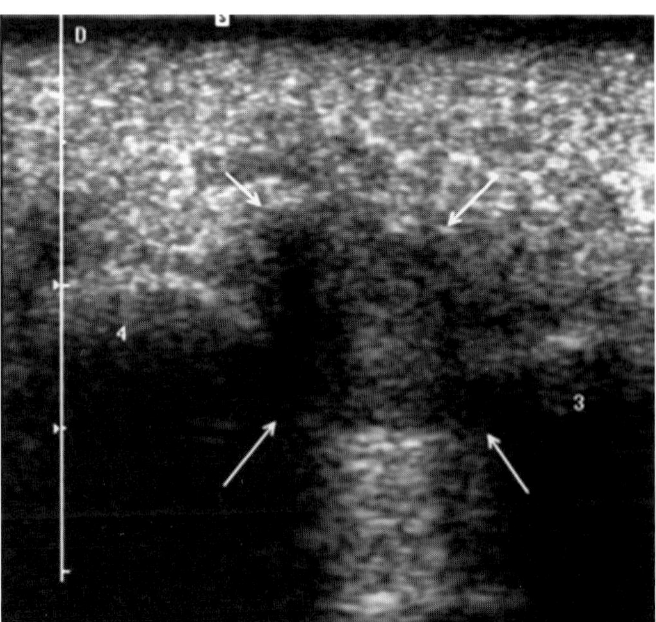

FIGURE 32 ■ Morton's neuroma. Sonogram of third intermetatarsal space in coronal plane shows round, hypoechoic mass (*arrows*) between the metatarsal heads (3 and 4).

Diffuse nerve swelling may be encountered in a rare disorder such as Charcot-Marie-Tooth disease, and US has been used to evaluate median nerve hypertrophy in such patients (53).

Nerve Flattening

US is accurate in the diagnosis of carpal tunnel syndrome (54). The diagnosis is made on the basis of three criteria: nerve swelling, flattening ratio, and palmar bowing of the flexor retinaculum. These criteria are assessed quantitatively using the mean flattening ratio, mean cross-sectional area, and palmar displacement of the flexor retinaculum.

In the nerve entrapment neuropathies (mentioned above as causes of nerve swelling), there may be abrupt flattening of the nerve at the compression site and fusiform hypoechoic swelling more proximally.

Nerve Displacement or Compression

The causes of mass effect on peripheral nerves may be detected by US. Soft-tissue mass, cystic lesions, and tenosynovitis are readily diagnosed by US.

REFERENCES

1. Schmid-Wendtner MH, Burgdorf W. Ultrasound scanning in dermatology. Arch Dermatol 2005; 141:217–224.

2. Chhem RK, Cardinal E. Guidelines and Gamuts in Musculoskeletal Ultrasound. New York: Wiley-Liss, 1999.
3. Peetrons P. Ultrasound of muscles. Eur Radiol 2002; 12(1):35–43.
4. Chhem RK, Beauregard G. Synovial diseases. In: Fornage BD, ed. Musculoskeletal Ultrasound. New York, Churchill Livingstone, 1995:43.
5. van Holsbeeck MT, Introcaso JH. Musculoskeletal Ultrasound. 2nd ed. St Louis: Mosby, 2001.
6. Finlay K, Ferry M, Friedman L. Ultrasound of the elbow. Skeletal Radiol 2004; 33(2):63–79.
7. Pfirrmann CW, Chung CB, Theumann NH, et al. Greater trochanter of the hip: attachment of the abductor mechanism and a complex of three bursae—MR imaging and MR bursography in cadavers and MR imaging in asymptomatic volunteers. Radiology 2001; 221(2):469–477.
8. Kim SM, Shin MJ, Kim KS, et al. Imaging features of ischial bursitis with an emphasis on ultrasonography. Skeletal Radiol 2002; 31(11):631–636.
9. Boutry N, Lapegue F, Masi L, et al. Ultrasonographic evaluation of normal extrinsic and intrinsic carpal ligaments: preliminary experience. Skeletal Radiol 2005; 34(9):513–521.
10. Court-Payen M. Sonography of the knee: intra-articular pathology. J Clin Ultrasound 2004; 32(9):481–490.
11. Peetrons P, Creteur V, Bacq C. Sonography of ankle ligaments. J Clin Ultrasound 2004; 32(9):491–499.
12. Schnur DP, DeLone FX, McClellan RM, et al. Ultrasound: a powerful tool in the diagnosis of ulnar collateral ligament injuries of the thumb. Ann Plast Surg 2002; 49(1):19–22.
13. Miller TT, Adler RS, Friedman L. Sonography of injury of the ulnar collateral ligament of the elbow-initial experience. Skeletal Radiol 2004; 33(7):386–391.
14. Martinoli C, Bianchi S, Dahmane, et al. Ultrasound of tendons and nerves. Eur Radiol 2002; 12(1):44–55.
15. Szkudlarek M, Narvestad E, Klarlund M, et al. Ultrasonography of the metatarsophalangeal joints in rheumatoid arthritis: comparison with magnetic resonance imaging, conventional radiography, and clinical examination. Arthritis Rheum 2004; 50(7):2103–2112.
16. Martinoli C, Bianchi S, Derchi LE. Ultrasonography of peripheral nerves. Semin Ultrasound CT MR 2000; 21(3):205–213.
17. Jacob D, Creteur V, Courthaliac C, et al. Sonoanatomy of the ulnar nerve in the cubital tunnel: a multicentre study by the GEL. Eur Radiol 2004; 14(10):1770–1773.
18. Martinoli C, Bianchi S, Pugliese F, et al. Sonography of entrapment neuropathies in the upper limb (wrist excluded). J Clin Ultrasound 2004; 32(9):438–450.
19. Martinoli C, Bianchi S, Gandolfo N, et al. US of nerve entrapments in osteofibrous tunnels of the upper and lower limbs. Radiographics 2000; 20:S199–S217.
20. Fornage BD. The hypoechoic normal tendon: a pitfall. J Ultrasound Med 1987; 6:19–22.
21. Norris MA, Scanlan KA. Hypoechoic fat: another location. AJR Am J Roentgenol 1996; 166:214.
22. Hall JC, Sauer GC. Sauer's Manual of Skin Diseases. 8th ed. Philadelphia: Lippincott Williams & Williams, 2000.
23. Harland CC, Kale SG, Jackson P, et al. Differentiation of common benign pigmented skin lesions from melanoma by high-resolution ultrasound. Br J Dermatol 2000; 143(2):281–289.
24. Bessoud B, Lassau N, Koscielny S, et al. High-frequency sonography and color Doppler in the management of pigmented skin lesions. Ultrasound Med Biol 2003; 29(6):875–879.
25. Fornage BD, Tassin GB. Sonographic appearances of superficial soft tissue lipomas. J Clin Ultrasound 1991; 19:215.
26. Inampudi P, Jacobson JA, Fessell DP, et al. Soft-tissue lipomas: accuracy of sonography in diagnosis with pathologic correlation. Radiology 2004; 233(3):763–767.
27. Soudack M, Nachtigal A, Gaitini D. Clinically unsuspected foreign bodies: the importance of sonography. J Ultrasound Med 2003; 22(12):1381–1385.
28. Torriani M, Etchebehere M, Amstalden E. Sonographically guided core needle biopsy of bone and soft tissue tumors. J Ultrasound Med 2002; 21(3):275–281.
29. Blankstein A, Cohen I, Heiman Z, et al. Localization, detection and guided removal of soft tissue in the hands using sonography. Arch Orthop Trauma Surg 2000; 120(9):514–517.
30. Cardinal E, Bureau NJ, Aubin B, et al. Role of ultrasound in musculoskeletal infections. Radiol Clin North Am 2001; 39:191–201.
31. Fornage BD, Nerot C. Sonographic diagnosis of rhabdomyolysis. J Clin Ultrasound 1986; 14(5):389–392.
32. Beggs I. Sonography of muscle hernias. AJR Am J Roentgenol 2003; 180(2):395–399.
33. Fessell JP, Jacobson JA, Craig J, et al. Using sonography to reveal and aspirate joint effusions. AJR Am J Roentgenol 2000; 174(5):1353–1362.
34. Narvaez JA, Narbaez J, Aguilera C, et al. MR imaging of synovial tumors and tumor-like lesions. Eur Radiol 2001; 11(12): 2549–2560.
35. McCarthy CL, McNally EG. The MRI appearance of cystic lesions around the knee. Skeletal Radiol 2004; 33(4):187–209.
36. Tsouli SG, Kiortsis DN, Argyropoulou MI, et al. Pathogenesis, detection and treatment of Achilles tendon xanthomas. Eur J Clin Invest 2005; 35(4):236–244.
37. Bond JR, Sim FH, Sundaram M. Radiologic case study. Gouty tophus involving the distal quadriceps tendon. Orthopedics 2004; 27(1):18:90–92.
38. Neustadter J, Raikin SM, Nazarian LN. Dynamic sonographic evaluation of peroneal tendon subluxation. AJR Am J Roentgenol 2004; 183(4):985–988.
39. Jacobson JA, Lancaster S, Prasad A, et al. Full-thickness and partial-thickness supraspinatus tendon tears: value of US signs in diagnosis. Radiology 2004; 230(1):234–242.
40. Fox MG, Krandsdorf MJ, Bancroft LW, et al. MR imaging of fibroma of the tendon sheath. AJR Am J Roentgenol 2003; 180(5): 1449–1453.
41. Martinoli C, Bianchi S, Prato N, et al. US of the shoulder: non-rotator cuff disorders. Radiographics 2003; 23(2):381–401.
42. Cardinal E, Buckwalter KA, Braunstein EM, et al. Amyloidosis of the shoulder in patients on chronic hemodialysis: sonographic findings. Am J Roentgenol 1996; 166:153.
43. Wunderbaldinger P, Bremer C, Schellenberger E, et al. Imaging features of iliopsoas bursitis. Eur Radiol 2002; 12(2):409–415.
44. Chau CL, Griffith JF. Musculoskeletal infections: ultrasound appearances. Clin Radiol 2005; 60(2):149–159.
45. Wenaden AE, Szyszko TA, Saifuddin A. Imaging of periosteal reactions associated with focal lesions of bone. Clin Radiol 2005; 60(4):439–456.
46. Simanovsky N, Hiller N, Liebner E, et al. Sonographic detection of radiographically occult fractures in paediatric ankle injuries. Pediatr Radiol 2005 Nov; 35(11):1062–1065.
47. Senall JA, Failla JM, Bouffard JA, et al. Ultrasound for the early diagnosis of clinically suspected scaphoid fracture. J Hand Surg [Am] 2004; 29(3):400–405.
48. Guermazi A, Taouli B, Lynch JA, et al. Imaging of bone erosion in rheumatoid arthritis. Semin Musculoskelet Radiol 2004; 8(4): 269–285.
49. Patten RM, Mack LA, Wang KY, et al. Nondisplaced fractures of the greater tuberosity of the humerus: sonographic detection. Radiology 1992; 182:201.
50. Quinn TJ, Jacobson JA, Craig JG, et al. Sonography of Morton's neuromas. AJR Am J Roentgenol 2000; 174(6):1723–1728.
51. Reynolds DL Jr, Jacobson JA, Inampudi P, et al. Sonographic characteristics of peripheral nerve sheath tumors. AJR Am J Roentgenol 2004; 182(3):741–744.
52. Lin J, Martel W. Cross-sectional imaging of peripheral nerve sheath tumors: characteristic signs on CT, MR imaging, and sonography. AJR Am J Roentgenol 2001; 176:75–82.
53. Martinoli C, Schenone A, Bianchi S, et al. Sonography of the median nerve in Charcot-Marie-Tooth disease. AJR Am J Roentgenol 2002; 178(6):1553–1556.
54. Koyuncuoglu HR, Kutluhan S, Yesildag A, et al. The value of ultrasonographic measurement in carpal tunnel syndrome in patients with negative electrodiagnostic tests. Eur J Radiol 2005 Dec; 56(3): 365–369.

Index

An f following an entry indicates a page containing a figure; a t indicates a page containing a table.
This is a cumulative index for both volumes (Volume 1, pages 1–770; Volume 2, pages 771–1408).

An f following an entry indicates a page containing a figure; a t indicates a page containing a table.
This is a cumulative index for both volumes (Volume 1, pages 1–770; Volume 2, pages 771–1408).

An f following an entry indicates a page containing a figure; a t indicates a page containing a table.
This is a cumulative index for both volumes (Volume 1, pages 1–770; Volume 2, pages 771–1408).

An f following an entry indicates a page containing a figure; a t indicates a page containing a table.
This is a cumulative index for both volumes (Volume 1, pages 1–770; Volume 2, pages 771–1408).

An f following an entry indicates a page containing a figure; a t indicates a page containing a table.
This is a cumulative index for both volumes (Volume 1, pages 1–770; Volume 2, pages 771–1408).

An f following an entry indicates a page containing a figure; a t indicates a page containing a table.
This is a cumulative index for both volumes (Volume 1, pages 1–770; Volume 2, pages 771–1408).

An f following an entry indicates a page containing a figure; a t indicates a page containing a table.
This is a cumulative index for both volumes (Volume 1, pages 1–770; Volume 2, pages 771–1408).

An f following an entry indicates a page containing a figure; a t indicates a page containing a table. This is a cumulative index for both volumes (Volume 1, pages 1–770; Volume 2, pages 771–1408).

An f following an entry indicates a page containing a figure; a t indicates a page containing a table.
This is a cumulative index for both volumes (Volume 1, pages 1–770; Volume 2, pages 771–1408).

An f following an entry indicates a page containing a figure; a t indicates a page containing a table.
This is a cumulative index for both volumes (Volume 1, pages 1–770; Volume 2, pages 771–1408).

An f following an entry indicates a page containing a figure; a t indicates a page containing a table.
This is a cumulative index for both volumes (Volume 1, pages 1–770; Volume 2, pages 771–1408).

An f following an entry indicates a page containing a figure; a t indicates a page containing a table.
This is a cumulative index for both volumes (Volume 1, pages 1–770; Volume 2, pages 771–1408).

An f following an entry indicates a page containing a figure; a t indicates a page containing a table.
This is a cumulative index for both volumes (Volume 1, pages 1–770; Volume 2, pages 771–1408).

An f following an entry indicates a page containing a figure; a t indicates a page containing a table.
This is a cumulative index for both volumes (Volume 1, pages 1–770; Volume 2, pages 771–1408).

An f following an entry indicates a page containing a figure; a t indicates a page containing a table.
This is a cumulative index for both volumes (Volume 1, pages 1–770; Volume 2, pages 771–1408).

An f following an entry indicates a page containing a figure; a t indicates a page containing a table.
This is a cumulative index for both volumes (Volume 1, pages 1–770; Volume 2, pages 771–1408).

An f following an entry indicates a page containing a figure; a t indicates a page containing a table.
This is a cumulative index for both volumes (Volume 1, pages 1–770; Volume 2, pages 771–1408).

An f following an entry indicates a page containing a figure; a t indicates a page containing a table.
This is a cumulative index for both volumes (Volume 1, pages 1–770; Volume 2, pages 771–1408).

An f following an entry indicates a page containing a figure; a t indicates a page containing a table.
This is a cumulative index for both volumes (Volume 1, pages 1–770; Volume 2, pages 771–1408).

An f following an entry indicates a page containing a figure; a t indicates a page containing a table.
This is a cumulative index for both volumes (Volume 1, pages 1–770; Volume 2, pages 771–1408).

An f following an entry indicates a page containing a figure; a t indicates a page containing a table.
This is a cumulative index for both volumes (Volume 1, pages 1–770; Volume 2, pages 771–1408).

An f following an entry indicates a page containing a figure; a t indicates a page containing a table.
This is a cumulative index for both volumes (Volume 1, pages 1–770; Volume 2, pages 771–1408).

An f following an entry indicates a page containing a figure; a t indicates a page containing a table.
This is a cumulative index for both volumes (Volume 1, pages 1–770; Volume 2, pages 771–1408).

An f following an entry indicates a page containing a figure; a t indicates a page containing a table.
This is a cumulative index for both volumes (Volume 1, pages 1–770; Volume 2, pages 771–1408).

An f following an entry indicates a page containing a figure; a t indicates a page containing a table.
This is a cumulative index for both volumes (Volume 1, pages 1–770; Volume 2, pages 771–1408).